PRINCIPLES OF NEURAL SCIENCE

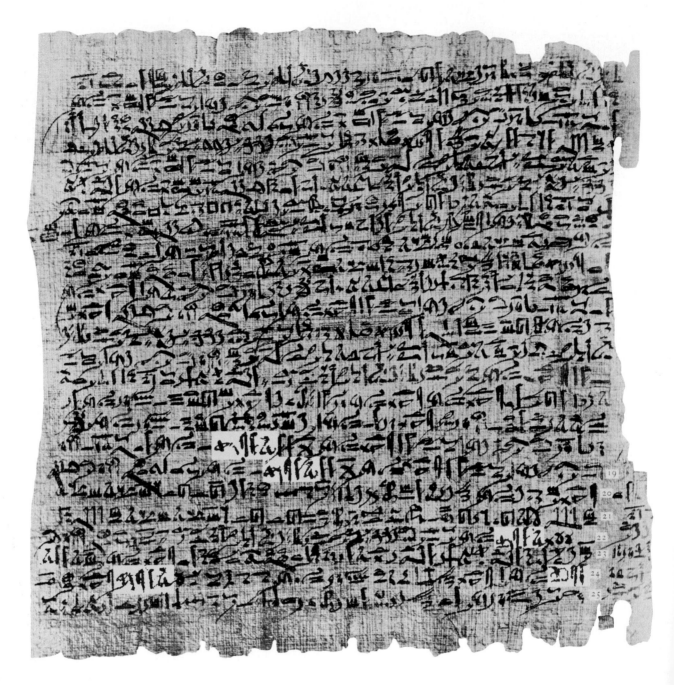

Columns II (left) and IV (right) of the Edwin Smith Surgical Papyrus

This papyrus, written in the seventeenth century B.C., contains the earliest reference to the brain anywhere in human records. According to James Breasted, who translated and published the document in 1930, the word brain 𓄹𓏏𓏤 occurs only eight times in ancient Egyptian records, six of them in these pages, which describe the symptoms, diagnosis, and prognosis of two patients, with compound fractures of the skull. The entire treatise is now in the Rare Book Room of the New York Academy of Medicine.

From James Henry Breasted, 1930. *The Edwin Smith Surgical Papyrus,* 2 volumes, Chicago: The University of Chicago Press.

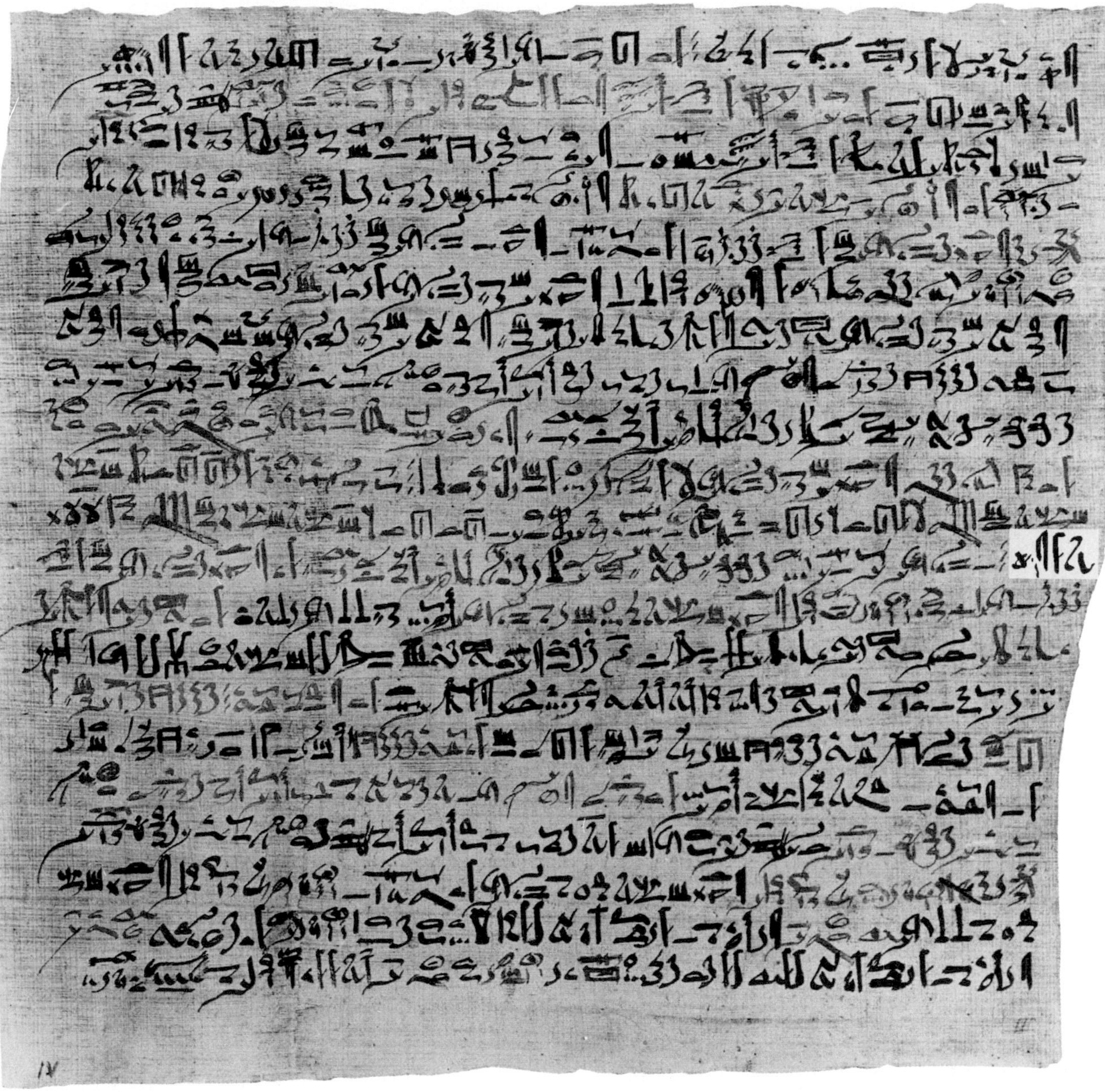

Men ought to know that from the brain, and from the brain only, arise our pleasures, joys, laughter and jests, as well as our sorrows, pains, griefs and tears. Through it, in particular, we think, see, hear, and distinguish the ugly from the beautiful, the bad from the good, the pleasant from the unpleasant. . . . It is the same thing which makes us mad or delirious, inspires us with dread and fear, whether by night or by day, brings sleeplessness, inopportune mistakes, aimless anxieties, absent-mindedness, and acts that are contrary to habit. These things that we suffer all come from the brain, when it is not healthy, but becomes abnormally hot, cold, moist, or dry, or suffers any other unnatural affection to which it was not accustomed. Madness comes from its moistness. When the brain is abnormally moist, of necessity it moves, and when it moves neither sight nor hearing are still, but we see or hear now one thing and now another, and the tongue speaks in accordance with the things seen and heard on any occasion. But when the brain is still, a man can think properly.

attributed to Hippocrates
Fifth Century, B.C.

From *Hippocrates*, Vol.2, translated by W.H.S. Jones, London and New York: William Heinemann and Harvard University Press. 1923.

PRINCIPLES OF NEURAL SCIENCE

Fourth Edition

Edited by

ERIC R. KANDEL

JAMES H. SCHWARTZ

THOMAS M. JESSELL

Center for Neurobiology and Behavior
College of Physicians & Surgeons of Columbia University
and
The Howard Hughes Medical Institute

Art direction by
Sarah Mack and Jane Dodd

McGraw-Hill
Health Professions Division

New York St. Louis San Francisco Auckland Bogotá Caracas Lisbon London
Madrid Mexico City Milan Montreal New Delhi San Juan
Singapore Sydney Tokyo Toronto

McGraw-Hill

A Division of The McGraw·Hill Companies

This book was set in Palatino by Clarinda Prepress, Inc.
The editors were John Butler and Harriet Lebowitz.
The production supervisor was Shirley Dahlgren.
The art manager was Eve Siegel.
The illustrators were Precision Graphics.
The designer was Joellen Ackerman.
The index was prepared by Judy Cuddihy.
R. R. Donnelley & Sons, Inc. was printer and binder.

This book is printed on acid-free paper.

Cataloging-in-Publication Data is on file for this title at the Library of Congress.

Notice

Medicine is an ever-changing science. As new research and clinical experience broaden our knowledge, changes in treatment and drug therapy are required. The editors and the publisher of this work have checked with sources believed to be reliable in their efforts to provide information that is complete and generally in accord with the standards accepted at the time of publication. However, in view of the possibility of human error or changes in medical sciences, neither the editors nor the publisher nor any other party who has been involved in the preparation or publication of this work warrants that the information contained herein is in every respect accurate or complete, and they are not responsible for any errors or omissions or for the results obtained from use of such information. Readers are encouraged to confirm the information contained herein with other sources. For example and in particular, readers are advised to check the product information sheet included in the package of each drug they plan to administer to be certain that the information contained in this book is accurate and that changes have not been made in the recommended dose or in the contraindications for administration. This recommendation is of particular importance in connection with new or infrequently used drugs.

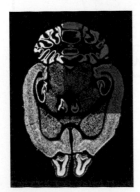

Cover image: The autoradiograph illustrates the widespread localization of mRNA encoding the NMDA-R1 receptor subtype determined by in situ hybridization. Areas of high NMDA receptor expression are shown as light regions in this horizontal section of an adult rat brain.

From Moriyoshi K, Masu M, Ishi T, Shigemoto R, Mizuno N, Nakanishi S. 1991. Molecular cloning and characterization of the rat NMDA receptor. Nature 354:31–37.

Contents in Brief

Part VI

Movement

Part VII

Arousal, Emotion, and Behavior Homeostasis

Part VIII

The Development of the Nervous System

Part IX

Language, Thought, Mood, and Learning, and Memory

Appendices

Contents

Part IV
The Neural Basis of Cognition

17 The Anatomical Organization
of the Central Nervous System 317
David G. Amaral

18 The Functional Organization
of Perception and Movement 337
David G. Amaral

Part V

Perception

Part VI
Movement

Part VII

Arousal, Emotion, and Behavioral
Homeostasis

Part VIII

The Development of the Nervous System

55 The Formation and Regeneration of Synapses 1087

Joshua R. Sanes, Thomas M. Jessell

56 Sensory Experience and the Fine-Tuning of Synaptic Connections   1115

Eric R. Kandel, Thomas M. Jessell, Joshua R. Sanes

Part IX

Language, Thought, Mood, and Learning, and Memory

63 Cellular Mechanisms of Learning and the Biological Basis of Individuality 1247

Eric R. Kandel

Appendices

A Current Flow in Neurons   1280

John Koester

Preface

The goal of neural science is to understand the mind—how we perceive, move, think, and remember. As in the earlier editions of this book, in this fourth edition we emphasize that behavior can be examined at the level of individual nerve cells by seeking answers to five basic questions: How does the brain develop? How do nerve cells in the brain communicate with one another? How do different patterns of interconnections give rise to different perceptions and motor acts? How is communication between neurons modified by experience? How is that communication altered by diseases?

When we published the first edition of this book in 1981, these questions could be addressed only in cell biological terms. By the time of the third edition in 1991, however, these same problems were being explored effectively at the molecular level.

In the eight years intervening between the third and the present edition, molecular biology has continued to facilitate the analysis of neurobiological problems. Initially molecular biology enriched our understanding of ion channels and receptors important for signaling. We now have obtained the first molecular structure of an ion channel, providing us with a three-dimensional understanding of the ion channel pore. Structural studies also have deepened our understanding of the membrane receptors coupled to intracellular second-messenger systems and of the role of these systems in modulating the physiological responses of nerve cells.

Molecular biology also has greatly expanded our understanding of how the brain develops and how it generates behavior. Characterizations of the genes encoding growth factors and their receptors, transcriptional regulatory factors, and cell and substrate adhesion molecules have changed the study of neural development from a descriptive discipline into a mechanistic one. We have even begun to define the molecular mechanisms underlying the developmental processes responsible for assembling functional neural circuits. These processes include the specification of cell fate, cell migration, axon growth, target recognition, and synapse formation.

In addition, the ability to develop genetically modified mice has allowed us to relate single genes to signaling in nerve cells and to relate both of these to an organism's behavior. Ultimately, these experiments will make it possible to study emotion, perception, learning, memory, and other cognitive processes on both a cellular and a molecular level. Molecular biology has also made it possible to probe the pathogenesis of many diseases that affect neural function, including several devastating genetic disorders: muscular dystrophy, retinoblastoma, neurofibromatosis, Huntington disease, and certain forms of Alzheimer disease.

Finally, the 80,000 genes of the human genome are nearly sequenced. With the possible exception of trauma, every disease that affects the nervous system has some inherited component. Information about the human genome is making it possible to identify which genes contribute to these disorders and thus to predict an individual's susceptibility to particular illnesses. In the long term, finding these genes will radically transform the practice of medicine. Thus we again stress vigorously our view, advocated since the first edition of this book, that the future of clinical neurology and psychiatry depends on the progress of molecular neural science.

Advances in molecular neural science have been matched by advances in our understanding of the biology of higher brain functions. The present-day study of visual perception, emotion, motivation, thought, language, and memory owes much to the collaboration of cognitive psychology and neural science, a collaboration at the core of the new cognitive neural science. Not long ago, ascribing a particular aspect of behavior to an unobservable mental process—such as planning a movement or remembering an event—was thought to be reason for removing the problem from experimental analysis. Today our ability to visualize functional changes in the brain during normal and abnormal mental activity permits even complex cognitive processes to be studied directly. No longer are we constrained simply to infer mental functions from observable behavior. As a result, neural science during the next several decades may develop the tools needed to probe the deepest of biological mysteries—the biological basis of mind and consciousness.

Despite the growing richness of neural science, we have striven to write a coherent introduction to the nervous system for students of behavior, biology, and medicine. Indeed, we think this information is even more necessary now than it was two decades ago. Today neurobiology is central to the biological sciences—students of biology increasingly want to become familiar with neural science, and more students of psychology are interested in the biological basis of behavior. At the same time, progress in neural science is providing clearer guidance to clinicians, particularly in the treatment of behavioral disorders. Therefore we believe it is particularly important to clarify the major principles and mechanisms governing the functions of the nervous system without becoming lost in details. Thus this book provides the detail necessary to meet the interests of students in particular fields. It is organized in such a way,

however, that excursions into special topics are not necessary for grasping the major principles of neural science. Toward that end, we have completely redesigned the illustrations in the book to provide accurate, yet vividly graphic, diagrams that allow the reader to understand the fundamental concepts of neural science.

With this fourth and millennial edition, we hope to encourage the next generation of undergraduate, graduate, and medical students to approach the study of behavior in a way that unites its social and its biological dimensions. From ancient times, understanding human behavior has been central to civilized cultures. Engraved at the entrance to the Temple of Apollo at Delphi was the famous maxim "Know thyself." For us, the study of the mind and consciousness defines the frontier of biology. Throughout this book we both document the central principle that all behavior is an expression of neural activity and illustrate the insights into behavior that neural science provides.

Eric R. Kandel
James H. Schwartz
Thomas M. Jessell

Acknowledgments

We are again fortunate to have had the creative editorial assistance of Howard Beckman, who read several versions of the text, demanding clarity of style and logic of argument. We owe a special debt to Sarah Mack, who rethought the whole art program and converted it to color. With her extraordinary insights into science, she produced remarkably clear diagrams and figures. In this task, she was aided by our colleague Jane Dodd, who as art editor supervised the program both scientifically and artistically.

We again owe much to Seta Izmirly: she undertook the demanding task of coordinating the production of this book at Columbia as she did its predecessor. We thank Harriet Ayers and Millie Pellan, who typed the many versions of the manuscript; Veronica Winder and Theodore Moallem, who checked the bibliography; Charles Lam, who helped with the art program; Lalita Hedge who obtained permissions for figures; and Judy Cuddihy, who prepared the index. We also are indebted to Amanda Suver and Harriet Lebowitz, our development editors, and to the manager of art services, Eve Siegel, for their help in producing this edition. Finally we want to thank John Butler, for his consistent and thoughtful support of this project throughout the work on this fourth edition.

Many colleagues have read portions of the manuscript critically. We are especially indebted to John H. Martin for helping us, once again, with the anatomical drawings. In addition, we thank the following colleagues, who made constructive comments on various chapters: George Aghajanian, Roger Bannister, Robert Barchi, Cornelia Bargmann, Samuel Barondes, Elizabeth Bates, Dennis Baylor, Ursula Bellugi, Michael V.L. Bennett, Louis Caplan, Dennis Choi, Patricia Churchland, Bernard Cohen, Barry Connors, W. Maxwell Cowan, Hanna Damasio, Michael Davis, Vincent Ferrera, Hans Christian Fibinger, Mark Fishman, Jeff Friedman, Joacquin M. Fuster, Daniel Gardner, Charles Gilbert, Mirchell Glickstein, Corey Goodman, Jack Gorman, Robert Griggs, Kristen Harris, Allan Hobson, Steven Hyman, Kenneth Johnson, Edward Jones, John Kalaska, Maria Karayiorgou, Frederic Kass, Doreen Kimura, Donald Klein, Arnold Kriegstein, Robert LaMotte, Peretz Lavie, Joseph LeDoux, Alan Light, Rodolfo Llinas, Shawn Lockery, John Mann, Eve Marder, C.D. Marsden, Richard Masland, John Maunsell, Robert McCarley, David McCormick, Chris Miller, George Miller, Adrian Morrison, Thomas Nagel, William Newsome, Roger Nicoll, Donata Oertel, Richard Palmiter, Michael Posner, V.S. Ramachandran, Elliott Ross, John R. Searle, Dennis Selkoe, Carla Shatz, David Sparks, Robert Spitzer, Mircea Steriade, Peter Sterling, Larry Swanson, Paula Tallal, Endel Tulving, Daniel Weinberger, and Michael Young.

Contributors

David G. Amaral, PhD
Professor, Department of Psychiatry, Center for
Neuroscience, University of California, Davis

Allan I. Basbaum, PhD
Professor and Chair, Department of Anatomy,
University of California, San Francisco; Member W.M.
Keck Foundation Center for Integrative Neuroscience

John C. M. Brust, MD
Professor, Department of Neurology, Columbia
University College of Physicians & Surgeons; Director
of Neurology Service, Harlem Hospital

Linda Buck, PhD
Associate Professor, Department of Neurobiology,
Harvard Medical School; Associate Investigator,
Howard Hughes Medical Institute

Pietro De Camilli, MD
Professor and Chairman; Department of Cell Biology,
Yale University Medical School

Antonio R. Damasio, MD, PhD
M.W. Van Allen Professor and Head, Department of
Neurology, University of Iowa College of Medicine;
Adjunct Professor Salk Institute for Biological Studies

Mahlon R. DeLong, MD
Professor and Chairman, Department of Neurology,
Emory University School of Medicine

Nina F. Dronkers, PhD
Chief, Audiology and Speech Pathology VA Northern
California Health Care System; Departments of Neurology
and Linguistics, University of California, Davis

Richard S.J. Frackowiak, MD, DSc
Dean, Institute of Neurology, University College
London; Chair, Wellcome Department of Cognitive
Neurology; The National Hospital for Neurology &
Neurosurgery, London

Esther P. Gardner, PhD
Professor, Department of Physiology and
Neuroscience, New York University School of Medicine

Claude P. J. Ghez, MD
Professor, Department of Neurology and Department
of Physiology and Cellular Biophysics; Center for
Neurobiology and Behavior; Columbia University
College of Physicians & Surgeons; New York State
Psychiatric Institute

T. Conrad Gilliam, PhD
Professor, Department of Genetics and Development,
Columbia University College of Physicians & Surgeons

Michael E. Goldberg, MD
Chief, Section of Neuro-opthalmological Mechanisms,
Laboratory of Sensorimotor Research; National Eye
Institute, National Institutes of Health

Gary W. Goldstein, MD
President, The Kennedy Krieger Research Institute;
Professor, Neurology and Pediatrics, The Johns
Hopkins University School of Medicine

James Gordon, EdD
Professor of Practice, Program Director, Physical
Therapy, Graduate School of Health Sciences, New
York Medical College

Roger A. Gorski, PhD
Professor, Department of Neurobiology, UCLA School
of Medicine

A. J. Hudspeth, MD, PhD
Professor and Head, Laboratory of Sensory
Neuroscience, Rockefeller University; Investigator,
Howard Hughes Medical Institute

Leslie L. Iversen, PhD
Professor, Department of Pharmacology, Oxford
University

Susan D. Iversen, PhD
Professor, Department of Experimental Psychology,
Oxford University

Thomas M. Jessell, PhD
Professor, Department of Biochemistry and Molecular
Biophysics; Center for Neurobiology and Behavior;
Investigator, The Howard Hughes Medical Institute,
Columbia University College of Physicians & Surgeons

Eric R. Kandel, MD
University Professor, Departments of Biochemistry and
Molecular Biophysics, Physiology and Cellular
Biophysics, and Psychiatry; Center for Neurobiology
and Behavior; Senior Investigator, The Howard Hughes
Medical Institute, Columbia University College of
Physicians & Surgeons

John Koester, PhD
Professor of Clinical Neurobiology and Behavior in
Psychiatry; Acting Director, Center for Neurobiology
and Behavior, New York State Psychiatric Institute,
Columbia University College of Physicians & Surgeons

John Krakauer, MD
Assistant Professor, Department of Neurology,
Columbia University College of Physicians & Surgeons

Irving Kupfermann, PhD
Professor, Department of Psychiatry and Department
of Physiology and Cellular Biophysics, Center for
Neurobiology and Behavior, Columbia University
College of Physicians & Surgeons

John Laterra, MD, PhD
Associate Professor of Neurology, Oncology, and
Neuroscience; The Kennedy Krieger Research Institute,
Johns Hopkins University School of Medicine

Peter Lennie, PhD
Professor of Neural Science, Center for Neural Science,
New York University

Gerald E. Loeb, MD
Professor, Department of Physiology, Member, MRC
Group in Sensory-Motor Neuroscience, Queen's
University, Canada

John H. Martin, PhD
Associate Professor, Department of Psychiatry; Center
for Neurobiology and Behavior, Columbia University
College of Physicians & Surgeons

Geoffrey Melvill Jones, MD
Professor, Department of Clinical Neurosciences,
Faculty of Medicine, University of Calgary, Canada

Keir Pearson, PhD
Professor, Department of Physiology, University of
Alberta

Steven Pinker, PhD
Professor, , Department of Brain and Cognitive
Sciences, Massachusetts Institute of Technology;
Director, McDonnell-Pew Center for Cognitive
Neuroscience

Donald L. Price, MD
Professor, Neuropathology Laboratory, The Johns
Hopkins University School of Medicine

Allan Rechtshaffen, PhD
Professor Emeritus, Department of Psychiatry, and
Department of Psychology, University of Chicago

Timothy Roehrs, PhD
Director of Research, Henry Ford Sleep Disorders Center

Thomas Roth, PhD
Director, Sleep Disorders and Research Center, Henry
Ford Hospital; University of Michigan

Lewis P. Rowland, MD
Professor, Department of Neurology; Columbia
University College of Physicians & Surgeons

Joshua R. Sanes, PhD
Professor, Department of Anatomy and Neurobiology;
Washington University School of Medicine

Clifford B. Saper, MD, PhD
Professor and Chairman, Department of Neurology;
Beth Israel Deaconess Medical Center, Harvard
Medical School

James H. Schwartz, MD, PhD
Professor, Departments of Physiology and Cellular
Biophysics, Neurology and Psychiatry, Center for
Neurobiology and Behavior, Columbia University
College of Physicians and Surgeons.

Jerome M. Siegel, PhD
Professor of Psychiatry, UCLA Medical Center; Chief
Neurobiology Research, Sepulveda VA Medical Center

Steven A. Siegelbaum, PhD
Professor, Department of Pharmacology, Center for
Neurobiology and Behavior Investigator, Howard
Hughes Medical Institute, Columbia University
College of Physicians and Surgeons

Marc T. Tessier-Lavigne, PhD
Professor, Departments of Anatomy and of
Biochemistry and Biophysics, University of California,
San Francisco; Investigator, Howard Hughes Medical
Institute

W. Thomas Thach, Jr., MD
Professor, Department of Anatomy and Neurobiology,
Washington University School of Medicine

Gary L. Westbrook, MD
Senior Scientist and Professor of Neurology, Vollum
Institute, Oregon Health Sciences University

Robert H. Wurtz, PhD
Chief, Laboratory of Sensorimotor Research, National
Eye Institute; National Institutes of Health

Part I

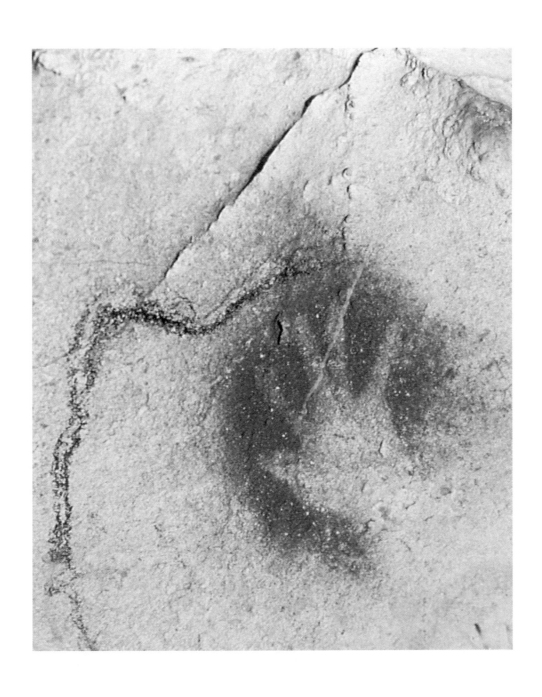

Preceding page

Cave Paintings Contain the First Human Signatures. A paleolithic cave painting from the Chauvet cave in the Ardèche region of France showing a negative image of a right human hand. Cave paintings, found in France and Spain in the regions at the borders of the two countries, primarily show game animals—bison, reindeer, horses, deer, oxen, rhinoceros, and mammoths. Although the purpose of the paintings cannot be known for certain, it is believed that they were used in magical or religious rituals to ensure a good hunt. Images of hands occur either in the negative, as shown here, or in the positive, and always in red. While their meaning is uncertain, it is tempting to think that this hand, which is over 30,000 years old, is early evidence of human cognition. (Reproduced with permission from Chauvet J-M, Deschamps EB, Hillare C. 1996. *Dawn of Art: The Chauvet Cave*, p. 120. New York: Harry N. Abrams, Incorporated.)

I

The Neurobiology of Behavior

T HE TASK OF NEURAL SCIENCE is to understand the mental processes by which we perceive, act, learn, and remember. How does the brain produce the remarkable individuality of human action? Are mental processes localized to specific regions of the brain, or do they represent emergent properties of the brain as an organ? If specific mental processes are represented locally in different brain regions, what rules relate the anatomy and physiology of a region to its specific role in mentation? Can these rules be understood better by examining the region as a whole or by studying its individual nerve cells?

To what extent are mental processes hard-wired into the neural architecture of the brain? What do genes contribute to behavior, and how is gene expression in nerve cells regulated by developmental and learning processes? How does experience alter the way the brain processes subsequent events? This book attempts to address these questions. In so doing it describes how neural science is attempting to link molecules to mind—how proteins responsible for the activities of individual nerve cells are related to the complexity of mental processes.

Today, it is possible to link the molecular dynamics of individual nerve cells to representations of perceptual and motor acts in the brain and to relate these internal mechanisms to observable behavior. New imaging techniques permit us to see the human brain in action—to identify specific regions of the brain associated with particular modes of thinking and feeling.

In the first part of this book we consider the degree to which mental functions can be located in specific regions of the brain. We also examine the extent to which a behavior can be understood in terms of the properties of specific nerve cells and their interconnections in one region of the brain.

The human brain is a network of more than 100 billion individual nerve cells interconnected in systems that construct our perceptions of the external world, fix our attention, and control the machinery of our actions. A first step toward understanding the mind, therefore, is to learn how neurons are organized into signaling pathways and how they communicate by means of synaptic transmission. One of the chief ideas we shall develop in this book is that the specificity of the synaptic connections established during development underlie perception, action, emotion, and learning. We must also understand both the innate (genetic) and environmental determinants of behavior. Specifically, we want to know how genes contribute to behavior. Of course, behavior itself is not inherited—what is inherited is DNA. Genes encode proteins that are important for the development and regulation of the neural circuits that underlie behavior. The environment, which begins to exert its influence in utero, becomes of prime importance after birth.

Modern neural science represents a merger of molecular biology, neurophysiology, anatomy, embryology, cell biology, and psychology. Along with astute clinical observation, neural science has reinforced the idea first proposed by Hippocrates over two millennia ago that the proper study of mind begins with the study of the brain. Cognitive psychology and psychoanalytic theory have emphasized the diversity and complexity of human mental experience. Both disciplines recognize the importance of genetic as well as learned factors in determining behavior. By emphasizing functional mental structure and internal representation, psychoanalysis served as a source of modern cognitive psychology, a psychology that has stressed the logic of mental operations and of internal representations. Experimental cognitive psychology and clinical psychotherapy can now be strengthened by insights into the cellular neurobiology of behavior. The task for the years ahead is to produce a psychology that—though still concerned with problems of how internal representations are generated, with psychodynamics, and with subjective states of mind—is firmly grounded in empirical neural science.

Part I

1

The Brain and Behavior

THE LAST FRONTIER OF THE biological sciences—their ultimate challenge—is to understand the biological basis of consciousness and the mental processes by which we perceive, act, learn, and remember. In the last two decades a remarkable unity has emerged within biology. The ability to sequence genes and infer the amino acid sequences for the proteins they encode has revealed unanticipated similarities between proteins in the nervous system and those encountered elsewhere in the body. As a result, it has become possible to establish a general plan for the function of cells, a plan that provides a common conceptual framework for all of cell biology, including cellular neurobiology. The next and even more challenging step in this unifying process within biology, which we outline in this book, will be the unification of the study of behavior—the science of the mind—and neural science, the science of the brain. This last step will allow us to achieve a unified scientific approach to the study of behavior.

Such a comprehensive approach depends on the view that all behavior is the result of brain function. What we commonly call the mind is a set of operations carried out by the brain. The actions of the brain underlie not only relatively simple motor behaviors such as walking or eating, but all the complex cognitive actions that we believe are quintessentially human, such as thinking, speaking, and creating works of art. As a corollary, all the behavioral disorders that characterize psychiatric illness—disorders of affect (feeling) and cognition (thought)—are disturbances of brain function.

The task of neural science is to explain behavior in terms of the activities of the brain. How does the brain marshal its millions of individual nerve cells to produce behavior, and how are these cells influenced by the environment, which includes the actions of other people? The progress of neural science in explaining human behavior is a major theme of this book.

Like all science, neural science must continually confront certain fundamental questions. Are particular mental processes localized to specific regions of the brain, or does the mind represent a collective and emergent property of the whole brain? If specific mental processes can be localized to discrete brain regions, what is the relationship between the anatomy and physiology of one region and its specific function in perception, thought, or movement? Are such relationships more likely to be revealed by examining the region as a whole or by studying its individual nerve cells? In this chapter we consider to what degree mental functions are located in specific regions of the brain and to what degree such local mental processes can be understood in terms of the properties of specific nerve cells and their interconnections.

To answer these questions, we look at how modern neural science approaches one of the most elaborate cognitive behaviors—language. In doing so we necessarily focus on the cerebral cortex, the part of the brain concerned with the most evolved human behaviors. Here we see how the brain is organized into regions or brain compartments, each made up of large groups of neurons, and how highly complex behaviors can be traced to specific regions of the brain and understood in terms of the functioning of groups of neurons. In the next chapter we consider how these neural circuits function at the cellular level, using a simple reflex behavior to examine the way sensory signals are transformed into motor acts.

Two Opposing Views Have Been Advanced on the Relationship Between Brain and Behavior

Our current views about nerve cells, the brain, and behavior have emerged over the last century from a convergence of five experimental traditions: anatomy, embryology, physiology, pharmacology, and psychology.

Before the invention of the compound microscope in the eighteenth century, nervous tissue was thought to function like a gland—an idea that goes back to the Greek physician Galen, who proposed that nerves convey fluid secreted by the brain and spinal cord to the body's periphery. The microscope revealed the true structure of the cells of nervous tissue. Even so, nervous tissue did not become the subject of a special science until the late 1800s, when the first detailed descriptions of nerve cells were undertaken by Camillo Golgi and Santiago Ramón y Cajal.

Golgi developed a way of staining neurons with silver salts that revealed their entire structure under the microscope. He could see clearly that neurons had cell bodies and two major types of projections or processes: branching dendrites at one end and a long cable-like axon at the other. Using Golgi's technique, Ramón y Cajal was able to stain individual cells, thus showing that nervous tissue is not one continuous web but a network of discrete cells. In the course of this work, Ramón y Cajal developed some of the key concepts and much of the early evidence for the *neuron doctrine*—the principle that individual neurons are the elementary signaling elements of the nervous system.

Additional experimental support for the neuron doctrine was provided in the 1920s by the American embryologist Ross Harrison, who demonstrated that the two major projections of the nerve cell—the dendrites and the axon—grow out from the cell body and that they do so even in tissue culture in which each neuron is isolated from other neurons. Harrison also confirmed Ramón y Cajal's suggestion that the tip of the axon gives rise to an expansion called the *growth cone*, which

leads the developing axon to its target (whether to other nerve cells or to muscles).

Physiological investigation of the nervous system began in the late 1700s when the Italian physician and physicist Luigi Galvani discovered that living excitable muscle and nerve cells produce electricity. Modern electrophysiology grew out of work in the nineteenth century by three German physiologists—Emil DuBois-Reymond, Johannes Müller, and Hermann von Helmholtz—who were able to show that the electrical activity of one nerve cell affects the activity of an adjacent cell in predictable ways.

Pharmacology made its first impact on our understanding of the nervous system and behavior at the end of the nineteenth century, when Claude Bernard in France, Paul Ehrlich in Germany, and John Langley in England demonstrated that drugs do not interact with cells arbitrarily, but rather bind to specific receptors typically located in the membrane on the cell surface. This discovery became the basis of the all-important study of the chemical basis of communication between nerve cells.

The psychological investigation of behavior dates back to the beginnings of Western science, to classical Greek philosophy. Many issues central to the modern investigation of behavior, particularly in the area of perception, were subsequently reformulated in the seventeenth century first by René Descartes and then by John Locke, of whom we shall learn more later. In the mid-nineteenth century Charles Darwin set the stage for the study of animals as models of human actions and behavior by publishing his observations on the continuity of species in evolution. This new approach gave rise to ethology, the study of animal behavior in the natural environment, and later to experimental psychology, the study of human and animal behavior under controlled conditions.

In fact, by as early as the end of the eighteenth century the first attempts had been made to bring together biological and psychological concepts in the study of behavior. Franz Joseph Gall, a German physician and neuroanatomist, proposed three radical new ideas. First, he advocated that all behavior emanated from the brain. Second, he argued that particular regions of the cerebral cortex controlled specific functions. Gall asserted that the cerebral cortex did not act as a single organ but was divided into at least 35 organs (others were added later), each corresponding to a specific mental faculty. Even the most abstract of human behaviors, such as generosity, secretiveness, and religiosity were assigned their spot in the brain. Third, Gall proposed that the center for each mental function grew with use, much as a muscle bulks up with exercise. As each center grew, it purportedly caused the overlying skull to bulge, creating a pattern of bumps and ridges on the skull that indicated which brain regions were most developed (Figure 1-1). Rather than looking within the brain, Gall sought to establish an anatomical basis for describing character traits by correlating the personality of individuals with the bumps on their skulls. His psychology, based on the distribution of bumps on the outside of the head, became known as *phrenology*.

In the late 1820s Gall's ideas were subjected to experimental analysis by the French physiologist Pierre Flourens. By systematically removing Gall's functional centers from the brains of experimental animals, Flourens attempted to isolate the contributions of each "cerebral organ" to behavior. From these experiments he concluded that specific brain regions were not responsible for specific behaviors, but that all brain regions, especially the cerebral hemispheres of the forebrain, participated in every mental operation. Any part of the cerebral hemisphere, he proposed, was able to perform all the functions of the hemisphere. Injury to a specific area of the cerebral hemisphere would therefore affect all higher functions equally.

In 1823 Flourens wrote: "All perceptions, all volitions occupy the same seat in these (cerebral) organs; the faculty of perceiving, of conceiving, of willing merely constitutes therefore a faculty which is essentially one." The rapid acceptance of this belief (later called the *aggregate-field* view of the brain) was based only partly on Flourens's experimental work. It also represented a cultural reaction against the reductionist view that the human mind has a biological basis, the notion that there was no soul, that all mental processes could be reduced to actions within different regions in the brain!

The aggregate-field view was first seriously challenged in the mid-nineteenth century by the British neurologist J. Hughlings Jackson. In his studies of focal epilepsy, a disease characterized by convulsions that begin in a particular part of the body, Jackson showed that different motor and sensory functions can be traced to different parts of the cerebral cortex. These studies were later refined by the German neurologist Karl Wernicke, the English physiologist Charles Sherrington, and Ramón y Cajal into a view of brain function called *cellular connectionism*. According to this view, individual neurons are the signaling units of the brain; they are generally arranged in functional groups and connect to one another in a precise fashion. Wernicke's work in particular showed that different behaviors are produced by different brain regions interconnected by specific neural pathways.

The differences between the aggregate-field theory and cellular-connectionism can best be illustrated by an

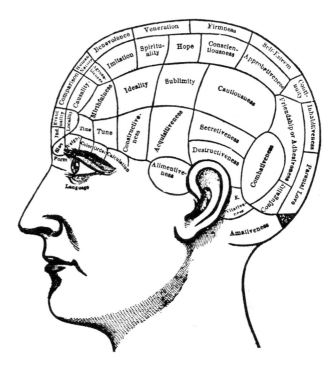

Figure 1-1 According to the nineteenth-century doctrine of phrenology, complex traits such as combativeness, spirituality, hope, and conscientiousness are controlled by specific areas in the brain, which expand as the traits develop. This enlargement of local areas of the brain was thought to produce characteristic bumps and ridges on the overlying skull, from which an individual's character could be determined. This map, taken from a drawing of the early 1800s, purports to show 35 intellectual and emotional faculties in distinct areas of the skull and the cerebral cortex underneath.

analysis of how the brain produces language. Before we consider the relevant clinical and anatomical studies concerned with the localization of language, let us briefly look at the overall structure of the brain. (The anatomical organization of the nervous system is described in detail in Chapter 17.)

The Brain Has Distinct Functional Regions

The central nervous system is a bilateral and essentially symmetrical structure with seven main parts: the spinal cord, medulla oblongata, pons, cerebellum, midbrain, diencephalon, and the cerebral hemispheres (Box 1-1 and Figures 1-2 and 1-3). Radiographic imaging techniques have made it possible to visualize these structures in living subjects. Through a variety of experimental methods, such images of the brain can be made while subjects are engaged in specific tasks, which then can be related to the activities of discrete regions of the brain. As a result, Gall's original idea that different regions are

Box 1-1 The Central Nervous System

The central nervous system has seven main parts (Figure 1-2A).

1. The **spinal cord,** the most caudal part of the central nervous system, receives and processes sensory information from the skin, joints, and muscles of the limbs and trunk and controls movement of the limbs and the trunk. It is subdivided into cervical, thoracic, lumbar, and sacral regions. The spinal cord continues rostrally as the *brain stem,* which consists of the medulla, pons, and midbrain (see below). The brain stem receives sensory information from the skin and muscles of the head and provides the motor control for the muscles of the head. It also conveys information from the spinal cord to the brain and from the brain to the spinal cord, and regulates levels of arousal and awareness, through the reticular formation. The brain stem contains several collections of cell bodies, the *cranial nerve nuclei.* Some of these nuclei receive information from the skin and muscles of the head; others control motor output to muscles of the face, neck, and eyes. Still others are specialized for information from the special senses: hearing, balance, and taste.

2. The **medulla oblongata,** which lies directly above the spinal cord, includes several centers responsible for vital autonomic functions, such as digestion, breathing, and the control of heart rate.

3. The **pons,** which lies above the medulla, conveys information about movement from the cerebral hemisphere to the cerebellum.

4. The **cerebellum** lies behind the pons and is connected to the brain stem by several major fiber tracts called *peduncles.* The cerebellum modulates the force and range of movement and is involved in the learning of motor skills.

5. The **midbrain,** which lies rostral to the pons, controls many sensory and motor functions, including eye movement and the coordination of visual and auditory reflexes.

6. The **diencephalon** lies rostral to the midbrain and contains two structures. One, the *thalamus,* processes most of the information reaching the cerebral cortex from the rest of the central nervous system. The other, the *hypothalamus,* regulates autonomic, endocrine, and visceral function.

7. The **cerebral hemispheres** consist of a heavily wrinkled outer layer—the *cerebral cortex*—and three deep-lying structures: the *basal ganglia,* the *hippocampus,* and the *amygdaloid nuclei.* The basal ganglia participate in regulating motor performance; the hippocampus is involved with aspects of memory storage; and the amygdaloid nuclei coordinate the autonomic and endocrine responses of emotional states. The cerebral cortex is divided into four lobes: frontal, parietal, temporal, and occipital (Figure 1-2B).

The brain is also commonly divided into three broader regions: the *hindbrain* (the medulla, pons, and cerebellum), *midbrain,* and *forebrain* (diencephalon and cerebral hemispheres). The hindbrain (excluding the cerebellum) and midbrain comprise the brain stem.

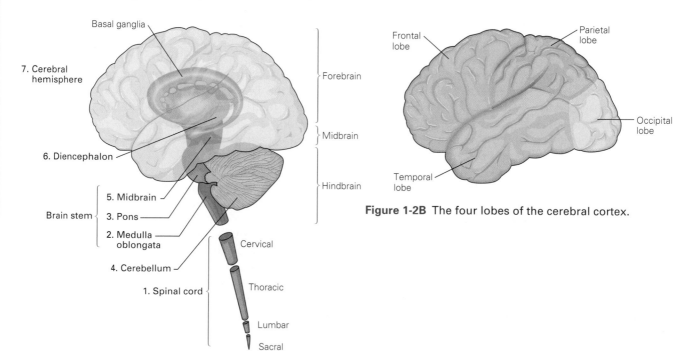

Figure 1-2A The central nervous system can be divided into seven main parts.

Figure 1-2B The four lobes of the cerebral cortex.

A

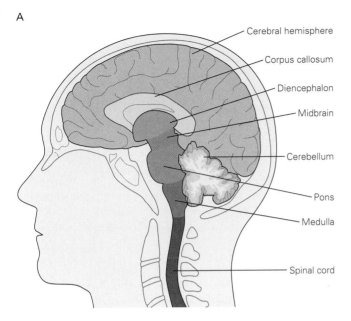

Cerebral hemisphere

Corpus callosum

Diencephalon

Midbrain

Cerebellum

Pons

Medulla

Spinal cord

B

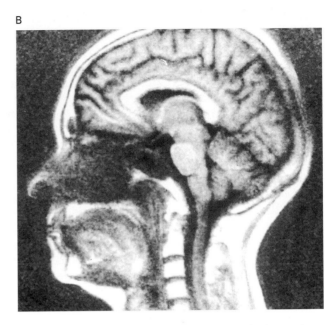

Figure 1-3 The main divisions are clearly visible when the brain is cut down the midline between the two hemispheres.

A. This schematic drawing shows the position of major structures of the brain in relation to external landmarks. Students of

brain anatomy quickly learn to distinguish the major internal landmarks, such as the corpus callosum, a large bundle of nerve fibers that connects the left and right hemispheres.

B. The major brain divisions drawn in **A** are also evident here in a magnetic resonance image of a living human brain.

specialized for different functions is now accepted as one of the cornerstones of modern brain science.

One reason this conclusion eluded investigators for so many years lies in another organizational principle of the nervous system known as *parallel distributed processing*. As we shall see below, many sensory, motor, and cognitive functions are served by more than one neural pathway. When one functional region or pathway is damaged, others may be able to compensate partially for the loss, thereby obscuring the behavioral evidence for localization. Nevertheless, the neural pathways for certain higher functions have been precisely mapped in the brain.

Cognitive Functions Are Localized Within the Cerebral Cortex

The brain operations responsible for our cognitive abilities occur primarily in the *cerebral cortex*—the furrowed gray matter covering the cerebral hemispheres. In each of the brain's two hemispheres the overlying cortex is divided into four anatomically distinct lobes: *frontal*, *parietal*, *temporal*, and *occipital* (see Figure 1-2B), originally named for the skull bones that encase them. These lobes have specialized functions. The frontal lobe is largely concerned with planning future action and with

the control of movement; the parietal lobe with somatic sensation, with forming a body image, and with relating one's body image with extrapersonal space; the occipital lobe with vision; the temporal lobe with hearing; and through its deep structures—the hippocampus and the amygdaloid nuclei—with aspects of learning, memory, and emotion. Each lobe has several characteristic deep infoldings (a favored evolutionary strategy for packing in more cells in a limited space). The crests of these convolutions are called *gyri*, while the intervening grooves are called *sulci* or *fissures*. The more prominent gyri and sulci are quite similar in everyone and have specific names. For example, the *central sulcus* separates the *precentral gyrus*, which is concerned with motor function, from the *postcentral gyrus*, which is concerned with sensory function (Figure 1-4A).

The organization of the cerebral cortex is characterized by two important features. First, each hemisphere is concerned primarily with sensory and motor processes on the *contralateral* (opposite) side of the body. Thus sensory information that arrives at the spinal cord from the left side of the body—from the left hand, say—crosses over to the right side of the nervous system (either within the spinal cord or in the brain stem) on its way to the cerebral cortex. Similarly, the motor areas in the right hemisphere exert control over the movements of the left half of the body. Second, although the hemispheres are similar in appearance, they are not completely symmetrical in structure nor equivalent in function.

To illustrate the role of the cerebral cortex in cognition, we will trace the development of our understanding of the neural basis of language, using it as an example of how we have progressed in localizing mental functions in the brain. The neural basis of language is discussed more fully in Chapter 59.

Much of what we know about the localization of language comes from studies of *aphasia*, a language disorder found most often in patients who have suffered a stroke (the occlusion or rupture of a blood vessel supplying blood to a portion of the cerebral hemisphere). Many of the important discoveries in the study of aphasia occurred in rapid succession during the last half of the nineteenth century. Taken together, these advances form one of the most exciting chapters in the study of human behavior, because they offered the first insight into the biological basis of a complex mental function.

The French neurologist Pierre Paul Broca was much influenced by Gall and by the idea that functions could be localized. But he extended Gall's thinking in an important way. He argued that phrenology, the attempt to localize the functions of the mind, should be based on examining damage to the brain produced by clinical lesions rather than by examining the distribution of bumps on the outside of the head. Thus he wrote in 1861: "I had thought that if there were ever a phrenological science, it would be the phrenology of convolutions (in the cortex), and not the phrenology of bumps (on the head)." Based on this insight Broca founded *neuropsychology,* a new science of mental processes that he was to distinguish from the phrenology of Gall.

In 1861 Broca described a patient named Leborgne, who could understand language but could not speak. The patient had none of the conventional motor deficits (of the tongue, mouth, or vocal cords) that would affect speech. In fact, he could utter isolated words, whistle, and sing a melody without difficulty. But he could not speak grammatically or create complete sentences, nor could he express ideas in writing. Postmortem examination of this patient's brain showed a lesion in the posterior region of the frontal lobe (now called *Broca's area;* Figure 1-4B). Broca studied eight similar patients, all with lesions in this region, and in each case found that the lesion was located in the left cerebral hemisphere. This discovery led Broca to announce in 1864 one of the most famous principles of brain function: *"Nous parlons avec l'hémisphère gauche!"* ("We speak with the left hemisphere!")

Broca's work stimulated a search for the cortical sites of other specific behavioral functions—a search

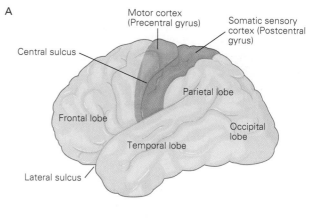

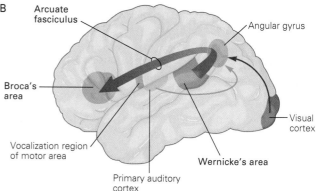

Figure 1-4 The major areas of the cerebral cortex are shown in this lateral view of the of the left hemisphere.

A. Outline of the left hemisphere.

B. Areas involved in language. **Wernicke's area** processes the auditory input for language and is important to the understanding of speech. It lies near the primary auditory cortex and the angular gyrus, which combines auditory input with information from other senses. **Broca's area** controls the production of intelligible speech. It lies near the region of the motor area that controls the mouth and tongue movements that form words. Wernicke's area communicates with Broca's area by a bidirectional pathway, part of which is made up of the **arcuate fasciculus.** (Adapted from Geschwind 1979.)

soon rewarded. In 1870 Gustav Fritsch and Eduard Hitzig galvanized the scientific community by showing that characteristic and discrete limb movements in dogs, such as extending a paw, can be produced by electrically stimulating a localized region of the precentral gyrus of the brain. These discrete regions were invariably located in the contralateral motor cortex. Thus, the right hand, the one most humans use for writing and skilled movements, is controlled by the left hemisphere, the same hemisphere that controls speech. In most people, therefore, the left hemisphere is regarded as *dominant.*

The next step was taken in 1876 by Karl Wernicke. At age 26 Wernicke published a now classic paper, "The

Symptom-Complex of Aphasia: A Psychological Study on an Anatomical Basis." In it he described another type of aphasia, one involving a failure to comprehend language rather than to speak (a *receptive* as opposed to an *expressive* malfunction). Whereas Broca's patients could understand language but not speak, Wernicke's patient could speak but could not understand language. Moreover, the locus of this new type of aphasia was different from that described by Broca: the critical cortical lesion was located in the posterior part of the temporal lobe where it joins the parietal and occipital lobes (Figure 1-4B).

On the basis of this discovery, and the work of Broca, Fritsch, and Hitzig, Wernicke formulated a theory of language that attempted to reconcile and extend the two theories of brain function holding sway at that time. Phrenologists argued that the cortex was a mosaic of functionally specific areas, whereas the aggregate-field school argued that mental functions were distributed homogeneously throughout the cerebral cortex. Wernicke proposed that only the most basic mental functions, those concerned with simple perceptual and motor activities, are localized to single areas of the cortex. More complex cognitive functions, he argued, result from interconnections between several functional sites. In placing the principle of localized function within a connectionist framework, Wernicke appreciated that different components of a single behavior are processed in different regions of the brain. He was thus the first to advance the idea of *distributed processing,* now central to our understanding of brain function.

Wernicke postulated that language involves separate motor and sensory programs, each governed by separate cortical regions. He proposed that the motor program, which governs the mouth movements for speech, is located in Broca's area, suitably situated in front of the motor area that controls the mouth, tongue, palate, and vocal cords (Figure 1-4B). And he assigned the sensory program, which governs word perception, to the temporal lobe area he discovered (now called Wernicke's area). This area is conveniently surrounded by the auditory cortex as well as by areas collectively known as *association cortex,* areas that integrate auditory, visual, and somatic sensation into complex perceptions.

Thus Wernicke formulated the first coherent model for language organization that (with modifications and elaborations we shall soon learn about) is still of some use today. According to this model, the initial steps in the processing of spoken or written words by the brain occur in separate sensory areas of the cortex specialized for auditory or visual information. This information is then conveyed to a cortical association area specialized for both visual and auditory information, the angular gyrus. Here, according to Wernicke, spoken or written words are transformed into a common neural representation shared by both speech and writing. From the angular gyrus this representation is conveyed to Wernicke's area, where it is recognized as language and associated with meaning. Without that association, the ability to comprehend language is lost. The common neural representation is then relayed from Wernicke's to Broca's area, where it is transformed from a sensory (auditory or visual) representation into a motor representation that can potentially lead to spoken or written language. When the last-stage transformation from sensory to motor representation cannot take place, the ability to express language (either as spoken words or in writing) is lost.

Based on this premise, Wernicke correctly predicted the existence of a third type of aphasia, one that results from disconnection. Here the receptive and motor speech zones themselves are spared but the neuronal fiber pathways that connect them are destroyed. This *conduction aphasia,* as it is now called, is characterized by an incorrect use of words (*paraphasia*). Patients with conduction aphasia understand words that they hear and read and have no motor difficulties when they speak. Yet they cannot speak coherently; they omit parts of words or substitute incorrect sounds. Painfully aware of their own errors, they are unable to put them right.

Inspired in part by Wernicke, a new school of cortical localization arose in Germany at the beginning of the twentieth century led by the anatomist Korbinian Brodmann. This school sought to distinguish different functional areas of the cortex based on variations in the structure of cells and in the characteristic arrangement of these cells into layers. Using this *cytoarchitectonic* method, Brodmann distinguished 52 anatomically and functionally distinct areas in the human cerebral cortex (Figure 1-5).

Thus, by the beginning of the twentieth century there was compelling biological evidence for many discrete areas in the cortex, some with specialized roles in behavior. Yet during the first half of this century the aggregate-field view of the brain, not cellular connectionism, continued to dominate experimental thinking and clinical practice. This surprising state of affairs owed much to the arguments of several prominent neural scientists, among them the British neurologist Henry Head, the German neuropsychologist Kurt Goldstein, the Russian behavioral physiologist Ivan Pavlov, and the American psychologist Karl Lashley, all advocates of the aggregate-field view.

The most influential of this group was Lashley, who was deeply skeptical of the cytoarchitectonic approach to functional delineation of the cortex. "The 'ideal' architectonic map is nearly worthless," Lashley wrote.

"The area subdivisions are in large part anatomically meaningless, and misleading as to the presumptive functional divisions of the cortex." Lashley's skepticism was reinforced by his attempts, in the tradition of Flourens's work, to find a specific seat of learning by studying the effects of various brain lesions on the ability of rats to learn to run a maze. But Lashley found that the severity of the learning defect seemed to depend on the size of the lesions, not on their precise site. Disillusioned, Lashley—and, after him, many other psychologists—concluded that learning and other mental functions have no special locus in the brain and consequently cannot be pinned down to specific collections of neurons.

On the basis of his observations, Lashley reformulated the aggregate-field view into a theory of brain function called *mass action,* which further belittled the importance of individual neurons, specific neuronal connections, and brain regions dedicated to particular tasks. According to this view, it was brain mass, not its neuronal components, that was crucial to its function. Applying this logic to aphasia, Head and Goldstein asserted that language disorders could result from injury to almost any cortical area. Cortical damage, regardless of site, caused patients to regress from a rich, abstract language to the impoverished utterances of aphasia.

Lashley's experiments with rats, and Head's observations on human patients, have gradually been reinterpreted. A variety of studies have demonstrated that the maze-learning task used by Lashley is unsuited to the study of local cortical function because the task involves so many motor and sensory capabilities. Deprived of one sensory capability (such as vision), a rat can still learn to run a maze using another (by following tactile or olfactory cues). Besides, as we shall see, many mental functions are handled by more than one region or neuronal pathway, and a single lesion may not eliminate them all.

In addition, the evidence for the localization of function soon became overwhelming. Beginning in the late 1930s, Edgar Adrian in England and Wade Marshall and Philip Bard in the United States discovered that applying a tactile stimulus to different parts of a cat's body elicits electrical activity in distinctly different subregions of the cortex, allowing for the establishment of a precise map of the body surface in specific areas of the cerebral cortex described by Brodmann. These studies established that cytoarchitectonic areas of cortex *can* be defined unambiguously according to several independent criteria, such as cell type and cell layering, connections, and—most important—physiological function. As we shall see in later chapters, local functional specialization has emerged as a key principle of cortical organiza-

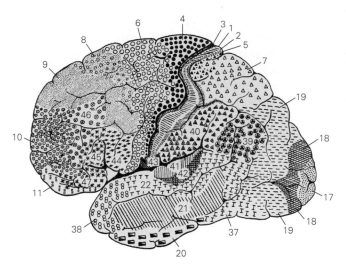

Figure 1-5 In the early part of the twentieth century Korbinian Brodmann divided the human cerebral cortex into 52 discrete areas on the basis of distinctive nerve cell structures and characteristic arrangements of cell layers. Brodmann's scheme of the cortex is still widely used today and is continually updated. In this drawing each area is represented by its own symbol and is assigned a unique number. Several areas defined by Brodmann have been found to control specific brain functions. For instance, area 4, the motor cortex, is responsible for voluntary movement. Areas 1, 2, and 3 comprise the primary somatosensory cortex, which receives information on bodily sensation. Area 17 is the primary visual cortex, which receives signals from the eyes and relays them to other areas for further deciphering. Areas 41 and 42 comprise the primary auditory cortex. Areas not visible from the outer surface of the cortex are not shown in this drawing.

tion, extending even to individual columns of cells within a functional area. Indeed, the brain is divided into many more functional regions than even Brodmann envisaged!

More refined methods have made it possible to learn even more about the function of different brain regions involved in language. In the late 1950s Wilder Penfield, and more recently George Ojemann used small electrodes to stimulate the cortex of awake patients during brain surgery for epilepsy (carried out under local anesthesia), in search of areas that produce language. Patients were asked to name objects or use language in other ways while different areas of the cortex were stimulated. If the area of the cortex was critical for language, application of the electrical stimulus blocked the patient's ability to name objects. In this way Penfield and Ojemann were able to confirm—in the living conscious brain—the language areas of the cortex described by Broca and Wernicke. In addition, Ojemann discovered other sites essential for language, indicating that the neural networks for language are larger than those delineated by Broca and Wernicke.

Our understanding of the neural basis of language has also advanced through brain localization studies that combine linguistic and cognitive psychological approaches. From these studies we have learned that a brain area dedicated to even a specific component of language, such as Wernicke's area for language comprehension, is further subdivided functionally. These modular subdivisions of what had previously appeared to be fairly elementary operations were first discovered in the mid 1970s by Alfonso Caramazza and Edgar Zurif. They found that different lesions within Wernicke's area give rise to different failures to comprehend. Lesions of the frontal-temporal region of Wernicke's area result in failures in *lexical processing,* an inability to understand the meaning of words. By contrast, lesions in the parietal-temporal region of Wernicke's area result in failures in *syntactical processing,* the ability to understand the relationship *between* the words of a sentence. (Thus syntactical knowledge allows one to appreciate that the sentence "Jim is in love with Harriet" has a different meaning from "Harriet is in love with Jim.")

Until recently, almost everything we knew about the anatomical organization of language came from studies of patients who had suffered brain lesions. Positron emission tomography (PET) and functional magnetic resonance imaging (MRI) have extended this approach to normal people (Chapter 20). PET is a noninvasive imaging technique for visualizing the local changes in cerebral blood flow and metabolism that accompany mental activities, such as reading, speaking, and thinking. In 1988, using this new imaging form, Michael Posner, Marcus Raichle, and their colleagues made an interesting discovery. They found that the incoming sensory information that leads to language production and understanding is processed in more than one pathway.

Recall that Wernicke believed that both written and spoken words are transformed into a representation of language by both auditory and visual inputs. This information, he thought, is then conveyed to Wernicke's area, where it becomes associated with meaning before being transformed in Broca's area into output as spoken language. Posner and his colleagues asked: Must the neural code for a word that is read be translated into an auditory representation before it can be associated with a meaning? Or can visual information be sent directly to Broca's area with no involvement of the auditory system? Using PET, they determined how individual words are coded in the brain of normal subjects when the words are read on a screen or heard through earphones. Thus, when words are heard Wernicke's area

becomes active, but when words are seen but not heard or spoken Wernicke's area is not activated. The visual information from the occipital cortex appears to be conveyed directly to Broca's area without first being transformed into an auditory representation in the posterior temporal cortex. Posner and his colleagues concluded that the brain pathways and sensory codes used to see words are different from those used to hear words. They proposed, therefore, that these pathways have independent access to higher-order regions of the cortex concerned with the meaning of words and with the ability to express language (Figure 1-6).

Not only are reading and listening processed separately, but the act of thinking about a word's *meaning* (in the absence of sensory inputs) activates a still different area in the left frontal cortex. Thus language processing is *parallel* as well as serial; as we shall learn in Chapter 59, it is considerably more complex than initially envisaged by Wernicke. Indeed, similar conclusions have been reached from studies of behavior other than language. These studies demonstrate that information processing requires many individual cortical areas that are appropriately interconnected—each of them responding to, and therefore coding for, only some aspects of specific sensory stimuli or motor movement, and not for others.

Studies of aphasia afford unusual insight into how the brain is organized for language. One of the most impressive insights comes from a study of deaf people who lost their ability to speak American Sign Language after suffering cerebral damage. Unlike spoken language, American signing is accomplished with hand gestures rather than by sound and is perceived by visual rather than auditory pathways. Nonetheless, signing, which has the same structural complexities characteristic of spoken languages, is also localized to the left hemisphere. Thus, deaf people can become aphasic for sign language as a result of lesions in the left hemisphere. Lesions in the right hemisphere do not produce these defects. Moreover, damage to the left hemisphere can have quite specific consequences, affecting either sign comprehension (following damage in Wernicke's area) or grammar (following damage in Broca's area) or signing fluency.

These observations illustrate three points. First, the cognitive processing for language occurs in the left hemisphere and is independent of pathways that process the sensory or motor modalities used in language. Second, speech and hearing are not necessary conditions for the emergence of language capabilities in the left hemisphere. Third, spoken language represents only one of a family of cognitive skills mediated by the left hemisphere.

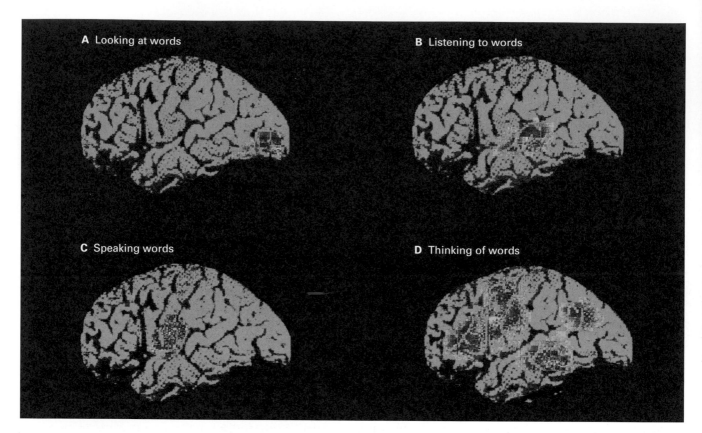

Figure 1-6 Specific regions of the cortex involved in the recognition of a spoken or written word can be identified with PET scanning. Each of the four images of the human brain shown here (from the left side of the cortex) actually represents the averaged brain activity of several normal subjects. (In these PET images white represents the areas of highest activity, red and yellow quite high activity, and blue and gray the areas of minimal activity.) The "input" component of language (reading or hearing a word) activates the regions of the brain shown in **A** and **B**. The motor "output" component of language (speech or thought) activates the regions shown in **C** and **D**. (Courtesy of Cathy Price.)

A. The reading of a single word produces a response both in the primary visual cortex and in the visual association cortex (see Figure 1-5).

B. Hearing a word activates an entirely different set of areas in the temporal cortex and at the junction of the temporal-

parietal cortex. (To control for irrelevant differences, the same list of words was used in both the reading and listening tests.) A and B show that the brain uses several discrete pathways for processing language and does not transform visual signals for processing in the auditory pathway.

C. Subjects were asked to repeat a word presented either through earphones or on a screen. Speaking a word activates the supplementary motor area of the medial frontal cortex. Broca's area is activated whether the word is presented orally or visually. Thus both visual and auditory pathways converge on Broca's area, the common site for the motor articulation of speech.

D. Subjects were asked to respond to the word "brain" with an appropriate verb (for example, "to think"). This type of thinking activates the frontal cortex as well as Broca's and Wernicke's areas. These areas play a role in all cognition and abstract representation.

Affective Traits and Aspects of Personality Are Also Anatomically Localized

Despite the persuasive evidence for localized language-related functions in the cortex, the idea nevertheless persisted that affective (emotional) functions are not localized. Emotion, it was believed, must be an expression of whole-brain activity. Only recently has this view been modified. Although the emotional aspects of behavior have not been as precisely mapped as sensory, motor,

and cognitive functions, distinct emotions can be elicited by stimulating specific parts of the brain in humans or experimental animals. The localization of affect has been dramatically demonstrated in patients with certain language disorders and those with a particular type of epilepsy.

Aphasia patients not only manifest cognitive defects in language, but also have trouble with the affective aspects of language, such as intonation (or *prosody*). These affective aspects are represented in the right hemisphere and, rather strikingly, the neural organization of the affective elements of language mirrors the organization of the logical content of language in the left hemisphere. Damage to the right temporal area corresponding to Wernicke's area in the left temporal region leads to disturbances in *comprehending* the emotional quality of language, for example, appreciating from a person's tone of voice whether he is describing a sad or happy event. In contrast, damage to the right frontal area corresponding to Broca's area leads to difficulty in *expressing* emotional aspects of language.

Thus some linguistic functions also exist in the right hemisphere. Indeed, there is now considerable evidence that an intact right hemisphere may be necessary to an appreciation of subtleties of language, such as irony, metaphor, and wit, as well as the emotional content of speech. Certain disorders of affective language that are localized to the right hemisphere, called *aprosodias,* are classified as sensory, motor, or conduction aprosodias, following the classification used for aphasias. This pattern of localization appears to be inborn, but it is by no means completely determined until the age of about seven or eight. Young children in whom the left cerebral hemisphere is severely damaged early in life can still develop an essentially normal grasp of language.

Further clues to the localization of affect come from patients with chronic temporal lobe epilepsy. These patients manifest characteristic emotional changes, some of which occur only fleetingly during the seizure itself and are called *ictal phenomena* (Latin *ictus,* a blow or a strike). Common ictal phenomena include feelings of unreality and déjà vu (the sensation of having been in a place before or of having had a particular experience before); transient visual or auditory hallucinations; feelings of depersonalization, fear, or anger; delusions; sexual feelings; and paranoia.

More enduring emotional changes, however, are evident when patients are not having seizures. These *interictal phenomena* are interesting because they represent a true psychiatric syndrome. A detailed study of such patients indicates they lose all interest in sex, and the decline in sexual interest is often paralleled by a rise in social aggressiveness. Most exhibit one or more distinctive personality traits: They can be intensely emotional, ardently religious, extremely moralistic, and totally lacking in humor. In striking contrast, patients with epileptic foci outside the temporal lobe show no abnormal emotion and behavior.

One important structure for the expression and perception of emotion is the amygdala, which lies deep within the cerebral hemispheres. The role of this structure in emotion was discovered through studies of the effects of the irritative lesions of epilepsy within the temporal lobe. The consequences of such irritative lesions are exactly the opposite of those of destructive lesions resulting from a stroke or injury. Whereas destructive lesions bring about loss of function, often through the disconnection of specialized areas, the electrical storm of epilepsy can increase activity in the regions affected, leading to excessive expression of emotion or over-elaboration of ideas. We consider the neurobiology of emotion in Part VIII of this book.

Mental Processes Are Represented in the Brain by Their Elementary Processing Operations

Why has the evidence for localization, which seems so obvious and compelling in retrospect, been rejected so often in the past? The reasons are several.

First, phrenologists introduced the idea of localization in an exaggerated form and without adequate evidence. They imagined each region of the cerebral cortex as an independent mental organ dedicated to a complete and distinct mental function (much as the pancreas and the liver are independent digestive organs). Flourens's rejection of phrenology and the ensuing dialectic between proponents of the aggregate-field view (against localization) and the cellular connectionists (for localization) were responses to a theory that was simplistic and overweening. The concept of localization that ultimately emerged—and prevailed—is more subtle by far than anything Gall (or even Wernicke) ever envisioned.

In the aftermath of Wernicke's discovery that there is a modular organization for language in the brain consisting of a complex of serial and parallel processing centers with more or less independent functions, we now appreciate that all cognitive abilities result from the interaction of many simple processing mechanisms distributed in many different regions of the brain. Specific brain regions are not concerned with *faculties* of the mind, but with elementary processing operations. Perception, movement, language, thought, and memory are all made possible by the serial and parallel interlinking of several brain regions, each with specific functions. As a result, damage to a single area need not result in the loss of an entire faculty as many earlier neurologists predicted. Even if a behavior initially disappears, it may partially return as undamaged parts of the brain reorganize their linkages.

Thus, it is not useful to represent mental processes as a series of links in a chain, for in such an arrangement the entire process breaks down when a single link is disrupted. The better, more realistic metaphor is to think of mental processes as several railroad lines that all feed into the same terminal. The malfunction of a single link on one pathway affects the information carried by that pathway, but need not interfere permanently with the system as a whole. The remaining parts of the system can modify their performance to accommodate extra traffic after the breakdown of a line.

Models of localized function were slow to be accepted because it is enormously difficult to demonstrate which components of a mental operation are represented by a particular pathway or brain region. Nor has it been easy to analyze mental operations and come up with testable components. Only during the last decade, with the convergence of modern cognitive psychology and the brain sciences, have we begun to appreciate that *all* mental functions are divisible into subfunctions. One difficulty with breaking down mental processes into analytical categories or steps is that our cognitive experience consists of instantaneous, smooth operations. Actually, these processes are composed of numerous independent information-processing components, and even the simplest task requires coordination of several distinct brain areas.

To illustrate this point, consider how we learn about, store, and recall the knowledge that we have in our mind about objects, people, and events in our world. Our common sense tell us that we store each piece of our knowledge of the world as a single representation that can be recalled by memory-jogging stimuli or even by the imagination alone. Everything we know about our grandmother, for example, seems to be stored in one complete representation of "grandmother" that is equally accessible to us whether we see her in person, hear her voice, or simply think about her. Our experience, however, is not a faithful guide to the knowledge we have stored in memory. Knowledge is not stored as complete representations but rather is subdivided into distinct categories and stored separately. For example, the brain stores separately information about animate and inanimate objects. Thus selected lesions in the left temporal lobe's association areas can obliterate a patient's knowledge of living things, especially people, while leaving the patient's knowledge of inanimate objects quite intact. Representational categories such as "living people" can be subdivided even further. A small lesion in the left temporal lobe can destroy a patient's ability to recognize people by name without affecting the ability to recognize them by sight.

The most astonishing example of the modular nature of representational mental processes is the finding that our very sense of ourselves as a self-conscious coherent being—the sum of what we mean when we say "I"—is achieved through the connection of independent circuits, each with its own sense of awareness, that carry out separate operations in our two cerebral hemispheres. The remarkable discovery that even consciousness is not a unitary process was made by Roger Sperry and Michael Gazzaniga in the course of studying epileptic patients in whom the corpus callosum—the major tract connecting the two hemispheres—was severed as a treatment for epilepsy. Sperry and Gazzaniga found that each hemisphere had a consciousness that was able to function independently of the other. The right hemisphere, which cannot speak, also cannot understand language that is well-understood by the isolated left hemisphere. As a result, opposing commands can be issued by each hemisphere—each hemisphere has a mind of its own! While one patient was holding a favorite book in his left hand, the right hemisphere, which controls the left hand but cannot read, found that simply looking at the book was boring. The right hemisphere commanded the left hand to put the book down! Another patient would put on his clothes with the left hand, while taking them off with the other. Thus in some commissurotomized patients the two hemispheres can even interfere with each other's function. In addition, the dominant hemisphere sometimes comments on the performance of the nondominant hemisphere, frequently exhibiting a false sense of confidence regarding problems in which it cannot know the solution, since the information was projected exclusively to the nondominant hemisphere.

Thus the main reason it has taken so long to appreciate which mental activities are localized within which regions of the brain is that we are dealing here with biology's deepest riddle: the neural representation of consciousness and self-awareness. After all, to study the relationship between a mental process and specific brain regions, we must be able to identify the components of the mental process that we are attempting to explain. Yet, of all behaviors, higher mental processes are the most difficult to describe, to measure objectively, and to dissect into their elementary components and operations. In addition, the brain's anatomy is immensely complex, and the structure and interconnections of its many parts are still not fully understood. To analyze how a specific mental activity is represented in the brain, we need not only to determine which aspects of the activity are represented in which regions of the brain, but also how they are represented and how such representations interact.

Only in the last decade has that become possible. By combining the conceptual tools of cognitive psychology with new physiological techniques and brain imaging methods, we are beginning to visualize the regions of the brain involved in particular behaviors. And we are just beginning to discern how these behaviors can be broken down into simpler mental operations and mapped to specific interconnected modules of the brain. Indeed, the excitement evident in neural science today is based on the conviction that at last we have in hand the proper tools to explore the extraordinary organ of the mind, so that we can eventually fathom the biological principles that underlie human cognition.

Eric R. Kandel

Selected Readings

Bear DM. 1979. The temporal lobes: an approach to the study of organic behavioral changes. In: MS Gazzaniga (ed). *Handbook of Behavioral Neurobiology*, Vol. 2, *Neuropsychology*. pp. 75–95. New York: Plenum.

Caramazza A. 1995. The representation of lexical knowledge in the brain. In: RD Broadwell (ed). *Neuroscience, Memory, and Language*, Vol. 1, *Decade of the Brain*, pp. 133–147. Washington, DC: Library of Congress.

Churchland PS. 1986. *Neurophilosophy, Toward a Unified Science of the Mind-Brain*. Cambridge, MA: MIT Press.

Cooter R. 1984. *The Cultural Meaning of Popular Science: Phrenology and the Organization of Consent in Nineteenth-Century Britain*. Cambridge: Cambridge Univ. Press.

Cowan WM. 1981. Keynote. In: FO Schmitt, FG Worden, G Adelman, SG Dennis (eds). *The Organization of the Cerebral Cortex: Proceedings of a Neurosciences Research Program Colloquium*, pp. xi–xxi. Cambridge, MA: MIT Press.

Ferrier D. 1890. *The Croonian Lectures on Cerebral Localisation*. London: Smith, Elder.

Geschwind N. 1974. *Selected Papers on Language and the Brain*. Dordrecht, Holland: Reidel.

Harrington A. 1987. *Medicine, Mind, and the Double Brain: A Study in Nineteenth-Century Thought*. Princeton, NJ: Princeton Univ. Press.

Harrison RG. 1935. On the origin and development of the nervous system studied by the methods of experimental embryology. Proc R Soc Lond B Biol Sci 118:155–196.

Jackson JH. 1884. The Croonian lectures on evolution and dissolution of the nervous system. Br Med J 1:591–593; 660–663; 703–707.

Kandel ER. 1976. The study of behavior: the interface between psychology and biology. In: *Cellular Basis of Behavior: An Introduction to Behavioral Neurobiology*, pp. 3–27. San Francisco: Freeman.

Kosslyn SM. 1988. Aspects of a cognitive neuroscience of mental imagery. Science 240:1621–1626.

Marshall JC. 1988. Cognitive neurophysiology: the lifeblood of language. Nature 331:560–561.

Marshall JC. 1988. Cognitive neuropsychology: sensation and semantics. Nature 334:378.

Ojemann GA. 1995. Investigating language during awake neurosurgery. In: RD Broadwell (ed). *Neuroscience, Memory, and Language*, Vol. 1, *Decade of the Brain*, pp. 117–131. Washington, DC: Library of Congress.

Petersen SE. 1995. Functional neuroimaging in brain areas involved in language. In: RD Broadwell (ed). *Neuroscience, Memory, and Language*, Vol. 1, *Decade of the Brain*, pp. 109–116. Washington DC: Library of Congress.

Posner MI, Petersen SE, Fox PT, Raichle ME. 1988. Localization of cognitive operations in the human brain. Science 240:1627–1631.

Ross ED. 1984. Right hemisphere's role in language, affective behavior and emotion. Trends Neurosci 7:342–346.

Shepherd GM. 1991. *Foundations of the Neuron Doctrine*. New York: Oxford Univ. Press.

Sperry RW. 1968. Mental unity following surgical disconnection of the cerebral hemispheres. Harvey Lect 62:293–323.

Young RM. 1970. *Mind, Brain and Adaptation in the Nineteenth Century*. Oxford: Clarendon.

References

Adrian ED. 1941. Afferent discharges to the cerebral cortex from peripheral sense organs. J Physiol (Lond) 100: 159–191.

Bernard C. 1878–1879. *Leçons sur les Phénomènes de la vie Communs aux Animaux et aux Végétaux*. Vols. 1, 2. Paris: Baillière.

Boakes R. 1984. *From Darwin to Behaviourism: Psychology and the Minds of Animals*. Cambridge, England: Cambridge Univ. Press.

Broca P. 1865. Sur le siége de la faculté du langage articulé. Bull Soc Anthropol 6:377–393.

Brodmann K. 1909. *Vergleichende Lokalisationslehre der Grosshirnrinde in ihren Prinzipien dargestellt auf Grund des Zeelenbaues*. Leipzig: Barth.

Darwin C. 1872. *The Expression of the Emotions in Man and Animals*. London: Murray.

Descartes R. [1649] 1984. *The Philosophical Writings of Descartes*. Cambridge: Cambridge Univ. Press.

DuBois-Reymond E. 1848–1849. *Untersuchungen über thierische Elektrizität*. Vols. 1, 2. Berlin: Reimer.

Ehrlich P. 1913. Chemotherapeutics: scientific principles, methods, and results. Lancet 2:445–451.

Flourens P. 1824. Recherches expérimentales. Archiv Méd 2:321–370; Cited and translated by P Flourens, JMD Olmsted. In: EA Underwood (ed). 1953. *Science, Medicine and History*, 2:290–302. London: Oxford Univ. Press.

Flourens P. 1824. *Recherches Expérimentales sur les Propriétés et les Fonctions du Système Nerveux, dans les Animaux Vertébrés*. Paris: Chez Crevot.

Fritsch G, Hitzig E. 1870. Über die elektrische Erregbarkeit des Grosshirns. Arch Anat Physiol Wiss Med, pp. 300–332; 1960. Reprinted in: G. von Bonin (transl). *Some Papers on the Cerebral Cortex*, pp. 73–96. Springfield, IL: Thomas.

Gall FJ, Spurzheim G. 1810. *Anatomie et Physiologie du Système Nerveux en Général, et du Cerveau en Particulier, avec des Observations sur la Possibilité de Reconnoître Plusieurs Dispositions Intellectuelles et Morales de l'Homme et des Animaux, par la Configuration de leurs Têtes.* Paris: Schoell.

Galvani L. [1791] 1953. *Commentary on the Effect of Electricity on Muscular Motion.* RM Green (transl). Cambridge, MA: Licht.

Gazzaniga MS, LeDoux JE. 1978. *The Integrated Mind.* New York: Plenum.

Geschwind N. 1979. Specializations of the human brain. Sci Am 241(3):180–199.

Goldstein K. 1948. *Language and Language Disturbances: Aphasic Symptom Complexes and Their Significance for Medicine and Theory of Language.* New York: Grune & Stratton.

Golgi C. [1906] 1967. The neuron doctrine: theory and facts. In: *Nobel Lectures: Physiology or Medicine, 1901–1921,* pp. 189–217. Amsterdam: Elsevier.

Head H. 1921. Release of function in the nervous system. Proc R Soc Lond B Biol Sci 92:184–209.

Head H. 1926. *Aphasia and Kindred Disorders of Speech.* Vols. 1, 2. Cambridge: Cambridge Univ. Press; 1963. Reprint. New York: Hafner.

Heilman KM, Scholes R, Watson RT. 1975. Auditory affective agnosia. Disturbed comprehension of affective speech. J Neurol Neurosurg Psychiatry 38:69–72.

Langley JN. 1906. On nerve endings and on special excitable substances in cells. Proc R Soc Lond B Biol Sci 78:170–194.

Lashley KS. 1929. *Brain Mechanisms and Intelligence: A Quantitative Study of Injuries to the Brain.* Chicago: Univ. Chicago Press.

Lashley KS, Clark G. 1946. The cytoarchitecture of the cerebral cortex of *Ateles*: a critical examination of architectonic studies. J Comp Neurol 85:223–305.

Locke J. 1690. An essay concerning humane understanding. In: *Four Books.* London.

Loeb J. 1918. *Forced Movements, Tropisms and Animal Conduct.* Philadelphia: Lippincott.

Marshall WH, Woolsey CN, Bard P. 1941. Observations on cortical somatic sensory mechanisms of cat and monkey. J Neurophysiol 4:1–24.

McCarthy RA, Warrington EK. 1988. Evidence for modality-specific meaning systems in the brain. Nature 334: 428–430.

Müller J. 1834–1840. *Handbuch der Physiologie des Menschen für Vorlesungen.* Vols 1, 2. Coblenz: Hölscher.

Nieuwenhuys R, Voogd J, van Huijzen, Chr. 1988. *The Human Central Nervous System: A Synopsis and Atlas,* 3rd rev. ed. Berlin: Springer.

Pavlov IP. 1927. *Conditioned Reflexes: An Investigation of the Physiological Activity of the Cerebral Cortex.* GV Anrep (transl). London: Oxford Univ. Press.

Penfield W. 1954. Mechanisms of voluntary movement. Brain 77:1–17.

Penfield W, Rasmussen T. 1950. *The Cerebral Cortex of Man: A Clinical Study of Localization of Function.* New York: Macmillan.

Penfield W, Roberts L. 1959. *Speech and Brain-Mechanisms.* Princeton, NJ: Princeton Univ. Press.

Petersen SE, Fox PT, Posner MI, Mintun M, Raichle ME. 1989. Positron emission tomographic studies of the processing of single words. J Cogn Neurosci 1(2):153–170.

Posner MI, Carr TH. 1992. Lexical access and the brain: anatomical constraints on cognitive models of word recognition. Am J Psychol 105:1–26.

Ramón y Cajal S. [1892] 1977. A new concept of the histology of the central nervous system. DA Rottenberg (transl). (See also historical essay by SL Palay, preceding Ramón y Cajal's paper.) In: DA Rottenberg, FH Hochberg (eds). *Neurological Classics in Modern Translation,* pp. 7–29. New York: Hafner.

Ramón y Cajal S. [1906] 1967. The structure and connexions of neurons. In: *Nobel Lectures: Physiology or Medicine, 1901–1921,* pp. 220–253. Amsterdam: Elsevier.

Ramón y Cajal S. [1908] 1954. *Neuron Theory or Reticular Theory? Objective Evidence of the Anatomical Unity of Nerve Cells.* MU Purkiss, CA Fox (transl). Madrid: Consejo Superior de Investigaciones Científicas Instituto Ramón y Cajal.

Ramón y Cajal S. 1937. *1852–1934. Recollections of My Life.* EH Craigie (transl). Philadelphia: American Philosophical Society; 1989. Reprint. Cambridge, MA: MIT Press.

Rose JE, Woolsey CN. 1948. Structure and relations of limbic cortex and anterior thalamic nuclei in rabbit and cat. J Comp Neurol 89:279–347.

Ross ED. 1981. The aprosodias: functional-anatomic organization of the affective components of language in the right hemisphere. Arch Neurol 38:561–569.

Sherrington C. 1947. *The Integrative Action of the Nervous System,* 2nd ed. Cambridge: Cambridge Univ. Press.

Spurzheim JG. 1825. *Phrenology, or the Doctrine of the Mind,* 3rd ed. London: Knight.

Swazey JP. 1970. Action proper and action commune: the localization of cerebral function. J Hist Biol 3:213–234.

von Helmholtz H. 1850. On the rate of transmission of the nerve impulse. Monatsber Preuss Akad Wiss Berlin, pp. 14–15. Translated in: W Dennis (ed). 1948. *Readings in the History of Psychology,* pp. 197–198. New York: Appleton-Century-Crofts.

Wernicke C. 1908. The symptom-complex of aphasia. In: A Church (ed), *Diseases of the Nervous System,* pp. 265–324. New York: Appleton.

Zurif E. 1974. Auditory lateralization, prosodic and syntactic factors. Brain Lang 1:391–401.

2

Nerve Cells and Behavior

HUMANS ARE VASTLY superior to other animals in their ability to exploit their physical environment. The remarkable range of human behavior—indeed, the complexity of the environment humans have been able to create for themselves—depends on a sophisticated array of sensory receptors connected to a highly flexible neural machine—a brain—that is able to discriminate an enormous variety of events in the environment. The continuous stream of information from these receptors is organized by the brain into perceptions (some of which are stored in memory for future reference) and then into appropriate behavioral responses. All of this is accomplished by the brain using nerve cells and the connections between them.

Individual nerve cells, the basic units of the brain, are relatively simple in their morphology. Although the human brain contains an extraordinary number of these cells (on the order of 10^{11} neurons), which can be classified into at least a thousand different types, all nerve cells share the same basic architecture. The complexity of human behavior depends less on the specialization of individual nerve cells and more on the fact that a great many of these cells form precise anatomical circuits. One of the key organizational principles of the brain, therefore, is that nerve cells with basically similar properties can nevertheless produce quite different actions because of the way they are connected with each other and with sensory receptors and muscle.

Since relatively few principles of organization give rise to considerable complexity, it is possible to learn a great deal about how the nervous system produces behavior by focusing on four basic features of the nervous system:

1. The mechanisms by which neurons produce signals.
2. The patterns of connections between nerve cells.
3. The relationship of different patterns of interconnection to different types of behavior.
4. The means by which neurons and their connections are modified by experience.

In this chapter we introduce these four features by first considering the structural and functional properties of neurons and the glial cells that surround and support them. We then examine how individual cells organize and transmit signals and how signaling between a few interconnected nerve cells produces a simple behavior, the knee jerk reflex. Finally, we consider how changes in the signaling ability of specific cells can modify behavior.

The Nervous System Has Two Classes of Cells

There are two main classes of cells in the nervous system: nerve cells (neurons) and glial cells (glia).

Glial Cells Are Support Cells

Glial cells far outnumber neurons—there are between 10 and 50 times more glia than neurons in the central nervous system of vertebrates. The name for these cells derives from the Greek for glue, although in actuality glia do not commonly hold nerve cells together. Rather, they surround the cell bodies, axons, and dendrites of neurons. As far as is known, glia are not directly involved in information processing, but they are thought to have at least seven other vital roles:

1. Glial cells support neurons, providing the brain with structure. They also separate and sometimes insulate neuronal groups and synaptic connections from each other.
2. Two types of glial cells (oligodendrocytes and Schwann cells) produce the myelin used to insulate nerve cell axons, the cell outgrowths that conduct electrical signals.
3. Some glial cells are scavengers, removing debris after injury or neuronal death.
4. Glial cells perform important housekeeping chores that promote efficient signaling between neurons (Chapter 14). For example, some glia also take up chemical transmitters released by neurons during synaptic transmission.
5. During the brain's development certain classes of glial cells ("radial glia") guide migrating neurons and direct the outgrowth of axons.
6. In some cases, as at the nerve-muscle synapse of vertebrates, glial cells actively regulate the properties of the presynaptic terminal.
7. Some glial cells (astrocytes) help form an impermeable lining in the brain's capillaries and venules— the *blood-brain barrier*—that prevents toxic substances in the blood from entering the brain (Appendix B).
8. Other glial cells apparently release growth factors and otherwise help nourish nerve cells, although

this role has been difficult to demonstrate conclusively.

Glial cells in the vertebrate nervous system are divided into two major classes: *microglia* and *macroglia.*

Microglia are phagocytes that are mobilized after injury, infection, or disease. They arise from macrophages outside the nervous system and are physiologically and embryologically unrelated to the other cell types of the nervous system. Not much is known about what microglia do in the resting state, but they become activated and recruited during infection, injury, and seizure. The activated cell has a process that is stouter and more branched than that of inactivated cells, and it expresses a range of antigens, which suggests that it may serve as the major antigen presenting cell in the central nervous system. Microglia are thought to become activated in a number of diseases including multiple sclerosis and AIDS-related dementia, as well as various chronic neurodegenerative diseases such as Parkinson's disease and Alzheimer's disease.

Three types of macroglial cells predominate in the vertebrate nervous system: oligodendrocytes, Schwann cells, and astrocytes.

Oligodendrocytes and *Schwann cells* are small cells with relatively few processes. Both types carry out the important job of insulating axons, forming a myelin sheath by tightly winding their membranous processes around the axon in a spiral. Oligodendrocytes, which are found in the central nervous system, envelop an average of 15 axonal internodes each (Figure 2-1A). By contrast, Schwann cells, which occur in the peripheral nervous system, each envelop just one internode of only one axon (Figure 2-1B). The types of myelin produced by oligodendrocytes and Schwann cells differ to some degree in chemical makeup.

Astrocytes, the most numerous of glial cells, owe their name to their irregular, roughly star-shaped cell bodies (Figure 2-1C). They tend to have rather long processes, some of which terminate in end-feet. Some astrocytes form end-feet on the surfaces of nerve cells in the brain and spinal cord and may play a role in bringing nutrients to these cells. Other astrocytes place end-feet on the brain's blood vessels and cause the vessel's endothelial (lining) cells to form tight junctions, thus creating the protective blood-brain barrier (Figure 2-1C).

Astrocytes also help to maintain the right potassium ion concentration in the extracellular space between neurons. As we shall learn below and in Chapter 7, when a nerve cell fires, potassium ions flow out of the cell. Repetitive firing may create an excess of extracellular potassium that could interfere with signaling between cells in the vicinity. Because astrocytes are highly

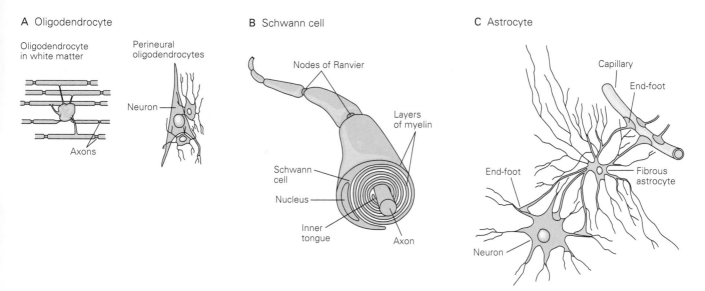

A Oligodendrocyte

Oligodendrocyte in white matter

Perineural oligodendrocytes

Neuron

Axons

B Schwann cell

Nodes of Ranvier

Layers of myelin

Schwann cell

Nucleus

Inner tongue

Axon

C Astrocyte

Capillary

End-foot

End-foot

Fibrous astrocyte

Neuron

Figure 2-1 The principal types of glial cells in the central nervous system are astrocytes and oligodendrocytes and in the peripheral nervous system, Schwann cells.

A. Oligodendrocytes are small cells with relatively few processes. In white matter (left) they provide the myelin, and in gray matter (right) perineural oligodendrocytes surround and support the cell bodies of neurons. A single oligodendrocyte can wrap its membranous processes around many axons, insulating them with a myelin sheath.

B. Schwann cells furnish the myelin sheaths that insulate axons in the peripheral nervous system. Each of several Schwann cells, positioned along the length of a single axon, forms a segment of myelin sheath about 1 mm long. The sheath assumes its form as the inner tongue of the Schwann cell turns around the axon several times, wrapping it in concentric layers of membrane. The intervals between segments of myelin are known as the nodes of Ranvier. In living cells the layers of myelin are more compact than what is shown here. (Adapted from Alberts et al. 1994.)

C. Astrocytes, the most numerous of glial cells in the central nervous system, are characterized by their star-like shape and the broad end-feet on their processes. Because these end-feet put the astrocyte into contact with both capillaries and neurons, astrocytes are thought to have a nutritive function. Astrocytes also play an important role in forming the blood-brain barrier.

permeable to potassium, they can take up the excess potassium and so protect those neighboring neurons. In addition, astrocytes take up neurotransmitters from synaptic zones after release and thereby help regulate synaptic activities by removing transmitters. But the role of astrocytes is largely a supporting one.

There is no evidence that glia are *directly* involved in electrical signaling. Signaling is the function of nerve cells.

Nerve Cells Are the Main Signaling Units of the Nervous System

A typical neuron has four morphologically defined regions: the cell body, dendrites, the axon, and presynaptic terminals (Figure 2-2). As we shall see later, each of these regions has a distinct role in the generation of signals and the communication of signals between nerve cells.

The cell body (*soma*) is the metabolic center of the cell. It contains the nucleus, which stores the genes of the cell, as well as the endoplasmic reticulum, an extension of the nucleus where the cell's proteins are synthesized. The cell body usually gives rise to two kinds of processes: several short *dendrites* and one, long, tubular *axon*. Dendrites branch out in tree-like fashion and are the main apparatus for receiving incoming signals from other nerve cells. In contrast, the axon extends away from the cell body and is the main conducting unit for carrying signals to other neurons. An axon can convey electrical signals along distances ranging from 0.1 mm to 3 m. These electrical signals, called *action potentials*, are rapid, transient, all-or-none nerve impulses, with an amplitude of 100 mV and a duration of about 1 ms (Figure 2-3). Action potentials are initiated at a specialized trigger region at the origin of the axon called the *axon hillock* (or *initial segment* of the axon); from there they are conducted down the axon without failure or distortion at rates of 1–100 m per second. The amplitude of an action potential traveling down the axon remains constant because the action potential is an all-or-none impulse that is regenerated at regular intervals along the axon.

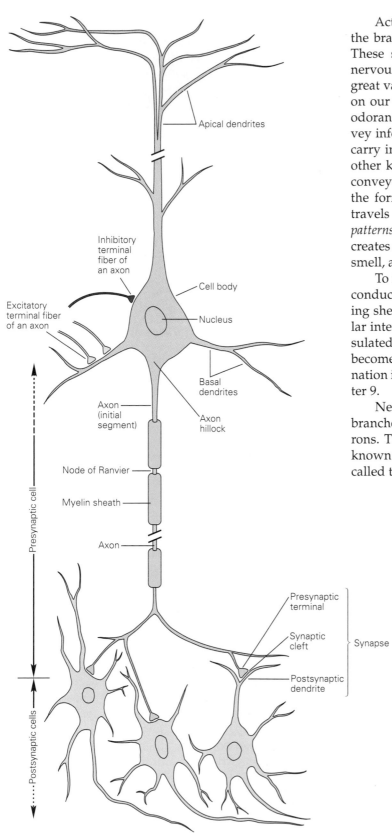

Action potentials constitute the signals by which the brain receives, analyzes, and conveys information. These signals are highly stereotyped throughout the nervous system, even though they are initiated by a great variety of events in the environment that impinge on our bodies—from light to mechanical contact, from odorants to pressure waves. Thus, the signals that convey information about vision are identical to those that carry information about odors. Here we encounter another key principle of brain function. The information conveyed by an action potential is determined not by the form of the signal but by the pathway the signal travels in the brain. The brain analyzes and interprets *patterns* of incoming electrical signals and in this way creates our everyday sensations of sight, touch, taste, smell, and sound.

To increase the speed by which action potentials are conducted, large axons are wrapped in a fatty, insulating sheath of myelin. The sheath is interrupted at regular intervals by the nodes of Ranvier. It is at these uninsulated spots on the axon that the action potential becomes regenerated. We shall learn more about myelination in Chapter 4 and about action potentials in Chapter 9.

Near its end, the tubular axon divides into fine branches that form communication sites with other neurons. The point at which two neurons communicate is known as a *synapse.* The nerve cell transmitting a signal is called the *presynaptic cell.* The cell receiving the signal is

Figure 2-2 Structure of a neuron. Most neurons in the vertebrate nervous system have several main features in common. The cell body contains the nucleus, the storehouse of genetic information, and gives rise to two types of cell processes, axons and dendrites. Axons, the transmitting element of neurons, can vary greatly in length; some can extend more than 3 m within the body. Most axons in the central nervous system are very thin (between 0.2 and 20 μm in diameter) compared with the diameter of the cell body (50 μm or more). Many axons are insulated by a fatty sheath of myelin that is interrupted at regular intervals by the nodes of Ranvier. The action potential, the cell's conducting signal, is initiated either at the axon hillock, the initial segment of the axon, or in some cases slightly farther down the axon at the first node of Ranvier. Branches of the axon of one neuron (the presynaptic neuron) transmit signals to another neuron (the postsynaptic cell) at a site called the synapse. The branches of a single axon may form synapses with as many as 1000 other neurons. Whereas the axon is the output element of the neuron, the dendrites (apical and basal) are input elements of the neuron. Together with the cell body, they receive synaptic contacts from other neurons.

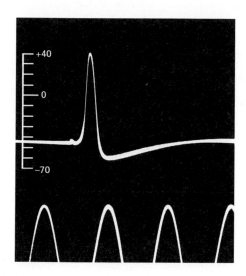

Figure 2-3 This historic tracing is the first published intracellular recording of an action potential. It was obtained in 1939 by Hodgkin and Huxley from the squid giant axon, using glass capillary electrodes filled with sea water. Time marker is 500 Hz. The vertical scale indicates the potential of the internal electrode in millivolts, the sea water outside being taken as zero potential. (From Hodgkin and Huxley 1939.)

the *postsynaptic cell.* The presynaptic cell transmits signals from the swollen ends of its axon's branches, called *presynaptic terminals.* However, a presynaptic cell does not actually touch or communicate anatomically with the postsynaptic cell since the two cells are separated by a space, the *synaptic cleft.* Most presynaptic terminals end on the postsynaptic neuron's dendrites, but the terminals may also end on the cell body or, less often, at the beginning or end of the axon of the receiving cell (Figure 2-2).

As we saw in Chapter 1, Ramón y Cajal provided much of the early evidence for the now basic understanding that neurons are the signaling units of the nervous system and that each neuron is a discrete cell with distinctive processes arising from its cell body (the neuron doctrine). In retrospect, it is hard to appreciate how difficult it was to persuade scientists of this elementary idea. Unlike other tissues, whose cells have simple shapes and fit into a single field of the light microscope, nerve cells have complex shapes; the elaborate patterns of dendrites and the seemingly endless course of some axons made it extremely difficult initially to establish a relationship between these elements. Even after the anatomists Jacob Schleiden and Theodor Schwann put forward the cell theory in the early 1830s—when the idea that cells are the structural units of all living matter became a central dogma of biology—most anatomists would not accept that the cell theory applied to the brain, which they thought of as a continuous web-like reticulum.

The coherent structure of the neuron did not become clear until late in the nineteenth century, when Ramón y Cajal began to use the silver staining method introduced by Golgi. This method, which continues to be used today, has two advantages. First, in a random manner that is still not understood, the silver solution stains only about 1% of the cells in any particular brain region, making it possible to study a single nerve cell in isolation from its neighbors. Second, the neurons that do take up the stain are delineated in their entirety, including the cell body, axon, and full dendritic tree. The stain shows that (with rare exceptions we shall consider later) there is no cytoplasmic continuity between neurons, even at the synapse between two cells. Thus, neurons do not form a syncytium; each neuron is clearly segregated from every other neuron.

Ramón y Cajal applied Golgi's method to the embryonic nervous systems of many animals, including the human brain. By examining the structure of neurons in almost every region of the nervous system and tracing the contacts they made with one another, Ramón y Cajal was able to describe the differences between classes of nerve cells and to map the precise connections between a good many of them. In this way Ramón y Cajal grasped, in addition to the neuron doctrine, two other principles of neural organization that would prove particularly valuable in studying communication in the nervous system.

The first of these has become known as the *principle of dynamic polarization.* It states that electrical signals within a nerve cell flow only in one direction: from the receiving sites of the neuron (usually the dendrites and cell body) to the trigger region at the axon. From there, the action potential is propagated unidirectionally along the entire length of the axon to the cell's presynaptic terminals. Although neurons vary in shape and function, the operation of most follows this rule of information flow. Later in this chapter we shall describe the physiological basis of this principle.

The second principle, the *principle of connectional specificity,* states that nerve cells do not connect indiscriminately with one another to form random networks; rather each cell makes specific connections—at particular contact points—with certain postsynaptic target cells but not with others. Taken together, the principles of dynamic polarization and connectional specificity form the cellular basis of the modern connectionist approach to the brain discussed in Chapter 1.

Ramón y Cajal was also among the first to realize that the feature that most distinguishes one neuron from another is *shape*—specifically, the number and form of the processes arising from the cell body. On the basis of shape, neurons are classified into three large groups: unipolar, bipolar, and multipolar.

Figure 2-4 Neurons can be classified as unipolar, bipolar, or multipolar according to the number of processes that originate from the cell body.

A. Unipolar cells have a single process, with different segments serving as receptive surfaces or releasing terminals. Unipolar cells are characteristic of the invertebrate nervous system.

B. Bipolar cells have two processes that are functionally specialized: the dendrite carries information to the cell, and the axon transmits information to other cells.

C. Certain neurons that carry sensory information, such as information about touch or stretch, to the spinal cord belong to a subclass of bipolar cells designated as pseudo-unipolar. As such cells develop, the two processes of the embryonic bipolar cell become fused and emerge from the cell body as a single process. This outgrowth then splits into two processes, *both* of which function as axons, one going to peripheral skin or muscle, the other going to the central spinal cord.

D. Multipolar cells have an axon and many dendrites. They are the most common type of neuron in the mammalian nervous system. Three examples illustrate the large diversity of these cells. Spinal motor neurons (left) innervate skeletal muscle fibers. Pyramidal cells (middle) have a roughly triangular cell body; dendrites emerge from both the apex (the apical dendrite) and the base (the basal dendrites). Pyramidal cells are found in the hippocampus and throughout the cerebral cortex. Purkinje cells of the cerebellum (right) are characterized by the rich and extensive dendritic tree in one plane. Such a structure permits enormous synaptic input. (Adapted from Ramón y Cajal 1933.)

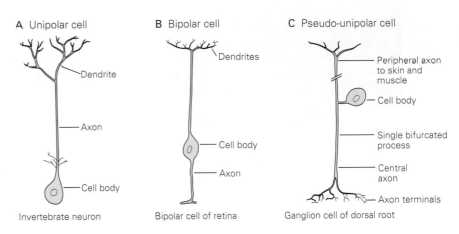

A Unipolar cell

Invertebrate neuron

B Bipolar cell

Bipolar cell of retina

C Pseudo-unipolar cell

Ganglion cell of dorsal root

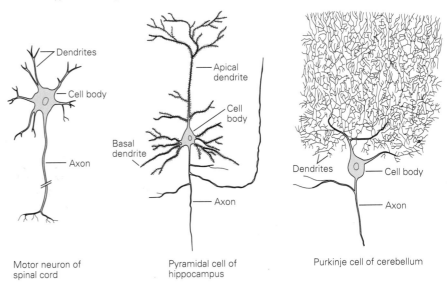

D Three types of multipolar cells

Motor neuron of spinal cord

Pyramidal cell of hippocampus

Purkinje cell of cerebellum

Unipolar neurons are the simplest nerve cells because they have a single primary process, which usually gives rise to many branches. One branch serves as the axon; other branches function as dendritic receiving structures (Figure 2-4A). These cells predominate in the nervous systems of invertebrates; in vertebrates they occur in the autonomic nervous system.

Bipolar neurons have an oval-shaped soma that gives rise to two processes: a dendrite that conveys information from the periphery of the body, and an axon that carries information toward the central nervous system (Figure 2-4B). Many sensory cells are bipolar cells, including those in the retina of the eye and in the olfactory epithelium of the nose. The mechanoreceptors that convey touch, pressure, and pain to the spinal cord are variants of bipolar cells called *pseudo-unipolar* cells. These cells develop initially as bipolar cells; later the two cell processes fuse to form one axon that emerges from the cell body. The axon then splits into two; one branch runs to the periphery (to sensory receptors in the skin, joints, and muscle), the other to the spinal cord (Figure 2-4C).

Multipolar neurons predominate in the nervous system of vertebrates. They have a single axon and, typically, many dendrites emerging from various points around the cell body (Figure 2-4D). Multipolar cells vary greatly in shape, especially in the length of their axons and in the number, length, and intricacy of dendrite branching. Usually the number and extent of their dendrites correlate with the number of synaptic contacts that other neurons make onto them. A spinal motor cell with a relatively modest number of dendrites receives about 10,000 contacts—2000 on its cell body and 8000 on its dendrites. The dendritic tree of a Purkinje cell in the cerebellum is much larger and bushier, as well it might be—it receives approximately 150,000 contacts!

Neurons are also commonly classified into three major functional groups: sensory, motor, and interneuronal. *Sensory neurons* carry information from the body's periphery into the nervous system for the purpose of both perception and motor coordination.[1] *Motor neurons* carry commands from the brain or spinal cord to muscles and glands. *Interneurons* constitute by far the largest class, consisting of all nerve cells that are not specifically sensory or motor. Interneurons are subdivided into two classes. *Relay* or *projection interneurons* have long axons and convey signals over considerable distances, from one brain region to another. *Local interneurons* have short axons and process information within local circuits.

Nerve Cells Form Specific Signaling Networks That Mediate Specific Behaviors

All the behavioral functions of the brain—the processing of sensory information, the programming of motor and emotional responses, the vital business of storing information (memory)—are carried out by specific sets of interconnected neurons. Here we shall examine in general terms how a behavior is produced by considering a simple stretch reflex, the knee jerk. We shall see how a transient imbalance of the body, which puts a stretch on the extensor muscles of the leg, produces sensory information that is conveyed to motor cells, which in turn convey commands to the extensor muscles to contract so that balance will be restored.

The anatomical components of the knee jerk are shown in Figure 2-5. The tendon of the quadriceps femoris, an extensor muscle that moves the lower leg, is attached to the tibia through the tendon of the kneecap, the patellar tendon. Tapping this tendon just below the

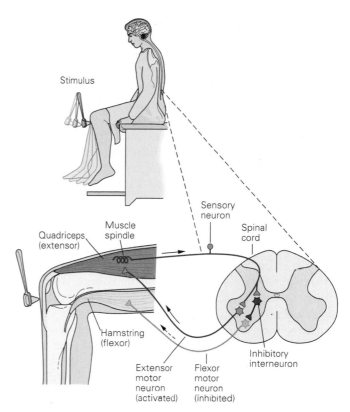

Figure 2-5 **The knee jerk is an example of a monosynaptic reflex system, a simple behavior controlled by direct connections between sensory and motor neurons.** Tapping the kneecap with a reflex hammer pulls on the tendon of the quadriceps femoris, an extensor muscle that extends the lower leg. When the muscle stretches in response to the pull of the tendon, information regarding this change in the muscle is conveyed by afferent (sensory) neurons to the central nervous system. In the spinal cord the sensory neurons act directly on extensor motor neurons that contract the quadriceps, the muscle that was stretched. In addition, the sensory neurons act indirectly, through interneurons, to inhibit flexor motor neurons that would otherwise contract the opposing muscle, the hamstring. These actions combine to produce the reflex behavior. In this schematic drawing each extensor and flexor motor neuron represents a population of many cells.

patella will pull (stretch) the quadriceps femoris. This initiates a reflex contraction of the quadriceps muscle to produce the familiar knee jerk, an extension of the leg smoothly coordinated with a relaxation of the hamstrings, the opposing flexor muscles. By increasing the tension of a selected group of muscles, the stretch reflex changes the position of the leg, suddenly extending it outward. (The regulation of movement by the nervous system is discussed in Section VI.)

Stretch reflexes like the knee jerk are a special type of reflex called *spinal reflexes*, behaviors mediated by neural circuits that are entirely confined to the spinal

---

[1.] Some primary sensory neurons are also commonly called afferent neurons, and we use these two terms interchangeably in the book. The term *afferent* (carried *toward* the nervous system) applies to all information reaching the central nervous system from the periphery, whether or not this information leads to sensation. The term *sensory* should, strictly speaking, be applied only to afferent input that leads to a perception.

cord. As we shall see later in the book, such spinal circuits relieve the major motor systems of the brain of having to micromanage elementary behavioral actions. Stretch reflexes are mediated in good part by *monosynaptic circuits*, in which the sensory neurons and motor neurons executing the action are directly connected to one another, with no interneuron intervening between them. Most other reflexes, including most spinal reflexes, use polysynaptic circuits that include one or more sets of interneurons. Polysynaptic circuits are more amenable to modification by the brain's higher processing centers.

The cell bodies of the mechanoreceptor sensory neurons involved in the knee jerk are clustered near the spinal cord in a *dorsal root ganglion* (Figure 2-5). They are pseudo-unipolar cells; one branch of the cell's axon goes to the quadriceps muscle at the periphery, while the other runs centrally into the spinal cord. The branch that innervates the quadriceps makes contact with stretch-sensitive receptors called *muscle spindles* and is excited when the muscle is stretched. The branch in the spinal cord forms excitatory connections with the motor neurons that innervate the quadriceps and control its contraction. In addition, this branch contacts local interneurons that inhibit the motor neurons controlling the *opposing* flexor muscles. These local interneurons are not involved in the stretch reflex itself, but by coordinating motor action they increase the stability of the reflex response. Thus, the electrical signals that produce the stretch reflex convey four kinds of information:

1. Sensory information is conveyed to the central nervous system (the spinal cord) from the body's surface.
2. Motor commands from the central nervous system are issued to the muscles that carry out the knee jerk.
3. Complementary, inhibitory commands are issued to motor neurons that innervate opposing muscles, providing coordination of muscle action.
4. Information about local neuron activity related to the knee jerk is conveyed to higher centers of the central nervous system, thus permitting the brain to coordinate behavioral commands.

The stretching of just one muscle, the quadriceps, activates several hundred sensory neurons, each of which makes direct contact with 100–150 motor neurons (Figure 2-6A). This pattern of connection, in which one neuron activates many target cells, is called *neuronal divergence*; it is especially common in the input stages of the nervous system. By distributing its signals to many target cells, a single neuron can exert wide and diverse

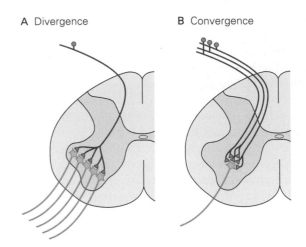

Figure 2-6 Diverging and converging neuronal connections are a key organizational feature of the brain.

A. In the sensory systems receptor neurons at the input stage usually branch out and make multiple, divergent connections with neurons that represent the second stage of processing. Subsequent connections diverge even more.

B. By contrast, motor neurons are the targets of progressively converging connections. With convergence, the target cell receives the sum of information from many presynaptic cells.

influence. For example, sensory neurons involved in a stretch reflex also contact projection interneurons that transmit information about the local neural activity to higher brain regions concerned with coordinating movements. In contrast, because there are usually five to 10 times more sensory neurons than motor neurons, a single motor cell typically receives input from many sensory cells (Figure 2-6B). This pattern of connection, called *convergence*, is common at the output stages of the nervous system. By receiving signals from numerous neurons, the target motor cell is able to integrate diverse information from many sources.

A stretch reflex such as the knee jerk is a simple behavior produced by two classes of neurons connecting at excitatory synapses. But not all important signals in the brain are excitatory. In fact, half of all neurons produce inhibitory signals. Inhibitory neurons release a transmitter that reduces the likelihood of firing. As we have seen, even in the knee-jerk reflex, the sensory neurons make both excitatory connections and connections through inhibitory interneurons. Excitatory connections with the leg's extensor muscles cause these muscles to contract, while connections with certain inhibitory interneurons prevent the antagonist flexor muscles from being called to action. This feature of the circuit is an example of *feed-forward inhibition* (Figure 2-7A). Feed-forward inhibition in the knee-jerk reflex is *reciprocal*, ensuring that the flexor and extensor pathways always

A Feed-forward inhibition

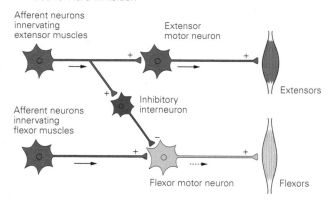

B Feedback inhibition

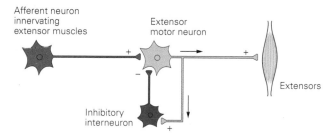

Figure 2-7 Inhibitory interneurons can produce either feed-forward or feedback inhibition.

A. Feed-forward inhibition is common in monosynaptic reflex systems, such as the knee-jerk reflex (see Figure 2-5). Afferent neurons from extensor muscles excite not only the extensor motor neurons, but also inhibitory neurons that prevent the firing of the motor cells in the opposing flexor muscles. Feed-forward inhibition enhances the effect of the active pathway by suppressing the activity of other, opposing, pathways.

B. Negative feedback inhibition is a self-regulating mechanism. The effect is to dampen activity within the stimulated pathway and prevent it from exceeding a certain critical maximum. Here the extensor motor neurons act on inhibitory interneurons, which feed back to the extensor motor neurons themselves and thus reduce the probability of firing by these cells.

inhibit each other, so only muscles appropriate for the movement, and not those that oppose it, are recruited.

Neurons can also have connections that provide *feedback inhibition*. For example, an active neuron may have excitatory connections with both a target cell and an inhibitory interneuron that has its own feedback connection with the active neuron. In this way signals from the active neuron simultaneously excite the target neuron and the inhibitory interneuron, which thus is able to limit the ability of the active neuron to excite its target (Figure 2-7B). We will encounter many examples of feed-forward and feedback inhibition when we examine more complex behaviors in later chapters.

Signaling Is Organized in the Same Way in All Nerve Cells

To produce a behavior, a stretch reflex for example, each participating sensory and motor nerve cell sequentially generates four different signals at different sites within the cell: an input signal, a trigger signal, a conducting signal, and an output signal. Regardless of cell size and shape, transmitter biochemistry, or behavioral function, almost all neurons can be described by a model neuron that has four functional components, or regions, that generate the four types of signals (Figure 2-8): a local input (receptive) component, a trigger (summing or integrative) component, a long-range conducting (signaling) component, and an output (secretory) component. This model neuron is the physiological representation of Ramón y Cajal's principle of dynamic polarization.

The different types of signals used by a neuron are determined in part by the electrical properties of the cell membrane. At rest, all cells, including neurons, maintain a difference in the electrical potential on either side of the plasma (external) membrane. This is called the *resting membrane potential*. In a typical resting neuron the electrical potential difference is about 65 mV. Because the net charge outside of the membrane is arbitrarily defined as zero, we say the resting membrane potential is −65 mV. (In different nerve cells it may range from about −40 to −80 mV; in muscle cells it is greater still, about −90 mV.) As we shall see in Chapter 7, the difference in electrical potential when the cell is at rest results from two factors: (1) the unequal distribution of electrically charged ions, in particular, the positively charged Na^+ and K^+ ions and the negatively charged amino acids and proteins on either side of the cell membrane, and (2) the selective permeability of the membrane to just one of these ions, K^+.

The unequal distribution of positively charged ions on either side of the cell membrane is maintained by a membrane protein that pumps Na^+ out of the cell and K^+ back into it. This *Na^+-K^+ pump*, which we shall learn more about in Chapter 7, keeps the Na^+ ion concentration in the cell low (about 10 times lower than that outside the cell) and the K^+ ion concentration high (about 20 times higher than that outside).

At the same time, the cell membrane is selectively permeable to K^+ because the otherwise impermeable membrane contains *ion channels*, pore-like structures that span the membrane and are highly permeable to K^+ but considerably less permeable to Na^+. When the cell is at rest, these channels are open and K^+ ions tend to leak out. As K^+ ions leak from the cell, they leave behind a cloud of unneutralized negative charge on the inner surface of the membrane, so that the net charge in-

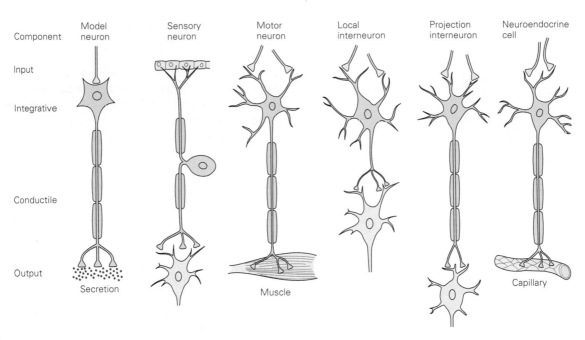

Component	Model neuron	Sensory neuron	Motor neuron	Local interneuron	Projection interneuron	Neuroendocrine cell
Input						
Integrative						
Conductile						
Output	Secretion		Muscle			Capillary

Figure 2-8 Most neurons, regardless of type, have four functional regions in common: an input component, a trigger or integrative component, a conductile component, and an output component. Thus, the functional organization of most neurons can be schematically represented by a model neuron. Each component produces a characteristic signal: the input, integrative, and conductile signals are all electrical, while the output signal consists of the release of a chemical transmitter into the synaptic cleft. Not all neurons share all these features; for example, local interneurons often lack a conductile component.

side the membrane is more negative than on the outside (Figure 2-9).

Excitable cells, such as nerve and muscle cells, differ from other cells in that their membrane potential can be significantly and quickly altered; this change can serve as a signaling mechanism. Reducing the membrane potential by say 10 mV (from −65 mV to −55 mV) makes the membrane much more permeable to Na^+ than to K^+. This influx of positively charged Na^+ ions tends to neutralize the negative charge inside the cell and results in an even greater reduction in membrane potential—the action potential. The action potential is conducted down the cell's axon to the axon's terminals which end on other cells (neurons or muscle), where the action potential initiates communication with the other cells. As noted earlier, the action potential is an all-or-none impulse that is actively propagated along the axon, so that its amplitude is not diminished by the time it reaches the axon terminal. Typically, an action potential lasts about one millisecond, after which the membrane returns to its resting state, with its normal separation of charges and higher permeability to K^+ than to Na^+. We shall learn more about the mechanisms underlying the resting potential and action potential in Chapters 6–9.

In addition to the long-range signal of the action po-

tential, nerve cells also produce local signals, such as receptor potentials and synaptic potentials, that are not actively propagated and therefore typically decay within just a few millimeters. Both long-range and local signals result from changes in the membrane potential, either a decrease or increase from the resting potential. The resting membrane potential therefore provides the baseline against which all signals are expressed. A reduction in membrane potential (eg, from −65 mV to −55 mV) is called *depolarization*. Because depolarization enhances a cell's ability to generate an action potential, it is *excitatory*. In contrast, an increase in membrane potential (eg, from about −65 mV to −75 mV) is called *hyperpolarization*. Hyperpolarization makes a cell less likely to generate an action potential and is therefore *inhibitory*.

The Input Component Produces Graded Local Signals

In most neurons at rest no current flows from one part of the neuron to another, so the resting potential is the same throughout the cell. In sensory neurons current flow is typically initiated by a sensory stimulus, which activates specialized receptor proteins at the neuron's receptive surface. In our example of the knee jerk,

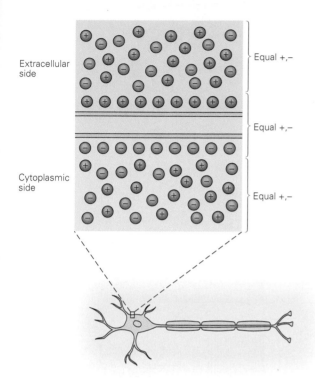

Figure 2-9 The membrane potential of a cell results from a difference in the net electrical charge on either side of its membrane. When a neuron is at rest there is an excess of positive charge outside the cell and an excess of negative charge inside it.

decreases in amplitude with distance and cannot be conveyed much farther than 1 or 2 mm. In fact, at about 1 mm down the axon the amplitude of the signal is only about one-third what it was at the site of generation. To be carried successfully to the rest of the nervous system, the local signal must be amplified—it must generate an action potential. In the knee jerk the receptor potential in the sensory neuron propagates to the first node of Ranvier in the axon, where, if it is large enough, it generates an action potential, which then propagates without failure (by a regenerative mechanism discussed in Chapter 9) to the axon terminals in the spinal cord. Here, at the synapse, between the sensory neuron and a motor neuron activating the leg muscles, the action potential produces a chain of events that result in an input signal to the motor neuron.

In our example of the knee jerk, the action potential in the sensory neuron releases a chemical signal (a neurotransmitter) across the synaptic cleft. The transmitter binds to receptor proteins on the motor neuron, and the resulting reaction transduces the potential chemical energy of the transmitter into electrical energy. This in turn alters the membrane potential of the motor cell, a change called the *synaptic potential.*

Like the receptor potential, the synaptic potential is graded. The amplitude of the synaptic potential depends on how much chemical transmitter is released, and its duration on how long the transmitter is active. The synaptic potential can be either depolarizing or hyperpolarizing, depending on the type of receptor molecule that is activated. Synaptic potentials, like receptor potentials, are local changes in membrane potential that spread passively along the neuron. The signal does not reach beyond the axon's initial segment unless it gives rise to an action potential. The features of receptor and synaptic potentials are summarized in Table 2-1.

The Trigger Component Makes the Decision to Generate an Action Potential

Charles Sherrington first pointed out that the quintessential action of the nervous system is its ability to weigh the consequences of different types of information and then decide on appropriate responses. This *integrative action* of the nervous system is clearly seen in the actions of the trigger component of the neuron.

Action potentials are generated by a sudden influx of Na^+ ions through voltage-sensitive channels in the cell membrane. When an input signal (a receptor potential or synaptic potential) depolarizes the cell membrane, the change in membrane potential opens the Na^+ ion channels, allowing Na^+ to flow down its concentration gradient, from outside the cell where the Na^+ con-

stretch of the quadriceps muscle activates specific proteins that are sensitive to stretch of the sensory neuron. The specialized receptor protein forms ion channels in the membrane, through which Na^+ and K^+ flow. These channels open when the cell is stretched, as we shall learn in Chapters 7 and 9, permitting a rapid influx of ions into the sensory cell. This ionic current disturbs the resting potential of the cell membrane, driving the membrane potential to a new level called the *receptor potential.* The amplitude and duration of the receptor potential depends on the intensity of the muscle stretch. The larger or longer-lasting the stretch, the larger and longer-lasting the resulting receptor potential (Figure 2-10A). Most receptor potentials are depolarizing (excitatory). However, hyperpolarizing (inhibitory) receptor potentials are found in the retina of the eye, as we shall learn in Chapter 26.

The receptor potential is the first representation of stretch to be coded in the nervous system. It is, however, a purely *local signal.* The receptor potential—the electrical activity in the sensory neuron initiated by a stimulus—spreads only passively along the axon. It therefore

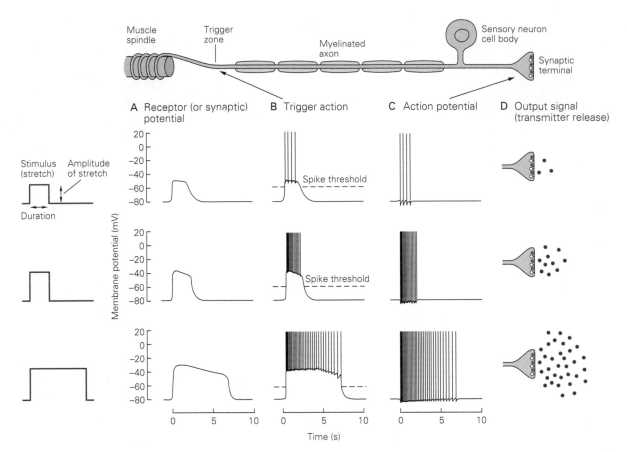

Figure 2-10 A sensory neuron transforms a physical stimulus (in our example, a stretch) into electrical activity in the cell. Each of the neuron's four signaling components produces a characteristic signal.

A. The input signal (a receptor or synaptic potential) is graded in amplitude and duration, proportional to the amplitude and duration of the stimulus.

B. The trigger zone integrates the input signal—the receptor potential in sensory neurons, or synaptic potential in motor neurons—into a trigger action that produces action potentials that will be propagated along the axon. An action potential is generated only if the input signal is greater than a certain *spike threshold*. Once the input signal surpasses this threshold, any further increase in amplitude of the input signal increases the *frequency* with which the action potentials are generated, not

their amplitude. The *duration* of the input signal determines the number of action potentials. Thus, the graded nature of input signals is translated into a frequency code of action potentials at the trigger zone.

C. Action potentials are all-or-none. Every action potential has the same amplitude and duration, and thus the same wave form on an oscilloscope. Since action potentials are conducted without fail along the full length of the axon to the synaptic terminals, the information in the signal is represented only by the frequency and number of spikes, not by the amplitude.

D. When the action potential reaches the synaptic terminal, the cell releases a chemical neurotransmitter that serves as the output signal. The total number of action potentials in a given period of time determines exactly how much neurotransmitter will be released by the cell.

centration is high to inside the cell where it is low. These voltage-sensitive Na$^+$ channels are concentrated at the initial segment of the axon, an uninsulated portion of the axon just beyond the neuron's input region. In sensory neurons the highest density of Na$^+$ channels occurs at the myelinated axon's first node of Ranvier; in interneurons and motor neurons the highest density occurs at the axon hillock, where the axon emerges from the cell body.

Because it has the highest density of voltage-

sensitive Na$^+$ channels, the initial segment of the axon has the lowest threshold for generating an action potential. Thus, an input signal spreading passively along the cell membrane is more likely to give rise to an action potential at the initial segment of the axon than at other sites in the cell. This part of the axon is therefore known as the impulse initiation zone, or *trigger zone*. It is here that the activity of all receptor (or synaptic) potentials is summed and where, if the size of the input signal reaches threshold, the neuron fires an action potential.

Table 2-1 Comparison of Local (Passive) and Propagated Signals

Signal type	Amplitude (mV)	Duration	Summation	Effect of signal	Type of propagation
Local (passive) signals					
Receptor potentials	Small (0.1–10)	Brief (5–100 ms)	Graded	Hyperpolarizing or depolarizing	Passive
Synaptic potentials	Small (0.1–10)	Brief to long (5 ms to 20 min)	Graded	Hyperpolarizing or depolarizing	Passive
Propagated (active) signals					
Action potentials	Large (70–110)	Brief (1–10 ms)	All-or-none	Depolarizing	Active

The Conductile Component Propagates an All-or-None Action Potential

The action potential, the conducting signal of the neuron, is all-or-none. This means that while stimuli below the threshold will not produce a signal, all stimuli above the threshold produce the *same* signal. However much the stimuli vary in intensity or duration, the amplitude and duration of each action potential are pretty much the same. In addition, unlike receptor and synaptic potentials, which spread passively and decrease in amplitude, the action potential does not decay as it travels along the axon to its target—a distance that can measure 3 m in length—because it is periodically regenerated. This conducting signal can travel at rates as fast as 100 meters per second.

The remarkable feature of action potentials is that they are highly stereotyped, varying only subtly (although in some cases importantly) from one nerve cell to another. This feature was demonstrated in the 1920s by Edgar Adrian, who was one of the first to study the nervous system at the cellular level. Adrian found that all action potentials have a similar shape or wave form on the oscilloscope (see Figure 2-3). Indeed, the voltage signals of action potentials carried into the nervous system by a sensory axon often are indistinguishable from those carried out of the nervous system to the muscles by a motor axon.

Only two features of the conducting signal convey information: the number of action potentials and the time intervals between them (Figure 2-10C). As Adrian put it in 1928, summarizing his work on sensory fibers: ". . . all impulses are very much alike, whether the message is destined to arouse the sensation of light, of touch, or of pain; if they are crowded together the sensation is intense, if they are separated by long intervals the sensation is correspondingly feeble." Thus, what determines the intensity of sensation or speed of movement is not the magnitude or duration of individual action potentials, but their *frequency*. Likewise, the duration of a sensation or movement is determined by the period over which action potentials are generated.

If signals are stereotyped and do not reflect the properties of the stimulus, how do neural signals carry specific behavioral information? How is a message that carries visual information distinguished from one that carries pain information about a bee sting, and how do both of these signals differ from messages that send commands for voluntary movement? As we have seen, and will learn to appreciate even more in later chapters, the message of an action potential is determined by the neural pathway that carries it. The visual pathways activated by receptor cells in the retina that respond to light are completely distinct from the somatic sensory pathways activated by sensory cells in the skin that respond to touch or to pain. The function of the signal—be it visual, tactile, or motor—is determined not by the signal itself but by the pathway along which it travels.

The Output Component Releases Neurotransmitter

When an action potential reaches a neuron's terminal it stimulates the release of a chemical transmitter from the cell. Transmitters can be small molecules, such as L-glutamate and acetylcholine, or they can be peptides like enkephalin (Chapter 15). Transmitter molecules are held in subcellular organelles called synaptic vesicles, which are loaded into specialized release sites in the presynaptic terminals called active zones. To unload their transmitter, the vesicles move up to and fuse with the neuron's plasma membrane, a process known as exocytosis. (We shall consider neurotransmitter release in Chapter 14.)

The release of chemical transmitter serves as a neuron's output signal. Like the input signal, the output signal is graded. The amount of transmitter released is

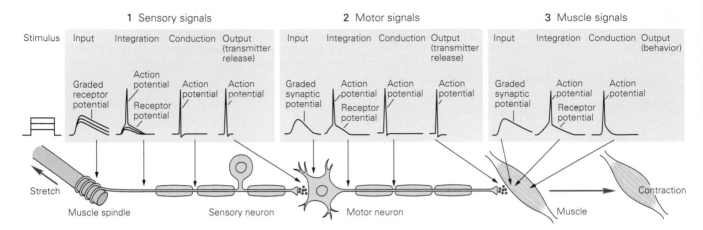

Figure 2-11 The sequence of signals that produces a reflex action.

1. The stretching of a muscle produces a receptor potential in the terminal fibers of the sensory neuron (the dorsal root ganglion cell). The amplitude of the receptor potential is proportional to the intensity of the stretch. This potential then spreads passively to the integrative segment, or trigger zone, at the first node of Ranvier. There, if the receptor potential is sufficiently large, it triggers an action potential, which then propagates actively and without change along the axon to the terminal region. At the terminal the action potential leads to an output signal: the release of a chemical neurotransmitter. The

transmitter diffuses across the synaptic cleft and interacts with receptor molecules on the external membranes of the motor neurons that innervate the stretched muscle. 2. This interaction initiates a synaptic potential in the motor cell. The synaptic potential then spreads passively to the trigger zone of the motor neuron axon, where it initiates an action potential that propagates actively to the terminal of the motor neuron. The action potential releases transmitter at the nerve-muscle synapse. 3. The binding of the neurotransmitter with receptors in the muscle triggers a synaptic potential in the muscle. This signal produces an action potential in the muscle, causing con-traction of the muscle fiber.

determined by the number and frequency of the action potentials in the presynaptic terminals (see Figure 2-10). After the transmitter is released from the presynaptic neuron, it diffuses across the synaptic cleft to receptors in the membrane of the postsynaptic neuron. The binding of transmitter to receptors causes the postsynaptic cell to generate a synaptic potential. Whether the synaptic potential has an excitatory or inhibitory effect will depend on the type of *receptors* in the postsynaptic cell, not on the particular neurotransmitter. The same transmitter can have different effects on different types of receptors.

The Transformation of the Neural Signal From Sensory to Motor Is Illustrated by the Stretch Reflex Pathway

We have seen that a signal is transformed as it is conveyed from one component of the neuron to the next and from one neuron to the next. This transformation—from input to output—can be seen in perspective by tracing the relay of signals for the stretch reflex.

When a muscle is stretched, the features of the stimulus—its amplitude and duration—are reflected in the amplitude and duration of the receptor potential in the sensory neuron. If the receptor potential exceeds the threshold for action potentials in that cell, the graded

signal is transformed at the trigger component into an action potential, an all-or-none signal. The more the receptor potential exceeds threshold, the greater the depolarization and consequently the greater the frequency of action potentials in the axon; likewise, the duration of the input signal determines the number of action potentials. (Several action potentials together are called a *train* of action potentials.) This information—the frequency and number of action potentials—is then faithfully conveyed along the entire axon's length to its terminals, where the frequency of action potentials determines how much transmitter is released.

These stages of transformation have their counterparts in the motor neuron. The transmitter released by a sensory neuron interacts with receptors on the motor neuron to initiate a graded synaptic potential, which spreads to the initial segment of the motor axon. If the membrane potential of the motor neuron reaches a critical threshold, an action potential will be generated and propagate without fail to the motor cell's presynaptic terminals. There the action potential causes transmitter release, which triggers a synaptic potential in the muscle. That in turn produces an action potential in the leg muscle, which leads to the final transformation—muscle contraction and an overt behavior. The sequence of transformations of a signal from sensory neuron to motor neuron to muscle is illustrated in Figure 2-11.

Nerve Cells Differ Most at the Molecular Level

The model of neuronal signaling we have outlined is a simplification that applies to most neurons, but there are some important variations. For example, some neurons do not generate action potentials. These are typically local interneurons without a conductile component—they have no axon, or such a short one that a conducted signal is not required. In these neurons the input signals are summed and spread passively to the nearby terminal region, where transmitter is released. There are also neurons that lack a steady resting potential and are spontaneously active.

Even cells with similar organization can differ in important molecular details, expressing different combinations of ion channels, for example. As we shall learn in Chapters 6 and 9, different ion channels provide neurons with various thresholds, excitability properties, and firing patterns. Thus, neurons with different ion channels can encode the same class of synaptic potential into different firing patterns and thereby convey different signals.

Neurons also differ in the chemical transmitters they use to transmit information to other neurons, and in the receptors they have to receive information from other neurons. Indeed, many drugs that act on the brain do so by modifying the actions of specific chemical transmitters or a particular subtype of receptor for a given transmitter. These differences not only have physiological importance for day-to-day functioning of the brain, but account for the fact that a disease may affect one class of neurons but not others. Certain diseases, such as amyotrophic lateral sclerosis and poliomyelitis, strike only motor neurons, while others, such as tabes dorsalis, a late stage of syphilis, affect primarily sensory neurons. Parkinson's disease, a disorder of voluntary movement, damages a small population of interneurons that use dopamine as a chemical transmitter. Some diseases are selective even within the neuron, affecting only the receptive elements, the cell body, or the axon. In Chapter 16 we shall see how research into myasthenia gravis, caused by a faulty transmitter receptor in the muscle membrane, has provided important insights into synaptic transmission. Indeed, because the nervous system has so many cell types and variations at the molecular level, it is susceptible to more diseases (psychiatric as well as neurological) than any other organ of the body.

Despite the differences among nerve cells, the basic mechanisms of electrical signaling are surprisingly similar. This simplicity is fortunate for those who study the brain. By understanding the molecular mechanisms that produce signaling in one kind of nerve cell, we are well on the way to understanding these mechanisms in many other nerve cells.

Nerve Cells Are Able to Convey Unique Information Because They Form Specific Networks

The stretch reflex illustrates how just a few types of nerve cells can interact to produce a simple behavior. But even the stretch reflex involves populations of neurons—perhaps a few hundred sensory neurons and a hundred motor neurons. Can the individual neurons implicated in a complex behavior be identified with the same precision? In invertebrate animals, and in some lower vertebrates, a single cell (the so-called *command cell*) can initiate a complex behavioral sequence. But, as far as we know, no complex human behavior is initiated by a single neuron. Rather, each behavior is generated by the actions of many cells. Broadly speaking, as we have seen, there are three neural components of behavior: sensory input, intermediate (interneuronal) processing, and motor output. Each of these components is mediated by a single group or several distinct groups of neurons.

As discussed in Chapter 1, one of the key strategies of the nervous system is localization of function: specific types of information are processed in particular brain regions. Thus, information for each of our senses is processed in a distinct brain region where the afferent connections typically form a precise map of the pertinent receptor sheet on the body surface—the skin (touch), the retina (sight), the basilar membrane of the cochlea (hearing), or the olfactory epithelium (smell). These maps are the first stage in creating a representation in the brain of the outside world in which we live. Similarly, areas of the brain concerned with movement contain an orderly arrangement of neural connections representing the musculature and specific movements. The brain, therefore, contains at least two types of neural maps: one for sensory perceptions and another for motor commands. The two maps are interconnected in ways we do not yet fully understand.

The neurons that make up these maps—motor, sensory, and interneuronal—do not differ greatly in their electrical properties. They have different functions because of the connections they make. These connections, established as the brain develops, determine the behavioral function of individual cells. Although our understanding of how sensory and motor information is processed and represented in the brain is based on the detailed studies of only a few regions, in those regions in which our understanding is particularly well advanced it is clear that the logical operations of a mental representation can be understood only by defining the flow of information through the connections that make up the various maps.

A single component of behavior sometimes recruits a number of groups of neurons that simultaneously provide the same or similar information. The deployment of several neuron groups or several pathways to convey similar information is called *parallel processing*. Parallel processing also occurs in a single pathway when different neurons in the pathway perform similar computations simultaneously. Parallel processing makes enormous sense as an evolutionary strategy for building a more powerful brain: it increases both the speed and reliability of function within the central nervous system.

The importance of abundant, highly specific parallel connections is now also being recognized by scientists attempting to construct computer models of the brain. Scientists working in this field, a branch of computer science known as *artificial intelligence,* first used serial processing to simulate the brain's higher-level cognitive processes—processes such as pattern recognition, learning, memory, and motor performance. They soon realized that although these serial models solved many problems rather well, including the challenge of playing chess, they performed poorly with other computations that the brain does almost instantaneously, such as recognizing faces or comprehending speech.

As a result, most computational neurobiologists have turned to systems with both serial and parallel (distributed) components, which they call *connectionist models*. In these models elements distributed throughout the system process related information simultaneously. Preliminary insights from this work are often consistent with physiological studies. Connectionist models show that individual elements of a system do not transmit large amounts of information. Thus, what makes the brain a remarkable information processing machine is not the complexity of its neurons, but rather its many elements and, in particular, the complexity of connections between them. Individual stereotyped neurons are able to convey unique information because they are wired together and organized in different ways.

The Modifiability of Specific Connections Contributes to the Adaptability of Behavior

That neurons make specific connections with one another raises an interesting question. How, if the nervous system is wired so precisely, is behavior modified? Even simple reflexes can undergo modification that lasts minutes, and much learning results in behavioral change that can endure for years. How can neural activity produce such long-term changes in the function of a set of prewired connections? A number of solutions for these dilemmas have been proposed. The proposal that has proven most farsighted is the *plasticity hypothesis,* first put forward at the turn of the century by Ramón y Cajal. A modern form of this hypothesis was advanced by the Polish psychologist Jerzy Konorski in 1948:

The application of a stimulus leads to changes of a twofold kind in the nervous system. . . . [T]he first property, by virtue of which the nerve cells *react* to the incoming impulse . . . we call *excitability,* and . . . changes arising . . . because of this property we shall call *changes due to excitability.* The second property, by virtue of which certain permanent functional transformations arise in particular systems of neurons as a result of appropriate stimuli or their combination, we shall call *plasticity* and the corresponding changes *plastic changes.*

There is now considerable evidence for plasticity at chemical synapses. Chemical synapses often have a remarkable capacity for short-term physiological changes (lasting hours) that increase or decrease the effectiveness of the synapse. Long-term changes (lasting days) can give rise to further physiological changes that lead to anatomical changes, including pruning of preexisting connections, and even growth of new connections. As we shall see in later chapters, chemical synapses can be modified functionally and anatomically during development and regeneration, and, most importantly, through experience and learning. Functional alterations are typically short term and involve changes in the effectiveness of existing synaptic connections. Anatomical alterations are typically long-term and consist of the growth of new synaptic connections between neurons. It is this potential for plasticity of the relatively stereotyped units of the nervous system that endows each of us with our individuality.

Eric R. Kandel

Selected Readings

Adrian ED. 1928. *The Basis of Sensation: The Action of the Sense Organs.* London: Christophers.

Gazzaniga MS (ed). 1995. *The Cognitive Neurosciences.* Cambridge, MA: MIT Press.

Jones EG. 1988. The nervous tissue. In: L Weiss (ed), *Cell and Tissue Biology: A Textbook of Histology,* 6th ed., pp. 277–351. Baltimore: Urban and Schwarzenberg.

Newan EA. 1993. Inward-rectifying potassium channels in retinal glial (Muller) cells. J Neurosci 13:3333–3345.

Perry VH. 1996. Microglia in the developing and mature central nervous system. In: KR Jessen, WD Richardson (eds). *Glial Cell Development: Basic Principles & Clinical Relevance,* pp. 123–140. Oxford: Bios.

Ramón y Cajal S. 1937. *1852–1937. Recollections of My Life.* EH Craigie (transl). Philadelphia: American Philosophical Society; 1989. Reprint. Cambridge, MA: MIT Press.

References

Adrian ED. 1932. *The Mechanism of Nervous Action: Electrical Studies of the Neurone.* Philadelphia: Univ. Pennsylvania Press.

Alberts B, Bray D, Lewis J, Raff M, Roberts K, Watson JD. 1994. *Molecular Biology of the Cell,* 3rd ed. New York: Garland.

Erlanger J, Gasser HS. 1937. *Electrical Signs of Nervous Activity.* Philadelphia: Univ. Pennsylvania Press.

Hodgkin AL, Huxley AF. 1939. Action potentials recorded from inside a nerve fiber. Nature 144:710–711.

Kandel ER. 1976. The study of behavior: the interface between psychology and biology. In: *Cellular Basis of Behavior: An Introduction to Behavioral Neurobiology,* pp. 3–27. San Francisco: WH Freeman.

Konorski J. 1948. *Conditioned Reflexes and Neuron Organization.* Cambridge: Cambridge Univ. Press.

Martinez Martinez PFA. 1982. *Neuroanatomy: Development and Structure of the Central Nervous System.* Philadelphia: Saunders.

Newman EA. 1986. High potassium conductance in astrocyte endfeet. Science 233:453–454.

Nicholls JG, Martin AR, Wallace BG. 1992. *From Neuron to Brain: A Cellular and Molecular Approach to the Function of the Nervous System,* 3rd ed. Sunderland, MA: Sinauer.

Penfield W (ed). 1932. *Cytology & Cellular Pathology of the Nervous System,* Vol. 2. New York: Hoeber.

Ramón y Cajal S. 1933. *Histology,* 10th ed. Baltimore: Wood.

Sears ES, Franklin GM. 1980. Diseases of the cranial nerves. In: RN Rosenberg (ed). *The Science and Practice of Clinical Medicine.* Vol. 5, *Neurology,* pp. 471–494. New York: Grune & Stratton.

Sherrington C. 1947. *The Integrative Action of the Nervous System,* 2nd ed. Cambridge: Cambridge Univ. Press

3

Genes and Behavior

ALL BEHAVIOR IS SHAPED BY the interplay of genes and the environment. Even the most stereotypic behaviors of simple animals can be influenced by the environment, while highly evolved behaviors in humans, such as language, are constrained by hereditary factors. In this chapter we review what is known about the role of genes in organizing behavior. Later in the book we discuss the role of environmental factors.

A striking illustration of how genes and environment interact is evident in phenylketonuria. This disease results in a severe impairment of cognitive function and affects 1 child in 15,000. Children who express this disease have two abnormal copies of the gene that codes for phenylalanine hydroxylase, the enzyme that converts the amino acid phenylalanine, a component of dietary proteins, to another amino acid, tyrosine. Many more children carry only one abnormal copy of the gene and have no symptoms. Children who lack both functional copies of the gene build up high blood levels of phenylalanine. High blood levels of phenylalanine in turn lead to the production of a toxic metabolite that interferes with the normal maturation of the brain.[1] Fortunately, the treatment for this disease is remarkably simple and effective: the mental retardation can be completely prevented by restricting protein intake, thereby reducing phenylalanine in the diet.

Phenylketonuria is a particularly clear example of how an individual's phenotype depends on the interaction between genes and environment (Figure 3-1). In phenylketonuria both heredity and environmental fac-

---

[1]The specific biochemical processes by which high levels of phenylalanine adversely affect maturation of the brain are still not understood.

Figure 3-1 Heredity and environment are both necessary for the expression of phenylketonuria. (From Barondes 1995.)

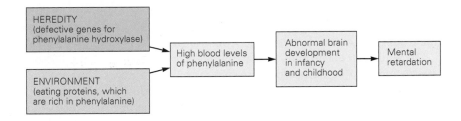

tors in the diet are clearly necessary for the expression of this form of mental retardation. A mere change in diet can rescue the genetic defect and the mental functioning.

In considering genetic factors that control behavior we need first to identify the components of behavior that are heritable. Clearly, behavior itself is not inherited; what is inherited is DNA, which encodes proteins. The genes expressed in neurons encode proteins that are important for development, maintenance, and regulation of the neural circuits that underlie all aspects of behavior. In turn, neural circuits are composed of many nerve cells, each of which expresses a special constellation of genes that direct the production of specific proteins. For the development and function of a single neural circuit, a wide variety of structural and regulatory proteins are required. In simple animals a single gene may control a behavioral trait by encoding a protein that affects the function of individual nerve cells in a specific neural circuit. In more complex animals the circuitry is also more complex and behavioral traits are generally shaped by the actions of many genes. Subtle differences in behavior can be achieved not only by the presence or absence of a given gene product or a set of products, but also by the *degree* to which different gene products are expressed, or by the specific contribution of gene products.

The interplay of the genes, proteins, and neural circuits underlying behavior has been studied in various organisms ranging in complexity from worms and flies to mice and humans. Molecular genetics provides the techniques to identify the genes involved in a particular behavior and to determine how the proteins they encode control behavior. In worms, flies, and even in vertebrate organisms such as mice and zebrafish, it is possible to examine directly how genes influence behavior because single-gene mutants of these organisms can be bred and isolated.

In this chapter we illustrate how the genetic dissection of behavior in simple animals can provide insight into the mechanisms that regulate human behavioral traits. We then discuss a few important examples of the effects of single-gene defects on human behavior. Finally, we consider complex behavioral traits that typically are determined by the actions of many genes.

Genetic Information Is Stored in Chromosomes

Genes contribute to the neural circuitry of behavior in two fundamental ways. First, through their ability to replicate reliably, each gene provides precise copies of itself to all cells in an organism as well as succeeding generations of organisms. Second, each gene that is expressed in a cell directs the manufacture of specific proteins that determine the structure, function, and other biological characteristics of the cell.

With rare exceptions, each cell in the human body contains precisely the same complement of genes, thought to be about 80,000. The reason cells differ from one another—why one cell becomes a liver cell and another a brain cell—is that a distinct set of genes is expressed (as messenger RNA) in each cell type. Which genes and proteins become activated in a particular cell depends on interactions between the molecules within the cell, between neighboring cells, and between the cell and the organism's external environment (see Chapter 52). More of the total genetic information encoded in DNA—perhaps 30,000 of the 80,000 genes—is expressed in brain cells than in any other tissue of the body. Genes vary in size from 1 to 200,000 kilobases; the average size is about 10 kilobases. The DNA of each gene that encodes a protein is made up of segments, called *exons*, which encode parts of the protein and these coding segments are interrupted by noncoding segments called *introns*.

DNA is not distributed randomly within the nucleus but arranged in an orderly way on structures called chromosomes. The number of chromosomes varies among different organisms. In addition, different types of organisms contain either one or two copies of each chromosome. With some exceptions, unicellular organisms are *haploid*; they have only a single copy of each chromosome. By contrast, most complex multicellular organisms (worms, fruit flies, mice, and humans) are *diploid;* in all their somatic cells they carry two homologous copies of each chromosome and each gene, one from the mother and the other from the father.

The number of chromosomes in the *germ,* or sex, cells (sperm and egg) is half that found in somatic cells. During the nuclear division that accompanies somatic cell division (the process of mitosis) the chromosomes are partitioned equally—each daughter cell receives one copy of each chromosome in the parent cell. However, during the two successive nuclear divisions that accompany division of the germ cells (meiosis), the number of chromosomes is reduced by half. Fertilization of the egg by the sperm restores the diploid number found in somatic cells, with homologous chromosomes contributed by each parent.

The 80,000 genes in the human genome are arranged in a precise order along the chromosomes. As a result, each gene is uniquely identifiable by its location at a characteristic position (locus) on a specific chromosome. The two copies of a gene at corresponding loci on a pair of homologous chromosomes commonly harbor sequence variations, or polymorphisms, at multiple sites throughout the gene. At any given site, the alternative gene versions are referred to as *alleles.* Alleles may be identical or, more commonly, differ to some degree because of polymorphisms or mutations, as discussed below.

If two alleles are identical, the organism is said to be *homozygous* at that locus. If the alleles vary in form (in their nucleotide sequence), the organism is said to be *heterozygous* at that locus. The recent DNA sequencing of a small number of human genes reveals large variance in the degree of intergenic polymorphism. In general, however, the rate of polymorphic variation between any two individuals is estimated to be 1 per 1000 base pairs in noncoding DNA and 1 per 2000 base pairs in coding DNA. Thus a 10 kilobase gene would harbor, on average, about 10 polymorphisms, including 1 or 2 in the coding sequence DNA. At each of these polymorphic sites, an individual will carry at most two different forms of the same allele, whereas the same allele may exist in many forms within a population. A difference within a population is called *allelic polymorphism,* or more generally, *genetic polymorphism.* Prominent examples of allelic polymorphism are the alleles of the genes responsible for hair and eye color.

Humans have 46 chromosomes: 22 pairs of autosomes and two sex chromosomes (two X chromosomes in females, one X and one Y chromosome in males). The parents contribute the sex chromosomes to their offspring differently from the manner they supply the autosomes. A spermatozoon carries either an X (female-determining) or a Y (male-determining) chromosome, whereas an ovum carries only an X chromosome. As a consequence, males inherit their single X chromosome from their mothers.

The 22 autosome pairs and the X and Y sex chromosomes vary in size and cytological banding pattern (Figure 3-2). Chromosome 1 is the largest autosome; it contains 8% of the human genome, or about 6400 genes. Chromosome 22 is the smallest, containing 1% or about 800 genes. Chromosomes also vary in the nucleotide sequence of their DNA, but paired autosomes are usually morphologically (cytogenetically) indistinguishable.

Gregor Mendel's Work Led to the Delineation of the Relationship Between Genotype and Phenotype

The existence of alternative allelic forms of genes were discovered in 1866 by Gregor Mendel, who demonstrated the difference between dominant and recessive alleles using garden peas as an experimental system. Mendel started out with self-breeding experiments on peas. These led to the creation of inbred strains of peas that bred true for given characteristics of the pea such as color or the shape of the pod. He then crossed these inbred strains with each other and observed how the various traits were manifested in the progeny of the pea plant. These crosses allowed Mendel to appreciate that the variability in heredity among the progeny lay in differences in discrete factors that are passed unchanged from one plant generation to another, factors we now call genes. Moreover, Mendel found that each pea had two sets of factors, one from the male parent and the other from the female.

Mendel carried out his studies before it was known how chromosomes behave during cell division. Forty years later it became clear that the segregation pattern of genes noted by Mendel paralleled, almost exactly, the behavior of chromosomes during meiotic cell division, the division that produces the male and female germ cells. These findings were used by Thomas Hunt Morgan to formulate the *chromosomal theory of heredity,* according to which each chromosome has a linear array of unique genes running from one end to the other, each gene having a definite location on a particular chromosome.

While studying Mendel's results, Wilhelm Johannsen later distinguished between the *genotype* of an organism (its genetic makeup) and the *phenotype* of an organism (its appearance). In the broad sense *genotype* refers to the entire set of alleles forming the genome of an individual; in the narrow sense it refers to the specific alleles of one gene. *Phenotype* denotes the functional expression or consequences of a gene or set of genes. The phenotype of an individual may change throughout life, whereas the genotype remains constant except for sporadic mutations.

Most mutations are simply allelic polymorphisms that are silent; that is, they do not have any effect on the phenotype. Some are not silent but are expressed in ways that nevertheless appear neutral and therefore be-

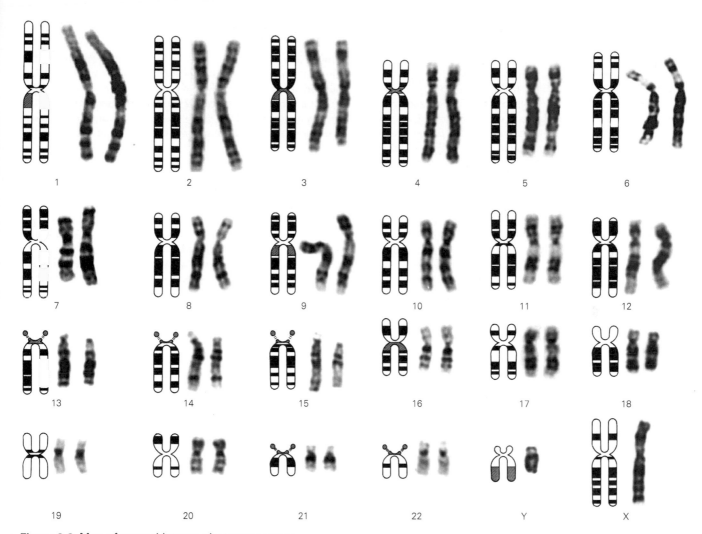

Figure 3-2 Map of normal human chromosomes at metaphase illustrating the distinctive morphology of each chromosome. (Adapted from Watson et al. 1983.)

nign (Box 3-1). Benign mutations are allelic polymorphisms that produce differences in body type, such as eye color or hair color, as well as differences in personality characteristics. The consequence of a mutation is often shaped by the environment. A mutation that favored a hunter-gatherer's survival during periodic food shortages might lead to pathological obesity in a modern-day environment. Many mutations that do not have benign consequences, such as those leading to excessive tallness, dwarfism, or color blindness, do not necessarily impair everyday functions. Some mutations may have significant consequences that are limited to the cell-biological level, without any functional effects. An example would be a mutation that results in the failure of a single type of cell to develop in an animal that can compensate for the loss of that cell type. Only rarely do mutations lead to significant changes in development, cell function, or overt behavior. Some mutations

are truly pathogenic, however, and these lead to human disease.

If a mutant phenotype results from one mutant allele in combination with one wild-type (normal) allele, the mutation or phenotypic trait is said to be *dominant*. Dominant mutations usually lead to the production of an abnormal protein by the mutant allele or to the expression of the wild-type gene product at an inappropriate time or place. Because they give rise to a new, perhaps toxic, variant of the protein or a new pattern of expression in the body, dominant mutations are often referred to as *gain of function* mutations. Some dominant mutations produce an inactive protein product that can nevertheless interfere with the function of the wild-type protein, thus leading to a complete loss of function of the gene. Such mutations are termed *dominant negative mutations*.

If a mutant phenotype is expressed only when both alleles of a gene are mutated (that is, only individuals

Box 3-1 The Origins of Genetic Diversity

Although DNA replication generally is carried out with high fidelity, spontaneous errors called *mutations* do occur. Mutations may result from damage to the purine and pyrimidine bases, mistakes during the DNA replication process, and recombinations that occur between two nonhomologous chromosomes as a result of errors in crossing over during meiosis. It is these mutations that give rise to genetic polymorphisms.

The rate of spontaneously occurring mutations is low. However, the frequency of mutations greatly increases when the organism is exposed to chemical mutagens or ionizing radiation. Chemical mutagens tend to induce *point mutations* involving changes in a single DNA base pair or the deletion of a few base pairs. By contrast, ionizing radiation can induce large insertions, deletions, or translocations. Both spontaneous and induced mutations can lead to changes in the structure of the protein encoded by the gene (as in a dominant mutation) or to a partial decrease or absence of gene function or expression (as in recessive mutations).

Changes in a single base pair involve one of three types of point mutations: (1) a *missense mutation*, where the point muta-

tion results in one amino acid in a protein being substituted for another; (2) a *nonsense mutation*, where a stop codon (triplet) is substituted for a codon within the coding region, thus resulting in a shortened (truncated) protein product; or (3) a *frameshift mutation*, in which small insertions or deletions change the reading frame, leading to the production of a truncated or abnormal protein.

Large-scale mutations involve changes in chromosome structure that can affect the function of many contiguous genes. Such mutations include rearrangement of genes without the addition or deletion of material (*inversion*), duplication of genes in a chromosome, or the exchange (*crossing over*) between segments of DNA. Sometimes large deletions of multiple genes occur. While these mutations are usually fatal if present in both copies of a gene (homozygous lethals), they can result in phenotypes in the heterozygous state (such as the mental retardation associated with the Wilms tumor deletion complex). Chromosomal translocation can also cause fusion between different (nonhomologous) chromosomes.

homozygous for the mutant allele will exhibit the phenotype), the mutation or phenotypic trait is said to be *recessive.* Recessive mutations usually result from the loss or reduction in amount of a functional protein. As a result, recessive mutations are often *loss of function* mutations. The reason both alleles need to be defective in a recessive mutation in order for a phenotype to become evident is that a 50% reduction of most proteins (such as most enzymes) usually does not cause serious (or even detectable) problems in cell function.

The Genotype Is a Significant Determinant of Human Behavior

Independent of Mendel's work, Francis Galton began to apply genetics to human behavior in 1869. In his book *Hereditary Genius*, Galton proposed that relatives of individuals with extremely high mental ability were more likely to be endowed with similar abilities than would be predicted by chance: the closer the family relationship, the higher the incidence of such gifted individuals.

Following Galton's initial insight, genetic studies of human behavior and disease have relied heavily on the analysis of kinship. Relatives share varying degrees of genetic information and are classified as first degree (parents, siblings, and offspring), second degree (grandparents, grandchildren, nephews and nieces, half-siblings), third degree (first cousins), and so on, depending on the number of steps, more precisely the number

of generations (meiotic events), separating the members of the family tree.

Despite the uncontrolled nature of this early study, Galton was among the first to address the interplay of inheritance (nature) and environment (nurture) in the determination of behavior. Galton was well aware that relatives of eminent individuals also share social, educational, and financial advantages, and that these environmental factors might also account for the correlation between eminence and familial relationship. He therefore endeavored to assess more accurately the relative contributions of heritable and environmental factors to behavioral traits. Thus, in 1883 he introduced the idea of the twin study, a method that today remains a primary strategy for evaluating the role of genes and environment in complex behavioral traits.

Identical twins are monozygotic; they develop from a single zygote that splits into two soon after fertilization. As a result, identical twins share all genes; they are as alike genetically as is possible for two individuals. In contrast, fraternal twins are dizygotic; they develop from two different fertilized eggs. Thus, dizygotic twins, like normal siblings, share on average half their genetic information. Systematic comparisons of pairs of identical versus fraternal twins can be used to assess the importance of genes in the development of a particular trait. If identical twins tend to be more similar (concordant) than fraternal twins, the trait is attributable, at least in part, to genes.

The findings from such twin studies are further sup-

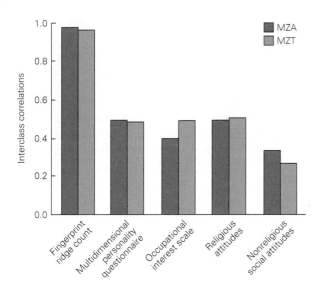

Figure 3-3 Correlations among monozygotic twins reared together (MZT) and those reared apart (MZA) for physiological characteristics, personality traits, interests, and attitudes. A score of zero represents no correlation—the average result for two random members of the population—while a score of 1.0 represents a perfect correlation. Fingerprint ridge count, which is not expected to be subject to significant environmental influence, is virtually identical in MZA and MZT pairs. Other characteristics, expected to be more subject to environmental influences, are not so highly correlated within each class. Although the correlations for these characteristics are low, the results for MZT and MZA are similar. The correlations for the multidimensional personality scale and religious attitudes among MZT and MZA are virtually identical, suggesting a significant, though not necessarily predominant, genetic influence on those traits. Correlations for the occupational interest scale and nonreligious social attitudes among MZA and MZT are more different between the two groups. (Based on Bouchard et al. 1990.)

ported by studies of identical twins that have been separated early in life and raised in different households. Despite sometimes great differences in their environment, such twins share a remarkable number of behavioral traits that we normally consider to be distinctive features of individuality, such as intellectual, religious, and vocational interests (Figures 3-3 and 3-4). Behavioral similarities between identical twins that have been separated at birth are attributable in part to genes, although environmental factors may also play a role. In general, twin studies reinforce the idea that human conduct is shaped by genetic factors but do not refute the role of environmental influences, which clearly exist.

The environmental contribution to behavioral traits is often divided into *shared* and *nonshared* components. Shared environmental influences, such as child-rearing practices or income, may underlie observed phenotypic similarities among family members. In contrast, non-

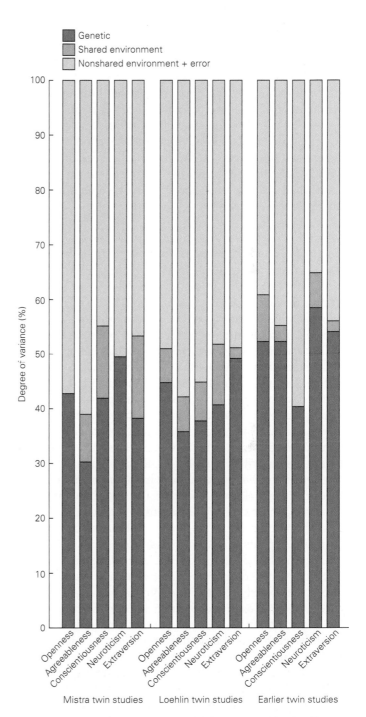

Figure 3-4 Variation in personality in studies of twins. The units express the degree of variance accounted for by various genetic and environmental influences. (Based on Bouchard 1994.)

shared influences, such as interactions with peers in school, can create differences among members of the same family. As discussed below, similarities in personality between biological relatives are due primarily to genetic components, with differences arising from genetic factors and nonshared environmental factors.

Although studies of identical twins and kinships provide strong support for the idea that human behavior has a significant hereditary component, they do not tell us how many genes are important, let alone how specific genes affect behavior. These questions can be addressed by genetic studies in experimental animals in which both the gene and the environment are strictly controlled and by studies of human genetic mutations that give rise to diseases.

Single Gene Alleles Can Encode Normal Behavioral Variations in Worms and Flies

A number of studies of natural populations of flies and worms have found that allelic polymorphisms in single genes can contribute to individual differences in naturally occurring behavior, including social behavior. The first example was provided by Ron Kondoka and his colleagues, who found variants in the circadian rhythm of flies as a result of molecular polymorphisms in the *period* gene. Wild-type flies vary in how well they can maintain their circadian rhythm in the presence of a temperature change, a feature called *temperature compensation*. As we will discuss below, the protein products of the *period* and *timeless* genes are involved in an autoregulatory feedback that is critical for circadian rhythms. The *per* gene has a repeat region of threonine-glycine that is polymorphic in length. Two of the major variants (with 17 repeats and 20 repeats) are found in Europe along a north-south cline. Flies with long repeats are better able to compensate for temperature shifts than those with short repeats.

A second example of such individual differences was discovered by Marta Sokolowski and her colleagues while examining the natural variation in the foraging behavior of fly larvae. Some larvae are rovers and others are sitters. Rovers follow longer foraging paths, whereas sitters use much smaller paths. The rover larvae also tend to move between patches of food, while the sitters tend to remain feeding within a food pack. This difference between rovers and sitters results from a single gene called *forager*. The rover allele has complete dominance over the sitter allele. In nature there are 70% rovers and 30% sitters. In fact, sitter larvae can be converted to rover larvae by expressing in them the gene encoding the rover phenotype. The forager gene encodes a cGMP-dependent protein kinase whose activities are higher in rover than in natural sitters, or sitter mutants, which suggests that the protein kinase may be regulated differently in the two natural variants.

Single genes can even account for differences in normal social behavior. In the course of studying 22 natural isolates of the nematode worm *Caenorhabditis elegans* collected from various locations around the world, Jonathan Hodgkin and Tabitha Doniach had found that, when grown on the surface of agar-filled Petri plates seeded with *Escherichia coli*, these natural isolates distributed themselves on the agar surface in two ways. Half the strains dispersed evenly across the bacterial patch, but the other strains spontaneously formed large, dense aggregates called *clumps*. This clumping arises, at least in part, from interaction among the worms in the clump. Mario deBono and Cornelia Bargmann realized that this reflected an example of individual differences in social behavior. They called the dispersing strains *solitary* and the clumping strains *social*.

Bargmann and deBono have identified natural variants in the behavior of worms feeding on *E. coli* in a Petri dish. Some worms are solitary foragers, moving across the food and feeding alone, while others are social foragers aggregating together on the food while they feed. More than 50 percent of the social foragers are found in groups, whereas less than two percent of the solitary foragers are found in groups. The social worms may aggregate due to the presence of a mutually attractive, as yet unidentified stimulus.

DeBono and Bargmann gathered social strains of worms that arose from mutagenesis screens of solitary strains in several laboratories and found that the mutation encodes for a gene that resembles the neuropeptide Y re-ceptor, a G protein-coupled receptor that is ubiquitous and important in mammals for feeding. Genetic analysis of normal, wild-type strains showed that the difference between social and solitary strains was due to the substitution of a single amino acid in a cytoplasmic loop of the neuropeptide Y receptor gene. Neuropeptides are found in the brain along with conventional small molecules and are often involved in regulating responses over long periods of time. Since neuropeptide Y receptors are associated with feeding and appetite in mammals, it raises the intriguing possibility that closely related peptides might control foraging and eating behaviors in a variety of organisms that are evolutionarily divergent.

Mutations in Single Genes Can Affect Certain Behaviors in Flies

The influence of genes on behavior can be explored most rigorously in simple animals, such as the fruit fly

Box 3-2 Introducing Transgenes in Flies and Mice

Genes can be manipulated in mice by injecting DNA into the nucleus of newly fertilized eggs (Figure 3-5). In some of the injected eggs the new gene, or transgene, is incorporated into a random site on one of the chromosomes and, since the embryo is at the one-cell stage, the incorporated gene is replicated and ends up in all (or nearly all) of the animal's cells, including the germline.

Gene incorporation is most easily detected by coinjecting the marker gene for pigment production into an egg obtained from an albino strain. Mice with patches of pigmented fur indicate successful expression of DNA. The transgene's presence is confirmed by testing a sample of DNA from the injected individuals.

A similar approach is used in flies. The DNA need not be injected directly into a nucleus since the vector used, called a *P element*, is capable of being incorporated into germ cell nuclei at the time the first cells form in the embryo. The development and function of the nervous system of flies can be altered using promoters that are expressed ubiquitously, such as the inducible heat-shock promoter *hsp70* in *Drosophila*. More specific patterns of expression in brain cells can be obtained using promoter and enhancer sequences from genes that are specific to a cell type.

Transgenes may be wild-type genes that rescue a mutant phenotype or novel "designer" genes that drive expression of a gene in new locations or produce a specifically altered gene product.

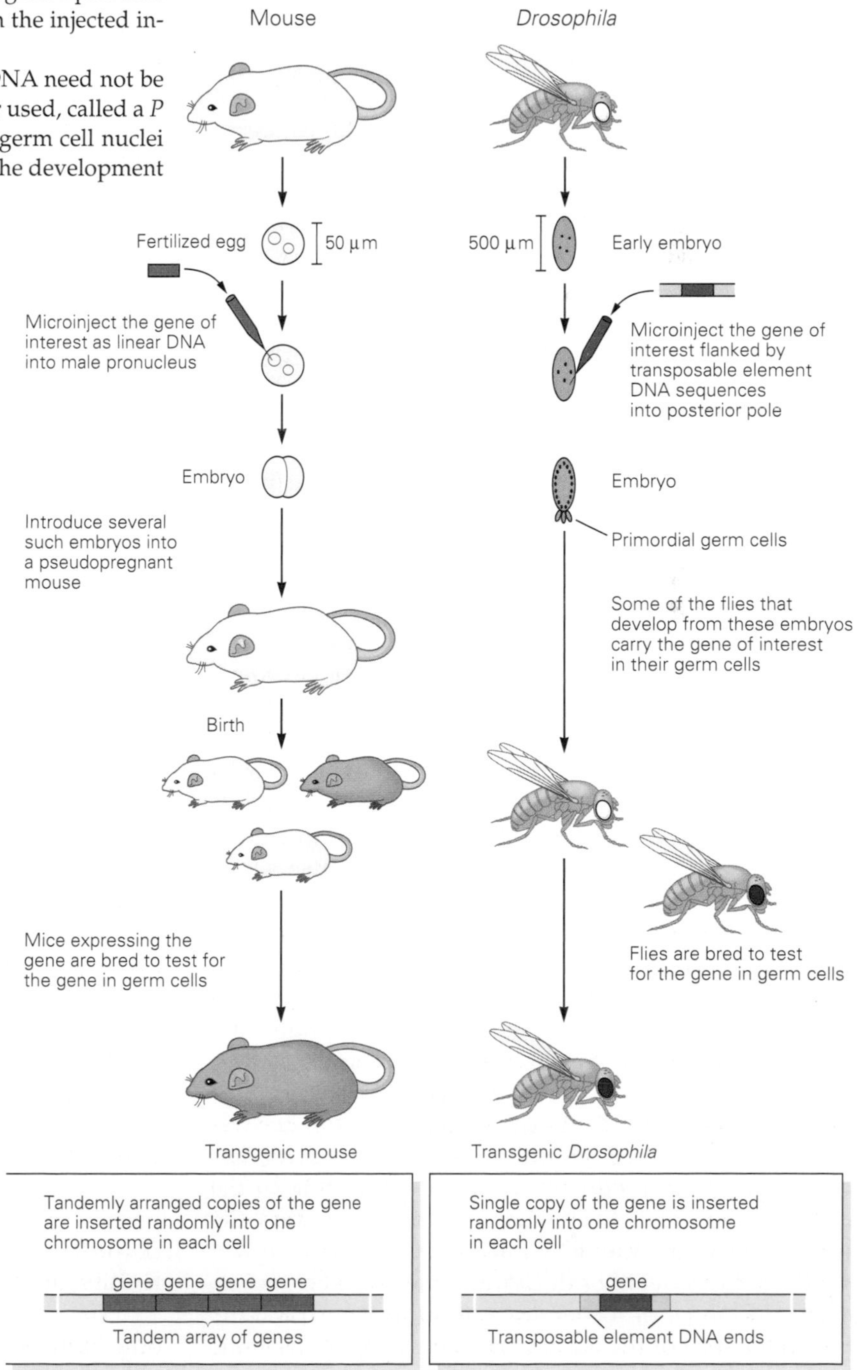

Figure 3-5 Standard procedures for generating transgenic mice and flies. Here the gene injected into the mouse causes a change in coat color, while the gene injected into the fly causes a change in eye color. In some transgenic animals of both species the DNA is inserted at different chromosomal sites in different cells (see illustration at bottom). (From Alberts et al. 1994.)

Drosophila. Mutations of single genes in *Drosophila* can produce abnormalities in learned as well as innate behaviors, such as courtship and circadian rhythms. Moreover, mutations that affect specific aspects of behavior can readily be induced in flies (Box 3-2).

The genetic analysis of the behavior of flies has its origins in the behavioral screens performed in the 1970s by Seymour Benzer and his colleagues. These screens detected and isolated mutations that affect circadian (daily) rhythms, courtship behavior, movement, visual perception, and memory. The powerful techniques of *Drosophila* molecular genetics have enabled investigators to identify these genes and characterize how their protein products act. Here we shall focus on one class of genes isolated by Benzer, those that affect circadian rhythms. In Chapter 63 we shall consider genes in *Drosophila* that influence memory.

Many aspects of animal physiology and behavior fluctuate in rhythmic cycles. Most of these rhythms follow a circadian period; others follow shorter-term (ultradian) periods. Circadian clocks are thought to have a significant adaptive advantage. For example, they provide a means of anticipating dawn and thereby coordinate physiological functions with environmental conditions. Circadian rhythms affect everything from locomotor activity to mood and play a major role in the biology of motivation (see Chapter 51). Because of the ubiquity of these clocks among animals (and even fungi), experimental advances in invertebrates should aid in our understanding of human circadian behaviors.

Clocks have three basic features. First, the core of the clock is an intrinsic *oscillator* capable of producing a circadian periodicity of approximately 24 hours. Second, this intrinsic oscillator can adapt its rhythm to changes in the duration of the day-night cycle throughout the year. This regulation is primarily achieved through various *light-driven signals* that are transmitted by the eye to the brain, where the signals in turn act on the oscillator. Third, there are a set of *output pathways* from the oscillator that control specific behaviors, such as sleep and wakefulness and locomotor activity.

Mutations altering biological rhythms have been isolated in several organisms. The greatest insight into the oscillator has been obtained from studies of two genes in *Drosophila*, the *period (per)* gene, identified originally by Benzer and his colleagues, and the *timeless (tim)* gene identified recently. The *period* and *timeless* genes appear to be devoted almost exclusively to the control of rhythms. Even when they are eliminated, the organism has no other major defects.

Mutations in either the *per* or *tim* gene affect the circadian rhythms of locomotor activity and eclosion (ie, the emergence of the adult from the pupa). Arrhythmic

per mutants exhibit no discernible rhythms in either of these behaviors. A long-day *per* allele produces 28-hour cycles for both locomotor activity and eclosion, whereas two short-day *per* alleles shorten the cycle (to 19 hours in one case and to 16 hours in the other; see Figure 3-6).

How do the *per* and *tim* genes keep time? The answer to this question has begun to emerge from genetic and molecular studies of the two genes and their protein products. The protein products of the *per* and *tim* genes (PER and TIM) are thought to shuttle between the cytoplasm and nucleus of cells, regulating expression of target genes, including themselves. As a result, the synthesis and accumulation of the messenger RNAs encoding PER and TIM follow a circadian cycle.

For the proteins to function, PER has to bind to TIM (Figure 3-7). Both genes are transcribed in the morning and their mRNAs accumulate during the day, during which the protein products appear not to be functional. A key step in the regulation of this cycle is the light-induced degradation of the TIM protein. During the day *tim* RNA is transcribed but the level of TIM protein remains low because of a high rate of degradation. In the absence of TIM, PER does not function. As a result, TIM and PER complexes are not formed. After dusk, when the levels of TIM and PER increase, the two proteins bind to one another, thus becoming functional, and enter the nucleus where they inhibit the transcription of their own genes as well as other, unidentified target genes. As a consequence, *per* and *tim* mRNA levels decrease and subsequently protein expression decreases. By morning, PER and TIM protein levels have fallen to low enough levels that they no longer repress transcription.

The finding that the *per* and *tim* transcripts are regulated by negative feedback raises the question of why the PER and TIM proteins do not immediately repress their own expression. The answer lies in a built-in delay in accumulation and translocation of the proteins to the nucleus. The PER protein cannot accumulate until sufficient TIM protein is present to bind to and stabilize it. TIM protein, on the other hand, cannot enter the nucleus unless it is bound to PER protein. Accurate time-keeping therefore depends on an oscillatory cycle in gene expression and inactivation by negative feedback.

What does this say for mechanisms in normal and short-cycle flies? In the long-day (28-hour) *per* mutants the binding affinity of PER proteins for TIM appears to be reduced. Binding thus cannot occur until the two proteins reach higher levels, causing a delay in the entry of the PER-TIM complex into the nucleus and thus extending the period of each cycle.

The mechanisms that control circadian rhythms in other organisms are likely to be similar in principle to

A

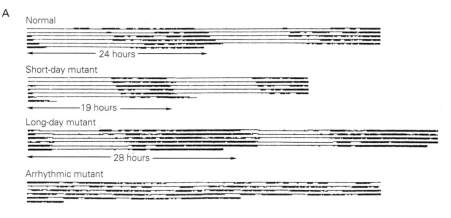

Normal

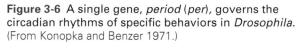

Short-day mutant

Long-day mutant

Arrhythmic mutant

B

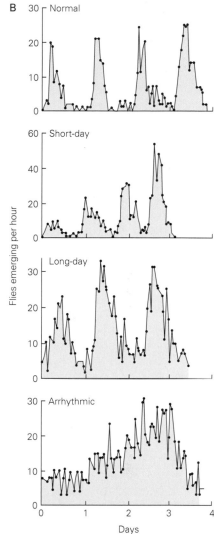

Figure 3-6 A single gene, *period* (*per*), governs the circadian rhythms of specific behaviors in *Drosophila*. (From Konopka and Benzer 1971.)

A. Locomotor rhythms in normal *Drosophila* and three *per* mutant strains: short-day, long-day, and arrhythmic. Flies were exposed to a cycle of 12 hours of light and 12 hours of darkness, and activity was then monitored under infrared light. Heavy lines indicate activity.

B. Normal adult fly populations emerge from their pupal cases in cyclic fashion, even in constant darkness. The plots show the number of flies (in each of four populations) emerging per hour over a 4-day period of constant darkness. The arrhythmic *per* mutant population emerges without any discernible rhythm.

the mechanism that controls the rhythmicity of the *per* and *tim* genes in *Drosophila*. In mammals circadian behavioral rhythms are governed by the suprachiasmatic nucleus in the hypothalamus (see Chapter 47). Because circadian behavior in mice is precise, it is easy to set up quantitative genetic screens for mutations that alter the circadian behavior. Joseph Takahashi took advantage of the regularity of this behavior to carry out a chemical mutagenesis screen. By this means he identified a semi-dominant autosomal mutation named *clock*. Mice homozygous for the *clock* mutation show extremely long circadian periods followed by a complete loss of circadian rhythmicity when transferred to constant darkness (Figure 3-8). The *clock* gene therefore appears to regulate two fundamental properties of the circadian rhythm in

mice: the circadian period itself and the persistence of circadian rhythmicity.

Since no anatomical defects have been observed with the *clock* mutation, the *clock* gene appears to encode a protein specific and essential for circadian rhythmicity in the mouse. When the *clock* gene was cloned it was found to encode a transcription factor, presumably involved in the basic regulation of genes important for the circadian rhythm. Particularly important is the fact that one of the domains of the clock protein (the PAS domain) is also found in PER. This raises the interesting possibility that the clock protein might bind to and interact with a mouse protein homologous to PER. Many mammalian genes related to *clock* have now been identified and implicated in the control of circadian rhythms.

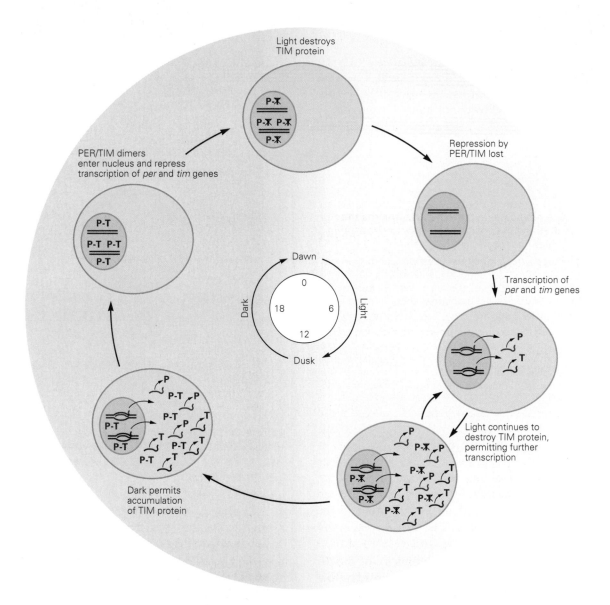

Figure 3-7 Light-dependent degradation of the TIM protein establishes the circadian control of biological rhythms in *Drosophila.* The genes that control the circadian clock are regulated by two nuclear proteins, PER and TIM, that slowly accumulate and then bind to one another to form dimers. Dimerization of PER and TIM is necessary for the complex to enter the nucleus and shut off the transcription of target genes, including the genes for PER and TIM themselves. During the hours of daylight TIM protein is degraded by light; thus PER cannot enter the nucleus and the transcription of target genes (including the *per* and *tim* genes) continues. After dark, TIM protein is no longer degraded, and the PER-TIM dimers enter the nucleus, where they repress transcription of target genes. In this way the day-night cycle regulates the expression of genes that control biological function. (Adapted from Barinaga 1996.)

Defects in Single Genes Can Have Profound Effects on Complex Behaviors in Mice

The use of chemical genetic techniques to identify circadian rhythm mutants in mice underscores the importance of this experimental mammal in behavioral genetic studies. Genetic studies of mouse behavior have begun to provide insight into the genetic bases of some human behavioral disorders. Here we discuss the evidence for a genetic basis for three disorders: obesity, impulsivity, and altered motivational state.

Mutations in the Gene Encoding Leptin Affect Feeding Behavior

Whether an individual is lean, obese, or of intermediate size is determined in large part by the balance between the amount of food consumed and energy expended, a balance governed by both psychological and physiological factors. Genetics studies of obese mice have provided the best insight into the physiological factors that control ingestive behavior.

The physical cloning and characterization of the region around a spontaneous obesity-causing mutation on mouse chromosome 6 led to the identification of the mouse *obese (ob)* gene and to a highly conserved (homologous) human gene. The mouse *ob* gene encodes the protein leptin, a small protein of 145 amino acids that is selectively expressed in adipose tissue and released into the bloodstream. Leptin contributes to the homeostatic mechanisms that permit an animal to maintain its weight within 5% of its normal weight for most of its life. Under normal conditions the amount of leptin secreted reflects the total mass of adipose tissue. When adipose tissue decreases, leptin levels decrease and the animal eats more; when adipose tissue increases, leptin levels increase and the animal eats less. Mice with homozygous mutations in the *ob* gene lack circulating leptin. This lack leads to marked obesity in these mutant animals. When leptin is supplied exogenously, however, food intake and body weight are reduced dramatically.

A receptor for leptin, called OB-R, encodes a protein that is related to a component of certain cytokine receptors that activate specific transcription factors. This leptin receptor is expressed at a high level in the hypothalamus, the part of the brain that controls appetite and feeding (Chapter 32). The gene encoding OB-R is located in the same region of mouse chromosome as the *diabetic* gene (*db*). This is interesting because obesity and diabetes are often linked in humans. In fact, *db/db* mice are also obese and exhibit a phenotype similar to the mice with a mutated *ob* gene. Moreover, there is good

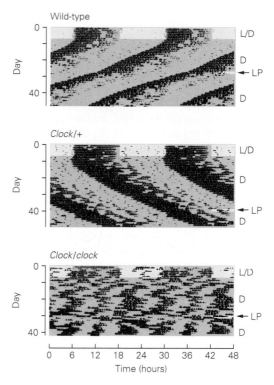

Figure 3-8 Locomotor activity records of *clock* mutant mice. The record shows periods of wheel-running activity by three offspring. All animals were kept on a light-dark cycle (**L/D**) of 12 hours for the first 7 days, then transferred to constant darkness (**D**). They later received a 6-hour light pulse (**LP**) to reset the rhythm. The activity rhythm for the wild-type mouse had a period of 23.1 hours. The period for the heterozygous *clock/+* mouse is 24.9 hours. The homozygous *clock/clock* mice experience a complete loss of circadian rhythmicity upon transfer to constant darkness and transiently express a rhythm of 28.4 hours after the light pulse. (From Takahashi et al. 1994.)

evidence that the *db* gene encodes the leptin receptor.

To what extent do these studies of mice provide insight into human disease? Most obese humans are not defective in leptin mRNA or protein levels and indeed produce higher levels than do nonobese individuals. Thus, it is likely that human obesity reflects not a lack of leptin but a failure to respond to normal or even elevated levels of leptin. Failure to respond to leptin could be a result of mutations of the leptin receptor or of molecules that interact with the receptor.

Leptin may affect feeding behavior by regulating neuropeptide and neurotransmitter expression in hypothalamic cells. Lesions of the hypothalamus affect body weight. For example, ablation of the ventromedial hypothalamus or the arcuate nucleus results in obesity. Leptin administration markedly inhibits the biosynthesis and release of neuropeptide Y, a peptide that stimulates food

Box 3-3 Generating Mutations in Flies and Mice

Flies

Genetic analysis of behavior in *Drosophila* relies on behavioral assays of animals in which individual genes have been mutated. Experimental mutations in *Drosophila* were originally produced through radiation-induced mutagenesis. This method, however, results in large-scale deletions or rearrangements in chromosomes; several genes are often affected, even when small deletions are the target, and molecular characterization of relevant genes is difficult. In contrast, the chemical ethyl methanesulfonate (EMS) induces point mutations and thus facilitates the characterization of mutations at specific loci.

Many spontaneous mutations and chromosomal rearrangements are produced by transposable elements. The most useful class of transposable elements in *Drosophila* is the P element. P elements encode a transposase enzyme that mediates the mobilization of the element and a repressor product that blocks transposition. P elements have become major tools of the modern *Drosophila* geneticist.

In one technique, P elements are used to isolate mutations in any *Drosophila* gene of interest. The investigator screens for mutants of the gene in progeny of crosses between *Drosophila* strains that carry P elements and those in which they are absent. New mutations result from the transposition of a P element into a gene. A vector is then constructed in which a P element is inserted. This vector is used as a probe to identify and isolate DNA segments that contain P elements; elements inserted into the gene of interest are found within a subset of these segments. The gene can then be cloned and studied.

Mice

Recent advances in molecular manipulation of mammalian genes have permitted *in situ* replacement of a known, normal gene with a mutant version. The process of generating a strain of mutant mice involves two separate manipulations: the replacement of a gene on a chromosome by homologous recombination in a special cell line known as embryonic stem cells (Figure 3-9), and the subsequent incorporation of this modified cell line into the germ cell population of the embryo (Figure 3-10).

The gene of interest must first be cloned. The gene is mutated, and a selectable marker, usually a drug-resistance gene,

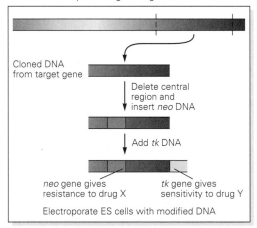

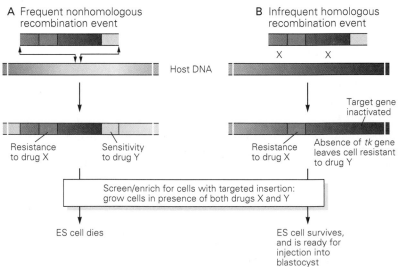

Figure 3-9. Experimentally controlled homologous recombination is the first step in creating mutant mice. Cloned DNA from the mouse gene to be mutated is modified by genetic engineering so that it contains a bacterial gene, *neo*. Integration of *neo* into a mouse chromosome makes the mouse cells resistant to drugs that otherwise would be lethal to the cells (drug X). A viral gene, *tk*, is also added, attached to one end of the mouse DNA. Integration of *tk* into a mouse chromosome makes the cells sensitive to a different drug (drug Y). (Adapted from Alberts et al. 1994.)

A. Most insertions occur at random sites in the mouse chromosome, and these nearly always include both ends of the engineered DNA fragment. Colonies of cells in which homologous recombination has incorporated the center of the engineered DNA fragment without the ends are obtained by selecting for those rare mouse cells that grow in the presence of both drugs.

B. Most of the cells that grow in the presence of both drugs will carry the targeted gene replacement.

is then introduced into the mutated fragment. The altered gene is then transfected into embryonic stem cells, and clones of cells that incorporate the altered gene are isolated. To identify a clone in which the mutated gene has been integrated into the homologous (normal) site, rather than some other random site, DNA samples of each clone are tested.

When a suitable clone has been obtained, cells are injected into a mouse embryo at the blastocyst stage (3–4 days after fertilization), when the embryo consists of approximately 100 cells. These embryos are then reintroduced into a female that has been hormonally prepared for implantation and allowed to come to term. Embryonic stem cells in the mouse have the capability of participating in all aspects of development, including the germline. Thus, injected cells can become germ cells and pass on the altered gene.

Since incorporated stem cells generally mix into other tissues besides the germline, their presence can be tested when the injected embryo is born. Initially, this can be done by using a stem cell line from a mouse strain with a fur color different from that of the strain used to obtain the embryo. The mixed (*chimeric*) offspring appear to have a patchy colored coat. These progeny are then mated to determine if any stem cells

have become germ cells. If so, their progeny will carry the altered gene on one of their chromosomes, detectable by analyzing DNA samples from each of the offspring. When the heterozygous individuals are mated together, one-fourth of the progeny will be homozygous mutant. This technique has been used to generate mutations in various genes crucial to development or function in the nervous system.

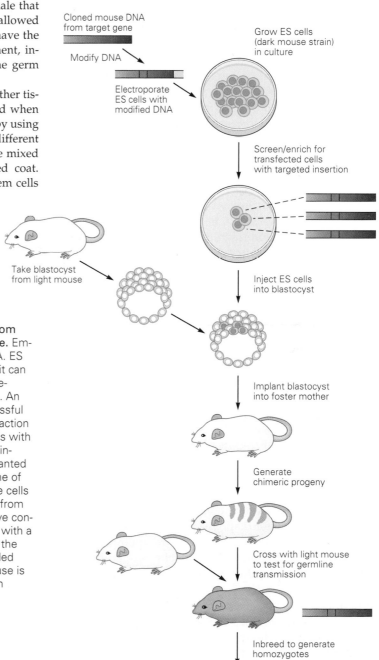

Figure 3-10. Altered embryonic stem cells derived from mouse blastocysts are used to create transgenic mice. Embryonic stem (ES) cells are transfected with altered DNA. ES cells that have integrated a transgene for a particular trait can be selected by using a donor that carries an additional sequence, such as a drug-resistance gene (see Figure 3-9). An alternative is to assay the transfected ES cells for successful integration of the donor DNA using polymerase chain reaction (PCR) technology. After obtaining a population of ES cells with a high proportion carrying the marker, the cells are then injected into a recipient blastocyst. This blastocyst is implanted into a foster mother to generate a chimeric mouse. Some of the tissues of the chimeric mice will be derived from the cells of the recipient blastocyst; other tissues will be derived from the injected ES cells. To determine whether ES cells have contributed to the germline, the chimeric mouse is crossed with a mouse that lacks the donor trait. Any progeny that have the trait must be derived from germ cells that have descended from the injected ES cells. By this means, an entire mouse is generated from the altered ES cell. (Adapted from Lewin 1994.)

intake when administered to rodents. Remarkably, as we have discussed earlier, the link between neuropeptide Y and food intake appears to have been conserved, in a general sense, between *C. elegans* and man.

Mutations in the Gene Encoding a Serotonergic Receptor Intensify Impulsive Behavior

Serotonin (5-hydroxytryptamine) is a monoamine that serves as a neurotransmitter in the brain. The level of serotonin is thought to be reduced in depressive illness. As we shall learn later (Chapter 44), neurons that synthesize serotonin are clustered in several nuclei in the brain stem, the most prominent of which are the *raphe nuclei*. Their axons project to many regions of the brain, notably the cerebral cortex. Neurons that synthesize serotonin modulate the activity of cortical and subcortical neurons in several ways by activating different receptor subtypes: some excitatory, some inhibitory, some both.

Because of its action on different receptors, serotonin has been implicated in the regulation of mood states, including depression, anxiety, food intake, and impulsive violence (see Chapter 61). Several animal studies have shown that aggressive behavior is often associated with decreased activity of serotonergic neurons. These studies are of particular interest because they provide a glimpse of how social and genetic factors interact to modify behavior.

Most animals, including humans, become aggressive when threatened, such as when their territory is invaded, their offspring are attacked, or sexual interactions are prevented. The importance of serotonergic transmission in aggressive behavior is clearly evident in studies of mice in which the gene for the serotonin 1B receptor has been ablated by targeted deletion (Box 3-3). When mice lacking the serotonin 1B receptor are isolated for four weeks and then exposed to a wild-type mouse, they are much more aggressive than wild-type animals under similar conditions. The mutant mice attack intruders faster than wild-type mice or mice lacking only one copy of the serotonin 1B receptor gene, and the number and intensity of attacks is significantly greater than that of wild-type mice. Thus, the serotonin 1B receptor plays a role in mediating aggressive behavior in mice.

Serotonin activity has been implicated as one of several important biological factors in determining the threshold for violence. People with a history of impulsive aggressive behavior (and of suicide)—and mouse strains that display increased aggressiveness—have low concentrations of serotonin in the brain. Inhibition of serotonin synthesis or destruction of serotonergic neu-

rons increases aggressiveness in mice and monkeys. Finally, certain serotonin agonists that act on the serotonin 1B receptor inhibit aggression.

In humans a variety of social stressors, such as social or sexual abuse during childhood, are thought to lower the biological thresholds for violence, including the level of serotonin in the brain. Indeed, male monkeys raised in isolation have reduced levels of serotonin in their brains, illustrating that both environmental and genetic factors can converge to influence the metabolism of serotonin.

The relationship of serotonin levels to aggression in humans is not simple, however. This complexity is evident in studies of a Dutch family that transmits an X-linked form of mental retardation. Fourteen of the affected males have a history of impulsive behavior that includes arson, rape, and attempted murder. Each of these men carries a point mutation in the gene that encodes the enzyme monoamine oxidase A, one of the two major enzymes that metabolizes monoamines. This class of neurotransmitter includes serotonin, norepinephrine, and dopamine (see Chapters 60 and 61). The mutation apparently leads to *increased* levels of serotonin, yet the affected people show enhanced impulsiveness. Thus, the relationship between serotonin and aggression is not simply that reduced serotonin causes aggression and enhanced serotonin causes placidity. Both increases *and* decreases in serotonin levels may enhance aggression. These findings suggest, not surprisingly, that in humans the relationship between serotonin and a complex trait such as aggression is not direct and may be quite subtle. Finally, although monoamines, in particular serotonin, are important in aggressive behavior, other transmitter systems also affect this behavior, as would be expected for a complex behavioral trait.

Deletion of a Gene That Encodes an Enzyme Important for Dopamine Production Disrupts Locomotor Behavior and Motivation

Dopamine, like serotonin, is a major monoaminergic transmitter in the central nervous system. The majority of dopaminergic neurons have their cell bodies in the substantia nigra while their axons project to the corpus striatum. Dopaminergic neurons have been implicated in the regulation of motor behavior—the degeneration of dopaminergic neurons underlies Parkinson's disease, a debilitating disorder of movement. Other dopaminergic pathways are thought to regulate motivated behaviors. Dysfunction of these pathways may contribute to schizophrenia (see Chapter 60).

The role of the dopaminergic system in mammalian

behavior has traditionally been studied through pharmacological techniques. Recently, however, gene knockout techniques have been applied to this system. In one set of experiments the ability of neurons to synthesize dopamine was blocked by selectively inactivating the gene that encodes tyrosine hydroxylase, one of the enzymes important in dopamine synthesis. The dopamine-deficient mice were born, began to nurse, and grew normally for about two weeks and then became inactive, failed to eat or drink, and died shortly thereafter. However, daily administration of L-DOPA, the product of tyrosine hydroxylase, restored normal feeding and produced increased activity.

Dopamine is cleared from the synapse by a high-affinity dopamine transporter. In mutant mice with a deficiency in this transporter the amount of extracellular dopamine is 100-fold greater than normal. The mutant mice exhibit spontaneous and excessive locomotion similar to that obtained in normal mice when the dopamine transporter is blocked pharmacologically (as with a psychostimulant such as cocaine).

Single Genes Are Critical Factors in Certain Human Behavioral Traits

Mutations in a Dopamine Receptor May Influence Novelty-Seeking Behavior

As we have seen, studies of identical twins suggest that a number of personality characteristics have a significant heritable component, but in no case has this finding been rigorously demonstrated by identifying a specific gene. One fascinating candidate is novelty-seeking behavior, a behavior characterized by exhilaration or excitement in response to stimuli that are novel. People who score high on tests of novelty seeking tend to be impulsive, exploratory, fickle, excitable, quick-tempered, and extravagant. They often do things for thrills, as opposed to thinking things through before coming to a decision.

Twin studies suggest that novelty-seeking behavior has a heritability of about 40%. A significant component (10% of the genetic component) seems to be due to a polymorphism in a single gene, the gene that encodes the D4 dopamine receptor. Dopamine is involved in exploratory and pleasure-seeking behavior. There are at least five known receptors for dopamine, called D1 to D5 (Chapter 60). The D4 receptor is expressed in the hypothalamus and the limbic areas of the brain concerned with emotion.

In general, the coding sequence of the receptors for dopamine are highly conserved (as are the coding sequence for other receptors to chemical transmitters), and polymorphisms are very rare. Nevertheless, an interesting polymorphism has been found in the D4 receptor. One form of the gene, called the short form, has a 48-base pair DNA sequence in one of its cytoplasmic domains. By contrast, the long form of the D4 receptor gene has seven repeats of this domain. Additionally, the long and short forms of the receptor appear to have slightly different signaling properties in response to dopamine. It appears that these slight differences in the long form of the receptor correlate with novelty seeking.

Mutations in Opsin Genes Influence Color Perception

Color vision is one of the few cases in which variation in normal human perception can be explained at a molecular level. Molecular cloning techniques have been used to identify and clone the genes encoding the proteins for the red, green, and blue pigments that transduce different wavelengths of light (see Chapter 29). Defects in one or more of the genes encoding red and green pigments lead to varying degrees of color blindness.

The genes for red and green pigments are arrayed head-to-tail, close to one another on the X chromosome and differ in only about 1 in 20 of their amino acid residues. Because of this tandem organization and similarity of sequence, crossing over between the red and green pigment genes occurs frequently, leading to gene rearrangement.[2] The resulting abnormality in both genes explains the origin of many cases of red-green color blindness.

Subtle variations in color perception occur even among individuals with normal color vision. This is attributable to polymorphism in the red pigment gene in humans. In 62% of the male population with normal color vision, amino acid 180 is a serine residue while in the remaining 38% it is an alanine residue. The effects of this sequence difference can be revealed in psychophysical tests in which subjects are asked to match the intensity of a mixture of red and green light. The intensity of red light needed to match a standard depends on the amino acid at position 180. Because females have two X chromosomes, they fall into three groups: homozygotes for Ser180, homozygotes for Ala180, and heterozygotes who display an intermediate phenotype. Thus, a major variation in human color perception can be explained by a small change in the coding sequence of a single gene.

---

[2]This gene rearrangement is the result of unequal crossing over between the X chromosomes in a female. This unequal crossover appears as a *hemizygous* condition in male offspring (genes on the male's X chromosome are called hemizygous because they exist only in one copy).

Box 3-4 Genetic Polymorphisms

If two genes are located very near one another they are likely to be inherited together. Thus, if an abnormality of one gene produces a disease and a nearby marker gene encodes a readily recognized phenotypic trait (such as hair or eye color) or a readily detectable gene product (such as a protein present in the blood), people who express the marker will likely also express the disease—even though the marker may have nothing to do with the disease. Both the phenotypic trait and the DNA sequence of the gene vary in the normal population.

In the past, genetic markers were used to distinguish variations in the protein coding regions of genes, such as blood group antigens, enzymes, and antigens of the histocompatibility complex. However, coding sequences represent only 5–10% of the total human genome; 90 or 95% of the genome contains noncoding regions. It is now possible to saturate the human genome with markers that distinguish variations that occur in otherwise homologous DNA sequences throughout the whole genome (including noncoding as well as coding sequences). This broad coverage has made it much easier to trace the inheritance of a disease to a specific region of a particular chromosome.

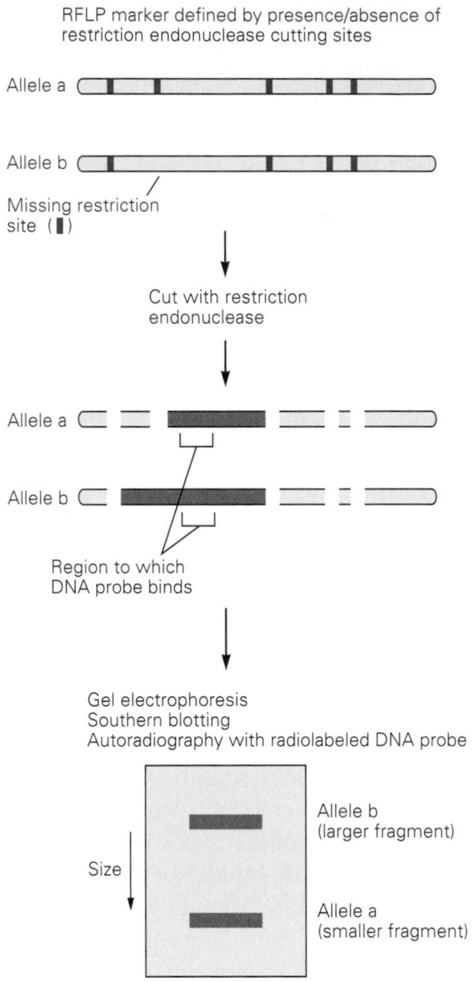

Figure 3-11A. The presence of a restriction fragment length polymorphism (RFLP) can be detected by analyzing DNA fragments cleaved by restriction endonucleases, enzymes that cut at specific restriction sites in nucleotide sequences. In this example chromosome *b* is missing a restriction site that is present on chromosome *a*. As a result, cutting chromosome *b* produces a larger than normal DNA fragment in this region. After cutting, the DNA from both chromosomes is separated according to size by means of gel electrophoresis and transferred to nylon filters (in a procedure called Southern blotting). Autoradiography is then used to reveal the polymorphism. Because the *b* fragment is larger, it is distinguishable from the *a* fragment. (Adapted from Alberts et al. 1994.)

Novelty seeking is a natural variation in human behavior. Color blindness is a similar variation in perception. It may be annoying to those who have it, but it interferes only marginally with life's function and not at all with longevity. These relatively neutral mutations differ importantly from mutations that produce serious disease.

Mutations in the Huntingtin Gene Result in Huntington Disease

One of the first complex human behavioral abnormalities to be traced to a single gene is Huntington disease, a degenerative disorder of the nervous system. Huntington disease affects both men and women with a frequency of about 5 per 100,000. It is characterized by four features: heritability, chorea (incessant, rapid, jerky movements), cognitive impairment (dementia), and death 15 to 20 years after the onset of symptoms. In most patients the onset of the disease occurs in the fourth to fifth decade of life. Thus, the disease often strikes after individuals have married and had children.

Huntington disease involves the death of neurons in the caudate nucleus, a part of the basal ganglia involved in regulating voluntary movement. The death of

One type of DNA marker, a *restriction fragment length polymorphism* (RFLP), is created by differences in DNA sequence in paired alleles. At one allele a cutting site for a particular restriction enzyme (an enzyme that cuts DNA only at a specific nucleotide sequence) is eliminated or an extra site added, while the other allele remains normal. As a result, the restriction enzyme produces DNA fragments of different lengths from the two alleles. These so-called restriction fragments can be separated by electrophoresis in agarose gels and distinguished by specific DNA probes (Figure 3-11A).

When such a polymorphic region of the DNA is closely linked to a particular gene, inheritance of the gene can be traced by following the inheritance of a particular pattern of restriction fragments. The method can be used to trace pathogenic genes (Figure 3-11B,C).

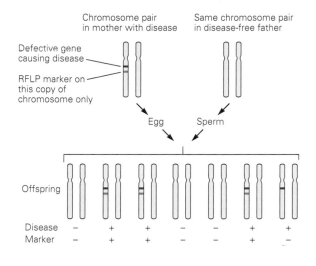

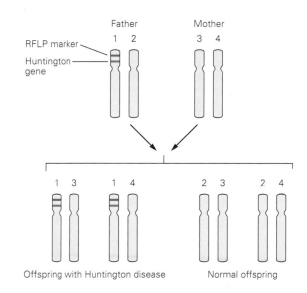

Figure 3-11B. Genetic linkage analysis detects the coinheritance of a mutated gene responsible for a human disease and a nearby restriction fragment length polymorphism (RFLP) marker. In this example the gene responsible for the disease is inherited in four offspring, three of which coinherit the marker. Thus, the gene responsible for the disease is located close to the RFLP marker on this chromosome. (Adapted from Alberts et al. 1994.)

Figure 3-11C. Inheritance of the gene responsible for Huntington disease can be traced by following the inheritance of a particular restriction fragment length on chromosome 4.

nerve cells in the caudate nucleus is thought to cause the chorea. The basis for the impaired cognitive functions and eventual dementia is less clear and is due either to a loss of cortical neurons or to the disruption of normal activity in the cognitive portion of the basal ganglia (see Chapter 43). The selective loss of neurons in the caudate nucleus can be demonstrated in living patients using imaging techniques.

Huntington disease is inherited as an autosomal dominant disorder and the mutation is highly penetrant.[3] The Huntington disease gene was identified on chromosome 4 using a technique based on DNA markers to map heritable disease mutations relative to genetic polymorphisms (Box 3-4). This gene encodes a large protein called Huntingtin, the function of which is as yet unknown.

---

[3]Penetrance refers to the frequency with which a heritable trait is manifested phenotypically by individuals carrying the mutant gene(s). Thus the Huntington disease gene is 100% penetrant.

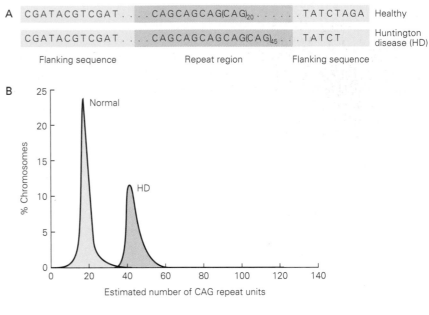

Figure 3-12. The DNA mutation in Huntington disease is an unstable CAG repeat.

A. The nucleotide sequence in the region of the unstable CAG repeat in the Huntingtin gene.

B. Distribution of CAG repeat lengths on normal and Huntington disease (HD) chromosomes. The percentages of normal and HD chromosomes containing different CAG repeat lengths (from 6 to 125) are compiled from several published studies.

C. A highly significant inverse correlation between age of onset of Huntington disease movements and CAG repeat length occurs across all HD alleles. (Modified from Gusella and MacDonald 1995.)

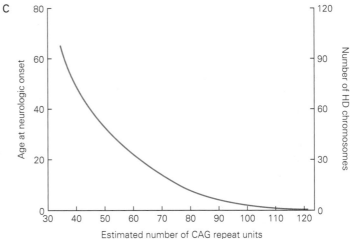

The mutated form of the Huntingtin protein contains a stretch of glutamine residues that is much longer than in the normal protein. The codon (CAG) that encodes glutamine is repeated 19–22 times in the normal gene but 48 or more times in the mutated gene (Figure 3-12A). This expansion results in abnormally long stretches of polyglutamine in the protein. The number of ways in which the abnormal stretch of glutamines affect protein function is not known.

Diseases that involve trinucleotide expansion have an additional feature: each successive generation of a family that harbors the mutant gene manifests the disease with greater severity at an earlier age (*genetic anticipation*). Thus, an individual may have a mild case of Huntington disease that was not manifested until age 60, whereas his great grandchild may develop more serious symptoms by age 40 (Figure 3-12B,C). This trend is due to the instability of the expanded trinucleotide repeat. As the repeat passes through the germline, the number of repeats tends to increase, particularly in the paternal line. These repeats are thought to create hairpin-like structures in DNA that interfere with its replication. As the repeats attain a certain length, the hairpin-like structures stabilize, leading to persistent mistakes in replication and consequently further expansion of the trinucleotide repeat. The polyglutamine structures appear to affect the protein in one of two ways: they may make the altered protein destructive to the cell, producing a gain-of-function mutation; or they may bind other proteins required for normal cellular function. Expanded tri-nucleotide repeat diseases are usually genetically dominant.

Table 3-1 Neurological Diseases Involving Trinucleotide Repeats[1]

Disease	Repeat	Repeat length[2]	Gene product
X-linked spinal and bulbar muscular atrophy	CAG	Normal: 11–34 Disease: 40–62	Androgen receptor
Fragile X mental retardation[3]	CGG	Normal: 6 to ~50 Premutation: 52–200 Disease: 200 to >1000	FMR-1 protein
Myotonic dystrophy[3]	CTG	Normal: 5–30 Premutation: 42–180 Disease: 200 to >1000	Myotonin protein kinase
Huntington disease	CAG	Normal: 11–34 Disease: 37–121	Huntingtin
Spinocerebellar ataxia type 1	CAG	Normal: 19–36 Disease: 43–81	Ataxin-1
FRAXE mental retardation[3]	GCC	Normal: 6–25 Disease: >200	?
Dentatorubral-pallidoluysian atrophy	CAG	Normal: 7–23 Disease: 49–75	?

[1]Eight diseases are now associated with the expansion of a trinucleotide CAG repeat in the coding region of the responsible gene: spinal and bulbar muscular atrophy (SBMA); Huntington disease (HD); dentatorubralpallidoluysian atrophy (DRPLA); spinocerebellar ataxia type 1 (SCA1); and SCA2, 3, 6, and 7. In addition, three congenital fragile X syndromes, each associated with hypermethylation and unstable trinucleotide repeats, have been identified: FRAXA (CGG); FRAXE (GCC), and FRAXF (GCC). For each of the *FRA* genes, expression is extinguished by expansion and methylation.
[2]Although individuals with repeat length in the "premutation" size range are phenotypically normal, the corresponding chromosomes are very likely to expand to the "disease-length" category in the next meiosis.
[3]CGG, CTG, and CGG expansions are transcribed into the noncoding region of the mRNAs, whereas the GAG expansions associated with neurodegenerative disorders are translated into glutamine tracts.
(Adapted from Warren 1996.)

Strikingly, many other hereditary diseases of the nervous system involve similar expansions in trinucleotide repeats within the coding region of the gene responsible for the disease. These diseases include Friedreich's ataxia type 1, spinocerebellar ataxia, and certain spinal and bulbar muscular dystrophies (Table 3-1; Figure 3-13). By contrast, fragile X mental retardation is an X-linked recessive disease that involves a trinucleotide repeat in the control region near the coding region of the gene, leading to the inactivation of the FMR (fragile X mental retardation) gene. As in Huntington disease, progressive death of specific subpopulations of neurons or muscle cells occurs in many of these diseases.

Most Complex Behavioral Traits in Humans Are Multigenic

So far we have considered examples of the effects of single genes on behavior. Classic genetic analysis focuses on Mendelian traits, which, as we have seen, are normally determined by allelic variation within a single gene. However, most behavioral traits as well as most common genetic disorders are multigenic; they are determined by several genes interacting with environmental factors.[4]

In contrast to single-locus Mendelian traits, multigenic traits do not have a simple recognizable pattern of inheritance (autosomal dominant, recessive, or X-linked), and thus the relative contributions of several genes to one trait is difficult to analyze. Nevertheless, determining which genes contribute to complex human traits has profound implications for the care and treatment of human disease.

Most common multigenic diseases, such as diabetes, coronary artery disease, asthma, schizophrenia,

---

[4]The term *multigenic* includes both oligogenic and polygenic traits. An *oligogenic* trait or disorder is determined by a small number of genes, each contributing to the phenotype in a significant way. In contrast, a *polygenic* trait is the result of many genes, each with a small effect on the phenotype.

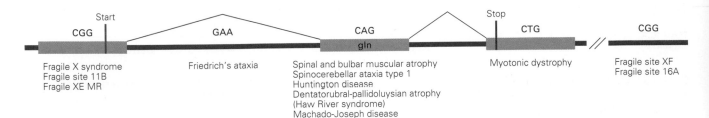

Figure 3-13 This model of a gene containing three exons and two introns (intervening blue line) depicts the location and type of expanded triplets involved in certain neurological diseases.

CGG repeats are found within the 5′ untranslated region of the first exons of the genes for fragile X syndrome, fragile XE mental retardation (MR), and fragile site 11B. CGG repeats are also found at two fragile sites, XF and 16A, which are not known to be in the vicinity of any genes and, like fragile site 11B, are not known to result in any disease phenotype. GAA repeats are found within the first exon of the X25 gene for Friedrich's ataxia. CAG repeats occur at five loci responsible for neurological diseases. These repeats are coding regions and thus result in the lengthening of a normal polyglutamine tract in their respective gene products. The repeats for Haw River syndrome are at the same locus as those for dentatorubral-pallidoluysian atrophy and similarly involve expansion of the same CAG repeat. A CTG repeat (CAG on the other strand) occurs in the 3′ untranslated region of the final exon of the protein kinase gene for myotonic dystrophy. (Adapted from Warren 1996.)

and manic-depressive disorder, are thought to represent a variety of disorders both etiologically and genetically. Thus, different mutant alleles and environmental factors are thought to produce indistinguishable phenotypes. In a typical multigenic disease, such as diabetes, there are scores of different alleles (among 10–12 different loci; see below) distributed throughout the human population of the world that are capable of contributing to the disease. In any one family three or four of these mutant alleles are likely to be sufficient to gives rise to the disease. In fact, it is possible that each of the alleles that contributes to a multigenic disease functions as a normal polymorphism when expressed by itself but gives rise to disease if expressed together with other alleles in a certain genetic background. Moreover, because mono-zygotic twins with identical genetic endowment are often discordant for multigenic traits, the role of nongenetic factors must be important.

Several techniques have facilitated the genome-wide search for multigenic disorders in humans. The most common genetic mapping strategy is *linkage analysis,* in which a gene's locus is determined by comparing the inheritance of the mutant gene with a precisely mapped polymorphic DNA marker in a family afflicted with the particular disease. A DNA marker is useful if it maps to a unique locus within the human genome and it identifies frequent polymorphic variations between individuals at this locus. Coinheritance of a particular DNA marker with a mutant phenotype (or disease state) suggests that the marker and the mutant gene are physically close together on the chromosome.

Until 1980 polymorphisms could only be detected by differences in the behavior of the protein, for example, by differences in enzyme activity or electrophoretic mo-

bility. In the early 1980s it was appreciated that the noncoding regions, which make up 90-95% of the DNA, are the sites of frequent DNA polymorphisms. Indeed, single base pair changes that give rise to variants are relatively frequent in the human genome, with rates perhaps as high as 1 in 500 base pairs, and most of these changes occur in noncoding regions. The method of restriction fragment length polymorphisms (see Box 3-4) is used to detect polymorphisms throughout the genome.

The coinheritance of a DNA marker and mutant gene can occur by chance, or it can occur because the two loci recombine infrequently during meiosis, a direct result of their physical proximity. The chance that any two unlinked loci—for example, loci from different chromosomes—will be inherited together is 1/2, and the chance that they will be coinherited in n siblings is $(1/2)^n$. Thus, if two loci are coinherited in all eight affected siblings from a single family, the odds against this being a random event would be $(1/2)^8 = 256:1$. In practice this is a more complicated event, one that is better analyzed by computer programs that calculate the ratio of the odds for and against linkage, while considering various statistical issues, and generate a value known as the *lod* (log of the *od*ds) score. (For practical purposes a lod score equal to or greater than 3 indicates that evidence for linkage between a gene marker is significant. This represents odds of 20:1 in favor of linkage between the two loci.)

A related method of identifying polymorphisms is the characterization of simple sequence repeats by the polymerase chain reaction (PCR). The construction of high-resolution human genetic maps composed of these markers and the application of semi-automated screening technologies have facilitated linkage analysis. A

Box 3-5 Analysis of Multigenic Traits

Quantitative trait locus (QTL) analysis is a method for identifying the multiple genes that condition a single behavioral trait. QTL analysis requires at least two strains of a species, each of which has been inbred until all members of the group are genetically identical and have two uniform sets of chromosomes. In the hypothetical example described here (Figure 3-14), two strains of mice have been selectively bred for aggressiveness (A) and docility (D).

1. Aggressive A-type mice are bred with docile D-type mice, producing a first generation (F_1) hybrid offspring in which every mouse has one set of chromosomes from each parent. In the F_1 generation the chromosomes in the cells that produce eggs and sperm exchange material. Segments of the mother's and father's DNA are recombined on individual chromosomes.
2. The F_1 generation is bred back to D-type mice, producing offspring with one recombinant set of chromosomes and one set that is pure D. In each offspring the recombinant chromosome will carry a unique mix of genes from both original strains.
3. Second-generation mice will show a range of aggressiveness because more than one gene determines aggressiveness and the mix of genes in the recombinant chromosome set varies. In Figure 3-14 the levels of aggressiveness in the second-generation mice are indicated by the different colors.
4. Sites in the genome that contain genes that contribute to aggression are identified by searching each mouse's DNA for genetic markers, landmarks scattered throughout the genome that are known to differ between the aggressive and docile strains. Each marker is examined to determine whether a mouse has inherited the A-type or D-type.
5. For each marker, the mice are sorted into those that have A-type DNA at that locus and those that have D-type DNA. The aggressiveness scores for the mice in the two groups are then compared. If the A-type group is significantly more aggressive than the D-type group, that marker represents a QTL that may contain a gene contributing to aggressiveness. Since each QTL interval contains many genes, additional methods must be used to find the one conditioning aggression.

(Modified from Barinaga 1994.)

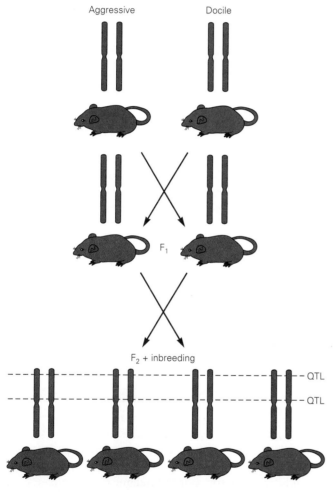

Figure 3-14.

gene that contributes to a multigenic trait is often called a *quantitative trait locus* (QTL) to indicate that it contributes to the genetic variance of a particular trait. QTL analysis is currently being used with mice and rats to track the genes that contribute to a number of behaviors (Box 3-5).

Linkage analysis is very sensitive to the model of transmission—dominant, recessive, X-linked, and others—and loses power when applied to multigenic traits where the mode of transmission is not known a priori. In the study of multigenic traits, therefore, researchers will often analyze the DNA marker data by linkage analysis (where genetic parameters must be specified prior to analysis) and by various nonparametric analyses that are much less dependent upon underlying genetic parameters. An example is sib-pair analysis where

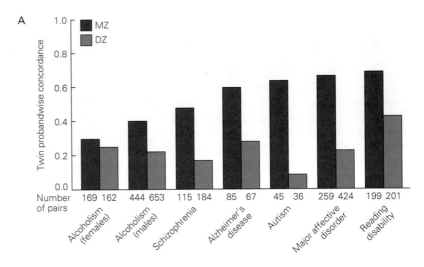

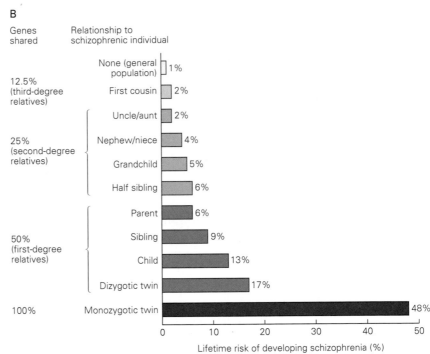

Figure 3-15. Many complex human behavioral disorders have a genetic component.

A. Concordance for disease phenotypes among monozygotic twins (MZ) and dizygotic twins (DZ) for some behavioral disorders. The proband is the family member through which the family was initially discovered and explored. (Modified from Plomin et al. 1994.)

B. The risk of developing schizophrenia is a function of pedigree.(Modified from Gottesman 1991.)

one evaluates whether particular alleles (or chromosomal segments) are shared among affected siblings more often than would be predicted by chance alone. When the degree of allele-sharing reaches statistical significance, one concludes that the causal or predisposing mutation is contained within the shared region.

Family, twin, and adoption studies indicate not only that patients who suffer from the major psychiatric disorders have a genetic predisposition to those disorders but also that in the normal population at large components of character and general cognitive abilities have important genetic components. In the past it was generally assumed that these genetic contributions to charac-

ter and cognitive functioning decline over the course of one's lifetime because of the accumulation over the years of social and environmental experience. However, a study of the cognitive capabilities of 240 pairs of twins in the ninth decade of their life showed that genes continue to account for 50% of the variance in later life, much as they do earlier in life. Thus, while environmental factors are important, genes clearly contribute to a variety of normal higher mental functions.

Similarly, bipolar affective disorder (manic-depressive illness) frequently occurs in both siblings if they are monozygotic twins, but it occurs less frequently in both siblings if they are dizygotic twins. The heritability of bipolar affective disorder, as well as that of schizophrenia, has been estimated to be about 50-60% (Figure 3-15). Thus, factors other than genes must play a critical role in determining the onset of disease in these multifactorial disorders.

Like other complex traits, schizophrenia and depression are most likely multigenic and multifactorial. It will be important to distinguish between various models of transmission. According to one (monogenic) model, many genes in the population can contribute to schizophrenia but each gene is rare and has a strong effect. Genetic linkage studies now indicate that such a monogenic model is likely to account for only a small fraction of schizophrenia patients. A second (oligogenic) model assumes that a small number of genes interact together to create a threshold of vulnerability for the disorder. Yet another (polygenic) model assumes that these disorders result from the cumulative effect of many genes, each with a minute effect. Several genetic forms of epilepsy most likely fit the monogenic model, whereas the major psychotic illnesses are thought to fit the oligogenic model. There may, however, be a subpopulation of people with major mental illness who suffer from the consequence of a powerful gene.

Schizophrenia and bipolar affective disorder were among the first multigenic traits to be analyzed by genetic linkage analysis. In fact, many of the early lessons learned from multigenic gene mapping came from mistakes made in these pioneering studies. Segregation analysis and genetic modeling studies indicate that both schizophrenia and bipolar disorder result from the effects of a small number of mutant genes. Thus, although mutations in a set of 10 or more genes may contribute to schizophrenia on a population basis (due to genetic heterogeneity), the combined effects of even a subset of these mutants would presumably be sufficient to place an individual at high risk for the disorder.

Furthermore, we know from twin studies that environmental and genetic factors together determine the overall likelihood of manifesting these disorders. According to this multifactorial model, a single mutation would produce a relatively small contribution to the overall predisposition to illness in the population and thus would be difficult to detect by genetic-linkage strategies. In any individual, however, one gene could actually be a quite strong contributor. For this reason, current psychiatric genetic studies usually involve international consortia cooperating in the systematic ascertainment and diagnosis of very large clinical samples, which lend sufficient power for the detection of small genetic contributions to illness. We shall see in Chapter 60 that the genotyping of several pedigrees has provided a possible genetic locus for susceptability to schizophrenia.

An Overall View

Most aspects of behavior are under genetic control. Evidence for this can be seen in the striking biological similarities of human twins and in our ability to select and breed domestic and laboratory animals for particular behavioral traits. Such breeding experiments generally indicate that behavioral traits are multigenic in origin. Only in rare instances has the source of natural variation been traceable to a single predominant genetic factor, as in the development of certain forms of obesity in mice.

Now, however, we are entering a new era in which it will be much easier to trace genes that control behavior. The availability of the complete genome for an organism will facilitate our understanding of how genes control genetic pathways important for cellular function, and this advance will allow much more effective and meaningful correlations with behavior. Several genomes are already completed: those of *Escherichia coli* and several other prokaryotic micro-organisms (5,000 genes, about 5 megabase (Mb) pairs), that of the yeast *Saccharomyces cervisiae* (6,000 genes, 12 Mb), and that of the worm *Caenorhabditis elegans* (20,000 genes, 97 Mb). The human genome—all 80,000 genes—is likely to be completed by the year 2003, and work on the genomes of *Drosophila* and mouse are well underway. From the several genomes that have been completed we have already learned a number of surprising facts.

First, the human genome seems to have undergone two major replications from the primitive genome of single-celled organisms.

Second, fully 40% of the genes in yeast and *C. elegans* are novel; their function is completely unknown.

Third, from *C. elegans* we have learned that genes fall into two large classes that perform different functions and have different positions on the chromosomes. One set of 5,000 genes performs the core or housekeeping functions of the cell, the genes encode the proteins for intermediary metabolism for the metabolism of DNA, RNA and protein, for cytoskeletal structures, transport and secretion. The housekeeping genes are highly conserved, in both number and structure, and their ancestors have been found in yeast. Most likely they occur in comparable number in all organisms. In *C. elegans* these core function genes are clustered together in the central region of the chromosomes where they appear to be protected from evolutionary change.

The second set of about 15,000 genes are more specialized, and newer from an evolutionary perspective; they are not found in yeast. These specialized genes are mostly concerned with intercellular signaling, transcription, and other forms of regulatory control unique to multicellular organisms. These newer genes are positioned at the two ends of the chromosomes, where they appear to be more susceptible to evolutionary pressures. They include genes for 400 protein kinases, 480 zinc finger proteins that appear to be transcription factors, and 790 membrane-spanning receptors. Genes have been identified in *C. elegans* for most classes of human transcription factors and signaling proteins. In fact, many genes in *C. elegans* are similar to human genes involved in disease. Indeed, 70% of human proteins so far identified can be related to orthologs—similar proteins with a presumed common ancestor—in *C. elegans*.

Finally, simple perturbations of a yeast cell, such as the action of a mating factor, affects not a few but a large number of genes. Thus, in the future the perspective of genetic analysis will change from examining how single genes and proteins work to examining how many genes and proteins interact to produce a patterned response.

It is expected that the complete human genome, and the genomes of still other key organisms, will be to biology what the periodic table of elements has been to chemistry. For any species the genome will define all the genetic elements on which life's processes depend. The ability to analyze entire genomes promises to provide us with new insights that should dramatically change our ability to analyze behavioral processes, thereby altering dramatically the theory and practice of all areas of medicine, including neurology and psychiatry.

For example, what we already know about the human genome has brought molecular geneticists to the brink of identifying the combinations of genes contributing to certain multigenic disorders. The wealth of genetic information derived from such genetic linkage studies has enormous practical benefits. Researchers recently identified 10 to 12 different genes that predispose individuals to insulin-dependent diabetes mellitus. In addition, a variation in the number of repeating sequences within the gene encoding the dopamine D4 receptor is thought to make an important contribution to the overall genetic variance that characterizes novelty-seeking behavior. In the future the detection of genes that produce only a small effect on phenotype is likely to have a major impact on the study of behavioral disorders.

These findings raise fascinating issues about natural genetic variations in humans that we should be able to confront soon. To what degree do genetically transmitted differences in behavioral traits reflect quantitative variation in the expression of benign alleles and therefore natural variations of a *normal* behavior, as opposed to mutations of the same gene that produce a disease state? To what degree do the genetic contributions to natural variations in behavior reflect variations in the level of expression of the same protein? The answers to

such questions will be essential for developing rational therapeutic strategies for treating psychiatric disorders.

Variations in genes—in DNA sequences—represent the basic material for evolutionary change. These variations also form the basis for individual differences in risk for the many genetically complex diseases that confront neurology and psychiatry.

T. Conrad Gilliam
Eric R. Kandel
Thomas M. Jessell

Selected Readings

Auwerx J, Staels B. 1998. Leptin. Lancet 351:737–742.

Bargmann CI. 1998. Neurobiology of the *Caenorhabditis elegans* genome. Science: 2028–2033.

Bouchard TJ, Jr. 1994. Genes, environment, and personality. Science 264:1700–1701.

Collins FS, Patrinos A, Jordan E, Chakravati A, Gesteland R, Walters L, and the members of the DOE and NIH planning groups. 1998. New goals for the U.S. human genome project: 1998–2003. Science 282:682–689.

Dunlap JC. 1998. Common threads in eukaryotic circadian systems. Curr Opin Genet Dev 8:400–406.

Hall JC. 1994. The mating of a fly. Science 264:1702–1714.

Hardin PE. 1998. Activating inhibitors and inhibiting activators: A day in the life of a fly. Curr Opin Neurobiol 8:642–647.

Houseknecht KL, Baile CA, Matteri RL, Spurlock ME. 1998. The biology of leptin: a review. J Anim Sci 76:1405–1420.

Jennings C. 1995. How trinucleotide repeats may function. Nature 378:127.

Mendel G. 1866. Versuche über Pflanzen-Hybriden. Verh Naturforsch 4:3–47; 1966. Translated in: C Stern, ER Sherwood (eds). *The Origin of Genetics: A Mendel Source Book.* San Francisco: WH Freeman.

Palmiter RD, Erickson JC, Hollopeter G, Baraban SC, Schwartz MW. 1998. Life without neuropeptide Y. Recent Prog Horm Res 53:163–199.

Plomin R, DeFries JC. 1998. The genetics of cognitive abilities and disabilities. Sci Am 278:62–69.

Plomin R, Owen MJ, McGuffin P. 1994. The genetic basis of complex human behaviors. Science 264:1733–1739.

Plomin R, Rutter M. 1998. Child development, molecular genetics, and what to do with genes once thay are found. Child Dev 69:1223–1242.

Suzuki DT, Griffiths AJF, Miller JH, Lewontin RC. 1989. *An Introduction to Genetic Analysis,* 4th ed. New York: WH Freeman.

Takahashi JS, Pinto LH, Vitaterna MH. 1994. Forward and reverse genetic approaches to behavior in the mouse. Science 264:1724–1733.

Wilsbacher LD, Takahashi JS. 1998. Circadian rhythms: molecular basis of the clock. Curr Opin Genet Dev 8:595–602.

Young MW. 1998. The molecular control of circadian behavioral rhythms and their entrainment in *Drosophila*. Annu Rev Biochem 67:135–152.

References

Alberts B, Bray D, Lewis J, Raff M, Roberts K, Watson JD. 1994. *Molecular Biology of the Cell*, 3rd ed. New York: Garland.

Baily DW. 1981. Recombinant inbred strains and bilineal congenic strains. In: HL Foster, JD Small, JG Fox (eds). *The Mouse in Biomedical Research*. Vol. 1, *Recombinant Inbred Strains and Bilineal Congenic Strains*, pp. 223–239. New York: Academic.

Barinaga M. 1994. Genes and behavior news report. Fruit flies, rats, mice: evidence of genetic influence. A new tool for examining multigenic traits. Science 264:1690–1693.

Barinaga M. 1995. New clock gene cloned. Science 270:732–733.

Barinaga M. 1996. Researchers find the reset button for the fruit fly clock. Science 271:1671–1672.

Benjamin J, Li L, Patterson C, Greenberg BD, Murphy DL, Hamer DH. 1996. Population and familial association between the D4 dopamine receptor gene and measures of novelty seeking. Nat Genet 12:81–84.

Bouchard TJ Jr., Lykken DT, McGue M, Segal NL, Tellegen A. 1990. Sources of human psychological differences: the Minnesota study of twins reared apart. Science 250:223–228.

Chakravarti A, 1999. Population genetics–making sense out of sequence. Nat Genet Suppl 21:56–60.

Chen H, Charlat O, Tartaglia LA, Woolf EA, Weng X, Ellis SJ, Lakey ND, Culpepper J, Moore KJ, Breitbart RE, Duyk GM, Tepper RI, Morgenstern JP. 1996. Evidence that the diabetes gene encodes the leptin receptor: identification of a mutation in the leptin receptor gene in *db/db* mice. Cell 84:491–495.

Cordell HJ, Todd JA. 1995. Multifactorial inheritance in type 1 diabetes. Trends Genet 11:499–504.

Cloninger CR, Adolfsson R, Svrakic NM. 1996. Mapping genes for human personality. Nat Genet 12:3–4.

Davies JL, Kawaguchi Y, Bennett ST, Copeman JB, Cordell HJ, Pritchard LE, Reed PW, Gough SC, Jenkins SC, Palmer SM, et al. 1994. A genome-wide search for human type 1 diabetes susceptibility genes. Nature 371:130–136.

de Bono M, Bargmann CI. 1998. Natural variation in a neuropeptide Y receptor homolog modifies social behavior and food response in *C. elegans*. Cell 94:679–689.

Ebstein RP, Novick O, Umansky R, Priel B, Osher Y, Blaine D, Bennett L, Nemanov M, Katz M, Belmaker RH. 1996. Dopamine D4 receptor (D4DR) exon III polymorphism associated with the human personality trait of novelty seeking. Nat Genet 12:78–80.

Galton F. 1869. *Hereditary Genius: An Inquiry into Its Laws and Consequences*. London: Macmillan; 1962. Reprint. Cleveland: Meridian Books.

Giros B, Jaber M, Jones SR, Wightman RM, Caron MG. 1996. Hyperlocomotion and indifference to cocaine and amphetamine in mice lacking the dopamine transporter. Nature 379:606–611.

Gottesman II 1991. *Schizophrenia Genesis. The Origins of Madness*. New York: WH Freeman.

Gusella JF, MacDonald ME. 1995. Huntington's disease. Semin Cell Biol 6:21–28.

Heath MJ, Hen R. 1995. Serotonin receptors. Genetic insights into serotonin function. Curr Biol 5:997–999.

The Huntington's Disease Collaborative Research Group. 1993. A novel gene containing a trinucleotide repeat that is expanded and unstable on Huntington's disease chromosomes. Cell 72:971–983.

King DP, Zhao Y, Sangoram AM, Wilsbacher LD, Tanka M, Antoch MP, Steeves TDL, Vitaterna MH, Kornhauser JM, Lowry PL, Turek FW, Takahashi JS. 1997. Positional cloning of the mouse circadian clock gene. Cell 69:641–653.

Konopka RJ, Benzer S. 1971. Clock mutants of *Drosophila melangaster*. Proc Natl Acad Sci U S A 68:2112–2116.

Lee C, Parikh V, Itsukaichi T, Bae K, Edery I. 1996. Resetting the *Drosophila* clock by photic regulation of PER and a PER-TIM complex. Science 271:1740–1744.

Lee GH, Proenca R, Montez JM, Carroll KM, Darvishzadeh JG, Lee JI, Friedman JM. 1996. Abnormal splicing of the leptin receptor in diabetic mice. Nature 379:632–635.

Lewin B. 1994. *Genes*, Vol. 5. Oxford: Oxford Univ. Press.

McClearn GE, Johansson B, Berg S, Pedersen NL, Ahern F, Petrill SA, Plonim R. 1997. Substantial genetic influence on cognitive abilities in twins 80 or more years old. Science 276:1560–1564.

Myers MP, Wager-Smith K, Rothenfluh-Hilfiker A, Young MW. 1996. Light-induced degradation of TIMELESS and entrainment of the *Drosophila* circadian clock. Science 271:1736–1740.

Nickelson DA, Taylor SL, Weiss KM, Clark AG, Hutchinson RG, Stengard J, Salomaa V, Vartiainen E, Boerwinkle E, Sing CF. 1998. DNA sequence diversity in a 9.7Kb region of the human lipoprotein lipase gene. Nat Genet 19:233–240.

Qu D, Ludwig DS, Gammeltoft S, Piper M, Pelleymounter MA, Cullen MJ, Mathes WF, Przypek R, Kanarek R, Maratos-Flier E. 1996. A role for melanin-concentrating hormone in the central regulation of feeding behaviour. Nature 380:243–247.

Risch N. 1990. Linkage strategies for genetically complex traits. I. Multilocus models. Am J Hum Genet 46:222–228.

Saudou F, Amara DA, Dierich A, LeMeur M, Ramboz S, Segu L, Buhot MC, Hen R. 1994. Enhanced aggressive behavior in mice lacking 5-HT$_{1B}$ receptor. Science 265:1875–1878.

Tecott LH, Barondes SH. 1996. Genes and aggressiveness. Behavioral genetics. Curr Biol 6:238–240.

Thomas SA, Matsumoto AM, Palmiter RD. 1995. Noradrenaline is essential for mouse fetal development. Nature 374:643–646.

Vosshall LB, Price JL, Sehgal A, Saez L, Young MW. 1994. Block in nuclear localization of period protein by a second clock mutation, timeless. Science 263:1606–1609.

Warren ST. 1996. The expanding world of trinucleotide repeats. Science 271:1374–1375.

Watson JD. 1997. Genes and Politics. Keynote Address. *Congress of Molecular Medicine. Berlin, Germany. Annual Report.* Cold Spring Harbor, NY: Cold Spring Harbor Laboratories.

Watson JD, Tooze J, Kurtz DT (eds). 1983. *Recombinant DNA: A Short Course.* New York: Scientific American; distr. by WH Freeman.

Zhang Y, Proenca R, Muffei M, Barone M, Leopold L, Friedman, JM. 1994. Positional cloning of the mouse obese gene and its human homologue. Nature 372:425–432.

Zhou QY, Palmiter RD. 1995. Dopamine-deficient mice are severely hypoactive, adipsic, and aphagic. Cell 83:1197–1209.

Zhou QY, Quaife CJ, Palmiter RD. 1995. Targeted disruption of the tyrosine hydroxylase gene reveals that catecholamines are required for mouse fetal development. Nature 374:640–643.

Part II

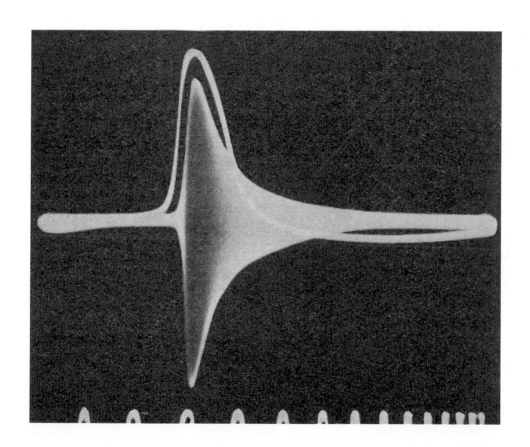

II

Cell and Molecular Biology of the Neuron

IN ALL BIOLOGICAL SYSTEMS, FROM THE most primitive to the most advanced, the basic building block is the cell. Cells are often organized into functional modules that are repeated in complex biological systems. The vertebrate brain is the most complex example of a modular system. Complex biological systems have another structural feature: they are *architectonic*—that is, their anatomy, fine structure, and biochemistry all reflect a specific physiological function. Thus, the construction of the brain and the cytology, biophysics, and biochemistry of its component neurons reflect its fundamental function—to mediate behavior.

The great diversity of nerve cells—the fundamental units from which the modules of the nervous systems are assembled—is derived from one basic cell plan. Three features of this plan give nerve cells the unique ability to communicate with one another precisely and rapidly over long distances. First, the neuron is polarized, possessing receptive dendrites on one end and axons with synaptic terminals at the other. This polarization of functional properties is commonly used to restrict the flow of impulses to one direction. Second, the neuron is electrically and chemically excitable. Its external membrane contains specialized proteins—ion channels and receptors—that permit the influx and efflux of specific inorganic ions, thus creating electrical currents. Third, the neuron's cell body contains proteins and organelles that endow it with specialized secretory properties.

In this part of the book we shall be concerned with the properties of the neuron that give it the ability to generate signals in the form of synaptic and action potentials. The initiation of a signal depends on ion channels in the cell membrane that open in response to changes in potential across the membrane and to neurotransmitters released by other nerve cells. Neurons use two classes of channels for signaling: (1) resting channels generate the resting potential and underlie the passive properties of neurons that determine the time course of synaptic potentials and the speed of conduction of the action potential and (2) voltage-gated channels are responsible for the active currents that generate the action potential.

Part II

4

The Cytology of Neurons

THE CELLS OF THE NERVOUS system vary more than those in any other part of the body. Nevertheless, all neurons have common features that distinguish them from cells in other tissues. For example, they typically are highly polarized. Furthermore, cell functions are compartmentalized, an arrangement that contributes significantly to the processing of electrical signals. The chief functional compartments of neurons—the cell body, dendrites, axons, and terminals—are usually separated by considerable distances, a feature that accounts for the functional polarization discussed in Chapter 2. In most neurons the cell body, which contains the nucleus

and the organelles for making RNA and protein, contains less than a tenth of the cell's total volume. The dendrites and axon that originate from the cell body make up the remainder. As discussed in Chapter 2, dendrites are thin processes that branch several times and are specially shaped to receive synaptic input from other neurons. The cell body usually gives off a single axon, another thin process that propagates electrical impulses, often over considerable distances, to the neuron's synaptic terminals on other nerve cells or on target organs.

Neurons also differ from most other cells in being excitable. Rapid shifts in electrical potential are made possible by specialized protein structures (ion channels and pumps) in the cell membrane that control the instantaneous flow of ions into and out of the cells.

Polarization and electrical excitability are not unique to neurons, however. Epithelial cells and other nonneuronal secretory cells also are polarized, with basolateral and apical surfaces that differ in structure and function. Some nonneural cells, notably muscle, are excitable, and like nerve cells their excitability depends on special protein molecules that allow ions to pass across the plasma membrane. In neurons, however, polarity and excitability are developed to a higher degree, permitting signals to be received, processed, and conducted over long distances.

Although built on a common plan, neurons are quite diverse—over 50 distinct types have been described. This cytological diversity, which results from developmental differentiation, is also apparent on a molecular level. Each neuron expresses a combination of general and specific molecules. The kinds of proteins a cell synthesizes depends on the genes expressed in the cell; each type of cell synthesizes certain macromolecules (enzymes, struc-

A

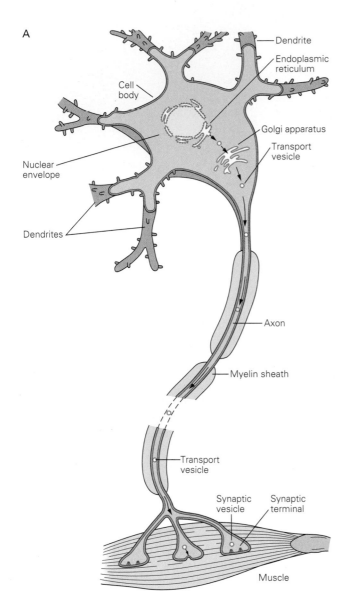

B

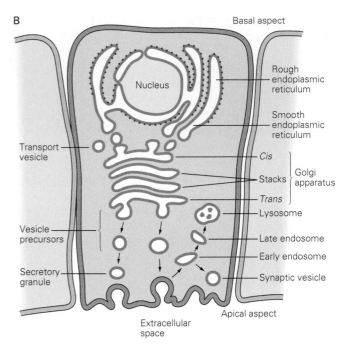

Figure 4-1 The epithelial blueprint of a neuron.

A. This diagram of a spinal motor neuron shows the cell body and the nucleus surrounded by the nuclear envelope, which is continuous with the rough and smooth endoplasmic reticulum. The space between the two membranes that constitute the nuclear envelope is continuous with the extracellular space. Dendrites emerge from the basal aspect of the neuron, the axon from the apical aspect. (Adapted from Williams et al. 1989.)

B. This diagram of an epithelial cell shows a membrane system called the *vacuolar apparatus,* which includes all the major organelles found in the neuron. Vesicles, which bud off the endoplasmic reticulum, shuttle to the *cis* face of the Golgi complex.

tural proteins, membrane constituents, and secretory products) and not others. In essence each cell *is* the macromolecules that it makes. Many of these molecules are common to all cells in the body; some are characteristic of all neurons, others of large classes of neurons, and still others are restricted to only a few nerve cells.

This chapter begins with an overview of the neuron, describing traits common to all neuronal types. We then discuss the differences among nerve cells. We have chosen to illustrate neuronal diversity with a detailed description of only three types of neurons: the sensory neurons of the dorsal root ganglion, the motor neurons of the spinal cord, and the pyramidal cells of the hip-

pocampus. Neuronal structure can be readily illustrated by comparing the sensory and motor neurons in the spinal cord that mediate the stretch reflex, responsible for the classic knee-jerk reflex. The distinctive features of the two neurons in this simple reflex circuit nicely illustrate the relationship between anatomy and function. The specialized features of nerve cells in complex neuronal circuits in the brain are illustrated by examining the pyramidal neurons of the CA3 and CA1 regions of the hippocampus. These cortical neurons belong to circuits thought to be responsible for memory storage (Chapters 62 and 63) and to be affected in certain forms of epilepsy (Chapter 46).

The Structural and Functional Blueprint of Neurons Is Similar to Epithelial Cells

Neurons develop from epithelial cells and retain fundamental epithelial features. For example, both cell types have distinctive poles: the epithelial cell's basolateral surface corresponds to the aspect of the neuron's cell body from which dendrites arise, while the apical surface corresponds to the aspect of the neuron from which the axon arises (Figure 4-1A).

The boundaries of the neuron are defined by the external cell membrane, or *plasmalemma*. Nerve cell membranes have the general asymmetric bilayer structure of all biological membranes and represent a hydrophobic barrier impermeable to most water-soluble substances. The cytoplasm has two main components: the cytosol (including the cytoskeletal matrix) and the membranous organelles.

The cytosol is the aqueous phase of the cytoplasm. In this phase only a very few proteins are freely soluble, mostly enzymes that catalyze various metabolic reactions. Many cytosolic proteins have general housekeeping functions and are common to all neurons. Others have specific roles in particular types of neurons; for example, the enzymes involved in the synthesis and degradation of the particular substance used as a neurotransmitter. Moreover, some cytosolic proteins are distributed unevenly in the cell because they interact to form aggregates, particles, or matrices. Many cytosolic proteins involved in signaling are concentrated at the cell's periphery in the cytoskeletal matrix immediately adjacent to the plasmalemma.

Membranous Organelles Are Selectively Distributed Throughout the Neuron

The membranous organelles of the cytoplasm include the mitochondria and peroxisomes as well as a complex system of tubules, vesicles, and cisternae (the vacuolar apparatus) that consists of the rough endoplasmic reticulum, the smooth endoplasmic reticulum, the Golgi complex, secretory vesicles, endosomes, lysosomes, and a multiplicity of transport vesicles that functionally interconnect these various compartments (Figures 4-1B and 4-2).

Membranes of the vacuolar apparatus are thought to be derived from deep invaginations of the cell's external membrane that become discrete organelles. Their lumen corresponds topologically to the outside of the cell; consequently the inner leaflet of their lipid bilayer corresponds to the outer leaflet of the plasmalemma (Figure 4-1B). Even though the major subcompartments of this system are anatomically discontinuous, membra-

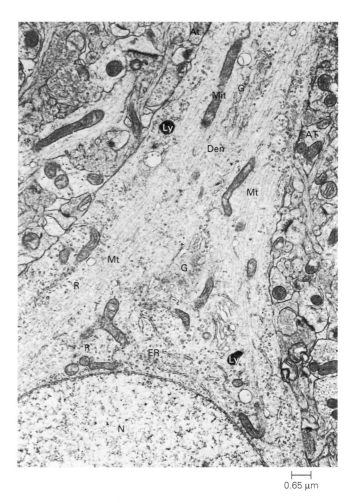

0.65 μm

Figure 4-2 Endoplasmic reticulum in a pyramidal cell. This micrograph of the basal pole of a pyramidal neuron's cell body, from which a single dendrite emerges, reveals the rough and smooth endoplasmic reticulum (**ER**) above the nucleus (**N**). A portion of the Golgi complex (**G**) appears at the base of the dendrite (**Den**); some Golgi cisternae have entered the dendrite, as have mitochondria (**Mit**), lysosomes (**Ly**), and ribosomes (**R**). Microtubules (**Mt**) are the prominent cytoskeletal filaments seen in the cytosol. Axon terminals (**AT**) are seen synapsing on the neuron. (From Peters et al. 1991.)

nous and lumenal material are moved from one compartment to another with great efficiency and specificity by means of transport vesicles. For example, proteins and phospholipids synthesized in the rough endoplasmic reticulum are transported to the Golgi complex and then to secretory vesicles destined to fuse with the plasmalemma by exocytosis (the secretory pathway). Conversely, membrane taken into the cell in the form of endocytic vesicles is incorporated into early endosomes, which are sorting compartments concentrated at the cell's periphery; the membrane is then either shuttled

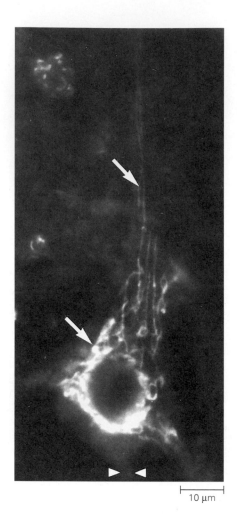

Figure 4-3 Under the light microscope the Golgi complex appears as a network of filaments that extend into dendrites (arrows), but not into the axon. The **arrowheads** at the bottom indicate the axon hillock. The Golgi complex in this micrograph is in a large neuron of the brain stem immunostained with antibodies specifically directed against this organelle. (From De Camilli et al. 1986.)

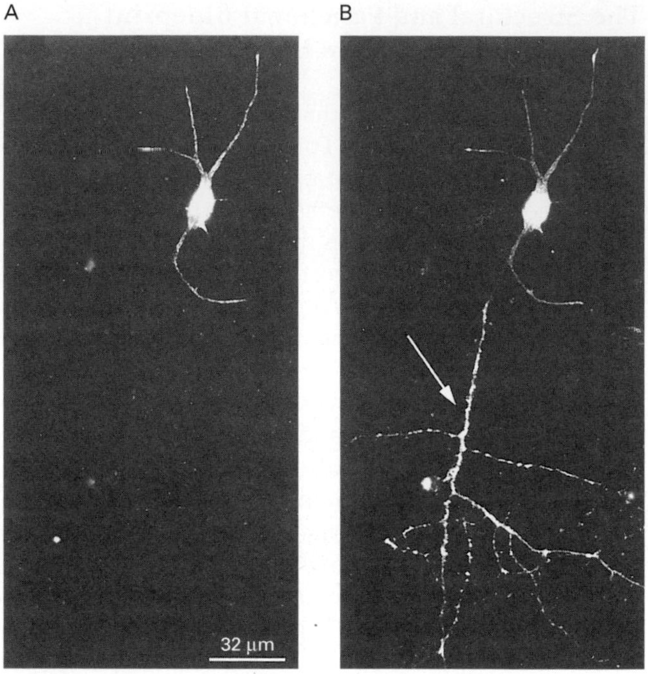

A   B

32 μm

Figure 4-4 Neurons develop two distinct types of processes, dendrites and axons, even when grown in isolation. The figure shows a hippocampal neuron grown in isolation in primary culture and stained by double immunofluorescence for the synaptic vesicle protein synaptophysin and the transferrin receptor, a protein involved in iron uptake. When photographed through an appropriate filter, immunofluorescence corresponding to the transferrin receptor is seen only in dendrites (**A**). When photographed for synapsin, synaptic vesicles are selectively concentrated in the axon (**arrow**) as revealed by synapsin immunofluorescence (**B**). (From Cameron et al. 1991.)

back to the plasmalemma by vesicle recycling or directed to late endosomes and eventually to lysosomes for degradation (the endocytic pathway).

A specialized portion of the rough endoplasmic reticulum forms a spherical flattened cisterna called the nuclear envelope, which surrounds the chromosomal DNA and its associated proteins and defines the nucleus (see Figure 4-1). This cisterna is continuous with other portions of the rough endoplasmic reticulum. Because of this continuity, the nuclear envelope is presumed to have evolved to ensheathe the chromosomes by an invagination of the plasmalemma. The nuclear envelope is interrupted by the nuclear pores, where fusion of the

inner and outer membrane of the nuclear envelope results in the formation of hydrophilic channels through which proteins and RNA are exchanged between the cytoplasm proper and the nuclear cytoplasm. Thus the nucleoplasm and cytoplasm can be considered functionally continuous domains of the cytosol.

Mitochondria and peroxisomes make use of molecular oxygen. Mitochondria generate ATP, the major molecule by which cellular energy is transferred or spent. Peroxisomes engage in detoxification through peroxidation reactions and also prevent the accumulation of the strong oxidizing agent hydrogen peroxide. These two organelles, which are thought to be derived from symbi-

Figure 4-5 Atlas of fibrillary structures.

A. Microtubules, the largest-diameter fibers (25 nm), are helical cylinders composed of 13 protofilaments each 5 nm in width. Protofilaments are linearly arranged pairs of alternating α- and β-tubulin subunits (each subunit has a molecular weight of about 50,000). A tubulin molecule is a heterodimer consisting of one α- and one β-tubulin subunit. **1.** In this exploded view up a microtubule the arrows indicate the direction of the right-handed helix. **2.** A side-view of a microtubule shows the alternating α- and β-subunits.

B. Neurofilaments are built with fibers that twist around each other to produce coils of increasing thickness. The thinnest units are monomers that form coiled-coil heterodimers. These dimers form a tetrameric complex that becomes the protofilament. Two protofilaments become a protofibril, and three protofibrils are helically twisted to form the 10 nm neurofilament. (Adapted from Bershadsky and Vasiliev 1988.)

C. Microfilaments, the smallest-diameter fibers (about 7 nm), are composed of two strands of polymerized globular (G) actin monomers arranged in a helix. Several isoforms of G-actin are encoded by families of actin genes. In mammals there are at least six different (but closely related) actins. Each variant is encoded by a separate gene. Microfilaments are polar structures; the globular monomers actually are asymmetric. The monomers look like arrowheads, with a pointed tip and chevron-shaped (barbed) end, and polymerize tip to tail.

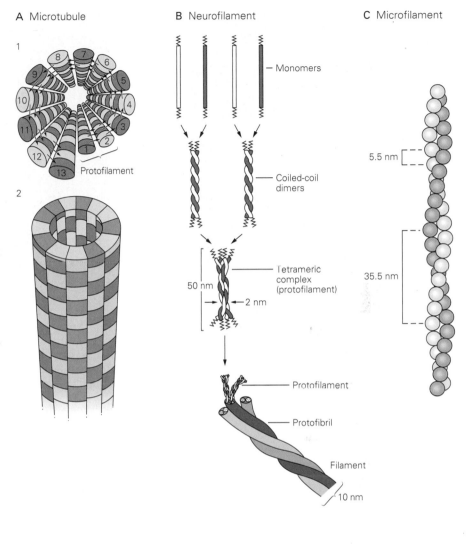

A Microtubule

B Neurofilament

C Microfilament

otic organisms that invaded eukaryotic cells early in evolution, are not functionally continuous with the vacuolar apparatus of the cell.

The cytoplasm of the cell body extends into the dendritic tree without any functional boundary. Generally, all organelles present in the cytoplasm of the cell body are also present in dendrites, although the concentrations of some organelles, such as the rough endoplasmic reticulum, the Golgi complex, and lysosomes, progressively diminish with distance from the cell body. In contrast, a sharp functional boundary exists at the axon hillock, the point of emergence of the axon. For example, ribosomes, the rough endoplasmic reticulum, and the Golgi complex—the organelles that represent the main protein biosynthetic machinery of the neuron—for the most part are excluded from axons (Figure 4-3). Lysosomes and certain proteins, which in epithelial cells are selectively targeted to the basolateral surface of the cell, also are excluded from axons. Axons are, however, rich in synaptic vesicles, synaptic vesicle precursor membranes, and endocytic intermediates involved in synaptic vesicle traffic (Figures 4-1 and 4-4).

Mitochondria and the smooth endoplasmic reticulum are present in all neuronal compartments, including the axon. The smooth endoplasmic reticulum is anatomically continuous with the rough endoplasmic reticulum. One of its functions is to act as a regulated Ca^{2+} store throughout the neuronal cytoplasm. It also performs a variety of enzymatic reactions and is involved in lipid metabolism.

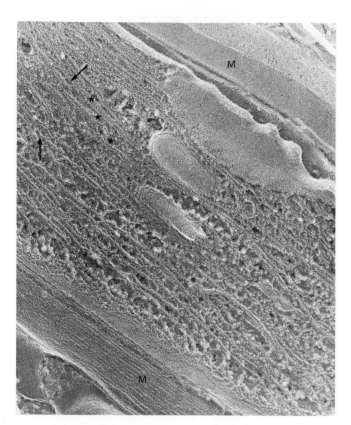

Figure 4-6 The cytoskeletal structure of an axon is visualized here by means of quick freezing and deep etching. The figure shows the dense packing of microtubules and neurofilaments linked by cross-bridges. Microtubules are indicated by **stars**. The arrows bracket the microtubule-rich domain of the axon through which organelles are transported both in the anterograde and the retrograde direction. **M** = myelin sheath. × 105,000. (Courtesy of B. Schnapp and T. Reese.)

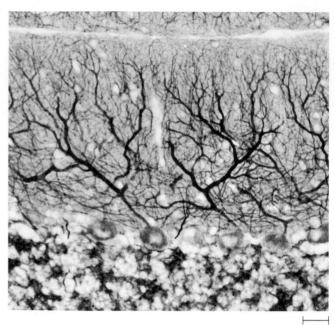

├──────┤
20 μm

Figure 4-7 The dendritic architecture in the cerebellar cortex is visualized here by immunoperoxidase staining for the microtubule-associated protein MAP2, a dendrite-specific MAP. Dendrites of all classes of neurons are stained. The field is dominated by the dendrites of Purkinje cells. (Courtesy of P. De Camilli.)

The Cytoskeleton Determines the Shape of the Neuron

The cytoskeleton is the major intrinsic determinant of the shape of a neuron and is responsible for the asymmetric distribution of organelles within the cytoplasm. It contains three main filamentous structures: microtubules, neurofilaments (called intermediate filaments in nonneuronal cells), and actin microfilaments (Figures 4-5 and 4-6). These filaments and their associated proteins account for about 25% of the total protein of the neuron.

Microtubules form long scaffolds that extend the full length of the neuron and play a key role in developing and maintaining the neuron's processes. A single microtubule can be as long as 0.1 mm. Microtubules are constructed of 13 protofilaments in a tubular array with an outside diameter of 25–28 nm (Figure 4-5A). Each protofilament consists of several pairs of α- and β-tubu-

lin subunits arranged linearly. The polar structure of the tubulin dimer creates a plus and a minus end of the polymer. The tubulins are encoded by a multigene family; at least six genes code for both the α- and β-subunits. More than 20 isoforms of tubulin are present in the brain because of the expression of different genes as well as post-translational modifications.

Tubulin is a GTPase and microtubules grow by the addition of GTP-bound tubulin dimers at their plus end. Shortly after polymerization GTP is hydrolyzed to GDP. When a microtubule stops growing its plus end becomes capped by GDP-bound tubulin. Given the low affinity of the GDP-bound tubulin for the polymer, this would lead to rapid catastrophic depolymerization unless the microtubule were stabilized by interaction with other proteins. In fact, microtubules undergo rapid cycles of polymerization and depolymerization in dividing cells, but they are much more stable in mature dendrites and axons. This stability is due to microtubule-associated proteins (MAPs), which promote the oriented polymerization and assembly of the microtubules. The MAPs in the axons differ from those in the dendrites. For example, MAP2 is present in dendrites but

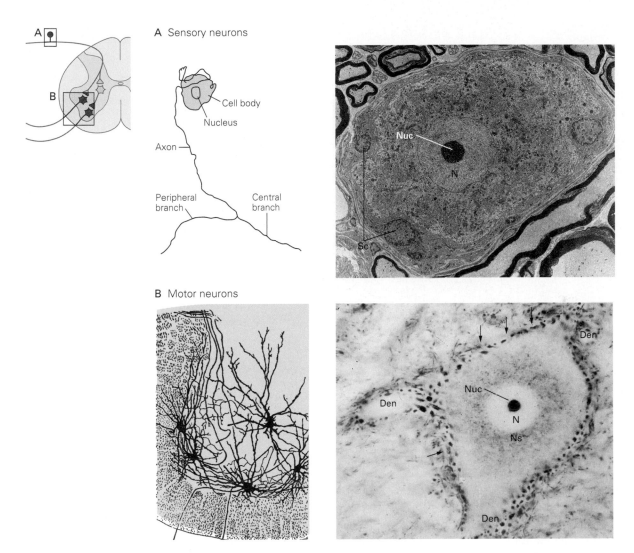

Figure 4-8 A sensory (dorsal root ganglion) cell and a spinal motor neuron form a monosynaptic circuit that controls the knee-jerk stretch reflex.

A. Sensory neuron. Left: The axon of the primary sensory neuron is typically quite convoluted before it bifurcates into a central and a peripheral branch. The cell body contains a prominent nucleus. (From Dogiel 1908.) **Right:** Low-power electron micrograph shows the cell body of a large dorsal root ganglion cell. A prominent nucleolus (**Nuc**) can be seen within the nucleus (**N**). The cell body of the neuron is surrounded by Schwann cells (**Sc**), the type of glial cells found in the peripheral nervous system. (Courtesy of R. E. Coggeshall and F. Mandriota.)

B. Motor neuron. Left: Many dendrites typically branch from the cell bodies of spinal motor neurons, as shown by five spinal motor neurons in the ventral horn of a kitten. (From Ramón y Cajal 1909.) **Right:** Detail of the cell body of a motor neuron is shown in this photomicrograph. An enormous number of nerve endings from presynaptic neurons (**arrows**) are visible. These terminals, called *synaptic boutons*, appear as knob-like enlargements on the cell membrane. The synaptic boutons are prominent in this micrograph because the tissue is specially impregnated with silver. Three dendrites (**Den**) are also shown. The nucleus and its nucleolus are surrounded by Nissl substance (**Ns**), clumps of ribosomes associated with the membrane of the endoplasmic reticulum. (Courtesy of G. L. Rasmussen.)

absent from axons (Figure 4-7), while tau and MAP3 are present in the axon.

Neurofilaments, 10 nm in diameter, are the bones of the cytoskeleton (see Figure 4-5B). They are the most abundant fibrillar components of the axon. (On average, there are 3–10 times more neurofilaments than microtubules in an axon.) Neurofilaments are related to the intermediate filaments of other cell types, all of which belong to a family of proteins called cytokeratins. (Other cytokeratins include vimentin, glial fibrillary acidic protein, desmin, and keratin.) Unlike microtubules, neurofilaments are very stable and almost totally polymerized

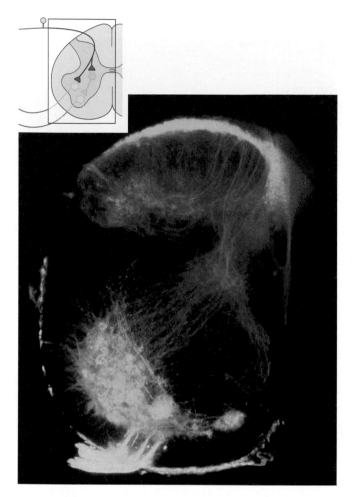

Figure 4-9 Connections between sensory neurons and motor neurons in the spinal cord of an embryonic rat are shown in this micrograph. The sensory axons (orange) enter the spinal cord through the dorsal root and then run longitudinally in the dorsal column. Collaterals descend from the dorsal column to the spinal gray matter, where they arborize and make synaptic contact with the dendrites of motor neurons (green). (Courtesy of W. Snider.)

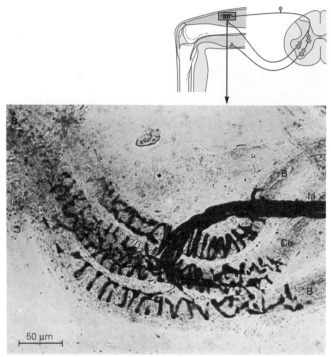

Figure 4-10 The ending of a sensory nerve in the muscle is shown in this photomicrograph of a cat soleus muscle. Numerous fibers of a single primary afferent axon (Ia) coil around specialized muscle fibers within the muscle spindle, the sensory organ for stretch. Specialized intrafusal fibers innervated by the IA afferent fibers include the bag fibers (B) and chain fibers (Ch). (From Boyd and Smith 1984.)

in the cell. In Alzheimer's disease and some other degenerative disorders they become modified and form a characteristic lesion called the neurofibrillary tangle (see Chapter 58).

Microfilaments, 3–5 nm in diameter, are the thinnest of the three main types of fibers that make up the cytoskeleton (see Figure 4-5C). Like the thin filaments of muscle, microfilaments are polar polymers of globular actin monomers (each bearing an ATP or ADP) wound into a double-stranded helix. Actin is a major constituent of all cells, perhaps the most abundant animal protein in nature. Several closely related molecular forms of actin, each encoded by a different gene, have

been identified: the α actin of skeletal muscle, and at least two other molecular forms, β and γ. Neural actin is a mixture of the β and γ species, which differ from muscle actin at a few amino acid residues. Most of the actin molecule is highly conserved, not only in different cells of an animal but also in organisms as distantly related as humans and protozoa.

Unlike the microtubules and neurofilaments, actin filaments form short polymers: they are concentrated at the cell's periphery in the cortical cytoplasm lying just underneath the plasmalemma, where, together with a very large number of actin-binding proteins (for example, spectrin-fodrin, ankyrin, talin, and actinin), they form a dense network. This matrix plays a key role in the dynamic function of the cell's periphery, such as the motility of growth cones during development, generation of specialized microdomains on the cell surface, and the formation of pre- and postsynaptic morphologic specializations.

Like microtubules, microfilaments are in a dynamic

A Peripheral   B Central   C Cortical

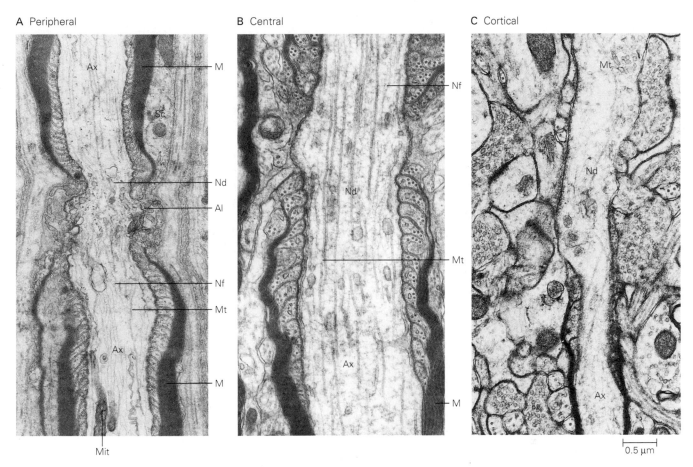

0.5 μm

Figure 4-11 The insulating myelin sheath of the axon has regularly spaced gaps called the nodes of Ranvier. Electron micrographs show the region of nodes in axons from the peripheral nervous system, spinal cord, and cerebral cortex. The axon (**Ax**) runs from the top to the bottom in all three micrographs. The axon is coated with many layers of myelin (**M**), which is lacking at the nodes (**Nd**), where the axolemma (**Al**) is exposed. (In the peripheral nervous system the support cell responsible for myelination is called a Schwann cell (**Sc**), and in the central nervous system it is an oligodendrocyte.) The elements of the cytoskeleton that can be seen within the axon are microtubules (**Mt**) and neurofilaments (**Nf**). Mitochondria (**Mit**) are also seen. (From Peters et al. 1991.)

state and undergo cycles of polymerization and depolymerization. At any one time about half the total actin in neurons can exist as unpolymerized monomers. The state of actin within the cell is controlled by binding proteins. These proteins facilitate assembly and block changes in polymer length by capping the rapidly growing end of the filament or by severing it. Other binding proteins cross-link or bundle microfilaments. The dynamic state of microtubules and microfilaments permit the mature neuron to retract old processes and extend new ones.

In addition to serving as cytoskeleton, microtubules and actin filaments act as tracks along which other organelles and proteins are driven by molecular motors. Since these filamentous polymers are polar, each motor drives its organelle cargo in one direction only. In the axon all microtubules are arranged in parallel, with the plus end pointing away from the cell body and the minus end facing the cell body. This regular orientation permits the orderly movement of distinct classes of organelles along the axon, thus maintaining the special distribution of organelles throughout the cell. In dendrites, however, microtubules with opposite polarities are mixed, and this explains why the organelles of the cell body and dendrites are similar. Actin motors, called *myosins*, mediate other types of cell motility, including extension of the cell's processes. Myosin is also thought to translocate membranous organelles within the cortical cytoplasm. Actomyosin in muscle is responsible for contraction (Chapter 34).

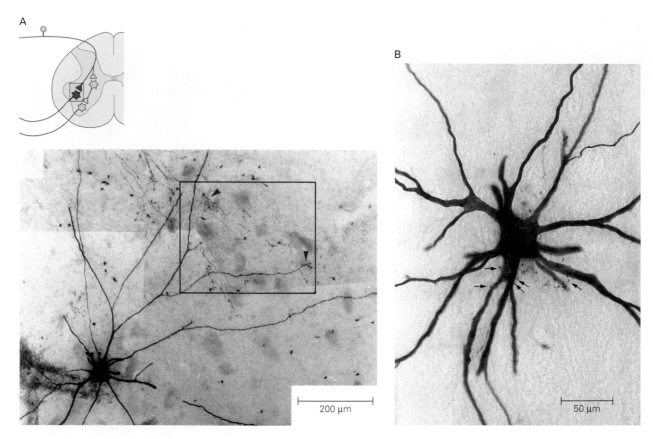

Figure 4-12 The dendritic structure of a spinal motor neuron.

A. Light micrograph of a motor neuron in the lumbosacral region of a cat's spinal cord. The cell body is shown in the lower left of the picture. The boxed area shows distal dendritic branches receiving contacts (**arrows**) from sensory (Ia afferent) neurons. Both sensory and motor neurons were identified by injection of the enzyme horseradish peroxidase, which serves as an intracellular marker. Because this is one of a set of serial

sections, the complete dendritic branching pattern of this motor neuron can be reconstructed. The **upper arrowhead** identifies a presynaptic contact on a fifth-order dendritic branch, and the **lower arrowhead** points to a contact on a third-order branch. (From Brown and Fyffe 1981.)

B. Presynaptic contacts (**arrows**) on primary dendrites within 45 μm of the cell body of the motor neuron shown in **A.** (From Brown and Fyffe 1984.)

The Neurons That Mediate the Stretch Reflex Differ in Morphology and Transmitter Substance

The relationship between neuronal structure and functions can be seen by comparing the sensory and motor neurons that mediate the stretch reflex. As described in Chapter 2, the monosynaptic component of the stretch reflex is a simple two-neuron circuit consisting of large sensory neurons that receive information from muscle cells and motor neurons that cause the skeletal muscles of the limb to contract (see Figure 2-5).

The Sensory Neuron Conducts Information From the Periphery to the Central Nervous System

Sensory neurons for the stretch reflex convey information about the state of muscle contraction. Their cell

bodies are round with large diameters (60–120 μm) and are located in dorsal root ganglia situated immediately adjacent to the spinal cord. At maturity these neurons possess a single axonal process that bifurcates into two branches a short distance from the cell body (Figure 4-8). The peripheral branch projects to muscle and the central branch to the spinal cord, where it forms synapses on the cell bodies and dendrites of motor neurons (Figure 4-9).

The peripheral branch of the sensory axon coils around a fine, specialized muscle fiber within the muscle spindle, a sensory receptor sensitive to stretch (Figure 4-10). The peripheral branch is 14–18 μm in diameter and is coated with an insulating sheath of myelin 8–10 μm thick. (Myelination is discussed in some detail later in the chapter.) The myelin sheath is regularly interrupted along the length of the axon. At these gaps, called nodes of Ranvier, the plasma membrane of the axon (the axolemma) is exposed to the extracellular space for about 0.5 μm (Figure 4-11). This arrangement greatly increases the speed at which the nerve impulse is conducted along the axon (in humans, 80 m/s) because the signal jumps from one unmyelinated node to the next by saltatory conduction (see Chapters 8 and 9).

The central branch of the sensory axon enters the spinal cord in the dorsal horn, where it bifurcates into branches that ascend and descend in the spinal cord. Collateral fibers from the axon form synapses on motor neurons in the ventral horn. When excited, the sensory neuron releases the excitatory amino acid neurotransmitter L-glutamate (see Chapter 15) that depolarizes the motor neurons.

The Motor Neuron Conveys Central Motor Commands to the Muscle Fiber

The axon of each sensory neuron directly contacts two classes of motor neurons: those that innervate the muscle within which the sensory ending is located (the *homonymous* muscle) and those that innervate other muscles that cooperate in stretching the knee joint (*synergistic* muscles). Both types of motor neurons are located in the ventral horn of the spinal cord. Motor neurons have large cell bodies, and their nucleus is distinctive because of its large and prominent nucleolus (see Figure 4-8B).

Unlike dorsal root ganglion cells, which have no dendrites, motor neurons have several dendritic trees that arise directly from the cell body. Each dendritic tree is complex, generated by extensive branching of primary dendrites (Figure 4-12). The total number of terminal dendritic branches per cell is often more than 100. The average length of a dendrite from the motor neuron's cell body to its end is about 20 cell-body diameters (1 mm), but some branches are twice as long. The branches project radially, so that the entire dendritic structure of a single motor neuron can extend within the spinal cord over an area about 2 to 3 mm in diameter. Such extensive dendritic structures are characteristic of central neurons, whose firing is regulated by input from many neurons. Short specialized dendritic extensions called *spines* serve to increase the area of the neuron available for synaptic inputs. Dendritic spines provide a biochemical and electrical compartment where incoming signals are initially received and processed; their morphology is discussed later in this chapter.

Messenger RNA is transported along dendrites and appears to be concentrated at the base of dendritic spines. Some protein synthesis occurs in dendrites, indicating that the dendrites are functional extensions of the

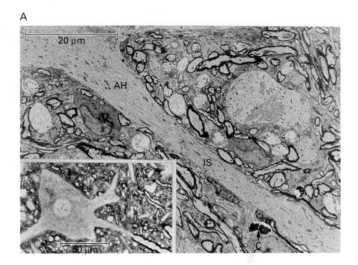

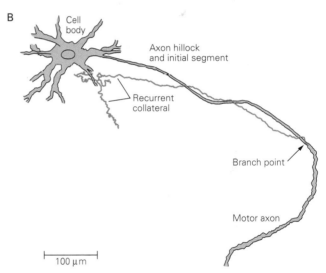

Figure 4-13 The axon of a spinal motor neuron has branches that make synaptic contact with several interneurons and, rarely, a recurrent (feedback) connection on the motor neuron.

A. An electron micrograph of a cat's spinal motor neuron shows the cell body, axon hillock (**AH**), initial segment (**IS**), and the first part of the myelinated portion of the axon. Glial cells surround the initial part of the axon. A cross-section of a capillary (**C**) is also visible. The inset shows two dendrites emerging from opposite sides of the cell body. (From Conradi 1969.)

B. The axons of motor neurons typically give off from one to five recurrent branches that usually make synaptic contact with inhibitory interneurons. In rare instances an axonal branch (a recurrent collateral) makes direct contact with its own cell body. (Courtesy of R. E. Burke.)

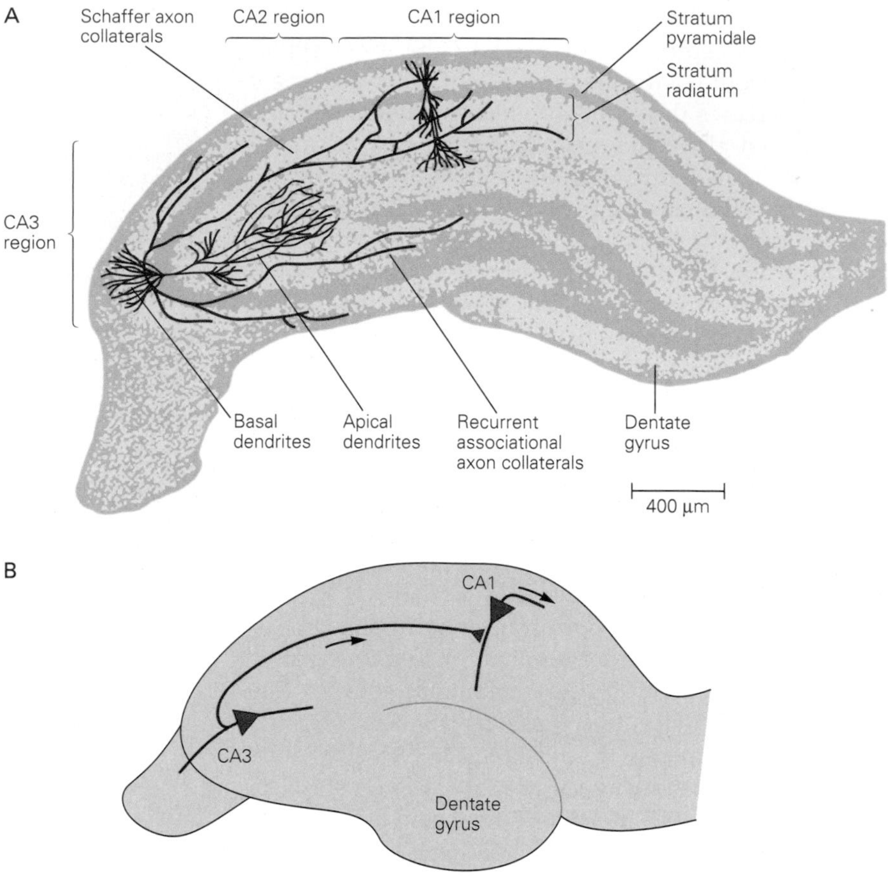

Figure 4-14 Pyramidal cells in the CA1 and CA3 regions of the hippocampus.

A. A composite illustration of the rat hippocampus and dentate gyrus. A major experimental advantage of the hippocampus for neuroscience research is its highly laminar organization. A Nissl-stained section shows dark bands representing accumulations of neuronal cell bodies in the pyramidal cell layer (stratum pyramidale) of the hippocampus. The hippocampus can be divided into three separate regions—CA1, CA2, CA3—based on the size and connections of the resident pyramidal cells. Typical CA3 and CA1 pyramidal cells are drawn on the Nissl-stained section. Each cell has been traced with an intracellular marker (horseradish peroxidase or *Phaseolus vulgaris* leukoagglutinin) through adjacent 400 μm slices and reconstructed by computer. The CA3 cell dendrites are shown as thin lines and the axon collaterals as thicker lines. The CA3 axon collaterals innervate other CA3 cells (the associational axon collaterals) and the CA1 pyramidal cells (the Schaffer collaterals). These axons run in the stratum radiatum. Only the dendrites of the CA1 pyramidal cell are illustrated. (Courtesy of D. G. Amaral.)

B. Schematic diagram of the hippocampus showing the connection between the two pyramidal neurons through the Schaffer axon collaterals.

cell body, where most proteins are synthesized. Consistent with this view, the cytoskeleton of dendrites more closely resembles that of the cell body than that of axons. Local protein synthesis at dendrites is thought to play an important role in synaptic plasticity.

Each motor neuron gives rise to only one axon, about 20 μm in diameter, from a specialized region of the cell body called the *axon hillock.* The axon hillock and the initial (unmyelinated) segment of the axon extend the length of about one cell-body diameter (Figure 4-13). About half the surface area of the axon hillock and cell body and three-quarters of the dendritic membrane are covered by *synaptic boutons,* the knob-like terminals of the axons of presynaptic neurons (see Figure 4-8B). The axon hillock and the initial segment of the axon function as a *trigger zone,* the site at which the many incoming signals from other neurons are integrated and the action potential, the output signal of the neuron, is generated (see Chapter 9).

Close to the cell body the axon gives off several *recurrent collateral* branches (Figure 4-13). These branches are called recurrent because many of them project back to

the motor neuron and modify the activity of the cell. More often, however, recurrent collaterals form synapses on a particular type of interneuron in the spinal cord, the Renshaw cell. These interneurons hyperpolarize the motor neurons, using the neurotransmitter L-glycine, and thus inhibit firing in the motor neurons.

In addition, motor neurons receive recurrent excitatory inputs from other motor neurons, and both excitatory and inhibitory inputs from interneurons driven by descending fibers from the brain that control and coordinate movement. These synaptic inputs, together with the excitatory input from the primary sensory neurons and inhibitory input from Renshaw cells, are integrated by mechanisms that are described in Chapter 12.

A Single Motor Neuron Forms Synapses With Several Muscle Cells

One striking difference between motor and sensory neurons is the location of their synaptic inputs. The sensory neuron has few if any boutons on its cell body or

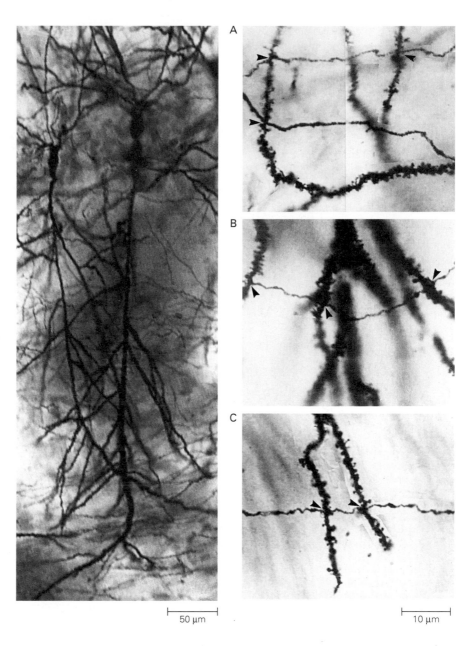

Figure 4-15 Pyramidal cells in the CA3 region of the hippocampus form synapses on the dendrites of CA1 cells in the stratum radiatum.

Left: Micrograph of a Golgi-stained CA1 pyramidal cell is shown with dendrites extending downward 350 μm into the stratum radiatum.

Right: Three micrographs show synapses formed on this CA1 cell by CA3 cells. **A.** Axons of two CA3 neurons form synapses on a dendrite 50 μm from the CA1 neuron's cell body. **B.** A single CA3 axon forms synapses on dendrites 259 μm from the cell body. **C.** A single CA3 axon forms synapses on two dendrites 263 μm from the cell body. (From Sorra and Harris 1993.)

50 μm

10 μm

along the peripheral branch of its axon. Its primary input is from sensory receptors at the terminal of the peripheral axon. In contrast, the motor neuron receives primary and modifying inputs throughout its dendrites and cell body. (Almost all presynaptic boutons on motor neurons are located on the dendritic branches; only 5% are located on the cell body.) The synapses on the motor neuron are distributed in a functional pattern. Most inhibitory synapses are on the cell body or close to it, whereas excitatory ones are located farther out along the dendrites. Inhibitory inputs are strategically placed close to the trigger zone to have maximal influence on the final tally of inputs to the neuron (see Chapter 12).

The information flow from sensory neurons to motor neurons is both divergent and convergent. Each sensory neuron contacts 500–1000 motor neurons and typically forms two to six synapses on a single motor neuron (divergence of information). At the same time each motor neuron receives input from many sensory neurons (convergence of information); inputs from more than 100 sensory neurons are needed for a motor neuron to reach the threshold for firing.

The axons that mediate the stretch reflex in the leg leave the lumbosacral region of the spinal cord and join the femoral nerve. (The motor axons and sensory fibers travel along the same peripheral path to the muscle.)

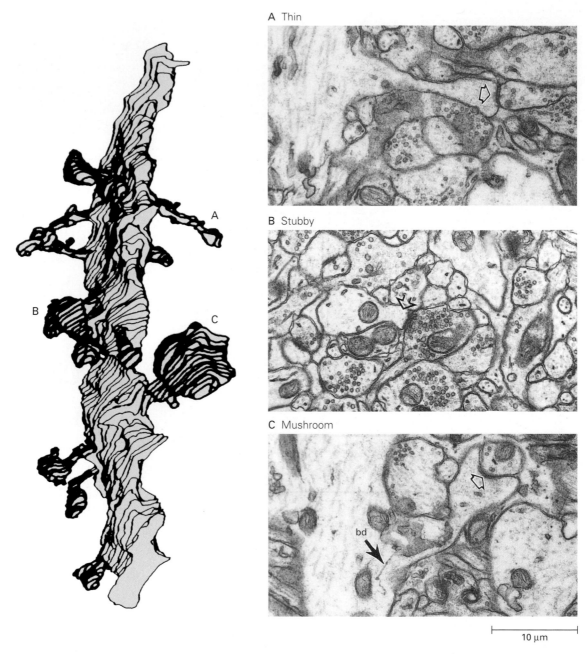

A Thin

B Stubby

C Mushroom

bd

10 µm

Figure 4-16 The dendrites of pyramidal cells in the CA1 region of the hippocampus bear a variety of spines.

Left: The diversity of dendritic spine shapes is evident along even a short segment of the mature dendrite in this three-dimensional reconstruction from a series of electron micrographs. (From Harris and Stevens 1989.)

Right: Three micrographs illustrate the details of different types of dendritic spines. **A.** A thin dendritic spine from the postnatal day-15 rat hippocampus. The postsynaptic density shows as the thickened receptive surface (**open arrow**) lo-

cated across from the presynaptic axon, which has round clear vesicles. **B.** Stubby spines containing postsynaptic densities (**open arrow**) are both small and rare in the mature hippocampus. Their larger counterparts (not shown) predominate in the immature brain. **C.** Mushroom-shaped spines have a larger head. These spines are present by day 15 as shown here. The immature spines contain flat cisternae of smooth endoplasmic reticulum, some with a beaded appearance (**bd**). Synapse with postsynaptic density is indicated by the **open arrow**. Branched spines did not occur in this dendritic segment. (From Harris et al. 1992.)

A Myelination in the central nervous system

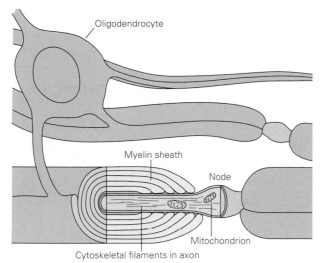

B Myelination in the peripheral nervous system

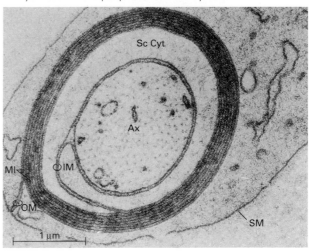

C Development of myelin sheath in the peripheral nervous system

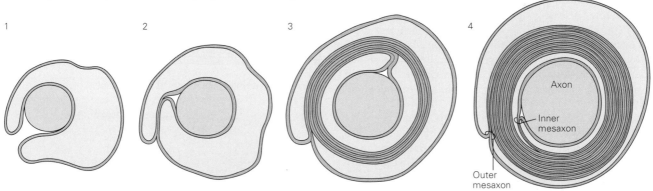

Figure 4-17 The axons of both central and peripheral neurons are insulated by a myelin sheath.

A. An axon in the central nervous system receives its myelin sheath from an oligodendrocyte. (Adapted from Bunge 1968.)

B. An electron micrograph of a transverse section through an axon (**Ax**) in the sciatic nerve of a mouse. The spiraling lamellae of the myelin sheath (**MI**) start at a structure called the inner

mesaxon (**IM**; circled). The spiraling sheath is still developing and is seen arising from the surface membrane (**SM**) of the Schwann cell, which is continuous with the outer mesaxon (**OM**; circled). The Schwann cell cytoplasm (**Sc Cyt**) is still present, next to the axon; eventually it is squeezed out and the sheath becomes compact. (From Dyck et al. 1984.)

C. A peripheral nerve fiber is myelinated by a Schwann cell. (Adapted from Williams et al. 1989.)

When the motor neuron enters the muscle it ramifies into many unmyelinated branches, each with a diameter of only a few micrometers. These terminal fibers run along the surface of a muscle fiber and form many synaptic contacts called *neuromuscular junctions*. These synapses are the most completely characterized and best understood of all synapses in the nervous system (see Chapter 11).

Each muscle fiber is contacted by only a single axon, but a single motor axon innervates several muscle fibers. The axon and the muscle fibers it innervates constitute a *motor unit*. The muscle fibers innervated by any one motor axon are widely spread, overlapping

muscle fibers of other motor units. The number of muscle fibers innervated by a single motor axon varies throughout the body, depending on the mass of the body part to be moved. Thus, in the leg a single motor axon innervates more than 1000 muscle fibers, while in the eye an axon contacts fewer than 100 muscle fibers. A lower innervation ratio permits greater precision of movement control.

The sensory and motor neurons that mediate the stretch reflex differ in appearance, location in the nervous system, the distribution of their axons and dendrites, and the inputs they receive. All of these cytologi-

Box 4-1 Defects in Myelin Proteins Disrupt Conduction of Nerve Signals

Because normal conduction of the nerve impulse depends on the insulating properties of the myelin sheath surrounding the axon, defective myelin can result in severe disturbances of motor and sensory function. Myelin in both the central and peripheral nervous systems contains a major class of proteins, myelin basic proteins (MBP), which have an important role in myelin compaction. At least seven related proteins are produced from a single MBP gene by alternative RNA splicing.

Myelin basic proteins are capable of eliciting a strong immune response. When injected into animals they cause experimental allergic encephalomyelitis, a syndrome characterized by local inflammation and by destruction of the myelin sheaths (*demyelination*) in the central nervous system. This experimental disease has been used as a model for multiple sclerosis, a common demyelinating disease in humans. Because demyelination slows down conduction of the action potential in the affected neurons' processes, multiple sclerosis and other demyelinating diseases (for example, Guillain-Barré syndrome) can have devastating effects on the function of neuronal circuits in the brain and spinal cord (see Chapter 35).

Many diseases that affect myelin, including some animal models of demyelinating disease, have a genetic basis. The *shiverer* (or *shi*) mutant mice have tremors and frequent convulsions and tend to die at young ages. In these mice the myelination of axons in the central nervous system is greatly deficient and the myelination that does occur is abnormal. The mutation that causes this disease is a deletion of five of the six exons of the gene for myelin basic protein, which in the mouse is located on chromosome 18. The mutation is recessive; a mouse will develop the disease only if it has inherited the defective gene from both parents. *Shiverer* mice that inherit both defective genes have only about 10% of the myelin basic protein found in normal mice.

When the wild-type gene is injected into fertilized eggs of the *shiverer* mutant with the aim of rescuing the mutant, the resulting transgenic mice express the wild-type gene but produce only 20% of the normal amounts of myelin basic proteins. Nevertheless, myelination of central neurons in the transgenic mice is much improved. Although they still have occasional tremors, the transgenic mice do not have convulsions and live a normal life span (Figure 4-18).

Central and peripheral myelin also contain a distinct protein termed myelin-associated glycoprotein (MAG). MAG belongs to a superfamily that is related to the immunoglobulins and includes several important cell surface proteins thought to be involved in cell-to-cell recognition (for example, the major histocompatibility complex of antigens, T-cell surface anti-

A

Normal mouse has abundant myelination

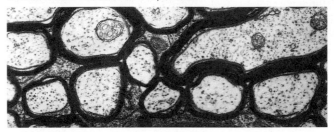

Shiverer mutant has scant myelination

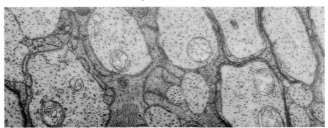

Transfected normal gene improves myelination

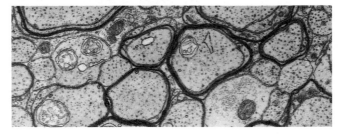

B

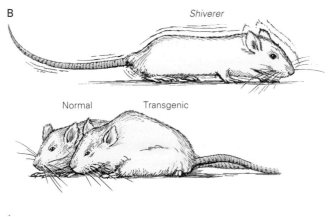

Figure 4-18 A genetic disorder of myelination in mice (*shiverer* mutant) can be partially cured by transfection of the normal gene that encodes myelin basic protein.

A. Electron micrographs show the state of myelination in the optic nerve of a normal mouse, a *shiverer* mutant, and a mutant transfected with the gene for myelin basic protein. (From Readhead et al. 1987.)

B. Myelination is incomplete in the *shiverer* mutant. As a result, the *shiverer* mutant exhibits poor posture and weakness. Injection of the wild-type gene into the fertilized egg of the mutant improves myelination. A normal mouse and a transfected *shiverer* mutant look perky.

gens, and the neural cell adhesion molecule or NCAM). MAG is expressed by Schwann cells early during peripheral myelination and eventually becomes a component of mature (compact) myelin. It is situated primarily at the margin of the mature myelin sheath just adjacent to the axon. Its early expression, subcellular location, and structural similarity to other surface recognition proteins suggest that it is an adhesion molecule important for the initiation of the myelination process. Two isoforms of MAG are produced from a single gene through alternative RNA splicing.

More than half of the total protein in central myelin is a characteristic proteolipid, PLP, which has five membrane-spanning domains. Proteolipids differ from lipoproteins in that they are insoluble in water. Proteolipids are soluble only in organic solvents because they contain long chains of fatty acids that are covalently linked to amino acid residues throughout the proteolipid molecule. In contrast, lipoproteins are noncovalent complexes of proteins with lipids so structured that many serve as soluble carriers of the lipid moiety in the blood.

Many mutations of the proteolipid PLP are known, in humans as well as in other mammals (for example, the *jimpy* mouse). Pelizaeus-Merzbacher disease, a heterogeneous X-linked disease in humans, results from a PLP mutation. Almost all of these mutations occur in a membrane-spanning domain of the molecule. All of these mutant animals have reduced amounts of the mutated protein and show hypomyelination and degeneration and death of oligodendrocytes. These observations suggest that the proteolipid is involved in the compaction of myelin.

The major protein in mature peripheral myelin, myelin protein zero (MPZ or P_0), spans the plasmalemma of the Schwann cell. It has a basic intracellular domain and, like myelin-associated glycoprotein, is a member of the immunoglobulin superfamily. The glycosylated extracellular part of the protein, which contains the immunoglobulin domain, functions as a homophilic adhesion protein during myelin spiraling and compaction by interacting with identical domains on the surface of the opposed membrane. Genetically engineered P_0 mice in which the function of myelin protein P_0 has been eliminated have poor motor coordination, tremors, and occasional convulsions.

Observation of *trembler* mouse mutants led to the identification of peripheral myelin protein 22 (PMP22). This Schwann cell protein spans the membrane four times and is normally present in compact myelin. PMP22 is altered by a single amino acid. A similar protein is found in humans, encoded by a gene on chromosome 17.

Although several hereditary peripheral neuropathies result from mutations of the PMP22 gene on chromosome 17, one form of Charcot-Marie-Tooth disease is caused by the DNA duplication of this gene (Figure 4-19). Charcot-Marie-Tooth disease, the most common inherited peripheral neuropathy, is characterized by progressive muscle weakness, greatly decreased conduction in peripheral nerves, and cycles of demyelination and remyelination. Since both duplicated genes are active, the disease results from *increased* production of PMP22 (a two- to three-fold increase in gene dosage) rather than from a reduction in a mutant protein.

(continued)

Box 4-1 Defects in Myelin Proteins Disrupt Conduction of Nerve Signals (continued)

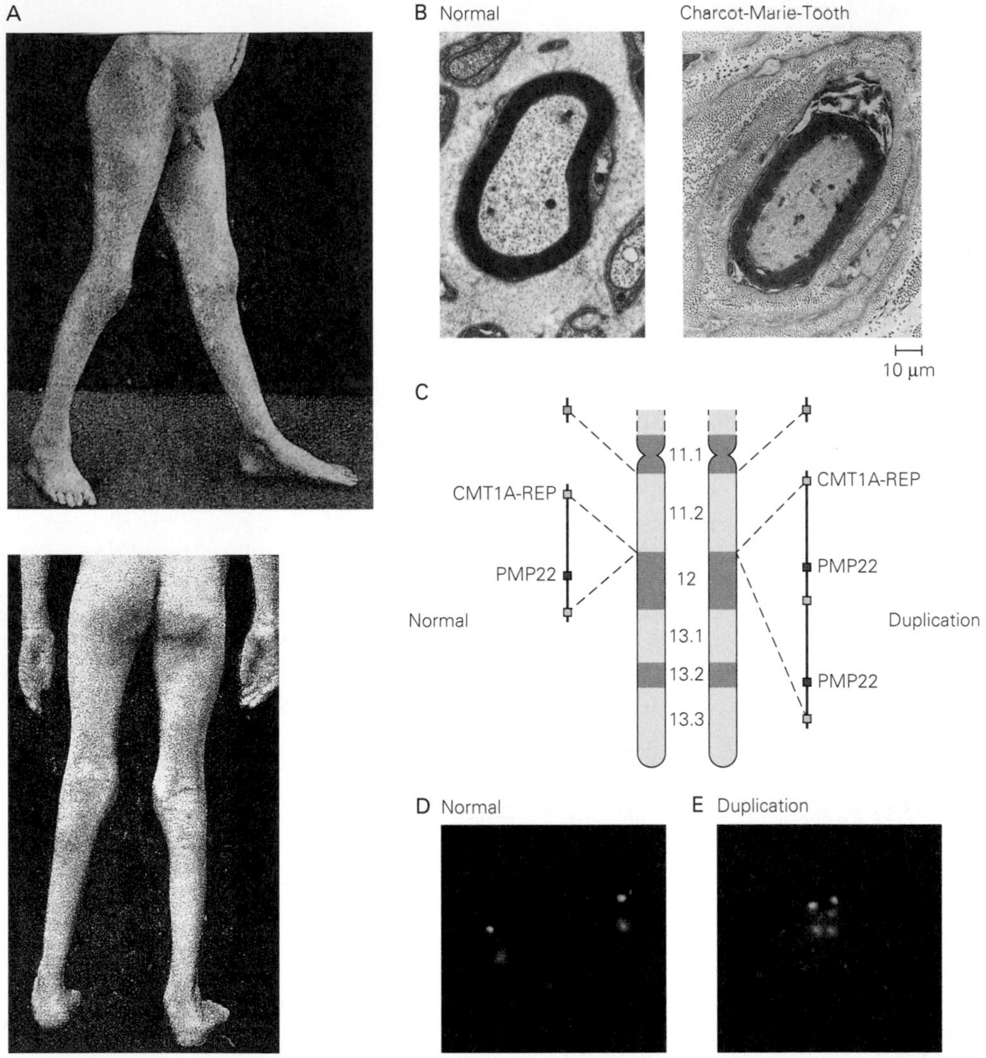

Figure 4-19 Charcot-Marie-Tooth disease (type 1A) results from gene dosage effects.

A. A patient with Charcot-Marie-Tooth shows impaired gait and deformities (from Charcot's original description of the disease, 1886).

B. Sural nerve biopsies from a normal individual (from AP Hays, Columbia University) and from a patient with Charcot-Marie-Tooth (from Lupski and Garcia 1993).

C. The disordered myelination in Charcot-Marie-Tooth disease results from the increased production of the peripheral myelin protein PMP22. The increase is caused by a duplication of a normal 1.5 megabase region of the DNA on the short arm of chromosome 17 at 17p11.2-p12. The PMP22 gene is flanked by two similar repeat sequences, as shown in the representation of a normal chromosome 17. Normal individuals have two normal chromosomes. In patients with the disease the duplication results in two functing PMP22 genes, each flanked by the repeat sequence. The normal and duplicated regions are shown in the expanded diagrams indicated by the dashed lines. (The repeats are thought to have given rise to the original duplica-

tion, which was then inherited. The presence of two similar flanking sequences with homology to a transposable element is believed to increase the frequency of unequal crossing-over in this region of chromosome 17 because the repeats enhance the probability of mispairing of the two parental chromosomes in a fertilized egg.)

D–E. Although a large duplication, 3 megabases cannot be detected in routine examination of chromosomes in the light microscope, but microscopic evidence for the duplication can be obtained using fluorescence *in situ* hybridization. With this technique, the PMP22 gene is detected with an oligonucleotide probe tagged with the dye Texas Red. An oligonucleotiede probe tagged with fluoroscein, a green fluorescent dye that hybridizes with DNA from region 11.2 (indicated in green closer to the centromere), is used for *in situ* hybridization on the same sample. A nucleus from a normal individual (**D**) shows a pair of chromosomes, each with one red site (PMP22 gene) for each green site. In a nucleus from a patient with the disease (**E**) there is one extra red site, indicating that one chromosome has one PMP22 gene and the other has two PMP22 genes.

cal features have important behavioral consequences. In addition, the two types of cells differ biochemically because they use different neurotransmitters (although both transmitters are excitatory). For example, the motor neuron, which uses acetylcholine as a transmitter, requires a set of macromolecules that includes the biosynthetic enzyme choline acetyltransferase and a specific membrane transporter for choline, an essential precursor in the synthesis of acetylcholine (Chapter 15).

Pyramidal Neurons in the Cerebral Cortex Have More Extensive Dendritic Trees Than Spinal Motor Neurons

Whereas motor neurons are the major excitatory projection neurons of the spinal cord, pyramidal cells are the excitatory projection neurons in the cerebral cortex. Pyramidal cells in different cortical regions are morphologically similar and use L-glutamate as a transmitter. We shall focus here on the pyramidal cells of the hippocampus, a structure important for memory storage.

The hippocampus is divided into two major regions, CA3 and CA1. In both regions the cell bodies of pyramidal cells are situated in a single continuous layer, the stratum pyramidale (Figure 4-14). In contrast to the motor neurons of the spinal cord, pyramidal cells have not one but two dendritic trees, and these emerge from opposite sides of the cell body: the basal dendrites arise from the side that gives rise to the axon, and the apical dendrites arise from the opposite side of the cell body.

Excitatory input to CA1 pyramidal neurons is extensive. About 5000 CA3 pyramidal cell axons—comprising the Schaffer collateral pathway—converge on a single CA1 cell. These Schaffer collaterals form synapses at all levels of the CA1 cell's dendritic tree close to the cell body and at more distant levels (Figure 4-15). The connections formed by the Schaffer collaterals are called *en passant* synapses because CA3 axons continue to pass through the stratum radiatum, making contact with the dendrites of many other CA1 pyramidal cells.

Most of the synapses are made on dendritic spines. In many parts of the brain, spines have two inputs, one excitatory and the other inhibitory. In area CA1, however, each pyramidal cell spine has only one synapse, which is excitatory. These spines have four principal shapes: thin, mushroom, branched, and stubby (Figure 4-16). The neck of the spine restricts diffusion between the head of the spine and the rest of the dendrite. Thus, each spine may function as a separate biochemical region. As we shall see later, this compartmentalization may be important for selectively altering the strength of synaptic connections during learning and memory.

Glial Cells Produce the Insulating Myelin Sheath Around Signal-Conducting Axons

The signal-conducting axons of both sensory and motor neurons are ensheathed in myelin along most of their length (see Figure 4-11). Acting as insulation, myelin speeds transmission along axons and thus is critical for quick reflex movements like the knee jerk. The myelin sheath is arranged in concentric bimolecular layers of lipids interspersed between protein layers (Figure 4-17). Biochemical analysis shows that myelin has a composition similar to that of plasma membranes, consisting of 70% lipid and 30% protein, with a high concentration of cholesterol and phospholipid.

Both the regular lamellar structure and biochemical composition of the myelin sheath are consequences of how myelin is formed from plasma membrane. In the development of the peripheral nervous system, before myelination takes place, the sensory cell axon lies along a peripheral nerve in a trough formed by a class of glia called Schwann cells. Schwann cells line up along the axon at intervals that will eventually become the nodes of Ranvier. The external cell membrane of each Schwann cell surrounds a single axon and forms a double-membrane structure called the *mesaxon*, which elongates and spirals around the axon in concentric layers (Figure 4-17C). The cytoplasm of the Schwann cell appears to be squeezed out during the ensheathing process when the Schwann cell's processes condense into the compact lamellae of the mature myelin sheath.

In the femoral nerve, which carries the sensory and motor axons that mediate the stretch reflex, the primary sensory axon is about 0.5 m long and the internodal distance is 1–1.5 mm; thus approximately 300–500 nodes of Ranvier occur along a primary afferent fiber between the thigh muscle and the dorsal root ganglion, where the cell body lies. Since each internodal segment is formed by a single Schwann cell, as many as 500 Schwann cells participate in the myelination of a single peripheral sensory axon.

In the central nervous system myelination of the central branch of dorsal root ganglion cell axons and the axons of motor neurons differs somewhat from myelination in the peripheral system. The glial cell responsible for elaborating central myelin is the *oligodendrocyte*, which typically ensheathes several axon processes. Schwann cells and oligodendrocytes differ developmentally and biochemically. The expression of myelin genes by Schwann cells in the peripheral nervous system is regulated by the contact between the axon and the myelinating Schwann cell. In contrast, the expression of myelin genes by oligodendrocytes in the central nervous system appears to depend on the presence of astrocytes, the other major type of glial cell in the central nervous system.

Specific diseases can arise from dysfunction of the specialized properties of neurons. In particular, defective myelination of the axon produces severe disturbances of motor and sensory function. Thus, understanding the biochemistry of myelin formation provides important insight into the basis of certain neurological diseases (Box 4-1).

An Overall View

Nerve cells have four distinctive compartments: dendrites, for receiving signals from other neurons; the cell body, which contains the DNA encoding neuronal proteins and the complex apparatus for synthesizing them; the axon, which projects over long distances to target cells (for example, other neurons or muscle); and nerve terminals, for release of neurotransmitters at synapses with targets.

In this chapter we have illustrated this basic cellular plan by describing three types of neurons. Although all of these cells conform to a basic plan, each type differs considerably, most obviously by location in the nervous system—peripheral or central, spinal cord, or brain. They also differ in the location of synaptic inputs on the cell and in the types of target cells to which they project. Furthermore, they differ in cell body size and shape, distribution of their dendritic trees and number of axon branches, and in their degree of myelination. Biochemically, they differ most obviously in transmitter type, and, as we shall see throughout this book, in many other constituents (for example, in the enzymes that synthesize neurotransmitters, the pumps that exchange ions or recapture neurotransmitter substances, and the receptors that transduce physical or biochemical inputs).

The functional significance of many morphological differences is plainly evident. For example, the dorsal root sensory neuron must extend a process in the peripheral nervous system, as must the spinal motor neuron. It also is clear why the motor neuron has a more complex dendritic tree than the sensory neuron: Even simple reflex activity requires coordination of inputs, both excitatory and inhibitory, to regulate specific motor units, and purposeful movements need still more integration because of inputs from the brain.

The functional significance of some other cytological differences is not so obvious, but can be understood in the context of the electrophysiological activities of the particular neurons. Thus the large number of dendrites and axonal branches in cortical pyramidal neurons must contribute to the complexity of information processing in the brain.

James H. Schwartz
Gary L. Westbrook

Selected Readings

Baldissera F, Hultborn H, Illert M. 1981. Integration in spinal neuronal systems. In: VB Brooks (ed). *Handbook of Physiology: A Critical, Comprehensive Presentation of Physiological Knowledge and Concepts*. Sect. 1, *The Nervous System*. Vol. 2, *Motor Control*, pp. 509–595. Bethesda, MD: American Physiological Society.

Burke RE. 1990. Spinal cord: ventral horn. In: GM Shepherd (ed). *The Synaptic Organization of the Brain*, 3rd ed., pp. 88–132. New York: Oxford University Press.

Dyck PJ, Thomas PK, Griffin JW, Low PA, Poduslo JF (eds). 1993. *Peripheral Neuropathy*, 3rd ed. Philadelphia: Saunders.

Lemke G. 1992. Myelin and myelination. In: Z Hall (ed). *An Introduction to Molecular Neurobiology*, pp. 281–312. Sunderland, MA: Sinauer.

Peters A, Palay SL, Webster H deF. 1991. *The Fine Structure of the Nervous System: Neurons and Their Supporting Cells*, 3rd ed. New York: Oxford Univ. Press.

Rothwell J. 1994. *Control of Human Voluntary Movement*, 2nd ed. London: Chapman & Hall.

Siegel GJ, Agranoff BW, Albers RW, Molinoff PB (eds). 1999. *Basic Neurochemistry: Molecular, Cellular, and Medical Aspects*, 6th ed. Philadelphia: Lippincott-Raven.

References

Amaral DG, Ishizuka N, Claiborne B. 1990. Neurons, numbers and the hippocampal network. Prog Brain Res 83:1–11.

Amaral DG. 1993. Emerging principles of intrinsic hippocampal organization. Curr Opin Neurobiol 3:225–229.

Bershadsky AD, Vasiliev JM. 1988. *Cytoskeleton*. New York: Plenum.

Boyd IA, Smith RS. 1984. The muscle spindle. In: PJ Dyck, PK Thomas, EH Lambert, R Bunge (eds). *Peripheral Neuropathy*, 2nd ed., 1:171–202. Philadelphia: Saunders.

Brown AG, Fyffe RE. 1981. Direct observations on the contacts made between Ia afferent fibres and α-motoneurones in the cat's lumbosacral spinal cord. J Physiol (Lond) 313:121–140.

Brown AG, Fyffe REW. 1984. *Intracellular Staining of Mammalian Neurones.* London: Academic.

Bunge RP. 1968. Glial cells and the central myelin sheath. Physiol Rev 48:197–251.

Burke RE. 1981. Motor units: anatomy, physiology, and functional organization. In: VB Brooks (ed). *Handbook of Physiology: A Critical, Comprehensive Presentation of Physiological Knowledge and Concepts.* Sect. 1, *The Nervous System.* Vol. 2, *Motor Control,* pp. 345–422. Bethesda, MD: American Physiological Society.

Burke RE, Dum RP, Fleshman JW, Glenn LL, Lev-Tov A, O'Donovan MJ, Pinter MJ. 1982. An HRP study of the relation between cell size and motor unit type in cat ankle extensor motoneurons. J Comp Neurol 209:17–28.

Cameron PL, Sudhof TC, Jahn R, De Camilli P. 1991. Colocalization of synaptophysin with transferrin receptors: implications for synaptic vesicle biogenesis. J Cell Biol 115:151–164.

Charcot J-M, Marie P. 1886. Sur une forme particulière d'atrophie musculaire progressive, souvent familiale, débutant par les pieds et les jambes et atteignant plus tard les mains. Rev Med 6:97–138.

Conradi S. 1969. Ultrastructure and distribution of neuronal and glial elements on the motoneuron surface in the lumbosacral spinal cord of the adult cat. Acta Physiol Scand 332:5–48 (Suppl.).

De Camilli P, Moretti M, Donini SD, Walter U, Lohmann SM. 1986. Heterogeneous distribution of the cAMP receptor protein RII in the nervous system: evidence for its intracellular accumulation on microtubules, microtubule-organizing centers, and in the area of the Golgi complex. J Cell Biol 103:189–203.

Dogiel AS. 1908. *Der Bau der Spinalganglien des Menschen und der Säugetiere.* Jena: Fischer.

Dyck PJ, Thomas PK, Lambert EH, Bunge R (eds). 1984. *Peripheral Neuropathy,* 2nd ed. Vols. 1, 2. Philadelphia: Saunders.

Gulyas AI, Miles R, Hájos N, Freund TF. 1993. Precision and variability in postsynaptic target selection of inhibitory cells in the hippocampal CA3 region. Eur J Neurosci 5:1729–1751.

Harris KM, Stevens JK. 1989. Dendritic spines of CA1 pyramidal cells in the rat hippocampus: serial electron microscopy with reference to their biophysical characteristics. J Neurosci 9:2982–2997.

Harris KM, Jensen FE, Tsao B. 1992. Three-dimensional structure of dendritic spines and synapses in rat hippocampus (CA1) at postnatal day 15 and adult ages: implications for the maturation of synaptic physiology and long-term potentiation. J Neurosci 12:2685–2705.

Ishizuka N, Weber J, Amaral DG. 1990. Organization of intrahippocampal projections originating from CA3 pyramidal cells in the rat. J Comp Neurol 295:580–623.

Lemke G. 1988. Unwrapping the genes of myelin. Neuron 1:535–543.

Lemke G. 1993. The molecular genetics of myelination: an update. Glia 7:263–271.

Lorente de Nó R. 1934. Studies on the structure of the cerebral cortex. II. Continuation of the study of the ammonic system. J Psychol Neurol 46:113–177.

Lupski JR, Garcia CA. 1992. Molecular genetics and neuropathology of Charcot-Marie-Tooth disease type 1A. Brain Pathol 2:337–349.

Lupski JR, de Oca-Luna RM, Slaugenhaupt S, Pentao L, Guzzetta V, Trask BJ, Saucedo-Cardenas O, Barker DF, Killian JM, Garcia CA, Chakravarti A, Patel PI. 1991. DNA duplication associated with Charcot-Marie-Tooth disease type 1A. Cell 66:219–232.

Ramón y Cajal S. [1901] 1988. Studies on the human cerebral cortex. IV. Structure of the olfactory cerebral cortex of man and mammals. In: J DeFelipe, EG Jones (eds, transl). *Cajál on the Cerebral Cortex,* pp. 289–362. New York: Oxford Univ. Press.

Ramón y Cajal S. [1909] 1995. *Histology of the Nervous System of Man and Vertebrates.* N Swanson, LW Swanson (transl). Vols. 1, 2. New York: Oxford Univ. Press.

Readhead C, Popko B, Takahashi N, Shine HD, Saavedra RA, Sidman RL, Hood L. 1987. Expression of a myelin basic protein gene in transgenic Shiverer mice: correction of the dysmyelinating phenotype. Cell 48:703–712.

Roa BB, Lupski JR. 1994. Molecular genetics of Charcot-Marie-Tooth neuropathy. Adv Human Genet 22:117–152.

Sorra KE, Harris KM. 1993. Occurrence and three-dimensional structure of multiple synapses between individual radiatum axons and their target pyramidal cells in hippocampal area CA1. J Neurosci 13:3736–3748.

Ulfhake B, Kellerth J-O. 1981. A quantitative light microscopic study of the dendrites of cat spinal α-motoneurons after intracellular staining with horseradish peroxidase. J Comp Neurol 202:571–583.

Williams PL, Warwick R, Dyson M, Bannister LH (eds). 1989. *Gray's Anatomy,* 37th ed, pp. 859–919. Edinburgh: Churchill Livingstone.

5

Synthesis and Trafficking of Neuronal Protein

The cell body is an important site of synaptic input in most neurons. As discussed in the preceding chapter, the cell body is close to the trigger zone, and inhibitory input is especially effective there. But in some neurons, such as the sensory neurons of the dorsal root ganglion, the cell body does not receive synaptic input. What then is the function of the cell body beyond its role as a postsynaptic site?

An answer to this question was suggested by Augustus Waller in the mid-nineteenth century. Waller cut the various roots and nerves of the spinal cord and observed which fibers degenerated as a result. From the patterns of degeneration Waller concluded that the cell body of a dorsal root ganglion cell maintains the vitality of its axons. In a lecture delivered to the Royal Institution of Great Britain in 1861, he said, "A nerve-cell would be to its effluent nerve fibers what a fountain is to the rivulet which trickles from it—*a centre of nutritive energy*." For the most part, this nourishment is provided in the form of proteins.

Almost all of the macromolecules of a neuron are synthesized in the cell body from mRNAs originating in the nucleus. Because the cell body is only one of the four critical regions of the neuron, and because the axons and terminals often lie at great distances from the cell body, transport mechanisms are crucial for the functioning of neurons. In this chapter we shall examine the synthesis of neuronal proteins and the mechanisms for distributing them to their proper destinations throughout the membranous organelles and functional compartments of the neuron.

Most Proteins Are Synthesized in the Cell Body

The cell body and the proximal portion of dendrites are the sites at which most macromolecules are assembled. Information for the synthesis of proteins is encoded in the DNA within the cell's nucleus. As we saw in Chapter 3, all nuclei contain the same genetic information and this information is passed from parent cell to daughter cell during cell division. Only a selected portion of this genetic information, however, is transcribed in a given cell to generate mRNAs and eventually proteins. Which proteins are expressed is determined by regulatory DNA-binding proteins (transcription factors)

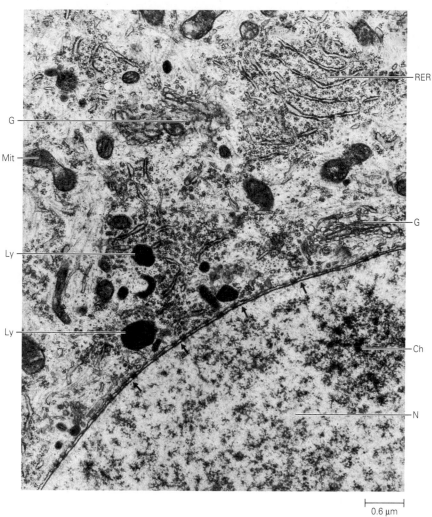

RER

G

Mit

G

Ly

Ch

Ly

N

0.6 µm

Figure 5-1 Some of the components of a spinal motor neuron that participate in the synthesis of macromolecules are shown in this electron micrograph. The nucleus (**N**), containing masses of chromatin (**Ch**), is bounded by a double-layered membrane, the nuclear envelope, which contains many nuclear pores (**arrows**). The mRNA leaves the nucleus through these pores and attaches to ribosomes that either remain free in the cytoplasm or attach to the membranes of the endoplasmic reticulum to form the rough endoplasmic reticulum (**RER**). Regulating proteins synthesized in the cytoplasm are imported into the nucleus through the pores. Several parts of the Golgi apparatus (**G**) are seen. Also present in the cytoplasm are lysosomes (**Ly**) and mitochondria (**Mit**). (From Peters et al. 1991.)

synthesized in the cytosol and taken up into the nucleus through the nuclear pores (Figure 5-1)

The brain expresses more of the total genetic information encoded in DNA than does any other organ in the body. About 200,000 distinct mRNA sequences are thought to be expressed, 10–20 times more than in the kidney or liver. In part, this diversity results from the greater number and variety of cell types in the brain as compared to cells in the more homogenous body tissues. But many neurobiologists also believe that each of the brain's 10^{11} nerve cells actually expresses a greater amount of its genetic information than does a liver or kidney cell.

Because cell division has stopped, in mature neurons the chromosomes no longer duplicate themselves and function only in gene expression. Because a large number of genes are being transcribed at any given time, the chromosomes are not arranged in compact structures but exist in a relatively uncoiled state. Thus,

the contents of the nucleus, when viewed in the electron microscope, have an amorphous appearance. Ribosomal RNA is transcribed in prominent nucleoli, a characteristic of all cells with a high rate of protein synthesis. Precursor RNA is transcribed and spliced within the nucleus to generate mature mRNA. Newly synthesized ribosomes and mRNA are exported from the nucleus through the nuclear pores.

Although most of the genetic information for the synthesis of proteins is encoded in the cell's nucleus, a small amount is contained in circular DNA within mitochondria. The human mitochondrial genome encodes information for mitochondrial transfer RNAs (tRNAs) and ribosomal RNAs (rRNAs), which differ from those in the rest of the cell, and for a few of the mitochondrion's proteins. The rest of the mitochondrion's proteins are encoded by genes in the nuclear chromosomes, synthesized on cytoplasmic ribosomes, and then imported into the mitochondrion.

A

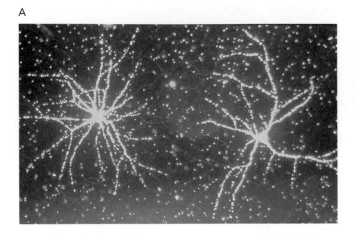

Figure 5-2 Ribosomes are present in the cell body and throughout the dendritic arbor but are absent in the axon.

A. This autoradiograph illustrates the distribution of ribosomal RNA (rRNA) in hippocampal neurons in low-density cultures as revealed by in situ hybridization. The photomicrograph is taken with dark field illumination, in which silver grains reflect light and thus appear as bright spots. Silver grains are heavily concentrated over cell bodies and dendrites, but there is no detectable labeling over the axons that criss-cross among the dendrites.

B. Polyribosomes in dendrites are selectively located beneath postsynaptic sites. In spine-bearing neurons clusters of polyribosomes are generally found just at the junction of the spine and the main dendritic shaft (**arrow**). This electron micrograph

B

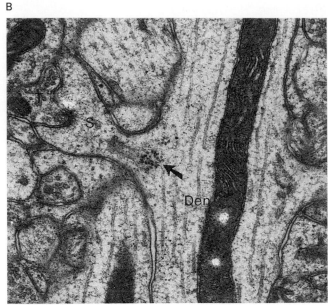

0.17 μm

shows a mushroom-shaped spine synapse in the hippocampal dentate gyrus. (**S** = spine head; **T** = presynaptic terminal; **Den** = main shaft of the dendrite containing a long mitchondrion.) Note the absence of polyribosomes in other parts of the dendritic shaft. × 60,000. (Courtesy of O. Steward, University of Virginia.)

Synthesis of proteins occurs almost exclusively in the cell body and in dendrites. Dendritic translation is made possible by active transport of ribosomes and mRNAs to dentritic spines (Figure 5-2). Most axonal protein is made in the cell body, but some selective translation does occur at nerve endings.

The synthesis of all proteins starts in the cytosol, where mRNA molecules become associated with free ribosomes that are generally linked into small clusters called *polysomes* by the mRNA (see Figures 5-3, 5-4, and 5-5). The final destination of the protein is encoded in its amino acid sequence. A major portion of newly synthesized proteins remain within the cytosol. Cytosolic proteins include the two most abundant groups of proteins in a neuron: the fibrillar elements that make up the cytoskeleton (Chapter 4) and numerous enzymes that catalyze the metabolic reactions of the cell.

Translation of mRNA into protein starts from the 5' end of the mRNA, which encodes the N-terminal end of the protein, and progresses codon by codon until the molecule is finished. Amino acid sequences at the N terminus,

or those within the protein molecule, often have special functions. Thus, certain sequences act as signals and, depending on the particular sequence, ticket the proteins for import into the endoplasmic reticulum, mitochondria, or peroxisomes. A special sequence within the molecule, the nuclear localization signal (NLS), targets the protein for passage into nucleoplasm through the nuclear pores. Other sequences make a protein suitable for posttranslational chemical modifications, which, for example, can direct the modified protein to the membrane. Examples are palmitoylation and isoprenylation, which anchor the protein to the inner leaflet of the plasmalemma. Ubiquitinylation, another post-translational modification, marks the protein for degradation. (These modifications are discussed below.)

Polysomes with nascent polypeptide chains destined to become secretory proteins or proteins of the external cell membrane and vacuolar apparatus attach to the endoplasmic reticulum because of an N-terminal signal sequence. This association gives the endoplasmic reticulum a rough appearance in the electron micro-

Motor neuron in spinal cord

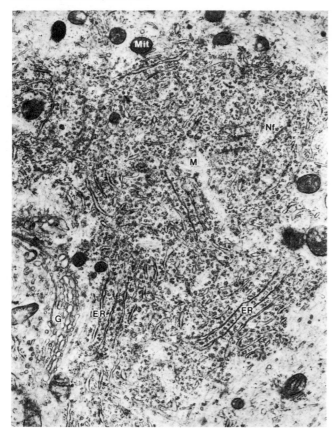

Dorsal root ganglion cell (sensory neuron)

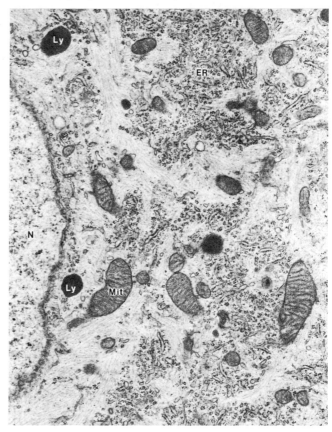

0.7 μm

Figure 5-3 The organelles in the cell body that are chiefly responsible for synthesis and processing of proteins are shown in these electron micrographs. Through the double-layered nuclear envelope that surrounds the nucleus (**N**), mRNA enters the cytoplasm, where it is translated into proteins. Free polysomes, strings of ribosomes attached to a single mRNA, generate cytosolic proteins and proteins to be imported into mitochondria (**Mit**) and peroxisomes. Proteins destined for the endoplasmic reticulum are formed after the polysomes attach to the membrane of the endoplasmic reticulum (**ER**). Both the motor neuron (**left**) and the dorsal root ganglion cell (**right**) have similar kinds of organelles. The particular

region of the motor neuron shown here also includes membranes of the Golgi apparatus (**G**), in which membrane and secretory proteins are further processed. Some of the newly synthesized proteins leave the Golgi apparatus into vesicles that move by rapid axonal transport down the axon to synapses; other membrane proteins are incorporated into lysosomes (**Ly**) and other membranous organelles. The vacuolar apparatus includes the nuclear envelope, the endoplasmic reticulum, the Golgi complex, the lysosomal system, and a variety of transport vesicles. Components of the neuronal cytoskeleton are microtubules (**M**) and neurofilaments (**Nf**). (From Peters et al. 1991.)

scope, hence the name *rough* endoplasmic reticulum.[1] While still undergoing synthesis, these proteins are translocated across the membrane of the endoplasmic reticu-

lum. All other proteins are synthesized on free ribosomes.

The proper function of a protein is defined not only by its primary amino acid sequence, but also by its secondary and tertiary structure, ie, by correct folding of the polypeptide chain. Although information for a protein's tertiary structure is encoded in its amino acid sequence, proper folding may not occur spontaneously. For many proteins, folding is catalyzed by interactions with *chaperones*, proteins that bind to unstructured, exposed regions of the newly synthesized polypeptide. (Two common chaperones are the heat shock proteins,

---

[1]Ribosomal RNA on the rough endoplasmic reticulum stains intensely with basic histological dyes (toluidine blue, cresyl violet, and methylene blue). When viewed under the light microscope, this basophilic material is called *Nissl substance* after the histologist who first described changes in the intensity and distribution of staining in neurons after their axons are cut. These changes, which reflect alterations in the patterns of protein synthesis in injured and regenerating neurons, are discussed in Chapter 55.

Figure 5-4 Protein synthesis on the ribosome. Translation begins at the 5' end of the messenger RNA. Peptide bonds are formed between the nascent polypeptide chain and an aminoacyl tRNA. The tRNA aligns amino acid moieties (**purple circles**) on the ribosome, acting as an adapter to bind its codon in the mRNA. The nascent polypeptide chain, the last (aminoacyl) residue of which remains bound to the mRNA through its tRNA, extends down a groove in the ribosome. When a bond is formed, the tRNA of the last residue of the chain is displaced, and the mRNA is moved in the direction of its 5' end (toward the right in the figure).

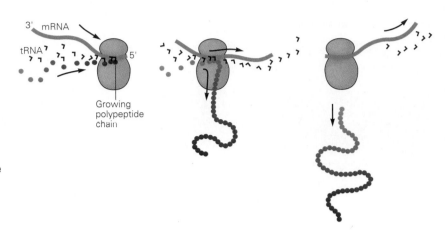

hsp70 and hsp60.) This binding prevents folding until appropriate regions of the protein become available to permit proper folding. Then, in an energy-dependent step, the chaperones are released from the polypeptide.

Proteins May Be Modified During or After Synthesis

Proteins may undergo several modifications by cytosolic enzymes either during synthesis (cotranslational) or afterward (post-translational). A common cotranslational modification is N-acylation, the transfer of an acyl group to the N terminus of the growing polypeptide chain. About 80% of a cell's proteins are acylated. Acylation by a myristoyl group, a 14-carbon saturated fatty acid, is a functionally important example because the modified protein can associate with membrane through the lipid chain:

In proteins that are N-myristoylated the initiator methionine is removed and the next residue becomes the N terminus of the growing chain. While the chain elongates, an acyl group is enzymatically transferred to the new N terminus. N-myristoylated proteins, in which a glycine must be the new N-terminal residue, include the small GTPase Arf; the α-subunit of some trimeric G proteins (the GTPases G_i and G_o); the catalytic subunit of the cAMP-dependent protein kinase; and calcineurin, a major calcium-dependent protein

phosphatase (see Chapter 13). Other fatty acids, notably palmitic acid (16-carbon, unsaturated), can also be conjugated to the sulfhydril group of cysteine residues within proteins:

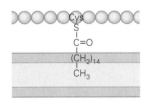

Thioacylation also anchors proteins to the cytosolic leaflet of membranes. This modification occurs, for example, in the GABA-synthesizing enzyme GAD; in the t-SNARE SNAP25, a protein that facilitates the fusion of vesicles with the plasma membranes; in the growth-associated protein GAP-43, which is enriched in growing axons (growth cones) and which binds both calmodulin and actin; and in some α-subunits of trimeric G proteins. Acylation may also occur on cytosolic domains of intrinsic membrane proteins.

Isoprenylation is another post-translational modification important for anchoring proteins to the cytosolic side of membranes. Isoprenylation happens shortly after synthesis is completed and involves a series of enzymatic steps that result in thioacylation by one of two long-chain hydrophobic polyisoprenyl moieties (farnesyl, with 15 carbons, or geranyl-geranyl, with 20) of the sulfhydril group of a cysteine at the C terminus of proteins. Farnesylation occurs on the GTPase Ras while geranyl-geranylation occurs on the Rab GTPases, which have an important role in vesicle transport reactions. These proteins cycle between membrane and cytosol. When soluble in the cytosol they are associated with other proteins that shield the geranyl-geranyl group in a hydrophobic pocket.

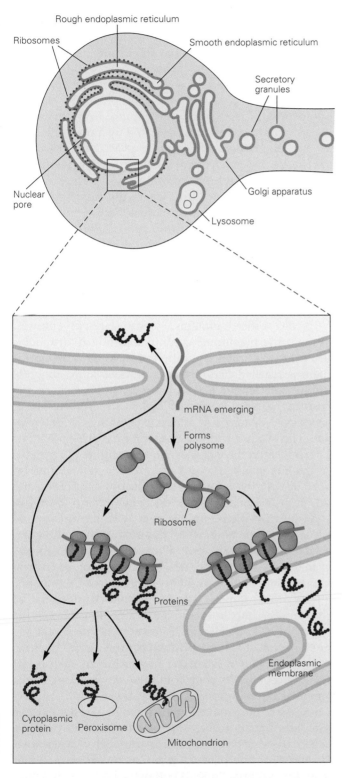

Figure 5-5 Free and membrane-bound polysomes translate mRNAs that encode proteins with a variety of destinations. Messenger RNAs, transcribed from genomic DNA in the neuron's nucleus, emerge through nuclear pores (enlargement) to form polysomes by attaching to ribosomes.

Some post-translational modifications are readily reversible and thus are used to regulate the function of a protein transiently. The most important of these modifications is phosphorylation of the hydroxyl group in Ser, Thr, or Tyr residues by protein kinases. Dephosphorylation is catalyzed by protein phosphatases. (These reactions are discussed in Chapter 13.) As with all post-translational modifications, the sites to be phosphorylated are determined by a particular sequence of amino acids around the residue that is being modified. Phosphorylation can change the properties of a protein (eg, its enzymatic activity or interaction properties) and is probably the most common mechanism for altering physiological processes in a reversible fashion. For example, protein phosphorylation-dephosphorylation reactions regulate the kinetics of ion channels, the activity of transcription factors, the assembly of the cytoskeleton, and the activity of enzymes.

Still another important post-translational modification is the addition of ubiquitin, a highly conserved protein with 76 amino acids, to the ε-amino group of Lys residues within the protein molecule:

Conjugation of ubiquitin requires the energy of ATP. Additional ubiquitin monomers are successively linked to the ε-amino group of a Lys residue within the previously added ubiquitin moiety. Addition of these multiubiquitin chains to a protein tags it for degradation by a proteasome, a large complex containing several different protease subunits. The ATP-ubiquitin-proteasome pathway, which is present in all regions of the neuron (dendrites, cell body, axon, and terminals), is a mechanism for the selective and regulated proteolysis of cytosolic proteins. Until recently proteolysis was thought to be primarily directed to poorly folded, denatured, or aged proteins. Recent evidence indicates, however, that ubiquitin-mediated proteolysis is important in many neuronal processes, including synaptogenesis and long-term memory storage.

Some Proteins Are Synthesized in the Cytosol and Actively Imported by the Nucleus, Mitochondria, and Peroxisomes

Nuclear and peroxisomal proteins, as well as the mitochondrial proteins that are encoded by the cell's nucleus, are formed in the cytosol on free polysomes and are imported only after their synthesis is completed. Import into the nucleus takes place through the nuclear pores and does not involve transport through a membrane. Although the cytosol and nucleoplasm are theoretically continuous, the nuclear pores prevent free intermixing between the two compartments.

Nuclear pores permit only molecules with a size smaller than 10 nm to pass. Most proteins involved in transcription of DNA (DNA polymerases) and in RNA processing (polymerases and splicing enzymes) have much higher molecular masses and thus cannot move passively through the pores. Nuclear uptake of these proteins depends on nuclear localization signals in the amino acid sequence of the proteins. For proteins that need to be returned to the cytosol, export signals are also required. Movement of proteins through nuclear pores requires the energy of ATP.

Proteins that are synthesized in the cytosol and destined for mitochondria and peroxisomes need to cross a phospholipid bilayer. Thus, unlike nuclear proteins, which are imported after they have been folded, these polypeptides reach their native conformation only after import into the target organelle, which occurs soon after the protein is synthesized. The signal for mitochondrial import is an N-terminal amino acid sequence 20–80 residues in length that can form an amphipathic helix, ie, a helix with basic, positively charged (hydrophilic) residues on one face and nonpolar (hydrophobic) residues on the other.

Import of the proteins occurs at special sites where the inner and outer mitochondrial membranes are in contact with each other, and proteins are therefore moved directly into the mitochondrial matrix. Movement of the polypeptide chain through the bilayer of the mitochondrial membranes requires special chaperones both in the cytosol and within the mitochondrion. Interactions with these chaperones result in the hydrolysis of ATP, and some of the energy released during those reactions is harvested for proper folding of the proteins within the mitochondrion.

Secretory Proteins and Proteins of the Vacuolar Apparatus and Plasmalemma Are Synthesized and Modified in the Endoplasmic Reticulum

Most proteins destined to become membrane or lumenal proteins of the vacuolar apparatus, as well as secretory proteins and proteins of the plasmalemma, are translocated across the membrane of the endoplasmic reticulum during synthesis (cotranslational transfer). As noted earlier, their mRNA is translated on polysomes at-

tached to the surface of this organelle (see Figure 5-5). These polysomes are formed from the same population of ribosomes that produce the other proteins in the cell.

A *signal sequence* in the nascent polypeptide induces the attachment of the ribosomes to the rough endoplasmic reticulum as soon as this portion of the nascent polypeptide chain starts protruding from the ribosomes. This attachment is mediated by a macromolecular complex called the *signal recognition particle*. In an energy-dependent process the growing peptide is transported through the lipid bilayer into the lumen of the endoplasmic reticulum, where the signal sequence usually is removed through proteolytic cleavage. The polypeptide continues to grow at its C-terminal end. If the protein does not contain hydrophobic sequences, cotranslational transfer continues until the C terminus itself is transferred across the membrane and the newly synthesized polypeptide becomes a free protein in the lumen (Figure 5-6A).

With other proteins, cotranslational transfer through the membrane continues until a hydrophobic *stop-transfer* segment within the nascent polypeptide chain is reached. Stop-transfer sequences are about 20 residues in length and contain hydrophobic, or uncharged, amino acids followed by several basic residues; they may occur anywhere along the polypeptide. The result is an integral membrane protein with its C terminus on the cytoplasmic side and its N terminus on the lumenal side of the endoplasmic reticulum (Figure 5-6B). If there is an alternating series of insertion and stop-transfer sequences within a single chain, the result is an integral membrane protein with multiple membrane-spanning regions because the polypeptide traversed the membrane several times as it grew. Examples of this type of intrinsic membrane proteins are neurotransmitter receptors and ion channels (see Chapter 6).

As with import into mitochondria, transfer of polypeptides into the endoplasmic reticulum requires the energy of ATP. Transfer is driven in part by the progressive addition of amino acids to the growing polypeptide. It is also assisted by chaperones in the lumen, such as BiP, a homolog of hsp70, which pulls the polypeptide into the lumen of the endoplasmic reticulum.

Some of the proteins synthesized in the endoplasmic reticulum remain in this organelle as resident proteins. Others are targeted to other compartments of the vacuolar apparatus, to the plasmalemma, or to the extracellular space by secretion. Proteins within the lumen of the endoplasmic reticulum are extensively modified. One important modification is the formation of intramolecular disulfide (Cys-S-S-Cys) linkages, a process that cannot occur in the reducing environment of the cytosol. Disulfide linkages are crucial to the tertiary structure of these proteins.

A   Formation of a secretory protein

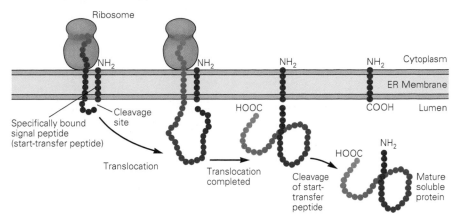

B   Formation of a transmembrane protein

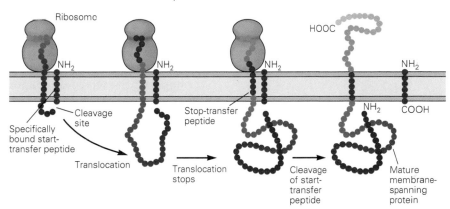

Figure 5-6 The configuration of proteins formed from polysomes attached to the endoplasmic reticulum is determined by the process of translocation through the reticulum's membrane. All of these proteins start with an N-terminal signal sequence with three functionally distinct portions. The first is a short hydrophilic segment that is important for the initiation of insertion but which plays little or no part in the association of the polysome to the signal receptor particle or its release from the docking protein on the membrane of the endoplasmic reticulum. This segment is not itself translocated through the membrane. The second segment is a stretch of 8–16 hydrophobic residues that is essential for translocation of the protein through the membrane. The mechanism of translocation is not yet well understood, but probably requires that some of this hydrophobic segment assume an α-helical structure and that part of it be extended because a stretch of eight hydrophobic residues is sufficient to span the 3 nm width of the membrane if fully extended but is too short in the helical configuration. The third segment, consisting of a few C-

terminal amino acids of the signal sequence, usually begins with glycine or proline (residues that interrupt α-helices) and is known to be important in the removal of the signal sequence by the *signal peptidase* located on the luminal side of the endoplasmic reticulum. (Adapted from Alberts et al. 1994.)

A. If the entire polypeptide chain is translocated through the membrane of the endoplasmic reticulum, a secretory protein results. Note that the N terminus is free because the signal sequence is cleaved, while the C terminus is free because the entire polypeptide chain is translocated.

B. If translocation of the polypeptide chain through the membrane is incomplete, a membrane-spanning protein results. Incomplete translocation occurs because of the presence of a stop-transfer sequence. As in the example shown in **A**, the N-terminal signal sequence is cleaved while the polypeptide chain is being synthesized. The C-terminal end of the completed protein remains within the cytosol.

Another important modification is glycosylation, which occurs on the amino groups of asparagine residues (N-linked glycosylation) and results in the addition *en bloc* of a complex polysaccharide chain. This complex chain is then trimmed and modified within the

lumen of the endoplasmic reticulum by a series of reactions controlled by chaperones, including calnexin and calreticulin. Because of the great chemical specificities of oligosaccharide moieties, these modifications can have important implications for cell function. For example, cell-to-cell interactions that occur during development rely on molecular recognition between glycoproteins present at the surface of the two interacting cells. Moreover, since the same protein can have somewhat different oligosaccharide chains, glycosylation can diversify the function of a protein. Thus, glycosylation increases the repertory of configurations a protein can have.

Some membrane-anchored proteins in the endoplasmic reticulum may also be conjugated to a glycolipid (glycosylphosphatidyl inositol or GPI), resulting in a lipid tail that is anchored to the inner leaflet of the vacuolar membrane:

This modification occurs soon after synthesis and transport through the membrane of the endoplasmic reticulum. These proteins bear a C-terminal recognition sequence 20–30 residues long. In the lumen of the endoplasmic reticulum this sequence is cleaved off, exposing a new C terminus. This free carboxyl group forms a peptide bond with phosphorylethanolamine, which in turn is anchored to the inner leaflet of the membrane through the diacylglycerol moiety of a complex inositol phospholipid. This type of membrane anchor is characteristic of several proteins destined for the outer leaflet of the plasmalemma, including a form of acetylcholinesterase and the neuronal cell adhesion molecule (NCAM). These proteins are destined to face the extracellular space because, as discussed in Chapter 4, the inner leaflet of the endoplasmic reticulum is functionally continuous with the outer leaflet of the plasmalemma.

Secretory Proteins Are Processed Further in the Golgi Complex and Then Exported

Proteins exported from the endoplasmic reticulum are carried to the Golgi complex in transport vesicles that bud off from the reticulum's membrane. There they are modified and then transported to other intracellular locations or secreted. In the electron microscope the Golgi complex appears as stacks of flattened cisternae aligned with one another in long ribbons (see Figures

5-1 and 5-3) and as filamentous structures when visualized by light microscopy with cytochemical markers (see Figure 4-3).

The mechanisms for vesicular transport at all stations of the secretory and endocytic pathways have been remarkably conserved from simple unicellular organisms (yeast) to complex cells (neurons). The generation of transport vesicles from a membrane is assisted by protein *coats*, which assemble at the cytosolic surface of the membrane patches that will form the vesicles. These coats are thought to have two functions. First, they mediate evagination of the membrane into a bud. Second, they select the protein cargo that will be incorporated into the vesicles. There are several types of coats. The clathrin coat assists in budding from the Golgi complex and from the plasmalemma. Two other coats, COPI and COPII, assist the vesicles involved in transport between the endoplasmic reticulum and the Golgi complex. The coats are rapidly lost once free vesicles have formed. Docking and fusion of vesicles with the target membrane is mediated by a hierarchy of molecular interactions, the most important of which is thought to be the reciprocal recognition of small proteins with short membrane anchors on the cytosolic surfaces of the two interacting membranes. The action of these small proteins, called v-SNARE (vesicular SNARE) and t-SNARE (target membrane SNARE), is discussed in Chapter 14 in connection with the role of synaptic vesicles in the release of neurotransmitter at synapses.

Vesicles derived from the endoplasmic reticulum arrive at the *cis* side of the Golgi complex, fuse with the membranes of Golgi cisternae, and thereby deliver their contents into the Golgi complex. The delivered proteins are then thought to travel from one cisterna to the next, from the *cis* to the *trans* side of this organelle, through a series of vesicular transport steps. Each subcompartment (cisterna or set of cisternae) of the Golgi complex is specialized for different types of enzymatic reactions. Several types of protein modifications occur within the lumen of the Golgi complex proper or within the transport station directly adjacent to its *trans* side, the so-called *trans-Golgi network*. These modifications include addition of more N-linked oligosaccharides, O-linked (on the hydroxyl groups of amino acids) glycosylation, phosphorylation, and sulfation. These changes are aimed at increasing the hydrophilicity of the protein (useful for secretory proteins), fine-tuning their ability to bind macromolecular partners, and delaying their degradation. In addition, many membrane and secretory proteins undergo proteolytic cleavage in the trans-Golgi network to generate smaller, biologically active proteins. Thus, in assembly-line fashion, the proteins undergo stepwise changes before leaving the Golgi complex at its *trans* side.

Proteins, both soluble and membrane-bound, that travel beyond the Golgi complex next bud off the trans-Golgi network in vesicles that have different molecular compositions and destinations. Traffic from the trans-Golgi network is responsible for secretion as well as for the delivery of newly synthesized components to the plasmalemma, endosomes, and other membranous organelles (see Figure 4-1B).

One class of vesicles carries newly synthesized plasmalemma proteins and proteins that are continuously secreted (constitutive secretion). These vesicles fuse with the plasmalemma in a nonregulated fashion. Neurons are thought to have at least two types of these vesicles, one targeted to dendrites and the other to the axon. Another class of vesicles, which bud from the trans-Golgi complex by being pinched off with a clathrin coat, delivers lysosomal enzymes to late endosomes.

Still other classes of vesicles transport secretory proteins that are released by an extracellular stimulus (regulated secretion). One type stores secretory products, primarily peptide neurohormones, in concentrated form. These vesicles, called *large dense-core vesicles* because of the electron-dense appearance of their core in the electron microscope, are similar in function and biogenesis to peptide-containing granules of endocrine cells. Large dense-core vesicles are targeted primarily to axons but can be seen in all regions of the neuron. They accumulate in cortical cytoplasm and are highly concentrated in axon terminals, where they undergo calcium-regulated exocytosis. The optimal stimulus for their secretion is a train of action potentials.

An important question that remains poorly understood is how the proteins that form synaptic vesicles, the small lucent vesicles responsible for the release of neurotransmitter, reach axon terminals. There is evidence to suggest that synaptic vesicles are not assembled in the trans-Golgi network but in the axon terminal, and that synaptic vesicle proteins are carried to endosomes and the plasmalemma of nerve terminals in precusor membranes. At the terminals these vesicle precursors would join existing synaptic vesicles as they pass through endosomes during the recycling process to be described in Chapter 14. Release of small-molecule neurotransmitters, stored in synaptic vesicles, occurs by an exocytotic process regulated by Ca^{2+} ion influx (see Chapters 14 and 15).

Surface Membrane and Extracellular Substances Are Taken Up Into the Cell by Endocytosis

Since the mature neurons does not grow, vesicular traffic toward the cell surface is continuously balanced by traf-

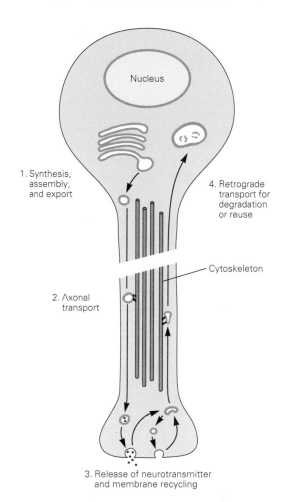

Figure 5-7 Membranes of organelles involved in synaptic transmission are returned to the cell body for reuse or degradation. **1.** Proteins and lipids of secretory organelles are synthesized in the endoplasmic reticulum and transported to the Golgi complex, where large dense-core vesicles (peptide-containing secretory granules) and synaptic vesicle precursor membranes are assembled. **2.** Large dense-core vesicles and transport vesicles that carry synaptic vesicle membrane proteins leave the Golgi complex and travel down the axon via axonal transport. **3.** In nerve terminals the synaptic vesicles are assembled and loaded with nonpeptide neurotransmitters. Synaptic vesicles and large dense-core vesicles release their contents by exocytosis. **4.** Following exocytosis, large dense-core vesicle membranes are returned to the cell body for reuse or degradation. Synaptic vesicle membranes undergo several cycles of exoendocytosis (see Chapter 14) and are eventually returned to the cell body for degradation.

fic back from the plasmalemma to internal organelles. This endocytic traffic, which is essential for maintaining the area of the plasmalemma in a steady state, has several other functions. It alters the activity of many important regulatory molecules on the cell surface (for example, re-

Box 5-1 Neuroanatomical Tracing Relies on Axonal Transport

In the past 20 years the study of neuroanatomy has been revolutionized by the use of a variety of labels to trace neural projections. Previously, the projections of neurons were mapped by cutting axons, allowing them to degenerate, and then locating the affected cell bodies or axons. These studies relied on difficult and sometimes unreliable histochemical staining procedures.

Axonal transport can distribute labeled material throughout the neuron. Neuroanatomists can now locate axons and terminals of specific nerve cell bodies by microinjection of dyes, expression of fluorescent proteins, or by autoradiographically tracing labeled protein soon after administering radioactively labeled amino acids, certain labeled sugars (fucose or amino sugars, precursors of glycoprotein), or specific transmitter substances. Similarly, the location of the cell bodies belonging to specific terminals can be identified by making use of particles, proteins, or dyes that are readily taken up at nerve terminals by endocytosis and transported back to cell bodies. Horseradish peroxidase has been most widely used for this type of study because it readily undergoes retrograde transport and its reaction product is conveniently visualized histochemically (Figure 5-8).

Axonal transport is also used by neuroanatomists to label material exchanged between neurons, making it possible to identify neuronal networks (Figure 5-9).

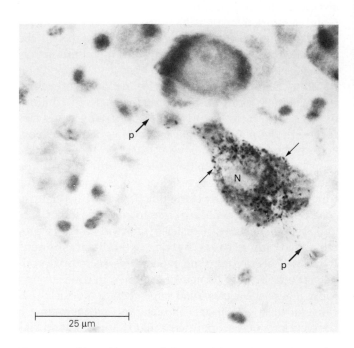

Figure 5-8 Use of horseradish peroxidase to investigate the sources of afferents to the inferior parietal lobule of the cerebral cortex in the rhesus monkey. A cell body in the magnocellular nucleus of the basal forebrain was found to be labeled two days after injection of horseradish peroxidase (HRP) into the cortex. The HRP was taken up by the cell's terminals in the cortex and transported to the cell body. **Thin arrows** indicate HRP reaction product in the cell body; **thick arrows** indicate processes (**p**) in which some reaction product can be seen. N = nucleus. (From Divac et al. 1977.)

ceptors and adhesion molecules). It also directs nutrients and molecules, such as expendable receptor ligands and aged membrane proteins, toward the degradative compartments of the cells. Finally, it is necessary for recycling synaptic vesicles at nerve terminals (Chapter 14).

A significant fraction of endocytic traffic is carried by clathrin-coated vesicles. Clathrin-mediated endocytosis is very selective, since components of the clathrin coat specifically interact via transmembrane receptor proteins with proteins in the extracellular space. For this reason clathrin-mediated internalization is often referred to as *receptor-mediated endocytosis*. Clathrin-coated vesicles eventually shed their coat and fuse with intracellular lysosomal vacuoles called early endosomes, where proteins to be recycled to the cell surface are separated from proteins destined for other intracellular organelles. Patches of plasmalemma membrane can also be internalized through larger, uncoated vacuoles that also fuse with early endosomes (*bulk endocytosis*). Early endosomes are also scattered throughout dendrites. Endocytosed material and membrane to be degraded are passed on to late endosomes. These organelles, which

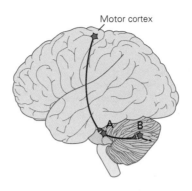

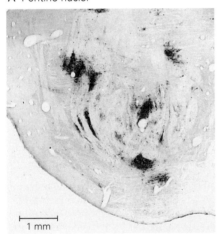

A Pontine nuclei

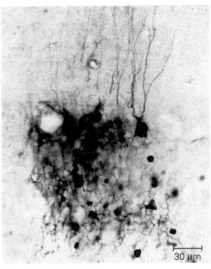

B Cerebellar cortex

Figure 5-9 Use of the herpes simplex virus to trace cortical pathways in monkeys. Depending on the strain, the virus moves in the anterograde or retrograde direction by axonal transport. In either direction it will enter a neuron with which the infected cell makes synaptic contact. Here an anterograde moving strain (HSV-1 [H129]) was used to trace the projections of cells in the primary motor cortex to the cerebellum in monkeys. Monkeys were injected in the region of the primary mo-

tor cortex representing the arm (Chapters 17 and 38). After four days the brain was sectioned and immunostained for viral antigen. The virus was transported from primary motor cortex to second-order neurons in pontine nuclei (**A**) and then to third-order neurons in the cerebellar cortex (**B**). A map of the connections demonstrated by this experiment is shown in the diagram of a brain. (Courtesy of Dr. P. L. Strick.)

are transported by retrograde axonal transport (see below), are concentrated in the proximal segments of dendrites and in the cell body where they fuse with lysosomes.

In the axon endocytosis occurs primarily at nerve terminals, mostly in the recycling of synaptic vesicles. Endocytosis of synaptic vesicles is mediated by the clathrin coat and dynamin. Although true endosomes exist in nerve terminals, they do not seem to play a role in synaptic vesicle recycling; rather, recycled synaptic vesicles are generated directly from clathrin-coated vesicles that lose their coat.

Proteins and Organelles Are Transported Along the Axon

The secretory process in neurons is formally similar to that in other cells. But the primary site of secretion, the axon terminal, is considerably distant from the cell body and dendrites, where secretory proteins are synthesized. For example, in a motor neuron that innervates the muscle of the leg in humans, the distance of the nerve terminals from the cell body can exceed 10,000 times its diameter. The distance between cell body and

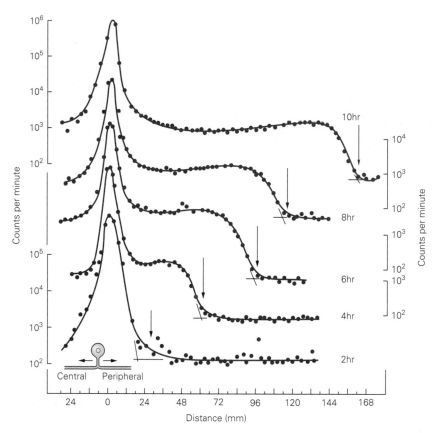

Figure 5-10 Early experiments on axonal transport used radioactive labeling of proteins. In the experiment illustrated here the distribution of radioactive proteins along the sciatic nerve of the cat was measured at various times after injection of [³H]-leucine into dorsal root ganglia in the lumbar region of the spinal cord. In order to show transport curves from various times (2, 4, 6, 8, and 10 hours after the injection) in one figure, several ordinate scales (in logarithmic units) are used. Large amounts of labeled protein stay in the ganglion cell bodies but with time protein moves out along axons in the sciatic nerve and the advancing front of the labeled proteins is displayed progressively farther from the cell body (**arrows**). The velocity of transport can be calculated from the distances displayed at the various times. From experiments of this kind, Sidney Ochs found that the rate of axonal transport is constant at 410 mm per day at body temperature. (Adapted from Ochs 1972.)

nerve terminals means that newly formed membrane and secretory products must be actively transported from the Golgi complex to the end of the axon (Figure 5-7).

In 1948 Paul Weiss tied off a sciatic nerve and observed that axoplasm in the nerve fiber accumulated with time on the proximal side of the ligature. He concluded that axoplasm moves at a slow, constant rate from the cell body toward the terminals in a process he called *axoplasmic flow*. Today we know that the flow Weiss observed consists of several kinetic components, both fast and slow.

Membranous organelles move toward the nerve terminal (anterograde direction) and back toward the cell body (retrograde direction) by *fast axonal transport*, a form of transport that is faster than 400 mm/day in warm-blooded animals. Cytosolic and cytoskeletal proteins move only in the anterograde direction by a much slower form of transport, *slow axonal transport*. Although these transport mechanisms are prominent in the axon, they represent adaptations of mechanisms that facilitate intracellular transport of organelles in all secretory cells. Because of their specialized function in axons, these transport mechanisms have proved to be convenient experimental models for elucidating how organelles are moved in other cells. They have also been used by neuroanatomists to label neurons (Box 5-1).

Fast Axonal Transport Carries Membranous Organelles

Large membranous organelles are transported in the axon, both to and from the cell body, by fast axonal

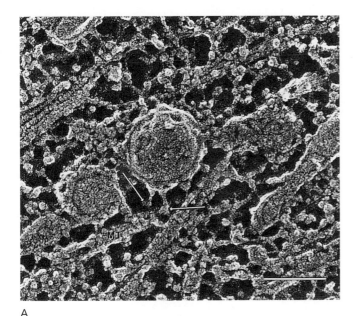

A

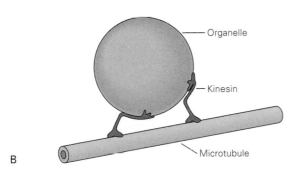

B

Figure 5-11 Kinesin is the motor molecule for anterograde transport in the axon.

A. This quick-freeze, deep-etched electron micrograph from rat spinal cord shows many rod-shaped structures bridging organelles (large round structures) and microtubules (**MT**). Several of these cross-bridges have globular ends that appear to contact the microtubules (**arrows**). Bar = 100 nm.

B. Model for how kinesin may move organelles along microtubules. Kinesin contains a pair of globular heads that bind to microtubules and a fan-shaped tail that binds the organelle to be moved. A hinge region is present near the center of the kinesin molecule. The similarities between kinesin and muscle myosin led to the idea that kinesin moves organelles by "walking" along microtubular tracks. (Adapted from Hirokawa et al. 1989.)

transport. These organelles include vesicles of the constitutive secretory pathway, synaptic vesicle precursor membranes, large dense-core vesicles, mitochondria, and elements of the smooth endoplasmic reticulum. Direct microscopic analysis of the movement of large particles in living axons in culture started as early as 1920. More recently, advances in video microscopy techniques have greatly helped in the visualization of this process. Continuous direct observation using video-enhanced light microscopy reveals that particles are actively transported in a stop-and-start (saltatory) fashion along linear tracks aligned with the main axis of the axon. These tracks have been convincingly shown to be microtubules.

Early experiments on axonal transport traced proteins synthesized in dorsal root ganglion cell bodies by labeling them with radioactive amino acids injected into the ganglion. The distribution of labeled protein along a nerve was obtained from different specimens at various times after the injection and the rate of movement was measured by counting the amount of radioactivity in uniform sequential segments along the nerve (Figure 5-10).

Studies using this system showed that anterograde transport depends critically on ATP, is not affected by inhibitors of protein synthesis (once the labeled amino acid is incorporated), and does not depend on the cell body, since it occurs in nerves actually severed from their cell bodies. In fact, transport occurs in reconstituted axoplasm. Studies with isolated axonal components (in vitro motility assays) have clarified how membranes and other cellular constituents move along nerve processes.

Anterograde transport in the axon depends on microtubules that provide an essentially stationary track on which specific organelles move by means of molecular motors. The saltatory nature of the movement is due to periodic dissociation of the organelle from the track or to collision with other structures. The idea that microtubules are involved first emerged from the finding that colchicine and vinblastine, alkaloids that cause the disruption of microtubules and block mitosis (which is known to depend on microtubules), also interfere with fast transport. About 30 years ago electron microscopists observed cross-bridges between microtubules and vesicular particles that were thought to play a role in moving the particles, and there is now evidence that some of these cross-bridges represent the motors.

The motor molecules for anterograde transport (toward the plus end of microtubules) are *kinesin* and a variety of kinesin-related proteins called KIFs—a large family of ATPases, each of which transports different membrane cargoes. Kinesin is a heterotetramer com-

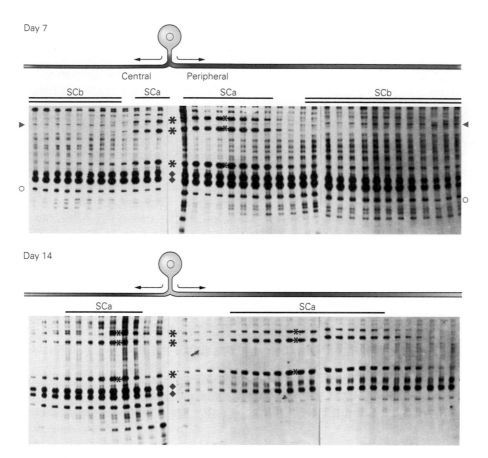

Figure 5-12 The two components of slow axonal transport in the axon of dorsal root ganglion (DRG) cells. Autoradiographs show the advance of different proteins in the axon 7 and 14 days after injecting [^{35}S]methionine into the L5 DRG cells of adult rats. Each lane in these autoradiographs represents the electrophoretic separation on a polyacrilamide gel of proteins in consecutive 2-mm segments of the central and peripheral branches of the axon of injected cells. The major proteins in the slower wave of axonal transport (**SCa**) are the neurofilament proteins (**large asterisks**), with molecular weights of 200,000, 145,000, and 68,000, and the tubulin subunits of the microtubule (**diamonds**), α-tubulin (mol wt 53,000) and β-tubulin (mol wt 57,000). The advance of the SCa wave over one week is indicated by the distance between the peaks of the radioactivity in the neurofilaments (**small asterisks**) at the two time intervals. The constituents of the faster component of axonal transport (**SCb**) are more complex. Three identified proteins are indicated: clathrin (**arrowhead**), actin (**open circle**), and tubulin (**diamonds**). (Courtesy of M. Oblinger.)

posed of two heavy chains and two light chains. Each heavy chain contains a globular head (the ATPase domain) that acts as the motor when attached to microtubules, a coil-coiled helical stalk responsible for dimerization with the other heavy chain, and a fan-like C terminus that interacts with the light chains and represents the organelle-interaction domain (Figure 5-11). These structures had suggested that kinesin moves organelles by "walking" along microtubules. However, the recent discovery of monomeric KIF motors (with only one "foot") has challenged this model.

Rapid transport also occurs in the retrograde direction, from nerve endings toward the cell body. The organelles transported in this direction are primarily endosomes generated by endocytic activity at nerve terminals (multivesicular bodies and other endosomes), mitochondria, and elements of the endoplasmic reticulum. Some of the material endocytosed in nerve endings is destined for the cell body (eg, the membranes of the large dense-core vesicle proteins that are shipped back for reuse). Although much of this material is degraded within lysosomes, retrograde transport is also used to deliver signals to the cell body. For example, activated growth factor receptors are thought to be carried along the axon to their site of action in the nucleus. Certain toxins (tetanus toxin) as well as pathogens (herpes simplex, rabies, and polio viruses) are also transported toward the cell body along the axon.

The rate of retrograde fast transport is about one-half to two-thirds that of fast transport in the antero-grade direction. As in anterograde transport, particles move along microtubules. The motor molecule for retro-grade transport is a microtubule-associated ATPase called MAP-1C. This axonal motor molecule is similar to the dyneins in cilia and flagella and consists of a multimeric protein complex with two globular heads on two stalks connected to a basal structure. The globular heads attach to microtubules and act as motors, moving toward the minus end of the polymer. Like kinesin, the rest of the complex is thought to associate with the or-ganelle being moved.

Slow Axonal Transport Carries Cytosolic Proteins and Cytoskeletal Elements

Whereas subcellular organelles are moved along the axon by fast transport, cytosolic proteins and elements of the cytoskeletal matrix are transported by slow ax-onal transport. Slow axonal transport occurs only in the anterograde direction (from the cell body). It consists of at least two kinetic components that transport different proteins and move at different rates along the axon.

A slower component travels at a rate of 0.2–2.5 mm per day and carries the proteins that make up the fibril-lar elements of the cytoskeleton: the subunits of neuro-filaments and the α- and β-tubulin subunits of micro-tubules (Figure 5-12). These fibrous proteins constitute about 75% of the total protein moved by the slower component. Microtubules move in polymerized form by a mechanism involving microtubule sliding. Rela-tively short preassembled microtubules are transported from the cell body down the axon by interacting with existing microtubules. Neurofilament subunits or short polymers are thought to move passively along with the microtubules because the two polymers are cross-linked by protein bridges.

The faster component of slow axonal transport is about twice as fast as the slower component. The pro-teins carried by this component are more complex, and include clathrin, actin, and actin-binding proteins as well as a variety of cytosolic enzymes and proteins.

An Overall View

Most neuronal proteins are synthesized in the cell body. The proper function of these proteins depends not only on their primary amino acid sequence, but also on cor-rect folding. Folding of proteins during or after synthe-sis is assisted by chaperones, and their final structure is often modified by permanent or reversible post-transla-tional modifications that may affect both the distribu-tion and function of the protein.

Proteins of the cytosol and of the cytoskeleton are made on free ribosomes and moved to all cell regions by diffusion or axonal transport. Proteins of mitochondria and peroxisomes, as well as proteins of the nucleus and some proteins of the vacuolar apparatus, are made in the cytosol and targeted post-translationally to their destination by signals in their amino acid sequence. Most secretory proteins, proteins of the plasmalemma, and proteins of the vacuolar apparatus are made on ribosomes of the rough endoplasmic reticulum and are translocated across the membrane during synthesis. From the rough endoplasmic reticulum they are trans-ported to other compartments of the vacuolar apparatus or to the cell surface by vesicular traffic (the secretory pathway).

Vesicular traffic from the plasmalemma (the endo-cytic pathway) carries proteins to degradative compart-ments or back to the secretory apparatus for reuse. Vesicular transport among intracellular membranes oc-curs with great specificity and results in the vectorial transport of selected membrane components. Since ma-ture neurons grow very little, vesicular transport to any type of membrane is balanced by traffic back to lyso-somes for degradation. Thus, material is transported from one compartment to another without modifying the steady-state composition of any organelle.

A variety of molecular motors drive organelles within the cytosol, resulting in their uneven distribution within the neuron. Concentration of dense-core and synaptic vesicles at axon terminals and their constant renewal is achieved by anterograde and retrograde ax-onal transport along cytoskeletal tracks, primarily microtubules.

James H. Schwartz
Pietro De Camilli

Selected Readings

Grafstein B. 1995. Axonal transport: function and mecha-nisms. In: SG Waxman, JD Kocsis, PK Stys (eds). *The Axon: Structure, Function and Pathophysiology*, pp. 185–199. New York: Oxford Univ. Press.

Hartl FU. 1996. Molecular chaperones in cellular protein folding. Nature 381:571–579.

Holtzman E. 1989. *Lysosomes*. New York: Plenum.

Kelly RB. 1993. Storage and release of neurotransmitters. Cell/Neuron 72/10:43–53.

Kreis T, Vale R (eds). 1999. *Guidebook to the Cytoskeletal and Motor Proteins,* 2nd ed. Oxford: Oxford Univ. Press.

Lodish H, Baltimore D, Berke A, Zipursky SL, Matsudaira P, Darnell T. 1995. *Molecular Cell Biology,* 3rd ed. New York: Scientific American Books.

Nigg EA. 1997. Nucleocytoplasmic transport: signals, mechanisms and regulation. Nature 386:779–787.

Peters A, Palay SL, Webster, H deF. 1991. *The Fine Structure of the Nervous System: Neurons and Their Supporting Cells,* 3rd ed. New York: Oxford Univ. Press.

Rothman JE, Wieland FT. 1996. Protein sorting by transport vesicles. Science 272:227–234.

Schatz G, Dobberstein B. 1996. Common principles of protein translocation across membranes. Science 271:1519–1526.

Schekman R, Orci L. 1996. Coat proteins and vesicle budding. Science 271:1526–1533.

Stryer L. 1995. *Biochemistry,* 4th ed. New York: WH Freeman.

Varshazsky A. 1997. The ubiquitin system. Trends Biochem Sci 22:283–287.

References

Alberts B, Bray D, Lewis J, Raff M, Roberts K, Watson JD. 1994. *Molecular Biology of the Cell,* 3rd ed. New York: Garland.

Benson DL, Cohen PA. 1996. Activity-dependent segregation of excitatory and inhibitory synaptic terminals in cultured hippocampal neurons. J Neurosci 16:6424–6432.

Brady ST. 1991. Molecular motors in the nervous system. Neuron 7:521–533.

Chain DG, Casadio A, Schacher S, Hedge AN, Valbrun M, Yamamoto N, Goldberg AL, Bartsch D, Kandel ER, Schwartz JH. 1999. Mechanisms for generating the autonomous cAMP-dependent protein kinase required for long-term facilitation in *Aplysia*. Neuron 22:147–156.

Cleveland DW, Hoffman PN. 1991. Slow axonal transport models come full circle: evidence that microtubule-sliding mediates axon elongation and tubulin transport. Cell 67:453–456.

Divac I, LaVail JH, Rakic P, Winston KR. 1977. Heterogeneous afferents to the inferior parietal lobule of the rhesus monkey revealed by the retrograde transport method. Brain Res 123:197–207.

Dokas LA. 1983. Analysis of brain and pituitary RNA metabolism: a review of recent methodologies. Brain Res Rev 5:177–218.

Görlich D, Mattaj IW. 1996. Nucleocytoplasmic transport. Science 271:1513–1518.

Hershko A, Ciechanover A. 1998. The ubiquitin system. Annu Revs Biochem 67:425–479.

Hirokawa N. 1997. The mechanisms of fast and slow transport in neurons: identification and characterization of the new Kinesin superfamily motors. Curr Op Neurobiol 7:605–614.

Hirokawa N, Pfister KK, Yorifuji H, Wagner MC, Brady ST, Bloom GS. 1989. Submolecular domains of bovine brain kinesin identified by electron microscopy and monoclonal antibody decoration. Cell 56:867–878.

Hoffman PN, Lasek RJ. 1975. The slow component of axonal transport: identification of major structural polypeptides of the axon and their generality among mammalian neurons. J Cell Biol 66:351–366.

Kreis T, Vale R (eds). 1999. *Guidebook to the Extracellular Matrix and Adhesion Proteins,* 2nd ed. Oxford: Oxford Univ. Press.

McIlhinney RAJ. 1990. The fats of life: the importance and function of protein acylation. Trends Biochem 15:387–391.

McNew JA, Goodman JM. 1996. The targeting and assembly of peroxisomal proteins: some old rules do not apply. Trends Biochem Sci 21:54–58.

Neupert W. 1997. Protein import into mitochondria. Annu Rev Biochem 66:863–917.

Oblinger MM, Lasek RJ. 1985. Selective regulation of two axonal cytoskeletal networks in dorsal root ganglion cells. In: P O'Lague (ed). *UCLA Symposium on Molecular and Cellular Biology.* Vol. 24, *Neurobiology: Molecular Biological Approaches to Understanding Neuronal Function and Development,* pp. 135–143. New York: Liss.

Ochs S. 1972. Fast transport of materials in mammalian nerve fibers. Science 176:252–260.

Ochs S. 1975. Waller's concept of the trophic dependence of the nerve fiber on the cell body in the light of early neuron theory. Clio Med 10:253–265.

Okada Y, Yamazaki H, Sekine-Aizawa Y, Hirokawa N. 1995. The neuron-specific kinesin superfamily protein KIFIA is a unique monomeric motor for anterograde axonal transport of synaptic vesicle precursors. Cell 81:769–780.

Schnapp BJ, Reese TS. 1982. Cytoplasmic structure in rapid-frozen axons. J Cell Biol 94:667–679.

Sossin, W. 1996. Mechanism for the generation of long-term memory: the implications of a requirement for transcription. Trends Neurosci 19:215–218.

Takei K, Mundigl O, Daniell L, De Camilli P. 1996. The synaptic vesicle cycle: a single vesicle budding step involving clathrin and dynamin. J Cell Biol 133:1237–1250.

Vale RD, Fletterick RJ. 1997. Design plan of kinesin motors. Annu Rev Cell Dev Biol 13:745–777.

Vallee RB, Bloom GS. 1991. Mechanisms of fast and slow axonal transport. Annu Rev Neurosci 14:59–92.

Weiss P, Hiscoe HB. 1948. Experiments on the mechanism of nerve growth. J Exp Zool 107:315–395.

Wells DG, Richter JD, Fallon JR. 2000. Molecular mechanisms for activity-regulated protein synthesis in the synapto-dendritic compartment. Curr Op Neurobiol. 10:132–137.

Zemanick MC, Strick PL, Dix RD. 1991. Direction of transneuronal transport of herpes simplex virus 1 in the primate motor system is strain-dependent. Proc Natl Acad Sci USA 88:8048–8051.

6

Ion Channels

NEURONAL SIGNALING DEPENDS on rapid changes in the electrical potential difference across nerve cell membranes. Individual sensory cells can generate changes in membrane potential in response to very small stimuli: receptors in the eye respond to a single photon of light; olfactory neurons detect a single molecule of odorant; and hair cells in the inner ear respond to tiny movements of atomic dimensions. Signaling in the brain depends on the ability of nerve cells to respond to these small stimuli by producing rapid changes in the electrical potential difference across nerve cell membranes.

During an action potential the membrane potential changes quickly, up to 500 volts per second. These rapid changes in membrane potential are mediated by ion channels, a class of integral membrane proteins found in all cells of the body. The ion channels of nerve cells are optimally tuned for rapid information processing. The channels of nerve cells are also heterogeneous, so that different types of channels in different parts of the nervous system can carry out specific signaling tasks.

Because of this selective distribution of finely tuned functional elements, malfunctioning of ion channels in nerve and skeletal muscle can cause a wide variety of neurological diseases (see Chapter 16). Diseases due to ion channel malfunction are not limited to the brain. Cystic fibrosis and certain types of cardiac arrhythmia, for example, are also caused by ion channel malfunction. Moreover, ion channels are often the site of action of drugs, poisons, or toxins. Thus ion channels have crucial roles in both the physiology and the pathophysiology of the nervous system.

Ion Channels Are Important for Signaling in the Nervous System

Ion channels have three important properties: (1) They conduct ions, (2) they recognize and select specific ions, and (3) they open and close in response to specific electrical, mechanical, or chemical signals. The channels in nerve and muscle conduct ions across the cell membrane at extremely rapid rates, thereby providing a large flow of ionic current: up to 100 million ions may pass through a single channel per second. This current flow causes the rapid changes in membrane potential required for signaling, as will be discussed in Chapter 9. The fast rate of flow of ions through channels—10^8 per second—is comparable to the turnover rate of the fastest

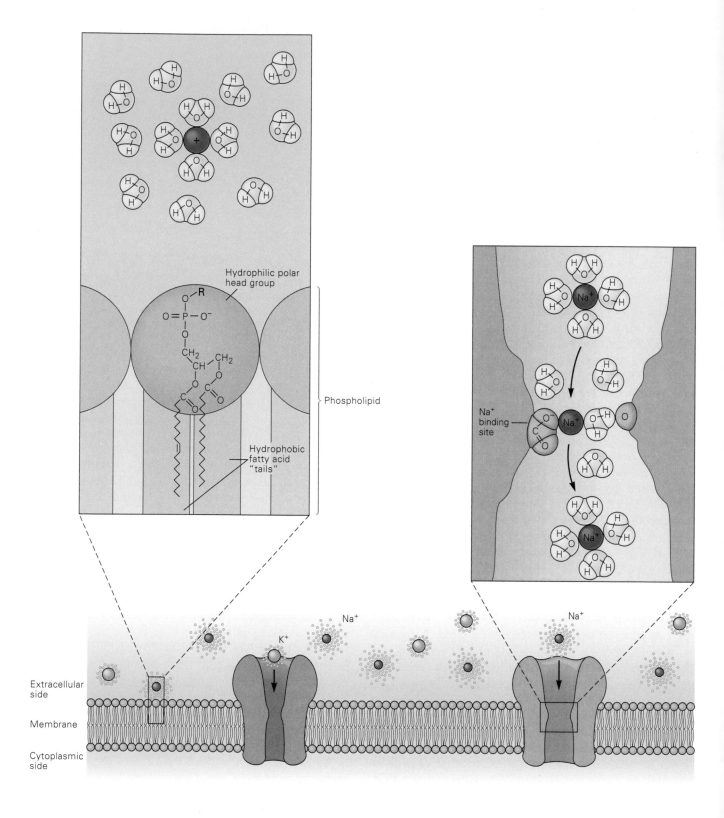

Hydrophilic polar
head group

Phospholipid

Hydrophobic
fatty acid
"tails"

Na+
binding
site

Na+

K+

Na+

Extracellular
side

Membrane

Cytoplasmic
side

enzymes, catylase and carbonic anhydrase, which are limited by diffusion of substrate. (The turnover numbers of most other enzymes are considerably slower, however, ranging from 10 to 1000 per second.)

Despite their ability to conduct ions at high rates, ion channels are surprisingly selective: Each type allows only one or a few types of ions to pass. For example, the membrane potential of nerve cells at rest is largely determined by channels that are selectively permeable to K^+. Typically, these channels are 100-fold more permeable to K^+ than to Na^+. During the action potential, however, ion channels 10- to 20-fold more permeable to Na^+ than to K^+ are activated. Thus, a key to the great versatility of neuronal signaling is the activation of different classes of ion channels, each of which is selective for specific ions.

Finally, many channels are regulated or gated; they open and close in response to various stimuli. *Voltage-gated channels* are regulated by changes in voltage, *ligand-gated channels* by chemical transmitters, and *mechanically gated channels* by pressure or stretch. An individual channel is usually most sensitive to one type of signal. In addition to the gated channels, there are nongated channels that are normally open in the cell at rest. These *resting channels* contribute significantly to the resting potential.

In this chapter we examine four questions: Why do nerve cells have channels? How can channels conduct ions at such high rates and still be selective? How are channels gated? How are the properties of these channels modified by various intrinsic and extrinsic conditions? In addition we compare the molecular structure of various channels and consider how they may have evolved. In succeeding chapters we consider how nongated channels generate the resting potential (Chapter 7), how voltage-gated channels generate the action potential (Chapter 9), and how ligand-gated channels produce synaptic potentials (Chapters 11, 12, and 13).

Ion Channels Are Proteins That Span the Cell Membrane

To appreciate why nerve cells use channels, we need to understand the nature of the plasma membrane and the physical chemistry of ions in solution. The plasma membrane of all cells, including nerve cells, is about 6–8 nm thick and consists of a mosaic of lipids and proteins. The surface of the membrane is formed by a double layer of phospholipids. Embedded within this continuous lipid sheet are integral membrane proteins, including ion channels.

The lipids of the membrane do not mix with water—they are hydrophobic. In contrast, the ions within the cell and those outside strongly attract water molecules—they are hydrophilic (Figure 6-1). The attraction between ions and water results because water molecules are dipolar: although the net charge on a water molecule is zero, charge is separated within the molecule. The oxygen atom in a water molecule tends to attract electrons and so bears a small net negative charge, while the hydrogen atoms tend to lose electrons and

Figure 6-1 (Opposite) The ionic permeability properties of the membrane are determined by the interactions of ions with water, the membrane lipid bilayer, and ion channels. Ion channels are integral membrane proteins that span the lipid bilayer, providing a pathway for ions to cross the membrane. Phospholipids form self-sealing lipid bilayers that are the basis for all cellular membranes. Phospholipids have a hydrophilic head and a hydrophobic tail. The hydrophobic tails join to exclude water and ions, while the polar hydrophilic heads face the aqueous environment of the extracellular fluid and cytoplasm.

Left enlargement: Ions in solution are surrounded by a cloud of water molecules (waters of hydration) that are attracted by the net charge of the ion. This cloud is carried along by the ion as it diffuses through solution, increasing the effective size of the ion. It is energetically unfavorable, and therefore improbable, for the ion to leave this polar environment to enter the nonpolar environment of the lipid bilayer. In the illustration, a positively charged ion (**red**) attracts the electronegative oxygen atoms of the surrounding water molecules. The inset also shows the structure of a phospholipid. It is composed of a backbone of glycerol in which two of its –OH groups are linked by ester bonds to fatty acid molecules. The third –OH group of glycerol is linked to phosphoric acid. The phosphate group is further linked to one of a variety of small, polar, alcohol head groups (**R**).

Bottom: A model showing how ion channels are able to select for either K^+ or Na^+ ions.

Potassium channel (left): Although a Na^+ ion itself is smaller than a K^+ ion, its effective diameter in solution is larger because its local field strength is more intense, causing it to attract a larger cloud of water molecules. Thus, a channel can select for K^+ over Na^+ by excluding hydrated ions whose diameter is larger than the pore.

Sodium channel (right): Sodium channels have a selectivity filter somewhere along the length of the channel, with a site that weakly binds Na^+ ions. According to the hypothesis developed by Bertil Hille and colleagues, a Na^+ ion binds transiently at an active site as it moves through the filter (**right enlargement**). At the binding site the positive charge of the ion is stabilized by a negatively charged amino acid residue on the channel wall and also by a water molecule that is attracted to a second polar amino acid residue on the other side of the channel wall. It is thought that a K^+ ion, because of its larger diameter, cannot be stabilized as effectively by the negative charge and therefore will be excluded from the filter. (Modified from Hille 1984.)

therefore carry a small net positive charge. As a result of this unequal distribution of charge, cations (positively charged ions) are strongly attracted electrostatically to the oxygen atom of water, and anions (negatively charged) are attracted to the hydrogen atoms. Similarly, ions attract water; in fact they become surrounded by electrostatically bound waters of hydration (Figure 6-1).

An ion cannot move away from water into the noncharged hydrocarbon tails of the lipid bilayer in the membrane unless a large amount of energy is expended to overcome the attractive forces between the ion and the surrounding water molecules. For this reason it is extremely unlikely that an ion will move from solution into the lipid bilayer, and therefore the bilayer itself is almost completely impermeable to ions. Ions cross the membrane only through specialized pores or openings in the membrane, such as ion channels, where as we shall see, the energetics favor ion movement.

Ion channels are not simply holes in the lipid membrane but are made up of protein. Although their molecular nature has been known with certainty for only about 15 years, the idea of ion channels dates to the end of the nineteenth century. At that time physiologists knew that, despite the barrier of the cell membrane, cells were nevertheless permeable to many small solutes, including some ions. To explain *osmosis*, the flow of water across biological membranes, Ernst Brücke proposed that membranes contain channels or pores that allow water but not larger solutes to flow across membranes. Later, William Bayliss suggested that a water-filled channel would permit ions to cross the cell membrane easily, since the ions would not need to be stripped of their waters of hydration.

The idea that ions move through channels leads to a question: How can a water-filled channel conduct at high rates and yet be selective? How, for instance, does a channel allow K^+ ions to pass while excluding Na^+ ions? Selectivity cannot be based solely on the diameter of the ion, because K^+, with a crystal radius of 0.133 nm, is larger than Na^+ (crystal radius of 0.095 nm). Because ions in solution are surrounded by waters of hydration, the ease with which an ion moves in solution (its mobility or diffusion constant) does not depend simply on the size of the ion; instead it depends on its size together with the shell of water surrounding it. The smaller an ion, the more highly localized is its charge and the stronger its electric field; smaller ions such as Na^+ have stronger effective electric fields than larger ions such as K^+. As a result, smaller ions attract water more strongly. Thus, as Na^+ moves through solution its strong electrostatic attraction for water causes it to have a larger water shell, which tends to slow it down relative to K^+. Because

of its larger water shell, Na^+ behaves as if it is larger than K^+. In fact, there is a precise relationship between the size of an ion and its mobility in solution: the smaller the ion, the lower its mobility. We therefore can construct a model of a channel that selects K^+ rather than Na^+ simply on the basis of the interaction of the two ions with water in a water-filled channel (Figure 6-1).

Although this model explains how a channel can select K^+ and exclude Na^+, it presents the puzzle of how a channel could select Na^+ and exclude K^+. This problem led many physiologists in the 1930s and 1940s to abandon the channel theory in favor of the idea that ions cross cell membranes by first binding to a specific carrier protein, which then transports the ion through the membrane. In this carrier model, selectivity is based on the chemical binding between the ion and the carrier protein, not on the mobility of the ion in solution.

Even though we now know that ions can cross membranes by means of transporters, the Na^+-K^+ pump being a well-characterized example (Chapter 7), many observations on ion conductance across the cell membrane do not fit the carrier model. Most important is the rapid rate of ion transfer across membranes. This transfer rate was first examined in the early 1970s by measuring the transmembrane current initiated by binding of acetylcholine (ACh) to its receptor in the cell membrane of skeletal muscle fibers at the synapse between nerve and muscle. Using measurements of membrane-current noise (small statistical fluctuations in the mean ionic current induced by ACh), Bernard Katz and Ricardo Miledi concluded that the current initiated by a single ACh receptor is 10 million ions per second. In contrast, the Na^+-K^+ pump is much slower; it can transport at most 100 ions per second. If the ACh receptor acted as a carrier, it would have to shuttle an ion across the membrane in 0.1 μs (one ten-millionth of a second), an implausibly fast rate. The 100,000-fold difference in rates strongly suggests that the ACh receptor (and other ligand-gated receptors) must conduct ions through a channel. Later measurements of current in many voltage-gated pathways selective for K^+, Na^+, and Ca^{2+} also demonstrate large unitary currents, indicating that they too are channels.

But we are still left with the original problem: What makes a channel selective? To explain selectivity, Bertil Hille extended the pore theory by proposing that channels have narrow regions that act as molecular sieves. At this selectivity filter an ion sheds most of its waters of hydration and, in their place, forms weak chemical bonds (electrostatic interactions) with polar (charged) amino acid residues that line the walls of the channel (Figure 6-1). Since it is energetically unfavorable for an ion to shed its waters of hydration, the ion will traverse a channel only if the energy of interaction with the selectivity filter compensates for the loss of waters of hydration. Ions traversing the channel are normally bound to the selectivity filter for only a short time (less than 1 μs), after which the electrostatic and diffusional forces propel the ion through the channel. In channels where the pore diameter is large enough to accommodate several water molecules, an ion need not be stripped completely of its water shell.

How is this chemical recognition and specificity established? One theory was developed in the early 1960s by George Eisenmann to explain the properties of ion-selective glass electrodes (which are similar to pH electrodes but select among the alkali metal cations). According to this theory, a binding site with a high negative field strength—for example, one formed by negatively charged carboxylic acid groups of glutamate or aspartate—will selectively bind Na^+ relative to K^+. This selectivity results because the electrostatic interaction between two charged groups, as governed by Coulomb's law, depends inversely on the distance between the two groups.

Since Na^+ has a smaller radius than K^+, Na^+ can approach a negative site more closely than K^+ and thus will derive a more favorable free-energy change upon binding. This highly favorable free energy of binding will compensate for the requirement that Na^+ lose some of its waters of hydration in order to traverse the narrow selectivity filter. In contrast, a binding site with a low field strength—one that is composed, for example, of polar carbonyl or hydroxyl oxygen atoms—would select K^+ over Na^+. At such a site the binding of Na^+ would not provide a sufficient free energy change to compensate for the loss of the ion's waters of hydration, which Na^+ holds strongly. Since the larger K^+ ions interact more weakly with water, a binding site with a low field strength would be able to compensate for the loss of a K^+ ion's associated water molecules. It is currently thought that ion channels are selective both because of specific chemical interactions and because of molecular sieving based on pore diameter.

Ion Channels Can Be Investigated Using Functional Methods

To understand fully how channels work, we ultimately will need three-dimensional structural information, which has been informative in the study of enzymes and other soluble proteins. X-ray crystallographic and other structural analyses have only recently begun to be applied to integral membrane proteins, such as ion channels, because their transmembrane hydrophobic regions make them difficult to crystallize. However, single-channel recording has provided important functional information that has led to interesting structural interpretations.

Before it became possible to resolve the small amount of current that flows through a single ion channel in biological membranes, channel function was studied in artificial lipid bilayers. In the early 1960s Paul Mueller and Donald Rudin developed a technique for forming functional lipid bilayers by painting a thin drop of phospholipid over a hole in a nonconducting barrier that separates two salt solutions. Although lipid membranes have a very high resistance to ions, ion flux across the membrane increases dramatically when certain peptide antibodies are added to the salt solution. Early studies with a 15–amino acid cyclic peptide, gramicidin A, were especially informative. Application of low concentrations of gramicidin A brings about small step-like changes in current flow across the membrane. These brief pulses of current reflect the all-or-none opening and closing of the single ion channel formed by the peptide.

The current through a single gramicidin channel varies with membrane potential in a linear manner, that is, the channel behaves as a simple resistor (Figure 6-2). The amplitude of the single-channel current can thus be obtained from Ohm's law, $i = V/R$, where i is the current through the single channel, V is the voltage across the channel, and R is the resistance of the open channel. The slope of the relation between i and V yields a value of R for a single open channel of around 8×10^{10} ohms (Figure 6-2B). In dealing with ion channels it is more useful to speak of the reciprocal of resistance or conductance ($\gamma = 1/R$), as this provides an electrical measure of ion permeability. Thus, Ohm's law can be expressed as $i = \gamma \times V$. The conductance of the gramicidin A channel is around 12×10^{-12} siemens, or 12 picosiemens (pS), where 1 siemen equals 1/ohm.

The insights into basic channel properties obtained from artificial membranes were later confirmed in biological membranes by the patch-clamp technique (Box 6-1). A glass micropipette containing ACh—the neurotransmitter that activates the transmitter-gated ion channels in the membrane of skeletal muscle—was pressed tightly against a frog muscle membrane. Small unitary current pulses representing the opening and closing of single ACh-activated ion channels were recorded from the area of the membrane under the pipette tip (Figure 6-3B). As with gramicidin A channels, the relation between current and voltage in these ACh-

A

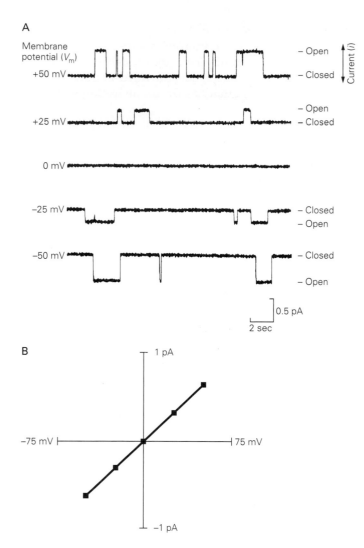

B

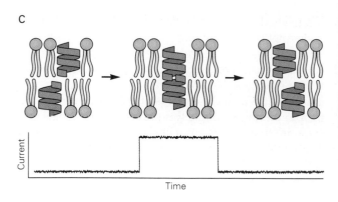

Figure 6-2 Characteristics of the current in a single ion channel. The data presented here were obtained from a channel formed by the addition of gramicidin A molecules to the solution bathing an artificial lipid bilayer.

A. The channel opens and closes in an all-or-none fashion, resulting in brief current pulses through the membrane. If the electrical potential (V_m) across the membrane is varied, the current through the channel (i) changes proportionally. V_m is measured in millivolts (mV); i is measured in picoamperes (pA).

B. A plot of the current through the channel versus the potential difference across the membrane reveals that the current is linearly related to the voltage; in other words, the channel behaves as an electrical resistor that follows Ohm's law ($i = V/R$ or $i = \gamma \times V$). (Data courtesy of Olaf Anderson and Lyndon Providence.)

C. Proposed structure of the gramicidin A channel. A functional channel is formed by end-to-end dimerization of two gramicidin peptides. (From Sawyer et al. 1989.)

activated channels is linear, with a single-channel conductance of around 25 pS.

Ion Channels in All Cells Share Several Characteristics

Most cells are capable of local intercellular signaling, but only nerve and muscle cells are specialized for rapid signaling over long distances. Although nerve and muscle cells have a particularly rich variety and high density of membrane ion channels, their channels do not appear to differ fundamentally from those of other cells in the body. In this section we describe the general properties of ion channels found in a wide variety of cells.

The Flux of Ions Through the Ion Channel Is Passive

The flux of ions through ion channels is passive, requiring no expenditure of metabolic energy by the channels. The direction and eventual equilibrium for this flux is determined not by the channel itself, but rather by the electrostatic and diffusional driving forces across the membrane.

Ion channels select the types of ions that they allow to cross the membrane, allowing either cations or anions to permeate. Some types of cation-selective channels allow the cations that are usually present in extracellular fluid—Na^+, K^+, Ca^{2+}, and Mg^{2+}—to pass almost indiscriminately. However, most cation-selective channels are primarily permeable to a single type of ion, whether it is Na^+, K^+, or Ca^{2+}. Most types of anion-selective

Box 6-1 Recording Current Flow in Single Ion Channels: The Patch Clamp

The patch-clamp technique is a refinement of voltage clamping (see Box 9-1) and was developed in 1976 by Erwin Neher and Bert Sakmann to record current flow from single ion channels. A small fire-polished glass micropipette with a tip diameter of around 1 μm is pressed against the membrane of a skeletal muscle fiber that has been treated with proteolytic enzymes to remove connective tissue from the muscle surface. The pipette is filled with a salt solution resembling that normally found in the extracellular fluid. A metal electrode in contact with the electrolyte in the micropipette connects the pipette to a special electrical circuit that measures the current flowing through channels in the membrane under the pipette tip.

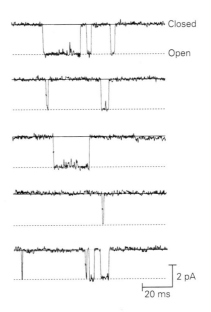

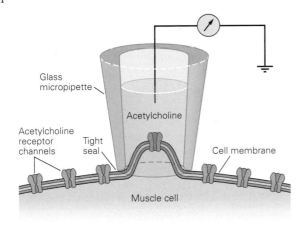

Figure 6-3A Patch-clamp setup. A pipette containing acetylcholine (ACh) is used to record transmitter-gated channels in skeletal muscle. (Adapted from Alberts et al. 1989.)

Figure 6-3B Patch-clamp record of the current flowing through a single ion channel as the channel switches between closed and open states. (Courtesy of B. Sakmann.)

In 1980 Neher discovered that applying a small amount of suction to the patch pipette greatly increased the tightness of the seal between the pipette and the membrane. The result was a seal with extremely high resistance between the inside and the outside of the pipette. The seal lowered the electronic noise and extended the utility of the technique to the whole range of channels involved in electrical excitability, including those with small conductances. Since this discovery, Neher and Sakmann, and many others, have used the patch-clamp technique to study all three major classes of ion channels—voltage-gated, transmitter-gated, and mechanically-gated—in a variety of neurons and other cells.

Christopher Miller independently developed a method for incorporating channels from biological membranes into planar lipid bilayers. With this technique, biological membranes are first homogenized in a laboratory blender; centrifugation of the homogenate then separates out a portion composed only of membrane vesicles. Under appropriate ionic conditions these membrane vesicles will fuse with a planar lipid membrane, incorporating any ion channel in the vesicle into the planar membrane. This technique has two experimental advantages. First, it allows recording from ion channels in regions of cells that are inaccessible to patch clamp; for example, Miller has successfully studied a K^+ channel isolated from the internal membrane of skeletal muscle (the sarcoplasmic reticulum). Second, it allows researchers to study how the composition of the membrane lipids influences channel function.

channels are also highly discriminating; they conduct only one physiological ion, chloride (Cl^-).

The kinetic properties of ion permeation are best described by the channel's conductance, which is determined by measuring the current (ion flux) that flows through the open channel in response to a given electrochemical driving force. The net electrochemical driving force is determined by two factors: the electrical potential difference across the membrane and the concentration gradient of the permeant ions across the membrane. Changing either one can change the net driving force (see Chapter 7).

As we have seen, in some channels the current flow varies linearly with driving force—that is, the channels behave as simple resistors. In others the current flow is a nonlinear function of driving force. This type of channel

Figure 6-4 In many ion channels the relation between current flow through the open channel and membrane voltage is linear. Such channels are said to be "ohmic," because they follow Ohm's law, $i = V_m/R$ or $V_m \times \gamma$, where γ is conductance (**left plot**). In other channels the relation between current and membrane potential is nonlinear (**right plot**). This kind of channel is said to "rectify," in the sense that it tends to conduct ions more readily in one direction (here positive current) than in the other.

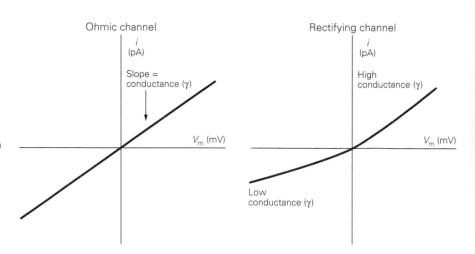

behaves as a rectifier—it conducts ions more readily in one direction than in the other. Whereas the conductance ($\Delta i/\Delta V$) of a resistor-like channel is constant—it is the same at all voltages—the conductance of a rectifying channel is variable and must be determined by plotting current versus voltage over the entire physiological range of membrane potential (Figure 6-4).

The rate of ion flux (current) through a channel depends on the concentration of the ions in the surrounding solution. At low concentrations the current increases almost linearly with concentration. At higher concentrations the current tends to reach a point beyond which it no longer increases with concentration. At this point the current is said to *saturate*.

This saturation effect is consistent with the idea that ion permeation does not strictly obey the laws of electrochemical diffusion in free solution but also involves the binding of ions to specific polar sites within the pore of the channel. A simple electrodiffusion model would predict that the ionic current should continue to increase as long as the ionic concentration also increases: the more charge carriers in solution, the greater the current flow.

The relation between current and ionic concentration for a wide range of ion channels is well described by a simple one-to-one binding equation, suggesting that a single ion binds to the channel during permeation. The ionic concentration at which current flow reaches half its maximum defines the *dissociation constant* for ion binding in the channel. The dissociation constant in plots of current vs concentration is typically quite high, around 100 mM, indicating weak binding. (In typical interactions between enzymes and substrates the dissociation constant is below 1 μM.) This weak interaction indicates that the bonds between the ion and the channel are rapidly formed and broken. In fact, an ion typically stays bound in the channel for less than

1 μs. The rapid off-rate for ion binding is necessary for the channel to achieve the very high conduction rates responsible for the rapid changes in membrane potential during signaling.

Some ion channels are susceptible to occlusion by various free ions or molecules in the cytoplasm or extracellular fluid. Passage through the channel can be blocked by particles that bind either to the mouth of the aqueous pore or somewhere within the pore. If the blocker is an ionized molecule that binds to a site within the pore, it will be influenced by the membrane electric field as it enters the channel. For example, if a positively charged blocker enters the channel from outside the membrane, then making the inside of the membrane more negative—which, according to convention, corresponds to a more negative membrane potential (see Chapter 7)—will drive the blocker into the channel, increasing the block. While blocking molecules are often toxins or drugs that originate outside the body, some are common ions present in the cell or its environment under normal physiological conditions, such as Mg^{2+}, Ca^{2+}, and Na^+, and polyamines such as spermine.

The Opening and Closing of a Channel Involve Conformational Changes

In all ion channels so far studied the channel protein has two or more conformational states that are relatively stable. Each of these stable conformations represents a different functional state. For example, each ion channel has at least one open state and one or two closed states. The transition of a channel between these different states is called *gating*.

Relatively little is known about the molecular mechanisms of gating, other than that they involve a temporary change in the channel's structure. Although the pic-

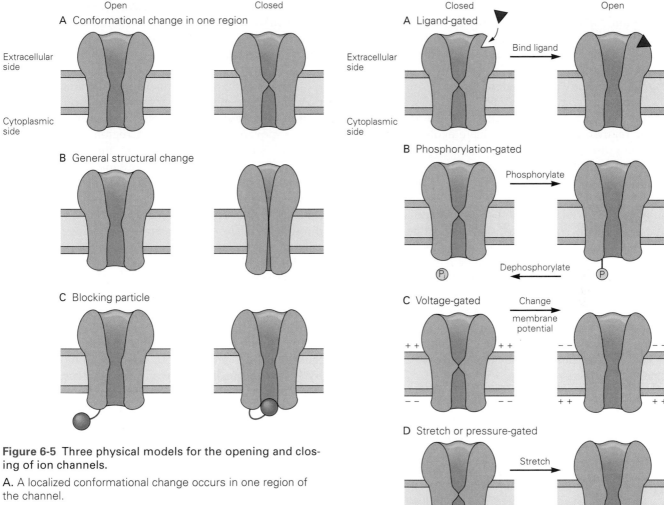

Figure 6-5 Three physical models for the opening and closing of ion channels.

A. A localized conformational change occurs in one region of the channel.

B. A generalized structural change occurs along the length of the channel.

C. A blocking particle swings into and out of the channel mouth.

ture of a gate swinging open and shut is a convenient image, it probably is accurate only for certain channels (for example the inactivation of Na^+ and K^+ channels, which we shall consider in Chapter 9). More commonly, channel gating involves widespread changes in the channel's conformation. For example, evidence from high-resolution electron microscopy and image analysis suggests that the opening and closing of gap junction channels (which we consider in Chapter 10) involve a concerted twisting and tilting of the six subunits that make up the channel. Similar evidence indicates that gating of the ACh-gated channels in skeletal muscle is achieved by a coordinated twisting and bending of the α-helices of each of the five subunits that form the channel pore. The molecular rearrangements that occur during

Figure 6-6 Several types of stimuli control the opening and closing of ion channels.

A. Ligand-gated channels open when the ligand binds to its receptor. The energy from ligand binding drives the channel toward an open state.

B. Protein phosphorylation and dephosphorylation regulate the opening and closing of some channels. The energy for channel opening comes from the transfer of the high-energy phosphate, P_i.

C. Changes in membrane voltage can open and close some channels. The energy for channel gating comes from a change in the electrical potential difference across the membrane, which causes a conformational change by acting on a component of the channel that has a net charge.

D. Channels can be activated by stretch or pressure. The energy for gating may come from mechanical forces that are passed to the channel through the cytoskeleton.

the transition from closed to open states appear to enhance ion conduction through the channel not only by creating a wider lumen, but also by shifting relatively more polar amino acid constituents into the surface that lines the aqueous pore. Three general physical models of channel gating are illustrated in Figure 6-5.

Because the primary function of ion channels in neurons is to generate transient electrical signals, three major regulatory mechanisms have evolved to control the amount of time a channel remains open and active (Figure 6-6). Some channels are regulated by chemical ligands. A ligand can bind directly to the channel—either at an extracellular site, in the case of transmitters, or at an intracellular site, in the case of certain cytoplasmic constituents such as Ca^{2+} and nucleotides. Alternatively, the ligand can activate cellular signaling cascades, which can covalently modify a channel through protein phosphorylation. Other ion channels are regulated by changes in membrane potential. Finally, some channels are regulated by mechanical stretch of the membrane. Under the influence of these regulators, channels enter one of three functional states: closed and activatable (resting), open (active), or closed and nonactivatable (refractory).

The rapid gating actions necessary for moment-to-moment signaling may be influenced by certain long-term changes in the metabolic state of the cell. For example, in some voltage-gated K^+ channels gating is sensitive to intracellular levels of ATP, while in others the gating properties change in response to the redox state of the cell.

For a stimulus to cause a channel to change from the closed to the open state, energy must be supplied. In the case of voltage-gated channels the energy is provided by the movement of a charged region of the channel protein, called the voltage-sensor, through the membrane's electric field. The voltage sensor contains a net electric charge because of the presence of basic (positively charged) or acidic (negatively charged) amino acids. The movement of the charged voltage-sensor through the electric field imparts a net change in free energy to the channel that alters the equilibrium between the closed and open states of the channel. In transmitter-gated channels, on the other hand, gating is driven by the change in chemical free energy that results when the transmitter binds to the receptor site on the channel. For mechanically activated channels the energy associated with membrane stretch is thought to be transferred to the channel either through the cytoskeleton or more directly by changes in tension of the lipid bilayer.

The signals that gate the channel also control the rate of transition between the open and closed states of a

Figure 6-7 Three mechanisms by which voltage-gated channels become closed and nonactivatable (the refractory state).

A. Many voltage-gated channels enter a refractory (inactivated) state after the transition from the resting (closed) state to a transient open state upon membrane depolarization. They recover from the refractory state and return to the resting state only after the membrane potential is restored to its original value.

B. When voltage-dependent Ca^{2+} channels are opened in response to depolarization, the internal Ca^{2+} level rises. The internal Ca^{2+} may then inactivate the channel by binding to a specific recognition site.

C. An increase in internal Ca^{2+} concentration in voltage-gated Ca^{2+} channels may produce inactivation through dephosphorylation of the channel. At pathologically high concentrations, Ca^{2+} may even produce an irreversible inactivation of the channel owing to the recruitment of protein-splitting enzymes activated by the Ca^{2+} ions.

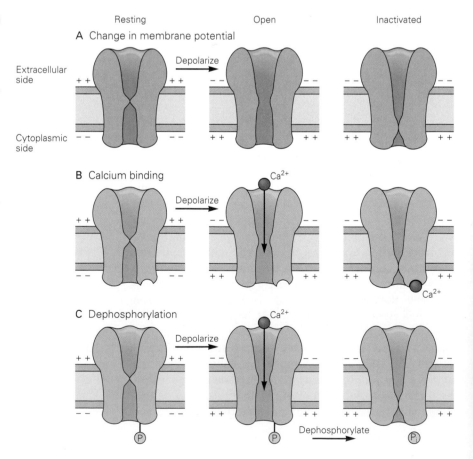

channel. For voltage-gated channels the rates are steeply dependent on membrane potential. Although the time scale can vary from several microseconds to a minute, the transition tends to require a few milliseconds on average. Thus, once a channel opens it stays open for a few milliseconds before closing, and after closing it stays closed for a few milliseconds before re-opening. Once the transition between open and closed states begins, it proceeds virtually instantaneously (in less than 10 μs, the present limit of experimental measurements), thus giving rise to abrupt, all-or-none step-like changes in current through the channel.

Transmitter-gated and voltage-gated channels enter refractory states through different processes. Ligand-gated channels can enter the refractory state when their exposure to the ligand is prolonged. This process, called *desensitization,* is discussed in Chapter 13. The mechanisms underlying desensitization of ion channels are not yet completely understood. In some channels desensitization appears to be an intrinsic property of the interaction between ligand and channel, while in others it is due to phosphorylation of the channel molecule by a protein kinase.

Many, but not all, voltage-gated channels can enter a refractory state after activation. This process is termed *inactivation.* In voltage-gated Na^+ and K^+ channels inactivation is thought to result from an intrinsic conforma-

tional change, controlled by a subunit or region of the channel separate from that which controls activation. (Applying certain proteolytic enzymes within the cell eliminates the ability of voltage-gated Na^+ channels to become inactivated without affecting the channel's ability to be activated.) In contrast, the inactivation of certain voltage-gated Ca^{2+} channels is thought to require Ca^{2+} influx. An increase in internal Ca^{2+} concentration inactivates the Ca^{2+} channel either directly, by binding to a control site on the inside of the channel, or indirectly, by activating an intracellular enzyme that inactivates the channel by protein dephosphorylation (Figure 6-7).

Exogenous factors, such as drugs and toxins, can affect the gating control sites of an ion channel. Most of these agents tend to close the channel; a few open it. Some compounds bind to the same site at which the endogenous gating ligand normally binds and thereby prevent the activator from exerting its usual effect. This binding can be weak and reversible, as in the blockade of the nicotinic ACh-gated channel in skeletal muscle by curare, a South American arrow poison (see Chapter 11). Or it can be strong and not reversible, as in the blockade of the same channel by the snake venom α-bungarotoxin. Other exogenous substances act in a noncompetitive manner and affect the normal gating mechanism without directly interacting with a ligand-binding site.

Figure 6-8 The binding of exogenous ligands, such as drugs, can make an ion channel favor either an open or a closed state through a variety of mechanisms.

A. In channels that are normally opened by the binding of an endogenous ligand (A_1, A_2), a drug or toxin may block the binding of the activator by means of either a reversible (A_3) or an irreversible (A_4) reaction.

B. Some exogenous regulators can make a channel favor the open state by binding to a regulatory site, distinct from the endogenous site that normally opens the channel.

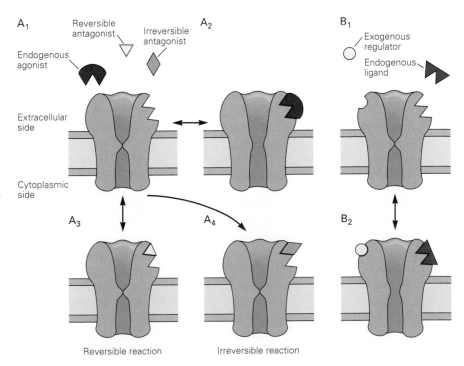

A

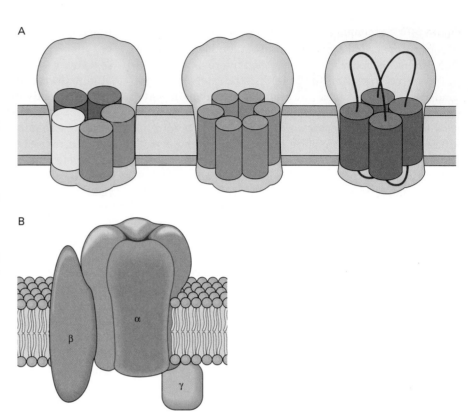

Figure 6-9 Ion channels are composed of several subunits.

A. Ion channels can be constructed as heterooligomers from distinct subunits (**left**), as homooligomers from a single type of subunit (**middle**), or from a single polypeptide chain organized into repeating motifs, where each motif functions as the equivalent of one subunit (**right**).

B. In addition to one or more pore-forming α subunits, which comprise a central core, some channels contain auxiliary subunits (β or γ), which modulate the inherent gating characteristics of the central core.

B

For example, binding of the drug valium to a regulatory site on GABA-gated Cl^- channels prolongs the opening of the channels in response to GABA. This type of indirect effect works not only on ligand-gating, but also on gating controlled by voltage or stretch (Figure 6-8).

The Structure of Ion Channels Is Inferred From Biophysical, Biochemical, and Molecular Biological Studies

What do ion channels look like? How does the channel protein span the membrane? What happens to the structure of the channel when it opens and closes? Where along the length of the channel do drugs and transmitters bind?

Biochemical and molecular biological approaches have resulted in considerable progress toward an understanding of channel structure and function. All ion channels have a basic glycoprotein component consisting of a large integral-membrane protein with carbohydrate groups attached to its surface. A central aqueous pore through the middle of the protein spans the entire width of the membrane. The pore-forming region of many channels is made up of two or more subunits, which may be identical or different (Figure 6-9). In addi-

tion, some channels have auxiliary subunits that modify their functional properties. These subunits may be cytoplasmic or embedded in the membrane.

The genes for most of the major classes of ion channels have now been cloned and sequenced. The primary amino acid sequence of the channel, inferred from its DNA sequence, has been used to create models of the structure of different channel proteins. These models rely on computer programs to predict regions of secondary structure, such as the arrangement of the amino acid residues into α-helices and β-sheets that are likely to correspond to membrane-spanning domains of the channel (Figure 6-10). The predictions, in turn, are based on existing information from proteins whose actual structure is known from electron and x-ray diffraction analysis.

The first membrane protein whose structure was well understood is bacteriorhodopsin, a photopigment in the cell membrane of *Halobacterium*. (Photopigment converts sunlight into electrochemical energy.) Bacteriorhodopsin contains regions with charged (hydrophilic) amino acids and other regions with uncharged (hydrophobic) amino acids. There are, in all, seven hydrophobic regions. Each of these is about 15–20 amino acids long and spans the membrane in the form of α-helices. These membrane-spanning regions are in turn

Figure 6-10 Secondary structure of membrane-spanning proteins.

A. A proposed secondary structure for a subunit of the nicotinic ACh-gated receptor channel. Each cylinder represents a putative membrane-spanning α-helix containing around 20 hydrophobic amino acid residues. The membrane segments are connected by cytoplasmic or extracellular segments (loops) of hydrophilic residues.

B. The membrane-spanning regions of an ion channel can be identified using a hydrophobicity plot. Here a running average of the hydrophobicity is plotted for the entire amino acid sequence for the α subunit of the nicotinic ACh receptor. Each point in the plot represents the average hydrophobic index of a 19–amino acid–long window plotted at the amino acid residue position corresponding to the midpoint of the window. This plot is based on the inferred amino acid sequence obtained from the nucleotide sequence of the cloned ACh receptor. Four of the hydrophobic regions (M1–M4) correspond to the membrane-spanning segments. The first hydrophobic region is the signal sequence that is required during protein synthesis to position the hydrophilic amino terminus of the protein on the extracellular surface of the cell. The signal sequence is cleaved from the mature protein. (From Schofield et al. 1987.)

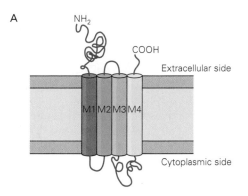

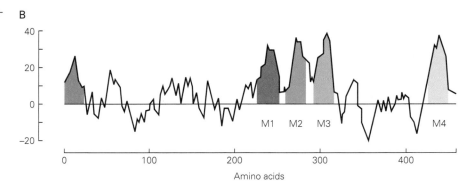

linked by six hydrophilic loops—three that extend outside the cell and three within it.

Additional insights into channel structure and function have been obtained by comparing the primary amino acid sequences of the same type of channel from different species. Regions that show a high degree of similarity (ie, have been highly conserved through evolution) are likely to be important in maintaining the effective structure and function of the channel. Likewise, conserved regions in different, but related, channels are likely to serve a common biophysical function in different channels. For example, all voltage-gated channels have a specific membrane-spanning domain that contains positively charged amino acids (lysine or arginine) spaced at every third position along an α-helix. This motif is observed in all voltage-gated channels, but not in transmitter-gated channels, suggesting that this charged region is important for voltage gating (see Chapter 9).

Once a structure for a channel has been proposed, it can be tested in several ways. For example, antibodies can be raised against synthetic peptides that correspond to different hydrophilic regions in the protein sequence. Immunocytochemistry can then be used to determine whether the antibody binds to the extracellular or cytoplasmic surface of the membrane, thus defining whether a particular region of the channel is extracellular or intracellular.

The functional consequences of changes in a channel's primary amino acid sequence can be explored through a variety of techniques. One particularly versatile approach is to use genetic engineering to construct channels in which various parts are derived from the genes of different species—so-called chimeric channels. This technique takes advantage of the fact that channels in different species have somewhat different properties. For example, the bovine ACh-gated receptor-channel has a slightly greater single-channel conductance than the same channel in electric fish. By comparing the properties of a chimeric channel to those of the two original channels, we can assess which regions of the channel are involved in which functions. This technique has been used to identify a specific membrane-spanning segment of the ACh-gated channel as the region that forms the lining of the pore (see Chapter 11).

The roles of different amino acid residues or stretches of residues can be tested using site-directed mutagenesis, a type of genetic engineering in which

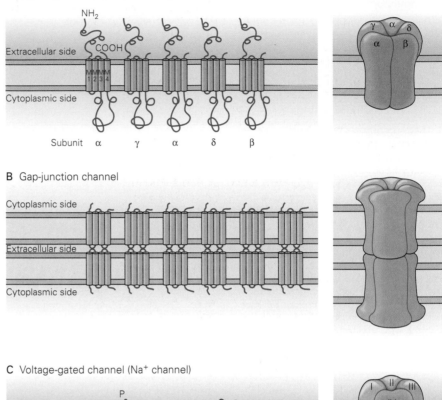

A Ligand-gated channel (ACh receptor)

Figure 6-11 Three families of ion channels.

A. Certain ligand-gated channels, including the nicotinic acetylcholine (ACh) receptor-channel, have five subunits, and each subunit consists of four transmembrane regions (M1–M4). Each cylinder represents a single transmembrane α-helix. A three-dimensional model of the channel is shown on the right.

B. The gap-junction channel, found at electrical synapses, is formed from a pair of hemichannels in the pre- and postsynaptic membranes that join in the space between two cells. Each hemichannel is made of six subunits, each with four transmembrane regions. A three-dimensional model of the two apposite hemichannels is illustrated on the **right**.

C. The voltage-gated Na⁺ channel is formed from a single (α) polypeptide chain that contains four homologous domains or repeats (motifs I–IV), each with six α-helical membrane-spanning regions (S1 to S6) and one P region thought to line the pore. The figure at the **right** shows a hypothetical model of the channel.

B Gap-junction channel

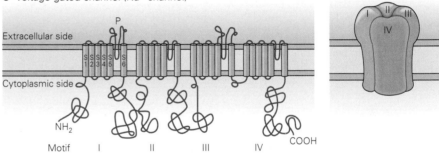

C Voltage-gated channel (Na⁺ channel)

specific amino acid residues are substituted or deleted. Finally, one can exploit the naturally occurring mutations in channel genes that underlie neurological diseases. Changes in functional phenotype are known to result from a number of spontaneously arising mutations in the genes that encode ion channels in nerve or muscle. Many of these effects have been localized to changes in single amino acids within channel proteins.

Ion Channels Can Be Grouped Into Gene Families

Most of the ion channels that have been described in nerve and muscle cells fall into a few gene families (Figure 6-11). Members of each gene family have similar amino acid sequences and transmembrane topology.

Each family is thought to have evolved from a common ancestral gene by gene duplication and divergence.

Genes that encode ligand-gated ion channels that are activated by acetylcholine, γ-aminobutyric acid (GABA), and glycine belong to one family. Each of these channels is composed of five closely related subunits. Each subunit has four transmembrane α-helixes (M1–M4). The members of the ligand-gated channel family can differ from each other in their ion selectivity in addition to their ligand specificity. The genes that encode the glutamate-activated channels may form a family distinct from other ligand-gated channels (see Chapter 12).

The genes coding for gap junction channels belong to a separate family. Each gap junction channel is composed of 12 identical subunits, each of which has four

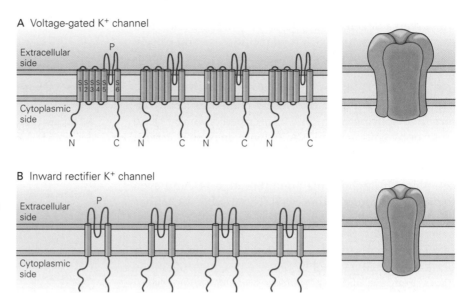

A Voltage-gated K⁺ channel

B Inward rectifier K⁺ channel

C Two-pore domain K⁺ channel

Figure 6-12 Three related families of K⁺-selective ion channels.

A. Voltage-gated K⁺ channels are composed of four polypeptide subunits. Each subunit corresponds to one repeated domain of a voltage-gated Na⁺ or Ca²⁺ channel, with six transmembrane segments and a loop through the extracellular face of the membrane (the so-called P region).

B. Inward-rectifier K⁺ channels are composed of four polypeptide subunits. Each subunit has only two transmembrane segments, connected by a P-region loop.

C. A third family of K⁺ channels has a characteristic subunit structure corresponding to two repeats of the inward-rectifier K⁺ channel architecture, with two P-regions in tandem. The subunit composition of these channels is not known.

membrane-spanning segments. These specialized channels bridge the cytoplasm of two cells at electrical synapses (see Chapter 10).

The genes that encode the voltage-gated ion channels responsible for generating the action potential all belong to a third family. These channels are activated by depolarization and are selective for Ca²⁺, Na⁺, or K⁺. All voltage-gated channels have a similar architecture. They contain four repeats of a basic motif composed of six transmembrane segments (S1–S6). The S5 and S6 segments are connected by a loop, through the extracellular face of the membrane, the P-region, that forms the selectivity filter of the channel. A single subunit of voltage-gated Na⁺ and Ca²⁺ channels contains four of these repeats. Potassium channels are composed of four separate subunits, each containing one repeat.

The major gene family encoding the voltage-gated K⁺ channels is more distantly related to two other families of K⁺-selective channels with distinctive properties and structure (Figure 6-12). One family consists of the genes encoding inward rectifying K⁺ channels, which are activated by hyperpolarization. Each channel subunit has only two transmembrane segments, connected by a pore-forming P-region. A second family of K⁺-selective channels is composed of subunits with two repeated pore-forming segments. These channels may also contribute to the resting K⁺ conductance.

The fast pace of molecular biological research is rapidly leading to the identification of additional ion channel gene families. These include Cl⁻ channels important for determining the resting potential of certain nerve and skeletal muscle cells and a class of ligand-gated channels activated by ATP, which functions as a neurotransmitter at certain synapses. As the genes for additional ion channels are sequenced, more channel families will likely be revealed.

Since most channels are made up of multiple subunits that can be combined in different permutations to produce channel with different functional properties, the number of different channel types is enormous.

More than a dozen basic types of channels are known to exist in neurons, and each type includes several closely related forms (isoforms) that differ in their rate of opening or closing and their sensitivity to different activators. This variability is produced either by differential expression of two or more closely related genes, by alternative splicing of mRNA transcribed from the same gene, or by editing of mRNA. As with enzyme isoforms, variants of a channel type are differentially expressed at specific developmental stages (Figure 6-13), in different cell types throughout the brain (Figure 6-14), and even in different regions within a cell. These subtle variations in structure and function presumably allow channels to perform highly specific functions

The complexity of ion channels in a multicellular organism is underscored by the recent sequencing of the entire genome of the nematode *Caenorhabditis elegans*. The genome contains five genes for voltage-gated Ca^+ channels, over 60 genes for K^+-selective channels, 90 genes for ligand-gated channels, and six genes for Cl^--selective channels. *C. elegans* has no voltage-gated Na^+ channels.

The rich variety of ion channels in different types of cells may make it possible to develop drugs that can activate or block channels in selected regions of the nervous system. Such drugs would, in principle, have maximum therapeutic effectiveness with a minimum of side effects.

The Structure of a Potassium-Selective Ion Channel Has Been Solved by X-ray Crystallography

Rod MacKinnon and his colleagues have recently provided the first high-resolution X-ray crystallographic analysis of the molecular architecture of an ion-selective channel. To overcome the difficulties inherent in obtaining crystals of integral membrane proteins, they used a bacterial K^+ channel that is a member of the inward-rectifier type of K^+ channels that are also present in higher organisms, including mammals. These channels have the advantage of having a relatively small size and a simple transmembrane topology (see Figure 6-12). The structure of the channel was further simplified using molecular engineering to truncate cytoplasmic regions that are not essential for forming the ion-selective pore.

The crystal structure determined from the resulting protein provides several important insights into the mechanisms by which the channel facilitates selectively the movement of K^+ ions across the hydrophobic lipid bilayer. The channel is made up of four identical subunits arranged symmetrically around a central pore (Figure 6-15). Each subunit contributes two membrane-spanning α-helices that are connected by a loop, the P region, that forms the selectivity filter of the channel.

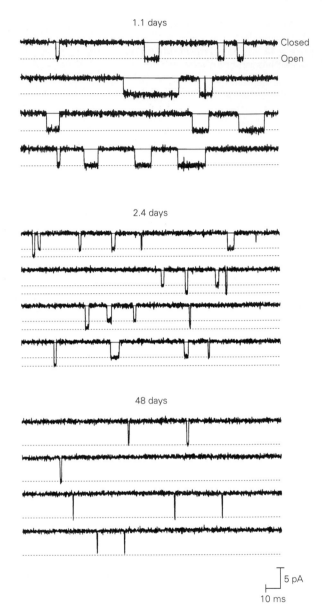

Figure 6-13 The functional properties of ion channels can change over the course of development. These examples of conductance in individual acetylcholine-activated channels were recorded from frog skeletal muscle at three stages of development: early (1.1 days), intermediate (2.4 days), and late (48 days). In immature muscle the single channels have a small conductance and a relatively long open time. In mature muscle the channel conductance is larger, and the average open time is shorter. At intermediate stages of development the population of channel variants is mixed; both long and short openings and both large and small classes of conductance are evident. (From Owens and Kullberg 1989.)

Figure 6-14 Variants of the voltage-gated potassium channel in the rat are expressed in different regions of the brain. When one of the genes *(KShIII)* that encodes voltage-gated K⁺ channels in the rat is transcribed, the pre-RNA molecule is alternatively spliced in four different versions. The four transcripts vary widely in their distributions throughout the nervous system **(A–D)**, thereby contributing to the regional specialization of neuronal function. Each panel shows the expression pattern for one transcript. Dark areas of these autoradiograms represent high densities of the corresponding mRNA transcript. The brain was sectioned at the level of the posterior thalamus. Thalamic nuclei: **VPL**, ventral posterior lateral; **VPM**, ventral posterior medial; **MD**, medial dorsal; **LD**, lateral dorsal; **VM**, ventromedial; **PO**, posterior; **RT**, reticular. Hippocampal regions **CA1, CA2, CA3**; **DG**, dentate gyrus; **ZI**, zona incerta.

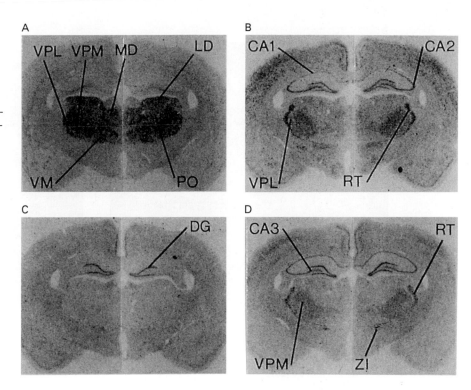

The two α-helices are tilted away from the central axis of the pore at the extracellular side of the channel. The resulting structure has the appearance of an inverted teepee.

The four inner α-helices from each of the subunits line the region of the pore on the cytoplasmic end. At the extracellular end of the channel the two helices from each subunit are connected by a region consisting of three elements: (1) a chain of amino acids that surrounds the mouth of the channel (the turret region); (2) an abbreviated α-helix (the pore helix) about 10 amino acids in length that projects into the membrane around the wall of the pore between the inner membrane-spanning helices; and (3) a 10-amino acid chain that forms a loop that lines the selectivity filter (Figure 6-15A, B).

The shape and structure of the pore determine its ion-conducting properties. Both the inner and outer mouths of the pore are lined by acidic amino acids, whose negative charge helps to attract selectively cations from the bulk solution. Going from inside to outside, the pore consists of a medium width, 18 Å-long tunnel, which leads into a wider (10 Å diameter) spherical inner chamber, both of which are lined predominantly by the side chains of hydrophobic amino acids. A high throughput rate is insured by the fact that the inner 28 Å of the channel lacks polar groups that could delay ion passage by binding and unbinding reactions with the channel wall. These relatively wide regions are followed by the very narrow selectivity filter, which is rate-limiting for the passage of ions and only 12 Å in length.

As an ion passes from the polar bulk solution into a nonpolar medium like the lipid bilayer, the energetically most unfavorable region is in the middle of the bilayer. This high energetic cost is minimized by two details of channel structure: the enlarged, water filled inner chamber provides a highly polar environment, which is enhanced by the fact that the pore helices provide a dipole whose electronegative carboxyl end is pointing towards this inner chamber (Figure 6-15C, D).

The selectivity filter is lined by three main-chain carbonyl atoms of the protein backbone of each of the four subunits. The negative polarization of these 12 carbonyl groups provides a highly polar environment for the K⁺ ions as they traverse the channel. The amino acid side groups of the selectivity filter, which are directed away from the central axis of the channel, help to stabilize the filter at a critical width, such that it provides optimal electrostatic interactions with K⁺ ions as they pass, but is too wide for smaller Na⁺ ions to interact effectively with all four carbonyl oxygens at any point along the length of the filter (Figure 6-15C).

X-ray analysis also shows that the channel is occu-

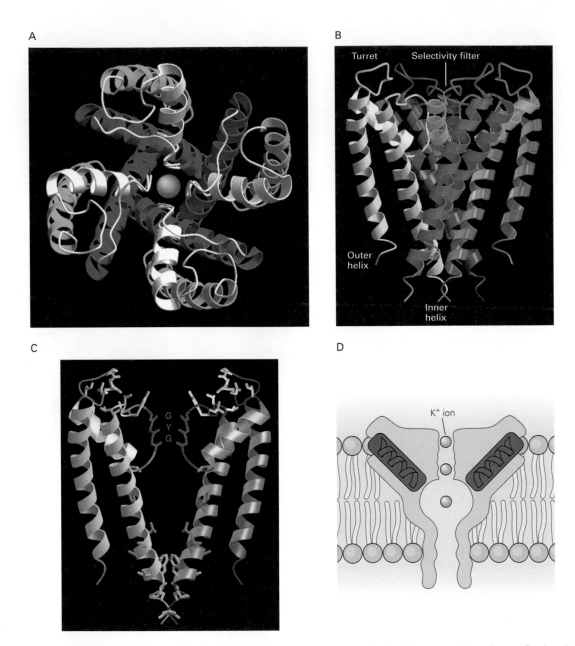

Figure 6-15 The X-ray crystal structure of a bacterial member of the inward rectifying K$^+$ channel family. (From Doyle et al., 1998)

A. A view looking down at the channel from the outside of the membrane. Each of the four subunits contributes two long membrane spanning helixes (in **blue** and **red**). The P-region is shown in **white**. It consists of a short α-helix (pore helix) and a loop that forms the selectivity filter of the channel. A K$^+$ ion is shown in the middle of the pore.

B. A view of the channel in cross section in the plane of the membrane. The four subunits are shown, with each subunit in a different color. The membrane-spanning helixes are arranged as an inverted teepee.

C. Another view in the same orientation as **B,** showing only two of the four subunits. The selectivity filter (**red** region) is formed by three carbonyl oxygen atoms from the main chain backbone of three amino acid residues—glycine (G), tyrosine (Y), and glycine (G). Other residues important for binding of channel-blocking toxins and drugs are labeled in **white.**

D. A side-view of the channel illustrating three K$^+$ sites within the channel. The pore helices contribute a negative dipole that helps stabilize the K$^+$ ion in the water-filled inner chamber. The two outer K$^+$ ions are loosely bound to the selectivity filter formed by the P-region.

pied by three K^+ ions. One K^+ ion is found in the wide, inner chamber. Up to two K^+ ions can occupy the selectivity filter at any one time (Figure 6-15D). If only one K^+ ion were in the channel the ion would be bound rather tightly, and the throughput rate for ion permeation would be compromised. But the mutual electrostatic repulsion that occurs when two K^+ ions occupy the two nearby sites insures that they can linger only briefly, thus ensuring a high overall K^+ conductance.

Thus we see that channels have developed multiple strategies for achieving both high selectivity and high throughput. Based on the homology of the bacterial K^+ channel pore with the pore in channels of higher organisms, we also find that this strategy has been conserved from prokaryotes through humans.

An Overall View

Ion channels regulate the flow of ions across the membrane in all cells. In nerve and muscle cells they are important for controlling the rapid changes in membrane potential associated with the action potential and with the postsynaptic potentials of target cells. In addition, the influx of Ca^{2+} ions controlled by these channels can alter many metabolic processes within cells, leading to the activation of various enzymes and other proteins, as well as release of neurotransmitter (see Chapter 15).

Channels differ from one another in their ion selectivity and in the factors that control their opening and closing, or gating. Ion selectivity is achieved through physical-chemical interaction between the ion and various amino acid residues that line the walls of the channel pore. Gating involves a change of the channel's conformation in response to an external stimulus, such as voltage, a ligand, or stretch or pressure.

Three methodological advances have greatly increased our understanding of channel function. First, the patch-clamp technique has made it possible to record the current flow through single open channels. Second, gene cloning and sequencing have determined the primary amino acid sequences of many genes that encode ion channels. From these results, many of the channels described so far can be grouped into three major gene families: voltage-gated channels and their related subfamilies, a large family of ligand-gated channels, and gap-junction channels. Finally, X-ray crystallography has provided a detailed view of the three-dimensional structure of one simple type of K^+-selective channel.

The activity of channels can be modified by cellular metabolic reactions, including protein phosphorylation; by various ions that act as blockers; and by toxins, poi-

sons, and drugs. Channels are also important targets in various diseases. Certain autoimmune neurological disorders, such as myasthenia gravis, result from the actions of specific antibodies that interfere with channel function (see Chapter 16). Other diseases, such as hyperkalemic periodic paralysis, involve ion channel defects resulting from genetic mutations. Detailed knowledge of the genetic basis of channel structure and function may one day make it possible to devise new pharmacological therapies for specific neurological and psychiatric disorders.

Steven A. Siegelbaum
John Koester

Selected Readings

Andersen OS, Koeppe RE II. 1992. Molecular determinants of channel function. Physiol Rev 72:S89–S158.

Catterall WA. 1993. Structure and function of voltage-gated ion channels. Trends Neurosci 16:500–506.

Eisenberg RS. 1990. Channels as enzymes. J Membr Biol 115:1–12.

Hille B. 1992. *Ionic Channels of Excitable Membranes*, 2nd ed. Sunderland, MA: Sinauer.

Miller C. 1987. How ion channel proteins work. In: LK Kaczmarek, IB Levitan (eds). *Neuromodulation: The Biological Control of Neuronal Excitability*, pp. 39–63. New York: Oxford Univ. Press.

References

Alberts B, Bray D, Lewis J, Raff M, Roberts K, Watson JD. 1994. *Molecular Biology of the Cell*, 3rd ed. New York: Garland.

Anderson CR, Stevens CF. 1973. Voltage clamp analysis of acetylcholine produced end-plate current fluctuations at frog neuromuscular junction. J Physiol (Lond) 235:655–691.

Armstrong CM. 1981. Sodium channels and gating currents. Physiol Rev 61:644–683.

Armstrong DL. 1989. Calcium channel regulation by calcineurin, a Ca^{2+}-activated phosphatase in mammalian brain. Trends Neurosci 12:117–122.

Bargmann, CI. 1998. Neurobiology of the *Caenorhabditis elegans* genome. Science 282:2028–2033.

Bayliss WM. 1918. *Principles of General Physiology*, 2nd ed., rev. New York: Longmans, Greene.

Brücke E. 1843. Beiträge zur Lehre von der Diffusion tropfbarflüssiger Korper durch poröse Scheidenwände. Ann Phys Chem 58:77–94.

Doyle DA, Cabral JM, Pfuetzner RA, Kuo A, Gulbis JM, Cohen SL, Chait BT, MacKinnon R. 1998. The structure of the potassium channel: molecular basis of K⁺ conduction and selectivity. Science 280:69–77.

Eisenman G. 1962. Cation selective glass electrodes and their mode of operation. Biophys J 2(Suppl 2):259–323.

Frech GC, VanDongen AM, Schuster G, Brown AM, Joho RH. 1989. A novel potassium channel with delayed rectifier properties isolated from rat brain by expression cloning. Nature 340:642–645.

Guharay F, Sachs F. 1984. Stretch-activated single ion channel currents in tissue-cultured embryonic chick skeletal muscle. J Physiol (Lond) 352:685–701.

Hamill OP, Marty A, Neher E, Sakmann B, Sigworth FJ. 1981. Improved patch-clamp techniques for high-resolution current recording from cells and cell-free membrane patches. Pflügers Arch 391:85–100.

Henderson R, Unwin PNT. 1975. Three-dimensional model of purple membrane obtained by electron microscopy. Nature 257:28–32.

Hladky SB, Haydon DA. 1970. Discreteness of conductance change in bimolecular lipid membranes in the presence of certain antibiotics. Nature 225:451–453.

Horn R, Patlak J. 1980. Single channel currents from excised patches of muscle membrane. Proc Natl Acad Sci U S A 77:6930–6934.

Huang K-S, Radhakrishnan R, Bayley H, Khorana HG. 1982. Orientation of retinal in bacteriorhodopsin as studied by cross-linking using a photosensitive analog of retinal. J Biol Chem 257:13616–13623.

Imoto K, Methfessel C, Sakmann B, Mishina M, Mori Y, Konno T, Fukuda K, Kurasaki M, Bujo H, Fujita Y, Numa S. 1986. Location of a δ-subunit region determining ion transport through the acetylcholine receptor channel. Nature 324:670–674.

Katz B, Miledi R. 1970. Membrane noise produced by acetylcholine. Nature 226:962–963.

Katz B, Thesleff S. 1957. A study of the 'desensitization' produced by acetylcholine at the motor end-plate. J Physiol (Lond) 138:63–80.

Kyte J, Doolittle RF. 1982. A simple method for displaying the hydropathic character of a protein. J Mol Biol 157:105–132.

MacKinnon R. 1995. Pore loops: an emerging theme in ion channel structure. Neuron 14:889–892.

Miller C (ed). 1986. Ion Channel Reconstitution. New York: Plenum.

Mueller P, Rudin DO, Tien HT, Wescott WC. 1962. Reconstitution of cell membrane structure in vitro and its transformation into an excitable system. Nature 194:979–980.

Mullins LJ. 1961. The macromolecular properties of excitable membrane. Ann NY Acad Sci 94:390–404.

Neher E, Sakmann B. 1976. Single-channel currents recorded from membrane of denervated frog muscle fibres. Nature 260:799–802.

Noda M, Takahashi H, Tanabe T, Toyosato M, Kikyotani S, Furutani Y, Hirose T, Takashima H, Inayama S, Miyata T, Numa S. 1983. Structural homology of Torpedo californica acetylcholine receptor subunits. Nature 302:528–532.

Owens JL, Kullberg R. 1989. In vivo development of nicotinic acetylcholine receptor channels in Xenopus myotomal muscle. J Neurosci 9:1018–1028.

Sawyer DB, Koeppe RE II, Andersen OS. 1989. Induction of conductance heterogeneity in gramicidin channels. Biochemistry 28:6571–6583.

Schofield PR, Darlison MG, Fujita N, Burt DR, Stephenson FA, Rodriguez H, Rhee LM, Ramachandran J, Reale V, Glencorse TA, Seeburg PH, Barnard EA. 1987. Sequence and functional expression of the GABA_A receptor shows a ligand-gated receptor super-family. Nature 328:221–227.

Tempel BL, Papazian DM, Schwarz TL, Jan YN, Jan LY. 1987. Sequence of a probable potassium channel component encoded at Shaker locus of Drosophila. Science 237:770–775.

Urry DW. 1971. The gramicidin A transmembrane channel: a proposed $\Pi_{(L,D)}$ helix. Proc Natl Acad Sci U S A 68:672–676.

Weiser M, Vega-Saenz de Miera E, Kentros C, Moreno H, Franzen L, Hillman D, Baker H, Rudy B. 1994. Differential expression of Shaw-related K⁺ channels in the rat central nervous system. J Neurosci 14:949–972.

7

Membrane Potential

INFORMATION IS CARRIED WITHIN and between neurons by electrical and chemical signals. Transient electrical signals are particularly important for carrying time-sensitive information rapidly and over long distances. These electrical signals—receptor potentials, synaptic potentials, and action potentials—are all produced by temporary changes in the current flow into and out of the cell that drive the electrical potential across the cell membrane away from its resting value.

This current flow is controlled by ion channels in the cell membrane. We can distinguish two types of ion channels—resting and gated—by their distinctive roles in neuronal signaling. Resting channels normally are open and are not influenced significantly by extrinsic factors, such as the potential across the membrane. They are primarily important in maintaining the resting membrane potential, the electrical potential across the membrane in the absence of signaling. Most gated channels, in contrast, are closed when the membrane is at rest. Their probability of opening is regulated by the three factors we considered in the last chapter: changes in membrane potential, ligand binding, or membrane stretch.

In this and succeeding chapters we consider how transient electrical signals are generated in the neuron. We begin by discussing how resting ion channels establish and maintain the resting potential. We also briefly describe the mechanism by which the resting potential can be perturbed, giving rise to transient electrical signals such as the action potential. In Chapter 8 we shall consider how the passive properties of neurons—their resistive and capacitive characteristics—contribute to local signaling within the neuron. In Chapter 9 we shall examine how voltage-gated Na^+, K^+, and Ca^{2+} channels generate the action potential, the electrical signal conveyed along the axon. Synaptic and receptor potentials are considered in Chapters 10–13 in the context of synaptic signaling between neurons.

The Resting Membrane Potential Results From the Separation of Charges Across the Cell Membrane

Every neuron has a separation of charges across its cell membrane consisting of a thin cloud of positive and negative ions spread over the inner and outer surfaces of the cell membrane (Figure 7-1). At rest a nerve cell has an excess of positive charges on the outside of the membrane and an excess of negative charges on the inside. This separation of charge is maintained because the lipid bilayer of the membrane blocks the diffusion of ions, as explained in Chapter 6. The charge separation gives rise to a difference of electrical potential, or voltage, across the membrane called the *membrane potential*. The membrane potential (V_m) is defined as

$$V_m = V_{in} - V_{out},$$

where V_{in} is the potential on the inside of the cell and V_{out} the potential on the outside.

The membrane potential of a cell at rest is called the *resting membrane potential*. Since, by convention, the potential outside the cell is defined as zero, the resting potential (V_r) is equal to V_{in}. Its usual range in neurons is −60 mV to −70 mV. All electrical signaling involves brief changes from the resting membrane potential due to alterations in the flow of electrical current across the cell membrane resulting from the opening and closing of ion channels.

The electric current that flows into and out of the cell is carried by ions, both positively charged (cations) and negatively charged (anions). The direction of current flow is conventionally defined as the direction of *net* movement of *positive charge*. Thus, in an ionic solution cations move in the direction of the electric current, anions in the opposite direction. Whenever there is a net flow of cations or anions into or out of the cell, the charge separation across the resting membrane is disturbed, altering the polarization of the membrane. A reduction of charge separation, leading to a less negative membrane potential, is called *depolarization*. An increase in charge separation, leading to a more negative membrane potential, is called *hyperpolarization*. Changes in membrane potential that do not lead to the opening of gated ion channels, are called *electrotonic potentials* and are said to be passive responses of the membrane. Hyperpolarizing responses are almost always passive, as are small depolarizations. However, when depolarization approaches a critical level, called the *threshold*, the cell responds actively with the opening of voltage-gated ion channels, which at threshold produces an all-or-none *action potential* (Box 7-1).

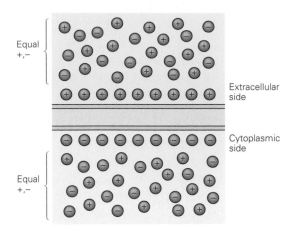

Figure 7-1 The membrane potential results from a separation of positive and negative charges across the cell membrane. The excess of positive charges (red circles) outside the membrane and negative charges (blue circles) inside the membrane of a nerve cell at rest represents a small fraction of the total number of ions inside and outside the cell.

We begin examining the membrane potential by analyzing how the passive flux of individual ion species through resting channels generates the resting potential. We shall then be able to understand how the selective gating of different types of ion channels generates the action potential, as well as the receptor and synaptic potentials.

The Resting Membrane Potential Is Determined by Resting Ion Channels

No single ion species is distributed equally on the two sides of a nerve cell membrane. Of the four most abundant ions found on either side of the cell membrane, Na^+ and Cl^- are more concentrated outside the cell, and K^+ and organic anions (A^-) are more concentrated inside. The organic anions are primarily amino acids and proteins. Table 7-1 shows the distribution of these ions inside and outside one particularly well-studied nerve cell process, the giant axon of the squid, whose blood has a salt concentration similar to sea water. Although the absolute values of the ionic concentrations for vertebrate nerve cells are two- to threefold lower than those for the squid giant axon, the concentration *gradients* (the ratio of the external ion concentration to internal ion concentration) are about the same.

The unequal distribution of ions raises several important questions. How do ionic gradients contribute to the resting membrane potential? How are they maintained? What prevents the ionic gradients from dissipating by diffusion of ions across the membrane through

Box 7-1 Recording the Membrane Potential

Reliable techniques for recording the electrical potential across cell membranes were developed in the late 1940s. These techniques allow accurate recordings of both the resting and the action potentials and make use of glass micropipettes filled with a concentrated salt solution that serve as electrodes. These microelectrodes are placed on either side of the cell membrane. Wires inserted into the back ends of the pipettes are connected via an amplifier to an oscilloscope, which displays the amplitude of the membrane potential in volts. Because the tip diameter of a microelectrode is very small ($<1\ \mu M$), it can be inserted into a cell with relatively little damage to the cell membrane.

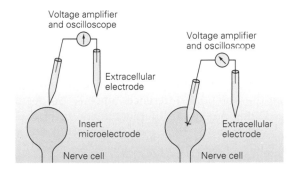

Figure 7-2A The recording setup.

When both electrodes are outside the cell no electrical potential difference is recorded. But as soon as one microelectrode is inserted into the cell the oscilloscope shows a steady voltage, the resting membrane potential. In most nerve cells at rest the membrane potential is around -65 mV.

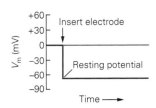

Figure 7-2B Oscilloscope display.

The membrane potential can be experimentally changed using a current generator connected to a second pair of electrodes—one intracellular and one extracellular. When the intracellular electrode is made positive with respect to the extracellular one, a pulse of positive current from the current generator will cause current to flow into the neuron from the intracellular electrode. This current returns to the extracellular electrode by flowing outward across the membrane. As a result, the inside of the membrane becomes more positive while the outside of the membrane becomes more negative. This progressive *decrease* in the normal separation of charge is called *depolarization*.

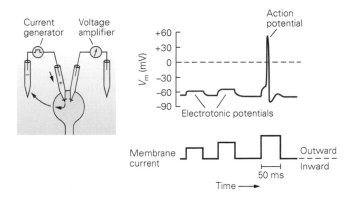

Figure 7-2C Depolarization.

Small depolarizing current pulses evoke purely electrotonic (passive) potentials in the cell—the size of the change in potential is proportional to the size of the current pulses. However, sufficiently large depolarizing current triggers the opening of voltage-gated ion channels. The opening of these channels leads to the action potential, which differs from electrotonic potentials not only in the way in which it is generated but also in magnitude and duration.

Reversing the direction of current flow—making the intracellular electrode negative with respect to the extracellular electrode—makes the membrane potential more negative. This *increase* in charge separation is called *hyperpolarization*.

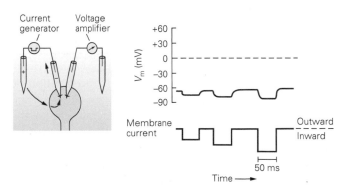

Figure 7-2D Hyperpolarization.

The responses of the cell to hyperpolarization are usually purely electrotonic—as the size of the current pulse increases, the hyperpolarization increases proportionately. Hyperpolarization does not trigger an active response in the cell.

Table 7-1 Distribution of the Major Ions Across a Neuronal Membrane at Rest: the Giant Axon of the Squid

Species of ion	Concentration in cytoplasm (mM)	Concentration in extracellular fluid (mM)	Equilibrium potential[1] (mV)
K^+	400	20	−75
Na^+	50	440	+55
Cl^-	52	560	−60
A^- (organic anions)	385	—	—

[1]The membrane potential at which there is no net flux of the ion species across the cell membrane.

the passive (resting) channels? These questions are interrelated, and we shall answer them by considering two examples of membrane permeability: the resting membrane of glial cells, which is permeable to only one species of ions, and the resting membrane of nerve cells, which is permeable to three. For the purposes of this discussion we shall consider only the resting ion channels, which are always open.

Resting Channels in Glial Cells Are Selective for Potassium Only

A membrane's overall selectivity for individual ion species is determined by the relative proportions of the various types of ion channels in the cell that are open. The simplest case is that of the glial cell, which has a resting potential of about −75 mV. Here, the vast majority of resting channels in the membrane are permeable only to K^+. As a result, the glial cell membrane at rest is almost exclusively permeable to K^+ ions. A glial cell has a high concentration of K^+ and negatively charged organic anions on the inside and a high concentration of Na^+ and Cl^- on the outside.

How do these ionic gradients generate the membrane potential of the glial cell? Because K^+ ions are present at a high concentration inside the cell and glial cells are selectively permeable to them, K^+ ions tend to diffuse from inside to outside the cell, down their chemical concentration gradient. As a result, the outside of the membrane accumulates a positive charge (due to the slight excess of K^+) and the inside a negative charge (because of the deficit of K^+ and the resulting slight excess of anions). Since opposite charges attract each other, the excess positive charges on the outside and the excess negative charges on the inside collect locally on either surface of the membrane (see Figure 7-1).

The diffusion of K^+ out of the cell is self-limiting.

The separation of charge resulting from the diffusion of K^+ gives rise to an electrical potential difference: positive outside, negative inside. The more K^+ continues to flow, the more charge will be separated and the greater will be the potential difference. Since K^+ is positively charged, this potential difference tends to oppose the further efflux of K^+. Thus, ions are subject to two forces driving them across the membrane: (1) a *chemical driving force* that depends on the concentration gradient across the membrane and (2) an *electrical driving force* that depends on the electrical potential difference across the membrane. Once K^+ diffusion has proceeded to a certain point, a potential develops across the membrane at which the electrical force driving K^+ into the cell exactly balances the chemical force driving K^+ ions out of the cell. That is, the outward movement of K^+ (driven by its concentration gradient) is equal to the inward movement of K^+ (driven by the electrical potential difference across the membrane). This potential is called the potassium equilibrium potential, E_K (Figure 7-3). In a cell permeable only to K^+ ions, E_K determines the resting membrane potential, which in most glial cells is about −75 mV.

The equilibrium potential for any ion X can be calculated from an equation derived in 1888 from basic thermodynamic principles by the German physical chemist Walter Nernst:

$$E_X = \frac{RT}{zF} \ln \frac{[X]_o}{[X]_i}, \quad \textbf{Nernst Equation}$$

where R is the gas constant, T the temperature (in degrees Kelvin), z the valence of the ion, F the Faraday constant, and $[X]_o$ and $[X]_i$ are the concentrations of the ion outside and inside of the cell. (To be precise, chemical activities should be used rather than concentrations.)

Since RT/F is 25 mV at 25°C (room temperature), and the constant for converting from natural logarithms

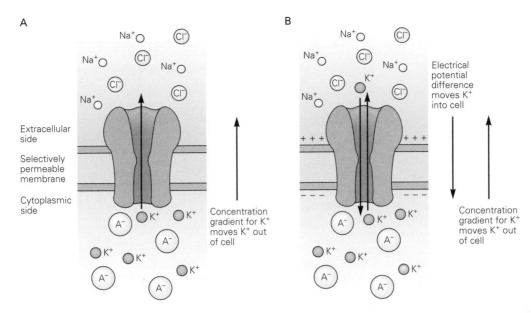

Figure 7-3 The flux of K$^+$ across the membrane is determined by both the K$^+$ concentration gradient and the electrical potential across the membrane.

A. In a cell permeable only to K$^+$ the resting potential is generated by the efflux of K$^+$ down its concentration gradient.

B. The continued efflux of K$^+$ builds up an excess of positive charge on the outside of the cell and leaves behind on the inside an excess of negative charge. This buildup of charge leads to a potential difference across the membrane that impedes the further efflux of K$^+$, so that eventually an equilibrium is reached: the electrical and chemical driving forces are equal and opposite, and as many K$^+$ ions move in as move out.

to base 10 logarithms is 2.3, the Nernst equation can also be written as:

$$E_X = \frac{58 \text{ mV}}{z} \log \frac{[X_o]}{[X_i]}.$$

Thus, for K$^+$, since $z = +1$ and given the concentrations inside and outside the squid axon in Table 7-1:

$$E_K = \frac{58 \text{ mV}}{1} \log \frac{[20]}{[400]} = -75 \text{ mV}.$$

The Nernst equation can be used to find the equilibrium potential of any ion that is present on both sides of a membrane permeable to that ion (the potential is sometimes called the *Nernst potential*). The Na$^+$, K$^+$, and Cl$^-$ equilibrium potentials for the distributions of ions across the squid axon are given in Table 7-1.

In our discussion so far we have treated the generation of the resting potential by the diffusion of ions down their chemical gradients as a passive mechanism, one that does not require the expenditure of energy by the cell, for example through hydrolysis of ATP. However, as we shall see below, energy (and ATP hydrolysis) *is* required to set up the initial concentration gradients and to maintain them during the activity of a neuron.

Resting Channels in Nerve Cells Are Selective for Several Ion Species

Measurements of the resting membrane potential with intracellular electrodes and flux studies using radioactive tracers show that, unlike glial cells, nerve cells at rest are permeable to Na$^+$ and Cl$^-$ ions in addition to K$^+$ ions. Of the abundant ion species in nerve cells only the large organic anions (A$^-$)—negatively charged proteins and amino acids—are unable to permeate the cell membrane. How can the concentration gradients for the three permeant ions (Na$^+$, K$^+$, and Cl$^-$) be maintained across the membrane of a single cell, and how do these three gradients interact to determine the cell's resting membrane potential?

To answer these questions, it will be easiest to examine first only the diffusion of K$^+$ and Na$^+$. Let us return to the simple example of a cell having only K$^+$ channels, with concentration gradients for K$^+$, Na$^+$, Cl$^-$, and A$^-$ as shown in Table 7-1. Under these conditions the resting membrane potential, V_r, is determined solely by the K$^+$ concentration gradient and will be equal to E$_k$ (-75 mV) (Figure 7-4A).

Now consider what happens if a few resting Na$^+$ channels are added to the membrane, making it slightly

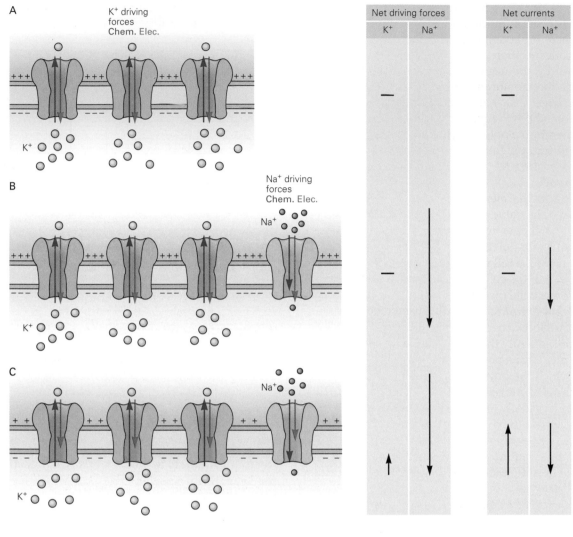

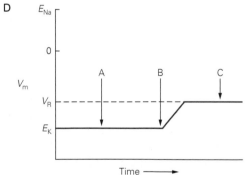

Figure 7-4 The resting potential of a cell is determined by the relative proportion of different types of ion channels that are open, together with the value of their equilibrium (Nernst) potentials. In this simplified diagram the channels shown represent the entire complement of K$^+$ or Na$^+$ channels in the cell membrane. The lengths of the arrows within the channels represent the relative amplitudes of the electrical (**red**) and chemical (**blue**) driving forces acting on Na$^+$ and K$^+$. The lengths of the arrows on the **right** denote the net driving

force on a particular ion (that is, the sum of the electrical and chemical driving forces) and the relative sizes of the different net ion fluxes. Three hypothetical situations are illustrated.

A. In a resting cell in which only K$^+$ permeant channels are present, K$^+$ ions are in equilibrium and $V_m = E_K$.

B. Adding a few Na$^+$ channels to the resting membrane at a given time allows Na$^+$ ions to diffuse into the cell, and this influx begins to depolarize the membrane.

C. The resting potential settles at a new resting potential, which is the value of V_m where $I_{Na} = -I_K$. In this example the aggregate conductance of the K$^+$ channels is much greater than that of the Na$^+$ channels because the K$^+$ channels are more numerous. As a result, a relatively small net driving force for K$^+$ ions drives a current equal and opposite to the Na$^+$ current driven by the much larger net driving force for Na$^+$ ions. This is a steady-state condition, in which neither Na$^+$ nor K$^+$ is in equilibrium but the net flux of charge is null.

D. Illustration of membrane voltage changes during the hypothetical situations considered in **A**, **B**, and **C**.

permeable to Na^+. Two forces act on Na^+ to drive it into the cell. First, Na^+ is more concentrated outside than inside and therefore it tends to flow into the cell down its chemical concentration gradient. Second, Na^+ is driven into the cell by the negative electrical potential difference across the membrane (Figure 7-4B). The influx of positive charge (Na^+) depolarizes the cell, but only slightly from the K^+ equilibrium potential (-75 mV). The new membrane potential does not come close to the Na^+ equilibrium potential of $+55$ mV because there are many more resting K^+ channels than Na^+ channels in the membrane.

As soon as the membrane potential begins to depolarize from the value of the K^+ equilibrium potential, K^+ flux is no longer in equilibrium across the membrane. The reduction in the negative electrical force driving K^+ into the cell means that there will be a net efflux of K^+ out of the cell, tending to counteract the Na^+ influx. The more the membrane potential is depolarized and moves away from the K^+ equilibrium potential, the greater is the electrochemical force driving K^+ out of the cell and consequently the greater is the K^+ efflux. Eventually, the membrane potential reaches a new resting potential at which the outward movement of K^+ just balances the inward movement of Na^+ (Figure 7-4C). This balance point (usually -60 mV) is far from the Na^+ equilibrium potential ($+55$ mV) and is only slightly more positive than the equilibrium potential for K^+ (-75 mV).

To understand how this balance point is determined, bear in mind that the magnitude of the flux of an ion across a cell membrane is the product of its *electrochemical driving force* (the sum of the electrical driving force and the chemical driving force due to the concentration gradient) and the conductance of the membrane to the ion:

$$\text{ion flux} = \text{(electrical driving force} \\ + \text{chemical driving force)} \\ \times \text{membrane conductance.}$$

A cell has relatively few resting Na^+ channels so at rest the conductance to Na^+ is quite low. Thus, despite the large chemical and electrical forces driving Na^+ into the cell, the influx of Na^+ is small. In contrast, since there are many resting K^+ channels, the membrane conductance of K^+ is relatively large. As a result, the small net outward force acting on K^+ at the resting membrane potential is enough to produce a K^+ efflux equal to the Na^+ influx.

Passive Flux of Sodium and Potassium Is Balanced by Active Pumping of the Ions

For a cell to have a steady resting membrane potential the charge separation across the membrane must be maintained constant over time. That is, the influx of positive charge must be balanced by the efflux of positive charge. If these fluxes were not equal, the charge separation across the membrane, and thus the membrane potential, would vary continually. As we have seen, the passive movement of K^+ out of the cell through resting channels balances the passive movement of Na^+ into the cell. However, these steady ion leaks cannot be allowed to continue unopposed for any appreciable length of time because the Na^+ and K^+ gradients would eventually run down, reducing the resting membrane potential.

Dissipation of ionic gradients is prevented by the Na^+-K^+ pump, which moves Na^+ and K^+ *against* their net electrochemical gradients: it extrudes Na^+ from the cell while taking in K^+. The pump therefore requires energy to run. The energy comes from the hydrolysis of ATP. Thus, at the resting membrane potential the cell is not in equilibrium but rather in a *steady state*: there is a continuous passive influx of Na^+ and efflux of K^+ through resting channels that is exactly counterbalanced by the Na^+-K^+ pump.

The Na^+-K^+ pump is a large membrane-spanning protein with catalytic binding sites for Na^+, K^+, and ATP. The sites for Na^+ and ATP are located on its intracellular surface and the sites for K^+ on its extracellular surface. With each cycle the pump hydrolyzes one molecule of ATP. It then uses this energy to extrude three Na^+ ions and bring in two K^+ ions. The unequal flux of Na^+ and K^+ ions causes the pump to generate a net outward ionic current. Thus, the pump is said to be *electrogenic*. This pump-driven outward flux of positive charge tends to hyperpolarize the membrane to a somewhat more negative potential than would be achieved by the simple passive-diffusion mechanisms discussed above.

Chloride Ions May Be Passively Distributed

So far we have ignored the contribution of chloride (Cl^-) to the resting potential, even though many nerve cells have Cl^- channels that are open in the resting membrane. This simplification is valid for nerve cells that do not have a mechanism for active transport of Cl^- against an electrochemical gradient. In these cells the resting potential is ultimately determined by K^+ and Na^+ fluxes because the intracellular concentrations of K^+ and Na^+ are fixed by active transport (the Na^+-K^+ pump), whereas the Cl^- concentration inside the cell is affected only by passive forces (electrical potential and concentration gradient). Therefore, the movement of Cl^- ions tends toward equilibrium across the membrane, so that E_{Cl} is equal to the resting potential, V_r, and there is no net Cl^- flux at rest.

In many nerve cells the Cl^- gradient is controlled by an integral membrane protein called a Cl^- transporter. Like the Na^+-K^+ pump it catalyzes the movement of ions across the membrane against an electrochemical gradient without forming a continuous pore. Unlike the Na^+-K^+ pump, the transport process does not require the hydrolysis of ATP. Although no chemical bond energy is utilized in the transport process, the Cl^- transporter can move Cl^- against its electrochemical gradient by utilizing the energy stored in a preexisting ionic concentration gradient for a different type of ion— a process known as *secondary active transport*. For example, one type of Cl^- transporter couples the outward movement of one Cl^- ion to the outward movement of one K^+ ion. Since the electrochemical gradient for K^+ is outward, the energetically favorable outward K^+ flux is able to drive the energetically unfavorable outward Cl^- flux. As a result, the outside-to-inside ratio of Cl^- is greater than would result from passive diffusion alone. The effect of increasing the Cl^- gradient is to make the equilibrium potential for Cl^- ions more negative than the resting membrane potential overall. (Remember, the valence (z) of Cl^- is -1.)

The Balance of Ion Fluxes That Gives Rise to the Resting Membrane Potential Is Abolished During the Action Potential

In the nerve cell at rest the steady Na^+ influx is balanced by a steady K^+ efflux, so that the membrane potential is constant. This balance changes, however, when the membrane is depolarized past the threshold for generating an action potential. Once the membrane potential reaches this threshold, voltage-gated Na^+ channels open rapidly. The resultant increase in membrane permeability to Na^+ causes the Na^+ influx to exceed the K^+ efflux, creating a net influx of positive charge that causes further depolarization. The increase in depolarization causes still more voltage-gated Na^+ channels to open, resulting in a greater influx of Na^+, which accelerates the depolarization even further.

This regenerative, positive feedback cycle develops explosively, driving the membrane potential toward the Na^+ equilibrium potential of +55 mV:

$$E_{Na} = \frac{RT}{F} \ln \frac{[Na]_o}{[Na]_i} = 58 \text{ mV} \log \frac{[440]}{[50]} = +55 \text{ mV}.$$

However, the membrane potential never quite reaches that point because K^+ efflux continues throughout the depolarization. A slight influx of Cl^- into the cell also counteracts the depolarizing tendency of the Na^+ influx. Nevertheless, so many voltage-gated Na^+ chan-

nels open during the rising phase of the action potential that the cell's permeability to Na^+ is much greater than to either Cl^- or K^+. Thus, at the peak of the action potential the membrane potential approaches the Na^+ equilibrium potential, just as at rest (when permeability to K^+ is predominant) the membrane potential tends to approach the K^+ equilibrium potential.

The membrane potential would remain at this large positive value near the Na^+ equilibrium potential indefinitely but for two processes that repolarize the membrane, thus terminating the action potential. First, as the depolarization continues, the population of voltage-gated Na^+ channels gradually closes by the process of inactivation (see Chapters 6 and 9). Second, opening of the voltage-gated K^+ channels causes the K^+ efflux to gradually increase. The increase in K^+ permeability is slower than the increase in Na^+ permeability because of the slower rate of opening of the voltage-gated K^+ channels. The delayed increase in K^+ efflux combines with a decrease in Na^+ influx to produce a net efflux of positive charge from the cell, which continues until the cell has repolarized to its resting membrane potential.

The Contributions of Different Ions to the Resting Membrane Potential Can Be Quantified by the Goldman Equation

Although Na^+ and K^+ fluxes set the value of the resting potential, V_m is not equal to either E_K or E_{Na} but lies between them. As a general rule, when V_m is determined by two or more species of ions, the influence of each species is determined not only by the concentrations of the ion inside and outside the cell but also by the ease with which the ion crosses the membrane. In terms of electrical current flow, the membrane's conductance (1/resistance) provides a convenient measure of how readily the ion crosses the membrane. Another convenient measure is the permeability (P) of the membrane to that ion in units of velocity, cm/s. This measure is similar to that of a diffusion constant, which measures the rate of solute movement in solution. The dependence of membrane potential on ionic permeability and concentration is given quantitatively by the Goldman equation:

$$V_m = \frac{RT}{F} \ln \frac{P_K[K^+]_o + P_{Na}[Na^+]_o + P_{Cl}[Cl^-]_i}{P_K[K^+]_i + P_{Na}[Na^+]_i + P_{Cl}[Cl^-]_o}.$$

Goldman Equation

This equation applies only when V_m is not changing. It states that the greater the concentration of a particular ion species and the greater its membrane permeability, the greater its role in determining the membrane potential. In the limit, when permeability to one ion is exceptionally high, the Goldman equation reduces to the Nernst equation for that ion. For example, if $P_K \gg P_{Cl}$ or P_{Na}, as in glial cells, the equation becomes

$$V_m \cong \frac{RT}{F} \ln \frac{[K^+]_o}{[K^+]_i}.$$

Alan Hodgkin and Bernard Katz used the Goldman equation to analyze changes in membrane potential. They first measured the variation in membrane potential of a squid giant axon while systematically changing the extracellular concentrations of Na^+, Cl^-, and K^+. They found that if V_m is measured shortly after the extracellular concentration is changed (before the internal ionic concentrations are altered), $[K^+]_o$ has a strong effect on the resting potential, $[Cl^-]_o$ has a moderate effect, and $[Na^+]_o$ has little effect. The data for the membrane at rest could be fit accurately by the Goldman equation using the following permeability ratios:

$$P_K : P_{Na} : P_{Cl} = 1.0 : 0.04 : 0.45.$$

At the peak of the action potential, however, the variation of V_m with external ionic concentrations was fit best

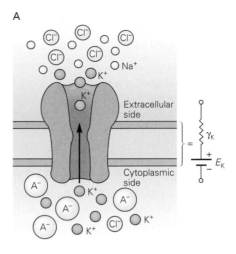

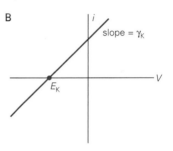

Figure 7-6 Chemical and electrical forces contribute to current flow.

A. A concentration gradient for K^+ gives rise to an electromotive force, with a value equal to the K^+ Nernst potential. This can be represented by a battery, E_K. In this circuit the battery is in series with a conductor, γ_K, representing the conductance of a channel that is selectively permeable to K^+ ions.

B. The current-voltage relation for a K^+ channel in the presence of both electrical and chemical driving forces. The potential at which the current is zero is equal to the K^+ Nernst potential.

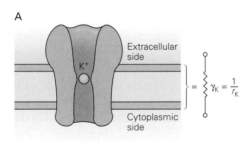

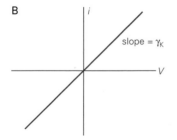

Figure 7-5. Electrical properties of a single K^+ channel.

A. A single K^+ channel can be represented as a conductor or resistor (conductance, γ, is the inverse of resistance, r).

B. The current-voltage relation for a single K^+ channel in the absence of a concentration gradient. The slope of the relation is equal to γ_K.

if a quite different set of permeability ratios were assumed:[1]

$$P_K : P_{Na} : P_{Cl} = 1.0 : 20 : 0.45.$$

For these values of permeabilities the Goldman equation approaches the Nernst equation for Na^+:

$$V_m \cong \frac{RT}{F} \ln \frac{[Na^+]_o}{[Na^+]_i} = +55 \text{ mV.}$$

Thus at the peak of the action potential, when the membrane is much more permeable to Na^+ than to any other ion, V_m approaches E_{Na}, the Nernst potential for Na^+.

---

[1] At the peak of the action potential there is an instant in time when V_m is not changing and the Goldman equation is applicable.

Figure 7-7 All of the passive K^+ channels in a nerve cell membrane can be lumped into a single equivalent electrical structure comprising a battery (E_K) in series with a conductor (g_K). The conductance is $g_K = N_K \times \gamma_K$, where N_K is the number of passive K^+ channels and γ_K is the conductance of a single K^+ channel.

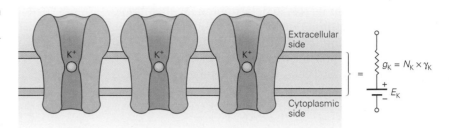

However, the finite permeability of the membrane to K^+ and Cl^- results in K^+ efflux and Cl^- influx that oppose Na^+ influx, thereby preventing V_m from quite reaching E_{Na}.

The Functional Properties of the Neuron Can Be Represented in an Electrical Equivalent Circuit

The Goldman equation is limited because it cannot be used to determine how rapidly the membrane potential changes in response to a change in permeability. Moreover, it is inconvenient for determining the magnitude of the individual Na^+, K^+, and Cl^- currents. This information can be obtained with a simple mathematical model derived from electrical circuits. Within this model, called an *equivalent circuit*, all of the important functional properties of the neuron are represented by an electrical circuit consisting only of conductors or resistors (representing the ion channels), batteries (representing the concentration gradients of relevant ions), and capacitors (the ability of the membrane to store charge). Equivalent circuits provide us with an intuitive understanding as well as a quantitative description of how current flow due to the movement of ions generates signals in nerve cells. The first step in developing a circuit is to relate the membrane's discrete physical properties to its electrical properties. (A review of elementary circuit theory in Appendix A may be helpful before proceeding to the discussion that follows.)

Each Ion Channel Acts as a Conductor and Battery in Series

As described in Chapter 6, the lipid bilayer of the membrane is a poor conductor of ionic current because it is not permeable to ions. Even a large potential difference will produce practically no current flow across a pure lipid bilayer. Consider the cell body of a typical spinal motor neuron, which has a membrane area of about 10^{-4} cm^2. If the membrane were composed solely of lipid bilayer, its electrical conductance would be only about 1 pS. In reality, however, the membrane contains thousands of resting ion channels through which ions constantly diffuse, so that the actual conductance of the membrane at rest is about 40,000 pS or 40×10^{-9} S, ie, 40,000 times greater than it would be if no ion channels were present.

In an equivalent circuit each K^+ channel can be represented as a resistor or conductor of ionic current with a single-channel conductance of γ_K (remember, conductance = 1/resistance) (Figure 7-5). If there were no K^+ concentration gradient, the current through the K^+ channel would be given by Ohm's law: $i_K = \gamma_K \times V_m$. Since there is normally a K^+ concentration gradient, there will be a chemical force driving K^+ across the membrane. In the equivalent circuit this chemical force is represented by a battery, whose electromotive force is given by the Nernst potential for K^+, E_K (Figure 7-6). (A source of electrical potential is called an *electromotive force* and an electromotive force generated by a difference in chemical potentials is called a *battery*.)

Figure 7-8 Each population of ion channels selective for Na^+, K^+, or Cl^- can be represented by a battery in series with a conductor. Note the directions of poles of batteries, indicating a negative electromotive force for K^+ and Cl^- and a positive one for Na^+.

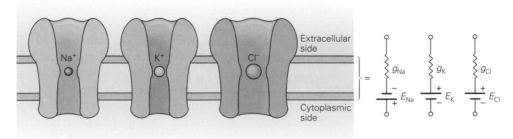

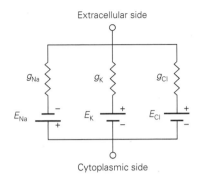

Figure 7-9 The passive current flow in a neuron can be modeled using an electrical equivalent circuit. The circuit includes elements representing the ion-selective membrane channels and the short-circuit pathways provided by the cytoplasm and extracellular fluid.

In the absence of voltage across the membrane the normal K^+ concentration gradient will cause an outward K^+ current flow. According to our conventions for electrical current flow an outward movement of positive charge corresponds to a positive electric current. From the Nernst equation, we also saw that when the concentration gradient for a positively charged ion, such as K^+, is directed outward (ie, there is a higher K^+ concentration inside than outside the cell), the equilibrium potential for that ion is negative. Thus, the K^+ current that flows solely because of its concentration gradient is given by $i_K = -\gamma_K \times E_K$ (the negative sign is required because a negative equilibrium potential produces a positive current).

Finally, for a real neuron that has both a membrane voltage and K^+ concentration gradient, the net K^+ current is given by the sum of the currents due to the electrical and chemical driving forces:

$$i_K = (\gamma_K \times V_m) - (\gamma_K \times E_K) = \gamma_K \times (V_m - E_K).$$

The term $V_m - E_K$ is called the *electrochemical driving force*. It determines the direction of ionic current flow and (along with the conductance) the magnitude of current flow. This equation is a modified form of Ohm's law that takes into account that ionic current flow through a membrane is determined not only by the voltage across the membrane but also by the ionic concentration gradients.

So far we have used two terms to indicate the ability of ions to cross membranes: permeability and conductance. Although they are related, we should be careful not to confuse them. The *permeability* of a membrane to

an ion is an intrinsic property of the membrane that is a measure of the ease with which the ion passes through the membrane (in units of cm/s). Permeability depends only on the types and numbers of ion channels present in the membrane. *Conductance*, on the other hand, measures the ability of the membrane (or channel) to carry electrical current (in units of 1/ohms). Since current is carried by ions, the conductance of a membrane will depend not only on the properties of the membrane but also on the concentration of ions in solution. A membrane can have a very high permeability to K^+ ions, but if there is no K^+ in solution there can be no K^+ current flow and so the conductance of the membrane will be zero. In practice, permeability is used in the Goldman equation whereas conductance is used in electrical measurements and equivalent circuits.

A cell membrane has many resting K^+ channels, all of which can be combined into a single equivalent circuit consisting of a conductor in series with a battery (Figure 7-7). In this equivalent circuit the total conductance of all the K^+ channels (g_K), ie, the K^+ conductance of the cell membrane in its resting state, is equal to the number N of resting K^+ channels multiplied by the conductance of an individual K^+ channel (γ_K):

$$g_K = N_K \times \gamma_K.$$

Since the battery in this equivalent circuit depends solely on the concentration gradient for K^+ and is independent of the number of K^+ channels, its value is the equilibrium potential for K^+, E_K (Figure 7-7).

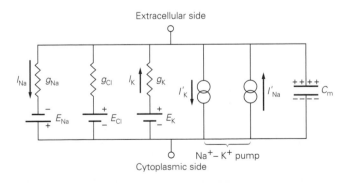

Figure 7-10 Under steady state conditions the passive Na^+ and K^+ currents are balanced by active Na^+ and K^+ fluxes (I'_{Na} and I'_K) driven by the Na^+-K^+ pump. The lipid bilayer endows the membrane with electrical capacitance (C_m). Note I'_{Na} is 50% greater than I'_K (and therefore I_{Na} is 50% greater than I_K) since the Na^+-K^+ pump transports three Na^+ ions out for every two K^+ ions it transports into the cell.

Box 7-2 Using the Equivalent Circuit Model to Calculate Resting Membrane Potential

The equivalent circuit model of the resting membrane can be used to calculate the resting potential. To simplify the calculation we shall initially ignore Cl^- channels and begin with just two types of passive channels, K^+ and Na^+, as illustrated in Figure 7-11. Moreover, we ignore the electrogenic influence of the Na^+-K^+ pump because it is small. Because we will consider only steady-state conditions, where V_m is not changing, we can also ignore membrane capacitance. (Membrane capacitance and its delaying effect on changes in V_m are discussed in Chapter 8.) Because there are more passive channels for K^+ than for Na^+, the membrane conductance for current flow carried by K^+ is much greater than that for Na^+. In the equivalent circuit in Figure 7-11, g_K is 20 times higher than g_{Na} (10×10^{-6} S compared to 0.5×10^{-6} S). Given these values and the values of E_K and E_{Na}, the membrane potential, V_m, is calculated as follows.

Since V_m is constant in the resting state, the net current must be zero, otherwise the separation of positive and negative charges across the membrane would change, causing V_m to change. Therefore I_{Na} is equal and opposite to I_K:

$$-I_{Na} = I_K$$

or

$$I_{Na} + I_K = 0 \qquad \text{(7-1)}$$

We can easily calculate I_{Na} and I_K in two steps. First, we add up the separate potential differences across the Na^+ and K^+ branches of the circuit. Going from the inside to the outside across the Na^+ branch, the total potential difference is the sum of the potential differences across E_{Na} and across g_{Na}:[*]

$$V_m = E_{Na} + I_{Na}/g_{Na}.$$

Similarly, for the K^+ conductance branch

$$V_m = E_K + I_K/g_K.$$

Next, we rearrange and solve for I:

$$I_{Na} = g_{Na} \times (V_m - E_{Na}) \qquad \text{(7-2a)}$$

$$I_K = g_K \times (V_m - E_K) \qquad \text{(7-2b)}$$

As these equations illustrate, the ionic current through each conductance branch is equal to the conductance of that branch multiplied by the net electrical driving force. For example, the conductance for the K^+ branch is proportional to the

---

[*]Because we have defined V_m as $V_{in} - V_{out}$, the following convention must be used for these equations. Outward current (in this case I_K) is positive and inward current is negative. Batteries with their positive poles toward the inside of the membrane (eg, E_{Na}) are given positive values in the equations. The reverse is true for batteries that have their negative poles toward the inside, such as the K^+ battery.

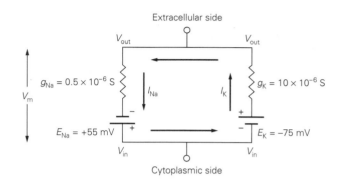

Figure 7-11 This electrical equivalent circuit omits the Cl^- pathway and Na^+-K^+ pump for simplicity in calculating the resting membrane potential.

number of open K^+ channels, and the driving force is equal to the difference between V_m and E_K. If V_m is more positive than E_K (-75 mV), the driving force is positive (outward); if V_m is more negative than E_K, the driving force is negative (inward).

In Equation 7-1 we saw that $I_{Na} + I_K = 0$. If we now substitute Equations 7-2a and 7-2b for I_{Na} and I_K in Equation 7-1, multiply through, and rearrange, we obtain the following expression:

$$V_m \times (g_{Na} + g_K) = (E_{Na} \times g_{Na}) + (E_K \times g_K).$$

Solving for V_m, we obtain an equation for the resting membrane potential that is expressed in terms of membrane conductances and batteries:

$$V_m = \frac{(E_{Na} \times g_{Na}) + (E_K \times g_K)}{g_{Na} + g_K}. \qquad \text{(7-3)}$$

From this equation, using the values in our equivalent circuit (Figure 7-11), we calculate $V_m = -69$ mV.

Equation 7-3 states that V_m will approach the value of the ionic battery that is associated with the greater conductance. This principle can be illustrated by considering what happens during the action potential. At the peak of the action potential g_K is essentially unchanged from its resting value, but g_{Na} increases as much as 500-fold. This increase in g_{Na} is caused by the opening of voltage-gated Na^+ channels. In the equivalent circuit example shown in Figure 7-11 a 500-fold increase would change g_{Na} from 0.5×10^{-6} S to 250×10^{-6} S. If we substitute this new value of g_{Na} into Equation 7-3 and solve for V_m, we obtain $+50$ mV, a value much closer to E_{Na} than to E_K. V_m is closer to E_{Na} than to E_K at the peak of the action potential because, since g_{Na} is now 25-fold greater than g_K, the Na^+ bat-

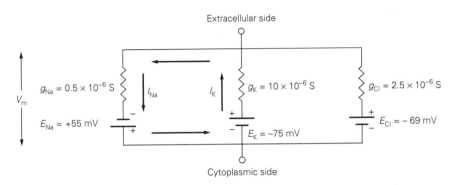

Figure 7-12 This electrical equivalent circuit includes the Cl⁻ pathway. However, no current flows through the Cl⁻ channels in this example because V_m is at the Cl⁻ equilibrium (Nernst) potential.

tery becomes much more important than the K⁺ battery in determining V_m.

The real resting membrane has open channels not only for Na⁺ and K⁺, but also for Cl⁻. One can derive a more general equation for V_m, following the steps outlined above, from an equivalent circuit that includes a conductance pathway for Cl⁻ with its associated Nernst battery (Figure 7-12):

$$V_m = \frac{(E_{Na} \times g_{Na}) + (E_K \times g_K) + (E_{Cl} \times g_{Cl})}{g_{Na} + g_K + g_{Cl}}. \quad (7\text{-}4)$$

This equation is similar to the Goldman equation presented earlier in this chapter. As in the Goldman equation, the contribution to V_m of each ionic battery is weighted in proportion to the conductance of the membrane for that particular ion. In the limit, if the conductance for one ion is much greater than that for the other ions, V_m will approach the value of that ion's Nernst potential.

The contribution of Cl⁻ ions to the resting potential can now be determined by comparing V_m calculated for the circuits for Na⁺ and K⁺ only (Figure 7-11) and for all three ions (Figure 7-12). For most nerve cells the value of g_{Cl} ranges from one-fourth to one-half of g_K. In addition, E_{Cl} is typically quite close to E_K, but slightly less negative. In the circuit in Figure 7-12, Cl⁻ ions are passively distributed across the membrane, so that E_{Cl} is equal to the value of V_m, which is determined by Na⁺ and K⁺. Note that if $E_{Cl} = V_m$ (-69 mV in this case), no net current flows through the Cl⁻ channels. If we include g_{Cl} and E_{Cl} from Figure 7-12 in the calculation of V_m, the calculated value of V_m does not differ from that for Figure 7-11. On the other hand, if Cl⁻ were not passively distributed but ac-

tively transported out of the cell, then E_{Cl} would be more negative than -69 mV. Adding the Cl⁻ pathway to the calculation would then shift V_m to a slightly more negative value.

The equivalent circuit can be further simplified by lumping the conductance of all the resting channels that contribute to the resting potential into a single conductance g_l and replacing the battery for each conductance channel with a single battery whose value, E_l, is that predicted by Equation 7-4 (Figure 7-13). This simplification will prove useful when we consider the effects of gated channels in later chapters.

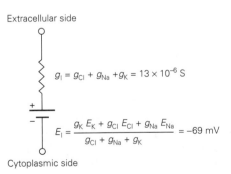

Figure 7-13 The complement of Na⁺, K⁺, and Cl⁻ resting channels can be represented by a single equivalent conductance and battery. In this simplified equivalent circuit the total resting membrane conductance $g_l = g_{Cl} + g_{Na} + g_K$, and the electromotive force or battery (E_l) is the resting potential predicted by Equation 7-4.

An Equivalent Circuit Model of the Membrane Includes Batteries, Conductors, a Capacitor, and a Current Generator

Like the population of resting K^+ channels, all the resting Na^+ channels can be represented by a single conductor in series with a single battery, as can the resting Cl^- channels (Figure 7-8). Since the K^+, Na^+, and Cl^- channels account for the bulk of the passive ionic current through the membrane in the cell at rest, we can calculate the resting potential by incorporating these three channels into a simple equivalent circuit of a neuron.

To construct this circuit we need only connect the elements representing each type of channel at their two ends with elements representing the extracellular fluid and cytoplasm. The extracellular fluid and cytoplasm are both excellent conductors because they have relatively large cross-sectional areas and many ions available to carry charge. Both can be approximated by a *short circuit*—a conductor with zero resistance (Figure 7-9).

The equivalent circuit of the neuron can be made more accurate by adding a current generator. As described earlier in this chapter, steady fluxes of Na^+ and K^+ ions through the passive membrane channels are exactly counterbalanced by active ion fluxes driven by the Na^+-K^+ pump, which extrudes three Na^+ ions from the cell for every two K^+ ions it pumps in. This electrogenic ATP-dependent pump, which keeps the ionic batteries charged, can be added to the equivalent circuit in the form of a current generator (Figure 7-10).

Finally, we can complete the equivalent circuit of the neuron by incorporating its *capacitance*, the third important passive electrical property of the neuron. Capacitance is the property of an electric nonconductor (insulator) that permits the storage of charge when opposite surfaces of the nonconductor are maintained at a difference of potential. For the neuron, the nonconductor (or capacitor) is the cell membrane, which separates the cytoplasm and extracellular fluid, both of which are highly conductive environments. Strictly speaking, the membrane is a leaky capacitor because it is penetrated by ion channels. However, since the density of the ion channels is low, the insulating portion of the membrane—the lipid bilayer—occupies at least 100 times the area of all the ion channels combined. Membrane capacitance is included in the equivalent circuit in Figure 7-10.

The electrical potential difference across a capacitor, V, is expressed as:

$$V = Q/C,$$

where Q is the excess of positive or negative charges on each side of the capacitor and C is the capacitance.

Capacitance is measured in units of farads, F, where a charge separation of 1 coulomb across a 1 farad capacitor produces a 1 volt potential difference.

A typical value of membrane capacitance for a nerve cell is about $1 \, \mu F/cm^2$ of membrane area. The excess of positive and negative charges separated by the membrane of a spherical cell body with a diameter of $50 \, \mu m$ and a resting potential of -60 mV is 29×10^6 ions. Although this number may seem large, it represents only a tiny fraction (1/200,000) of the total number of positive or negative charges in solution within the cytoplasm. The bulk of the cytoplasm and the bulk of the extracellular fluid are electroneutral.

The use of the equivalent circuit model of the neuron to analyze neuronal properties quantitatively is illustrated in Box 7-2.

An Overall View

The lipid bilayer, which is virtually impermeant to ions, is an insulator separating two conducting solutions, the cytoplasm and the extracellular fluid. Ions can cross the lipid bilayer only by passing through ion channels in the cell membrane. When the cell is at rest, the passive ionic fluxes into and out of the cell are balanced, so that the charge separation across the membrane remains constant and the membrane potential remains at its resting value.

The value of the resting membrane potential in nerve cells is determined primarily by resting channels selective for K^+, Cl^-, and Na^+. In general, the membrane potential will be closest to the equilibrium (Nernst) potential of the ion (or ions) with the greatest membrane permeability. The permeability for an ion species is proportional to the number of open channels that allow passage of that ion.

At rest, the membrane potential is close to the Nernst potential for K^+, the ion to which the membrane is most permeable. The membrane is also somewhat permeable to Na^+, however, and therefore an influx of Na^+ drives the membrane potential slightly positive to the K^+ Nernst potential. At this potential the electrical and chemical driving forces acting on K^+ are no longer in balance, so K^+ diffuses out of the cell. These two passive fluxes are each counterbalanced by active fluxes driven by the Na^+-K^+ pump.

Chloride is actively pumped out of some, but not all, cells. When it is not, it is passively distributed so as to be at equilibrium inside and outside the cell. Under most physiological conditions the bulk concentrations of Na^+, K^+, and Cl^- inside and outside the cell are constant. During signaling the changes in membrane potential (action potentials, synaptic potentials, and receptor potentials) are caused by substantial changes in the membrane's relative permeabilities to these three ions, not by changes in the bulk concentrations of ions, which are negligible. These changes in permeability, caused by the opening of gated ion channels, cause changes in the net charge separation across the membrane.

John Koester
Steven A. Siegelbaum

Selected Readings

Finkelstein A, Mauro A. 1977. Physical principles and formalisms of electrical excitability. In: ER Kandel (ed). *Handbook of Physiology: A Critical, Comprehensive Presentation of Physiological Knowledge and Concepts*, Sect. 1, *The Nervous System*. Vol. 1, *Cellular Biology of Neurons*, Part 1, pp. 161–213. Bethesda, MD: American Physiological Society.

Hille B. 1992. *Ionic Channels of Excitable Membranes*, 2nd ed. Sunderland, MA: Sinauer.

Hodgkin AL. 1992. *Chance and Design*. Cambridge: Cambridge Univ. Press.

References

Bernstein J. [1902] 1979. Investigations on the thermodynamics of bioelectric currents. Pflügers Arch 92:521–562. Translated in: GR Kepner (ed). *Cell Membrane Permeability and Transport*, pp. 184–210. Stroudsburg, PA: Dowden, Hutchinson & Ross.

Goldman DE. 1943. Potential, impedance, and rectification in membranes. J Gen Physiol 27:37–60.

Hodgkin AL, Katz B. 1949. The effect of sodium ions on the electrical activity of the giant axon of the squid. J Physiol (Lond) 108:37–77.

Nernst W. [1888] 1979. On the kinetics of substances in solution. Z Physik Chem. 2:613–622, 634–637. Translated in: GR Kepner (ed). *Cell Membrane Permeability and Transport*, pp. 174–183. Stroudsburg, PA: Dowden, Hutchinson & Ross.

Orkand RK. 1977. Glial cells. In: ER Kandel (ed). *Handbook of Physiology: A Critical, Comprehensive Presentation of Physiological Knowledge and Concepts*, Sect. 1, *The Nervous System*. Vol. 1, *Cellular Biology of Neurons*, Part 2, pp. 855–875. Bethesda, MD: American Physiological Society.

Siegel GJ, Agranoff BW, Albers RW (eds). 1999. *Basic Neurochemistry: Molecular, Cellular, and Medical Aspects*, 6th ed, Philadelphia: Lippincott-Raven.

8

Local Signaling: Passive Electrical Properties of the Neuron

WHILE ALL CELLS OF THE body have a membrane potential, only neurons (and muscle cells) generate electrical signals that can be conducted rapidly over long distances. In the last chapter we saw how these electrical signals are generated by the flux of ions across the cell membrane through specialized ion channels, and how to calculate the expected membrane potential for any set of ionic concentration gradients and membrane permeabilities using the Goldman equation.

This description does not, however, provide any information about *changes* in the membrane potential in response to a stimulus, since the Goldman equation applies only to the steady state when the voltage does not change. During signaling, when the neuron generates action potentials, synaptic potentials, or sensory generator potentials in response to a stimulus, the membrane voltage changes constantly. What determines the rate of change in potential? Will a brief synaptic current always produce a similar potential change, regardless of the size of the postsynaptic cell? What determines whether a stimulus will or will not produce an action potential?

Here we consider how a neuron's passive electrical properties and geometry, which are relatively constant, affect the cell's electrical signaling. In the next chapter we shall consider how the properties of the ion channels that generate the active ionic currents also help determine changes in membrane potential.

Neurons have three passive electrical properties that are important to electrical signaling: the resting membrane resistance, the membrane capacitance, and the intracellular axial resistance along axons and dendrites. Because these elements provide the return pathway to complete the electrical circuit when active currents flow into or out of the cell, they determine the time course and amplitude of the synaptic potential change generated by the synaptic current. They also determine whether a synaptic potential generated in a dendrite will result in a suprathreshold depolarization at the trigger zone on the axon hillock. Still further, the passive properties influence the speed at which an action potential is conducted.

Input Resistance Determines the Magnitude of Passive Changes in Membrane Potential

The difference between the effects of passive and active properties of neurons can be demonstrated by injecting

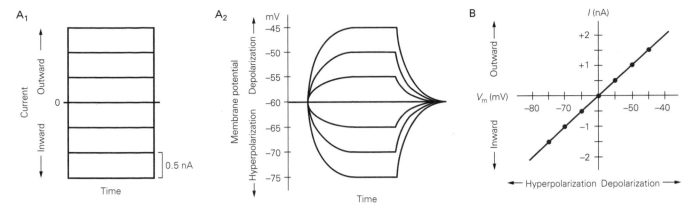

Figure 8-1 Current-voltage relationships. By passing sub-threshold, graded, inward and outward current pulses into a cell, one can determine the relationship between current injected into the cell and the resulting changes in membrane potential, V_m.

A. Increases in outward or inward current pulses (**A₁**) produce proportional and symmetrical changes in V_m (**A₂**). Note that the potential changes more slowly than the step current pulses.

B. An *I-V* curve is obtained by plotting the steady state voltage against the injected current. The slope of the *I-V* curve defines the input resistance of the neuron. The *I-V* curve shown here is linear; V_m changes by 10 mV for every 1 nA change in current, yielding a resistance of 10 mV/1 nA, or $10 \times 10^6 \, \Omega$ (10 MΩ).

current pulses into the cell body (see Box 7-1). Injecting a negative charge through an electrode increases the charge separation across the membrane, making the membrane potential more negative, or hyperpolarized. The larger the negative current, the greater is the hyperpolarization. In most neurons there is a linear relation between the size of the negative current and the steady-state hyperpolarization (Figure 8-1). The relation between current and voltage defines a resistance, R_{in}, the neuron's *input resistance.*

Likewise, when a positive charge is injected into the cell, producing depolarization, the neuron behaves as a simple resistor, but only over a limited voltage range. A large enough positive current will produce a depolarization that exceeds threshold, at which point the neuron generates an action potential. When this happens the neuron no longer behaves as a simple resistor because of the special properties of its voltage-gated channels considered in Chapter 9. Still, much of a neuron's behavior in the hyperpolarizing and subthreshold depolarizing range of voltages can be explained by simple equivalent circuits made up of resistors, capacitors, and batteries.

The input resistance of the cell determines how much the cell will depolarize in response to a steady current. The magnitude of the depolarization, ΔV, is given by Ohm's law:

$$\Delta V = I \times R_{in}.$$

Thus, of two neurons receiving identical synaptic current inputs, the cell with the higher input resistance will show a greater change in membrane voltage. For an idealized spherical neuron with no processes, the input resistance depends on both the density of the resting ion channels in the membrane (that is, the number of channels per unit area of membrane) and the size of the cell. The larger the neuron, the greater will be its membrane surface area and the lower the input resistance, since there will be more resting channels to conduct ions.

To compare the membrane properties of neurons of differing sizes, electrophysiologists often use the resistance of a unit area of membrane, the *specific membrane resistance*, R_m, measured in units of $\Omega \cdot cm^2$. The specific membrane resistance depends only on the density of the resting ion channels (the number of channels per square centimeter) and their conductance.

To obtain the total input resistance of the cell we *divide* the specific membrane resistance by the membrane area of the cell because the greater the area of a cell, the lower its resistance. For the spherical neuron we obtain

$$R_{in} = R_m/4\pi a^2,$$

where *a* is the radius of the neuron. Thus, for a spherical cell the input resistance is inversely proportional to the square of the radius. For a real neuron with extensive dendrites and axons, the input resistance also depends on the membrane resistance of its processes as well as on the intracellular cytoplasmic resistance between the cell body and those processes (discussed below).

Membrane Capacitance Prolongs the Time Course of Electrical Signals

In Figure 8-1 the magnitude of the steady state changes in the cell's voltage in response to subthreshold current resembles the behavior of a simple resistor, but the *time course* of the changes does not. A true resistor responds to a step change in current with a similar step change in voltage, but the cell in Figure 8-1 shows a voltage response that rises and decays more slowly than the step change in current. This property of the membrane is due to its *capacitance.*

To understand how the capacitance slows down the voltage response we need to recall that the voltage across a capacitor is proportional to the charge stored on the capacitor:

$$V = Q/C,$$

where Q is the charge in coulombs and C is the capacitance in farads. To alter the voltage, charge must either be added to or removed from the capacitor:

$$\Delta V = \Delta Q/C.$$

The change in charge (ΔQ) is the result of the flow of current across the capacitor (I_c). Since current is the flow of charge per unit time ($I_c = \Delta Q/\Delta t$), we can calculate the change in voltage across a capacitor as a function of current and the time that the current flows (Δt):

$$\Delta V = I_c \cdot \Delta t/C. \qquad (8\text{-}1)$$

The magnitude of the change in voltage across a capacitor in response to a current pulse depends on the duration of the current, as time is required to deposit and remove charge on the plates of the capacitor.

Capacitance is directly proportional to the area of the plates of the capacitor. The larger the area of a capacitor, the more charge it will store for a given potential difference. The value of the capacitance also depends on the insulation medium and the distance between the two plates of the capacitor. Since all biological membranes are composed of lipid bilayers with similar insulating properties that provide a similar separation between the two plates (4 nm), the specific capacitance per unit area of all biological membranes, C_m, has the same value, approximately 1 μF/cm^2 of membrane. The total input capacitance of a spherical cell, C_{in},

is therefore given by the capacitance per unit area multiplied by the area of the cell:

$$C_{in} = C_m(4\pi a^2).$$

Because capacitance increases with the size of the cell, more charge, and therefore current, is required to produce the same change in membrane potential in a larger neuron than in a smaller one.

According to Equation 8-1 the voltage across a capacitor continues to increase with time as long as a current pulse is applied. But in neurons the voltage levels off after some time (Figure 8-1) because the membrane of a neuron acts as a resistor (owing to its ion-conducting channels) and a capacitor (owing to the phospholipid bilayer) in parallel.

In the equivalent circuit developed in Chapter 7 to model current flow in the neuron, we placed the resistance and capacitance in parallel, since current crossing the membrane can flow either through ion channels (the resistive pathway) or across the capacitor (Figure 8-2). The resistive current carried by ions flowing across the membrane through ion channels—for example, Na$^+$ ions moving through Na$^+$ channels from outside to inside the cell—is called the *ionic membrane current*. The current carried by ions that change the net charge stored on the membrane is called the *capacitive membrane current*. An outward capacitive current, for example, adds positive charges to the inside of the membrane and re-

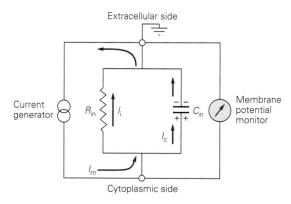

Figure 8-2 A simplified electrical equivalent circuit is used to examine the effects of membrane capacitance (C_{in}) on the rate of change of membrane potential in response to current flow. All resting ion channels are lumped into a single element (R_{in}). Batteries representing the electromotive forces generated by ion diffusion are not included because they affect only the absolute value of membrane potential, not the rate of change. This equivalent circuit represents the experimental setup shown in Box 7-1 (Figure 7-2C), in which pairs of electrodes are connected to the current generator and the membrane potential monitor.

moves an equal number of positive charges from the outside of the membrane. The total current crossing the membrane, I_m, is given by the sum of the ionic current (I_i) and the capacitive current:

$$I_m = I_i + I_c. \qquad \text{(8-2)}$$

The capacitance of the membrane has the effect of reducing the rate at which the membrane potential changes in response to a current pulse. If the membrane had only resistive properties, a step pulse of outward current passed across it would change the membrane potential instantaneously. On the other hand, if the membrane had only capacitive properties, the membrane potential would change linearly with time in response to the same step pulse of current. Because the membrane has *both* capacitive and resistive properties in parallel, the actual change in membrane potential combines features of the two pure responses. The initial slope of the relation between V_m and time reflects a purely capacitive element, whereas the final slope and amplitude reflect a purely resistive element (Figure 8-3).

It is now easy to explain why a step change in current produces the slowly rising voltage waveform seen in Figure 8-3. Since the resistance and capacitance of the membrane are in parallel, the voltage across each element must always be the same and equal to the membrane potential. Assume that the membrane potential starts off at 0 mV and that at time $t = 0$ a depolarizing current step is applied from a current generator with magnitude I_m. Initially the voltage across the resistor and capacitor are both equal to 0 mV. Since the ionic current through the resistor is given by Ohm's law ($I_i = V/R_{in}$), initially no current will flow through the resistor (since V starts off at 0 mV) and all the current will flow across the capacitor (ie, $I_c = I_m$). As a result of the large initial capacitive current, the potential across the capacitor, and hence the membrane potential, will rapidly become more positive.

As V_m increases, the voltage difference across the membrane begins to drive current across the membrane resistance. As the voltage across the membrane becomes more positive, more current flows through the resistor and less flows across the capacitor, since I_c plus I_i is constant (and equal to I_m). As a result, the membrane potential begins to rise more slowly. Eventually, the membrane potential reaches a value where all the membrane current flows through the resistor ($I_i = I_m$). From Ohm's law this voltage is given by $V_m = I_m \cdot R_{in}$. At this point the capacitative current is zero and, following Equation 8-1, the membrane potential no longer changes. Once the step of current is turned off, the total membrane current I_m equals zero, so that the positive ionic current flowing through the resistor must flow back into the cell

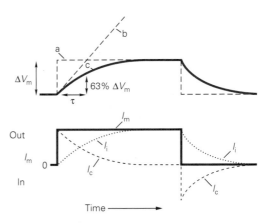

Figure 8-3 The rate of change in the membrane potential is slowed by the membrane capacitance. The response of the membrane potential (ΔV_m) to a step current pulse is shown in the **upper plot**. The actual shape of the response (**red line c**) combines the properties of a purely resistive element (**dashed line a**) and a purely capacitive element (**dashed line b**). The **lower plot** shows the total membrane current (I_m) and its ionic (I_i) and capacitive (I_c) components ($I_m = I_i + I_c$) in relation to the current pulse. The time taken to reach 63% of the final voltage defines the membrane time constant, τ. The time constants of different neurons typically range from 20 to 50 ms.

as an equal and opposite capacitive current, ie, $I_i = -I_c$. With no applied current, the charge on the capacitor dissipates by flowing in a loop around the circuit through the resistive pathway, and the membrane potential returns to zero.

The rising phase of the potential change can be described by the following equation:

$$\Delta V_m(t) = I_m R_{in}(1 - e^{-t/\tau}), \qquad \text{(8-3)}$$

where e, which has a value of around 2.72, is the base of the system of natural logarithms, and τ is the *membrane time constant*, the product of the input resistance and capacitance of the membrane ($R_{in}C_{in}$). The time constant can be measured experimentally (Figure 8-3). It is the time it takes the membrane potential to rise to $(1 - 1/e)$, about 63% of its steady state value. We shall return to the time constant when we consider the temporal summation of synaptic inputs in a cell in Chapter 12.

Membrane and Axoplasmic Resistance Affect the Efficiency of Signal Conduction

So far we have considered the effects of the passive properties of neurons on signaling only within the cell body. Because the neuron's soma can be approximated

Figure 8-4 A neuronal process can be represented by an electrical equivalent circuit. The process is divided into unit lengths. Each unit length of the process is a circuit with its own membrane resistance (r_m) and capacitance (c_m). All the circuits are connected by resistors (r_a), which represent the axial resistance of segments of cytoplasm, and a short circuit, which represents the extracellular fluid.

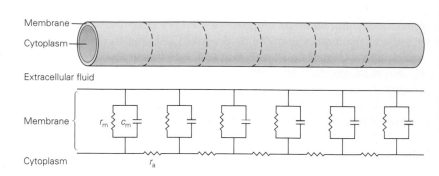

as a simple sphere, the effect of distance on the propagation of a signal does not matter. However, in electrical signaling along dendrites, axons, and muscle fibers, a subthreshold voltage signal decreases in amplitude with distance from its site of initiation. To understand how this attenuation occurs we will again have need of an equivalent circuit, one that shows how the geometry of a neuron influences the distribution of current flow.

Synaptic potentials that originate in dendrites are conducted along the dendrite toward the cell body and the trigger zone. The cytoplasmic core of a dendrite offers significant resistance to the longitudinal flow of current, because it has a relatively small cross-sectional area, and ions flowing down the dendrite collide with other molecules. The greater the length of the cytoplasmic core, the greater the resistance, since the ions experience more collisions the further they travel. Conversely, the larger the diameter of the cytoplasmic core, the lower will be the resistance in a given length, since the number of charge carriers at any cross section of dendrite increases with the diameter of the core.

To represent the incremental increase in resistance along the length of the dendritic core, the dendrite can be divided into unit lengths, each of which is a circuit with its own measurable membrane resistance and capacitance as well as an axial resistance within the cytoplasmic core. Because of its large volume, the extracellular fluid has only negligible resistance and therefore can be ignored. The equivalent circuit for this simplified model is shown in Figure 8-4.

If current is injected into the dendrite at one point, how will the membrane potential change with distance along the dendrite? For simplicity, consider the variation of membrane potential with distance after a constant-amplitude current pulse has been on for some time ($t \gg \tau$). Under these conditions the membrane potential will have reached a steady value, so capacitive current will be zero. When $I_c = 0$, all of the membrane current is ionic ($I_m = I_i$). The variation of the potential with distance thus depends solely on the relative values of the *membrane resis-*

tance, r_m (units of $\Omega \cdot cm$), and the *axial resistance,* r_a (units of Ω/cm), per unit length of dendrite.

The injected current flows out through several parallel pathways across successive membrane cylinders along the length of the process (Figure 8-5). Each of these current pathways is made up of two resistive components in series: the total axial resistance, r_x, and the membrane resistance, r_m, of the unit membrane cylinder. For each outflow pathway the total axial resistance is the resistance between the site of current injection and the site of the outflow pathway. Since resistors in series are added, $r_x = r_a x$, where x is the distance along the dendrite from the site of current injection. The membrane resistance, r_m, has the same value at each outflow pathway along the cell process.

More current flows across a membrane cylinder near the site of injection than at more distant regions because current always tends to follow the path of least resistance, and the total axial resistance, r_x, increases with distance from the site of injection (Figure 8-5). Because $V_m = I_m r_m$, the change in membrane potential produced by the current across a membrane cylinder at position x, $\Delta V_m(x)$, becomes smaller with distance down the dendrite away from the current electrode. This decay with distance is exponential (Figure 8-5) and expressed by

$$\Delta V(x) = \Delta V_0 e^{-x/\lambda},$$

where λ is the membrane *length constant,* x is the distance from the site of current injection, and ΔV_0 is the change in membrane potential produced by the current flow at the site of injection ($x = 0$). The length constant λ is defined as the distance along the dendrite to the site where ΔV_m has decayed to $1/e$, or 37% of its initial value (Figure 8-5), and it is determined as follows:

$$\lambda = \sqrt{(r_m/r_a)}.$$

The better the insulation of the membrane (that is, the greater r_m) and the better the conducting properties of the inner core (the lower r_a), the greater the length constant of the dendrite. That is, current is able to spread farther along the inner conductive core of the dendrite before leaking across the membrane.

To consider how neuronal geometry affects signaling, it will be helpful first to consider how the diameter of a process affects r_m and r_a . Both r_m and r_a are measures of resistance that apply to a 1 cm segment of an individual neuronal process with a certain radius α. The axial resistance of a neuronal process depends on the intrinsic resistive properties of the cytoplasm, expressed as the specific resistance, ρ, of a 1 cm^3 cube of cytoplasm (in units of $\Omega \cdot$cm), and the cross-sectional area of the process, which determines the total volume in a unit length of the process and hence the number of charge carriers. Thus, r_a is given by

$$r_a = \rho/\pi a^2, \qquad (8\text{-}4)$$

and r_a has the required units of $\Omega/$cm. The diameter of the process also affects r_m since the total number of channels in a unit length of membrane is directly proportional to both the channel density (number of channels per unit area) and the membrane area. Since r_m is inversely related to the total number of channels in a unit length of membrane and the area in a unit length of cylinder depends on the circumference, r_m is given by

$$r_m = R_m/2\pi a, \qquad (8\text{-}5)$$

where R_m is the specific resistance of a unit area of membrane (units of $\Omega \cdot$cm^2) and r_m has the units of $\Omega \cdot$cm.

Neuronal processes vary greatly in diameter, from as much as 1 mm for the giant axon of the squid down to 1 μm for fine dendritic branches in the mammalian brain. These variations in diameter control the efficiency of neuronal signaling because the diameter determines the length constant. For processes with similar intrinsic properties (that is with similar values of R_m and ρ), the larger the diameter of the process (dendrite or axon), the longer the length constant, because r_m/r_a is directly related to the radius (Equations 8-4 and 8-5). Thus, the length constant is expressed in terms of the intrinsic (size invariant) properties R_m and ρ as follows:

$$\lambda = \sqrt{\frac{R_m}{\rho} \cdot \frac{a}{2}}.$$

That is, the length constant is proportional to the square root of the radius (or diameter) of a process. Thus, thicker axons and dendrites will have longer length constants than do narrower processes and hence will transmit electrotonic signals for greater distances. Typical values for neuronal length constants range from 0.1 to 1.0 mm.

The length constant is a measure of the efficiency of the passive spread of voltage changes along the neuron, or *electrotonic conduction*. The efficiency of electrotonic

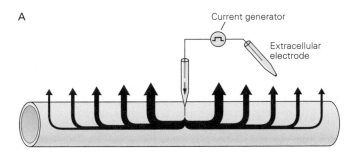

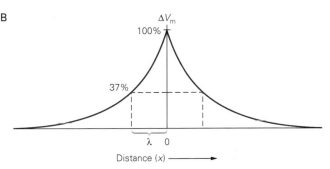

Figure 8-5 The voltage response in a passive neuronal process decays with distance due to electronic conduction. Current injected into a neuronal process by a microelectrode follows the path of least resistance to the return electrode in the extracellular fluid (**A**). The thickness of the arrows represents membrane current density at any point along the process. Under these conditions the change in V_m decays exponentially with distance from the site of current injection (**B**). The distance at which ΔV_m has decayed to 37% of its value at the point of current injection defines the length constant, λ.

conduction has two important effects on neuronal function. First, it influences *spatial summation*, the process by which synaptic potentials generated in different regions of the neuron are added together at the trigger zone, the decision-making component of the neuron (see Chapter 12).

Second, electrotonic conduction is a factor in the *propagation* of the action potential. Once the membrane at any point along an axon has been depolarized beyond threshold, an action potential is generated in that region in response to the opening of voltage-gated Na$^+$ channels (see Chapter 9). This local depolarization spreads electrotonically down the axon, causing the adjacent region of the membrane to reach the threshold for generating an action potential (Figure 8-6). Thus the depolarization spreads along the length of the axon by "local-circuit" current flow resulting from the potential difference between active and inactive regions of the axon membrane. In cells with longer length constants the local-circuit current has a greater spread and therefore the action potential propagates more rapidly.

A

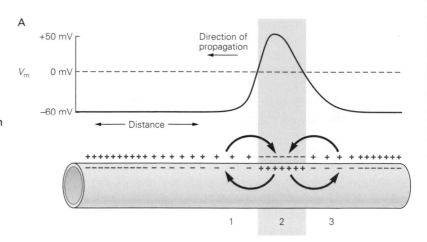

Figure 8-6 Passive conduction of depolarization along the axon contributes to propagation of the action potential.

A. The waveform of an action potential propagating from right to left. The difference in potential along the length of the axon creates a local-circuit current flow that causes the depolarization to spread passively from the active region (**2**) to the inactive region *ahead* of the action potential (**1**), as well as to the area *behind* the action potential (**3**). However, because there is also an increase in g_K in the wake of the action potential (see Chapter 9), the buildup of positive charge along the inner side of the membrane in area **3** is more than balanced by the local efflux of K^+, allowing this region of membrane to repolarize.

B. A short time later the voltage waveform and the current distributions have shifted down the axon and the process is repeated.

B

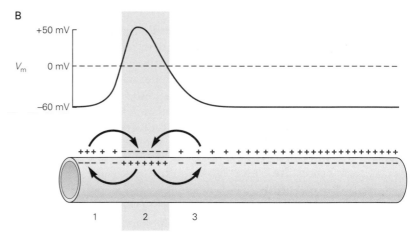

Large Axons Are More Easily Excited Than Small Axons by Extracellular Current Stimuli

In examination of a neurological patient for diseases of peripheral nerves the nerve often is stimulated by passing current between a pair of extracellular electrodes placed over the nerve, and the population of resulting action potentials (the *compound action potential*) is recorded farther along the nerve by a second pair of voltage-recording electrodes. In this situation the total number of axons that generate action potentials varies with the amplitude of the current pulse.

To drive a cell to threshold, the current must pass through the cell membrane. In the vicinity of the positive electrode, current flows across the membrane into the axon. It then flows along the axoplasmic core, eventually flowing out through more distant regions of axonal membrane to the second (negative) electrode in the extracellular fluid. For any given axon, most of the stimulating current bypasses the fiber, moving instead through other axons or through the low-resistance pathway provided by the extracellular fluid. The axons into which current can enter most easily are the most excitable.

In general, axons with the largest diameter have the lowest threshold for extracellular current. The larger the diameter of the axon, the lower the axial resistance to the flow of longitudinal current because of the greater number of intracellular charge carriers (ions) per unit length of the axon. Therefore a greater fraction of total current enters the larger axon, so it is depolarized more efficiently than a smaller axon. For these reasons, larger axons are recruited at low values of current; smaller-diameter axons are recruited only at relatively greater current strengths.

A

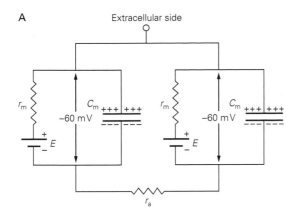

B

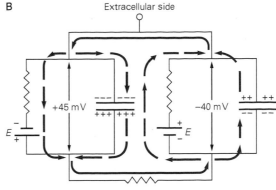

Figure 8-7 Axial resistance and membrane capacitance limit the rate of spread of depolarization during the action potential.

A. The electrical equivalent circuit represents two adjacent segments of the resting membrane of an axon connected by a segment of axoplasm (r_a).

B. An action potential is spreading from the membrane segment on the **left** to the segment on the **right**. Purple lines indicate pathways of current flow.

Passive Membrane Properties and Axon Diameter Affect the Velocity of Action Potential Propagation

The passive spread of depolarization during conduction of the action potential is not instantaneous. In fact, the electrotonic conduction is a rate-limiting factor in the propagation of the action potential. We can understand this limitation by considering a simplified equivalent circuit of two adjacent membrane segments connected by a segment of axoplasm (Figure 8-7). As described above, an action potential generated in one segment of membrane supplies depolarizing current to the adjacent membrane, causing it to depolarize gradually toward threshold. According to Ohm's law, the larger the axoplasmic resistance, the smaller the current flow around the loop ($I = V/R$) and the longer it takes to change the charge on the membrane of the adjacent segment.

Recall that since $\Delta V = \Delta Q/C$, the membrane potential changes slowly if the current is small because ΔQ changes slowly. Similarly, the larger the membrane capacitance, the more charge must be deposited on the membrane to change the potential across the membrane, so the current must flow for a longer time to produce a given depolarization. Therefore, the time it takes for depolarization to spread along the axon is determined by both the axial resistance, r_a, and the capacitance per unit length of the axon c_m (units F/cm). The rate of passive spread varies inversely with the product

$r_a c_m$. If this product is reduced, the rate of passive spread increases and the action potential propagates faster.

Rapid propagation of the action potential is functionally important, and two distinct mechanisms have evolved to increase it. One adaptive strategy is to increase conduction velocity by increasing the diameter of the axon core. Because r_a decreases in proportion to the square of axon diameter, while c_m increases in direct proportion to diameter, the net effect of an increase in diameter is a decrease in $r_a c_m$. This adaptation has been carried to an extreme in the giant axon of the squid, which can reach a diameter of 1 mm. No larger axons have evolved, presumably because of the opposing need to keep neuronal size small so that many cells can be packed into a limited space.

A second mechanism for increasing conduction velocity is myelination of the axon, the wrapping of glial cell membranes around an axon (see Chapter 4). This process is functionally equivalent to increasing the thickness of the axonal membrane by as much as 100 times. Because the capacitance of a parallel-plate capacitor such as the membrane is inversely proportional to the thickness of the insulation material, myelination decreases c_m and thus $r_a c_m$. Myelination results in a proportionately much greater decrease in $r_a c_m$ than does the same increase in the diameter of the axon core. For this reason, conduction in myelinated axons is typically faster than in nonmyelinated axons of the same diameter.

In a neuron with a myelinated axon the action potential is triggered at the nonmyelinated segment of membrane at the axon hillock. The inward current that flows through this region of membrane is then available to discharge the capacitance of the myelinated axon ahead of it. Even though the thickness of myelin makes the capacitance of the axon quite small, the amount of current flowing down the core of the axon from the trigger zone is not enough to discharge the capacitance along the *entire* length of the myelinated axon.

To prevent the action potential from dying out, the myelin sheath is interrupted every 1–2 mm by bare patches of axon membrane about 2 μm in length, the nodes of Ranvier (see Chapter 4). Although the area of membrane at each node is quite small, the nodal membrane is rich in voltage-gated Na^+ channels and thus can generate an intense depolarizing inward Na^+ current in response to the passive spread of depolarization down the axon. These regularly distributed nodes thus boost the amplitude of the action potential periodically, preventing it from dying out.

The action potential, which spreads quite rapidly along the internode because of the low capacitance of the myelin sheath, slows down as it crosses the high-capacitance region of each bare node. Consequently, as the action potential moves down the axon it jumps quickly from node to node (Figure 8-8A). For this reason, the action potential in a myelinated axon is said to move by *saltatory conduction* (from the Latin *saltare*, to jump). Because ionic membrane current flows only at the nodes in myelinated fibers, saltatory conduction is also favorable from a metabolic standpoint. Less energy must be expended by the Na^+-K^+ pump in restoring the Na^+ and K^+ concentration gradients, which tend to run down as a result of action-potential activity.

Various diseases of the nervous system, such as multiple sclerosis and Guillain-Barre syndrome, cause demyelination (see Box 4-1). Because the lack of myelin slows down the conduction of the action potential, these diseases can have devastating effects on behavior (Chapter 35). As an action potential goes from a myelinated region to a bare stretch of axon, it encounters a region of relatively high c_m and low r_m. The inward current generated at the node just before the demyelinated segment may be too small to provide the capacitive current required to depolarize the demyelinated membrane to threshold. In addition, this local-circuit current does not spread as far as it normally would because it is flowing into a segment of axon that, because of its low r_m, has a short length constant (Figure 8-8B). These two factors can combine to slow, and in some cases actually block, the conduction of action potentials.

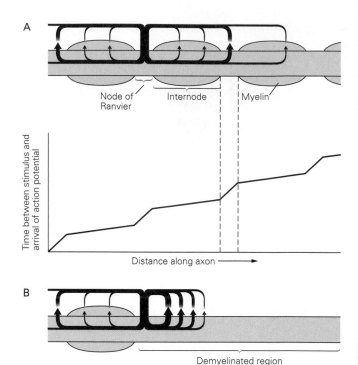

Figure 8-8 Action potentials in myelinated nerves are regenerated at the nodes of Ranvier.

A. In the axon capacitive and ionic membrane current densities (membrane current per unit area of membrane) are much higher at the nodes of Ranvier than in the internodal regions. The density of membrane current at any point along the axon is represented by the thickness of the **arrows**. Because of the higher capacitance of the axon membrane at the unmyelinated nodes, the action potential slows down as it approaches each node and thus appears to skip rapidly from node to node.

B. In regions of the axon that have lost their myelin, the spread of the action potential is slowed down or blocked. The local-circuit currents must charge a larger membrane capacitance and, because of the low r_m, they do not spread well down the axon.

An Overall View

Two competing needs determine the functional design of neurons. First, to maximize the computing power of the nervous system, neurons must be small so that large numbers of them can fit into the brain and spinal cord. Second, to maximize the ability of the animal to respond to changes in its environment, neurons must conduct signals rapidly. These two design objectives are constrained by the materials from which neurons are made.

Because the nerve cell membrane is very thin and is surrounded by a conducting medium, it has a very high capacitance, which slows down the conduction of voltage signals. In addition, the currents that change the charge on the membrane capacitance must flow through a relatively poor conductor—a thin column of cytoplasm. The ion channels that give rise to the resting potential also degrade the signaling function of the neuron. They make the cell leaky and, together with the high membrane capacitance, they limit the distance that a signal can travel passively.

As we shall see in the next chapter, neurons use voltage-gated channels to compensate for these physical constraints when generating all-or-none action potentials, which are continually regenerated and conducted without attenuation. For pathways in which rapid signaling is particularly important, the conduction velocity of the action potential is enhanced either by myelination or by an increase in axon diameter, or by both.

John Koester
Steven A. Siegelbaum

Selected Readings

Hodgkin AL. 1964. Chapter 4. In: *The Conduction of the Nervous Impulse*, pp. 47–55. Springfield, IL: Thomas.

Jack JJB, Noble D, Tsien RW. 1975. Chapters 1, 5, 7, and 9. In: *Electric Current Flow in Excitable Cells*, pp. 1–4, 83–97, 131–224, 276–277. Oxford: Clarendon.

Johnston D, Wu M-S. 1995. Functional properties of dendrites. In: *Foundations of Cellular Neurophysiology*, pp. 55–120. Cambridge: MIT Press.

Koch C. 1999. *Biophysics of Computation*, pp. 25–48. New York: Oxford University Press.

Moore JW, Joyner RW, Brill MH, Waxman SD, Najar-Joa M. 1978. Simulations of conduction in uniform myelinated fibers: relative sensitivity to changes in nodal and internodal parameters. Biophys J 21:147–160.

Rall W. 1977. Core conductor theory and cable properties of neurons. In: ER Kandel (ed). *Handbook of Physiology: A Critical, Comprehensive Presentation of Physiological Knowledge and Concepts*, Sect. 1, *The Nervous System*. Vol. 1, *Cellular Biology of Neurons*, Part 1, pp. 39–97. Bethesda, MD: American Physiological Society.

References

Hodgkin AL, Rushton WAH. 1946. The electrical constants of a crustacean nerve fibre. Proc R Soc Lond Ser B. 133:444–479.

Huxley AF, Stämpfli R. 1949. Evidence for saltatory conduction in peripheral myelinated nerve fibres. J Physiol 108:315–339.

9

Propagated Signaling: The Action Potential

NERVE CELLS ARE ABLE TO carry signals over long distances because of their ability to generate an action potential—a regenerative electrical signal whose amplitude does not attenuate as it moves down the axon. In Chapter 7 we saw how an action potential arises from sequential changes in the membrane's selective permeability to Na^+ and K^+ ions. In Chapter 8 we considered how the membrane's passive properties influence the speed at which action potentials are conducted. In this chapter we focus on the voltage-gated ion channels that are critical for generating and propagating action potentials and consider how these channels are responsible for many important features of a neuron's electrical excitability.

The Action Potential Is Generated by the Flow of Ions Through Voltage-Gated Channels

An important early clue about how action potentials are generated came from an experiment performed by Kenneth Cole and Howard Curtis. While recording from the giant axon of the squid they found that the ion conductance across the membrane increases dramatically during the action potential (Figure 9-1). This discovery provided the first evidence that the action potential results from changes in the flux of ions through the channels of the membrane. It also raised the question: Which ions are responsible for the action potential?

A key to this problem was provided by Alan Hodgkin and Bernard Katz, who found that the amplitude of the action potential is reduced when the external Na^+ concentration is lowered, indicating that Na^+ influx is responsible for the rising phase of the action potential. Their data also suggested that the falling phase of the action potential was caused by a later increase in K^+ permeability. Hodgkin and Katz proposed that depolarization of the cell above threshold causes a brief increase in the cell membrane's permeability to Na^+, during which Na^+ permeability overwhelms the dominant permeability of the resting cell membrane to K^+ ions.

Sodium and Potassium Currents Through Voltage-Gated Channels Are Recorded With the Voltage Clamp

To test this hypothesis, Hodgkin and Andrew Huxley conducted a second series of experiments. They systematically varied the membrane potential in the squid giant axon and measured the resulting changes in the membrane conductance to Na^+ and K^+ through voltage-gated Na^+ and K^+ channels. To do this they made use of a new apparatus, the voltage clamp. Prior to the availability of the voltage-clamp technique, attempts to measure Na^+ and K^+ conductance as a function of membrane potential had been limited by the strong interdependence of the membrane potential and the gating of Na^+ and K^+ channels. For example, if the membrane is depolarized sufficiently to open some of the voltage-gated Na^+ channels, inward Na^+ current flows through these channels and causes further depolarization. The additional depolarization causes still more Na^+ channels to open and consequently induces more inward Na^+ current:

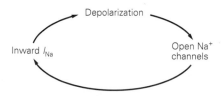

This positive feedback cycle, which eventually drives the membrane potential to the peak of the action potential, makes it impossible to achieve a stable membrane potential. A similar coupling between current and membrane potential complicates the study of the voltage-gated K^+ channels.

The basic function of the voltage clamp is to interrupt the interaction between the membrane potential and the opening and closing of voltage-gated ion channels. The voltage clamp does so by injecting a current into the axon that is equal and opposite to the current flowing through the voltage-gated membrane channels. In this way the voltage clamp prevents the charge separation across the membrane from changing. The amount of current that must be generated by the voltage clamp to keep the membrane potential constant provides a direct measure of the current flowing across the membrane (Box 9-1). Using the voltage-clamp technique, Hodgkin and Huxley provided the first complete description of the ionic mechanisms underlying the action potential.

One advantage of the voltage clamp is that it readily allows the total membrane current to be separated into its ionic and capacitive components. As described in Chapter 8, the membrane potential V_m, is proportional to the charge Q_m on the membrane capacitance (C_m). When V_m is not changing, Q_m is constant and no capacitive current ($\Delta Q_m / \Delta t$) flows. Capacitive current flows *only* when V_m is changing. Therefore, when the membrane potential changes in response to a very rapid step of command potential, capacitive current flows only at the beginning and end of the step. Since the capacitive current is essentially instantaneous, the ionic currents that flow through the gated membrane channels can be analyzed separately.

Measurements of these ionic membrane currents can be used to calculate the voltage and time dependence of changes in membrane conductances caused by the opening and closing of Na^+ and K^+ channels. This information provides insights into the properties of these two types of channels.

A typical voltage-clamp experiment starts with the membrane potential clamped at its resting value. If a 10 mV depolarizing potential step is commanded, we

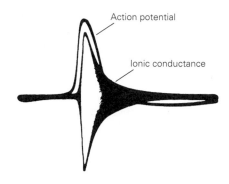

Figure 9-1 A net increase in ionic conductance in the membrane of the axon accompanies the action potential. This historic recording from an experiment conducted in 1938 by Kenneth Cole and Howard Curtis shows the oscilloscope record of an action potential superimposed on a simultaneous record of the ionic conductance.

Box 9-1 Voltage-Clamp Technique

The voltage-clamp technique was developed by Kenneth Cole in 1949 to stabilize the membrane potential of neurons for experimental purposes. It was used by Alan Hodgkin and Andrew Huxley in the early 1950s in a series of experiments that revealed the ionic mechanisms underlying the action potential.

The voltage clamp permits the experimenter to "clamp" the membrane potential at predetermined levels. The voltage-gated ion channels continue to open or close in response to changes in membrane potential, but the voltage clamp prevents the resultant changes in membrane current from influencing the membrane potential. This technique thus permits measurement of the effect of changes in membrane potential on the conductance of the membrane to individual ion species.

The voltage clamp consists of a source of current connected to two electrodes, one inside and the other outside the cell (Figure 9-2A). By passing current across the cell membrane, the membrane potential can be stepped rapidly to a predetermined level of depolarization.

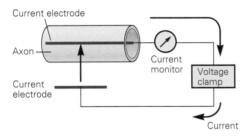

Figure 9-2 A

The voltage clamp is a current generator that is connected to a pair of electrodes. It is used to change the charge separation, and thus the electrical potential difference, across the membrane. Monitoring the additional current that is passed to clamp the membrane potential at its new value then provides a measure of the membrane current passing through the ion channels in the membrane.

These depolarizations open voltage-gated Na^+ and K^+ channels. The resulting movement of Na^+ and K^+ across the membrane would ordinarily change the membrane potential, but the voltage clamp maintains the membrane potential at its commanded level. When Na^+ channels open in response to a moderate depolarizing voltage step, an inward ionic current develops because Na^+ ions flow through these channels as a result of their electrochemical driving force. This Na^+ influx normally depolarizes the membrane by increasing the positive charge on the inside of the membrane and reducing the positive charge on the outside.

The voltage clamp intervenes in this process by simultaneously withdrawing positive charges from the cell and depositing them in the external solution. By generating a current that is equal and opposite to the ionic current, the voltage-clamp circuit automatically prevents the ionic current from changing the membrane potential from the commanded value (Figure 9-2A). As a result, the *net* amount of charge separated by the membrane does not change and therefore no significant change in V_m can occur.

The voltage clamp is a negative feedback system. A negative feedback system is one in which the value of the output of the system (V_m in this case) is "fed back" to the input of the system, where it is compared to a command signal for the desired output. Any difference between the command potential and the output signal activates a "controller" device that automatically reduces the difference. Thus the membrane potential *automatically* follows the command potential exactly (Figure 9-2B).

For example, assume that an inward Na^+ current through the voltage-gated Na^+ channels causes the membrane potential to become more positive than the command potential. The input to the feedback amplifier is equal to ($V_{command} - V_m$). Thus, both the input and the resulting output voltage at the feedback amplifier will be negative. This negative output voltage will make the internal current electrode negative, withdrawing net positive charge from the cell through the voltage-clamp circuit. As the current flows around the circuit, an equal amount of net positive charge will be deposited into the external solution through the other current electrode.

A refinement of the voltage clamp, the patch-clamp technique, allows the functional properties of *individual* ion channels to be analyzed (see Box 6-1).

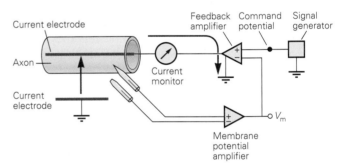

Figure 9-2 B

The negative feedback mechanism by which the voltage clamp operates. Membrane potential is measured by one amplifier connected to an intracellular electrode and to an extracellular electrode in the bath. The membrane potential signal is displayed on an oscilloscope and is also fed into one terminal of the "feedback" amplifier. This amplifier has two inputs, one for membrane potential (V_m) and the other for the command potential. The command potential, which comes from a signal generator, is selected by the experimenter and can be of any desired amplitude and waveform. The feedback amplifier subtracts the membrane potential from the command potential. Any difference between these two signals is amplified several thousand times at the feedback amplifier. The output of this amplifier is connected to a current electrode, a thin wire that runs the length of the axon. To accurately measure the current-voltage relationship of the cell membrane, the membrane potential must be uniform along the entire surface of the axon. This is achieved by using a highly conductive current electrode, which short circuits the axoplasmic resistance, reducing the axial resistance to zero (see Chapter 8). This low-resistance pathway within the axon eliminates all potential differences along the axon core.

observe that an initial, very brief outward current instantaneously discharges the membrane capacitance by the amount required for a 10 mV depolarization. This *capacitive current* (I_c) is followed by a smaller outward ionic current that persists for the duration of this pulse. At the end of the pulse there is a brief inward capacitive current, and the total membrane current returns to zero (Figure 9-3A). The steady ionic current that persists throughout the depolarization is the current that flows through the resting ion channels of the membrane (see Chapter 6) and is called the *leakage current, I_l*. The total conductance of this population of channels is called the *leakage conductance* (g_l). These resting channels, which are always open, are responsible for generating the resting membrane potential (see Chapter 7). In a typical neuron most of the resting channels are permeable to K^+ ions; the remaining channels are permeable to Cl^- or Na^+ ions.

If a larger depolarizing step is commanded, the current record becomes more complicated. The capacitive and leakage currents both increase in amplitude. In addition, shortly after the end of the capacitive current and the start of the leakage current, an inward current develops; it reaches a peak within a few milliseconds, declines, and gives way to an outward current. This outward current reaches a plateau that is maintained for the duration of the pulse (Figure 9-3B).

A simple interpretation of these results is that the depolarizing voltage step sequentially turns on active conductance channels for two separate ions: one type of channel for inward current and another for outward current. Because these two oppositely directed currents partially overlap in time, the most difficult task in analyzing voltage-clamp experiments is to determine their separate time courses.

Hodgkin and Huxley achieved this separation by changing ions in the bathing solution. By substituting a larger, impermeant cation (choline·H^+) for Na^+, they eliminated the inward Na^+ current. Subsequently, the task of separating inward and outward currents was made easier by selectively blocking the voltage-sensitive conductance channels with drugs or toxins. Tetrodotoxin, a poison from certain Pacific puffer fish, blocks the voltage-gated Na^+ channel with a very high potency in the nanomolar range of concentration. (Ingestion of only a few milligrams of tetrodotoxin from improperly prepared puffer fish, consumed as the Japanese sushi delicacy fugu, can be fatal.) The cation tetraethylammonium specifically blocks the voltage-gated K^+ channel (Figure 9-4).

When tetraethylammonium is applied to the axon to block the K^+ channels, the total membrane current (I_m) consists of I_c, I_l, and I_{Na}. The leakage conductance,

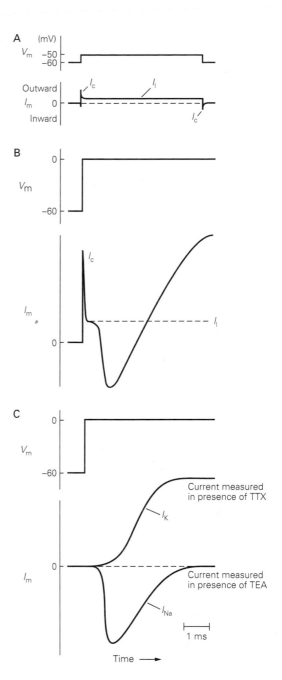

Figure 9-3 A voltage-clamp experiment demonstrates the sequential activation of two types of voltage-gated channels.

A. A small depolarization is accompanied by capacitive and leakage currents (I_c and I_l, respectively).

B. A larger depolarization results in larger capacitive and leakage currents, plus an inward current followed by an outward current.

C. Depolarizing the cell in the presence of tetrodotoxin (which blocks the Na^+ current) and again in the presence of tetraethylammonium (which blocks the K^+ current), reveals the pure K^+ and Na^+ currents (I_K and I_{Na}, respectively) after subtracting I_c and I_l.

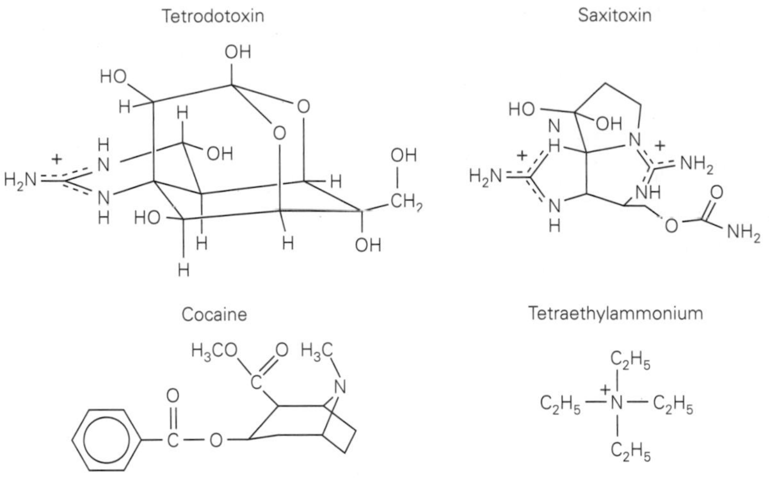

Figure 9-4 Drugs that block voltage-gated Na⁺ and K⁺ channels. Tetrodotoxin and saxitoxin both bind to Na⁺ channels with a very high affinity. **Tetrodotoxin** is produced by certain puffer fish, newts, and frogs. **Saxitoxin** is synthesized by the dinoflagellates *Gonyaulax* that are responsible for red tides. Consumption of clams or other shellfish that have fed on the dinoflagellates during a red tide causes paralytic shellfish poisoning. **Cocaine**, the active substance isolated from coca leaves, was the first substance to be used as a local anesthetic. It also blocks Na⁺ channels but with a lower affinity and specificity than tetrodotoxin. **Tetraethylammonium** is a cation that blocks certain voltage-gated K⁺ channels with a relatively low affinity. The red plus signs represent positive charge.

Tetrodotoxin

Saxitoxin

Cocaine

Tetraethylammonium

Voltage-Gated Sodium and Potassium Conductances Are Calculated From Their Currents

g_l, is constant; it does not vary with V_m or with time. Therefore, I_l, the leakage current, can be readily calculated and subtracted from I_m, leaving I_{Na} and I_c. Because I_c occurs only briefly at the beginning and end of the pulse, it can be easily isolated by visual inspection, leaving the pure I_{Na}. The full range of current flow through the voltage-gated Na⁺ channels (I_{Na}) is measured by repeating this analysis after stepping V_m to many different levels. With a similar process, I_K can be measured when the Na⁺ channels are blocked by tetrodotoxin (Figure 9-3C).

Voltage-Gated Sodium and Potassium Conductances Are Calculated From Their Currents

The Na⁺ and K⁺ currents depend on two factors: the conductance for each ion and the electrochemical driving force acting on the ion. Since the Na⁺ and K⁺ membrane conductance is directly proportional to the number of open Na⁺ and K⁺ channels, we can gain insight into how membrane voltage controls channel opening by calculating the amplitudes and time courses of the Na⁺ and K⁺ conductance changes in response to voltage-clamp depolarizations (Box 9-2).

Measurements of Na⁺ and K⁺ conductances at various levels of membrane potential reveal two functional similarities and two differences between the Na⁺ and K⁺ channels. Both types of channels open in response to depolarizing steps of membrane potential. Moreover, as the size of the depolarization increases, the probability and rate of opening increase for both types of channels. The Na⁺ and K⁺ channels differ, however, in their rates of opening and in their responses to prolonged depolar-

ization. At all levels of depolarization the Na⁺ channels open more rapidly than do the K⁺ channels (Figure 9-6). When the depolarization is maintained for some time, the Na⁺ channels begin to close, leading to a decrease of inward current. The process by which Na⁺ channels close during a maintained depolarization is termed *inactivation*. In contrast, the K⁺ channels in the squid axon do not inactivate; they remain open as long as the membrane is depolarized (Figure 9-7).

Thus, depolarization causes Na⁺ channels to undergo transitions among three different states, which represent three different conformations of the Na⁺ channel protein: resting, activated, or inactivated. Upon depolarization the channel goes from the resting (closed) state to the activated (open) state (see Figure 6-6C). If the depolarization is brief, the channels go directly back to the resting state upon repolarization. If the depolarization is maintained, the channels go from the open to the inactivated (closed) state. Once the channel is inactivated it cannot be opened by further depolarization. The inactivation can be reversed only by repolarizing the membrane to its negative resting potential, which allows the channel to switch from the inactivated to the resting state. This switch takes some time because channels leave the inactivated state relatively slowly (Figure 9-8).

These variable, time-dependent effects of depolarization on g_{Na} are determined by the kinetics of the gating reactions that control the Na⁺ channels. Each Na⁺ channel has two kinds of gates that must be opened simultaneously for the channel to conduct Na⁺ ions. An *activation gate* is closed when the membrane is at its negative resting potential and is rapidly opened by de-

Box 9-2 Calculation of Membrane Conductances From Voltage-Clamp Data

Membrane conductance can be calculated from voltage-clamp currents using equations derived from an equivalent circuit of the membrane that includes the membrane capacitance (C_m) and leakage conductance (g_l), as well as g_{Na} and g_K (Figure 9-5). In this context g_l represents the conductance of all of the resting K^+, Na^+, and Cl^- channels (see Chapter 7); g_{Na} and g_K represent the conductances of the voltage-gated Na^+ and K^+ channels. The ionic battery of the resting (leakage) channels, E_l, is equal to the resting potential. The voltage-sensitive Na^+ and K^+ conductances are in series with their appropriate ionic batteries.

The current through each class of voltage-gated channel may be calculated from Ohm's law:

$$I_K = g_K(V_m - E_K)$$

and

$$I_{Na} = g_{Na}(V_m - E_{Na}).$$

Rearranging and solving for g gives two equations that can be used to compute the conductances of the active Na^+ and K^+ channel populations:

$$g_K = \frac{I_K}{(V_m - E_K)}$$

and

$$g_{Na} = \frac{I_{Na}}{(V_m - E_{Na})}.$$

To solve these equations, one must know V_m, E_K, E_{Na}, I_K, and I_{Na}. The independent variable, V_m, is set by the experimenter. The dependent variables, I_K and I_{Na}, can be calculated from the records of voltage-clamp experiments (see Figure 9-3C). The remaining variables, E_K and E_{Na}, are constants; they can be determined empirically by finding the values of V_m at which I_K and I_{Na} reverse their polarities, that is, their *reversal potentials*. For example, as V_m is stepped to very positive values, the inward I_{Na} becomes smaller because of the smaller inward electrochemical driving force on Na^+. When V_m equals E_{Na}, I_{Na} is zero owing to the lack of a net driving force. At potentials that are positive to E_{Na}, I_{Na} becomes outward (corresponding to a net efflux of Na^+ ions from the axon) because of a net outward driving force on Na^+.

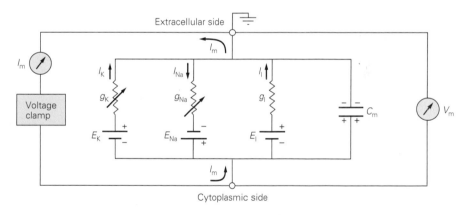

Figure 9-5 Electrical equivalent circuit of a nerve cell being held at a depolarized potential under voltage-clamp conditions. The voltage-gated conductance pathways (g_K and g_{Na}) are represented by the symbol for variable conductance— a conductor (resistor) with an arrow through it.

polarization; an *inactivation gate* is open at the resting potential and closes slowly in response to depolarization. The channel conducts only for the brief period during a depolarization when both gates are open. Repolarization reverses the two processes, closing the activation gate rapidly and opening the inactivation gate more slowly. After the channel has returned to the resting state, it can again be activated by depolarization (Figure 9-9).

The Action Potential Can Be Reconstructed From the Properties of Sodium and Potassium Channels

Hodgkin and Huxley were able to fit their measurements of membrane conductance changes to a set of empirical equations that completely describe variations in membrane Na^+ and K^+ conductances as functions of membrane potential and time. Using these equations

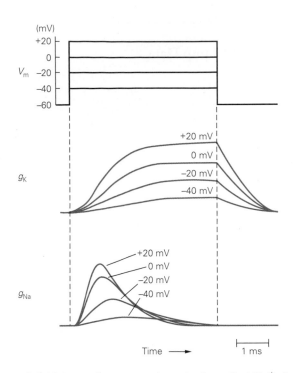

Figure 9-6 Voltage-clamp experiments show that Na+ channels turn on and off more rapidly than K+ channels over a wide range of membrane potentials. The increases and decreases in the Na+ and K+ conductances (g_{Na} and g_K) shown here reflect the shifting of thousands of voltage-gated channels between the open and closed states.

and measured values for the passive properties of the axon, they computed the expected shape and the conduction velocity of the propagated action potential. The calculated waveform of the action potential matched the waveform recorded in the unclamped axon almost perfectly! This close agreement indicates that the voltage and time dependence of the active Na+ and K+ channels, calculated from the voltage-clamp data, accurately describe the properties of the channels that are essential for generating and propagating the action potential. A half century later, the Hodgkin-Huxley model stands as the most successful quantitative computational model in neural science if not in all of biology.

According to the Hodgkin-Huxley model, an action potential involves the following sequence of events. A depolarization of the membrane causes Na+ channels to open rapidly (an increase in g_{Na}), resulting in an inward Na+ current. This current, by discharging the membrane capacitance, causes further depolarization, there-

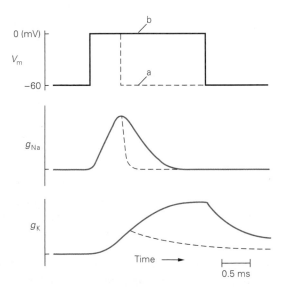

Figure 9-7 Sodium and potassium channels respond differently to long-term depolarization. If the membrane is repolarized after a brief depolarization **(line a)**, both g_{Na} and g_K return to their initial values. If depolarization is maintained **(line b)**, the Na+ channels close (or inactivate) before the depolarization is terminated, whereas the K+ channels remain open and g_K increases throughout the depolarization.

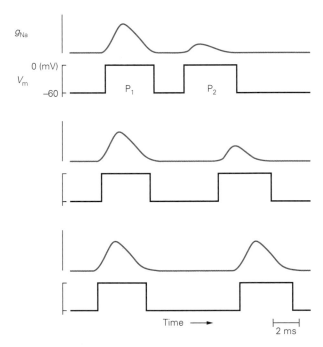

Figure 9-8 Sodium channels remain inactivated for a few milliseconds after the end of a depolarization. Therefore if the interval between two depolarizing pulses (P₁ and P₂) is brief, the second pulse produces a smaller increase in g_{Na} because many of the Na+ channels are inactivated. The longer the interval between pulses, the greater the increase in g_{Na}, because a greater fraction of channels will have recovered from inactivation and returned to the resting state when the second pulse begins. The time course of recovery from inactivation contributes to the time course of the refractory period.

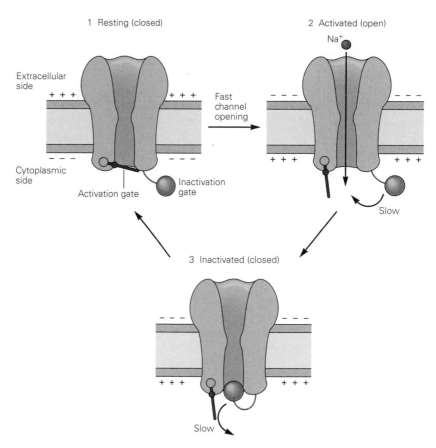

1 Resting (closed)

2 Activated (open)

Na⁺

Extracellular side

Fast channel opening

Cytoplasmic side

Activation gate   Inactivation gate

Slow

3 Inactivated (closed)

Slow

Figure 9-9 Voltage-gated Na^+ channels have two gates, which respond in opposite ways to depolarization. In the resting (closed) state the activation gate is closed and the inactivation gate is open (**1**). Upon depolarization a rapid opening of the activation gate allows Na^+ to flow through the channel (**2**). As the inactivation gates close, the Na^+ channels enter the inactivated (closed) state (**3**). Upon repolarization, first the activation gate closes, then the inactivation gate opens as the channel returns to the resting state (**1**).

by opening more Na^+ channels, resulting in a further increase in inward current. This regenerative process drives the membrane potential toward E_{Na}, causing the rising phase of the action potential.[1] The depolarizing state of the action potential then limits the duration of the action potential in two ways: (1) It gradually inactivates the Na^+ channels, thus reducing g_{Na}, and (2) it opens, with some delay, the voltage-gated K^+ channels, thereby increasing g_K. Consequently, the inward Na^+ current is followed by an outward K^+ current that tends to repolarize the membrane (Figure 9-10).

In most nerve cells the action potential is followed by a transient hyperpolarization, the *after-potential*. This brief increase in membrane potential occurs because the K^+ channels that open during the later phase of the action potential close some time after V_m has returned to its resting value. It takes a few milliseconds for all of the voltage-gated K^+ channels to return to the closed state. During this time, when the permeability of the membrane to K^+ is greater than during the resting state, V_m is hyperpolarized slightly with respect to its normal resting value, resulting in a V_m closer to E_K (Figure 9-10).

The action potential is also followed by a brief period of diminished excitability, or refractoriness, which can be divided into two phases. The *absolute refractory period* comes immediately after the action potential; during this period it is impossible to excite the cell no matter how great a stimulating current is applied. This phase is followed directly by the *relative refractory period*, during which it is possible to trigger an action potential but only by applying stimuli that are stronger than those normally required to reach threshold. These periods of refractoriness, which together last just a few milliseconds, are caused by the residual inactivation of Na^+ channels and increased opening of K^+ channels.

---

1. It may at first seem paradoxical that to depolarize the cell experimentally one passes *outward* current across the membrane (see Figure 7-2C), while at the same time attributing the depolarization during the upstroke of the action potential to an *inward* Na^+ current. However, in both cases the current flow across the passive components, the nongated leakage channels (g_l) and the capacitance of the membrane (C_m), is outward because positive charge is injected into the cell in one case through an intracellular electrode (see Figure 7-2) and in the other case by the opening of voltage-gated Na^+ channels. It is a matter of convention that when we refer to current injected through a microelectrode we refer to the direction in which the current crosses the membrane capacitance and leakage channels, whereas when we refer to current that flows through channels we refer to the direction of movement of charge through the channels.

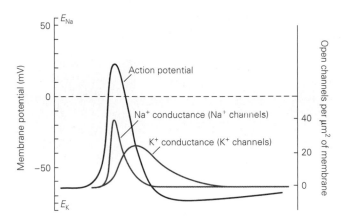

Figure 9-10 The sequential opening of voltage-gated Na$^+$ and K$^+$ channels generates the action potential. One of Hodgkin and Huxley's great achievements was to separate the total conductance change during an action potential, first detected by Cole and Curtis (see Figure 9-1) into separate components attributable to the opening of Na$^+$ and K$^+$ channels. The shape of the action potential and the underlying conductance changes can be calculated from the properties of the voltage-gated Na$^+$ and K$^+$ channels.

Another feature of the action potential predicted by the Hodgkin-Huxley model is its all-or-none behavior. A fraction of a millivolt can be the difference between a subthreshold depolarizing stimulus and a stimulus that generates an action potential. This all-or-none phenomenon may seem surprising when one considers that the Na$^+$ conductance increases in a strictly *graded* manner as depolarization is increased (see Figure 9-6). Each increment of depolarization increases the number of voltage-gated Na$^+$ channels that switch from the closed to the open state, thereby causing a gradual increase in Na$^+$ influx. Why then is there an abrupt threshold for generating an action potential?

Although a small subthreshold depolarization increases the inward I_{Na}, it also increases two *outward* currents, I_K and I_l, by increasing the electrochemical driving force on K$^+$ and Cl$^-$. In addition, the depolarization augments the K$^+$ conductance, g_K, by gradually opening more voltage-gated K$^+$ channels (see Figure 9-6). As I_K and I_l increase with depolarization, they tend to resist the depolarizing action of the Na$^+$ influx. However, because of the great voltage sensitivity and rapid kinetics of activation of the Na$^+$ channels, the depolarization eventually reaches a point where the increase in inward I_{Na} exceeds the increase in outward I_K and I_l. At this point there is a net inward current producing a further depolarization so that the depolarization becomes regenerative. The specific value of V_m at which the *net*

ionic current ($I_{Na} + I_K + I_l$) just changes from outward to inward, depositing a net positive charge on the inside of the membrane capacitance, is the threshold.

Variations in the Properties of Voltage-Gated Ion Channels Increase the Signaling Capabilities of Neurons

The basic mechanism of electrical excitability identified by Hodgkin and Huxley in the squid giant axon—whereby voltage-gated ion channels conduct an inward ionic current followed by an outward ionic current—appears to be universal in all excitable cells. However, dozens of different types of voltage-gated ion channels have been identified in other nerve and muscle cells, and the distribution of specific types varies not only from cell to cell but also from region to region within a cell. These differences in the pattern of ion channel expression have important consequences for the details of membrane excitability, as we shall now explore.

The Nervous System Expresses a Rich Variety of Voltage-Gated Ion Channels

Although the voltage-gated Na$^+$ and K$^+$ channels in the squid axon described by Hodgkin and Huxley have been found in almost every type of neuron examined, several other kinds of channels have also been identified. For example, most neurons contain voltage-gated Ca^{2+} channels that open in response to membrane depolarization. A strong electrochemical gradient drives Ca^{2+} into the cell, so these channels give rise to an inward I_{Ca}. Some neurons and muscle cells also have voltage-gated Cl$^-$ channels. Finally, many neurons have monovalent cation-permeable channels that are slowly activated by hyperpolarization and are permeable to both K$^+$ and Na$^+$. The net effect of the mixed permeability of these rather nonselective channels, called *h-type*, is the generation of an inward, depolarizing current in the voltage range around the resting potential.

Each basic type of ion channel has many variants. For example, there are four major types of voltage-activated K$^+$ channels that differ in their kinetics of activation, voltage activation range, and sensitivity to various ligands. These variants are particularly common in the nervous system. (1) The slowly activating channel described by Hodgkin and Huxley is called the *delayed rectifier*. (2) A *calcium-activated K$^+$ channel* is activated by intracellular Ca^{2+}, but its sensitivity to intracellular Ca^{2+} is enhanced by depolarization. It requires both a rise in internal Ca^{2+} (mediated by voltage-gated Ca^{2+} channels) and depolarization to achieve a maximum probability of opening. (3) The *A-type K⁺ channel* is activated rapidly by depolarization, almost as rapidly as the Na^+ channel; like the Na^+ channel, it also inactivates rapidly if the depolarization is maintained. (4) The *M-type K⁺ channel* is very slowly activated by small depolarizations from the resting potential. One distinctive feature of the M-type channels is that they can be closed by a neurotransmitter, acetylcholine (ACh).

Similarly, there are at least five subtypes of voltage-gated Ca^{2+} channels and two or more types of voltage-gated Na^+ channels. Moreover, each of these subtypes has several structurally and functionally different isoforms.

The squid axon can generate an action potential with just two types of voltage-gated channels. Why then are so many different types of voltage-gated ion channels found in the nervous system? The answer is that neurons with an expanded set of voltage-gated channels have much more complex information-processing abilities than those with only two types of channels. Some ways in which this large variety of voltage-gated channels influences neuronal function are described below.

Gating of Voltage-Sensitive Ion Channels Can Be Influenced by Various Cytoplasmic Factors

In a typical neuron the opening and closing of certain voltage-gated ion channels can be modulated by various cytoplasmic factors, resulting in increased flexibility of the neuron's excitability properties. Changes in such cytoplasmic modulator substances may result from the normal intrinsic activity of the neuron itself or from the influences of other neurons.

The flow of ionic current through membrane channels during an action potential generally does not result in appreciable changes in the intracellular concentrations of most ion species. Calcium is a notable exception to this rule. Changes in the intracellular concentration of Ca^{2+} can have important modulatory influences on the gating of various channels. The concentration of free Ca^{2+} in the cytoplasm of a resting cell is extremely low, about 10^{-7} M, several orders of magnitude below the external Ca^{2+} concentration. For this reason the intracellular Ca^{2+} concentration may increase significantly as a result of inward current flow through voltage-gated Ca^{2+} channels.

The transient increase in Ca^{2+} concentration near the inside of the membrane has several effects. It enhances the probability that Ca^{2+}-activated K^+ channels will open. Some Ca^{2+} channels are themselves sensitive to levels of intracellular Ca^{2+} and are inactivated when incoming Ca^{2+} binds to their intracellular surface. In other channels the influx of Ca^{2+} activates a Ca^{2+}-sensi-

tive protein phosphatase, calcineurin, which dephosphorylates the channel, thereby inactivating it (see Figure 6-7C).

Thus, in some cells the Ca^{2+} influx during an action potential can have two opposing effects: (1) The positive charge that it carries into the cell contributes to the regenerative depolarization, while (2) the increase in cytoplasmic Ca^{2+} concentration results in the opening of more K^+ channels and the closing of Ca^{2+} channels. Because of the opening of K^+ channels and the closing of Ca^{2+} channels, outward ionic current increases while inward ionic current decreases; the resulting net efflux of positive charge causes the cell to repolarize. In this way the depolarizing influx of Ca^{2+} through voltage-gated Ca^{2+} channels is self-limited by two processes that aid repolarization: an increase in K^+ efflux and a decrease in Ca^{2+} influx.

Calcium's role in modulating the gating of ion channels is the simplest example of a variety of second-messenger systems that control channel activity. Gating of ion channels can also be modulated by changes in the cytoplasmic level of small organic second-messenger compounds as a result of synaptic input from other neurons. The gating properties of several voltage-gated channels that are directly involved in generating action potentials are modified when their phosphorylation state is changed by a protein kinase (eg, the cAMP-dependent protein kinase) whose activity is controlled by changes in the concentration of synaptically activated second messengers (eg, cAMP). The importance of Ca^{2+} and other second messengers in the control of neuronal activity will become evident in many contexts throughout this book.

Excitability Properties Vary Between Regions of the Neuron

Different regions of the cell perform specific signaling tasks. The axon, for example, usually specializes in carrying signals faithfully over long distances. As such, it functions as a relatively simple relay line. In contrast, the input, integrative, and output regions of a neuron (see Figure 2-8) typically perform more complex processing of the information they receive before passing it along. The signaling function of a discrete region of the neuron depends on the particular set of ion channels that it expresses.

In many types of neurons the dendrites have voltage-gated ion channels, including Ca^{2+}, K^+, and in some cases Na^+ channels. When activated, these channels modify the passive, electrotonic conduction of synaptic potentials. In some neurons action potentials may be propagated from their site of initiation at the trigger zone back into the dendrites, thereby influencing synaptic integration in the dendrites. In other neurons the density of dendritic voltage-gated channels may even support the orthograde propagation of a dendritic impulse to the cell soma and axon hillock.

The trigger zone of the neuron has the lowest threshold for action potential generation, in part because it has an exceptionally high density of voltage-gated Na^+ channels. In addition, it typically has voltage-gated ion channels that are sensitive to relatively small deviations from resting potential. These channels are important in determining whether synaptic input will drive the membrane potential to spike threshold. They thus play a critical role in the transformation of graded, analog changes in synaptic or receptor potentials into a temporally patterned, digital train of all-or-none action potentials. Examples include the M-type and certain A-type K^+ channels, the hyperpolarization-activated h-type channels, and a class of low voltage-activated Ca^{2+} channels (see below).

As the action potential is carried down the axon it is mediated primarily by voltage-gated Na^+ and K^+ channels that function much like those in the squid axon. At the nodes of Ranvier of myelinated axons the mechanism of action potential repolarization is particularly simple—the spike is terminated by fast inactivation of Na^+ channels combined with a large outward leakage current. Voltage-gated K^+ channels do not play a significant role in action potential repolarization at the nodal membrane.

Presynaptic nerve terminals at chemical synapses commonly have a high density of voltage-gated Ca^{2+} channels. Arrival of an action potential in the terminal opens these channels, causing Ca^{2+} influx, which in turn triggers transmitter release.

Excitability Properties Vary Among Neurons

The computing power of an entire neural circuit is enhanced when cells in the circuit represent a wide range of functional properties, because specific functions within the circuit can be assigned to cells with the most appropriate dynamic properties. Thus, while the function of a neuron is determined to a great extent by its anatomical relationships to other neurons (its inputs and its outputs), the biophysical properties of the cell also play a critical role.

How a neuron responds to synaptic input is determined by the proportions of different types of voltage-gated channels in the cell's integrative and trigger zones. Cells with different combinations of channels respond to a constant excitatory input differently. Some cells respond with only a single action potential, others

with a constant-frequency train of action potentials, and still others with either an accelerating or decelerating train of action potentials. Some neurons even fire spontaneously in the absence of any external input because of the presence of h-type channels that generate endogenous pacemaker currents (Figure 9-11).

In certain neurons small changes in the strength of synaptic inputs produce a large increase in firing rate, whereas in other cells large changes in synaptic input are required to modulate the firing rate. In many neurons a steady hyperpolarizing input makes the cell less responsive to excitatory input by reducing the resting inactivation of the A-type K^+ channels. In other neurons such a steady hyperpolarization makes the cell *more* excitable, because it removes the inactivation of a particular class of voltage-gated Ca^{2+} channels. In many cases the firing properties of a neuron can be modulated by second messenger–mediated changes in the function of voltage-gated ion channels (Figure 9-11).

The Signaling Functions of Voltage-Gated Channels Can Be Related to Their Molecular Structures

The empirical equations derived by Hodgkin and Huxley are quite successful in describing how the flow of ions through the Na^+ and K^+ channels generates the action potential. However, these equations describe the process of excitation primarily in terms of changes in membrane conductance and current flow. They tell little about the molecular structure of the voltage-gated channels and the molecular mechanisms by which they are activated. Fortunately, technical advances such as those described in Chapter 6 have made it possible to examine the structure and function of the voltage-gated Na^+, K^+, and Ca^{2+} channels in detail at the molecular level.

One of the first clues that Na^+ channels are distinct physical entities came from studies that measured the binding of radiolabeled tetrodotoxin to nerve membranes. The density of voltage-gated Na^+ channels in different nerves was estimated by measuring the total amount of tritium-labeled tetrodotoxin bound when specific axonal binding sites are saturated. In nonmyelinated axons the density of channels is quite low, ranging from 35 to 500 Na^+ channels per square micrometer of axon membrane in different cell types. In myelinated axons, where the Na^+ channels are concentrated at the nodes of Ranvier, the density is much higher—between 1000 and 2000 channels per square micrometer of nodal membrane. The greater the density of Na^+ channels in the membrane of an axon, the greater the velocity at

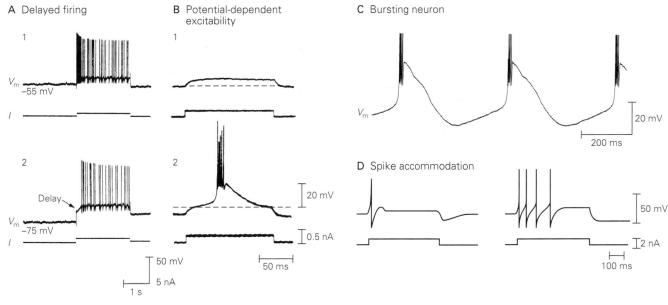

Figure 9-11 Repetitive firing properties vary widely among different types of neurons because the neurons differ in the types of voltage-gated ion channels they express.

A. Injection of a depolarizing current pulse into a neuron from the nucleus tractus solitarius normally triggers an immediate train of action potentials (**1**). If the cell is first held at a hyperpolarized membrane potential, the depolarizing pulse triggers a spike train after a delay (**2**). The delay is caused by the A-type K^+ channels, which are activated by depolarizing synaptic input. The opening of these channels generates a transient outward K^+ current that briefly drives V_m away from threshold. These channels typically are inactivated at the resting potential (−55 mV), but steady hyperpolarization removes the inactivation, allowing the channels to be activated by depolarization. (From Dekin and Getting 1987.)

B. When a small depolarizing current pulse is injected into a thalamic neuron at rest, only an electrotonic, subthreshold depolarization is generated (**1**). If the cell is held at a hyperpolarized level, the same current pulse triggers a burst of action potentials (**2**). The effectiveness of the current pulse is enhanced because the hyperpolarization causes a type of voltage-gated Ca^{2+} channel to recover from inactivation. The dashed line indicates the level of the resting potential. (From Llinás and Jahnsen 1982.)

The data in **A** and **B** demonstrate that steady hyperpolarization, such as might be produced by inhibitory synaptic input to a neuron, can profoundly affect the spike train pattern that a neuron generates. This effect varies greatly among cell types.

C. In the absence of synaptic input, thalamocortical relay neu-

rons can fire spontaneously in brief bursts of action potentials. These endogenously generated bursts are produced by current flow through two types of voltage-gated ion channels. The gradual depolarization that leads to a burst is driven by inward current flowing through the h-type channels, whose activation gates have the unusual property of opening in response to hyperpolarizing voltage steps. The burst is triggered by inward Ca^{2+} current through voltage-gated Ca^{2+} channels that are activated at relatively low levels of depolarization. This Ca^{2+} influx generates sufficient depolarization to reach threshold and drive a train of Na^+-dependent action potentials. The strong depolarization during the burst causes the h-type channels to close and inactivates the Ca^{2+} channels, allowing the interburst hyperpolarization to develop. This hyperpolarization then opens the h-type channels, initiating the next cycle in the rhythm. (From McCormick and Huguenard 1992.)

D. The firing properties of sympathetic neurons in autonomic ganglia are regulated by a neurotransmitter. A prolonged depolarizing current normally results in only a single action potential. This is because depolarization turns on a slowly activated K^+ current, the M current. The slow activation kinetics of the M-type channels allow the cell to fire one action potential before the efflux of K^+ through the M-type channels becomes sufficient to shift the membrane to more negative voltages and prevent the cell from firing more action potentials (a process termed *accommodation*). The neurotransmitter acetylcholine (ACh) closes the M-type channels, allowing the cell to fire many action potentials in response to the same stimulus. (From Jones and Adams 1987.)

which the axon conducts action potentials. A higher density of voltage-gated Na^+ channels allows more current to flow through the excited membrane and along the axon core, thus rapidly discharging the capacitance of the unexcited membrane downstream (see Figure 8-6).

Opening of Voltage-Gated Channels Is All-or-None

The current flow through a single channel cannot be measured in ordinary voltage-clamp experiments for two reasons. First, the voltage clamp acts on a large area of membrane in which thousands of channels are opening and closing randomly. Second, the background noise caused by the flow of current through passive membrane channels is much larger than the flow of current through any one channel. Both these problems can be circumvented by electrically isolating a tiny piece of membrane in a patch-clamp electrode (see Box 6-1).

Patch-clamp experiments demonstrate that voltage-gated channels generally have only two conductance states, open and closed. Each channel opens in an all-or-none fashion and, when open, permits a pulse of current to flow with a variable duration but constant amplitude (Figure 9-12). The conductances of single voltage-gated Na^+, K^+, and Ca^{2+} channels in the open state typically range from 1 to 20 pS, depending on channel type. One class of Ca^{2+}-activated K^+ channels has an unusually large conductance of about 200 pS.

Redistribution of Charges Within Voltage-Gated Sodium Channels Controls Channel Gating

In their original study of the squid axon, Hodgkin and Huxley suggested that a voltage-gated channel has a net charge, the *gating charge,* somewhere within its wall. They postulated that a change in membrane potential causes this charged structure to move within the plane of the membrane, resulting in a conformational change that causes the channel to open or close. They further predicted that such a charge movement would be measurable. For example, when the membrane is depolarized a positive gating charge would move from near the inner surface toward the outer surface of the membrane, owing to its interaction with the membrane electric field. Such a displacement of positive charge would reduce the net separation of charge across the membrane and hence tend to hyperpolarize the membrane. To keep the membrane potential constant in a voltage-clamp experiment, a small extra component of outward capacitive current, called *gating current,* would have to be generated by the voltage clamp. When the membrane current was examined by means of very sensitive techniques, the predicted gating current was found to flow at the beginning and end of a depolarizing voltage-clamp step prior to the opening or closing of the Na^+ channels (Figure 9-13).

Analysis of the gating current reveals that activation and inactivation of Na^+ channels are coupled processes. During a short depolarizing pulse net outward movement of gating charge within the membrane at the beginning of the pulse is balanced by an opposite inward movement of gating charge at the end of the pulse. However, if the pulse lasts long enough for Na^+ inactivation to take place, the movement of gating charge back across the membrane at the end of the pulse is delayed. The gat-

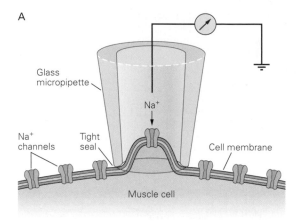

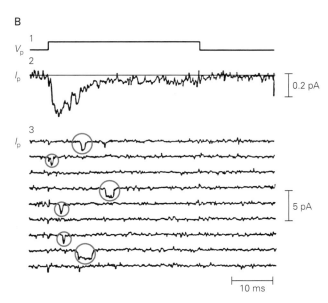

Figure 9-12 Individual voltage-gated channels open in an all-or-none fashion.

A. A small patch of membrane containing only a single voltage-gated Na^+ channel is electrically isolated from the rest of the cell by the patch electrode. The Na^+ current that enters the cell through these channels is recorded by a current monitor connected to the patch electrode.

B. Recordings of single Na^+ channels in cultured muscle cells of rats. **1.** Time course of a 10 mV depolarizing voltage step applied across the patch of membrane (V_p = potential difference across the patch). **2.** The sum of the inward current through the Na^+ channels in the patch during 300 trials (I_p = current through the patch of membrane). The trace was obtained by blocking the K^+ channels with tetraethylammonium and subtracting the capacitive current electronically. **3.** Nine individual trials from the set of 300, showing six individual Na^+ channel openings (**circles**). These data demonstrate that the total Na^+ current recorded in a conventional voltage-clamp record (see Figure 9-3C) can be accounted for by the all-or-none opening and closing of individual Na^+ channels. (From Sigworth and Neher 1980.)

Figure 9-13 Gating currents directly measure the changes in charge distribution associated with Na$^+$ channel activation.

A. When the membrane is depolarized the Na$^+$ current (I_{Na}) first activates and then inactivates. The activation of the Na$^+$ current is preceded by a brief outward gating current (I_g), reflecting the outward movement of positive charge within the Na$^+$ channel protein associated with the opening of the activation gate. To detect the small gating current it is necessary to block the flow of ionic current through the Na$^+$ and K$^+$ channels and mathematically subtract the capacitive current due to charging of the lipid bilayer.

B. Illustration of the position of the activation and inactivation gates when the channel is at rest (**1**), when the Na$^+$ channels have been opened (**2**), and when the channels have been inactivated (**3**). It is the movement of the positive charge on the activation gate through the membrane electric field that generates the gating current.

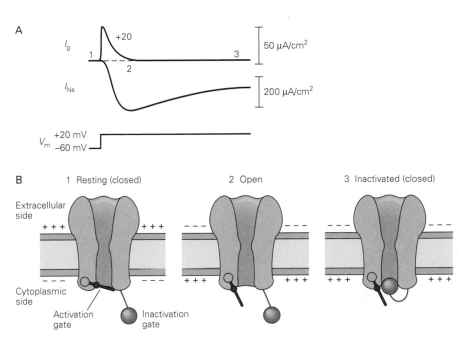

ing charge is thus temporarily immobilized; only as the Na$^+$ channels recover from inactivation is the charge free to move back across the membrane. This charge immobilization indicates that the gating charge cannot move while the channel is in the inactivated state, ie, while the inactivation gate is closed (see Figure 9-9).

To explain this phenomenon, Clay Armstrong and Francisco Bezanilla proposed that Na$^+$ channel inactivation occurs when the open (activated) channel is blocked by a tethered plug (the ball and chain mechanism), thereby preventing the closure of the activation gate. In support of this idea, exposing the inside of the axon to proteolytic enzymes selectively removes inactivation, causing the Na$^+$ channels to remain open during a depolarization, presumably because the enzymes clip off the inactivation "ball."

The Voltage-Gated Sodium Channel Selects for Sodium on the Basis of Size, Charge, and Energy of Hydration of the Ion

After the gates of the Na$^+$ channel have opened, how does the channel discriminate between Na$^+$ and other ions? The channel's selectivity mechanism can be probed by measuring the channel's relative permeability to several types of organic and inorganic cations that differ in size and hydrogen-bonding characteristics. As we

learned in Chapter 6, the channel behaves as if it contains a filter or recognition site that selects partly on the basis of size, thus acting as a molecular sieve (see Figure 6-3). The ease with which ions with good hydrogen-bonding characteristics pass through the channel suggests that part of the inner wall of the channel is made up of negatively polarized or charged amino acid residues that can substitute for water. When the pH of the fluid surrounding the cell is lowered, the conductance of the open channel is gradually reduced, consistent with the titration of important negatively charged carboxylic acid residues.

The selectivity filter of the Na$^+$ channel is made up of four loops within the molecule (the P region) that are similar in structure (see below). A glutamic acid residue is situated at equivalent points in two of these loops. A lysine and an alanine residue are situated at the equivalent site in the other two loops. The channel is thought to select for Na$^+$ ions by the following mechanism. The negatively charged carboxylic acid groups of the glutamic acid residues, which are located at the outer mouth of the pore, perform the first step in the selection process by attracting cations and repelling anions. The cations then encounter a constricted portion of the pore, the selectivity filter, with rectangular dimensions of 0.3×0.5 nm. This cross section is just large enough to accommodate one Na$^+$ ion contacting one water molecule. Cations that are larger in diameter cannot pass through the pore. Cations smaller than this critical size pass through the pore, but only after losing most of the waters of hydration they normally carry in free solution.

The negative carboxylic acid group, as well as other oxygen atoms that line the pore, can substitute for these waters of hydration, but the degree of effectiveness of this substitution varies among ion species. The more effective the substitution, the more readily ions can traverse the Na$^+$ channel. The Na$^+$ channel excludes K$^+$ ions, in part because the larger-diameter K$^+$ ion cannot interact as effectively with the negative carboxylic group. The lysine and alanine residues also contribute to the selectivity of the channel. When these residues are changed to glutamic acid residues by site-directed mutagenesis, the Na$^+$ channels can act as Ca^{2+}-selective channels! (The mechanism whereby K$^+$ selectivity is achieved was discussed in Chapter 6.)

Genes Encoding the Potassium, Sodium, and Calcium Channels Stem From a Common Ancestor

Since a change in two amino acid residues can cause a Na$^+$ channel to behave as a Ca^{2+} channel, it is reasonable to believe that the Na$^+$ and Ca^{2+} channels may be closely related. Detailed molecular studies have revealed that all voltage-gated ion channels—those for K$^+$, Na$^+$, and Ca^{2+}—share several functionally important domains and are indeed quite similar. In fact, there is now strong evidence from studies of bacteria, plants, invertebrates, and vertebrates that most voltage-sensitive cation channels stem from a common ancestral channel—perhaps a K$^+$ channel—that can be traced to a single-cell organism living over 1.4 billion years ago, before the evolution of separate plant and animal kingdoms. The amino acid sequences conserved through evolution help identify the domains within contemporary cation channels that are critical for function.

Molecular studies of the voltage-sensitive cation channels began with the identification of Na$^+$ channel molecules. Three subunits have been isolated: one large glycoprotein (α) and two smaller polypeptides (β1 and β2). The α-subunit is ubiquitous, and insertion of this subunit into an artificial lipid bilayer reconstitutes the basic features of Na$^+$ channel function. Therefore the α-subunit is presumed to form the aqueous pore of the channel. The smaller subunits, whose presence varies in different regions of the nervous system, regulate various aspects of α-subunit function.

Examination of the amino acid sequence encoded by the cloned gene for the α-subunit of the Na$^+$ channel reveals two fundamental features of the structure of the Na$^+$ channel. First, the α-subunit is composed of four internal repeats (domains I–IV), with only slight variations, of a sequence that is approximately 150 amino acids in length. Each of the four repeats of this sequence domain is believed to have six membrane-spanning hydrophobic regions (S1–S6) that are primarily α-helical in form. A seventh hydrophobic region the P region that connects the S5 and S6 segments, appears to form a loop that dips into and out of the membrane (Figure 9-14). The four repeated domains are thought to be arranged roughly symmetrically, with the P region and some of the membrane-spanning regions forming the walls of the water-filled pore (Figure 9-15).

The second structural feature of the Na$^+$ channel revealed by amino acid sequence analysis is that one of the six putative membrane-spanning regions, the S4 region, is structurally quite similar in the Na$^+$ channels of many different species. This strict conservation suggests that the S4 region is critical to Na$^+$ channel function. Moreover, the S4 region of the Na$^+$ channel is similar to corresponding regions of the voltage-gated Ca^{2+} and K$^+$ channels (Figure 9-14) but is lacking in K$^+$ channels that are not activated by voltage (see below). For this reason the S4 region may be the voltage sensor—that part of the protein that transduces depolarization of the cell membrane into a gating transition within the channel, thereby opening the channel. This idea is supported by the observation that the S4 region contains a distinctive pattern of amino acids. Every third amino acid along the S4 helix is positively charged (lysine or arginine) while the intervening two amino acids are hydrophobic. This highly charged structure is therefore likely to be quite sensitive to changes in the electric field across the membrane. Experiments using site-directed mutagenesis show that reducing the net positive charge in one of the S4 regions of the channel lowers the voltage sensitivity of Na$^+$ channel activation.

Structure-function studies based on genetic engineering of the α-subunit have led to a hypothesis about how the charges in the S4 region move across the membrane during channel gating. According to the scheme, at rest one of the charged residues on the S4 α-helix is completely buried in the wall of the channel, where its positive charge is stabilized by interaction with a negatively charged amino acid residue in one of the other membrane-spanning segments of the channel (Figure 9-16). The other positive charges are located on parts of the S4 helix that are within a water-filled lacuna in the wall of the channel that is continuous with the cytoplasm. When the membrane is depolarized the change in electrostatic force causes movement of the S4 helix relative to the surrounding channel wall, translocating some of the positively charged residues to the outside of

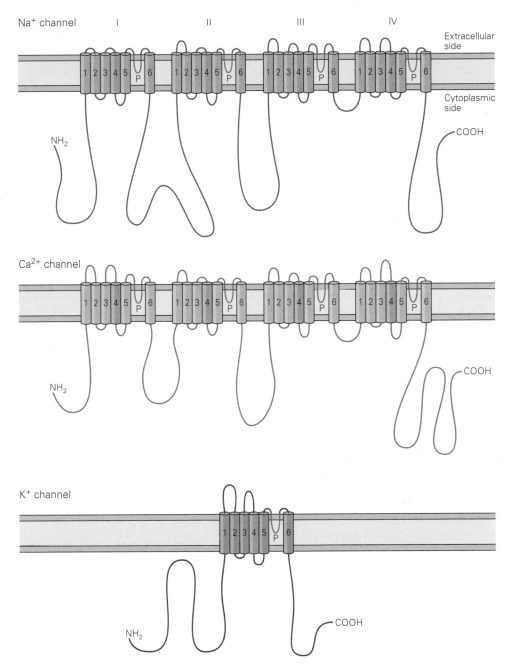

Figure 9-14 The pore-forming subunits of the voltage-gated Na⁺, Ca²⁺, and K⁺ channels are composed of a common repeated domain. The α-subunit of the Na⁺ and Ca²⁺ channels consists of a single polypeptide chain with four repeats (I-IV) of a domain that contains six membrane-spanning α-helical regions (S1-S6). A stretch of amino acids, the P region between α-helices 5 and 6, forms a loop that dips into and out of the membrane. The S4 segment is shown in red, representing its net positive charge. The fourfold repetition of the P region is believed to form a major part of the pore lining (see Figure 9–15). The K⁺ channel, in contrast, has only a single repeat of the six α-helices and the P region. Four K⁺ channel subunits are assembled to form a complete channel (see Figure 6–12). (Adapted from Catterall 1988, Stevens 1991.)

the membrane. This movement is somehow transduced into opening of the activation gate.

The genes encoding the major α-subunits of several voltage-gated Ca²⁺ channels have also been cloned. Their sequences reveal that the Ca²⁺ channels are also composed of four repeating domains, each with six hydrophobic transmembrane regions and one P loop, which have amino acid sequences homologous to those of the voltage-gated Na⁺ channel (see Figure 9-14).

The K⁺ channel genes contain only one copy of the domain that is repeated four times in the genes for Na⁺ and Ca²⁺ channels. Nevertheless, the basic channel structure is similar for the three channel types, as four α-subunits must aggregate symmetrically around a central pore to form a K⁺ channel. It is this striking homology among the voltage-gated Na⁺, Ca²⁺, and K⁺ channels that suggests that all three channels belong to the same gene family and have evolved by gene duplication and modification from a common ancestral structure, presumably a K⁺ channel.

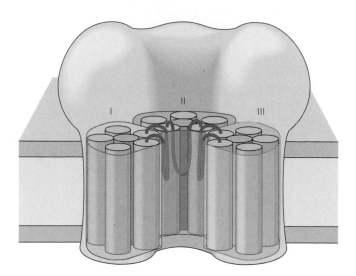

Figure 9-15 The four membrane-spanning domains of the α-subunit in voltage-gated Na⁺ and Ca²⁺ channels form the channel pore. The tertiary structure of the channels proposed here is based on the secondary structures shown in Figure 9-14. The central pore is surrounded by the four internally repeated domains (M-I to M-IV). (Only three of the domains are shown here for clarity.) Each quadrant of the channel includes six cylinders, which represent six putative membrane-spanning α-helices. The S4 segment (in red) is thought to be involved in gating because it contains a significant net charge. The protruding loop in each quadrant represents the P region segment that dips into the membrane to form the most narrow region of the wall of the pore.

The conservative mechanism by which evolution proceeds—creating new structural or functional entities by modifying, shuffling, and recombining existing gene sequences—is illustrated by the modular design of various members of the extended gene family that includes the voltage-gated Na⁺, K⁺, and Ca²⁺ channels. For example, the basic structures of both a Ca²⁺-activated K⁺ channel, an h-type cation channel activated by hyperpolarization and intracellular cycle neucleotides, and a voltage-independent cation channel activated by intracellular cyclic nucleotides are the same as the structures of other members of the gene family (six membrane-spanning α-helices and a P region), with some modifications. The functional differences between these two channels are due primarily to the addition of regulatory domains that bind Ca²⁺ or cyclic nucleotides, respectively, to the C-terminal ends of the proteins. As we saw in Chapter 6, the subunits that comprise the inward-rectifying K⁺ channels are truncated versions of the fundamental domain, consisting of the P region and its two flanking membrane-spanning regions. Four such subunits combine to form a functional channel (Figure 9-17).

The modular design of this extended gene family is also illustrated by a comparison of activation and inactivation mechanisms of various channels within the family. The S4 membrane-spanning region, which is thought to be the voltage sensor in channels of this family, has a relatively large net charge in the Na⁺, K⁺, and Ca²⁺ channels that open in response to depolarization. In contrast, the S4 regions in cyclic nucleotide-gated channels, which are only weakly sensitive to voltage, have significantly less net charge, and h-type channels lack certain conserved S4 residues. Moreover, inward-rectifying K⁺ channels, which have essentially no intrinsic voltage sensitivity, completely lack the S4 region. These inward-rectifying channels are activated by the effect of hyperpolarization on freely diffusible, positively charged blocking particles in the cytoplasm. Depending on the subspecies of channel, this blocker may be either Mg²⁺ or various organic polyamines. These channels open when the cation-blocking particle is electrostatically drawn out of the channel at negative potentials around the resting potential.

Inactivation of voltage-gated ion channels is also mediated by different molecular modules. For example, the rapid inactivation of both the A-type K⁺ channel and the voltage-gated Na⁺ channel can be attributed to a tethered plug that binds to the inner mouth of the channel when the activation gate opens. In the A-type K⁺ channel the plug is formed by the cytoplasmic N terminus of the channel, whereas in voltage-gated Na⁺ channels the cytoplasmic loop connecting domains III and IV of the α-subunit forms the plug.

Various Smaller Subunits Contribute to the Functional Properties of Voltage-Gated Sodium, Calcium, and Potassium Channels

Most, perhaps all, voltage-gated Na⁺, K⁺, and Ca²⁺ channels have β- and, in some cases, γ- and δ-subunits that modulate the functional properties of the channel-forming α-subunits. The modulatory function of these subunits, which may be either cytoplasmic or membrane-spanning, depends on the type of channel. For example, the subunits may enhance the efficiency of coupling of depolarization to activation or inactivation gating. They may also shift the gating functions to different voltage ranges. In some K⁺ channels in which the α-subunit lacks a tethered inactivation plug, addition of a set of β-subunits with their own N-terminal tethered plugs can endow the channel with the ability to rapidly inactivate. In contrast to the α-subunits, there is no known homology among the β-, γ-, and δ-subunits from the three-major subfamilies of voltage-gated channels.

A

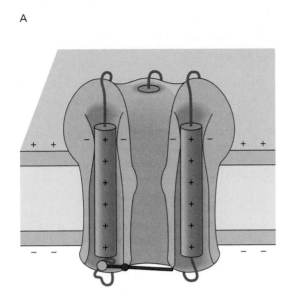

B

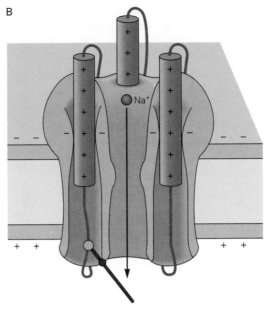

Figure 9-16 Gating of the Na$^+$ channel is thought to rely on redistribution of net charge in the S4 region.

A. At rest, the inside-negative electric field across the membrane biases the positively charged S4 helix toward the inside of the membrane. One of the positive charges is stabilized by interaction with a negative charge in another part of the channel. The remainder of the charged region lies in a water-filled

cavity in the channel wall that is continuous with the cytoplasm.

B. When the cell is depolarized the change in electrical field across the membrane drives the S4 region toward the extracellular face of the membrane. This change in configuration opens the activation gate by a mechanism that is not well understood. (Adapted from Yang et al. 1996.)

The Diversity of Voltage-Gated Channel Types Is Due to Several Genetic Mechanisms

A single ion species can cross the membrane through several distinct types of ion channels, each with its own characteristic kinetics, voltage sensitivity, and sensitivity to different modulators. In voltage-gated channels this diversity may be due to any of five genetic mechanisms: (1) More than one gene may encode related α-subunits within each class of channel. (2) A single gene product may be alternatively spliced in different classes of neurons, resulting in different variants of the mRNA that encodes the α-subunit. (3) The four α-subunits that coalesce to form a K$^+$ channel may be encoded by different genes. After translation the gene products are mixed and matched in various combinations, thus forming different subclasses of heteromultimeric channels. (4) A given α-subunit may be combined with different β-, γ- or δ-subunits to form functionally different channel types. (5) The diversity of some β-subunits is in-

creased either by alternative splicing of the pre-mRNA molecule or by the encoding of different variants of a basic β-subunit type on different genes. These various sources of diversity endow the nervous system with tremendous opportunities for regional diversity of functional properties.

Mutations in Voltage-Gated Channels Cause Specific Neurological Diseases

Several inherited neurological disorders are now known to be caused by mutations in voltage-gated ion channels. Patients with hyperkalemic periodic paralysis have episodes of muscle stiffness (myotonia) and muscle weakness (paralysis) in response to the elevation of K$^+$ levels in serum after vigorous exercise. Genetic studies have shown that the disease is caused by a point mutation in the α-subunit of the gene for the voltage-gated Na$^+$ channel found in skeletal muscle. Voltage-clamp

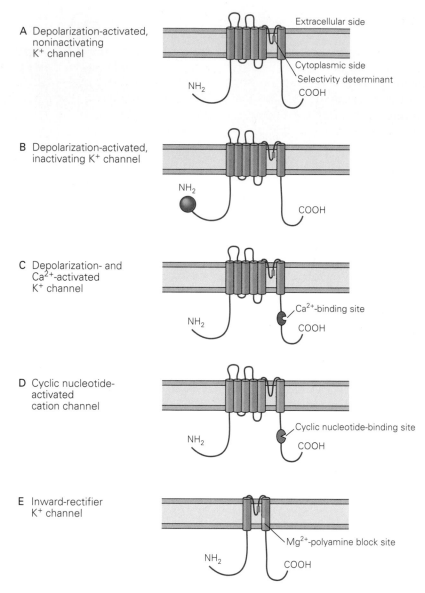

A Depolarization-activated, noninactivating K+ channel

Extracellular side

Cytoplasmic side
Selectivity determinant

NH₂
COOH

B Depolarization-activated, inactivating K+ channel

NH₂
COOH

C Depolarization- and Ca²⁺-activated K+ channel

Ca²⁺-binding site
NH₂
COOH

D Cyclic nucleotide-activated cation channel

Cyclic nucleotide-binding site
NH₂
COOH

E Inward-rectifier K+ channel

Mg²⁺-polyamine block site
NH₂
COOH

Figure 9-17 Ion channels belonging to the extended gene family of voltage-gated channels are variants of a common molecular design.

A. Depolarization-activated, noninactivating K+ channels are formed from four copies of an α-subunit, the basic building block of voltage-gated channels. The α-subunit is believed to have six membrane-spanning regions and one membrane-embedded region (the P region). The P region contains a K+-selective sequence (denoted by the rectangle).

B. Many K+ channels that are first activated and then inactivated by depolarization have a ball-and-chain segment on their N-terminal ends that inactivates the channel by plugging its inner mouth.

C. Potassium channels that are activated by both depolarization

and intracellular Ca²⁺ have a Ca²⁺-binding sequence attached to the C-terminal end of the channel.

D. Cation channels gated by cyclic nucleotides have a cyclic nucleotide-binding domain attached to the C-terminal end. One class of such channels is the voltage-independent, cyclic nucleotide-gated channels important in the transduction of olfactory and visual sensory signals. Another subclass consists of the hyperpolarization-activated h-type channels important for pacemaker activity (see Figure 9-11C).

E. Inward-rectifying K+ channels, which are gated by blocking particles available in the cytoplasm, are formed from truncated versions of the basic building block, with only two membrane-spanning regions and the P region.

studies of cultured skeletal muscle cells obtained from biopsies of patients with this disorder demonstrate that the voltage-gated Na^+ channels fail to completely inactivate. This defect is exacerbated by elevation of external K^+. The prolonged opening of the Na^+ channels is thought to cause muscles to fire repetitive trains of action potentials, thus producing the muscle stiffness. As the fraction of channels with altered inactivation increases (as a result of continued K^+ elevation), the muscle resting potential eventually reaches a new stable depolarized level (around -40 mV), at which point most Na^+ channels become inactivated so that the membrane fails to generate further action potentials (paralysis).

Patients with episodic ataxia exhibit normal neurological function except during periods of emotional or physical stress, which can trigger a generalized ataxia due to involuntary muscle movements. The disease has been shown to result from one of several point mutations in a delayed-rectifier, voltage-gated K^+ channel. These mutations decrease current through the channel, in part by enhancing the rate of inactivation. As a result, because less outward K^+ current is available for repolarization, the tendency of nerves and muscle cells to fire repetitively is enhanced. (Remarkably, the first K^+ channel gene to be cloned was identified based on a genetic strategy involving a similar mutation in a *Drosophila* K^+ channel gene, which gives rise to the so-called Shaker phenotype.) Muscle diseases involving mutations in Cl^- channels (myotonia congenita) and Ca^{2+} channels (hypokalemic periodic paralysis) have also been identified.

An Overall View

An action potential is produced by the movement of ions across the membrane through voltage-gated channels. This ion movement, which occurs only when the channels are open, changes the distribution of charges on either side of the membrane. An influx of Na^+, and in some cases Ca^{2+}, depolarizes the membrane, initiating an action potential. An outflow of K^+ then repolarizes the membrane by restoring the initial charge distribution. A particularly important subset of voltage-gated ion channels opens primarily when the membrane potential nears the threshold for an action potential; these channels have a profound effect on the firing patterns generated by a neuron.

We know something about how channels function from studies using variations on the voltage-clamp technique—these studies let us eavesdrop on a channel at work. And we know something from biochemical and molecular biology studies about the channel's

structure—about the primary amino acid sequence of the proteins that form them. Now these two approaches are being combined in a concerted effort to understand the relationship between structure and function in these channels: how they are put together, what their contours and surface map look like, how they interact with other molecules, what the structure of the channel pore is, and how its gate is opened.

Thus, we may soon be able to understand the molecular mechanism for the remarkable ability of voltage-gated channels to generate the action potential. These insights have two important implications: they will allow us to understand better the molecular bases of certain genetic diseases that involve mutations in ion channel genes, and they will enable us to design safer and more effective drugs to treat a variety of diseases that involve disturbances in electrical signaling (such as epilepsy, multiple sclerosis, myotonia, and ataxia).

John Koester
Steven A. Siegelbaum

Selected Readings

Armstrong CM. 1992. Voltage-dependent ion channels and their gating. Physiol Rev 72:S5–13.

Armstrong CM, Hille B. 1998. Voltage-gated ion channels and electrical excitability. Neuron 20:371–380.

Cannon SC. 1996. Ion-channel defects and aberrant excitability in myotonia and periodic paralysis. Trends Neurosci 19:3–10.

Catterall WA. 1994. Molecular properties of a superfamily of plasma-membrane cation channels. Curr Opin Cell Biol 6:607–615.

Hille B. 1991. *Ionic Channels of Excitable Membranes,* 2nd ed. Sunderland, MA: Sinauer.

Hodgkin AL. 1992. *Chance & Design: Reminiscences of Science in Peace and War.* Cambridge: Cambridge Univ. Press.

Isom LL, De Jongh KS, Catterall WA. 1994. Auxiliary subunits of voltage-gated ion channels. Neuron 12:1183–1194.

Jan LY, Jan YN. 1997. Cloned potassium channels from eukaryotes and prokaryotes. Annu Rev Neurosci 20:91–123.

Kukuljan M, Labarca P, Latorre R. 1995. Molecular determinants of ion conduction and inactivation in K^+ channels. Am J Physiol 268:C535–C556.

Llinás RR. 1988. The intrinsic electrophysiological properties of mammalian neurons: insights into central nervous system function. Science 242:1654–1664.

References

Armstrong CM, Bezanilla F. 1977. Inactivation of the sodium channel. II. Gating current experiments. J Gen Physiol 70:567–590.

Catterall WA. 1988. Structure and function of voltage-sensitive ion channels. Science 242:50–61.

Cole KS, Curtis HJ. 1939. Electric impedance of the squid giant axon during activity. J Gen Physiol 22:649–670.

Dekin MS, Getting PA. 1987. In vitro characterization of neurons in the vertical part of the nucleus tractus solitarius. II. Ionic basis for repetitive firing patterns. J Neurophysiol 58:215–229.

Hartmann HA, Kirsch GE, Drewe JA, Taglialatela M, Joho RH, Brown AM. 1991. Exchange of conduction pathways between two related K$^+$ channels. Science 251:942–944.

Heinemann SH, Terlau H, Stühmer W, Imoto K, Numa S. 1992. Calcium channel characteristics conferred on the sodium channel by single mutations. Nature 356:441–443.

Hodgkin AL, Huxley AF. 1952. A quantitative description of membrane current and its application to conduction and excitation in nerve. J Physiol (Lond) 117:500–544.

Hodgkin AL, Katz B. 1949. The effect of sodium ions on the electrical activity of the giant axon of the squid. J Physiol (Lond) 108:37–77.

Jones SW. 1985. Muscarinic and peptidergic excitation of bull-frog sympathetic neurones. J Physiol 366:63–87.

Llinás R, Jahnsen H. 1982. Electrophysiology of mammalian thalamic neurones in vitro. Nature 297:406–408.

MacKinnon R. 1991. Determination of the subunit stoichiometry of a voltage-activated potassium channel. Nature 350:232–235.

McCormick DA, Huguenard JR. 1992. A model of electrophysiological properties of thalamocortical relay neurons. J Neurophysiol 68:1384–1400.

Noda M, Shimizu S, Tanabe T, Takai T, Kayano T, Ikeda T, Takahashi H, Nakayama H, Kanaoka Y, Minamino N, Kangawa K, Matsuo H, Raferty MA, Hirose T, Inayama S, Hayashida H, Miyata T, Numa S. 1984. Primary structure of Electrophorus electricus sodium channel deduced from cDNA sequence. Nature 312:121–127.

Papazian DM, Schwarz TL, Tempel BL, Jan YN, Jan LY. 1987. Cloning of genomic and complementary DNA from Shaker, a putative potassium channel gene from Drosophila. Science 237:749–753.

Pongs O, Kecskemethy N, Müller R, Krah-Jentgens I, Baumann A, Kiltz HH, Canal I, Llamazares S, Ferrus A. 1988. Shaker encodes a family of putative potassium channel proteins in the nervous system of Drosophila. EMBO J 7:1087–1096.

Rosenberg RL, Tomiko SA, Agnew WS. 1984. Single-channel properties of the reconstituted voltage-regulated Na channel isolated from the electroplax of Electrophorus electricus. Proc Natl Acad Sci U S A 81:5594–5598.

Santoro B, Liu DT, Yao H, Bartsch D, Kandel ER, Siegelbaum SA, Tibbs GR. 1998. Identification of a gene encoding a hyperpolarization-activated pacemaker of brain. Cell 93:717–729.

Sigworth FJ, Neher E. 1980. Single Na$^+$ channel currents observed in cultured rat muscle cells. Nature 287:447–449.

Stühmer W, Conti F, Suzuki H, Wang X, Noda M, Yahagi N, Kubo H, Numa S. 1989. Structural parts involved in activation and inactivation of the sodium channel. Nature 339:597–603.

Takeshima H, Nishimura S, Matsumoto T, Ishida H, Kangawa K, Minamino N, Matsuo H, Ueda M, Hanaoka M, Hirose T, Numa S. 1989. Primary structure and expression from complementary DNA of skeletal muscle ryanodine receptor. Nature 339:439–445.

Vassilev PM, Scheuer T, Catterall WA. 1988. Identification of an intracellular peptide segment involved in sodium channel inactivation. Science 241:1658–1661.

Woodhull AM. 1973. Ionic blockage of sodium channels in nerve. J Gen Physiol 61:687–708.

Yang N, George AL Jr, Horn R. 1996. Molecular basis of charge movement in voltage-gated sodium channels. Neuron 16:113–122.

Yellen G, Jurman ME, Abramson T, MacKinnon R. 1991. Mutations affecting internal TEA blockade identify the probable pore-forming region of a K$^+$ channel. Science 251:939–942.

Yool AJ, Schwarz TL. 1991. Alteration of ionic selectivity of a K$^+$ channel by mutation of the H5 region. Nature 349:700–704.

Part III

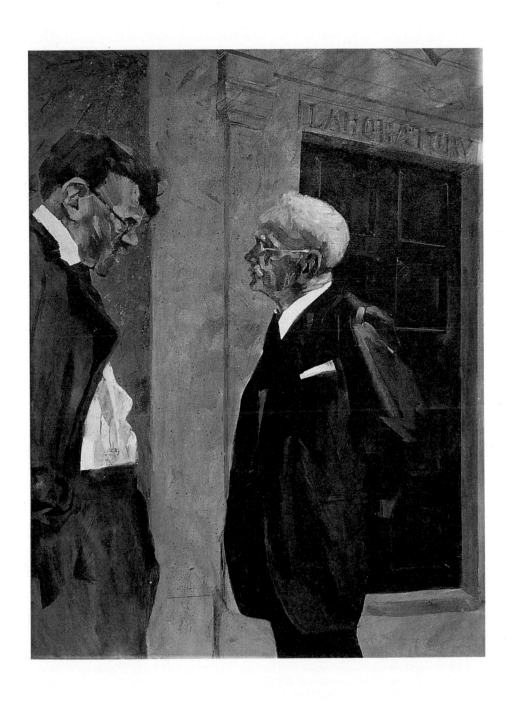

Charles Sherrington, John Eccles, and the Modern Study of Synaptic Transmission. This portrait of Charles Sherrington and John Eccles by the British painter Stan Smith hangs in the Laboratory of Physiology at the University of Oxford, which also preserves Sherrington's library, equipment, and other memorabilia. Sherrington coined the word *synapse* and initiated the experimental study of spinal reflexes as paradigms of neural integration. Eccles, his last student, was the first to study chemical synaptic transmission in the brain through intracellular microelectrode recording of single nerve cells. He stressed the importance of approaching the brain through nerve cells, its elementary units. (Reproduced with the permission of Stan Smith and Professor Colin Blakemore, University of Oxford.)

III

Elementary Interactions Between Neurons: Synaptic Transmission

I N PART II WE EXAMINED HOW ELECTRICAL signals are initiated and propagated within an individual neuron. We now turn to synaptic transmission, the process by which nerve cells signal one another. An average neuron forms and receives about 1000 synaptic connections and the human brain contains at least 10^{11} neurons. Thus 10^{14} synaptic connections are formed in the brain. There are more neurons and synapses in one brain than the several billion stars in our galaxy! Fortunately, only a few basic mechanisms underlie synaptic transmission at these many connections.

With some exceptions, the synapse consists of the terminus of a presynaptic axon apposed to a postsynaptic cell. Based on the structure of the apposition, synapses are categorized into two major groups: electrical and chemical. At electrical synapses, the presynaptic terminal and the postsynaptic cell are not completely separated and the current generated by an action potential in the presynaptic neuron flows directly into the postsynaptic cell through specialized channels called gap junctions, which physically connect the cytoplasm of the presynaptic and postsynaptic cells. At chemical synapses a cleft separates the two cells and the cells do not communicate through bridging channels. At the chemical synapse, a change in the membrane potential of the presynaptic cell leads to the release of a chemical transmitter from the nerve terminal. The transmitter diffuses across the synaptic cleft and binds to receptor molecules on the postsynaptic membrane, thus opening ion channels through which current flows.

Receptors for transmitters can be classified into two major groups depending on how they control ion channels in the postsynaptic cell. One type, the ionotropic receptor, is an ion channel that opens when the transmitter binds. The second type, the metabolic receptor, acts indirectly on ion channels by activating a second-messenger system within the postsynaptic cell. Both types of receptors can result in excitation or inhibition. The sign of the signal depends on the properties of the receptor with which the transmitter interacts, not on the identity of the transmitter. A single transmitter can produce several distinct effects by activating different types of receptors. Thus receptor diversity permits a relatively small number of transmitters to produce a wide variety of synaptic actions. Most transmitters are low-molecular-weight molecules, but certain peptides also can act as messengers at synapses. The methods of molecular biology are being used to characterize the receptors in postsynaptic cells that respond to these various chemical messengers. These methods have also clarified how second-messenger pathways transduce signals within cells.

In this part of the book we consider synaptic transmission in its most elementary forms: the communication between one presynaptic neuron and a single postsynaptic cell, and the processing by one postsynaptic cell of the signal it receives from a few presynaptic cells. Understanding the synapse at this level of resolution is necessary for considering how injury and disease interfere with synaptic transmission and thus disrupt neural function. Because the molecular architecture of chemical synapses is complex, many diseases can affect chemical synaptic transmission. One disorder that we consider in detail in this section is myasthenia gravis, a disease that disrupts transmission at synapses between spinal motor neurons and skeletal muscle. Analysis of abnormalities in synaptic transmission associated with human disease is important clinically. At the same time, clinical studies have provided critical insight into mechanisms that underlie normal synaptic function.

Part III

10

Overview of Synaptic Transmission

WHAT GIVES NERVE CELLS their special ability to communicate with one another so rapidly, over such great distances, and with such tremendous precision? We have already seen how signals are propagated *within* a neuron, from its dendrites and cell body to its axonal terminal. Beginning with this chapter we consider the cellular mechanisms for signaling *between* neurons. The point at which one neuron communicates with another is called a *synapse*, and synaptic transmission is fundamental to many of the processes we consider later in the book, such as perception, voluntary movement, and learning.

The average neuron forms about 1000 synaptic connections and receives even more, perhaps as many as 10,000 connections. The Purkinje cell of the cerebellum receives up to 100,000 inputs. Although many of these connections are highly specialized, all neurons make use of one of two basic forms of synaptic transmission:

electrical or chemical. Moreover, the strength of both forms of synaptic transmission can be enhanced or diminished by cellular activity. This *plasticity* in nerve cells is crucial to memory and other higher brain functions.

In the brain, electrical synaptic transmission is rapid and rather stereotyped. Electrical synapses are used primarily to send simple depolarizing signals; they do not lend themselves to producing inhibitory actions or making long-lasting changes in the electrical properties of postsynaptic cells. In contrast, chemical synapses are capable of more variable signaling and thus can produce more complex behaviors. They can mediate either excitatory or inhibitory actions in postsynaptic cells and produce electrical changes in the postsynaptic cell that last from milliseconds to many minutes. Chemical synapses also serve to amplify neuronal signals, so that even a small presynaptic nerve terminal can alter the response of a large postsynaptic cell. Because chemical synaptic transmission is so central to understanding brain and behavior, it is examined in detail in Chapters 11, 12, and 13.

Synapses Are Either Electrical or Chemical

The term *synapse* was introduced at the turn of the century by Charles Sherrington to describe the specialized zone of contact at which one neuron communicates with another; this site had first been described histologically (at the level of light microscopy) by Ramón y Cajal. Initially, all synapses were thought to operate by means of electrical transmission. In the 1920s, however, Otto Loewi showed that acetylcholine (ACh), a *chemical* compound, conveys signals from the vagus nerve to the

Table 10-1 Distinguishing Properties of Electrical and Chemical Synapses

Type of synapse	Distance between pre- and postsynaptic cell membranes	Cytoplasmic continuity between pre- and postsynaptic cells	Ultrastructural components	Agent of transmission	Synaptic delay	Direction of transmission
Electrical	3.5 nm	Yes	Gap-junction channels	Ion current	Virtually absent	Usually bidirectional
Chemical	20–40 nm	No	Presynaptic vesicles and active zones; postsynaptic receptors	Chemical transmitter	Significant: at least 0.3 ms, usually 1–5 ms or longer	Unidirectional

heart. Loewi's discovery in the heart provoked considerable debate in the 1930s over how chemical signals could generate electrical activities at other synapses, including nerve-muscle synapses and synapses in the brain.

Two schools of thought emerged, one physiological and the other pharmacological. Each championed a single mechanism for all synaptic transmission. The physiologists, led by John Eccles (Sherrington's student), argued that all synaptic transmission is electrical, that the action potential in the presynaptic neuron generates a current that flows passively into the postsynaptic cell. The pharmacologists, led by Henry Dale, argued that transmission is chemical, that the action potential in the presynaptic neuron leads to the release of a chemical substance that in turn initiates current flow in the postsynaptic cell.

When physiological techniques improved in the 1950s and 1960s it became clear that both forms of transmission exist. Although most synapses use a chemical transmitter, some operate purely by electrical means. Once the fine structure of synapses was made visible with the electron microscope, chemical and electrical synapses were found to have different morphologies. At chemical synapses neurons are separated completely by a small space, the *synaptic cleft*. There is no continuity between the cytoplasm of one cell and the next. In contrast, at electrical synapses the pre- and postsynaptic cells communicate through special channels, the *gap-junction channels*, that serve as conduits between the cytoplasm of the two cells.

The main functional properties of the two types of synapses are summarized in Table 10-1. The most important differences can be observed by injecting current

A Current flow at electrical synapses

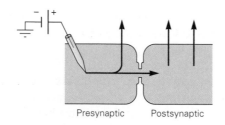

Presynaptic   Postsynaptic

B Current flow at chemical synapses

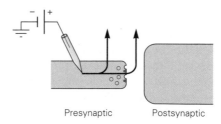

Presynaptic   Postsynaptic

Figure 10-1 Current flows differently at electrical and chemical synapses.

A. At an electrical synapse some of the current injected into a presynaptic cell escapes through resting ion channels in the cell membrane. However, some current also flows into the postsynaptic cell through specialized ion channels, called gap-junction channels, that connect the cytoplasm of the pre- and postsynaptic cells.

B. At chemical synapses all of the injected current escapes through ion channels in the presynaptic cell. However, the resulting depolarization of the cell activates the release of neurotransmitter molecules packaged in synaptic vesicles (**open circles**), which then bind to receptors on the postsynaptic cell. This binding opens ion channels, thus initiating a change in membrane potential in the postsynaptic cell.

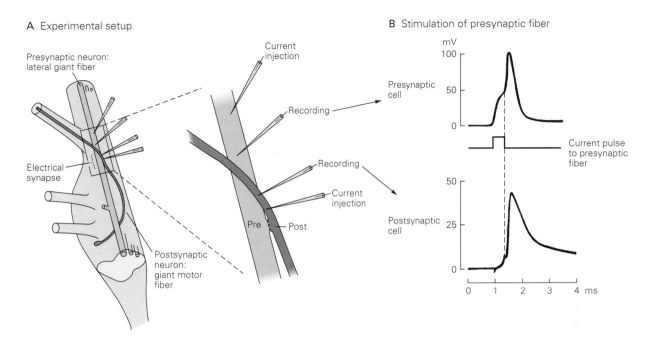

Figure 10-2 Electrical synaptic transmission was first demonstrated to occur at the giant motor synapse in the crayfish. (Adapted from Furshpan and Potter 1957 and 1959.)

A. The presynaptic neuron is the lateral giant fiber running down the nerve cord. The postsynaptic neuron is the motor fiber, which projects from the cell body in the ganglion to the periphery. The electrodes for passing current and for recording

voltage are placed within both the pre- and postsynaptic cells.

B. Transmission at an electrical synapse is virtually instantaneous—the postsynaptic response follows presynaptic stimulation in a fraction of a millisecond. The dashed line shows how the responses of the two cells correspond in time. In contrast, at chemical synapses there ia a delay between the pre- and postsynaptic potentials (see Figure 10–7).

into the presynaptic cell to elicit a signal (Figure 10-1). At both types of synapses the current flows outward across the presynaptic cell membrane. This current deposits a positive charge on the inside of the presynaptic cell membrane, reducing its negative charge and thereby depolarizing the cell (see Chapter 8).

At electrical synapses the gap-junction channels that connect the pre- and postsynaptic cells provide a low-resistance (high conductance) pathway for electrical current to flow between the two cells. Thus, some of the current injected in the presynaptic cell flows through these channels into the postsynaptic cell. This current deposits a positive charge on the inside of the membrane of the postsynaptic cell and depolarizes it. The current then flows out through resting ion channels in the postsynaptic cell (Figure 10-1A). If the depolarization exceeds threshold, voltage-gated ion channels in the postsynaptic cell will open and generate an action potential.

At chemical synapses there is no direct low-resistance pathway between the pre- and postsynaptic cells. Thus, current injected into a presynaptic cell flows out of the cell's resting channels into the synaptic cleft, the path of least resistance. Little or no current crosses the

external membrane of the postsynaptic cell, which has a high resistance (Figure 10-1B). Instead, the action potential in the presynaptic neuron initiates the release of a chemical transmitter, which diffuses across the synaptic cleft to interact with receptors on the membrane of the postsynaptic cell. Receptor activation causes the cell either to depolarize or to hyperpolarize.

Electrical Synapses Provide Instantaneous Signal Transmission

At electrical synapses the current that depolarizes the postsynaptic cell is generated directly by the voltage-gated ion channels of the presynaptic cell. Thus these channels not only have to depolarize the presynaptic cell above the threshold for an action potential, they must also generate sufficient ionic current to produce a change in potential in the postsynaptic cell. To generate such a large current, the presynaptic terminal has to be large enough for its membrane to contain a large number of ion channels. At the same time, the postsynaptic cell has to be relatively small. This is because a small cell has a higher input resistance (R_{in}) than a large cell and,

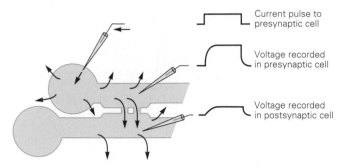

Current pulse to presynaptic cell

Voltage recorded in presynaptic cell

Voltage recorded in postsynaptic cell

Figure 10-3 Electrical transmission is graded and occurs even when the currents in the presynaptic cell are below the threshold for an action potential. This can be demonstrated by depolarizing the presynaptic cell with a small outward current pulse. Current is passed by one electrode while the membrane potential is recorded with a second electrode. A subthreshold depolarizing stimulus causes a passive depolarization in the presynaptic and postsynaptic cells. (Outward, depolarizing current is indicated by upward deflection.)

according to Ohm's law ($\Delta V = \Delta I \times R_{in}$), will undergo a greater voltage change (ΔV) in response to a given presynaptic current (ΔI).

Electrical synaptic transmission was first described in the giant motor synapse of the crayfish, where the presynaptic fiber is much larger than the postsynaptic fiber (Figure 10-2A). An action potential generated in the presynaptic fiber produces a depolarizing postsynaptic potential that is often large enough to discharge an action potential. The *latency*—the time between the presynaptic spike and the postsynaptic potential—is remarkably short (Figure 10-2B).

Such a short latency is incompatible with chemical transmission, which requires several biochemical steps: release of a transmitter from the presynaptic neuron, diffusion of the transmitter to the postsynaptic cell, binding of the transmitter to a specific receptor, and subsequent gating of ion channels (all described later in this chapter). Only current flowing directly from one cell to another can produce the near-instantaneous transmission observed at the giant motor synapse.

Further evidence for electrical transmission is that the change in potential of the postsynaptic cell is directly related to the size and shape of the change in potential of the presynaptic cell. At an electrical synapse any amount of current in the presynaptic cell triggers a response in the postsynaptic cell. Even when a subthreshold depolarizing current is injected into the presynaptic neuron, current flows into the postsynaptic cell

and depolarizes it (Figure 10-3). In contrast, at a chemical synapse the presynaptic current must reach the threshold for an action potential before the cell can release transmitter.

Most electrical synapses will transmit both depolarizing and hyperpolarizing currents. A presynaptic action potential that has a large hyperpolarizing afterpotential will produce a biphasic (depolarizing-hyperpolarizing) change in potential in the postsynaptic cell. Transmission at electrical synapses is similar to the passive electrotonic propagation of subthreshold electrical signals along axons (see Chapter 8) and therefore is often referred to as *electrotonic transmission*. Electrotonic transmission has been observed even at junctions where, unlike the giant motor synapse of the crayfish, the pre- and postsynaptic elements are similar in size. Because signaling between neurons at electrical synapses depends on the passive electrical properties at the synapse, such electrical synapses can be bidirectional, transmitting a depolarization signal equally well from either cell.

Gap-Junction Channels Connect Communicating Cells at an Electrical Synapse

Electrical transmission takes place at a specialized region of contact between two neurons termed the *gap junction*. At electrical synapses the separation between two neurons is much less (3.5 nm) than the normal, nonsynaptic space between neurons (20 nm). This narrow gap is bridged by the *gap-junction channels*, specialized protein structures that conduct the flow of ionic current from the presynaptic to the postsynaptic cell (Figure 10-4).

All gap-junction channels consist of a pair of *hemichannels*, one in the presynaptic and the other in the postsynaptic cell. These hemichannels make contact in the gap between the two cell membranes, forming a continuous bridge between the cytoplasm of the two cells (Figure 10-4A). The pore of the channel has a large diameter of around 1.5 nm, and this large size permits small intracellular metabolites and experimental markers such as fluorescent dyes to pass between the two cells.

Each hemichannel is called a *connexon*. A connexon is made up of six identical protein subunits, called *connexins* (Figure 10-4B). Each connexin is involved in two sets of interactions. First, each connexin recognizes the other five connexins to form a hemichannel. Second, each connexin of a hemichannel in one cell recognizes the extracellular domains of the apposing connexin of the hemichannel of the other cell to form the conducting channel that connects the two cells.

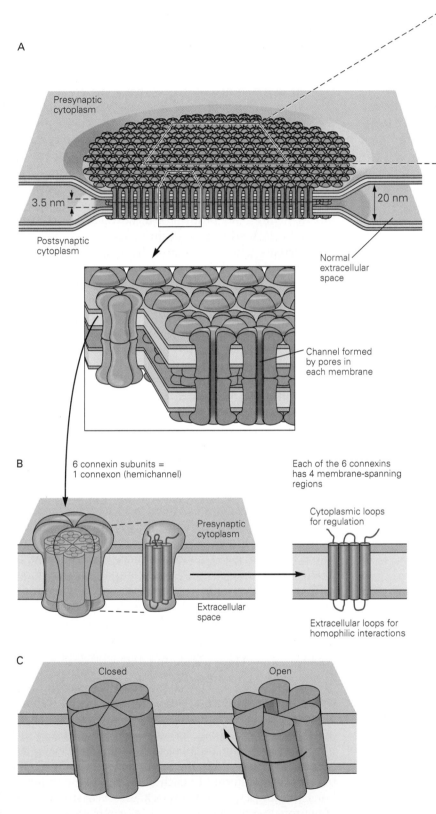

A

Presynaptic cytoplasm

3.5 nm

Postsynaptic cytoplasm

20 nm

Normal extracellular space

Channel formed by pores in each membrane

B

6 connexin subunits = 1 connexon (hemichannel)

Each of the 6 connexins has 4 membrane-spanning regions

Presynaptic cytoplasm

Extracellular space

Cytoplasmic loops for regulation

Extracellular loops for homophilic interactions

C

Closed   Open

Figure 10-4 A three-dimensional model of the gap-junction channel, based on X-ray and electron diffraction studies.

A. At electrical synapses two cells are structurally connected by gap-junction channels. A gap-junction channel is actually a pair of hemichannels, one in each apposite cell, that match up in the gap junction through homophilic interactions. The channel thus connects the cytoplasm of the two cells and provides a direct means of ion flow between the cells. This bridging of the cells is facilitated by a narrowing of the normal intercellular space (20 nm) to only 3.5 nm at the gap junction. (Adapted from Makowski et al. 1977.)

Electron micrograph: The array of channels shown here was isolated from the membrane of a rat liver. The tissue has been negatively stained, a technique that darkens the area around the channels and in the pores. Each channel appears hexagonal in outline. Magnification × 307,800. (Courtesy of N. Gilula.)

B. Each hemichannel, or connexon, is made up of six identical protein subunits called connexins. Each connexin is about 7.5 nm long and spans the cell membrane. A single connexin is thought to have four membrane-spanning regions. The amino acid sequences of gap-junction proteins from many different kinds of tissue all show regions of similarity. In particular, four hydrophobic domains with a high degree of similarity among different tissues are presumed to be the regions of the protein structure that traverse the cell membrane. In addition, two extracellular regions that are also highly conserved in different tissues are thought to be involved in the homophilic matching of apposite hemichannels.

C. The connexins are arranged in such a way that a pore is formed in the center of the structure. The resulting connexon, with an overall diameter of approximately 1.5–2 nm, has a characteristic hexagonal outline, as shown in the electron micrograph in **A.** The pore is opened when the subunits rotate about 0.9 nm at the cytoplasmic base in a clockwise direction. (From Unwin and Zampighi 1980.)

Connexins from different tissues all belong to one large gene family. Each connexin subunit has four hydrophobic domains thought to span the cell membrane. These membrane-spanning domains in the gap-junction channels of different tissues are quite similar, as are the two extracellular domains thought to be involved in the homophilic recognition of the hemichannels of apposite cells (Figure 10-4C). On the other hand, the cytoplasmic regions of different connexins vary greatly, and this variation may explain why gap junctions in different tissues are sensitive to different modulatory factors that control their opening and closing.

For example, most gap-junction channels close in response to lowered cytoplasmic pH or elevated cytoplasmic Ca^{2+}. These two properties serve to decouple damaged cells from other cells, since damaged cells contain elevated Ca^{2+} and proton concentrations. At some specialized gap junctions the channels have voltage-dependent gates that permit them to conduct depolarizing current in only one direction, from the presynaptic cell to the postsynaptic cell. These junctions are called *rectifying synapses.* (The crayfish giant motor synapse is an example.) Finally, neurotransmitters released from nearby chemical synapses can modulate the opening of gap-junction channels through intracellular metabolic reactions (see Chapter 13).

How do the channels open and close? One suggestion is that, to expose the channel's pore, the six connexins in a hemichannel rotate slightly with respect to one another, much like the shutter in a camera. The concerted tilting of each connexin by a few Ångstroms at one end leads to a somewhat larger displacement at the other end (Figure 10-4B). As we saw in Chapter 7, conformational changes in ion channels may be a common mechanism for opening and closing the channels.

Electrical Transmission Allows the Rapid and Synchronous Firing of Interconnected Cells

Why is it useful to have electrical synapses? As we have seen, transmission across electrical synapses is extremely rapid because it results from the direct flow of current from the presynaptic neuron to the postsynaptic cell. And speed is important for certain escape responses. For example, the tail-flip response of goldfish is mediated by a giant neuron (known as Mauthner's cell) in the brain stem, which receives input from sensory neurons at electrical synapses. These electrical synapses rapidly depolarize the Mauthner's cell, which in turn activates the motor neurons of the tail, allowing the fish to escape quickly from danger.

Electrical transmission is also useful for connecting large groups of neurons. Because current flows across the membranes of all electrically coupled cells at the same time, several small cells can act coordinately as one large cell. Moreover, because of the electrical coupling between the cells, the effective resistance of the coupled network of neurons is smaller than the resistance of an individual cell. As we have seen from Ohm's law ($\Delta V = \Delta I \times R$), the lower the resistance of a neuron, the smaller the depolarization produced by an excitatory synaptic current. Thus, electrically coupled cells require a larger synaptic current to depolarize them to threshold, compared with the current that would be necessary to fire an individual cell. This property makes it difficult to cause them to fire action potentials. Once this high threshold is surpassed, however, electrically coupled cells tend to fire synchronously because active Na^+ currents generated in one cell are rapidly transmitted to the other cells.

Thus, a behavior controlled by a group of electrically coupled cells has an important adaptive advantage: It is triggered explosively in an all-or-none manner. For example, when seriously perturbed, the marine snail *Aplysia* releases massive clouds of purple ink that provide a protective screen. This stereotypic behavior is mediated by three electrically coupled, high-threshold motor cells that innervate the ink gland. Once the threshold for firing is exceeded in these cells, they fire synchronously (Figure 10-5). In certain fish, rapid eye movements (called saccades) are also mediated by electrically coupled motor neurons acting synchronously.

In addition to providing speed or synchrony in neuronal signaling, electrical synapses also may transmit *metabolic signals* between cells. Because gap-junction channels are relatively large and nonselective, they readily allow inorganic cations and anions to flow through. In fact, gap-junction channels are large enough to allow moderate-sized organic compounds (less than 1000 molecular weight)—such as the second messengers IP_3 (inositol triphosphate), cAMP, and even small peptides—to pass from one cell to the next.

Gap Junctions Have a Role in Glial Function and Disease

Gap junctions are found between glial cells as well as between neurons. In glia the gap junctions seem to mediate both intercellular and intracellular communication. The role of gap junctions in signaling between glial cells is best observed in the brain, where individual astrocytes are connected to each other through gap junctions, forming a glial cell network. Electrical stimulation of neuronal pathways in brain slices can trigger a rise of intracellular Ca^{2+} in certain astrocytes. This produces a wave of intracellular Ca^{2+} throughout the astrocyte net-

Figure 10-5 Electrically coupled motor neurons firing together can produce instantaneous behaviors. The behavior illustrated here is the release of a protective cloud of ink by the marine snail *Aplysia*. (Adapted from Carew and Kandel 1976.)

A. Sensory neurons from the tail ganglion form synapses with three motor neurons that project to the ink gland. The motor neurons are interconnected by means of electrical synapses.

B. A train of stimuli applied to the tail produces a synchronized discharge in all three motor neurons. **1.** When the motor neurons are at rest the stimulus triggers a train of identical action potentials in all three cells. This synchronous activity in the motor neurons results in the release of ink. **2.** When the cells are hyperpolarized the stimulus cannot trigger action potentials, because the cells are too far from their threshold level. Under these conditions the inking response is blocked.

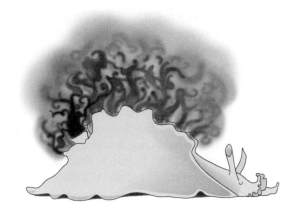

A Neural circuit of the inking response

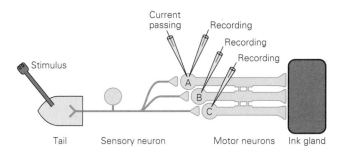

B Motor cell responses to tail stimulation

1 Cells at rest

2 Cells hyperpolarized

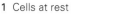
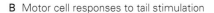

work, traveling at a rate of around 1 μm/ms. These Ca^{2+} waves are believed to propagate by diffusion through gap-junction channels. Although the precise function of such Ca^{2+} waves is not known, their existence clearly suggests that glia may play an active role in signaling in the brain.

Evidence that gap junctions enhance communication within a single glial cell is found in Schwann cells of the myelin sheath. As we have seen in Chapter 4, successive layers of myelin are connected by gap junctions, which may serve to hold the layers of myelin together. However, they may also be important for passing small metabolites and ions across the many intervening layers of myelin, from the outer perinuclear region of the Schwann cell down to the inner periaxonal region. The importance of these gap-junction channels is underscored by certain neurological genetic diseases. For example, the X chromosome–linked form of Charcot-Marie-Tooth disease, which causes demyelination, results from single mutations in one of the connexin genes (connexin32) expressed in the Schwann cell. Such mutations prevent this connexin from forming functional gap-junction channels essential for the normal flow of metabolites in the Schwann cell.

Chemical Synapses Can Amplify Signals

In contrast to the situation at electrical synapses, there is no structural continuity between pre- and postsynaptic neurons at chemical synapses. In fact, at chemical synapses the region separating the pre- and postsynaptic cells—the *synaptic cleft*—is usually slightly wider (20–40 nm), sometimes substantially wider, than the adjacent nonsynaptic intercellular space (20 nm). As a result, chemical synaptic transmission depends on the release of a neurotransmitter from the presynaptic neuron. A *neurotransmitter* is a chemical substance that will bind to specific receptors in the postsynaptic cell membrane. At most chemical synapses transmitter release occurs from *presynaptic terminals,* specialized swellings of the axon. The presynaptic terminals contain discrete collections of *synaptic vesicles,* each of which is filled with several thousand molecules of a specific transmitter (Figure 10-6).

The synaptic vesicles cluster at regions of the membrane specialized for releasing transmitter called *active zones.* During discharge of a presynaptic action potential Ca^{2+} enters the presynaptic terminal through voltage-gated Ca^{2+} channels at the active zone. The rise in intracellular Ca^{2+} concentration causes the vesicles to fuse with the presynaptic membrane and thereby release their neurotransmitter into the synaptic cleft, a process

termed *exocytosis.*

The transmitter molecules then diffuse across the synaptic cleft and bind to their receptors on the postsynaptic cell membrane. This in turn activates the receptors, leading to the opening or closing of ion channels. The resulting ionic flux alters the membrane conductance and potential of the postsynaptic cell (Figure 10-7).

These several steps account for the synaptic delay at chemical synapses, a delay that can be as short as 0.3 ms but often lasts several milliseconds or longer. Although chemical transmission lacks the speed of electrical synapses, it has the important property of *amplification.* With the discharge of just one synaptic vesicle, several thousand molecules of transmitter stored in that vesicle are released. Typically, only two molecules of transmitter are required to open a single postsynaptic ion channel. Consequently, the action of one synaptic vesicle can open thousands of ion channels in the postsynaptic cell. In this way a small presynaptic nerve terminal, which generates only a weak electrical current, can release thousands of transmitter molecules that can depolarize even a large postsynaptic cell.

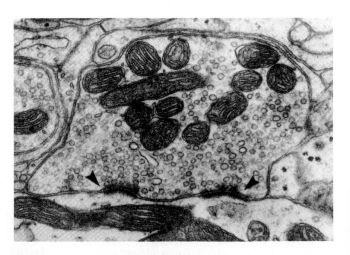

Figure 10-6 The synaptic cleft separates the presynaptic and postsynaptic cell membranes at chemical synapses. This electron micrograph shows the fine structure of a presynaptic terminal in the cerebellum. The large dark structures are mitochondria. The many round bodies are vesicles that contain neurotransmitter. The fuzzy dark thickenings along the presynaptic side of the cleft (**arrows**) are specialized areas, called active zones, that are thought to be docking and release sites for vesicles. (Courtesy of J. E. Heuser and T. S. Reese.)

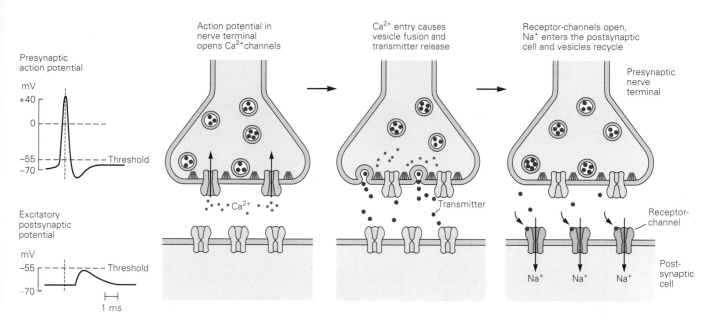

Presynaptic
action potential

mV
+40
0
−55 ‑‑‑‑‑‑‑ Threshold
−70

Excitatory
postsynaptic
potential

mV
−55 ‑‑‑‑‑‑ Threshold
−70
⊢ 1 ms ⊣

Figure 10-7 Synaptic transmission at chemical synapses in-volves several steps. An action potential arriving at the termi-nal of a presynaptic axon causes voltage-gated Ca^{2+} channels at the active zone to open. The influx of Ca^{2+} produces a high concentration of Ca^{2+} near the active zone, which in turn causes vesicles containing neurotransmitter to fuse with the presynaptic cell membrane and release their contents into the synaptic cleft (a process termed exocytosis). The released neurotransmitter molecules then diffuse across the synaptic cleft and bind to specific receptors on the post-synaptic mem-brane. These receptors cause ion channels to open (or close), thereby changing the membrane conductance and membrane potential of the postsynaptic cell. The complex process of chemical synaptic transmission is responsible for the delay be-tween action potentials in the pre- and post-synaptic cells com-pared with the virtually instantaneous transmission of signals at electrical synapses (see Figure 10-2B). The gray filaments rep-resent the docking and release sites of the active zone.

Chemical Transmitters Bind to Postsynaptic Receptors

Chemical synaptic transmission can be divided into two steps: a *transmitting* step, in which the presynaptic cell releases a chemical messenger, and a *receptive* step, in which the transmitter binds to the receptor molecules in the postsynaptic cell.

The transmitting process resembles the release process of an endocrine gland, and chemical synaptic transmission can be seen as a modified form of hormone secretion. Both endocrine glands and presynaptic termi-nals release a chemical agent with a signaling function, and both are examples of regulated secretion (Chapter 4). Similarly, both endocrine glands and neurons are usually some distance from their target cells. There is one important difference, however. The hormone re-leased by the gland travels through the blood stream until it interacts with all cells that contain an appropri-ate receptor. A neuron, on the other hand, usually com-municates only with specific cells, the cells with which it forms synapses. Communication consists of a presynap-tic neuron sending an action potential down its axon to the axon terminal, where the electrical signal triggers the focused release of the chemical transmitter onto a target cell. Thus the chemical signal travels only a small distance to its target. Neuronal signaling, therefore, has two special features: It is fast and precisely directed.

To accomplish this highly directed or focused re-lease, most neurons have specialized secretory machin-ery, the active zones. In neurons without active zones the distinction between neuronal and hormonal trans-mission becomes blurred. For example, the neurons in the autonomic nervous system that innervate smooth muscle reside at some distance from their postsynaptic cells and do not have specialized release sites in their terminals. Synaptic transmission between these cells is slower and more diffuse. Furthermore, at one set of ter-minals a transmitter can be released at an active zone, as a conventional transmitter acting directly on neighbor-ing cells; at another locus it can be released in a less fo-cused way as a modulator, producing a more diffuse ac-tion; and at a third locus it can be released into the blood stream as a neurohormone.

Although a variety of chemicals serve as neuro-transmitters, including both small molecules and pep-tides (see Chapter 15), the action of a transmitter in the

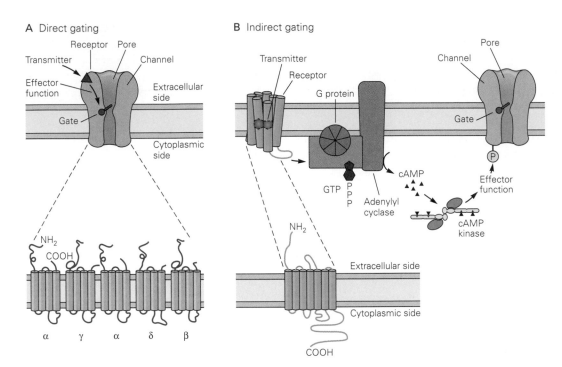

Figure 10-8 Neurotransmitters act either directly or indirectly on ion channels that regulate current flow in neurons.

A. Direct gating of ion channels is mediated by ionotropic receptors. This type of receptor is an integral part of the same macromolecule that forms the channel it regulates and thus is sometimes referred to as a receptor-channel or ligand-gated channel. Many ionotropic receptors are composed of five subunits, each of which is thought to contain four membrane-spanning α-helical regions (see Chapters 11, 12).

B. Indirect gating is mediated by activation of metabotropic receptors. This type of receptor is distinct from the ion channels it regulates. The receptor activates a GTP-binding protein (G protein), which in turn activates a second-messenger cascade that modulates channel activity. Here the G protein stimulates adenylyl cyclase, which converts ATP to cAMP. The cAMP activates the cAMP-dependent protein kinase (cAMP-kinase), which phosphorylates the channel (P), leading to a change in function. (The action of second messengers in regulating ion channels is described in detail in Chapter 13.) The typical metabotropic receptor is composed of a single subunit with seven membrane-spanning α-helical regions that bind the ligand within the plane of the membrane.

postsynaptic cell does not depend on the chemical properties of the transmitter but rather on the properties of the receptors that recognize and bind the transmitter. For example, acetylcholine (ACh) can excite some postsynaptic cells and inhibit others, and at still other cells it can produce both excitation and inhibition. It is the receptor that determines whether a cholinergic synapse is excitatory or inhibitory and whether an ion channel will be activated directly by the transmitter or indirectly through a second messenger.

Within a group of closely related animals a given transmitter substance binds to conserved families of receptors and is associated with specific physiological functions. For example, in vertebrates ACh produces synaptic excitation at the neuromuscular junction by acting on a special type of excitatory ACh receptor. It also slows the heart by acting on a special type of inhibitory ACh receptor.

The notion of a receptor was introduced in the late nineteenth century by the German bacteriologist Paul Ehrlich to explain the selective action of toxins and other pharmacological agents and the great specificity of immunological reactions. In 1900 Ehrlich wrote, "Chemical substances are only able to exercise an action on the tissue elements with which they are able to establish an intimate chemical relationship. . . . [This relationship] must be specific. The [chemical] groups must be adapted to one another . . . as lock and key." In 1906 the English pharmacologist John Langley postulated that the sensitivity of skeletal muscle to curare and nicotine was caused by a "receptive molecule." A theory of receptor function was later developed by Langley's students (in particular, Eliot Smith and Henry Dale), a development that was based on concurrent studies of enzyme kinetics and cooperative interactions between small molecules and proteins. As we shall see in the next chapter, Langley's "receptive molecule" has been isolated and characterized as the ACh receptor of the neuromuscular junction.

All receptors for chemical transmitters have two biochemical features in common:

1. They are membrane-spanning proteins. The region exposed to the external environment of the cell recognizes and binds the transmitter from the presynaptic cell.
2. They carry out an effector function within the target cell. The receptors typically influence the opening or closing of ion channels.

Postsynaptic Receptors Gate Ion Channels Either Directly or Indirectly

Chemical neurotransmitters act either directly or indirectly in controlling the opening of ion channels in the postsynaptic cell. The two classes of transmitter actions are mediated by receptor proteins derived from different gene families.

Receptors that gate ion channels directly, such as the nicotinic ACh receptor at the neuromuscular junction, are integral membrane proteins. Several subunits comprise a single macromolecule that contains both an extracellular domain that forms the receptor for transmitter and a membrane-spanning domain that forms an ion channel (Figure 10-8A). Such receptors are often referred to as *ionotropic receptors*. Upon binding neurotransmitter the receptor undergoes a conformational change that results in the opening of the channel. The actions of ionotropic receptors, also called receptor-channels or ligand-gated channels, are discussed in greater detail in Chapter 11.

Receptors that gate ion channels indirectly, like the several types of norepinephrine or serotonin receptors at synapses in the cerebral cortex, are macromolecules that are distinct from the ion channels they affect. These receptors act by altering intracellular metabolic reactions and are often referred to as *metabotropic receptors*. Activation of these receptors very often stimulates the production of second messengers, small freely diffusible intracellular metabolites such as cAMP and diacylglycerol. Many such second messengers activate protein kinases, enzymes that phosphorylate different substrate proteins. In many instances the protein kinases directly phosphorylate ion channels, leading to their opening or closing. The actions of the metabotropic receptor are examined in detail in Chapter 13.

Ionotropic and metabotropic receptors have different functions. The ionotropic receptors produce relatively fast synaptic actions lasting only milliseconds. These are commonly found in neural circuits that mediate rapid behaviors, such as the stretch receptor reflex. The metabotropic receptors produce slower synaptic ac-

tions lasting seconds to minutes. These slower actions can modulate behavior by altering the excitability of neurons and the strength of the synaptic connections of the neural circuitry mediating behavior. Such modulatory synaptic pathways often act as crucial reinforcing pathways in the process of learning.

Eric R. Kandel
Steven A. Siegelbaum

Selected Readings

Bennett MV. 1997. Gap junctions as electrical synapses. J Neurocytol 26:349–366.

Eccles JC. 1976. From electrical to chemical transmission in the central nervous system. The closing address of the Sir Henry Dale Centennial Symposium. Notes Rec R Soc Lond 30:219–230.

Furshpan EJ, Potter DD. 1959. Transmission at the giant motor synapses of the crayfish. J Physiol (Lond) 145:289–325.

Goodenough DA, Goliger JA, Paul DL. 1996. Connexins, connexons, and intercellular communication. Ann Rev Biochem 65:475–502.

Jessell TM, Kandel ER. 1993. Synaptic transmission: a bidirectional and a self-modifiable form of cell-cell communication. Cell 72(Suppl):1–30.

Unwin N. 1993. Neurotransmitter action: opening of ligand-gated ion channels. Cell 72(Suppl):31–41.

References

Beyer EC, Paul DL, Goodenough DA. 1987. Connexin43: a protein from rat heart homologous to a gap junction protein from liver. J Cell Biol 105:2621–2629.

Bruzzone R, White TW, Scherer SS, Fischbeck KH, Paul DL. 1994. Null mutations of connexin 32 in patients with x-linked Charcot-Marie-Tooth disease. Neuron 13:1253–1260.

Carew TJ, Kandel ER. 1976. Two functional effects of decreased conductance EPSP's: synaptic augmentation and increased electrotonic coupling. Science 192:150–153.

Cornell-Bell AH, Finkbeiner SM, Cooper MS, Smith SJ. 1990. Glutamate induces calcium waves in cultured astrocytes: long-range glial signaling. Science 247:470–473.

Dale H. 1935. Pharmacology and nerve-endings. Proc R Soc Med (Lond) 28:319–332.

Eckert R. 1988. Propagation and transmission of signals. In: *Animal Physiology: Mechanisms and Adaptations*, 3rd ed, pp. 134–176. New York: Freeman.

Ehrlich P. 1900. On immunity with special reference to cell life. Croonian Lect Proc R Soc Lond 66:424–448.

Furshpan EJ, Potter DD. 1957. Mechanism of nerve-impulse transmission at a crayfish synapse. Nature 180:342–343.

Heuser JE, Reese TS. 1977. Structure of the synapse. In: ER Kandel (ed), *Handbook of Physiology: A Critical, Comprehensive Presentation of Physiological Knowledge and Concepts*, Sect. 1, *The Nervous System*. Vol. 1, *Cellular Biology of Neurons*, Part 1, pp. 261–294. Bethesda, MD: American Physiological Society.

Jaslove SW, Brink PR. 1986. The mechanism of rectification at the electrotonic motor giant synapse of the crayfish. Nature 323:63–65.

Langley JN. 1906. On nerve endings and on special excitable substances in cells. Proc R Soc Lond B Biol Sci 78:170–194.

Loewi O, Navratil E. 1926. Über humorale Übertragbarkeit der Herznervenwirkung. X. Mitteilung: über das Schicksal des Vagusstoffs. Pflügers Arch. 214:678–688; 1972. Translated in: On the humoral propagation of cardiac nerve action. Communication X. The fate of the vagus substance. In: I Cooke, M Lipkin Jr (eds). *Cellular Neurophysiology: A Source Book*, pp. 478–485. New York: Holt, Rinehart and Winston.

Makowski L, Caspar DLD, Phillips WC, Baker TS, Goodenough DA. 1984. Gap junction structures. VI. Variation and conservation in connexon conformation and packing. Biophys J 45:208–218.

Pappas GD, Waxman SG. 1972. Synaptic fine structure—morphological correlates of chemical and electrotonic transmission. In: GD Pappas, DP Purpura (eds). *Structure and Function of Synapses*, pp. 1–43. New York: Raven.

Ramón y Cajal S. 1894. La fine structure des centres nerveux. Proc R Soc Lond 55:444–468.

Ramón y Cajal S. 1911. *Histologie du Système Nerveux de l'Homme & des Vertébrés*, Vol. 2. L Azoulay (transl). Paris: Maloine; 1955. Reprint. Madrid: Instituto Ramón y Cajal.

Sherrington C. 1947. *The Integrative Action of the Nervous System*, 2nd ed. New Haven: Yale Univ. Press.

Unwin PNT, Zampighi G. 1980. Structure of the junction between communicating cells. Nature 283:545–549.

11

Signaling at the Nerve-Muscle Synapse: Directly Gated Transmission

SYNAPTIC COMMUNICATION in the brain relies mainly on chemical mechanisms. Before we examine the complexities of chemical synaptic transmission in the brain, however, it will be helpful to examine the basic features of chemical synaptic transmission at the site where they were first studied and remain best understood—the nerve-muscle synapse, the junc-

tion between a motor neuron and a skeletal muscle fiber.

The nerve-muscle synapse is an ideal site for studying chemical signaling because it is relatively simple and also very accessible to experimentation. The muscle cell is large enough to accommodate the two or more microelectrodes needed to make electrical measurements. Also, the postsynaptic muscle cell is normally innervated by just one presynaptic axon, in contrast to the convergent connections on central nerve cells. Most importantly, chemical signaling at the nerve-muscle synapse involves a relatively simple mechanism. Release of neurotransmitter from the presynaptic nerve directly opens a single type of ion channel in the post-synaptic membrane.

The Neuromuscular Junction Is a Well-Studied Example of Directly Gated Synaptic Transmission

The axon of the motor neuron innervates the muscle at a specialized region of the muscle membrane called the *end-plate* (see Figure 11-1). At the region where the motor axon approaches the muscle fiber, the axon loses its myelin sheath and splits into several fine branches. The ends of the fine branches form multiple expansions or varicosities, called *synaptic boutons,* from which the motor neuron releases its transmitter (Figure 11–1). Each bouton is positioned over a *junctional fold,* a deep depression in the surface of the postsynaptic muscle fiber that contains the transmitter receptors (Figure 11–2). The transmitter released by the axon terminal is acetylcholine (ACh), and the receptor on the muscle mem-

Figure 11-1 The neuromuscular junction is readily visible with the light microscope. At the muscle the motor axon ramifies into several fine branches approximately 2 μm thick. Each branch forms multiple swellings called presynaptic boutons, which are covered by a thin layer of Schwann cells. The boutons lie over a specialized region of the muscle fiber membrane, the *end-plate,* and are separated from the muscle membrane by a 100 nm *synaptic cleft.* Each presynaptic bouton contains mitochondria and synaptic vesicles clustered around *active zones,* where the acetylcholine (ACh) transmitter is released. Immediately under each bouton in the endplate are several *junctional folds,* which contain a high density of ACh receptors at their crests. The muscle fiber is covered by a layer of connective tissue, the *basement membrane* (or basal lamina), consisting of collagen and glycoproteins. Both the presynaptic terminal and the muscle fiber secrete proteins into the basement membrane, including the enzyme acetylcholinesterase, which inactivates the ACh released from the presynaptic terminal by breaking it down into acetate and choline. The basement membrane also organizes the synapse by aligning the presynaptic boutons with the postsynaptic junctional folds. (Adapted in part from McMahan and Kuffler 1971.)

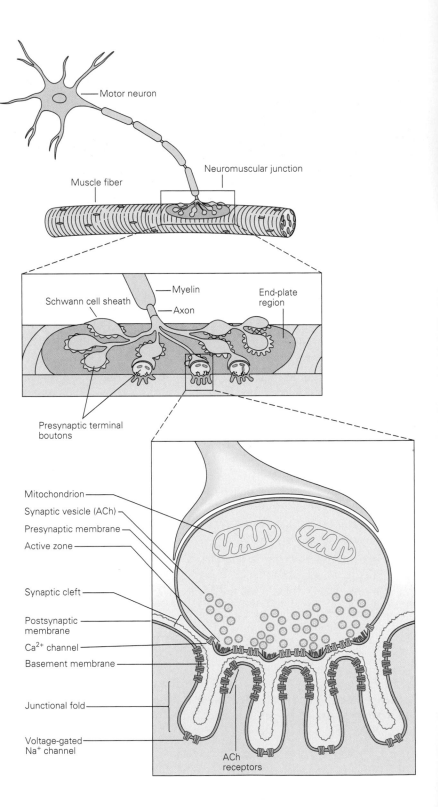

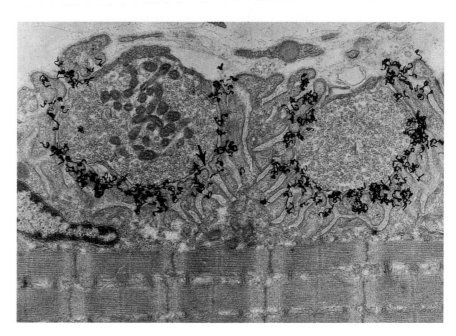

Figure 11-2 Electron microscope autoradiograph of the vertebrate neuromuscular junction, showing localization of ACh receptors (black developed grains) at the top one-third of the postsynaptic junctional folds. This receptor-rich region is characterized by an increased density of the postjunctional membrane (**arrow**). The membrane was incubated with radiolabeled α-bungarotoxin, which binds to the ACh receptor. Radioactive decay results in the emittance of a radioactive particle, causing silver grains to become fixed (**dark grains**). Magnification × 18,000. (From Salpeter 1987.)

brane is the nicotinic type of ACh receptor (Figure 11–3).[1]

The presynaptic and postsynaptic membranes are separated by a synaptic cleft around 100 nm wide. Within the cleft is a basement membrane composed of collagen and other extracellular matrix proteins. The enzyme acetylcholinesterase, which rapidly hydrolyzes ACh, is anchored to the collagen fibrils of the basement membranes. In the muscle cell, in the region below the crest of the junctional fold and extending into the fold, the membrane is rich in voltage-gated Na^+ channels.

Each presynaptic bouton contains all the machinery required to release neurotransmitter. This includes the *synaptic vesicles*, which contain the transmitter ACh, and the *active zone*, a part of the membrane specialized for vesicular release of transmitter (see Figure 11-1). Every active zone in the presynaptic membrane is positioned opposite a junctional fold in the postsynaptic cell. At the crest of each fold the receptors for ACh are clustered in a lattice, with a density of about 10,000 receptors per square micrometer (Figures 11-2 and 11-3). In addition, each active zone contains voltage-gated Ca^{2+} channels

that permit Ca^{2+} to enter the terminal with each action potential (see Figure 11-1). This influx of Ca^{2+} triggers fusion of the synaptic vesicles in the active zones with the plasma membrane, and fusion leads to release of the vesicle's content into the synaptic cleft.

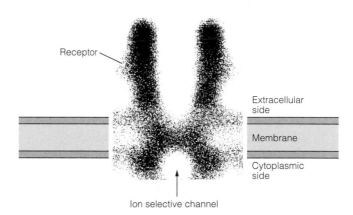

Figure 11-3 Reconstructed electron microscope image of the ACh receptor-channel complex in the fish *Torpedo californica*. The image was obtained by computer processing of negatively stained images of ACh receptors. The resolution is 1.7 nm, fine enough to see overall structures but too coarse to resolve individual atoms. The overall diameter of the receptor and its channel is about 8.5 nm. The pore is wide at the external and internal surfaces of the membrane but narrows considerably within the lipid bilayer. The channel extends some distance into the extracellular space. (Adapted from Toyoshima and Unwin 1988.)

---

[1] There are two basic types of receptors for ACh: nicotinic and muscarinic. The nicotinic receptor is an ionotropic receptor while the muscarinic receptor is a metabotropic receptor (see Chapter 10). The two receptors can be distinguished further because certain drugs that simulate the actions of ACh—that is, nicotine and muscarine—bind exclusively to one or the other type of ACh receptor. We shall learn about muscarinic ACh receptors in Chapter 13.

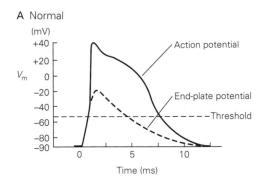

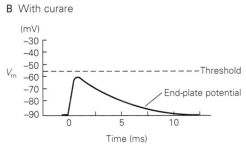

Figure 11-4 The end-plate potential can be isolated pharmacologically for study.

A. Under normal circumstances stimulation of the motor axon produces an action potential in a skeletal muscle cell. The **dashed line** shows the inferred time course of the end-plate potential that triggers the action potential.

B. The end-plate potential can be isolated in the presence of curare, which blocks the binding of ACh to its receptor and so prevents the end-plate potential from reaching the threshold for an action potential (**dashed line**). In this example, a low concentration of curare, which blocks only a fraction of the ACh receptors, is used. In this way the currents and channels that contribute to the end-plate potential, which are different from those producing an action potential, can be studied. The values for the resting potential (−90 mV), end-plate potential, and action potential shown in these intracellular recordings are typical of a vertebrate skeletal muscle.

The Motor Neuron Excites the Muscle by Opening Ion Channels at the End-Plate

Upon release of ACh from the motor nerve terminal, the membrane at the end-plate depolarizes rapidly. The excitatory postsynaptic potential in the muscle cell is called the *end-plate potential*. The amplitude of the end-plate potential is very large; stimulation of a single motor cell produces a synaptic potential of about 70 mV. This change in potential usually is large enough to rapidly activate the voltage-gated Na^+ channels in the junctional folds. This converts the end-plate potential into an action potential, which propagates along the muscle fiber. (In contrast, in the central nervous system most presynaptic neurons produce postsynaptic poten-

tials less than 1 mV in amplitude, so that input from many presynaptic neurons is needed to generate an action potential there.)

The Synaptic Potential at the End-Plate Is Produced by Ionic Current Flowing Through Acetylcholine-Gated Channels

The end-plate potential was first studied in detail in the 1950s by Paul Fatt and Bernard Katz using intracellular voltage recordings. Fatt and Katz were able to isolate the end-plate potential using the drug curare[2] to reduce the amplitude of the end-plate potential below the threshold for the action potential (Figure 11-4). They found that the synaptic potential in muscle cells was largest at the end-plate, decreasing progressively with distance from the end-plate region (Figure 11-5). They concluded that the synaptic potential is generated by an inward ionic current confined to the end-plate region, which then spreads passively away from the end-plate. (Remember, an inward current corresponds to an influx of positive charge, which will depolarize the inside of the membrane.) Current flow is confined to the end-plate because the ACh-activated ion channels are localized there, opposite the presynaptic terminal from which transmitter is released.

The synaptic potential at the end-plate rises rapidly but decays more slowly. The rapid rise is due to the sudden release of ACh into the synaptic cleft by an action potential in the presynaptic nerve terminal. Once released, ACh diffuses rapidly to the receptors at the end-plate. Not all the ACh reaches postsynaptic receptors, however, because it is quickly removed from the synaptic cleft by two processes: hydrolysis and diffusion out of the synaptic cleft.

The current that generates the end-plate potential was first studied in voltage-clamp experiments (see Box 9-1). These studies revealed that the end-plate current rises and decays more rapidly than the resultant end-plate potential (Figure 11-6). The time course of the end-plate current is directly determined by the rapid opening and closing of the ACh-gated ion channels. Because it takes time for an ionic current to charge or discharge the muscle membrane capacitance, and thus alter the membrane voltage, the end-plate potential lags behind the synaptic current (see Figure 8-3 and the Postscript at the end of this chapter).

---

[2] Curare is a mixture of plant toxins used by South American Indians, who apply it to arrowheads to paralyze their quarry. Tubocurarine, the purified active agent, blocks neuromuscular transmission by binding to the nicotinic ACh receptor, preventing its activation by ACh.

Figure 11-5 The synaptic potential in muscle is largest at the end-plate region and passively propagates away from it. (Adapted from Miles 1969.)

A. The amplitude of the synaptic potential decays and the time course of the potential slows with distance from the site of initiation in the end-plate.

B. The decay results from leakiness of the muscle fiber membrane. Since current flow must complete a circuit, the inward synaptic current at the end-plate gives rise to a return flow of outward current through resting channels and across the membrane (the capacitor). It is this return flow of outward current that produces the depolarization. Since current leaks out all along the membrane, the current flow decreases with distance from the end-plate. Thus, unlike the regenerative action potential, the local depolarization produced by the synaptic potential of the membrane decreases with distance.

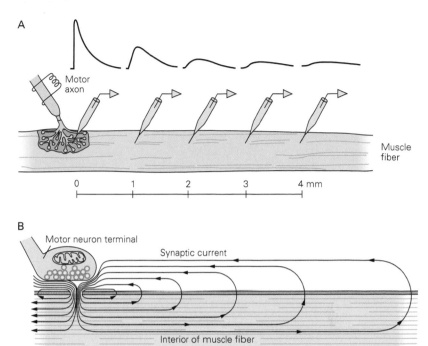

The Ion Channel at the End-Plate Is Permeable to Both Sodium and Potassium

Why does the opening of the ACh-gated ion channels lead to an inward current flow that produces the depolarizing end-plate potential? And which ions move through the ACh-gated ion channels to produce this inward current? One important clue to the identity of the ion (or ions) responsible for the synaptic current can be obtained from experiments that measure the value of the chemical driving force propelling ions through the channel. Remember, from Chapter 7, the current flow through a membrane conductance is given by the product of the membrane conductance and the electrochemical driving force on the ions conducted through the channels. The end-plate current that underlies the excitatory postsynaptic potential (EPSP) is defined as

$$I_{EPSP} = g_{EPSP} \times (V_m - E_{EPSP}), \qquad (11\text{-}1)$$

where I_{EPSP} is the end-plate current, g_{EPSP} is the conductance of the ACh-gated channels, V_m is the membrane potential, and E_{EPSP} is the chemical driving force, or battery, that results from the concentration gradients of the ions conducted through the ACh-gated channels. The fact that current flowing through the end-plate is inward at the normal resting potential of a muscle cell (−90 mV) indicates that there is an inward (negative) electrochemical driving force on the ions that carry current through the ACh-gated channels at this potential. Thus, E_{EPSP} must be positive to −90 mV.

From Equation 11-1 we see that the value of E_{EPSP} can be determined by altering the membrane potential in a voltage-clamp experiment and determining its effect on the synaptic current. Depolarizing the membrane reduces the net inward electrochemical driving force, causing a decrease in the magnitude of the inward end-plate current. If the membrane potential is set equal to the value of the battery representing the chemical driving force (E_{EPSP}), no net synaptic current will flow through the end-plate because the electrical driving force (due to V_m) will exactly balance the chemical driving force (due to E_{EPSP}). The potential at which the net ionic current is zero is the *reversal potential* for current flow through the synaptic channels. By determining the reversal potential we can experimentally measure the value of E_{EPSP}, the chemical force driving ions through the ACh-gated channels at the end-plate. If the membrane potential is made more positive than E_{EPSP}, there will be a net outward driving force. In this case stimulation of the motor nerve leads to an outward ionic current, by opening the ACh-gated channels, and this outward ionic current hyperpolarizes the membrane.

If an influx of Na^+ were solely responsible for the end-plate potential, the reversal potential for the excitatory postsynaptic potential would be the same as the equilibrium potential for Na^+, or +55 mV. Thus, if the membrane potential is experimentally altered from −100 to +55 mV, the end-plate current should diminish progressively because the electrochemical driving force

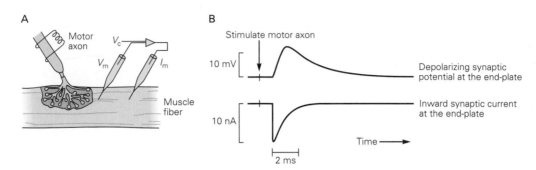

Figure 11-6 The end-plate current rises and decays more rapidly than the end-plate potential.

A. The membrane at the end-plate is voltage-clamped by inserting two microelectrodes into the muscle at the end-plate. One electrode measures membrane voltage (V_m) and the second passes current (I_m). Both electrodes are connected to a feedback amplifier, which ensures that the proper amount of current (I_m) is delivered so that V_m will be clamped at the command potential V_c. The synaptic current evoked by stimulating

the motor nerve can then be measured at a constant membrane potential, for example −90 mV (see Box 9-1).

B. The end-plate potential, measured when the voltage clamp is not active, changes relatively slowly, following in time the inward synaptic current measured under voltage-clamp conditions. This is because synaptic current must first alter the charge on the membrane capacitance of the muscle before the muscle membrane is depolarized (see Chapter 8 and Postscript in this chapter).

on Na^+ ($V_m - E_{Na}$) is reduced. At +55 mV the inward current flow should be abolished, and at potentials more positive than +55 mV the end-plate current should reverse in direction and flow outward.

Instead experiments at the end-plate showed that as the membrane potential is reduced, the inward current rapidly becomes smaller and is abolished at 0 mV! At values more positive than 0 mV the end-plate current reverses direction and begins to flow outward (Figure 11-7). This particular value of membrane potential is not equal to the equilibrium potential for Na^+, or for that matter any of the major cations or anions. In fact, this potential is produced not by a single ion species but by a combination of ions. The synaptic channels at the end-plate are almost equally permeable to both major cations, Na^+ and K^+. Thus, during the end-plate potential Na^+ flows into the cell and K^+ flows out. The reversal potential is at 0 mV because this is a weighted average of the equilibrium potentials for Na^+ and K^+ (Box 11-1). At the reversal potential the influx of Na^+ is balanced by an equal efflux of K^+.

Why are the ACh-gated channels at the end-plate not selective for a single ion species like the voltage-gated channels selective for either Na^+ or K^+? The pore diameter of the ACh-gated channel is thought to be substantially larger than that of the voltage-gated channels. Electrophysiological measurements suggest that the pore may be up to 0.8 nm in diameter in mammals. This estimate is based on the size of the largest organic cation that can permeate the channel. For example, the perme-

ant cation tetramethylammonium (TMA) is around 0.6 nm in diameter. In contrast, the voltage-gated Na^+ channel is only permeant to organic cations that are smaller than 0.5 × 0.3 nm in cross section, and voltage-gated K^+ channels will only conduct ions less than 0.3 nm in diameter. The relatively large diameter of the ACh pore is thought to provide a water-filled environment that allows cations to diffuse through the channel, much as they would in free solution. This explains why the pore does not discriminate between Na^+ and K^+. It also explains why even divalent cations, such as Ca^{2+}, can permeate the channel. Anions are excluded, however, by the presence of fixed negative charges in the channel, as described later in this chapter.

The Current Flow Through Single Ion Channels Can Be Measured by the Patch Clamp

The current for an end-plate potential flows through several hundred thousand channels. Recordings of the current flow through single ACh-gated ion channels, using the patch clamp technique (see Box 6-1), have provided us with insight into the molecular events underlying the end-plate potential. Before the introduction of the patch clamp physiologists held two opposing views as to what the time course of the single-channel current should look like. Some thought that the single-channel currents were a microscopic version of the end-plate current recorded with the voltage clamp, having a rapid

Figure 11-7 The end-plate potential is produced by the simultaneous flow of Na$^+$ and K$^+$ through the same ACh-gated channels.

A. The ionic currents responsible for the end-plate potential can be determined by measuring the reversal potential of the end-plate current. The voltage of the muscle membrane is clamped at different potentials, and the synaptic current is measured when the nerve is stimulated. If Na$^+$ flux alone were responsible for the end-plate current, the reversal potential would occur at +55 mV, the equilibrium potential for Na$^+$ (E_{Na}). The arrow next to each current record reflects the magnitude of the net Na$^+$ flux at that membrane potential.

B. The end-plate current actually reverses at 0 mV because the ion channel is permeable to both Na$^+$ and K$^+$, which are able to move into and out of the cell simultaneously (see Box 11-1). The net current is the sum of the Na$^+$ and K$^+$ fluxes through the end-plate channels. At the reversal potential (E_{EPSP}) the inward Na$^+$ flux is balanced by an outward K$^+$ flux so that no net current flows.

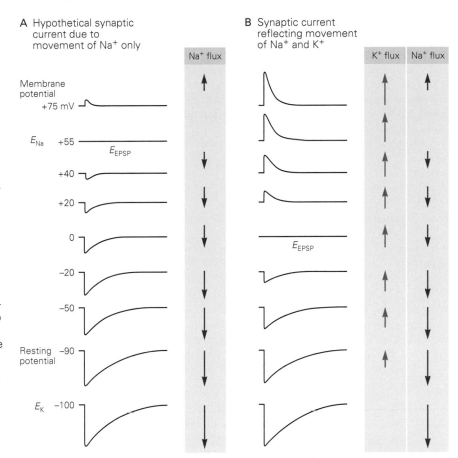

rising phase and a more slowly decaying falling phase. Others thought that the channels opened in an all-or-none manner, producing step-like currents similar to that seen with gramicidin (see Chapter 6).

Individual Acetylcholine-Gated Channels Conduct a Unitary Current

The first successful recordings of single ACh-gated channels from skeletal muscle cells, by Erwin Neher and Bert Sakmann in 1976, showed that the channels open and close in a step-like manner, generating very small rectangular steps of ionic current (Figure 11-8). At a constant membrane potential a channel generates a similar-size current pulse each time it opens. At a resting potential of −90 mV the current steps are around −2.7 pA in amplitude. Although this is a very small current, it corresponds to a flow through an open channel of around 17 million ions per second!

The unitary current steps change in size with membrane potential. This is because the single-channel

current depends on the electrochemical driving force ($V_m - E_{EPSP}$). Recall that Ohm's law applied to synaptic current is

$$I_{EPSP} = g_{EPSP} \times (V_m - E_{EPSP}).$$

For single ion channels the equivalent expression is

$$i_{EPSP} = \gamma_{EPSP} \times (V_m - E_{EPSP}),$$

where i_{EPSP} is the amplitude of current flow through one channel and γ_{EPSP} is the conductance of a single channel. The relationship between i_{EPSP} and membrane voltage is linear, indicating that the single-channel conductance is constant and does not depend on membrane voltage; that is, the channel behaves as a simple resistor. From the slope of this relation the channel is found to have a conductance of 30 pS. The reversal potential of 0 mV, obtained from the intercept of the voltage axis, is identical to that for the end-plate current (Figure 11-9).

Although the amplitude of the current flowing through a single ACh channel is constant from opening

Box 11-1 Reversal Potential of the End-Plate Potential

The reversal potential of a membrane current carried by more than one ion species, such as the end-plate current through the ACh-gated channel, is determined by two factors: (1) the relative conductance for the permeant ions (g_{Na} and g_K in the case of the end-plate current) and (2) the equilibrium potentials of the ions (E_{Na} and E_K).

At the reversal potential for the ACh-gated current, inward current carried by Na^+ is balanced by outward current carried by K^+:

$$I_{Na} + I_K = 0. \tag{11-2}$$

The individual Na^+ and K^+ currents can be obtained from

$$I_{Na} = g_{Na} \times (V_m - E_{Na}) \tag{11-3a}$$

and

$$I_K = g_K \times (V_m - E_K). \tag{11-3b}$$

Remember that these currents do not result from Na^+ and K^+ flowing through separate channels (as occurs during the action potential) but represent Na^+ and K^+ movement through the same ACh-gated channel. Since at the reversal potential $V_m = E_{EPSP}$, we can substitute Equations 11-3a and 11-3b for I_{Na} and I_K in Equation 11-2:

$$g_{Na} \times (E_{EPSP} - E_{Na}) + g_K \times (E_{EPSP} - E_K) = 0. \tag{11-4}$$

Solving this equation for E_{EPSP} yields

$$E_{EPSP} = \frac{(g_{Na} \times E_{Na}) + (g_K \times E_K)}{g_{Na} + g_K}. \tag{11-5}$$

If we divide the top and bottom of the right side of this equation by g_K, we obtain

$$E_{EPSP} = \frac{E_{Na}(g_{Na}/g_K) + E_K}{(g_{Na}/g_K) + 1}. \tag{11-6}$$

Thus, if $g_{Na} = g_K$, then $E_{EPSP} = (E_{Na} + E_K)/2$.

These equations can also be used to solve for the ratio g_{Na}/g_K if one knows E_{EPSP}, E_K, and E_{Na}. Thus, rearranging Equation 11-4 yields

$$\frac{g_{Na}}{g_K} = \frac{E_{EPSP} - E_K}{E_{Na} - E_{EPSP}}. \tag{11-7}$$

At the neuromuscular junction $E_{EPSP} = 0$ mV, $E_K = -100$ mV, and $E_{Na} = +55$ mV. Thus, from Equation 4, g_{Na}/g_K has a value of approximately 1.8, indicating that the conductance of the ACh-gated channel for Na^+ is slightly higher than for K^+. A comparable approach can be used to analyze the reversal potential and the movement of ions during excitatory and inhibitory synaptic potentials in central neurons (Chapter 12).

---

to opening, the duration of openings and the time between openings of an individual channel vary considerably. These variations occur because channel openings and closings are stochastic. They obey the same statistical law that describes radioactive decay. Because of the random thermal motions and fluctuations that a channel experiences, it is impossible to predict exactly how long it will take any one channel to encounter ACh or how long that channel will stay open before the ACh dissociates and the channel closes. However, the average length of time a particular type of channel stays open is a well-defined property of that channel, just as the half-life of radioactive decay is an invariant property of a particular isotope. The mean open time for ACh-gated channels is around 1 ms. Thus each channel opening is associated with the movement of about 17,000 ions.

Unlike the voltage-gated channels, the ACh-gated channels are not opened by membrane depolarization. Instead a ligand (ACh) causes the channels to open. Each channel is thought to have two binding sites for ACh; to open, a channel must bind two molecules of ACh. Once a channel closes, the ACh molecules dissociate and the channel remains closed until it binds ACh again.

Four Factors Determine the End-Plate Current

Stimulation of a motor nerve releases a large quantity of ACh into the synaptic cleft. The ACh rapidly diffuses across the cleft and binds to the ACh receptors, causing more than 200,000 ACh receptor-channels to open almost simultaneously. (This number is obtained by comparing the total end-plate current, around −500 nA, with the current through a single ACh-gated channel, around −2.7 pA). How do small step-like changes in current flowing through 200,000 individual ACh-gated channels produce the smooth waveform of the end-plate current?

The rapid and large rise in ACh concentration upon stimulation of the motor nerve causes a large increase in the total conductance of the end-plate membrane, g_{EPSP}, and produces the rapid rise in end-plate current (Figure 11-10). The ACh in the cleft falls to zero rapidly (in less than 1 ms) because of enzymatic hydrolysis and diffusion. After the fall in ACh concentration, the channels begin to close in the random manner described above. Each closure produces a small step-like decrease in end-plate current because of the all-or-none nature of single-channel currents. However, since each unitary current step is

A

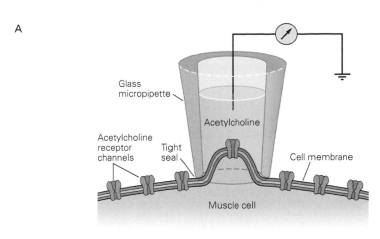

Glass micropipette

Acetylcholine

Acetylcholine receptor channels

Tight seal

Cell membrane

Muscle cell

Figure 11-8 Individual ACh-gated channels open in an all-or-none fashion.

A. The patch-clamp technique is used to record currents from single ACh-gated channels. The patch electrode is filled with salt solution that contains a low concentration of ACh and is then brought into close contact with the surface of the muscle membrane (see Box 6-1).

B. Single-channel currents from a patch of membrane on a frog muscle fiber were recorded in the presence of 100 nM ACh at a resting membrane potential of −90 mV. **1.** The opening of a channel results in the flow of inward current (recorded as a downward step). The patch contained a large number of ACh-gated channels so that successive openings in the record probably arise from distinct channels. **2.** A histogram of the amplitudes of these rectangular pulses has a single peak. This distribution indicates that the patch of membrane contains only a single type of active channel and that the size of the elementary current through this channel varies randomly around a mean of −2.7 pA (1 pA = 10^{-12} A). This mean, the *elementary current,* is equivalent to an elementary conductance of about 30 pS. (Courtesy of B. Sakmann.)

C. When the membrane potential is increased to −130 mV, the individual channel currents give rise to all-or-none increments of −3.9 pA, equivalent to 30 pS. Sometimes more than one channel opens simultaneously. In this case, the individual current pulses add linearly. The record shows one, two, or three channels open at different times in response to transmitter. (Courtesy of B. Sakmann.)

B_1 Single-channel currents

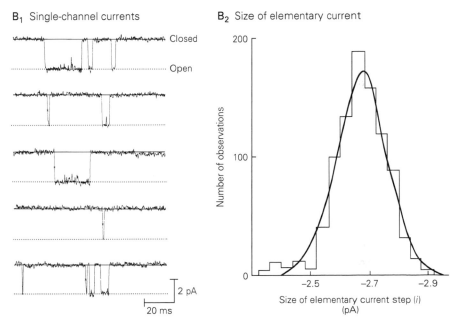

Closed

Open

2 pA

20 ms

B_2 Size of elementary current

Number of observations

200

100

0

−2.5   −2.7   −2.9

Size of elementary current step (i)
(pA)

C Total ionic current in a patch of membrane

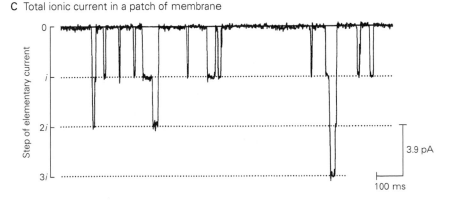

Step of elementary current

0

i

$2i$

$3i$

3.9 pA

100 ms

A

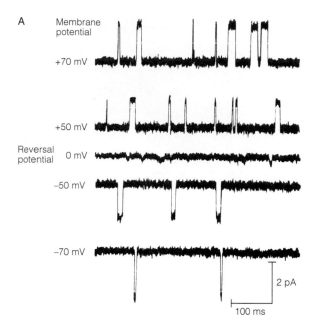

B

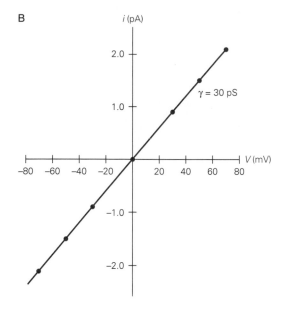

Figure 11-9 Single open ACh-gated channels behave as simple resistors.

A. The voltage across a patch of membrane was systematically varied during exposure to 2 μM ACh. The current recorded at the patch is inward at voltages negative to 0 mV and outward at voltages positive to 0 mV, defining the reversal potential for the channels.

B. The current flow through a single ACh-activated channel depends on membrane voltage. The linear relation shows that the channel behaves as a simple resistor with a conductance of about 30 pS.

tiny relative to the large current carried by many thousands of channels, the random closing of a large number of small unitary currents causes the total end-plate current to appear to decay smoothly (Figure 11-10).

The summed conductance of all open channels in a large population of ACh channels is the total synaptic conductance, $g_{EPSP} = n \times \gamma$, where n is the average number of channels opened by the ACh transmitter and γ is the conductance of a single channel. For a large number of ACh channels, $n = N \times p_o$, where N is the total number of ACh channels in the end-plate membrane and p_o is the probability that any given ACh channel is open. The probability that a channel is open depends largely on the concentration of the transmitter at the receptor, not on the value of the membrane potential, because the channels are opened by the binding of ACh, not by voltage. The total end-plate current is therefore given by

$$I_{EPSP} = N \times p_o \times \gamma \times (V_m - E_{EPSP})$$

or

$$I_{EPSP} = n \times \gamma \times (V_m - E_{EPSP}).$$

This equation shows that the current for the end-plate potential depends on four factors: (1) the total number of end-plate channels (N); (2) the probability that a

channel is open (p_o); (3) the conductance of each open channel (γ); and (4) the driving force that acts on the ions ($V_m - E_{EPSP}$).

The relationships between single-channel current, total end-plate current, and end-plate potential are shown in Figure 11-11 for a wide range of membrane potentials.

The Molecular Properties of the Acetylcholine-Gated Channel at the Nerve-Muscle Synapse Are Known

Ligand-Gated Channels for Acetylcholine Differ From Voltage-Gated Channels

Ligand-gated channels such as the ACh-gated channels that produce the end-plate potential differ in two important ways from the voltage-gated channels that generate the action potential at the neuromuscular junction. First, two distinct classes of voltage-gated channels are activated sequentially to generate the action potential, one selective for Na^+ and the other for K^+. In contrast, the ACh-gated channel alone generates end-plate potentials, and it allows both Na^+ and K^+ to pass with nearly equal permeability.

A second difference between ACh-gated and voltage-gated channels is that Na$^+$ flux through voltage-gated channels is regenerative: the increased depolarization of the cell caused by the Na$^+$ influx opens more voltage-gated Na$^+$ channels. This regenerative feature is responsible for the all-or-none property of the action potential. In contrast, the number of ACh-activated channels opened during the synaptic potential varies according to the amount of ACh available. The depolarization produced by Na$^+$ influx through these channels does not lead to the opening of more transmitter-gated channels; it is therefore limited and by itself cannot produce an action potential. To trigger an action potential, a synaptic potential must recruit neighboring voltage-gated channels (Figure 11-12).

As might be expected from these two differences in physiological properties, the ACh-gated and voltage-gated channels are formed by distinct macromolecules that exhibit different sensitivities to drugs and toxins. Tetrodotoxin, which blocks the voltage-gated Na$^+$ channel, does not block the influx of Na$^+$ through the nicotinic ACh-gated channels. Similarly, α-bungarotoxin, a snake venom protein that binds tightly to the nicotinic receptors and blocks the action of ACh, does not interfere with voltage-gated Na$^+$ or K$^+$ channels (α-bungarotoxin has proved useful in the biochemical characterization of the ACh receptor).

In Chapter 12 we shall learn about still another type of ligand-gated channel, the N-methyl-D-aspartate or NMDA–type glutamate receptor, which is found in most neurons of the brain. This channel is doubly gated, responding both to voltage *and* to a chemical transmitter.

A Single Macromolecule Forms the Nicotinic Acetylcholine Receptor and Channel

The nicotinic ACh-gated channel at the nerve-muscle synapse is a directly gated or ionotropic channel: the pore in the membrane through which ions flow and the binding site for the chemical transmitter (ACh) that regulates the opening of the pore are all formed by a single macromolecule. Where in the molecule is the binding site located? How is the pore formed? What are its properties? Insights into these questions have been obtained from molecular studies of the ACh-gated receptor-channel proteins and their genes.

Biochemical studies by Arthur Karlin and Jean-Pierre Changeux indicate that the mature nicotinic ACh receptor is a membrane glycoprotein formed from five subunits: two α-subunits and one β-, one γ-, and one δ-subunit (Figure 11-13). The amino terminus of each of the subunits is exposed on the extracellular surface of the membrane. The amino terminus of the α-subunit

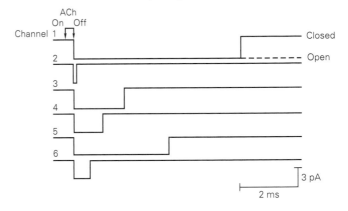

A Idealized time course of opening of six ion channels

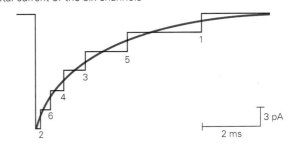

B Total current of the six channels

Figure 11-10 The time course of the total current at the end-plate results from the summed contributions of many individual ACh-gated channels. (Adapted from D. Colquhoun 1981.)

A. Individual ACh-gated channels open in response to a brief pulse of ACh. All channels (1-6) open rapidly and nearly simultaneously. The channels then remain open for varying durations and close at different times.

B. The stepped trace shows the sum of the six records in **A.** It reflects the sequential closing of each channel (the number indicates which channel has closed) at a hypothetical end-plate containing only six channels. In the final period of net current flow only channel 1 is open. In a current record from a whole muscle fiber, with thousands of channels, the individual channel closings are not visible because the total end-plate current (hundreds of nanoamperes) is so much larger than the single-channel current amplitude (−2.7 pA). As a result, the total end-plate current appears to decay smoothly.

contains a site that binds ACh with high affinity. Karlin and his colleagues have demonstrated the presence of two extracellular binding sites for ACh on each channel. Those sites are formed in a cleft between each α-subunit and its neighboring γ- or δ-subunits. One molecule of ACh must bind to each of the two α-subunits for the channel to open efficiently (Figure 11-13). The inhibitory snake venom α-bungarotoxin also binds to the α-subunit.

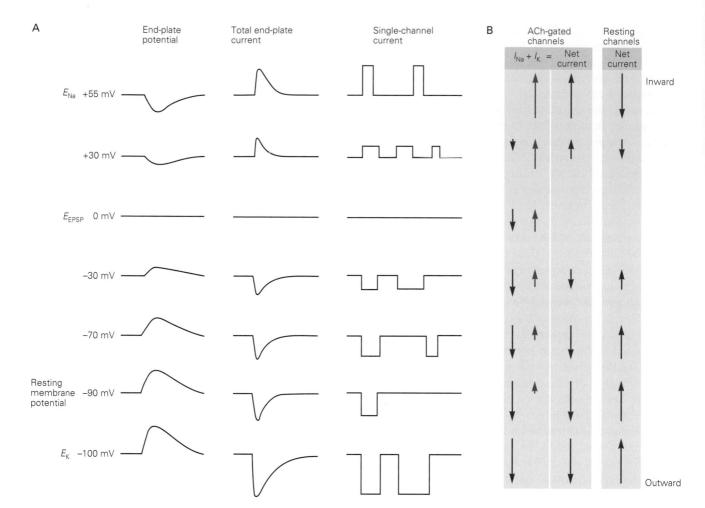

Figure 11-11 Membrane potential affects the end-plate potential, total end-plate current, and ACh-gated single-channel current in a similar way.

A. At the normal muscle resting potential of −90 mV the single-channel currents and total end-plate current (made up of currents from more than 200,0000 channels) are large and inward because of the large inward driving force on current flow through the ACh-gated channels. This large inward current produces a large depolarizing end-plate potential. At more positive levels of membrane potential (increased depolarization), the inward driving force on Na$^+$ is less and the outward driving force on K$^+$ is greater. This results in a decrease in the size of the single-channel currents and in the magnitude of the end-plate currents, thus reducing the size of the end-plate potential. At the reversal potential (0 mV) the inward Na$^+$ flux is balanced by the outward K$^+$ flux, so there is no net current flow at the end-

plate and no change in V_m. Further depolarization to +30 mV inverts the direction of the end-plate current, as there is now a large outward driving force on K$^+$ and a small inward driving force on Na$^+$. As a result, the outward flow of K$^+$ hyperpolarizes the membrane. On either side of the reversal potential the end-plate current drives the membrane potential toward the reversal potential.

B. The direction of Na$^+$ and K$^+$ fluxes in individual channels is altered by changing V_m. The algebraic sum of the Na$^+$ and K$^+$ currents, I_{Na} and I_K, gives the *net current* that flows through the ACh-gated channels. This net synaptic current is equal in size, and opposite in direction, to that of the net extrasynaptic current flowing in the return pathway of the resting channels and membrane capacitance. (The length of each arrow represents the relative magnitude of a current.)

Insight into the structure of the channel pore has come from analysis of the primary amino acid sequences of the receptor-channel subunits as well as from biophysical studies. The work of Shosaku Numa and his colleagues demonstrated that the four subunit types are encoded by distinct but related genes. Sequence comparison of the subunits shows a high degree of similarity among them: half of the amino acid residues are identical or conservatively substituted. This similarity suggests that all subunits have a similar structure. Furthermore, all four of the genes for the sub-units are homologous; that is, they are derived from a common ancestral gene.

The distribution of the polar and nonpolar amino acids of the subunits provides important clues as to how the subunits are threaded through the membrane bi-layer. Each subunit contains four hydrophobic regions of about 20 amino acids called M1–M4, each of which is thought to form an α-helix traversing the membrane. The amino acid sequences of the subunits suggest that the subunits are symmetrically arranged to create the pore through the membrane (Figure 11-14).

The walls of the channel pore are thought to be formed by the M2 region and by the segment connect-ing M2 to M3 (Figure 11-14B). Certain drugs that bind to one ring of serine residues and two rings of hydropho-bic residues on the M2 region within the channel pore are able to inhibit current flow through the pore. More-over, three rings of negative charge that flank the M2 re-gion (Figure 11-15B) contribute to the channel's selectiv-ity for cations. Each ring is made up of three or four aligned negatively charged residues contributed by dif-ferent subunits.

A three-dimensional model of the ACh receptor has been proposed by Arthur Karlin and Nigel Unwin based on neutron scattering and electron diffraction im-ages respectively (see Figure 11-3). The receptor-channel complex is divided into three regions: a large vestibule at the external membrane surface, a narrow transmem-brane pore that determines cation selectivity, and a larger exit region at the internal membrane surface (Fig-ure 11-15A). The region that extends into the extracellu-lar space is surprisingly large, about 6 nm in length. At the external surface of the membrane the channel has a wide mouth about 2.5 nm in diameter. Within the bi-layer of the membrane the channel gradually narrows.

This narrow region is quite short, only about 3 nm in length, corresponding to the length of both the M2 seg-ment and the hydrophobic core of the bilayer (Figure 11-15B). In the open channel, the M2 segment appears to slope inward toward the central axis of the channel, so that the pore narrows continuously from the outside of the membrane to the inside (Figure 11-15C). Near the inner surface of the membrane the pore reaches its narrowest di-ameter, around 0.8 nm, in reasonable agreement with esti-mates from electrophysiological measurements. This site may correspond to the selectivity filter of the channel. At the selectivity filter, polar threonine residues extend their side chains into the lumen of the pore. The electronegative oxygen atom of the hydroxyl group may interact with the permeant cation to compensate for loss of waters of hy-dration. At the inner surface of the membrane, the pore suddenly widens again.

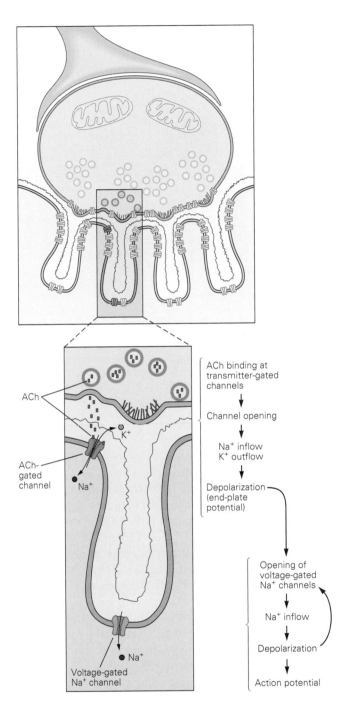

Figure 11-12 The binding of ACh in a postsynaptic muscle cell opens channels permeable to both Na$^+$ and K$^+$. The flow of these ions into and out of the cell depolarizes the cell membrane, producing the end-plate potential. This depolariza-tion opens neighboring voltage-gated Na$^+$ channels in the mus-cle cell. To trigger an action potential, the depolarization pro-duced by the end-plate potential must open a sufficient number of Na$^+$ channels to exceed the cell's threshold. (After Alberts et al. 1989.)

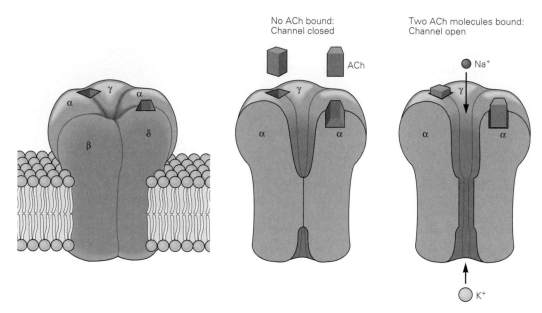

Figure 11-13 Three-dimensional model of the nicotinic ACh–gated ion channel. The receptor-channel complex consists of five subunits, all of which contribute to forming the pore. When two molecules of ACh bind to portions of the α-subunits exposed to the membrane surface, the receptor-channel changes conformation. This opens a pore in the portion of the channel embedded in the lipid bilayer, and both K+ and Na+ flow through the open channel down their electrochemical gradients.

On the basis of images of ACh receptors in the presence and absence of transmitter, Unwin has proposed that the M2 helix may be important for channel gating, as well as for ion permeation. His studies indicate that the M2 helix is not straight but rather has a bend or kink in its middle (Figure 11-15C). When the channel is closed, this kink projects inward toward the central axis of the pore, thereby occluding it. When the channel opens, the M2 helix rotates so that the kink lies along the wall of the channel.

A somewhat different view of the pore and gate has been provided by Karlin, who studied the reactions of small, charged reagents with amino acid side chains in the M2 segment. By comparing the ability of these compounds to react in the open and closed states of the

A A single subunit in the ACh receptor-channel

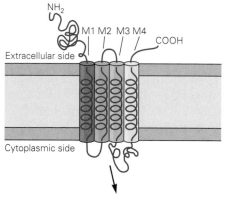

B Hypothetical arrangement of subunits in one channel

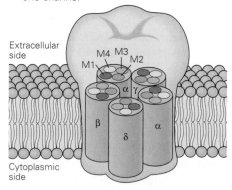

Figure 11-14 A molecular model of the transmembrane subunits of the nicotinic ACh receptor-channel.

A. Each subunit is composed of four membrane-spanning α-helices (labeled M1 through M4).

B. The five subunits are arranged such that they form an aqueous channel, with the M2 segment of each subunit facing inside and forming the lining of the pore (see turquoise cylinders, Figure 11-15A). Note that the γ-subunit lies between the two α-subunits.

A Functional model of ACh
   receptor-channel

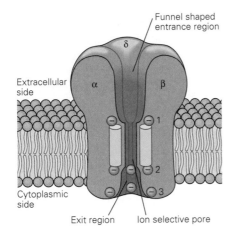

B Amino acid sequence of channel
   subunits

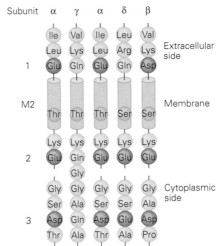

C Structural model for channel gating

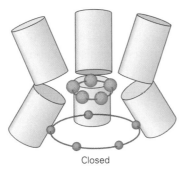

Closed   Open

Figure 11-15 A functional model of the nicotinic ACh receptor-channel.

A. According to this model negatively charged amino acids on each subunit form three rings of charge around the pore (see part B). As an ion traverses the channel it encounters this series of negatively charged rings. The rings at the external (**1**) and internal (**3**) surfaces of the cell membrane may serve as prefilters and divalent blocking sites. The central ring (**2**) within the bilayer may contribute to the selectivity filter for cations, along with a ring of threonine and serine residues that contribute an electronegative oxygen. (Dimensions are not to scale.)

B. The amino acid sequences of the M2 and flanking regions of each of the five subunits. The horizontal series of amino acids

numbered **1, 2,** and **3** identify the three rings of negative charge (see part **A**). The position of the aligned serine and threonine residues within M2, which help form the selectivity filter, is indicated.

C. A model for gating of the ACh receptor-channel. Three of the five M2 transmembrane segments are shown. Each M2 segment is split into two cylinders, one on top of the other. **Left:** In the closed state each M2 cylinder points inward toward the central axis of the channel. A ring of five hydrophobic leucine residues (large spheres, one from each M2 segment) occludes the pore. **Right:** In the open state the cylinders tilt, thus enlarging the ring of leucines. A ring of hydrophilic threonine residues (small spheres) may form the selectivity filter near the inner mouth of the channel. (Based on Unwin 1995).

channel, Karlin concluded that the gate was at the cytoplasmic end of M2.

An Overall View

The terminals of motor neurons form synapses with muscle fibers at specialized regions in the muscle mem-

brane called end-plates. When an action potential reaches the terminals of a presynaptic motor neuron, it causes release of ACh. The transmitter diffuses across the synaptic cleft and binds to nicotinic ACh receptors in the end-plate, thus opening channels that allow Na^+, K^+, and Ca^{2+} to flow across the postsynaptic muscle. A net influx of Na^+ ions produces a depolarizing synaptic potential called the end-plate potential.

Because the ACh-activated channels are localized to the end-plate, the opening of these channels produces only a local depolarization that spreads passively along the muscle fibers. But by depolarizing the postsynaptic cell past threshold, the transmitter-gated channels activate voltage-dependent Na^+ channels near the end-plate region. As the postsynaptic cell becomes progressively depolarized, more and more voltage-gated Na^+ channels open. In this way the Na^+ channels can quickly generate enough current to produce an actively propagated action potential.

The protein that forms the nicotinic ACh-activated channel has been purified, its genes cloned, and its amino acids sequenced. It is composed of five subunits, two of which—the α-subunits that recognize and bind ACh—are identical. Each subunit has four hydrophobic regions that are thought to form membrane-spanning α-helices.

The protein that forms the nicotinic ACh-gated channel also contains a site for recognizing and binding the ACh. This channel is thus gated directly by a chemical transmitter. The functional molecular domains of the ACh-gated channel have been identified, and the steps that link ACh-binding to the opening of the channel are now being investigated. Thus, we may soon be able to see in atomic detail the molecular dynamics of this channel's various physiological functions.

The large number of ACh-gated channels at the end-plate normally ensures that synaptic transmission will proceed with a high safety factor. In the autoimmune disease myasthenia gravis, antibodies to the ACh receptor decrease the number of ACh-gated channels, thus seriously compromising transmission at the neuromuscular junction (see Chapter 16).

Acetylcholine is only one of many neurotransmitters in the nervous system, and the end-plate potential is just one example of chemical signaling. Do transmitters in the central nervous system act in the same fashion, or are other mechanisms involved? In the past such questions were virtually unanswerable because of the small size and great variety of nerve cells in the central nervous system. However, advances in experimental technique—in particular, patch clamping—have made synaptic transmission at central synapses easier to study. Already it is clear that many neurotransmitters operate in the central nervous system much as ACh operates at the end-plate, while other transmitters produce their effects in quite different ways. In the next two chapters we shall explore some of the many variations of synaptic transmission that characterize the central and peripheral nervous systems.

Postscript: The End-Plate Current Can Be Calculated From an Equivalent Circuit

Although the flow of current through a population of ACh-activated end-plate channels can be described by Ohm's law, to understand fully how the flow of electrical current generates the end-plate potential we also need to consider all the resting channels in the surrounding membrane. Since channels are proteins that span the bilayer of the membrane, we must also take into consideration the capacitive properties of the membrane and the ionic batteries determined by the distribution of Na^+ and K^+ inside and outside the cell.

The dynamic relationship of these various components can be explained using the same rules we used in Chapter 8 to analyze the flow of current in passive electrical devices that consist only of resistors, capacitors, and batteries. We can represent the end-plate region with an equivalent circuit that has three parallel branches: (1) a branch representing the flow of synaptic current through the transmitter-gated channels; (2) a branch representing the return current flow through resting channels (the nonsynaptic membrane); and (3) a branch representing current flow across the lipid bilayer, which acts as a capacitor (Figure 11-16).

Since the end-plate current is carried by both Na^+ and K^+, we could represent the synaptic branch of the equivalent circuit as two parallel branches, each representing the flow of a different ion species. At the end-plate, however, Na^+ and K^+ flow through the same ion channel. It is therefore more convenient (and correct) to combine the Na^+ and K^+ current pathways into a single conductance, representing the channel gated by ACh. The conductance of this pathway depends on the number of channels opened, which in turn depends on the concentration of transmitter. In the absence of transmitter no channels are open and the conductance is zero. When a presynaptic action potential causes the release of transmitter, the conductance of this pathway rises to a value of around 5×10^{-6} S (or a resistance of $2 \times 10^5\ \Omega$). This is about five times the conductance of the parallel branch representing the resting or leakage channels (g_l).

The end-plate conductance is in series with a battery (E_{EPSP}), whose value is given by the reversal potential for synaptic current flow (0 mV) (Figure 11-16). This value is the weighted algebraic sum of the Na^+ and K^+ equilibrium potentials (see Box 11-1).

The current flowing during the excitatory postsynaptic potential (I_{EPSP}) is given by

$$I_{EPSP} = g_{EPSP} \times (V_m - E_{EPSP}).$$

Using this equation and the equivalent circuit of Figure 11-17 we can now analyze the end-plate potential in

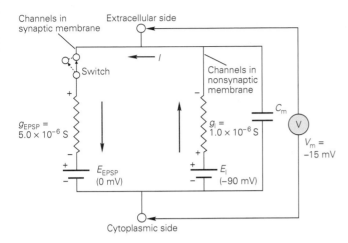

Figure 11-16 The equivalent circuit of the end-plate with two parallel current pathways. One pathway representing the synapse consists of a battery, E_{EPSP}, in series with a conductance through ACh-gated channels, g_{EPSP}. The other pathway consists of the battery representing the resting potential (E_l) in series with the conductance of the resting channels (g_l). In parallel with both of these conductance pathways is the membrane capacitance (C_m). The voltmeter (V) measures the potential difference between the inside and the outside of the cell.

When no ACh is present, the gated channels are closed and no current flows through them. This state is depicted as an open electrical circuit in which the synaptic conductance is not connected to the rest of the circuit. The binding of ACh opens the synaptic channel. This event is electrically equivalent to throwing the switch that connects the gated conductance pathway (g_{EPSP}) with the resting pathway (g_l). In the steady state current flows inward through the gated channels and outward through the resting channels. With the indicated values of conductances and batteries, the membrane will depolarize from −90 mV (its resting potential) to −15 mV (the peak of the end-plate potential).

terms of the flow of ionic current. At the onset of the excitatory synaptic action (the dynamic phase), an inward current (I_{EPSP}) flows through the ACh-activated channels because of the increased conductance to Na^+ and K^+ and the large inward driving force on Na^+ at the initial resting potential (−90 mV). Since current flows in a closed loop, the inward synaptic current must leave the cell as outward current. From the equivalent circuit we see that there are two parallel pathways for outward current flow: a conductance pathway (I_l) representing current flow through the resting (or leakage) channels and a capacitive pathway (I_c) representing current flow across the membrane capacitance. Thus,

$$I_{EPSP} = -(I_l + I_c).$$

During the earliest phase of the end-plate potential the membrane potential, V_m, is still close to its resting

value, E_l. As a result, the outward driving force on current flow through the resting channels ($V_m - E_l$) is small. Therefore, most of the current leaves the cell as capacitive current and the membrane depolarizes rapidly (phase 2 in Figure 11-17). As the cell depolarizes, the outward driving force on current flow through the resting channels increases, while the inward driving force on synaptic current flow through the ACh-gated channels decreases. Concomitantly, as the concentration of ACh in the synapse falls, the ACh-gated channels begin to close, and eventually the flow of inward current through the gated channels is exactly balanced by outward current flow through the resting channels ($I_{EPSP} = -I_l$). At this point no current flows into or out of the capacitor, that is, $I_c = 0$. Since the rate of change of membrane potential is directly proportional to I_c,

$$I_c = C_m \times \Delta V / \Delta t,$$

the membrane potential will have reached a peak steady-state value, $\Delta V / \Delta t = 0$ (phase 3 in Figure 11-17).

As the gated channels close, I_{EPSP} decreases further. Now I_{EPSP} and I_l are no longer in balance and the membrane potential starts to repolarize, because the outward current flow due to I_l becomes larger than the inward synaptic current. During most of the declining phase of the synaptic action, current no longer flows through the ACh-gated channels since all these channels are closed. Instead, current flows out only through the resting channels and in across the capacitor (phase 4 in Figure 11-17).

When the end-plate potential is at its peak or steady-state value, $I_c = 0$ and therefore the value of V_m can be easily calculated. The inward current flow through the gated channels (I_{EPSP}) must be exactly balanced by outward current flow through the resting channels (I_l):

$$I_{EPSP} + I_l = 0. \tag{11-8}$$

The current flowing through the active ACh-gated channels (I_{EPSP}) and through the resting channels (I_l) is given by Ohm's law:

$$I_{EPSP} = g_{EPSP} \times (V_m - E_{EPSP}),$$

and

$$I_l = g_l \times (V_m - E_l).$$

By substituting these two expressions into Equation 11-8, we obtain

$$g_{EPSP} \times (V_m - E_{EPSP}) + g_l \times (V_m - E_l) = 0.$$

To solve for V_m we need only expand the two products in the equation and rearrange them so that all terms in

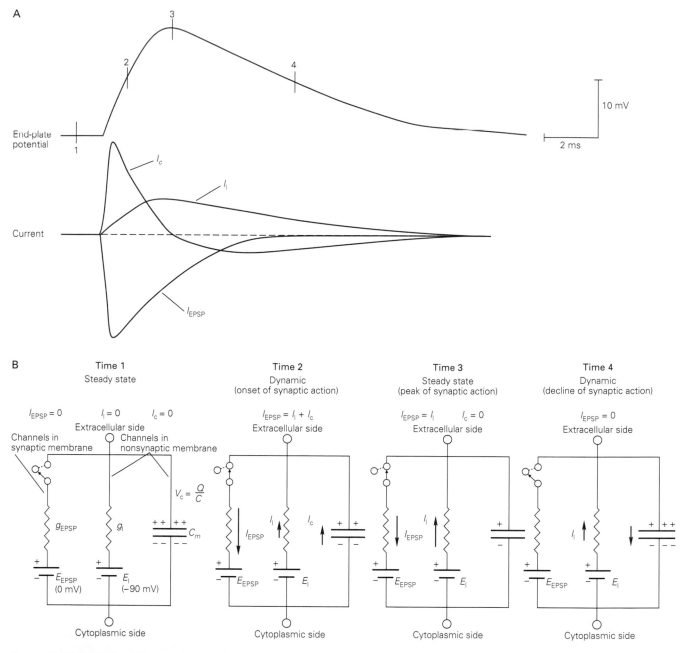

Figure 11-17 Both the ACh-gated synaptic conductance and the passive membrane properties of the muscle cell determine the time course of the end-plate potential.

A. Comparison of the time course of the end-plate potential (**top trace**) with the time courses of the component currents through the ACh-gated channels (I_{EPSP}), the resting (or leakage) channels (I_l), and the capacitor (I_c). Capacitive current flows only when the membrane potential is changing. In the steady state, such as at the peak of the end-plate potential, the inward flow of ionic current through the ACh-gated channels is exactly balanced by the outward flow of ionic current across the resting channels, and there is no flow of capacitive current.

B. Equivalent circuits for the current at times 1, 2, 3, and 4 shown in part **A.** (The relative magnitude of a current is represented by the length of the arrows.)

voltage (V_m) appear on the left side:

$$(g_{EPSP} \times V_m) + (g_l \times V_m) = (g_{EPSP} \times E_{EPSP}) + (g_l \times E_l).$$

By factoring out V_m on the left side, we finally obtain

$$V_m = \frac{(g_{EPSP} \times E_{EPSP}) + (g_l \times E_l)}{g_{EPSP} + g_l}. \qquad \textbf{(11-9)}$$

This equation is similar to that used to calculate the resting and action potentials (Chapter 7). According to Equation 11-9, the peak voltage of the end-plate potential is a weighted average of the electromotive forces of the two batteries for gated and resting currents. The weighting factors are given by the relative magnitude of the two conductances. If the gated conductance is much smaller than the resting membrane conductance ($g_{EPSP} \ll g_l$), $g_{EPSP} \times E_{EPSP}$ will be negligible compared with $g_l \times E_l$. Under these conditions, V_m will remain close to E_l. This situation occurs when only a few channels are opened by ACh (because its concentration is low). On the other hand, if g_{EPSP} is much larger than g_l, Equation 11-9 states that V_m approaches E_{EPSP}, the synaptic reversal potential. This situation occurs when the concentration of ACh is high and a large number of ACh-activated channels are open. At intermediate ACh concentrations, with a moderate number of ACh-activated channels open, the peak end-plate potential lies somewhere between E_l and E_{EPSP}.

We can now use this equation to calculate the peak end-plate potential for the specific case shown in Figure 11-16, where $g_{EPSP} = 5 \times 10^{-6}$ S, $g_l = 1 \times 10^{-6}$ S, $E_{EPSP} = 0$ mV, and $E_l = -90$ mV. Substituting these values into Equation 11-9 yields

$$V_m =$$

$$\frac{[(5 \times 10^{-6}\,S) \times (0\,mV)] + [(1 \times 10^{-6}\,S) \times (-90\,mV)]}{(5 \times 10^{-6}\,S) + (1 \times 10^{-6}\,S)}.$$

or

$$V_m = \frac{(1 \times 10^{-6}\,S) \times (-90\,mV)}{(6 \times 10^{-6}\,S)}$$

$$= -15\,mV.$$

The peak amplitude of the end-plate potential is then

$$\Delta V_{EPSP} = V_m - E_l$$

$$= -15\,mV - (-90\,mV)$$

$$= 75\,mV.$$

As a check for consistency we can see whether, at the peak of the end-plate potential, the synaptic current is equal and opposite to the nonsynaptic current so that the net membrane current is indeed equal to zero:

$$I_{EPSP} = (5 \times 10^{-6}\,S) \times (-15\,mV - 0\,mV)$$

$$= -75 \times 10^{-9}\,A$$

and

$$I_l = (1 \times 10^{-6}\,S) \times [-15\,mV - (-90\,mV)],$$

$$= 75 \times 10^{-9}\,A.$$

Here we see that Equation 11-9 ensures that $I_{EPSP} + I_l = 0$.

Eric R. Kandel
Steven A. Siegelbaum

Selected Readings

Fatt P, Katz B. 1951. An analysis of the end-plate potential recorded with an intra-cellular electrode. J Physiol (Lond) 115:320–370.

Heuser JE, Reese TS. 1977. Structure of the synapse. In: ER Kandel (ed), *Handbook of Physiology: A Critical, Comprehensive Presentation of Physiological Knowledge and Concepts*, Sect. 1, *The Nervous System*. Vol. 1, *Cellular Biology of Neurons*, Part 1, pp. 261–294. Bethesda, MD: American Physiological Society.

Hille B. 1992. In: *Ionic Channels of Excitable Membranes*, 2nd ed, pp. 140–169. Sunderland, MA: Sinauer.

Imoto K, Busch C, Sakmann B, Mishina M, Konno T, Nakai J, Bujo H, Mori Y, Fukuda K, Numa S. 1988. Rings of negatively charged amino acids determine the acetylcholine receptor-channel conductance. Nature 335:645–648.

Karlin A, Akabas MH. 1995. Toward a structural basis for the function of nicotinic acetylcholine receptors and their cousins. Neuron 15:1231–1244.

Neher E, Sakmann B. 1976. Single-channel currents recorded from membrane of denervated frog muscle fibres. Nature 260:799–802.

Unwin N. 1993. Neurotransmitter action: opening of ligand-gated ion channels. Cell 72(Suppl):31–41.

References

Akabas MH, Kaufmann C, Archdeacon P, Karlin A. 1994. Identification of acetylcholine receptor-channel–lining residues in the entire M2 segment of the α-subunit. Neuron 13:919–927.

Alberts B, Bray D, Lewis J, Raff M, Roberts K, Watson JD. 1989. *Molecular Biology of the Cell*, 2nd ed. New York: Garland.

Charnet P, Labarca C, Leonard RJ, Vogelaar NJ, Czyzyk L, Gouin A, Davidson N, Lester HA. 1990. An open channel blocker interacts with adjacent turns of α-helices in the nicotinic acetylcholine receptor. Neuron 4:87–95.

Claudio T, Ballivet M, Patrick J, Heinemann S. 1983. Nucleotide and deduced amino acid sequences of *Torpedo californica* acetylcholine receptor γ-subunit. Proc Natl Acad Sci U S A 80:1111–1115.

Colquhoun D. 1981. How fast do drugs work? Trends Pharmacol Sci 2:212–217.

Dwyer TM, Adams DJ, Hille B. 1980. The permeability of the endplate channel to organic cations in frog muscle. J Gen Physiol 75:469–492.

Fertuck HC, Salpeter MM. 1974. Localization of acetylcholine receptor by ^{125}I-labeled α-bungarotoxin binding at mouse motor endplates. Proc Natl Acad Sci U S A 71:1376–1378.

Heuser JE, Salpeter SR. 1979. Organization of acetylcholine receptors in quick-frozen, deep-etched, and rotary-replicated *Torpedo* postsynaptic membrane. J Cell Biol 82:150–173.

Ko C-P. 1984. Regeneration of the active zone at the frog neuromuscular junction. J Cell Biol 98:1685–1695.

Kuffler SW, Nicholls JG, Martin AR. 1984. *From Neuron to Brain: A Cellular Approach to the Function of the Nervous System,* 2nd ed. Sunderland, MA: Sinauer.

McMahan UJ, Kuffler SW. 1971. Visual identification of synaptic boutons on living ganglion cells and of varicosities in postganglionic axons in the heart of the frog. Proc R Soc Lond B Biol Sci 177:485–508.

Miles FA. 1969. *Excitable Cells.* London: Heinemann.

Noda M, Furutani Y, Takahashi H, Toyosato M, Tanabe T, Shimizu S, Kikyotani S, Kayano T, Hirose T, Inayama S, Numa S. 1983. Cloning and sequence analysis of calf cDNA and human genomic DNA encoding α-subunit precursor of muscle acetylcholine receptor. Nature 305:818–823.

Noda M, Takahashi H, Tanabe T, Toyosato M, Kikyotani S, Furutani Y, Hirose T, Takashima H, Inayama S, Miyata T, Numa S. 1983. Structural homology of *Torpedo californica* acetylcholine receptor subunits. Nature 302:528–532.

Palay SL. 1958. The morphology of synapses in the central nervous system. Exp Cell Res Suppl 5:275–293.

Raftery MA, Hunkapiller MW, Strader CD, Hood LE. 1980. Acetylcholine receptor: complex of homologous subunits. Science 208:1454–1457.

Revah F, Galzi J-L, Giraudat J, Haumont PY, Lederer F, Changeux J-P. 1990. The noncompetitive blocker [3H]chlorpromazine labels three amino acids of the acetylcholine receptor gamma subunit: implications for the alpha-helical organization of regions MII and for the structure of the ion channel. Proc Natl Acad Sci U S A 87:4675–4679.

Salpeter MM (ed). 1987. *The Vertebrate Neuromuscular Junction,* pp. 1–54. New York: Liss.

Takeuchi A. 1977. Junctional transmission. I. Postsynaptic mechanisms. In: ER Kandel (ed), *Handbook of Physiology: A Critical, Comprehensive Presentation of Physiological Knowledge and Concepts,* Sect. 1, *The Nervous System.* Vol. 1, *Cellular Biology of Neurons,* Part 1, pp. 295–327. Bethesda, MD: American Physiological Society.

Toyoshima C, Unwin N. 1988. Ion channel of acetylcholine receptor reconstructed from images of postsynaptic membranes. Nature 336:247–250.

Verrall S, Hall ZW. 1992. The N-terminal domains of acetylcholine receptor subunits contain recognition signals for the initial steps of receptor assembly. Cell 68:23–31.

Villarroel A, Herlitze S, Koenen M, Sakmann B. 1991. Location of a threonine residue in the alpha-subunit M2 transmembrane segment that determines the ion flow through the acetylcholine receptor-channel. Proc R Soc Lond B Biol Sci 243:69–74.

Unwin N. 1995. Acetylcholine receptor-channel imaged in the open state. Nature 373:37–43.

12

Synaptic Integration

L IKE SYNAPTIC TRANSMISSION at the neuromuscular junction, most rapid signaling between neurons in the central nervous system involves ionotropic receptors in the cell membrane. Thus, many principles that apply to synaptic connections at the neuromuscular junction also apply in the central nervous system.

Synaptic transmission between central neurons is more complex, however, for several reasons. First, whereas most muscle fibers are innervated by only one motor neuron, a central nerve cell (such as the motor neuron in the spinal cord) receives connections from hundreds of neurons. Second, muscle fibers receive only excitatory inputs, while central neurons receive both excitatory and inhibitory inputs. Third, all synaptic actions on muscle fibers are mediated by one neurotransmitter, acetylcholine (ACh), which activates only one type of receptor (the nicotinic ACh receptor-channel), whereas in the central nervous system the inputs to a single cell are mediated by a variety of transmitters that alter the activity of a variety of ion channels. These channels include not only many that are directly gated by transmitters, much like the nicotinic ACh receptor, but others that are gated indirectly by metabotropic receptors and the second messengers they activate. As a result, unlike muscle fibers, central neurons must integrate diverse inputs into one coordinated response.

Finally, the nerve-muscle synapse is a model of efficiency—every action potential in the motor neuron produces an action potential in the muscle fiber. In comparison, connections made by a presynaptic neuron onto the motor neuron are only modestly effective—perhaps 50–100 excitatory neurons must fire together to produce a synaptic potential large enough to trigger an action potential in a motor cell.

The first insight into synapses in the central nervous system mediated by ionotropic receptors came from experiments by John Eccles and his colleagues in the 1950s on the synaptic mechanisms of the spinal motor neu-

A Stretch reflex circuit for knee jerk

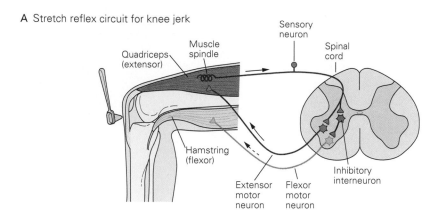

B Experimental setup for recording from cells in the circuit

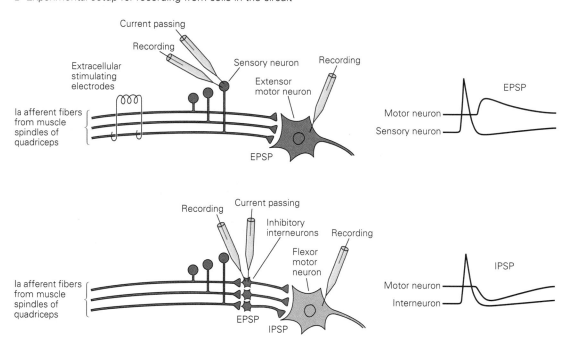

Figure 12-1 The combination of excitatory and inhibitory synaptic connections mediating the stretch reflex of the quadriceps muscle is typical of circuits in the central nervous system.

A. The stretch-receptor sensory neuron at the quadriceps muscle makes an excitatory connection with the motor neuron innervating this same muscle group (the extensor motor neuron). It also makes an excitatory connection with an interneuron. This interneuron, in turn, makes an inhibitory connection with the motor neuron innervating the antagonist biceps muscle group (the flexor motor neuron). Conversely, an afferent fiber from the biceps excites an interneuron that makes an inhibitory synapse on the extensor motor neuron (not shown).

B. This idealized experimental setup shows the approaches to studying the inhibition and excitation of an extensor motor neuron in the pathway illustrated in **A. Top:** Two alternatives for eliciting excitatory potentials in the extensor motor neuron. (1) The whole afferent nerve from the quadriceps can be stimulated electrically with extracellular electrodes, or (2) single axons can be stimulated with an intracellular current-passing electrode inserted into the sensory neuron cell body. An action potential stimulated in the afferent neuron from the quadriceps triggers an excitatory (depolarizing) postsynaptic potential, or EPSP, in the extensor motor neuron. **Bottom:** The setup for eliciting and measuring inhibitory potentials in the flexor motor neuron. The inhibitory interneurons receiving input from the quadriceps pathway are stimulated intracellularly. An action potential stimulated in the inhibitory interneuron in the quadriceps (extensor) pathway causes an inhibitory (hyperpolarizing) postsynaptic potential, or IPSP, in the flexor motor neuron.

rons that control the stretch reflex, the simple behavior we considered in Chapters 2 and 4. The spinal motor neurons remain particularly useful for examining central synaptic mechanisms because they have large, accessible cell bodies and, most important, they receive both excitatory and inhibitory connections and therefore allow us to study the integrative action of the nervous system on the cellular level.

A Central Neuron Receives Both Excitatory and Inhibitory Signals

To analyze the synapses that mediate the stretch reflex, Eccles activated a large population of axons of the sensory cells that innervate the stretch receptor organs in the quadriceps muscle. Nowadays the same experiments can be done by stimulating a single sensory neuron. Passing sufficient current through a microelectrode into the cell body of a stretch-receptor neuron in the dorsal root ganglion generates an action potential in the sensory cell. This in turn produces a small excitatory postsynaptic potential (EPSP) in the motor neuron innervating the same muscle monitored by the sensory neuron (Figure 12-1). The EPSP produced by the one sensory cell depolarizes the motor neuron by less than 1 mV, often only 0.2–0.4 mV, far below the threshold for generating an action potential (typically, a depolarization of 10 mV or more is required to reach threshold).

Stimulating a stretch-receptor neuron that innervates the biceps (hamstrings), a muscle group antagonistic to the quadriceps, produces a small inhibitory postsynaptic potential (IPSP) in the motor neuron of the quadriceps (Figure 12-1). This hyperpolarizing action is mediated by an inhibitory interneuron, which receives excitatory input from the sensory neurons of the biceps and in turn connects with the quadriceps motor neurons. The interneurons can also be stimulated intracellularly.

Although a single EPSP in the motor neuron is not nearly large enough to elicit an action potential, the convergence of many excitatory synaptic potentials from many afferent fibers can be integrated by the neuron to initiate an action potential. At the same time, inhibitory synaptic potentials, if strong enough, can counteract the sum of the excitatory actions and prevent the membrane potential from reaching threshold.

In addition to counteracting synaptic excitation, synaptic inhibition can exert powerful control over spontaneously active nerve cells. Many cells in the brain are spontaneously active, as are the pacemaker cells of the heart. By suppressing the spontaneous generation of action potentials in these cells, synaptic inhibition can

shape the pattern of firing in a cell. This function, called the *sculpturing* role of inhibition, is illustrated in Figure 12-2.

Excitatory and Inhibitory Synapses Have Distinctive Ultrastructures

As we learned in Chapter 10, the effect of a synaptic potential—whether it is excitatory or inhibitory—is determined not by the type of transmitter released from the presynaptic neuron but by the type of ion channels gated by the transmitter in the postsynaptic cell. Although most transmitters are recognized by types of receptors that mediate either excitatory or inhibitory potentials, some act predominantly on receptors that are of one or another sign. For example, in the vertebrate brain neurons that release glutamate typically act on receptors that produce excitation; neurons that release γ-aminobutyric acid (GABA) or glycine act on ionotropic inhibitory receptors. (An exception is found in the vertebrate retina, which we discuss in a later chapter, and there are many exceptions in invertebrates.) The synaptic terminals of excitatory and inhibitory neurons can sometimes be distinguished by their morphology.

There are two common morphological types of synaptic connections in the brain, Gray type I and type II (named after E. G. Gray, who described them). Type I synapses are often glutamatergic and therefore excitatory, whereas type II synapses are often GABA-ergic and therefore inhibitory. In type I synapses the cleft is

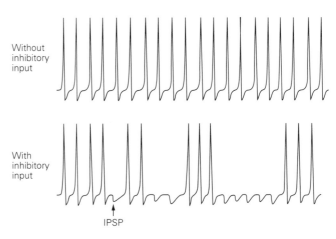

Without inhibitory input

With inhibitory input

IPSP

Figure 12-2 Inhibition can shape the firing pattern of a spontaneously active neuron. Without inhibitory input the neuron fires continuously at a fixed interval. With inhibitory input some action potentials are inhibited, resulting in a distinctive pattern of impulses. This effect of inhibition on the firing of a neuron is called *sculpturing.*

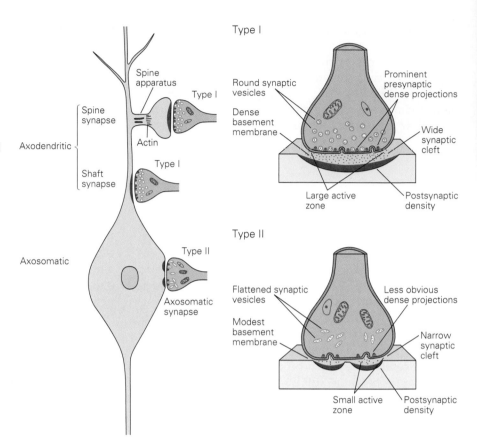

Figure 12-3 The two most common morphologic types of synapses in the central nervous system are Gray type I and type II. Type I is usually excitatory, exemplified by glutamatergic synapses; type II is usually inhibitory, exemplified by GABA-ergic synapses. Differences include the shape of vesicles, prominence of presynaptic densities, total area of the active zone, width of the synaptic cleft, and presence of a dense basement membrane. Type I synapses typically contact specialized projections on the dendrites, called spines, and less commonly contact the shafts of dendrites. Type II synapses often contact the cell body.

Figure 12-4 (Opposite) Excitatory actions at chemical synapses result from the opening of channels permeable to both Na⁺ and K⁺. This can be demonstrated by determining the reversal potential for the EPSP.

A. Intracellular electrodes are used to stimulate and record from the neurons. Current is passed in the postsynaptic motor neuron either to alter the level of the resting membrane potential prior to presynaptic stimulation (a method of membrane control called current clamping) or to keep the membrane potential fixed during the flow of synaptic current (voltage clamping).

B. A weak stimulus to the afferent nerve from the quadriceps recruits only a few Ia afferent fibers, resulting in a subthreshold postsynaptic potential. A strong stimulus recruits more afferent fibers, resulting in a suprathreshold synaptic potential that drives the membrane potential more effectively toward its reversal potential, which is beyond the threshold (-55 mV) for initiating an action potential.

C. The reversal potential for the synaptic potential can be determined using a current clamp. When the membrane potential is at its resting value (-65 mV), a presynaptic action potential pro-

duces a depolarizing EPSP, which increases in amplitude when the membrane is hyperpolarized to -70 and -80 mV. In contrast, when the membrane is depolarized to -20 mV, the EPSP becomes smaller; when the membrane potential reaches the reversal potential (0 mV), the EPSP is nullified. Further depolarization to $+20$ mV inverts the synaptic potential, causing hyperpolarization. Thus synaptic action, whether hyperpolarizing or depolarizing, always drives the membrane potential toward the reversal potential, E_{EPSP}.

D. The reversal potential for the synaptic current can be determined using a voltage clamp. At the resting membrane potential and at more negative clamped potentials (-70 and -80 mV) the synaptic current is large and inward because the electrochemical driving force is inward. This inward current generates the EPSP. When the membrane potential is made less negative (-20 mV), the magnitude of the inward synaptic current decreases; at the reversal potential (0 mV) it becomes zero. When the membrane potential is made more positive than the reversal potential ($+20$ or $+55$ mV), the synaptic current is outward. The magnitude and sign of the synaptic current is determined by the sum of the fluxes of K⁺ and Na⁺ through the synaptic conductance.

A Experimental setup

B Excitatory synaptic actions

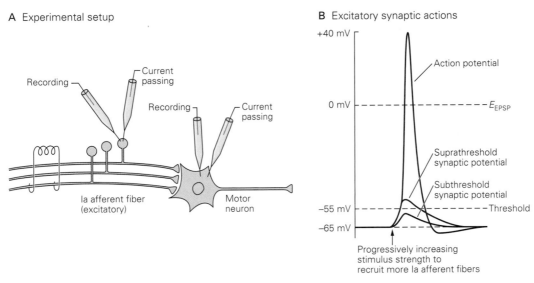

C Reversal potential for synaptic potential

D Reversal potential for synaptic current

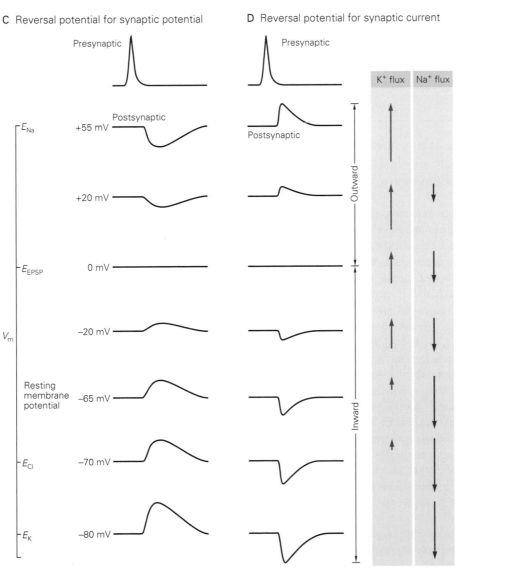

slightly widened to approximately 30 nm; the presynaptic active zone is 1–2 μm^2 in area; and dense regions on the presynaptic membrane, the presumed sites for vesicular release, are prominent. The synaptic vesicles tend to assume a characteristic round shape when treated with certain electron microscope fixatives. The postsynaptic membrane also includes extensive dense regions, and amorphous dense basement-membrane material appears in the synaptic cleft. In type II synapses the synaptic cleft is 20 nm across; the active zone is smaller (less than 1 μm^2); the presynaptic membrane specializations and dense regions are less obvious; and there is little or no basement membrane within the cleft. Characteristically, the vesicles of type II synapses tend to be oval or flattened (Figure 12-3).

Although type I synapses are often excitatory and type II inhibitory, the morphological distinctions between the two types of synapses have proved to be only a first approximation of transmitter biochemistry. As we shall learn in Chapter 15, much more reliable distinctions between transmitter types have been gained through the use of immunocytochemistry, based on the biochemical nature of the transmitters or the enzymes involved in their synthesis.

Excitatory Synaptic Action Is Mediated by Glutamate-Gated Channels That Conduct Sodium and Potassium

The excitatory transmitter released from the stretch-receptor neurons is the amino acid L-glutamate, the major excitatory transmitter in the brain and spinal cord. Eccles and his colleagues discovered that the excitatory postsynaptic potential in spinal motor cells results from the opening of glutamate-gated channels permeable to both Na^+ and K^+. This ionic mechanism is similar to that produced by ACh at the neuromuscular junction described in Chapter 11. Like the ACh-gated channels, the glutamate-gated channels conduct both Na^+ and K^+, with nearly equal permeability. As a result, the reversal potential for current flow through these channels lies at 0 mV (Figure 12-4C,D). As the strength of the extracellular stimulus is increased, more afferent fibers are excited, and the depolarization produced by the excitatory synaptic potential becomes larger. The depolarization eventually becomes large enough to bring the membrane potential of the axon hillock (the integrative component of the motor neuron) to the threshold for generation of an action potential.

The glutamate receptors can be divided into two broad categories: the ionotropic receptors that directly gate channels and the metabotropic receptors that indirectly gate channels through second messengers (Figure 12-5). There are three major subtypes of ionotropic glutamate receptors: AMPA, kainate, and NMDA, named according to the types of synthetic agonists that activate them (α-amino-3-hydroxy-5-methylisoxazole-4-propionic acid, kainate, and N-methyl-D-aspartate, respectively). The NMDA glutamate receptor is selectively blocked by the drug APV (2-amino-5-phosphonovaleric acid). The AMPA and kainate receptors are not affected by APV, but both are blocked by the drug CNQX (6-cyano-7-nitroquinoxaline-2,3-dione). Thus the AMPA and kain-ate receptors are sometimes referred to together as the non-NMDA receptors. The metabotropic glutamate receptors can be selectively activated by trans-(1S,3R)-1-amino-1,3-cyclopentanedicarboxylic acid (ACPD) (Figure 12-5). The action of glutamate on the ionotropic receptors is always excitatory, while activation of the metabotropic receptors can produce either excitation or inhibition.

The motor neuron has both non-NMDA and NMDA receptors. At the normal resting potential the non-NMDA ionotropic receptors generate the large early component of the EPSP in motor neurons (as well as in most other central neurons) in response to stimulation of the primary afferent sensory fibers (see Figure 12-7). These receptors gate cation channels with relatively low conductances (≤ 20 pS) that are permeable to both Na^+ and K^+ but are usually not permeable to Ca^{2+}.

The NMDA receptor-channel, which contributes to the late component of the EPSP, has three exceptional properties. First, the receptor controls a cation channel of high conductance (50 pS) that is permeable to Ca^{2+} as well as to Na^+ and K^+ (Figure 12-5). Second, opening of the channel requires extracellular glycine as a cofactor; the channel will only function in the presence of glycine. Under normal conditions the concentration of glycine in the extracellular fluid is sufficient to allow the NMDA receptor-channel to function efficiently. Third, the channel is unique among transmitter-gated channels thus far characterized because its opening depends on membrane voltage as well as a chemical transmitter.

The voltage-dependence is due to a mechanism that is quite different from that employed by the voltage-gated channels that generate the action potential. In the latter, changes in membrane potential are translated into conformational changes in the channel by an intrinsic voltage-sensor. In the NMDA-activated channels an extrinsic blocking particle, extracellular Mg^{2+}, binds to a site in the pore of the open channel and acts like a plug, blocking current flow. At the resting membrane potential (-65 mV) Mg^{2+} binds tightly to the channel. But when the membrane is depolarized (for example, by the action of glutamate on the non-NMDA receptors), Mg^{2+} is expelled from the channel by electrostatic repulsion, allowing Na^+ and Ca^{2+} to enter. Thus, maximal current flows through the NMDA-type channel only when two conditions are met: glutamate is present and the cell is depolarized (Figure 12-6). The NMDA receptor has the further interesting property that it is inhibited by the hallucinogenic drug phencyclidine (PCP, also known as angel dust) and by MK801, both of which bind to a site within the open channel pore that is distinct from the Mg^{2+} binding site. Blockade of NMDA receptors produces symptoms that resemble the hallucinations associated with schizophrenia, while certain antipsychotic drugs enhance current flow through the NMDA receptor-channels. This has led to the hypothesis that schizophrenia may involve a defect in NMDA receptor function.

Most cells have both NMDA and non-NMDA glutamate receptors. However, because Mg^{2+} is present in the NMDA receptor-channel at the resting membrane potential, this channel does not normally contribute significantly to the EPSP. Thus the EPSP generated at the resting level depends largely on the activation of the non-NMDA receptors. As the depolarization of the neuron increases, Mg^{2+} is driven out of the mouth of the NMDA receptor-channels, more NMDA-type channels are opened, and more current flows through these channels.

The NMDA-type channel has a further characteristic property: It opens and closes relatively slowly in response to glutamate and thus contributes to the late phase of the EPSP (Figure 12-7). This late phase of the EPSP is normally small after a single presynaptic action potential, because of Mg^{2+} blockade of the channel. However, when the presynaptic neuron fires repeatedly so that the EPSPs summate to depolarize the postsynaptic cell by 20 mV or more, the NMDA receptor gives rise to a much larger current. This current is carried, to an important degree, by Ca^{2+}. Thus activation of the NMDA receptor leads to the activation of calcium-dependent enzymes and certain second messenger–dependent protein kinases in the postsynaptic cell (see Chapter 13). These biochemical reactions are important for triggering signal transduction pathways that contribute to certain long-lasting modifications in the synapse that are thought to be important for learning and memory (Chapter 63). Because the NMDA receptors require a significant level of presynaptic activity before they can function maximally, long-term synaptic modification mediated by the NMDA receptor is often referred to as *activity-dependent synaptic modification*.

Surprisingly, an imbalance in excitatory transmitters such as glutamate may, under certain circumstances, contribute to disease. Excessive amounts of glutamate are highly toxic to neurons. Most cells in the

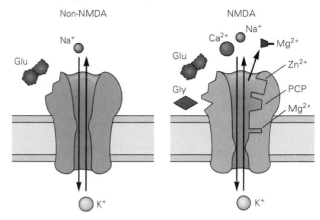

A Ionotropic glutamate receptor

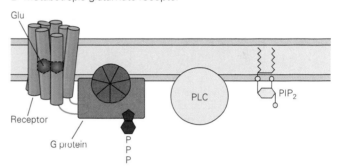

B Metabotropic glutamate receptor

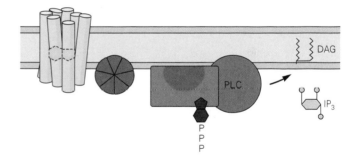

Figure 12-5 Three classes of glutamate receptors regulate excitatory synaptic actions in neurons in the spinal cord and brain.

A. Two types of ionotropic glutamate receptors directly gate ion channels. Two subtypes of non-NMDA receptors bind the glutamate agonists kainate or AMPA and regulate a channel permeable to Na^+ and K^+. The NMDA (*N*-methyl-D-aspartate) receptor regulates a channel permeable to Ca^{2+}, K^+, and Na^+ and has binding sites for glycine, Zn^{2+}, phencyclidine (PCP, or "angel dust"), MK801 (an experimental drug), and Mg^{2+}, which regulate the functioning of this channel in different ways.

B. The metabotropic glutamate receptors indirectly gate ion channels by activating a second messenger. The binding of glutamate to certain types of metabotropic glutamate receptors stimulates the activity of the enzyme phospholipase C (PLC), leading to the formation of two second messengers derived from phosphatidylinositol 4,5-bisphosphate (PIP_2): inositol 1,4,5-triphosphate (IP_3) and diacylglycerol (DAG) (see Chapter 13).

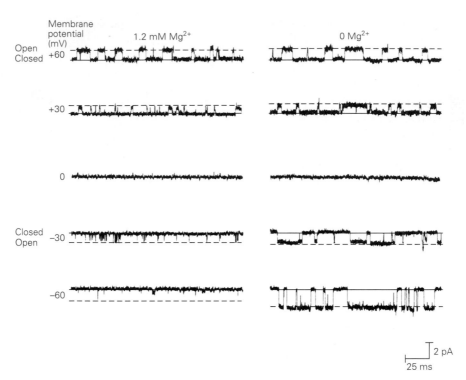

Figure 12-6 Current flow through the NMDA-type gluta-mate receptor-channel is dependent on voltage. These recordings are from individual channels activated by NMDA (from rat hippocampal cells in culture). When Mg^{2+} is present in normal concentration (1.2 mM) in the extracellular solution, the channel is largely blocked at the resting potential (-60 mV) (recordings on the left). At negative potentials only brief, flickery openings are seen due to the Mg^{2+} block. Upon substantial depolarization (to $+30$ mV or $+60$ mV) the Mg^{2+} block is relieved, revealing longer lasting outward pulses of current through the channel. When Mg^{2+} is removed from the extracellular solution the opening and closing of the channel does not depend on voltage (recording on the right). The channel is open at the resting potential of -60 mV, and the synaptic current reverses near 0 mV, like the total membrane current (see Figure 12-4D). (Courtesy of J. Jen and C. F. Stevens.)

brain have receptors that respond to L-glutamate. In tissue culture even a brief exposure to high concentrations of glutamate will kill many neurons, an action called *glutamate excitotoxicity*. In many cell types glutamate excitotoxicity is thought to result predominantly from excessive inflow of Ca^{2+} through NMDA-type channels. High concentrations of intracellular Ca^{2+} may activate calcium-dependent proteases and phospholipases and may produce free radicals that are toxic to the cell. Glutamate toxicity may contribute to cell damage after stroke, to the cell death that occurs with episodes of rapidly repeated seizures experienced by people who have status epilepticus, and to degenerative diseases such as Huntington disease. Agents that selectively block the NMDA receptor may protect against the toxic effects of glutamate and are currently being tested clinically.

Inhibitory Synaptic Action Is Usually Mediated by GABA- and Glycine-Gated Channels That Conduct Chloride

Inhibitory postsynaptic potentials in spinal motor neurons and most central neurons are generated by the inhibitory amino acid neurotransmitters GABA and glycine. GABA is a major inhibitory transmitter in the brain and spinal cord. It acts on two receptors, $GABA_A$ and $GABA_B$. The $GABA_A$ receptor is an ionotropic receptor that gates a Cl^- channel. The $GABA_B$ receptor is a metabotropic receptor that activates a second-messenger cascade, which often activates a K^+ channel (see Chapter 13). Glycine, a less common inhibitory transmitter, also activates ionotropic receptors that gate to Cl^- channels. Glycine is released in the spinal cord by interneurons that inhibit antagonist muscles.

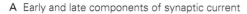

A Early and late components of synaptic current

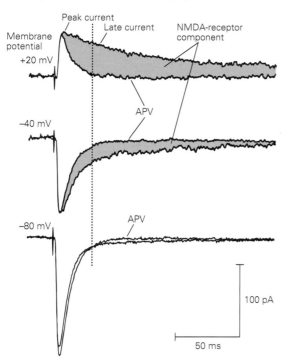

B Current-voltage relationship of the synaptic current

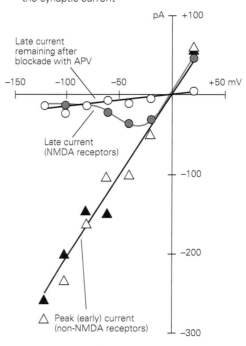

Figure 12-7 The NMDA-type glutamate receptor-channel contributes only a small late component to the normal excitatory postsynaptic current. These records are from a cell in the hippocampus. Similar receptor-channels are present in motor neurons and throughout the brain. (After Hestrin et al. 1990.)

A. The contribution of the NMDA receptor-channel to the excitatory postsynaptic current is revealed by the drug APV, which selectively binds to and blocks the NMDA receptor. The records show the excitatory postsynaptic current before and during application of 50 μM APV at three different membrane potentials. The difference between the traces **(blue region)** represents the APV-sensitive current, which yields the NMDA receptor-channel contribution. The current that remains in the presence of APV is the non-NMDA receptor-channel contribution to the synaptic current. At −80 mV there is no current through the NMDA receptor-channels because of pronounced Mg^{2+} block. At −40 mV a small late inward current is evident. At +20 mV the late component is more prominent and has reversed to become an outward current. The vertical **dotted line** indicates a time 25 ms after the peak of the synaptic current

and is used for the calculations of late current in **B**.

B. The relation between excitatory postsynaptic current through the NMDA and non-NMDA receptor-channels and postsynaptic membrane potential. The current through the non-NMDA receptors was measured at the peak of the synaptic current and is plotted as a function of membrane potential **(filled triangles)**. The current through the NMDA receptors was measured 25 ms after the peak of the synaptic current (dotted line in **A**; a time at which the non-NMDA component has decayed to zero) and is shown as **filled circles**. Note that the non-NMDA receptor-channels behave as simple resistors; current and voltage have a linear relationship. In contrast, current through the NMDA receptors is non-linear and increases as the membrane is depolarized from −80 to −40 mV, owing to progressive relief of Mg^{2+} block. The reversal potential of both receptor-channel types is at 0 mV. The **open symbols** show the components of the excitatory post-synaptic current mediated by the non-NMDA receptors (triangles) and NMDA receptors (circles) in the presence of 50 μm APV. Note how APV blocks the late (NMDA) component but not the early (non-NMDA) component of the EPSP.

Eccles and his colleagues determined the ionic mechanism of the IPSP in spinal motor neurons by systematically changing the level of the resting membrane potential in a motor neuron while stimulating an inhibitory presynaptic interneuron to fire an action potential (Figure 12-8). When the motor neuron membrane was held at the resting potential (−65 mV), a small hyperpolarizing potential was generated when the in-

terneuron was stimulated. When the membrane was held at −70 mV, no change in potential was recorded when the interneuron was stimulated. At potentials more negative than −70 mV, stimulating the inhibitory interneuron generated a depolarizing response in the motor neuron. The reversal potential of −70 mV corresponds to the Cl^- equilibrium potential in spinal motor neurons (the extracellular concentration of Cl^- is much

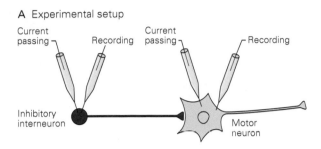

A Experimental setup

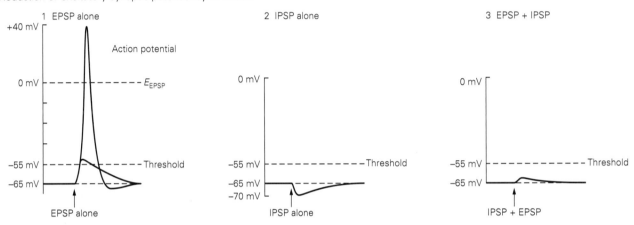

B Reduction of excitatory synaptic potential by inhibition

Figure 12-8 Inhibitory actions at chemical synapses result from the opening of ion channels selective for Cl⁻.

A. In this hypothetical experiment two electrodes are placed in the presynaptic interneuron and two in the postsynaptic motor neuron. The current-passing electrode in the presynaptic cell is used to produce an action potential; in the postsynaptic cell it is used to alter the membrane potential systematically (using a current clamp) prior to the presynaptic input.

B. Inhibitory actions counteract excitatory actions. **1.** A large EPSP occurring alone moves the membrane potential toward E_{EPSP} and exceeds the threshold for generating an action potential. **2.** An IPSP occurring alone moves the membrane potential away from the threshold toward E_{Cl}, the Nernst potential for Cl⁻ (−70 mV). **3.** When inhibitory and excitatory potentials occur together, the effectiveness of the EPSP is reduced, preventing it from reaching threshold.

C. The IPSP and inhibitory synaptic current reverse at the equilibrium potential for Cl⁻. **1.** At the resting membrane potential (−65 mV) a presynaptic spike produces a hyperpolarizing IPSP, which increases in amplitude when the membrane is artificially depolarized to −40 mV. However, when the membrane potential is hyperpolarized to −70 mV, the IPSP is nullified. This reversal potential for the IPSP occurs at E_{Cl}, the Nernst potential for Cl⁻. With further hyperpolarization the IPSP is inverted to a depolarizing postsynaptic potential (at −80 and −100 mV) because the membrane potential is negative to E_{Cl}. Even this depolarizing action has an inhibitory effect, however, because the inhibitory input tends to hold the membrane potential at or below −70 mV, a considerable distance from threshold (−55 mV). **2.** The reversal potential of the inhibitory postsynaptic current measured under voltage clamp. An inward (negative) current flows at membrane potentials negative to the reversal potential (corresponding to an efflux of Cl⁻) and an outward (positive) current flows at membrane potentials positive to the reversal potential (corresponding to an influx of Cl⁻).

C Reversal of inhibitory synaptic potential

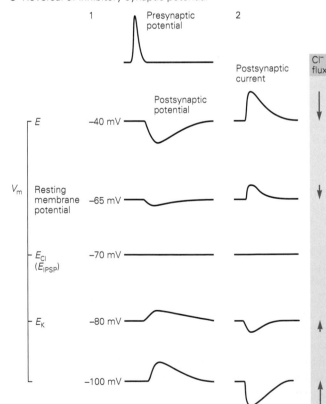

greater than the intracellular concentration). Subsequent experiments using the voltage-clamp technique also demonstrated that the ionic current reverses at the Cl^- equilibrium potential. Thus, the inhibitory IPSP results from an increase in conductance to Cl^-.

Currents Through Single GABA- and Glycine-Gated Channels Can Be Recorded

The unitary currents through single GABA and glycine receptor-channels have been measured using the patch-clamp technique. Both transmitters activate Cl^- channels that show all-or-none step-like openings, similar to the ACh- and glutamate-activated current. The conductance of a glycine-gated channel (46 pS) is larger than that of a GABA-gated channel (30 pS) so that the unitary current steps activated by glycine are somewhat larger than the current steps activated by GABA (Figure 12-9). This difference in single-channel conductance is due to the larger pore diameter of the glycine-gated channel compared with that of the GABA-gated channel.

The inhibitory action upon the opening of these Cl^- channels can be demonstrated by comparing the reversal potential of single-channel inhibitory currents induced by activation of $GABA_A$ receptors to that of single-channel excitatory currents induced by glutamate. The excitatory current reverses at 0 mV. Therefore, opening of glutamate-gated channels will generate an inward current at the normal resting potential, driving the membrane past threshold. In contrast, the inhibitory current becomes nullified and begins to reverse at values more negative than -60 mV. Thus opening of GABA-gated channels will normally generate an outward (hyperpolarizing) current at typical resting potentials, preventing the membrane from reaching threshold (Figure 12-9).

How Does the Opening of Chloride Channels Inhibit the Postsynaptic Cell?

In a typical neuron the resting potential (-65 mV) is slightly more positive than E_{Cl} (-70 mV). Thus, at the resting potential the electrochemical driving force on Cl^- (given by $V_m - E_{Cl}$) will be positive. As a result, the opening of Cl^- channels leads to a positive (outward) current. In the case of the IPSP, the charge carrier is actually the negatively charged Cl^- ion. Thus, the positive current corresponds to an influx of Cl^- down its electrochemical gradient. This causes a net increase in the total negative charge on the inside of the membrane's capacitance so the membrane hyperpolarizes.

Some central neurons have a resting potential that is equal to E_{Cl}. In these cells synaptic actions that increase Cl^- conductance do not change the postsynaptic membrane potential at all—the cell does not become hyperpolarized. How then does the opening of Cl^- channels prevent a cell from firing?

One way of viewing the effects of an inhibitory synaptic input is to consider how it will affect the magnitude of a simultaneous EPSP. The ability of an excitatory input to drive the membrane toward threshold depends on the conductance of the excitatory synaptic channels and on the batteries driving current flow through these channels (chemical driving force) as well as on the conductance of all the other ion channels in the postsynaptic membrane and the batteries for these channels, including the resting channels and any inhibitory synaptic channels that are open. Since the battery of the inhibitory synaptic channels (E_{Cl}) lies at or slightly negative to the resting potential, we can combine the resting channels and inhibitory synaptic channels into a single pathway. As we saw in Chapter 11 (Postscript), the depolarization produced by an excitatory input depends on a weighted average of the batteries for the excitatory synaptic conductance and the resting channels. Since the weighting factor depends on the relative magnitudes of the synaptic and resting conductances, the opening of inhibitory synaptic channels will help hold the membrane near its negative resting potential during the EPSP by increasing the total resting conductance of the membrane.

Another way of looking at the effect that the opening of Cl^- channels has on the magnitude of an EPSP is based on Ohm's law. According to this view, the amplitude of the depolarization during an EPSP, ΔV_{EPSP}, is given by

$$\Delta V_{EPSP} = I_{EPSP}/g_l,$$

where I_{EPSP} is the excitatory synaptic current and g_l is the magnitude of the resting conductance channels, including any contributions from inhibitory synaptic channels. Because the opening of the inhibitory synaptic channels will increase the resting conductance, the size of the depolarization during the EPSP will be decreased. This consequence of synaptic inhibition is called the *short-circuiting* or *shunting* effect of an increased conductance IPSP (see Figure 12-16).

In some cells, such as those with $GABA_B$ receptors, inhibition is associated with the opening of K^+ channels. Since the K^+ equilibrium potential of neurons ($E_K = -80$ mV) is always negative to the resting potential, the opening of K^+ channels will inhibit the postsynaptic cell even more profoundly than the opening of Cl^- channels (assuming a similar-size postsynaptic conductance).

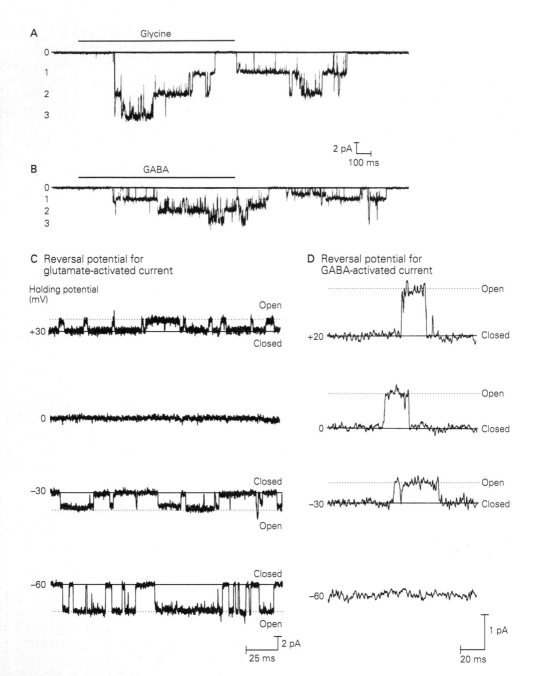

Figure 12-9 Comparison of single-channel currents activated by the excitatory transmitter glutamate and those activated by the inhibitory transmitters GABA and glycine. In the recordings shown here, downward deflection indicates pulses of inward (negative) current; upward deflection indicates outward (positive) current.

A. Currents through three glycine-activated channels in a patch from a mouse spinal neuron.

B. Single-channel currents activated by GABA in the same patch. In **A** and **B** the membrane was held at a voltage negative to the reversal potential, so channel openings generate an inward current owing to an efflux of Cl⁻.

C. Excitatory current through a single NMDA-type glutamate-gated channel in a rat hippocampal neuron. As the membrane

potential is moved in a depolarizing direction (from −60 to −30 mV), the current pulses become smaller. At 0 mV (the reversal potential for the EPSP) the current pulses are nullified, and at +30 mV they invert and are outward. The reversal potential at 0 mV is the weighted average of equilibrium potentials for Na^+, Ca^{2+}, and K^+, the three ions responsible for generating this current. (Courtesy of J. Jen and C. F. Stevens.)

D. Inhibitory current through a single GABA-activated channel in a rat hippocampal neuron. The current is nullified at approximately −60 mV (the reversal potential for the IPSP). At more depolarized levels the current pulses are outward (corresponding to the influx of Cl⁻). This reversal potential lies near the equilibrium potential for Cl⁻, the only ion contributing to this current. (Courtesy of B. Sakmann.)

Paradoxically, under some conditions the opening of GABA-gated Cl^- channels in brain cells can cause excitation. After intense periods of stimulation the influx of Cl^- into the cell can be so great that the intracellular Cl^- concentration increases. It may even double. As a result, the Cl^- equilibrium potential will become more positive than the resting potential. Under these conditions opening of Cl^- channels will depolarize the neuron. Such depolarizing Cl^- responses are particularly prominent in newborn animals. But they can occur in adults and may contribute to epileptic discharges in which very large, synchronized, depolarizing GABA-gated responses are recorded. Depolarizing GABA-gated responses may also play a role in generating an oscillatory activity in the brain, where neurons tend to fire repetitively at a frequency of around 40 action potentials per second. This rhythm may be important for allowing synchronous discharges in neurons in widely separated areas of the brain, enabling the brain to bind individual neuronal signals into a coherent, overall percept.

Synaptic Receptors for Glutamate, GABA, and Glycine Are Transmembrane Proteins

Many of the genes coding for the ionotropic glutamate, $GABA_A$, and glycine receptors have been cloned. Surprisingly, the GABA and glycine receptors are structurally related to the nicotinic acetylcholine receptors, even though the channels select for different ions. Thus, these receptors are thought to be members of one large genetic family. In contrast, the glutamate receptors appear to have evolved from a different class of proteins and thus represent a second genetic family of ligand-gated channels.

GABA and Glycine Receptors

Like the ACh-gated receptor-channels, the $GABA_A$- and glycine-gated receptor-channels are each composed of five subunits, coded by a related family of genes (Figure 12-10B). The GABA receptor-channels are likely composed of two α-, two β-, and one γ-subunit. The different subunits appear to be more closely related to each other than are those of the ACh receptor-channels since GABA can bind to any of the receptor's subunits. The glycine receptor-channels are composed of three α- and two β-subunits. Glycine binds primarily to the α-subunit.

Each subunit of the GABA and glycine receptor-channels contains a large extracellular domain at its amino terminus that contains the ligand-binding site. Two molecules of GABA and up to three molecules of glycine are required to activate their respective channels.

The extracellular ligand-binding domain of the subunits is followed by four hydrophobic transmembrane domains (labeled M1, M2, M3, and M4). As in the ACh receptor-channels, the second transmembrane domain (M2) is thought to form the lining of the channel pore. However, the amino acids flanking the M2 domain are strikingly different from those of the ACh receptor-channel. As was discussed in the previous chapter, the pore of the ACh-gated channel contains rings of negatively charged acidic residues that help the channel select for cations over anions. The GABA and glycine receptor-channels contain either neutral or positively charged basic residues, which are thought to contribute to the selectivity of these channels for anions.

The GABA- and glycine-gated channels play important roles in disease and in the actions of drugs. The GABA-gated channel is the target for three types of drugs that are at once clinically important and socially abused: the benzodiazepines, barbiturates, and alcohol. The benzodiazepines are anti-anxiety agents and muscle relaxants that include diazepam (Valium), lorazepam (Ativan), and clonazepam (Klonopin). The barbiturates comprise a group of hypnotics that includes phenobarbital and secobarbital. The four classes of compounds—GABA, benzodiazepine, barbiturates, and alcohol—act at different sites to increase the opening of the channel and hence enhance inhibitory synaptic transmission. The presence of any one of the four influences the binding of the others. For example, a benzodiazepine (or a barbiturate) will bind more strongly to the receptor when GABA also is bound. Although all four sites can influence one another, each is distinct.

Missense mutations in the α-subunit of the glycine receptor underlie an inherited neurological disorder called *startle disease* (*hyperekplexia*) characterized by abnormally high muscle tone and exaggerated responses to noise. These mutations decrease the function of the glycine receptor and so reduce the normal levels of inhibitory transmission in the spinal cord.

Glutamate Receptors

The amino acid sequence of the glutamate receptor family bears little resemblance to that of the family of ACh, GABA, and glycine receptors. The ionotropic glutamate receptors belong to a separate genetic family of ligand-gated channels. Two branches of the glutamate receptor-gene family, closely related to each other, include the AMPA and kainate receptors. A more distantly related branch of the family codes for the NMDA type of receptors.

The glutamate-gated channels are all multimeric proteins, now thought to be composed of four subunits.

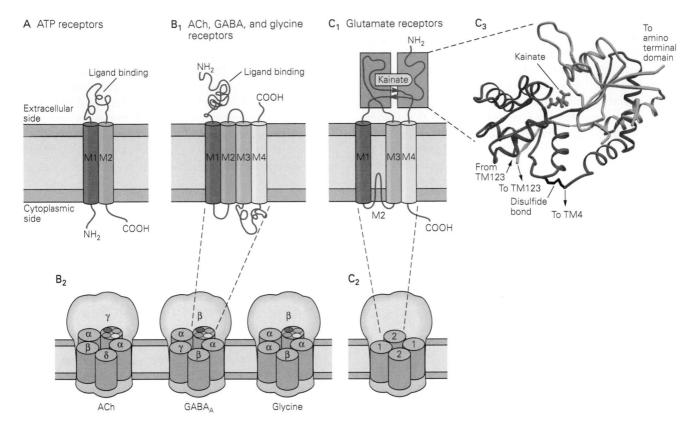

Figure 12-10 The three families of ligand-gated channels.

A. The ATP-gated channels possess two membrane-spanning domains (M1 and M2) and a large extracellular loop. Their subunit stoichiometry is not known.

B₁. The nicotinic ACh, GABA_A, and glycine receptor-channels are all pentamers composed of several types of related subunits (**B₂**). As shown here (**B₁**), each subunit has four transmembrane domains (M1-M4). The M2 domain lines the channel pore.

C. The glutamate receptor-channels are thought to be tetramers composed of two different types of closely related subunits (here denoted 1 and 2) (**C₂**). The subunits have three transmembrane domains (M1, M3, and M4) and one region

(M2) that forms a loop that dips into the membrane. The M2 loop lines the channel pore. The glutamate binding site is formed by residues in the extracellular amino terminus preceding the M1 domain and in the extracellular loop connecting the M3 and M4 domains. The three-dimensional structure of the extracellular glutamate binding domain of a subunit of the AMPA-type of glutamate receptor (GluR₂) has been solved by X-ray crystallography. The binding site is a bilobed "clamshell" structure (**C₃**) formed by the extracellular NH₂ terminal portion of a subunit (domain 1, **green**) and the extracellular loop connecting the M3 and M4 segments (domain 2, **purple**). Here the subunit has bound a molecule of kainate (which ia a weak agonist at AMPA receptors). (From Armstrong et al. 1998.)

Compelling evidence suggests that these channels have a transmembrane topology that is very different from that of other ionotropic channels. Each channel subunit is thought to contain only three transmembrane α-helices (Figure 12-10C). The channel pore may be formed by a loop connecting the first and second transmembrane segments, like the pore-lining P region of voltage-gated K⁺ channels (see Figure 9-14). This fascinating possibility suggests a potential relationship between the structures of ligand-gated and voltage-gated channels.

Based on the homology of the glutamate receptors to certain bacterial amino acid binding proteins and on mutagenesis studies, the glutamate binding site was thought to be formed as two lobes: One lobe formed by the large extracellular amino terminus of a subunit and the other by the extracellular loop connecting the M3 and M4 membrane-spanning segments. This structure has recently been elegantly confirmed by X-ray analysis of crystals formed from extracellular regions of the GluR2 subunit of the AMPA receptor (Figure 12-10C).

The AMPA and NMDA receptors have different

pore properties that have been attributed to a single amino acid residue in the pore-forming M2 region (Figure 12-11). All NMDA receptor subunits contain the neutral but polar residue asparagine at a certain position in the M2 region. In most types of AMPA receptor subunits this residue is the uncharged polar amino acid glutamine, but in the GluR2 subunit it is an arginine. Peter Seeburg and his colleagues have made the remarkable discovery that the DNA of the GluR2 gene encodes a glutamine residue at this position in the M2 region, but the codon for glutamine is replaced with one for arginine through editing of the mRNA.

This editing has a dramatic effect on the properties of the AMPA receptors. AMPA receptor-channels formed from subunits that all contain glutamine have permeability properties similar to those of the NMDA receptors in that they readily conduct Ca^{2+}. In contrast, if just one subunit of the receptor contains an arginine, the permeability to Ca^{2+} is abolished (Figure 12-11). Presumably, one positively charged arginine is sufficient to exclude the divalent cation Ca^{2+}, perhaps through electrostatic repulsion. Some cells actually express AMPA receptors that lack the GluR2 subunit and therefore generate a significant Ca^{2+} influx.

Glutamate receptor-channels like most transmitter-gated channels, are normally clustered at postsynaptic sites in the membrane, opposed to glutamatergic presynaptic terminals. Certain postsynaptic sites appear to contain both the NMDA and AMPA types of glutamate receptors, whereas other sites in the same cell may contain only the NMDA type. At early stages of development, synapses containing only NMDA type receptors are particularly common. How are synaptic receptors clustered and targeted to appropriate sites? How can a cell determine whether to cluster the NMDA or AMPA types of receptors at a particular site in the cell? One postsynaptic protein important for the clustering of glutamate receptors is PSD-95 (postsynaptic density protein of 95 kD MW). PSD-95 is a cytoplasmic protein that contains three repeated domains, important for protein-protein interaction. These so-called PDZ domains (named for the three proteins in which they were first identified: PSD-95, the DLG tumor suppressor protein in *Drosophila,* and a protein termed ZO-1) bind a number of cellular proteins. In PSD-95 the PDZ domains bind the NMDA type receptor and the Shaker type of voltage-gated K^+ channel, thereby localizing and concentrating these proteins together at postsynaptic sites. AMPA receptors interact with a distinct PDZ domain protein called GRIP, and metabotropic glutamate receptors interact with yet another PDZ domain protein called HOMER. In addition to interacting with receptors

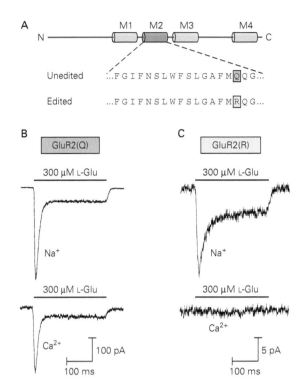

Figure 12-11 Determinants of Ca^{2+} permeability in the AMPA-type glutamate receptors.

A. Comparison of amino acid sequences in the M2 region coded by unedited and edited transcripts of the GluR2 type of AMPA receptor. The unedited transcript codes for the polar residue glutamine (Q, using the single-letter amino acid notation), whereas the edited transcript codes for the positively charged residue arginine (R).

B, C. Channels expressed from unedited subunits (**B**) are permeable to Ca^{2+}. Those expressed from edited subunits (**C**) do not conduct Ca^{2+}. In the adult the GluR2 receptor exists exclusively in the edited form. **Top traces** are currents elicited by glutamate with extracellular Na^+ as the predominant cation. **Lower traces** are currents elicited by glutamate with extracellular Ca^{2+} as the predominant cation. (From Sackman 1992.)

regulating ion channels, proteins with PDZ domains interact with a number of other cellular proteins, acting as a scaffold around which a complex of postsynaptic proteins may be constructed.

Other Receptor-Channels in the Central Nervous System

Certain fast excitatory actions of the neurotransmitter serotonin (5-HT) are mediated by the 5-HT$_3$ class of ligand-gated channels. These ionotropic receptors have four transmembrane segments and are structurally similar to the nicotinic ACh receptors. Like the ACh-gated channels, the 5-HT$_3$-gated channels are permeable to monovalent cations and display a reversal potential near 0 mV. They are thought to participate in rapid excitatory synaptic transmission in certain areas of the brain.

A third family of transmitter-gated ion channels is defined by receptors for adenosine triphosphate (ATP), which serves as a transmitter at certain synapses. These so-called purinergic receptors occur on smooth muscle cells innervated by sympathetic neurons of the autonomic ganglia as well as on certain central and peripheral neurons. At these synapses ATP activates an ion channel that is permeable to both monovalent cations and Ca^{2+}, with a reversal potential near 0 mV. Several genes coding for this family of ATP receptors (the P$_{2x}$ receptors) have been cloned. The amino acid sequence of these ATP receptors is different from the other two ligand-gated channel families. Although their transmembrane topology has not yet been fully delineated, these channels appear to contain only two transmembrane domains connected by a large extracellular loop (see Figure 12-10A).

Excitatory and Inhibitory Signals Are Integrated Into a Single Response by the Cell

Each neuron in the central nervous system, whether in the spinal cord or in the brain, is constantly bombarded by synaptic input from other neurons. A single motor neuron, for example, may be innervated by as many as 10,000 different presynaptic endings. Some are excitatory, others inhibitory; some strong, others weak. Some inputs contact the motor cell on the tips of its apical dendrites, others on proximal dendrites, some on the dendritic shaft, others on dendritic spines. The different inputs can reinforce or cancel one another.

The synaptic potentials produced by a single presynaptic neuron typically are small and are not capable of exciting a postsynaptic cell sufficiently to reach the threshold for an action potential. The EPSPs produced in a motor neuron by most stretch-sensitive afferent neurons are only 0.2–0.4 mV in amplitude. If the EPSPs generated in a single motor neuron were to sum linearly (which they do not), at least 25 afferent neurons would have to fire together in order to depolarize the trigger zone by the 10 mV required to reach threshold. At the same time the postsynaptic cell is receiving excitatory inputs, it may also be receiving inhibitory inputs that tend to prevent the firing of action potentials. The net effect of the inputs at any individual excitatory or inhibitory synapse will therefore depend on several factors: the location, size, and shape of the synapse, and the proximity and relative strength of other synergistic or antagonistic synapses.

These competing inputs are integrated in the postsynaptic neuron by a process called neuronal integration. Neuronal integration reflects at the level of the cell the task that confronts the nervous system as a whole: decision making. A cell at any given moment has two options: to fire or not to fire an action potential. Charles Sherrington described the brain's ability to choose between competing alternatives as the *integrative action of the nervous system*. He regarded this decision-making as the brain's most fundamental operation.

In motor neurons and most interneurons the decision to initiate an action potential is made at the initial segment of the axon, the axon hillock (see Chapter 2). This region of cell membrane has a lower threshold for action potentials than the cell body or dendrites because it has a higher density of voltage-dependent Na$^+$ channels. For each increment of membrane depolarization, more Na$^+$ channels open and thus more inward current flows at the axon hillock than elsewhere in the cell. The depolarization increment required to reach the threshold at the axon hillock (-55 mV) is only 10 mV (from the resting level of -65 mV). In contrast, the membrane of the cell body has to be depolarized by 30 mV before its threshold (-35 mV) is reached. Synaptic excitation will therefore first discharge the region of membrane at the axon hillock. The action potential generated at the axon hillock then brings the membrane of the cell body to threshold and at the same time is propagated along the axon. Thus the membrane potential of the axon hillock serves as the readout for the integrative action of a neuron (Figure 12-12).

Because neuronal integration involves the summation of synaptic potentials that spread passively to the trigger zone, it is critically affected by two passive membrane properties of the neuron (Chapter 8). First, the *time constant* helps to determine the time course of the synaptic potential and thereby affects *temporal summation*, the process by which consecutive synaptic potentials at the same site are added together in the postsynaptic cell. Neurons with a large time constant have a greater capacity for temporal summation than do neurons with a smaller time constant (Figure 12-13A). As a result, the larger the time constant, the greater the likelihood that two consecutive inputs from an excitatory presynaptic neuron will summate to bring the cell membrane to its threshold for an action potential.

Second, the *length constant* of the cell determines the degree to which a depolarizing current decreases as it spreads passively. In cells with a larger length constant, signals spread to the trigger zone with minimal decrement; in cells with a small length constant the signals

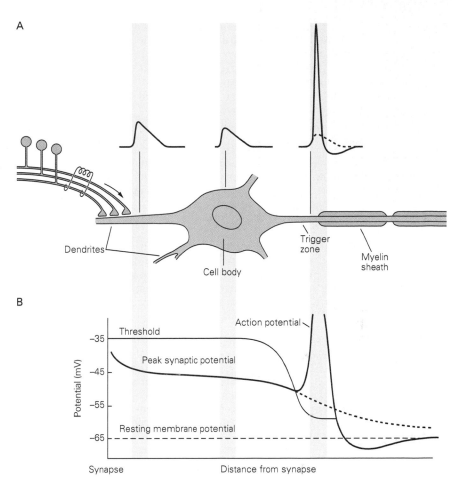

Figure 12-12 A synaptic potential in a dendrite can generate an action potential at the axon hillock. (Adapted from Eckert et al., 1988.)

A. An excitatory synaptic potential originating in the dendrites decreases with distance as it propagates passively in the cell. Nevertheless, an action potential can be initiated at the trigger zone (the axon hillock) because the density of the Na^+ channels in this region is high, and thus the threshold is low.

B. Comparison of the threshold for initiation of the action potential at different sites in the neuron (corresponding to drawing **A**). An action potential is generated when the amplitude of the synaptic potential exceeds the threshold. The **dashed line** shows the spatial decay of the synaptic potential if no action potential were generated at the axon hillock.

decay rapidly with distance. Since the depolarization produced at one synapse is almost never sufficient to trigger an action potential at the trigger zone, the inputs from many presynaptic neurons acting at different sites on the postsynaptic neuron must be added together. This process is called *spatial summation*. Neurons with a large length constant are more likely to be brought to threshold by two different inputs arising from different sites than are neurons with a short space constant (Figure 12-13B).

Originally, propagation of signals down dendrites was thought to be purely passive. However, we now know that the dendrites of most neurons contain voltage-gated Na^+, K^+, and Ca^{2+} channels, in addition to the ligand-gated channels. One function of the voltage-gated Na^+ and Ca^{2+} channels is to amplify the small EPSP. In some neurons there are sufficient concentrations of voltage-gated channels in the dendrites to serve as a local trigger zone. This can further amplify weak excitatory input that arrives at remote parts of the dendrite. When a cell has several dendritic trigger zones, each one sums the local excitation and inhibition

produced by nearby synaptic inputs and, if the net input is above threshold, an action potential may be generated, usually by voltage-dependent Ca^{2+} channels. Nevertheless, the number of voltage-gated Na^+ or Ca^{2+} channels in the dendrites is usually not sufficient to support the regenerative propagation of these action potentials to the cell body. Rather, action potentials generated in the dendrites propagate electrotonically to the cell body and axon hillock, where they are integrated with all other input signals in the cell.

The dendritic voltage-gated channels also permit action potentials generated at the axon hillock to propagate backwards into the dendritic tree. These back-propagating action potentials are largely generated by dendritic voltage-gated Na^+ channels. Although the precise role of back-propagating action potentials is not clear, they may provide a temporally precise mechanism for regulating current flow through the NMDA receptor by the depolarization-dependent relief of Mg^{2+} block. Indeed, Ca^{2+} imaging studies have shown that when a back-propagating action potential is paired with presynaptic stimulation, a large dendritic Ca^{2+} signal is

Figure 12-13 Central neurons are able to integrate a variety of synaptic inputs through temporal and spatial summation of synaptic potentials.

A. The time constant of a postsynaptic cell (see Figure 8-3) affects the amplitude of the depolarization caused by consecutive EPSPs produced by a single presynaptic neuron (A). Here the synaptic current generated by the presynaptic neuron is nearly the same for both EPSPs. In a cell with a *long* time constant the first EPSP does not decay totally by the time the second EPSP is triggered. Therefore the depolarizing effects of both potentials are additive, bringing the membrane potential above the threshold and triggering an action potential. In a cell with a *short* time constant the first EPSP decays to the resting potential before the second EPSP is triggered. The second EPSP alone does not cause enough depolarization to trigger an action potential.

B. The length constant of a postsynaptic cell (see Figure 8-5) affects the amplitudes of two excitatory postsynaptic potentials produced by two presynaptic neurons (A and B). For illustrative purposes, both synapses are the same distance from the postsynaptic cell's trigger zone in the initial axon segment, and the current produced by each synaptic contact is the same. If the distance between the site of synaptic input and the trigger zone in the postsynaptic cell is only one length constant (the postsynaptic cell has a *long* length constant of 1 mm), the synaptic potentials produced by each of the two presynaptic neurons will decrease to 37% of their original amplitude by the time they reach the trigger zone. Summation of the two potentials results in enough depolarization to exceed threshold, triggering an action potential. If the distance between the synapse and the trigger zone is equal to three length constants (the postsynaptic cell has a *short* length constant of 0.33 mm), each synaptic potential will be barely detectable when it arrives at the trigger zone, and even the summation of two potentials is not sufficient to trigger an action potential.

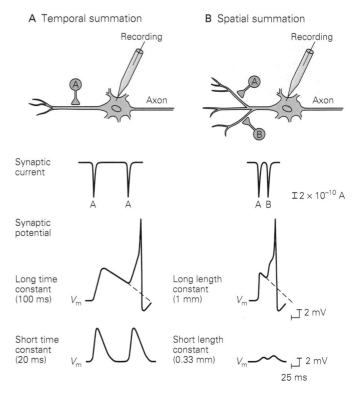

observed that is greater than the sum of the individul Ca^{2+} signals from synaptic stimulation alone or action potential stimulation alone.

Thus, our current view is that dendrites are complex, integrative compartments in nerve cells that can exert powerful orthograde effects on the propagation of synaptic potentials to the cell body as well as powerful retrograde effects on the relay of activity-dependent information from the cell body and axon hillock back to the dendritic synapses.

Synapses On a Single Central Neuron Are Grouped According to Function

All four regions of the nerve cell—axon, terminals, cell body, and dendrites—can be presynaptic or postsynaptic sites. The most common types of contact, illustrated in Figure 12-14, are axo-axonic, axosomatic, and axodendritic (by convention, the presynaptic element is

identified first). Axodendritic synapses can occur at the shaft or spine of the dendrite. Dendrodendritic and somasomatic contacts are also found, but they are rare.

The proximity of a synapse to the trigger zone of the postsynaptic cell is obviously important to its effectiveness. Synaptic current generated at an axosomatic site has a stronger signal and therefore a greater influence on the outcome at the trigger zone than does current from the more remote axodendritic contacts (Figure 12-15).

Synapses on Cell Bodies Are Often Inhibitory

The location of inhibitory inputs in relation to excitatory ones is also critical for their functional effectiveness. Inhibitory short-circuiting actions, which we discussed earlier in the chapter, are more significant when they are initiated at the cell body near the initial axon segment. The depolarization produced by an excitatory current from a dendrite must pass through the cell body as it moves to-

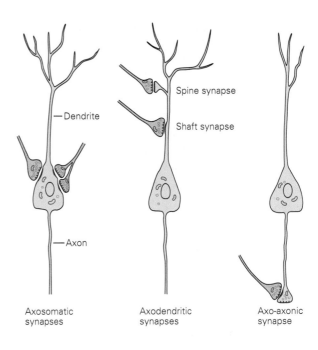

Figure 12-14 Synaptic contact can occur on the cell body, the dendrites, or the axon of the postsynaptic cell. The names of various kinds of synapses—axosomatic, axodendritic, and axo-axonic—identify the contacting regions of both the presynaptic and postsynaptic neurons (the presynaptic element is identified first). Note that axodendritic synapses can occur on either the main shaft of a dendrite branch or on a specialized input zone, the spine.

Figure 12-15 The impact of an inhibitory current in the postsynaptic neuron depends on the distance the current travels from the synapse to the cell's trigger zone. In this hypothetical experiment the inputs from inhibitory axosomatic and axodendritic synapses are compared by means of recordings from both the cell body (V_1) and the dendrite (V_2) of the postsynaptic cell. Stimulating cell B at the axosomatic synapse produces a large IPSP in the cell body. Because the synaptic potential is initiated in the cell body it will not decay before arriving at the trigger zone in the initial segment of the axon. Stimulating cell A at the axodendritic synapse produces only a small IPSP in the cell body because the potential is initiated so far from the axon hillock; it decays as it spreads to the cell body.

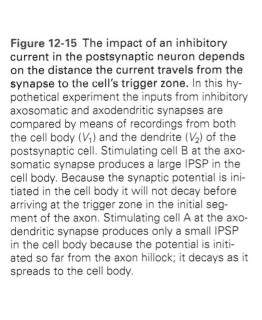
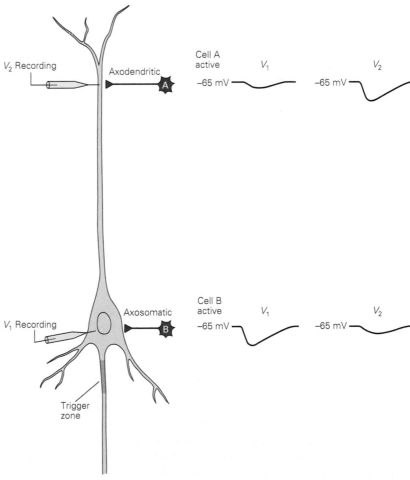

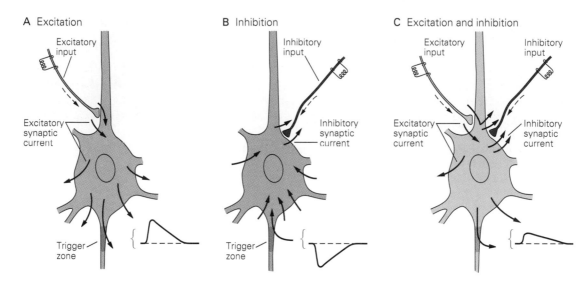

Figure 12-16 Excitatory and inhibitory currents have competitive effects in a single nerve cell. (Adapted from Eckert et al., 1988.)

A. An excitatory input at the base of a dendrite causes inward current to flow through cation-selective channels (Na^+ and K^+). This current flows outward across the membrane capacitance at the initial segment where it produces a large depolarizing synaptic potential.

B. An inhibitory input causes an outward (Cl^-) current at the synapse on the cell body and an inward current across the membrane capacitance at other regions of the cell, producing a large hyperpolarization at the initial segment.

C. The shunting action of inhibition. When the cell receives both excitatory and inhibitory synaptic current, the channels opened by the inhibitory pathway shunt the excitatory current, thereby reducing the excitatory synaptic potential.

ward the initial axon segment. Inhibitory actions at the cell body open Cl^- channels, thus increasing Cl^- conductance and reducing, by shunting, much of the depolarization produced by the spreading excitatory current. As a result, the influence of the excitatory current on the membrane potential at the trigger zone is strongly curtailed (Figure 12-16). In contrast, inhibitory actions at a remote part of a dendrite are much less effective in shunting excitatory actions or in affecting the more distant trigger zone. Thus, in the brain significant inhibitory input frequently occurs on the cell body of neurons.

Synapses on Dendritic Spines Are Often Excitatory

Central neurons often have as many as 20–40 main dendrites that branch into finer dendritic processes (see Figure 4-15). Each branch has two major sites for synaptic inputs: the main shaft and the spines. The spine is a highly specialized input zone, connected to the main shaft by a thin neck and ending in a more bulbous head (see Figure 12-3). Every spine forms at least one synapse. In certain cortical neurons, such as the pyramidal cells of the CA1 region of the hippocampus, the spine head contains both non-NMDA and NMDA types of glutamate receptors. These postsynaptic receptors are

embedded in a material that appears dense in electromicrographic sections and is therefore called the postsynaptic density. The dense region of the membrane is rich in Ca^{2+}/calmodulin–dependent protein kinase II. This kinase can therefore be activated selectively when Ca^{2+} flows through the NMDA receptor-channels located in the spine. The thin neck of the spine is thought to restrict the rise in Ca^{2+} concentration to the spine in which it is generated. Thus each spine represents a distinct biochemical compartment.

Synapses on Axon Terminals Are Often Modulatory

In contrast to axodendritic and axosomatic input, most axo-axonic synapses have no direct effect on the trigger zone of the postsynaptic cell. Instead, they affect the activity of the postsynaptic neuron by controlling the amount of transmitter released from its terminals onto the cell postsynaptic to it (see Chapter 14).

An Overall View

While many of the principles of synaptic transmission at the neuromuscular junction also apply in the central nervous system, peripheral and central synaptic actions differ in some essential ways. In the central nervous system synaptic transmission can be either excitatory or inhibitory. Excitatory postsynaptic potentials in the central nervous system tend to be less than 1 mV in amplitude, as compared to 70 mV in skeletal muscle. However, central neurons receive input from hundreds of presynaptic neurons, whereas a single muscle fiber is innervated by just one motor neuron.

The main excitatory transmitter in the brain and spinal cord is glutamate, and several classes of postsynaptic ionotropic receptors for glutamate have been identified. The non-NMDA (AMPA and kainate) receptors are so similar to one another that they are often grouped together. Like the nicotinic ACh receptor, most of these receptors form channels permeable to both Na^+ and K^+ and have reversal potentials near 0 mV. Rapid ion flux through these channels contributes to the fast early peak of the excitatory postsynaptic potential (EPSP).

A second type of glutamate receptor, the NMDA receptor, forms a channel that is permeable to Ca^{2+} as well as to Na^+ and K^+. This receptor-channel is unique among ionotropic channels in that it is also voltage-dependent: It is blocked by extracellular Mg^{2+} when the membrane is in the resting state and relieved from Mg^{2+} block when the membrane is depolarized. Thus, both glutamate and depolarization are needed to open the NMDA receptor-channels. Because the kinetics of activation of the NMDA receptor-channels are relatively slow, the ion flow through these channels contributes only to the late component of the EPSP. However, the Ca^{2+} that flows through NMDA receptor-channels is thought to play a particularly significant role in both health and disease. In normal amounts, Ca^{2+} apparently triggers signaling pathways essential for certain types of memory; in excess, Ca^{2+} is thought to cause brain damage. A third class of glutamate receptors, the metabotropic receptors, indirectly acts on channels through second messengers.

A neuron integrates information from thousands of excitatory and inhibitory inputs before deciding whether the threshold for an action potential (-55 mV) has been reached. The summation of all these inputs within a single cell depends critically on the cell's passive properties, namely on its time and length constants. A synapse's location can also be key to its efficacy. Excitatory synapses tend to be located on the dendrites, but inhibitory synapses predominate on the cell body, where they can effectively interrupt and override the excitatory inputs traveling down the cell's dendrites to the axon. The final summing of inputs to the cell is made at the axon hillock, which contains the highest density of

Na^+ channels in the cell and thus has the lowest threshold for spike initiation.

Although the sign of the synaptic potential is determined by the receptor, not by the transmitter, particular transmitters are more likely to gate either inhibitory or excitatory receptors. The most common transmitters in the central nervous system that activate inhibitory receptors are GABA and glycine. GABA can activate two types of inhibitory receptors: ionotropic $GABA_A$ receptors, which form channels permeable to Cl^-, and metabotropic $GABA_B$ receptors, which couple to G proteins and either increase K^+ permeability or inhibit voltage-gated Ca^{2+} channels. Gating of the $GABA_A$ channels permits Cl^- to flow into the cell, which hyperpolarizes the membrane. In addition, opening these channels increases the resting membrane conductance, which also short-circuits any excitatory current flowing into the cell. Three important classes of drugs—benzodiazepines, barbiturates, and alcohol—bind to portions of these $GABA_A$ receptors to enhance Cl^- flow through the channels in response to GABA.

The transmitter-gated channels so far cloned fall into one of three major gene families. The nicotinic ACh receptor, the GABA and glycine receptors, and the $5\text{-}HT_3$ receptor belong to one family. They are all composed of multiple subunits (most likely five), with each subunit containing four membrane-spanning segments. The GABA and glycine receptors, which conduct anions, are more similar to each other than to the ACh receptor, which conducts cations. The glutamate receptors constitute a separate family. These receptors also have multiple subunits, with each subunit likely to have three membrane-spanning domains and a channel-lining loop. The ATP-gated receptors form a third gene family whose members contain only two membrane-spanning segments.

Much of the discussion in this chapter has been based on the schematic model of the neuron outlined in Chapters 2 and 3. According to this model, the dendritic tree is specialized as the receptive pole of the neuron, the axon is the signal-conducting portion, and the axon terminal is the transmitting pole. This model implies that the neuron, the signaling unit of the nervous system, merely sends and receives information. In reality, neurons in most brain regions are not quite that simple. As we shall see when considering the sensory and motor systems, cells in many brain regions transform information in addition to receiving and transmitting it.

Eric R. Kandel

Steven A. Siegelbaum

Selected Readings

Choi DW. 1994. Calcium and excitotoxic neuronal injury. Ann NY Acad Sci. 747:162–71.

Edwards FA. 1995. Anatomy and electrophysiology of fast central synapses lead to a structural model for long-term potentiation. Physiol Rev 75:759–787.

Hollmann M, Heinemann S. 1994. Cloned glutamate receptors. Annu Rev Neurosci 17:31–108.

Kuhse J, Betz H, Kirsch J. 1995. The inhibitory glycine receptor: architecture, synaptic localization, and molecular pathology of a postsynaptic ion channel complex. Curr Opin Neurobiol 5:318–323.

Magee J, Hoffman D, Colbert C, Johnston D. 1998. Electrical and calcium signaling in dendrites of hippocampal pyramidal neurons. Annu Rev Physiol 60:327–46.

Nicoll RA, Malenka RC, Kauer JA. 1990. Functional comparison of neurotransmitter receptor subtypes in mammalian central nervous system. Physiol Rev 70:513–565.

O'Brien RJ, Lau LF, Huganir RL. 1998. Molecular mechanisms of glutamate receptor clustering at excitatory synapses. Curr Opin Neurobiol 8:364–369.

Peters A, Palay SL, Webster HD. 1991. *The Fine Structure of the Nervous System.* New York: Oxford Univ. Press.

Sakmann B. 1992. Elementary steps in synaptic transmission revealed by currents through single ion channels. Neuron 8:613–629.

Smith GB, Olsen RW. 1995. Functional domains of GABA$_A$ receptors. Trends Pharmacol Sci 16:162–168.

Wo ZG, Oswald RE. 1995. Unraveling the modular design of glutamate-gated ion channels. Trends Neurosci 18:161–168.

References

Armstrong N, Sun Y, Chen GQ, Gouaux E. 1998. Structure of a glutamate-receptor ligand-binding core in complex with kainate. Nature 395:913–917.

Coombs JS, Eccles JC, Fatt P. 1955. The specific ionic conductances and the ionic movements across the motoneuronal membrane that produce the inhibitory post-synaptic potential. J Physiol (Lond) 130:326–373.

Eccles JC. 1964. *The Physiology of Synapses.* New York: Academic.

R Eckert, D Randall, G Augustine. 1988. Propagation and transmission of signals. *Animal Physiology: Mechanisms and Adaptations,* 3rd ed, pp. 134–176. New York: Freeman.

Finkel AS, Redman SJ. 1983. The synaptic current evoked in cat spinal motoneurones by impulses in single group Ia axons. J Physiol (Lond) 342:615–632.

Gray EG. 1963. Electron microscopy of presynaptic organelles of the spinal cord. J Anat 97:101–106.

Grenningloh G, Rienitz A, Schmitt B, Methsfessel C, Zensen M, Beyreuther K, Gundelfinger ED, Betz H. 1987. The strychnine-binding subunit of the glycine receptor shows homology with nicotinic acetylcholine receptors. Nature 328:215–220.

Hamill OP, Bormann J, Sakmann B. 1983. Activation of multiple-conductance state chloride channels in spinal neurones by glycine and GABA. Nature 305:805–808.

Hestrin S, Nicoll RA, Perkel DJ, Sah P. 1990. Analysis of excitatory synaptic action in pyramidal cells using whole-cell recording from rat hippocampal slices. J Physiol (Lond) 422:203–225.

Heuser JE, Reese TS. 1977. Structure of the synapse. In: ER Kandel (ed), *Handbook of Physiology: A Critical, Comprehensive Presentation of Physiological Knowledge and Concepts,* Sect. 1, *The Nervous System.* Vol. 1, *Cellular Biology of Neurons,* Part 1, pp. 261–294. Bethesda, MD: American Physiological Society.

Hollmann M, O'Shea-Greenfield A, Rogers SW, Heinemann S. 1989. Cloning by functional expression of a member of the glutamate receptor family. Nature 342:643–648.

Masu M, Tanabe Y, Tsuchida K, Shigemoto R, Nakanishi S. 1991. Sequence and expression of a metabotropic glutamate receptor. Nature 349:760–765.

Moriyoshi K, Masu M, Ishii T, Shigemoto R, Mizuno N, Nakanishi S. 1991. Molecular cloning and characterization of the rat NMDA receptor. Nature 354:31–37.

Palay SL. 1958. The morphology of synapses in the central nervous system. Exp Cell Res Suppl 5:275–293.

Pritchett DB, Sontheimer H, Shivers BD, Ymer S, Kettenmann H, Schofield PR, Seeburg PH. 1989. Importance of a novel GABA$_A$ receptor subunit for benzodiazepine pharmacology. Nature 338:582–585.

Redman S. 1979. Junctional mechanisms at group Ia synapses. Progr Neurobiol 12:33–83.

Sherrington CS. 1897. The central nervous system. In: M Foster. *A Text Book of Physiology,* 7th ed. London: Macmillan.

Stuart G, Spruston N, Häuser M (eds). 1999. *Dendrites.* Oxford, England and New York: Oxford Univ. Press.

Surprenant A, Buell G, North RA. 1995. P$_{2x}$ receptors bring new structure to ligand-gated ion channels. Trends Neurosci 18:224–229.

13

Modulation of Synaptic Transmission: Second Messengers

S YNAPTIC RECEPTORS HAVE two major functions: the recognition of specific transmitters and the activation of effectors. The receptor first recognizes and binds a transmitter in the external environment of the cell; then, as a consequence of binding, the receptor alters the cell's membrane potential and biochemical state.

The synaptic receptors so far identified can be divided into two major types according to how the receptor and effector functions are coupled. One type, the *ionotropic receptor*, gates ion channels directly: The receptor and effector functions of gating are carried out by different domains of a single macromolecule (Figure 13-1A). The molecular mechanisms underlying the action of the ionotropic receptors were discussed in Chapters 11 and 12.

The other major type of receptor, the *metabotropic receptor*, gates ion channels only indirectly: The receptor and effector functions of gating are carried out by separate molecules. This receptor type consists of two families: the G protein-coupled receptors and the receptor tyrosine kinases. The *G protein-coupled receptors* are coupled to an effector component by a guanine nucleotide-binding protein, or G protein (Figure 13-1B). This family contains the α- and β-adrenergic receptors, the muscarinic acetylcholine (ACh) receptors, the GABA_B receptors, certain glutamate and serotonin receptors, receptors for neuropeptides, as well as the odorant receptors and rhodopsin (the protein that reacts to light, initiating visual signals).

Activation of the effector component of G protein-coupled receptors requires the participation of several distinct proteins. Typically the effector is an enzyme that produces a diffusible second messenger. These second messengers in turn trigger a biochemical cascade, either by activating specific protein kinases that phosphorylate a variety of the cell's proteins (on serine or threonine residues) or by mobilizing Ca^{2+} ions from intracel-

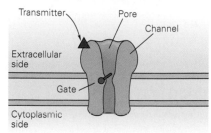

A Direct gating (ionotropic receptor)

B Indirect gating

1 G protein–coupled receptor

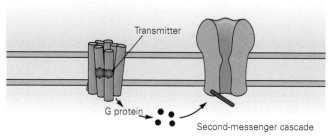

2 Receptor tyrosine kinase

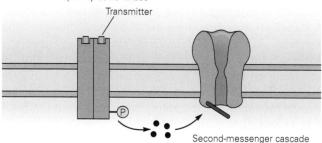

Figure 13-1 All known neurotransmitter receptors can be divided into two groups according to the way in which receptor and effector functions are coupled.

A. Ionotropic receptors directly gate ion channels as part of a single macromolecule that also forms the ion channel. The receptor, located on the extracellular side, and the ion channel pore, embedded in the cell membrane, are formed within the same protein.

B. Receptors that indirectly gate ion channels fall into two families. **1.** Metabotropic G protein-coupled receptors activate ion channels and other substrates indirectly by activating a GTP-binding protein that often engages a second-messenger cascade. **2.** Receptor tyrosine kinases modulate the activity of ion channels indirectly through a cascade of protein phosphorylation reactions, beginning with autophosphorylation of the kinase itself on tyrosine residues.

lular stores and thus initiating the reactions that change the cell's biochemical state. In some instances, however, either the G protein or the second messenger can act directly on an ion channel.

The second family of receptors that gate ion channels indirectly consists of the *receptor tyrosine kinases.* The cytoplasmic domain of a receptor tyrosine kinase is an enzyme that phosphorylates itself and other proteins on tyrosine residues. Phosphorylation of the cytoplasmic domain of the receptor allows it to bind and thereby activate other proteins, including other kinases that are capable of acting on ion channels. Receptor tyrosine kinases are typically activated by hormones, growth factors, and neuropeptides.[1]

Second-Messenger Pathways Activated by Metabotropic Receptors Share a Common Molecular Logic

The number of substances known to act as second messengers in synaptic transmission is far fewer than the number of transmitters. Approximately 100 substances serve as transmitters, each of which activates several different receptors on the cell surface. The few second messengers that have been well characterized fall into two categories, nongaseous and gaseous.

The best understood nongaseous second messenger is cyclic adenosine monophosphate (cAMP). The work on cAMP has greatly influenced our thinking about second-messenger mechanisms in general. Another class of nongaseous second messengers is produced by hydrolysis of phospholipids in the cell's plasma membrane; inositol polyphosphates and diacylglycerol are liberated by the action of phospholipase C, while arachidonic acid is released by phospholipase A_2. Intracellular calcium can also serve as a second messenger. These are the nongaseous second-messenger pathways that we shall examine in this chapter.

Gaseous second messengers are highly diffusible. The two best studied are nitric oxide (NO) and carbon monoxide (CO). The enzyme nitric oxide synthetase generates NO, while heme oxygenase generates CO. These messengers will also be examined in this chapter.

Despite their differences, second-messenger pathways share many basic features (Figure 13-2). All G protein-coupled receptors consist of a single subunit with seven characteristic membrane-spanning regions (Figure 13-3). The binding of transmitter to these re-

---

1. Most tyrosine kinases are cytoplasmic proteins that are not receptors and do not have a ligand-recognition site, nor do they have a transmembrane component. These kinases are therefore classified as *nonreceptor* tyrosine kinases. They often associate with either G protein-coupled or tyrosine kinase receptors and therefore are responsive (albeit indirectly) to neurotransmitters and hormones. Some nonreceptor tyrosine kinases also play a role in signal transduction events that occur during growth and development.

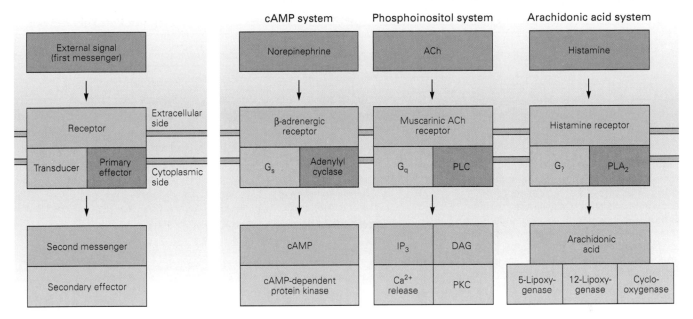

Figure 13-2 The synaptic second-messenger systems identified so far all follow a common plan. The signal-transduction pathways illustrated here follow a common sequence of steps **(left)**. Chemical transmitters arriving at receptor molecules in the plasma membrane activate a closely related family of transducer proteins that activate primary effector enzymes. These enzymes produce a second messenger that activates a secondary effector or acts directly on a target (or regulatory) protein.

Cyclic AMP system. This pathway can be activated by a β-adrenergic receptor. The second messenger cAMP is produced by adenylyl cyclase, which is activated by a G protein, so called because it requires guanosine triphosphate (GTP) to function. The G protein here is termed G_s because it *stimulates* the cyclase. Some receptors activate a G protein that *inhibits* the cyclase.

Phosphoinositol system. This pathway, activated by a muscarinic acetylcholine (**ACh**) receptor, uses another kind of G protein (G_q) to activate the primary effector, the enzyme phospholipase C (**PLC**). This enzyme yields a pair of second messengers, diacylglycerol (**DAG**) and inositol 1,4,5-trisphosphate (**IP$_3$**). In turn, IP$_3$ mobilizes Ca^{2+} from internal stores. DAG activates protein kinase C (**PKC**).

Arachidonic acid system. This pathway is activated by a histamine receptor. An unidentified G protein activates phospholipase A$_2$ (**PLA$_2$**), which in turn releases the second messenger arachidonic acid. Subsequently, arachidonic acid is metabolized in a cascade that involves several enzymes, including 5- and 12-lipoxygenase and cyclooxygenase.

ceptors activates a transducing trimeric G protein. (G proteins are discussed in detail later.) The activated G protein then binds to an effector enzyme: adenylyl cyclase in the cAMP pathway, phospholipase C in the diacylglycerol–inositol polyphosphate pathway, and phospholipase A$_2$ in the arachidonic acid pathway. Each of these signaling pathways initiates changes in specific target proteins within the cell, either by generating second messengers that bind to the target (or regulator) protein directly or by activating a protein kinase that phosphorylates the target protein. In some pathways, G proteins couple directly to ion channels to regulate their opening.

The phosphorylation mediated by protein kinases is central to understanding the action of second-messenger pathways. Cyclic AMP, Ca^{2+}, and diacylglycerol exert a major part of their effect on cells through the actions of protein kinases. Since a single protein kinase can phosphorylate many different target proteins, thereby altering their activities in dramatic ways, protein kinases often lead to the amplification and distribution of signals.

The Cyclic AMP Pathway Involves a Polar and Diffusible Cytoplasmic Messenger

The cAMP pathway is the prototype of an intracellular signaling pathway that makes use of a water-soluble second messenger that diffuses within the cytoplasm. This pathway illustrates the typical steps in a neuronal second-messenger pathway.

The binding of transmitter to receptors linked to the cAMP cascade leads to the activation of a stimulatory G protein called G_s, first identified by Martin Rodbell and Al Gilman and their colleagues. In its resting, inactive

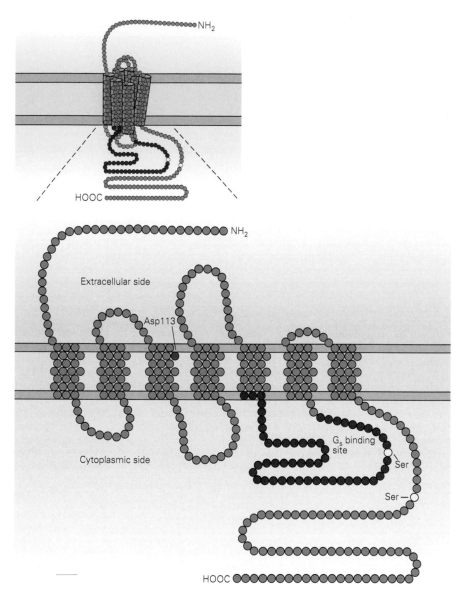

Figure 13-3 A G protein-coupled receptor contains seven membrane-spanning domains. The β_2-adrenergic receptor shown here is structurally similar to other G protein-coupled metabotropic receptors, including the β_1-adrenergic and muscarinic ACh receptors and rhodopsin. An important functional feature is that the binding site for the neurotransmitter lies in a cleft in the receptor that is embedded in the lipid bilayer accessible from the extracellular surface of the cell. The amino acid residue aspartic acid–113 (**Asp113, in dark blue**) participates in binding. The part of the receptor indicated in **brown** is the part with which G protein associates. The two serine residues (**yellow**) are sites for phosphorylation, which is involved in inactivating the receptor. (Adapted from Frielle et al. 1989.)

state G_s normally has a molecule of GDP bound to it. On activation, G_s binds a molecule of GTP in exchange for the GDP, thereupon activating the G protein. The activated G protein then stimulates adenylyl cyclase. This enzyme, an integral membrane protein that spans the plasma membrane 12 times, in turn catalyzes the conversion of ATP to cAMP. The GTP–G protein complex and the catalytic subunit of the cyclase together constitute the active form of the enzyme.

When associated with the catalytic cyclase subunit, G_s also acts as a GTPase, hydrolyzing its bound GTP to GDP. As a result, the G protein dissociates from the cyclase, inactivating the cyclase to stop the synthesis of cAMP (Figure 13-4). The receptor and the cyclase thus do not interact directly but are coupled by the trans-

Figure 13-4 (Opposite) The cAMP cycle. The binding of a transmitter to the receptor allows the stimulatory G protein (G_s) bearing GDP to bind to an intracellular domain of the receptor. This association causes GTP to exchange with GDP, which causes the α_s-subunit of G_s, now bearing GTP, to dissociate from the $\beta\gamma$-subunits. The α_s-subunit next associates with an intracellular domain of adenylyl cyclase, thereby activating the enzyme to produce many molecules of cAMP from ATP. The α_s-subunit, when bound to the cyclase, is a GTPase. The hydrolysis of GTP to GDP and inorganic phosphate (P_i) leads to the dissociation of the α_s-subunit from the cyclase and its reassociation with the $\beta\gamma$-subunits. The cyclase then stops producing the second messenger. Sometime during this cycle the transmitter dissociates from the receptor. The system returns to an inactive state when the transmitter-binding site on the receptor is empty, the three subunits of the G protein have reassociated, and the guanine nucleotide-binding site on the α-subunit is occupied by GDP. (Adapted from Alberts et al. 1994.)

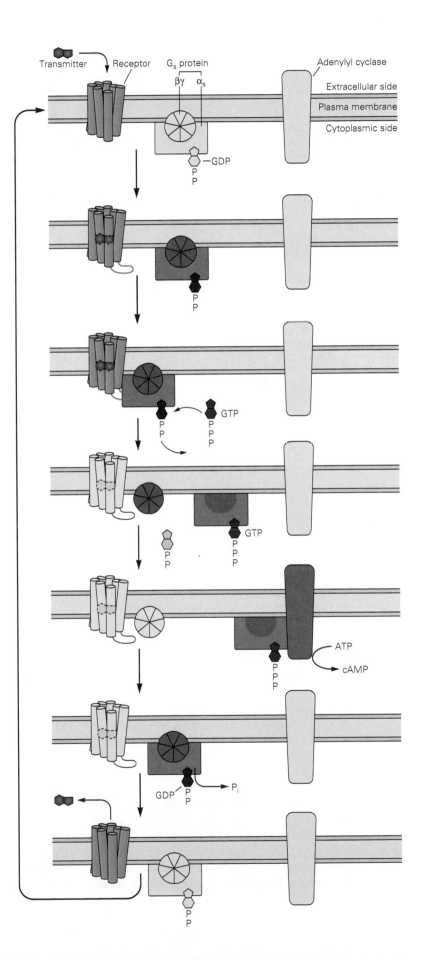

Transmitter binding alters conformation of receptor, exposing binding site for G_s protein

Diffusion in the bilayer leads to association of transmitter receptor complex with G_s protein, thereby activating it for GTP-GDP exchange

Displacement of GDP by GTP causes the α-subunit to dissociate from the G_s complex, exposing a binding site for adenylyl cyclase on the α-subunit

α-subunit binds to and activates cyclase to produce many molecules of cAMP

Hydrolysis of the GTP by the α-subunit returns the subunit to its original conformation, causing it to dissociate from the cyclase (which becomes inactive) and reassociate with a βγ complex

The activation of cyclase is repeated until the dissociation of transmitter returns the receptor to its original conformation

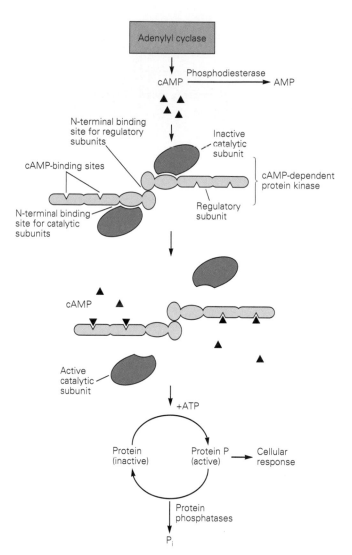

Figure 13-5 The cAMP pathway is typical of neuronal second-messenger pathways. Adenylyl cyclase converts ATP into cAMP. Four cAMP molecules bind to the two regulatory subunits of the cAMP-dependent protein kinase, liberating the two catalytic subunits, which are then free to phosphorylate specific substrate proteins that regulate a cellular response. Two kinds of enzymes regulate this pathway. Phosphodiesterases convert cAMP to AMP (which is inactive), and protein phosphatases remove phosphate groups from the regulator (substrate) proteins releasing inorganic phosphate, P_i.

brane, although they are associated with the internal leaflet of the plasma membrane. Gilman and his colleagues found that G proteins consist of three subunits: α, β, and γ. The α-subunit is only loosely associated with the membrane and is usually the coupling agent between receptors and primary effector enzymes. In contrast, the $\beta\gamma$ complex is much more tightly fixed to the membrane than is the α-subunit. As we shall learn later in this chapter, the $\beta\gamma$-subunits of G proteins can also affect ion channels directly. More than a dozen types of α-subunits have been identified. G proteins with different α-subunits have different actions and therefore different names. For example, the β-adrenergic receptor activates adenylyl cyclase by acting on G_s, a G protein that contains an α_s-type subunit, while other receptors inhibit the cyclase by acting on the G_i proteins, which contain an inhibitory α_i-type subunit. Still other G proteins activate phospholipases A_2 and C (Figure 13-2) and probably many other signal transduction mechanisms not yet identified. Compared with other organs of the body, the brain contains an exceptionally large proportion of these other G proteins.

G protein molecules outnumber the receptor molecules to which they are coupled in a cell. Since a single liganded receptor can activate many G proteins, the G proteins serve to amplify a small synaptic signal (represented by relatively few chemical transmitter and receptor molecules) into the larger number of activated cyclase complexes needed to catalyze the synthesis of an effective concentration of cAMP within the cell. Further amplification occurs with the protein kinase reaction, the next step in the cAMP cascade.

The major target of action of cAMP in most cells is the cAMP-dependent protein kinase, or PKA. This protein kinase, identified and characterized by Edward Krebs and colleagues, is a multisubunit enzyme consisting of two regulatory subunits and two catalytic subunits. In the absence of cAMP the regulatory subunits bind to and inhibit the catalytic subunits. In the presence of cAMP each regulatory subunit binds two cAMP molecules, leading to a conformational change that causes the regulatory and catalytic subunits to dissociate (Figure 13-5). This then frees the active catalytic subunits and allows them to transfer the γ-phosphoryl group of ATP to the hydroxyl groups of specific serine and threonine residues in substrate proteins. The other serine and threonine protein kinases that we shall consider here—the cGMP-dependent and Ca^{2+}/calmodulin-dependent protein kinases as well as protein kinase C—have regulatory and catalytic domains within the same polypeptide (Figure 13-6).

In addition to inhibiting enzymatic activity, the regulatory subunits of PKA may also serve to localize and

ducer protein, G_s. The duration of cAMP synthesis is regulated by the GTPase activity of G_s. In the continued presence of transmitter, after the GTP is hydrolyzed, G_s is able to bind a new transmitter-receptor complex at the surface of the cell, thereby activating the cyclase again.

G proteins are not integral components of the mem-

Figure 13-6 All protein kinases are related and are regulated in a similar way. In the absence of an activator the kinases are enzymatically inactive because their catalytic domains are inhibited. With the serine and threonine protein kinases (**A–D**), the catalytic domains are actually covered by regulatory domains that have amino acid sequences similar to those that are phosphorylated in substrate proteins. However, unlike the substrate proteins, the serine or threonine residue to which a phosphoryl group would be transferred is absent. These inhibitory domains, known as *pseudosubstrates,* therefore bind to the catalytic domain but cannot become phosphorylated.

A. In the cAMP-dependent protein kinase two identical regulatory subunits associate with each other at site **A** and with the catalytic subunits at site **R**. Each regulatory subunit also contains two binding sites for cAMP. When cAMP is bound the regulatory domains of the subunits change conformation and dissociate from the two catalytic subunits. Dissociated catalytic subunits can then phosphorylate substrate proteins.

B–D. In the other major protein kinases the regulatory domains (**R**) and the catalytic domains (**C**) are part of the same polypeptide chain. The cGMP-dependent protein kinase is similar to the cAMP-dependent protein kinase in amino acid sequence and, to a great degree, in the catalytic domain. The Ca²⁺/calmodulin-dependent protein kinase (**D**), unlike other kinases, is present in the cell as a complex of several molecules, each with similar biochemical properties. In all these enzymes the binding of second messenger is thought to unfold the molecule, thereby exposing and activating the catalytic region.

E. Activation of receptor tyrosine kinases is somewhat different. The regulatory domains are extracellular while the catalytic domains are intracellular. The binding of a transmitter, hormone, or growth factor to the regulatory domain causes two monomeric receptors to associate. This leads to the auto-phosphorylation of the receptor on its cytoplasmic domain. The autophosphorylated receptor then phosphorylates and activates other downstream targets.

A cAMP-dependent protein kinase

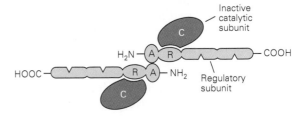

B cGMP-dependent protein kinase

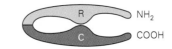

C Protein kinase C

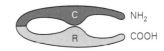

D Ca²⁺/calmodulin-dependent protein kinase

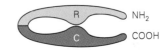

E Tyrosine kinase

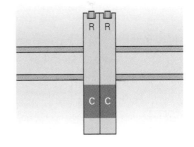

target the catalytic subunits to distinct sites within cells. A class of proteins termed the A kinase attachment proteins (AKAPs) specifically bind to one type of regulatory subunit isoform (R_{II}). Some AKAPs are thought to localize PKA next to ion channels. Localizing a particular kinase next to a particular substrate can increase the specificity, speed, and efficiency of second messenger–mediated signaling.

The specificity of protein kinases also depends critically on the fact that specific kinases can only phosphorylate proteins on serine or threonine residues that are contained within the context of a specific *phosphory-*

lation sequence of amino acids around the residue to be phosphorylated. For example, PKA phosphorylation usually requires a phosphorylation sequence of two contiguous basic amino acids (lysine or arginine), followed by any amino acid, followed by a serine or threonine residue (eg, Arg-Arg-Phe-Thr). Other residues near this sequence also contribute to the affinity of the protein substrate for the kinase.

Several important substrates for PKA have been identified in neurons. These include both voltage-gated and ligand-gated ion channels, synaptic vesicle proteins, enzymes involved in transmitter synthesis, and proteins that regulate gene transcription. As a result, the cAMP pathway (as well as other second-messenger pathways) can have widespread effects on the electrophysiological and biochemical properties of neurons. We shall consider some of these actions later in this chapter.

IP₃, Diacylglycerol, and Arachidonic Acid Are Generated Through Hydrolysis of Phospholipids

In addition to the cAMP pathway, many important second messengers are generated through the hydrolysis of phospholipids in the inner leaflet of the plasma membrane (Figure 13-7). This hydrolysis is catalyzed by two specific enzymes, phospholipase C and phospholipase A_2, each of which can be activated by different G proteins that are coupled to different receptors. These two phospholipases are named for the ester bonds that they hydrolyze in the phospholipid. Although these two enzymes can target multiple phospholipids, the most commonly hydrolyzed phospholipid is phosphatidylinositol 4,5-bisphosphate (PIP_2). PIP_2 typically contains the fatty acid stearate esterified to the glycerol backbone in the first position and the unsaturated fatty acid arachidonate in the second position:

PIP₂

Phospholipase C hydrolyzes the phosphodiester bond that links the glycerol backbone to the polar head group, leading to the formation of diacylglycerol (DAG) and inositol 1,4,5-trisphosphate (IP_3). Both DAG and IP_3 are second messengers. Diacylglycerol, which is hydrophobic, remains on the membrane, where it activates protein kinase C (Figure 13-7B and Box 13-1). In its inactive form this kinase is localized in the cytoplasm. When DAG is generated, the enzyme is moved to the membrane to form the active complex that can phosphorylate many protein substrates in the cell, both membrane-associated and cytoplasmic. Activation of protein kinase C requires membrane phospholipids and often require elevated levels of cytoplasmic Ca^{2+} in addition to DAG (Box 13–1).

IP_3, the second limb of the phospholipase C pathway, leads to the release of Ca^{2+} from internal membrane stores into the cytoplasm (Figure 13-7A). These membrane stores contain a high concentration of Ca^{2+} in their lumen and possess a type of Ca^{2+} channel in their membrane. This Ca^{2+} channel is a large protein that contains a receptor on its cytoplasmic surface for IP_3. Binding of IP_3 to its receptor leads to the opening of the Ca^{2+} channel and release of Ca^{2+} into the cytoplasm. The rise in intracellular Ca^{2+} in turn can trigger many biochemical reactions as well as the opening of calcium-activated ion channels in the plasma membrane.

An important aspect of the bifurcating second-messenger pathway that stems from phospholipase C is that the two products of hydrolysis (IP_3 and DAG) can act independently as well as together. Some transmitter receptors cause the production of IP_3 alone, without activating protein kinase C.

Calcium often acts when it forms a complex with the small protein calmodulin. An important example is the activation of the Ca^{2+}/calmodulin–dependent protein kinase (Figure 13-7C). This enzyme is made up of a complex containing many similar subunits, with each subunit containing regulatory and catalytic domains within the same polypeptide chain. Each subunit can be autophosphorylated by an intramolecular reaction at many sites in the enzyme molecule. When Ca^{2+} and calmodulin are absent, the C-terminal regulatory domain binds to and inactivates the catalytic portion of this kinase. Binding of the Ca^{2+}-calmodulin complex causes conformational changes of the kinase molecule that unfetter the catalytic domain for action. The autophosphorylation of this enzyme has an important functional effect: It converts the enzyme into a Ca^{2+}-independent form that is persistently active even in the absence of Ca^{2+}. PKA and PKC also can become active in the absence of a second messenger, due to the action of proteases that degrade the regulatory regions of these enzymes. Constitutively active kinases are thought to be important for triggering long-term changes in synaptic plasticity associated with certain forms of learning and memory.

Arachidonic Acid Is Metabolized to Produce Other Second Messengers

Receptors that activate phospholipase A_2 cause the release of arachidonic acid from the cell membrane (Figure 13-8), whereupon the arachidonic acid is rapidly converted into one of a family of active metabolites, named *eicosanoids* for their 20 (Greek *eicosa*) carbon atoms. Arachidonic acid is metabolized by three types of enzymes: (1) cyclooxygenases, producing prostaglandins and thromboxanes; (2) several lipoxygenases, pro-

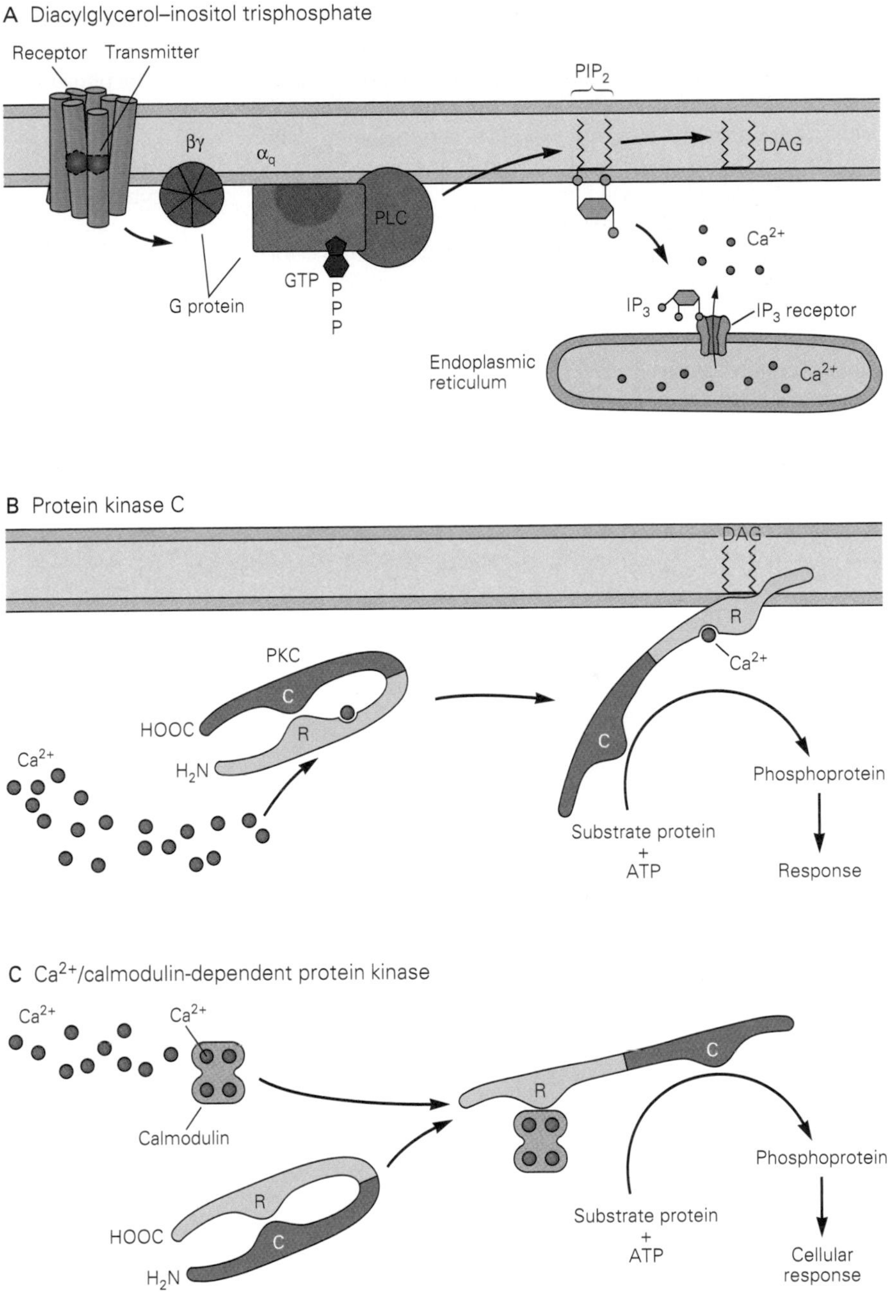

A Diacylglycerol–inositol trisphosphate

Figure 13-7 Hydrolysis of phospholipids in the cell membrane activates three major second-messenger cascades.

A. In the inositol-lipid pathway the binding of transmitter to a receptor activates a G protein, which in turn activates phospholipase C (**PLC**). This phospholipase cleaves phosphatidylinositol 1,4,5-bisphosphate (**PIP$_2$**) into two second messengers, inositol 1,4,5-trisphosphate (**IP$_3$**) and diacylglycerol (**DAG**). Inositol 4,5-trisphosphate is water soluble and can diffuse into the cytoplasm. There it binds to a receptor on the endoplasmic reticulum to release Ca^{2+} from internal stores.

B. Diacylglycerol, the other second messenger produced by the cleavage of PIP$_2$, remains in the membrane where it activates protein kinase C (**PKC**). Membrane phospholipid is also necessary for this activation. Thus, PKC is active only when translocated from the cytoplasm to the membrane. Some isoforms of PKC also require Ca^{2+} for activation.

C. Calcium bound to calmodulin activates the calcium/calmodulin-dependent protein kinase.

B Protein kinase C

C Ca^{2+}/calmodulin-dependent protein kinase

ducing a variety of metabolites to be discussed below; and (3) the cytochrome P450 heme-containing complex, which oxidizes arachidonic acid itself as well as cyclooxygenase and lipoxygenase metabolites.

The cyclooxygenase and lipoxygenase pathways in nervous tissue have been the most thoroughly studied. Metabolites of arachidonic acid were first characterized in other tissues because of their potent actions in inflammation, injury, and the control of smooth muscle tone in blood vessels and lung. In the brain the synthesis of prostag-

landins and thromboxanes is dramatically increased by nonspecific stimulation such as electroconvulsive shock, trauma, or acute cerebral ischemia (localized loss of blood). Many of the actions of prostaglandins are mediated by a family of G protein-linked prostaglandin receptors present in the plasma membrane. These receptors, which have seven transmembrane segments, can activate or inhibit adenylyl cyclase or activate phospholipase C.

Lipoxygenases introduce an oxygen molecule into the arachidonic acid molecule, resulting in hydroper-

Box 13-1 Isoforms of Protein Kinase C

At least nine isoforms of protein kinase C (PKC) exist, and all have been found in nervous tissue. Rather than having different proteins as regulatory and catalytic elements, each enzyme contains regulatory and catalytic domains in a single continuous polypeptide chain (see Figure 13-6C).

Two functionally interesting differences have thus far been found among these isoforms. The so-called major forms (α, β_I, β_{II}, and γ) all have a calcium-binding site and are activated by Ca^{2+} ions together with diacylglycerol. The minor forms (eg, δ, ϵ, and ζ) lack the calcium-binding domain, and therefore their activity is independent of Ca^{2+}. The second interesting difference is that, of the major forms, only PKCγ is activated by low concentrations of arachidonic acid, a membrane fatty acid, while all the isoforms respond to diacylglyc-

erol or phorbol esters (plant toxins that bind to PKC and promote tumors).

All PKC isoforms also contain a site that is sensitive to proteolysis between the regulatory and catalytic domains of the enzyme. Elevation of cytoplasmic Ca^{2+} levels associated with prolonged activation of PKC can lead to activation of proteases that cleave the kinase at this site. This releases a form of PKC called PKM, which is constitutively active because it lacks the regulatory domain. A PKC ζ lacking a regulatory domain can be synthesized during the induction of long-term potentiation in hippocampal neurons. Persistent PKMs are thought to prolong changes in synaptic plasticity that may contribute to certain forms of learning and memory.

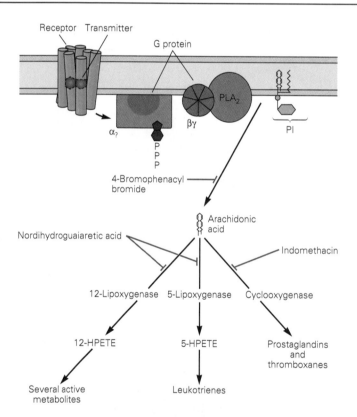

Figure 13-8 Arachidonic acid is released when a phospholipase is activated by a histamine receptor. The $\beta\gamma$ subunits of the G protein activate phospholipase A_2 (**PLA$_2$**), which hydrolyzes phosphatidylinositol (**PI**) in the plasma membrane. This enzyme can be inhibited by alkylation with 4-bromophenacyl bromide. Once released, arachidonic acid is metabolized through several pathways, three of which are shown. The 12- and 5-lipoxygenase pathways both produce several active metabolites. Lipoxygenases are inhibited by nordihydroguaiaretic acid (NDGA). The cyclooxygenase pathway produces prostaglandins and thromboxanes. This enzyme is inhibited by indomethacin, aspirin, and other nonsteroidal anti-inflammatory drugs.

oxyeicosatetraenoic acid (HPETE). Depolarization of brain slices with high concentrations of extracellular K^+ ions, glutamate, or N-methyl-D-aspartate (NMDA) greatly increases 12-lipoxygenase activity. 12-HPETE and some of its metabolites have been shown to modulate ion channels at specific synapses.

Arachidonic acid and its metabolites are highly lipid soluble and readily diffuse through membranes. They can be active both within the cell in which they are produced and in neighboring cells, including the presynaptic neuron. These substances can therefore act as transcellular synaptic messengers (Figure 13-9).

The Tyrosine Kinase Pathway Utilizes Both Receptor and Cytoplasmic Kinases

Receptor tyrosine kinases bind various peptides, including epidermal growth factor (EGF), fibroblast growth factor (FGF), nerve growth factor (NGF), brain derived growth factor (BDNF), and insulin. They differ from G protein-coupled receptors in two ways. First, they span the membrane only once. Second, their cytoplasmic domain contains a protein kinase activity that phosphorylates proteins on tyrosine residues (see Figure 13-1B). Like the serine-threonine protein kinases described earlier in this chapter, tyrosine kinases also regulate the function of the neuronal proteins they phosphorylate. The substrates for tyrosine kinase often belong to a special class of proteins that are thought to be dedicated to producing long-term changes in neuronal function.

In addition to the membrane-spanning domain and the cytoplasmic kinase domain, tyrosine kinase receptors have an extracellular binding domain for a peptide ligand. On binding a ligand, a monomeric tyrosine kinase receptor protein associates with another to form a dimer.

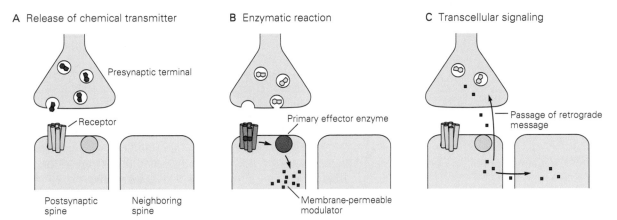

Figure 13-9 There is evidence for transcellular signaling from the post- to the presynaptic neuron (retrograde transmission) and between postsynaptic cells. Until recently synaptic transmission was thought to occur only in one direction, from the presynaptic neuron to the postsynaptic target cell. A presynaptic terminal releases a neurotransmitter at the synapse and the transmitter reacts with a G protein-coupled receptor in a postsynaptic dendritic spine (**A**). The receptor activates an enzyme that produces a membrane-permeable modulator, for example the gas nitric oxide (**B**). The modulator is able to cross over to neighboring postsynaptic spines as well as to presynaptic terminals where it can produce second messenger-like effects (**C**). A transcellular modulator of the presynaptic terminal is now called a retrograde messenger rather than a second messenger. There is some evidence that transcellular signaling occurs in long-term potentiation in the hippocampus (Chapter 64).

Dimerization causes the intracellular kinase to be active. Each monomer phosphorylates its counterpart on a tyrosine residue. This phosphorylation then further activates the kinase so that it becomes capable of phosphorylating other proteins in the cytoplasm.

The best characterized action of the receptor tyrosine kinases is the initiation of a cascade of reactions, involving several adaptor proteins and protein kinases, that ultimately leads to changes in gene transcription. Adaptor proteins serve to assemble a multiprotein signaling complex. They contain one domain (SH2) that binds to regions of activated tyrosine kinase receptors that contain the phosphotyrosine residues and a second domain (SH3) that binds to proline-rich regions of effector proteins, thus coupling receptor to effector function. These relatively slow actions are thought to promote neuronal survival and regulate neuronal differentiation and development. Recently, however, it has become apparent that receptor tyrosine kinases can also produce shorter-term modulatory actions, including the modulation of ion channels and control of transmitter release.

The Gaseous Second Messengers, Nitric Oxide and Carbon Monoxide, Stimulate cGMP Synthesis

Nitric oxide (NO) is produced in neurons by a Ca^{2+}/calmodulin-dependent enzyme, NO synthase, in response to glutamate, apparently acting through NMDA-receptors and requiring an influx of Ca^{2+} ions. Carbon monoxide (CO) is produced by the enzyme heme oxy-genase. Like other second messengers, NO and CO are not unique to neurons but operate in other cells of the body. For example, NO is a local hormone released from the endothelial cells of blood vessels, causing relaxation of the smooth muscle of vessel walls and thus allowing the vessels to dilate.

Like the metabolites of arachidonic acid, NO and CO have three distinctive properties: (1) They pass through membranes readily; (2) they affect nearby cells without acting through a surface receptor; and (3) they are extremely short-lived. Thus these substances also may serve as transcellular messengers (see Figure 13-9).

How do NO and CO produce their actions? Both of these gaseous messengers stimulate the synthesis of cGMP. Cyclic GMP, like cyclic AMP, is another freely diffusible cytoplasmic second messenger that activates a specific protein kinase. However, the mechanism of activation of guanylyl cyclase, the enzyme that converts GTP to cGMP, is very different from the cAMP cascade. Two forms of guanylyl cyclase have been identified. One form is an integral membrane protein with an extracellular receptor domain and an intracellular catalytic domain that synthesizes cGMP. A second form is a cytoplasmic enzyme, and this cyclase is the one activated by NO. Thus, in both cases production of cGMP is not directly linked to G protein activation.

Cyclic GMP acts directly on specific ion channels in the outer segment of retinal rod cells, an important regulatory role that is described in Chapter 26 in detail. The cGMP-dependent protein kinase differs from the cAMP-

Table 13-1 Comparison of Synaptic Excitation Produced by the Opening and Closing of Ion Channels

	Ion channels involved	Effect on total membrane conductance	Contribution to action potential	Time course	Second messenger	Nature of synaptic action
EPSP[1] due to opening of channels	Cation channel for Na^+ and K^+	Increase	None	Usually fast (milliseconds)	None	Mediating
EPSP due to closing of channels	Channel for K^+	Decrease	Modulates current of action potential	Slow (seconds or minutes)	Cyclic AMP (or other second messengers)	Modulating

[1]Excitatory postsynaptic potential.

dependent protein kinase in that it is a single polypeptide that contains both regulatory (cGMP-binding) and catalytic domains. As we have seen, these domains are similar to those in other protein kinases with similar function, especially those responsible for catalysis. Because of the similarities among the cAMP-dependent, cGMP-dependent, and Ca^{2+}/calmodulin-dependent protein kinases, all of these second-messenger enzymes are believed to be related to an ancestral enzyme.

The greatest amounts of cGMP-dependent protein phosphorylation occur in Purkinje cells of the cerebellum, large neurons with copiously branching dendrites. In these neurons the cGMP cascade contributes to a long-term depression of synaptic transmission (LTD), a form of synaptic plasticity that may underlie certain forms of motor learning.

The Physiological Actions of Ionotropic and Metabotropic Receptors Differ: Second Messengers Can Close As Well As Open Ion Channels

The structural differences between the metabotropic and ionotropic receptors are reflected in their physiological functions (Table 13-1). For example, neurobiologists often classify the actions of transmitters on receptors as being fast or slow, a distinction that refers both to speed of onset and the duration of the postsynaptic effect. Direct gating of ion channels through ionotropic receptors usually is rapid—on the order of milliseconds—because it involves a change in the conformation of only a single macromolecule. In contrast, indirect gating of ion channels through metabotropic receptors is slower in onset (tens of milliseconds to seconds) and longer lasting (seconds to minutes) because it involves a cascade of reactions, each of which takes time.

A second important functional difference is the physiological actions of the two classes of receptors. Ligand-gated channels function as simple on-off switches. Their main job is either to excite a neuron to fire an action potential or to inhibit the neuron from firing an action potential. Because these channels open only when they bind a transmitter available in the synaptic cleft, they are normally localized to the postsynaptic membrane. Ligand-gated channels do not participate in setting the resting potential of a cell or in generating and conducting an action potential.

In contrast, metabotropic receptors, by virtue of their ability to recruit freely diffusible intracellular second messengers, can act on channels that are located throughout the cell soma, dendrites, axons, and even presynaptic terminals and growth cones. As a result, a variety of channel types are affected by these indirect-acting receptors, including resting channels, voltage-gated channels that generate the action potential and that provide Ca^{2+} influx for neurotransmitter release, and ligand-gated channels. A third important difference is that metabotropic synaptic actions can not only *increase* channel opening, they can also *decrease* channel opening.

By themselves, the slow synaptic actions of metabotropic receptors normally are insufficient to cause a cell to fire an action potential. Consequently, they do not normally mediate rapid behaviors, as do the ligand-gated channels. However, they can greatly influence the electrophysiological properties of a cell, including changes in resting potential, input resistance, length and time constants, threshold potential, action potential duration, and repetitive firing characteristics. Thus, the actions of metabotropic receptors are often referred to as *modulatory synaptic actions*.

We can distinguish three broad classes of modulatory synaptic actions based on the site of action within a neuron and the normal function of the channel that is modulated (Figure 13-10):

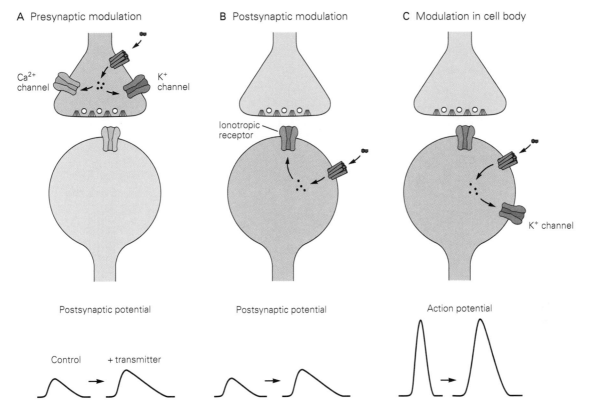

Figure 13-10 Modulatory synaptic actions involving second messengers occur at three sites.

A. Synaptic action at presynaptic terminals can activate second messengers that regulate presynaptic K$^+$ and Ca^{2+} channels, thus regulating transmitter release and the size of the postsynaptic potential.

B. Synaptic action at the postsynaptic membrane can activate second messengers that alter the size of fast postsynaptic potentials by modulating ionotropic receptors.

C. Second messengers can affect the function of resting and voltage-gated channels in the cell soma, thus altering a variety of electrical properties, including threshold, space and time constants, and action potential duration.

1. Modulation of transmitter release through actions on channels in presynaptic terminals;
2. Modulation of fast synaptic potentials through modulation of transmitter-gated channels;
3. Modulation of electrical excitability and neuronal firing properties through modulation of resting and voltage-gated channels in the cell body.

The distinction between direct and indirect transmitter actions is nicely illustrated by cholinergic synaptic transmission in neurons of the autonomic ganglia. Stimulation of the presynaptic nerve releases ACh, which produces a fast excitatory postsynaptic potential (EPSP) in the postsynaptic neuron by binding to and activating ionotropic nicotinic ACh receptors. This fast EPSP is then followed by a slow EPSP that requires 100 ms to develop but then lasts for several seconds

(Figure 13-11). The slow EPSP is due to the stimulation by ACh of metabotropic muscarinic ACh receptors.

The muscarinic ACh receptor is one of two basic types of receptors for ACh, the other being the nicotinic ACh receptor. The nicotinic ACh receptors in neurons are much like those in muscle, which we considered in Chapter 11; they directly gate an ion channel. Muscarinic ACh receptors are members of the family of G protein-coupled receptors. David Brown and Paul Adams found that this action of ACh in autonomic ganglia is due to a decrease in a K$^+$ current that contributes to and helps set the resting potential. This current is carried by a slowly activating, voltage-gated K$^+$ channel called the *M-type* (for muscarine-sensitive) K$^+$ channel (Figure 13-11B). It is also distinguished from other delayed-rectifier K$^+$ channels by its slower time course of activation; the M-type K$^+$ channels require several hundred milliseconds to open upon depolarization.

A Fast and slow synaptic transmission

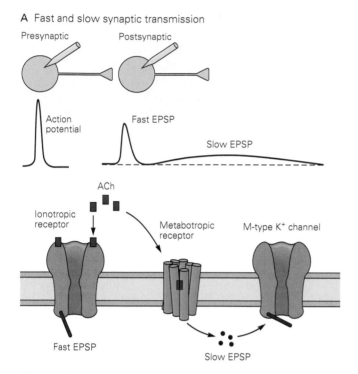

B The effect of muscarine on the M current

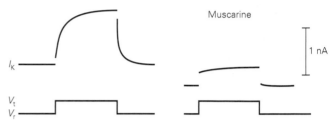

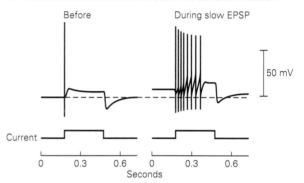

C The anti-accommodation effect of M current inhibition

Figure 13-11 Both fast and slow synaptic transmission occur in the same autonomic ganglion neurons.

A. The release of ACh onto a postsynaptic neuron produces a fast EPSP owing to activation of ionotropic (nicotinic) ACh receptors and a slow EPSP owing to activation of G protein-coupled (muscarinic) ACh receptors. The second messenger involved in the latter action has not yet been identified.

B. Voltage clamp recordings indicate that ACh decreases the magnitude of a slowly activating voltage-gated K$^+$ current, carried by the M-type K$^+$ channel. The traces show membrane current (I_K) recorded in response to depolarizing voltage-clamp pulses. The membrane was stepped from the holding potential (V_r) to the test potential (V_t) for 1 second. Currents were

recorded under control conditions (left) and after application of muscarine (right). Muscarine produces a decrease in outward K$^+$ current at the holding potential by closing the M-type K$^+$ channels, which are open at rest (note shift in current baseline). In addition, closure of the M-type K$^+$ channels decreases the magnitude of the slowly activating outward current in response to the step depolarization.

C. The slow voltage-dependent activation of the M-type channel normally helps keep the membrane near its resting potential during prolonged depolarizing stimuli. When the M-type channel is shut during the slow EPSP, the membrane fires a train of action potentials in response to a prolonged current pulse—it no longer shows accommodation.

Whereas the fast EPSP is generated by the opening of channels that conduct Na$^+$ and K$^+$, the slow EPSP is generated by the closure of the M-type K$^+$ channels. When M-type channels close, less K$^+$ leaves the cell. As a result, the continuous small influx of Na$^+$ through resting channels will lead to a net inward current that depolarizes the membrane to a new potential. How far will the membrane depolarize? Membrane depolarization near the resting potential has two main effects: It decreases the inward driving force on Na$^+$ and increases the outward driving force on K$^+$. The membrane thus depolarizes until the decrease in K$^+$ conductance, which results from the closure of the M-type channel, is offset by the increase in the outward driving force on K$^+$ and the decrease in the inward driving force on Na$^+$. At the new resting potential, the

outward K$^+$ current and inward Na$^+$ current are once again in balance.

This modulatory synaptic action, involving closure of channels, contrasts with the actions of ionotropic receptors, where transmitter always increases channel opening. What are the special properties of decreased-conductance, slow EPSPs? One important feature is that the decrease in resting conductance due to closure of the M-type channels not only increases cell excitability by causing a depolarization, but also decreases the current necessary to depolarize a cell by a certain amount. From Ohm's law ($\Delta V = \Delta I/g_1$), whenever the resting conductance, g_1, decreases, less excitatory current will be needed to depolarize a cell to threshold. A decrease in outward current can have other important actions in certain instances, such as helping to prolong the action potential (see below).

The decrease in outward K^+ current through the M-type channels also has pronounced effects on the accommodation of neurons to prolonged depolarizing stimuli (Figure 13-11C). In response to a prolonged excitatory stimulus that is just above threshold, a ganglionic neuron will fire rapidly one or two action potentials and then *accommodate* or adapt to the increased stimulus and stop firing. However, when the same cell is given a prolonged stimulus during the slow EPSP mediated by the M-type K^+ channels, the closure of the M-type K^+ channels allows the cell to fire a continuous burst of impulses (called *anti-accommodation*).

As this modulation by ACh illustrates, the M-type K^+ channels do more than help set the resting potential—they also control excitability. In the absence of ACh the opening of the M-type channels increases in response to small depolarizations from the resting potential. This slow voltage-dependent gating underlies the role of these channels in determining the accommodation properties of the neurons in the absence of ACh. Thus, at the resting potential only a fraction of all M-type channels are active. A prolonged depolarizing current is initially able to depolarize the membrane past threshold, and the cell fires one or two action potentials. However, the steady excitation slowly activates the M-type current. This eventually generates enough of an outward K^+ flux to offset the depolarizing current that is driving the cell to fire action potentials. As a result, the cell repolarizes toward its initial resting potential and it stops firing, or accommodates. Another way of looking at this effect is that the opening of M-type channels leads to a decrease in the membrane resistance. From Ohm's law, the same stimulating current now produces a smaller depolarization, leading to a sag in the membrane potential.

Cyclic AMP–Dependent Protein Kinase Can Close Potassium Channels

How does a transmitter, acting through a G protein-coupled receptor, elicit the closure of an ion channel? Synaptic actions mediated by cAMP were among the first second messenger-dependent synaptic potentials to be studied and are still perhaps the best understood at the molecular level.

Stimulation of certain serotonergic interneurons in the abdominal ganglion of the marine mollusk *Aplysia* produces a slow EPSP in mechanoreceptor sensory neurons. These sensory neurons mediate a gill-withdrawal reflex by firing action potentials in response to tactile stimuli and making fast, excitatory connections onto motor neurons that innervate the animal's gill and siphon. Serotonin sensitizes this reflex, enhancing the animal's response to a stimulus (see Chapter 62). The

slow EPSP in the sensory neurons is mediated by the release of serotonin, which acts on metabotropic receptors to cause a rise in cAMP in the sensory neurons (Figure 13-12). Similar to the slow EPSP in autonomic ganglion neurons, the serotonin-mediated response is associated with a decrease in the sensory neuron membrane conductance. Single-channel recordings reveal that serotonin acts by closing a class of resting K^+ channels, called the S-type (serotonin-sensitive) channels (Figures 13-12 and 13-13). Similar to the cholinergic modulation of the M-type channel, closure of the S-type channels decreases the resting K^+ efflux from the cell, thereby depolarizing it. These effects of serotonin on the S-type channel are mediated by cAMP through activation of the cAMP-dependent protein kinase (PKA). Application of the purified catalytic subunit of PKA to the inside (cytoplasmic) surface of a cell-free patch of membrane also closes the S-type channel, suggesting that the channel itself or a protein closely associated with the channel is directly regulated by phosphorylation.

In other instances it has been possible to purify ion channels biochemically to show that the ion channel is directly phosphorylated by the kinase. For example, in vertebrate nerve and muscle cells cAMP decreases the magnitude of a voltage-gated Na^+ current by directly phosphorylating the Na^+ channel.

Arachidonic Acid Metabolites Open the Same Channels Closed by cAMP

The same S-type K^+ channels in *Aplysia* sensory neurons that are closed by a serotonin-activated cAMP cascade are activated by a neuropeptide, Phe-Met-Arg-Phe-amide (FMRFamide). By increasing the probability of opening the S-type channels, FMRFamide hyperpolarizes the membrane and increases the resting membrane conductance, thus increasing the threshold for firing an action potential (Figure 13-14). These actions of FMRFamide are due to the activation of a G protein that stimulates phospholipase A_2, leading to the release of arachidonic acid from membrane lipids. The arachidonic acid is then metabolized by the 12-lipoxygenase pathway to 12-HPETE and other downstream products. 12-HPETE (or one of its metabolites) appears to act directly on the channel, since it increases the opening of S-type K^+ channels in cell-free patches. Lipoxygenase metabolites also operate in vertebrate neurons. In the mammalian hippocampus the neuropeptide somatostatin inhibits neurons by increasing the opening of M-type K^+ channels through the 5-lipoxygenase pathway and its leukotriene metabolites.

Thus different transmitters acting through different receptors can engage distinct second-messenger path-

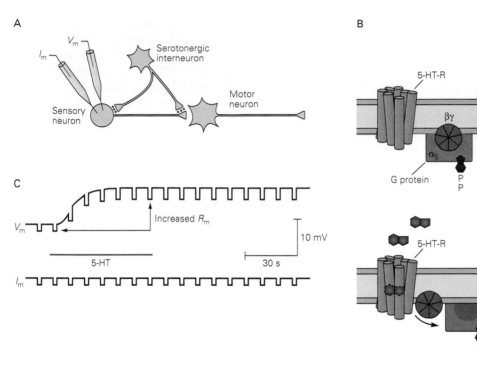

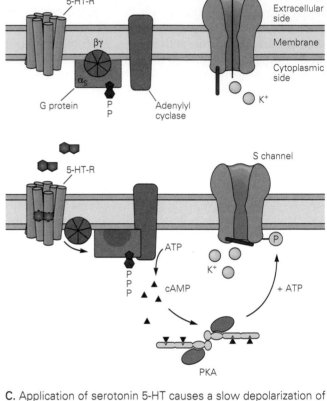

Figure 13-12 A slow synaptic action mediated by serotonin closes the S-type K$^+$ channel in *Aplysia* sensory neurons.

A. A serotonergic interneuron makes modulatory synaptic connections on the axon terminals and cell body of a mechanoreceptor sensory neuron. The sensory neuron makes a fast, excitatory glutamatergic connection onto a motor neuron.

B. Serotonin binds to a metabotropic receptor (5-HT-R) that acts through cAMP and cAMP-dependent protein kinase (PKA) to close the S-type (resting) K$^+$ channels in the sensory neurons.

C. Application of serotonin 5-HT causes a slow depolarization of the sensory neuron and a decrease in resting membrane conductance (ie, an increase in membrane resistance) due to closure of the S-type K$^+$ channels. The top trace shows the sensory neuron membrane voltage and the bottom trace shows the current injected into the sensory neuron through a microelectrode. The brief hyperpolarizing current pulses produce brief hyperpolarizing voltage responses. The magnitude of the voltage response is related to the membrane conductance by Ohm's law ($\Delta V = \Delta T_m / g_l$). The decrease in membrane conductance leads to an increase in the size of the voltage pulse.

ways to regulate the same ion channels in opposite ways, producing either slow excitation or slow inhibition. As in the case with serotonin and FMRFamide in the sensory neurons of *Aplysia*, the actions of different modulatory transmitters are often represented within neurons through the particular molecular cascades that they activate. The interaction of these cascades provides a molecular means by which neurons may integrate the biochemical signals initiated by their synaptic actions just as the initial segment of a neuron provides a site for integration of electrical signals (see the discussion of cross-talk below).

G Proteins Can Modulate Ion Channels Directly

Although second-messenger systems commonly alter the activity of ion channels by phosphorylating the channel protein, this is not the only way in which metabotropic receptors affect ion channels. G proteins can themselves directly act on an ion channel, causing it to open or close without the intervention of a freely diffusible second messenger or a protein kinase (Figure 13-15).

Activation of muscarinic receptors in the heart and in certain neurons causes a hyperpolarization mediated by the direct action of a G protein that opens a K$^+$ chan-

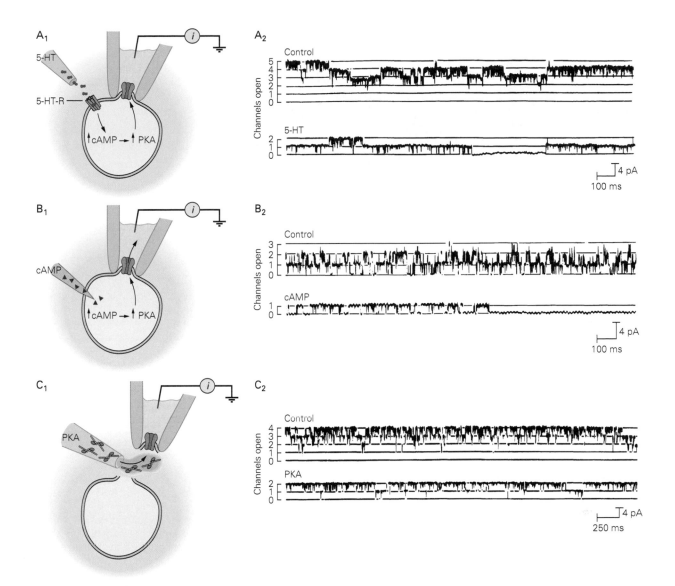

Figure 13-13 Patch-clamp recordings of S-type K$^+$ channel activity.

A. Application of serotonin (5-HT) to the bath (**1**) closes three of five S-type K$^+$ channels that were active in this cell-attached patch (**2**). The experiment implicates a diffusible messenger since the serotonin applied in the extracellular solution bathing the cell has no direct access to the S-type channels under the patch pipette. The numbers to the left of the traces indicate the number of channels open at any instant. Each channel opening

contributes an outward (positive) current pulse.

B. Injection of cAMP into a sensory neuron through a microelectrode closes three out of three active S-type channels in this patch.

C. Application of the purified catalytic subunit of cAMP-dependent protein kinase (PKA) to the inside (cytoplasmic) surface of the membrane closes two out of four active S-type channels in this cell-free patch. ATP was also present in this experiment to provide a source of high-energy phosphate.

nel. The muscarinic activation of this K$^+$ current contributes to a slowing of the heart beat and was among the first modulatory transmitter actions to be described. Yet for many years it presented a puzzle in that it seemed to show properties of both direct and indirect receptor-mediated transmitter actions.

Studies of the time course of muscarinic ACh activation of K$^+$ currents showed a distinct delay, requiring

over one hundred milliseconds for complete activation. While this is slow compared to directly gated transmitter actions, it is faster than many effects mediated by protein kinases, which can take several seconds. Patch-clamp experiments were able to demonstrate that ACh activates the K$^+$ channels without recruitment of a diffusible second messenger (Figure 13-15C). Yet other studies clearly demonstrated that the actions of ACh re-

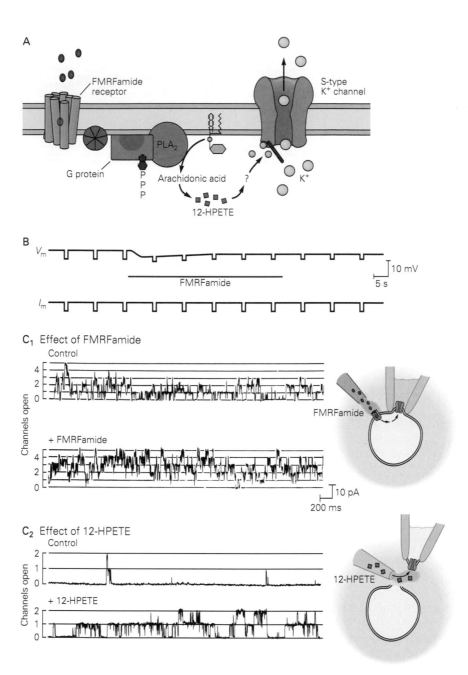

Figure 13-14 A slow synaptic action mediated by FMRF-amide opens the same S-type K$^+$ channel closed by serotonin.

A. The neuropeptide FMRFamide acts through the arachidonic acid pathway (here involving the 12-HPETE metabolite) to open the S-type K$^+$ channel in *Aplysia* sensory neurons.

B. Application of FMRFamide produces a slow hyperpolarization of the sensory neuron resting potential and an increase in resting membrane conductance. The latter effect is seen as a decrease in the size of the voltage response (V_m) to a series of

hyperpolarizing current pulses (I_m) delivered through a microelectrode.

C. Patch-clamp recordings of S-type K$^+$ channels and their modulation by FMRFamide. **1.** Application of FMRFamide to the bath increases the opening of S-type channels in cell-attached patches. **2.** Application of 12-HPETE to the bath also increases the opening of S-type channels in cell-free, outside-out patches. Both FMRFamide and 12-HPETE increase the fraction of time that an individual channel is open without increasing the total number of active channels in the membrane.

A Model of G protein activation of a K⁺ channel

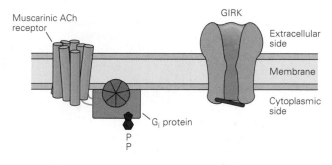

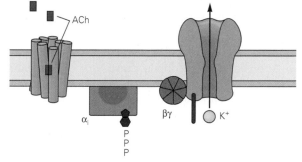

Figure 13-15 G proteins can open ion channels directly without employing second messengers.

A. The G protein-coupled, inward-rectifying K⁺ (GIRK) channel is activated by ACh acting on a muscarinic receptor. The Gᵢ protein is not coupled to an effector that produces a second messenger but instead acts directly on the ion channel. The βγ-subunits of the Gᵢ protein are thought to bind to a region on the cytoplasmic domain of the channel, causing it to open.

B. Acetylcholine, acting at metabotropic muscarinic receptors, hyperpolarizes cardiac muscle cells by activating GIRK channels. This helps slow the heart.

C. Three single-channel records show that the activation of GIRK channels does not involve a freely diffusible second messenger. Application of ACh in the bath solution (outside the pipette) does not activate channels in the patch of membrane under the pipette (see middle record). The ACh must be in the patch pipette to activate the channel (bottom record). (In this experiment the patch pipette contained a high K⁺ concentration, so opening of K⁺ channels causes an inward current to flow, shown as a downward deflection.)

B ACh hyperpolarizes cardiac muscle cells

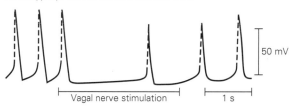

C ACh opens a K⁺ channel

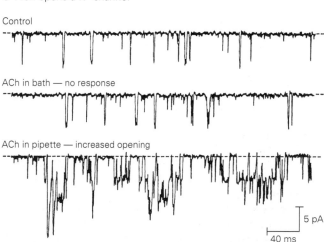

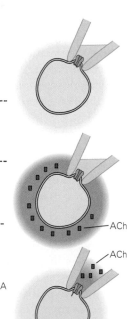

Figure 13-16 Activation of the cAMP cascade through a variety of metabotropic receptors leads to phosphorylation of a different receptor, the ACh receptor-channel. Phosphorylation causes the ACh receptor to respond less effectively to ACh, a process called desensitization. Phosphorylation of the ACh receptor can also result from the action of protein kinase C (PKC) and a tyrosine kinase. (Adapted from Huganir and Greengard 1990.)

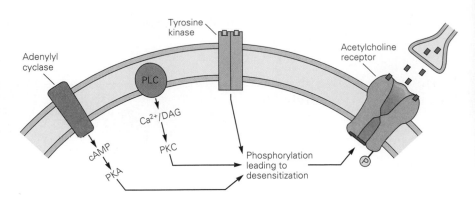

quire the activation of a G protein. To reconcile these findings, Paul Pfaffinger, Bertil Hille and their colleagues proposed that ACh may act through a G protein that is directly coupled to the K^+ channel, so that the K^+ channel would serve as the effector for the G protein. David Clapham and his colleagues were able to demonstrate this action using biochemically purified G proteins. Surprisingly, the action is not mediated by the α-subunit but by the $\beta\gamma$-subunits of the G protein (see Figure 13-15A).

The K^+ channel activated by ACh is called GIRK (G protein–regulated inward-rectifying K^+ channel). It is a member of the family of inward rectifier channels because it passes current more readily in the inward direction than in the outward direction. Like other members of the inward-rectifier channel family it resembles a truncated voltage-gated K^+ channel in having two transmembrane regions connected by a loop that resembles the P region of voltage-gated channels (see Figure 9-14). The $\beta\gamma$ subunits appear to act by binding directly to cytoplasmic regions of the GIRK channel protein.

Second-Messenger Pathways Interact With One Another

The regulatory effects of the various second-messenger systems, including those mediated directly by G proteins as well as those mediated indirectly by second messengers, can be broadened through interaction between these pathways. Such interaction can take one of several forms: parallel actions, convergent actions, and antagonistic actions. Opportunities for interaction (also called *cross-talk*) occur at many sites where individual signaling pathways converge. For example, convergence can occur with phosphorylation of common substrates, such as channels, receptors, enzymes, or cytoskeletal proteins.

One example involves the modulation of the nicotinic ACh receptor. Many transmitter receptors exhibit a property called *desensitization*, the progressive inactivation of a receptor due to the continuous presence of the transmitter. For example, during a prolonged application of ACh, the current carried by nicotinic ACh receptor-channels rapidly declines within a few seconds. Although the mechanism of desensitization of the nicotinic ACh receptor is not well understood, the rate of desensitization can be modulated by several second-messenger pathways, each activating distinct protein kinases. These multiple protein kinases phosphorylate the nicotinic ACh receptor at distinct sites (Figure 13-16).

Richard Huganir, Paul Greengard, and their colleagues have shown that the nicotinic ACh receptor is a substrate for PKA, PKC, and tyrosine kinase. PKA phosphorylates the γ- and δ-subunits of the nicotinic ACh receptor. PKC phosphorylates the α- and δ-subunits, and tyrosine kinase phosphorylates the β-, γ-, and δ-subunits. In all, three different kinases phosphorylate the ACh receptor at seven different sites, all of which are located in the major cytoplasmic loop of each subunit. Not all of these phosphorylations are known to have functional consequences, but the cAMP-dependent phosphorylation of the γ- and δ-subunits, as well as tyrosine phosphorylation, does increase the rate at which the receptor desensitizes in response to ACh.

Other types of cross-talk involve antagonistic modulatory actions, in which one pathway opposes or overrides a different pathway. The classic example of antagonistic modulation is the action of transmitters that activate the G_i protein and therefore inhibit the production of cAMP in response to transmitters that act through G_s. We have already encountered a second type of antagonistic modulation in which the opening of the S-type K^+ channel is up-regulated by FMRFamide (acting through the 12-lipoxygenase pathway) and down-regulated by serotonin (acting through cAMP). Next we consider a third type of antagonistic cross-talk involving the regulation of protein dephosphorylation by the second messenger Ca^{2+}.

Phosphoprotein Phosphatases Regulate the Levels of Phosphorylation

Synaptic actions mediated by phosphorylation are terminated by enzymes called phosphoprotein phosphatases, which remove the phosphate group and thereby generate inorganic phosphate (Figure 13-17). One class of phosphatases, the serine-threonine phosphatases, dephosphorylates proteins on serine or threonine residues and hence can reverse the actions of PKA, PKC, and Ca^{2+}/calmodulin kinase. A second class of phosphatases, the protein phosphotyrosine phosphatases, dephosphorylates proteins on tyrosine residues.

The actions of neurotransmitters were initially thought to focus on the activation of the protein kinases, and the phosphoprotein phosphatases were considered to be housekeeping enzymes that were not subject to regulation. However, we now know that several phosphatases are powerfully regulated. One of the major serine-threonine phosphatases in cells, phosphatase-1, is under the control of a regulatory protein called inhibitor-1 (Figure 13-17). Inhibitor-1 binds to and inhibits the activity of phosphatase-1. However, this action only occurs after inhibitor-1 has itself been phosphorylated by PKA. A rise in cAMP therefore both increases the forward rate of phosphorylation due to activation of PKA and decreases the reverse rate of dephosphorylation due to inhibition of phosphatase-1 activity (which results from phosphorylation of inhibitor-1). This provides a positive-feedback mechanism for controlling phosphorylation levels in cells.

A further regulatory step is provided by calcineurin, another serine-threonine phosphatase. Calcineurin, when activated by the Ca^{2+}/calmodulin complex, dephosphorylates inhibitor-1 (rendering it inactive). This complex system allows for potent interactions between Ca^{2+} influx and protein phosphorylation. In dopaminergic neurons of the basal ganglia, dopamine (acting through metabotropic D1 receptors) activates PKA, which in turn phosphorylates inhibitor-1 (called DARPP-32 in these cells). The resulting inhibition of phosphatase-1 leads to an overall enhancement of phosphorylation in the neuron. In these cells inhibitor-1 can be dephosphorylated when calcineurin becomes activated by Ca^{2+} influx via NMDA-type glutamate receptors, leading to a stimulation of phosphatase activity.

As we shall learn later (Chapter 63), a similar cascade is thought to underlie a long-lasting depression of synaptic transmission in the hippocampus. In this case

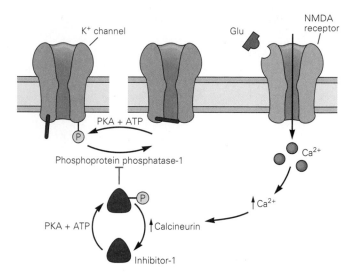

Figure 13-17 Phosphoprotein phosphatases terminate the actions of protein kinases. The forward and reverse rates of phosphorylation are controlled by protein kinases and phosphoprotein phosphatases, respectively. The extent and duration of phosphorylation can be controlled by inhibiting phosphatase activity through a protein termed inhibitor-1. Phosphorylation of inhibitor-1 by the cAMP-dependent protein kinase (PKA) reduces the activity of phosphoprotein phosphatase-1. The extent of phosphorylation of inhibitor-1 is controlled by calcineurin, a Ca^{2+}-activated phosphatase, which dephosphorylates inhibitor-1 in the presence of Ca^{2+} and calmodulin. Calcium can enter the cell through activation of the NMDA-type glutamate receptor. (Modified from Halpain et al. 1990.)

Ca^{2+} influx through NMDA receptors activates calcineurin; this dephosphorylates inhibitor-1, increasing the activity of phosphatase-1 and resulting in reduced phosphorylation in the hippocampal neurons.

Second Messengers Can Endow Synaptic Transmission With Long-Lasting Consequences

So far we have considered two types of chemically mediated synaptic actions. In one type transmitters act directly on postsynaptic receptor channels and thus produce fast direct synaptic actions lasting milliseconds. In the other type transmitters act through second messengers to modify ion channels and other substrate proteins and thus produce slow synaptic actions lasting seconds to minutes.

In a third kind of synaptic action transmitters act through second messengers to phosphorylate transcriptional proteins and thereby alter the cell's gene expression (Figure 13-18). Thus, protein kinases activated by

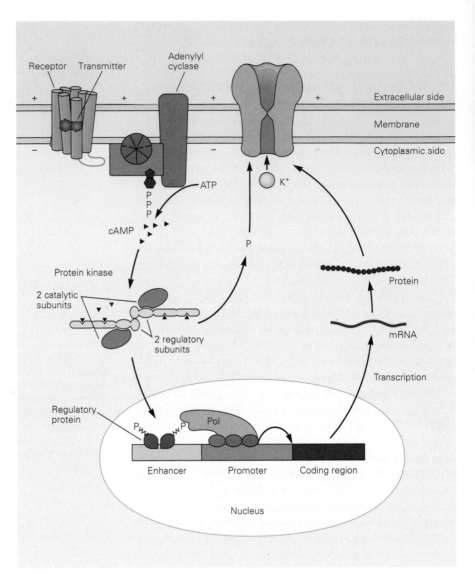

Figure 13-18 A single chemical transmitter can have either short-term or long-term effects on an ion channel. In this example a single exposure to the transmitter activates the cAMP second-messenger system, which in turn activates the cAMP-dependent protein kinase (PKA). The kinase phosphorylates a K$^+$ channel to produce a synaptic potential that modifies neuronal excitability for minutes. With repeated activation, the transmitter, acting through PKA, will phosphorylate one or more transcriptional regulatory proteins that activate gene expression. Gene activation results in a protein that produces more enduring closure of the channel and changes in neuronal excitability lasting days or weeks.

second messengers not only can modify preexisting proteins, but also can induce the synthesis of new proteins by altering gene expression. This third kind of synaptic action can lead to other changes lasting days or even longer. These long-term changes are likely to be important for neuronal development and for long-term memory.

Finally, transmitters can act through second messengers to stimulate local protein synthesis in specific dendritic spines of postsynaptic neurons. This is thought to be a mechanism that contributes to long-term synapse-specific changes.

An Overall View

Signaling between neurons occurs through the interactions of neurotransmitters with three distinct classes of receptors. These receptors, in turn, produce effects in the postsynaptic cell that differ widely in their biochemical mechanism, duration of action, and physiological function. Activation of ionotropic receptors directly opens an ion channel that is part of the receptor macromolecule. These transmitter-gated channels produce the fastest and briefest type of synaptic action, lasting only a few milliseconds, on average. This fast synaptic transmission mediates most motor actions and perceptual processing within the nervous system.

Longer-lasting effects of transmitters are mediated by activation of the G protein-coupled receptors and the receptor tyrosine kinases. G protein-coupled receptors are proteins with seven transmembrane segments that are members of a large genetic superfamily. These receptors all act through guanine nucleotide-binding proteins (G proteins), which either activate second-messenger cascades or directly alter ion channel activity. Prominent second messengers include cyclic AMP and the products of hydrolysis of phospholipids: IP_3, diacylglycerol, and arachidonic acid.

Many second-messenger actions depend on activation of protein kinases, leading to phosphorylation of a variety of cellular proteins, including ion channels, which changes their functional state. These second messenger actions generally last from seconds to minutes. They therefore do not mediate rapid behaviors but rather serve to modulate the strength and efficacy of fast synaptic transmission—by modulating transmitter release, the sensitivity of ionotropic receptors, or the electrical excitability of the postsynaptic cell.

These actions are implicated in emotional states, mood, arousal, and certain simple forms of learning and memory. Second-messenger actions not only open ion channels, as do the transmitter-gated receptors, but can also close channels that normally open in the absence of transmitter, producing decreases in membrane conductance.

The longest-lasting form of synaptic transmission involves changes in gene transcription, changes that can persist for days or weeks. These more permanent actions are thought to involve many of the same types of receptors and second-messenger pathways involved in the shorter-term modulatory actions of transmitters. However, they may require repeated stimulation and more prolonged action of the second messengers. As we shall see in Chapter 63, synaptically induced activation of gene expression is critical for the storage of long-term memory.

Steven A. Siegelbaum
James H. Schwartz
Eric R. Kandel

Selected Readings

Cooper JR, Bloom FE, Roth RH. 1996. *The Biochemical Basis of Neuropharmacology,* 7th ed. New York: Oxford Univ. Press.

Gilman AG. 1995. Nobel lecture. G proteins and regulation of adenylyl cyclase. Biosci Rep 15(2):65–97.

Hille B. 1994. Modulation of ion-channel function by G-protein-coupled receptors. Trends Neurosci 17:531–536.

Huganir RL, Greengard P. 1990. Regulation of neurotransmitter receptor desensitization by protein phosphorylation. Neuron 5:555–567.

Levitan IB. 1994. Modulation of ion channels by protein phosphorylation and dephosphorylation. Annu Rev Physiol 56:193–212.

Levitan IB, Kaczmarek LK. 1987. *Neuromodulation: The Biochemical Control of Neuronal Excitability.* New York: Oxford Univ. Press.

Marrion NV. 1997. Control of M-current. Annu Rev Physiol 59:483–504.

Schulman H, Hyman SE. 1998. Intracellular Signalling. In Zigmond MJ, Bloom FE, Landis SC, Squire, LR (eds). Fundamental Neuroscience. New York: Academic Press.

Schwartz JH. 1991. Arachadonic acid metabolism: potential for diverse signalling within the same neuron. Biochem Soc Trans 19:387–390.

Schwartz JH. 1993. Cognitive kinases. Proc Natl Acad Sci U S A 90:8310–8313.

Siegelbaum SA, Tsien RW. 1983. Modulation of gated ion channels as a mode of neurotransmitter action. Trends Neurosci 6:307–313.

Strader CD, Fong TM, Tota MR, Underwood D, Dixon RA. 1994. Structure and function of G protein–coupled receptors. Annu Rev Biochem 63:101–132.

Wickman KD, Clapham DE. 1995. G-protein regulation of ion channels. Curr Opin Neurobiol 5(3):278–285.

References

Alberts B, Bray D, Lewis J, Raff M, Roberts K, Watson JD. 1994. *Molecular Biology of the Cell,* 3rd ed. New York: Garland.

Belardetti F, Kandel ER, Siegelbaum SA. 1987. Neuronal inhibition by the peptide FMRFamide involves opening of S K^+ channels. Nature 325:153–156.

Brown D. 1988. M-currents: an update. Trends Neurosci 11:294–299.

Buttner N, Siegelbaum SA, Volterra A. 1989. Direct modulation of *Aplysia* S-K channel by a 12-lipoxygenase metabolite of arachidonic acid. Nature 342:553–555.

Chain DG, Casadio A, Schacher S, Hedge AN, Valbrun M, Yamamoto N, Goldberg AL, Bartsch D, Kandel ER, Schwartz JH. 1999. Mechanisms for generating the autonomous cAMP-dependent protein kinase required for long-term facilitation in *Aplysia*. Neuron: 22:147–156.

Colledge M, Scott JD. 1999. AKAPs: Structure to function, Trends Cell Biol.9:216–221.

Comb M, Hyman SE, Goodman HM. 1987. Mechanisms of trans-synaptic regulation of gene expression. Trends Neurosci 10:473–478.

Edelman AM, Blumenthal DK, Krebs EG. 1987. Protein serine/threonine kinases. Annu Rev Biochem 56:567–613.

Fantl WJ, Johnson DE, Williams LT. 1993. Signalling by receptor tyrosine kinases. Annu Rev Biochem 62:453–481.

Francis SH, Corbin JD. 1994. Structure and function of cyclic nucleotide–dependent protein kinases. Annu Rev Physiol 56:237–272.

Frielle T, Kobilka B, Dohlman H, Caron MG, Lefkowitz RJ. 1989. The β-adrenergic receptor and other receptors coupled to guanine nucleotide regulatory proteins. In: S Chien (ed). *Molecular Biology in Physiology*, pp. 79–91. New York: Raven.

Greenberg SM, Castellucci VF, Bayley H, Schwartz JH. 1987. A molecular mechanism for long-term sensitization in *Aplysia*. Nature 329:62–65

Halpain S, Girault JA, Greengard P. 1990. Activation of NMDA receptors induces dephosphorylation of DARPP-32 in rat striatal slices. Nature 343:369–372.

Hanson PI, Schulman H. 1992. Neuronal Ca^{2+}/calmodulin–dependent protein kinases. Annu Rev Biochem 61:559–601.

Logothetis DE, Kurachi Y, Galper J, Neer EJ, Clapham DE. 1987. The βγ subunits of GTP-binding proteins activate the muscarinic K^+ channel in heart. Nature 325:321–326.

Majerus PW. 1992. Inositol phosphate biochemistry. Annu Rev Biochem 61:225–250.

Murphy RC, Fitzpatrick FA (eds). 1990. Arachidonate related lipid mediators. Methods Enzymol 187:1–683.

Needleman P, Turk J, Jakschik BA, Morrison AR, Lefkowith JB. 1986. Arachidonic acid metabolism. Annu Rev Biochem 55:69–102.

Osten P, Valsamis L, Harris A, Sacktor TC. 1996. Protein synthesis-dependent formation of protein kinase Mzeta in long-term potentiation. J Neurosci 16:2444–2451.

Pfaffinger PJ, Martin JM, Hunter DD, Nathanson NM, Hille B. 1985. GTP-binding proteins couple cardiac muscarinic receptors to a K channel. Nature 317:536–538.

Piomelli D, Volterra A, Dale N, Siegelbaum SA, Kandel ER, Schwartz JH, Belardetti F. 1987. Lipoxygenase metabolites of arachidonic acid as second messengers for presynaptic inhibition of *Aplysia* sensory cells. Nature 328:38–43.

Schwartz JH, Greenberg SM. 1987. Molecular mechanism for memory: second messenger-induced modifications of protein kinases in nerve cells. Ann Rev Neurosci 10:459–476.

Siegel GJ, Agranoff BW, Albers RW, Molinoff PB (eds). 1994. *Basic Neurochemistry: Molecular, Cellular and Medical Aspects*, 5th ed. New York: Raven-Press.

Siegelbaum SA, Camardo JS, Kandel ER. 1982. Serotonin and cyclic AMP close single K^+ channels in *Aplysia* sensory neurones. Nature 299:413–417.

Soejima M, Noma A. 1984. Mode of regulation of the ACh-sensitive K-channel by the muscarinic receptor in rabbit atrial cells. Pflugers Arch 400:424–431.

Steel, DJ, Tieman TL, Schwartz JH, Feinmark SJ. 1997. Identification of an 8-lipoxygenase pathway in neurons of *Aplysia*. J Biol Chem 272:18673–18681.

Tanaka C, Nishizuka Y. 1994. The protein kinase C family for neuronal signaling. Annu Rev Neurosci 17:551–567.

14

Transmitter Release

SOME OF THE BRAIN'S MOST remarkable feats, such as learning and memory, are thought to emerge from the elementary properties of chemical synapses. The distinctive feature of these synapses is that action potentials in the presynaptic terminals lead to the release of chemical transmitters. In the past three chapters we saw how postsynaptic receptors for these transmitters control the ion channels that generate the postsynaptic potential. Now we return to the presynaptic cell and consider how electrical events in the terminal are coupled to the secretion of neurotransmitters. In the

next chapter we shall examine the chemistry of the neurotransmitters themselves.

Transmitter Release Is Regulated by Depolarization of the Presynaptic Terminal

How does an action potential in the presynaptic cell lead to the release of transmitter? The importance of depolarization of the presynaptic membrane was demonstrated by Bernard Katz and Ricardo Miledi using the giant synapse of the squid. This synapse is large enough to permit the insertion of two electrodes into the presynaptic terminal (one for stimulating and one for recording) and an electrode into the postsynaptic cell for recording the synaptic potential, which provides an index of transmitter release.

The presynaptic cell typically produces an action potential with an amplitude of 110 mV, which leads to transmitter release and the generation of a large synaptic potential in the postsynaptic cell. The action potential is produced by voltage-gated Na^+ influx and K^+ efflux. Katz and Miledi found that when the voltage-gated Na^+ channels are blocked upon application of tetrodotoxin, successive presynaptic action potentials become progressively smaller, owing to the progressive blockade of Na^+ channels during the onset of tetrodotoxin's effect. The postsynaptic potential is reduced accordingly. When the Na^+ channel blockade becomes so profound as to reduce the amplitude of the presynaptic spike below 40 mV, the synaptic potential disappears altogether (Figure 14-1B). Thus, transmitter release (as measured by the size of the postsynaptic potential) shows a steep dependence on presynaptic depolarization.

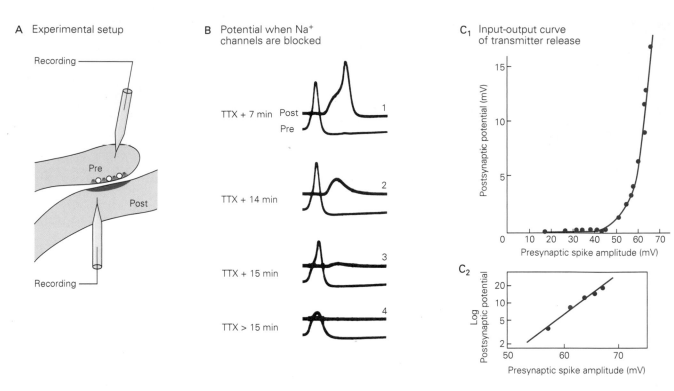

A Experimental setup

B Potential when Na$^+$ channels are blocked

C$_1$ Input-output curve of transmitter release

C$_2$

Figure 14-1 The contribution of voltage-gated Na$^+$ channels to transmitter release is tested by blocking the channels and measuring the amplitude of the presynaptic action potential and the resulting postsynaptic potential. (Adapted from Katz and Miledi 1967a.)

A. Recording electrodes are inserted in both the pre- and postsynaptic fibers of the giant synapse in the stellate ganglion of a squid.

B. Tetrodotoxin (**TTX**) is added to the solution bathing the cell in order to block the voltage-gated Na$^+$ channels. The amplitudes of both the presynaptic action potential and the postsynaptic potential gradually decrease. After 7 min the presynaptic action potential can still produce a suprathreshold synaptic potential that triggers an action potential in the postsynaptic cell (**1**). After 14 and 15 min the presynaptic spike gradually becomes smaller and produces smaller synaptic potentials (**2** and

3). When the presynaptic spike is reduced to 40 mV or less, it fails to produce a synaptic potential (**4**).

C. An input-output curve for transmitter release can be inferred from the dependence of the amplitude of the synaptic potential on the amplitude of the presynaptic action potential. This is obtained by stimulating the presynaptic nerve as the Na$^+$ channels for the presynaptic action potential are progressively blocked. **1.** A 40 mV presynaptic depolarization is required to produce a synaptic potential. Beyond this threshold there is a steep increase in amplitude of the synaptic potential in response to small changes in the amplitude of the presynaptic potential. **2.** The semilogarithmic plot of the data in the input-output curve illustrates that the relationship between the presynaptic spike and the postsynaptic potential is logarithmic. A 10 mV increase in the presynaptic spike produces a 10-fold increase in the synaptic potential.

How does membrane depolarization cause transmitter release? One possibility, suggested by the above experiment, is that Na$^+$ influx may be the important factor. However, Katz and Miledi were able to show that such influx is not necessary. While the Na$^+$ channels were still fully blocked by tetrodotoxin, Katz and Miledi directly depolarized the presynaptic membrane by passing depolarizing current through the second intracellular microelectrode. Beyond a threshold of about 40 mV from the resting potential, progressively greater amounts of transmitter are released (as judged by the appearance and amplitude of the postsynaptic potential). In the range of depolarization at which chemical

transmitter is released (40–70 mV above the resting level), a 10 mV increase in depolarization produces a 10-fold increase in transmitter release. Thus, the presynaptic terminal is able to release transmitter without an influx of Na$^+$. The Na$^+$ influx is important only insofar as it depolarizes the membrane enough to generate the action potential necessary for transmitter release.

Might the voltage-gated K$^+$ efflux triggered by the action potential be responsible for release of transmitter? To examine the contribution of K$^+$ efflux to transmitter release, Katz and Meledi blocked the voltage-gated K$^+$ channels with tetraethylammonium at the same time they blocked the voltage-sensitive Na$^+$ chan-

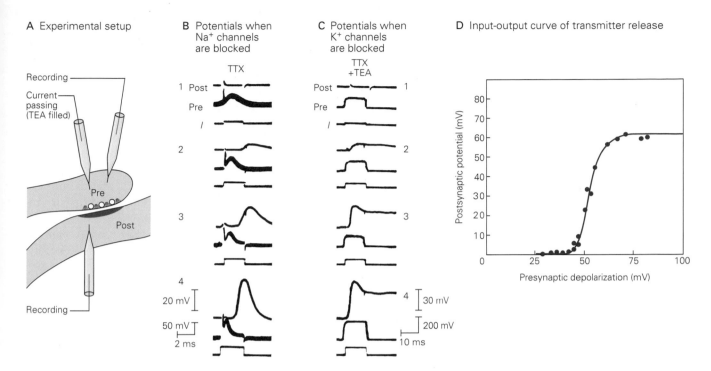

A Experimental setup

B Potentials when Na⁺ channels are blocked

C Potentials when K⁺ channels are blocked

D Input-output curve of transmitter release

Figure 14-2 Blocking the voltage-sensitive Na⁺ channels and K⁺ channels in the presynaptic terminals affects the amplitude and duration of the presynaptic action potential and the resulting postsynaptic potential, but does not block the release of transmitter. (Adapted from Katz and Miledi 1967a.)

A. The experimental arrangement is the same as in Figure 14-1, except that a current-passing electrode has been inserted into the presynaptic cell. (**TEA** = tetraethylammonium.)

B. The voltage-gated Na⁺ channels are completely blocked by adding tetrodotoxin (**TTX**) to the cell-bathing solution. Each set of three traces represents (from bottom to top) the depolarizing current pulse injected into the presynaptic terminal (**I**), the resulting potential in the presynaptic terminal (**Pre**), and the postsynaptic potential generated as a result of transmitter release onto the postsynaptic cell (**Post**). Progressively stronger current pulses are applied to produce correspondingly greater depolarizations of the presynaptic terminal (**2–4**). These presynaptic depolarizations cause postsynaptic potentials even in the absence of Na⁺ flux. The greater the presynaptic depolarization, the larger the postsynaptic potential, indicating that membrane potential exerts a direct control over transmitter release. The presynaptic depolarizations are not maintained throughout the duration of the depolarizing current pulse because of the delayed activation of the voltage-gated K⁺ channels, which causes repolarization.

C. After the voltage-gated Na⁺ channels of the action potential have been blocked, tetraethylammonium (**TEA**) is injected into the presynaptic terminal to block the voltage-gated K⁺ channels as well. Each set of three traces represents current pulse, presynaptic potential, and postsynaptic potential as in part B. Because the presynaptic K⁺ channels are blocked, the presynaptic depolarization is maintained throughout the current pulse. The large sustained presynaptic depolarizations produce large sustained postsynaptic potentials (**2–4**). This indicates that neither Na⁺ nor K⁺ channels are required for effective transmitter release.

D. Blocking both the Na⁺ and K⁺ channels permits the measurement of a more complete input-output curve than that in Figure 14-1. In addition to the steep part of the curve, there is now a plateau. Thus, beyond a certain level of presynaptic depolarization, further depolarization does not cause any additional release of transmitter. The initial level of the presynaptic membrane potential was about −70 mV.

nels with tetrodotoxin. They then passed a depolarizing current through the presynaptic terminals and found that the postsynaptic potentials nonetheless were of normal size, indicating that normal transmitter release occurred (Figure 14-2). Indeed, under the conditions of this experiment, the presynaptic potential is maintained throughout the current pulse because the K⁺ current that normally repolarizes the presynaptic membrane is blocked. As a result, transmitter release is sustained (Figure 14-2C). Increases in the presynaptic potential above an upper limit produce no further increase in postsynaptic potential (Figure 14-2D). Thus, neither Na⁺ nor K⁺ flux is required for transmitter release.

Transmitter Release Is Triggered by Calcium Influx

Katz and Miledi then turned their attention to Ca²⁺ ions. Earlier, José del Castillo and Katz had found that

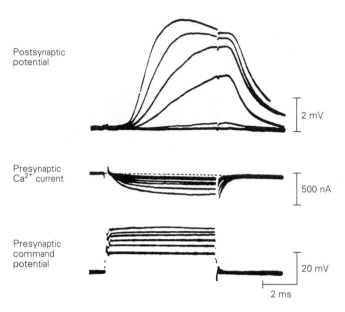

Postsynaptic potential

2 mV

Presynaptic Ca²⁺ current

500 nA

Presynaptic command potential

20 mV

2 ms

Figure 14-3 A simple experiment demonstrates that transmitter release is a function of Ca²⁺ influx into the presynaptic terminal. The voltage-sensitive Na⁺ and K⁺ channels in a squid giant synapse are blocked by tetrodotoxin and tetraethylammonium. The presynaptic terminal is voltage-clamped and the membrane potential is stepped to six different command levels of depolarization (**bottom traces**). The amount of presynaptic inward Ca²⁺ current (**middle traces**) that accompanies the depolarization correlates with the amplitude of the resulting postsynaptic potential (**top traces**). This is because the amount of Ca²⁺ current through voltage-gated channels determines the amount of transmitter released, which in turn determines the size of the postsynaptic potential. The notch in the postsynaptic potential trace is an artifact that results from turning off the presynaptic command potential. (Adapted from Llinás and Heuser 1977.)

increasing the extracellular Ca²⁺ concentration enhanced transmitter release; lowering the extracellular Ca²⁺ concentration reduced and ultimately blocked synaptic transmission. However, since transmitter release is an intracellular process, these findings implied that Ca²⁺ must enter the cell to influence transmitter release.

Previous work on the squid giant axon had identified a class of voltage-gated Ca²⁺ channels. As there is a very large inward electrochemical driving force on Ca²⁺—the extracellular Ca²⁺ concentration is normally four orders of magnitude greater than the intracellular concentration—opening of voltage-gated Ca²⁺ channels would result in a large Ca²⁺ influx. These Ca²⁺ channels are, however, sparsely distributed along the main axon. Katz and Miledi proposed that the Ca²⁺ channels might be much more abundant at the presynaptic terminal and that Ca²⁺ might serve dual functions: as a carrier of de-

polarizing charge during the action potential (like Na⁺) and as a special signal conveying information about changes in membrane potential to the intracellular machinery responsible for transmitter release.

Direct evidence for the presence of a voltage-gated Ca²⁺ current at the squid presynaptic terminal was provided by Rodolfo Llinás and his colleagues. Using a microelectrode voltage clamp, Llinás depolarized the terminal while blocking the voltage-gated Na⁺ and K⁺ channels with tetrodotoxin and tetraethylammonium, respectively. He found that graded depolarizations activated a graded inward Ca²⁺ current, which in turn resulted in graded release of transmitter (Figure 14-3). The Ca²⁺ current is graded because the Ca²⁺ channels possess voltage-dependent activation gates, like the voltage-gated Na⁺ and K⁺ channels. The Ca²⁺ channels in the squid terminals differ from Na⁺ channels, however, in that they do not inactivate quickly but stay open as long as the presynaptic depolarization lasts. One striking feature of transmitter release at all synapses is its steep and nonlinear dependence on Ca²⁺ influx—a two-fold increase in Ca²⁺ influx can increase transmitter release up to 16-fold. This relationship indicates that at some site—called the *calcium sensor*—the binding of up to four Ca²⁺ ions is required to trigger release.

Even in the axon terminal Ca²⁺ currents are small and are normally masked by Na⁺ and K⁺ currents, which are 10–20 times larger. However, in the region of the active zone (the site of transmitter release) Ca²⁺ influx is 10 times greater than elsewhere in the terminal. This localization is consistent with the distribution of intramembranous particles seen in freeze-fracture electron micrographs and thought to be the Ca²⁺ channels (see Figure 14-7 in Box 14-2).

The localization of Ca²⁺ channels at active zones provides a high, local rise in Ca²⁺ concentration at the site of transmitter release during the action potential. Indeed, during an action potential the Ca²⁺ concentration at the active zone can rise more than a thousandfold (to ~100 μM) within a few hundred microseconds. This large and rapid increase is required for the rapid synchronous release of transmitter. The calcium sensor responsible for fast transmitter release is thought to have a low affinity for Ca²⁺. On the order of 50–100 μM intracellular Ca²⁺ is required to trigger release, whereas only ~1 μM of Ca²⁺ is required for many enzymatic reactions. Because of the low-affinity calcium sensor, release only takes place in a narrow region surrounding the intracellular mouth of a Ca²⁺ channel, the only location where the Ca²⁺ concentration is sufficient to trigger release. The requirement for a high concentration of Ca²⁺ also ensures that release will be rapidly terminated upon repolarization. Once the Ca²⁺ channels close, the high local Ca^{2+} concentration dissipates rapidly (within 1 ms) because of diffusion.

Calcium channels open somewhat more slowly than the Na^+ channels and therefore Ca^{2+} influx does not occur until the action potential in the presynaptic cell has begun to repolarize (Figure 14-4). The delay that is characteristic of chemical synaptic transmission—the time from the onset of the action potential in the presynaptic terminals to the onset of the postsynaptic potential—is due in large part to the time required for Ca^{2+} channels to open in response to depolarization. However, because the voltage-dependent Ca^{2+} channels are located very close to the transmitter release sites, Ca^{2+} needs to diffuse only a short distance, permitting transmitter release to occur within 0.2 ms of Ca^{2+} entry!

As we shall see later in this chapter, the duration of the action potential is an important determinant of the amount of Ca^{2+} that flows into the terminal. If the action potential is prolonged, more Ca^{2+} flows into the cell and therefore more transmitter is released, causing a greater postsynaptic potential.

Calcium channels are found in all nerve cells as well as in cells outside the nervous system, such as skeletal and cardiac muscle cells, where the channels are important for excitation-contraction coupling, and endocrine cells, where they mediate release of hormones. There are many types of Ca^{2+} channels—called L, P/Q, N, R, and T—with specific biophysical and pharmacological properties and different physiological functions. The distinct properties of these channel types are determined by the identity of their pore-forming subunit (termed the $\alpha1$-subunit), which is encoded by a family of related genes (Table 14-1). Calcium channels also have associated subunits (termed $\alpha2$, β, γ, and δ) that modify the properties of the channel formed by the $\alpha1$-subunits. All $\alpha1$-subunits are homologous to the voltage-gated Na^+ channel α-subunits, consisting of four repeats of a basic domain containing six transmembrane segments (including an S4 voltage-sensor) and a pore-lining P region (see Figure 9-14).

Most nerve cells contain more than one type of Ca^{2+} channel. Channels formed from the different $\alpha1$-subunits can be distinguished by their different voltage-dependent gating properties, their distinctive sensitivity to pharmacological blockers, and their specific physiological function. The *L-type channels* are selectively blocked by the dihydropyridines, a class of clinically important drugs used to treat hypertension. The *P/Q-type channels* are selectively blocked by ω-agatoxin IVA, a component of the venom of the funnel web spider. The *N-type channels* are blocked selectively by a toxin obtained from the venom of the marine cone snail, the ω-conotoxin GVIA. The L-type, P/Q-type, N-type,

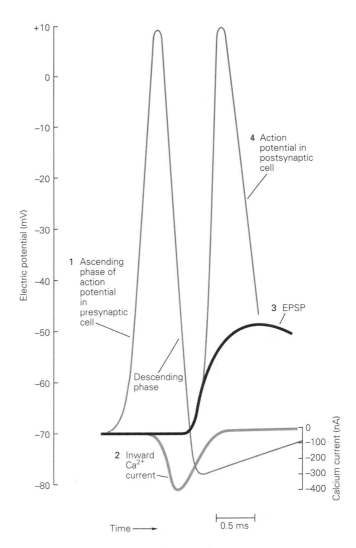

Figure 14-4 The time course of Ca^{2+} influx in the presynaptic cell determines the onset of synaptic transmission. An action potential in the presynaptic cell (**1**) causes voltage-gated Ca^{2+} channels in the terminal to open and a Ca^{2+} current (**2**) to flow into the terminal. (Note that the Ca^{2+} current is turned on during the descending phase of the presynaptic action potential owing to delayed opening of the Ca^{2+} channels.) The Ca^{2+} influx triggers release of neurotransmitter. The postsynaptic response to the transmitter begins soon afterward (**3**) and, if sufficiently large, will trigger an action potential in the postsynaptic cell (**4**). (**EPSP** = excitatory postsynaptic potential.) (Adapted from Llinás 1982.)

and R-type channels all require fairly strong depolarizations for their activation (voltages positive to -40 to -20 mV are required), and are thus often referred to as *high-voltage-activated* Ca^{2+} channels. In contrast, T-type Ca^{2+} channels are *low-voltage-activated* Ca^{2+} channels that open in reponse to small depolarizations around the threshold for generating an action potential (-60 to -40 mV). Because they are activated by small changes in membrane potential, the T-type channels help control

Table 14-1 Molecular Bases for Calcium Channel Diversity

Gene[1]	Ca^{2+} channel type	Tissue	Selective blockers	Function
A	P/Q	Neurons	ω-agatoxin (spider venom)	Fast release
B	N	Neurons	ω-conotoxin (snail venom)	Fast release
C/D/S	L	Neurons, endocrine	Dihydropyridines	Slow release
		Heart, skeletal muscle		(Peptides)
E	R	Neurons	?	Fast release
G/H	T	Neurons, heart	?	Excitability

[1]The gene for the main pore-forming type of α1-subunit.

excitability at the resting potential and are an important source of the excitatory current that drives the rhythmic pacemaker activity of certain cells, both in the brain and the heart.

In neurons the rapid release of conventional transmitters associated with fast synaptic transmission is mediated by three main classes of Ca^{2+} channels: the P/Q-type, the N-type, and R-type channels. The L-type channels do not contribute to fast transmitter release but are important for the slower release of neuropeptides from neurons and of hormones from endocrine cells. The fact that Ca^{2+} influx through only certain types of Ca^{2+} channels, can control transmitter release is presumably due to the fact that these channels are concentrated at active zones. Localization of the N-type Ca^{2+} channels at the active zones has been visualized with fluorescently labeled ω-conotoxin at the frog neuromuscular junction (Figure 14-5). By contrast, L-type channels may be excluded from active zones, limiting their participation to slow synaptic transmission.

Transmitter Is Released in Quantal Units

How and where does Ca^{2+} influx trigger release? To answer that question we must first consider how transmitter substances are released. Even though the release of synaptic transmitter appears smoothly graded, it is actually released in discrete packages called *quanta*. Each quantum of transmitter produces a postsynaptic potential of fixed size, called the *quantal synaptic potential*. The total postsynaptic potential is made up from an integral number of quantal responses (Figure 14-6). Synaptic potentials seem smoothly graded in recordings only because each quantal (or unit) potential is small relative to the total potential.

Paul Fatt and Bernard Katz obtained the first clue as to the quantal nature of synaptic transmission when they made recordings from the nerve-muscle synapse of the frog without presynaptic stimulation and observed small spontaneous postsynaptic potentials of about 0.5 mV. Like the nerve-evoked end-plate potentials, these small depolarizing responses were largest at the site of nerve-muscle contact and decayed electronically with distance (see Figure 11-5). Similar results have since been obtained in mammalian muscle and in central neurons. Because the synaptic potentials at vertebrate nerve-muscle synapses are called end-plate potentials, Fatt and Katz called these spontaneous potentials *miniature end-plate potentials*.

The time course of the miniature end-plate potentials and the effects of various drugs on them are indistinguishable from the properties of the end-plate potential evoked by nerve stimulation. Because acetylcholine (ACh) is the transmitter at the nerve-muscle synapse, the miniature end-plate potentials, like the end-plate potentials, are enhanced and prolonged by prostigmine, a drug that inhibits the hydrolysis of ACh by acetylcholinesterase. Likewise, the miniature end-plate potentials are reduced and finally abolished by agents that block the ACh receptor. In the absence of stimulation the miniature end-plate potentials occur at random intervals; their frequency can be increased by depolarizing the presynaptic terminal. They disappear if the presynaptic motor nerve degenerates but reappear when a new motor synapse is formed, indicating that these events represent small amounts of transmitter that are continuously released from the presynaptic nerve terminal.

What could account for the fixed size (around 0.5 mV) of the miniature end-plate potential? Del Castillo and Katz first tested the possibility that each quantum represented a fixed response due to the opening of a *single* ACh receptor-channel. By applying small amounts of

Figure 14-5 Calcium channels are concentrated at the neuromuscular junction in regions of the presynaptic nerve terminal opposite clusters of acetylcholine (ACh) receptors on the postsynaptic membrane. The fluorescent image shows the presynaptic Ca^{2+} channels in **red**, after labeling with a Texas red–coupled marine snail toxin that binds to Ca^{2+} channels. Postsynaptic ACh receptors are labeled in **green** with boron-dipyromethane difluoride-labeled α-bungarotoxin, which binds selectively to ACh receptors. The two images are normally superimposed but have been separated for clarity. The patterns of labeling with both probes are in almost precise register, indicating that the active zone of the presynaptic neuron is in almost perfect alignment with the postsynaptic membrane containing the high concentration of ACh receptors. (From Robitaille et al. 1990.)

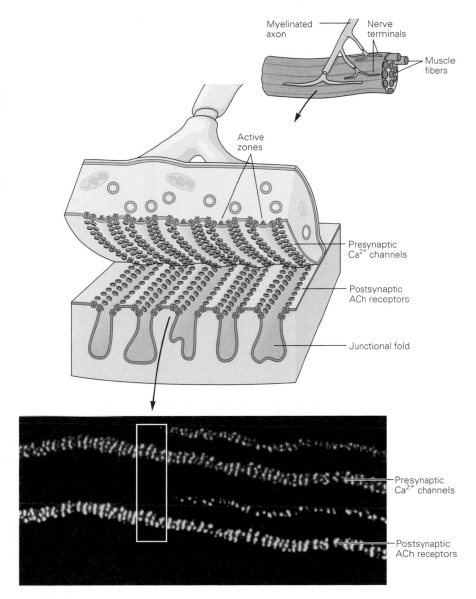

ACh to the frog muscle end-plate they were able to elicit depolarizing responses much smaller than 0.5 mV. From this it became clear that the miniature end-plate potential must reflect the opening of more than one ACh receptor-channel. In fact, Katz and Miledi were later able to estimate the elementary current through a single ACh receptor-channel as being only about 0.3 μV (see Chapter 6). This is about 1/2000 of the amplitude of a spontaneous miniature end-plate potential. Thus a miniature end-plate potential of 0.5 mV requires summation of the elementary currents of about 2000 channels. This estimate was later confirmed when the currents through single ACh-activated channels were measured directly using patch-clamp techniques (see Box 6-2).

Since the opening of a single channel requires the binding of two ACh molecules to the receptor (one molecule to each of the two α-subunits), and some of the released ACh never reaches the receptor molecules (either because it diffuses out of the synaptic cleft or is lost through hydrolysis), about 5000 molecules are needed to produce one miniature end-plate potential. This number has been confirmed by direct chemical measurement of the amount of ACh released with each quantal synaptic potential.

We can now ask some important questions. Is the normal postsynaptic potential evoked by nerve stimulation also composed of quantal responses that correspond to the quanta of spontaneously released transmit-

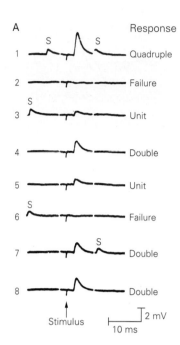

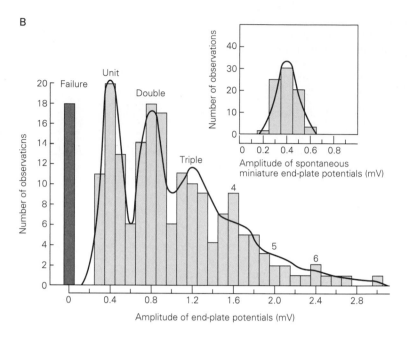

Figure 14-6 Neurotransmitter is released in fixed increments, or quanta. Each quantum of transmitter produces a unit postsynaptic potential of fixed amplitude. The amplitude of the postsynaptic potential evoked by nerve stimulation is equal to the unit amplitude multiplied by the number of quanta of transmitter released.

A. Intracellular recordings from a muscle fiber at the endplate show the postsynaptic change in potential when eight consecutive stimuli of the same size are applied to the motor nerve. To reduce transmitter output and to keep the end-plate potentials small, the tissue was bathed in a Ca^{2+}-deficient (and Mg^{2+}-rich) solution. The postsynaptic responses to the stimulus vary. Two presynaptic impulses elicit no postsynaptic response (failures); two produce unit potentials; and the others produce responses that are approximately two to four times the amplitude of the unit potential. Note that the spontaneous miniature end-plate potentials **(S)** are the same size as the unit potential. (Adapted from Liley 1956.)

B. After many end-plate potentials were recorded, the number of responses at each amplitude was counted and then plotted

in the histogram shown here. The distribution of responses falls into a number of peaks. The first peak, at 0 mV, represents failures. The first peak of responses, at 0.4 mV, represents the unit potential, the smallest elicited response. This unit response is the same amplitude as the spontaneous miniature end-plate potentials **(inset)**. The other peaks in the histogram occur at amplitudes that are integral multiples of the amplitude of the unit potential. The **red line** shows a theoretical distribution composed of the sum of several Gaussian functions fitted to the data of the histogram. In this distribution each peak is slightly spread out, reflecting the fact that the amount of transmitter in each quantum, and hence the amplitude of the postsynaptic response, varies randomly about the peak. The number of events under each peak divided by the total number of events in the histogram is the probability that the presynaptic terminal releases the corresponding number of quanta. This probability follows a Poisson distribution (see Box 14-1). The distribution of amplitudes of the spontaneous miniature potentials, shown in the inset, is also fit by a Gaussian curve. (Adapted from Boyd and Martin 1956.)

ter? If so, what determines the number of quanta of transmitter released by a presynaptic action potential? Does Ca^{2+} alter the number of ACh molecules that make up each quantum or does it affect the number of quanta released by each action potential?

These questions were addressed by del Castillo and Katz in a study of synaptic signaling at the nerve-muscle synapse when the external concentration of Ca^{2+} is decreased. When the neuromuscular junction is bathed in a solution low in Ca^{2+}, the evoked end-plate potential (normally 70 mV in amplitude) is reduced markedly, to about 0.5–2.5 mV. Moreover, the amplitude

of successively evoked end-plate potentials varies randomly from one stimulus to the next, and often no responses can be detected at all (termed *failures*). However, the minimum response above zero—the unit synaptic potential in response to a presynaptic potential—is identical in size (about 0.5 mV) and shape to the spontaneous miniature end-plate potentials. All end-plate potentials larger than the quantal synaptic potential are integral multiples of the unit potential (Figure 14-6).

Del Castillo and Katz could now ask: How does the rise of intracellular Ca^{2+} that accompanies each action potential affect the release of transmitter? They found

Box 14-1 Calculating the Probability of Transmitter Release

The release of a quantum of transmitter is a random event. The fate of each quantum of transmitter in response to an action potential has only two possible outcomes—a quantum is or is not released. This event resembles a binomial or Bernoulli trial (similar to tossing a coin in the air to determine whether it comes up heads or tails). The probability of a quantum being released by an action potential is independent of the probability of other quanta being released by that action potential. Therefore, for a population of releasable quanta, each action potential represents a series of independent binomial trials (comparable to tossing a handful of coins to see how many coins come up heads).

In a binomial distribution p stands for the average probability of success (ie, the probability that any given quantum will be released) and q (or $1 - p$) stands for the mean probability of failure. Both the average probability (p) that an individual quantum will be released and the store (n) of readily releasable quanta are assumed to be constant. (Any reduction in the store is assumed to be quickly replenished after each stimulus.) The product of n and p yields an estimate, m, of the mean number of quanta that are released to make up the end-plate potential. This mean is called the *quantal content* or *quantal output*.

Calculation of the probability of transmitter release can be illustrated with the following example. Let us consider a terminal that has a releasable store of five quanta ($n = 5$). If we assume that $p = 0.1$, then q (the probability that an individual quantum is not released from the terminals) is $1 - p$, or 0.9. We can now determine the probability that a stimulus will release no quanta (failure), a single quantum, two quanta, three quanta, or any number of quanta (up to n). The probability that none of the five available quanta will be released by a given stimulus is the product of the individual probabilities that each quantum will not be released: $q^5 = (0.9)^5$, or 0.59. We would thus expect to see 59 failures in a hundred stimuli. The probabilities of observing zero, one, two, three, four, or five quanta are represented by the successive terms of the binomial expansion:

$$(q + p)^5 = q^5 \text{(failures)} + 5\,q^4 p\,(1 \text{ quantum})$$
$$+ 10\,q^3 p^2\,(2 \text{ quanta}) + 10\,q^2 p^3\,(3 \text{ quanta})$$
$$+ 5\,qp^4\,(4 \text{ quanta}) + p^5\,(5 \text{ quanta}).$$

Thus, in 100 stimuli the binomial expansion would predict 33 unit responses, 7 double responses, 1 triple response, and 0 quadruple and quintuple responses.

Values for m vary, from about 100–300 at the vertebrate nerve-muscle synapse, the squid giant synapse, and *Aplysia* central synapses, to as few as 1–4 in the synapses of the sympathetic ganglion and spinal cord of vertebrates. The probability of release p also varies, ranging from as high as 0.7 at the neuromuscular junction in the frog and 0.9 in the crab down to around 0.1 at some central synapses. Estimates for n range from 1000 (at the vertebrate nerve-muscle synapse) to 1 (at single terminals of central neurons).

The parameters n and p are statistical terms; the physical processes represented by them are not yet known. Although the parameter n is assumed to refer to the number of readily releasable (or available) quanta of transmitter, it may actually represent the number of *release sites* or *active zones* in the presynaptic terminals that are loaded with vesicles. Although the number of release sites is thought to be fixed, the fraction that is loaded with vesicles is thought to be variable. The parameter p probably represents a compound probability depending on at least two processes: the probability that a vesicle has been loaded or docked onto a release site (a process referred to as vesicle mobilization) and the probability that an action potential will discharge a quantum of transmitter from a docked active zone. The parameter p is thought to depend on the presynaptic Ca^{2+} influx during an action potential.

The quantal size (a) is the response of the postsynaptic membrane to a single quantum of transmitter. Quantal size depends largely on the properties of the postsynaptic cell, such as the input resistance and capacitance (which can be independently estimated) and the sensitivity of the postsynaptic membrane to the transmitter substance. This can also be measured by the postsynaptic membrane's response to the application of a constant amount of transmitter.

that when the external Ca^{2+} concentration is increased, the amplitude of the unit synaptic potential does not change. However, the number of failures decreases and the incidence of higher-amplitude responses (composed of multiple quantal units) increases. These observations illustrate that alterations in external Ca^{2+} concentration do not affect the *size* of a quantum of transmitter (the number of ACh molecules) but rather affect the average

number of quanta that are released in response to a presynaptic action potential (Box 14-1). The greater the Ca^{2+} influx into the terminal, the larger the number of quanta released.

The findings that the amplitude of the end-plate potential varies in a stepwise manner at low levels of ACh release, that the amplitude of each step increase is an integral multiple of the unit potential, and that the unit potential has the same mean amplitude as that of the spontaneous miniature end-plate potentials led del Castillo and Katz to conclude that transmitter is released in fixed packets or quanta. When the external Ca^{2+} concentration is normal, an action potential in the presynaptic terminal releases about 150 quanta, each about 0.5 mV in amplitude, resulting in a large end-plate potential. In the absence of an action potential, the rate of quantal release is very low—only one quantum per second is released spontaneously at the end-plate. The rate of quantal release increases 100,000-fold when Ca^{2+} enters the presynaptic terminal with an action potential, bringing about the synchronous release of about 150 quanta in one or two milliseconds.

Transmitter Is Stored and Released by Synaptic Vesicles

What morphological features of the cell might account for the quantum of transmitter? The physiological observations indicating that transmitter is released in fixed quanta coincided with the discovery, through electron microscopy, of accumulations of small vesicles in the presynaptic terminal. The electron micrographs suggested to del Castillo and Katz that the vesicles were organelles for the storage of transmitter. They also argued that each vesicle stored one quantum of transmitter (amounting to several thousand molecules) and that each vesicle releases its entire contents into the synaptic cleft when the vesicle fuses with the inner surface of the presynaptic terminal at specific release sites.

At these sites, *the active zones*, a band of synaptic vesicles cluster above a fuzzy electron-dense material attached to the internal face of the presynaptic membrane, directly above the junctional folds in the muscle (see Figure 11-1). As we saw in Chapter 11, the neuromuscular junction in frogs contains about 300 active zones with a total of about 10^6 vesicles. Here, and at central synapses, the vesicles are typically clear, small, and ovoid, with a diameter of about 50 nm.

Neuropeptides and certain transmitters released from neuroendocrine cells are packaged in larger vesicles that contain an electron-dense material. These large dense-core vesicles are not localized at active zones. They can be released from anywhere within a neuron, including the cell body. Release of transmitter from large dense-core vesicles is associated with slow modulatory synaptic actions (see Chapter 13).

Quantal transmission has been demonstrated at all chemical synapses so far examined, with one exception, in the retina, which we shall examine in Chapter 26. At most synapses in the central nervous system each action

potential releases only between 1 and 10 quanta, many fewer than the 150 quanta released at the nerve-muscle synapse. Whereas the surface area of a presynaptic motor terminal ending on a muscle fiber is large (about 2000–6000 μm^2) and contains about 300 active zones, a typical excitatory afferent fiber from a dorsal root ganglion cell forms only about four synapses on a motor neuron, each of which is about 2 μm^2 and contains only one active zone.

Quantal analysis of transmitter release from these afferent neurons indicates that release from each active zone is all-or-none. That is, any given active zone releases either one quantum or none at all in response to a presynaptic action potential. The probability of release depends on the amount of Ca^{2+} influx during the action potential. Similar results have been obtained for other central synapses. Thus, variations in the response of a central neuron to a single presynaptic neuron result from the all-or-none release of one quantum from each of a few terminals, each usually with only one active zone.

Not all chemical signaling between neurons depends on vesicular storage and release. Some membrane-permeable substances, such as prostaglandins, the metabolites of arachidonic acid, and the gases CO and NO (see Chapter 13), can traverse the lipid bilayer of the membrane by diffusion. These substances may act at synapses either as chemical messengers or as retrograde signals that diffuse from the postsynaptic neuron back to the presynaptic neuron to regulate transmitter release. Other substances can be moved out of nerve endings by carrier proteins if their intracellular concentration is sufficiently high. In certain retinal glial cells, transporters for glutamate or GABA that normally take up transmitter into a cell from the extracellular space can reverse direction and release transmitter into the extracellular space. Still other substances simply leak out of nerve terminals at a low rate. For example, about 90% of the ACh that leaves the presynaptic terminal at the neuromuscular junction can be traced to continuous leakage. However, because this leakage is so diffuse and not targeted to receptors at the end-plate region, and because it is continuous and low level rather than synchronous and concentrated, it is ineffective functionally.

Synaptic Vesicles Discharge Transmitter by Exocytosis

Direct evidence that exocytosis of a single synaptic vesicle is responsible for the release of one quantum of transmitter was at first difficult to obtain, because the chance of finding a vesicle in the act of being discharged

Box 14-2 Freeze-Fracture Technique

Figure 14-7A. Freeze-fracture exposes the intramembranous area to view. The path of membrane cleavage is along the hydrophobic interior of the lipid bilayer, resulting in two complementary fracture faces. The **P face** (corresponding to the cytoplasmic-facing leaflet of the bilayer) contains most of the integral membrane proteins (particles), because these are anchored to cytoskeletal structures. The **E face** (corresponding to the extracellular-facing leaflet of the bilayer) shows pits complementary to the integral protein particles. (Adapted from Fawcett 1981.)

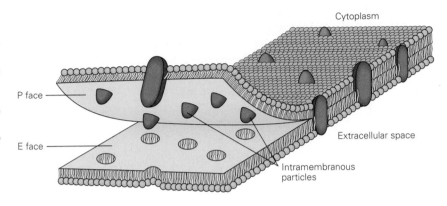

Figure 14-7B. This idealized three-dimensional view of pre- and postsynaptic membranes shows the active zones with adjacent rows of synaptic vesicles, as well as places where the vesicles are undergoing exocytosis. The rows of particles on either side of the active zone are intramembranous proteins thought to be Ca^{2+} channels. (Adapted from Kuffler et al. 1984.)

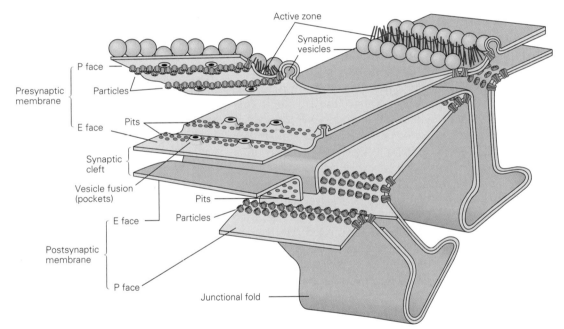

Freeze fracture reveals the structural details of synaptic membranes. In this technique frozen tissue is broken open under a high vacuum and coated with platinum and carbon. Frozen membrane tends to break at the weakest plane, which is between the two molecular layers of lipids. Two complementary faces of the membrane are thus exposed: The leaflet nearest the cytoplasm (the interior half) is the protoplasmic (P) face, while the leaflet that borders the extracellular space is the external (E) face (Figure 14-7A).

Freeze-fracture exposes a large expanse of the presynaptic intramembranous area (Figure 14-7B). Deformations of the membrane that occur at the active zone, where vesicles are attached, are readily apparent. The advantage of the freeze-fracture technique is best appreciated by comparing a freeze-fracture electron micrograph with a conventional thin-section electron micrograph of the active zone (see Figure 14-8).

is extremely small. A thin section through a conventionally fixed terminal at the neuromuscular junction of the frog shows only 1/4000 of the total presynaptic membrane. Moreover, the exocytotic opening of each small vesicle is of the same dimension as the thickness of the ultrathin (50–100 nm) sections required for transmission electron microscopy. To overcome such problems, freeze-fracture techniques began to be applied to the synapse in the 1970s (Box 14-2).

Using these techniques, Thomas Reese and John Heuser made three important observations. First, they found one or two rows of unusually large intramembranous particles along the presynaptic density, on both margins (Figure 14-8A). Although the function of these particles is not yet known, they are thought to be voltage-gated Ca^{2+} channels. Their density (about 1500 per μm^2) is approximately that of the voltage-gated Ca^{2+} channels essential for transmitter release. Moreover, the proximity of the particles to the release site is consistent with the short time interval between the onset of the Ca^{2+} current and the release of transmitter. Second, they noted the appearance of deformations alongside the rows of intramembranous particles during synaptic activity (Figure 14-8B). They interpreted these deformations as representing invaginations of the cell membrane during exocytosis. Finally, Reese and Heuser found that these deformations do not persist after the transmitter has been released; they seem to be transient distortions that occur only when vesicles are discharged.

To catch vesicles in the act of exocytosis, Heuser, Reese, and their colleagues had to quick-freeze the tissue with liquid helium at precisely defined intervals after the presynaptic nerve had been stimulated. The neuromuscular junction can thus be frozen just as the action potential invades the terminal and exocytosis occurs. In addition, they applied the drug 4-aminopyridine— a compound that blocks certain voltage-gated K^+ channels—to broaden the action potential and increase the number of quanta of transmitter discharged with each nerve impulse. These techniques provided clear images of synaptic vesicles during exocytosis.

The electron micrographs revealed a number of omega-shaped (Ω) structures that correspond to vesicles that have just fused with the membrane. Varying the concentration of 4-aminopyridine altered the amount of transmitter release. Moreover, there was an increase in the number of Ω-shaped structures that was directly correlated with the size of the postsynaptic response. These morphological studies therefore provide independent evidence that transmitter is released by exocytosis from synaptic vesicles.

The fusion of the synaptic vesicles with the plasma membrane during exocytosis increases the surface area of the plasma membrane. In certain favorable cell types this increase in area can be detected in electrical measurements as increases in membrane capacitance, providing further support for exocytosis. As we saw in Chapter 8, the capacitance of the membrane is proportional to its surface area. In adrenal chromaffin cells (which release epinephrine) and in mast cells of the rat peritoneum (which release histamine), individual large dense-core vesicles are large enough to permit measurement of the increase in capacitance associated with fusion of a single vesicle. Release of transmitter in these cells is accompanied by stepwise increases in capacitance, which in turn are followed somewhat later by stepwise decreases in capacitance, which presumably reflect the retrieval and recycling of the excess membrane (Figure 14-9B). Capacitance increases can be detected at fast synapses after a rise in Ca^{2+} due to the fusion of a large number of small synaptic vesicles (Figure 14-9C). However, the increase in capacitance associated with the fusion of a single small synaptic vesicle is too small to resolve.

Exocytosis Involves the Formation of a Fusion Pore

Exactly how fusion of the synaptic vesicle membrane with the plasma membrane occurs and the role that Ca^{2+} plays in catalyzing this reaction is under intensive study. Morphological studies from mast cells using rapid freezing suggested that exocytosis depends on the temporary formation of a *fusion pore* that spans the membranes of the vesicle and plasma membrane. Subsequent studies of capacitance increases in mast cells showed that prior to complete fusion a channel-like fusion pore could be detected in the electrophysiological recordings (Figure 14-10). This fusion pore starts out with a single-channel conductance of around 200 pS, similar to that of gap-junction channels, which also bridge two membranes. During exocytosis the pore rapidly dilates, probably from around 1 nm to 50 nm, and the conductance increases dramatically (Figure 14-10A). In some instances the fusion pore flickers open and closed several times prior to complete fusion (Figure 14-10B).

Since transmitter release is so fast, fusion must occur within a fraction of a millisecond. Therefore, the proteins that fuse synaptic vesicles to the plasma membrane are most likely preassembled into a fusion pore that bridges the vesicle and plasma membranes before fusion occurs. Much like the gap-junction channels we learned about in Chapter 10, the fusion pore may consist of two hemichannels, one each in the vesicle membrane and the plasma membrane, which then join in the course of vesicle docking (Figure 14-10C). Calcium influx would then simply cause the preexisting pore to

Cytoplasmic half of presynaptic membrane (freeze fracture)

Presynaptic membrane (thin section)

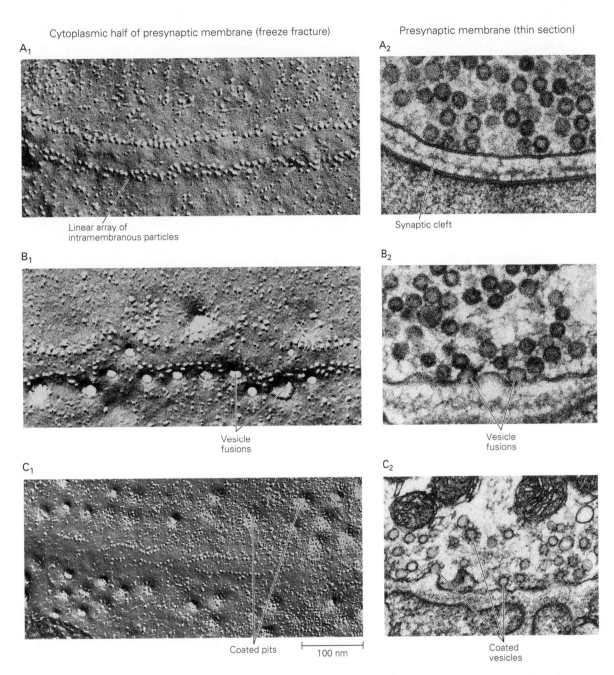

Figure 14-8 The events of exocytosis at the presynaptic terminal are revealed by electron microscopy. The images on the left are freeze-fracture electron micrographs of the cytoplasmic half (P face) of the presynaptic membrane (compare Figure 14-7). Thin-section electron micrographs of the presynaptic membrane are shown on the right. (Adapted from Alberts et al. 1989.)

A. Parallel rows of intramembranous particles arrayed on either side of an active zone may be the voltage-gated Ca^{2+} channels essential for transmitter release.

B. Synaptic vesicles begin fusing with the plasma membrane within 5 ms after the stimulus. Fusion is complete within another 2 ms. Each opening in the plasma membrane represents

the fusion of one synaptic vesicle. In thin-section micrographs, vesicle fusion events are observed in cross section as Ω-shaped structures.

C. Membrane retrieval becomes apparent as coated pits form within about 10 s after fusion of the vesicles with the presynaptic membrane. After another 10 s the coated pits begin to pinch off by endocytosis to form coated vesicles. These vesicles include the original membrane proteins of the synaptic vesicle and also contain molecules captured from the external medium. The vesicles are recycled at the terminals or are transported to the cell body, where the membrane constituents are degraded or recycled (see Chapter 4).

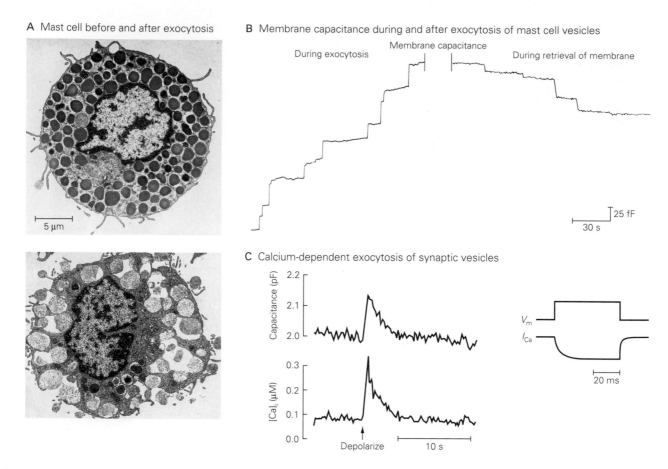

A Mast cell before and after exocytosis

B Membrane capacitance during and after exocytosis of mast cell vesicles

During exocytosis   Membrane capacitance   During retrieval of membrane

5 µm

25 fF
30 s

C Calcium-dependent exocytosis of synaptic vesicles

Capacitance (pF)
2.2
2.1
2.0

[Ca]$_i$ (µM)
0.3
0.2
0.1
0.0

Depolarize   10 s

V_m
I_{Ca}

20 ms

Figure 14-9 Capacitance measurements allow direct study of exocytosis and endocytosis.

A. Exocytosis from mast cells. Electron micrographs of a mast cell before (top) and after (bottom) inducing exocytosis. Mast cells are secretory cells of the immune system that contain large dense-core vesicles filled with the transmitter histamine. Exocytosis of mast cell secretory vesicles is normally triggered by the binding of antigen complexed to an immunoglobulin (IgE). Under experimental conditions massive exocytosis can be triggered by the inclusion of a nonhydrolyzable analog of GTP in an intracellular recording electrode. (From Lawson et al., 1977.)

B. Stepwise increases in capacitance reflect the successive fusion of individual secretory vesicles with the cell membrane. The step increases are unequal because of a variability in the diameter (and thus membrane area) of the vesicles. After exocytosis the membrane added through fusion is retrieved through endocytosis. Endocytosis of individual vesicles gives rise to the stepwise decreases in membrane capacitance. In

this way the cell maintains a constant size. (The units are in femtofarads, fF, where 1 fF = 0.1 µm^2 of membrane area.) (Adapted from Fernandez et al. 1984.)

C. Exocytosis and membrane retrieval from a neuronal presynaptic terminal. Recordings were obtained from isolated synaptic terminals of bipolar neurons in the retina of the goldfish. Transmitter release was triggered by a depolarizing voltage-clamp step (applied at **arrow**), which elicited a large sustained Ca^{2+} current (**inset**). The Ca^{2+} influx causes a transient rise in the cytoplasmic Ca^{2+} concentration (**bottom trace**). This results in the exocytosis of several thousand small synaptic vesicles, leading to an increase in total capacitance (**top trace**). The increments in capacitance due to fusion of a single small synaptic vesicle are too small to resolve. As the internal Ca^{2+} concentration falls back to its resting level upon repolarization, the extra membrane area is rapidly retrieved and capacitance returns to its baseline value. (Adapted from von Gersdorff and Matthews 1994.)

open and then dilate, allowing the release of transmitter.

Recent advances in chemical detection suggest that transmitter may be released through the fusion pore itself, prior to full dilation and vesicle fusion (Figure 14-10C). An electrochemical method termed *voltametry* permits the detection of certain amine-containing transmitters, such as serotonin, using an extracellular

carbon-fiber electrode (Figure 14-11). A large voltage is applied to the electrode, which leads to the oxidation of the released transmitter. This oxidation reaction releases free electrons, which can be detected as a transient electrical current that is proportional to the amount of transmitter released. In response to action potentials large transient increases in transmitter release are observed,

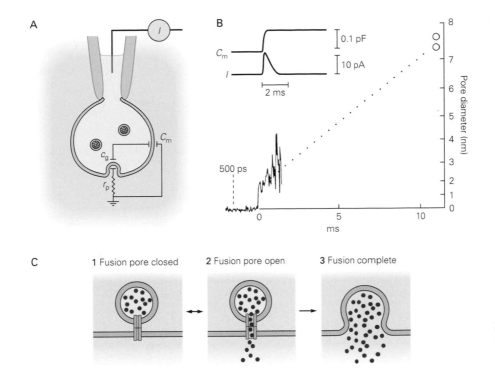

Figure 14-10 Transmitter is released from synaptic vesicles through the opening of a fusion pore that connects a secretory vesicle with the presynaptic membrane.

A. Patch-clamp recording setup for recording current through the fusion pore. As a vesicle fuses with the plasma membrane, the capacitance of the vesicle (C_g) is initially connected to the capacitance of the rest of the cell (C_m) through the high resistance (r_p) of the fusion pore. (From Monck and Fernandez 1992.)

B. Electrical events associated with the opening of the fusion pore. Since the membrane potential of the vesicle (lumenal side negative) is normally much more negative than the membrane potential of the cell, there will be a transient flow of charge (current) from the vesicle to the cell membrane associated with fusion. This generates a transient current (I) associated with the increase in membrane capacitance (C_m). The magnitude of the conductance of the fusion pore (g_p) can be

calculated from the time constant of the transient current according to $\tau = C_g r_p = C_g/g_p$. The fusion pore diameter can be calculated from the fusion pore conductance, assuming that the pore spans two lipid bilayers and is filled with a solution whose resistivity is equal to that of the cytoplasm. The fusion pore shows an initial conductance of around 200 pS, similar to the conductance of a gap-junction channel, corresponding to a pore diameter of around 2 nm. The conductance rapidly increases within a few milliseconds as the pore dilates to around 7–8 nm (**dotted line**). (From Spruce et al. 1990.)

C. Steps in exocytosis through a fusion pore. **1.** A docked vesicle contains a preassembled fusion pore ready to open. **2.** During the initial stages of exocytosis the fusion pore rapidly opens, allowing transmitter to leak out of the vesicle. **3.** In most cases the fusion pore rapidly dilates as the vesicle undergoes complete fusion with the plasma membrane.

corresponding to the exocytosis of the contents of a single large dense-core vesicle. Often, these large transient increases are preceded by a smaller longer-lasting signal, corresponding to a period of release at a low rate (Figure 14-11C). Such events are thought to reflect leakage of transmitter through the fusion pore, prior to complete exocytotic fusion. A good deal of fast transmitter release may involve release through fusion pores without the requirement for complete fusion.

Synaptic Vesicles Are Recycled

If there were no process to compensate for the fusion of successive vesicles to the plasma membrane during continued nerve activity, the membrane of a synaptic terminal would enlarge and the number of synaptic vesicles would decline. This does not occur, however, because the vesicle membrane added to the terminal membrane is retrieved rapidly and recycled, generating new synaptic vesicles (Figure 14-12).

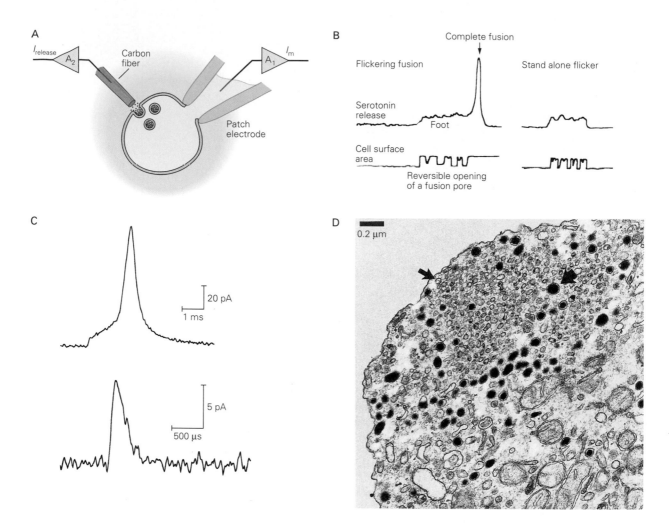

Figure 14-11 Transmitter release through the fusion pore can be measured using electrochemical detection methods.

A. Setup for recording transmitter release by voltametry. A cell is voltage-clamped with an intracellular patch electrode while an extracellular carbon fiber is pressed against the cell surface. A large voltage applied to the tip of the electrode oxidizes certain amine-containing transmitters (such as serotonin or norepinephrine). This oxidation reaction generates one or more free electrons, which results in an electrical current that can be recorded through an amplifier (A₂) connected to the carbon electrode. The current is proportional to the amount of transmitter release. Membrane current and capacitance are recorded through the intracellular patch electrode amplifier (A₁).

B. Recordings of transmitter release and capacitance measurements from mast cell secretory vesicles indicate that the fusion pore may "flicker" (open and close several times) prior to complete membrane fusion. During these brief openings transmitter can diffuse out through the pore, producing a "foot" of low-level release that precedes a large spike of transmitter release

upon a full fusion event. Sometimes the reversible fusion pore opening and closing is not followed by full fusion, resulting in "stand alone flicker" in which transmitter is released only by diffusion through the fusion pore. (From Neher 1993.)

C–D. Similar patterns of release of the transmitter serotonin are observed from Retzius neurons of the leech. The electron micrograph shows that these neurons package serotonin in both large, dense-core vesicles and small, clear synaptic vesicles (**arrow**). Amperometry measurements show that Ca²⁺ elevation triggers both large spikes of serotonin release (**top trace**) and smaller release events (**bottom trace**) (note the difference in current scales). These correspond to fusion of the large dense-core vesicles and synaptic vesicles, respectively. The synaptic vesicles release their contents rapidly, in less than 1 ms. This rapid time course is consistent with the expected rate of diffusion of transmitter through a fusion pore of 300 pS. Each large vesicle contains around 15,000–300,000 molecules of serotonin. Each small vesicle contains approximately 5000 molecules of serotonin. (From Bruns and Jahn 1995.)

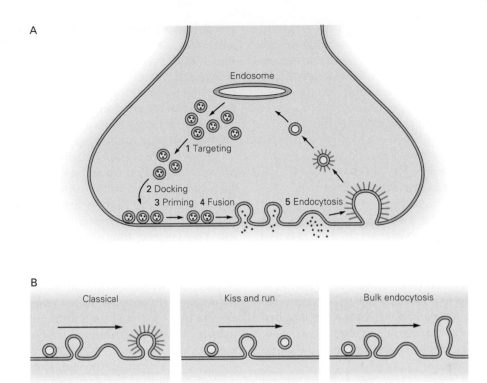

Figure 14-12 The cycling of synaptic vesicles at nerve terminals involves several distinct steps.

A. Free vesicles must be *targeted* to the active zone (**1**) and then dock at the active zone (**2**). The docked vesicles must become primed so that they can undergo exocytosis (**3**). In response to a rise in Ca^{2+} the vesicles undergo fusion and release their contents (**4**). The fused vesicle membrane is taken up into the interior of the cell by endocytosis (**5**). The endocytosed vesicles then fuse with the endosome, an internal membrane compartment. After processing, new synaptic vesicles bud off the endosome, completing the recycling process.

B. Retrieval of vesicles after exocytosis is thought to occur via three distinct mechanisms. In the first, **classical pathway** excess membrane is retrieved by means of clathrin-coated pits. These coated pits concentrate certain intramembranous parti-cles into small packages. The pits are found throughout the terminal except at the active zones. As the plasma membrane enlarges during exocytosis, more membrane invaginations are coated on the cytoplasmic surface. (The path of the coated pits is shown by arrows after step 5.) This pathway may be important at normal to high rates of release. In the **kiss-and-run pathway** the vesicle does not completely integrate itself into the plasma membrane. This corresponds to release through the fusion pore. This pathway may predominate at lower to normal release rates. In the **bulk endocytosis pathway** excess membrane reenters the terminal by budding from uncoated pits. These uncoated cisternae are formed primarily at the active zones. This pathway may be reserved for retrieval after very high rates of release and may not be used during the usual functioning of the synapse. (Adapted from Schweizer et al. 1995.)

Although the number of vesicles in a nerve terminal does decrease transiently during release, the total amount of membrane in vesicles, cisternae, and plasma membrane remains constant, indicating that membrane is retrieved from the surface membrane into the internal organelles. How the synaptic vesicles are recycled has not yet been resolved, but the process is known to involve clathrin-coating of the vesicle and the protein dynamin (Chapter 4 and below) and is thought to be similar to known mechanisms in epithelial cells (Figure 14-12). According to this view, the excess membrane from synaptic vesicles that have undergone exocytosis is recycled through endocytosis into an intracellular organelle called the endosome. Endocytosis and recycling takes about 30 seconds to one minute to be completed.

More rapid components of membrane recovery have been detected with capacitance measurements. Importantly, the rate of membrane recovery appears to depend on the extent of stimulation and exocytosis. With relatively weak stimuli that release only a few vesicles, membrane retrieval is rapid and occurs within a few seconds (for example, see Figure 14-9B). Stronger stimuli that release more vesicles lead to a slowing of membrane recovery. The fastest form of vesicle cycling involves the release of transmitter through the transient opening and closing of the fusion pore without full membrane fusion. The advantage of such "kiss-and-run" release is that it rapidly recycles the vesicle for subsequent release because it requires only closure of the fusion pore. Thus, different types of retrieval processes may operate under different conditions (Figure 14-12).

A Variety of Proteins Are Involved in the Vesicular Release of Transmitter

What is the nature of the molecular machinery that drives vesicles to cluster near synapses, to dock at active zones, to fuse with the membrane in response to Ca^{2+} influx, and then to recycle? Proteins have been identified that are thought to (1) restrain the vesicles so as to prevent their accidental mobilization, (2) target the freed vesicles to the active zone, (3) dock the targeted vesicles at the active zone and prime them for fusion, (4) allow fusion and exocytosis, and (5) retrieve the fused membrane by endocytosis (Figure 14-13).

We first consider proteins involved in restraint and mobilization. The vesicles outside the active zone represent a reserve pool of transmitter. They do not move about freely in the terminal but rather are restrained or anchored to a network of cytoskeletal filaments by the synapsins, a family of four proteins (Ia, Ib, IIa, and IIb). Of these four, synapsins Ia and Ib are the best studied. These two proteins are substrates for both the cAMP-dependent protein kinase and the Ca^{2+}/calmodulin-dependent kinase. When synapsin I is not phosphorylated, it is thought to immobilize synaptic vesicles by linking them to actin filaments and other components of the cytoskeleton. When the nerve terminal is depolarized and Ca^{2+} enters, synapsin I is thought to become phosphorylated by the Ca^{2+}/calmodulin-dependent protein kinase. Phosphorylation frees the vesicles from the cytoskeletal constraint, allowing them to move into the active zone (Figure 14-14).

The targeting of synaptic vesicles to docking sites for release may be carried out by Rab3A and Rab3C, two members of a class of small proteins, related to the ras proto-oncogene superfamily, that bind GTP and hydrolyze it to GDP and inorganic phosphate (Figure 14-14B). These Rab proteins bind to synaptic vesicles through a hydrophobic hydrocarbon group that is covalently attached to the carboxy terminus of the Rab protein. Hydrolysis of the GTP bound to Rab, converting it to GDP, may be important for the efficient targeting of synaptic vesicles to their appropriate sites of docking. During exocytosis the Rab proteins are released from the synaptic vesicles into the cytoplasm.

Following the targeting of a vesicle to its release site a complex set of interactions occurs between proteins in the synaptic vesicle membrane and proteins in the presynaptic membrane. Such interactions are thought to complete the docking of vesicles and to prime them so they are ready to undergo fusion in response to Ca^{2+} influx. Similar interactions are important for exocytosis in all cells, not only in the synaptic terminals of neurons.

As we have seen in Chapter 4, all secretory proteins are synthesized on ribosomes and injected into the lumen of the endoplasmic reticulum (ER). When these proteins leave the ER they are targeted to the Golgi apparatus in vesicles formed from the membrane of the ER. The vesicles then dock and fuse with the Golgi membrane, discharging their protein into the lumen of the Golgi, where the protein is modified. Other vesicles shuttle the secretory protein between the cis and the trans compartments (the different cisternae) of the Golgi apparatus until the protein becomes fully modified and mature. The mature protein is packaged in vesicles that bud off the Golgi and migrate to the cell surface, where the protein is released through exocytosis. This type of release is constitutive (that is the release is continuous and occurs independently of Ca^{2+}) in contrast to regulated release, which occurs at synapses in response to Ca^{2+} entry into the presynaptic terminal.

One prominent hypothesis for how membrane vesicles are docked and readied for exocytosis has been proposed by James Rothman, Richard Scheller, and Reinhard Jahn. According to this theory, specific integral proteins in the vesicle membrane (vesicle-SNARES, or v-SNARES) bind to specific receptor proteins in the target membrane (target membrane or t-SNARE) (Figure 14-15). In the brain two t-SNARES have been identified: syntaxin, a nerve terminal integral membrane protein, and SNAP-25, a peripheral membrane protein of 25 kDa mass. In the synaptic vesicle the integral membrane protein VAMP (or synaptobrevin) has been identified as the v-SNARE.

The importance of the SNARE proteins in synaptic transmission is emphasized by the finding that all three proteins are targets of various clostridial neurotoxins. All of these toxins act by inhibiting synaptic transmission. One such toxin, tetanus toxin, a zinc endoprotease, specifically cleaves VAMP. Three other zinc endoproteases, botulinum toxins A, B, and C, specifically cleave SNAP-25, VAMP, and syntaxin, respectively. VAMP has the additional feature that it resembles a viral fusion peptide.

Reconstitution studies of purified proteins in lipid vesicles indicate that VAMP, syntaxin, and SNAP-25 may form the minimal functional unit that mediates membrane fusion. Moreover a detailed structural model

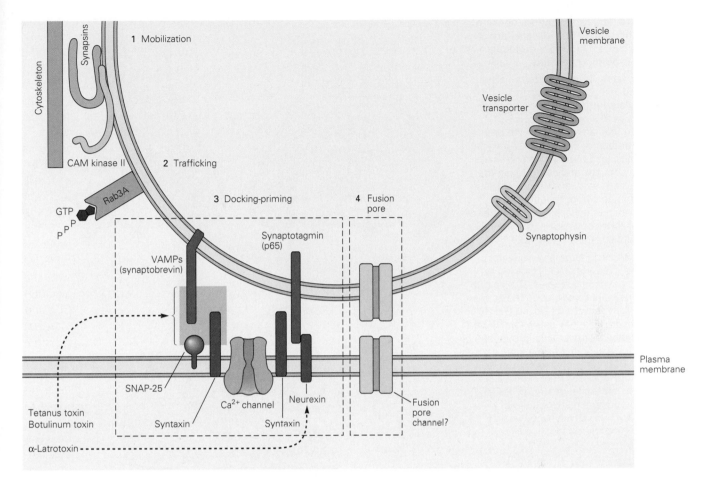

Figure 14-13 This diagram depicts characterized synaptic vesicle proteins and some of their postulated receptors and functions. Separate compartments are assumed for (**1**) storage (where vesicles are tethered to the cytoskeleton), (**2**) trafficking and targeting of vesicles to active zones, (**3**) the docking of vesicles at active zones and their priming for release, and (**4**) release. Some of these proteins represent the targets for neurotoxins that act by modifying transmitter release. VAMP (synaptobrevin), SNAP-25, and syntaxin are the targets for tetanus and botulinum toxins, two zinc-dependent metalloproteases, and are cleaved by these enzymes. α-Latrotoxin, a spider toxin that generates massive vesicle depletion and transmitter release, binds to the neurexins. **1.** Synapsins are vesicle-associated proteins that are thought to mediate interactions between the synaptic vesicle and the cytoskeletal elements of the nerve ter-

minal. **2.** The Rab proteins (see Figure 14-14B) appear to be involved in vesicle trafficking within the cell and also in targeting of vesicles within the nerve terminal. **3.** The docking, fusion, and release of vesicles appears to involve distinct interactions between vesicle proteins and proteins of the nerve terminal plasma membrane: VAMP (synaptobrevin) and synaptotagmin (p65) on the vesicle membrane, and syntaxins and neurexins on the nerve terminal membrane. Arrows indicate potential interactions suggested on the basis of in vitro studies. **4.** The identity of the vesicle and plasma membrane proteins that comprise the fusion pore remains unclear. Synaptophysin, an integral membrane protein in synaptic vesicles, is phosphorylated by tyrosine kinases and may regulate release. Vesicle transporters are involved in accumulation of neurotransmitter within the synaptic vesicle (see Chapter 15).

has been proposed for how these proteins interact to promote membrane fusion (Figure 14-15B).

The ternary complex of VAMP, syntaxin, and SNAP-25 is extraordinarily stable. For efficient vesicle recycling to occur this complex must be disassembled by the binding of two soluble cytoplasmic proteins: the *N*-ethylmaleimide-sensitive fusion (NSF) protein

and the soluble NSF attachment protein (SNAP—this protein is unrelated to SNAP-25; the similar names are coincidental). The v-SNARES and t-SNARES serve as receptors for SNAP (hence their name *SNAP receptors*), which then binds NSF. The NSF is an ATPase, utilizing the energy released upon hydrolysis of ATP to unravel the SNARE assembly.

Figure 14-14 The mobilization, docking, and function of synaptic vesicles are controlled by Ca^{2+} and low-molecular-weight GTP-binding proteins.

A. Synaptic vesicles in nerve terminals are sequestered in a *storage compartment* where they are tethered to the cytoskeleton, as well as in a *releasable* compartment where they are docked to the presynaptic membrane. Entry of Ca^{2+} into the nerve terminal leads to the opening of the fusion pore complex and neurotransmitter release. Calcium entry also frees vesicles from the storage compartment through phosphorylation of synapsins, thus increasing the availability of vesicles for docking at the presynaptic plasma membrane.

B. The Rab3A cycle targets vesicles to their release sites. Rab3A complexed to GTP binds to synaptic vesicles. During the targeting of synaptic vesicles to the active zone, Rab3A hydrolyzes its bound GTP to GDP. GTP hydrolysis may serve to make a reversible reaction irreversible, preventing vesicles from leaving the active zone once they arrive. During fusion and exocytosis, Rab3A-GDP dissociates from the vesicle. There is then an exchange of GTP for GDP. This is followed by the association of Rab3A-GTP with a new synaptic vesicle, thus completing the cycle.

A Calcium control of vesicle fusion and mobilization

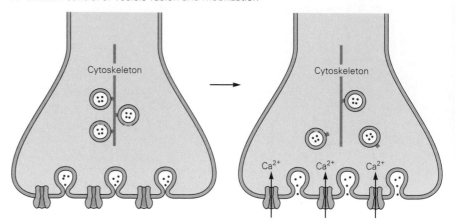

B Rab3A control of vesicle fusion

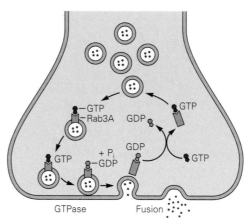

One additional integral membrane protein of the synaptic vesicle, thought to be important for exocytosis, is *synaptotagmin* (or p65). Synaptotagmin contains two domains (the C2 domains) homologous to the regulatory region of protein kinase C. The C2 domains bind to phospholipids in a calcium-dependent manner. This property suggests that synaptotagmin might insert into the presynaptic phospholipid bilayer in response to Ca^{2+} influx, thus serving as the calcium sensor for exocytosis (see Figure 14-12). Synaptotagmin may also function as a v-SNARE since it binds syntaxin and a SNAP isoform.

Several mutant animals that lack synaptotagmin have been created to test this protein's role in synaptic transmission. Based on these experiments two models have been proposed for the role of synaptotagmin. According to one view synaptotagmin acts as a fusion clamp or negative regulator of release (preventing exocytosis in the absence of Ca^{2+}). In this view, the influx of Ca^{2+} rapidly frees this clamp, allowing synchronous re-

lease. This hypothesis is attractive since the same machinery involved in synaptic vesicle fusion (the SNAP-SNARE complex) also functions in constitutive release that is independent of external Ca^{2+}. This model is based on results from experiments with *Drosophila* and nematode mutants lacking synaptotagmin, which show greatly impaired synaptic transmission in response to an action potential in the presynaptic terminal. Moreover, in *Drosophila* the rate of spontaneous miniature end-plate potentials is increased, suggesting that synaptotagmin has an inhibitory role.

The second hypothesis is that synaptotagmin serves as a positive regulator of release, actively promoting vesicle fusion. This view is based on the observation that in mutant mice that lack a major isoform of synaptotagmin, fast synaptic transmission is blocked without an increase in spontaneous release. Since there are several isoforms of synaptotagmin in mammals, but only one isoform in invertebrates, it is possible that the different mammalian isoforms have different roles: One

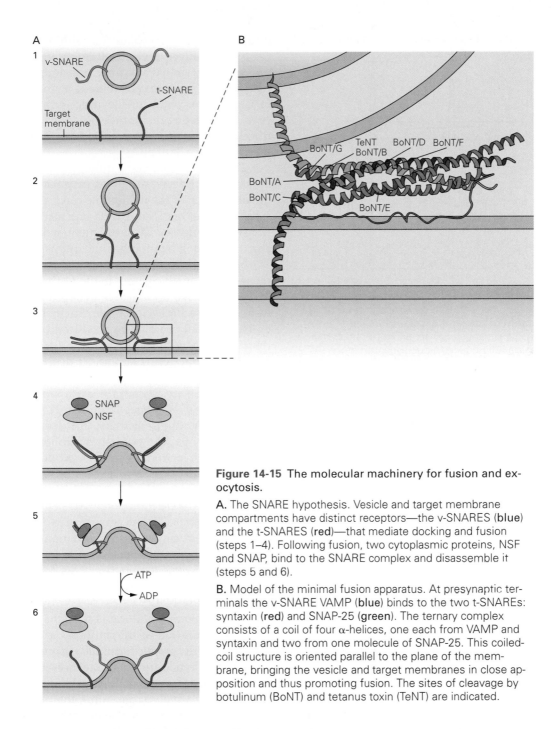

Figure 14-15 The molecular machinery for fusion and exocytosis.

A. The SNARE hypothesis. Vesicle and target membrane compartments have distinct receptors—the v-SNARES (**blue**) and the t-SNARES (**red**)—that mediate docking and fusion (steps 1–4). Following fusion, two cytoplasmic proteins, NSF and SNAP, bind to the SNARE complex and disassemble it (steps 5 and 6).

B. Model of the minimal fusion apparatus. At presynaptic terminals the v-SNARE VAMP (**blue**) binds to the two t-SNAREs: syntaxin (**red**) and SNAP-25 (**green**). The ternary complex consists of a coil of four α-helices, one each from VAMP and syntaxin and two from one molecule of SNAP-25. This coiled-coil structure is oriented parallel to the plane of the membrane, bringing the vesicle and target membranes in close apposition and thus promoting fusion. The sites of cleavage by botulinum (BoNT) and tetanus toxin (TeNT) are indicated.

may mediate regulated fast release and another may control constitutive release.

Synaptotagmin may also play an additional role in endocytosis. Following exocytosis the fused membrane is retrieved by endocytosis. Excess membrane anywhere in the terminal except at the active zone leads to the formation of a pit that is coated with clathrin. The binding of clathrin to the membrane is enhanced by certain adaptor proteins. Synaptotagmin serves as a receptor

for the clathrin adaptor protein AP-2. The clathrin coat forms a regular lattice around the pit, which finally pinches off as a small coated vesicle. The pinching off of the vesicle depends on a cytoplasmic GTPase called dynamin, which forms a constricting helical ring around the neck of the vesicle during endocytosis. A *Drosophila* mutant defective in dynamin is impaired in synaptic transmission owing to an inhibition of vesicle recycling.

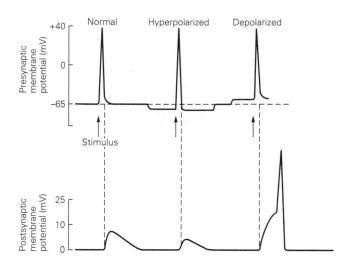

Figure 14-16 Changes in membrane potential of the presynaptic terminal affect the intracellular concentration of Ca^{2+} and thus the amount of transmitter released. When the presynaptic membrane is at its normal resting potential, an action potential (**top trace**) produces a postsynaptic potential of a given size (**bottom**). Hyperpolarizing the presynaptic terminal by 10 mV prior to an action potential decreases the steady state Ca^{2+} influx, so that the same-size action potential produces a smaller postsynaptic potential. In contrast, *depolarizing* the presynaptic neuron by 10 mV *increases* the steady state Ca^{2+} influx, so that the same-size action potential produces a postsynaptic potential large enough to trigger an action potential in the postsynaptic cell.

The Amount of Transmitter Released Can Be Modulated by Regulating the Amount of Calcium Influx During the Action Potential

The effectiveness of chemical synapses can be modified for both short and long periods. This modifiability, or *synaptic plasticity*, is controlled by two types of processes: (1) processes within the neuron that result from changes in the resting potential or the firing of action potentials and (2) extrinsic processes, such as the synaptic input from other neurons.

Long-term changes in chemical synaptic action are crucial to development and learning, and we consider these changes in detail later in the book. Here we shall first discuss the short-term changes—changes in the amount of transmitter released due to either changes within the presynaptic terminal or extrinsic factors.

Intrinsic Cellular Mechanisms Regulate the Concentration of Free Calcium

As we saw at the beginning of this chapter, transmitter release depends strongly on the intracellular Ca^{2+} concentration. Thus, mechanisms within the presynaptic neuron that affect the concentration of free Ca^{2+} in the presynaptic terminal also affect the amount of transmitter released. In some cells there is a small steady influx of Ca^{2+} through the presynaptic terminal membrane, even at the resting membrane potential. This Ca^{2+} flows through the L-type voltage-gated Ca^{2+} channels, which inactivate little, if at all.

The steady state Ca^{2+} influx is enhanced by depolarization and decreased by hyperpolarization. A slight depolarization of the membrane can increase the steady state influx of Ca^{2+} and thus enhance the amount of transmitter released by subsequent action potentials. A slight hyperpolarization has the opposite effect (Figure 14-16). By altering the amount of Ca^{2+} that flows into the terminal, small changes in the resting membrane potential can make an effective synapse inoperative or a weak synapse highly effective. Such changes in membrane potential can also be produced by other neurons releasing transmitter at axo-axonic synapses that regulate presynaptic ion channels, as described later. They can also be produced experimentally by injecting current.

Synaptic effectiveness can also be altered in most nerve cells by intense activity. In these cells a high-frequency train of action potentials is followed by a period during which action potentials produce successively larger postsynaptic potentials. High-frequency stimulation of the presynaptic neuron (which in some cells can generate 500–1000 action potentials per second) is called *tetanic stimulation*. The increase in size of the postsynaptic potentials during tetanic stimulation is called *potentiation;* the increase that persists after tetanic stimulation is called *posttetanic potentiation*. This enhancement usually lasts several minutes, but it can persist for an hour or more (Figure 14-17).

Posttetanic potentiation is thought to result from a transient saturation of the various Ca^{2+} buffering systems in the presynaptic terminals, primarily the smooth endoplasmic reticulum and mitochondria. This leads to a temporary excess of Ca^{2+}, called *residual* Ca^{2+}, the result of the relatively large influx that accompanies the train of action potentials. The increase in the resting concentration of free Ca^{2+} enhances synaptic transmission for many minutes or longer by activating certain enzymes that are sensitive to the enhanced levels of resting Ca^{2+}, for example, the Ca^{2+}/calmodulin-dependent protein kinase. Activation of such calcium-dependent enzymatic pathways is thought to increase the mobilization of synaptic vesicles in the terminals, for example through phosphorylation of the synapsins. Phosphorylation of synapsin allows synaptic vesicles to be freed from their cytoskeletal restraint and to be mobilized into and docked at release sites. As a result, each action potential sweeping into the terminals of the presynaptic neuron will release more transmitter than before.

Here then is a simple kind of cellular memory! The presynaptic cell stores information about the history of its activity in the form of residual Ca^{2+} in its terminals. The storage of biochemical information in the nerve cell, after a brief period of activity, leads to a strengthening of the presynaptic connection that persists for many minutes. In Chapter 62 we shall see how posttetanic potentiation at certain synapses is followed by an even longer-lasting process (also initiated by Ca^{2+} influx), called *long-term potentiation*, which can last for many hours or even days.

Axo-axonic Synapses on Presynaptic Terminals Regulate Intracellular Free Calcium

Synapses are formed on axon terminals as well as the cell body and dendrites of neurons (see Chapter 12). Whereas axosomatic synaptic actions affect all branches of the postsynaptic neuron's axon (because they affect the probability that the neuron will fire an action potential), axo-axonic actions selectively control individual branches of the axon. One important action of axo-axonic synapses is to control Ca^{2+} influx into the presynaptic terminals of the postsynaptic cell, either depressing or enhancing transmitter release.

As we saw in Chapter 12, when one neuron hyperpolarizes the cell body (or dendrites) of another, it decreases the likelihood that the postsynaptic cell will fire; this action is called *postsynaptic inhibition*. In contrast, when a neuron contacts the axon terminal of another cell, it can reduce the amount of transmitter that will be released by the second cell onto a third cell; this action is called *presynaptic inhibition* (Figure 14-18A). Likewise, axo-axonic synaptic actions can increase the amount of transmitter released by the postsynaptic cell; this action is called *presynaptic facilitation* (Figure 14-18B). For reasons that are not well understood, presynaptic modulation usually occurs early in sensory pathways.

The best-analyzed mechanisms of presynaptic inhibition and facilitation are in the neurons of invertebrates and in the mechanoreceptor neurons (whose cell bodies lie in dorsal root ganglia) of vertebrates. Three mechanisms for presynaptic inhibition have been identified in these cells. One is mediated by activation of metabotropic receptors that leads to the simultaneous closure of Ca^{2+} channels and opening of voltage-gated K^+ channels, which both decreases the influx of Ca^{2+} and enhances repolarization of the cell. The second mechanism is mediated by activation of ionotropic GABA-gated Cl^- channels, resulting in an increased

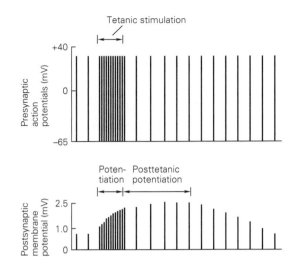

Figure 14-17 A high rate of stimulation of the presynaptic neuron produces a gradual increase in the amplitude of the postsynaptic potentials. This enhancement in the strength of the synapse represents storage of information about previous activity, an elementary form of memory. The time scale of the experimental record here has been compressed (each presynaptic and postsynaptic potential appears as a simple line indicating its amplitude). To establish a baseline (control), the presynaptic neuron is stimulated at a rate of 1 per second, producing a postsynaptic potential of about 1 mV. The presynaptic neuron is then stimulated for several seconds at a higher rate of 5 per second. During this *tetanic stimulation* the postsynaptic potential increases in size, a phenomenon known as *potentiation*. After several seconds of stimulation the presynaptic neuron is returned to the control rate of firing (1 per second). However, the postsynaptic potentials remain enhanced for minutes, and in some cells for several hours. This persistent increase is called *posttetanic potentiation*.

conductance to Cl^-, which decreases (or short-circuits) the amplitude of the action potential in the presynaptic terminal. As a result, less depolarization is produced and fewer Ca^{2+} channels are activated by the action potential. The third mechanism is also mediated by activation of metabotropic receptors and involves direct inhibition of the transmitter release machinery, independent of Ca^{2+} influx. This is thought to work by decreasing the Ca^{2+} sensitivity of one or more steps involved in the release process.

Presynaptic facilitation, in contrast, can be caused by an enhanced influx of Ca^{2+}. In certain molluscan neurons serotonin acts through cAMP-dependent protein phosphorylation to close K^+ channels, thereby broadening the action potential and allowing the Ca^{2+} influx to persist for a longer period (see Chapter 13). In

A Presynaptic inhibition

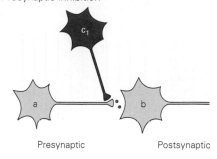

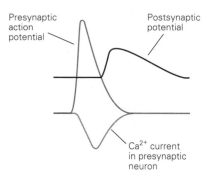

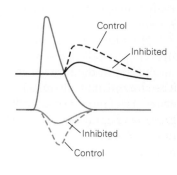

B Presynaptic facilitation

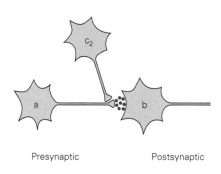

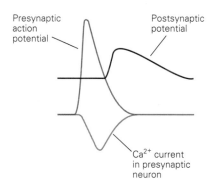

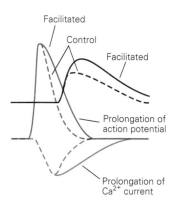

Figure 14-18 Axo-axonic synapses can inhibit or facilitate transmitter release by the postsynaptic cell.

A. An inhibitory neuron (c_1) contacts the terminal of a second presynaptic neuron (a). Release of transmitter by cell c_1 depresses the Ca^{2+} current in cell a, thereby reducing the amount of transmitter released by cell a. As a result, the postsynaptic potential in cell b is depressed.

B. A facilitating neuron (c_2) contacts the terminal of a second presynaptic neuron (a). Release of transmitter by cell c_2 depresses the K^+ current in cell a, thereby prolonging the action potential in cell a and increasing the Ca^{2+} influx through voltage-gated Ca^{2+} channels. As a result, the postsynaptic potential in cell b is increased.

addition, the cAMP-dependent protein kinase also acts directly on the machinery of exocytosis to enhance release in a manner that is independent of the amount of Ca^{2+} influx. In other cells activation of presynaptic ligand-gated channels, such as nicotinic ACh receptors or the kainate type of glutamate receptors, increases transmitter release, possibly by depolarizing the presynaptic terminals and enhancing Ca^{2+} influx.

Thus, regulation of the free Ca^{2+} concentration in the presynaptic terminal is an important factor in a variety of mechanisms that endow chemical synapses with plastic capabilities. Although we know a fair amount about short-term changes in synaptic effectiveness—changes that last minutes and hours—we are only beginning to learn about changes that persist days, weeks, and longer. These long-term changes often require alteration in gene expression and growth of synapses in ad-

dition to alteration in Ca^{2+} influx and enhancement of release from preexisting synapses.

An Overall View

In his book *Ionic Channels of Excitable Membranes*, Bertil Hille summarizes the importance of calcium in neuronal function:

Electricity is used to gate channels and channels are used to make electricity. However, the nervous system is not primarily an electrical device. Most excitable cells ultimately translate their electrical excitation into another form of activity. As a broad generalization, excitable cells translate their electricity into action by Ca^{2+} fluxes modulated by voltage-sensitive Ca^{2+} channels. Calcium ions are intracellular messengers capable of activating many cell functions. Calcium channels. . . serve as the only link to transduce depolarization into all the nonelectrical activities controlled by excitation. Without Ca^{2+} channels our nervous system would have no outputs.

Neither Na^+ influx nor K^+ efflux is required to release neurotransmitters at a synapse. Only Ca^{2+}, which enters the cell through voltage-gated channels in the presynaptic terminal, is essential. Synaptic delay—the time between the onset of the action potential and the release of transmitter—largely reflects the time it takes for voltage-gated Ca^{2+} channels to open and for Ca^{2+} to trigger the discharge of transmitter from synaptic vesicles.

Transmitter is packaged in vesicles and each vesicle contains approximately 5000 transmitter molecules. Release of transmitter from a single vesicle results in a quantal synaptic potential. Spontaneous miniature synaptic potentials result from the spontaneous fusion of single synaptic vesicles. Synaptic potentials evoked by nerve stimulation are composed of integral multiples of the quantal potential. Increasing the extracellular Ca^{2+} does not change the size of the quantal synaptic potential. Rather, it increases the probability that a vesicle will discharge its transmitter. As a result, there is an increase in the number of vesicles released and a larger postsynaptic potential.

Rapid freezing experiments have shown that the vesicles fuse with the presynaptic plasma membrane in the vicinity of the active zone. Freeze-fracture studies have also revealed rows of large intramembranous particles along the active zone that are thought to be Ca^{2+} channels. These highly localized channels may be responsible for the rapid increase, as much as a thousand-fold, in the Ca^{2+} concentration of the axon terminal during an action potential. One hypothesis about how Ca^{2+} triggers vesicle fusion is that this ion permits the formation of a fusion pore that traverses both the vesicle and the plasma membrane. This pore allows the contents of the vesicle to be released into the extracellular space and may further dilate so that the entire vesicle fuses with the presynaptic plasma membrane.

Calcium also regulates the mobilization of the synaptic vesicles to the active zone. These vesicles appear to be bound to the cytoskeleton by synapsin, and Ca^{2+} is thought to free the vesicles by activating the Ca^{2+}/calmodulin–dependent protein kinase, which phosphorylates the synapsins.

Several molecular candidates have been identified that could account for the two other components of release: targeting and docking. Targeting is thought to be mediated by the small GTP-binding Rab3A and Rab3C proteins. Docking and fusion is thought to involve the synaptic vesicle v-SNARE VAMP (or synaptobrevin) and the plasma membrane t-SNARES, syntaxin and SNAP-25. Calcium binding to synaptotagmin may actively promote vesicle fusion or remove an inhibitory clamp that normally blocks fusion.

Finally, the amount of transmitter released from a neuron is not fixed but can be modified by both intrinsic and extrinsic modulatory processes. High-frequency stimulation produces an increase in transmitter release called posttetanic potentiation. This (intrinsic) potentiation, which lasts a few minutes, is caused by Ca^{2+} left in the terminal after the large Ca^{2+} influx that occurs during the train of action potentials. Tonic depolarization or hyperpolarization of the presynaptic neuron can also modulate release by altering steady state Ca^{2+} influx. The extrinsic action of neurotransmitters on receptors in the axon terminal of another neuron can facilitate or inhibit transmitter release by altering the steady state level of resting Ca^{2+} or the Ca^{2+} influx during the action potential.

In the next chapter we shall carry our discussion of synaptic transmission further by examining the nature of the transmitter molecules that are used for chemical transmission.

Eric R. Kandel
Steven A. Siegelbaum

Selected Readings

Dunlap K, Luebke JI, Turner TJ. 1995. Exocytotic Ca^{2+} channels in mammalian central neurons. Trends Neurosci 18:89–98.

Hanson PI, Heuser JE, Jahn R. 1997. Neurotransmitter release—four years of SNARE complexes. Curr Opin Neurobiol 7(3):310–315.

Jessell TM, Kandel ER. 1993. Synaptic transmission: a bidirectional and self-modifiable form of cell-cell communication. Cell 72:1–30.

Katz B. 1969. *The Release of Neural Transmitter Substances.* Springfield, IL: Thomas.

Lindau M, Almers W. 1995. Structure and function of fusion pores in exocytosis and ectoplasmic membrane fusion. Curr Opin Cell Biol 7:509–517.

Matthews G. 1996. Synaptic exocytosis and endocytosis: capacitance measurements. Curr Opin Neurobiol 6(3):358–364.

Schweizer FE, Betz H, Augustine GJ. 1995. From vesicle

docking to endocytosis: intermediate reactions of exocytosis. Neuron 14(4):689–696.

Smith SJ, Augustine GJ. 1988. Calcium ions, active zones and synaptic transmitter release. Trends Neurosci 11:458–464.

Südhof TC. 1995. The synaptic vesicle cycle: a cascade of protein-protein interactions. Nature 375:645–653.

References

Alberts B, Bray D, Lewis J, Raff M, Roberts K, Watson JD. 1994. *Molecular Biology of the Cell*, 3rd ed. New York: Garland.

Almers W, Tse FW. 1990. Transmitter release from synapses: Does a preassembled fusion pore initiate exocytosis? Neuron 4:813–818.

Bähler M, Greengard P. 1987. Synapsin I bundles F-actin in a phosphorylation-dependent manner. Nature 326:704–707.

Baker PF, Hodgkin AL, Ridgway EB. 1971. Depolarization and calcium entry in squid giant axons. J Physiol (Lond) 218:709–755.

Boyd IA, Martin AR. 1956. The end-plate potential in mammalian muscle. J Physiol (Lond) 132:74–91.

Breckenridge LJ, Almers W. 1987. Currents through the fusion pore that forms during exocytosis of a secretory vesicle. Nature 328:814–817.

Bruns D, Jahn R. 1995. Real-time measurement of transmitter release from single synaptic vesicles. Nature 377:62–65.

Couteaux R, Pecot-Dechavassine M. 1970. Vésicules synaptiques et poches au niveau des "zones actives" de la jonction neuromusculaire. C R Hebd Séances Acad Sci Sér D Sci Nat 271:2346–2349.

Del Castillo J, Katz B. 1954. The effect of magnesium on the activity of motor nerve endings. J Physiol (Lond) 124:553–559.

Erulkar SD, Rahamimoff R. 1978. The role of calcium ions in tetanic and post-tetanic increase of miniature end-plate potential frequency. J Physiol (Lond) 278:501–511.

Faber DS, Korn H. 1988. Unitary conductance changes at teleost Mauthner cell glycinergic synapses: a voltage-clamp and pharmacologic analysis. J Neurophysiol 60:1982–1999.

Fatt P, Katz B. 1952. Spontaneous subthreshold activity at motor nerve endings. J Physiol (Lond) 117:109–128.

Fawcett DW. 1981. *The Cell*, 2nd ed. Philadelphia: Saunders.

Fernandez JM, Neher E, Gomperts BD. 1984. Capacitance measurements reveal stepwise fusion events in degranulating mast cells. Nature 312:453–455.

Geppert M, Sudhof TC. 1998. RAB3 and synaptotagmin: the yin and yang of synaptic membrane fusion. Annu Rev Neurosci 21:75–95.

Heuser JE, Reese TS. 1977. Structure of the synapse. In: ER Kandel (ed). *Handbook of Physiology: A Critical, Comprehensive Presentation of Physiological Knowledge and Concepts*, Sect. 1, *The Nervous System*. Vol. 1, *Cellular Biology of Neurons*, Part 1, pp. 261–294. Bethesda, MD: American Physiological Society.

Heuser JE, Reese TS. 1981. Structural changes in transmitter release at the frog neuromuscular junction. J Cell Biol 88:564–580.

Hille B. 1992. *Ionic Channels of Excitable Membranes*, 2nd ed. Sunderland, MA: Sinauer.

Hirning LD, Fox AP, McCleskey EW, Olivera BM, Thayer SA, Miller RJ, Tsien RW. 1988. Dominant role of N-type Ca^{2+} channels in evoked release of norepinephrine from sympathetic neurons. Science 239(4835):57–61.

Jones SW. 1998. Overview of voltage-dependent Ca channels. J Bionerg Biomembr 30(4):299–312.

Kandel ER. 1976. *The Cellular Basis of Behavior: An Introduction to Behavioral Neurobiology*. San Francisco: Freeman.

Kandel ER. 1981. Calcium and the control of synaptic strength by learning. Nature 293:697–700.

Katz B, Miledi R. 1967a. The study of synaptic transmission in the absence of nerve impulses. J Physiol (Lond) 192:407–436.

Katz B, Miledi R. 1967b. The timing of calcium action during neuromuscular transmission. J Physiol (Lond) 189:535–544.

Kelly RB. 1993. Storage and release of neurotransmitters. Cell 72:43–53.

Klein M, Shapiro E, Kandel ER. 1980. Synaptic plasticity and the modulation of the Ca^{2+} current. J Exp Biol 89:117–157.

Kretz R, Shapiro E, Connor J, Kandel ER. 1984. Post-tetanic potentiation, presynaptic inhibition, and the modulation of the free Ca^{2+} level in the presynaptic terminals. Exp Brain Res Suppl 9:240–283.

Kuffler SW, Nicholls JG, Martin AR. 1984. *From Neuron to Brain: A Cellular Approach to the Function of the Nervous System*, 2nd ed. Sunderland, MA: Sinauer.

Lawson D, Raff MC, Gomperts B, Fewtrell C, Gilula NB. 1977. Molecular events during membrane fusion. A study of exocytosis in rat peritoneal mast cells. Cell Biol 72:242–59.

Liley AW. 1956. The quantal components of the mammalian end-plate potential. J Physiol (Lond) 133:571–587.

Llinás RR. 1982. Calcium in synaptic transmission. Sci Am 247(4):56–65.

Llinás RR, Heuser JE. 1977. Depolarization-release coupling systems in neurons. Neurosci Res Progr Bull 15:555–687.

Llinás R, Steinberg IZ, Walton K. 1981. Relationship between presynaptic calcium current and postsynaptic potential in squid giant synapse. Biophys J 33:323–351.

Martin AR. 1977. Junctional transmission. II. Presynaptic mechanisms. In: ER Kandel (ed). *Handbook of Physiology: A Critical, Comprehensive Presentation of Physiological Knowledge and Concepts*, Sect. 1, *The Nervous System*. Vol. 1, *Cellular Biology of Neurons*, Part 1, pp. 329–355. Bethesda, MD: American Physiological Society.

Monck JR, Fernandez JM. 1992. The exocytotic fusion pore. J Cell Biol 119:1395–1404.

Neher E. 1993. Cell physiology. Secretion without full fusion. Nature 363:497–498.

Nicoll RA. 1982. Neurotransmitters can say more than just "yes" or "no." Trends Neurosci 5:369–374.

Peters A, Palay SL, Webster H deF. 1991. *The Fine Structure of the Nervous System: Neurons and Supporting Cells*, 3rd ed. Philadelphia: Saunders.

Redman S. 1990. Quantal analysis of synaptic potentials in neurons of the central nervous system. Physiol Rev 70:165–198.

Robitaille R, Adler EM, Charlton MP. 1990. Strategic location of calcium channels at transmitter release sites of frog neuromuscular synapses. Neuron 5:773–779.

Scheller RH. 1995. Membrane trafficking in the presynaptic nerve terminal. Neuron 14:893–897.

Smith SJ, Augustine GJ, Charlton MP. 1985. Transmission at voltage-clamped giant synapse of the squid: evidence for cooperativity of presynaptic calcium action. Proc Natl Acad Sci U S A 82:622–625.

Söllner T, Whiteheart SW, Brunner M, Erdjument-Bromage H, Geromanos S, Tempest P, Rothman JE. 1993. SNAP receptors implicated in vesicle targeting and fusion. Nature 362:318–324.

Spruce AE, Breckenridge LJ, Lee AK, Almers W. 1990. Properties of the fusion pore that forms during exocytosis of a mast cell secretory vesicle. Neuron 4:643–654.

Südhof TC, Czernik AJ, Kao H-T, Takei K, Johnston PA, Horiuchi A, Kanazir SD, Wagner MA, Perin MS, De Camilli P, Greengard P. 1989. Synapsins: mosaics of shared and individual domains in a family of synaptic vesicle phosphoproteins. Science 245:1474–1480.

Sutton RB, Fasshauer D, Jahn R, Brunger AT. 1998. Crystal structure of a SNARE complex involved in synaptic exocytosis at 2.4 A resolution. Nature 395(6700):347–353.

von Gersdorff H, Matthews G. 1994. Dynamics of synaptic vesicle fusion and membrane retrieval in synaptic terminals. Nature 367:735–739.

Weber T, Zemelman BV, McNew JA, Westermann B, Gmachl M, Parlati F, Sollner TH, Rothman JE. 1998. SNAREpins: minimal machinery for membrane fusion. Cell 92(6): 759–772.

Wernig A. 1972. Changes in statistical parameters during facilitation at the crayfish neuromuscular junction. J Physiol (Lond) 226:751–759.

Zucker RS. 1973. Changes in the statistics of transmitter release during facilitation. J Physiol (Lond) 229:787–810.

15

Neurotransmitters

C HEMICAL TRANSMISSION at synapses can be divided into four steps—two presynaptic and two post-synaptic. These steps are (1) the synthesis of a transmitter substance, (2) the storage and release of the transmitter, (3) the transmitter's interaction with a receptor in the postsynaptic membrane, and (4) the removal of transmitter from the synaptic cleft. In the previous chapter we considered steps 2 and 3, the release of transmitters and how they interact with postsynaptic receptors. We now turn to the initial and final steps of chemical synaptic transmission—the synthesis of the molecules used as transmitters and their removal from the synaptic cleft after synaptic action.

Chemical Messengers Must Fulfill Four Criteria to Be Considered Transmitters

Before considering the biochemical processes involved in synaptic transmission in detail, it is important to make clear what is meant by a *chemical transmitter*. The concept had become familiar by the early 1930s, after Otto Loewi demonstrated the release of acetylcholine (ACh) from vagus terminals in frog heart and Henry Dale reported his work on cholinergic and adrenergic transmission. The terms *cholinergic* and *adrenergic* were introduced to indicate that a neuron uses ACh or norepinephrine (or epinephrine) as neurotransmitter. Since that time many other substances have been discovered to act as transmitters. Furthermore, because of the work of Bernard Katz in the 1950s on quantal release (see Chapter 14), it is usually taken for granted that substances acting as transmitters are stored in vesicles at synapses and released by exocytosis. Nevertheless, some substances acknowledged as neurotransmitters are released into the synaptic cleft directly from the cytoplasm as well as by exocytosis. Thus, ideas about neurotransmitters have had to be continually modified to accommodate new information about the cell biology of neurons and the pharmacology of receptors.

As a first approximation, we can define a transmitter as a substance that is released at a synapse by one neuron and that affects a postsynaptic cell, either a neuron or effector organ, such as a muscle cell or gland, in a specific manner. As with many other operational con-

Table 15-1 Small-Molecule Transmitter Substances and Their Key Biosynthetic Enzymes

Transmitter	Enzymes	Activity
Acetylcholine	Choline acetyltransferase	Specific
Biogenic amines		
Dopamine	Tyrosine hydroxylase	Specific
Norepinephrine	Tyrosine hydroxylase and dopamine β-hydroxylase	Specific
Epinephrine	Tyrosine hydroxylase and dopamine β-hydroxylase	Specific
Serotonin	Tryptophan hydroxylase	Specific
Histamine	Histidine decarboxylase	Specificity uncertain
Amino acids		
γ-Aminobutyric acid	Glutamic acid decarboxylase	Probably specific
Glycine	Enzymes operating in general metabolism	Specific pathway undetermined
Glutamate	Enzymes operating in general metabolism	Specific pathway undetermined

cepts in biology, the concept of a transmitter is not precise. Typically, neurotransmitters differ from *hormones* in that the postsynaptic cell is close to the site of transmitter release, whereas hormones are released into the bloodstream to act on distant targets. Transmitters can act on targets that are at some distance from the site of release, however.

Transmitters also differ from *autocoids* in that a transmitter typically acts on a target other than the releasing neuron itself, whereas an autocoid acts on the cell from which it was released. Nevertheless, at some synapses many acknowledged transmitters activate not only receptors in the postsynaptic cell but also *autoreceptors,* receptors on the terminal from which the transmitter is released. Autoreceptors usually modulate synaptic transmission in progress, for example, by limiting further release of the transmitter. An important characteristic of neurotransmitters is that their effects are transient, lasting from milliseconds to minutes. Nevertheless, neurotransmitter action can result in long-term changes in target cells lasting hours or days.

Despite these difficulties in arriving at a comprehensive definition, a limited number of substances of low molecular weight are generally accepted as neurotransmitters. Even for these substances, however, it is often difficult to demonstrate a transmitter function at a particular synapse. Because of these difficulties, many neurobiologists believe that a substance should not be accepted as a neurotransmitter unless the following four criteria are met:

1. It is synthesized in the neuron.
2. It is present in the presynaptic terminal and is released in amounts sufficient to exert a defined action on the postsynaptic neuron or effector organ.
3. When administered exogenously (as a drug) in reasonable concentrations, it mimics the action of the endogenously released transmitter exactly (for example, it activates the same ion channels or second-messenger pathway in the postsynaptic cell).
4. A specific mechanism exists for removing it from its site of action (the synaptic cleft).

The nervous system makes use of two main classes of chemical substances for signaling: small-molecule transmitters and neuroactive peptides, which are short polymers of amino acids. Both classes of neurotransmitters are contained in vesicles, large and small. Neuropeptides are packaged in large dense-core vesicles, which release their contents by an exocytotic mechanism similar to that seen in secretory glands and mast cells. Small-molecule transmitters are packaged in small lucent vesicles, which release their contents through exocytosis at active zones closely associated with specific Ca^{2+} channels (see Chapter 14). Large dense-core vesicles can also contain small-molecule transmitters as well as neuropeptides. Most neurons contain both types of vesicles, but in different proportions. Small synaptic vesicles are characteristic of neurons that use acetylcholine, glutamine, GABA, and glycine as transmitters, while large dense-core vesicles are typical of catecholaminergic and serotonergic neurons. The adrenal medulla, often used as a model for studying exocytosis, contains only secretory granules that are similar to the large dense-core vesicles. Since dense-core vesicles can contain both small-molecule transmitters and neuropeptides, they are important in cotransmission, which is discussed later in this chapter.

Only a Few Small-Molecule Substances Act as Transmitters

Nine low-molecular-weight substances are generally accepted as neurotransmitters. Eight are amines; of these eight, seven are amino acids or their derivatives (Table 15-1). The ninth is ATP or its metabolites. The amine chemical messengers share many biochemical similarities. All are charged small molecules that are formed in relatively short biosynthetic pathways, and all are synthesized from precursors derived from the major carbohydrate substrates of intermediary metabolism. Like other pathways of intermediary metabolism, synthesis of these neurotransmitters is catalyzed by enzymes that, almost without exception, are cytosolic. ATP, which originates in mitochondria, is abundantly present throughout the cell.

As in any biosynthetic pathway, the overall synthesis of amine transmitters typically is regulated at one enzymatic reaction. The controlling enzyme often is characteristic of one type of neuron and usually is absent in other types of mature neurons.

Acetylcholine

Acetylcholine is the only accepted low-molecular-weight amine transmitter substance that is not an amino acid or derived directly from one. The biosynthetic pathway for ACh has only one enzymatic reaction, that catalyzed by choline acetyltransferase (step 1 in the reaction shown below). This transferase is the characteristic enzyme in ACh biosynthesis. Nervous tissue cannot synthesize choline, which is derived from the diet and delivered to neurons through the blood stream. The co-substrate, acetyl coenzyme A (acetyl CoA), participates in many general metabolic pathways and is not restricted to cholinergic neurons.

Acetylcholine is the transmitter used by the motor neurons of the spinal cord and therefore is released at all vertebrate neuromuscular junctions (Chapter 11). In the autonomic nervous system it is the transmitter for all preganglionic neurons and for parasympathetic postganglionic neurons as well (Chapter 49). It is used at many synapses throughout the brain. In particular, cell bodies synthesizing ACh are numerous in the nucleus basalis, which has widespread projections to the cerebral cortex.

Biogenic Amine Transmitters

The term *biogenic amine*, although chemically imprecise, has been used for decades to designate certain neurotransmitters. This group includes the catecholamines and serotonin. Histamine, an imidazole, is also often referred to as a biogenic amine, although its biochemistry is remote from the catecholamines and the indolamines.

The catecholamine transmitters—dopamine, norepinephrine, and epinephrine—are all synthesized from the essential amino acid tyrosine in a common biosynthetic pathway containing five enzymes: tyrosine hydroxylase, aromatic amino acid decarboxylase, dopamine β-hydroxylase, pteridine reductase, and phenylethanolamine-N-methyl transferase. Catecholamines have a catechol nucleus, a 3,4-dihydroxylated benzene ring.

The first enzyme, tyrosine hydroxylase (step 1, below), is an oxidase that converts tyrosine to L-dihydroxyphenylalanine (L-DOPA). This enzyme is rate-limiting for the synthesis of both dopamine and norepinephrine. It is present in all cells producing catecholamines and requires a reduced pteridine cofactor, Pt-2H, which is regenerated from pteridine (Pt) by another enzyme, pteridine reductase, which uses NADH (step 4, below). (This reductase is not specific to neurons.)

L-DOPA is next decarboxylated by a decarboxylase (step 2, below) to give dopamine and CO_2:

The third enzyme in the sequence, dopamine β-hydroxylase (step 3, below), converts dopamine to norepinephrine. Unlike all other enzymes in the biosynthetic pathways of small-molecule neurotransmitters, dopamine β-hydroxylase is membrane-associated. The hydroxylase is bound tightly to the inner surface of aminergic vesicles as a peripheral protein. Consequently, norepinephrine is synthesized within vesicles and is the only transmitter synthesized in this way.

In the central nervous system norepinephrine is

Norepinephrine

used as a transmitter by neurons whose cell bodies are located in the locus ceruleus, a nucleus of the brain stem with many complex modulatory functions (Chapter 61). Although these adrenergic neurons are relatively few in number, they project diffusely throughout the cortex, cerebellum, and spinal cord. In the peripheral nervous system norepinephrine is the transmitter in the postganglionic neurons of the sympathetic nervous system (Chapter 49).

In addition to these four catecholaminergic biosynthetic enzymes, a fifth enzyme, phenylethanolamine-N-methyl transferase (step 5, below), methylates norepinephrine to form epinephrine (adrenaline) in the adrenal medulla. This reaction requires S-adenosylmethionine as a methyl donor. The transferase is a cytoplasmic enzyme. Thus, for epinephrine to be formed, its immediate precursor, norepinephrine, must exit from vesicles into the cytoplasm. For epinephrine to be released, it must first be taken up into vesicles. A small number of neurons in the brain are thought to use epinephrine as a transmitter.

Epinephrine

Not all cells that release catecholamines express all five of these biosynthetic enzymes, although cells that release epinephrine do. Neurons that use norepinephrine do not express the methyltransferase, and neurons releasing dopamine do not express the transferase or dopamine β-hydroxylase. Thus, during development the expression of the genes encoding the enzymes that synthesize catecholamines can be regulated independently.

Of the four major dopaminergic tracts, three arise in the substantia nigra of the midbrain (Chapter 43). One, the nigrostriatal pathway, is important for the control of movement and is affected in Parkinson's disease and other disorders of movement (Chapter 43). The other two, the mesolimbic and mesocortical tracts, are important for affect, emotion, and motivation and are affected in schizophrenia (Chapter 60). The fourth dopaminergic

tract originates in the arcuate nucleus of the hypothalamus and projects to the pituitary gland, where it regulates secretion of hormones (Chapter 49).

The synthesis of biogenic amines is highly regulated. As a result, the amounts of transmitter available for release can keep up with wide variations in neuronal activity (Box 15-1).

Several other naturally occurring amines derived from catecholamines also may be transmitters. Tyramine and octopamine have both been found to be active in invertebrate nervous systems.

Serotonin (5-hydroxytryptamine or 5-HT) and the essential amino acid tryptophan from which it is derived belong to a group of aromatic compounds called indoles, with a five-member ring containing nitrogen joined to a benzene ring. Two enzymes are needed to synthesize serotonin: tryptophan (Try) hydroxylase (step 1, below), an oxidase similar to tyrosine hydroxylase, and 5-hydroxytryptophan (5-HTP) decarboxylase (step 2, below).

Serotonin

The controlling reaction is catalyzed by the first enzyme in the pathway, tryptophan hydroxylase. Tryptophan hydroxylase is similar to tyrosine hydroxylase not only in catalytic mechanism but also in amino acid sequence. The two enzymes are thought to stem from a common ancestral protein by gene reduplication, because the two hydroxylases are syntenic, that is, they are encoded by genes that are close together on the same chromosome (tryptophan hydroxylase, 11p15.3-p14; tyrosine hydroxylase, 11p15.5). The second enzyme in the pathway, 5-hydroxytryptophan decarboxylase, seems to be identical to L-DOPA decarboxylase. Enzymes with similar activity, L–aromatic amino acid decarboxylases, are present in many nonnervous tissues.

Cell bodies of serotonergic neurons are found in and around the midline raphe nuclei of the brain stem, which are involved in regulating attention and other complex cognitive functions. The projections of these cells (like those of noradrenergic cells in the locus ceruleus) are widely distributed throughout the brain and spinal cord. Serotonin (and possibly norepinephrine) is implicated in depression, the major disorder of mood (Chapter 61).

Histamine, like the essential amino acid histidine from which it is derived, contains a characteristic five-member ring with two nitrogen atoms. It has long been

Box 15-1 Norepinephrine Production Varies With Neuronal Activity

The production of norepinephrine is able to keep up with wide variations in neuronal activity because its synthesis is highly regulated. In autonomic ganglia the amount of norepinephrine is regulated transynaptically. With moderate activity in the presynaptic neurons, which are both cholinergic and peptidergic (VIP), the chemical messengers first induce short-term changes in second messengers in the postsynaptic adrenergic cells. These changes increase the supply of norepinephrine through the cAMP-dependent phosphorylation of tyrosine hydroxylase, the first enzyme in the biosynthetic pathway. Phosphorylation enhances the affinity of the hydroxylase for the pteridine cofactor and diminishes feedback inhibition by end products such as norepinephrine. In the short term, phosphorylation of tyrosine hydroxylase lasts only as long as cAMP remains elevated, since the phosphorylated hydroxylase is quickly dephosphorylated by protein phosphatases.

If the presynaptic activity is sufficiently prolonged, however, longer-term changes in the production of norepinephrine will occur. Severe stress to an animal results in intense presynaptic activity and persistent firing of the postsynaptic adrenergic neuron, placing a greater demand on transmitter synthesis. To meet this challenge, the tyrosine hydroxylase gene is induced to increase production of the enzyme protein. Elevated amounts of tyrosine hydroxylase are observed in the cell body within hours and at nerve endings days later.

The persistent release of chemical messengers from the presynaptic neuron leads to prolonged activation of the cAMP pathway in the adrenergic cell. The cAMP-dependent protein kinase phosphorylates not only existing tyrosine hydroxylase molecules, but also a transcriptional activator protein. Once phosphorylated, this transcription activator, called CREB (cAMP-recognition element–binding protein), binds to a specific DNA enhancer sequence (called the cAMP-recognition element, CRE), which lies upstream (5') to the gene for the hydroxylase. Binding of the transcriptional activator to CRE facilitates the binding of RNA polymerase to the gene's promotor and thus increases the frequency of transcriptional initiation. Historically, the induction of tyrosine hydroxylase was the first example of a neurotransmitter altering gene expression.

There is a high degree of similarity in amino acid sequence and in the nucleic acid sequences encoding three of the biosynthetic enzymes: tyrosine hydroxylase, dopamine β-hydroxylase, and phenylethanolamine-N-methyltransferase. This similarity suggests that the three enzymes arose from a common ancestral protein. Moreover, long-term changes in the synthesis of these enzymes are coordinately regulated in adrenergic neurons. At first, coordinate regulation suggested that the genes encoding these enzymes might be located sequentially along the same chromosome and be controlled by the same promoter, as are genes in a bacterial operon. But in humans the genes for the biosynthetic enzymes for norepinephrine are not located on the same chromosome. Therefore, coordinate regulation is likely to be achieved by parallel activation through similar transcription activator systems.

---

recognized as an autocoid, active when released from mast cells in the inflammatory reaction and in the control of vasculature, smooth muscle, and exocrine glands (eg, secretion of gastric juice of high acidity). Histamine is a transmitter in both invertebrates and vertebrates. It is concentrated in the hypothalamus, one of the centers for regulating the secretion of hormones (Chapter 49). It is synthesized from histidine by decarboxylation. Although not extensively analyzed, the decarboxylase (step 1, below) catalyzing this step appears to be characteristic of histaminergic neurons.

$$\text{Histidine} \xrightarrow{\;(1)\;} \underset{\text{Histamine}}{\left[\underset{HN \diagdown N}{}\right]} CH_2 - CH_2 - NH_2 + CO_2$$

Histamine also is a precursor of two dipeptides found in nervous tissue. A synthetase catalyzes the formation of carnosine (β-alanyl histidine) from the amino acid β-alanine and ATP. (Although β-alanine is normally present in tissues, only α–amino acids, with both carboxyl and amino groups on the α-carbon, can be incorporated into proteins.) The same enzyme forms homocarnosine (β-aminobutyrylhistidine) from histidine and γ-aminobutyric acid (GABA). The roles of these peptides are not known, but carnosine may have a special function in olfactory areas of the brain, where it is highly concentrated.

Amino Acid Transmitters

While acetylcholine and the biogenic amines are not intermediates in general biochemical pathways and are produced only in certain neurons, amino acids that function as neurotransmitters are also universal cellular constituents. Since they can be synthesized in neurons, none are essential amino acids. These include glutamate and glycine.

Glutamate, the neurotransmitter most frequently used throughout the central nervous system, is produced from α-ketoglutarate, an intermediate in the tricarboxylic acid cycle of intermediary metabolism, which we shall not review here. After it is released, glutamate (and other transmitters) is taken up from the synaptic cleft by both neurons and glia, as we shall see later in this chapter. The glutamate taken up by astrocytes is converted to glutamine by the enzyme glutamine synthase. This glutamine then diffuses back into neurons that use glutamate as a transmitter where it is hydrolyzed back to glutamate. A specific glutaminase, which is present at high concentrations in these neurons, is responsible for salvaging the molecule for reuse as a transmitter. Glutamate is excitatory at ionotropic receptors and modulatory at metabotropic receptors.

Glycine is the major transmitter in inhibitory interneurons of the spinal cord and is probably synthesized from serine. Its specific biosynthesis in neurons has not been studied, but its biosynthetic pathway in other tissues is well known. The amino acid γ-aminobutyric acid (GABA) is synthesized from glutamate in a reaction catalyzed by glutamic acid decarboxylase (step 1, below):

$$
\begin{array}{ccc}
\text{COOH} & & \text{COOH} \\
| & & | \\
\text{CH}_2 & & \text{CH}_2 \\
| & & | \\
\text{CH}_2 & \xrightarrow{\text{(1)}} & \text{CH}_2 \quad + \text{CO}_2 \\
| & & | \\
\text{H}_2\text{N}-\text{CH} & & \text{H}_2\text{N}-\text{CH}_2 \\
| & & \\
\text{COOH} & & \\
\text{Glutamate} & & \text{GABA}
\end{array}
$$

GABA is present at high concentrations throughout the central nervous system and is also detectable in other tissues (especially islet cells of the pancreas and the adrenal gland). It is used as a transmitter by an important class of inhibitory interneurons in the spinal cord. In the brain GABA is the major transmitter in various inhibitory interneurons, for example, in basket cells of both the cerebellum and the hippocampus, in Purkinje cells of the cerebellum, in the granule cells of the olfactory bulb, and in amacrine cells of the retina.

ATP and Adenosine

ATP and its degradation products (for example, adenosine) act as transmitters at some synapses. Adenine and guanine and their derivatives are called purines; the evidence for *purinergic* transmission is especially strong for autonomic neurons to the vas deferens, bladder, and muscle fibers of the heart; for nerve plexuses on smooth muscle in the gut; and for some neurons in the brain. Purinergic transmission is particularly important in the generation of pain (Chapter 24). ATP released by tissue damage excites the naked endings of the peripheral

C-fiber axon of dorsal root ganglion cells through one type of ionotropic purine receptor. ATP released from the terminal of the central axon of the dorsal root ganglion cell excites another type of ionotropic purine receptor on neurons in the dorsal horn of the spinal cord.

Small-Molecule Transmitters Are Actively Taken Up Into Vesicles

It might at first seem puzzling that common amino acids can act as transmitters in some neurons but not in others. This phenomenon shows that the presence of a substance in a neuron, even in substantial amounts, is not in itself sufficient evidence that the substance is used as a transmitter. To illustrate this point, let us consider the following example. GABA is inhibitory at the neuromuscular junction of the lobster (and of other crustacea and insects), and glutamate is excitatory. The concentration of GABA is about 20 times greater in inhibitory cells than in excitatory cells, and this supports the idea that GABA is the inhibitory transmitter at the lobster neuromuscular junction. But the concentration of glutamate, the excitatory transmitter, is the same in both excitatory and inhibitory cells. Glutamate therefore must be compartmentalized within these neurons; that is, *transmitter* glutamate must be kept separate from *metabolic* glutamate. Transmitter glutamate is compartmentalized in synaptic vesicles.

Although the presence of a specific set of biosynthetic enzymes can determine whether a small molecule can be used as a transmitter by a neuron, it does not guarantee that the molecule will be used. Typically, before a substance can be released as a transmitter, it must be concentrated into vesicles. Transmitter concentrations within vesicles are high, on the order of 50–100 mM. The molecular mechanism for concentrating neurotransmitter substances involves a transporter specific to a given neuron and a vesicular-ATPase (V-ATPase) common to neurons of all types (and found also in glandular tissue, such as the adrenal medulla). Using the energy generated by the hydrolysis of cytoplasmic ATP, the V-ATPase creates a pH, or chemiosmotic, gradient by promoting the influx of protons into the vesicle. (A similar ATPase, F-ATPase, operates in mitochondria to produce ATP.) Transporters then use this proton gradient to drive the transmitter molecules into the vesicles against their concentration gradient. Four different vesicle transporters have been identified: one for acetylcholine, a second for amine transmitters, a third for glutamate, and a fourth for GABA and glycine. All of these proteins span the vesicle membrane 12 times, and all are thought to be distantly related to a class of bacterial drug-resistance transporters. (Although similar in function, vesicular transporters differ from the transporters in the external membrane, which are discussed later in the chapter.)

In each of the four types of vesicular transporters, the ionized transmitter molecule is exchanged for two protons (Figure 15-1A). Because the maintenance of the pH gradient requires the hydrolysis of ATP, the uptake of transmitter into vesicles is energy-dependent. The uptake of transmitters must be fast, since recycling of synaptic vesicles must be quite rapid to maintain the supply of transmitter available for release (see Chapter 14). While the specificity of transporters is quite marked—the acetylcholine transporter does not transport choline or any other transmitter, and the glutamate transporter hardly carries any aspartate at all—the affinity for their transmitters can be quite low. For example, the K_m for acetylcholine or glutamate is about 0.3 mM, and for GABA 5–10 mM. This low affinity presumably does not limit synaptic transmission, however, because the concentrations of these substances in the cytoplasm is normally high. In contrast, the amine transporter has a much greater affinity for monoamines ($K_m \sim 1$–15 μM) and the low cytoplasmic concentrations of these transmitters can be limiting, as it is with the transsynaptic regulation of norepinephrine (see Box 15-1). As further evidence that uptake of monoamines is an important regulatory step, the mRNA for the amine transporter is up-regulated under the stressful conditions that result in a long-term increase in the production of norepinephrine.

Transporters and V-ATPases are present in the membranes both of small synaptic vesicles and of large dense-core vesicles. As with any specific mechanism that controls a physiological process, vesicular transporters are the targets of pharmacological agents. Most of the drugs thus far examined target the amine transporter. Reserpine and tetrabenazine both inhibit uptake of amine transmitters by binding to the transporter, and both have been used as antipsychotic drugs. The psychostimulants amphetamine and 3,4-methylenedioxymethanphetamine ("ecstasy") are thought to deplete vesicles of amine transmitters by dissipating the pH gradient. Ecstasy also competes with the amine transmitter and therefore is presumed to interact directly with the transporter.

Drugs that are sufficiently similar to the normal transmitter substance can act as *false transmitters*. These are packaged in the vesicles and released as if they were true transmitters, but they often bind only weakly or not at all to the postsynaptic receptor for the natural transmitter. Therefore, their release decreases the efficacy of transmission. Several drugs used to treat hypertension, such as phenylethylamines, are taken up into adrenergic terminals and replace norepinephrine in synaptic vesicles. When released, these drugs are not as potent as norepinephrine at postsynaptic adrenergic receptors. Some of these drugs must be actively taken up into neurons by transporters that are present in the external membrane of the cell. These transporter molecules will be discussed later in this chapter.

Many Neuroactive Peptides Serve as Transmitters

With one exception (dopamine β-hydroxylase) the enzymes that catalyze the synthesis of the low-molecular-weight neurotransmitters are found in the cytoplasm. These enzymes are synthesized on free polysomes in the cell body and are distributed throughout the neuron by slow axoplasmic flow. Thus, small-molecule transmitter substances can be formed in all parts of the neuron; most importantly, these transmitters can be synthesized at the nerve terminals where they are released.

In contrast, the neuroactive peptides are derived from secretory proteins that are formed in the cell body. Like other secretory proteins, neuroactive peptides or their precursors are first processed in the endoplasmic reticulum and then move to the Golgi apparatus to be processed further. They leave the Golgi apparatus within secretory granules that are destined to become large dense-core vesicles and are moved to terminals by fast axonal transport.

More than 50 short peptides are pharmacologically active in nerve cells (Table 15-2). These peptides cause inhibition or excitation, or both, when applied to appropriate target neurons. Some of these peptides had been previously identified as hormones with known targets outside the brain (for example, angiotensin and gastrin), or as products of neuroendocrine secretion (for example, oxytocin, vasopressin, somatostatin, luteinizing hormone, and thyrotropin-releasing hormone). These peptides, in addition to being hormones in some tissues, also act as transmitters when released close to the site of intended action. The study of neuroactive peptides is particularly important because some have been implicated in modulating sensory perception and emotions. For example, some peptides (substance P and enkephalins) are preferentially located in many regions of the central nervous system involved in the perception of pain; others regulate complex responses to stress (γ-melanocyte-stimulating hormone, adrenocorticotropin, and β-endorphin).

Although the diversity of neuroactive peptides is enormous, as a class these chemical messengers share a common cell biology. A striking generality is that neuroactive peptides are grouped in families whose members

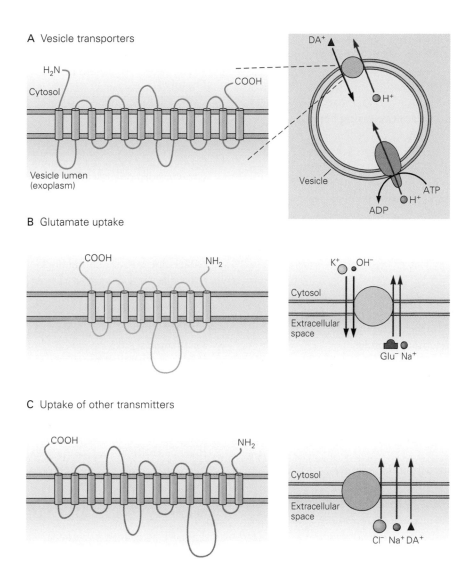

Figure 15-1 Transport of small-molecule transmitters from the cytosol into vesicles or from the synaptic cleft to the cytosol requires energy. Energy is required because transport is typically from a region containing a low concentration to one with a higher concentration. Transport is achieved by transporters, large membrane-spanning proteins that carry a molecule across the membrane rather than allowing it to pass through a pore, as in ion channels. Thus, transporters are similar to enzymes in mechanism.

A. Neurotransmitters are packaged in synaptic vesicles by vesicle transporters. These proteins span the vesicle membrane 12 times and catalyze the uptake of charged neurotransmitter molecules (here shown as dopamine, DA$^+$) in exchange for protons. Since the concentration of dopamine within vesicles is usually much greater than that in the surrounding cytosol, energy is required and is drawn from the proton gradient established by the vesicle ATPase (V-ATPase). This ATPase causes the influx of H$^+$ ions into the vesicles, producing a pH gradient (cytosol pH 7.2; vesicles 5.5). The energy to maintain

this chemiosmotic gradient is derived from the hydrolysis of ATP.

B. Transmitter glutamate is taken up from the synaptic cleft into the cytosol by a transporter protein thought to have six or eight membrane-spanning domains. Here the energy required to move glutamate from the extracellular space, where it is greatly diluted, is derived from the cotransport of Na$^+$ into the terminal. The electrochemical gradient for Na$^+$ influx is generated by the difference between the Na$^+$ concentration (much higher outside the cell than in the cytosol) and the negative resting potential. Uptake of glutamate requires the cotransport of Na$^+$ and the countertransport of K$^+$ and a hydroxyl ion.

C. Other transmitters are removed from the synaptic cleft by a transporter specific for each transmitter. These proteins span the membrane 12 times and are closely related to each other, unrelated to the glutamate transporters, and very distantly related to the vesicular transporters. All require the cotransport of Na$^+$ and Cl$^-$. As with glutamate uptake, they are driven by the energy drawn from the Na$^+$ gradient.

Table 15-2 Neuroactive Mammalian Brain Peptides Categorized According to Tissue Localization. (Expanded from Krieger 1983.)

Category	Peptide
Hypothalamic releasing hormone	Thyrotropin-releasing hormone
	Gonadotropin-releasing hormone
	Somatostatin
	Corticotropin-releasing hormone
	Growth hormone-releasing hormone
Neurohypophyseal hormones	Vasopressin
	Oxytocin
Pituitary peptides	Adrenocorticotropic hormone
	β-Endorphin
	α-Melanocyte-stimulating hormone
	Prolactin
	Luteinizing hormone
	Growth hormone
	Thyrotropin
Invertebrate peptides	FMRFamide[1]
	Hydra head activator
	Proctolin
	Small cardiac peptide
	Myomodulins
	Buccalins
	Egg-laying hormone
	Bag cell peptides
Gastrointestinal peptides	Vasoactive intestinal polypeptide
	Cholecystokinin
	Gastrin
	Substance P
	Neurotensin
	Methionine-enkephalin
	Leucine-enkephalin
	Insulin
	Glucagon
	Bombesin
	Secretin
	Somatostatin
	Thyrotropin-releasing hormone
	Motilin
Heart	Atrial naturetic peptide
Other	Angiotensin II
	Bradykinin
	Sleep peptide(s)
	Calcitonin
	CGRP[2]
	Neuropeptide Y
	Neuropeptide Yy
	Galanin
	Substance K (neurokinin A)

[1]Phe-Met-Arg-Phe-NH$_2$.
[2]Calcitonin gene–related peptide.

have similar sequences of amino acid residues. At least 10 have been identified; the seven main families are listed in Table 15-3. How is relatedness between peptides determined? The most direct way is to compare either the amino acid sequences of the peptides or the nucleotide base sequences in the genes that encode them.

Usually, in the production of neurotransmitter peptides several different neuroactive peptides are encoded by a single continuous mRNA, which is translated into one large protein precursor, or *polyprotein* (Figure 15-2). (Polyproteins are often called *prohormones* or *preprohormones*.) Production from a large precursor sometimes can serve as a mechanism for amplification, since more than one copy of the same peptide can be produced from the one polyprotein. Examples can be found in the opioid peptide family, where several distinct peptides with opioid activity are cleaved from one precursor. (Opioid peptides arise from three different polyprotein precursors, each of which is the product of a distinct gene. These genes, although related, are not syntenic in humans, each being on a different chromosome.) Another example is the precursor of glucagon, which contains two copies of the hormone. Sometimes the biological purposes served are more complicated, since peptides with either related or antagonistic functions can be generated from the same precursor.

The processing of more than one functional peptide from a single polyprotein is by no means unique to peptide chemical messengers. The mechanism was first described for proteins encoded by small RNA viruses. Several viral polypeptides are produced from the same viral polyprotein, and all contribute to the generation of new virus particles. As with the virus, where the different proteins obviously serve a common biological purpose (formation of new viruses), a neuronal polypeptide will in many instances yield peptides that work together to serve a common behavioral goal.

A particularly striking example of this form of synergy is the group of peptides formed from the ELH (egg-laying hormone) precursor protein, a set of neuropeptides that govern reproductive behavior in the marine mollusk *Aplysia*. *Aplysia* eggs, contained in chitinous cases, are extruded in long strings, each containing more than a million eggs. An egg string is extruded by the contraction of muscles in the reproductive duct. As the egg string is extruded, the animal's heartbeat quickens, its respiration increases, and it grasps the emerging string in its mouth. The animal then rears up its head and waves it back and forth, thus helping to draw the string out of the duct and weave it into a single skein, which the animal fixes onto a rock or some other solid support. These diverse behaviors are all regulated

by at least four peptide fragments cut from the same polyprotein precursor as ELH. ELH can act as a hormone causing the contraction of duct muscles; it can also act as a neurotransmitter on several neurons involved in the behaviors, as do the other peptides cut from the polyprotein.

The processing of polyprotein precursors to neuroactive peptides takes place within the neuron's major intracellular membrane system and in vesicles. Several peptides are produced from a single polyprotein by limited and specific proteolytic cleavages that are catalyzed by proteases present within these internal membrane systems. Some of these enzymes are serine proteases, a class that includes the pancreatic enzymes trypsin and chymotrypsin. They are called serine proteases because they all have a serine residue at the catalytic center whose hydroxyl group participates in the cleavage reaction. As with trypsin, the peptide bond cleaved is determined by the presence of one or two dibasic amino acid residues (lysine and arginine). Cleavage occurs between residue X and the pair of dibasic residues (eg, -X-Lys-Lys, -X-Lys-Arg, -X-Arg-Lys, or -X-Arg-Arg). Although cleavage at dibasic residues is common, cleavage usually occurs at single basic residues, and polyproteins sometimes are cleaved at peptide bonds between amino acids in sequences other than -X–basic amino acid residue.

Other types of peptidases also catalyze the limited proteolysis required for processing polyproteins into neuroactive peptides. Among these are thiol endopeptidases (with catalytic mechanisms like that of pepsin), amino peptidases (which remove the N-terminal amino acid of the peptide), and carboxypeptidase B (an enzyme that removes an amino acid from the N-terminal end of the peptide if it is basic).

Processing of polyprotein precursors is a critical step in determining which peptides will be released by a peptidergic neuron. Neurons with the same gene encoding a polyprotein may release different neuropeptides because of differences in the way each of the neurons processes the polyprotein. An example is proopiomelanocortin (POMC), one of the three branches of the opioid family. The same mRNA for POMC is found in the anterior and intermediate lobes of the pituitary, in the hypothalamus and several other regions of the brain, as well as in the placenta and the gut, but different peptides are produced and released in each of these tissues. It is not yet known how differential processing occurs, but current information on the biochemistry of membrane proteins and secretory products (see Chapter 5) suggests two plausible mechanisms. Two neurons might process the same polyprotein differently because they contain proteases with different specificities within

Table 15-3 Some Families of Neuroactive Peptides

Family	Peptide members
Opioids	Opiocortins, enkephalins, dynorphin, FMRFamide
Neurohypophyseal hormones	Vasopressin, oxytocin, neurophysins
Tachykinins	Substance P, physalaemin, kassinin, uperolein, eledoisin, bombesin, substance K
Secretins	Secretin, glucagon, vasoactive intestinal peptide, gastric inhibitory peptide, growth hormone–releasing factor, peptide histidine isoleucineamide
Insulins	Insulin, insulin-like growth factors I and II
Somatostatins	Somatostatins, pancreatic polypeptide
Gastrins	Gastrin, cholecystokinin

the lumina of the internal endoplasmic reticulum and Golgi apparatus and vesicles. Alternatively, the two neurons might contain the same processing proteases, but each cell might glycosylate the common polyprotein at different sites, thereby protecting different regions of the polypeptide from cleavage.

Peptides and Small-Molecule Transmitters Differ in Several Ways

Some peptides satisfy many of the four established criteria for a substance to be a neurotransmitter, and several peptides satisfy all of the criteria. Nevertheless, the metabolism of peptides differs from that of the accepted small-molecule transmitters in several important ways: in their site of synthesis, in the type of vesicle in which they are stored, and in the mechanism of exocytotic release. Neuroactive peptides are made only in the cell body because their synthesis requires peptide bond formation on ribosomes, whereas the small-molecule transmitters are chiefly synthesized locally at terminals. No uptake mechanisms exist for neuropeptides, but small-molecule transmitters are rapidly concentrated by vesicles.

Peptides are stored in large dense-core vesicles, which originate from the *trans*-Golgi network through a pathway different from that of small-molecule synaptic vesicles. Large dense-core vesicles are homologous with the secretory granules of nonneuronal cells and follow the "regulated" secretory pathway. The membrane of the synaptic vesicles, on the other hand, follows the "constitutive" secretory pathway, as early endosomes; when it reaches nerve terminals this membrane does not function directly but must be processed into synaptic vesicles before actually operating in the release of neurotransmitter. While both types of vesicles contain many similar proteins, dense-core vesicles lack several pro-

teins that are needed for localized release at active zones and subsequent recycling. Thus, while the membranes of the synaptic vesicles are recycled, membranes from dense-core vesicles are used only once. Because synaptic vesicles can be refilled rapidly with the small-molecule transmitters that are resynthesized at terminals, release can be both rapid and sustained. With peptides, however, once release occurs, a new supply of the peptide must arrive from the cell body before release can take place again.

Large secretory vesicles release their contents by an exocytotic mechanism that is not specialized to nerve cells and can take place anywhere along the terminal's membrane. As in other examples of regulated secretion, exocytosis of large vesicles depends on a general elevation of intracellular Ca^{2+}, whereas exocytosis of the synaptic vesicles depends on a local increase in Ca^{2+} at domains near the active zone. Therefore, release of neuropeptides from dense-core vesicles typically requires greater stimulation frequencies than does release of transmitters from synaptic vesicles.

Peptides and Small-Molecule Transmitters Can Coexist and Be Coreleased

Neuroactive peptides, small-molecule transmitters, and other neuroactive molecules can coexist in the same neuron. In mature neurons the combination usually consists of one of the small-molecule transmitters and one or more peptides derived from one kind of polyprotein. For example, ACh and vasoactive intestinal peptide (VIP) can be released together by a presynaptic neuron and work synergistically on the same target cells.

Another example is calcitonin gene-related peptide (CGRP), which is present in most spinal motor neurons

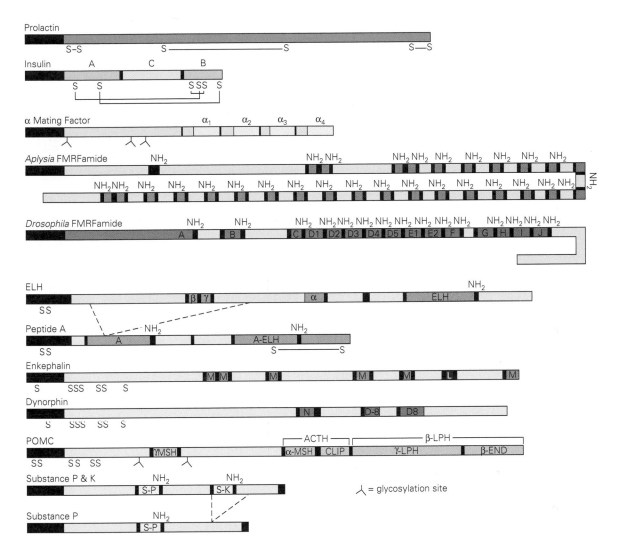

Figure 15-2 Structures of several hormone and neuropeptide precursors. Translation of each preprohormone is initiated by a hydrophobic signal sequence (**black bars**). Internal cleavages at basic residues are indicated by the **vertical lines** within the sequence. Several of the active peptides are named, and cysteine (**S**) and sugar (**inverted Y-shapes**) residues are indicated below the schematic.

For **prolactin** the mature hormone arises from the removal of the signal sequence and formation of three pairs of disulfide bonds. The **insulin** precursor is cleaved at two internal sites, resulting in the disulfide-linked A and B chains of mature insulin and the C peptide. The **α-mating factor** from yeast is processed by endoproteolytic cleavage at dibasic residues, followed by diaminopeptidyl peptidase trimming to generate four copies of the mating factor (α_1–α_4). The *Aplysia* FMRFamide precursor encodes 28 copies of the tetrapeptide (**light purple**) and a single copy of a peptide closely related to FMRFamide (**dark purple**). The *Drosophila* FMRFamide precursor encodes at least 15 predicted peptides with 10 different structures. The **egg-laying hormone (ELH)** precursor encodes at least four physiologically active peptides: α, β, and γ bag cell peptides, as well as ELH. The **peptide A** precursor is quite similar to the ELH precursor; the major differences are deletion of a 240–amino acid sequence encompassing the β and γ bag cell peptides (indicated by **dashed lines**) and single base changes that affect the patterns of cleavage, amidation, and disulfide linkage.

The family of peptides giving rise to the opioid peptides is also illustrated. The **enkephalin** precursor gives rise to six Met (**M**) and one Leu (**L**) enkephalin peptides. The **dynorphin** precursor is cleaved into at least three peptides, which are related to Leu enkephalin. The **proopiomelanocortin (POMC)** precursor is processed differently in different lobes of the pituitary gland, resulting in α–melanocyte stimulating hormone (α–MSH) and γ-MSH, corticotropin-like intermediate lobe peptide (CLIP), and β-lipotropin (β-LPH). β-LPH is cleaved to yield γ-LPH and β-endorphin (β-END). The endoproteolytic cleavages within adrenocorticotropic hormone (ACTH) and β-LPH take place in the intermediate lobe but not the anterior lobe. Alternative RNA splicing generates two prohormones that give rise to either **substance P (S-P)** alone or both S-P and **substance K (S-K)**. (Adapted from Sossin et al. 1989.)

Box 15-2 Histochemical Detection of Chemical Messengers Within Neurons

A major task in studying how neurons function is to identify the chemical messengers they use. Powerful histochemical techniques are available for detecting both small-molecule transmitter substances and neuroactive peptides in histological sections of nervous tissue.

Catecholamines and serotonin, when reacting with formaldehyde vapor, form fluorescent derivatives. In an early example of transmitter histochemistry, the Swedish neuroanatomists Bengt Falck and Nils Hillarp found that the reaction can be used to locate transmitters with the fluorescent (light) microscope under properly controlled conditions. Because individual vesicles are too small to be resolved by the light microscope, histofluorescence can only localize transmitters relatively imprecisely in a nerve cell (eg, cytoplasm versus nucleus). The exact position of the vesicles can be inferred by comparing the distribution of fluorescence under the light miscroscope with the position of vesicles under the electron microscope.

Histochemical analysis can be extended to the ultrastructural level under special conditions. Fixation of nervous tissue in the presence of potassium permanganate, chromate, or silver salts intensifies the electron density of vesicles containing biogenic amines and thus brings out the large number of dense-core vesicles that are characteristic of aminergic neurons.

It is also possible to identify neurons that express the gene for a particular transmitter enzyme or peptide precursor. Many methods for detecting specific mRNA depend on the phenomenon of nucleic acid hybridization. One particularly elegant method is in situ hybridization. Two single strands of a nucleic acid polymer will pair if their sequence of bases is complementary. With in situ hybridization, the strand of noncoding DNA (negative or antisense strand or its corresponding RNA) is applied to tissue sections under conditions suitable for hybridizing with endogenous (sense) mRNA. If the probes are radiolabeled, autoradiography reveals the locations of neurons that contain the complex formed between the labeled complementary nucleic acid strand and the mRNA. When oligonucleotides synthesized with nucleotides containing chemically tagged or immunoreactive base analogs are used, the hybrid can be localized cytochemically. Both labels can be used at once, as shown in Figure 15-3.

Transmitter substances can also be localized by immunocytochemistry. Amino acid transmitters, biogenic amines, and neuropeptides can be successfully located by autoradiography because they have a primary amino group that permits their covalent fixation in place within the neurons; this group becomes cross-linked to proteins by aldehydes, the usual fixatives used in microscopy.

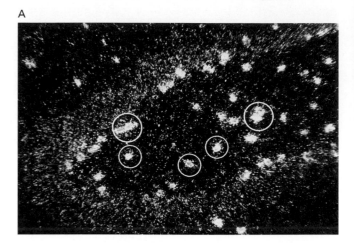

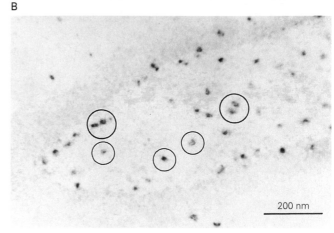

Figure 15-3 In situ hybridization reveals the distribution of the mRNA for glutamic acid decarboxylase (GAD), the specific biosynthetic enzyme for GABA, and GAT-1, a transporter for GABA, in a light miscroscope section of the hippocampus of the rat.

A. The probe for GAT-1 was end-labeled with α-^{35}S-dATP. The GAT-1 probe was visualized by clusters of silver grains in the overlying autoradiographic photographic emulsion. Neurons expressing both transcripts are labeled by the phosphatase reaction product and by silver grains. **Circles** enclose nerve cell bodies that contain both labels.

B. In situ hybridization of the mRNA for GAD was carried out with an oligonucleotide probe linked to the enzyme alkaline phosphatase. The GAD probe was visualized by accumulation of colored alkaline phosphatase reaction product in the cytoplasm. **Circles** enclose areas containing cells with the greatest reactivity. (Courtesy of Sara Augood.)

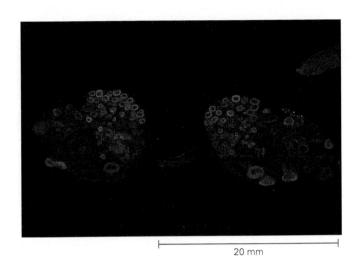

20 mm

Figure 15-4 An immunochemical technique visualizes a neuropeptide. The buccal ganglion of *Aplysia* contains the sensory, motor, and interneurons that control the rhythmic movements of the feeding apparatus of the animal. A cryostat section of the bilaterally symmetrical buccal ganglion is labeled with an antibody raised against FMRFamide. The staining shows the presence of FMRFamide immunoreactivity in the subset of neurons that includes both sensory neurons (most of the cells with the small-diameter cell bodies) as well as motor neurons (cells with larger-diameter cell bodies). Some of these cells contain one or more other peptides or conventional transmitters such as acetylcholine. (Courtesy of P. E. Lloyd, M. Frankfurt, P. Stevens, I. Kupfermann, and K. R. Weiss.)

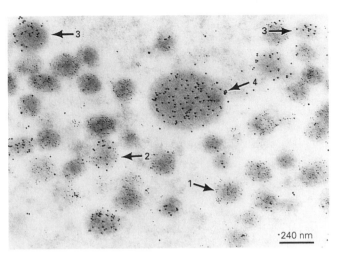

·240 nm

Figure 15-5 Immunogold (electron-opaque gold particles complexed to antibody) is used to locate two antigens in a single electron miscroscope tissue section. The electron micrograph shows a section through an *Aplysia* bag cell body, treated with two antibodies against different regions of the prohormone. The bag cells, which control reproductive behavior by releasing a group of neuropeptides cleaved from the ELH prohormone (see Figure 15-2), contain several kinds of dense-core vesicles. One of the antibodies was raised in rabbits and the other in rats. These antibodies were detected with antirabbit or antirat immunoglobulins (secondary antibodies) raised in goats. Each secondary antibody was coupled to colloidal gold particles of a distinct size. The specific fragments cleaved from the prohormone are seen to be localized in different vesicles, since vesicles indicated by numbered **arrows 1 and 2** are labeled with gold particles smaller than vesicles indicated by **arrows 3 and 4.** (From Fisher et al. 1988.)

For immunohistochemical localization, specific antibodies to the transmitter substances are necessary. Specific antibodies have been raised to serotonin, histamine, and many neuroactive peptides. These transmitter-specific antibodies can be detected by a second antibody (in a technique called *indirect immunofluorescence*). As an example, if the first antibody is rabbit antipeptide, the second antibody can be goat antibody raised against rabbit immunoglobulin. These commercially available antibodies are labeled with fluorescent dyes. They can be used under the fluorescence microscope to locate antigens to regions of individual neurons—cell bodies, axons, and sometimes terminals (Figure 15-4).

Ultrastructure localization can be achieved by immunohistochemical techniques, usually involving a peroxidase-antiperoxidase system. Another method is to use antibodies linked to gold particles, which are electron-dense (Figure 15-5). Spheres of colloidal gold can be generated with precise diameters in the nanometer range and, because they are electron-dense, can be seen in the electron microscope. This technique has the additional useful feature that more than one specific antibody can be used to examine the same tissue section if each of the antibodies is linked to gold particles of a different size.

together with ACh, the transmitter used at the neuromuscular synapse. CGRP activates adenylyl cyclase, raising cAMP and cAMP-dependent protein phosphorylation in the muscles (see Chapter 11). Increased protein phosphorylation results in an increase in the force of contraction. Thus, at the neuromuscular junction a small-molecule transmitter (ACh) and a peptide (CGRP) are both released from the same presynaptic neuron. One other example is the co-release of glutamate and dynorphin in the hippocampus, where glutamate is excitatory and the opioid peptide inhibitory. Since nearby postsynaptic cells have receptors for both chemical messengers, all of these examples of co-release are also examples of *cotransmission*.

Neurons that contain peptides processed from a single polyprotein can release several neuroactive peptides with potentially different postsynaptic actions. As already described, the vesicles that release peptides differ from those that release small-molecule transmitters. The peptide-containing vesicles may or may not contain small-molecule transmitter, but both types of vesicles contain ATP, and ATP is released by exocytosis of both large dense-core vesicles and synaptic vesicles.

The co-release of ATP (which after release can be degraded to adenosine) is an important illustration that coexistence and corelease do not necessarily signify cotransmission. ATP, like many other substances, can be released from neurons but still not be effective if there are no appropriate receptors close by: It is like the unheard falling of a tree in a forest.

Recall that one criterion for judging whether a particular substance is used as a transmitter is that the substance is present in sufficient amounts to be released. Histochemistry provides an important method for detecting chemical messengers in neurons (Box 15-2).

Removal of Transmitter From the Synaptic Cleft Terminates Synaptic Transmission

Timely removal of transmitters from the synaptic cleft is critical to synaptic transmission. If transmitter molecules released in one synaptic action were allowed to remain in the cleft after release, they would prevent new signals from getting through and the synapse would become refractory, mainly because of receptor desensitization resulting from continued exposure to transmitter. Transmitters are removed from the cleft by three mechanisms: diffusion, enzymatic degradation, and re-uptake. Diffusion removes some fraction of *all* chemical messengers.

Enzymatic degradation of transmitter is used primarily by cholinergic synapses. At the neuromuscular

junction, the active zones of the presynaptic nerve terminal are located just above the junctional folds of the muscle membrane. The ACh receptors are situated at the surface of the muscle and do not extend deep into the folds (see Figure 11-1), while acetylcholinesterase is anchored to the basement membrane within the folds. This anatomical arrangement of transmitter and enzyme serves two functions. First, since any ACh after dissociation from a receptor most likely will be hydrolyzed to choline and acetate by the esterase, the transmitter molecules are used only once. That is, one function of the esterase is to punctuate the synaptic message. The second function is to recapture the choline that otherwise might be lost by diffusion away from the synaptic cleft. Once hydrolyzed by the esterase, the choline is held at a low concentration in the reservoir provided by the junctional folds and is later taken back up into cholinergic nerve endings by a high-affinity choline transporter.

Many other enzymatic pathways that degrade released transmitter are not involved in terminating synaptic transmission but can be important for controlling the concentration of the transmitter within the neuron or for inactivating transmitter molecules that have diffused away from the synaptic cleft. Many are important clinically—they provide sites for drug action and serve as diagnostic indicators. For example, monoamine oxidase inhibitors, which block the degradation of amine transmitters, are used to treat high blood pressure and depression. Concentrations of the metabolites of catechol-*O*-methyltransferase, which is important for degrading biogenic amines and is found in the cytoplasm of most cells, indicate the efficacy of drugs that affect the synthesis or degradation of the biogenic amines in nervous tissue.

Neuroactive peptides are removed more slowly than small-molecule transmitters from the synaptic cleft. Probably the only mechanisms of peptide removal are diffusion and proteolysis by extracellular peptidases. The slow removal of neuropeptides contributes to the long duration of their effects.

Re-uptake of transmitter substance is the most common mechanism for inactivation. This mechanism serves the dual purposes of terminating the synaptic action of the transmitter and recapturing the transmitter molecule for possible reuse. High-affinity uptake, with binding constants of 25 μM or less for the released transmitter, is mediated by *transporter molecules* in the membranes of nerve terminals and glial cells.

Specific neurons each have their own characteristic uptake mechanisms; as an example, noncholinergic neurons do not take up choline with high affinity. Certain powerful psychotropic drugs can block uptake processes; for example, cocaine blocks the uptake of norepinephrine, and the tricyclic antidepressants and selective serotonin re-uptake inhibitors, such as fluoxetine (Prozac), block that of serotonin. The application of appropriate drugs to block transporter molecules can prolong and enhance the action of the biogenic amines and GABA. In some instances drugs act both on the transporter molecules and on the vesicular transporters described earlier in this chapter. For example, amphetamines must be actively taken up by the dopamine transporter in the external membrane of the neuron before they can operate on the vesicular transporter for amine transmitters.

Transporter molecules have been cloned and belong to two distinct groups that are different in both structure and mechanism. One group consists of the transporters of glutamate, the other transporters of GABA, glycine, norepinephrine, dopamine, serotonin, and choline. Transporters in the second group belong to a superfamily of membrane-spanning proteins that thread through the plasmalemma 12 times (see Figure 15-1). The topology of the glutamate group, which contains at least three different members, is not yet certain because the results of hydropathy analyses of their inferred amino acid sequences are ambiguous as to whether six or eight membrane-spanning domains are present.

The 12-membrane-spanning group includes several transporters for each transmitter; for example, there are at least four for GABA. As inferred from DNA sequence alignments, all of the members of this group are related, stemming from an ancestor protein that gave rise to bacterial permeases. They are more remotely related to the vesicular transporters, however.

The two groups can be distinguished functionally. Although both are driven by the electrochemical potential provided by the Na^+ gradient, transport of glutamate requires the countertransport of K^+, and transport by the 12-membrane-spanning transporters requires the cotransport of a Cl^- ion. Thus, during transport of glutamate one negatively charged molecule of the transmitter is imported with two Na^+ ions into the cell (symport) in exchange for one K^+ and one pH-changing ion (OH^- or HCO_3^-). The 12-membrane-spanning transporters symport one to three Na^+ ions and one Cl^- ion and have no requirement for countertransport.

The concentration of transmitter is much higher in the terminal than in the synaptic cleft, typically by four orders of magnitude. Nevertheless, the electrochemical potential is sufficient for transporters to take up the dilute transmitter into the cell. Under certain conditions, however, a transporter can operate in the reverse direction, thereby releasing transmitter. This release is voltage-dependent (the electrochemical Na^+ gradient driving the transporter is diminished by depolarization) but it does not depend on Ca^{2+}. Nonvesicular release, ie, released by transporters, is used by amacrine cells of the retina to release GABA and has been described for several other kinds of neurons as well. Since transmitter released in this manner activates postsynaptic receptors, it no longer can be taken for granted that a substance must be stored in vesicles to act as a neurotransmitter.

Several membrane-soluble molecules with profound effects on nerve cells have been classified as neurotransmitters. These molecules diffuse through neuronal membranes and therefore are released without being packaged in vesicles. The most prominent of these are the gas nitric oxide (NO) and the fatty acid arachidonic acid (Chapter 13). Nitric oxide is formed through the oxidation of the amino acid arginine by the enzyme nitric oxide synthase (of which there are three isoforms) together with an electron donor such as flavin adenine dinucleotide (FAD). Arachidonate is released from membrane phospholipid by receptor-mediated activation of phospholipase A_2. It has been suggested that these membrane-soluble molecules may act as retrograde messengers at some synapses, carrying information from the postsynaptic neuron to the presynaptic cell. NO produces its effects on receptors *within* target neurons. Thus the major action of NO is to stimulate the production of cGMP by the intracellular enzyme guanylyl cyclase. The actions of both NO and arachidonic acid on the vascular system and in the inflammatory reaction have been extensively studied.

An Overall View

Information carried by a neuron is encoded in electrical signals that travel along its axon and into the nerve terminal. At the synapse these signals are carried across the synaptic cleft by one or more chemical messengers. None of these chemical messengers carries unique information, as RNA and DNA do. Indeed, some are also metabolites in a variety of biochemical pathways within the cell: amino acids are polymerized into proteins; glutamate and GABA act as substrates in intermediary metabolism; and ATP is the principal means of transferring metabolic energy.

These molecules become signals when they bind to receptor proteins in the membrane of another cell causing them to change shape. Once the molecules of transmitter are bound, the receptor generates electrical or metabolic signals in the postsynaptic cell. The co-release of several neuroactive substances onto appropriate postsynaptic receptors permits an extraordinary diversity of information to be transferred in a single synaptic action.

These chemical messengers are packaged in vesicles within the neuron. Vesicles play different roles in the life cycle of the two major classes of chemical messengers—small-molecule transmitters and neuroactive peptides. After their synthesis in the cytoplasm small-molecule transmitters are taken up and concentrated in vesicles, where they are protected from degradative enzymes that maintain a constant level of transmitter substance in the cytoplasm.

Nerve endings contain a high concentration of synaptic vesicles. Because the contents of the synaptic vesicles are continuously released, much of the small-molecule transmitter in the neuron must be synthesized at the terminals. In contrast, the protein precursors of neuroactive peptides are synthesized only in the cell body; there they become packaged in secretory granules and synaptic vesicles that are transported from the cell body to the terminals. Unlike the vesicles that contain small-molecule transmitters, these vesicles are not refilled at the terminal. The physiology of the two types of transmitters is also different as well, as discussed in Chapter 13.

Can we arrive at a comprehensive and precise definition of a neurotransmitter? Probably not. The first step in understanding the molecular strategy of chemical transmission usually involves identifying the contents of synaptic vesicles. Except for those rare neurons in which transmitter is released by transporter molecules, only molecules suitably packaged in vesicles can be released from a neuron's terminals. But not all molecules released by a neuron are chemical messengers—only those that can bind to appropriate receptors and thus initiate changes in the activity of the postsynaptic cell can be considered transmitters. Typically, vesicles mediate the release of a chemical messenger through exocytosis, but in some instances transmitters are released by other mechanisms.

James H. Schwartz

Selected Readings

Amara SG, Arriza JL. 1993. Neurotransmitter transporters: three distinct gene families. Curr Opin Neurobiol 3:337–344.

Cooper JR, Bloom FE, Roth RH. 1996. *The Biochemical Basis of Neuropharmacology*, 7th ed. New York: Oxford Univ. Press.

Edwards RH. 1992. The transport of neurotransmitters into synaptic vesicles. Curr Opin Neurobiol 2:586–594.

Hall ZW. 1992. *An Introduction to Molecular Neurobiology.* Sunderland, MA: Sinauer.

Koob GF, Sandman CA, Strand FL (eds). 1990. A decade of neuropeptides: past, present and future. Ann NY Acad Sci 579:1–281.

Kupfermann I. 1991. Functional studies of cotransmission. Physiol Rev 71:683–732.

Nicholls DG. 1994. *Proteins, Transmitters and Synapses.* Oxford: Blackwell.

Siegel GJ, Agranoff BW, Albers RW, Molinoff PB (eds). 1998. *Basic Neurochemistry: Molecular, Cellular, and Medical Aspects,* 6th ed. Philadelphia: Lippincott.

References

Augood SJ, Herbison AE, Emson PC. 1995. Localization of GAT-1 GABA transporter mRNA in rat striatum: cellular coexpression with GAD_{67} mRNA, GAD_{67} immunoreactivity, and paravalbumin mRNA. J Neurosci 15:865–874.

Burnstock G. 1986. Purines as cotransmitters in the adrenergic and cholinergic neurones. In: T Hökfelt, K Fuxe, P Pernow (eds). Coexistence of neuronal messengers: a new principle in chemical transmission. Progr Brain Res 68:193–203.

Dale H. 1935. Pharmacology and nerve-endings. Proc R Soc Med (Lond) 28:319–332.

Falck B, Hillarp N-Å, Thieme G, Torp A. 1982. Fluorescence of catecholamines and related compounds condensed with formaldehyde. Brain Res Bull 9(1–6):11–15.

Fisher JM, Sossin W, Newcomb R, Scheller RH. 1988. Multiple neuropeptides derived from a common precursor are differentially packaged and transported. Cell 54:813–822.

Iversen LL. 1995. Neuropeptides: promise unfulfilled? Trends Neurosci 18(2):49–50.

Kaneko T, Mizuno N. 1994. Glutamate-synthesizing enzymes in GABAergic neurons of the neocortex: a double immunofluorescence study in the rat. Neuroscience 61:839–849.

Kanner BI. 1994. Sodium-coupled neurotransmitter transport: structure, function and regulation. J Exp Biol 196:237–249.

Katz B. 1969. *The Release of Neural Transmitter Substances.* Springfield IL: Thomas.

Krieger DT. 1983. Brain peptides: what, where, and why? Science 222:975–985.

Lloyd PE, Frankfurt M, Stevens P, Kupfermann I, Weiss KR. 1987. Biochemical and immunocytological localization of the neuropeptides FMRFamide SCP_A, SCP_B, to neurons involved in the regulation of feeding in *Aplysia*. J Neurosci 7:1123–1132.

Loewi O. 1960. An autobiographic sketch. Perspect Biol Med 4:3–25.

Myers RD. 1994. Neuroactive peptides: unique phases in research on mammalian brain over three decades. Peptides 15(2):367–381.

Nelson N, Lill H. 1994. Porters and neurotransmitter transporters. J Exp Biol 196:213–228.

Otsuka M, Kravitz EA, Potter DD. 1967. Physiological and chemical architecture of a lobster ganglion with particular reference to γ-aminobutyrate and glutamate. J Neurophysiol 30:725–752.

Scheller RH, Axel R. 1984. How genes control an innate behavior. Sci Am 250(3):54–62.

Sossin WS, Fisher JM, Scheller RH. 1989. Cellular and molecular biology of neuropeptide processing and packaging. Neuron 2:1407–1417.

Thoenen H. 1974. Trans-synaptic enzyme induction. Life Sci 14:223–235.

Tuček S. 1988. Choline acetyltransferase and the synthesis of acetylcholine. In: VP Whittaker (ed). *The Cholinergic Synapse. Handbook of Experimental Pharmacology*, 86: 125–165. Berlin: Springer.

Weisskopf MG, Zalutsky RA, Nicoll RA. 1993. The opioid peptide dynorphin mediates heterosynaptic depression of hippocampal mossy fibre synapses and modulates long-term potentiation. Nature 362:423–427.

16

Diseases of Chemical Transmission at the Nerve-Muscle Synapse: Myasthenia Gravis

IN THE PRECEDING CHAPTERS we examined the mechanisms by which chemical transmitters are synthesized and released by neurons and the functional consequences of activating neurotransmitter receptors. Chemical transmission between neurons and their target cells is disrupted by many diseases. By analyzing such abnormalities in transmission, researchers have shed light on the mechanisms underlying normal synaptic function. The most common and most thoroughly studied disease affecting transmission is *myas-*

thenia gravis, a disorder of function at the synapse between cholinergic motor neurons and skeletal muscle.

There are two major forms of myasthenia gravis (the term means severe weakness of muscle). The most prevalent by far, and the only one known until about two decades ago, is the autoimmune form. Myasthenia gravis is the prototypical human autoimmune disease, fulfilling all the criteria proposed by Daniel Drachman. (1) An antibody is present in almost all cases. (2) The antibody reacts with an antigen that is important in the pathophysiology of the disease. (3) Features of the disease can be reproduced by transferring the antibodies to experimental animals. (4) An experimental form of the illness can be induced by immunizing animals with the antigen. (5) Therapeutic reduction of antibody levels ameliorates symptoms. The prevalence of autoimmune myasthenia is estimated to be 50–125 patients per million population, or about 25,000 affected people in the United States at any time.

The second form of myasthenia is congenital and heritable; it is not autoimmune and is heterogeneous. Fewer than 100 cases have been identified, but analysis of the congenital syndromes has provided information about the organization and function of the human neuromuscular junction. We will discuss this form later in the chapter.

In autoimmune myasthenia gravis, antibodies are produced against the nicotinic acetylcholine (ACh) receptor in muscle. These antibodies interfere with synaptic transmission by reducing the number of functional receptors or by impeding the interaction of ACh with its receptors. As a result, the skeletal muscle becomes weakened. This weakness has four special characteristics:

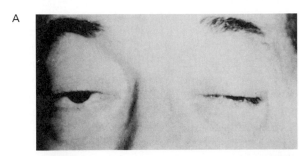

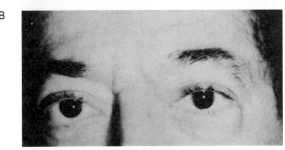

Figure 16-1 Myasthenia gravis typically affects the cranial muscles. (From Rowland et al. 1960.)

A. Severe drooping of the eyelids, or ptosis, is characteristic of myasthenia gravis. This patient also could not move his eyes to look to either side.

B. One minute after an intravenous injection of 10 mg edrophonium, an inhibitor of acetylcholinesterase, both eyes are open and can be moved freely.

1. It almost always affects cranial muscles—eyelids, eye muscles, and oropharyngeal muscles (Figure 16-1A)—as well as limb muscles.
2. The severity of symptoms varies in the course of a single day, from day to day, or over longer periods (giving rise to periods of remission or exacerbation), making myasthenia gravis unlike any other disease of muscle or nerve.
3. There are no conventional clinical signs of denervation, and there is no electromyographic evidence of denervation. In addition to weakness, the clinical signs of denervation include atrophy of the weak muscles, visible fasciculation, and loss of tendon reflexes. These signs are seen in diseases of the motor unit, especially those that affect the motor neuron itself.
4. The weakness is reversed by drugs that inhibit acetylcholinesterase, the enzyme that degrades ACh (Figure 16-1B).

Abnormal fatigability is an additional characteristic recognized by many experts. It is certainly true that the physiologic abnormality of transmission at the endplate can be regarded as excessive fatigability; repetitive stimulation of the nerve produces a decremental response of the evoked motor action potential. Moreover, when the eyelids are affected, gazing upward for long periods aggravates the ptosis. However, an emphasis on symptomatic fatigue can be misleading. For one thing, weak muscles, regardless of the cause, are likely to fatigue more rapidly than normal. And patients with myasthenia generally complain of weakness, not fatigue in the sense of tiredness or lack of energy.

Myasthenia Gravis Affects Transmission at the Nerve-Muscle Synapse

The first well-documented example of myasthenia gravis was reported in 1877 by Samuel Wilks. By 1900 neurologists had described the important clinical characteristics of the disease. At that time, however, diseases were still defined primarily in terms of lesions observed by microscopy at postmortem examination rather than in terms of physiological or etiological factors. In patients with myasthenia, the brain, spinal cord, peripheral nerves, and muscles all appeared normal at autopsy, and the disease was therefore considered a disorder of *function*.

Physiological Studies Showed a Disorder of Neuromuscular Transmission

Two discoveries in the mid 1930s helped to identify myasthenia as a disease of neuromuscular signal transmission. First, Henry Dale, Wilhelm Feldberg, and Marthe Vogt demonstrated that transmission at the neuromuscular junction is mediated by a chemical transmitter that they identified as ACh. Second, Mary Walker found that inhibitors of acetylcholinesterase, such as physostigmine and neostigmine, reverse the symptoms of myasthenia gravis.

In the years between 1945 and 1960 A. McGhee Harvey and his colleagues described in detail the physiological basis of the disorder. When a motor nerve is stimulated electrically, the summed electrical activity of a population of muscle fibers (known as the *compound action potential*) can be measured with surface electrodes. At stimulation rates of 2–5 per second the amplitude of the compound action potential evoked in normal human muscle remains constant. Harvey found that in myasthenia gravis the amplitude of evoked compound action potentials decreases rapidly. This abnormality resembles the pattern induced in normal muscle by *d*-tubocurarine (curare), which blocks ACh receptors and inhibits the action of ACh at the neuromuscular junction. Neostigmine (Prostigmin), an inhibitor of

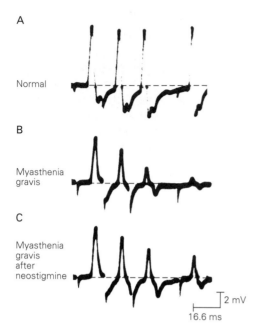

Figure 16-2 Neostigmine increases the duration of action of ACh and thus can compensate for the reduced ACh activity in myasthenia. (From Harvey et al. 1941.)

A. In a normal person the amplitude of action potentials evoked by a train of four stimuli at 16.6 ms intervals remains constant.

B. In the myasthenic patient there is a rapid decrease in amplitude.

C. After injection of 2 mg neostigmine into the brachial artery of the myasthenic patient, the decrease in amplitude was partially reversed.

cholinesterase that increases the duration of action of ACh at the neuromuscular junction, reverses the decrease in amplitude of evoked compound action potentials in myasthenic patients (Figure 16-2).

Immunological Studies Indicated That Myasthenia Is an Autoimmune Disease

Soon after the clinical syndrome had been identified it was recognized that about 15% of adult patients with myasthenia had a benign tumor of the thymus (thymomas). In 1939 Alfred Blalock first reported that the symptoms in myasthenic patients were improved by removal of the thymoma. Based on this finding, Blalock and Harvey, in the 1950s, found that removing the thymus in patients with myasthenia gravis also resulted in a reduction in symptoms, even in the absence of a thymoma. This procedure, known as *thymectomy*, has become standard treatment for patients with generalized myasthenia gravis.

In the 1950s, it was not clear why these tumors were associated with myasthenia or why thymectomy was beneficial, because the immunological role of the thymus was not established until the 1960s. The neurologist John Simpson was one of the first to suggest that myasthenia was an immunological disorder; he pointed out that myasthenia gravis often affects people who have other autoimmune diseases, such as rheumatoid arthritis, systemic lupus erythematosus, or Graves disease (hyperthyroidism).

Identification of Antibodies to the Acetylcholine Receptor Initiated the Modern Period of Research

The modern concept of myasthenia emerged with the isolation and characterization of the nicotinic ACh receptor. The breakthrough came in 1966. Two chemists, C. C. Chang and C.-Y. Lee, were concerned with a local public health problem in Taiwan—poisonous snake bites. One of the toxins they isolated from snake venom, α-bungarotoxin, was found to cause paralysis by binding essentially irreversibly to ACh receptors at the motor end-plate. By 1971 Lee and Jean-Pierre Changeux in Paris as well as Ricardo Miledi and Lincoln Potter in London had used the toxin to isolate and purify ACh receptors from the electric organ of the electric eel.

In 1973 Douglas Fambrough and Daniel Drachman used radioactive α-bungarotoxin to label the ACh receptors in human end-plates. They found fewer binding sites in myasthenic muscle than in controls (Figure 16-3). In the same year James Patrick and Jon Lindstrom injected ACh receptors purified from eel electroplax (which is related to the skeletal muscles of higher vertebrates) into rabbits, intending to use the resulting antibodies to study the properties of eel ACh receptors. Strikingly, the generation of the antibodies was accompanied by the onset of myasthenia-like symptoms in the rabbit. The weakness was reversed by the cholinesterase inhibitors neostigmine or edrophonium. As in humans with myasthenia gravis, the animals were abnormally sensitive to neuromuscular blocking agents, such as curare, and the evoked compound action potentials in muscle decreased with repetitive stimulation. It was later found that a similar syndrome can be induced in mice and other mammals by immunization with ACh receptor protein (Figure 16-4).

By 1975 all the essential characteristics of the human disease had been reproduced in experimental autoimmune myasthenia gravis. These characteristics included a reduction in the amplitude of the miniature end-plate potentials; a smoothing of the normal convo-

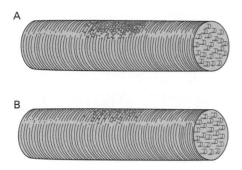

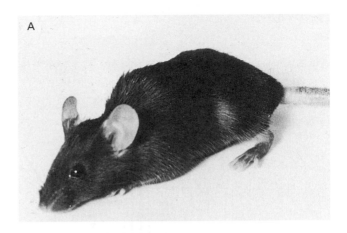

Figure 16-3 In myasthenia gravis the density of ACh receptors in human muscle fibers is reduced. ACh receptors are marked with ^{125}I-labeled α-bungarotoxin and detected in autoradiograms (drawn here). (Adapted from Fambrough et al. 1973.)

A. In normal fibers there is a dense accumulation of silver grains in a limited junctional area, the end-plate, and a paucity of grains outside this region.

B. In myasthenic fiber the grains are also localized in the end-plate region, but the number per unit area is markedly reduced, indicating a reduced density of functional reactive sites.

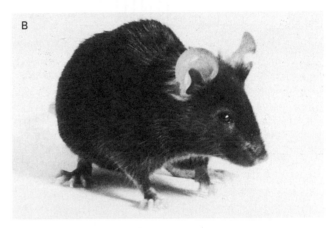

Figure 16-4 Posture of a myasthenic mouse before and after treatment with neostigmine. To produce the syndrome the mouse was immunized with 15 μg of ACh receptors from *Torpedo californica* and received a booster shot 45 days later with 15 μg of the receptor. (From Berman and Patrick 1980.)

A. Before treatment the mouse is inactive.

B. Twelve minutes after receiving an intraperitoneal injection of 37.5 μg/kg neostigmine bromide, the mouse is standing.

luted appearance of the postjunctional folds; loss of ACh receptors from the tips of postjunctional folds (see Figure 16-6); and the deposition at postjunctional sites of antibody and complement, a serum protein that participates in antibody-mediated cell lysis. ACh receptors from electric fish induced experimental autoimmune myasthenia gravis in mice, rats, and monkeys, suggesting that the structure of ACh receptors is highly conserved across species.

After experimental myasthenia gravis was characterized, antibodies directed against ACh receptors were found in the serum of patients with myasthenia. When B-lymphocytes from patients with myasthenia were cultured, the lymphocytes produced antibodies to ACh receptors. The idea that the human antibodies actually cause the symptoms of myasthenia was also supported by other observations. Repeated injections of serum from patients with myasthenia into mice reproduced the electrophysiological abnormalities in the recipients by reducing the number of available ACh receptors in their end-plates. A similar reduction in ACh receptors occurs with monoclonal antibodies to ACh receptors.

Further support for the role of antibodies against ACh receptors was provided by the detection of antibodies in infants with neonatal myasthenia. These children of myasthenic mothers have difficulty swallowing and their limb movements are impaired. The syndrome lasts from 7 to 10 days; as the symptoms abate, the level of antibodies declines. Similarly, draining lymph from the thoracic lymph ducts improves symptoms of myasthenia in adults. The symptoms recur when the patient's own lymphatic fluid is injected back into the patient, but not when the patient's lymphocytes are given separately. The causative factor is therefore in the plasma, rather than a function of the lymphocytes themselves. Furthermore, symptoms improve and antibody levels decline when patients are subjected to plasmapheresis, a procedure in which blood is removed from a patient, cells are separated from plasma, and the cells alone are returned to the patient. The plasma, which contains the antibodies, is discarded.

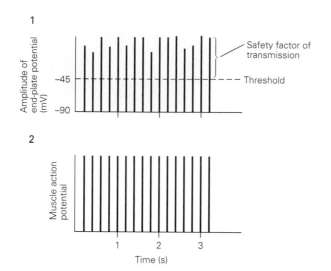

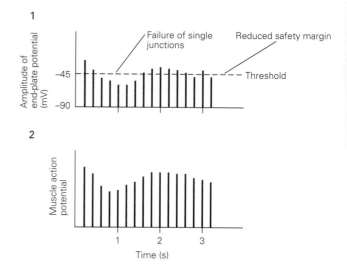

Figure 16-5 Failure of transmission at the neuromuscular junction in myasthenia gravis. (From Lisak and Barchi, 1982.)

A. In the normal neuromuscular junction the amplitude of the end-plate potential is so large that all fluctuations in the efficiency of transmitter release occur well above the threshold for a muscle action potential (1). Therefore, the amplitude of a compound muscle action potential during repetitive stimulation is constant and invariant (2).

B. In the myasthenic neuromuscular junction, postsynaptic changes reduce the amplitude of the end-plate potential in response to presynaptic release of a given amount of ACh, so

that under optimal circumstances the end-plate potential may be just sufficient to produce a muscle action potential. Fluctuations in transmitter release that normally accompany repeated stimulation now cause the end-plate potential to drop below this threshold, leading to conduction failure at that junction (1). When the action potential is recorded from the surface of a myasthenic muscle, the amplitude of the compound action potential—a measure of contributions from all fibers in which synaptic transmission is successful—shows a progressive decline and only a small and variable recovery (2) and indicates why the safety factor is reduced in myasthenia.

Immunological Changes Cause the Physiological Abnormality

How do the immunological observations that we have just considered account for the characteristic decrease in the response of myasthenic muscle to repetitive stimulation?

Normally, an action potential in a motor axon releases enough ACh from synaptic vesicles to induce an excitatory end-plate potential with an amplitude of about 70–80 mV (see Chapter 11). Thus the normal end-plate potential is greater than the threshold needed to initiate an action potential, about –45 mV. In normal muscle the difference between the threshold and the actual end-plate potential amplitude—*the safety factor*—is therefore quite large (Figure 16-5A). In fact, in many muscles the amount of ACh released during synaptic transmission can be reduced by 75%, to as little as 25% of normal before it fails to initiate an action potential.

Most of the ACh released into the synaptic cleft by an action potential is rapidly hydrolyzed by acetylcholinesterase. When the density of ACh receptors is re-

duced, as it is in myasthenia, the probability that a molecule of ACh will find a receptor before it is hydrolyzed is reduced. Moreover, the geometry of the end-plate is also disturbed in myasthenia. The normal infolding at the junctional folds is reduced and the synaptic cleft is enlarged (Figure 16-6). These morphological changes increase the diffusion of ACh away from the synaptic cleft and thus further reduce the probability of ACh interacting with the few remaining functional receptors. As a result, the amplitude of the end-plate potential is reduced to the point where it is barely above threshold (Figure 16-5B). Thus, transmission is readily blocked even though the vesicles in the presynaptic terminals contain normal amounts of ACh and the processes of exocytosis and release are intact. Both the physiological abnormality (the decremental response) and the clinical symptoms (muscle weakness) are partially reversed by drugs that inhibit active cholinesterase because the released ACh molecules remain unhydrolyzed for a longer time, and this increases the probability that they will interact with receptors.

The reduced efficacy of neuromuscular transmission in myasthenia can be assessed by the clinical tech-

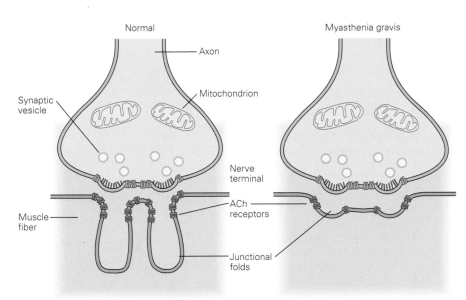

Figure 16-6 Morphological abnormalities characteristic of the myasthenic junction. At neuromuscular junctions vesicles release ACh at specialized release sites in the nerve terminal. Acetylcholine crosses the synaptic space to reach receptors that are concentrated at the peaks of junctional folds. Acetylcholinesterase in the cleft rapidly terminates transmission by hydrolyzing ACh. The myasthenic junction has reduced numbers of ACh receptors, simplified synaptic folds, a widened synaptic space, but a normal nerve terminal.

nique of single-fiber electromyography, which measures the intervals between discharges of different muscle fibers innervated by the same motor neuron. The normal variation in intervals is called *jitter.* The extent of jitter depends on the velocity of conduction in nerve terminals, transmitter release, and activation of the postsynaptic membrane. Jitter may therefore increase in nonmyasthenic neurogenic diseases but is especially pronounced in myasthenia gravis.

Antibody Binds to the α-Subunit of the Acetycholine Receptor in Myasthenia Gravis

As discussed in Chapter 11, the genes for each of the subunits of mammalian ACh receptor have been cloned and sequenced, and peptides corresponding to specific domains of ACh receptor subunits have been synthesized. In experimental animals antibodies that cause myasthenia are usually active against either of two peptide sequences on the native receptor—the bungarotoxin-binding site or an area on the α-subunit called the *main immunogenic region.* Circulating antibodies in humans are often directed against the main immunogenic region.

Even though it has been well established that antibodies to the α-subunit of ACh receptors have a central role in the pathogenesis of myasthenia—so much so that myasthenia is now the prototype of human autoimmune disease—several questions remain unanswered. What, for example, initiates the production of antibodies to the ACh receptor? One possibility is that persistent viral infection could alter the properties of the

surface membrane, rendering it immunogenic, but this has not been shown. Another possibility is that viral or bacterial antigens may share epitopes with the ACh receptor. Thus, when a person is infected, the antibodies generated against the foreign organism may also recognize the ACh receptor. The molecular similarity of the antigens is called *molecular mimicry.*

How do antibodies cause the symptoms of myasthenia? The antibodies do not occupy the receptor site alone. This conclusion emanates from the test used to detect antireceptor antibodies in human serum. The circulating antibodies will even react with purified ACh receptors that have been labeled with radioactive α-bungarotoxin. Because the toxin itself occupies and blocks the ligand binding site, the antibody must react with epitopes elsewhere on the receptor molecule.

One effect of the antibodies might be to interfere with the interaction of ACh and the receptor. The loss of receptors is, however, probably due to an increase in turnover and degradation of ACh receptors. Myasthenic antibodies are able to bind and cross-link ACh receptors, in this way triggering the internalization and degradation of the receptor (Figure 16-7). In addition, some antibodies to ACh receptors in myasthenic patients bind proteins of the complement cascade, which may result in lysis of the postsynaptic membrane.

Although the evidence implicating ACh receptor antibodies in myasthenic symptoms is compelling, the antibodies are not found in all myasthenic patients. Moreover, there is no consistent relationship between the serum concentration of antibodies directed against ACh receptors and the severity of symptoms. One explanation of this dissociation is that the antibodies found in the serum of myasthenic patients or in animals

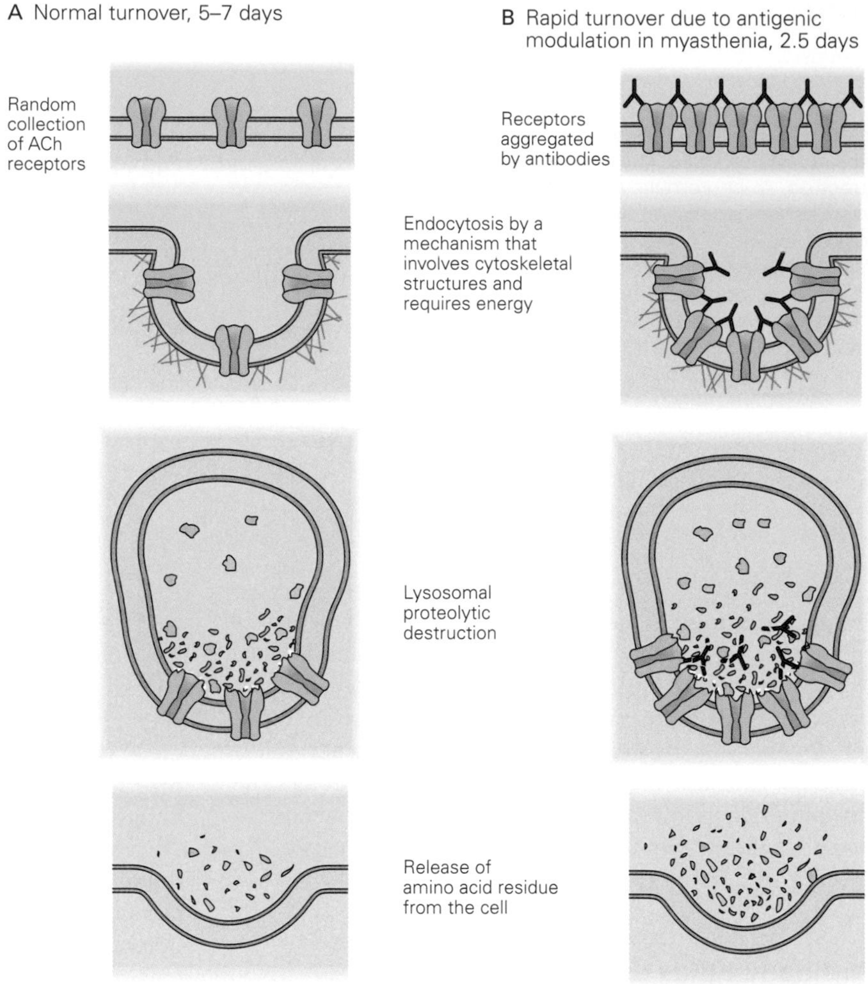

Figure 16-7 The rate of destruction of ACh receptors increases in myasthenia. (Adapted from Lindstrom 1983, and Drachman 1983.)

A. Normal turnover of randomly spaced ACh receptors takes place every 5–7 days.

B. In myasthenia gravis and in experimental myasthenia gravis the cross-linking of ACh receptors by the antibody facilitates the normal endocytosis and phagocytic destruction of the receptors, which leads to a two- to threefold increase in the rate of receptor turnover. Binding of antireceptor antibody activates the complement cascade, which is involved in focal lysis of the postsynaptic membrane. This focal lysis is probably primarily responsible for the characteristic alterations of postsynaptic membrane morphology observed in myasthenia (see Figure 16-6).

with experimentally induced myasthenia gravis are polyclonal; they are produced by different B cells in response to different antigenic determinants, and therefore the serum of each patient contains antibodies with distinct specificities. As a consequence, some people with high titers of antibodies to the receptor but few or no clinical symptoms might have a type of antibody that is limited in its ability to interfere with synaptic transmission or to influence ACh receptor turnover. In contrast, other patients with severe myasthenia might have low titers of antibodies that are effective in interfering with the function of the receptor and its turnover.

The Molecular Basis of the Autoimmune Reaction Has Been Defined

The autoimmune reaction depends on interactions within a trimolecular complex comprising the following: (1) the antigen, the immunogenic peptide of the ACh receptor or a peptide that mimics the receptor; (2) an antigen-specific T-cell receptor; and (3) class II molecules of the major histocompatibility complex (MHC) that are expressed on the antigen-presenting cell (Figure 16-8A). The T cells become reactive against the ACh receptor. This could result from an infection in which a viral protein includes a peptide homologous to one in the ACh receptor, a form of molecular mimicry. Once activated, the T cells could recognize the ACh receptor on myoid cells in the thymus. Antigen-specific T cells have actually been identified in the thymus glands of patients with myasthenia.

The class II MHC genes also play a major role in determining susceptibility. Patients with myasthenia gravis have more of the histocompatibility subtypes DR3 and DQ2. The relative risk of people with human leukocyte antigen (HLA)–DQ for myasthenia is 32 times more than that of people with other HLA haplotypes.

A Activation of autoimmune T lymphocytes

C The ACh receptor

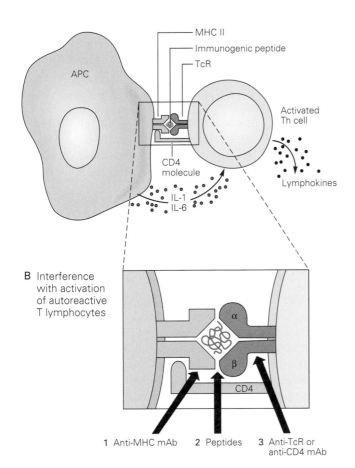

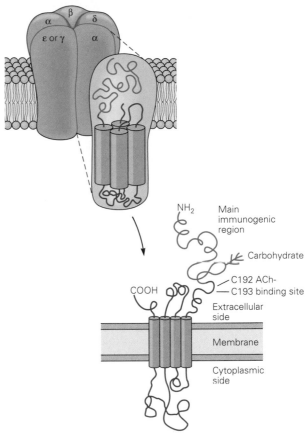

Figure 16-8 Mechanisms of the autoimmune reaction directed against the ACh receptor. Abbreviations: **APC** = antigen-presenting cell; **Th** = thymocyte; **MHC** = major histocompatibility complex; **TcR** = T-cell receptor; **IL** = interleukin; **mAb** = monoclonal antibody. (Adapted from Steinman and Mantegazza 1990.)

A. Activation of autoimmune T lymphocytes requires three molecules: an immunogenic peptide in the ACh receptor (AChR) or one that mimics it, a specific class II molecule of the major histocompatibility complex (MHC) on the antigen-

presenting cell, and an antigen-specific T-cell receptor (TcR).

B. Treatment of myasthenia gravis may be improved by molecular therapy designed to inhibit MHC recognition by **(1)** using antibodies to MHC, **(2)** administering peptides that compete with ACh receptors and so block the T cells, or **(3)** using antibodies directed against the T cells themselves.

C. Molecular structure of the ACh receptor. The main immunogenic region is in the extracellular portion of the α-subunit. The ACh binding site is not located within the immunogenic region.

The specific immunogenic peptides of human ACh receptors have also been identified.

These findings open new approaches to therapy for patients who do not improve sufficiently with anticholinesterase drug therapy or thymectomy. For instance, it might be possible to make antibodies against

the anti-ACh receptor antibodies or anti-idiotype antibodies. However, this has proven difficult in experimental myasthenia. Another approach is to develop peptide competitors for ACh receptors that might block T-cell recognition of ACh receptors or MHC binding of ACh receptor fragments (Figure 16-8B). Alternatively, antibodies might be developed against either MHC class II molecules of the antigen-presenting cells or receptors on the T cells that recognize ACh receptors.

Current Therapy for Autoimmune Myasthenia Gravis Is Effective But Not Ideal

Treatment of a patient with myasthenia is based upon the altered physiology and the autoimmune pathogenesis. Anticholinesterases, especially pyridostigmine, are used to provide symptomatic relief but this is rarely complete and does not alter the basic disease. Immunosuppressive therapies include corticosteroids and azathioprine or related drugs that suppress antibody synthesis. Plasmapheresis, removing the plasma and the antibodies to the ACh receptor, often ameliorates symptoms within days or a few weeks, but the benefit is transient. The temporary benefit may be sufficient to prepare a patient for thymectomy or to support the patient through more severe episodes. Intravenous administration of immunoglobulins also reduces the titer of antibodies to the ACh receptor by mechanisms that are not clear.

Twenty-five years ago the mortality rate of myasthenia was about 33%. Now, few patients die of the disease and life expectancy is almost normal. This change is largely due to advances in intensive care, including mechanical ventilation and antibiotics. Years ago respiratory-care units of hospitals were populated by many patients in myasthenic "crisis," defined by the use of a mechanical ventilator for a patient in respiratory distress. Now the number of patients in crisis has declined drastically. Many investigators attribute this change to the practice of thymectomy. After thymectomy about half of the patients are in "remission"—they have no symptoms of myasthenia and take no drugs. It is not clear how thymectomy is beneficial; it removes a source of antigen (ACh receptors are present on the myoid cells found in normal thymus), and it also removes a major source of lymphocytes that synthesize the antibodies. The thymus must also play a role in immunoregulation, including the pathophysiology of myasthenia gravis. Further improvement in therapy will have to be directed toward patients who are not helped by thymectomy.

Congenital Forms of Myasthenia Gravis

It had long been recognized that symptoms of myasthenia may be present from birth. Congenital myasthenia differs from neonatal myasthenia; in the neonatal syndrome the mothers themselves have myasthenia, whereas with congenital myasthenia the mothers are unaffected. Moreover, there seems to be a disproportionate number of familial cases among those with congenital myasthenia. When the antibodies to ACh were found in autoimmune myasthenia, another difference emerged: children with the congenital forms do not show this antibody activity. The pathophysiology must therefore differ, too.

In 1977 Andrew Engel and his colleagues studied a patient with congenital myasthenia and concluded that there was a *deficiency of acetylcholinesterase* at the endplate. Since then they have described several other abnormalities, including abnormalities of presynaptic nerve terminals resulting in impaired release of ACh from the terminals. Other conditions are attributed to postsynaptic disorders, such as congenital lack of acetylcholinesterase (AChE), impaired capacity of ACh receptors to interact with ACh, or abnormally low numbers of ACh receptors.

The studies involve standard electromyography, cytochemical localization of AChE, immunocytochemical analysis of that enzyme and the receptors as well as the deposition of immunoglobulins, labeled bungarotoxin binding, electron microscopy and electron cytochemistry, microelectrode analysis of miniature endplate amplitude and frequency as well as end-plate current and quantal release of transmitter, analysis of ACh-induced current noise to identify kinetic abnormalities, and single-channel patch clamp studies. Needless to say, these investigations require a combination of skills found in only a few laboratories worldwide.

The identification of numerous syndromes has been a tour de force for Engel and his associates. Even so, the patients within any group show differences that imply further heterogeneity, and there is much to be done to identify the specific abnormalities. For instance, John Newsom-Davis, Angela Vincent, and their associates found that few of the 22 patients they studied fit neatly into the categories identified by Engel. Even so, two congenital disorders can be described to provide examples of the pathophysiology of congenital myasthenia.

In deficiency of acetylcholinesterase there is a decremental response of the compound action potential evoked in muscle by repetitive stimulation of the nerve at 2 Hz, as in autoimmune myasthenia, but the muscle responds repetitively to a single stimulus, a feature not seen in other conditions. End-plate potentials and miniature end-plate potentials are not small, as in autoimmune myasthenia, but are markedly prolonged, which could explain the reiterative response of the evoked muscle potential. Cytochemical studies indicate that AChE is absent from the postsynaptic membranes.

In contrast, ACh receptors, as visualized by labeling with radioactive bungarotoxin, are preserved.

The *slow-channel syndrome* is characterized by prominent limb weakness with little weakness of cranial muscles (the reverse of the pattern usually seen in autoimmune myasthenia, where muscles of the eyes and oropharynx are almost always affected). The end-plate potentials of the slow-channel syndrome are prolonged in a manner similar to that observed in AChE deficiency, and spontaneous miniature end-plate potentials are also prolonged. In contrast, however, AChE is present and shows normal kinetics. These features suggest that the opening of the ACh receptor channel is abnormally prolonged. In addition, miniature end-plate potentials are of abnormally low amplitude, which could result from the degeneration of junctional folds and loss of ACh receptors.

It is not certain how the slow-channel syndrome arises. However, the ACh receptor-channel is similarly slow in newly formed end-plates in normal mammalian muscle. It is possible that the developmental transition from slow to fast channels (which is accompanied by replacement of the γ-subunit of the ACh receptor by an ϵ-subunit) is prevented. It is also possible that a mutation has altered the ACh receptor in a way that modifies the time the channel spends in the open state.

Because the genes for all its subunits have been cloned, it is now possible to identify the specific mutations of the ACh receptor. This has not yet been achieved, but progress is being made. For instance, immunocytochemical analysis has revealed the absence of the long cytoplasmic loop of the ϵ-subunit in one form of congenital myasthenia. Molecular DNA analysis tends to confirm this interpretation.

Anticholinesterase inhibitors are effective in some of these disorders, not in others. Some patients seem to benefit from 3,4-diaminopyridine, which blocks K^+ conductance and promotes the release of ACh at nerve terminals.

Other Disorders of Neuromuscular Transmission: Lambert-Eaton Syndrome and Botulism

Some patients with cancer, especially small-cell cancer of the lung, have a syndrome of proximal limb weakness and a neuromuscular disorder with characteristics that are the opposite of those seen in myasthenia gravis. Instead of a decline in synaptic response to repetitive nerve stimulation, the amplitude of the evoked potential increases, a state called *facilitating neuromuscular block.* Here the first postsynaptic potential is abnormally small, but subsequent responses increase in amplitude so that the final summated potential produced by a train of five spikes per second is two to four times the amplitude of the first potential. This disorder, the *Lambert-Eaton syndrome,* is attributed to the action of antibodies against voltage-gated Ca^{2+} channels in the presynaptic terminals.

It has not yet been possible to identify which subtype of Ca^{2+} channel is affected, but an assay has been developed with the ligand ω-conotoxin, which is isolated from a snail and binds to the N-type channel. Serum from patients with the syndrome binds to the ω-conotoxin receptor. Although the assay is convenient and sensitive, it is not specific and there are many false positive responses in people who do not have the Lambert-Eaton syndrome. Also, serum from patients reacts with L-, T-, and P-type voltage-gated Ca^{2+} channels. Nevertheless, it is thought that the antibody reacts with an antigen in the channel and that, in parallel with the process in myasthenia, the antibody-antigen complex is internalized and the receptors are degraded. Similar Ca^{2+} channels are found in cultured cells from the small-cell carcinoma of the lung; development of antibodies against these antigens in the tumor might be followed by pathogenic action against nerve terminals, another kind of molecular mimicry.

This theory emerged from passive transfer experiments. Mice injected with serum from Lambert-Eaton patients showed electrophysiological abnormalities typical of the human syndrome; electron microscope evidence showed loss of the presynaptic active zones and active zone particles thought to be Ca^{2+} channels (see Chapter 13). Loss of the voltage-gated Ca^{2+} channels at the active zones would be expected to reduce the entry of Ca^{2+} when nerve terminals are depolarized, impairing the release of transmitter.

Confirmation of the autoimmune theory has come from therapeutic responses of the patients to plasmapheresis, intravenous immunoglobulin therapy, and long-term immunosuppressive drug therapy. In some patients the neurological disorder has disappeared with successful treatment of the cancer. Some patients with the Lambert-Eaton syndrome have no recognized tumor, even at autopsy. In these patients the pathogenesis is not known.

A similar facilitating neuromuscular block is found in human botulism; the botulinum toxin also impairs release of ACh from nerve terminals. Both botulism and the Lambert-Eaton syndrome are ameliorated by administration of calcium gluconate or guanidine, agents that promote the release of ACh, but these drugs are less effective than immunosuppressive treatments for long-term control of the Lambert-Eaton syndrome, which is chronic. Botulism, on the other hand, is transient, and if the patient is kept alive during the acute phase by treating symptoms, the disorder disappears in weeks as the infection is controlled and botulinum toxin is inactivated.

An Overall View

Studies of autoimmune myasthenia, congenital myasthenia, and the Lambert-Eaton syndrome are good examples of the useful synergy between clinical and basic neuroscience, and the fruitful interactions of both approaches with molecular genetics and molecular immunology. All three of these illnesses have been elucidated by advances in basic neuroscience. In turn, the clinical disorders have provided information about the normal structure and function of the neuromuscular junction. A combination of clinical and basic science has also led to more effective therapy. Nevertheless, the symptoms of these diseases cannot always be alleviated and some patients remain disabled, so more advances through research are essential.

Lewis P. Rowland

Selected Readings

Cherington M. 1998. Clinical spectrum of botulism. Muscle Nerve 21:701–10.

DeBaets M, Oosterhuis HJGH (eds). 1993. *Myasthenia Gravis.* Boca Raton, FL: CRC.

Drachman DB (ed). 1987. Myasthenia gravis: biology and treatment. Ann NY Acad Sci 505:1–914.

Drachman DB. 1994. Myasthenia gravis. N Engl J Med 330:1797–1810.

Engel AG, (ed). 1999. *Myasthenia Gravis and Myasthenic Syndromes.* New York: Oxford Univ. Press.

Lewis RA, Selwa JF, Lisak RP. 1995. Myasthenia gravis: immunological mechanisms and immunotherapy. Ann Neurol 37:(Suppl 1):S51–S62.

Lindstrom J. 1983. Using monoclonal antibodies to study acetylcholine receptors and myasthenia gravis. Neurosci Comment 1:139–156.

Lisak RP (ed). 1994. *Handbook of Myasthenia Gravis and Myasthenic Syndromes.* New York: Marcel Dekker.

Lisak RP, Barchi RL. 1982. *Myasthenia Gravis.* Philadelphia: Saunders.

Newsom-Davis J. 1997. Autoantibody-mediated channelopathies at the neuromuscular junction. Neuroscientist 3:337-346.

Maselli RA. 1998. Pathogenesis of human botulism. Ann NY Acad Sci 841:122–39.

Newsom-Davis N. 1997. Antibody-mediated channelopathies at the neuromuscular junction. Neuroscientist 3:337–346.

Newsom-Davis J. 1998. A treatment algorithm for Lambert-Eaton myasthenic syndrome. Ann NY Acad Sci 841:817–822.

Numa S. 1989. Molecular structure and function of acetylcholine receptors and sodium channels. In: S Chien (ed). *Molecular Biology in Physiology,* pp. 93–118. New York: Raven.

Pachner AR. 1988. Myasthenia gravis. Immunol Allerg Clin North Am 8:277–293.

Rowland LP. 1980. Controversies about the treatment of myasthenia gravis. J Neurol Neurosurg Psychiatry 43:644–659.

Seybold ME. 1995. Myasthenia gravis: diagnosis and therapeutic perspectives in the 1990s. Neurologist 1:345–360.

Shapiro RL. Hatheway C, Serdlow DL. 1998. Botulism in the United States: a clinical and epidemiologic review. Ann Intern Med 129:221–228.

Swift TR. 1981. Disorders of neuromuscular transmission other than myasthenia gravis. Muscle Nerve 4:334–353.

Tim RW et al. 1998. Lamber-Eaton myasthenic syndrome (LEMS). Clinical and electrodiagnostic features and response to therapy in 59 patients. Ann NY Acad Sci 841:823–826.

Verchuuren JJ, Dalmau J, Tunkel R, Lang B, Graus F, Schramm L, Posner JB, Newsom-Davis J, Rosenfeld MR. 1998. Antibodies against the calcium channel beta-subunit in Lambert-Eaton myasthenic syndrome. Neurology 50:475–479.

Voltz R, Carrpentier AF, Rosenfeld MR, Posner JB, Dalmau J. 1999. P/Q-type voltage-gated calcium channel antibodies in paraneoplastic disorder of the central nervous system. Muscle Nerve 22:119–122.

Wilks S. 1883. *Lectures on Diseases of the Nervous System Delivered at Guy's Hospital,* 2nd ed. Philadelphia: P. Blakiston, Son & Co.

Younger DS (ed). 1997. Advances in the diagnosis, pathogenesis, and treatment of myasthenia gravis. Neurology 48(Suppl 5):S1–S81.

References

Berman PW, Patrick J. 1980. Experimental myasthenia gravis: a murine system. J Exp Med 151:204–223.

Berman PW, Patrick J, Heinemann S, Klier FG, Steinbach JH. 1981. Factors affecting the susceptibility of different strains of mice to experimental myasthenia gravis. Ann NY Acad Sci 377:237–257.

Blalock A, Mason MF, Morgan HJ, Riven SS. 1939. Myasthenia gravis and tumors of the thymic region. Report of a case in which the tumor was removed. Ann Surg 110:544–561.

Chang CC, Lee C-Y. 1966. Electrophysiological study of neuromuscular blocking action of cobra neurotoxin. Br J Pharm Chemother 28:172–181.

Changeux J-P, Kasai M, Lee C-Y. 1970. Use of a snake venom toxin to characterize the cholinergic receptor protein. Proc Natl Acad Sci USA 67:1241–1247.

Cull-Candy SG, Miledi R, Trautmann A. 1979. End-plate currents and acetylcholine noise at normal and myasthenic human end-plates. J Physiol (Lond) 287:247–265.

Dale HH, Feldberg W, Vogt M. 1936. Release of acetylcholine at voluntary motor nerve endings. J Physiol (Lond) 86:353–380.

Drachman DB. 1983. Myasthenia gravis: immunology of a receptor disorder. Trends Neurosci 6:446–451.

Dwyer JM. 1992. Manipulating the immune system with immune globulin. N Engl J Med 326:107–116.

Eaton LM, Lambert EH. 1957. Electromyography and electric stimulation of nerves in diseases of the motor unit: observations on myasthenic syndrome associated with malignant tumors. JAMA 163:1117–1124.

Engel AG, Ohno K, Sine SM. 1999. Congenital myasthenic syndromes: recent advances. Arch Neurol 56:163–71.

Engel AG, Ohno K, Wang HL, Milone M, Sine SM. 1998. Molecular basis of congenital myasthenic syndrome: mutations in the acetylkcholine receptor. The Neuroscientist 4:185–94.

Fambrough DM, Drachman DB, Satyamurti S. 1973. Neuromuscular junction in myasthenia gravis: decreased acetylcholine receptors. Science 182:293–295.

Gomez CM, Bhattacharya BB, Charnet P, Day JW, Labarca C, Wollmann RL, Lambert EH. 1996. A transgenic mouse model of the slow-channel syndrome. Muscle Nerve 19:79–87.

Harcourt GC, Sommer N, Rothbard J, Willcox HNA, Newsom-Davis J. 1988. A juxta-membrane epitope on the human acetylcholine receptor recognized by T cells in myasthenia gravis. J Clin Invest 82:1295–1300.

Harvey AM, Lilienthal JL Jr, Talbot SA. 1941. Observations on the nature of myasthenia gravis: the phenomena of facilitation and depression of neuromuscular transmission. Bull Johns Hopkins Hosp 69:547–565.

Hohlfeld R, Toyka KV, Miner LL, Walgrave SL, Conti-Tronconi BM. 1988. Amphipathic segment of the nicotinic receptor alpha subunit contains epitopes recognized by T lymphocytes in myasthenia gravis. J Clin Invest 81:657–660.

Jaretzki A III, Penn AS, Younger DS, Wolff M, Olarte MR, Lovelace RE, Rowland LP. 1988. "Maximal" thymectomy for myasthenia gravis. Results. J Thorac Cardiovasc Surg 95:747–757.

Kim YI, Neher E. 1988. IgG from patients with Lambert-Eaton syndrome blocks voltage-dependent calcium channels. Science 239:405–408.

Lennon VA, Kryzer TJ, Griesmann GE, O'Suilleabhain PE, Windebank AJ, Woppman A, Miljanich GP, Lambert EH.

1995. Calcium-channel antibodies in the Lambert-Eaton syndrome and other paraneoplastic syndromes. N Engl J Med 332:1467–1474.

Mason WP, Graus F, Lang B, Honnorat J, Delattre J-Y, Valldeoriola F, Antonine JC, Rosenblum MK, Rosenfield MR, Newsom-Davis J, Posner JB, Dalman J. 1997. Small-cell lung cancer, paraneoplastic cerebellar degeneration and the Lambert-Eaton myasthenic syndrome. 120:1279–1300.

Middleton LT. 1996. Congenital myasthenic syndromes. 34th ENMC International Workshop, 10–11 June 1995. Neuromusc Disord 6:133–136.

Miledi R, Molinoff P, Potter LT. 1971. Isolation of the cholinergic receptor protein of Torpedo electric tissue. Nature 229:554–557.

Palace J, Wiles CM, Newsom-Davis J. 1991. 3,4-Diaminopyridine in the treatment of congenital (hereditary) myasthenia. J Neurol Neurosurg Psychiatry 54:1069–1072.

Palmisani MT, Evoli A, Battochi AP, Provenzano C, Tolnali P. 1994. Myasthenia gravis associated with thymoma: clinical characteristics and long-term outcome. Eur Neurol 34:78–82.

Patrick J, Lindstrom J. 1973. Autoimmune response to acetylcholine receptor. Science 180:871–872.

Penn AS, Richman DP, Ruff VA, Lennon VA (eds). 1993. Myasthenia gravis and related disorders. Ann NY Acad Sci 681:16–22.

Rowland LP, Hoefer PFA, Aranow H Jr. 1960. Myasthenic syndromes. Res Publ Assoc Res Nerv Ment Dis 38:548–600.

Simpson JA. 1960. Myasthenia gravis: a new hypothesis. Scott Med J 4:419–436.

Soliven BC, Lange DJ, Penn AS, Younger D, Jaretzki A III, Lovelace RE, Rowland LP. 1988. Seronegative myasthenia gravis. Neurology 38:514–517.

Steinman L, Mantegazza R. 1990. Prospects for specific immunotherapy in myasthenia gravis. FASEB J 4:2726–2731.

Thomas CE, Mayer SA, Gungor Y, Swarup R, Webster EA, Chang I, Brannagan TH, Fink ME, Rowland LP. 1997. Myasthenic crisis: clinical features, mortality, complications, and risk factors for prolonged intubation. Neurology 48:1253–1260.

Toyka KV, Drachman DB, Pestronk A, Kao I. 1975. Myasthenia gravis: passive transfer from man to mouse. Science 190:397–399.

Vincent A, Pinching AJ, Newsom-Davis JM. 1977. Circulating anti-acetylcholine receptor antibody in myasthenia gravis treated by plasma exchange. Neurology 27:364.

Walker MB. 1934. Treatment of myasthenia gravis with physostigmine. Lancet 1:1200–1201.

Weinberg D. 1994. Discussion of Lambert-Eaton syndrome. Case Records of the Massachusetts General Hospital,

Part IV

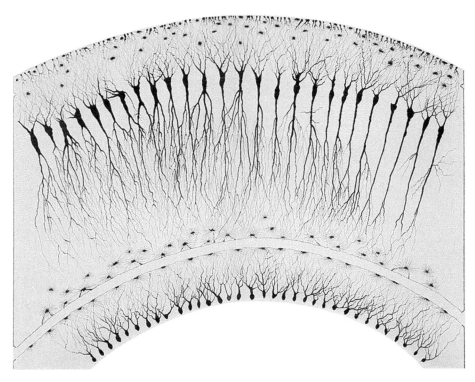

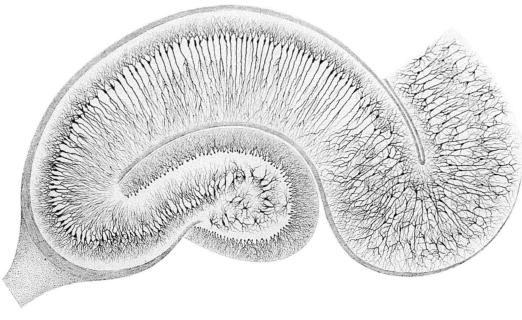

Preceding page

Histological Section of the Hippocampus. The hippocampus is important for the conversion of short- to long-term memory. These drawings were published in 1903 in *Camillo Golgi's Opera Omnia* (Milan: Ulrico Hoepli), probably in celebration of Golgi's sixtieth birthday. Golgi, who not only invented the silver chromate staining method so important to neurocytology but also used it so beautifully as shown here, shared the Nobel prize with Ramón y Cajal in 1926. The top section depicts the hippocampus of the rabbit and the bottom section, that of the neonatal kitten.

IV   The Neural Basis of Cognition

S O FAR IN THIS BOOK WE HAVE examined the properties of individual nerve cells and how they communicate at synapses to produce simple reflex behaviors. We now begin to consider larger, interconnected networks of neurons, the complex circuits that give rise to mental activity: perception, planned action, and thought. Understanding how these networks produce the cognitive functions of the brain is one of the ultimate challenges of science. We need to know how sensory information is perceived and how perceptions are assembled into inner representations and formulated into plans for immediate behavior or concepts for future actions. It is still unclear how complex memories are made and how percepts, ideas, and feelings are transformed into language.

These questions have been asked since the beginning of recorded history. For centuries philosophers have been at work developing a coherent epistemology. Several modern disciplines—psychology, linguistics, information theory—have focused on the problem of how we think. Why then do we now need a new discipline called cognitive neural science?

Neural science, the modern science of the brain, emerged in the mid 1970s with the development of powerful techniques for exploring the cellular dynamics of the nervous system and with the convergence of several previously separate disciplines concerned with the brain: molecular biology, neuroanatomy, electrophysiology, cell biology, and developmental biology. Now, with the development of techniques that permit us to observe the system properties of the brain directly in controlled behavior experiments, neural science is able to address testable hypotheses about how the brain thinks. Cognitive neural science is a pragmatic attempt to merge neural science with psychology.

The aim of cognitive neural science is to examine classical philosophical and psychological questions about mental functions in the light of cell and molecular biology. This is a bold undertaking. How do we begin to think about perception, ideas, and feelings in biological terms? So far progress in understanding the major functional systems of the brain—the sensory, motor, motivational, memory, and attentional systems—has benefited from a reductionist approach to mental function, an approach based on the assumption that these functions will emerge from the biological properties of nerve cells and of their pattern of interconnections. According to this view, which was introduced in Chapter 1, the mind can be considered a set of operations carried out by the brain, an information-processing organ made powerful by the enormous number, variety, and interactions of its nerve cells and by the complexity of interconnection among these cells. In this and later parts of this book we describe the attempt to extend this cell biological approach to the cognitive functions of the brain. We focus specifically on the major domains of cognitive neural science: perception, action, emotion, motivation, language, learning, and memory.

An understanding of the biological basis of cognitive functions also requires an appreciation of the anatomy of the neural systems that subserve these functions in the brain. In the same way that the detailed structure of a protein reveals important principles of its action, knowledge of neuroanatomy, seemingly a static science, can provide profound insight into how the nervous system functions. Just as many contemporary ideas about the dynamic mechanisms underlying the development of connectivity in the nervous system were anticipated a century ago by Ramón y Cajal on the basis of Golgi images of neurons in histological specimens, we predict that much of our understanding of higher brain function will depend on refined mapping of neuronal circuits.

Modern anatomical and imaging techniques are defining how neural circuits are organized. For example, the sensory pathways from one brain region to the next are organized in such a way that neighboring groups of neurons in the brain maintain the spatial relationship of sensory receptors in the periphery of the body. This topological organization is an important way of conveying spatial information about sensory events. In recent years the study of brain anatomy has been advanced even further with new imaging techniques that have revolutionized the study of cognitive functions. These techniques have made visible the neuroanatomy of the living human brain during specific behaviors. As a consequence, a much clearer idea of the brain regions involved in many complex cognitive functions is emerging.

In this part of the book we first review the anatomical organization of the three major functional subdivisions of the nervous system: sensory, motor, and modulatory. We then take a closer look at the structural organization of the central nervous system by following the flow of sensory information from the periphery into the spinal cord and brain, the transformation of that information into a motor command, and the effect of that command on muscle, the organ of movement. We then examine the cognitive processes of the brain that are concerned with attention, memory, visual perception, and planned action. Many of these activities are represented in higher-order association regions of the cerebral cortex, areas that bring together information from various sensory systems to provide coordinated plans for action. One of the important questions that we shall examine in this section is how mental functions are represented in different regions of the brain. How is that representation processed on the cellular level? What are the cellular mechanisms for cognition?

In later parts of the book we shall explore each functional system of the brain in detail, examining how the specific structure and cellular interconnections of a system determine its particular function.

Part IV

17

The Anatomical Organization of the Central Nervous System

IN THE EARLIER PARTS OF THIS book we learned that neurons in different regions of the vertebrate nervous system, and indeed in all nervous systems, are quite similar. What distinguishes one brain region from another and one brain from the next are the number and types of its neurons and how they are interconnected. It is from the patterns of interconnections that the distinctiveness of behavior emerges. Whether it be a simple reflex response or a complex mental act, behavior results from the pattern of signaling between appropriately interconnected cells.

This fundamental simplicity in the organization of neuronal circuits is more than counterbalanced by numerical complexity. Even a relatively simple behavior recruits the activity of many neurons. Consider the act of hitting a tennis ball (Figure 17-1). For this task several sensory systems are called into play. Visual information about the motion of the approaching ball is processed in the visual system, which identifies the flying object and computes its direction and velocity. Proprioceptive information about the position of the player's arms, legs, and trunk in space are also computed by the brain to plan the appropriate positioning of the body for interception of the ball. All of this sensory information ulti-

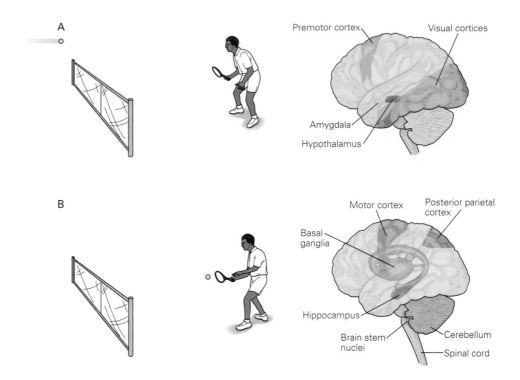

Figure 17-1 Even simple behaviors use many parts of the brain.

A. The tennis player is watching the approaching ball. He uses his visual cortex to identify the ball and judge its size, direction, and velocity. His premotor cortex develops a motor program that will allow him to approach the ball and hit it back. The amygdala adjusts the heart rate, respiration, and other homeostatic mechanisms to allow successful performance of the behavior. The amygdala also activates the hypothalamus to motivate the player to hit a good shot.

B. To execute the shot the player must use all of the structures illustrated in **A** as well as others. The player's motor cortex must send signals to the spinal cord that will activate and inhibit many muscles in the arms and legs. The basal ganglia become involved in initiating motor patterns and perhaps in recall-

ing learned movements to hit the ball properly. The cerebellum fine tunes the movements based on proprioceptive information from peripheral sensory receptors. The posterior parietal cortex provides the player with a sense of where his body is located in three-dimensional space and where his racket arm is located with respect to the rest of the body. During this entire process, brain stem nuclei are involved in regulating heart rate, respiration, and arousal. The hippocampus is not involved in hitting the ball, but it is involved in recording in memory all of the details of the point so that the player can brag about it later. In fact, many other brain regions are also active during this simple behavior. The common sense notion that only a fraction of the brain is used at any one time is clearly wrong. It is more likely that virtually all of the brain is active in even simple behaviors such as hitting a tennis ball.

mately reaches multisensory processing regions in the cerebral cortex called association areas, where the information is combined to elicit the memory of earlier attempts to hit a tennis ball.

In addition, the afferent information for the planned behavior recruits activity in the amygdala, a structure concerned with emotion and social behavior. The amygdala in turn activates the autonomic nervous system to prepare the body for action. Finally, brain systems concerned with voluntary movement are recruited to initiate the behavior. The multisensory association areas make connections with higher-order motor centers that compute a program for moving the racket into position.

This program is then passed on to the primary motor cortex for execution. The motor commands from the brain must be targeted to the correct muscles in the back, shoulder, arm, and hand. They must also be timed so that contraction and relaxation of appropriate muscle groups are coordinated, and they must regulate body posture as a whole.

Once the behavior is initiated the job of the brain is not over. As the arm is raised and the ball approaches, many minor adjustments of the initial motor program are made based on more recent sensory information about the exact trajectory of the approaching ball before the arm moves the racket against the ball. Of course, as the behavior is being executed, the brain is also engaged in maintaining the player's heart rate, respiration, and other autonomic functions that are typically outside the awareness of the player.

As this example illustrates, our behavior is shaped in response to stimuli in our environment, and the environment that we know is created in the brain from our senses: sight, sound, smell, taste, touch, pain, and the sensation of body movements. Perception begins with receptor cells at the periphery that are sensitive to one or another kind of stimulus and encode information about the stimulus, such as its location and intensity. The receptors in turn excite sensory neurons that form connections with discrete sets of neurons in the spinal cord. The information from each receptor is then analyzed in the brain stem, thalamus, and cerebral cortex in the context of information from all other receptors. For example, when we hold something in the hand, touch receptors produce action potentials in afferent fibers from the hand. These signals eventually reach the processing centers of the somatic sensory system—in the dorsal column nuclei, the thalamus, and several connected areas of the cortex—where they cause certain populations of cells to discharge.

Initially, sensory information is processed in a series of relays, each of which involves more complex information processing than the preceding relay. Sensory fibers project in an orderly pattern from the periphery to the central nervous system, and from one part of the brain to the next, thereby creating a topographically organized neural map of the receptive surface in the brain. In fact, most sensory systems have several serial pathways that process different types of information simultaneously. This *parallel processing* of sensory information by different components of one sensory system, and by all sensory systems together, is the way our brain first analyzes sensory information. In addition, the perceptions generated by the sensory systems recruit the amygdala, which colors perception with emotion, and the hippocampus, which stores aspects of perception in long-term memory. Finally, our sensory experiences initiate and guide our actions: The ascending stream of sensory information connects with the motor systems, which convey signals down motor pathways to the spinal cord for reflexive and volitional movement.

Thus, to understand behavior, it is necessary to break down a behavior into component behaviors, identify the regions of the brain that contribute to each component, and analyze how the participating regions connect. Although the anatomy of the brain and the pattern of its interconnections appear complex, the functional organization of the nervous system is governed by a relatively simple set of principles that make the many details of brain anatomy comprehensible. In this chapter we review the major anatomical components of the central nervous system and outline the organizational principles of the major functional systems. In the next chapter we shall use the somatosensory system to examine the principles underlying the neural basis of perception and movement.

The Central Nervous System Has Seven Major Divisions

All behavior is mediated by the central nervous system, which consists of the spinal cord and the brain. The brain is composed of six regions, each of which can be further subdivided into several anatomically and functionally distinct areas. The six major brain divisions are the medulla, pons, cerebellum, midbrain, diencephalon, and cerebral hemispheres or telencephalon (Figure 17-2). Each of these divisions is found in both hemispheres of the brain, but may differ in size and shape. The orientation of components of the central nervous system within the body is described with reference to three axes (Figure 17-3).

Spinal Cord

The spinal cord is the most caudal part of the central nervous system and, in many respects, the simplest part. It extends from the base of the skull to the first lumbar vertebra. The spinal cord receives sensory information from the skin, joints, and muscles of the trunk and limbs and contains the motor neurons responsible for both voluntary and reflex movements.

Along its length the spinal cord varies in size and shape, depending on whether the emerging motor nerves innervate the limbs or trunk. The cord is divided into gray matter and surrounding white matter. The gray matter, which contains nerve cell bodies, is typically divided into dorsal and ventral horns (so-called because the gray matter appears H-shaped in transverse sections). The *dorsal horn* contains an orderly arrangement of sensory relay neurons that receive input from the periphery, while the *ventral horn* contains motor nuclei that innervate specific muscles. The white matter is made up of longitudinal tracts of myelinated axons that form the ascending pathways through which sensory information reaches the brain and the descending pathways that carry motor commands and modulatory influences from the brain (see Figure 18-1).

The nerve fibers that link the spinal cord with muscles and sensory receptors in the skin are bundled in 31 pairs of spinal nerves, each of which has a sensory divi-

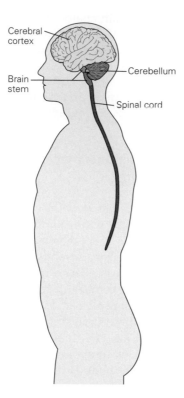

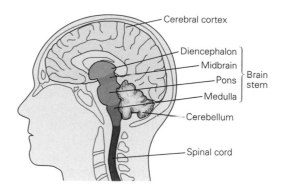

Figure 17-2 Major divisions of the central nervous system.

Left: The brain is illustrated within an outline of the human body; the lateral surface of the brain is visible.

Right: The medial surface of the brain is shown along with the spinal cord. The major subdivisions of the brain and spinal cord are indicated. (Adapted from Nieuwenhuys et al. 1988.)

sion that emerges from the dorsal aspect of the cord (the *dorsal root*) and a motor division that emerges from the ventral aspect (the *ventral root*). The dorsal roots carry sensory information into the spinal cord from muscles and skin. Different classes of axons coursing in the dorsal roots mediate sensations of pain, temperature, and touch. The cord also receives sensory information from internal organs. The ventral roots are bundles of the outgoing axons of motor neurons that innervate muscles. The motor neurons of the spinal cord comprise the "final common pathway," since all higher brain levels controlling motor activity must ultimately act through these neurons in the ventral horn and their connections to muscles. Ventral roots from certain levels of the spinal cord also include sympathetic and parasympathetic axons.

The next three divisions of the central nervous system rostral to the spinal cord—the medulla, pons, and midbrain—are collectively termed the *brain stem.* The brain stem is continuous with the spinal cord and contains distinct nerve cell clusters that contribute to a variety of sensory and motor systems. The sensory input and motor output of the brain stem is carried by 12 cranial nerves that are functionally analogous to the 31 spinal nerves. Whereas the spinal cord mediates sensation and motor control of the trunk and limbs, the brain

stem is concerned with sensation from and motor control of the head, neck, and face.

The brain stem is also the site of entry for information from several specialized senses, such as hearing, balance, and taste. Motor neurons in the brain stem control the muscles of the head and neck. Neurons in the brain stem also mediate many parasympathetic reflexes, such as decreases in cardiac output and blood pressure, increased peristalsis of the gut, and constriction of the pupils. The brain stem contains ascending and descending pathways that carry sensory and motor information to other divisions of the central nervous system. In addition, a relatively diffuse network of neurons distributed throughout the core of the brain stem, known as the *reticular formation,* receives a summary of much of the sensory information that enters the spinal cord and brain stem and is important in influencing the arousal level of an organism.

Medulla

The medulla is the direct rostral extension of the spinal cord and resembles the spinal cord both in organization and function. Neuronal groups in the medulla participate in regulating blood pressure and respiration. The

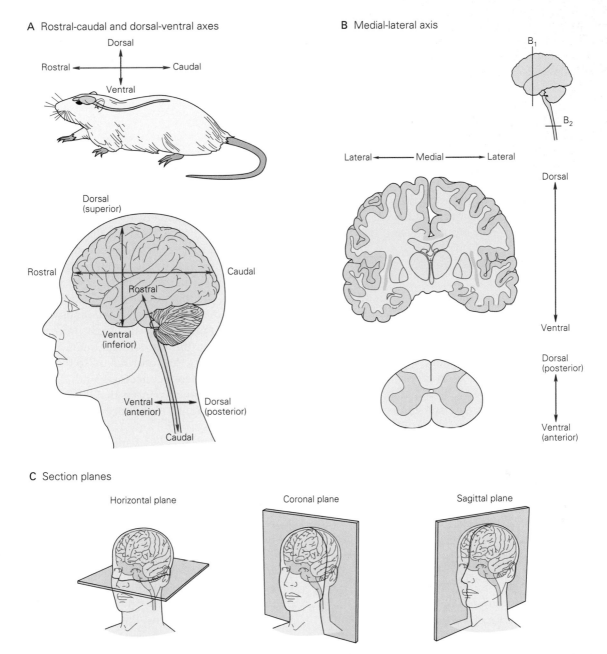

A Rostral-caudal and dorsal-ventral axes

Dorsal

Rostral ◄────────► Caudal

Ventral

Dorsal
(superior)

Rostral

Caudal

Rostral

Ventral
(inferior)

Ventral
(anterior)

Dorsal
(posterior)

Caudal

B Medial-lateral axis

B₁

B₂

Lateral ◄──── Medial ────► Lateral

Dorsal

Ventral

Dorsal
(posterior)

Ventral
(anterior)

C Section planes

Horizontal plane

Coronal plane

Sagittal plane

Figure 17-3 The central nervous system—the brain and the spinal cord—is organized along three major axes. (Adapted from Martin 1996.)

A. *Rostral* means toward the nose and *caudal* toward the tail. *Dorsal* means toward the back of the animal and *ventral* toward the belly. In lower mammals the orientations of these two axes are maintained through development into adult life. In humans and other higher primates the longitudinal axis flexes in the brain stem by approximately 110°. Because of this flexure positional terms are used slightly differently depending on whether the part of the mature human central nervous system is below or above the flexure. Below the flexure, in the spinal cord, rostral means toward the head; caudal means toward the coccyx

(the lower end of the spinal column); ventral (anterior) means toward the belly; and dorsal (posterior) means toward the back. Above the flexure, rostral means toward the nose; caudal means toward the back of the head; ventral means toward the jaw; and dorsal means toward the top of the head. The term *superior* is often used synonymously with dorsal, and *inferior* means the same as ventral.

B. *Medial* means toward the middle of the brain and *lateral* toward the side.

C. When brains are sectioned for analysis, slices are typically made in one of three cardinal planes: horizontal, coronal, or sagittal.

medulla also contains neuronal cell groups that form some of the early relay nuclei involved in taste, hearing, and maintenance of balance as well as the control of neck and facial muscles.

Pons

The pons lies rostral to the medulla and protrudes from the ventral surface of the brain stem. The ventral portion of the pons contains a large number of neuronal clusters, the pontine nuclei, that relay information about movement and sensation from the cerebral cortex to the cerebellum. The dorsal portion of the pons contains structures involved in respiration, taste, and sleep.

Midbrain

The midbrain, the smallest part of the brain stem, lies rostral to the pons. Neurons in the midbrain provide important linkages between components of the motor systems, particularly the cerebellum, the basal ganglia, and the cerebral hemispheres. For example, the substantia nigra, a distinct nucleus of the midbrain, provides important input to a portion of the basal ganglia that regulates voluntary movements. The substantia nigra is the focus of intense clinical and research interest since its dopaminergic neurons are damaged in Parkinson's disease, resulting in the pronounced motor disturbances that are associated with the disease (Chapter 43). The midbrain also contains components of the auditory and visual systems. Finally, several regions of the midbrain are connected to the extraocular muscles of the eye and provide the major pathway for controlling eye movements.

Cerebellum

The cerebellum, which lies over the pons, contains a far greater number of neurons than any other single subdivision of the brain, including the cerebral hemispheres. Nevertheless, it contains relatively few neuronal types, and as a result, its circuitry is well understood.

The surface, or cortex, of the cerebellum is divided into several lobes separated by distinct fissures. The cerebellum receives somatosensory input from the spinal cord, motor information from the cerebral cortex, and input about balance from the vestibular organs of the inner ear. It is important for maintaining posture and for coordinating head and eye movements and is also involved in fine tuning the movements of muscle and in learning motor skills. In the past, the cerebellum was considered to be purely a motor structure, but mod-

ern functional imaging studies of the human brain reveal that it is also involved in language and other cognitive functions. Underlying these functions is substantial input from sensory association regions of the neocortex to the pontine nuclei.

Diencephalon

The diencephalon contains two major subdivisions: the thalamus and hypothalamus. The *thalamus* is an essential link in the transfer of sensory information (other than olfactory) from receptors in the periphery to sensory processing regions of the cerebral hemispheres. It was previously thought that the thalamus acted only as a relay station for sensory information traveling to the neocortex, but it is now clear that it plays a gating and modulatory role in relaying sensory information. In other words, the thalamus determines whether sensory information reaches conscious awareness in the neocortex. The thalamus participates in the integration of motor information from the cerebellum and the basal ganglia and transmits this information to the regions of the cerebral hemispheres concerned with movement. The diencephalon also has regions that, like the reticular formation, are thought to influence levels of attention and consciousness.

The *hypothalamus* lies ventral to the thalamus and regulates several behaviors that are essential for homeostasis and reproduction. For example, it controls a variety of bodily functions, including growth, eating, drinking, and maternal behavior, by regulating the hormonal secretions of the pituitary gland. The hypothalamus also influences behavior through its extensive afferent and efferent connections with practically every region of the central nervous system. It is an essential component of the motivational system of the brain, initiating and maintaining behaviors the organism finds rewarding. One part of the hypothalamus, the suprachiasmatic nucleus, regulates circadian rhythms, cyclical behaviors that are entrained to the daily light-dark cycle.

Cerebral Hemispheres

The cerebral hemispheres form the largest region of the human brain. They consist of the cerebral cortex, the underlying white matter, and three deep-lying structures: the basal ganglia, the amygdala, and the hippocampal formation. The cerebral hemispheres are concerned with perceptual, motor, and cognitive functions, including memory and emotion. The two hemispheres are interconnected by the corpus callosum, a prominent set of fibers that connect symmetrical regions in both hemispheres. The corpus callosum, which is visible on the medial surface of the hemispheres, is the largest of the commissures, structures that contain fibers that mainly link similar regions of the left and right sides of the brain. The amygdala is concerned with social behavior and the expression of emotion, the hippocampus with memory, and the basal ganglia with the control of fine movement.

Five Principles Govern the Organization of the Major Functional Systems

The central nervous system consists of several discrete functional systems. There are, for example, discrete systems for each of the modalities of sensation (touch, vision, hearing, taste, smell) and for action.

Each Functional System Involves Several Brain Regions That Carry Out Different Types of Information Processing

The neural circuits of several functional systems course through some of the same brain structures. In a number of sensory systems, for example, receptors in the periphery project to one or more regions in the spinal cord, brain stem, and thalamus. The thalamus projects to the primary sensory cortices, which in turn project to other regions of the cerebral cortex. Thus one structure may contain components of several functional systems.

The components of a functional system are often called relays because of their serial organization. The term *relay* is misleading, however, since it implies passage of information without modification. In fact, information is transformed at every step, and the output of one stage of a functional system is rarely the same as its input. Information may be amplified at one stage of the system or it may be attenuated, depending, for example, on the arousal level of the animal. At each stage a single neuron typically receives inputs from thousands of presynaptic neurons, and it is the summation of all of these influences that governs the output of the neuron to the next stage.

Although a variety of neurons are involved at each stage in information processing, these neurons generally fall into two functional classes: principal (or projection) neurons and local interneurons. The axons of principal neurons convey information to the next stage in the system. Interneurons may receive inputs from the same sources as the principal cells, but they contact only local cells involved in the same processing stage. Whereas principal neurons tend to excite the neurons to which they project, interneurons often inhibit their target neurons (see Chapters 2 and 4).

Identifiable Pathways Link the Components of a Functional System

Axons leaving one component of a functional system are bundled together in a *pathway* that projects to the next component. Each pathway is located in approximately the same region in every brain. Thus many large bundles of axons can be seen with the unaided eye in the gross brain and were named by the classical neuroanatomists. The pyramidal tracts, for example, project conspicuously from the cerebral cortex to the spinal cord. The corpus callosum is another prominent fiber bundle. Most pathways are not nearly as prominent but can be demonstrated with modern neuroanatomical tracing techniques (see Box 5-1). These more subtle pathways, too, are typically found in the same position in all individuals.

Each Part of the Brain Projects in an Orderly Fashion Onto the Next, Thereby Creating Topographical Maps

One of the most striking features of the organization of most sensory systems is that the peripheral receptive surface—the retina of the eye, the cochlea of the inner ear, and the surface of the skin—is represented *topographically* throughout successive stages of processing. Neighboring groups of cells in the retina, for example, project to neighboring groups of cells in the visual portion of the thalamus, which in turn project to neighboring regions of the visual cortex. In this way an orderly *neural map* of information from the receptive surface is retained at each successive level in the brain.

Such neural maps reflect not only the position of receptors but also their density, since density of innervation determines the degree of sensitivity to sensory stimuli. For example, the central region of the retina, the fovea, has the highest density of receptors and thus affords the greatest visual acuity. Correspondingly, in the visual cortex the area devoted to information from the fovea is greater than the area representing the peripheral portion of the retina, where the density of receptors (and visual acuity) is lower.

In the motor system, neurons that regulate particular body parts are clustered together to form a motor map; the most well-defined motor map is in the primary motor cortex. The motor map, like the sensory maps, does not represent every part of the body equally. The extent of the representation of an individual body part reflects the density of innervation of that part and thus the fineness of control required for movements in that part.

Functional Systems Are Hierarchically Organized

In most brain systems information processing is organized hierarchically. In the visual system, for example, each neuron in the lateral geniculate nucleus (within the thalamus) is responsive to a spot of light in a particular region of the visual field. The axons of several adjacent thalamic neurons converge on cells in the primary visual cortex, where each cell fires only when a particular arrangement of presynaptic cells is active. For example, a cortical cell may fire only when the inputs signal a bar of light with a particular orientation.

In turn, cells in the primary visual cortex converge on individual cells in the association cortex. These cells respond even more selectively to information, for example a bar of light moving in a certain direction. Information passes both serially and in parallel through as many as 35 or more cortical regions dedicated to the processing of visual information. At very advanced stages of visual information processing in the cortex, individual neurons are responsive to highly complex information, such as the shape of a face.

Functional Systems on One Side of the Brain Control the Other Side of the Body

An important, but as yet unexplained, feature of the organization of the central nervous system is that most neural pathways are bilaterally symmetrical and cross over to the opposite (contralateral) side of the brain or spinal cord. As a result, sensory and motor activities on one side of the body are mediated by the cerebral hemisphere on the opposite side. Thus, movement on the left side of the body is largely controlled by neurons in the right motor cortex.

The pathways of different systems cross at different anatomical levels within the brain. For example, the ascending pathway for pain crosses in the spinal cord almost immediately upon entering the central nervous system. The pathway for fine touch, however, ascends on the same side of the spinal cord that it enters and ascends to the medulla, where it makes its first synapse. There, second-order fibers cross over to the thalamus on the contralateral side. Crossings of this kind within the brain stem and spinal cord are called *decussations*.

The Cerebral Cortex Is Concerned With Cognitive Functioning

While many life-sustaining functions are mediated by regions of the spinal cord, brain stem, and diencephalon, it is the cerebral cortex—the thin outer layer of the cerebral hemispheres—that is responsible for much of the planning and execution of actions in everyday life. Phylogenetically, humans have the most elaborated cerebral cortex, and much of modern neuroscience is directed at understanding the functions and disorders of the human cortex.

The cerebral cortex has a highly convoluted shape, formed by grooves (*sulci*) that separate elevated regions (*gyri*). The precise reason for this convoluted shape is not known. It is likely that it arose during evolution to accommodate an increase in the number of neurons. The thickness of the cortex does not vary substantially in different species; it is always around 2 to 4 mm thick. The surface area, however, is dramatically larger in higher primates, particularly in the human brain. The number of neurons in the cerebral cortex is one of the crucial determinants of the cortex's capacity for information processing. As we shall see shortly, the neocortex is organized in functional layers. Information in the neocortex is processed *across* the layers in an inter-

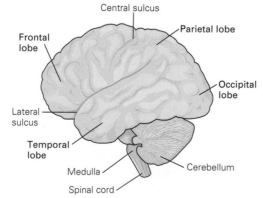

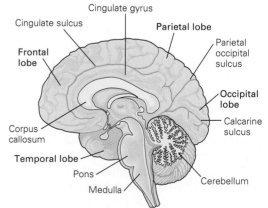

Figure 17-4 The major lobes of the cerebral cortex, some prominent sulci, and other brain regions are illustrated in lateral (left) and medial (right) views of the human brain. (Adapted from Martin 1989.)

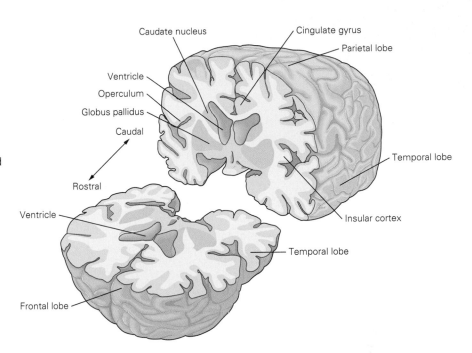

Figure 17-5 Some structures of the cerebral hemispheres cannot be seen from the surface of the brain. For example, the basal ganglia (caudate nucleus and globus pallidus) and insular cortex can be seen only after the brain has been sectioned. Large cavities in the brain called *ventricles* are filled with cerebrospinal fluid. (Adapted from England and Wakely 1991.)

connected set of neurons called *columns,* or *modules* (see Chapter 23). An increase in the surface area of the cortex permits a greater number of modules and thus provides greater capacity for processing information.

The Cerebral Cortex Is Anatomically Divided Into Four Lobes

The cerebral cortex is divided into four major lobes named after the overlying cranial bones: frontal, parietal, temporal, and occipital (Figures 17-4 and 17-5). Each lobe includes many distinct functional domains. The temporal lobe, for example, has distinct regions that carry out auditory, visual, or memory functions. Two additional regions of the cerebral cortex are the cingulate cortex, which surrounds the dorsal surface of the corpus callosum, and the insular cortex (insula), which is not visible on the surface owing to the overgrowth of the frontal, parietal, and temporal lobes. (The overhanging portion of the cerebral cortex that buries the insula within the lateral sulcus is called the operculum.)

The four lobes are conspicuously defined by particularly prominent sulci of the cortex that have a relatively consistent position in human brains. One of the most prominent indentations of the cerebral cortex—the lateral sulcus or sylvian fissure—separates the temporal lobe from the frontal and parietal lobes. The insular cortex forms the medial limit of the lateral sulcus. Another prominent indentation, the central sulcus, runs medially and laterally on the dorsal surface of the hemisphere and separates the frontal and parietal lobes (Figure 17-4).

Pierre Paul Broca first drew attention to the continuity of medial portions of the cerebral hemispheres, where portions of the frontal, parietal, and temporal lobes encircle and border the fluid-filled ventricles of the brain. Broca called this region the limbic lobe (Latin *limbus,* border). The limbic lobe is no longer considered one of the major subdivisions of the cerebral cortex. However, the cingulate cortex, which surrounds the corpus callosum (Figure 17-4), is considered a separate division of the neocortex, much like the insular cortex.

The Cerebral Cortex Has Functionally Distinct Regions

Many areas of the cerebral cortex are concerned primarily with processing sensory information or delivering motor commands. In addition, an area dedicated to a particular sensory modality or motor function includes several specialized areas that have different roles in processing information. These areas are known as primary, secondary, or tertiary sensory or motor areas, depend-

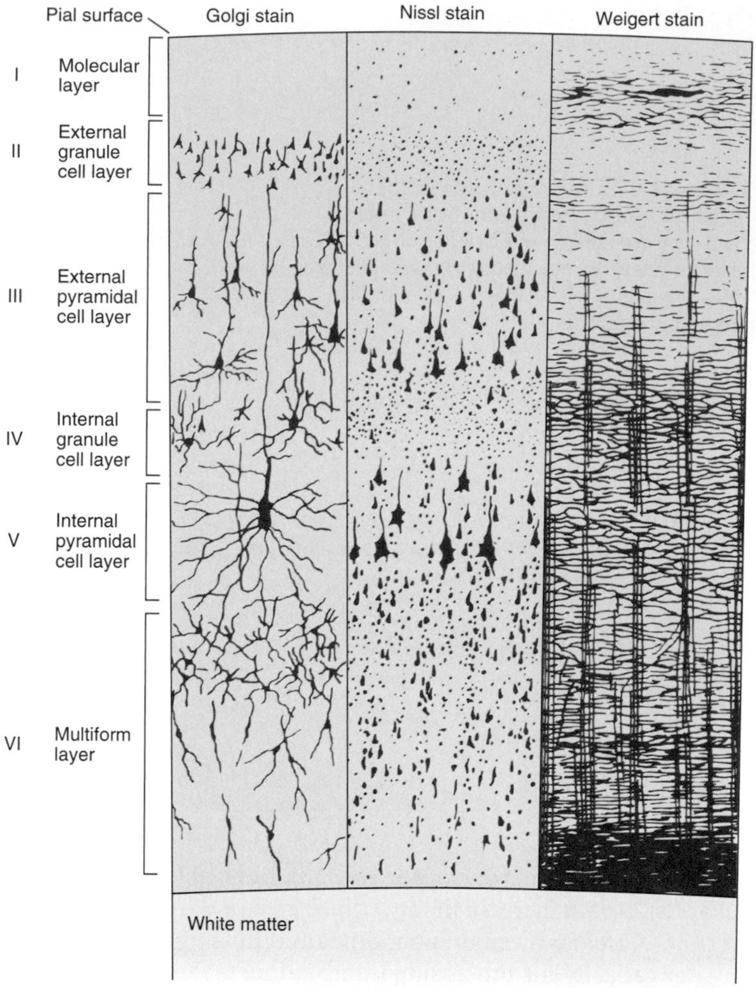

Figure 17-6 The neurons of the cerebral cortex are arranged in distinctive layers. The appearance of the cortex depends on what is used to stain it. The Golgi stain reveals neuronal cell bodies and dendritic trees. The Nissl method shows cell bodies and proximal dendrites. A Weigert stain for myelinated fibers reveals the pattern of axonal distribution. (From Heimer 1994.)

ing on their proximity to the peripheral sensory and motor pathways. For example, the primary motor cortex mediates voluntary movements of the limbs and trunk; it is called *primary* because it contains neurons that project directly to the spinal cord to activate somatic motor neurons. The primary sensory areas receive most of their information directly from the thalamus; only a few synaptic relays are interposed between the thalamus and the peripheral receptors.

The primary visual cortex is located caudally in the occipital lobe and is predominantly associated with the prominent calcarine sulcus (Figure 17-4). The primary auditory cortex is located in the temporal lobe, where it is associated with a series of gyri (Heschl's gyri) on the lateral sulcus. The primary somatosensory cortex is located caudal to the central sulcus on the postcentral gyrus, in the parietal lobe.

Each primary sensory area conveys information to an adjacent, higher-order area (or unimodal association area), which refines the information of a single sensory modality. Each higher-order area sends its outputs to one or another of three major multimodal association areas that integrate information from two or more sensory modalities and coordinate this information with plans for action (see Chapter 19).

The primary motor cortex, located just rostral to the central sulcus, is intimately associated with the motor systems of the spinal cord. Cortical cells influence neurons in the ventral horn of the spinal cord responsible for muscle movements. Whereas the primary sensory areas of cortex are the *initial* site of cortical processing of sensory information, the primary motor cortex is the *final* site in the cortex for processing motor commands. Higher-order motor areas, located rostral to the primary motor cortex in the frontal lobe, compute programs of movement that are conveyed to the primary motor cortex for implementation.

The Cerebral Cortex Is Organized in Layers

The cerebral cortex is organized into cell layers. The number of layers and the details of their functional organization vary throughout the cortex. The most typical form of neocortex contains six layers, numbered from the outer surface (pia mater) of the cortex to the white matter (Figure 17-6).

Layer I is an acellular layer called the *molecular layer*. It is occupied by dendrites of the cells located deeper in the cortex and axons that travel through or form connections in this layer.

Layer II is comprised mainly of small spherical cells called granule cells and therefore is called the *external granule cell layer*.

Layer III contains a variety of cell types, many of which are pyramidally shaped; the neurons located deeper in layer III are typically larger than those located more superficially. Layer III is called the *external pyramidal cell layer*.

Layer IV, like layer II, is made up primarily of granule cells and is called the *internal granule cell layer*.

Layer V, the *internal pyramidal cell layer*, contains mainly pyramidally shaped cells that are typically larger than those in layer III.

Layer VI is a fairly heterogeneous layer of neurons and is thus called the *polymorphic or multiform layer*. It blends into the white matter that forms the deep limit of the cortex and carries axons to and from the cortex.

Although each layer of the cerebral cortex is defined primarily by the presence or absence of neuronal cell bodies, each layer also contains additional elements. Thus, layers I–III contain the apical dendrites of neurons that have their cell bodies in layers V and VI, while layers V and VI contain the basal dendrites of neurons with cell bodies in layers III and IV. The profile of inputs to a particular cortical neuron depends more on the distribution of its dendrites than on the location of its cell body.

Not all cortical regions have the same laminar organization. For example, the precentral gyrus, which functions as the primary motor cortex, has essentially no internal granule cell layer (layer IV) and thus is called agranular cortex. In contrast, the region of the occipital cortex that functions as the primary visual cortex has an extremely prominent layer IV that typically is further subdivided into at least three sublayers (Figure 17-7). These two cortical areas are among the easiest to identify in histological sections.

The prominence or lack of prominence of layer IV can be understood in relation to its connections with the thalamus. Layer IV is the main target of sensory information arriving from the thalamus. In highly visual animals, such as humans, the lateral geniculate nucleus provides a large and highly organized input to layer IV of the primary visual cortex. The motor cortex, on the other hand, is primarily an output region of the neocortex and thus receives little sensory information directly from the thalamus.

The distinctive laminar structure of the primary visual or motor cortices is not typical of the neocortical surface. However, early students of the cerebral cortex, such as Korbinian Brodmann, used the relative prominence of the layers above and below layer IV or the distinctive cell size or packing characteristics in cortical regions to define borders between cortical areas. Based on such differences, Brodmann in 1909 divided the cerebral cortex into 47 cytoarchitectonic regions (Figure 17-7).

While Brodmann's demarcation appears to coincide in part with more recent information on the functions of the neocortex, the cytoarchitectonic method alone does not capture the subtlety or variety of function of all the distinct regions of the cortex. For example, Brodmann listed five regions (areas 17–21) as being concerned with visual function in the monkey. In contrast, modern connectional neuroanatomy and electrophysiology have identified more than 35 functionally distinct cortical regions within the region studied by Brodmann.

The Layers Organize Inputs and Outputs

What is the functional significance of the layered organization? The neocortex receives inputs from the thalamus, from other cortical regions on both sides of the brain, and from a variety of other sources. The output of the neocortex is also directed to several brain regions, including other regions of the neocortex on both sides of the brain, the basal ganglia, the thalamus, the pontine nuclei, and the spinal cord. Different inputs to the neocortex appear to be processed in different ways and the outputs of the neocortex arise from different populations of neurons. The layering of neurons provides an efficient means of organizing the input-output relationships of neocortical neurons (Figure 17-8).

Within the neocortex information passes serially from one processing center to another. In the visual system, for example, the connections between the primary visual cortex and secondary and tertiary visual areas, called associational or feed-forward connections, origi-

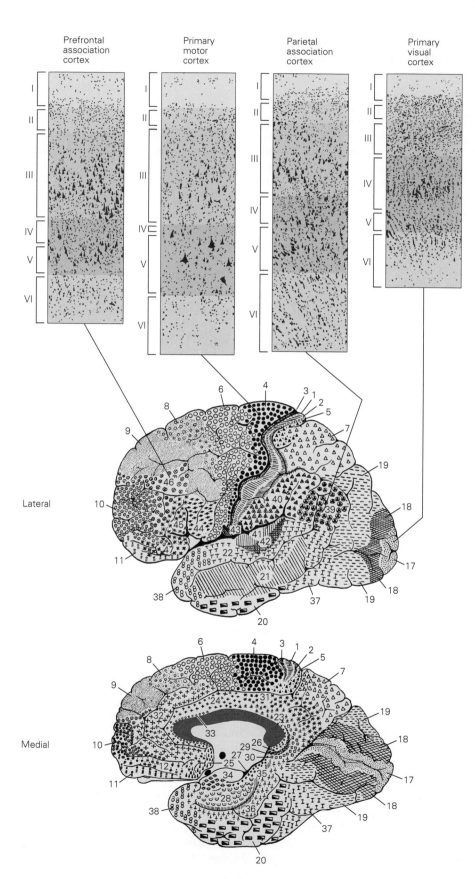

Figure 17-7 The prominence of particular cell layers of the cerebral cortex varies throughout the cortex. Sensory cortices, such as the primary visual cortex, tend to have very prominent internal granule cell layers. Motor cortices, such as the primary motor cortex, have a very meager layer IV but prominent output layers, such as layer V. These differences led Brodmann and others working at the turn of the century to divide the brain into various cytoarchitectonic regions. The subdivision by Brodmann (1909) seen in the **bottom half** of this illustration is a classic analysis but was based on a single human brain! (From Martin 1996.)

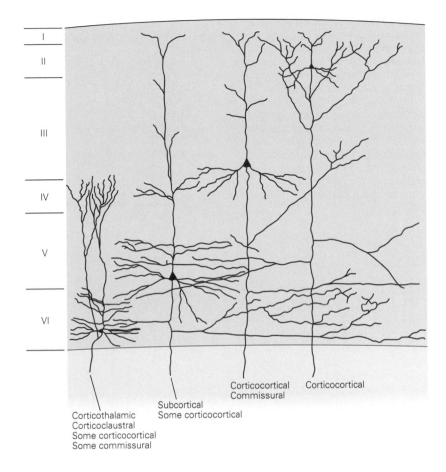

Figure 17-8 Neurons in different layers of the neocortex project to different parts of the brain. Projections to other parts of the neocortex, the so-called corticocortical or associational connections, arise primarily from neurons in layers II and III. Projections to subcortical regions arise mainly from layers V and VI. (From Jones 1986.)

nate mainly from cells in layer III and terminate mainly in layer IV. Feedback projections from later to earlier stages of processing are also typical; these originate from cells in layers V and VI and terminate in layers I/II and VI (Figure 17-9).

The Cerebral Cortex Has Two Major Neuronal Cell Types: Projection Neurons and Interneurons

The neurons of the cortex have a variety of shapes and sizes. Raphael Lorente de Nó, a student of Santiago Ramón y Cajal, used the Golgi method to identify more than 40 different types of cortical neurons based only on the distribution of their dendrites and axons. In general, the neurons of the cortex, as elsewhere, can be broadly defined as projection neurons and local interneurons. *Projection neurons* typically have pyramidally shaped cell bodies (Figure 17-10). They are located mainly in layers III, V, and VI and use the excitatory amino acid glutamate as their primary transmitter. *Local interneurons* use the inhibitory neurotransmitter γ-amino-

butyric acid (GABA), constitute 20–25% of the neurons in the neocortex, and are located in all layers.

Several types of GABA-ergic interneurons have been distinguished based on their pattern of connections and the cotransmitters they contain (Figure 17-11). Some have axons that terminate on the cell bodies of target neurons; these are typically called *basket cells*. Others have axons that terminate exclusively on the axons of target neurons; the multiple arrays of synaptic terminals formed by these GABA-ergic axons resemble a chandelier, and these cell types are typically called *chandelier cells*. Some GABA-ergic neurons contain other neuroactive peptides, such as somatostatin, cholecystokinin, or the opiate peptides. The neocortex also has a population of excitatory interneurons, located primarily in layer IV. These cells have a stellate plexus of dendrites, use the amino acid glutamate as a transmitter, and form synapses with neurons near the cell body. These excitatory interneurons are the primary recipients of sensory information received in the neocortex from the thalamus.

Neurons in the neocortex are not only distributed in layers but also in columns that traverse the layers, although the columnar organization is not particularly

Figure 17-9 Information is processed in the neocortex in a series of relays that produce progressively more complex information. How does one know that a particular cortical area is higher or lower in the hierarchy? This illustration demonstrates that ascending or feed-forward projections generally originate in superficial layers of the cortex and invariably terminate in layer IV. Descending or feedback projections generally originate from deep layers and terminate in layers I and VI. (Adapted from Felleman and Van Essen 1991.)

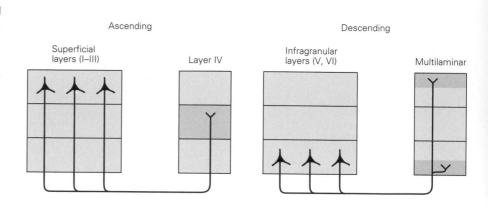

Figure 17-10 A projection neuron (P) and interneuron (I) in the somatic sensory cortex of a monkey are shown in these photomicrographs made at different depths of focus through the same Golgi-stained preparation. The pyramidal cell (Golgi type I) is seen better on the left, while the interneuron (Golgi type II) is seen better on the right. (From Jones and Peters, Vol. 1, 1986.)

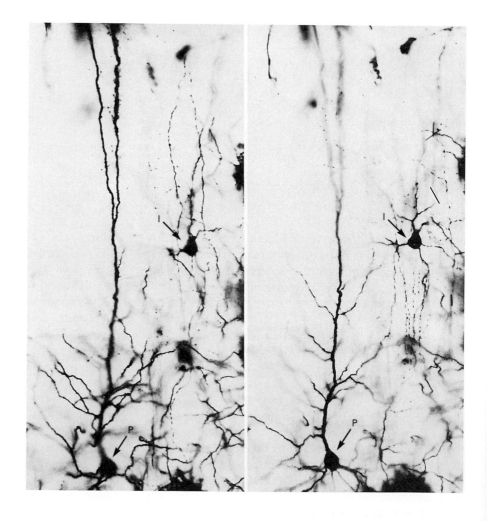

evident in standard histological preparations. A cortical column would fit within a cylinder a fraction of a millimeter in diameter. Neurons within a particular column tend to have very similar response properties, presumably because they form a local processing network. Columns are thought to be the fundamental computational modules of the neocortex (see Chapter 21).

As we have seen, the thickness of the neocortex is always found to be between 2 and 4 mm. In fact, the number of neurons stacked on top of each other through the thickness of the cortex is remarkably similar in different cortical regions and in different species. The one exception is the primary visual cortex, which has about twice as many neurons in a column. Thus, what mainly differentiates the cerebral cortex of a human from that of a rat is not the thickness of the cortex or the organization of the cortical columns, but the total number of columns. The massive expansion of the surface area of the cerebral cortex in humans accommodates many more columns and thus provides greater computational power.

Subcortical Regions of the Brain Contain Functional Groups of Neurons Called Nuclei

The ability of the cerebral cortex to process sensory information, to associate it with emotional states, to store it as memory, and to initiate action is modulated by three structures that lie deep within the cerebral hemispheres: the basal ganglia, the hippocampal formation, and the amygdala. The major components of the basal ganglia are the caudate nucleus, putamen, and globus pallidus (Figure 17-12). Neurons in the basal ganglia regulate movement and contribute to certain forms of cognition such as the learning of skills. They receive input from all parts of the cerebral cortex but send their output only to the frontal lobe through the thalamus.

The hippocampus and associated cortical regions form the floor of the temporal horn of the lateral ventricle. Together these structures are responsible for the formation of long-term memories about our daily experiences. The hippocampus is not the permanent storage site of memories, however (see Chapter 62). Damage to the hippocampus causes people to become unable to form new memories but does not significantly impair old memories.

The amygdala, which lies just rostral to the hippocampus, is involved in analyzing the emotional or motivational significance of sensory stimuli and in coordinating the actions of a variety of brain systems to allow an individual to make an appropriate response. The amygdala receives input directly from the major sensory systems. In turn, it projects back to the neocortex, to the basal ganglia, the hippocampus, and a variety of subcortical structures including the hypothalamus. Through its projections to the brain stem the amygdala can modulate somatic and visceral components of the peripheral nervous system and thus orchestrate the body's response to a particular situation. Responses to danger—the sense of fear and the change in heart rate and respiration that result from seeing a snake, for example—are mediated by the amygdala and its connections.

In thin histological sections through the brain stem stained by any of the common methods to demonstrate neuronal cell bodies, the neuronal cell bodies appear to be grouped in clusters of different sizes and shapes. These clusters of neurons are commonly called *nuclei* (see lateral geniculate nucleus in Figure 17-13).

Most nuclei are not homogeneous populations of cells but instead include a variety of cells organized into

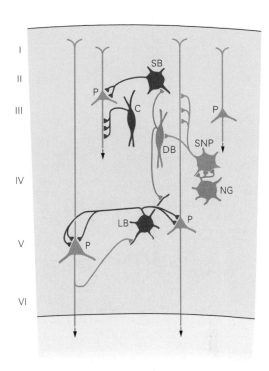

Figure 17-11 Different types of GABA-ergic neurons (dark gray) and putative GABA-ergic neurons (light gray) have different connections with pyramidal (**P**) and spiny non-pyramidal (**SNP**) cells in the neocortex. The GABA-ergic cells include chandelier cells (**C**), which terminate exclusively on the axons of other neurons, and the large and small basket cells (**LB, SB**), whose axons terminate mainly on other cell bodies. Double bouquet (**DB**) and neurogliaform cells (**NG**) may also be GABA-ergic. (Adapted from Houser et al. 1986.)

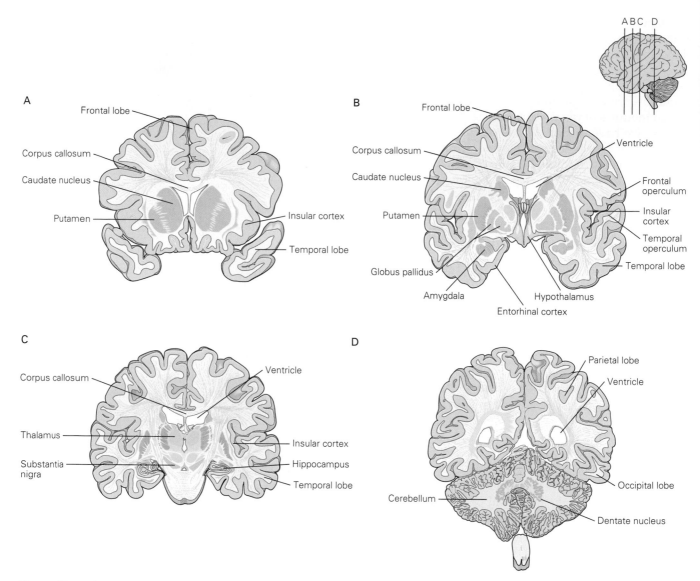

Figure 17-12 Several brain regions are shown in these coronal sections of the human brain. The sections are arranged from rostral (**A**) to caudal (**D**) and the approximate lo- cation of these sections are shown on the lateral surface view of the brain shown above. (From Nieuwenhuys et al. 1988.)

subnuclei, divisions, or layers. Neurons in the lateral geniculate nucleus of the thalamus, for example, are grouped into alternating bands of smaller or larger neu- rons with different functions (Figure 17-14). Even within a nucleus that appears homogeneous when viewed with the nonspecific Nissl method (Figure 17-13), the use of other stains that highlight the structure of den- drites (such as the Golgi technique) or the chemical composition of the neurons (such as histochemistry or immunohistochemistry) reveal substantial heterogene- ity of neuronal cell types.

The definition of nuclei in the brain is thus depen-

dent on the method by which the neurons are visualized. And, in fact, modern neuroanatomy has made great progress in adding new differential criteria to the defini- tion of brain regions and brain types. One particularly telling example occurred in the 1970s when Bengt Falck and Nils Hillarp developed a histofluorescence tech- nique for staining monoamine neurotransmitters. This histofluorescence technique allowed groupings of sero- tonergic, adrenergic, or dopaminergic neurons to be rec- ognized in the reticular formation, a region of the brain stem so named because of its diffuse and relatively non- nuclear appearance. Many other powerful techniques

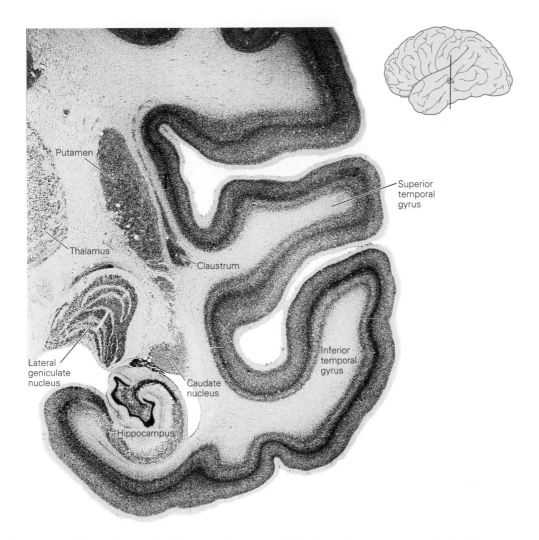

Figure 17-13 Several nuclei can be seen in this coronal section through the right hemisphere of a Macaque monkey brain. Nissl stains mark neuronal and glial cell bodies and make up the grainy dark appearance of much of the section. In this low-magnification photograph individual neuronal cell bodies are difficult to distinguish. Several nuclei are visible. The lateral geniculate nucleus of the thalamus is subdivided into layers.

Other layered neurons appear in the hippocampus and the neocortex of the temporal lobe. Other nuclei are more homogeneous, such as the caudate nucleus, putamen, and claustrum. The white regions between the cellular staining constitute the white matter where unstained axons run from one brain region to the next.

for defining the chemical or genetic composition of neuronal cell types have emerged in the last two decades. For example, in situ hybridization allows neurons to be visualized based on the genes they express.

The cellular organization of the brain would be of far less functional significance if it varied greatly from individual to individual. However, the types of neurons within a particular brain nucleus and the connections they make are the end result of a stereotypical developmental program of cellular proliferation, migration, and differentiation and therefore are similar in every individual. This regularity of the position and components

of brain nuclei provides support for the notion that the spatial location of neurons, their relationship to other neurons within a nucleus, and the three-dimensional distribution of their axons and dendrites within the nervous system are all crucial for normal brain function.

Modulatory Systems in the Brain Influence Motivation, Emotion, and Memory

Some areas of the brain are neither purely sensory nor purely motor but instead are modulatory. These modu-

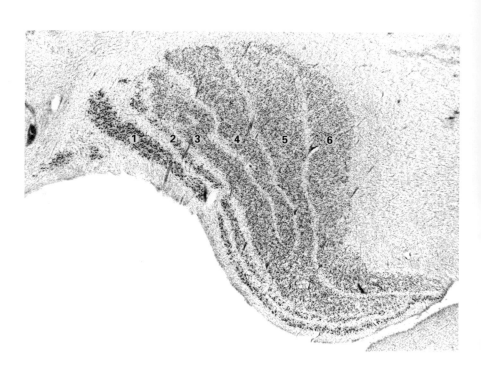

Figure 17-14 Most nuclei are not homogeneous populations of cells. The organizational complexity of the lateral geniculate nucleus can be seen in this Nissl-stained coronal section of the right hemisphere of a human brain. Axons from neurons in the retina terminate in different layers (1–6) of the nucleus. Layers 1 and 2 contain much larger neurons (magnocellular) than layers 3–6 (parvocellular), and the two types of cells have different functions. Each layer contains both projection neurons and interneurons.

latory systems are nevertheless essential components of the neural circuitry underlying complex behaviors. Complex behaviors are often directed toward filling a primary need such as hunger, thirst, or sleep. Thus, sensory and modulatory systems in the hypothalamus determine blood glucose levels. Once blood sugar drops below a certain critical level, we feel hunger. To satisfy hunger, perceptual and modulatory processes must first be brought into play. Thus, when a predator surveys the environment for clues of prey, including sights, sounds, or odors, modulatory systems in the brain focus the sensory apparatus on stimuli that are relevant to feeding.

The neural basis of arousal and selective attention is not well understood. We know, however, that distinct modulatory systems within the brain stem participate in these functions. Small groups of modulatory neurons in the brain stem contain noradrenaline and serotonin, and these neurotransmitters set the general arousal level of an animal through their modulatory influences on forebrain structures. Another group of modulatory neurons involved in arousal or attention is the basal nucleus of Meynert, located beneath the basal ganglia in the basal forebrain portion of the telencephalon. Cholinergic neurons in the basal nucleus send connections to essentially all portions of the neocortex, where they participate in attentional mechanisms that sharpen cognitive or perceptual processes.

If a predator finds potential prey, a variety of cortical and subcortical structures determines whether the prey is edible. Once food is recognized, other cortical and subcortical systems initiate a comprehensive voli-

tional motor program to bring the animal into contact with the prey, capture it and place it in the mouth, and chew and swallow.

Finally, the physiological satisfaction the animal experiences in consuming food reinforces the behaviors that led to the successful predation. Modulatory systems of dopaminergic neurons in the midbrain mediate these rewarding aspects of behavior. The power of these systems has been demonstrated by experiments with rats. When electrodes were implanted into the animals' reward regions and the animals were allowed to press a lever to electrically stimulate their brains, the rats preferred self-stimulating their brains to obtaining food or water, engaging in sexual behavior, or any other naturally rewarding activity.

How the brain's modulatory systems concerned with reward, attention, and motivation interact with the sensory and motor systems remains one of the most interesting questions in neuroscience, one that is fundamental to our understanding of learning and memory storage. We take up this question in Chapters 44 and 45.

The Peripheral Nervous System Is Anatomically But Not Functionally Distinct From the Central Nervous System

In this chapter we have outlined the anatomy of the central nervous system—the brain and spinal cord—and its functional systems because the focus of this book is on how the brain mediates behavior. As we shall see throughout the book, however, the brain processes a continuous stream of information about the environment—both the external environment and the internal environment of the body. This information is supplied by the peripheral nervous system, which, though anatomically separate from the central nervous system, is functionally intertwined with it.

The peripheral nervous system is divided into somatic and autonomic divisions. The *somatic division* includes the sensory neurons that innervate the skin, muscles, and joints. The cell bodies of these sensory neurons lie in the dorsal root ganglia and the cranial ganglia. Receptors associated with dorsal root and cranial ganglion cells provide sensory information to the central nervous system about muscle and limb position and about touch and pressure at the body surface. In Part V (Perception) we shall see how remarkably specialized the sensory receptors are in transducing the variety of physical energies (stimuli) into a code used universally throughout the nervous system. In Part VI (Movement) we shall see that sensory receptors in the muscles and joints are crucial to shaping coherent action that allows us to move about the world and exploit its resources.

The *autonomic division* of the peripheral nervous system mediates visceral sensation as well as motor control of the viscera, smooth muscles, and exocrine glands. It consists of the sympathetic, parasympathetic, and enteric systems. The sympathetic system participates in the body's response to stress, while the parasympathetic system acts to conserve body resources and restore homeostasis. The enteric nervous system controls the function of smooth muscle of the gut. The functional organization of the autonomic nervous system is described in Chapter 49 and its role in emotion and motivation in Chapters 50 and 51.

An Overall View

The nervous system obtains sensory information from the environment, evaluates the significance of the information, and generates appropriate behavioral responses. Accomplishing these tasks requires an anatomical plan of considerable complexity. The human nervous system is comprised of several hundreds of billions of neurons, each of which receives and gives rise to tens of thousands of connections. Some of these connections are located nearly a meter from the cell bodies of origin.

Despite this complexity, the structure of the nervous system is similar from individual to individual within a species. Knowledge of neuronal structure and the pathways of information flow in the brain is important not only for understanding the normal function of the brain but also for identifying specific regions that are disturbed during neurological illness.

The nervous system has two anatomically distinct components: the central nervous system, consisting of the brain and the spinal cord, and the peripheral nervous system, composed of specialized clusters of neurons (ganglia) and peripheral nerves. The peripheral nervous system relays information to the central nervous system and executes motor commands generated in the brain and spinal cord. The simplest action involves the integrated activity of multiple sensory, motor, and motivational pathways in the central nervous system. Each pathway contains a series of relay nuclei and each nucleus has several functional subdivisions. Most neurons are precisely arranged into functional pathways that have the same anatomical arrangement in every individual. Many pathways cross from one side of the nervous system to the other. These basic principles govern the organization of the nervous system from the spinal cord through the brain stem to the highest levels of the cerebral cortex.

While neuroanatomy may seem to provide only a static picture of the nervous system, it can provide profound insight into how the nervous system functions, in the same way that the detailed structure of proteins reveals important principles of protein function. Many of the prevailing ideas about the dynamic mechanisms in the nervous system were forecast a century ago by Ramón y Cajal on the basis of images of neurons in stained histological specimens. Indeed, many of the established properties of neuronal connectivity were first discovered using the methods of classical anatomy. Golgi staining first showed the existence of two major classes of nerve cells in the brain: projection neurons, whose axons connect the major regions of the nervous system, and local interneurons, which integrate information within specific nuclei of the brain. Later staining techniques demonstrated the considerable convergence and divergence of projections between brain regions.

The introduction of electron microscopic methods to neuroanatomy in the 1950s revealed the structure of synapses and illustrated that different classes of neurons form synapses with quite different features. Some synaptic terminals are located on dendrites, others on axon terminals, and still others on the soma of the postsynaptic cell. The location of synapses on the neuronal surface critically affects the function of the cell.

Today, our understanding of higher brain function depends on refined mapping of neuronal circuits using new anatomical and imaging techniques. Modern neuroanatomical labeling techniques have revealed the topographic organization of projections from one brain region to the next.

As we shall see in later chapters, modern imaging techniques have revolutionized the study of the cognitive functions of the brain and thereby placed neurology and psychiatry on a firmer empirical footing. Positron emission tomography (PET) and magnetic resonance imaging (MRI) have made the functional organization of the human brain visible during behavioral experiments. These techniques, in addition to being important tools for diagnosing diseases of the central nervous system, have given us a much clearer idea of the brain regions involved in many complex cognitive functions.

David G. Amaral

Selected Readings

Brodal A. 1981. *Neurological Anatomy in Relation to Clinical Medicine*, 3rd ed. New York: Oxford Univ. Press.

England MA, Wakely J. 1991. *Color Atlas of the Brain and Spinal Cord: An Introduction to Normal Neuroanatomy*. St. Louis: Mosby Year Book.

Martin JH. 1996. *Neuroanatomy: Text and Atlas*, 2nd ed. Stamford, CT: Appleton & Lange.

Nauta WJH, Feirtag D. 1986. *Fundamental Neuroanatomy*. New York: Freeman.

Nieuwenhuys R, Voogd J, van Huijzen Chr. 1988. *The Human Central Nervous System: A Synopsis and Atlas*, 3rd rev. ed. Berlin: Springer-Verlag.

Paxinos G. 1990. *The Human Nervous System*. San Diego: Academic Press.

References

Broca P. 1878. Anatomie compárée des circonvolutions cérébrales. Le grand lobe limbique et le scissure limbique dans le serie des mammitères. Rev Anthropol 12:646–657.

Brodmann K. 1909. *Vergleichende Lokalisationslehre der Grosshirnrinde in ihren Prinzipien dargestellt auf Grund des Zellenbaues*. Leipzig: Barth.

Dahlström A, Carlsson A. 1986. Making visible the invisible. In: MJ Parnam, J Bruinnvels (eds). *Discoveries in Pharmacology*. Vol. 3, *Pharmacological Methods, Receptors and Chemotherapy*, pp. 97–125. Amsterdam: Elsevier.

Falck B, Hillarp NÅ, Thieme G, Torp A. 1962. Fluorescence of catecholamines and related compounds condensed with formaldehyde. J Histochem Cytochem 10:348–354.

Felleman DJ, Van Essen DC. 1991. Distributed hierarchical processing in the primate cerebral cortex. Cereb Cortex 1:1–47.

Heimer L. 1994. *The Human Brain and Spinal Cord: Functional Neuroanatomy and Dissection Guide*, 2nd ed. New York: Springer.

Houser CR, Vaughn JE, Hendry SHC, Jones EG, Peters, A. 1986. GABA neurons in the cerebral cortex. In: EG Jones, A Peters (eds). *Cerebral Cortex*. Vol. 2, Chapter 3. *Functional Properties of Cortical Cells*, pp. 63–89. New York/London: Plenum.

Jones EG. 1986. Connectivity of the primate sensory-motor cortex. In: EG Jones, A Peters (eds). *Cerebral Cortex*. Vol. 5, Chapter 4. *Sensory-Motor Areas and Aspects of Cortical Connectivity*, pp. 113–183. New York/London: Plenum.

Lorente de Nó R. 1949. Cerebral cortex. Architecture, intracortical connections, motor projections. In: JF Fulton (ed). *Physiology of the Nervous System*, 3rd ed., pp. 288–330. New York: Oxford Univ. Press.

Ramón y Cajal S. 1995. *Histology of the Nervous System of Man and Vertebrates*, 2 vols. N Swanson, LW Swanson (transl). New York: Oxford Univ. Press.

West MJ. 1990. Stereological studies of the hippocampus: a comparison of the hippocampal subdivisions of diverse species including hedgehogs, laboratory rodents, wild mice and men. Progr Brain Res 83:13–36.

18

The Functional Organization of Perception and Movement

S TUDIES OF ARTIFICIAL intelligence have shown that the human brain recognizes objects and carries out actions in ways no current computer can even begin to approach. Merely to see—to look onto the world and recognize a face or enjoy a landscape—entails amazing computational achievements. Indeed, all our perceptions—seeing, hearing, smelling, tasting, and touching—are analytical triumphs. Similarly all of our voluntary actions are triumphs of engineering. The brain accomplishes these computational feats because its many components—its nerve cells—are wired together in very precise ways.

In this chapter we outline the principles essential for understanding perception and action. We shall focus on touch because the somatosensory system is particularly well understood and because touch clearly illustrates the interaction of sensory and motor systems—how information from the body surface ascends through the sensory relays of the nervous system to the cerebral cortex and is transformed into motor commands that descend to the spinal cord to produce movements.

There is now a fairly complete understanding of how the physical energy of a tactile stimulus is transduced by mechanoreceptors in the skin into electrical activity, and how this activity at different relays in the brain correlates with specific aspects of the experience of touch. Since the central paths are well delineated, we now can see how this electrical information is processed at different relay points.

Trying to comprehend the functional organization of the brain might at first seem daunting. But as we saw in the last chapter, the organization of the brain is simplified by three anatomical considerations. First, there are relatively few types of neurons. Each of the many thousands of spinal motor neurons or millions of neocortical pyramidal cells has a similar structure and serves a similar function. Second, neurons in the brain and spinal cord are clustered into discrete cellular groups called nuclei, which are connected to form functional systems. Third, local regions of the cerebral cortex are specialized for sensory, motor, or associational functions. We begin by examining these three anatomical principles in the context of the perception of touch.

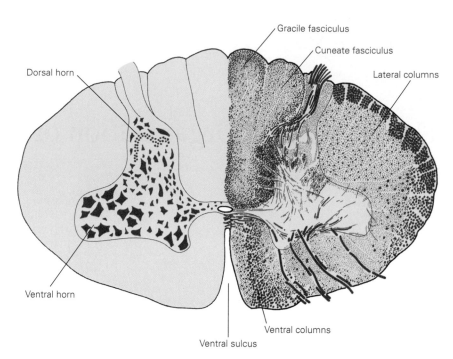

Figure 18-1 The major anatomical features of the spinal cord. The **left** side depicts a cell stain of the gray matter and the **right** side a fiber-stained section. The ventral horn contains large motor neurons, whereas the dorsal horn contains small neurons. Fibers of the gracile fasciculus carry somatosensory information from the lower limbs. Fibers of the cuneate fasciculus carry somatosensory information from the upper body. Fiber bundles of the lateral and ventral columns include both ascending and descending fiber bundles.

Sensory Information Processing Is Illustrated in the Somatosensory System

Complex behaviors such as tactile perception generally require the integrated action of several nuclei and cortical regions. A general principle of brain information processing is that it is carried out in a hierarchical fashion. Stimulus information is conveyed through a succession of subcortical and then cortical regions. To increase the computational capacity of the brain, information processing, even within a single sensory modality, is carried out simultaneously in several anatomically discrete pathways. In the somatosensory system a light touch and a painful stimulus to the same area of skin are mediated by different pathways in the brain.

Somatosensory Information From the Trunk and Limbs Is Conveyed to the Spinal Cord

Sensory information from the trunk and limbs enters the spinal cord, which is composed of a central core region of gray matter surrounded by white matter. The gray matter is shaped like the letter H, with each side subdivided into dorsal (or posterior) and ventral (or anterior) horns (Figure 18-1). In cross sections of the cord, the gray matter of the dorsal horn contains the sensory nuclei, or groups of sensory neurons, whose axons receive stimulus information from the body's surface. The ventral horn contains the motor nuclei, or groups of motor neurons, whose axons exit the spinal cord and innervate skeletal muscles. The motor cells do not actually form discrete clusters, like the sensory nuclei, but instead are arranged in columns that run along the length of the spinal cord. Interneurons of various types in the gray matter modulate information flowing from the sensory neurons toward the brain and the commands from higher centers in the brain to the motor neurons, as well as information passed between groups of motor neurons.

The white matter surrounding the gray matter is divided into dorsal, lateral, and ventral columns (Figure 18-1). Each of these columns includes a variety of bundles of ascending or descending axons. The dorsal columns, which lie between the two dorsal horns of the gray matter, contain only ascending axons that carry somatic sensory information to the brain stem. The lateral columns include both ascending axons and axons descending from the brain stem and neocortex that innervate interneurons and motor neurons in the spinal cord. The ventral columns also include ascending and descending axons. The ascending somatic sensory axons in the lateral and ventral columns constitute parallel pathways that convey information about pain and thermal sensation to higher levels of the central nervous system. The descending motor axons control axial muscles and posture.

The spinal cord is divided into four major regions: cervical, thoracic, lumbar, and sacral (Figure 18-2).

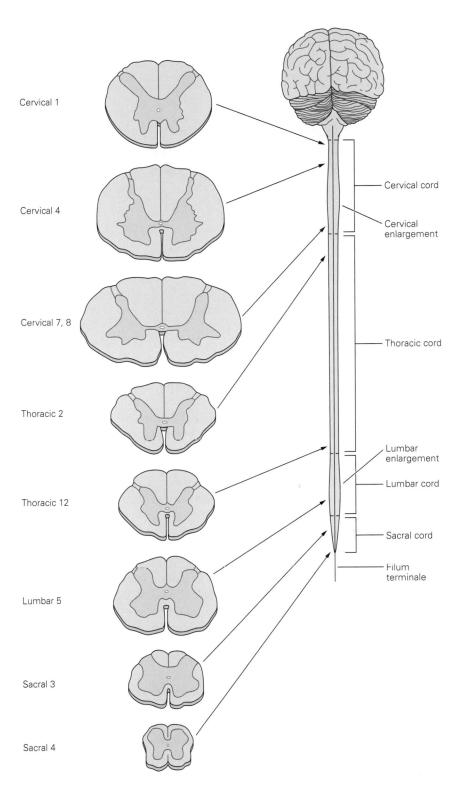

Figure 18-2 The internal and external appearances of the spinal cord vary at different levels. The proportion of gray matter to white matter is greater at sacral levels than at cervical levels. At sacral levels very few incoming sensory fibers have joined the spinal cord, whereas most of the motor fibers have already terminated at higher levels of the spinal cord. The cross-sectional area of the spinal cord shows enlargements at the lumbar and cervical levels, regions where the large number of fibers innervating the limbs enter or leave the spinal cord.

Cervical 1

Cervical 4

Cervical 7, 8

Thoracic 2

Thoracic 12

Lumbar 5

Sacral 3

Sacral 4

Cervical cord

Cervical enlargement

Thoracic cord

Lumbar enlargement

Lumbar cord

Sacral cord

Filum terminale

These regions are related to the embryological somites from which muscles, bones, and other components of the body develop (Chapters 52 and 53). Axons leaving the spinal cord to innervate body structures that develop at the same segmental level join together in the intervertebral foramen with axons entering the spinal cord to form spinal nerves. Spinal nerves at the cervical level are involved with sensory perception and motor function of the back of the head, neck, and arms. Nerves at the thoracic level innervate the upper trunk, while

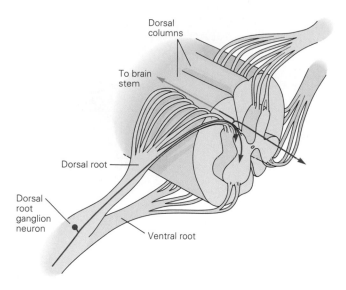

Figure 18-3 Dorsal root ganglia and spinal nerve roots.

lumbar and sacral spinal nerves innervate the lower trunk, back, and legs.

Each of the four regions of the spinal cord contains several segments characterized by the number and location of the dorsal and ventral roots that enter or exit the cord. There are 8 cervical segments, 12 thoracic segments, 5 lumbar segments, and 5 sacral segments. Although the actual substance of the mature spinal cord does not look segmented, the spinal cord varies in size and shape along its rostrocaudal axis because of two organizational features. First, relatively few sensory axons enter the cord at the sacral level. At higher (lumbar, thoracic, and cervical) levels the number of sensory axons entering the cord increases progressively. Conversely, most descending axons from the brain terminate at cervical levels, with progressively fewer descending to lower levels of the spinal cord. Thus the number of fibers in the white matter is highest at cervical levels (where there are the highest numbers of both ascending and descending fibers) and lowest at sacral levels. As a result, sacral levels of the spinal cord have much less white matter than gray matter whereas the cervical cord has more white matter than gray matter (Figure 18-2).

The second feature that differentiates the shape of the spinal cord along its rostrocaudal axis is variation in the size of the ventral and dorsal horns. The ventral horn is larger where the motor nerves that innervate the arms and legs exit the spinal cord because of the larger number of motor neurons needed to innervate the greater number of muscles and to regulate the greater complexity of movement in the limbs as compared with the trunk.

Likewise, the dorsal horn is larger where sensory nerves from the limbs enter the cord because the limbs have a greater density of sensory receptors and thus send more fibers to the cord. These regions of the cord are known as the lumbosacral and cervical *enlargements*.

The Primary Sensory Neurons of the Trunk and Limbs Are Clustered in the Dorsal Root Ganglia

The sensory neurons that convey information from the skin, muscles, and joints of the limbs and trunk to the spinal cord are clustered together in dorsal root ganglia within the vertebral column immediately adjacent to the spinal cord (Figure 18-3). These neurons are pseudo-unipolar neurons; they have a bifurcated axon with central and peripheral branches (see Figures 52-4 and 4-8). The peripheral branch terminates in skin, muscle, or other tissue as a free nerve ending or in association with specialized receptors.

The central process enters the spinal cord close to the tip of the dorsal horn. Upon entry the axon forms branches that either terminate within the spinal gray matter or ascend to nuclei located at the junction of the spinal cord with the medulla (Figure 18-3). These local and ascending branches provide two functional pathways for somatosensory information entering the spinal cord from dorsal root ganglion cells. The local branches can activate local reflex circuits while the ascending branches carry information into the brain, where this information becomes the basis of the perception of touch, position sense, or pain.

The Central Axons of Dorsal Root Ganglion Neurons Are Arranged to Produce a Map of the Body Surface

The central axons of the dorsal root ganglion cells form a neural map of the body surface when they terminate in the spinal cord. This orderly distribution of inputs from different portions of the body surface is called *somatotopy* and is maintained throughout the entire ascending somatosensory pathway.

Axons that enter the cord in the sacral region ascend in the dorsal column near the midline, while those that enter at successively higher levels ascend at progressively more lateral positions within the dorsal columns. Thus, in the cervical cord, where axons from all portions of the body have already entered the cord, sensory fibers from the lower body are carried medially in the dorsal column; fibers from the trunk, the arm and shoulder, and finally the neck occupy progressively more lateral areas. At the cervical levels of the cord the axons forming the dorsal columns are divided into two bundles: a medially situated gracile funiculus and a more laterally situated cuneate funiculus (Figure 18-4).

Each Somatic Submodality Is Processed in a Distinct Subsystem From the Periphery to the Brain

The submodalities of somatic sensation—touch, pain, and position sense—are processed in the brain through different pathways that end in different brain regions. To illustrate the specificity of these parallel pathways, we will follow the path of information for the submodality of touch.

The primary afferent fibers that carry information about touch enter the ipsilateral dorsal column and, without crossing to the contralateral column, ascend to the medulla. Fibers from the *lower* body run in the gracile funiculus and terminate in the gracile nucleus, while fibers from the *upper* body run in the cuneate funiculus and terminate in the cuneate nucleus. Neurons in the gracile and cuneate nuclei give rise to axons that cross to the other side of the brain and ascend to the thalamus in a long fiber bundle called the medial lemniscus (Figure 18-4). As in the dorsal columns of the spinal cord, the fibers of the medial lemniscus are arranged somatotopically. Because the sensory fibers cross the midline to the other side of the brain, the right side of the brain receives sensory information from the left side of the body, and vice versa. The fibers of the medial lemniscus end in a specific subdivision of the thalamus called the ventral posterior nucleus. The fibers maintain their somatotopic organization in the thalamus; fibers from the lower body end laterally, and those from the upper body and face end medially.

The Thalamus Is an Essential Link Between Sensory Receptors and the Cerebral Cortex for All Modalities Except Olfaction

The thalamus is an oval-shaped structure that constitutes the dorsal portion of the diencephalon. It conveys sensory input to the primary sensory areas of the cerebral cortex but is more than simply a relay. It acts as a gatekeeper for information to the cerebral cortex, preventing or enhancing the passage of specific information depending on the behavioral state of the animal.

The thalamus is a good example of a brain region made up of several well-defined nuclei. As many as 50 thalamic nuclei have been identified. Some nuclei receive information specific to a sensory modality and project to a specific area of the neocortex. Thus, the axons of cells in the ventral posterior lateral nucleus

(where the medial lemniscus terminates) project to the primary somatosensory cortex in the postcentral gyrus (Figure 18-4). Others participate in motor functions, transmitting information from the cerebellum and basal ganglia to the motor regions of the frontal lobe.

Axons from cells of the thalamus that project to the neocortex travel in the internal capsule, a large fiber bundle that carries most of the axons running to and from the cerebral hemisphere. Through its connections with the frontal lobe the thalamus may also play a role in cognitive functions, such as memory. Some nuclei that may play a role in attention project diffusely to large but distinctly different regions of cortex. The reticular nucleus, which forms the outer shell of the thalamus, does not project to the neocortex at all. It receives inputs from other fibers as they exit the thalamus en route to the neocortex and in turn projects to the other thalamic nuclei, thus providing feedback to the output nuclei of the thalamus.

The nuclei of the thalamus are most commonly classified into four groups—anterior, medial, ventrolateral, and posterior—with respect to the internal medullary lamina, a sheet-like bundle of fibers that runs the rostrocaudal length of the thalamus (Figure 18-5). Thus, the medial group of nuclei is located medial to the internal medullary lamina, while the ventrolateral and posterior groups are located lateral to it. At the rostral pole of the thalamus the internal medullary lamina splits and surrounds the anterior group. The caudal pole of the thalamus is occupied by the posterior nuclear group, comprised mainly of the pulvinar nucleus. Groups of neurons are also located within the fibers of the internal medullary lamina and are collectively referred to as the intralaminar nuclei.

The *anterior group* in humans consists of only one nucleus, which receives its major input from the mammillary nuclei of the hypothalamus and from the presubiculum of the hippocampal formation. The role of the anterior thalamic group is uncertain, but it is thought to participate in memory and emotion. The anterior thalamic group is also interconnected with regions of the cingulate and frontal cortices.

The *medial group* consists mainly of the mediodorsal nucleus. This large thalamic nucleus has three subdivisions, each of which is connected to a particular portion of the frontal cortex. The nucleus receives inputs from portions of the basal ganglia, the amygdala, and midbrain and has been implicated in memory.

The nuclei of the *ventral group* are named according to their position within the thalamus. The ventral anterior and ventral lateral nuclei are important for motor control and carry information from the basal ganglia and cerebellum to the motor cortex. The ventral post-

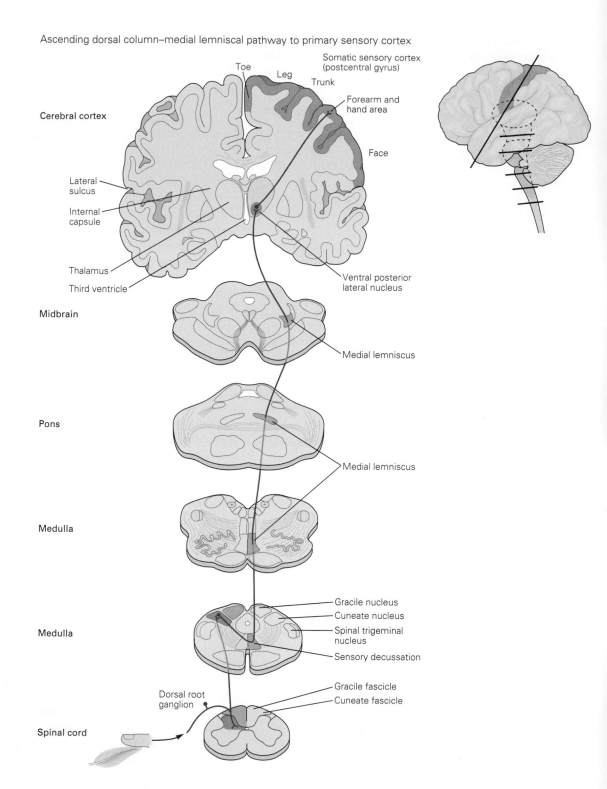

Ascending dorsal column–medial lemniscal pathway to primary sensory cortex

Figure 18-4 The medial lemniscus is a major afferent pathway for somatosensory information. Somatosensory information enters the nervous system through the dorsal root ganglion cells. The flow of information ultimately leads to excitation of the somatosensory cortex. Fibers representing differ- ent parts of the body maintain an orderly relationship to each other and form a neural map of the body surface that is maintained at each stage of information processing and ultimately in the neocortex.

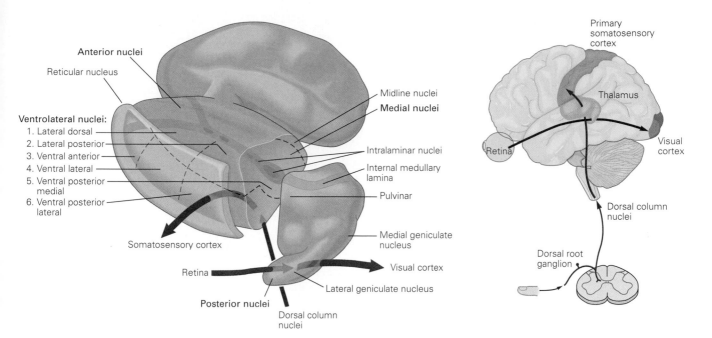

Figure 18-5 The major subdivisions of the thalamus. The thalamus is the critical relay for the flow of sensory information to the neocortex. Somatosensory information from the dorsal root ganglia reaches the ventral posterior lateral nucleus, which relays it to the primary somatosensory cortex. Visual informa- tion from the retina reaches the lateral geniculate nucleus, which conveys it to the primary visual cortex in the occipital lobe. Each of the sensory systems, except olfaction, has a simi- lar processing step within a distinct region of the thalamus.

erior lateral nucleus conveys somatosensory informa- tion to the neocortex.

The *posterior group* includes the medial and lateral geniculate nucleus, lateral posterior nucleus, and the pulvinar. The medial and lateral geniculate nuclei are lo- cated near the posterior part of the thalamus. The medial geniculate nucleus is a component of the auditory sys- tem and conveys tonotopically organized auditory infor- mation to the superior temporal gyrus of the temporal lobe. The lateral geniculate nucleus receives information from the retina and conveys it to the primary visual cor- tex in the occipital lobe. The pulvinar is most enlarged in the primate brain, especially in the human brain, and its development seems to parallel the enlargement of the as- sociation regions of the parietal-occipital-temporal cor- tex (Chapter 19). It has been divided into at least three subdivisions and is extensively interconnected with widespread regions of the parietal, temporal, and occipi- tal lobes, as well as with the superior colliculus and other nuclei of the brain stem related to vision.

The thalamus not only projects to the visual areas of the neocortex but also receives a return projection from the neocortex. The return projection from the occipital cortex actually accounts for a greater number of synapses in the lateral geniculate nucleus than does the retinal in- put! Most nuclei of the thalamus receive a similarly prominent return projection from the cerebral cortex.

The thalamic nuclei described thus far are called the *relay* (or *specific*) *nuclei* because they have a specific and selective relationship with a particular portion of the neocortex. Other thalamic nuclei, called *diffusely project- ing* (or *nonspecific*) *nuclei,* project to several cortical and subcortical regions. These nuclei are located either on the midline of the thalamus (the midline nuclei) or within the internal medullary lamina (the intralaminar nuclei). The largest of the midline nuclei are the para- ventricular, parataenial, and reuniens nuclei; the largest of the intralaminar cell groups is the centromedian nu- cleus. The intralaminar nuclei project to limbic struc- tures, such as the amygdala and hippocampus, but also send projections to components of the basal ganglia. These nuclei receive inputs from a variety of sources in the spinal cord, brain stem, and cerebellum and are thought to mediate cortical arousal and perhaps to par- ticipate in the integration of sensory submodalities that we shall learn about in Chapters 20 and 28.

Finally, the outer covering of the thalamus is formed by a unique sheet-like structure, the *reticular nu-*

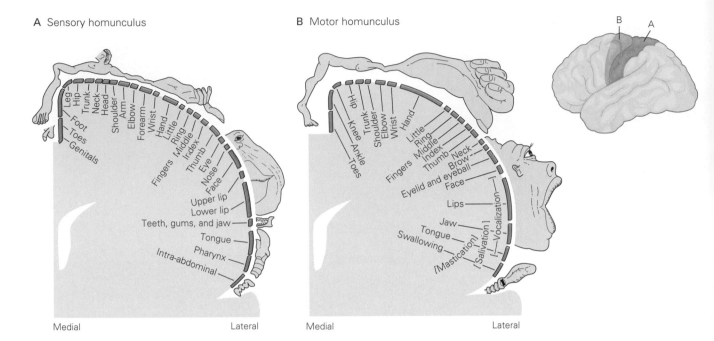

A Sensory homunculus

B Motor homunculus

Medial   Lateral   Medial   Lateral

Figure 18-6 The homunculus is a way of illustrating the location and amount of cortical area dedicated to a particular function. The entire body surface is represented in an orderly array of somatosensory inputs to the cortex. The area of cortex dedicated to processing information from a particular part of the body is not proportional to the mass of the body part but instead reflects the degree of innervation of that part. Thus, sensory input from the lips and hands occupies more area of cortex than, say, that from the elbow. Output from the motor cortex is organized in a similar fashion; the amount of cortical surface dedicated to a part of the body is related to the degree of motor control exercised in that part. Thus, in humans much of the motor cortex is dedicated to moving the muscles of the fingers and the muscles related to speech. (Adapted from Penfield and Rasmussen 1950.)

cleus. The majority of its neurons utilize the inhibitory transmitter γ-aminobutyric acid (GABA), whereas most of the neurons in the other thalamic nuclei utilize the excitatory transmitter glutamate. Moreover, the neurons of the reticular nucleus are not interconnected with the neocortex. Rather, their axons terminate on the other nuclei of the thalamus. These other nuclei also provide the input to the reticular nucleus via collaterals of their axons that exit the thalamus through the reticular nucleus. Thus, the reticular nucleus modulates activity in other thalamic nuclei based on its monitoring of the entirety of the thalamocortical stream of information.

We see, then, that the thalamus is not a relay station where information is simply passed on to the neocortex. Rather it is a complex brain region where substantial information processing is possible. To give but one example, the output of somatosensory information from the ventral posterior lateral nucleus is subject to four types of processing: (1) local processing within the nucleus; (2) modulation by brain stem inputs, such as the noradrenergic and serotonergic monoamine systems; (3) inhibitory feedback from the reticular nucleus; and (4) excitatory feedback from the neocortex.

Sensory Information Processing Culminates in the Cerebral Cortex

After the ventral posterior lateral nucleus of the thalamus, what is the next relay in the processing of somatic sensory information? The axons of cells in the ventral posterior lateral nucleus terminate primarily in the primary somatosensory cortex in Brodmann's area 3b. The neurons here are exquisitely sensitive to tactile stimulation of the skin surface. As in the other processing organs of the somatosensory system, the neurons in different parts of the cortex are somatotopically organized. When Wilder Penfield stimulated the surface of the somatic sensory cortex in patients undergoing brain surgery, he found that sensation from the lower limbs is mediated by neurons located near the midline of the brain, while sensations from the upper body, hands and fingers, the face, lips, and tongue are mediated by neurons located laterally.

As we shall learn in more detail in Chapter 20, Penfield and Jasper found that all portions of the body are represented in the cortex somatotopically, but not in proportion to body mass. Instead, each part of the body

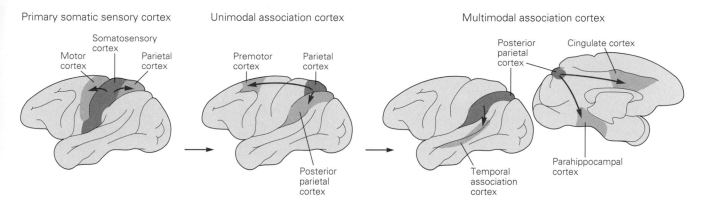

Figure 18-7 The processing of sensory information in the cerebral cortex begins with primary sensory cortices, continues in unimodal association cortices, and is completed in **multimodal association areas.** In each brain shown here the dark colored areas indicate the origin of a projection and the light colored areas the termination. Sensory systems also project to portions of the motor cortex. In the somatosensory sys-

tem, for example, the primary somatosensory cortex projects to the motor area in addition to the somatosensory association area. The somatosensory association area, in turn, projects to higher-order somatosensory association areas and to the premotor cortex. Information from different sensory systems converges in the multimodal association areas, which include the parahippocampal, temporal association, and cingulate cortices.

is represented in the cortex in proportion to its degree of innervation. Thus the area of cortex devoted to the fingers is larger than that for the arms. Likewise, the representation of the lips and tongue occupies more cortical surface than that of the remainder of the face (Figure 18-6A). Because the cerebral cortex is organized functionally into columns of cells extending from the white matter to the surface of the cortex, the larger the area of cortex dedicated to a function, the greater the number of computational columns that are involved in that function (Chapter 17). Our highly discriminative sense of touch in the fingers is thus due to the large area of cortex dedicated to the processing of somatosensory information from this part of the body.

A second major insight from the early electrophysiological studies was that the somatosensory cortex contains not one but several topographically organized sets of inputs from the skin and therefore several somatotopic maps of the body surface. The primary somatosensory cortex (anterior parietal cortex) has four complete maps of the skin, one each in areas 3a, 3b, 1, and 2. Basic processing of tactile information takes place in area 3, while more complex or higher-order processing occurs in area 1. In area 2 both tactile information and information concerning limb position are combined to mediate the tactile recognition of objects. Neurons in the primary somatosensory cortex project to neurons in adjacent areas, which in turn project to other adjacent cortical

regions (Figure 18-7). At higher levels of the hierarchy, somatosensory information is used in motor control, eye-hand coordination, and memory related to tactile experience and touch.

The cortical areas involved in the early stages of processing somatosensory information are concerned only (or primarily) with the processing of somatosensory information. These cortical regions are called unimodal association areas. Ultimately, however, somatosensory information from the unimodal association areas converges on multimodal association areas of the cortex concerned with combining sensory modalities. As we shall learn in the next two chapters and again in Chapter 62, these multimodal associational areas, which are heavily interconnected with the hippocampus, appear to be particularly important for two tasks: (1) the production of a unified percept and (2) the representation of the percept in memory.

Thus, from the mechanical pressure on a receptor in the skin to the perception that a finger has been touched by a friend shaking your hand, somatosensory information is processed in a series of steps as it ascends in serial and parallel pathways from the dorsal root ganglia to the somatosensory cortex, to unimodal association areas, and finally to multimodal association areas. One of the primary purposes of somatosensory information is to guide directed movement. As one might imagine, there is a close linkage between the somatosensory and motor functions of the cortex.

Descending lateral corticospinal pathway

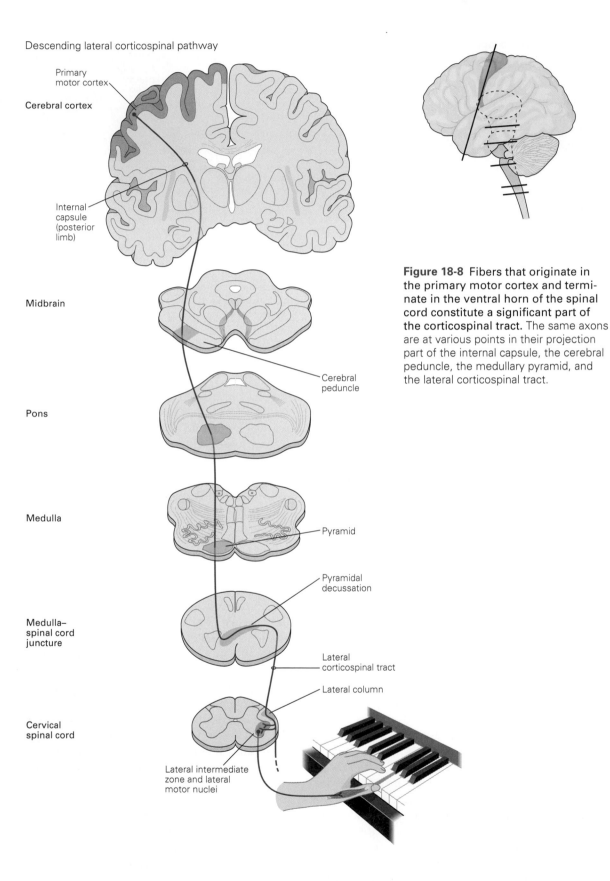

Primary
motor cortex

Cerebral cortex

Internal
capsule
(posterior
limb)

Midbrain

Pons

Medulla

Medulla–
spinal cord
juncture

Cervical
spinal cord

Cerebral
peduncle

Pyramid

Pyramidal
decussation

Lateral
corticospinal tract

Lateral column

Lateral intermediate
zone and lateral
motor nuclei

Figure 18-8 Fibers that originate in the primary motor cortex and terminate in the ventral horn of the spinal cord constitute a significant part of the corticospinal tract. The same axons are at various points in their projection part of the internal capsule, the cerebral peduncle, the medullary pyramid, and the lateral corticospinal tract.

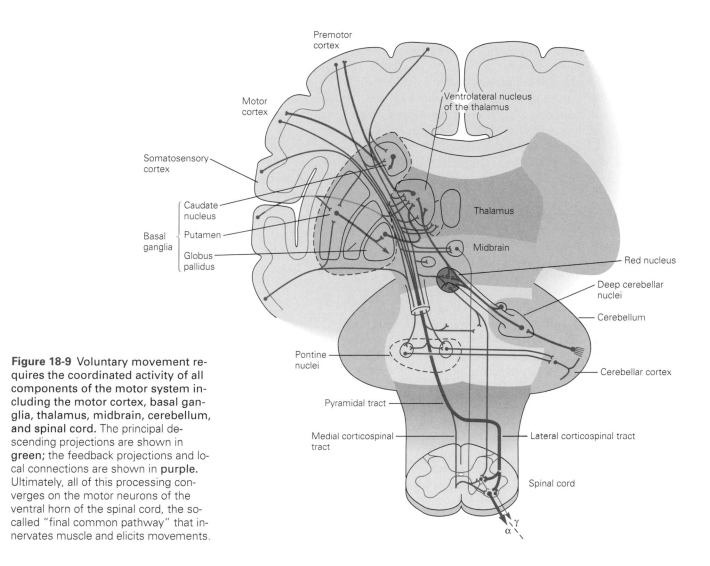

Figure 18-9 Voluntary movement requires the coordinated activity of all components of the motor system including the motor cortex, basal ganglia, thalamus, midbrain, cerebellum, and spinal cord. The principal descending projections are shown in **green**; the feedback projections and local connections are shown in **purple**. Ultimately, all of this processing converges on the motor neurons of the ventral horn of the spinal cord, the so-called "final common pathway" that innervates muscle and elicits movements.

Voluntary Movement Is Mediated by Direct Connections Between the Cortex and Spinal Cord

A major function of the perceptual systems is to provide the sensory information necessary for the actions mediated by the motor systems of the brain and spinal cord. The primary motor cortex is organized somatotopically like the somatic sensory cortex (see Figure 18-6B). Specific regions of the motor cortex influence the activity of specific muscle groups. Neurons in layer V of the primary motor cortex project their axons directly to motor neurons, or interneurons, in the ventral horn of the spinal cord via the corticospinal tract.

The human corticospinal tract consists of about one million axons, of which about 40% originate in the motor cortex. These axons descend through the subcortical

white matter, the internal capsule, and the cerebral peduncle (Figure 18-8). As the fibers of the corticospinal tract descend they form the medullary pyramids, prominent protuberances on the ventral surface of the medulla, and thus the entire projection is sometimes called the pyramidal tract.

Like the ascending somatosensory system, the descending corticospinal tract crosses to the opposite side of the spinal cord. Most of the corticospinal fibers cross the midline in the medulla at a location known as the pyramidal decussation. However, about 10% of the fibers do not cross until they reach the level of the spinal cord at which they will terminate.

The corticospinal tract makes monosynaptic connections with motor neurons, connections that are particularly important for individuated finger movements. It also forms synapses with interneurons in the spinal cord. These indirect connections are important for coordinating larger groups of muscles in behaviors such as reaching and walking.

The motor information carried in the corticospinal tract is significantly modulated by both sensory information and information from other motor regions. This includes a continuous stream of tactile, visual, and proprioceptive information needed to make voluntary movement both accurate and properly sequenced. In addition, the output of the motor cortex is under the substantial influence of other motor regions of the brain, including the cerebellum and basal ganglia, structures that are essential for smoothly executed movements.

The basal ganglia receive direct projections from much of the neocortex, which supplies it with both sensory information and information about movement, and the cerebellum receives somatosensory information directly from spinal afferents as well as from corticospinal axons descending from the neocortex (Figure 18-9). The cerebellum can influence posture and movement through its connection to the red nucleus, which can directly modulate descending projections to the brain stem and spinal cord. However, the major influence of the cerebellum on movement is through its connections to the ventral nuclear group of the thalamus, which connects directly to the motor cortex. Interestingly, the fibers of the medial lemniscus, basal ganglia, and cerebellum terminate in distinctly different portions of the ventral nuclear complex and ultimately influence different portions of both the somatosensory and motor regions of the cortex.

An Overall View

Sensory and motor information is processed in the brain in a variety of discrete pathways that are active simultaneously. Each pathway is formed by the serial connection of identifiable groups of neurons with each group processing progressively more complex or specific information. Thus, the sensations of touch and pain are mediated by different pathways that run through the spinal cord, brain stem, and into the cortex. All sensory and motor systems follow the pattern of hierarchical and parallel processing.

As we shall see in later chapters, contrary to an intuitive analysis of our personal experience, perceptions are not precise copies of the world around us. Sensation is an abstraction, not a replication, of the world around us. The brain constructs an internal representation of external physical events after first analyzing various features of those events. When we hold an object in the hand, the shape, movement, and texture of the object are simultaneously but separately analyzed according to the brain's own rules, and the results are integrated in a conscious experience.

As we shall see in the next two chapters, how this integration occurs—the *binding problem*—and how conscious experience emerges from the brain's *selective attention* to incoming sensory information are two of the most pressing questions in the neural and cognitive sciences and are likely to be solved only through the combined efforts of both fields.

David G. Amaral

Selected Readings

Brodal A. 1981. *Neurological Anatomy in Relation to Clinical Medicine*, 3rd ed. New York: Oxford Univ. Press.

Carpenter MB. 1991. *Core Text of Neuroanatomy*, 4th ed. Baltimore: Williams and Wilkins.

England MA, Wakely J. 1991. *Color Atlas of the Brain and Spinal Cord: An Introduction to Normal Neuroanatomy*. St. Louis: Mosby Year Book.

Felleman DJ, Van Essen DC. 1991. Distributed hierarchical processing in the primate cerebral cortex. Cereb Cortex 1:1–47.

Martin JH. 1996. *Neuroanatomy: Text and Atlas*, 2nd ed. Stamford, CT: Appleton & Lange.

Nieuwenhuys R, Voogd J, van Huijzen Chr. 1988. *The Human Central Nervous System: A Synopsis and Atlas*, 3rd rev. ed. Berlin: Springer-Verlag.

Peters A, Jones EG (eds). 1984. *Cerebral Cortex*. Vol. 1, *Cellular Components of the Cerebral Cortex*. New York/London: Plenum.

Peters A, Palay S, Webster H deF. 1991. *The Fine Structure of the Nervous System*, 3rd ed. New York: Oxford Univ. Press.

References

Brodmann K. 1909. *Vergleichende Lokalisationslehre der Grosshirnrinde in ihren Prinzipien dargestellt auf Grund des Zellenbaues*. Leipzig: Barth.

Penfield W, Boldrey E. 1937. Somatic motor and sensory representation in the cerebral cortex of man as studied by electrical stimulation. Brain 60:389–443.

Penfield W, Rasmussen T. 1950. *The Cerebral Cortex of Man: A Clinical Study of Localization of Function*. New York: Macmillan.

Ramón y Cajal S. 1995. *Histology of the Nervous System of Man and Vertebrates*. 2 vols. N Swanson, LW Swanson (transl). New York/Oxford: Oxford Univ. Press.

19

Integration of Sensory and Motor Function: The Association Areas of the Cerebral Cortex and the Cognitive Capabilities of the Brain

B Y 1950 IT WAS WELL ESTABLISHED that different sensory modalities are mediated by distinct sensory systems and that different actions recruit distinct components of the motor system. But it was still unclear whether this specificity of neural action applied to higher cognitive functions. Indeed, many scientists thought that cognitive functions, because of their complexity, required the operation of the brain as a whole. Only in the last 40 years has strong support been obtained for the idea that all mental functions are localizable to specific areas of the brain (see Chapter 1). But it also has become clear that complex mental functions require integration of information from several cortical areas. This in turn has raised the question: How is this parallel and distributed processing of cognitive information brought together? In which cortical area does the integration occur? And how is the integration brought about?

A prescient answer to these questions was provided in the 1870s by John Hughlings Jackson, the founder of modern British neurology. He proposed that the cortex is organized hierarchically and that some cortical areas serve higher-order integrative functions that are neither purely sensory nor purely motor, but associative. These higher-order areas of cortex, which we now call *association areas,* serve to associate sensory inputs to motor response and perform those mental processes that intervene between sensory inputs and motor outputs. The mental processes that Jackson attributed to these areas include interpretation of sensory information, association of perceptions with previous experience, focusing of attention, and exploration of the environment. Jackson supported his proposal with clinical evidence that certain cortical lesions,

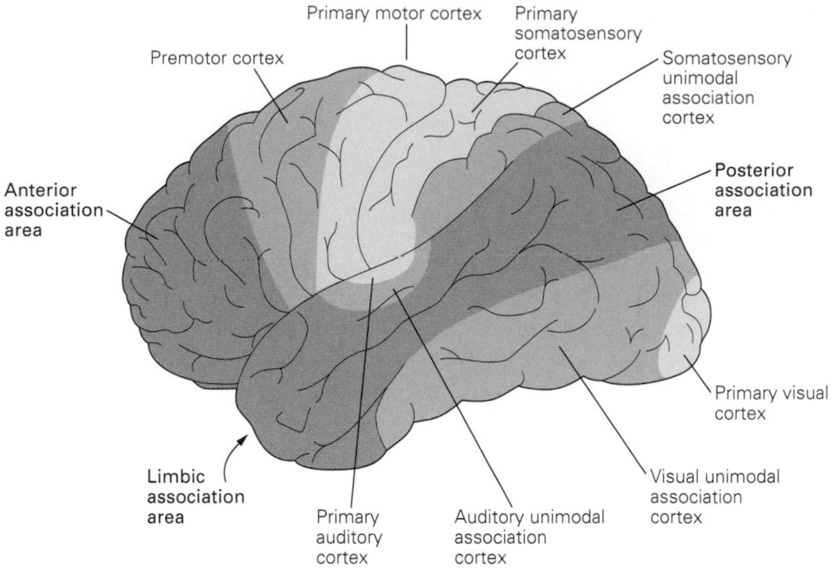

Figure 19-1 The association cortices occupy large areas on the exposed surfaces of the brain. The lateral surface of the human brain shows the regions of the primary sensory and motor cortices, the higher-order motor and sensory cortices, and the three association cortices.

although limited in extent, produced surprisingly complex disturbances in behavior.

How then do the association cortices achieve their integrative action? As we shall learn in this chapter, the association areas are capable of mediating complex cognitive processes because they receive information from different higher-order sensory areas and convey the information to higher-order motor areas that organize planned actions after appropriate processing and transformation.

Three Multimodal Association Areas Are Concerned With Integrating Different Sensory Modalities and Linking Them to Action

Jackson's view of the association areas has now been firmly established experimentally. We now know that each primary sensory cortex projects to nearby higher-order areas of sensory cortex, called *unimodal association areas*, that integrate afferent information for a single sensory modality. For example, the visual association cortex integrates information about form, color, and motion that arrives in the brain in separate pathways. The unimodal association areas in turn project to *multimodal sensory association areas* that integrate information about more than one sensory modality. Finally, the multimodal sensory association areas project to *multimodal motor association areas* located rostral to the primary motor cortex in the frontal lobe. The higher-order motor areas transform sensory information into planned move-

ment and compute the programs for these movements, which are then conveyed to the premotor and primary motor cortex for implementation. The term *primary cortex* therefore has two different meanings: the primary sensory areas are the *initial* sites of cortical processing of sensory information, while the primary motor areas are the *final* sites for the cortical processing of motor commands.

Because the multimodal association areas integrate sensory modalities and link sensory information to the planning of movement, they are thought to be the anatomical substrates of the highest brain functions—conscious thought, perception, and goal-directed action. Consistent with this idea, lesions to these association areas result in profound cognitive deficits.

The major primary and higher-order sensory and motor cortical areas as well as the multimodal association areas of the cerebral cortex are listed in Table 19-1. Three multimodal association areas are particularly important (Figure 19-1):

1. The *posterior association area*, at the margin of the parietal, temporal, and occipital lobes, links information from several sensory modalities for perception and language.
2. The *limbic association area*, along the medial edge of the cerebral hemisphere, is concerned with emotion and memory storage.
3. The *anterior association area* (prefrontal cortex), rostral to postcentral gyrus, is concerned with planning movement.

Table 19-1 Major Functional Areas of the Cerebral Cortex

Functional designation	Lobe	Specific location
Primary sensory cortex		
Somatosensory	Parietal	Postcentral gyrus
Visual	Occipital	Banks of calcarine fissure
Auditory	Temporal	Heschl's gyrus
Unimodal sensory association areas		
Somatosensory	Parietal	Posterior parietal
Visual	Occiptotemporal	Inferolateral surface of occipital and temporal lobes
Auditory	Temporal	Superior temporal gyrus
Multimodal sensory association areas		
Posterior multimodal sensory integration (including visuospatial localization, language, attention)	Parietotemporal	Junction between lobes
Anterior multimodal motor integration (including motor planning, language production, judgment)	Frontal	Prefrontal cortex, rostral to premotor areas on dorsal and lateral surfaces
Limbic (emotion, memory)	Temporal, parietal, frontal	Cingulate gyrus, hippocampal formation, parahippocampal gyrus, amygdala
Motor association cortex		
Premotor (motor preparation and programs)	Frontal	Rostral to primary motor cortex
Primary motor cortex		
Motor cortex (movement of a joint along a vector)	Frontal	Precentral gyrus

Much of what we know about the function of the three association areas has come from observing humans with selective injuries to the cerebral cortex resulting from trauma, tumor, or stroke, or in some cases resulting from surgery for an underlying neurological or behavioral disorder. Surgical cases can be particularly instructive, because the lesions are well-defined and limited. Experimental studies with monkeys also provide detailed neuroanatomical and cellular physiological information on specific regions of the cerebral cortex. Finally, sophisticated radiological imaging techniques are being used to localize brain function in humans performing cognitive tasks.

Nowhere in the brain is the link between specific mental functions and brain structure more obvious than in the *posterior parietal cortex*. Lesions in this area inter-

fere with awareness of one's body and of the space in which it moves. Gordon Holmes in England and Aleksander Luria in Russia studied soldiers who had been wounded in the First and Second World Wars (Figure 19-2A). They found that the posterior parietal association area is concerned with extrapersonal space (with defining spatial relationships in the world around us), and with binding the elements of a visual scene into a coherent whole. For example, Holmes and Luria found that soldiers with bilateral injuries to the posterolateral parietal lobe had normal visual acuity but were unable to scan visually or reach for an object of interest. When asked to describe what they saw, the wounded soldiers could not put together the elements of a visual scene. These studies showed that the posterior association areas are critical for integrating different sensory modali-

A₁

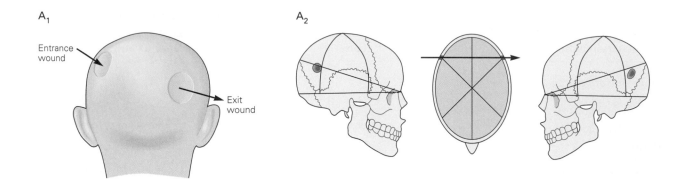

A₂

B₁ H.M.

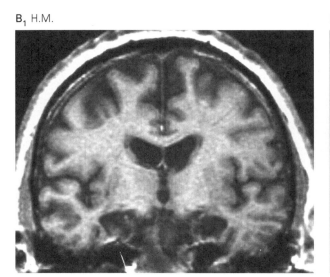

B₂ Control

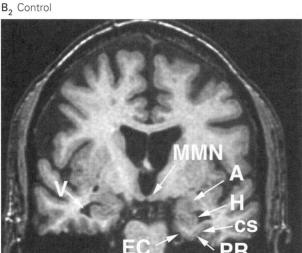

C

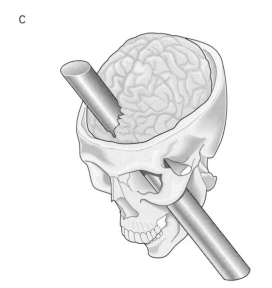

Figure 19-2 Important insights into the function of cortical association areas has come from observations on patients with specific injuries of the cerebral cortex.

A.1. The drawing shows the path of a bullet in a soldier wounded in World War I. The bullet entered the skull over the dorsolateral parietal lobe on the left and exited through the ventrolateral parietal lobe on the right. This patient was studied by Gordon Holmes, an English neurologist, who derived the importance of the parietal lobe in visuospatial integration from his observations. **2.** Drawing from the work of Aleksander Luria showing the path taken by a bullet through the parietal lobes of a Russian soldier in World War II. The soldier's visuospatial deficit was nearly identical to Holmes's patient.

B. This magnetic resonance (MR) image shows the bilateral removal of the medial temporal lobe including the hippocampus in patient H.M. **1.** Scan of H.M.'s brain. **2.** Scan of a control subject's brain. **A** = amygdala; **H** = hippocampus; **EC** = entorhinal cortex; **CS** = collateral sulcus; **PR** = perirhinal sulcus; **MMN** = medial mammillary nucleus. (Courtesy of D. Amaral.)

C. A drawing of a computer reconstruction of the passage of a tamping iron through the brain of Phineas Gage over a century ago. This injury resulted in severe personality changes that illuminated our understanding of the function of the frontal lobes. (Adapted from Damasio et al. 1994.)

ties and for using that integrated information to direct behavior. Later experiments with intact awake monkeys (to be considered in the next chapter) demonstrated that neurons in the dorsolateral posterior parietal cortex receive both visual and somatosensory information and are concerned with directing vision and exploratory behavior toward stimuli in the contralateral visual field.

The dual functions of the *limbic association area*, notably those of emotional expression and memory formation, may seem disparate unless one realizes that the emotional impact of an event is an important determinant of whether the event is remembered. Study of the now famous patient H.M. after both medial temporal lobes had been removed (Figure 19-2B) first demonstrated the remarkably selective role of this part of the brain in converting short-term into long-term memory (Chapter 62). Neuroanatomical and cellular physiological studies of monkeys have helped establish that association areas in the medial temporal lobe, including the hippocampal formation, receive information from virtually every other association area. These connections allow the hippocampal formation to sample the entire stream of ongoing cognitive activity and thereby to relate different aspects of a single event so that they can be recalled as a coherent experience.

Finally, the executive functions of behavior—judgment, planning for the future, and holding and organizing events from memory for prospective action—are the responsibility of the *anterior association area* (prefrontal cortex). Interest was drawn to this part of the brain in the nineteenth century by the curious case of a railroad foreman, Phineas Gage. A tamping iron was driven through Gage's frontal lobes by an explosion, but, surprisingly, he survived the accident (Figure 19-2C). After recovering, his personality was remarkably changed. Before the accident he had been reliable and industrious, but afterward his colleagues complained that "Gage was not Gage." He became unreliable and often drank excessively. He was unable to manage his work or personal life, and eventually became a homeless drifter. More recent studies of patients with frontal lobe lesions confirm that the frontal lobes play a critical role in long-term planning and judgment. Parallel studies in monkeys, which we shall consider later, indicate that neurons in the dorsolateral prefrontal cortex provide continuity of behavioral planning. For example, an individual neuron that may fire when a specific behavioral response has been cued will continue to fire, sometimes for minutes, until the response is executed. If the neuron fails to fire, the monkey will not complete the task.

What is the relationship of the primary sensory and motor cortices to the association regions? According to the *hierarchical model* of information processing in the cerebral cortex, sensory information is first received and interpreted by the primary sensory areas, then sent to the unimodal association areas, and finally to the multimodal sensory areas. At each successive stage of this stream more complex analysis is achieved, culminating eventually, as with vision, for example, in object and pattern recognition in the inferotemporal cortex (Chapters 27 and 28).

Three Principles Govern the Function of the Association Areas

Studies of afferent sensory pathways and association areas in the cortex have led to three important principles of sensory information processing:

1. Sensory information is processed in a series of relays along several parallel pathways from peripheral receptors through primary sensory cortex and unimodal association cortex to the multimodal association cortex of the posterior part of the hemisphere: the posterior parietal and temporal cortices.
2. Sensory information representing different modalities converges upon areas of cortex that integrate that information into a polysensory event.
3. The posterior association areas that process sensory information are highly interconnected with the frontal association areas responsible for planning motor actions. These anterior association areas convert plans about future behaviors to concrete motor responses, such as satisfying hunger by eating.

Sensory Information Is Processed Both Sequentially and in Parallel

Cortical processing of sensory information has been studied most extensively in the visual and somatosensory systems, but the general principles derived from these studies apply to the other sensory modalities as well. In the chapters on the visual system (Chapters 25–29) we shall examine the cortical mechanisms that process incoming sensory signals into coherent information to construct visual perceptions. We shall learn how the axons of neurons in the primary visual cortex conveying simple sensory information converge on cells in adjacent secondary visual areas (Figure 19-3).

The secondary visual areas are unimodal association areas. Even though neurons in these areas respond selectively to an array of inputs and are able to signal more complex aspects of the visual image, the information they process is entirely visual. In the monkey specific neurons in the visual association areas of the tem-

Primary sensory cortex   Unimodal association cortex   Multimodal association cortex

Somatosensory

Visual

Auditory

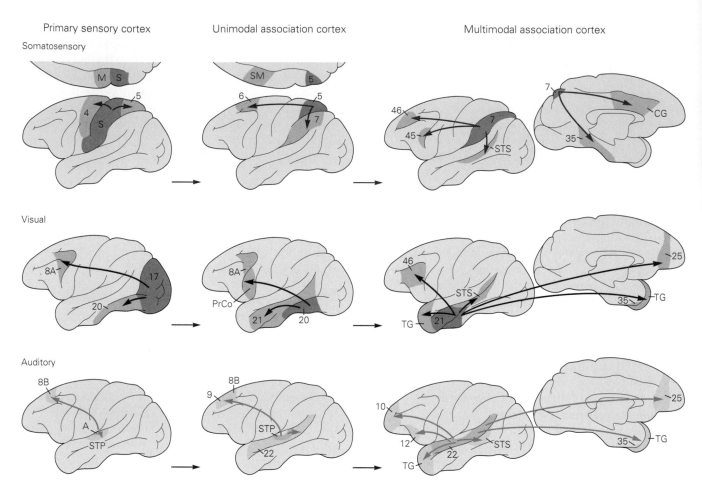

Figure 19-3 Pathways to the somatosensory, visual, and auditory association areas. Connections between cortical areas represent stages of information processing. At each stage progressively more abstract information is extracted from the sensory stimulus. Sensory information flows from the primary sensory areas (**orange** = primary somatosensory cortex; **purple** = primary visual cortex; **yellow** = primary auditory cortex) to adjacent unimodal association cortex. (From Jones EG, Powell TPS. 1970. Brain 93:793–820.)

poral lobe respond preferentially to a particular complex shape, such as a hand; some may respond selectively to specific faces. Damage to secondary sensory areas or to unimodal association cortex impairs the processing of specific types of sensory information, a condition called *agnosia* (Greek, "not knowing"). Injury to ventral areas of extra-striate cortex in humans may destroy the ability to recognize objects presented visually without affecting the ability to identify the same object by touch (*apperceptive agnosia*). Some patients can perceive an object and draw it accurately but cannot name it (*associative agnosia*).

Sensory Information From Unimodal Areas of Cortex Converges in Multimodal Areas

Sensory pathways dedicated solely to visual, auditory,

or somatic information converge in multimodal association areas in the prefrontal, parietotemporal, and limbic cortices (Figure 19-4). Neurons in these areas respond to combinations of signals representing different sensory modalities by constructing an internal representation of the sensory stimulus concerned with a specific aspect of behavior.

For example, the multimodal sensory association cortex in the inferior parietal lobule is concerned with directing visual attention to objects in the contralateral visual field. Neurons in this area receive information about the position of a stimulus in the world as well as its spatial relationship to the individual's personal space. In monkeys, neurons in this area may respond to sight of a reward if the reward is within arm's reach (personal space) but not if it is across the room (extrapersonal space). These neurons also receive highly spe-

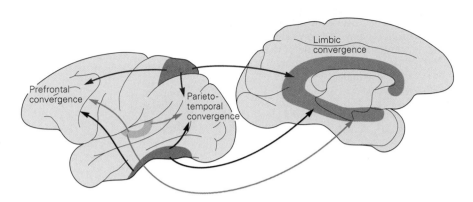

Figure 19-4 Unimodal sensory inputs converge on multimodal association areas in the prefrontal, the parietotemporal, and limbic cortices. (The limbic cortices form an unbroken stretch along the medial edge of the hemisphere, surrounding the corpus callosum and the diencephalon.) **Orange** = somatosensory association cortex; **purple** = visual association cortex; **yellow** = auditory association cortex.

cific information from the cingulate cortex (the limbic association area), such that emotional state is a factor in their firing. For example, if a monkey is presented with a syringe filled with juice, neurons in the inferior parietal lobule may respond more vigorously if the monkey is thirsty than if it is sated.

As we shall see in Chapter 20, unilateral damage to the inferior parietal lobule results in sensory neglect of the contralateral world. Bilateral injury impairs the ability to explore the world on either side (Balint syndrome). Patients with Balint syndrome live as if they see only what is directly in front of them. They cannot locate objects in their visual world or construct an internal representation of the world around them (*amorphosynthesis*).

In Chapter 59, we shall learn about a region in the angular gyrus that is concerned with language and receives both visual input (reading) and somatosensory input (Braille). Injury to this area produces *alexia* (inability to read). Damage to the superior temporal lobe region (Wernicke's area), where the meaning of spoken words is analyzed, produces sensory aphasia. These difficulties in extracting language information from the ongoing sensory stream are also agnosias, but of a complex order.

The Sequence of Information Processing Is Reversed in the Motor System

The posterior association areas are heavily interconnected with the association cortex of the frontal lobe. To understand these relationships we must first recognize that information processing in the motor system is essentially the reverse of the sequence in the sensory systems (Figure 19-5). Motor planning begins with a general outline of behavior and is translated into concrete motor responses through processing in the motor pathways. Within the frontal cortex individual neurons are not hard-wired to specific motor responses. Rather, individual cells fire during a range of related behaviors. Individual movements as well as complex motor actions derive from the patterns of firing of large networks of neurons in the frontal lobe.

The final motor pathways leaving the cerebral cortex originate primarily from the primary motor cortex, which occupies the precentral gyrus. As we shall learn in Chapter 38, individual neurons in the primary motor cortex of normal, active monkeys fire just before a group of muscles contract to move a specific joint in a particular direction.

The premotor cortex is a set of interconnected areas in the frontal lobe just rostral to the motor cortex. Premotor cortex includes areas 6 and 8 and the supplementary motor cortex on the medial surface of the hemisphere. Neurons there are active during preparation for movement. For example, some neurons fire while the animal is planning for movement, far in advance of the actual motor response. Whereas lesions of the primary motor cortex in humans produce contralateral hemiplegia—the complete absence of voluntary movement, although some postural and stereotyped involuntary movements may persist—lesions of the premotor cortex result in the inability to use the contralateral limbs (even though the strength of elemental movements such as grip and pulling may be largely preserved). The patient behaves as if the motor programs for moving the contralateral limbs have been lost, a condition known as *limb kinetic apraxia*. If the lesion is in the dominant hemisphere, even movement of the ipsilateral limbs, which depend upon the learned motor programs in the dominant hemisphere, will be impaired (*sympathetic apraxia*).

The premotor cortex receives inputs mainly from three sources: (1) the motor nuclei in the ventroanterior and ventrolateral thalamus (which receive input from

Figure 19-5 The flow of information in the frontal lobe motor control system is essentially the reverse of that in the sensory systems. Information is processed in polymodal prefrontal areas (A) that are involved in motor planning and project to the premotor cortex. The premotor cortex generates motor programs (B) that it actuates by means of its projections to the motor cortex. Neurons in the motor cortex primarily fire to produce movements in particular directions around specific joints.

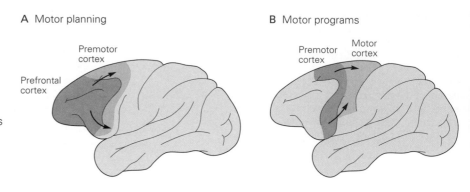

the basal ganglia and the cerebellum); (2) the primary somatosensory cortex and parietal association cortex (which provide information about the ongoing motor response); and (3) the prefrontal association cortex.

In the next section we discuss the prefrontal association cortex in detail to illustrate how a multimodal association area functions. The posterior parietal association areas are considered in Chapter 20 and the posterior, temporal, and occipital areas in Chapter 28 in the context of visual perception. The limbic association areas are discussed in Chapter 50 in connection with emotion and again in Chapter 62 in connection with learning and memory.

The Prefrontal Association Areas Illustrate the Function of Association Cortex

The prefrontal cortex has three main regions: the lateral prefrontal cortex (Figure 19-6), the medial prefrontal cortex, and the orbitofrontal cortex. All three regions are very large in primates, and all receive prominent afferent input from the mediodorsal thalamic nucleus, which terminates in the granule cell layer. The three regions are therefore sometimes referred to as the *frontal granular cortex*, distinguishing them from the agranular cortex of the motor and premotor areas. All three association areas carry out executive functions.

The orbitofrontal cortex and medial prefrontal cortex are related to the limbic association cortex and connect directly to limbic structures such as the amygdala and cingulate cortex (Chapter 50). The most important functions of the prefrontal association area are to weigh the consequences of future actions and to plan and organize actions accordingly. To select appropriate motor responses, the frontal association areas must integrate sensory information from both the outside world and the body.

Cellular recordings from neurons in the prefrontal association area indicate that the neurons are concerned with such executive functions as planning and regulating behavior and finding solutions to novel problems. The prefrontal association area is specifically concerned with the sequencing of behaviors over time. Two of its functions are short-term "working" memory and planning. Thus, the prefrontal association area is engaged in tasks that require a delay between a stimulus and a behavioral response or that depend heavily upon recent experience for completion (Box 19-1).

Lesions of the Prefrontal Association Area in Monkeys Interfere With Motor Planning

In the 1930s Carlyle Jacobsen showed that the prefrontal association area is concerned with the memory and planning of motor actions. He removed the prefrontal association area in two monkeys and studied their behavior using a variety of tasks that involved delayed action. In a *delayed alternation task* the monkey had to choose between two containers, one on the right and one on the left, with a time delay between each choice. In a *delayed-response task* the experimenter showed food to a hungry animal and, while the animal watched, the food was placed randomly under one of two identical opaque containers, one on the left, the other on the right. After a delay of 5 s or longer the monkey was permitted to select one of the containers (Figure 19-8). Normal animals quickly learned to perform the two tasks correctly, but the animals with frontal damage did poorly on both. Most important, the lesioned animals performed well only when there was no delay.

Jacobsen's experiments suggested that the frontal association area is needed for executing complex motor tasks when the essential cues are not present in the environment at the time of the response and must be recalled by short-term memory. Therefore the prefrontal association cortex is involved in short-term memory. Later research showed, however, that the lesions do not produce a generalized deficit involving all aspects of short-term memory. Rather, the deficit is specific for *working memory*, a temporary storing of information used to guide future actions. Working memory is a form of motor planning, and it refers to the active maintenance of information relevant to an ongoing behavior.

The idea of working memory was introduced in 1974 by the cognitive psychologist Alan Baddeley. He suggested that apparently simple aspects of everyday life—carrying on a conversation, adding a list of numbers, driving a car—depend on a short-term memory mechanism that integrates moment-to-moment perceptions across time, rehearses them, and combines them with simultaneous access to archival information about past experience, actions, or knowledge. According to Baddeley, working memory has three distinct components: one for verbal memories; a parallel component for visual memories; and a third component that functions as a central executive, coordinating the flow of attention from one component of working memory to another. Neuropsychologists have developed several tests of working memory and have used them to activate the frontal lobe in imaging studies in order to demonstrate aspects of working memory that are impaired by lesions of the frontal lobe (Box 19-2).

The Cortex Surrounding the Principal Sulcus Is Concerned With Tasks That Require Working Memory

The association areas of the dorsal prefrontal cortex can be subdivided into three regions with respect to the principal sulcus: (1) the cortex around the sulcus, (2) the region ventral to the sulcus, and (3) the region dorsal to the sulcus (Figure 19-6). Each of these areas is concerned with working memory and motor planning.

The cortex surrounding the principal sulcus has been studied in greatest detail. In a monkey even a relatively small lesion to this area produces a deficit in working memory, as reflected in the delayed response tasks. In 1971 Joaquin Fuster and Garret Alexander first recorded from neurons in the cortex surrounding the principal sulcus and discovered that these neurons respond only to stimuli at a particular position in the visual field, usually in the contralateral hemifield, and only during delayed-response tasks requiring directed eye or limb movements toward that site. A prefrontal neuron begins firing when the visual stimulus is presented and continues firing during the delay period of the task (even when the stimulus is turned off) when the monkey is presumably maintaining in working memory

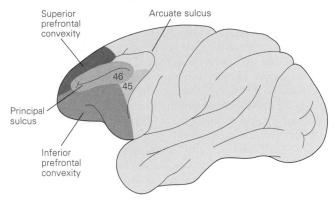

A Lateral view of monkey brain

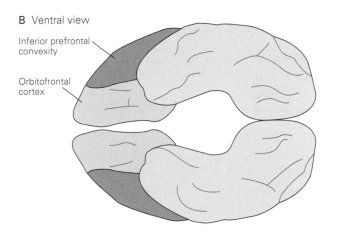

B Ventral view

Figure 19-6 Basic subdivisions of the prefrontal cortex of the monkey. (From Rosenkilde 1979.)

A. A lateral view shows the cortex surrounding the principal sulcus, whose role in visual working memory has been studied extensively, with respect to the superior and inferior prefrontal convexity. Brodmann areas 45 and 46 are indicated for comparison with the human brain.

B. A ventral view illustrates the relationship of the inferior prefrontal convexity with the orbitofrontal cortex on the undersurface of the frontal lobe.

a particular location in the visual field in anticipation of reaching for that place. If on a given trial the prefrontal neuron stops firing before the animal is directed to attend to a predetermined site in the visual field (either by reaching or fixating), this signals that the monkey has forgotten the spatial location and will fail on that trial. Activity of these prefrontal neurons therefore seems to provide the necessary neural processing to establish the behavioral continuity required for executing the task.

Patricia Goldman-Rakic, Charles Bruce, and their colleagues extended these findings by demonstrating that prefrontal neurons not only remember particular places within the visual field but do so in order to guide eye movements to those places. Thus, eye movements

Box 19-1 Tests of Frontal Lobe Function

Patients with damage to the frontal lobe have difficulty performing tasks that involve planning. Planning behavior is often evaluated with the "Tower" tasks. In the Tower of London task (Figure 19-7A), the subject is shown three moveable colored balls in an initial position and asked to move them to specified positions with as few movements as possible. The balls must remain on the pegs and the subject must look ahead to determine the order of moves necessary to rearrange the balls. The difficulty is graded in terms of the minimal number of moves required to complete the task.

The same strategic principles apply in the Tower of Hanoi task (Figure 19-7A) in which the rings are of different sizes. The object is to transfer all of the rings from the first peg to the third, but no ring may be placed on top of a smaller one, and at the finish the rings have to be in the same order as they were at the start.

Planning often requires the ability to be flexible and change strategy in the face of changing circumstances. The Wisconsin Card Sorting Test emphasizes this aspect of cognitive behavior (Figure 19-7B). Subjects are given a pack of 60 cards on which are printed one to four symbols (triangle, star, cross, or circle) in one of four colors (red, green, yellow, or blue). No two are the same. Subjects are told to place the cards one by one under four sample cards. The subject must deduce the sorting rule from the tester's approval or disapproval after each card is laid down. The sorting order that is required for the subject is color first, then form, and then number. Once the subject has transformed the correct strategy and 10 correct placements have been made in the middle pile, the rule is changed and the subject must find the next correct strategy. Proficiency is measured by how many correct sorting strategies are deduced with the pack of cards.

Patients with frontal lobe lesions fail all of these planning tasks, and imaging studies confirm the activation of dorsal aspects of the frontal cortex in normal controls during performance on the tasks.

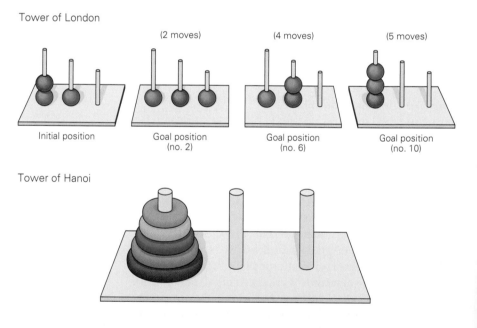

Tower of London

(2 moves)   (4 moves)   (5 moves)

Initial position   Goal position (no. 2)   Goal position (no. 6)   Goal position (no. 10)

Tower of Hanoi

Figure 19-7A The Tower tasks. In the Tower of London task the subject is shown the initial position and goal to be achieved, whereas in the Tower of Hanoi task the subject is told what the goal is. (From Shallice, 1982, reproduced by permission.)

Figure 19-7B Cards used in the Wisconsin test. The task is frequently presented on a touch-sensitive computer screen.

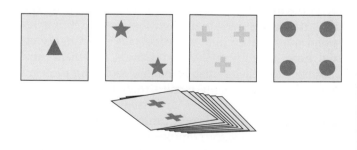

can be used as a precise monitor of the animal's working memory. Monkeys were trained to fix their gaze on a circular spot on a screen while they used their peripheral vision to detect a square cue that was flashed briefly at one of eight positions in the visual field. After a delay of several seconds the animal was directed to turn its eyes to where the cue had been. Thus the animal had to keep information about the position of the square cue in working memory for several seconds.

Many neurons in the prefrontal region increase their rate of firing when a cue is presented and continue to fire throughout the delay period, when the visual cue is no longer there (Figure 19-10). Thus, neurons in the principal sulcus have *memory fields*. They can use stored knowledge to guide appropriate motor responses at a later time.

Moreover, different points in space activate different neurons. For example, a neuron may fire after a brief presentation of a stimulus at a location of 135° with a delay of 5 s. The neuron's activity then increases sharply during the delay and remains high until the response is initiated, even in the absence of a stimulus. The neuron is active only when the animal has to remember the location at 135° but not when the animal has to remember targets presented at other locations (Figure 19-11). The firing of the neurons takes place over a short range of delays, usually less than 30 s. Information that is retained over longer delays, such as tens of seconds, enters intermediate or short-term memory stores and is thought to depend on mechanisms other than working memory.

This pattern of cellular response suggests that the prefrontal region contains a complete map of the contralateral visual field that can be used for visual working memory. Consistent with this idea, a small lesion of the cortex surrounding the principal sulcus interferes with the monkey's capacity to remember the position of an object in specific regions of the visual field contralateral to the side of the lesion. These highly focal effects are described as blind spots (or *scotomas*) of visual memory.

In accord with Baddeley's suggestion based on cognitive psychological studies in humans, recent studies with monkeys and humans indicate that working memory is modular and that different regions of the prefrontal association area are important for different aspects of visual memory. As we shall learn in Chapter 25, the brain's analysis of a visual scene is carried out in at least two major parallel pathways: a ventral pathway through the inferior temporal lobe that processes information about color and shape of objects (information that relates to *what* the visual image is about) and a dorsal pathway through the posterior parietal cortex that processes information about location of objects (infor-

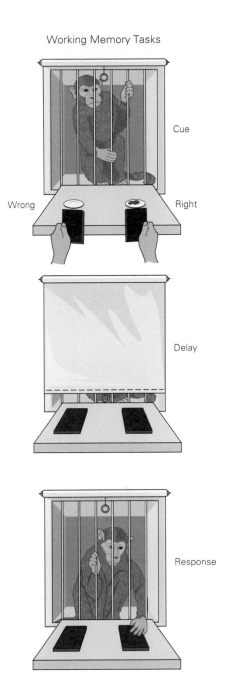

Working Memory Tasks

Cue

Wrong   Right

Delay

Response

Figure 19-8 A delayed response task tests the functioning of the prefrontal cortex. A monkey briefly views a target stimulus, in this case a morsel of food. After a delay the animal is allowed to retrieve the food. The experimenter randomly varies the location of the food between trials, so that each response tests only the animal's short-term retention of visual and spatial information. The relevant information is not present at the time the response is made. Behavior is guided by the internal representation of the rewarded location. (From Goldman-Rakic 1992.)

Box 19-2 Verbal Working Memory

People are capable of keeping a small amount of verbal information in mind for almost indefinite periods. We commonly use working memory to remember telephone numbers for short periods of time until we can write them down or consign them to long-term memory. Alan Baddeley proposed a model of working memory based on observations in normal subjects carrying out specific tasks that interfere with components of this system. This model conceives of an "articulatory loop" with two components: (1) a silent speech or subvocal rehearsal system the phonological logs that can be accessed by reading words or numbers, and (2) a short-term memory store activated directly by speech (the phonological store).

This theoretical model now has a biological basis in neuroanatomy, supported by imaging studies. Areas of brain activation are indexed by changes of cerebral blood flow observed when subjects perform tasks known to isolate these two components of verbal working memory.

In one task subjects were told to rehearse silently a list of consonants presented on a screen and then indicate if a probe letter had been seen previously. This task engaged both components of the articulatory loop. In a second task subjects were required to make rhyming judgments. Letters again appeared on the screen, and the subjects were required to indicate when a letter that rhymed with the letter B appeared. This task is known to engage the subvocal rehearsal system but not the phonological store. The results show that the phonological store involves the left supramarginal gyrus whereas the subvocal rehearsal system involves Broca's area (Figure 19-9A,B).

Nonverbal working memory has a similar dichotomy between a visuospatial scratch pad and short-term visuospatial memory system (Figure 19-9C). Baddeley stressed that the various components of verbal and nonverbal memory are controlled through a central executive function. The frontal lobes play a crucial role in this process, which ensures that complex behavior can be planned and remains flexible in the face of changing circumstances. One marked feature of central executive function is the ability to remember what one has done recently.

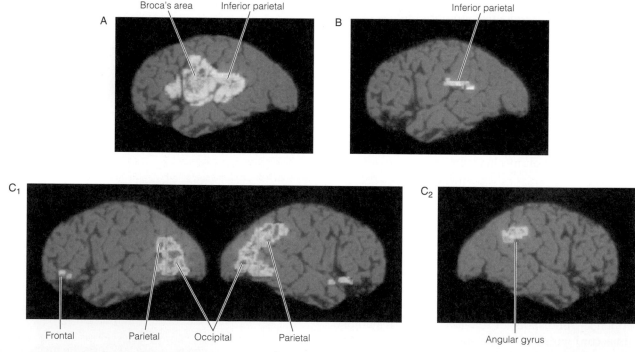

Figure 19-9 Imaging of working memory. Statistical parametric maps (SPMs) rendered onto the lateral brain surface **(green)** demonstrate the functional anatomy of the verbal and visuospatial short-term working-memory systems. Areas of significant changes in blood flow associated with a comparison of experimental and control blood-flow distributions are shown as **yellow, red, or white areas.** The **blue lines** indicate sulci. (Courtesy of E. Paulesu.)

A. Scans were recorded during a short-term verbal memory task for letters and compared with scans from a similar nonverbal task. The "phonological loop" localizes to Broca's area and the left inferior parietal cortex.

B. Comparison of scans from a short-term memory task with those from a rhyming task with no memory demands enables identification of the inferior parietal lobule as the anatomical site of the "phonological store."

C. Comparison of scans from a task in which a series of line drawings were remembered with those from a control task reveal that the "visuospatial sketchpad" localizes to the right occipital, parietal, and prefrontal cortices. **1.** The visuospatial "buffer" in this experiment localized to the inferior parietal lobe in the region of the angular gyrus on the right (**2**).

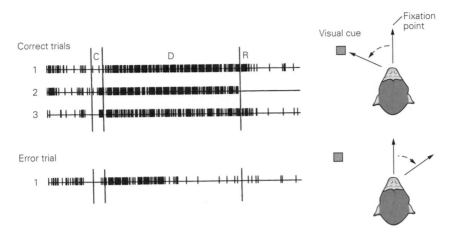

Figure 19-10 Neurons in the cortex around the principal sulcus track working memory. The records show the firing of a neuron in the right principal sulcus of a monkey during an oculomotor delayed-response task. While the animal fixated at the center of the visual field a visual cue was presented in the left visual hemifield for 0.5 s (indicated by the letter **C**). The animal was required to continue to stare at the center of the visual field during the delay period (**D**) following the presentation of the cue. At the end of the delay period a signal was given for the animal to turn its eyes to where the cue had been (response, **R**). On trials in which the monkey correctly turned its eyes to the left (**upper traces**), the neuron fired throughout the delay period. On the trial in which the animal incorrectly turned its eyes to the right (**lower trace**), the neuron began to fire but then almost completely stopped firing after 3 s. Some neurons failed to show any increase in firing during the delay when the animal made an incorrect response. (Adapted from Funahashi et al. 1989.)

mation that relates to *where* the visual image is located in space).

The region ventral to the principal sulcus stores information in working memory about what the object is—the object's shape and color. The region dorsal to the sulcus holds information about *where* the object is—its location in space. In addition, some neurons in the prefrontal cortex respond to both object shape and object location, suggesting that they may integrate information about an object and spatial information, which is necessary to guide behavior. These neurons presumably receive input from both dorsolateral and ventrolateral regions of the prefrontal cortex. Moreover, in addition to these regions concerned with visuospatial memory, positron emission tomography (PET) studies have demonstrated that the human brain has a separate locus for verbal memory, as predicted by the earlier cognitive experiments.

As we shall learn in the next chapter and in Chapter 25, the posterior parietal association cortex, which is concerned with spatial perception, projects to the prefrontal cortex and makes connections with the regions involved in working memory and with the motor regions concerned with motor planning and execution of eye and hand movements. To plan and execute complex behavior under everyday conditions, the frontal association areas must in turn call upon the posterior parietal and limbic association areas. Indeed, anatomical studies suggest that the prefrontal association areas work reciprocally with the posterior parietal association areas.

Lesions of the Prefrontal Association Area Disturb Behavioral Planning in Humans

As might be expected, patients with damaged frontal lobes do not respond to environmental stimuli in the same way as normal individuals. Patients with damaged prefrontal association areas achieve little in life—their behavior suggests that their ability to plan and organize everyday activities is diminished. Nevertheless, general intelligence, perception, and long-term memory are surprisingly intact.

The prefrontal area of humans and other animals has a particularly prominent dopaminergic innervation, and depletion of dopamine from this area has effects similar to those of lesions. Performance of delayed-response tasks is disrupted in monkeys when dopamine in the cortex surrounding the principal sulcus is depleted by means of a localized injection of the drug 6-hydroxydopamine, which selectively destroys cate-

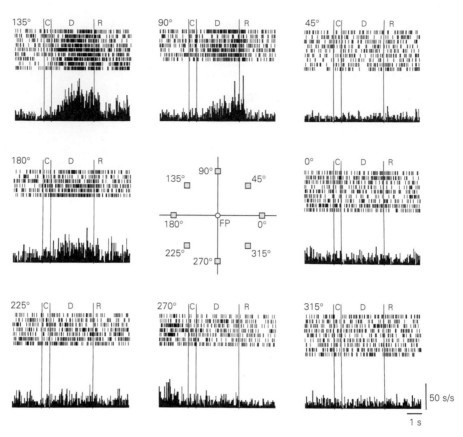

Figure 19-11 Recordings from one neuron during many trials in which a monkey performed an oculomotor delayed-response task. Over the course of a testing session the monkey's ability to make correct memory-guided responses was tested approximately 10–12 times per target location. The neuron's activity in all trials for a given target location (135°, 45°, etc) is plotted as a histogram of the average response per unit time for that location. The activity is shown in relation to the timed events in the task for each target location (C = cue; D = delay; R = response). The neuron's rate of discharge increases maximally during the delay when the target at the 135° location is no longer present and the monkey is simply maintaining fixation; the neuronal activation is maintained throughout the delay period until the response is made. Activity is also observed during the delay period for the 90° and 180° targets but is less than that exhibited for the neuron's "best direction," indicating that the neuron's tuning is rather broad. However, this neuron codes the same location trial after trial. Different neurons code different spatial locations, providing a spatial map in working memory. (From Goldman-Rakic 1989.)

cholaminergic terminals. Disturbances of this dopaminergic system are thought to contribute to the symptoms of schizophrenia, which include prominent disorders of thought. As we shall learn in Chapter 60, imaging studies of the brains of schizophrenic patients show prefrontal hypofunction. When challenged by a task that engages prefrontal functions, such as the Wisconsin Card Sorting Test (see Box 19-1), blood flow into the prefrontal areas of schizophrenic subjects who perform poorly in the task increases much less than that of normal subjects. However, if the schizophrenic subjects are rewarded for their performance in the task, they show a disproportionate increase in prefrontal blood flow. These observations underscore the importance of the prefrontal cortex for executive function and suggest that the cognitive deficits in schizophrenia may involve difficulty in appropriately activating these prefrontal areas.

Interaction Among Association Areas Leads to Comprehension, Cognition, and Consciousness

The dorsolateral prefrontal association cortex and parietal association cortex are among the most densely interconnected regions of association cortex, and both project to numerous common cortical and subcortical structures (Figure 19-12).

Figure 19-12 Common output targets of parietal and prefrontal association areas in cortical and subcortical areas. The connections of the posterior parietal (intraparietal sulcus) and caudal principal sulcus are based on double-label studies in which one anterograde tracer was injected into the prefrontal cortex and another into the parietal cortex of the same animal. Superimposition of adjacent sections shows these areas projecting to common target areas including (**1**) limbic areas on the medial surface, (**2**) opercular and superior temporal cortices on the lateral surface, and (**3**) a range of subcortical sites. (Adapted from Goldman-Rakic 1987.)

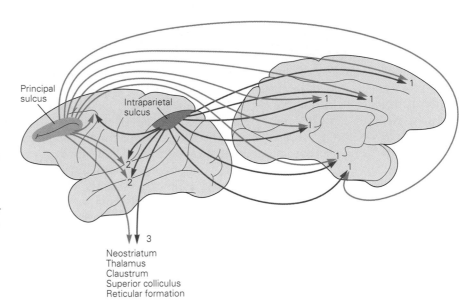

Neostriatum
Thalamus
Claustrum
Superior colliculus
Reticular formation

The interactions between the posterior and anterior association areas are critical in guiding behaviors. Neurons in the posterior association areas often also continue firing after the stimulus has ceased. They may also respond to a particular stimulus only when the stimulus is involved in a behavior, and not when the stimulus is not involved. For example, they might fire in response to a light if it is a cue to explore the nearby space (to obtain a reward). These neurons fire regardless of the type of behavioral response required, such as an eye or hand movement, and may even fire when the animal is prevented from making any exploratory movement but merely required to attend to a part of space from the periphery of its vision to obtain a reward. Hence, neurons in the posterior association area are most tightly linked to the sensory rather than motor aspects of a complex behavior. Neurons in the premotor cortex may have similarly selective responses to sensory stimuli, but they fire only if action (motor output) is required. The interactions between the posterior and anterior association areas determine whether an action will occur and what the temporal pattern of motor responses will be.

More than a century ago John Hughlings Jackson expressed the view that the conscious sense of a coherent self is not the outcome of a distinct system in the brain. Rather, he argued, consciousness emerges from the operation of the association cortices. Patients with focal lesions of association areas have selective and quite restricted loss of self-awareness for certain classes of stimuli while maintaining awareness for others. For example, a patient with a large lesion in the right (nondominant) parietal lobe may be unaware of the contralateral world. Lacking the concept of "left," the patient will eat only the food on the right side of the tray and, if still hungry, will learn to rotate to the right in order to position the remaining food on the right side. Similarly, a patient with language disturbance resulting from damage to Wernicke's area will be unaware of the symbolic content of language. The patient will prattle on in response to a question, without understanding the question. Because the patient's "speech" is inflected normally with emotional tone, it appears from the patient's behavior as if words are merely an adornment to gestural communication.

Similar dissociation is found in the so-called split-brain patient, in whom the cerebral hemispheres have been separated (by surgically sectioning the corpus callosum and anterior commissure) in order to control chronic epileptic seizures. Split-brain patients seem to have two independent conscious selves. Because the nondominant (usually right) hemisphere is "mute," some might assume that only the dominant (left) hemisphere, which "talks," is conscious. However, as we shall see next, by forcing behavioral choices that rely upon information available only to the right hemisphere, it is possible to identify a broad range of cognitive functions that are mediated by the right hemisphere alone.

Consciousness and the Sensory Processing Streams Are Not Distributed Symmetrically in the Two Cerebral Hemispheres

Although some asymmetries of sensory processing in the cerebral hemispheres probably exist in most mammals, such asymmetry is accentuated in humans by our reliance upon complex *symbolic* behavior. Language, mathematics, and the reading of musical scores are obvious examples of the use of symbols, but symbolic representation is an important component of virtually all human behavior. Nevertheless, most activities engage both hemispheres to some extent. Even speech involves both hemispheres. The dominant (usually left) hemisphere is more concerned with the significance of words, whereas the nondominant hemisphere is more concerned with tonal inflection, emotional gesturing, and facial expression (see Chapter 59).

The importance of the nondominant hemisphere in the analysis of space is revealed by its critical role in attention. Damage to the left inferior parietal lobe usually produces only a minor degree of sensory neglect of the right side of space. When the right parietal lobe is damaged, sensory neglect is much greater. As we shall see in Chapter 20, patients with such damage may fail to recognize the existence of contralateral space and deny their left limbs as their own. In the most extreme cases, patients cannot even comprehend

that their left limbs are paralyzed and will deny that they are ill, even though they cannot sit up in bed unaided.

The functional differentiation of the two hemispheres is also apparent in movement. Unlike the behavior of other animals, much of human behavior consists of motor acts whose intended result is not immediately evident in each act. When a monkey is thirsty it runs to a stream, puts its face near the water, and splashes or lifts water into its mouth. A human may walk into a specific room in the house, reach into a cabinet, take a glass, turn a faucet, fill the glass, and lift the water to drink. No part of the behavior except the very last (lifting the glass) is immediately related to drinking. All of the other actions are learned motor acts that could be performed for a variety of other purposes (eg, turning a knob can turn on the stove, turn on the lights in a car, or open a door).

The dominant hemisphere, therefore, has the major role of coordinating and managing actions that *together* constitute an intentional behavior. Damage to the posterior part of area 5 in the parietal lobe of the dominant hemisphere impairs performance of learned motor responses (apraxia) to a much greater degree than does similar damage in the nondominant hemisphere. Similarly, injury to the frontal portions of the dominant hemisphere can result in the inability to perform fine, learned movements with either hand.

Almost all right-handed people have left-hemisphere speech.[1] Surprisingly, although most left-handed people also have left-hemisphere speech, 25% have right-hemisphere speech. Roger Sperry, Michael Gazzaniga, and Joseph Bogen, using a tachistoscope, demonstrated the independence of vision and language by presenting visual stimuli to either the right or left visual field of split-brain subjects. Tachistoscopic visual stimuli project only to the opposite hemisphere of split-brain patients because, in the absence of callosal fibers, the briefly presented visual information is unable to gain access to the ipsilateral hemisphere (Figure 19-13).

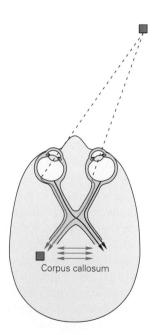

Figure 19-13 An image in the right visual field stimulates the left temporal retina and right nasal retina. Because signals from the nasal retina are conveyed contralaterally and those from the temporal retina ipsilaterally (as shown here in a superior view of the brain), information from the right of the visual field goes to the left hemisphere, although it can secondarily reach the right hemisphere if the corpus callosum is intact. (Adapted from Sperry 1968.)

---

[1]This hemispheric distinction was revealed by the Wada test. The Wada test is used to determine the dominant hemisphere for speech functions in order to avoid neurosurgical procedures that might destroy language ability. In this test the patient is instructed to count aloud or speak. Meanwhile, sodium Amytal, a rapidly acting barbiturate, is injected into the left or right internal carotid artery. The drug is preferentially carried to the hemisphere on the same side as where it is injected and produces a brief dysfunction of that hemisphere. When the hemisphere dominant for speech is affected, the patient stops speaking and does not respond to a command to continue.

When a split-brain subject was presented with an apple in the right visual field and questioned about what he saw, he said—not surprisingly—apple. When however, the apple was presented to the left visual field, the patient denied having seen anything or, if prompted to give an answer, guessed or confabulated. This failure is not because the right hemisphere is blind or is unable to remember a simple stimulus. The patient could readily identify the object with the left hand if he could point to it and, using tactile cues, could pick it out from several others presented under a cover (Figure 19-14). Thus, when visual stimuli were limited to the right hemisphere, the patient could not *name* what he saw but was able to identify it by nonverbal means. This anomia suggests that although the right hemisphere cannot talk, it indeed can perceive, learn, remember, and issue commands for motor tasks.

Nevertheless, the right hemisphere may have a primitive understanding of language. For example, many words projected only to the right hemisphere can be read and understood. When the letters D-O-G were flashed to the right hemisphere (the left visual field) of split-brain patients, subjects selected a model of a dog with the left hand. More complicated verbal input to the right hemisphere, such as commands, were comprehended poorly. Thus, although the right hemisphere appears to be almost totally incapable of talking, it is able to understand very simple language.

The right hemisphere is not merely a copy of the left hemisphere without verbal capacity, however. On certain perceptual tasks the right hemisphere performs better than the left. For example, in a block-design task involving fitting together pieces of colored wooden blocks to make a pattern, split-brain patients performed better with the left hand than with the right. Thus, as indicated earlier, the nonspeech hemisphere is superior in spatial-perceptual problems.

In the normal brain, there is communication between the two hemispheres through the commissures, and this interaction may be essential to certain functions controlled by one hemisphere. In fact, there is now evidence that the capacity of one hemisphere to perform a particular task may *deteriorate* after commissurotomy. For example, Gazzaniga has described a patient who could discriminate the detailed shapes of wire figures with either hand before split-brain surgery. Even though experimental evidence indicates that this task may be mediated primarily by the right hemisphere, after the surgery the patient could not perform the task with either hand, suggesting that interaction between the hemispheres is needed for this task. Thus, despite dramatic differences in the capacities of the isolated

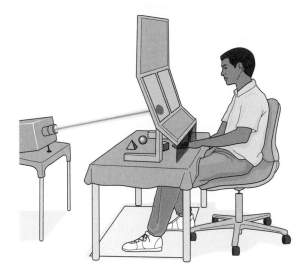

Figure 19-14 An experiment tests the independent functions of the left and right cerebral hemispheres. A commissurotomized subject's gaze is fixed between two screens. Words or images of objects are briefly flashed on one of the screens, one in the left or one in the right visual field of the subject. The subject is asked to name what he saw. The subject can identify an image either verbally or by touching objects hidden behind the screen and pointing to the object that had been represented on the screen either as a word or image. (Adapted from Sperry 1968.)

hemispheres, when interconnected they seem to aid one another in a variety of tasks, both verbal and nonverbal.

An Overall View

The neurobiological analysis of cognitive processes indicates that even the most complex functions of the brain are localized to specific combinations of regions. Localization has great clinical importance and explains why certain syndromes are characteristic of disease in specific regions of the brain. Nevertheless, the question of whether function is a localized or an ensemble property of the nervous system appears to be a dialectical issue.

No part of the nervous system functions in the same way alone as it does in concert with other parts. When a part of the brain is removed in a lesion study, the behavior of the animal afterward is more a reflection of the adjusted capacities of the remaining brain than of the capacities of the part of the brain that was removed.

It is unlikely, therefore, that the neural basis of any cognitive function—thought, memory, perception, and language—will be understood by focusing on one region of the brain without considering the relationship of that region to the others.

Postscript: Functional Imaging Offers a Unique Window on Cognitive Function

Many of the most interesting new insights into cognitive functioning have come from the development during the last two decades of methods for imaging functional activity in the living human brain. As a result, we now have, for the first time, efficient means of addressing many central questions in the study of human cognition: How is sensory input mapped onto the brain and how is a complex sensory representation built up? How do sensory and motor representations interact to guide motor actions? How are complex cognitive functions such as memory, language, and emotion organized? Brain imaging allows us to explore these questions at the level of large neuronal groupings, networks, and systems in living, active brains. Imaging, therefore, explores how functional systems are embodied in the physical structure of the brain.

As we saw in Chapter 18, the primary sensory input and the final motor output are conveyed in pathways that are topographically organized so as to constitute topographic maps of both the receptor surface and of the muscles for movement. Modern imaging has significantly improved the precision with which these maps can be located in the normal human brain. Prior to the advent of imaging we were limited to localizing functions through inferences drawn from clinical observations of patients with brain damage (and from parallel functional studies in the primate brain). Now the functions of different regions of the normal human brain can be examined directly with a variety of different imaging techniques.

Three-dimensional brain imaging began with *X-ray computerized tomography* (CT scanning) and *magnetic resonance imaging* (MRI) in the 1970s and 1980s. These two methods are still widely used today as diagnostic tools. CT and MRI provide detailed three-dimensional anatomical images of the brain in a living patient, but they are static. CT scanning uses an X-ray tube that emits a narrow beam of X-rays and rotates around the head of the subject. Many X-ray detectors are positioned at opposite sides of the tube and detect the X-ray beams coming through the other side of the subject's head. CT scanning detects different brain structures that vary in density and therefore attenuate the passage of X-rays to different degrees. Because the tube has a number of detectors and rotates around the subject's head, the CT scan obtains information from many positions of the subject's head and thereby reconstructs a three-dimensional image of the brain by using mathematical techniques that take advantage of the fact that the narrow beam of X-rays is passed through the head at many different angles.

MRI provides even more detailed anatomical images of the brain (Figures 19-15, 19-16, and 19-17). MRI generates images that result from the effects of changing strong magnetic fields applied to brain tissue. When placed in a magnetic field, nuclei of certain atoms, for example hydrogen atoms (protons), can be made to resonate if a radio frequency pulse is applied to them (Box 19-3).

Different brain structures can be imaged because their protons have different properties; for example, protons in fat differ from protons in water. In addition, protons in different structures can be distinguished on the basis of two relaxation parameters, T_1 and T_2, associated with different behaviors of protons after a radio frequency pulse. Thus, proton resonance differs in fat and water and also depends upon whether water is intracellular or extracellular, in the blood, or in cerebral spinal fluid. As a result, it is possible to distinguish gray and white matter as well as cerebrospinal fluid with high contrast. Certain physical properties of the tissue can also be imaged. For example, diffusion-weighted imaging shows free hydrogen ions that diffuse abnormally in water, and ions that enter injured neurons after ischemia or hypoxia. This technique is now being developed as an accurate way to assess progression of stroke damage.

By using detectors that are sensitive to the radio frequencies emitted by the oscillating nuclei of the hydrogen atom and the computational techniques developed earlier for CT scanning, images of the living human brain can be obtained with remarkable resolution. In contrast to CT scans, MRI images can be obtained from *any* desired angle. For example, it is possible with MRI to obtain images of the living brain in slices in any desired plane—coronal, sagittal, or horizontal—and at any level. As a result, any deep structure can be studied using imaging parameters that are optimal for its visualization.

The resolution of routine MRI is about 1 mm. Resolution is determined mostly by the strength of the magnetic field and in part by MRI pulse technique. Until recently the available magnets had a field strength of 1.5 tesla. Now magnets with field strengths of up to 4 tesla, are beginning to be used and these provide images with resolution of less than 1 mm.

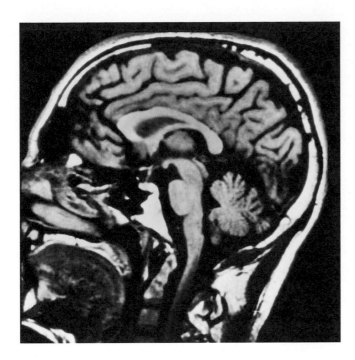

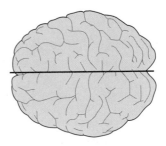

Figure 19-15 This MRI scan of a midsagittal section through the cerebral hemispheres, corpus callosum, brain stem, and spinal cord reveals all major regions of the central nervous system as well as components of the ventricular system. Whereas dense bone is not seen on MRI, marrow is. The diagram shows the detail visible in the MRI scan. The cingulate gyrus, a prominent gyrus on the medial surface, overlies the corpus callosum and fornix. These three structures each have a C-shape. The cingulate gyrus and fornix are both part of the limbic system. The corpus callosum contains the axons of neurons that interconnect the two halves of the cerebral cortex. The fornix curves around the dorsal part of the thalamus, a major constituent of the diencephalon. The other major component of the diencephalon, the hypothalamus, can be seen ventral to the thalamus. The two lobes of the pituitary gland are also clearly revealed. The posterior lobe is distinguished from the anterior by the presence of antidiuretic hormone in the terminals of neurosecretory cells, which produces an intense signal on MRI. The imaging plane in the scan cuts through the third ventricle. The cerebral aqueduct can be seen connecting the third and fourth ventricles.

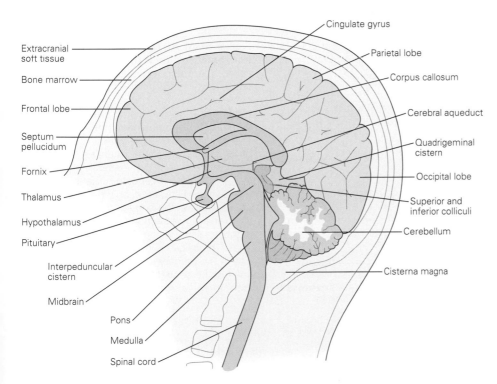

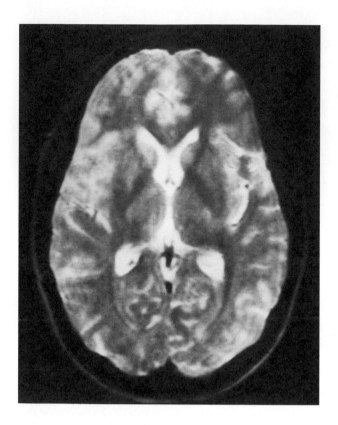

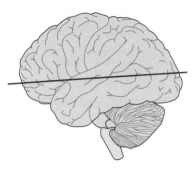

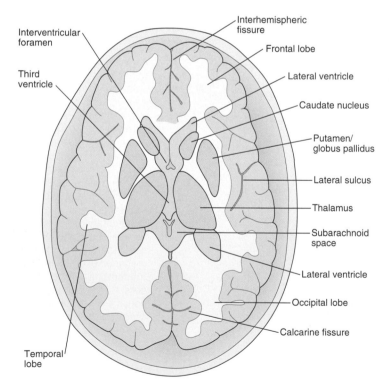

Interventricular foramen

Third ventricle

Temporal lobe

Interhemispheric fissure

Frontal lobe

Lateral ventricle

Caudate nucleus

Putamen/ globus pallidus

Lateral sulcus

Thalamus

Subarachnoid space

Lateral ventricle

Occipital lobe

Calcarine fissure

Figure 19-16 An MRI scan of a horizontal section through the cerebral hemisphere and diencephalon. The MRI scan shows some aspects of the nuclear organization of the thalamus. The caudate nucleus and putamen, the two major components of the basal ganglia, are clearly seen, as are components of the ventricular system. While the caudate nucleus is a C-shaped structure, only the head is visible; the body is above the plane of the section and the tail is too small to be seen on MR images. The calcarine fissure—the site of the primary visual cortex—can also be seen in the occipital lobe.

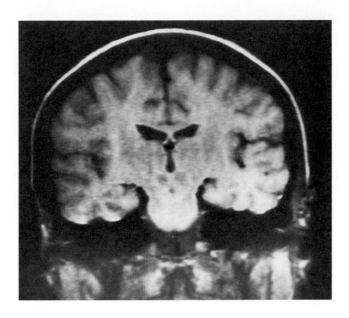

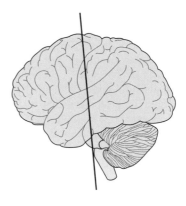

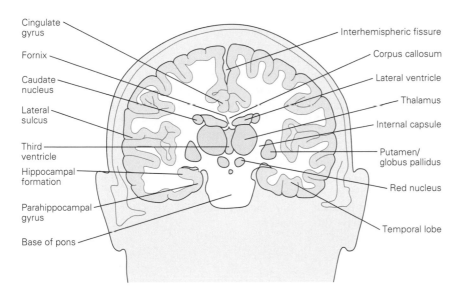

Cingulate gyrus

Fornix

Caudate nucleus

Lateral sulcus

Third ventricle

Hippocampal formation

Parahippocampal gyrus

Base of pons

Interhemispheric fissure

Corpus callosum

Lateral ventricle

Thalamus

Internal capsule

Putamen/ globus pallidus

Red nucleus

Temporal lobe

Figure 19-17 An MRI scan of a coronal section through the cerebral hemisphere and diencephalon. The scan shows many of the structures that appear in the horizontal section in Figure 19-16. In addition, the hippocampal formation, a common site of epileptic seizures, can be seen. Two other key features of the internal structure of the brain are revealed in this section and Figure 19-16: the *third ventricle,* which separates the two halves of the thalamus, and the *internal capsule,* which separates the thalamus from components of the basal ganglia. In horizontal section the internal capsule appears as an arrow-head, with its point, the genu, flanked by the anterior and posterior limbs. The internal capsule is particularly important clinically. Damage to this region is often devastating because axons descending from the motor regions of the cortex form a relatively compact bundle of fibers in this area. Occlusion of the vascular supply of the internal capsule, a common form of stroke, can result in paralysis of the opposite side of the body. The ascending sensory and descending motor axons course in the posterior limb of the internal capsule.

Box 19-3 Magnetic Resonance Imaging

The magnetic properties of tissue can be used to obtain information about the structure and function of the living brain. In MRI, signals are produced by protons in brain tissue. The proton is the nucleus of the hydrogen atom and responds to applied magnetic fields by emitting characteristic radio waves. Each proton rotates around its axis, acting as a small magnet with its own dipole. Normally, protons are directed at random so the tissue essentially has no net dipole, but when placed in a magnetic field the protons become aligned (Figure 19-18).

A second magnetic field formed by a radio frequency pulse is applied to the tissue and causes the protons to start wobbling around their axes, much as a spinning top wobbles around its axis when the force of gravity competes with its spin. This wobbling is called *precession*. Precession creates a rotating magnetic field that changes in time, which according to Faraday's law generates an electric current. Ultimately it is this electric current that is measured in MRI. When the radio frequency pulse is turned off, protons in the tissue relax. The protons that were rotating together begin to fall out of synchrony with one another; they precess less dramatically; and their axes become aligned with the original magnetic field.

MRI measures the rates of two relaxation processes characterized by time constants T_1 and T_2. These changes in the tissue take place as the excited protons relax back to their lower energy state after the radio frequency pulse is turned off.

The relaxation component emphasized in the T_1 weighted image is the "righting" of tipped protons as they realign with the original magnetic field. The rate of this relaxation is influenced by nonexcited molecules in the surrounding tissue.

In a T_2 weighted image the falling out of synchrony or the "dephasing" of rotating protons is emphasized. Dephasing occurs relatively quickly and results largely from the loss of energy to spinning nuclei nearby (it is also influenced by such factors as the quality of the magnets used). Protons have dif-

ferent relaxation rates and corresponding T_1 and T_2 time constants depending on whether they are embedded in fat, cerebrospinal fluid, white matter, etc (Table 19-2). The signals expected for protons in different tissue environments can be compared with calibrated MRI images (Figure 19-19).

One of the most important developments in magnetic resonance imaging is the ability to localize the signal in the three-dimensional volume of the brain. This is accomplished by using magnetic gradients—magnetic fields in which the strength of the field changes gradually along an axis. Applying gradients along three axes subdivides the tissue: one magnetic gradient is used to excite a single "slice" of the subject's brain, two more gradients subdivide that slice into rows and columns (Figure 19-20).

Functional MRI (fMRI), like PET scanning, is sensitive to the increased blood flow that is associated with neural activity. This technique has several advantages over PET scanning, however. Its spatial and temporal resolution are greater, and it requires no injection of foreign contrast material into the bloodstream (fMRI uses endogenous hemoglobin for a marker).

When neurons are activated, the supply of blood to the active region increases. For reasons that are still unclear, the delivery of oxygenated hemoglobin to the region is greater than local oxygen consumption, resulting in a greater proportion of oxygenated to deoxygenated hemoglobin. Oxygenated and deoxygenated hemoglobin have different magnetic properties. Deoxyhemologlobin causes more dephasing than does oxyhemoglobin, so a decrease in its concentration results in less dephasing and a stronger MRI signal (Figure 19-21). Functional MRI has shown activation of primary sensory cortices in simple sensory activation tasks and now can be used to examine the activation of association cortices during cognitive tasks.

Figure 19-18 (Opposite) The magnetic resonance signal.

A. In unperturbed tissue protons spin around their axes, creating individual magnetic fields with random directions (1). When a vertical magnetic field is applied to the tissue the protons align with it to create a net magnetic field that is also vertical but is very small and difficult to detect (2). A radio frequency pulse applied in a second (horizontal) direction makes the protons wobble, or precess, around their vertical axes (3). This creates a magnetic field that changes in time and gives rise to an electric current that is ultimately measured in MRI. The net magnetic field can be divided into a vertical and a horizontal component (4). MRI measures the changes in these two components as the protons respond to the applied magnetic fields and radio frequency pulses.

B. A typical MRI sequence begins by placing the subject in a

vertical magnetic field. With the protons aligned vertically, a horizontal radio frequency pulse is applied to tip the protons so that they rotate in the horizontal plane synchronously, or "in phase," with one another (1). The horizontal pulse is then turned off (2) and the rotating protons begin to move out of phase with one another—they "dephase" (top graph at right). Dephasing occurs relatively quickly and leads to a loss of horizontal magnetization and a weakened dephasing signal in the horizontal field. The time constant of this decay is T_2. After withdrawal of the horizontal pulse the protons realign with the vertical magnetic field, with restoration of vertical magnetization (3–5). This "righting" of the protons occurs more slowly than the dephasing (bottom graph at right) and is measured indirectly. The time constant of the recovery of longitudinal magnetization is T_1.

A Magnetic resonance

1

2

Vertical external
magnetic field

Net internal
magnetic field

3

Horizontal
magnetic field
(RF pulse)

4

Vertical component
of magnetic field

Horizontal component
of magnetic field

B Relaxation processes emphasized in MRI

1

2

Horizontal
pulse
turned off

Horizontal magnetization
decay curve
(T_2 time constant)

Signal intensity

Time

3

4

5

Vertical magnetization
recovery curve
(T_1 time constant)

Signal intensity

Time

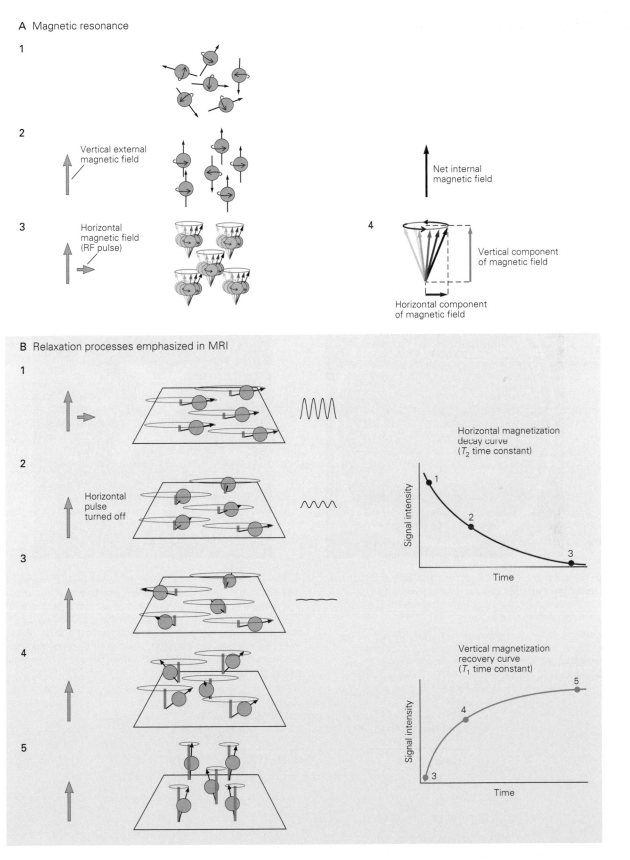

(continued)

Box 19-3 Magnetic Resonance Imaging (continued)

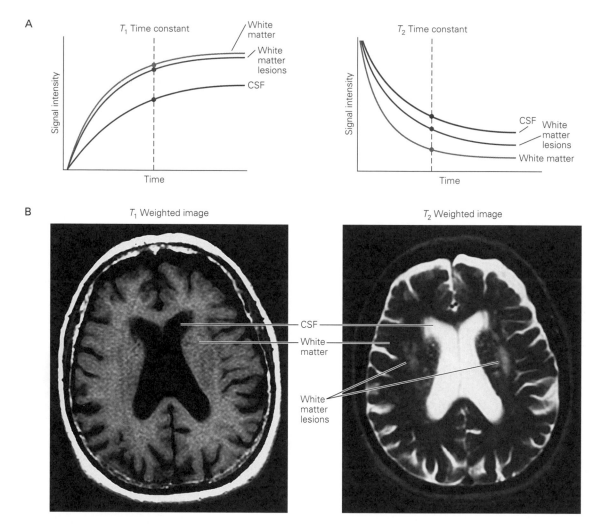

Figure 19-19 Different T_1 and T_2 time constants provide the contrast that distinguishes tissues in the MR image. T_1 and T_2 weighted images together provide a range of information about the structure of the brain.

A. The relaxation rates of cerebrospinal fluid (CSF) are slower than those of white matter for both T_1 and T_2 time constants. The CSF signal at a given point in time is weaker than that of the white matter in T_1 and stronger in T_2.

B. The resulting images show a weak (**black**) CSF signal in T_1 and a strong (**white**) CSF signal in T_2. In this example the T_2 image reveals white matter lesions that are not prominent in the T_1 weighted image. The lesions and the surrounding white matter have similar T_1 rates and their corresponding signals are indistinguishable. On the other hand their T_2 relaxation rates are more distinct, providing sufficient contrast in their signals to reveal the lesions.

Table 19-2 Time Constants (ms) of Different Tissues at a Field Strength of 1 Tesla.

Tissue	T_1	T_2
Fat	241	85
Brain, white matter	683	90
Brain, gray matter	813	100
CSF	2500	1400

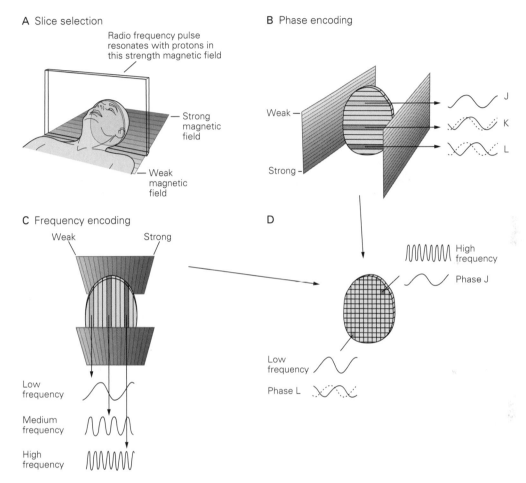

Figure 19-20 Three-dimensional encoding of the MR signal. The signals emitted from a three-dimensional volume are encoded by first exciting a single "slice" of tissue, then applying two different gradients to divide it into rows and columns of pixels. A patient is placed in a magnetic field whose strength is graded along an axis. (When MRI is performed the patient is placed in a tube-like structure surrounded by magnetic coils, but for simplicity the magnets are shown here as planes.) This gradient effectively divides the tissue into "slices." A slice is selected for imaging by using a specific radio frequency pulse to excite or "tip" the protons in the desired magnetic field (**A**).

The slice is then subdivided into rows by grading the strength of the magnetic field along a second axis. Protons in each row will be at a different place or phase in their precessional rotation. When the second magnetic gradient is turned off each row maintains this unique phase (**B**). The slice is further divided into columns by grading the vertical magnetic fields so that protons in each column precess at a different frequency (**C**). With this encoding, each pixel in a slice will have a unique signal (**D**); a mathematical operation called a Fourier transform identifies the signal coming from each pixel.

(continued)

Box 19-3   Magnetic Resonance Imaging (continued)

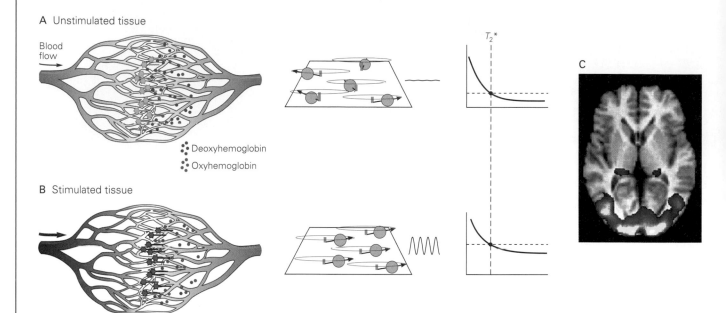

Figure 19-21 Functional MRI study of the visual cortex.
Functional MRI (fMRI) locates neural activity by examining regional blood flow in the brain. In a region of neuronal activity the supply of oxygenated blood is greater than its consumption, leading to a higher than normal ratio of oxygenated to deoxygenated blood. Because the two forms of hemoglobin have different effects on the dephasing of protons, they produce different magnetic resonance signals.

A. In the unstimulated condition visual information is kept to a minimum. There is little activation of neurons; blood flow is not increased; and a relatively large proportion of the hemoglobin is in the deoxy form. Because deoxyhemoglobin promotes

efficient dephasing of the rotating protons, the T_2^* curve that characterizes fMRI is relatively steep and the magnetic resonance signal weak.

B. In the stimulated condition the patient is exposed to a flashing checkerboard pattern. Neurons become active; blood flow increases; and the proportion of deoxyhemoglobin decreases. As a result, the dephasing of the protons is slower, the T_2^* curve less steep, and the corresponding magnetic resonance signal stronger.

C. An image showing the increased signal in the visual cortex is generated from a comparison of the images of the stimulated and unstimulated cortex.

Functional MRI Is an Adaptation of MRI That Records Changes Related to Tissue Function in Successive Images

There are several methods of functional MRI (fMRI) scanning, but the most important makes use of blood oxygen level detection (BOLD), an index of brain activity composed of several variables, some of which are still incompletely understood. The BOLD signal reflects changes in the ratio of oxyhemoglobin to deoxyhemoglobin, the levels of which in turn vary with blood volume, flow, metabolism, and perfusion.

Deoxyhemoglobin is paramagnetic, while oxyhemoglobin is not. Increased blood flow to activated brain regions supplies more oxygenated blood than is immediately necessary for local metabolism, leading to a reduction in the concentration of deoxyhemoglobin. The resulting change in the local magnetic properties of surrounding tissue alters the image intensity on the MRI scan. BOLD is a sensitive method for measuring cerebral cortical activity that has considerably greater spatial resolution than PET scanning (Figure 19-22). Because it depends on blood volume as well as oxygenation, which changes relatively slowly, the temporal resolution of BOLD is on the order of seconds.

Use of Radioactive Tracers Yields Images of Biochemical Processes in the Living Brain

Positron emission tomography (PET) is a sensitive method of imaging based on the detection of trace amounts of radioactive isotopes. These isotopes tag molecules of biological interest by emitting positrons. The tagged tracers reach the brain after being injected into the bloodstream and permit imaging of regional changes in blood flow and changes in the metabolism of glucose in different regions of the brain. Both of these measures indicate changes in neural activity. In addition, appropriate tracers such as radioisotopically labeled transmitters allow imaging of the binding or uptake of specific transmitters (Box 19-4).

For imaging glucose metabolism, the isotope ^{18}F-deoxyglucose is used (Figure 19-24). Although deoxyglucose is taken up by neurons like glucose, it is not metabolized. It accumulates within the cell because it is phosphorylated by hexokinase but is not metabolized further, and the amount accumulated reflects the rate of glucose metabolism. Louis Sokoloff and his colleagues first showed that local glucose consumption, measured by radioactive deoxyglucose accumulation, is a reliable index of local neuronal activity. Most of the energy derived from glucose is used to reestablish ionic gradients across the membranes of neurons that have fired (through the Na$^+$-K$^+$ ATPase). Activity-dependent glucose uptake is therefore localized to synapses that have been active rather than cell bodies.

Local change in blood flow is linearly related to glucose consumption and thus also indicates local neuronal activity (Figure 19-25). Several isotopes have been used for imaging blood flow, in particular H$_2$^{15}O. Increased blood flow, necessary for increased uptake of glucose and O$_2$, appears not to be caused by ions or metabolites from the activated neurons. Rather it is thought that some mediator—perhaps NO—that is released by active neurons causes dilation of cerebral blood vessels. It is important to keep in mind that energy is consumed by the activity of both excitatory and inhibitory synapses, and thus neural excitation and inhibition should not be confused with activation and deactivation of cerebral energy consumption. In some pathological conditions, such as ischemia, the normally tight correlation between blood flow and metabolism breaks down.

Other radiotracers are used to label analogs of ligands for specific receptors (Figures 19-23 and 19-26). These positron-emitting isotopes are safe. For example, ^{15}O has a short half-life of two minutes, so that with

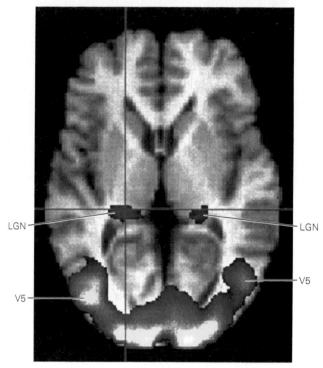

Occipital lobes

Figure 19-22 Blood oxygen level is an index of brain activity. The blood oxygen level detection (BOLD) signal is superimposed on a transverse slice of the brain imaged by anatomical MRI through the basal ganglia and thalamus. **Colored areas** correspond to areas that have been activated by a visual stimulus, compared with imaging obtained with the eyes closed. Visual areas are activated bilaterally, including the visual motion area (V5) in the occipitotemporal region on the lateral convexity of the brain. The lateral geniculate nucleus (**LGN**) behind the thalamus is also activated bilaterally. The changes in signal in response to a strong sensory stimulus are large, particularly in the initial processing areas of the visual system.

modern equipment regional blood flow in the whole brain can be imaged with H$_2$^{15}O in 12 scanning sessions of 40–90 s with a safe and acceptable exposure to radiation. Detection of positron emission is achieved with equal sensitivity in both deep and superficial regions of the brain. The PET method is, however, limited to a few research centers because the short-lived radioisotopes must be generated locally in a cyclotron.

The related technique of single photon emission computerized tomography (SPECT) does not require short-lived isotopes and therefore is more widely available. SPECT makes use of radioisotopes that emit single photon radiation, typically in the form of gamma rays (eg, xenon-133, iodine-123, and technetium-99). The method is limited by relatively low spatial resolution

Box 19-4 Positron Emission Tomography

PET imaging requires the introduction into the brain of substances tagged with radionuclides that emit positrons (positively charged electrons). Commonly used are ^{11}C, ^{18}F, ^{15}O, and ^{13}N. The synthesis of compounds with these isotopes does not result in the loss of biological activity; thus $H_2^{15}O$ behaves like $H_2^{16}O$ and ^{18}F-deoxyglucose like deoxyglucose. The isotopes are produced in a cyclotron by accelerating protons into the nuclei of nitrogen, oxygen, carbon, and fluorine. These nuclei normally contain protons and neutrons in equal numbers. Incorporation of an extra proton into the nucleus produces an unstable isotope; half-lives of such isotopes range from minutes to hours.

These unstable isotopes are then used to synthesize a tracer that can be detected when a proton is broken down into two particles: (1) a neutron, which remains within the nucleus because a stable nucleus can contain extra neutrons, and (2) a positron, an unstable particle that travels away from the nucleus with the speed of light, dissipating energy as it goes. The positron eventually collides with an electron, and the collision leads to their mutual annihilation and the emission of two gamma rays (also called photons) at 180° from one another. The site where the positron is annihilated is the site detected by the scanner. The distance between the site of annihilation and the emitting nucleus, which can be several millimeters, limits the spatial resolution of the method (Figure 19-23A).

Neuroimaging PET scanners contain arrays of gamma ray detectors (scintillation crystals coupled to photomultiplier tubes) encircling the subject's head (Figure 19-23B). The two gamma rays emitted by the annihilation of a positron and electron ultimately reach pairs of coincidence detectors that will record an event when, and only when, two simultaneous detections are made. Emission is detected along a line or slice in one plane. Multiple slices are obtained and reconstructed to localize the position of the source of the emission in the three-dimensional brain. The method of coincident detection permits precise localization of the site of gamma emission.

The spatial resolution of PET, between 3 and 8 mm, is greater than that of electroencephalograms and event-related electric potentials, the other major methods available for probing the dynamics of human brain activity (see Chapter 46). Integration of signals over tens of seconds can generate images that theoretically have an optimal spatial resolution of approximately $3 \times 3 \times 3$ mm and a typical resolution of 6–8 mm.

Figure 19-23 (Opposite) Gamma ray detection.

A. The nucleus of an unstable radionuclide emits a positron, which travels a certain distance before it collides with an electron and is annihilated emitting two gamma rays, which then travel in precisely opposite directions. The site of positron annihilation that is imaged (1) may be a few millimeters from the site of origin (2). For example, the distance between sites of origin and annihilation is 2 mm for ^{18}F and 3 mm for ^{15}O. The distance between the emitting nucleus and the site where the positron is annihilated is an absolute limit on the spatial resolution of PET scan images.

B. Gamma rays are detected by an array of crystals and photomultipliers that surround the head. Only signals that are detected simultaneously by diagonally placed photomultipliers are recorded. (Adapted from Oldendorf 1980.)

Figure 19-24 (Opposite) The normal resting pattern of glucose consumption within the human brain as measured with PET and ^{18}F-labeled fluorodeoxyglucose (an analog of glucose). These images were taken with a PET camera in three-dimensional mode, giving high sensitivity and a resolution approximating 3 mm. Deoxyglucose is not metabolized but accumulates in neurons, and the amount accumulated is an index of the rate of glucose metabolism. Changes in local glucose metabolism reflect changes in local synaptic activity, whether as a result of normal function or disease. This series of PET scans shows the patterns of local metabolism of glucose in the brain of a normal person at rest. Glucose consumption is highest in gray matter because this tissue contains the cell bodies and dendrites of neurons and their synaptic contacts. White matter is less active because it contains myelinated axons. The brain is sectioned in the horizontal plane from the dorsal (top left image) to the ventral (bottom right) surface. The cerebellum, basal ganglia, cortex, and white matter are readily distinguished. (Images courtesy of Dr. David Townsend.)

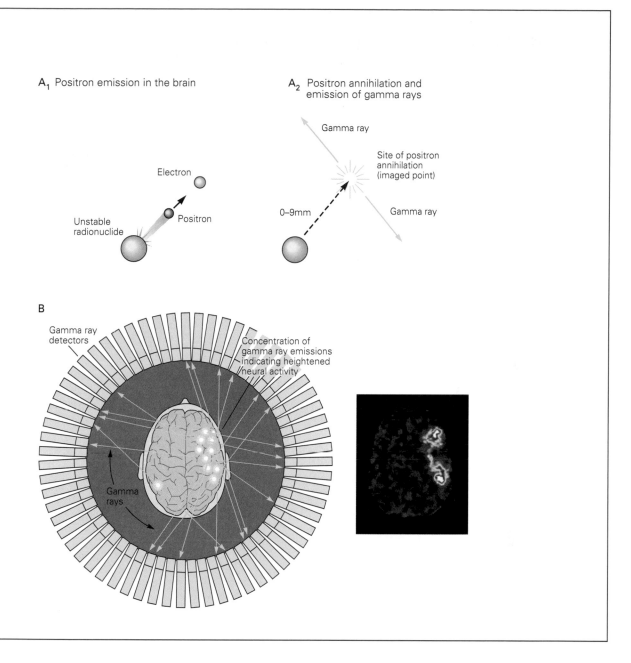

A₁ Positron emission in the brain

Electron

Unstable radionuclide   Positron

A₂ Positron annihilation and emission of gamma rays

Gamma ray

Site of positron annihilation (imaged point)

0–9mm

Gamma ray

B

Gamma ray detectors

Concentration of gamma ray emissions indicating heightened neural activity

Gamma rays

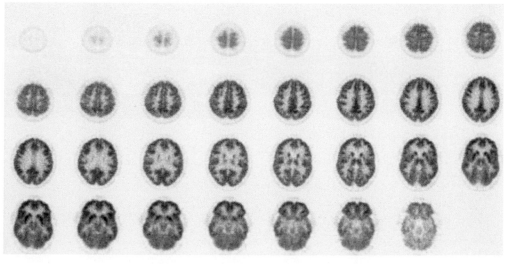

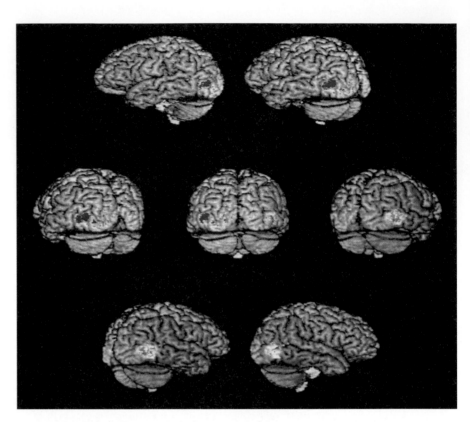

Figure 19-25 Local changes in cerebral blood flow measured by PET reveal regions of the brain involved in processing visual information. These images show areas in the occipital region that were activated when a subject looked at either moving or static visual stimuli. The stimulus was a display of approximately 600 small black squares on a white ground presented as a stationary stimulus or changing in 1 of 8 directions every 5 s. The activated area (red) is projected onto MRI scans of the surface of the brain in different orientations and involves V5, a region that encodes moving visual stimuli.

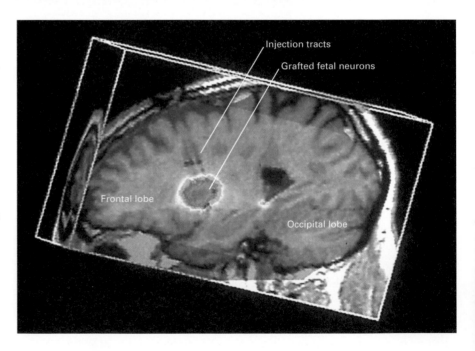

Figure 19-26 Imaging fetal dopaminergic cells surgically implanted in the brain of patients with Parkinson's disease. In this PET scan the precursor of dopamine, dihydroxy-phenylalanine (DOPA), labeled with ^{18}F (F-DOPA) was used to identify dopaminergic fetal mesencephalic cells that had been implanted in the putamen of a patient with Parkinson disease. The exogenous cells are meant to supplement the patient's decreased brain dopamine. The PET images here are super-imposed on an anatomical MRI image. The site of the craniotomy and the three needle tracks left from the surgical implantation of the cells can also be seen.

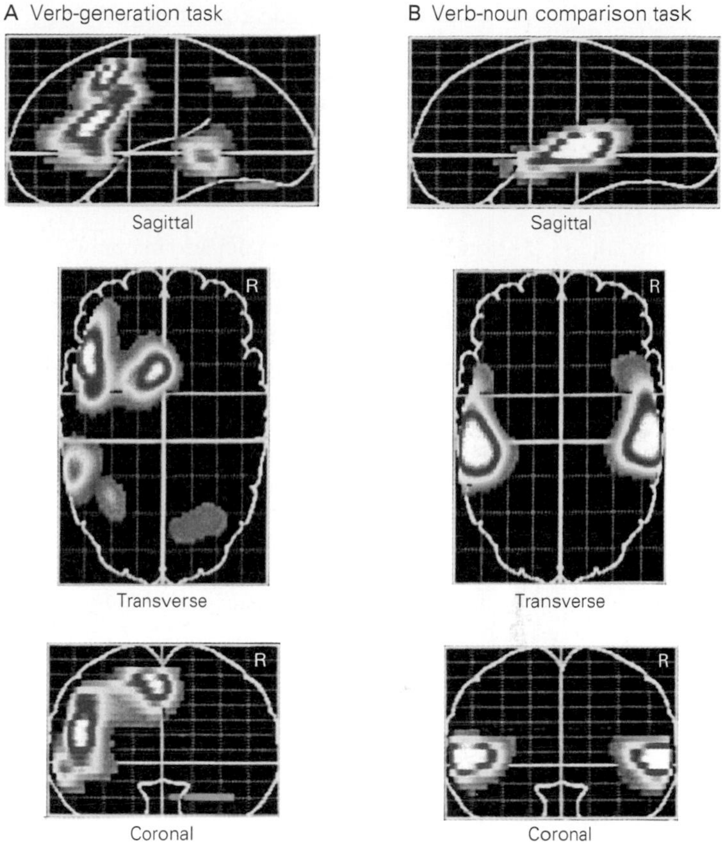

A Verb-generation task

Sagittal

Transverse

Coronal

B Verb-noun comparison task

Sagittal

Transverse

Coronal

Figure 19-27 PET imaging is used to study human language. The differences in color indicate different levels of significance of change in regional cerebral blood flow between control and experimental states. Experimental subjects were instructed to think without vocalization of as many verbs as possible that would correspond to a noun presented to them. For example, the word "apple" might elicit the verbs eat, pick, slice, peel. Control subjects spoke the verbs they chose. The pattern of activation was completely different under the two conditions.

A. Broca's area, supplementary motor areas, and parts of the posterior superior temporal cortex in the dominant (left) hemisphere are activated in the verb-generation task (silent thinking).

B. The two auditory and periauditory cortices are primarily activated in the control group doing verb-noun comparison (vocalized thinking).

and sensitivity, but it can provide valuable information on cerebral blood flow and the distribution of radiolabeled ligands. Because MR images are sharp, PET and other functional techniques are often done concomitantly with MRI to take advantage of MRI's ability to locate within the brain the site of the isotope signal detected by PET scanning.

As we shall see in Chapters 60, 61, and 62, functional imaging techniques can be used to identify and correlate metabolic abnormalities in particular brain areas with behavioral deficits. They are also used for studies of normal subjects performing well-controlled tasks that involve cognitive processes such as attention, perception, memory, or language (Figure 19-27). At present PET gives reliable, readily interpreted state-dependent maps of brain function that are formed by integrating activity during different brain states during 90 s of scanning. Functional MRI provides equally rapid, noninvasive state-dependent functional maps with greater spatial resolution and also promises to yield maps of brain

function that can be related to specific behavioral events.

Clifford B. Saper
Susan Iversen
Richard Frackowiak

Selected Readings

Andersen RA. 1987. Inferior parietal lobule function in spatial perception and visuomotor integration. In: F Plum (ed). *Handbook of Physiology.* Sect 1. *The Nervous System.* Vol. 5, *Higher Functions of the Brain,* Part 2, pp. 483–518. Bethesda, MD: American Physiological Society.

Andreasen NC. 1988. Brain imaging: applications in psychiatry. Science 239:1381–1388.

Damasio H. 1995. *Human Brain Anatomy in Computerized Images.* New York: Oxford Univ. Press.

Damasio H, Grabowski T, Frank R, Galaburda AM, Damasio AR. 1994. The return of Phineas Gage: clues about the brain from the skull of a famous patient. Science 264:1102–1105.

Frackowiak RSJ, Friston KJ. 1994. Functional neuroanatomy of the human brain: positron emission tomography—a new neuroanatomical technique. J Anat 184:211–225.

Funahashi S, Bruce CJ, Goldman-Rakic PS. 1989. Mnemonic coding of visual space in the monkey's dorsolateral prefrontal cortex. J Neurophysiol 61:331–349.

Fuster JM. 1997. *The Prefrontal Cortex: Anatomy, Physiology, and Neuropsychology of the Frontal Lobe,* 3rd ed. Philadelphia/New York: Lippincott-Raven.

Goldman-Rakic PS. 1996. Regional and cellular fractionation of working memory. Proc Natl Acad Sci U S A 93:13473–13480.

Kolb B, Whishaw IQ. 1990. *Fundamentals of Human Neuropsychology,* 3rd ed. New York: Freeman.

Krasuki J, Horowitz B, Rumsey JM. 1996. A survey of functional and anatomical neuroimaging techniques. In: GR Lyon, JM Rumsey (eds). *Neuroimaging, A Window to the Neurological Foundations of Learning and Behavior in Children,* pp. 25–52. Baltimore, MD: PH Brookes.

Milner B. 1974. Hemispheric specialization: scope and limits. In: FO Schmitt, FG Worden (eds). *The Neurosciences: Third Study Program,* pp. 75–89. Cambridge, MA: MIT Press.

Pandya DN, Seltzer B. 1982. Association areas of the cerebral cortex. Trends Neurosci 5:386–390.

Passingham RE. 1993. *The Frontal Lobes and Voluntary Action.* Oxford: Oxford Univ. Press.

References

Baddeley A. 1988. Cognitive psychology and human memory. Trends Neurosci 11(4):176–181.

Bonda E, Petrides M, Evans A. 1996. Neural systems for tactual memories. J Neurophysiol 75:1730–1737.

Décety J, Perani D, Jeannerod M, Bettinardi V, Tadary B, Woods R, Mazziotta JC, Fazio F. 1994. Mapping motor representations with positron emission tomography. Nature 371:600–602.

Fox PT, Miezin FM, Allman JM, Van Essen DC, Raichle ME. 1987. Retinotopic organization of human visual cortex mapped with positron emission tomography. J Neurosci 7:913–922.

Friston KJ, Frith CD, Lidall PF, Frackowiak RS. 1991. Comparing functional (PET) images: the assessment of significant change. J Cereb Blood Flow Metab 11:690–699.

Friston KJ, Frith CD, Lidall PF, Frackowiak RS. 1991. Plastic transformation of PET images. J Comput Assist Tomogr 15:634–639.

Frostig RD, Lieke EE, Ts'o DY, Grinvald A. 1990. Cortical functional architecture and local coupling between neuronal activity and the microcirculation revealed by in vivo high-resolution optical imaging of intrinsic signals. Proc Natl Acad Sci U S A 87:6082–6086.

Funchashi S, Bruce CJ, Goldman-Rakic PS. 1989. Mnemonic coding of visual space in the monkey's dorsolateral prefrontal cortex. J Neurophysiol 61:331–349.

Gazzaniga MS. 1989. Organization of the human brain. Science 245:947–952.

Goldman-Rakic PS. 1987. Circuitry of primate prefrontal cortex and regulation of behavior by representational memory. In: F Plum, VB Mountcastle (eds). *Handbook of Physiology.* Sect 1, *The Nervous System.* Vol. 5, *Higher Functions of the Brain,* Part 1, pp. 373–417. Bethesda, MD: American Physiological Society.

Goldman-Rakic PS. 1992. Working memory and the mind. Sci Am 267:111–117.

Holmes G. 1931. Mental symptoms associated with brain tumors. Lancet 1:408–410.

Jackson JH. 1915. On affections of speech from diseases of the brain. Brain 38:107–174.

Jacobsen CF, Nissen HW. 1937. Studies of cerebral function in primates. The effects of frontal lobe lesions on the delayed alteration habit in monkeys. J Comp Physiol Psychol 23:101–112.

Lezak MD. 1976. *Neuropsychological Assessment,* 3rd ed. New York: Oxford Univ. Press.

Luria A. 1966. *Higher Cortical Function in Man.* New York: Basic Books.

Oldendorf W, Oldendorf W Jr. 1991. *MRI Primer.* New York: Raven.

Oldendorf WH. 1980. *The Quest for an Image of Brain: Computerized Tomography in the Perspective of Past and Future Imaging Methods.* New York: Raven.

Rosenkilde CE. 1979. Functional heterogeneity of the prefrontal cortex in the monkey: a review. Behav Neural Biol 25:301–345.

Shallice T. 1982. Specific impairments of planning. Philosophical Transactions of the Royal Society of London 298:199–209.

Sokoloff L. 1984. Metabolic probes of central nervous system activity in experimental animals and man. Sunderland, MA: Sinauer.

Sperry RW. 1968. Mental unity following surgical disconnection of the cerebral hemispheres. Harvey Lect 62:293–323.

Tanaka K. 1992. Inferotemporal cortex and higher visual functions. Curr Opin Neurobiol 2:502–505.

Toga AW, Mazziotta JC. 1996. *Brain Mapping the Methods.* San Diego: Academic.

Ungerleider LG. 1995. Functional brain imaging studies of cortical mechanisms for memory. Science 270:769–775.

Van Hoesen GW. 1993. The modern concept of association cortex. Curr Opin Neurobiol 3:150–154.

Zeki S. 1993. *A Vision of the Brain.* Oxford: Blackwell.

20

From Nerve Cells to Cognition:
The Internal Cellular Representation
Required for Perception and Action

It has been said that beauty is in the eye of the beholder. As a hypothesis . . . it points clearly enough to the central problem of cognition: . . . the world of experience is produced by the man who experiences it. . . . There certainly is a real world of trees and people and cars and even books, and it has a great deal to do with our experience of these objects. However, we have no direct immediate access to the world, nor to any of its properties. . . .

Whatever we know about reality has been *mediated* not only by the organs of sense but by complex systems which interpret and reinterpret sensory information. . . . The term "cognition" refers to all the processes by which the sensory input is transformed, reduced, elaborated, stored, recovered and used.

Ulric Neisser, 1967

CONSIDERING THAT THE BRAIN has a hundred billion nerve cells, it is remarkable how much can be learned about mental activity by examining one nerve cell at a time. Progress has been particularly good when we understand the anatomy and the connections of the functionally important pathways. Cellular studies of the sensory systems, for example, provide important insight into how stimuli at the body's surface are translated by the brain into sensations and planned action. Analyses of vision, the sensory modality most thoroughly studied at the cellular level, show that information arrives in the brain from the retina in separate, parallel pathways, each dedicated to analyzing a different aspect of the visual image (form, movement, or color), and that these separate inputs are integrated into coherent images according to the brain's own rules.

Different modalities of perception—an object seen, a face touched, or a melody heard—are processed similarly by different sensory systems. Receptors in each system first analyze and deconstruct stimulus information. Receptors at the periphery of the body for each system are sensitive to a particular kind of physical event—light, pressure, tone, or chemical odorants. When a receptor is stimulated—when, for example, a receptor cell in the retina is excited by an image—it responds with a distinct pattern of firing that represents certain properties of the image. Each sensory system obtains information from the stimulus in this way and transmits this information along a pathway of cells leading to a specific region of cerebral cortex. In the cortex different unimodal regions representing different sensory modalities communicate through specific intracortical pathways with multimodal association areas, which select and combine signals into an apparently seamless perception.

The brain thus produces an integrated perception because nerve cells are wired together in precise and orderly ways according to a general plan that does not vary greatly among normal individuals. Nevertheless, the connections are not exactly the same in all individuals. As we shall learn in later chapters, connections between cells can be altered by activity and by learning. We remember specific events because the structure and function of the connections between nerve cells are modified by those events.

Neural scientists believe that a cellular approach is necessary to understand how the brain works. But it is also their conviction that this approach is not sufficient. To understand how people think, behave, feel, and act, it also is essential to understand how the integrative action of the brain—the simultaneous activity of discrete sets of neurons—produces cognition. A combination of methods from a variety of fields—cell biology, systems neural science, brain imaging, cognitive psychology, behavioral neurology, and computer science—has given rise to a functional approach to the brain called *cognitive neural science.*

In this chapter we first discuss the emergence of cognitive neural science as an integrative approach for studying behavior. We then illustrate the success of the approach by considering what has been learned about a complex mental state: the experience, both real and imagined, of the body in space and the space around it. Finally, because such experiences rely on conscious awareness and selective attention, we discuss the feasibility of a scientific approach to understanding consciousness. In subsequent parts of this book we take up in turn the five major areas of cognitive neural science: perception, action, emotion, language, and memory.

The Major Goal of Cognitive Neural Science Is to Study the Neural Representations of Mental Acts

The academic study of normal mental activity was a subfield of philosophy until the end of the nineteenth century, and the chief method for understanding the mind was introspection. By the middle of the nineteenth century this tactic had given way to experimental approaches and eventually the formation of the independent discipline of experimental psychology. In its early years experimental psychology was concerned primarily with the study of sensation: the sequence of events by which a stimulus gives rise to a behavioral response. By the turn of the century the interests of psychologists turned to the behaviors themselves—learning, memory, attention, perception, and voluntary action.

The discovery of simple experimental means for studying learning and memory—first in humans by Hermann Ebbinghaus in 1885, and a few years later in experimental animals by Ivan Pavlov and Edgar Thorndike—led to a rigorous empirical school of psychology called *behaviorism.* Behaviorists, notably J. B. Watson and B. F. Skinner, argued that behavior could be studied with the same precision achieved in the physical sciences but only if students of behavior abandoned speculation about what goes on in the mind (the brain) and focused instead on *observable* aspects of behavior. For behaviorists, unobservable mental processes, especially anything as abstract as conscious awareness, was simply deemed inaccessible to scientific study. Instead, they concentrated on evaluating—objectively and precisely—the relationship between specific physical stimuli and observable responses in intact animals. Their early successes in rigorously studying simple forms of behavior and learning encouraged them to treat all processes that intervene between the stimulus (input) and behavior (output) as *irrelevant* to a scientific study of behavior.

Thus, behaviorism largely ignored mental processes. In fact, during behaviorism's most influential period, the 1950s, many psychologists accepted the most radical behaviorist position, that observable behavior is *all* there is to mental life. As a result, the scientific concept of behavior was largely defined in terms of the limited techniques used to study it. This emphasis reduced the domain of experimental psychology to a restricted set of problems, and it excluded from study some of the most fascinating features of mental life.

Therefore it was not difficult in the 1960s for the founders of *cognitive psychology*—Frederick Bartlett, Edwin Tolman, George Miller, Noam Chomsky, Ulric

Neisser, Herbert Simon, and others—to convince the scientific community of the narrowness of behaviorism. These early cognitive psychologists, building on the evidence from Gestalt psychology, psychoanalysis, and European neurology, sought to demonstrate that our knowledge of the world is based on our biological apparatus for perceiving the world, that perception is a *constructive* process that depends not only on the information inherent in a stimulus but also on the mental structure of the perceiver.

Thus, cognitive psychology is concerned not simply with specifying the input and output for a particular behavior, but also with analyzing the process by which sensory information is transformed into perception and action—that is, with evaluating how a stimulus leads to a particular behavioral response. Only in this way, cognitive psychologists argue, can we hope to understand the relationship between a person's actions and what that person sees, remembers, or believes. It is now clear that the behavior studied by behaviorists was largely restricted to simple reflex actions that do not require conscious mental activity. Any approach to the study of more complex behavior that fails to address mental activity is simply inadequate to account for all but the simplest components of behavior.

In redirecting scientific attention to complex mental operations, cognitive psychologists have focused on *information processing,* on the flow of sensory information from sensory receptors to its eventual use in memory and action. The cognitive approach to behavior assumes that each perceptual or motor act has an *internal representation* in the brain. Since the brain is a physical organ, an internal representation for a perceptual or motor act must have the form of a distinctive pattern of neural activity in a specific set of interconnected nerve cells that encodes the percept or the action. Looked at in this way, an internal representation is a neural representation: a representation of neural activity.

An empirical approach to internal representations, which looks at them as neural representations, has not been without its own problems, however. Once psychologists acknowledged that internal representations are an essential component of behavior, they had to come to terms with the serious problem that most mental processes are still largely inaccessible to experimental analysis. Without direct access to the neural substrates of internal representations it is difficult, if not impossible, to distinguish between rival theories. Fortunately, significant progress in the cellular analysis of the visual, somatosensory, and motor systems in intact behaving primates has allowed a beginning in the neurobiological analysis of mental processes. We now know how neural

activity in different sensory and motor pathways encodes different sensory stimuli and planned actions. As we saw in Chapter 19, sophisticated radiological imaging methods also permit direct visualization of the various regions of active human brain pathways in controlled behavioral experiments. By comparing the results of cellular recordings in primates with imaging in humans, we now have the power to study directly the neural representation of sensory stimuli and motor actions.

Cognitive Neural Science Integrates Five Major Approaches to the Study of Cognitive Function

Cognitive neural science is an integrative approach to the study of mental activity that emerged from five major technical and conceptual developments. First, in the 1960s and 1970s techniques for studying the activity of single cells in the brains of intact and behaving animals, including primates, were developed by Ed Evarts and by Vernon Mountcastle. Soon these techniques were used to correlate the actions of individual cells under controlled behavioral conditions. It then also became possible to stimulate small groups of cells and to increase their activity or to lesion them so as to reduce their activity. By correlating individual cells with behavior, seeing the effects of introducing activity (stimulation) and reducing activity (lesion), these studies made it possible to examine perceptual and motor processes at the cellular level while animals were engaged in typical sensory or motor behaviors. As a result, we know that the mechanisms of perception are much the same in humans and monkeys and other simpler animals.

Second, cellular studies in monkeys also led to the ability to correlate the patterns of firing of individual cells in specific brain regions with higher cognitive processes, such as attention and decision making. This changed the way behavior is studied in both experimental animals and humans. Unlike the behaviorists, we no longer focus only on the stimulus response properties of behavior; instead, we focus on the information processing in the brain that leads to a behavior.

Third, developments in systems neural science and cognitive psychology stimulated a renewed interest in the behavioral analysis of patients with lesions of the brain that interfere with mental functioning. This field had remained strong in Europe but was neglected in the United States. Patients with lesions of specific regions of the brain exhibit quite specific cognitive deficits. The behavioral consequences of brain lesions thus tell us much

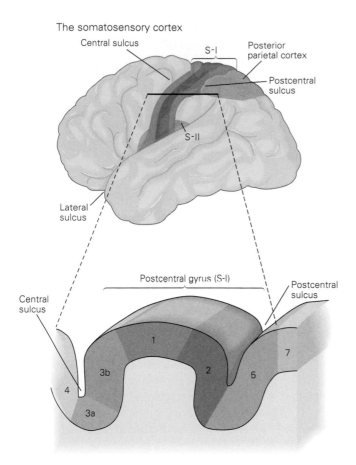

Figure 20-1 The neural architecture of the somatosensory system.

Top: A lateral view of a cerebral hemisphere illustrates the location of the primary somatic sensory cortices in the parietal lobe. The somatic sensory cortex has three major divisions: the primary (S-I) and secondary (S-II) somatosensory cortices and the posterior parietal cortex. The relationship of S-I to S-II and to the posterior parietal cortex is seen best from a lateral perspective of the surface of the cerebral cortex. **Bottom:** A section shows the four distinct cytoarchitectonic regions of S-I (Brodmann's areas 3a, 3b, 1, and 2) and their spatial relationship to area 4 of the motor cortex and areas 5 and 7 of the posterior parietal cortex.

about the function of specific areas and pathways in the brain. Lesion studies have shown that cognition is not a unitary process but that there are several cognitive systems, each with many independent information-processing modules. For example, the visual system, a prototype of a cognitive system concerned with sensory perception, has specialized pathways for processing information about color, form, and movement.

Fourth, new radiological imaging techniques—positron emission tomography (PET), magnetic reso-

nance imaging (MRI), magnetoencephalography, and voltage-sensitive dyes—have made it possible to relate changes in activity in entire populations of neurons to specific mental acts in living humans (see Chapter 19).

Finally, computer science has made a distinctive contribution to cognitive neural science. Computers have made it possible to model the activity of large populations of neurons and to begin to test ideas about the role of specific components of the brain in particular behaviors. To understand the neural organization of a complex behavior such as speech, we must understand not only the properties of individual cells and pathways but also the *network properties* of functional circuits in the brain. Network properties, although dependent on the properties of individual neurons in the network, need not be identical or even similar to the properties of individual cells in the network. Computational approaches, especially when combined with *psychophysics,* the analysis of the relationship between the physical attributes of a stimulus and perception, are helpful in characterizing the system as whole, in specifying what the system is capable of doing, and in determining how the properties of the constituent cells account for system properties.

To illustrate a cognitive neural science approach to a particular problem in cognition, we consider in this chapter how objects accessible to touch are represented internally (neurally). We shall begin with the representation of *personal space,* the neural representation of the body surface. We examine how this representation arises in primary and higher-order somatosensory cortices from a map of the tactile sensibilities of the body surface, and how modification of this map by the loss of a body part can create a phantom representation. We also consider how representations of personal space are elaborated in unimodal and multimodal association cortices into a more complex *peripersonal space,* the space within arm's reach, and *extrapersonal space,* the larger environment around the body. Finally, we consider how representations of spatial relations in the association cortex of the posterior parietal lobe can give rise to *imagined* and *remembered space.*

The Brain Has an Orderly Representation of Personal Space That Can Be Studied on the Cellular Level

When we say internal representations are neural representations, it is important to note that the term "neural representation" is used in two ways. First, the term can refer simply to the anatomical organization of afferent sensory pathways in the cerebral cortex, ie, to the fact

Evoked potentials in the somatosensory cortex

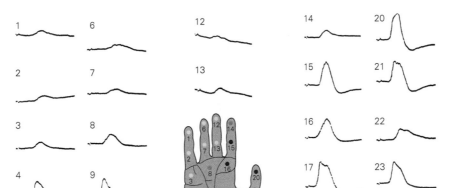

Figure 20-2 The first maps of neural representation of specific areas of the body in the somatosensory cortex were based on patterns of evoked potentials. This figure shows the evoked potentials of one large group of neurons in the left postcentral gyrus of a monkey elicited by a light tactile stimulus applied to different points on the right palm. The evoked potentials are strongest when the stimulus is applied to the thumb and forefinger (**points 15, 16, 17, 20, 21, and 23**). They are weakest when the stimulus is applied to the middle or the small finger (**points 1, 2, 3, 12, and 13**). (Adapted from Marshall et al. 1941.)

that afferent fibers throughout each sensory system are arranged to form topographic maps of the receptor surface. Second, the term can refer to the more complex and conceptual case of the cortical representation of the space surrounding the body. Here the representation is not topographical but dynamic, and the representation is encoded in the pattern of firing of cells that need not have any specific topographic relation to one another with respect to the receptor surface.

Perhaps the simplest examples of internal representations are those of the body surface (personal space). This has been extensively explored in the study of touch and proprioception, two modalities mediated by the somatic sensory system. Touch provides us with information about our body surface as well as the properties of objects, such as their shape, texture, and solidity (see Chapter 23). Proprioception provides us with information on the static position and movement of our fingers and limbs (see Chapter 23).

In the case of touch, primary sensory neurons with receptors in the skin translate stimulus energy into neural events that initiate activity in precise pathways that include several processing stages before they terminate in the somatosensory areas of the parietal lobe of the cerebral cortex. At each processing stage in the somatosensory system—where afferent axons terminate on the cells of a nucleus—the arrangement of the inputs preserves the spatial relations of the receptors on the body surface. This topographic constancy thus creates a *neural map* of the body surface at each processing point in the somatosensory system so that neighborhood relations are preserved: information from receptors that are close to each other in the skin is conveyed to neighboring cells in each relay. In this way each bit of information in each relay is associated with activity in a specific point on the body.

Neural maps of the body surface were first obtained using gross recording and stimulation techniques on the surface of the postcentral gyrus, which was the only portion of the brain readily accessible to experimentation with the techniques available (Figure 20–1). In the late 1930s Wade Marshall found that he could produce an *evoked potential* in the cortex (Figure 20-2) by touching a specific part of the animal's body surface. Evoked potentials are recorded electrical signals that represent the summed activity of thousands of cells and are often obtained by using macroelectrodes. The evoked response method was used by Marshall, Clinton Woolsey, and

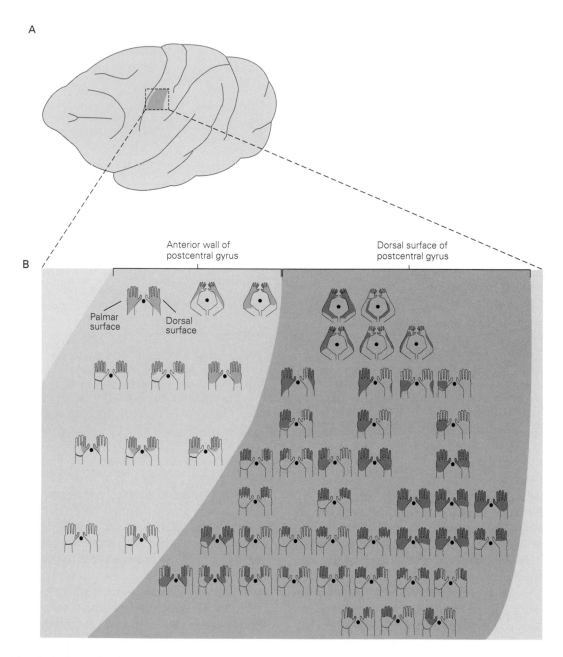

Figure 20-3 An early map of cortical responses to tactile stimulation in monkeys.

Recordings were made in the primary somatic sensory cortex (S-I). The lateral view of the brain shows the recording site (**A**). Two maps show the sites (**black dots**) in Brodmann's areas 3a and 1 that responded to stimulation of the palmar and dorsal surfaces of the right hand (**B**). At each site the **colored** areas of the hand indicate areas of stimulation that evoke a response at that site. The sites on the left side of the figure are in the anterior wall of the postcentral gyrus, corresponding roughly to areas 3b and 3a in S-I. The sites on the right side of the figure are on the dorsal surface of the postcentral gyrus, corresponding roughly to area 1 in S-I. (Adapted from Marshall et al. 1941.)

Figure 20-4 Somatic sensory and motor projections from and to the body surface and muscle are arranged in an orderly way in the cortex. The sensory map illustrated here is for Brodmann's area 1 in the postcentral gyrus of the parietal cortex. Each area within the somatosensory cortex (areas 3a, 3b, 1, and 2) contains a full representation of the body (see Figure 20-5). Parts of the body that are important for tactile discrimination, such as the tip of the tongue, the fingers, and the hand, have disproportionately large representations reflecting greater degrees of innervation. (Adapted from Penfield and Rasmussen 1950.)

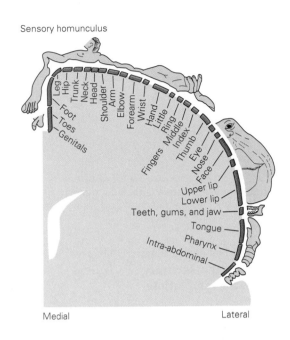

Sensory homunculus

Medial   Lateral

Philip Bard to map the neural representation of the body surface in the postcentral gyrus of monkeys (Figure 20-3).

The human somatosensory cortex was similarly mapped by the neurosurgeon Wilder Penfield during operations for epilepsy and other brain disorders. Working with locally anesthetized patients, Penfield stimulated various points in the primary somatosensory cortex (on the surface of the postcentral gyrus) and asked the patients what they felt. (This procedure is necessary to ascertain where the epilepsy started and therefore to avoid unnecessary damage to normal brain tissue during surgery.) Penfield found that stimulation of specific populations of cells in the postcentral gyrus served as a reasonable simulation of natural activation of these populations, producing tactile sensations in discrete parts of the opposite side of the body. From these studies Penfield constructed a map of the neural representation of the body in the primary somatosensory cortex of humans that was homologous to that obtained by Marshall, Woolsey, and Bard for the monkey.

As shown in Figure 20-4, in humans the leg is represented most medially at the crown of the skull, followed by the trunk, arms, face, and finally, most laterally (near the ear), the teeth, tongue, and esophagus. Note that in Figure 20-4 each part of the body is drawn in proportion to its relative importance in sensory perception. The face is large compared with the back of the head; the index finger is gigantic compared with the big toe, and the torso has the smallest area of all. This distortion reflects differences in innervation density in different areas of the body. Similar distortions are observed in the body representations of other animals. In rabbits, for example, the face and snout have the largest representation because they are the primary way a rabbit explores its environment (Figure 20-5).

The Cortex Has a Map of the Body for Each Submodality of Sensation

The early efforts at constructing a somatosensory map of the cortex probed only a limited area of the postcentral gyrus using techniques that had poor spatial resolution. This work led to the conclusion that there was a single large representation of the body surface in the cortex. Later studies, using microelectrodes to record the responses of individual cortical neurons, revealed that there are actually four fairly complete maps in the primary somatosensory cortex, one each in Brodmann areas 3a, 3b, 1, and 2 (Figure 20-6).

Although each of the areas has essentially the same body map, each represents different types of information. Sensory information from muscles and joints, important for limb proprioception, is represented in area 3a. Information from the skin, important for touch, is represented in area 3b. This information from the skin is further processed within area 1 and then combined with information from muscles and joints in area 2. This explains why a small discrete lesion in area 1 impairs tactile discrimination, whereas a small lesion in area 2 impairs the ability to recognize the size and shape of a grasped object.

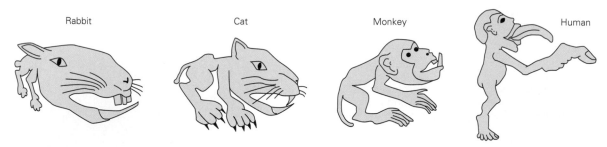

Figure 20-5 Different species rely on different parts of the body for adaptive somatosensory information. These drawings show the relative importance of body regions in the so- matic sensibilities of four species, based on studies of evoked potentials in the thalamus and cortex.

The Orderliness of the Cortical Maps of the Body Is the Basis of the Accuracy of Clinical Neurological Examinations

The precision of the brain's sensorial map of the body surface, its map to the retina, the cochlea, and the olfactory epithelium (Figure 20-4), and its parallel motor map explains why clinical neurology has long been an accurate diagnostic discipline, even though for many decades it relied on only the simplest tools—a wad of cotton, a safety pin, a tuning fork, and a reflex hammer. Disturbances within the somatic sensory system can be located with remarkable accuracy because there is a direct relationship between the anatomical organization of the functional pathways in the brain and specific perceptual and motor behaviors.

A dramatic example of this relationship is the Jacksonian march, a characteristic sensory seizure first described by the neurologist John Hughlings Jackson. In this type of epileptic attack the numbness and paresthesia (inappropriate sensations such as burning or prickling) begin in one place and spread throughout the body. For example, numbness might begin at the fingertips, spread to the hand, up the arm, across the shoulder, into the back, and down the leg on the same side. This sequence is explained by the arrangement of inputs from the body in the somatosensory cortex; the seizure starts in the lateral region of the cortex, in the area where the hand is represented, and propagates across the cortex toward the midline (see Figure 20-4).

The Internal Representation of Personal Space Is Modifiable by Experience

Until recently it was simply assumed that the cortical maps of the body surface were hard wired, that the pathways from the receptors in the skin to the cortex were fixed early in development. But the cortical maps do change, even in adults, with the *use* of the afferent pathways. Two studies were particularly important in demonstrating this. First, a study of normal animals showed that the details of topographic maps vary considerably from one individual to another. Since this study did not separate the effects of experience from genetic endowment, a second set of experiments was carried out to determine the relative contributions of genes and experience to this variability.

In this experiment monkeys were trained to touch a rotating disk with the tips of the middle finger to obtain food pellets. After several months of touching the disk, the area in the cortex devoted to the tips of these middle fingers was greatly expanded at the expense of the adjacent proximal phalanges, which did not contact the moving surface. These results suggest that use of the finger tips strengthens the connections, somewhere along the somatosensory pathway, between the stimulated skin regions and the cortex (Figure 20-7).

Intense use or disuse produces even more dramatic changes in these connections. Several monkeys have been studied 10 years or more after an upper limb was completely deafferented by severing all sensory nerves serving the arm. In all of these monkeys the cortical representation of the face (where innervation remained intact) has expanded into the adjacent area that had represented the hand before deafferentation, so now stimulation of the face evokes responses in the area that normally represents the hand. These changes occur over a wide area of cortex: In fully one third of the map devoted to the body surface, an area of about 10 mm of cortex, the connections representing the hands and arms have been replaced by those representing the face.

What mechanisms underlie these changes? Recent evidence suggests that afferent connections to neurons in the somatic sensory cortex are formed on the basis of correlated firing. It is thought that cells that fire together wire together! Michael Merzenich and his colleagues tested this idea by surgically connecting the skin surfaces of the fingers of two adjacent digits on the hand of

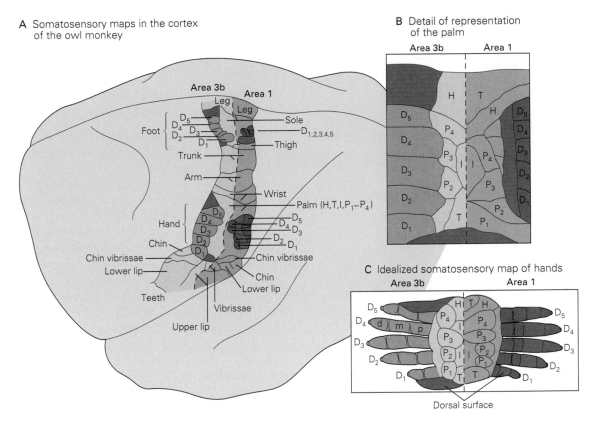

A Somatosensory maps in the cortex
   of the owl monkey

B Detail of representation
   of the palm

C Idealized somatosensory map of hands

Dorsal surface

Figure 20-6 Each of the four areas of the primary somatic sensory cortex (Brodmann's areas 3a, 3b, 1, and 2) has its own complete representation of the body surface. (Adapted from Kaas et al. 1981.)

A. Somatosensory maps in areas 3b and 1 are shown in this dorsolateral view of the brain of an owl monkey. The two maps are roughly mirror images. Each digit of the hands and feet is individually represented (D₁ to D₅).

B. A more detailed illustration of the representation of the

glabrous pads of the palm in areas 3b and 1. These include the palmar pads (numbered in order, P₄ to P₁), two insular pads (I), two hypothenar pads (H), and two thenar pads (T).

C. An idealized map of the hands based on studies of a large number of monkeys. The representations of the palm and digits reflect the extent of innervation of each palmar area in the cortex. The five digital pads (D₁ to D₅) include distal, middle, and proximal segments (d, m, p).

a monkey. This procedure ensures that the connected fingers are always used together and therefore increases the correlation of inputs from the skin surfaces of the adjacent fingers. Increasing the correlation of activity from adjacent fingers in this way abolishes the sharp discontinuity normally evident between the zones in the somatosensory cortex that receive inputs from these digits (Figure 20-8). Thus, the demarcation in the pattern of connections not only is genetically programmed, but also develops *normally* through learning, by temporal correlations in patterns of input.

The Cortical Representation of the Human Hand Area Can Be Modified

Does reorganization of afferent fibers also occur in the human brain? Magnetoencephalography can now be used to construct functional maps of the hand in normal subjects with a precision of millimeters. This imaging technique has been used to compare the hand area in the cortex of normal adult humans to that of patients with a congenital fusion of the fingers (syndactyly). Patients with this syndrome do not have individual fingers—their hand is much like a fist—so that neural activity in one part of the hand is always correlated with activity in all other parts of the hand. The size of the representation in the cortex of the syndactylic hand is considerably less than that of a normal person, and within this shrunken representation the fingers are not organized somatotopically, as are separate fingers (Figure 20-9).

When the fingers of one patient were surgically separated, however, each of the newly separate fingers became individually represented in the cortex within weeks. The new representation of the hand occupied

A Cortical representation of fingers

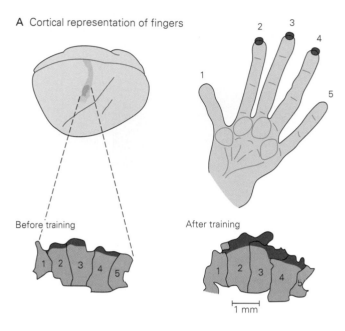

Before training   After training

1 mm

B Cortical receptive fields of fingers

Before training   After training

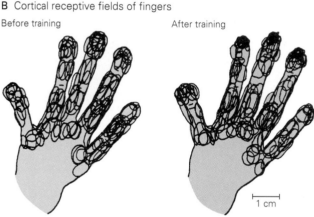

1 cm

Figure 20-7 Increased use of selected fingers enlarges the cortical representation of those fingers. (Adapted from Jenkins et al. 1990).

A. The regions in cortical area 3b representing the surfaces of the digits of an adult monkey are shown before training and after training. During the period of training the monkey performed a task that required repeated use, for one hour per day, of the tips of the distal phalanges of digits 2, 3, and occasionally 4. There is a substantial enlargement of the cortical representation of the stimulated fingers after training (**brown**).

B. Cells with receptive fields on the surfaces of the digits were identified before and after training. The receptive field for a cortical neuron is the area on the skin where a tactile stimulation either excites or inhibits a cell. After training, the number of receptive fields in the distal phalanges of digits 2, 3, and 4 is larger than before learning (as indicated by the denser outlines).

3–9 mm of cortex, almost corresponding to the normal representation of the hand and the normal distance between each digit (Figure 20-10).

The Phantom Limb Syndrome May Result From Rearrangements of Cortical Inputs

Many patients with amputated limbs continue to have a vivid sensory experience of the missing limb, a phenomenon known as the *phantom limb syndrome*. The patient senses the presence of the missing limb, feels it move around, and even feels it try to shake hands when greeting someone. People often feel terrible pain in the phantom limb. Phantom limb sensation and the pain associated with it have been attributed to impulses entering the spinal cord from the scar of nervous tissue in the stump. In fact, removing the scar or cutting the sensory nerves just above it does relieve pain in some cases.

However, recent imaging studies by Vilayanur Ramachandran of the somatosensory cortex of patients who have lost a hand suggest another explanation for phantom limb sensations. These studies show that phantom sensations are due to a rearrangement of cortical circuits. The afferent pathways adjacent to the area normally occupied by afferents from the hand expands into the latter area, just as they do in monkeys with deafferented limbs. More than half a dozen patients have now been examined, and in all of them the area of cortex that represented the hand before amputation now receives afferents from at least one other site on the skin. Ramachandran has called this *remapping of referred sensations*. These referred sensations are not distributed randomly on the body. Some of the patients have two sites of referred sensation of the lost hand, one on the face and two on the upper arm (Figure 20-11).

These referred sensations are entirely predictable from the fact that afferents from the face and upper arm, which normally lie next to those from the hand, now occupy the cortical territory previously occupied by the afferents from the amputated hand. Magnetoencephalography has been used to map the inputs to the cortex from the face, hand, and foot of some of these patients. In each there is a precise, direct correspondence between a point on the face and an individual digit (Figure 20-11A). In normal individuals afferents from an intact hand are situated between those of the face and arm. However, in the hemisphere representing the amputated limb the areas representing the face and arm abut each other in the region that formerly represented the hand. Thus, touch receptors in the face and arm form connections with neurons in the cortex normally contacted by receptors in the missing hand.

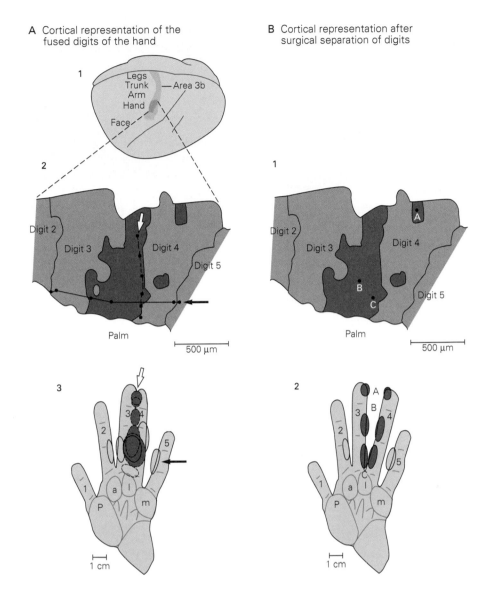

A Cortical representation of the fused digits of the hand

B Cortical representation after surgical separation of digits

Figure 20-8 The normal discontinuities in the cortical representation of the digits of an adult owl monkey become blurred after surgical fusion of the digits. (Adapted from Clark et al. 1988.)

A. 1. A dorsolateral view of the cortex of an owl monkey shows the representation of the animal's body in area 3b of the primary somatosensory cortex. **2.** This detailed drawing of portions of the representation of the hand shows the areas for digits 3 and 4 and surrounding skin surfaces 5.5 months after surgical fusion of these digits. The areas of representation that changed after digit fusion are indicated in **brown**. Instead of the normal discontinuity between the two digits, 3 and 4, a large common area (340–1000 μm in width) now represents the parts of the digits that are fused. Stimulation of the surface of either one of the two fused digits evokes responses in cortical cells within this zone. In contrast, the discontinuity in the

areas representing the fused digits and the two adjacent free digits (2 and 5) remains sharp. Evoked potentials were obtained in two series of sites corresponding to sequential stimulation of the digits in two axes: a rostral-to-caudal axis (**dashed line**) and medial-to-lateral (**solid line**). **3.** The receptive fields for the neurons at the recording sites shown in part 2. The **solid** and **white arrows** indicate sequences of stimulation corresponding to the sequences of recording sites shown in part 2.

B. Even after the fused digits are separated, the common area of representation remains. Thus, the intermingling of the representation of digits 3 and 4 is achieved centrally and does not result from peripheral regeneration that spares the site of contact. Evoked potentials were obtained at points A, B, and C in area 3b of the cortex (**1**) by stimulation of digits 3 and 4 at discrete sites (**2**).

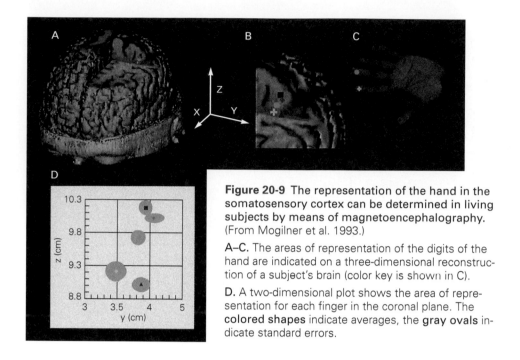

Figure 20-9 The representation of the hand in the somatosensory cortex can be determined in living subjects by means of magnetoencephalography. (From Mogilner et al. 1993.)

A–C. The areas of representation of the digits of the hand are indicated on a three-dimensional reconstruction of a subject's brain (color key is shown in C).

D. A two-dimensional plot shows the area of representation for each finger in the coronal plane. The **colored shapes** indicate averages, the **gray ovals** indicate standard errors.

Figure 20-10 The area of representation of the hand in the somatosensory cortex changes after surgical correction of syndactyly of digits 2–5. (From Mogilner et al. 1993.)

A. A preoperative map of a patient with syndactyly shows that the cortical representation of the thumb, index, middle, and little fingers is abnormal and lacks any somatotopic organization. For example, the distance between sites of representation of the thumb and little finger is significantly smaller than normal.

B. Twenty-six days after surgical separation of the digits 2–5 the organization of the inputs from the digits is somatotopic. The distance between the sites of representation of the thumb and little finger has increased to 1.06 cm.

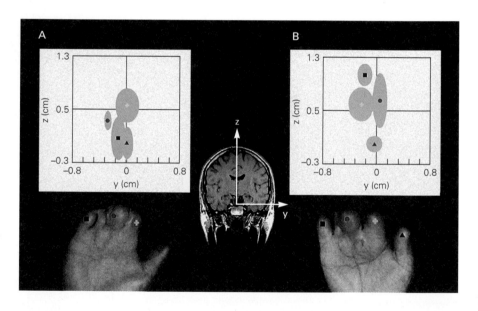

Real as Well as Imagined and Remembered Extrapersonal Space Is Represented in the Posterior Parietal Association Cortex

Neurons in the primary somatosensory cortex project to higher-order somatosensory areas of the anterior parietal lobe and to the multimodal association areas in the posterior parietal cortex (Brodmann's areas 5 and 7). The posterior parietal association areas also receive inputs from the visual and auditory systems and from the hippocampus. These posterior parietal areas thus integrate somatic

sensory information with other sensory modalities, an integration that is necessary for three-dimensional perception and planned manipulation of objects.

The connection between higher mental processes and signaling in nerve cells is no more clearly evident than in the posterior parietal cortex. Lesions in this area do not produce simple sensory deficits such as blindness, deafness, or loss of tactile sensibility. Rather, damage to the posterior parietal lobe produces agnosia, an inability to perceive objects through otherwise normally functioning sensory channels. The deficits with agnosia

A
B
C

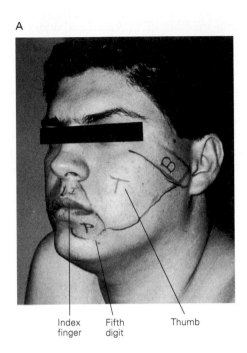
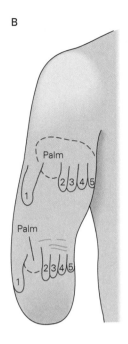
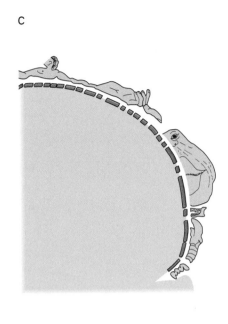

Index   Fifth   Thumb
finger   digit

Figure 20-11 Phantom limb sensations can be evoked by stimulating body surfaces. (From Ramachandran 1993.)

A. A subject whose arm was amputated above the left elbow shows sites on his face where stimulation (brushing the face with a cotton swab) elicits sensation referred to the phantom digits. Regions of the body that evoke referred sensations are called *reference fields.* Stimulation of the region labeled T always evoked sensations in the phantom thumb. Stimulation of facial areas marked I, P, and B evoked sensation in the phantom index finger, pinkie, and ball of the thumb, respectively. This patient was tested four weeks after amputation.

B. The upper arm of a subject who experienced referred sensation in the face and in two distinct areas on the arm—one area

close to the line of amputation and a second area 6 cm above the elbow crease. Each area is a precise spatial map of the lost digits; the maps are almost identical except for the absence of fingertips in the upper map. When the patient imagined pronating his phantom lower arm, the entire upper map shifted in the same direction by about 1.5 cm. Stimulating the skin region between these two maps did not elicit sensations in the phantom limb.

C. Portion of sensory homunculus showing how the cortical area receiving inputs from the hand is flanked by the regions devoted to the face and the arm. Rearrangement of these cortical inputs is thought to be responsible for some types of phantom limb sensation.

---

are complex, such as defects in spatial perception, visuomotor integration, and selective attention. The agnosias most commonly seen with lesions of the right posterior parietal visuocortex are among the most remarkable that can be seen in neurological patients. A particularly dramatic agnosia is *astereognosis,* an inability to recognize the form of objects through touch. This agnosia is commonly accompanied by a left-sided paralysis.

Patients with astereognosis show a striking deficit in the self-image of the left side of their body as well as a deficit in perceiving the external world on the left. For example, some patients will not dress, undress, or wash the affected side (*personal neglect syndrome*). Patients may even deny or disown their left arm or leg, going so far as to say, "Who put this arm in bed with me?" Because the idea of having a left limb is completely foreign to them, patients also appear to deny the existence of any paralysis in this limb and may attempt to leave the

hospital prematurely since they believe nothing is wrong with them. These patients, then, seem to lose a discrete part of self-awareness.

In some patients with neglect syndrome the sensory neglect extends from personal space (the self-image of the body) to peri- and extrapersonal space (*spatial neglect*). In such cases, for example, the ability to copy the left side of a drawing is severely disturbed. The patient may draw a flower with petals on only the right side of the plant. When asked to copy a clock, the patient may ignore the numbers on the left, or try to cram all the numbers into the right half of the clock, or draw them on one side running off the clock face (Figure 20-12).

A particularly dramatic example of spatial neglect is seen in self-portraits painted by a German artist who suffered a stroke that affected his right posterior parietal cortex (Figure 20-13). The portraits done at two months and three and a half months after the stroke showed a

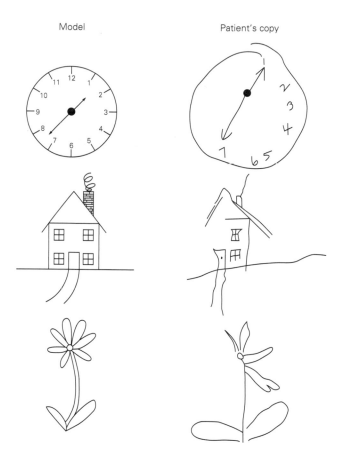

Model   Patient's copy

Figure 20-12 The three drawings on the right were made from the models on the left by patients with unilateral visual neglect following lesion of the right posterior parietal cortex. (From Bloom and Lazerson 1988.)

profound neglect of the left side of the face. The neglect persisted, albeit in a minor way, even when the patient had essentially recovered at nine months.

The spatial neglect of stimuli can be remarkably selective. Studies of patients with neglect syndrome following right hemisphere damage have revealed important selective deficits in the perception of the forms of objects. Such patients are unable to "see" all the parts of an object, even though the visual pathways are intact, but nevertheless are able to recognize the object (Figure 20-14). These clinical findings provided some of the first evidence that normal perceptual pathways include discrete circuits for attending to (1) the global shape of an object and (2) local components of the global shape (Figure 20-15).

Perhaps the most fascinating form of sensory neglect is *representational neglect*, in which the left or right visual field is neglected in an internal representation of a scene. This was first observed by Edoardo Bisiach in a

group of patients in Milan, all of whom had injury to the right parietal lobe. As the patients were sitting in the hospital's examining room they were asked to imagine that they were standing opposite the cathedral in the city's main public square, the Piazza del Duomo, and to describe from memory the key buildings around the square. These subjects were able to identify all the buildings on the right side of the square (ipsilateral to the lesion) but could not recall the buildings on the left, even though these buildings were thoroughly familiar to them. The patients were next asked to imagine that they were standing on the steps of the cathedral, so that right and left were reversed. In this imagined position the patients were able to name the buildings they previously had been unable to identify but could not now identify the buildings they had previously named (Figure 20-16).

This suggests that memory of extrapersonal space is stored with a *body-centered* frame of reference (see Box 25-1 for a discussion of retinotopic head-centered and body-centered frames of reference). The Milan patients clearly have a complete memory of the entire public square and complete access to that memory. However, they neglect the left half of the remembered space, just as they neglect the left half of the visual field in reality, because they are unable to access and recall images associated with their left side, contralateral to the side of the lesion. Thus, memories for each half of the visual field are accessed through the contralateral hemisphere.

Recent PET scanning studies of normal subjects indicate that when subjects close their eyes and visualize an object such as the letter "a," the visualization recruits activity in the primary visual cortex, in much the same way as an actual object seen with the eyes. That is, imagined visual images are generated by the same components of the visual system as are real images produced by external stimuli. Thus, damage to the posterior parietal cortex, which impairs real-time visual perception, also impairs remembered or imagined visual imagery. Moreover, many tasks that require visual imagery from memory recruit very strong activation of the posterior parietal cortex, suggesting that in their imagination individuals orient their body with respect to the imagined figure! It is presumably this imagined orientation that is lacking in patients with representational neglect.

Figure 20-13 (Opposite) Self-portraits by an artist after damage to his right posterior parietal cortex. The portraits were drawn 2 months after a stroke (upper left), at 3.5 months (upper right), at 6 months (lower left), and at 9 months (lower right), by which time the artist had largely recovered. The early portraits show severe neglect of the side of the face opposite the lesion. (From Jung 1974.)

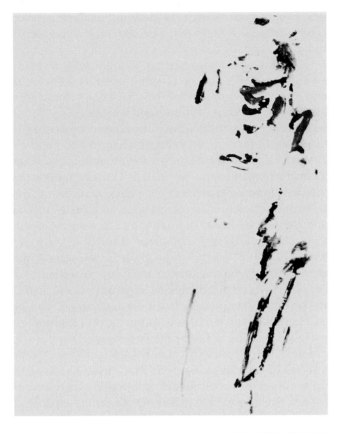

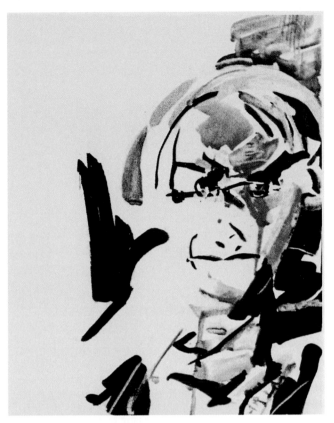

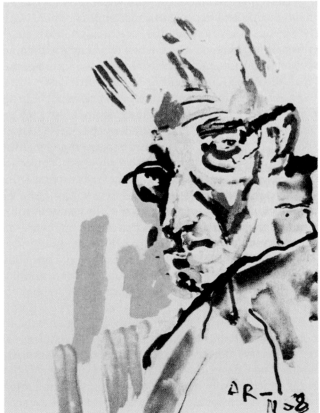

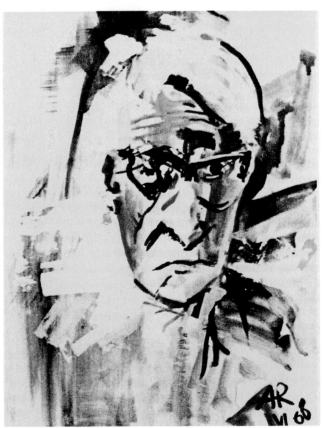

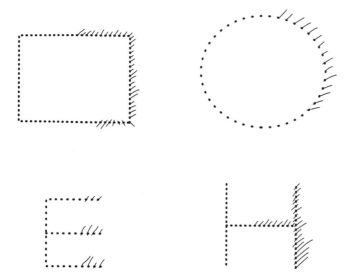

Figure 20-14 The neglect of space on the left after injury to the right posterior parietal cortex may be remarkably selective. A patient may not be visually aware of all parts of an object but still able to recognize the object. Patients with neglect after a right hemisphere stroke were shown drawings in which the shape of an object is drawn in dots (or other tiny forms). The patient was then asked to mark with a pencil each dot. In the figure here the patient was able to report accurately each shape (rectangle, circle, letter E, letter H) but when required to mark each dot with a pencil she neglected the left half of each object. (Adapted from Marshall and Halligan 1995.)

Is Consciousness Accessible to Neurobiological Analysis?

Consciousness Poses Fundamental Problems for a Biological Theory of the Mind

In studying visual neglect we are beginning to address one of the great mysteries of cognitive neural science, in fact of all science: the nature of consciousness. The special character of consciousness attracts fierce interest and debate among philosophers of mind because it is difficult for some to see how consciousness might be explained in reductionist physical terms.

To begin with, how does one define consciousness? At the beginning of this book we stated that what we commonly call the mind is simply the entire set of operations of the brain. In this sense, consciousness is fundamentally a function of the brain and therefore in principle we should be able to identify neural mechanisms that give rise to consciousness. This, of course, does not begin to tell us what to look for in the brain. We must first come to terms with the defining characteristics of consciousness if we are to develop productive neural theories of consciousness.

Consciousness is ordinarily thought of as a state of awareness. Philosophers of mind such as John Searle and Thomas Nagel ascribe three dominant features to awareness: subjectivity, unity, and intentionality.

The *subjectivity* of conscious experience is seen by Searle and Nagel as its defining characteristic and the characteristic that poses the greatest scientific challenge. Each of us experiences a world of private and unique sensations. Our own experience seems much more *real* to us than the experiences of others. Our own ideas, moods, and sensations—our successes and disappointments, joys and pains—are experienced directly, whereas we can only appreciate other people's ideas, moods, and sensations by referring to our own direct experience. Are the blue you see and the lavender you smell identical to the blue that I see and the lavender that I smell? The fact that conscious experience is uniquely personal and intensely subjective raises the question of whether it is even possible to determine objectively some common characteristics of consciousness in different individuals. If the senses ultimately produce only subjective experience, we cannot, the argument goes, use those same senses to arrive at an objective understanding of experience.

The *unitary nature* of consciousness refers to the fact that our experiences come to us as a unified whole: All of the various sensory modalities are melded into a single conscious experience. Thus, when we sit down to dinner we feel the chair against our back, hear the sound of music in the background, and taste the fruity flavor of the wine as a single experience. Our perceptions not only appear whole for the instant of the experience, but they appear to be whole and continuous over time. When we speak to our dinner partners we do so in whole sentences and pay little if any attention to the process of constructing the sentence, yet we are aware that we are completing an idea. Finally, consciousness has *intentionality*. Our experiences have meaning beyond the physical sensations of the moment. Our mind can connect with and represent the range of our experiences.

In earlier times these special features of consciousness led many philosophers to a dualistic view of mind, a view that the body had a physical existence but the mind did not, and therefore the mind was not a proper subject of the natural sciences. Now almost all contemporary philosophers of mind agree that what we call consciousness derives from physical properties of the brain. Since consciousness has properties that other brain functions do not (subjectivity, unity, and intentionality), a physicalist explanation of consciousness poses a formidable scientific problem.

Some philosophers of mind, such as Colin McGinn, believe that consciousness is simply not accessible to empirical study because there are limits to human cognitive capacities that reflect inherent and insurmountable limitations in the architecture of the brain. Searle and Nagel, on the other hand, believe that consciousness is accessible to analysis by human mental processes and that we have been unable to account for it because it is an *emergent property* of the brain and therefore unlike any property of the brain that we understand—indeed unlike any other subject of scientific inquiry. Finally, some philosophers, for example Daniel Dennett, deny that there is any problem at all. Dennett argues, much as did the neurologist John Hughlings Jackson a century earlier, that consciousness is not a discrete operation of the brain but is simply the outcome of the computational workings of the association areas of the brain.

Of the three features of consciousness, the major difficulty, as we have said, derives from its subjective qualities. The precise difficulty is illustrated by Nagel and Searle in the following way. Assume we succeed in studying a person's consciousness by recording the electrical activity of neurons in a region known to be important for consciousness while that person carries out a particular task requiring conscious attention. How do we then analyze the results? Can we say that the firing of a group of neurons *causes* a private subjective experience? Can we say that a burst of action potentials in the thalamus and somatic sensory cortices causes someone to consciously perceive an object in his or her hand and to tell whether the object is round or square, hard or malleable? What empirical grounds do we have for believing that when a mother looks at her infant child, the firing of cells in the inferotemporal cortex concerned with face recognition give rise to her perception of her child's face?

We as yet do not know how the firing of specific neurons leads to conscious perception even in the most simple case. In fact, according to Searle, we completely lack an adequate theoretical model of how an *objective* phenomenon—electrical signals in a person's brain—can cause a *subjective* experience such as pain. Because consciousness is irreducibly subjective, it lies beyond the reach of science as we *currently* practice it.

Since science, as we currently practice it, is essentially a reductionist approach to events, it cannot, according to Nagel, address consciousness without a significant change in method, one that would allow the demonstration and analysis of the *elements* of subjective experience. These elements are likely to be basic components of brain function much as atoms and molecules are basic components of matter. According to Nagel,

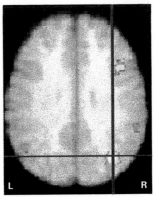

Divided attention

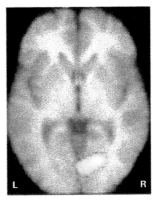

Globally directed attention

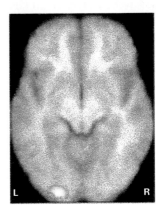

Locally directed attention

Figure 20-15 The visual system has separate circuits for focusing attention on the global or on the local features of an object. The letter L composed of Ds (**upper left**) has global features (the shape of the letter L) and local features (the Ds) to which attention can be selectively directed. When subjects direct attention to the global features of the figure, activity increases in visual area V3 (**lower left**). Attention to the local features activates visual area V2 (**lower right**). Area V3 is less retinotopically organized than visual area V2. There also appears to be hemispheric specialization; attention to global features causes greater activity in the visual cortex in the right hemisphere, while attention to local features produces more activity in the visual cortex in the left hemisphere. When the subject repeatedly switches attention from local to global features, areas in the parietal and prefrontal cortex are activated (**upper right**). These three images demonstrate the existence of a system that is responsible for directed visual attention. In the early stages of visual processing the parietal (and possibly prefrontal) regions modulate activity to focus attention on the global components of the visual scene. (Adapted from Fink et al. 1996.)

object-to-object reductions are not problematic because we understand, at least in principle, how the properties of a given type of matter arise from the molecules of which it is made. What we lack in a science of consciousness are rules for extrapolating subjective properties (consciousness) from the properties of objects (interconnected nerve cells). Nagel argues that our complete lack of insight into the elements of subjective experience should not prevent us from discovering rules that relate conscious phenomena with cellular processes in the brain. In fact, it is only through the accumulation of cell-biological information that we will have the data necessary to think intelligently about a more fundamental type of reduction, from the physical to the subjective. It is only after we have developed a theory that supports this more fundamental reduction that we will be able to tackle the problem of relating specific neural activity to specific subjective experiences. To arrive at that theory, we will first have to discover the elementary components of subjective consciousness. This discovery, Nagel argues, will be of enormous magnitude and implication and one that may require a revolution in biology and most likely a complete transformation of scientific thought.

Despite Philosophical Cautions, Neurobiologists Have Adopted a Reductionist Approach to Consciousness

The aim of most neural scientists working on consciousness is more modest than that envisaged by Nagel. They are not necessarily working toward a revolution in scientific thought. Although neural scientists must struggle with the difficulties of defining consciousness experimentally, these difficulties do not appear to be totally forbidding. This optimism is due in part to the fact that neural scientists are not immediately concerned with the subjective and unitary nature of consciousness.

This attitude of most neural scientists is perhaps best expressed by the physicist Steven Weinberg: "I don't see how anyone but George will ever know how it feels to be George. On the other hand, I can readily believe that at least in principle we will be able to explain all of George's behavior reductively, including what he says about what he feels, and that consciousness will be one of the emergent higher-level concepts appearing in this equation."

Indeed, neural scientists have been able to make considerable progress in understanding the neurobiology of perception without having to account for individual experience. The philosopher Patricia Churchland reminds us that cognitive neural scientists have made progress in understanding the neural basis of perception of color without addressing whether each of us sees the same blue. Since considerable progress has been made in understanding color perception without having to account for its subjective qualities, or *qualia*, perhaps the question about qualia is itself not so meaningful within a neurobi-

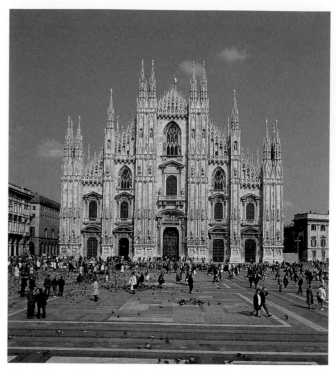

Figure 20-16 When patients with lesions of the right posterior parietal cortex were asked to recall from memory landmarks bordering the Piazza del Duomo in Milan, they were able to describe those on the right but neglected those on the left. The **blue** circles in the map on the opposite page represent landmark buildings recalled from **perspective A**, the point opposite Duomo; the **green** circles represent landmark buildings recalled from **perspective B** on the steps of the Duomo. (Based on Bisiach and Luzzatti 1978.)

ological approach to behavior. As we shall learn in later chapters, the brain does indeed *construct* our perception of an object, but the resulting perception is not *arbitrary* and appears to correspond to independently determined physical properties of the objects. What we do not understand is how action potentials give rise to meaning. Why is it that you see a *face* when the neurons of the inferotemporal cortex fire action potentials?

Although Churchland concedes that the subjectivity of consciousness makes the neurobiology of consciousness especially difficult, she does not believe the problem is in principle insurmountable. To begin with, although most simple percepts, such as the shape of an object felt in the hand, are subjective to some degree, the subjective quality of perception does not prevent a third person from objectively evaluating experimental data about what the perceiver actually is perceiving. Some characteristics of perception, even specific qualia, can therefore be correlated with the same patterns of neuronal activity in different subjects and under a variety of circumstances. If one can discern a detailed correlation

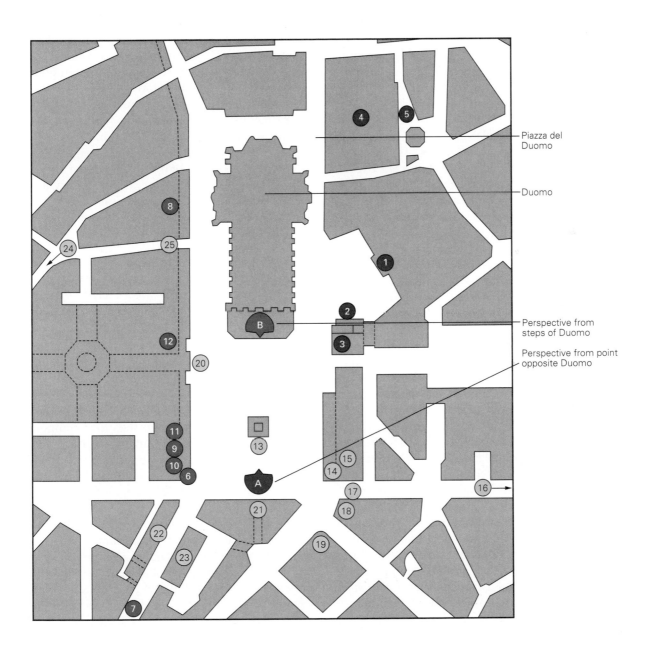

Piazza del
Duomo

Duomo

Perspective from
steps of Duomo

Perspective from point
opposite Duomo

between a particular neural event and a mental event, that description should be a sufficient first approximation of how neural events can give rise to a mental event by any reasonable standards of scientific explanation.

Thus the initial task is to focus on neural correlates of consciousness, by locating within the brain neurons whose activity correlates best with conscious experience, and to determine the neural circuits to which they belong. Having done that, we may be in a position eventually to meet Searle's and Nagel's higher demands: to develop a theory of the correlations we discover empirically in order to state the *laws of correlation* between neural phenomena and subjective experience.

The unitary nature of consciousness emphasized by Searle and Nagel may also not be an obstacle to fashioning a neurobiology of the mind. The unity of consciousness—our continuous and connected experience of events—must depend on the brain's ability to link discrete spatial or temporal events into a single experience. If that is so, is there a difference in principle between the sequencing of notes in a birdsong and the sequencing of words in a sentence? In each case the brain has a template of a unified sequence of utterances. If the neural representation of a sequence like a birdsong can be successfully analyzed, why should a sequence like a sentence be, in principle, less tractable to neurobiological analysis?

Finally, neurobiologists believe that consciousness has many forms, presumably mediated by a different neural system. For example, the *alert state*—the change that occurs when a person awakens or when a person who could not respond to commands becomes able to respond to commands—is thought to involve activation of the thalamus and cortex by neurons of the brain stem and its reticular formation. Alertness itself is thought to be a family of states that differ by degrees of alertness (heightened attention, indifference, inattention, sleepiness) and are influenced by mood (surprise, anger). As we shall learn in Chapter 45, variations in alertness may, in part, be mediated by the components of the major modulatory systems of the brain stem—the cholinergic, dopaminergic, serotonergic, and noradrenergic systems—acting on the thalamus and cerebral cortex. Finally, alertness can be general or focused, as when we selectively attend to one object in the external world to the exclusion of others.

We will likely gain a general understanding of the neurobiology of consciousness by studying these distinct states in their simplest form and by relating well-defined characteristics of one state to the cellular changes that parallel the state. Thus, rather than grapple with the broad concept of consciousness, neurobiology approaches the problem of consciousness by studying tractable, well-

defined components of consciousness, such as selective attention, to which we now turn. (See also Appendix D.)

Selective Attention Is a Testable Component of Consciousness

The phenomenon of selective attention is a particularly useful starting point for the scientific study of consciousness. At any given moment we are aware of only a small fraction of the sensory stimuli that impinge upon us. As we look out on the world we focus on specific objects or scenes that have particular interest and exclude others. Let us say you raise your eyes from this book to look at someone entering the room. Now you are no longer attending to the words on this page. Nor are you attending to the decor of the room or other people in the room. This selective focusing of the sensory apparatus on one element out of many is an essential feature of all sensory processing, as William James first noted in his *Principles of Psychology* (1890):

Millions of items . . . are present to my senses which never properly enter my experience. Why? Because they have no *interest* for me. *My experience is what I agree to attend to*. . . . Everyone knows what attention is. It is the taking possession by the mind, in clear and vivid form, of one out of what seem several simultaneously possible objects of trains of thought. Focalization, concentration of consciousness are of its essence. It implies withdrawal from some things in order to deal effectively with others.

Research on visual perception has shown that selective attention is actually a series of behaviors. For example, Michael Posner distinguishes four components of selective attention when an organism orients to a novel stimulus: (1) disengagement or release from the present focus of attention, (2) movement to a new location, (3) engagement at the new location, and usually (4) a sustained state of alertness.

Cellular studies of the posterior parietal cortex in monkeys have provided important insight into the neural mechanisms of selective attention. Like neurons in other visual areas, parietal neurons respond to the presence of a visual stimulus in the receptive field (see Chapter 27 for a description of visual receptive fields). A remarkable observation by Robert Wurtz, Michael Goldberg, and their colleagues indicates that the strength of this response depends on whether the animal is paying attention to the stimulus (Figure 20-17). When the animal's gaze is fixed away from the stimulus, there is a moderate response to the appearance of a visual stimulus. But when the monkey has to attend to the stimulus, the same retinal input elicits a much larger response. This enhancement is consistent with observa-

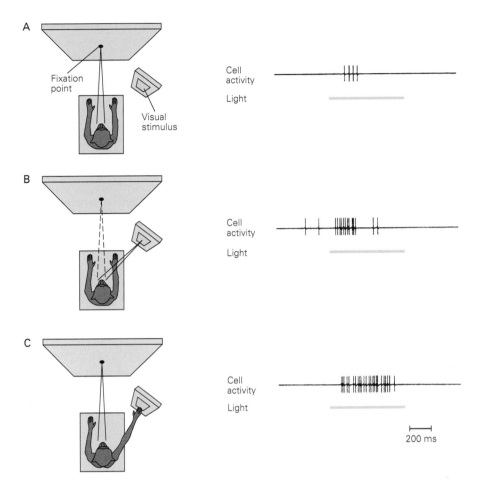

Figure 20-17 Neurons in the posterior parietal cortex of a monkey respond more effectively to a stimulus when the animal is attentive to the stimulus. (From Wurtz and Goldberg 1989.)

A. A spot of light elicits only a few action potentials in a cell when the animal's gaze is fixed away from the stimulus.

B. The same cell's activity is enhanced when the animal takes visual notice of the stimulus through saccadic eye movement.

C. The cell's activity is further enhanced when the monkey touches the spot but without moving his eyes.

tions that the parietal cortex contributes to selective attention to the location of objects in space. It occurs independently of the type of response the animal makes to the stimulus. The firing rate of the neuron increases by the same amount whether the animal merely looks at the stimulus or reaches toward it while looking elsewhere.

This independence indicates that the increase in firing rate is related specifically to attention rather than to the preparation of a motor response. However, the posterior parietal cortex does make connections with structures in the prefrontal cortex that are involved in the planning and execution of movements of the eyes and the hands. Studies by Richard Anderson indicate that one of the functions of selective attention is the intention to direct a movement of the hand or eye to a location.

Here we see a central issue in the study of cognition: how a percept leads to a voluntary act.

Selective attention enhances the responses of neurons in many brain areas. Neurons in the frontal cortex and superior colliculus, for example, discharge more briskly when the animal attends to the stimulus. Cells in the visual processing area of the temporal cortex also respond more strongly to attended objects. These effects of attention are evident throughout the visual system.

This type of evidence suggests that selective attention sharpens our sensory machinery, an obvious advantage in planning movement. Following up on this view, Francis Crick and Christof Koch have proposed that the attentional signals that modulate neurons in the visual system originate in the prefrontal cortex, the multimodal association area concerned with planning and motor strategies.

Neural scientists are thus beginning to address aspects of the fundamental question of consciousness by focusing on a specific, testable problem: What neural mechanisms are responsible for focusing visual attention? The solution to this specific problem, which is on the horizon, will most certainly enhance our understanding of sensory perception in general but may also contribute to the development of a biological theory of consciousness.

An Overall View

To come to grips with the biological processes of cognition we must move beyond the individual neuron and consider how information is processed in neural networks. This requires not only the methods and approaches of cellular and systems neuroscience but also the insights of cognitive psychology.

Studies of the sense of touch and its cortical representation in the anterior regions of the parietal lobe provide elementary examples of the internal representation of the body surface and of peripersonal space. This representation is not fixed, but can be modified by experience. Analysis of modifications of this representation in the posterior parietal association cortex indicates that attentiveness is a factor in integrating the representation of the body with vision and movement, an integration that allows a representation of personal space to be further integrated with a representation of extrapersonal space. Thus, the representation of the body becomes related to the representation of visual space, whether actual, imagined, or remembered, and it is within this integrated representation that the conscious self functions. It is therefore perhaps not surprising that the Russian neuropsychologist A. R. Luria suggested that portions of the parietal lobe constitute the most distinctly human aspects of cortical organization.

Eric R. Kandel

Selected Readings

Beaumont JG. 1983. *Introduction to Neuropsychology.* New York: Guilford.

Block N, Flanagan O, Güzeldere G (eds). 1997. *The Nature of Consciousness, Philosophical Debates.* Cambridge, MA: MIT Press.

Edelman GM. 1989. *The Remembered Present: A Biological Theory of Consciousness.* New York: Basic Books.

Feinberg TE, Farah M. 1997. *Behavioral Neurology and Neuropsychology.* New York: Mc Graw-Hill.

Farber IB, Churchland PS. 1995. Consciousness and the neurosciences: philosophical and theoretical issues. In: M Gazzaniga (ed). *The Cognitive Neurosciences,* pp. 1295–1306. Cambridge, MA: MIT Press.

Kolb B, Whishaw IQ. 1995. *Fundamentals of Human Neuropsychology,* 4th ed. New York: Freeman.

McCarthy RA, Warrington EK. 1990. *Cognitive Neuropsychology: A Clinical Introduction.* San Diego: Academic.

McGinn C. 1999. Can we ever understand consciousness? New York Review of Books XLVI:44–48.

Neisser U. 1967. *Cognitive Psychology.* Englewood Cliffs, NJ: Prentice-Hall.

Ramachandran VS, Blakeslee S. 1998. *Phantom in the Brain: Probing the Mysteries of the Human Mind.* New York: William Morrow.

Weiskrantz L. 1997. *Consciousness Lost and Found.* Oxford: Oxford Univ. Press.

References

Andersen RA. 1987. Inferior parietal lobule function in spatial perception and visuomotor integration. In: F Plum (ed). *Handbook of Physiology.* Sect. 1, *The Nervous System.* Vol. 5, *Higher Functions of the Brain,* Part 2, pp. 483–518. Bethesda, MD: American Physiological Society.

Bisiach E, Luzzatti C. 1978. Unilateral neglect of representational space. Cortex 14:129–133.

Bloom F, Lazerson A. 1988. *Brain, Mind and Behavior,* 2nd ed, p. 300. New York: W. H. Freeman.

Bushnell MC, Goldberg ME, Robinson DL. 1981. Behavioral enhancement of visual responses in monkey cerebral cortex. I. Modulation in posterior parietal cortex related to selective visual attention. J Neurophysiol 46:755–772.

Chomsky N. 1968. Language and the mind. Psychol Today 1(9):48–68.

Clark SA, Allard T, Jenkins WM, Merzenck MM. 1988. Receptive fields in the body surface map in adult cortex defined by temporally correlated inputs. Nature 332:444–445.

Corbetta M, Miezin FM, Shulman GL, Petersen SE. 1993. A PET study of visuospatial attention. J Neurosci 13:1202–1226.

Crick F, Koch C. 1990. Towards a neurobiological theory of consciousness. Semin Neurosci 2:263–275.

Darian-Smith I. 1982. Touch in primates. Annu Rev Psychol 33:155–194.

Dennett D. 1991. *Consciousness Explained.* Boston: Little Brown.

Fink GR, Halligan PW, Marshall JC, Frith CD, Frackowiak RS, Dolan RJ. 1996. Where in the brain does visual attention select the forest and the trees? Nature 382:626–628.

Gardner EP, Hamalainen HA, Palmer CI, Warren S. 1989. Touching the outside world: representation of motion and direction within primary somatosensory cortex. In: JS

Lund (ed). *Sensory Processing in the Mammalian Brain: Neural Substrates and Experimental Strategies*, pp. 49–66. New York: Oxford Univ. Press.

Hyvärinen J, Poranen A. 1978. Movement-sensitive and direction- and orientation-selective cutaneous receptive fields in the hand area of the post-central gyrus in monkeys. J Physiol (Lond) 283:523–537.

Jackson JH. 1915. On affections of speech from diseases of the brain. Brain 38:107–174.

James W. [1890] 1950. *The Principles of Psychology*. New York: Dover.

Jenkins WM, Merzenich MM, Ochs MT, Allard T, Guic-Robles E. 1990. Functional reorganization of primary somatosensory cortex in adult owl monkeys after behaviorally controlled tactile stimulation. J Neurophysiol 63:83–104.

Jung R. 1974. Neuropsychologie und Neurophysiologie Des Contour–und Farmsehens in Zeidineeng und Malerei. In: HH Wieck (ed). *Psycho-pathologie Musischer bestaltungen*, pp. 29–88. Stattgatt, Frt: Schaltauer.

Kaas JH, Nelson RJ, Sur M, Lin CS, Merzenich MM. 1979. Multiple representations of the body within the primary somatosensory cortex of primates. Science 204:521–523.

Kaas JH, Nelson RJ, Sur M, Merzenich MM. 1981. Organization of somatosensory cortex in primates. In: FO Schmitt, FG Worden, G Adelman, SG Dennis (eds). *The Organization of the Cerebral Cortex: Proceedings of a Neurosciences Research Program Colloquium*, pp. 237–261. Cambridge, MA: MIT Press.

Kolb B, Whishaw IQ. 1990. *Fundamentals of Human Neuropsychology*, 3rd ed. New York: Freeman.

Luria A. 1980. *Higher Cortical Functions in Man*. New York: Basic Books.

Marshall JC, Halligan PW. 1995. Seeing the forest but only half the trees? Nature 373:521–523.

Marshall WH, Woolsey CN, Bard P. 1941. Observations on cortical somatic sensory mechanisms of cat and monkey. J Neurophysiol 4:1–24.

McGinn C. 1997. Consciousness. In: *The Character of Mind*, 2nd ed, pp. 40–48. Oxford: Oxford Univ Press.

Mesulam M-M. 1985. *Principles of Behavioral Neurology*. Philadelphia: F.A. Davis.

Mogilner A, Grossman JA, Ribraly V, Joliot M, Volkmann J, Rappaport D, Beasley RW, Llinas RR. 1993. Somatosensory cortical plasticity in adult humans revealed by magneto-encephalography. Proc Natl Acad Sci U S A 9:3593–3597.

Mountcastle VB. 1984. Central nervous mechanisms in mechanoreceptive sensibility. In: I Darian-Smith (ed). *Handbook of Physiology*. Sect. 1, *The Nervous System*. Vol. 3, *Sensory Processes*, Part 2, pp. 789–878. Bethesda, MD: American Physiological Society.

Nagel T. 1993. What is the mind-brain problem? In: *Experimental and Theoretical Studies of Consciousness*, 174:1–13. New York: Wiley Interscience/CIBA Foundation.

Pandya DN, Seltzer B. 1982. Association areas of the cerebral cortex. Trends Neurosci 5:386–390.

Pavlov IP. 1927. *Conditioned Reflexes: An Investigation of the Physiological Activity of the Cerebral Cortex*. GV Anrep (transl). London: Oxford Univ. Press.

Pons TP, Garraghty PE, Friedman DP, Mishkin M. 1987. Physiological evidence for serial processing in somatosensory cortex. Science 237:417–420.

Posner MI, Dahaene S. 1994. Attentional networks. Trends Neurosci 17:75–79.

Ramachandran VS. 1993. Behavioral and magnetoencephalographic correlates of plasticity in the adult human brain. Proc Natl Acad Sci U S A 90:10413–10420.

Searle JR. 1993. The problem of consciousness. In: *Experimental and Theoretical Studies of Consciousness*, 174:61–80. New York: Wiley Interscience/CIBA Foundation.

Searle JR. 1998. How to study consciousness scientifically. In: Fuxe K, Grillner S, Hökfelt T, Olson L, Agnati LF (eds). *Towards an Understanding of Integrative Brain Function*, pp. 379–387. Amsterdam: Elsevier.

Shadlen M. 1997. Look but don't touch or vice versa. Nature 386:122–123.

Skinner BF. 1938. *The Behavior of Organisms: An Experimental Analysis*. New York: Appleton-Century.

Snyder LH, Batista AP, Andersen RA. 1997. Coding for intention in the posterior parietal cortex. Nature 386:167–170.

Thorndike EL. 1911. *Animal Intelligence: Experimental Studies*. New York: Macmillan.

Tolman EC. 1932. *Purposive Behavior in Animals and Men*. New York: Century.

Vallbo ÅB, Olsson KÅ, Westberg KG, Clark FJ. 1984. Microstimulation of single tactile afferents from the human hand. Sensory attributes related to unit type and properties of receptive fields. Brain 107:727–749.

Watson JB. 1930. *Behaviorism*. Chicago: Univ. Chicago Press.

Weinberg S. 1995. Reductionism redux. New York Review of Books. 42:39–42.

Wurtz RH, Goldberg ME, Robinson DL. 1982. Brain mechanisms of visual attention. Sci Am 246(6):124–135.

Part V

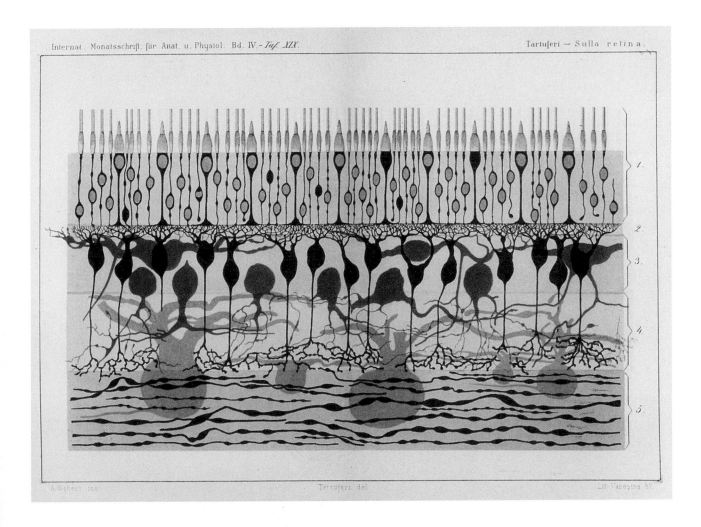

Internat. Monatsschrift für Anat. u. Physiol. Bd. IV.—Taf. XIX.   Tartuferi — Sulla retina.

A. Usheri inc.   Tartuferi del.   Lit. Varesina 87.

Preceding page

A schematic diagram of a radial section showing the various layers of the retina published in 1887 by Ferrucio Tartuferi. Tartuferi was Professor of Ophthalmology at the University of Messina in Sicily and was interested primarily in clinical eye diseases. This study, "Sull anatomia della retina" (International Monatsschrift Anatomie Physiolgie 4:421–441), appeared a year before Ramón y Cajal's first work on the retina. Courtesy of Robert Rodieck.

V   Perception

. . . one day in winter, on my return home, my mother, seeing that I
was cold, offered me some tea, a thing I did not ordinarily take. I declined at first, and then, for no particular reason, changed my mind.
She sent for one of these squat, plump little cakes called "petites
madeleines," which look as though they had been moulded in the
fluted valve of a scallop shell. And soon, mechanically, dispirited after a dreary day with the prospect of a dreary morrow, I raised to my
lips a spoonful of the tea in which I had soaked a morsel of the cake.
No sooner had the warm liquid mixed with the crumbs touched my
palate than a shudder ran through me and I stopped, intent upon the
extraordinary thing that was happening to me. An exquisite pleasure
had invaded my senses, something isolated, detached, with no suggestion of its origin. And at once the vicissitudes of life had become
indifferent to me, its disasters innocuous, its brevity illusory—this
new sensation having had on me the effect which love has of filling
me with a precious essence; or rather this essence was not in me, it
was me.*

HE TASTE OF THE MADELEINE dipped in tea is one of the most famous evocations of sensory experience in literature. Proust's
description of the conscious nature of sensation and memory
provides profound insights into some of the subjects that we shall explore in the next few chapters. His description of the shape of the pas-
tries on the plate, the feel of the cup in his hand, the warmth of the
tea, and the mingled flavors of tea and cake remind us that knowledge of the world comes through the senses.

Perceptions begin in receptor cells that are sensitive to one or another kind of stimuli. Most sensations are identified with a particular
type of stimulus. Thus, light of short wavelength falling on the eye is
seen as blue, and sugar on the tongue tastes sweet. How the quantitative aspects of physical stimuli correlate with the sensations they
evoke is the subject of psychophysics. Important additional information about perception can be obtained from studying the various sensory receptors and the stimuli to which they respond as well as the
major sensory pathways that carry information from these receptors
to the cerebral cortex. Specific neurons in the sensory system, both peripheral receptors and central cells, encode certain critical attributes
of sensations, such as location and intensity. Other attributes of sensation are encoded by the pattern of activity in a population of sensory

---

*Proust M. [1913] 1934. *Swann's Way*. CK Scott-Moncrieff (transl), p. 34. New York: Random
House.

neurons. Determining the extent to which receptor specificity and patterns of neural activity are used in different sensory systems to encode information is a major task of current research in sensory physiology. We know, for example, that taste depends greatly on receptor specificity. In contrast, the differentiation of sounds depends, in large part, on pattern coding.

Each sensory modality is mediated by a distinct neural system, and it is important to know what each component of a sensory system contributes to perception. Sensory pathways include neurons that link the receptors at the periphery with the spinal cord, brain stem, thalamus, and cerebral cortex. A touch on the hand is perceived when a touch receptor causes a population of afferent fibers to discharge action potentials, thus setting up a propagated response in the dorsal column nuclei of the thalamus and then in several areas in the cortex. An illusion of sensation in the hand, albeit a slightly blunted one, can be elicited by electrical stimulation of the cortical area that represents the hand.

In this part of the book we examine the principles essential for understanding how perception occurs in the brain. Contrary to our intuitive understanding based on personal experience, perceptions are not direct copies of the world around us. The brain is not a camera that passively records the external world; instead it constructs representations of external events based on its functional anatomy and the molecular dynamics of populations of nerve cells. Throughout each sensory system, from the peripheral receptors to the cerebral cortex, information about physical stimuli is edited in stages according to computational rules that reflect the functional properties of the neurons and their interconnections at each stage.

In the visual system, for example, there is now a fairly complete understanding of how photons are transduced by photoreceptors in the retina into electrical activity and how the retina processes this activity in parallel pathways. Since the central pathways have, at least in part, been delineated, we now have some insight into how visual information is processed at the cellular level along several parallel pathways.

Clearly, one of the major goals of cognitive neural science is to determine how the information that reaches the cortex by means of parallel afferent pathways is "bound" together to form a unified conscious perception. Indeed, one of the hopes driving cognitive neural science is that progress in understanding the binding problem will yield our first insights into the biological basis of attention and ultimately consciousness.

Part V

21

Coding of Sensory Information

SENSATION AND PERCEPTION provided the starting points for modern research into our mental processes. In the early nineteenth century the French philosopher Auguste Comte argued that the study of behavior should become a branch of the biological sciences and that the laws governing the mind should be derived from objective observation. Comte's new philosophy, which he called *positivism*, was influenced by the British empiricists John Locke, George Berkeley, and David Hume, who maintained that all knowledge is obtained through sensory experience—from what we see, hear, feel, taste, and smell. At birth, Locke proposed, the human mind is a *tabula rasa*, a blank slate upon which experience leaves its mark.

Let us then suppose the Mind to be, as we say, white Paper void of all Characters without any Ideas: How comes it to be furnished? Whence comes it by that vast store, which the busie and boundless Fancy of Man has painted on it with an almost endless variety? Whence has it all the materials of Reason and Knowledge? To this I answer, in one word, From *Experience*. In that all of our Knowledge is founded; and from that it ultimately derives itself.

It was this empiricist view that led to the emergence of psychology as a separate discipline apart from philosophy, which had long monopolized the study of the human mind. Thus, in its early days, psychology came to focus on the experimental study of mental processes by emphasizing sensation as the key to the mind. How does a stimulus lead to subjective experience? By what sequence of physiological events? For the fathers of experimental psychology—Ernst Weber, Gustav Fechner, Hermann Helmholtz, and Wilhelm Wundt—those were the central questions.

These researchers soon found that while the senses

differed in their modes of reception, all the senses shared three common steps: (1) a physical stimulus, (2) a set of events transforming the stimulus into nerve impulses, and (3) a response to this signal in the form of a perception or conscious experience of sensation. Their findings gave rise to the fields of psychophysics and sensory physiology. Psychophysics focused on the relationship between the physical characteristics of a stimulus and the attributes of the sensory experience. Sensory physiology examined the neural consequences of a stimulus—how the stimulus is transduced by sensory receptors and processed in the brain. Some of the most exciting advances in our understanding of perception have come from merging these two approaches in, for example, recent human experiments that use positron emission tomography (PET) and functional magnetic resonance imaging (fMRI) to scan brain function.

Early findings in psychophysics and sensory physiology, however, exposed one weakness in the empiricist argument: A newborn's mind is not blank, nor is our perceptual world formed simply from passive encounters with the physical properties of objects and stimuli. In fact, our perceptions differ qualitatively from the physical properties of stimuli because the nervous system extracts only *certain* pieces of information from each stimulus, while ignoring others, and then interprets this information in the context of the brain's intrinsic structure and previous experience. Thus we *receive* electromagnetic waves of different frequencies, but we *perceive* them as the colors red, blue, and green. We receive pressure waves from objects vibrating at different frequencies, but we hear sounds, words, and music. We encounter chemical compounds floating in the air or water, but we experience them as smells and tastes.

Colors, tones, smells, and tastes are mental creations constructed by the brain out of sensory experience. They do not exist, as such, outside the brain. Thus we can now answer the old riddle: Does a falling tree make a sound if no one is near enough to hear it? Sound, as we know it, occurs only when pressure waves from the falling tree are perceived by the brain of a living being.

Although our perceptions of the size, shape, and color of objects are derived entirely from patterns of light that strike our retinas, our perceptions nevertheless appear to correspond to the physical properties of objects. In most instances we can use our perceptions to manipulate an object and to predict aspects of its behavior. Perception, we can show, organizes an object's essential properties well enough to let us handle the object appropriately.

In short, our perceptions are not direct records of the world around us. Rather, they are constructed internally according to constraints imposed by the architecture of the nervous system and its functional abilities. The philosopher Immanuel Kant referred to these inherent brain properties as *a priori* knowledge. In Kant's view the mind was not the passive receiver of sense impressions envisaged by empiricists. Rather the human mind was built to conform with certain preexisting conditions, such as space, time, and causality. The existence of these ideals was *independent* of any physical stimuli coming from beyond the body. So knowledge, according to Kant, was based not simply on sensory experience but on the brain's properties that organize sensory experience.

As we shall see later, the dialectical tension between Kant's idealism and Comte's empirical positivism continues to reverberate in studies of perception. Kant's concept of a priori knowledge left its mark on *Gestalt psychology*, which holds that aspects of perception are the product of the brain's inborn capacity to order simple sensations in characteristic ways. Positivism, meanwhile, influenced *behaviorist psychology*, with its focus on the observable components of behavior—a person's motor response to the physical properties of a stimulus.

In this chapter we consider, in general, how a stimulus impinges on the body and how sensation leads to conscious awareness of events in our world. Specifically we shall consider how stimuli are transduced by sensory receptors and encoded into neural signals. While succeeding chapters will explore in detail the individual coding mechanisms for touch, pain, vision, hearing, balance, smell, and taste, here we shall emphasize the organizational principles that are universal to all sensory systems. Indeed, it is striking how sensory systems—not just in humans but in animals—rely on the same basic principles of information processing. The extent to which these features have been conserved in the course of evolution seems nothing short of astonishing.

Sensory Systems Mediate Four Attributes of a Stimulus That Can Be Correlated Quantitatively With a Sensation

The modern study of sensation began in the nineteenth century with the pioneering work of Weber and Fechner in sensory psychophysics. They discovered that despite the diversity of sensations we experience, all sensory systems convey four basic types of information when stimulated—modality, location, intensity, and timing. Together, these four elementary attributes of a stimulus yield sensation. The fact that all sensory systems convey the same type of information may be one reason why they have such similar organization.

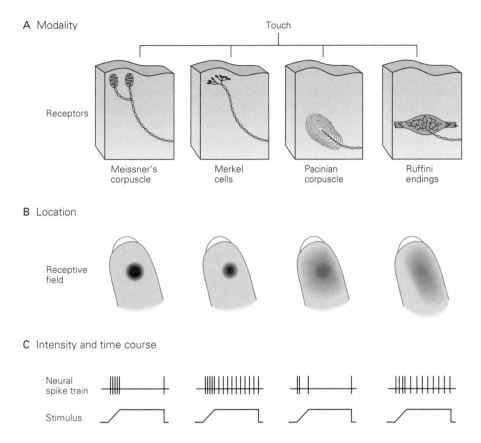

Figure 21-1 The sensory systems encode four elementary attributes of stimuli—modality, location, intensity, and timing—which are manifested in sensation. The four attributes of sensation are illustrated in this figure for the somatosensory modality of touch.

A. In the human hand the submodalities of touch are sensed by four types of mechanoreceptors. Specific tactile sensations occur when distinct types of receptors are activated. Firing of all four receptors produces the sensation of contact with an object. Selective activation of Merkel cells and Ruffini endings produces sensations of steady pressure on the skin above the receptor. When the same patterns of firing occur only in Meissner's and Pacinian corpuscles, the tingling sensation of vibration is perceived.

B. Location and other spatial properties of a stimulus are encoded by the spatial distribution of the population of activated receptors. Each receptor fires action potentials only when the skin close to its sensory terminals is touched, ie, when a stimulus impinges on the receptor's *receptive field* (see Figure 21-5). The receptive fields of mechanoreceptors—shown as **red** areas on the finger tip—differ in size and response to touch. Merkel cells and Meissner's corpuscles provide the most precise localization of touch, as they have the smallest receptive fields and are also more sensitive to pressure applied by a small probe.

C. The intensity of stimulation is signaled by the firing rates of individual receptors, and the duration of stimulation is signaled by the time course of firing. The spike trains below each finger indicate the action potentials evoked by pressure from a small probe at the center of the receptive field. Two of these receptors (Meissner's and Pacinian corpuscles) adapt rapidly to constant stimulation, while the other two adapt slowly (see Figure 21-8).

The four fundamental attributes of sensory experience are encoded within the nervous system by specialized subgroups of neurons. *Modality* defines a general class of stimulus, determined by the type of energy transmitted by the stimulus and the receptors specialized to sense that energy (Figure 21-1). Receptors, together with their central pathways and target areas in the brain, comprise a sensory system, and activity within a system gives rise to specific types of sensations such as touch, taste, vision, or hearing.

The *location* of the stimulus is represented by the set of sensory receptors within the sensory system that are active. Receptors are distributed topographically in a sense organ so that their activity signals not only the modality of the stimulus but also its position in space and its size. As a stimulus activates many receptors simulta-

Table 21-1 Sensory Systems and Modalities

Sensory system	Modality	Stimulus energy	Receptor class[1]	Receptor cell types[2]
Visual	Vision	Light	Photoreceptor	Rods, cones
Auditory	Hearing	Sound	Mechanoreceptor	Hair cells (cochlea)
Vestibular	Balance	Gravity	Mechanoreceptor	Hair cells (vestibular labyrinth)
Somatosensory	Somatic senses:			Dorsal root ganglion neurons
	Touch	Pressure	Mechanoreceptor	Cutaneous mechanoreceptors
	Proprioception	Displacement	Mechanoreceptor	Muscle and joint receptors
	Temperature sense	Thermal	Thermoreceptor	Cold and warm receptors
	Pain	Chemical, thermal, or mechanical	Chemoreceptor, thermoreceptor, or mechanoreceptor	Polymodal, thermal, and mechanical nociceptors
	Itch	Chemical	Chemoreceptor	Chemical nociceptor
Gustatory	Taste	Chemical	Chemoreceptor	Taste buds
Olfactory	Smell	Chemical	Chemoreceptor	Olfactory sensory neurons

[1]See Figures 21-2 and 21-3.

[2]Receptor cell types are further specialized, forming the cellular basis for submodalities. These cell types are described in the chapters on individual sensory systems.

neously, the distribution of the active population provides important information to the brain about sensation.

The *intensity* of the stimulus is signaled by the response amplitude of each receptor, which reflects the total amount of stimulus energy delivered to the receptor. The *timing* of stimulation is defined by when the response in the receptor starts and stops and is determined by how quickly the energy is received or lost by the receptor. Therefore, both the intensity and time course of stimulation are represented by the firing patterns of active sensory neurons.

Sensory Modality Is Determined by the Stimulus Energy

Since ancient times five major sensory modalities have been recognized: vision, hearing, touch, taste, and smell. In addition to these classical senses we also consider the somatic senses of pain, temperature, itch, and proprioception (posture and the movement of parts of the body) and the vestibular sense of balance (the position of the body in the gravitational field).

An early insight into the neuronal basis of sensation came in 1826, when Johannes Müller advanced his "laws of specific sense energies." Müller proposed that modality is a property of the sensory nerve fiber. Each nerve fiber is activated primarily by a certain type of stimulus and each makes specific connections to struc-

tures in the central nervous system whose activity gives rise to specific sensations. Thus Müller's laws of specific sense energies identified the most important mechanism for neural coding of stimulus modality.

Modality Is Encoded by a Labeled Line Code

In each sensory system the initial contact with the external world occurs through specialized neural structures called *sensory receptors*. The sensory receptor is the first cell in each sensory pathway and transforms stimulus energy into electrical energy, thus establishing a common signaling mechanism in all sensory systems. The electrical signal produced by the receptor is termed the *receptor potential*. The amplitude and duration of the receptor potential are related to the intensity and time course of stimulation of the particular receptor. The process by which specific stimulus energy is converted into an electrical signal is called *stimulus transduction*.

Receptors are morphologically specialized to transduce specific forms of energy. Each receptor has a specialized anatomical region where stimulus transduction occurs. Most sensory receptors are optimally selective for a single stimulus energy, a property termed *receptor specificity*. The unique stimulus that activates a specific receptor at a low energy level was called an *adequate stimulus* by Charles Sherrington.

The specificity of response in receptors underlies the *labeled line code,* the most important coding mecha-

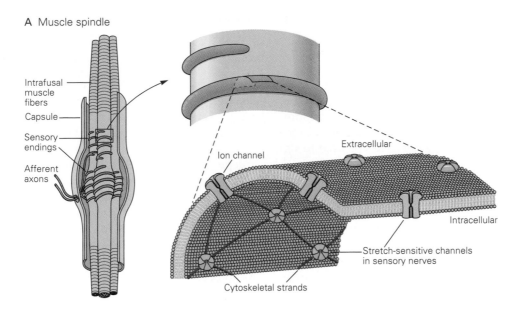

A Muscle spindle

Intrafusal muscle fibers

Capsule

Sensory endings

Afferent axons

Ion channel

Extracellular

Intracellular

Stretch-sensitive channels in sensory nerves

Cytoskeletal strands

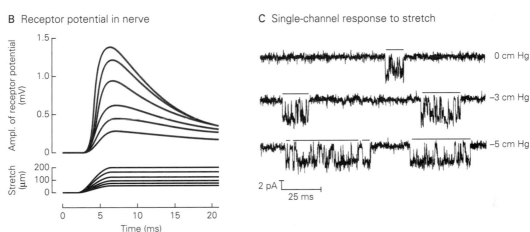

B Receptor potential in nerve

C Single-channel response to stretch

0 cm Hg

−3 cm Hg

−5 cm Hg

2 pA

25 ms

Figure 21-2 Mechanoreceptors are depolarized by stretch of the cell membrane and the depolarization is proportional to the stimulus amplitude.

A. The spindle organ in skeletal muscle mediates limb proprioception. These receptors signal muscle length and the speed at which the muscle is stretched. The receptor consists of a bundle of specialized (intrafusal) muscle fibers enclosed by a capsule. The sensory nerve endings respond to stretch of the muscle fibers. Stretch-sensitive ion channels in the nerve membrane are linked to the cytoskeleton by the protein spectrin. Mechanical deformation of the membrane opens these cation-selective channels. The influx of Na^+ and possibly Ca^{2+} depolarizes the nerve ending, producing the receptor potential. (Adapted from Sachs 1990.)

B. Response of an isolated muscle spindle to stretch. **Upper records** show the depolarizing receptor potentials recorded from the sensory axon when the muscle spindle is stretched to different lengths. **Lower records** show the amplitude and rate of stretch. Action potentials in this nerve have been blocked

with tetrodotoxin to allow analysis of the receptor potentials. The initial depolarization of the muscle spindle in response to change in muscle length (dynamic response) is proportional to both the rate and amplitude of stretch. When stretch is maintained at a fixed length, the receptor potential decays to a lower value proportional only to the amount of stretch (static response). (Adapted from Ottoson and Shepherd 1971.)

C. Patch clamp records of a single stretch-sensitive channel recorded from skeletal myocytes. Pressure is applied to the receptor cell membrane by suction. At rest (**top record**) the stretch-sensitive channel opens sporadically for short time intervals, producing a transient depolarizing current. As the pressure on the membrane is increased (**lower records**), the channel opens more often and remains in the open state for longer time intervals (indicated by the bar above the channel openings). Each channel opening increases the membrane conductance to cations. The increase in the probability of opening and open time produces longer and larger depolarizations. (Adapted from Sachs 1990.)

nism for stimulus modality. The fact that the receptor is selective for a particular type of stimulus energy means that the axon of the receptor functions as a modality-specific line of communication; activity in the axon necessarily conveys information about a particular type of stimulus. Excitation of a particular sensory neuron, whether naturally or artificially by direct electrical stimulation, elicits the same sensation. For example, electrical stimulation of the auditory nerve can be used to signal tones of different frequencies in patients with deafness caused by damage to receptors in the inner ear.

Each class of sensory receptors makes connections with distinctive structures in the central nervous system, at least in the early stages of information processing. Thus, sight or touch is experienced because a particular central nervous structure is activated. Modality is therefore represented by the ensemble of neurons connected to a specific class of receptors. Such ensembles of neurons are referred to as *sensory systems* and comprise the somatosensory system, visual system, auditory system, vestibular system, olfactory system, and gustatory system.

Receptors Transduce Specific Types of Energy Into an Electrical Signal

Humans have four classes of receptors, each of which is sensitive primarily to one form of physical energy—mechanical, chemical, thermal, or electromagnetic (Table 21-1). The mechanoreceptors of the somatosensory system mediate the sense of touch, proprioceptive sensations (muscle stretch or contraction), and the sense of joint position, whereas the mechanoreceptors of the inner ear mediate hearing and the sense of balance. Chemoreceptors are involved in the senses of pain, itch, taste, and smell. Thermoreceptors in the skin sense the body temperature and also the temperature of the ambient air and the objects that we touch. Humans possess only one type of receptor for electromagnetic energy: the photoreceptors in the retina.

The mechanisms for transducing stimulus energy into the receptor potential vary with the types of physical stimuli. Mechanoreceptors sense physical deformation of the tissue in which they reside. Mechanical pressure, such as pressure on the skin or stretch of muscles, is transduced into electrical energy by the physical impact of the stimulus on cation channels in the membrane that are linked to the cytoskeleton (Figure 21-2A). Mechanical stimulation deforms the receptor membrane, thus opening the stretch-sensitive channels and increasing ion conductances that depolarize the receptor (Figure 21-2B). The depolarizing receptor potential is therefore similar in mechanism to the excitatory postsynaptic

potential (see Chapter 10). The amplitude of the receptor potential is proportional to the stimulus intensity; by opening more ion channels for a longer time, strong pressure produces a greater depolarization than does weak pressure. Removal of the stimulus relieves mechanical stress on the receptor membrane and causes stretch-sensitive channels to close.

The mechanoreceptors of the inner ear demonstrate directional responses to mechanical stimulation. These receptors respond to bending of sensory cilia on their apical membrane. When the sensory hairs are deflected in one direction by a sound of the appropriate frequency, the receptor cell depolarizes, whereas deflection of the hairs in the opposite direction hyperpolarizes the receptor cell (Chapter 31).

Receptor potentials in chemoreceptors and photoreceptors are generated by intracellular second messengers activated when the stimulus agent binds to membrane receptors coupled to G proteins (Figure 21-3). The second messengers produce conductance changes locally or at remote sites. Chemoreceptors normally respond to the appropriate ligand with a depolarizing potential. Photoreceptors, by contrast, respond to light with hyperpolarization. As we have seen in Chapter 13, the great advantage of the second-messenger mechanism is that the sensory signal becomes amplified. A few quanta of light-activating photopigments, or a few odorant molecules binding to the receptor sites on olfactory neurons, can affect the conductance of many ionic channels in the receptor cell.

Each Receptor Responds to a Narrow Range of Stimulus Energy

Each of the major modalities has several constituent qualities or *submodalities*. For example, taste can be sweet, sour, salty, or bitter; objects that we see differ in color, shape, and movement; and touch has qualities of temperature, texture, and rigidity. Submodalities exist because each class of receptors—chemoreceptors, mechanoreceptors, thermoreceptors, and photoreceptors—is not homogenous. Instead, each class contains a variety of specialized receptors that respond to a limited range of stimulus energies.

The receptor behaves as a filter for a narrow range, or *bandwidth,* of energy. For example, individual photoreceptors are not sensitive to all wavelengths of light but to only a small part of the spectrum. We say that receptors are *tuned* to an adequate stimulus, the unique stimulus that activates a receptor at low energy. As a result, we can plot a tuning curve for each receptor based on physiological experiments. The tuning curve shows the receptor's range of sensitivity, including the preferred

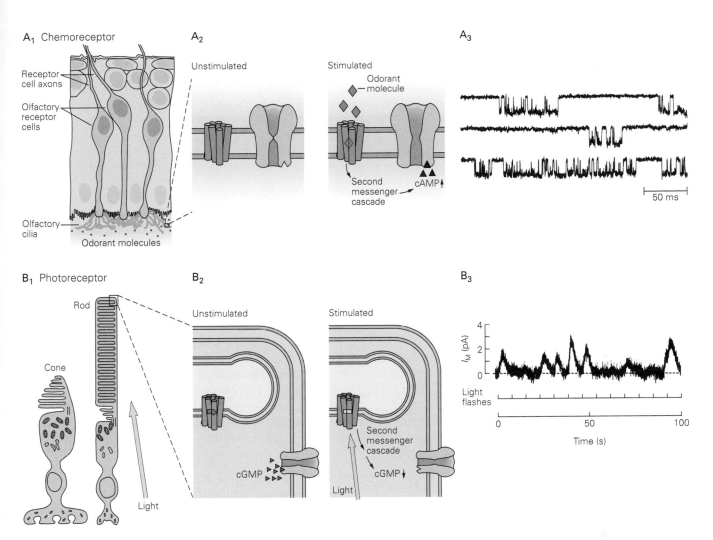

Figure 21-3 Transduction of stimulus energy into neural activity by chemoreceptors and photoreceptors requires intracellular second messengers. (Adapted from Shepherd 1994.)

A.1. The olfactory hair cell is a chemoreceptor that mediates the sense of smell. The olfactory cilia on the mucosal surface bind specific odorant molecules and depolarize the sensory nerve via a second-messenger system. The firing rate signals the concentration of odorant in the inspired air. **2.** Chemoelectric transduction is produced when the appropriate odorant binds to a receptor protein on the cell membrane, which activates G proteins linked to the receptor. Channel opening and depolarization in olfactory receptors and certain gustatory receptors are mediated by a second messenger (cAMP) stimu-

lated by G protein activation. **3.** Receptor currents evoked by the appropriate odorant. (Reproduced with permission from Maue and Dionne 1987).

B.1. Rod and cone photoreceptors are the sensory receptors of the retina. The outer segment of both receptors contains the photopigment rhodopsin, which changes configuration when it absorbs light. **2.** Stimulation of the chromophore by light reduces the concentration of cGMP in the cytoplasm. This hyperpolarizes the photoreceptor by closing cation channels, decreasing the transmitter released by the photoreceptor terminals in the inner segment. **3.** Receptor currents evoked by light flashes. (Reproduced with permission from Baylor et al. 1979.)

Figure 21-4 Tuning curves of sensory receptors measure the minimum amplitude of stimulation needed to activate a sensory receptor over a range of stimulus energies. Each sensory receptor responds optimally to a narrow range of intensities of a single type of energy. The tuning curve shown here is for an auditory receptor most sensitive to sound at 2.0 kHz. Higher and lower frequencies require stronger amplitude stimuli to evoke a response from the receptor. The tuning curve also illustrates the range of stimulus energies that can excite the receptor when presented at a given intensity. In this example, as the loudness of the tone rises, the receptor responds to a greater range of auditory frequencies. However, the receptor provides a stronger response at the preferred frequency than at other frequencies. Graded responses over the energy bandwidth provide a mechanism for sensory neurons to signal the particular type of stimulus energy that is presented. The auditory system tunes receptors in distinct parts of the sensory epithelium to different frequencies of sound. The relative response amplitude of these receptors to tones signals the sound frequency.

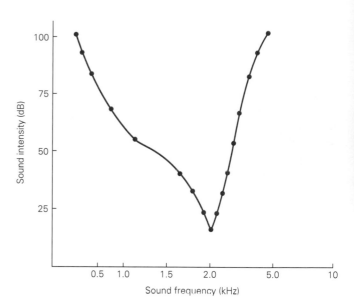

stimulus energy band at which it is activated by the smallest amplitude stimulus. At greater or lesser values, the stimulus intensity must be substantially increased to excite the receptor (Figure 21-4).

Under normal circumstances each sensory neuron is sensitive primarily to one type of stimulus. However, the sensitivity of a sensory nerve fiber to a particular type of stimulus is not absolute; if a stimulus is strong enough, it can activate several kinds of nerve fibers. For example, the retina is relatively insensitive to mechanical stimulation but very sensitive to light. Nevertheless, photoreceptors will respond to a blow to the eye, producing a perceptible flash of light (termed a phosphene). The mechanical stimulus produces a visual image because the receptor is connected to the visual centers of the central nervous system—an illustration of the principle that each sensory pathway conveys a specific modality.

The Spatial Distribution of Sensory Neurons Activated by a Stimulus Conveys Information About the Stimulus Location

The spatial arrangement of activated receptors within a sense organ conveys important information concerning the stimulus. In the modalities of somatic sensation and vision the spatial distribution of receptors conveys information about the location of the stimulus on the body or in the external world. In these modalities spatial awareness involves three distinct perceptual abilities: (1) locating the site of stimulation on the body or the stimulus source in space, (2) discriminating the size and shape of objects, and (3) resolving the fine detail of

the stimulus or environment. These spacial abilities are linked to the structure of the *receptive field* of each sensory neuron—that area within the receptive sheet where stimulation excites the cell. The position of the receptive field is an important factor in the perception of the location of a stimulus on the body.

The Receptive Fields of Sensory Neurons in the Somatosensory and Visual Systems Define the Spatial Resolution of a Stimulus

The receptive field of a sensory neuron in somatic sensation and vision assigns a specific topographic location to the sensory information. For example, the receptive field of a mechanoreceptor for touch is the region of skin directly innervated by the terminals of the receptor neuron and thus includes the entire area of skin through which a tactile stimulus can be conducted to reach the nerve terminals (Figure 21-5). The receptive field of a photoreceptor in the retina is the region of the visual field projected by the lens of the eye onto the portion of the retina in which the photoreceptor is located.

Each receptor responds only to stimulation within its receptive field. A stimulus that affects an area larger than the receptive field of one receptor will activate adjacent receptors. The size of a stimulus therefore influences the total number of receptors that are stimulated. A large object, such as a basketball, held between both hands will contact and activate more touch receptors than a pencil grasped between the thumb and index finger.

The density of receptors in a given part of the body determines how well the sensory system can resolve the detail of stimuli in that area. A dense population of re-

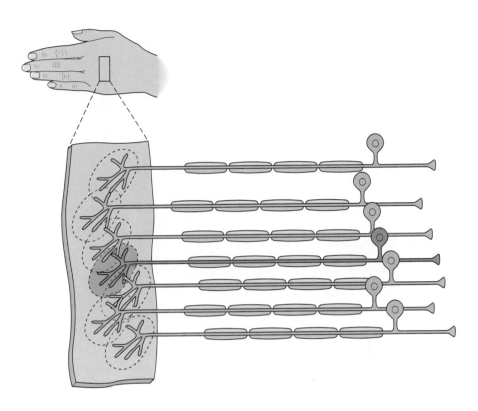

Figure 21-5 Structural basis of the receptive field of receptors for the sense of touch. The receptive field of a touch-sensitive neuron in the skin includes the sensory transduction apparatus in the nerve terminals and the surrounding skin in which the terminals are located. A patch of skin contains many overlapping receptive fields innervated by individual sensory nerve fibers. When this region is touched, spikes are initiated at the node of Ranvier closest to the nerve terminals in the skin. They are conducted past the cell body, located in the dorsal root ganglion, to the synaptic terminals in the spinal cord or medulla.

ceptors leads to finer resolution of spatial detail because the receptors have smaller receptive fields (Figure 21-6). The spatial resolution of a sensory system is not uniform throughout the receptor sheet, however. For example, spatial discrimination is very acute in the finger tips and the central retina (or *fovea*), where sensory receptors are plentiful and the receptive fields are small. In other regions, such as the trunk or the outer margins of the retina, the spatial information signaled by individual nerves is less precise because receptors in those areas are fewer and thus have larger receptive fields. These differences in receptor density are reflected in the central nervous system in the maps of the body created by the topographic arrangement of afferent inputs. In each map the most densely innervated regions of the body occupy the largest areas while sparsely innervated regions occupy smaller areas because of the smaller number of inputs.

The Sensory Neurons for Hearing, Taste, and Smell Are Spatially Organized According to Sensitivity

For hearing and the chemical senses (taste and smell), the receptors are spatially distributed following the energy spectrum for these modalities. For example, auditory receptors are arranged according to the sound frequencies to which they respond. Receptors at a specific location vibrate most strongly when stimulated by a particular range of sounds, with high frequencies located at the base of the cochlea and low frequencies at the apex. Thus the organization of the inner ear's receptor sheet represents the spectrum of sound, not the location of the sounds in space.

For taste and smell, receptors that have particular chemical sensitivities are located in different parts of the receptive surface of the tongue and inside the nose. For example, specific regions of the tongue contain receptors sensitive to salts, sugars, acids, bases, or proteins. Different foods will excite specific combinations of these receptors to evoke their characteristic tastes. The spatial distribution of activity in the chemoreceptor population allows the brain to differentiate salty from sweet or bitter tastes.

Intensity of Sensation Is Determined by the Stimulus Amplitude

Historically, the early scientific studies of the mind focused not on subjective perceptions of qualities such as color or taste but on phenomena that could be *measured* precisely: the size, shape, amplitude, velocity, and timing of stimuli. Psychophysics had its beginnings in the systematic study of the intensity of sensations produced by stimuli of defined magnitude.

Natural stimuli vary greatly in intensity. For example, we experience a range of sounds, from a whisper to a

A 400 receptors

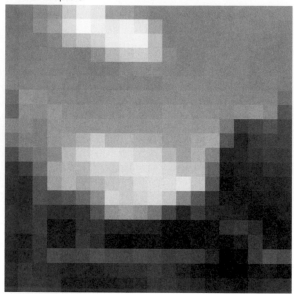

B 3,600 receptors

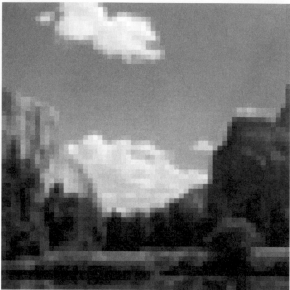

C 14,400 receptors

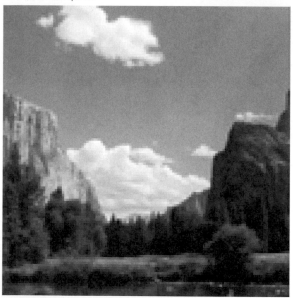

D 160,000 receptors

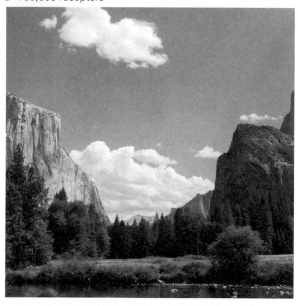

Figure 21-6 The density of sensory receptors in the retina and the size of the receptive field for each receptor determine the resolution of a visual image. Each square or pixel in these images represents a receptive field. The gray scale is proportional to the average light intensity in that region of the image. White pixels represent receptors with the highest firing rate, while black pixels represent receptors with the lowest firing rate. If there are a small number of receptors and each spans a large area of the scene, the result is a fuzzy, very schematic representation of the scene (**A**). There is no cue from this representation what the picture actually shows. As the density of receptors increases, and the size of the receptive field of each receptor decreases, the spatial detail becomes clearer (**B–D**). Clouds, mountains, trees, grasslands, and water emerge, until the scenery is identifiable as Yosemite val-

ley. However, the increased resolution comes at the cost of enlarging the total size of the receptor population.

The brain resolves the conflict between information overload from a huge number of receptors and the need for resolution of spatial detail by having a higher density of receptors in regions of the body where high resolution of detail is behaviorally important and using progressively lower numbers of receptors in surrounding regions. Spatial resolution for vision and touch parallels the density of receptors in the retina and skin. Spatial resolution on the fingertips approaches that of the image in **D**. Receptor density and tactile sensitivity on the palm is similar to the resolution in **C**. Resolution of spatial detail on the forearm approaches that in image **B**, while on the trunk it is similar to that in image **A**. (Photographs courtesy of Daniel Gardner.)

shout. The intensity or amount of a sensation depends on the strength of the stimulus. The capacity of sensory systems to extract information about the magnitude of the stimulus is important for two aspects of sensory discrimination: (1) distinguishing among stimuli that differ only in strength (as opposed to those that differ in modality or location) and (2) evaluating stimulus amplitude.

Psychophysical Laws Govern the Perception of Stimulus Intensity

The first psychophysicists—Weber, Fechner, Helmholz, and von Frey—developed simple experimental paradigms to compare how two stimuli of different amplitudes are distinguished. They quantitated the intensity of sensations in the form of mathematical laws that allowed them to predict the relationship between stimulus magnitude and sensory discrimination. For example, in 1834 Weber demonstrated that the sensitivity of the sensory system to differences depends on the absolute strength of the stimuli. We easily perceive that 1 kg is different from 2 kg, but it is difficult to distinguish 50 kg from 51 kg! Yet both sets differ by 1 kg! This relationship is expressed in the equation now known as Weber's law:

$$\Delta S = K \times S,$$

where ΔS is the minimal difference in strength between a reference stimulus S and a second stimulus that can be discriminated, and K is a constant. This is termed the *just noticeable difference* or difference limen. It follows that the difference in magnitude necessary to discriminate between a reference stimulus and a second stimulus increases with the strength of the reference stimulus.

Fechner extended Weber's law in 1860 to describe the relationship between the stimulus strength (S) and the intensity of the sensation (I) experienced by a subject:

$$I = K \log S/S_0,$$

where S_0 is the threshold amplitude of the stimulus and K is a constant. In 1953 Stanley Stevens noted that, over an extended range of stimulation, the intensity of a sensation is best described by a power function rather than by a logarithmic relationship.

$$I = K(S - S_0)^n.$$

For some sensory experiences, such as the sense of pressure on the hand, there is a linear relationship between the stimulus magnitude and the perceived intensity. This represents an example of a power function with a unity exponent (ie, $n = 1$).

The lowest stimulus strength a subject can detect is termed the *sensory threshold*. Thresholds are normally determined statistically by presenting a subject with a series of stimuli of random amplitude. The percentage of times the subject reports detecting the stimulus is plotted as a function of stimulus amplitude, forming a relation called the *psychometric function* (Box 21-1). By convention, threshold is defined as the stimulus amplitude detected in half of the trials. Thresholds can also be determined by the method of limits, in which the subject reports the intensity at which a progressively decreasing stimulus is no longer detectable or an increasing stimulus is detectable.

The measurement of sensory thresholds is a useful diagnostic technique for determining sensory function in individual modalities. Elevation of threshold may signal an abnormality in sensory receptors (such as loss of hair cells in the inner ear caused by aging or exposure to very loud noise), deficits in nerve conduction properties (as in multiple sclerosis), or a lesion in sensory processing areas of the brain. Sensory thresholds may also be altered as a result of emotional or psychological factors related to the conditions in which stimulus detection is measured (Box 21-1).

The sensory threshold for a modality is limited by the sensitivity of receptors. The threshold energy is related to the minimum stimulus amplitude that generates action potentials in a sensory nerve. We define thresholds in terms of action potentials because receptor potentials are local signals; they are propagated passively, as are synaptic potentials, and therefore are not transmitted over distances greater than 1 mm. To convey a sensory message to the brain, the stimulus information must be represented as a series of action potentials.

Stimulus Intensity Is Encoded by the Frequency of Action Potentials in Sensory Nerves

The quantitative features of sensory stimuli measured in psychophysical studies are signaled by the firing patterns of the activated population of sensory neurons. The details of neuronal activity—how long a neuron fires, how fast, and how many neurons are firing—encode the intensity and time course of sensory experience. In the 1920s Edgar Adrian and Yngve Zotterman first noted that the discharge frequency of an afferent fiber increases with increasing stimulus intensity. This is because the activity of sensory receptors changes in relation to the stimulus amplitude. The change in membrane potential produced by the sensory stimulus is transformed into a digital pulse code, in which the frequency of action potentials reflects the amplitude of the receptor potential. Strong stimuli evoke larger receptor potentials, which generate a greater number and a higher frequency of action potentials (Figure 21-8A).

Box 21-1 Sensory Thresholds Are Modified by Psychological and Pharmacological Factors

Sensory thresholds depend upon psychological factors and the context in which the stimulus occurs. The threshold for pain is often heightened during competitive sports or in childbirth, as reflected in a shift in the psychometric function to higher stimulus intensities (Figure 21-7B, curve c). Similarly, sensory thresholds can be lowered. Consider a runner at the starting line prepared to respond to the starter's shot. It is advantageous to respond as rapidly as possible, and the slightest noise resembling the start gun may trigger a leap to action. The runner's response to a lower stimulus intensity is represented as a shift in the psychometric function to lower stimulus intensities (Figure 21-7B, curve a).

The modifiability of sensory thresholds can be understood by considering two aspects of sensation: (1) the absolute detectability of the stimulus and (2) the criterion the subject uses to evaluate whether a stimulus is present. Detectability measures the capacity of a sensory system to process a stimulus, whereas the response criterion reflects an attitude or bias of the subject toward the sensory experience.

In the 1950s Wilson Tanner and John Swets developed the signal detection theory to explain the observation that subjects often report a sensory experience (ie, detection of a stimulus) when no stimulus is actually presented. A consequence of this decrease in response criterion (or bias) is that a subject is more likely to make mistakes. For example, the runner at the starting block is likely to make a false start in a crucial race. Similarly, elderly patients with sensory loss may falsely report feeling stimuli tested in a neurological examination as a denial of aging. The opposite condition—ignoring the occurrence of a stimulus such as pain—is also common.

The separate measures of stimulus detectability and response criterion can be combined with the concept of threshold to explain the mechanisms of drug action. For example, morphine, a potent analgesic, elevates the pain threshold both by reducing the detectability of a painful stimulus and by elevating the criterion the subject uses to determine whether a stimulus is painful or not. Marijuana also increases pain thresholds, but does so by increasing the response criterion rather than decreasing stimulus detectability—the stimulus is just as painful but the subject is more tolerant.

A

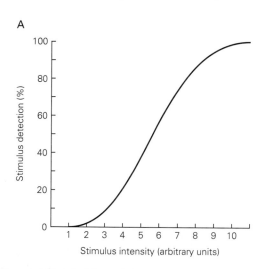

B

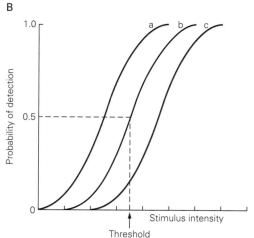

Figure 21-7 Sensory thresholds and the just noticeable difference (JND) between stimuli that differ in intensity, frequency, or other parametric features are quantifiable.

A. The psychometric function plots the percentage of stimuli detected by a human observer as a function of stimulus intensity. Threshold is defined as the stimulus intensity detected on 50% of the trials.

B. The absolute sensory threshold (curve b) is an idealized relationship between stimulus intensity and the probability of stimulus detection. If the sensory system's ability to detect the stimulus is increased or the subject's response criterion is decreased, curve a would be observed; curve c illustrates the converse.

A Neural code of stimulus magnitude

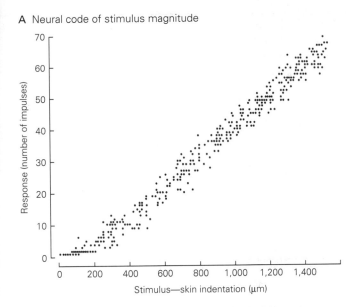

B Perceived sensation intensity

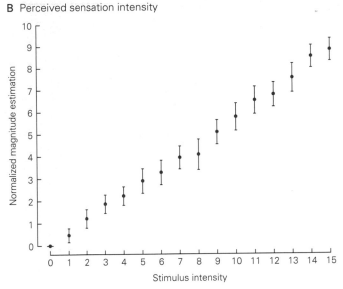

Figure 21-8 The firing rates of sensory nerves encode the stimulus magnitude. (Adapted from Mountcastle et al. 1966.)

A. The number of action potentials per second in a slowly adapting mechanoreceptor action the amount of skin indentation. This receptor required a minimum indentation of 80 μm to respond. The relationship between increases in frequency of firing and pressure on the skin is linear.

B. Estimates made by a human subject of the magnitude of

sensation produced by pressure on the hand increase linearly as a function of skin indentation. The relation between a subject's estimate of the intensity of the stimulus and its strength resembles the relation between the discharge frequency of a sensory neuron and the stimulus strength. These data suggest that the neural coding of stimulus intensity is faithfully transmitted from the peripheral receptors to the cortical centers that mediate sensation.

The translation of the receptor potential amplitude into a frequency code is similar to the process governing repetitive firing of neurons in response to synaptic potentials. The timing of action potentials following depolarization of a neuron depends on the neuron's threshold for firing, which in turn varies depending on the neuron's previous firing. Immediately after the action potential there is an absolute refractory period, lasting 0.8–1.0 ms, during which action potentials cannot be generated because Na^+ channels are inactivated. The upper limit on neuronal firing is about 1000–1200 spikes per second.

The nerve fires a second impulse when the amplitude of the receptor potential exceeds the neuronal threshold. Receptor potentials of small amplitude are only slightly larger than the resting threshold. Therefore, the second impulse is generated late in the refractory period or at its end, resulting in a long interval between the first and second spikes fired by the receptor's axon. However, a large-amplitude receptor potential produced by a strong stimulus allows the threshold to be reached earlier in the refractory period, reducing the time between impulses. Thus, a large depolarization produces a short interspike interval and high firing

rates, whereas a small depolarization results in long interspike intervals and low firing rates.

In addition to increasing the frequency of firing of individual sensory neurons, stronger stimuli also activate a greater number of receptors. Therefore, the intensity of a stimulus is also encoded in the size of the responding receptor population. These *population codes* depend on the fact that individual receptors in a sensory system differ in their sensory thresholds. Most sensory systems have at least two kinds of receptors: low- and high-threshold receptors. When the stimulus intensity is increasing from weak to strong, low-threshold receptors are first recruited, followed by high-threshold receptors.

The Duration of a Sensation Is Determined in Part by the Adaptation Rates of Receptors

The temporal properties of a stimulus are encoded as changes in the frequency of sensory neuron activity. Stimuli appear, rise in intensity, fluctuate or remain steady, and eventually disappear. Many receptors signal the rate at which the stimulus increases or decreases in

A   Slowly adapting receptor

B   Rapidly adapting receptor

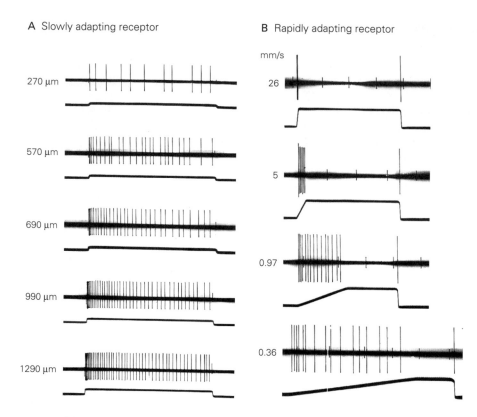

Figure 21-9 Measurements of firing rates quantify how sensory neurons represent the intensity of stimulation over time.

A. Slowly adapting mechanoreceptors respond throughout a continuous stimulus. Each successive trace illustrates the response to increases in the pressure applied to the skin; the trace below each spike record illustrates the amplitude and time course of the stimulus. As the pressure increases, the total number of action potentials discharged rises, leading to higher firing rates. The firing rate is higher at the beginning of skin contact than during steady pressure, as these receptors also sense how rapidly pressure is applied to the skin. When the probe is removed from the skin, the spike activity ceases. (Adapted from Mountcastle et al. 1966.)

B. Rapidly adapting mechanoreceptors respond only at the beginning and end of the stimulus, signaling the rate at which the stimulus is applied or removed. The slope of the pressure pulse indicates the speed of skin indentation in millimeters per second; all the stimuli have the same final amplitude. Slowly applied pressure evokes a long-lasting burst of low frequency firing; rapid indentation produces a very brief burst of high frequency firing. Motion of the probe against the skin is signaled by both the rate and duration of firing of this receptor. The receptor is silent when the indentation is maintained at a fixed amplitude and fires again when the probe is removed from the skin. (Adapted from Talbot et al. 1968.)

intensity by rapidly changing their firing rate. For example, when a probe touches the skin, the initial spike discharge is proportional to both the speed at which the skin is indented and the total amount of pressure (Figure 21-9A). During steady pressure the firing rate slows to a level proportional to skin indentation. Firing stops when the probe is retracted. Thus, neurons signal important properties of stimuli not only when they fire but also when they stop firing.

Although the continuous firing of a sensory neuron encodes the intensity of the stimulus, if the stimulus persists for several minutes without a change in posi-

tion or amplitude, its intensity diminishes and sensation is lost. This decrease is called *adaptation*. All sensory receptors adapt to constant stimulation. Receptor adaptation is thought to be an important neural basis of perceptual adaptation in which a constant stimulus fades from consciousness.

Receptors can adapt slowly or rapidly. Receptors that respond to prolonged and constant stimulation are designated *slowly adapting receptors*. These receptors are able to signal stimulus magnitude for several minutes. The stimulus duration is signaled by persistent depolarization and generation of action potentials throughout the period of stimulation (Figure 21-9A). These receptors adapt gradually to a stimulus as a result of slow inactivation of Na$^+$ or Ca^{2+} channels by the depolarizing receptor potential, or as a result of activation of calcium-dependent K$^+$ channels.

Some receptors *cease* firing in response to constant-amplitude stimulation and are active only when the stimulus intensity increases or decreases. These *rapidly adapting receptors* respond only at the beginning and end of a stimulus, signaling the rate or velocity of stimulation (Figure 21-9B). Adaptation of rapidly adapting receptors depends on two factors. First, in many of these receptors the prolonged depolarization of the receptor potential inactivates the spike generation mechanism in the axon. Second, the receptor structure filters the steady components of the stimulus by changing shape, thus decreasing the electrical signal generated by the receptor (Figure 21-10).

The existence of two kinds of receptors—rapidly and slowly adapting sensors—shows another important principle of sensory coding. Sensory systems detect *contrasts* in discrete stimuli, ie, changes in the pattern of stimulation in time and space. Rapidly adapting receptors sense the time derivatives of stimuli (velocity and acceleration) that signal motion. The firing rates of these receptors are proportional to the speed of motion; they stop firing when the stimulus comes to rest. Activation of rapidly adapting receptors at the beginning and end of stimulation conveys information about the changing sensory environment to the brain.

Many sensory receptors also sense spatial contrasts. In Chapters 22 and 25 we will learn that certain neurons mediating touch and vision are particularly sensitive to edges. These neurons fire much faster if the spatial properties of a stimulus in their receptive field change abruptly than if the stimulus has uniform spatial properties.

Sensory Systems Have a Common Plan

We have learned that the various sensory systems use similar neural codes for the properties of modality, location, intensity, and timing of physical stimuli. When a sensory neuron fires, it communicates to the brain that a certain form of energy has been received at a specific location in the sense organ. The details of the action potential code tell the brain how much energy was received at that place, when it began, when it stopped, and how quickly the energy changed in intensity. All sensory systems also have similar central processing mechanisms, which are briefly reviewed in this section and more fully described in later chapters.

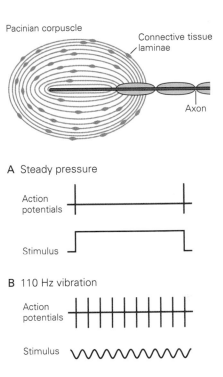

Figure 21-10 Receptor morphology influences adaptation in rapidly adapting mechanoreceptors. The Pacinian corpuscle is a rapidly adapting mechanoreceptor located in the skin, in joint capsules, and in the mesentary of the abdominal wall. The receptor consists of concentrically arranged, fluid-filled lamellae of connective tissue that form a capsule surrounding the sensory nerve terminal. Because of this capsule, the sensory endings specialize in the detection of motion.

A. The capsule of the Pacinian corpuscle deflects steady pressure. The receptor responds with one or two action potentials at the beginning and end of a pressure stimulus but is silent when the stimulus is constant in intensity. When a stimulus first impinges on the skin, the capsule is deformed, compressing the nerve terminal. The pressure pulse activates stretch-sensitive channels in the nerve terminal, producing the response to stimulus onset. During steady pressure the capsule changes shape, reducing stretch of the nerve membrane. The outer lamellae of the capsule are compressed, absorbing the static load and preventing the deformation from being transmitted to the inner core of the capsule and the nerve terminal. When the pressure is removed, the capsule resumes its initial shape, and the resultant tissue movement stimulates the nerve terminal again, producing an "off" response.

B. Pacinian corpuscles are sensitive to vibration. Rapid movements are transmitted through the lamellae to the nerve terminal, generating a receptor potential and action potential for each vibratory cycle.

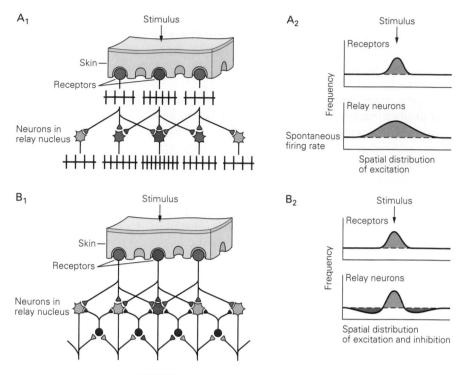

Figure 21-11 The functional and anatomical organization of sensory processing networks is hierarchical. Stimulation of a population of receptors initiates signals that are transmitted through a series of relay nuclei to higher centers in the brain (only one relay is shown). At each processing stage the signals are integrated into more complex sensory information. (Adapted from Dudel 1983.)

A. In the somatosensory system excitatory synaptic connections from each receptor in the skin are widely distributed to a large group of postsynaptic neurons at each relay nucleus. **1.** Each relay neuron receives sensory input from a large group of receptors and therefore has a bigger receptive field than any of the input neurons. **2.** Receptors closest to the stimulus respond more vigorously than distant receptors.

B.1. The addition of inhibitory interneurons (**gray**) narrows the discharge zone. **2.** On either side of the excitatory region the discharge rate is driven below the resting level by feedback inhibition.

Sensory Information Is Conveyed by Populations of Sensory Neurons Acting Together

The richness of sensory experience—the complexity of sounds in a Mahler symphony, the subtle layering of color and texture in views of the Grand Canyon, or the multiple flavors of a salsa—is obviously conveyed not by a single receptor or sensory axon but by populations of nerve fibers. The activity of whole populations of sensory neurons is orchestrated by the myriad of stimuli that typically impinge on receptors at once. The messages of individual sensors are integrated, not merely added up, as the signals converge on processing centers in the central nervous system. Understanding how sensory information conveyed by simultaneously activated receptors is processed in parallel pathways before it is combined in the highest centers of the cerebral cortex is key to understanding sensory perception.

Parallel processing is of particular importance in vision, where nearly all of the photoreceptors of the retina simultaneously receive light of varying hue and brightness. To make sense of a scene, the visual system needs to group the signals produced by individual objects, separate them, and distinguish objects of interest from the background. Thus in humans, of all sensory modalities, vision is the most highly developed; over half of the cortex processes visual information.

Specific submodalities, such as the color turquoise or the taste of a nectarine, depend upon the combined activity of populations of receptors sensitive to overlapping energy ranges rather than the unique firing of a single type of receptor. The subjective experience of a particular color or taste is constructed by the brain by integrating the inputs from these diverse receptors.

Sensory Systems Process Information in a Series of Relay Nuclei

The constituent pathways of sensory systems have a serial organization. Receptors project to first-order neurons in the central nervous system, which in turn project to second- and higher-order neurons. This sequence of connections gives rise to a distinct functional hierarchy. In the somatic sensory system, for example, primary afferent fibers converge onto second-order neurons, usually located in the central nervous system, and then onto third- and higher-order neurons (Figure 21-11).

The relay nuclei serve to preprocess sensory information and determine whether it is transmitted to the cortex. They filter out noise or sporadic activity in single fibers by transmitting only strong sequences of repetitive activity from individual sensory fibers or activity transmitted simultaneously by multiple receptors. The convergent connections from sensory receptors within the relay nucleus allow each of the higher-order neurons to interpret the sensory message in the context of activity in neighboring input channels.

Like receptor neurons, neurons in each sensory relay nucleus have a receptive field. The receptive field of each relay neuron is defined by the population of presynaptic cells that converge on it. The receptive fields of second-order and higher-order sensory neurons are larger and more complex than those of receptor neurons. They are larger because they receive convergent input from many hundreds of receptors, each with a slightly different but overlapping receptive field. They are more complex because they are sensitive to specific stimulus features, such as movement in a particular direction in the visual field.

Inhibitory Interneurons Within Each Relay Nucleus Help Sharpen Contrast Between Stimuli

Unlike the uniformly excitatory receptive field of the sensory receptor, the receptive field of higher-order sensory neurons in the visual and somatosensory systems usually has both excitatory and inhibitory regions. Inhibition is produced by inhibitory interneurons in the relay nuclei. The inhibitory region in a receptive field is an important way of enhancing the contrast between stimuli and thus gives the sensory systems additional power to resolve spatial detail.

Inhibitory interneurons are activated by three distinct pathways (Figure 21-12). The most important is the one in which the afferent fibers of receptors or lower-order relay neurons make connections with inhibitory interneurons which have connections with nearby projection neurons in the nucleus. This *feed-forward inhibition* by afferent fibers allows the most active afferents to reduce the output of adjacent, less active projection neurons. It permits what Sherrington called a singleness of action, a winner-take-all strategy, which ensures that only one of two or more competing responses is expressed.

The inhibitory interneurons can also be activated by the projection neurons in the relay nucleus through recurrent axon collaterals from the projection neurons. This *feedback inhibition* allows the most active output neurons to limit the activity of less active neurons. Such inhibitory networks create zones of contrasting activity within the

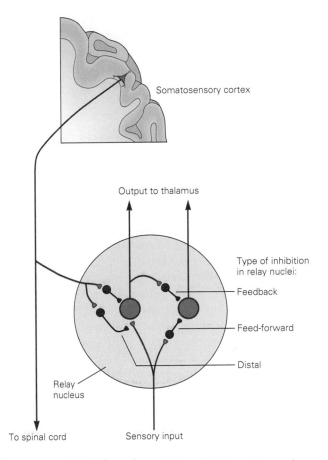

Figure 21-12 Inhibition of selected projection neurons in a sensory relay nucleus enhances the contrast between stimuli. The illustration shows three inhibitory pathways in the circuitry of the dorsal column nuclei, the first relay in the system for touch. The projection (or relay) cells (**brown**) send their axons to the thalamus. They receive excitatory input from touch receptor axons traveling in the dorsal columns. These afferent fibers also excite inhibitory interneurons (**gray**) that make *feed-forward* inhibitory connections onto adjacent projection cells. In addition, activity in the projection cells can inhibit surrounding cells by means of *feedback* connections. Finally, neurons in the cerebral cortex can modulate the firing of projection cells by *distal* inhibition of either the terminals of primary sensory neurons or the cell bodies of projection neurons.

central nervous system: a central zone of active neurons surrounded by a ring of less active neurons (Figure 21-11B). As we shall see, in the visual system these cellular interactions contribute to selective attention, by which we attend to one stimulus and not to another.

In addition to the local feed-forward and feedback circuits for inhibition in a relay nucleus, the inhibitory interneurons can be activated by neurons in more distant sites, such as the cerebral cortex. In this way higher brain centers can control the flow of information through relay nuclei. Unlike the local feed-forward and feedback mechanisms, inhibition from distant regions of the brain is not necessarily related to the intensity of the sensory-evoked responses.

An Overall View

Our sensory systems are the way in which we perceive the external world, remain alert, form a body image, and regulate our movements. Sensations occur when external stimuli interact with receptors. Sensory information is conveyed to the brain as trains of action potentials traveling along individual sensory neurons and by populations of such neurons acting together. All sensory systems respond to four elementary features of stimuli—modality, location, intensity, and duration. The diverse sensations we experience, the sensory modalities, reflect different forms of energy that are transduced by receptors into depolarizing or hyperpolarizing electrical signals called receptor potentials. Receptors specialized for particular forms of energy, and sensitive to particular ranges of the energy bandwidth, allow humans to sense many kinds of mechanical, thermal, chemical, and electromagnetic events. To maintain the specificity of each modality within the nervous system, receptor axons are segregated into discrete anatomical pathways and processing areas.

The location and spatial dimensions of a stimulus are conveyed topographically, through each activated receptor's position in the sensory epithelium, called its receptive field. The identity of the active sensory neurons therefore signals not only the modality of a stimulus, but also the place where it occurs. The intensity and duration of stimulation, meanwhile, are reflected by the amplitude and time course of the receptor potential and by the total number of receptors activated. In the brain, intensity is conveyed by an action potential code in which the frequency of firing is proportional to the strength of the stimulus. The temporal features of a stimulus, such as duration and changes in magnitude, are signaled by the dynamics of the spike train.

The complex qualities of sounds, visual images, shapes, textures, tastes, and odors require the activation of large ensembles of receptors acting in parallel, each one signaling a particular stimulus attribute. For us to savor the richness and diversity of perception, the central nervous system must integrate the activity of an entire sensory population.

Sensory information in the central nervous system is processed in stages, in the sequential relay nuclei of the spinal cord, brain stem, thalamus, and cerebral cortex. Each of these processing stations brings together sensory inputs from adjacent receptors and—using networks of inhibitory neurons—transforms the information to emphasize the strongest signals.

Esther P. Gardner
John H. Martin

Selected Readings

Bell J, Bolanowski S, Holmes MH. 1994. The structure and function of Pacinian corpuscles: a review. Progr Neurobiol 42:79–128.

Corey DP, Roper SD (eds). 1992. *Sensory Transduction: Society of General Physiologists, 45th Annual Symposium. Marine Biological Laboratory, Woods Hole, Massachusetts, 5–8 September 1991.* New York: Rockefeller Univ. Press.

Miller GA. 1962. *Psychology: The Science of Mental Life.* New York: Harper & Row.

Mountcastle VB. 1975. The view from within: pathways to the study of perception. Johns Hopkins Med J 136:109–131.

Mountcastle VB. 1980. Sensory receptors and neural encoding: introduction to sensory processes. In: VB Mountcastle (ed). *Medical Physiology,* 14th ed., 1:327–347. St. Louis: Mosby.

Perkel DH, Bullock TH. 1969. Neural coding. Neurosci Res Symp Summ 3:405-527.

Stevens SS. 1961. The psychophysics of sensory function. In: WA Rosenblith (ed). *Sensory Communication,* pp. 1–33. Cambridge, MA: MIT Press.

Stevens SS. 1975. *Psychophysics: Introduction to Its Perceptual, Neural, and Social Prospects.* New York: Wiley.

References

Adrian ED. 1928. *The Basis of Sensation: The Action of the Sense Organs.* London: Christophers.

Adrian ED, Zotterman Y. 1926. The impulses produced by sensory nerve-endings. Part 2. The response of a single end-organ. J Physiol (Lond) 61:151–171.

Andres KH, von Düring M. 1973. Morphology of cutaneous receptors. In: A Iggo (ed). *Handbook of Sensory Physiology.* Vol. 2, *Somatosensory System,* pp. 3–28. Berlin: Springer-Verlag.

Berkeley G. 1957. *A Treatise Concerning the Principles of Human Knowledge.* K Winkler (ed). Indianapolis: Bobbs-Merrill.

Boring EG. 1942. *Sensation and Perception in the History of Experimental Psychology.* New York: Appleton-Century.

Comte A. 1896. *Cours de philosophie positive* (The positive philosophy of Auguste Comte). H Martineau (transl). London: G. Bell & Sons.

Cowey A, Stoerig P. 1995. Blindsight in monkeys. Nature 373:247–249.

Dudel J. 1983. General sensory physiology. In: RF Schmidt, G Thews (eds), MA Biederman-Thorsen (transl). *Human Physiology*, pp. 177–192. Berlin: Springer

Fechner G. [1860] 1966. *Elements of Psychophysics*, Vol. 1. DH Howes, EG Boring (eds), HE Adler (transl). New York: Holt, Rinehart and Winston.

Helmholtz HLF. 1859. Über physikalische Ursuche der Harmonie und Disharmonie. Gesellsch Deutsch Naturf Aerzte Amtl Ber 34:157–159.

Hensel H. 1973. Cutaneous thermoreceptors. In: A Iggo (ed). *Handbook of Sensory Physiology*. Vol. 2, *Somatosensory System*, pp. 79–110. Berlin: Springer-Verlag.

Hudspeth AJ. 1989. How the ear's works work. Nature 341:397–404.

Hume D. 1984. *A Treatise of Human Nature*. EC Mossner (ed). London: Viking Penguin; New York: Penguin Books.

Humphrey NK, Weiskrantz L. 1967. Vision in monkeys after removal of the striate cortex. Nature 215:595–597.

Kant I. [1781/1787] 1961. *Critique of Pure Reason*. NK Smith (transl). London: Macmillan.

LaMotte RH, Mountcastle VB. 1975. Capacities of humans and monkeys to discriminate vibratory stimuli of different frequency and amplitude: a correlation between neural events and psychological measurements. J Neurophysiol 38:539–559.

Locke J. 1690. Chapter 1. In: *An Essay Concerning Human Understanding: In Four Books*, Book 2. London.

Loewenstein WR, Mendelson M. 1965. Components of receptor adaptation in a Pacinian corpuscle. J Physiol (Lond) 177:377–397.

Martin JH. 1996. *Neuroanatomy: Text and Atlas*, 2nd ed. Stamford, CT: Appleton & Lange.

Maue RA, Dionne VE. 1987. Patch-clamp studies of isolated mouse olfactory receptor neurons. J Gen Physiol 90:95–125.

Mountcastle VB, Talbot WH, Kornhuber HH. 1966. The neural transformation of mechanical stimuli delivered to the monkey's hand. In: AVS de Reuck, J Knight (eds). *Ciba Foundation Symposium: Touch, Heat and Pain*, pp. 325–351. London: Churchill.

Müller J. 1833–1840. *Handbuch der Physiologie des Menschen für Vorlesungen*. 2 vols. Coblenz: Hölscher.

Ottoson D, Shepherd GM. 1971. Transducer properties and integrative mechanisms in the frog's muscle spindle. In:

WR Loewenstein (ed). *Handbook of Sensory Physiology*. Vol. 1, *Principles of Receptor Physiology*, pp. 442–499. Berlin: Springer-Verlag.

Sachs F. 1990. Stretch-sensitive ion channels. Sem Neurosci 2:49–57.

Savage CW. 1970. *The Measurement of Sensation: A Critique of Perceptual Psychophysics*. Berkeley: Univ. California Press.

Shepherd GM. 1994. *Neurobiology*, 3rd ed. New York: Oxford Univ. Press.

Sherrington C. 1947. *The Integrative Action of the Nervous System*, 2nd ed. New Haven: Yale Univ. Press.

Somjen G. 1972. *Sensory Coding in the Mammalian Nervous System*. New York: Appleton-Century-Crofts.

Stevens SS. 1953. On the brightness of lights and the loudness of sounds. Science 118:576.

Talbot WH, Darian-Smith I, Kornhuber HH, Mountcastle VB. 1968. The sense of flutter-vibration: comparison of the human capacity with response patterns of mechanoreceptive afferents from the monkey hand. J Neurophysiol 31:301–334.

Tanner WP Jr, Swets JA. 1954. A decision-making theory of visual detection. Psychol Rev 61:401–409.

Vallbo ÅB. 1995. Single-afferent neurons and somatic sensation in humans. In: MS Gazzaniga (ed). *The Cognitive Neurosciences*, pp. 237–252. Cambridge, MA: MIT Press.

Vallbo ÅB, Hagbarth K-E, Torebjörk HE, Wallin BG. 1979. Somatosensory, proprioceptive, and sympathetic activity in human peripheral nerves. Physiol Rev 59:919–957.

von Frey M. 1894. Beiträge zur Physiologie des Schmerzsinns. Ber Kgl Sächs Ges Wiss Leipzig, pp. 185–196.

von Frey M. 1895. Beiträge zue Sinnesphysiologie der Haut. III. Ber Sächs Ges (Akad) Wiss 47:166–184.

Weber EH. 1846. Der Tastsinn und das Gemeingefühl. In: R Wagner (ed). *Handwörterbuch der Physiologie*, vol. 3, part 2, pp. 481–588, 709–728. Braunschweig: Vieweg.

Weiskrantz L. 1986. *Blindsight: A Case Study and Implications*. Oxford: Clarendon.

Weiskrantz L, Warrington EK, Sanders MD, Marshall J. 1974. Visual capacity in the hemianopic field following a restricted occipital ablation. Brain 97:709–728.

Wundt WM. 1893–1895. *Logik. Eine Untersuchung der Prinzipien der Erkenntnis under der Methoden Wissenschaftlicher Forschung*. Stuttgart: Enke.

Wundt WM. 1896. *Lectures on Human and Animal Psychology*. Translated from 2nd German ed. by JE Creighton, EB Titchener. London/New York: S Sonnenschein/ Macmillan.

22

The Bodily Senses

TUDY OF THE NEUROPHYSIOLOGICAL mechanisms of sensation began in 1925, when Edgar Adrian and Yngve Zotterman first recorded action potentials in a sensory nerve innervating the muscle spindle receptor. They discovered that the nerve transmits information from the receptor by modulation of the frequency of electrical impulses. Subsequently, Zotterman and other investigators clearly established the notion of specific nerve energies articulated by Johannes Müller in the early nineteenth century. This concept, as we have seen, states that morphologically distinct receptors transduce particular forms of energy and transmit this information to the brain through nerve fibers dedicated to that modality. Zotterman's studies demonstrated, for example, that pain is not the result of overstimulation of a generalized cutaneous receptor but results from electrical activity transmitted by specific sensory receptors called *nociceptors*.

We begin the study of the individual sensory systems with somatic sensation, the modality that was the subject of the first electrophysiological studies of sensation. Somatic sensibility arises from information provided by a variety of receptors distributed throughout the body. Somatic sensibility has four major modalities: *discriminative touch* (required to recognize the size, shape, and texture of objects and their movement across the skin), *proprioception* (the sense of static position and movement of the limbs and body), *nociception* (the signaling of tissue damage or chemical irritation, typically perceived as pain or itch), and *temperature sense* (warmth and cold).

Each of these modalities is mediated by a distinct system of receptors and pathways to the brain. However all share a common class of sensory neurons: the dorsal root ganglion neurons. Individual dorsal root ganglion neurons respond selectively to specific types of stimuli because of morphological and molecular specialization of their peripheral terminals.

In this chapter we describe in general the sensory response properties of dorsal root ganglion neurons that innervate the skin and mediate the senses of touch, temperature, pain, and itch. We consider how specialization of the nerve terminals allows these receptors to sense specific forms of energy. We will learn why some receptors sense light touch and others pressure, and why a painful stimulus, such as burning the skin, activates small-diameter sensory nerve fibers but not those neurons with thicker myelinated fibers that respond to light touch. In addition, we briefly consider nociceptors, proprioceptors, and visceral receptors, which are discussed in detail in later chapters when we consider, respectively, pain perception, voluntary movement, and the autonomic nervous system. Finally, we review the two major anatomical pathways that convey somatosensory information to the forebrain. Understanding the anatomy of these pathways is necessary to appreciate why certain lesions of the spinal cord may interrupt ipsilateral sensations of touch but not pain or temperature, while contralaterally producing the opposite deficits. In the next chapter, where we concentrate on touch, we will see how these afferent pathways convey somatosensory information to the cerebral cortex and how the cortex processes and integrates this information.

The Dorsal Root Ganglion Neuron Is the Sensory Receptor in the Somatic Sensory System

Irrespective of modality, all somatosensory information from the limbs and trunk is conveyed by dorsal root ganglion neurons. Somatosensory information from cranial structures (the face, lips, oral cavity, conjunctiva, and dura mater) is transmitted by the trigeminal sensory neurons, which are functionally and morphologically homologous to dorsal root ganglion neurons. As we have seen in Chapter 5, the dorsal root ganglion neuron is well suited to its two principal functions: (1) stimulus transduction and (2) transmission of encoded stimulus information to the central nervous system. The cell body lies in a ganglion on the dorsal root of a spinal nerve. The axon has two branches, one projecting to the periphery and one projecting to the central nervous system (Figure 22-1). The terminal of the peripheral branch of the axon is the only portion of the dorsal root ganglion cell that is sensitive to natural stimuli. The properties of the nerve terminal determine the sensory function of

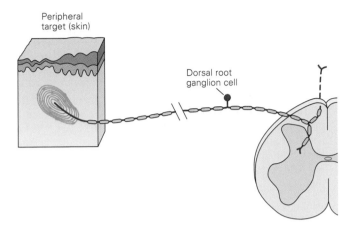

Figure 22-1 The morphology of a dorsal root ganglion cell. The cell body lies in a ganglion on the dorsal root of a spinal nerve. The axon has two branches, one projecting to the periphery, where its specialized terminal is sensitive to a particular form of stimulus energy, and one projecting to the central nervous system.

each dorsal root ganglion neuron. The remainder of the peripheral branch, together with the central branch, is called the *primary afferent fiber;* it transmits the encoded stimulus information to the spinal cord or brain stem.

The peripheral terminals of dorsal root ganglion neurons are of two types. The terminal may be a bare nerve ending or the nerve ending may be encapsulated by a nonneural structure (Figure 22-2). Dorsal root ganglion neurons with encapsulated terminals mediate the somatic modalities of touch and proprioception (Table 22-1). They sense stimuli that indent or otherwise physically deform the receptive surface. In contrast, dorsal root ganglion neurons with bare nerve endings mediate painful or thermal sensations. Mechanoreceptors and proprioceptors are innervated by dorsal root ganglion neurons with large-diameter, myelinated axons that conduct action potentials rapidly. Thermal receptors and nociceptors have small-diameter axons that are either unmyelinated or thinly myelinated; these nerves conduct impulses more slowly.

Neurologists distinguish between two classes of somatic sensation: epicritic and protopathic. *Epicritic sensations* involve fine aspects of touch and are mediated by encapsulated receptors. These sensations include the ability to (1) detect gentle contact of the skin and localize the position that is touched (*topognosis*); (2) discern vibration and determine its frequency and amplitude; (3) resolve by touch spatial detail, such as the texture of surfaces, and the spacing of two points touched simultaneously (two-point discrimination); and (4) recognize

Table 22-1 Receptor Types Active in Somatic Sensation

Receptor type	Fiber group[1]	Fiber name[1]	Modality
Cutaneous and subcutaneous mechanoreceptors			Touch
Meissner's corpuscle	Aα,β	RA	Stroking, fluttering
Merkel disk receptor	Aα,β	SAI	Pressure, texture
Pacinian corpuscle[2]	Aα,β	PC	Vibration
Ruffini ending	Aα,β	SAII	Skin stretch
Hair-tylotrich, hair-guard	Aα,β	G1, G2	Stroking, fluttering
Hair-down	Aδ	D	Light stroking
Field	Aα,β	F	Skin stretch
Thermal receptors			Temperature
Cool receptors	Aδ	III	Skin cooling (25°C)
Warm receptors	C	IV	Skin warming (41°C)
Heat nociceptors	Aδ	III	Hot temperatures (>45°C)
Cold nociceptors	C	IV	Cold temperatures (<5°C)
Nociceptors			Pain
Mechanical	Aδ	III	Sharp, pricking pain
Thermal-mechanical	Aδ	III	Burning pain
Thermal-mechanical	C	IV	Freezing pain
Polymodal	C	IV	Slow, burning pain
Muscle and skeletal mechanoreceptors			Limb proprioception
Muscle spindle primary	Aα	Ia	Muscle length and speed
Muscle spindle secondary	Aβ	II	Muscle stretch
Golgi tendon organ	Aα	Ib	Muscle contraction
Joint capsule mechanoreceptors	Aβ	II	Joint angle
Stretch-sensitive free endings	Aδ	III	Excess stretch or force

[1]See Table 22–2.

[2]Pacinian corpuscles are also located in the mesentery, between layers of muscle, and on interosseous membranes.

the shape of objects grasped in the hand (*stereognosis*). *Protopathic sensations* involve pain and temperature senses (as well as itch and tickle) and are mediated by receptors with bare nerve endings. Distinguishing between epicritic and protopathic sensation helps explain changes in sensation that take place following peripheral nerve damage. Protopathic sensations are considered to be cruder than epicritic sensations, in part because, more intense stimuli are needed to evoke pain. Nevertheless, the coding mechanisms for pain are very sensitive to the noxious or tissue-damaging aspects of the stimulus.

Touch Is Mediated by Mechanoreceptors in the Skin

Tactile sensitivity is greatest on the hairless (*glabrous*) skin on the fingers, the palmar surface of the hand, the sole of the foot, and the lips. Glabrous skin is characterized by a regular array of ridges formed by folds of the epidermis. The ridges are arranged in circular patterns called *fingerprints* and contain a dense matrix of mechanoreceptors. These receptors mediate the sense of touch; they are excited by indentation of the skin or by motion across its surface. When an object presses against the hand, the skin conforms to its contours. The depth of indentation depends on the force exerted by the object on the skin as well as its geometry. All mechanoreceptors sense these changes in skin contour but differ morphologically in important ways that affect their physiological function (Figure 22-2).

Mechanoreceptors Differ in Morphology and Skin Location

Virtually all mechanoreceptors have specialized end organs surrounding the nerve terminal. Although the sensitivity of these receptors to mechanical displacement is a property of the nerve terminal membrane, their dynamic response to stimulation is shaped by the specialized capsule. These nonneural structures must be de-

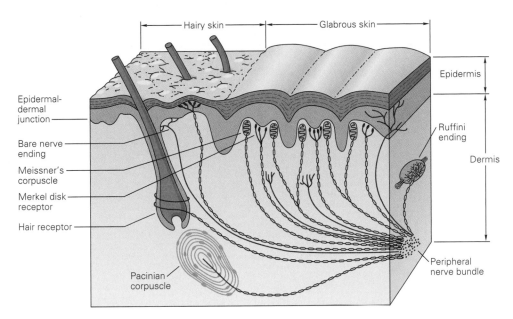

Figure 22-2 The location and morphology of mechano-receptors in hairy and hairless (glabrous) skin of the human hand. Receptors are located in the superficial skin, at the junction of the dermis and epidermis, and more deeply in the dermis and subcutaneous tissue. The receptors of the glabrous skin are Meissner's corpuscles, located in the dermal papillae; Merkel disk receptors, located between the dermal papillae; and bare nerve endings. The receptors of the hairy skin are hair receptors, Merkel's receptors (having a slightly different orga- nization than their counterparts in the glabrous skin), and bare nerve endings. Subcutaneous receptors, beneath both glabrous and hairy skin, include Pacinian corpuscles and Ruffini endings. Nerve fibers that terminate in the superficial layers of the skin are branched at their distal terminals, innervating several nearby receptor organs; nerve fibers in the subcutaneous layer innervate only a single receptor organ. The structure of the receptor organ determines its physiological function.

formed in particular ways in order to excite the sensory nerve. Histological and physiological studies have identified four major types of mechanoreceptors in glabrous skin. Two of these receptors are located in the superficial layers of the skin, and two are situated in the subcutaneous tissue (see Figure 22-2). The small superficial receptors sense deformation of the papillary ridges in which they reside. The larger subcutaneous receptors sense deformation of a wider area of skin that extends beyond the overlying ridges.

The two principal mechanoreceptors in the superficial layers of the skin are the Meissner's corpuscle and the Merkel disk receptor. The *Meissner's corpuscle*, a rapidly adapting receptor, is coupled mechanically to the edge of the papillary ridge, a relationship that confers fine mechanical sensitivity. The receptor is a globular, fluid-filled structure that encloses a stack of flattened epithelial cells; the sensory nerve terminal is entwined between the various layers of the corpuscle. The *Merkel disk* receptor, a slowly adapting receptor, is a small epithelial cell that surrounds the nerve terminal. The Merkel cell encloses a semirigid structure that transmits compressing strain from the skin to the sen- sory nerve ending, evoking sustained, slowly adapting responses. Merkel disk receptors are normally found in clusters at the center of the papillary ridge.

The two mechanoreceptors found in the deep subcutaneous tissue are the Pacinian corpuscle and the Ruffini ending. These receptors are much larger than the Merkel cells and Meissner's corpuscles, and less numerous. The *Pacinian corpuscle* is physiologically similar to the Meissner's corpuscle. It responds to rapid indentation of the skin but not to steady pressure because of the connective tissue lamellae that surround the nerve ending (see Figure 21-10). The large capsule of this receptor is flexibly attached to the skin, allowing the receptor to sense vibration occurring several centimeters away. These receptors are activated selectively by the common neurological test of touching a tuning fork (oscillating at 200–300 Hz) to the skin or bony prominence. *Ruffini endings* are slowly adapting receptors that link the subcutaneous tissue to folds in the skin at the joints and in the palm or to the fingernails. These receptors sense stretch of the skin or bending of the fingernails as these stimuli compress the nerve endings. Mechanical information sensed by Ruffini endings contributes to our perception

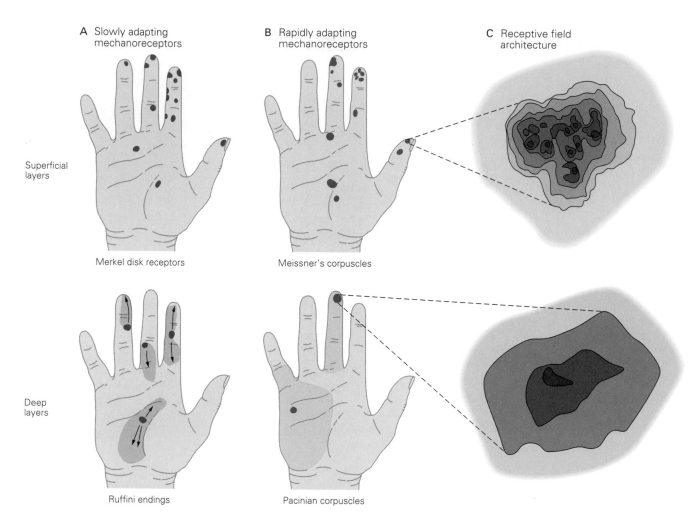

Figure 22-3 Mechanoreceptors in glabrous skin vary in the size and structure of their receptive fields. Each colored area on the hands indicates the receptive field of a different sensory nerve fiber in the human median nerve. (Adapted from Johansson and Vallbo 1983.)

A. The Merkel disk receptor in the superficial skin and the subcutaneous Ruffini ending are slowly adapting receptors (see Figure 21-9A). The Merkel disk receptor has a small, highly localized receptive field, whereas the Ruffini ending has a large field (**light purple**) with a central zone of maximal sensitivity (**dark purple**). Depending on their location, individual Ruffini endings are excited by stretch of the skin in specific directions as indicated by arrows.

B. The Meissner's corpuscle in the superficial skin and the subcutaneous Pacinian corpuscle are rapidly adapting receptors (see

Figure 21-9B). Meissner's corpuscles on the fingertips have receptive fields averaging 2–3 mm in diameter, while receptive fields on the palm average 10 mm in diameter. The receptive fields of Pacinian corpuscles cover larger continuous surfaces on the fingers or palm (**light pink**) but have a central zone of maximal sensitivity located directly above the receptor (**red**).

C. Expanded view of the receptive fields of mechanoreceptors in the superficial and deep layers of glabrous skin. The relative sensitivity to pressure is shown as a contour map in which the most sensitive regions are indicated in **red** and the least sensitive areas in **pale pink**. Receptive fields in the superficial layers of the skin have many points of high sensitivity, marking the positions of the Meissner's corpuscles or Merkel disk receptors. Receptive fields in the deep layers have a single point of maximal sensitivity overlying the Pacinian or Ruffini receptor.

of the shape of grasped objects. The anatomical arrangement of mechanoreceptors in glabrous skin is shown in Figure 22-2.

Similar mechanoreceptors are found in the hairy skin that covers most of the body surface. The principal rapidly adapting mechanoreceptors of the hairy skin are

the hair follicle receptor and the field receptor. Hair follicle receptors respond to hair displacement. The three separate classes of these receptors (down, guard, and tylotrich hairs) differ in sensitivity to hair movement and conduction velocity (see Table 22-1). Field receptors are located primarily over the joints of the fingers, wrist,

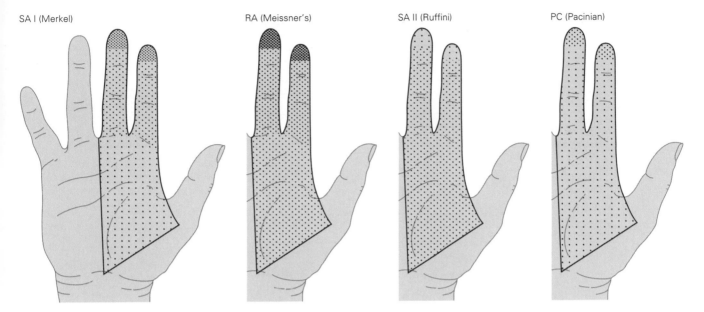

Figure 22-4 The distribution of receptor types in the human hand varies. The number of sensory nerve fibers innervating an area is indicated by the stippling density, with the highest density of receptors shown by the heaviest stippling. (**RA** = rapidly adapting, **SA** = slowly adapting.) Meissner's corpuscles (RA) and Merkel disk receptors (SA I) are the most numerous receptors; they are distributed preferentially on the distal half of the fingertip. Pacinian corpuscles (PC) and Ruffini endings (SA II) are much less common; they are distributed more uniformly on the hand, showing little differentiation of the distal and proximal regions. The fingertips are the most densely innervated region of skin in the human body, receiving approximately 300 mechanoreceptive nerve fibers per square centimeter. The number of mechanoreceptive fibers is reduced to 120/cm^2 in the proximal phalanges, and to 50/cm^2 in the palm. (Adapted from Vallbo and Johansson 1978.)

and elbow. They sense skin stretch when the joint is flexed or when the skin is rubbed.

Mechanoreceptors in the Superficial and Deep Layers of Skin Have Different Receptive Fields

Each individual dorsal root ganglion neuron conveys sensory information from a limited area of skin determined by the location of its receptive endings. As we saw in Chapter 21, the region of skin from which a sensory neuron is excited is called its receptive field.

The size and structure of receptive fields differ for receptors in the superficial and deep layers of the skin. A single dorsal root ganglion cell innervating the superficial layers receives input from a cluster of 10–25 Meissner's corpuscles or Merkel disk receptors. The afferent fiber has a receptive field that spans a small circular area with a diameter ranging from 2 to 10 mm (Figure 22-3). These receptive fields are at least an order of magnitude greater in diameter than that of an individual receptor. Therefore, nerve fibers innervating the superficial layers of the skin sample the activity of many different sensory receptors of one particular sort. In contrast, each nerve fiber innervating the deep layers of skin innervates a

single Pacinian corpuscle or Ruffini ending. Consequently, the receptive fields of these receptors cover large areas of skin, and their borders are indistinct (Figure 22-3). Usually, these receptive fields have a single "hot spot" where sensitivity to touch is greatest; this point is located directly above the receptor. The large receptive fields result from the ability of these receptors to sense mechanical displacement at some distance from the end organ.

The difference in size of the receptive fields of receptors in the superficial and deep layers of the skin plays an important role in the functions of the receptors. Meissner's corpuscle and Merkel disk receptors in the superficial layers resolve fine spatial differences because they transmit information from a restricted area of skin. As these receptors are smaller in diameter than the fingerprint ridges of glabrous skin, individual receptors can be stimulated by very small bumps on a surface. This very fine spatial resolution allows humans to perform fine tactile discrimination of surface texture and to read Braille. Pacinian corpuscles and Ruffini endings in the deep layers resolve only coarse spatial differences. They are poorly suited for accurate spatial localization or for resolution of fine spatial detail. Mechanoreceptors

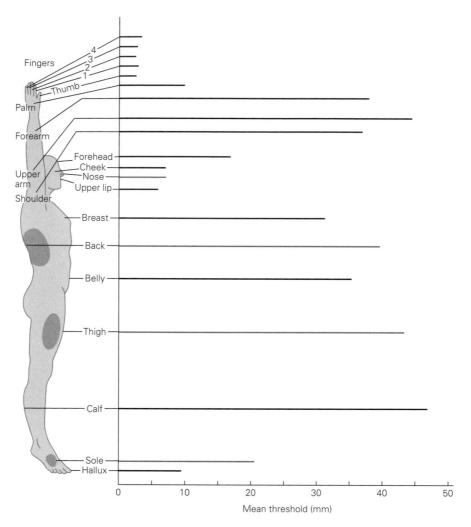

Figure 22-5 Two-point discrimination varies throughout the body surface. The two-point threshold measures the minimum distance at which two stimuli are resolved as distinct. At smaller separations the stimuli are blurred into a single continuous sensation spanning the distance between the points. Two-point thresholds are measured clinically using a calibrated compass in which the separation of the tips is accurately scaled. Two-point thresholds can also be determined from measurements of the ability of subjects to discriminate the orientation of grating ridges as a function of their spacing. This method measures spatial acuity more accurately. The two-point threshold varies for different body regions; it is about 2 mm on the finger tip but increases to 10 mm on the palm and 40 mm on the arm. The two-point thresholds highlighted in **pink** match the diameter of the corresponding receptive fields shown in pink on the body. The greatest discriminative capacity is afforded in the finger tips, lips, and tongue, which have the smallest receptive fields. (Adapted from Weinstein 1968.)

in the deep layers of the skin sense more global properties of objects and detect displacements from a wide area of skin.

The Spatial Resolution of Stimuli on the Skin Varies Throughout the Body Because the Density of Mechanoreceptors Varies

In addition to the differences in spatial resolution between receptor classes due to differences in receptive field size,

the skin area enclosed within receptive fields varies throughout the body. The smallest receptive fields are found on the tips of the fingers. Receptive fields are slightly larger on the proximal phalanges and even bigger on the palm. The receptive fields on hairy skin also increase in area as stimuli are moved proximally from the wrist to the trunk. These variations in receptive field size reflect the density of mechanoreceptors in the different regions of skin. Although individual dorsal root ganglion neurons innervate approximately the same number of sensory recep-

Box 22-1   Vibration Sense Is Coded by Spike Trains in Mechanoreceptors in the Skin

Vibration is the sensation produced by sinusoidal oscillation of objects placed against the skin. Vibration may be produced by the hum of an electric motor, the strings of a musical instrument, or a tuning fork used in the neurological examination. Mechanoreceptors in the skin respond to these oscillations by a pulse code in which each action potential signals one cycle of the sinusoidal wave (Figure 22-6A). The vibratory frequency is signaled by the frequency of action potentials fired by the sensory nerves.

Individual mechanoreceptors differ in their threshold sensitivity to vibration (Figure 22-6B). Merkel disk receptors are most responsive to extremely low frequencies (5–15 Hz); Meissner's corpuscles are most sensitive to midrange stimuli (20–50 Hz). The Pacinian corpuscles have the lowest thresholds for high frequencies (60–400 Hz); at 250 Hz they detect vibrations as small as 1 μm but at 30 Hz require stimuli with much larger amplitudes.

The receptor tuning thresholds determine the ability to sense vibration. Humans are most sensitive to vibration at frequencies of 200–250 Hz. To be felt, lower and higher frequencies must have proportionately larger amplitude vibrations.

The perception of vibration as a series of repeating events results from the fact that the receptors under the probe are activated synchronously and therefore fire action potentials simultaneously. The intensity of vibration is signaled by the total number of sensory nerve fibers that are active rather than the frequency of firing, which codes the vibratory frequency. If a patient is tested with a 250 Hz vibration near sensory threshold, only Pacinian corpuscles right under the contact point in the skin are activated. As the vibratory amplitude is increased, more distant Pacinian corpuscles as well as Meissner's corpuscles under the vibrator become activated. The total number of active sensory nerves is linearly related to the amplitude of vibration.

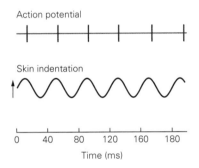

Figure 22-6A A rapidly adapting mechanoreceptor responds to sinusoidal mechanical stimuli with a single action potential for each cycle. The record here is for a receptor stimulated with a 25 Hz vibratory stimulus; the firing frequency of the receptor is 25 action potentials per second. The lowest stimulus intensity that evokes one action potential per cycle of the sinusoidal stimulus is called the receptor's "tuning threshold." (Adapted from Talbot et al. 1968.)

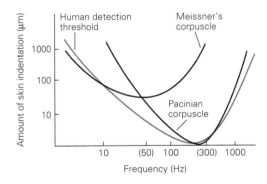

Figure 22-6B The threshold for detecting vibration corresponds to the tuning threshold of the mechanoreceptor. The sensitivity threshold for Meissner's corpuscles is lowest for frequencies of 20–50 Hz. Pacinian corpuscles sense higher frequencies. (Adapted from Mountcastle et al. 1972.)

tors in the skin, there are far more Meissner's corpuscles and Merkel disk receptors in the fingertip skin than on the palm. The spacing of mechanoreceptors is therefore smallest on the fingertips and widens proximally on the palm, where receptors are less densely packed (Figure 22-4).

The size of the receptive fields in a particular region of skin delimits the capacity to determine whether one or more points are stimulated. A sensory neuron innervating Meissner's corpuscles and Merkel disk receptors transmits information about the *largest* skin in-

dentation within its receptive field. If two points within the same receptive field are stimulated, the neuron will signal only the larger indentation. But if the points are located in the receptive fields of two different nerve fibers, then information about both points of stimulation will be signaled. The farther apart the points lie on the surface, the greater the likelihood that the two active nerves will be separated by silent nerve fibers. The contrast between active and inactive nerve fibers seems to be necessary for resolving spatial detail.

Spatial resolution of stimuli on various regions of the skin can be quantified in humans by measuring their ability to perceive a pair of nearby stimuli as two distinct entities. The minimum distance between two detectable stimuli is called the *two-point threshold*. The two-point threshold varies for different body regions (Figure 22-5). These variations are correlated with the size of sensory receptive fields and the innervation density of mechanoreceptors in the superficial layers of the skin. Thus, measurements of sensory function of the human hand reveal important information concerning the organization of peripheral sense organs.

Mechanoreceptors Differ in Adaptation Properties and Sensory Thresholds

Why is each layer of the skin endowed with two different sets of mechanoreceptors with similar receptive fields? The answer lies in their physiological function. Although all four types of mechanoreceptor are excited by indentation of the skin, they signal different information. As we learned in Chapter 21, mechanoreceptors respond to touch with sustained slowly adapting responses or with rapidly adapting bursts at the beginning and end of contact. The slowly adapting receptors signal the pressure and shape of objects by their average firing rate (see Figure 21-9A). The total number of action potentials evoked per second is proportional to the indentation force applied to the receptor. Rapidly adapting receptors sense motion of objects on the skin (see Figure 21-9B). These receptors respond during the period when the position of a stimulus changes, and they stop firing when it comes to rest. Their firing rates are proportional to the speed of motion, and the duration of activity signals the duration of the motion. They sense vertical impact such as the pressure wave produced when the hand contacts an object and vibration when the object oscillates (see Box 22-1). Rapidly adapting receptors are also stimulated by lateral motion such as stroking, rubbing, or palpation.

Mechanoreceptors also differ in sensory thresholds, the minimum intensity of stimulation required to generate an action potential in the nerve. Rapidly adapting receptors have lower touch thresholds than slowly adapting receptors. The Pacinian corpuscle is the most sensitive mechanoreceptor (Figure 22-6). These receptors are able to detect the minute vibrations produced by impacts on a surface on which the hand rests or caused by the hum of an electric motor. Pacinian corpuscles also sense the frictional displacement of the skin when the hand moves across an object, regardless of whether the surface is smooth or rough. The Meissner's corpuscle is particularly sensitive to abrupt changes in the shape of objects

that occur at the edges or corners and to small irregularities on the surface sensed during palpation by the hand. Meissner's corpuscles are used to detect and localize small bumps or ridges on an otherwise smooth surface.

More salient bumps or edges are required to activate the slowly adapting Merkel disk receptors. However, once stimulated, the Merkel receptors provide a clearer image of contours by changes in the frequency of firing. If the surface is flat, these receptors fire continuously at relatively low rates. Convexities that indent the skin increase firing rates, whereas concavities silence these receptors. Responses are proportional to the surface curvature; large-diameter, gently curved objects evoke weaker responses than small-diameter objects (Figure 22-7). The strongest responses occur when sharp edges or punctate probes, such as a pencil point, contact the receptive field. These changes in receptor activity are reflected in the corresponding perceptions of object shape experienced when we grasp spheres of different diameters between the thumb and index finger. A tiny sphere, such as a ball bearing, feels relatively sharp, whereas a ping-pong ball feels blunt.

The Spatial Characteristics of Objects Are Signaled by Populations of Mechanoreceptors

If the firing rate of slowly adapting receptors signals both pressure and shape, how does the brain decipher which parameter is signaled by an individual receptor? In fact, one receptor cannot signal both of these properties unambiguously. Information about size and shape is signaled by populations of receptors that are stimulated by different portions of the object. A small-diameter object, which indents the skin at a small localized spot, produces a sharply peaked response in which a small number of adjacent receptors fire at high rates. A gently rounded object, which contacts a large region of skin, evokes weak responses in a large population of receptors, forming a broad, low-amplitude profile (Figure 22-7A).

Information about texture is also mediated by populations of mechanoreceptors. Humans are able to sense the roughness of surfaces as well as the spacing and orientation of texture patterns, such as gratings or arrays of Braille dots. When the hand is rubbed over a set of Braille dots, the Merkel disk receptors and Meissner's corpuscles fire bursts of action potentials as each dot in the pattern crosses their receptive fields and are silent as the smooth regions between dots pass. The periodic firing of these receptors signals the spatial arrangement of the texture pattern (Figure 22-8).

However, each receptor axon is stimulated by only a small portion of the pattern. The overall picture is not contained in the firing patterns of any one individual

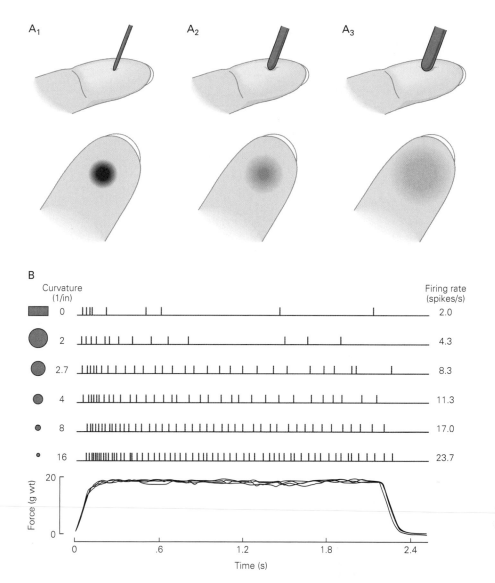

Figure 22-7 The shape and size of objects touching the hand are encoded by populations of Merkel disk receptors.

A. The area of contact on the skin determines the total number of stimulated Merkel disk receptors in the population. The **pink region** on the fingertip shows the spread of excitation when probes of different diameters are pressed upon the skin with constant force. The intensity of color is proportional to the firing rates of the stimulated receptors. **1.** A small-diameter, sharp probe activates a small population of Merkel receptors. However, the active receptors fire intensely because all of the force is concentrated at the small probe tip. **2.** An intermediate-size probe excites more receptors but the peak firing rate in the population is reduced. The probe does not feel as sharp as the small-diameter probe. **3.** A gently rounded, large-diameter probe stimulates a large population of receptors spread across the width of the finger. These receptors fire at low rates because the force is spread over a larger area of skin. (Adapted from Goodwin et al. 1995.)

B. The firing rate of individual Merkel disk receptors signals the probe diameter. These recordings of action potentials fired by a Merkel disk receptor illustrate the responses evoked when probes of decreasing size are pressed on the center of the receptive field. All of the probes evoke a strong initial response as contact is made with the skin. The firing rate of the neuron during steady pressure is proportional to the curvature of each probe. The weakest responses are evoked by flat surfaces and gently rounded (large diameter) probes. The firing rate increases as the probe diameter becomes smaller. (Adapted from Srinivasan and LaMotte 1991.)

Figure 22-8 The firing patterns of mechanoreceptors in the superficial layers of the skin encode the texture of objects rubbed across the skin.

A. 1. The nerve responses to textures are measured with the hand immobilized. The receptive field of a single receptor on a monkey's finger is stimulated with an embossed array of raised dots on a rotating drum. The pattern moves horizontally over the receptive field as the drum rotates. The experimenter thus controls the speed of movement and the location of the dot pattern in the receptive field. The pattern is moved laterally on successive rotations to allow the dots to cross the medial, central, and lateral portions of the receptive field on successive rotations. The composite response of an individual nerve fiber to successive views of the raised dots simulates the distribution of active and inactive nerve fibers in the population. 2. Sequential action potentials discharged by individual receptors during each revolution of the drum are represented in spatial event plots in which each action potential is a small dot, and each horizontal row of dots represents a scan with the pattern shifted laterally on the finger.

B. Spatial event plots of three types of mechanoreceptors to dot patterns with different spacing. Slowly adapting Merkel disk receptors and rapidly adapting Meissner's corpuscles differentiate between dots and blank space when the spacing of the dots exceeds the receptive field diameter. A receptor fires bursts of action potentials for each dot, spaced by silent intervals. As the dots are brought closer together, the resolution of individual dots blurs. Pacinian corpuscles do not distinguish texture patterns because their receptive fields are larger than the dot spacing. (Reproduced from Connor et al. 1990.)

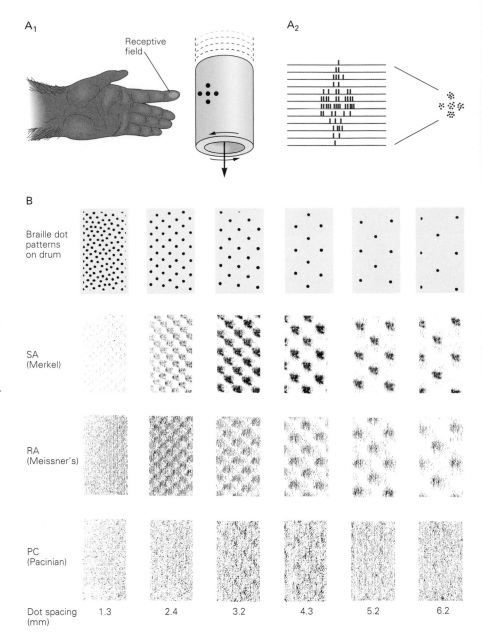

nerve fiber but in the total ensemble of inputs provided by the active and inactive sensory nerves. The distribution of active and inactive nerve fibers represents the spacing and arrangement of the dots in the texture pattern. Therefore, a representation of the texture pattern is transmitted by a group of activated receptor axons in the peripheral nerve innervating the finger. We will learn in Chapter 23 how the central nervous system uses convergent connections to compare activity among members of the population to abstract the arrangement of dots comprising the textured surface.

The spatial resolution of detail within a pattern depends on the total area of skin innervated by each sensory nerve (see Figure 21-6). The Merkel disk receptors provide the sharpest resolution of spatial pattern, as each receptor axon monitors a single dot. Meissner's corpuscles also resolve individual dots but the image of the pattern that they provide is not as sharp because they have slightly larger receptive fields. Pacinian corpuscles do not signal changes in surface contour because their large receptive fields encompass several dots in the textured surface. Instead they fire continuously, measuring the speed at which the hand moves across the surface. The activity of Pacinian corpuscles provides timing information that allows the brain to convert the number of bursts per second fired by Meissner's corpuscles and Merkel disk receptors into spatial information about the number of dots per centimeter on the textured surface.

The pure sensory experiences evoked by the stimuli used in the neurological examination—a light tap, pressure from a pin, or a sinusoidal vibratory stimulus—are quite different from the tactile sensations evoked by the complex natural stimuli that we usually encounter. Natural stimuli rarely activate a single type of receptor; rather they activate different combinations of mechanoreceptors that act synergistically. For example, when we grasp, lift, and replace an object on a surface, the four classes of receptors signal important phases of the movement. Meissner's corpuscles are highly active during the initial period of contact as grasp force increases; these receptors also fire a second burst when the grip is released. Merkel disk receptors are also stimulated during the initial grip, but they continue to fire as the object is lifted, signaling grip force; they cease firing when the grip is released. Pacinian corpuscles are most sensitive to transient mechanical pressures at the start and stop of motion, when the object is lifted off and replaced on the surface. The vertical gravitational forces applied to the skin as the object is lifted are signaled by Ruffini endings. The coordinated sensory information from these receptors provides important signals to the motor system controlling the hand, which we shall study in Chapter 38.

Other Somatic Sensations Are Mediated by a Variety of Specialized Receptors

Warmth and Cold Are Mediated by Thermal Receptors

Although the size, shape, and texture of objects are also sensed by vision, the thermal qualities of objects are uniquely somatosensory. Humans recognize four distinct types of thermal sensation: cold, cool, warm, and hot. These thermal sensations result from differences between the external temperature of the air or of objects contacting the body and the normal skin temperature of 34°C.

Thermal receptors modulate their firing as a function of temperature. At constant temperatures they have tonic discharges, firing action potentials at a steady rate governed by the actual temperature sensed. Unlike mechanoreceptors, which are silent in the absence of tactile stimuli, cold receptors and warmth receptors fire action potentials continuously at low rates (2–5 spikes per second) when the skin temperature is set at its normal value of 34°C (Figure 22–9A). The steady-state firing rate

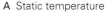
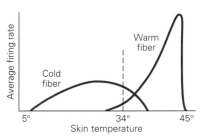
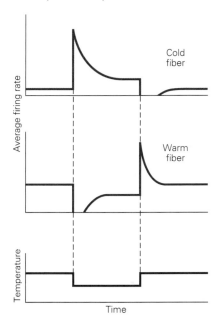

Figure 22-9 Skin temperature is coded by warmth receptors and cold receptors.

A. Static temperatures. Cold receptors and warmth receptors differ in the range of steady-state temperatures to which they respond and in their peak temperature sensitivities. Cold receptors respond to steady-state temperatures of 5–40°C. Warmth receptors are tonically active at steady temperatures of 29–45°C. Cold receptors fire at highest rates at a skin temperature of 25°C, while warmth receptors are most active at 45°C. At the normal skin temperature of 34°C, cold receptors are more active than warmth receptors. (Adapted from Darian-Smith 1973.)

B. Dynamic temperatures. Both receptors are more sensitive to changes in skin temperature than to constant temperatures. Cooling the skin below the resting level evokes a sharp rise in the firing rate of cold receptors and silences warmth receptors. If the cold temperature is maintained, the firing rates of the cold receptors adapt. When the skin temperature is rewarmed to the resting level, cold receptors are briefly silenced, whereas warmth receptors fire a burst of impulses. Warming the skin produces the opposite firing patterns in warmth and cold receptors. (Adapted from Hensel 1973.)

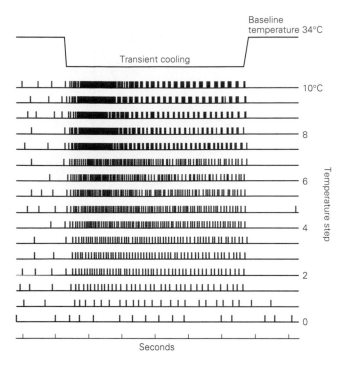

Figure 22-10 The rate and amplitude of cooling the skin is coded by the firing rates of cold receptors. Action potentials were recorded from a cold fiber when the skin was cooled rapidly. Each successive trace shows a smaller cooling pulse. The cold fiber shows a sharp rise in firing rate when the skin is cooled by 10° from 34°C to 24°C. Smaller cooling steps (eg, from 34°C to 30°C) evoke a smaller rise in the firing rate of the cold fiber. The frequency of discharge of cold fibers is linearly related to the size of the cooling step. Warming the skin at the end of the stimulus silences the cold fiber. (Reproduced from Darian-Smith et al. 1973.)

does not increase or decrease monotonically if the skin is slowly warmed or cooled. Instead, each class of thermal receptor shows peak firing at a preferred skin temperature. Cold receptors fire most vigorously at skin temperatures of 25°C, whereas warmth receptors are most active at 45°C. Temperatures above or below these values evoke progressively weaker responses. Therefore, individual cold and warmth receptors do not give a precise reading of the skin temperature, as the same firing rate can be evoked by stimuli greater than or less than the preferred value. Rather, the code for skin temperature involves comparing the relative activity of the different populations of thermal receptors and nociceptors.

The coding of object temperature is analogous to the representation of color in the visual system. In each of these modalities there are populations of receptors sensitive to limited ranges of the energy bandwidth. Each population has a peak sensitivity in a specific posi-

tion of the energy band. The perceived temperature or color is determined by the relative activity of each of the responding populations of receptors.

Thermal receptors are very sensitive to differences between the temperature of the skin and the temperature of objects that are touched. Rapid changes in skin temperature evoke dynamic responses, with increases in temperature signaled by warmth receptors and decreases by cold receptors (Figure 22-9B). If contact with the object is maintained for several seconds, the firing rate of the receptor drops to a lower rate (Figure 22-10). The adaptation of the spike discharge corresponds to the phenomenon of sensory adaptation.

Warmth receptors respond proportionally to increases in skin temperature above the resting value of 34°C. However, if the stimulus temperature exceeds 45°C, warmth fibers fire an intense burst of impulses and then cease firing even if the heat stimulus is maintained. Warmth receptors are unresponsive to hot temperatures, as stimuli above 50°C fail to excite them. At these high temperatures humans perceive heat pain rather than sensations of warmth.

Pain Is Mediated by Nociceptors

The receptors that respond selectively to stimuli that can damage tissue are called *nociceptors* (Latin *nocere*, to injure). They respond directly to some noxious stimuli and indirectly to others by means of one or more chemicals released from cells in the traumatized tissue. A variety of substances have been proposed to act as the chemical intermediary for pain in humans: histamine, K^+ released from injured cells, bradykinin, substance P and other related peptides, acidity (ie, decreases in the local pH around the nerve terminals), ATP, serotonin, and acetylcholine. Humans experience burning pain when these substances stimulate nociceptors. Therefore, it is likely that most nociceptors are really chemoreceptors sensitive to the concentration of irritant chemicals released in the surrounding tissue by noxious thermal or mechanical stimuli, or to exogenous chemicals that may penetrate the skin and bind to their sensory endings. Some nociceptors respond to chemicals such as histamine, yielding itching sensations. These fibers become tonically active in inflamed tissue owing to the release of histamine, peptides, or certain exogenous chemicals such as allergens.

Three classes of nociceptors can be distinguished on the basis of the type of stimulus: mechanical and thermal nociceptors are activated by particular forms of noxious stimuli, whereas polymodal nociceptors, the largest class, are sensitive to the destructive effects of a stimulus rather than to its physical properties.

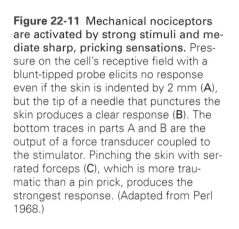

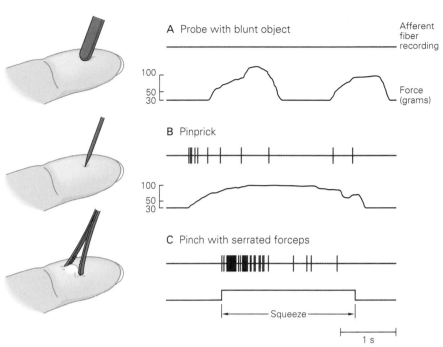

A Probe with blunt object   Afferent fiber recording

100
50
30

Force (grams)

B Pinprick

100
50
30

C Pinch with serrated forceps

|←——— Squeeze ———→|

|—— 1 s ——|

Figure 22-11 Mechanical nociceptors are activated by strong stimuli and mediate sharp, pricking sensations. Pressure on the cell's receptive field with a blunt-tipped probe elicits no response even if the skin is indented by 2 mm (**A**), but the tip of a needle that punctures the skin produces a clear response (**B**). The bottom traces in parts A and B are the output of a force transducer coupled to the stimulator. Pinching the skin with serrated forceps (**C**), which is more traumatic than a pin prick, produces the strongest response. (Adapted from Perl 1968.)

Mechanical nociceptors require strong, often painful tactile stimuli, such as a pinch, in order to respond. They are also excited by sharp objects that penetrate, squeeze, or pinch the skin (Figure 22-11), and therefore mediate sensations of sharp or pricking pain. Their firing rates increase with the destructiveness of mechanical stimuli, from near-damaging to overtly destructive of the skin. The afferent fibers for mechanical nociceptors have bare nerve endings and, because they are myelinated, are the fastest-conducting nociceptive afferents.

Thermal nociceptors are excited by extremes of temperature as well as by strong mechanical stimuli. One group of thermal nociceptors is excited by noxious heat (temperatures above 45°C). A second group responds to noxious cold (cooling the skin below 5°C).

Polymodal nociceptors respond to a variety of destructive mechanical, thermal, and chemical stimuli. They are activated by noxious mechanical stimuli, such as pinch or puncture, by noxious heat and noxious cold, and by irritant chemicals applied to the skin. These receptors are insensitive to gentle mechanical stimuli, such as stroking the skin or light pressure. Stimulation of these receptors in humans evokes sensations of slow, burning pain. Polymodal nociceptors provide the major sensory innervation of the tooth pulp.

Proprioception Is Mediated by Mechanoreceptors in Skeletal Muscle and Joint Capsules

Proprioception (Latin *proprius,* belonging to one's own self) is the sense of position and movement of one's own limbs and body without using vision. There are two submodalities of proprioception: the sense of stationary position of the limbs (limb-position sense) and the sense of limb movement (kinesthesia). These sensations are important for controlling limb movements, manipulating objects that differ in shape and mass, and maintaining an upright posture.

Three types of mechanoreceptors in muscle and joints signal the stationary position of the limb and the speed and direction of limb movement: (1) specialized stretch receptors in muscle termed *muscle spindle receptors;* (2) Golgi tendon organs, receptors in the tendon that sense contractile force or effort exerted by a group of muscle fibers; and (3) receptors located in joint capsules that sense flexion or extension of the joint. The morphology and physiology of these proprioceptors will be discussed in detail in conjunction with their role in spinal reflex pathways (Chapter 36).

In addition, stretch-sensitive receptors in the skin (Ruffini endings, Merkel cells in hairy skin, and field receptors) also signal postural information. Cutaneous proprioception is particularly important for control of lip movements in speech and facial expression.

The Viscera Have Mechanosensory and Chemosensory Receptors

Although humans normally do not experience conscious sensations from the viscera, sensory innervation plays an important role in the neural control of visceral function. (Gastrointestinal discomfort is mediated by re-

Table 22-2 Afferent Fiber Groups in Peripheral Nerves

	Muscle nerve*	Cutaneous nerve*	Fiber diameter (μm)	Conduction velocity (m/s)
Myelinated				
Large	I	Aα	12–20	72–120
Medium	II	Aβ	6–12	36–72
Small	III	Aδ	1–6	4–36
Unmyelinated	IV	C	0.2–1.5	0.4–2.0

*Sensory nerves in muscle are classified according to their fiber diameters. Sensory afferents in cutaneous nerves are classified by conduction velocities. The types of receptors innervated by each type of afferent are listed in Table 22-1.

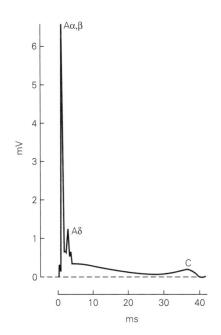

Figure 22-12 Conduction velocities of peripheral nerves are measured clinically from compound action potentials. By electrically stimulating a peripheral nerve at varying intensities different populations of nerve fibers are activated. The action potentials of all the nerves activated by a particular level of current are summed to create the compound action potential. The example in this figure has two major deflections corresponding to action potentials conducted by large and small myelinated fibers (Aα, β, and Aδ fibers). The conduction velocity of each fiber group is computed by dividing the latency of the peaks (the time between the electric shock and the appearance of the neural response) by the distance along the nerve between the stimulating and recording electrodes. Although there are approximately equal numbers of large- and small-diameter myelinated fibers in this nerve, the Aδ peak of the compound action potential is smaller because the spike amplitude of each nerve fiber is proportional to the fiber diameter. Action potentials in unmyelinated nerves (C fibers) are conducted slowly and produce a small late peak. (Reproduced from Gasser 1941).

ceptors in the peritoneal lining of the gut.) The viscera are innervated by dorsal root ganglion neurons with free nerve endings. The morphology of mechanosensory visceral afferents is similar to that of mechanical nociceptors in the skin. They are activated by distention and stretching of visceral muscle, which may evoke sensations of pain. Chemosensory nerve endings in the viscera play important roles in monitoring visceral function and provide the afferent limb for many autonomic reflexes. These sensory functions are described in more detail in our discussion of the autonomic nervous system (Chapter 49).

The Afferent Fibers of Different Receptors Conduct Action Potentials at Different Rates

The diverse modalities of somatic sensation—touch, proprioception, pain, and temperature sense—are mediated by the terminals of dorsal root ganglion cells that differ in the morphology of their terminals and stimulus selectivity. They also differ in the size and conduction velocity of their axons. Mechanoreceptors and proprioceptors are innervated by large-diameter myelinated axons, whereas thermal receptors and nociceptors have small myelinated or unmyelinated axons. These differences in fiber size are important physiologically, because they affect the speed at which action potentials are conducted to the brain (Table 22-2).

Large fibers conduct action potentials more rapidly because the internal resistance to current flow along the axon is low and the nodes of Ranvier are more widely spaced along its length (see Chapter 8). The conduction velocity of large myelinated fibers is approximately six times the axon diameter, while that of thinly myelinated fibers is five times the axon diameter. The factor for converting axon diameter to conduction velocity is much smaller for unmyelinated fibers (1.5–2.5).

Box 22-2 Mapping the Innervation of the Dorsal Roots

The area of skin innervated by a single dorsal root, known as a dermatome, can be identified in experimental animals by probing the skin with different stimuli and observing the response of the fibers within the root. The dermatomes follow a highly regular pattern on the body (Figure 22-13).

Dermatomal maps are an important diagnostic tool for locating the site of injury to the spinal cord and dorsal roots. For example, on the basis of the dermatomal map for the human forearm, we can predict that sensory changes limited to the distal forearm and the fourth and fifth fingers are the result of injury to the C8 and T1 dorsal roots.

In actuality, the boundaries of the dermatomes are less distinct than shown here because the axons making up a dor-

sal root originate from several different peripheral nerves. Similarly, individual peripheral nerves contribute axons to several adjacent dorsal roots, leading to overlap in the area innervated by each segment. Pain dermatomes mapped with a pinprick overlap less than tactile dermatomes mapped with light mechanical stimuli.

The merging of axons from several peripheral nerves has important clinical consequences. Damage to a dorsal root often results in a small sensory deficit throughout the broad area innervated by that root. In contrast, cutting the distal portion of a peripheral cutaneous nerve results in a complete loss of sensory receptors in the circumscribed area innervated by the nerve.

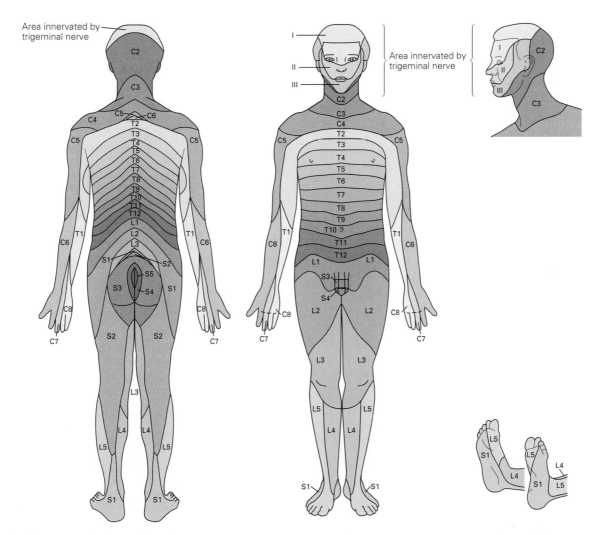

Figure 22-13 The distribution of dermatomes. The 31 pairs of dorsal roots are labeled by the corresponding vertebral foramen through which the root enters the spinal cord. There are 7 cervical (C), 12 thoracic (T), 5 lumbar (L), and 5 sacral (S) roots, which are numbered rostrally to caudally for each division of

the vertebral column. Note that there is no dorsal root at C1, only a ventral (or motor) root, and that the S5 dermatome located in the perianal region is not shown. The facial skin is innervated by the three branches of the trigeminal nerve: the ophthalmic (I), maxillary (II), and mandibular (III) branches.

The clinician takes advantage of the known distribution of conduction velocities of afferent fibers in peripheral nerves to diagnose diseases that result in degeneration of the fibers. In certain conditions there is a selective loss of axons; in diabetes, for example, large sensory fibers degenerate (large-fiber neuropathy). This selective loss is reflected in a reduction in the peak of the compound action potential (Figure 22-12), a slowing of nerve conduction, and a corresponding diminution of sensory capacity. Similarly, in multiple sclerosis the myelin sheath of large-diameter fibers degenerates, producing slowing of nerve conduction or failure of impulse transmission.

Afferent Fibers Conveying Different Somatic Sensory Modalities Have Distinct Terminal Patterns in the Spinal Cord and Medulla

The topographic arrangement of receptors in the skin is preserved as the central processes of the dorsal root ganglion neurons enter the spinal cord through the dorsal roots. The area of skin innervated by the nerve fibers comprising a dorsal root is called a *dermatome*. The distribution of dermatomes for all spinal segments has been mapped by studying sensation and reflex responsiveness that remain after injury to dorsal roots (Box 22-2). Dermatomes are arranged in a caudal-rostral sequence, with the anus and genitalia most caudally and the shoulder, neck, and dorsum of the head rostrally. The three branches of the trigeminal nerve also preserve the topographic arrangements of receptors in the face through their projections to the trigeminal nuclei of the brain stem.

Upon entry to the spinal cord the central axons of dorsal root ganglion neurons branch extensively and project to nuclei in the spinal gray matter and brain stem. The spinal gray matter is divided into three functionally distinct regions: the dorsal horn, the intermediate zone, and the ventral horn. Based on its cytoarchitecture, the spinal gray matter is also divided into 10 layers (laminae). Each layer contains functionally distinct nuclei that have different patterns of projections. Laminae I-VI correspond to the dorsal horn, lamina VII is roughly equivalent to the intermediate zone, and laminae VIII and IX comprise the ventral horn. Lamina X consists of the gray matter surrounding the central canal.

The sensory specialization of dorsal root ganglion neurons is preserved in the central nervous system through distinct ascending pathways for the various somatic modalities. The modalities of touch and proprioception are transmitted directly to the medulla through the ipsilateral dorsal columns. Pain and temperature sense are relayed through synapses in the spinal cord to the contralateral anterolateral quadrant, where axons of dorsal horn neurons ascend to the brain stem and thalamus.

The Dorsal Column–Medial Lemniscal System Is the Principal Pathway for Perception of Touch and Proprioception

The principal central branch of the axon of neurons mediating tactile sensation and proprioception from the limbs and trunk ascends in the spinal cord in the ipsilateral dorsal columns to the medulla. Secondary branches terminate in the dorsal horn. Axons that enter the cord in the sacral region are found near the midline of the dorsal columns; axons that enter the cord at successively higher levels are added in progressively more lateral positions.

At upper spinal levels the dorsal columns are divided into two bundles (fascicles) of axons: the *gracile fascicle* and the *cuneate fascicle*. The gracile fascicle is located medially and contains fibers that ascend from the

Figure 22-14 (Opposite) Sensory information from the limbs and trunk is conveyed to the thalamus and cerebral cortex by two ascending pathways. The anatomy of the pathways is shown on a series of brain slices. The top slice is a schematic oblique section through the postcentral gyrus, which is the location of the primary somatic sensory cortex. The bottom five slices are schematic transverse sections through the brain stem and spinal cord at levels marked on the neuraxis.

Tactile sensation and limb proprioception are transmitted to the thalamus by the dorsal column–medial lemniscal system (**orange**). Painful and thermal sensations are transmitted to the thalamus by the anterolateral system (**brown**).

In the spinal cord the large-diameter dorsal root ganglion axons mediating touch and proprioception diverge from the smaller sensory afferents for pain and temperature sense. The large fibers ascend in ipsilateral dorsal columns to the brain stem where they terminate in the cuneate nucleus. The small fibers terminate on second-order neurons in the dorsal horn of the spinal cord, and the axons of these neurons cross the midline of the spinal cord to form the anterolateral tract. Thus touch and proprioception ascend *ipsilaterally* in the spinal cord, whereas pain and temperature sense ascend *contralaterally*.

The second-order neurons in the dorsal column nuclei send axons across the midline in the medulla, where they form the medial lemniscus. As these axons ascend through the brain stem they shift laterally, joining fibers of the spinothalamic tract in the midbrain, before terminating in the ventral posterior lateral nucleus of the thalamus. Spinothalamic fibers terminate in other thalamic nuclei that are not illustrated in this brain slice. Thalamic neurons mediating touch and proprioception send their axons to the primary somatic sensory cortex in the postcentral gyrus. Thalamic neurons sensitive to painful or thermal stimuli project to the primary somatic sensory cortex, to the dorsal anterior insular cortex, and to the anterior cingulate gyrus rostral to this section. (Adapted from Carpenter and Sutin 1983.)

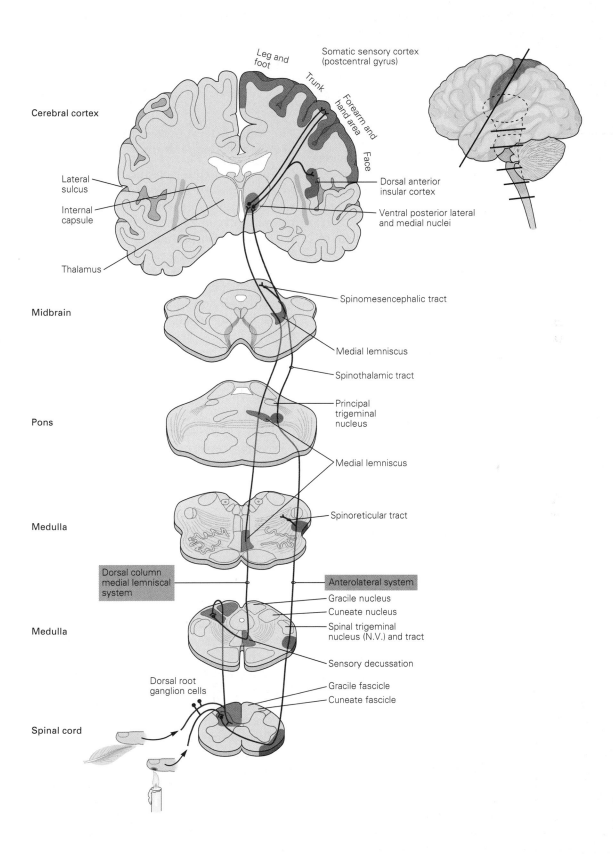

Somatic sensory cortex
(postcentral gyrus)

Leg and foot

Trunk

Forearm and hand area

Face

Cerebral cortex

Lateral sulcus

Internal capsule

Thalamus

Dorsal anterior insular cortex

Ventral posterior lateral and medial nuclei

Midbrain

Spinomesencephalic tract

Medial lemniscus

Spinothalamic tract

Pons

Principal trigeminal nucleus

Medial lemniscus

Medulla

Spinoreticular tract

Dorsal column medial lemniscal system

Anterolateral system

Gracile nucleus

Cuneate nucleus

Medulla

Spinal trigeminal nucleus (N.V.) and tract

Sensory decussation

Dorsal root ganglion cells

Gracile fascicle

Cuneate fascicle

Spinal cord

ipsilateral sacral, lumbar, and lower thoracic segments. The cuneate fascicle is located laterally and contains fibers from the upper thoracic and cervical segments. Axons in the two bundles terminate in the lower medulla in the gracile nucleus and cuneate nucleus, respectively (Figure 22-14A). Mechanosensory information from the face and scalp is transmitted to the principal trigeminal nucleus (Figure 22-14), which is in the pons rostral to the dorsal column nuclei.

The somatotopic organization of the axons relaying input from receptors in the skin and joints is maintained throughout the entire ascending somatosensory pathway, through the thalamus, to the somatosensory areas in the postcentral gyrus of the cerebral cortex. In Chapter 23 we will see how the topographic arrangement of sensory nerve fibers creates sensory maps of the body at each sensory relay nucleus. These maps are the basis for integrating information from receptors in adjoining areas of the skin, or from agonist or antagonist muscle pairs.

Sensory information from the cuneate, gracile, and principal trigeminal nuclei is transmitted directly to the thalamus. The axons of the neurons in the cuneate and gracile nuclei cross to the other side of the brain stem and ascend to the ventral posterior lateral nucleus of the thalamus in a fiber bundle called the *medial lemniscus* (Figure 22-14). As the medial lemniscal fibers cross, the body map becomes reversed: The sacral segments are located most laterally and the cervical segments medially. An adjacent parallel pathway from the principal trigeminal nucleus, the *trigeminal lemniscus,* conveys tactile and proprioceptive information from the face and terminates in the ventral posterior medial nucleus. The trigeminal lemniscus later joins axons from the arm and back of the head in the medial lemniscus.

Because of the crossing of the fibers in the medulla, and pons, the right side of the brain receives sensory input from the limbs and trunk on the left side of the body, and vice versa. As sensory information ascends in the brain stem, the topographic arrangement of the axons changes, so that when the axons enter the thalamus they have the same mediolateral organization as the ventral posterior nuclei. Inputs from the legs are located most laterally, while those from the arm are located more medially. Inputs from the face are most medial.

Although the dorsal columns contain both tactile and proprioceptive axons, these two submodalities remain segregated anatomically. The axons from proprioceptors are positioned more ventrally in the dorsal columns than those of tactile receptors, which are located dorsally. Furthermore, proprioceptors terminate more rostrally in the gracile and cuneate nuclei. A similar segregation of cutaneous and proprioceptive axons

exists in the spinal cord. Neurons mediating the sense of touch terminate in the nucleus proprius (laminae III and IV) of the dorsal horn, whereas proprioceptive afferents terminate more ventrally in the nucleus of Clarke's column (located in lamina VII), on interneurons in laminae V and VI, and on motor neurons in lamina IX.

The Anterolateral System Mediates Sensations of Pain and Temperature

Neurons mediating sensations of pain or temperature from the limbs and trunk terminate in the ipsilateral dorsal horn of the spinal cord. These dorsal root ganglion neurons have much smaller axons and cell bodies than the neurons transmitting sensations of touch or proprioception, and most are unmyelinated. These small fibers branch extensively in the white matter, forming the *tract of Lissauer,* and terminate in the most superficial regions of the dorsal horn. Thus neurons in the marginal zone and substantia gelatinosa (laminae I and II) respond almost exclusively to painful or thermal stimuli. Trigeminal sensory afferents that carry sensations of pain and temperature from the head and face form the descending *spinal trigeminal tract* that terminates in the spinal trigeminal nucleus (a portion of which is also called the medullary dorsal horn). The spinal trigeminal nucleus contains a marginal zone and substantia gelatinosa that receive nociceptive information and a magnocellular division that is innervated by mechanoreceptors and corresponds to the nucleus proprius.

Like the information on touch and proprioception conveyed in the dorsal column–medial lemniscal system, pain and temperature information also ascends to the thalamus, in an anatomical pathway located in the anterolateral quadrant of the contralateral spinal cord (Figure 22-14). The anterolateral pathway originates from neurons in the marginal zone (lamina I), the nucleus proprius (lamina IV), the deep layers of the dorsal horn (laminae V and VI), and the intermediate zone (lamina VII). These spinal neurons send their axons across the midline of the spinal cord and ascend in the anterolateral column of the opposite side of the body. The axons of trigeminal neurons also decussate in the brain stem and join ascending fibers from the most rostral spinal segments.

Like axons in the dorsal columns, the axons of the anterolateral tract are also arranged somatotopically. At each successive spinal segment entering axons lie adjacent to those ascending from lower portions of the spinal cord. Thus, anterolateral fibers from sacral segments are located most laterally, with lumbar fibers slightly more medially, and cervical segments occupying the most medial locations. This somatotopic arrangement of ascending fibers is important clinically for diagnosing and treating pain disorders.

Unlike the medial lemniscus, which transmits sensory information directly to the thalamus, the anterolateral system has both direct and indirect paths to the thalamus. The anterolateral tract consists of three ascending pathways: the spinothalamic, spinoreticular, and spinomesencephalic. The spinothalamic tract conveys information about painful and thermal stimuli directly to the ventral posterior lateral nucleus of the thalamus. Axons in the spinoreticular tract synapse on neurons in the reticular formation of the medulla and pons, which then relay information to the intralaminar and posterior nuclei of the thalamus and to other structures in the diencephalon, such as the hypothalamus.

An Overall View

The somatic sensory system transmits information about four major modalities: touch, proprioception, pain, and temperature sense. Although the four modalities share the same type of sensory neuron—the dorsal root ganglion cell—the receptors for each modality have distinct morphological and molecular specializations that allow them to sense specific types of stimuli.

Discriminative touch and limb proprioception depend on encapsulated mechanoreceptors sensitive to physical deformation produced by indentation or lateral motion across the skin, stretch or contraction of muscles, or the angle of individual joints. Mechanoreceptors in the skin are further specialized to transduce pressure or motion, allowing them to sense the shape and surface texture of objects. Spatial resolution depends on the receptive fields of these receptors and is greatest on the finger tips and lips, where the receptors are most abundant.

The sense of temperature is mediated by the bare endings of thinly myelinated or unmyelinated nerves sensitive to specific ranges of thermal energy. Separate classes of thermal receptors sense temperatures that are perceived as cold, cool, warm, and hot, as they differ in their peak sensitivities and temperature ranges. Painful sensations are mediated by free nerve endings, called nociceptors, that sense destructive mechanical stimuli that squeeze, pinch, or puncture the skin; extremely hot or cold temperatures that might burn or freeze the skin; or chemical substances released from cells as a result of tissue damage.

The four modalities are conveyed in separate ascending pathways to the thalamus and cerebral cortex. Touch and proprioception are transmitted by large-diameter axons with fast conduction velocities to the dor-sal horn of the spinal cord and then to the brain stem and thalamus through the dorsal column–medial lemniscal system. Pain and temperature sense are conveyed by thinly myelinated and unmyelinated nerves that terminate in the most superficial layers of the spinal or trigeminal dorsal horn. These modalities are conveyed directly, and through multisynaptic networks, to the thalamus through the contralateral anterolateral pathway.

The somatic sensory stimuli we encounter in everyday life are complex, cover large areas of skin, and have many characteristics. Each type of receptor is selectively activated by distinct spatial and qualitative properties of a stimulus. Different types of information about an object are transmitted by populations of different types of sensory neurons, and conveyed in parallel pathways to the primary somatosensory cortex, where all the information is combined into a unified somatic percept. How this occurs is the subject of the next chapter.

Esther P. Gardner
John H. Martin
Thomas M. Jessell

Selected Readings

Burgess PR, Perl ER. 1973. Cutaneous mechanoreceptors and nociceptors. In: A Iggo (ed). *Handbook of Sensory Physiology.* Vol. 2, *Somatosensory System,* pp. 29–78. Berlin/New York: Springer-Verlag.

Darian-Smith I. 1984. The sense of touch: performance and peripheral neural processes. In: I Darian-Smith (ed). *Handbook of Physiology: A Critical, Comprehensive Presentation of Physiological Knowledge and Concepts.* Sect. 1, *The Nervous System.* Vol. 3, *Sensory Processes,* Part 2, pp. 739–788. Bethesda, MD: American Physiological Society.

Darian-Smith I. 1984. Thermal sensibility. In: I Darian-Smith (ed). *Handbook of Physiology: A Critical, Comprehensive Presentation of Physiological Knowledge and Concepts.* Sect. 1, *The Nervous System.* Vol. 3, *Sensory Processes,* Part 2, pp. 879–913. Bethesda, MD: American Physiological Society.

Dellon AL. 1981. *Evaluation of Sensibility and Re-Education of Sensation in the Hand.* Baltimore, MD: Williams and Wilkins.

Iggo A, Andres KH. 1982. Morphology of cutaneous receptors. Annu Rev Neurosci 5:1–31.

Johnson KO, Hsiao SS. 1992. Neural mechanisms of tactual form and texture perception. Annu Rev Neurosci 15: 227–250.

Light AR, Perl ER. 1984. Peripheral sensory systems. In: PJ Dyck, PK Thomas, EH Lambert, R Burge (eds). *Peripheral Neuropathy*, 2nd ed. 1:210–230. Philadelphia: Saunders.

Vallbo ÅB. 1995. Single-afferent neurons and somatic sensation in humans. In: MS Gazzaniga (ed). *The Cognitive Neurosciences*, pp. 237–252. Cambridge, MA: MIT Press.

Vallbo ÅB, Hagbarth K-E, Torebjörk HE, Wallin BG. 1979. Somatosensory, proprioceptive, and sympathetic activity in human peripheral nerves. Physiol Rev 59:919–957.

Willis WD, Coggeshall RE. 1978. *Sensory Mechanisms of the Spinal Cord.* New York: Plenum.

References

Adrian ED. 1928. *The Basis of Sensation: The Action of the Sense Organs.* London: Christophers.

Adrian ED, Zotterman Y. 1926. The impulses produced by sensory nerve-endings. Part 2. The response of a single end-organ. J Physiol (Lond) 61:151–171.

Adrian ED, Zotterman Y. 1926. The impulses produced by sensory nerve-endings. Part 3. Impulses set up by touch and pressure. J Physiol (Lond) 61:465–483.

Carpenter MB, Sutin J. 1983. *Human Neuroanatomy*, 8th ed. Baltimore, MD: Williams and Wilkins.

Connor CE, Hsiao SS, Phillips JR, Johnson KO. 1990. Tactile roughness: neural codes that account for psychophysical magnitude estimates. J Neurosci 10:3823–3836.

Connor CE, Johnson KO. 1992. Neural coding of tactile texture: comparison of spatial and temporal mechanisms for roughness perception. J Neurosci 12:3414–3426.

Darian-Smith I, Johnson KO, Dykes R. 1973. "Cold" fiber population innervating palmar and digital skin of the monkey: responses to cooling pulses. J Neurophysiol 36:325–346.

Edin BB, Abbs JH. 1991. Finger movement responses of cutaneous mechanoreceptors in the dorsal skin of the human hand. J Neurophysiol 65:657–670.

Gardner EP, Palmer CI. 1990. Simulation of motion on the skin. III. Mechanisms used by rapidly adapting cutaneous mechanoreceptors in the primate hand for spatiotemporal resolution and two-point discrimination. J Neurophysiol 63:841–859.

Gasser HS. 1941. The classification of nerve fibers. Ohio J Sci 41:145.

Goodwin AW, Browning AS, Wheat HE. 1995. Representation of curved surfaces in responses of mechanoreceptive afferent fibers innervating the monkey's fingerpad. J Neurosci 15:798–810.

Goodwin AW, John KT, Sathian JK, Darian-Smith I. 1989. Spatial and temporal factors determining afferent fiber responses to a grating moving sinusoidally over the monkey's fingerpad. J Neurosci 9:1280–1293.

Hensel H. 1973. Cutaneous thermoreceptors. In: A Iggo (ed). *Handbook of Sensory Physiology.* Vol. 2, *Somatosensory System*, pp. 79–110. Berlin/New York: Springer-Verlag.

Hensel H, Zotterman Y. 1951. The response of the cold receptors to constant cooling. Acta Physiol Scand 22:96–113.

Johansson RS, Vallbo ÅB. 1983. Tactile sensory coding in the glabrous skin of the human hand. Trends Neurosci 6:27–32.

Kimura J. 1989. *Electrodiagnosis in Diseases of Nerve and Muscle: Principles and Practice*, 2nd ed. Philadelphia: FA Davis.

LaMotte RH, Srinivasan MA. 1987. Tactile discrimination of shape: responses of slowly adapting mechanoreceptor afferents to a step stroked across the monkey fingerpad. J Neurosci 7:1655–1671.

Mountcastle VB, LaMotte RH, Carli G. 1972. Detection thresholds for stimuli in humans and monkeys: comparison with threshold events in mechanoreceptive afferent nerve fibers innervating the monkey hand. J Neurophysiol 35:122–136.

Müller J. 1838–1840. *Handbüch der Physiologie des Menschen für Vorlesungen*, 2 vols. Coblenz: J Hölscher.

Perl ER. 1968. Myelinated afferent fibres innervating the primate skin and their response to noxious stimuli. J Physiol (Lond) 197:593–615.

Phillips JR, Johansson RS, Johnson KO. 1992. Responses of human mechanoreceptive afferents to embossed dot arrays scanned across fingerpad skin. J Neurosci 12:827–839.

Srinivasan MA, LaMotte RH. 1991. Encoding of shape in the responses of cutaneous mechanoreceptors. In: O Franzen, J Westman (eds). *Wenner-Gren International Symposium Series: Information Processing in the Somatosensory System*, pp. 59–69. London: Macmillan.

Talbot WH, Darian-Smith I, Kornhuber HH, Mountcastle VB. 1968. The sense of flutter-vibration: comparison of the human capacity with response patterns of mechanoreceptive afferents from the monkey hand. J Neurophysiol 31:301–334.

Vallbo ÅB, Johansson RS. 1978. The tactile sensory innervation of the glabrous skin of the human hand. In: G Gordon (ed). *Active Touch*, pp. 29–54. New York: Pergamon.

Vallbo ÅB, Olausson H, Wessberg J, Kakuda N. 1995. Receptive field characteristics of tactile units with myelinated afferents in hairy skin of human subjects. J Physiol (Lond) 483:783–795.

Vallbo ÅB, Olsson KÅ, Westberg K-G, Clark FJ. 1984. Microstimulation of single tactile afferents from the human hand: sensory attributes related to unit type and properties of receptive fields. Brain 107:727–749.

Van Boven RW, Johnson KO. 1994. A psychophysical study of the mechanism of sensory recovery following nerve injury in humans. Brain 117:149–167.

Weinstein S. 1968. Intensive and extensive aspects of tactile sensitivity as a function of body part, sex, and laterality. In: DR Kenshalo (ed). *The Skin Senses*, pp. 195–222. Springfield, IL: Thomas.

Westling G, Johansson RS. 1987. Responses in glabrous skin mechanoreceptors during precision grip in humans. Exp Brain Res 66:128–140.

Zotterman Y. 1933. Studies in the peripheral nervous mechanism of pain. Acta Med Scand 80:185–242.

Zotterman Y. 1935. Action potentials in the glossopharyngeal nerve and in the chorda tympani. Skand Arch Physiol 72:73–77.

23

Touch

INFORMATION TRANSMITTED to the brain from mechanoreceptors in the fingers enables us to feel the shape and texture of objects and permits us to read braille, play musical instruments, type on computer keyboards, or perform fine surgical dissections. In this chapter we shall examine how neuronal activity of mechanoreceptors in the skin gives rise to perception of discriminative touch and why the fingertips are best suited to this task.

Since this chapter is the first in which we discuss, in cell-physiological detail, the central projections of a sensory system to the cerebral cortex, we also address two key questions about the cerebral cortex. How does it work on the cellular level? How does it integrate and transform sensory information coming from the periphery? Thus, we describe how the cortex constructs an image of objects we touch from the fragmented information provided by the receptors of the skin. Moreover, in this chapter we use the sense of touch as a model for deriving principles of cortical organization that give rise to conscious perception. Specifically, we examine the degree to which the various somatic modalities are functionally segregated in the central nervous system and how they are recombined for coherent perception of tactile information. We have chosen the modality of touch to introduce the principles of cortical function because these principles were first established for the somatosensory cortex and later extended to other sensory and motor cortical areas, as we shall see in subsequent chapters.

Tactile Information About an Object is Fragmented by Peripheral Sensors and Must Be Integrated by the Brain

The ability to recognize objects placed in the hand on the basis of touch alone is one of the most important and complex functions of the somatosensory system. By holding an object in the hand we can perceive its size, shape, texture, mass, and temperature. These properties together give rise to the percept of a coherent object. Neurologists call the ability to perceive form through touch *stereognosis*. Stereognosis not only tests the ability of the dorsal column–medial lemniscal system to transmit sensations from the hand but also measures the ability of cognitive processes in the brain to integrate that information.

Many familiar objects such as an apple, a screwdriver, or a set of keys are much larger than the receptive field of any one receptor in the hand. These objects stimulate a large population of sensory nerve fibers, each of which scans a small portion of the object. The peripheral sensory apparatus deconstructs the object into tiny segments because, as we saw in Chapter 22, a sensory nerve fiber conveys information from only a small area of the receptor sheet. When a particular nerve fiber fires an action potential, it signals that its territory has been contacted at an intensity sufficient to cause it to fire. By analyzing which nerve fibers have been excited, the brain reconstructs the pattern made by the object.

In addition, objects excite more than one kind of receptor. For example, a textured surface such as an array of Braille dots stimulates Merkel disk receptors, Meissner's corpuscles, and Pacinian corpuscles but evokes a different discharge pattern in each type of receptor because each signals a special feature of the stimulus. Similarly, the shape of an object is signaled by the firing patterns of Merkel disk receptors, which sense the curvature of the object's surface; by Meissner's corpuscles, which signal edges (where the curvature changes abruptly); and by the postural information provided by receptors in the muscles and joints of the hand.

Thus, no single sensory axon, or even class of sensory axons, signals all of the relevant information. Spatial properties are processed by populations of receptors that form many parallel pathways to the brain. It is the job of the central nervous system to construct a coherent image of an object from fragmented information conveyed in multiple pathways. In this chapter we shall examine how neural circuits in the dorsal column–medial lemniscal system and the somatosensory areas of the cerebral cortex integrate information from neighboring areas of skin and different populations of receptors in order to form a *percept*.

The Primary Somatic Sensory Cortex Integrates Information About Touch

The anatomical plan of the somatic sensory system reflects an organizational principle common to all sensory systems: Sensory information is processed in a series of relay regions within the brain. We learned in Chapter 22 that there are only three synaptic relay sites between sensory receptors in the skin and the cerebral cortex (see Figure 22-14). Mechanoreceptors in the skin send their axons to the caudal medulla, where they terminate in the gracile or cuneate nuclei. These second-order neurons project directly to the contralateral thalamus, terminating in the ventral posterior lateral nucleus. A parallel pathway from the principal trigeminal nucleus, which represents the face, ascends to the ventral posterior medial nucleus. The third-order neurons in the thalamus send axons to the primary somatic sensory cortex (S-I), located in the postcentral gyrus of the parietal lobe.

As we learned in Chapter 20, the primary somatic cortex S-I contains four cytoarchitectural areas: Brodmann's areas 3a, 3b, 1, and 2 (Figure 23-1). Most thalamic fibers terminate in areas 3a and 3b, and the cells in areas 3a and 3b project their axons to areas 1 and 2. Thalamic neurons also send a small projection directly to Brodmann's areas 1 and 2. These four regions of the cortex differ functionally. Areas 3b and 1 receive information from receptors in the skin, whereas areas 3a and 2 receive proprioceptive information from receptors in muscles and joints. However, the four areas of the cortex are extensively interconnected, so that both serial and parallel processing are involved in higher-order elaboration of sensory information.

The *secondary somatic sensory cortex* (S-II), located on the superior bank of the lateral fissure, is innervated by neurons from each of the four areas of S-I (Figure 23-1C). The projections from S-I are required for the function of S-II. For example, when the neural connections from the hand area of S-I are removed, stimuli applied to the skin of the hand do not activate neurons in S-II. In contrast, removal of parts of S-II has no effect on the response of neurons in S-I. The S-II cortex projects to the *insular cortex*, which in turn innervates regions of the temporal lobe believed to be important for tactile memory.

Finally, as we have seen in Chapters 19 and 20, other important somatosensory cortical areas are located in the *posterior parietal cortex* (Brodmann's areas 5 and 7). These areas receive input from S-I as well as input from the pulvinar and thus have an associational function. They are also connected bilaterally through the corpus callosum. Area 5 integrates tactile information from mechanoreceptors in the skin with proprio-

A The somatosensory cortex

B Coronal section

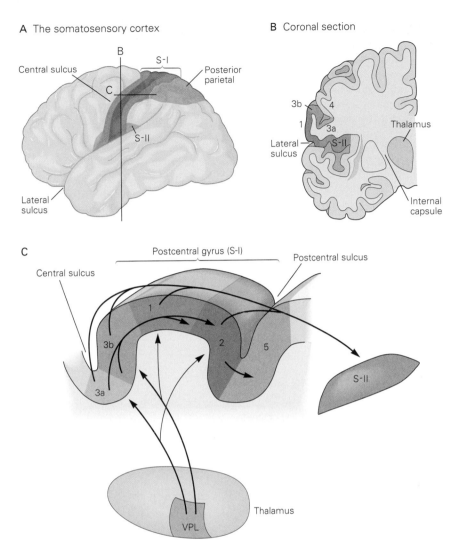

C

Figure 23-1 The somatic sensory cortex has three major divisions: the primary and secondary somatosensory cortices and the posterior parietal cortex.

A. The anatomical location of the three divisions of the somatic sensory cortex is seen best from a lateral perspective of the surface of the cerebral cortex. The *primary somatic sensory cortex* (S-I) forms the most rostral portion of the parietal lobe. It covers the postcentral gyrus, beginning at the bottom of the central sulcus and extending posteriorly to the postcentral and intraparietal sulci. The postcentral gyrus also extends into the medial wall of the hemisphere to the cingulate gyrus. The *posterior parietal cortex* (Brodmann's areas 5 and 7) lies immediately posterior to S-I. The *secondary somatic sensory cortex* (S-II) is located on the parietal operculum of the lateral sulcus (fissure of Sylvius).

B. The relationship of the S-I to the S-II cortex is illustrated in a

coronal section through the cortex. The S-II cortex lies lateral to S-I, and extends laterally to the insular cortex, forming the superior bank of the lateral sulcus. The numbers on the section indicate Brodmann's cytoarchitectural areas.

C. S-I is subdivided into four distinct cytoarchitectonic regions (Brodmann's areas). This sagittal section illustrates the spatial relationship of these four regions to area 5 of the posterior parietal cortex. Somatosensory input to the cortex originates from the ventral posterior lateral nucleus of the thalamus. Neurons in this nucleus project to all areas in S-I, mainly to Brodmann's areas 3a and 3b but also to areas 1 and 2. In turn, neurons in areas 3a and 3b project to areas 1 and 2, and all of these project to S-II and to posterior parietal cortex. These higher-order somatosensory areas also contain distinct cytoarchitectonic and functional subregions that are not illustrated here. (Modified from Jones and Friedman 1982.)

ceptive inputs from the underlying muscles and joints. This region also integrates information from the two hands. Area 7 receives visual as well as tactile and proprioceptive inputs, allowing integration of stereognostic

and visual information. The posterior parietal cortex projects to the motor areas of the frontal lobe and plays an important role in sensory initiation and guidance of movement.

Box 23-1   Extracellular Recordings Are Used to Study Neurons in the Central Nervous System

Much of what we know about the processing of somatic sensory information in the brain, particularly in the cerebral cortex, has been learned from studies of monkeys. The monkey has proven so useful because primates have sensory receptors identical to those of humans. Furthermore, psychophysical measurements of somatosensory discriminative abilities indicate that humans and monkeys experience the same tactile sensations in their hands when they feel vibration, palpate objects, or touch a textured surface.

The techniques for studying the physiology of the cerebral cortex at the cellular level were developed by Vernon Mountcastle and his colleagues in the 1950s. Using extracellular microelectrodes (which had just become available) they recorded the electrical responses of individual neurons. Extracellular recordings reveal only the action potentials of the cell

and thus, do not show synaptic activity except under certain circumstances. (Extracellular recording, however, is much simpler than intracellular recording in the intact brain because the brain pulsates, making it difficult to maintain intracellular penetrations.) Nevertheless, extracellular recording has been a useful tool in defining how sensory stimuli modulate the firing patterns of single cells.

Microelectrode recording allows the receptive fields of several neurons at adjacent locations in the brain to be examined in sequence (Figure 23-2). By systematically moving the electrode in steps of thousandths of a millimeter, one can reconstruct a three-dimensional map of the cerebral cortex. This technique, termed micromapping, forms the experimental foundation for what we know about the columnar and somatotopic organization of the cortex.

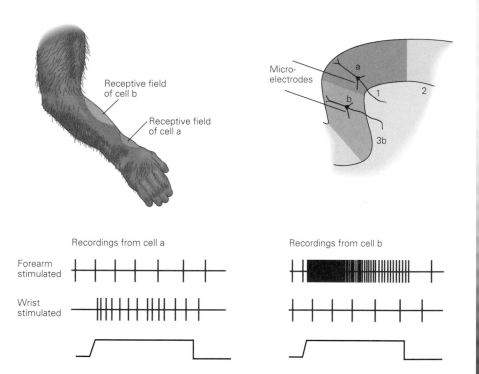

Figure 23-2 Three-dimensional functional maps of the cerebral cortex are created by examining the receptive fields of adjacent cortical neurons in sequence. In this example a pair of microelectrodes are advanced into the S-I cortex. The neuron recorded at location **a** in area 1 has a sustained, slowly adapting response to pressure applied to the wrist with a small blunt probe and ceases firing when the probe is removed from the skin. It does not respond to pressure on the forearm. The neuron recorded at location **b** in area 3b responds vigorously to pressure on the forearm but not on the wrist. Note that cortical neurons, unlike sensory afferents, fire action potentials at low rates in the absence of stimuli.

Cortical Neurons Are Defined by Their Receptive Fields As Well As by Modality

To understand the function of these different regions of the cortex, we begin by examining the properties of individual cortical neurons. The neurons in the primary somatic sensory cortex are at least three synapses beyond the peripheral receptors. Thus their response properties reflect information processing in the dorsal column nuclei, the thalamus, and in the cortex itself.

Cortical neurons, like neurons elsewhere in the brain, are usually studied using the technique of extracellular recording (see Box 23-1). Microelectrodes are inserted into the cortex to record both the spike trains that occur spontaneously and those evoked by appropriate stimuli.

Like mechanoreceptors, the cortical neurons receiving sensory information from the skin are either slowly adapting or rapidly adapting neurons, signaling either

Figure 23-3 The receptive fields of neurons in the primary somatic sensory cortex are larger than those of the sensory afferents. Each of the hand figurines shows the receptive field of an individual neuron in areas 3b, 1, 2, and 5 of the primary somatic sensory cortex, based on recordings made in alert monkeys. The colored regions indicate the region of the hand where light touch elicits action potentials from the neuron. Neurons that participate in later stages of cortical processing (Brodmann's areas 1 and 2) have larger receptive fields and more specialized inputs than neurons in area 3b. The neuron illustrated from area 2 is directionally sensitive to motion toward the fingertips. Neurons in area 5 often have symmetric bilateral receptive fields at mirror image locations on the contralateral and ipsilateral hand. (Adapted from Gardner 1988, Iwamura et al. 1994.)

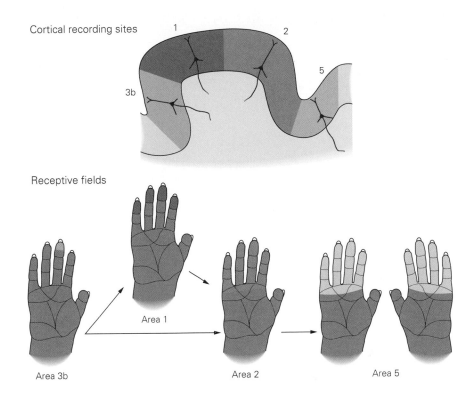

the amplitude or rate of the peripheral skin indentation. Moreover, since each cortical neuron receives inputs from receptors in a specific area of the skin, central neurons also have receptive fields. Thus, each cortical neuron is defined by its receptive field as well as by its sensory modality. Any point on the skin is represented in the cortex by a population of cortical cells connected to the afferent fibers that innervate that point on the skin. When a point on the skin is touched, the population of cortical neurons connected to the receptors at that location is excited. Stimulation of another point on the skin activates another population of cortical neurons. We perceive contact at a particular location on the skin because a specific population of neurons in the brain is activated. Conversely, as we saw in Chapter 19, when a point on the cortex is stimulated electrically, we experience tactile sensations on a specific part of the skin. We shall show later in this chapter that cortical neurons are grouped by function and that their receptive fields are arranged in an orderly topographic sequence that forms a map of the body.

The receptive fields of cortical neurons are much larger than those of dorsal root ganglion neurons. For example, the receptive fields of sensory neurons innervating a finger cover tiny spots on the skin, while those of the cortical cells receiving these inputs are large areas covering an entire fingertip, or several adjacent fingers,

or the palmar surface of the contralateral hand (Figure 23-3). The receptive field of a neuron in area 3b represents a composite of inputs from about 300–400 mechanoreceptive afferents. Receptive fields in higher cortical areas are even larger. In the posterior parietal cortex, receptive fields are often bilateral, located at symmetric positions on the contralateral and ipsilateral hands.

Cortical receptive fields encompass functional regions of skin that are activated simultaneously during motor activity. The size and position of cortical receptive fields on the skin are not fixed permanently but can be modified by experience or by injury to sensory nerves. Cortical receptive fields appear to be formed during development and maintained by simultaneous activation of the input pathways.

Although the receptive fields of cortical neurons cover a large area of skin, a cortical neuron is nevertheless able to discriminate fine detail because it responds best to excitation in the middle of its receptive field. As the stimulation site is moved toward the periphery of the field, responses become progressively weaker until eventually no spikes are recorded. Thus, a stimulus applied to the tip of the index finger strongly excites some neurons, while others fire weakly or not at all. If a more proximal spot on the finger is touched, many of the same cells are activated but in different proportions. In-

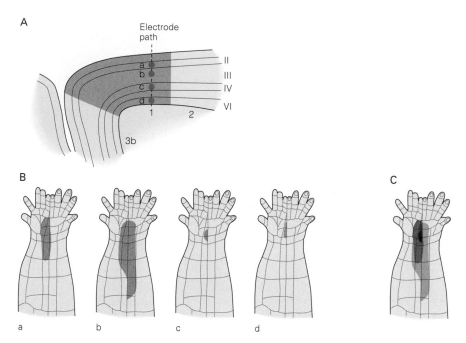

Figure 23-4 The receptive fields of cells in a column in Brodmann's area 1 share a common central location on the skin. The columns representing a given skin location are approximately 300–600 μm wide. (Adapted from Favorov and Whitsel 1988.)

A. Sagittal section through S-I cortex illustrating the recording sites of a group of neurons located in a single column. The most superficial neuron (**a**) is located in layer II, and the deepest neuron (**d**) is located in layer VI. Neuron **b** is located in layer III, and neuron **c** is situated in layer IV.

B. Receptive fields of the four neurons shown in A. The neurons in this column share receptive fields on the ulnar portion of the forearm, wrist, and hand. The dorsal and volar surfaces of the hand and arm have been juxtaposed to illustrate the continuity of receptive fields along the ulnar margin. The receptive

fields are labeled according to depth in the cortex. Neuron **c** has the smallest receptive field, localized near the wrist; it is located in layer IV where the thalamic afferents terminate. Pyramidal neurons in layers II and III have larger receptive fields because their large basal dendritic fields extend into the neighboring columns.

C. Superimposition of the receptive fields illustrated in B. The darkest region in the center is shared by all receptive fields of the neurons in the column; this region is used to reconstruct the representation area of the column in the somatotopic map. The skin areas surrounding the central focus are shared by most, but not all, of the neurons in the column. The skin locations at the outer margins of the column's global receptive field are represented in only a few cells' receptive fields.

formation provided by the entire population of excited cells localizes a stimulus on the skin.

The Properties of Cortical Receptive Fields Are Due to Convergent and Divergent Connections in the Relay Nuclei

The increase in area of the receptive fields of cortical neurons reflects the anatomical circuitry within the relay nuclei. Relay nuclei, such as the dorsal column or thalamic nuclei, are composed of projection (or relay) neurons that send their axons to the next nucleus in the pathway and inhibitory interneurons that terminate upon relay neurons. Sensory inputs to the relay nucleus are characterized by extensive convergence and divergence. Each sensory afferent has a branched terminal that innervates several postsynaptic neurons, so that

each projection neuron receives synaptic input from many sensory axons. This pattern of divergent presynaptic connections and convergent postsynaptic connections is repeated at each relay in the pathway.

Inputs to the Somatic Sensory Cortex Are Organized in Columns by Receptive Field and Modality

Although convergence of sensory afferents enlarges the receptive fields of projection neurons at successive relay nuclei, the topographic arrangement of the receptive fields is preserved. In a series of pioneering studies Mountcastle discovered that the cortex is organized into vertical columns or slabs, 300–600 μm wide, spanning all six layers from the cortical surface to the white matter. All of the neurons within a column receive inputs

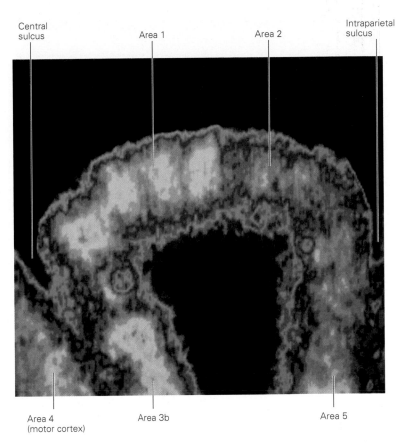

Figure 23-5 Columns of neurons in the primary somatic sensory cortex comprise the elementary functional modules of cortical processing of somatosensory information. This autoradiograph shows the pattern of ^{14}C 2-deoxyglucose (2-DG) labeling of neurons in a sagittal section through the hand area of the S-I cortex after 45 minutes of stroking the hand and wrist with a brush. Uptake of 2-DG in the brain is proportional to neuronal activity. Stimulation of the hand produces dense patches of labeled neurons in both area 3b and in area 1. Active neurons are found in vertical columns extending from layer II through layer V, with the strongest responses seen in layer IV (pale **red**). Columns are continuous in area 3b, but form distinct modules in area 1. Very little activity is seen in area 2, which receives input from deep receptors. (Photograph courtesy of S. Juliano, P. Hand, and B. Whitsel.)

from the same local area of skin and respond to a single class of receptors. Although the receptive fields of the neurons comprising a column are not precisely congruent, they do share a common center, which is most clearly evident in layer IV (Figure 23-4). A column therefore provides an anatomical structure that preserves the properties of location and modality. Neurons lying within a column comprise an elementary functional module of the cortex (Figure 23-5). We shall see in later chapters that columnar organization is a basic organizational and structural principle of the cerebral cortex.

The columnar organization of the cortex is a direct consequence of cortical circuitry. The pattern of intrinsic connections within the cerebral cortex is oriented vertically, perpendicular to the surface of the cortex (Figure 23-6). Thalamic afferents to the cortex terminate mainly on clusters of stellate cell neurons in layer IV. The axons of the stellate cells project vertically toward the surface of the cortex. Similarly, both the apical dendrites and axons of the pyramidal cells are oriented vertically, parallel to the stellate cell axons. The thalamocortical input is therefore relayed to a narrow vertical column of pyramidal cells whose apical dendrites are contacted by the stellate cell axons. This means that the same information

is relayed up and down through the thickness of the cortex in columnar fashion.

In addition to sharing a common focal location on the skin, all of the neurons in a column usually respond to only one modality: touch, pressure, temperature, or pain. This is not surprising, as we have seen that the various somatosensory modalities are conveyed by anatomically separate pathways. The cells that make up these pathways have distinctive response properties inasmuch as each pathway conveys information from a different class of receptor. Sensory receptors and primary sensory neurons responsive to one submodality, such as pressure or vibration, are connected to clusters of cells in the dorsal column nuclei and thalamus that receive inputs only for that submodality. These relay neurons in turn project to modality-specific cells in the cortex.

Although each of the four areas of the primary somatic sensory cortex (3a, 3b, 1, and 2) receives input from all areas of the body surface, one modality tends to dominate in each area. In area 3a the dominant input is from proprioceptors signaling muscle stretch. Area 3b receives input primarily from cutaneous mechanoreceptors. Here the inputs from a discrete site on the skin are

Figure 23-6 The columnar organization of cortical neurons is a consequence of the pattern of connections between neurons in different layers of cortex. (Modified from Jones 1981.)

A. The dendrites and axons of most cortical neurons extend vertically from the surface to white matter, forming the anatomical basis of the columnar structure of the cortex.

B. Morphology of the relay neurons of layers III–V. Stellate neurons (small spiny cell) are located in layer IV. These neurons are the principal target of thalamocortical axons. The axons of the stellate neurons project vertically toward the surface of the cortex, terminating on the apical dendrites of a narrow beam of pyramidal cells whose somas lie in layers II, III, and V above or below them. Stellate cell axons also terminate on the basal branches of pyramidal cells in layers II and III. The axons of pyramidal neurons project vertically to deeper layers of the cortex and to other cortical or subcortical regions; they also send horizontal branches within the same cortical region to activate columns of neurons sharing similar physiological properties.

C. Schematic diagram of intracortical excitatory circuits. The principal connections are made vertically between neurons in different layers.

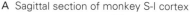

A Sagittal section of monkey S-I cortex

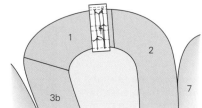

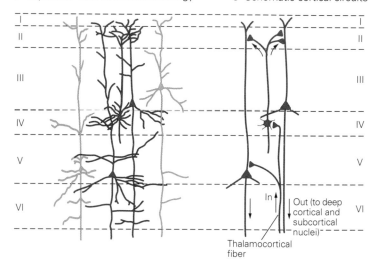

B Expanded view of cortical histology   C Schematic cortical circuits

Thalamocortical fiber

In | Out (to deep cortical and subcortical nuclei)

divided into two sets of columns, one each for inputs from rapidly adapting and slowly adapting receptors (Figure 23-7). In area 1 rapidly adapting cutaneous receptors predominate, and the receptive fields of these cells are considerably larger than those of cells in area 3b, often covering several adjacent fingers. In area 2 and higher cortical areas the modality segregation is much weaker. Columns of neurons in area 2 receive convergent input from slowly and rapidly adapting cutaneous receptors or from cutaneous receptors and proprioceptors in the underlying muscles and joints. Thus, the receptive fields and response properties of neurons in areas 1 and 2 represent convergent input from regions of the hand and fingers that are represented separately in areas 3a and 3b.

How does the layering of the cortex contribute to the functional organization of the cortex? As described in Chapter 19, each layer of cells has connections with different parts of the brain: Layer IV receives input from the thalamus; layer VI projects back to the thalamus; layers II and III project to other cortical regions; and layer V projects to subcortical structures. As a result, the information on stimulus location and modality processed in each column is conveyed to different regions of the brain.

The Body Surface Is Represented in the Brain by the Somatotopic Arrangement of Sensory Inputs

The columns of neurons in the somatic sensory cortex are arranged such that there is a complete topographic representation of the body in each of the four areas (3a, 3b, 1, and 2). The cortical map of the body corresponds to the spinal dermatomes defined by the afferent fibers entering the spinal cord at successively rostral levels (see Box 22-2). Sacral segments are represented medially, lumbar and thoracic segments centrally, cervical segments more laterally, and the trigeminal representation at the most lateral portion of the S-I cortex (Figure 23-8). The maps in adjacent cytoarchitectonic areas are rough mirror images of the distal-proximal or dorsal-ventral axes of each dermatome.

Topographic maps of the human parietal cortex have been constructed from measurements of sensory-evoked potentials or by using electrical stimulation of the cortex. These techniques, together with more modern noninvasive diagnostic tools such as magnetoencephalography (MEG), functional magnetic resonance imaging (fMRI), and positron emission tomography

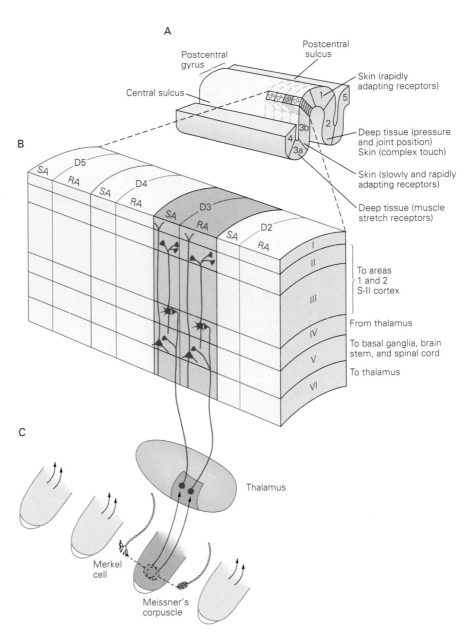

Figure 23-7 Each region of the somatic sensory cortex receives inputs from primarily one type of receptor.

A. In each of the four regions of the somatic sensory cortex—Brodmann's areas 3a, 3b, 1, and 2—inputs from one type of receptor in specific parts of the body are organized in columns of neurons that run from the surface to the white matter. (Adapted from Kaas et al. 1981.)

B. Detail of the columnar organization of inputs from digits 2, 3, 4, and 5 in a portion of Brodmann's area 3b. Alternating columns of neurons receive inputs from rapidly adapting (**RA**) and slowly adapting (**SA**) receptors in the superficial layers of skin. (Adapted from Sur et al. 1984.)

C. Overlapping receptive fields from RA and SA receptors project to distinct columns of neurons in area 3b.

(PET scan), allow neurologists to image the somatotopic functioning of the cortex in individual patients. While these imaging methods are less precise than the microelectrode maps made in animals, they are useful diagnostic tools in clinical neurology.

Spatial Resolution in the Cortex Is Correlated With the Innervation Density of the Skin

The somatotopic arrangement of somatosensory inputs in the human cortex is called a *homunculus;* it corresponds closely to the somatotopic maps of cortical columns determined by single neuron recordings in

monkeys. However, the internal representation of the body within the homunculus does not duplicate the spatial topography of the skin exactly. Rather, the image of the body in the brain exaggerates certain body regions, particularly the hand, foot, and mouth and compresses more proximal body parts.

Each part of the body is represented in the brain in proportion to its relative importance to sensory perception. The map represents the *innervation density* of the skin rather than its total surface area. In humans a large number of cortical columns receive input from the hands, particularly from the fingers. About 100 times as much cortical tissue is devoted to a square centimeter of

A

B

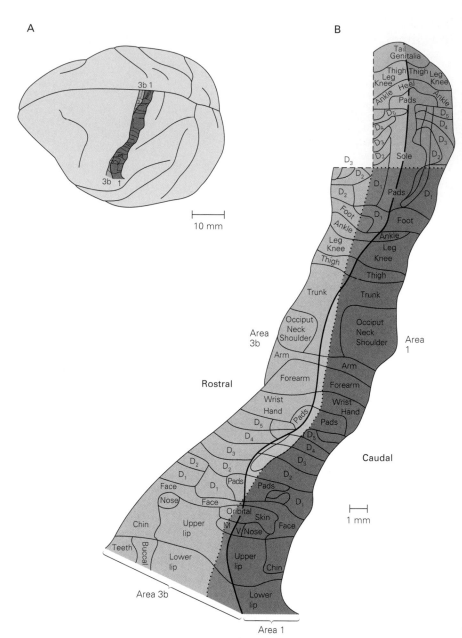

Figure 23-8 Each of the four regions of the primary somatic sensory cortex contains a complete map of the body surface. (Adapted from Nelson et al. 1980.)

A. Location of the primary somatosensory cortex in the brain of the macaque monkey. The body surface is mapped to the surface of the cortex as rostrocaudal strips arranged in the order of the spinal dermatomes.

B. Enlarged view of the body maps in areas 3b and 1 of the macaque primary somatic sensory cortex. The cortex is unfolded in this diagram along the central sulcus (**dotted line,** which parallels the border between 3b and 1), and at the medial wall of the hemisphere (**dashed line** at the edge of the foot representation). The sacral and lower lumbar segments are represented on the medial wall of the hemisphere. More rostral segments are mapped more laterally; the most lateral portions of the cortex contain the representation of the neck, face, mouth, and tongue. The largest portion of the cortical map is devoted to the glabrous surface of the hand and foot; each finger has its own separate representation along the medial-to-lateral axes of the cortex. The maps in areas 3b and 1 form mirror images of the distal-proximal or dorsal-ventral axes of each dermatome. (**M** = mandible or lower jaw, **V** = maxilla or upper jaw.)

skin on the fingers as to a square centimeter of skin on the abdomen. Similarly, large numbers of cortical neurons receive input from the foot and face. More than any other part of the body, the hands, face, and feet are important sensors of the properties of objects and thus have the highest density of touch receptors. The proximal portions of the limbs and trunk are much less densely innervated; correspondingly, fewer cortical neurons receive inputs from these regions.

In lower species the hand representation in the brain is smaller than in primates, as these animals use other body parts to probe the environment. For exam-

ple, rodents use their whiskers for tactile exploration rather than their hands. The representation of the whisker fields in the cortex is larger than that of the paw, forming distinct morphological structures called barrels (Box 23-2).

An important consequence of the magnification of the hand representation in the cortex is that the size of individual peripheral receptive fields on the hand cover a much smaller area of skin than receptive fields on the arm, which are smaller than receptive fields on the trunk. For example, receptive fields in the hand region may cover the tips of one or more fingers (Figure 23-3)

Box 23-2 The Cortical Representation of Whiskers in Rodents Is Precisely the Same From Animal to Animal

In rodents the whiskers are the principal tactile receptors. Thus the region surrounding the mouth is more extensively represented in the cortex than are the paws. Each whisker is innervated by a separate vibrissal nerve containing about 100 myelinated fibers, which are activated by movements of the whiskers in specific directions.

The cortical representation of the whiskers has a unique structure. The neurons of layer IV are arranged in discrete functional units called barrels, so-called because when the cortex is cut tangentially, parallel to the cortical surface, the cell bodies of layer IV appear to form barrel-shaped arrays around a neuropil of axons and dendrites (Figure 23-9). Each barrel processes tactile input principally from a single whisker. The number of barrels is the same as the number of vibrissae on the contralateral side of the face, and the barrels are arranged in a pattern that corresponds to the topography of the whiskers.

The fact that each barrel represents a morphologically distinct group of tactile receptors makes it useful for studying plasticity of the cortical maps. Selective removal of vibrissae or vibrissal follicles, or distinctive patterns of stimulation of specific vibrissae, result in alterations in neuronal firing patterns in both the test and adjacent barrel fields. There is also a dynamic interaction between adjacent whiskers in the supragranular and infragranular layers of the cortex.

The unique morphology of the rodent barrel fields allows experimenters to correlate specific cortical locations with function without having to perform direct electrophysiological recordings. Thus measurements can be made of cytochemical, morphological, and metabolic changes related to altered sensory input.

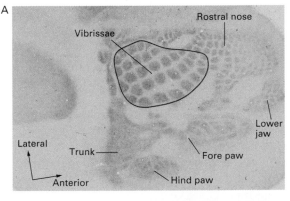

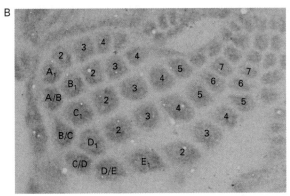

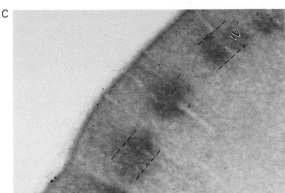

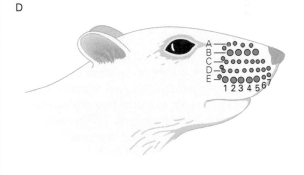

Figure 23-9 The representation of whiskers in the somatosensory cortex of the rat. (Adapted from Bennett-Clarke et al. 1997).

A. Photomicrograph of a horizontal section through layer IV of the somatosensory cortex of a juvenile rat that has been stained for serotonin. The dark immunoreactive patches correspond to the cortical representations of specific parts of the body. The largest part of the cortical map is devoted to the face representation (whiskers, nose, and lower jaw).

B. Enlarged view of the whisker representation. Neurons that receive projections from the whisker fields are arranged in discrete circular units called *barrels*. Each barrel is most responsive to a single whisker.

C. Coronal section through the rat somatosensory cortex. The barrels form dense patches localized to layer IV of the cortex.

D. The topographic arrangement of the barrels in the cortex corresponds to the spatial arrangement of the whiskers in discrete rows and columns on the face.

whereas receptive fields on the forearm may span the entire ulnar surface (Figure 23-4). The large receptive fields for proximal portions of the body (due to the low innervation density) grow proportionally greater at each successive relay.

Cortical Receptive Fields Are Altered by Use of the Hand

An important feature of somatotopic maps is that they are not fixed but can be altered by experience. While the general medial-to-lateral and rostral-to-caudal arrangement of cortical columns is the same in all individuals, the details of the map vary between individuals. A tennis champion will develop a larger proportion of cortical neurons devoted to sensory inputs from the arm than a pianist, who needs to differentiate inputs from individual fingers. As we saw in Chapter 20, the configuration of the map in individual animals can be altered experimentally by fusing adjacent digits or by increased stimulation of a particular finger.

Inhibitory Networks Sharpen Spatial Resolution by Restricting the Spread of Excitation

For somatotopic mapping of cortical function it is enough to know which neurons respond to a stimulus at a particular site on the body. For this purpose the receptive fields of individual neurons are identified by touching the skin with a small probe. A more complex receptive field structure emerges when the skin is touched at two or more points simultaneously. Stimulation of regions of skin surrounding the excitatory region of the receptive field of a cortical neuron may reduce the responsiveness of the neuron to an excitatory stimulus because afferent inputs surrounding the excitatory region are inhibitory. These regions of the receptive field of a cortical neuron are called the *inhibitory surround*. This spatial distribution of excitatory and inhibitory activity serves to sharpen the peak of activity within the brain.

The inhibitory responses observed in the cortex are generated by interneurons in the dorsal column nuclei, the ventral posterior lateral nucleus of the thalamus, and the cortex itself. Inhibitory interneurons in relay nuclei form circuits that tend to limit the spatial spread of excitation through divergent connections (see Figure 21-12). Peripheral receptors in the somatic sensory system are not themselves inhibited (Figure 23-10A). At the first relay point in the somatic sensory system the afferent fibers inhibit the activity of cells in the dorsal col-

umn nuclei that surround the cells they excite (Figure 23-10B). Inhibition generated by activity of the most intensely activated receptors reduces the output of projection neurons that are less strongly excited. It permits a winner-take-all strategy, which ensures that the strongest of two or more competing responses is expressed. In addition, the most active output neurons use recurrent collateral fibers to limit the activity of adjacent neurons. This lateral inhibition further sharpens the contrast between the active cells and their neighbors (Figure 23-10C).

Lateral Inhibition Can Aid in Two-Point Discrimination

Inhibitory interactions are particularly important for fine tactile discrimination such as reading Braille. We can understand how this is accomplished by considering the simplest example of spatial discrimination: the ability to distinguish two closely placed point stimuli. We are able to perceive two points rather than one because two distinct populations of neurons are activated. Stimuli applied to two widely spaced positions on the skin set up excitatory gradients of activity in two cell populations at every relay nucleus.

If the two stimuli are brought close together, the activity in the two populations tends to overlap, and the distinction between the two peaks might become blurred. However, the inhibition produced by each stimulus also summates in the zone of overlap. As a result of this more effective inhibition, the peaks of activity in the two responding populations become sharpened, thereby separating the two active populations spatially (Figure 23-11B). This sculpturing role of the inhibition thus preserves the spatial distinction between the two stimuli.

Spatial Detail Is Accurately Represented in the Cortex

How far does this fidelity of the sensory stimulus extend? Studies of cortical neurons using Braille dot patterns, or embossed letters touched by the fingers, indicate that the signal transmitted to the cortex faithfully reproduces the stimulus features encoded by the receptors in the skin. As we saw in Chapter 22, both Merkel disk receptors and Meissner's corpuscles transmit a faithful neural image of such patterns (see Figure 22-8). These sharp sensory images are preserved up to the first stage of cortical processing in area 3b of the somatic sensory cortex. Neurons in area 3b fire bursts as each line segment of a letter is scanned across the receptive field and together faithfully signal its shape (Figure 23-12).

Figure 23-10 The receptive field of a higher-order neuron in the dorsal column nuclei has a characteristic pattern of excitation and inhibition that increases spatial resolution.

A. Many peripheral receptors converge onto a single second-order sensory neuron in the dorsal column nuclei. As a consequence, the excitatory receptive field of the central neuron is made up of the receptive fields of all the presynaptic cells.

B. The receptive field of a neuron in the dorsal column nuclei and in the ventral posterior nuclei of the thalamus typically has a central excitatory receptive field surrounded or flanked by an inhibitory region. The addition of inhibitory interneurons (**gray**) narrows the discharge zone. Feed-forward inhibition sharpens the representation of a punctate stimulus by limiting the spread of excitation through convergent neural networks. On either side of the excitatory region the discharge rate is driven below the resting level by inhibition.

C. The asymmetric distribution of inhibitory interneurons produces lateral inhibition. In this schematic network, stimulation in the upper portion of the receptive field produces strong excitation of the relay neuron. Stimulation of the lower portion of the receptive field inhibits firing because the interneurons produce feed-forward inhibition. Stimulation in the zone of overlap of excitation and inhibition reduces the responsiveness of the relay neuron to the stimulus. Lateral inhibition is particularly important for feature detection.

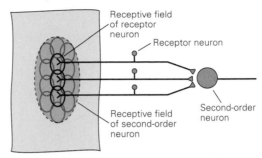

A Convergent excitation

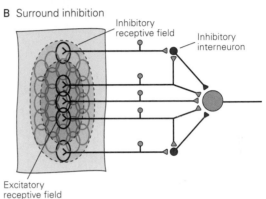

B Surround inhibition

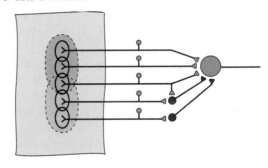

C Lateral inhibition

The cortical representation of each letter is further sharpened by a pause in firing as the moving edges exit the excitatory receptive field and enter its inhibitory surround. The contrast between the spike bursts and subsequent silent intervals permits the letters to stand out from the noisy background activity.

Neurons in area 3b are able to signal the precise shape of the letters moved over the finger because their receptive fields are smaller than the letters. The individual line segments that characterize each letter are viewed one at a time as they cross the neuron's receptive field. The spatial arrangement of stimulated and unstimulated regions of skin is represented in the cortex in columns of active and silent neurons.

In later stages of cortical processing, however, the responses are more abstract. For example, activity in neurons in area 1 does not reproduce the shape of the letters but instead signals specific features common to groups of letters, such as the presence of vertical or horizontal line segments. Since certain cortical neurons represent letter stimuli faithfully and neurons at a later stage do not, it should be possible to determine the intermediate step by which the initial representation becomes abstracted.

Neurons in Higher Cortical Areas Have Complex Feature-Detecting Properties

To produce a coherent sensation of an object the nervous system must integrate information from a large number and variety of receptors as well as the modalities of touch, proprioception, and temperature. How is this integration accomplished? At least four factors are in-

A One-point stimulus

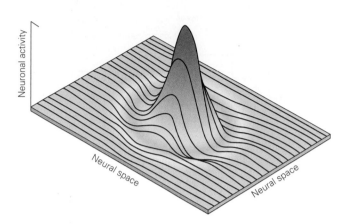

B Two-point stimulus

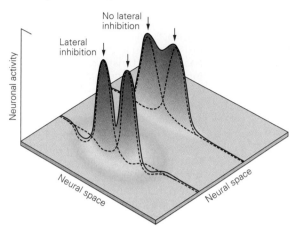

Figure 23-11 Two-point discrimination depends on separation of the signals from each source. (Adapted from Mountcastle and Darian-Smith 1968.)

A. Stimulation of a single point on the skin activates one population of cells in the cortex. Maximal activity is in the center of the population. These neurons are surrounded by a band of neurons whose firing rates are depressed below normal tonic levels by the actions of interneurons that form lateral inhibitory networks.

B. Stimulation of two adjacent points activates two populations of receptors, each with a peak of activity (**dotted lines**). Normally the convergence of the two active populations in the central nervous system would result in a single large group of undistinguished inputs (all excitatory). However, lateral inhibitory networks suppress excitation of the neurons between the points, sharpening the central focus and preserving the spatial clarity of the original stimulus (**solid line**).

volved: (1) The size of the receptive field becomes larger at each level of processing, so that eventually the entire object rather than a single edge is sensed by a neuron. (2) The profile of activity in the active population of neurons changes through the action of inhibitory networks. (3) At successive levels of sensory processing in the cortex individual neurons respond to more complex inputs. (4) The submodalities converge on individual neurons in association cortical areas.

We have seen that neurons in area 3b provide a detailed representation of the properties of an individual object such as an embossed letter. They respond to a particular form and amount of energy at a specific location in space and together reproduce its shape. As information flows from the initial stages of cortical processing toward higher-order cortical areas, specific combinations of stimuli or stimulus patterns are needed to excite individual neurons. Neurons in areas 1 and 2 are concerned with more abstract properties of tactile stimuli than simply the site of stimulation. These cells ignore many of the myriad details of a stimulus and instead detect regularities amid the confusion. Their firing patterns signal features such as the orientation of edges, the direction of motion across the skin, the surface curvature of objects, or the spatial arrangement of repeated patterns that form textures. Feature detection is a basic principle of cortical processing that allows the brain to

find patterns common to stimuli of a particular class.

Experiments using alert animals have revealed a variety of feature-detection neurons in the cortex. Some cortical neurons in area 2 respond preferentially to specific combinations of simultaneously stimulated receptors. Such *orientation-sensitive* neurons sense the angle of edges contacted by the skin (Figure 23-13A). This information is extremely important in reconstructing the shapes of objects. Other cells are *direction sensitive*. They respond vigorously when the skin is stroked in a preferred direction and are unresponsive when the same region of skin is stroked in the opposite direction (Figure 23-13B). Some neurons in area 2 are even more specialized, sensing the spacing or alignment of ridges in a grating when the hand is rubbed over its surface.

The ability of a cortical neuron to detect the orientation of an edge or direction of motion results from the spatial arrangement of its input neurons (Figure 23-14). The excitatory receptive fields of the input neurons are aligned along the preferred axis and produce a strong excitatory response when the stimulus orientation matches that of the receptive fields. In addition, the inhibitory receptive fields are placed to one side of the excitatory fields, suppressing inputs with the "wrong" orientation or approaching from the "wrong" direction.

The convergent projections from areas 3a and 3b onto areas 1 and 2 permit neurons in area 2 to respond

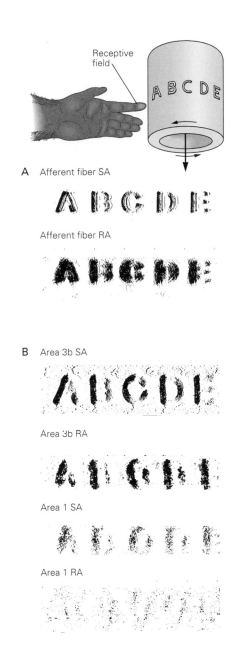

Figure 23-12 The spatial characteristics of embossed letters are accurately represented by neurons in area 3b of the primary somatic sensory cortex but not in area 1. (Adapted from Phillips et al. 1988.)

A. Spatial event plots (see Figure 22–8A) for the principal tactile afferent fibers of the hand: the slowly adapting (**SA**) Merkel disk receptors and rapidly adapting (**RA**) Meissner's corpuscles. Both SA and RA receptors accurately encode the shape of each letter.

B. Spatial event plots for neurons in areas 3b and 1 of an awake monkey. In area 3b slowly adapting (SA) receptors continue to signal the shape of the letters, but rapidly adapting (RA) neurons are more sensitive to the vertical leading edges. In area 1 SA neurons sense particular features of the letter (in this case the vertical but not horizontal components) while the RA neuron illustrated failed to represent form.

to other complex features, such as the shape of objects. Whereas neurons in 3b and 1 respond only to touch, and neurons in areas 3a respond only to position sense, certain neurons in area 2 have both inputs. These neurons respond best when an object of a specific shape is grasped by the hand. Some of these cells respond more vigorously to round objects than to objects with distinct edges, while others are activated selectively by rectangular objects. As we shall see below, this information is thought to provide the necessary tactile clues for skilled movement of the fingers.

Detection of the direction of movement and of other features of the stimulus is not apparent in neurons in the dorsal column nuclei, in the thalamus, or even in areas 3a and 3b. Feature-detecting neurons sensitive to stimulus direction and orientation are first found in area 1 and are represented more extensively in area 2, the areas concerned with stereognosis (the three-dimensional perception of objects) and with discriminating the direction of movement of objects on the skin. Thus, these complex stimulus properties arise not from thalamic input but from cortical processing of more elementary inputs.

In the posterior parietal cortex (areas 5 and 7) the somatosensory responses are even more complex and are often integrated with other sensory modalities. These association cortical areas play an important role in the sensory guidance of movement and are consequently organized functionally rather than topographically (Chapter 19). Many neurons in area 5 receive inputs from several adjacent joints or groups of muscles that provide information about the posture of the entire hand or arm, particularly when monkeys reach out their hands to grasp objects. Other cells integrate tactile and postural information and are most vigorously activated when the monkey preshapes the hand to grasp and acquire objects, or plucks food morsels from a small container.

Neurons in area 7 of the posterior parietal cortex integrate tactile and visual stimuli that overlap in space and play an important role in eye-hand coordination. They respond more vigorously when the monkey is able to observe its hand while manipulating objects of interest than when simply looking at the object or handling it in the dark. Such neurons are used to monitor visually guided hand movements rather than to convey detailed sensory information concerning the exact position or intensity of touch.

Stimulus Features Are Processed in Parallel by Distinct Areas of Cortex

We have seen that specific stimulus features are represented in discrete somatosensory cortical areas. Neu-

A Orientation-sensitive neuron

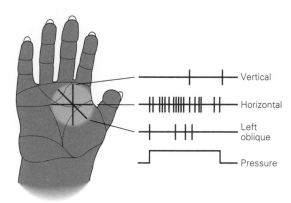

B Direction-sensitive neuron

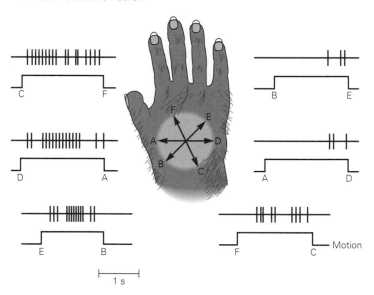

1 s

Figure 23-13 Feature-detection neurons in area 2 of the primary somatic sensory cortex respond to highly specific features of a stimulus. The examples shown here are from a macaque monkey.

A. This orientation-sensitive neuron distinguishes horizontal and vertical edges pressed on the palm. The neuron responds vigorously when the edge is oriented horizontally but is nearly silent when the edge is oriented vertically. Responses to the oblique orientation are weaker than those to the horizontal position. (Adapted from Hyvärinen and Poranen 1978.)

B. This direction-sensitive neuron responds most vigorously to movement across the hand toward the thumb and index finger. The neuron displays its strongest responses to motion in the radial direction (D to A and E to B); the weakest responses occur in the ulnar direction (A to D and B to E). Responses to distal movements toward the fingers (C to F) are more vigorous than responses to proximal movements toward the wrist (F to C). The trace below each cell record shows the duration of motion and the start and end points of the path. (Adapted from Costanzo and Gardner 1980.)

rons in area 3b with small receptive fields sense which finger is contacted and indeed which individual phalanx touches the object. Neurons in area 1 with multifinger receptive fields sense the object size; they fire at higher rates if several fingers are touched and at lower rates if only a small portion of the receptive field is contacted. Neurons in area 2 sense even more complex features, such as the direction of motion across the hand, the curvature of surfaces, the orientation of edges, or the spacing of ridges on textured surfaces. Neurons in area 5 integrate tactile inputs from the skin with proprioceptive postural information from the fingers to encode the shape of objects grasped in the hand. Neurons in the posterior parietal cortex integrate the tactile and proprioceptive information with visual properties of the objects touched.

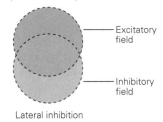

A Relay neuron receptive field

Excitatory field

Inhibitory field

Lateral inhibition

B Convergence of relay neurons produces direction sensitivity

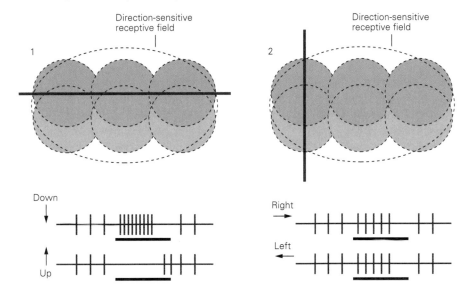

Figure 23-14 The spatial arrangement of presynaptic inputs to a cortical neuron determined which specific features of a stimulus will activate the neuron.

A. Stimuli moving across the receptive field of a relay neuron receiving lateral inhibition (see Figure 23–10) are more effective when the excitatory field is stimulated first because the inhibitory responses are longer in duration than the excitatory responses. Stimuli starting from the excitatory field produce a burst of action potentials followed by inhibition as the stimulus moves into the inhibitory field. Motion in the opposite direction is less effective because the long-lasting inhibitory postsynaptic potential evoked from the inhibitory field decreases the ability of the cell to respond when the stimulus moves into the excitatory field.

B. Convergence of three relay neurons with the same arrange-

ment of excitatory and inhibitory fields confers direction sensitivity on a cortical neuron. In this example the preferred stimulus is a horizontal bar moving downward. **1.** Motion of a horizontal bar across the cortical receptive field (**solid line** below the spike trace). Downward motion of the bar produces a strong excitatory response because it crosses the excitatory fields of all three relay neurons simultaneously. Upward motion of the bar strongly inhibits firing because it enters all three inhibitory fields first. The neuron responds poorly to upward motion through the excitatory field because the initial inhibition outlasts the stimulus. **2.** Motion of a vertical bar across the cortical receptive field evokes a weak response because it crosses excitatory and inhibitory fields of the relay neurons simultaneously. Motion to the left and right are not distinguished in this example.

The somatosensory information necessary for stereognosis is processed in parallel in these areas because palpation involves repetitive touching of the object for several seconds. Such information is not simply relayed from point to point in the brain, as are the somatosensory evoked potentials after a brief shock to the nerve. Instead, tactile sensory information transmitted to higher cortical areas must be compared with more re-

cent information being processed at the early stages. Thus, the activity that occurs simultaneously in different cortical areas is produced by events that happen at different moments in time. Responses in areas 3a and 3b occur 20 ms after touch or movement and therefore reflect stimuli in the immediate past. The more posterior cortical areas receive sensory information at longer latencies, processing stimuli presented 30–100 ms earlier.

How does the brain put together all of these features to form a coherent percept of an object? The firing patterns of neurons in separate cortical areas interact in ways we do not fully understand. The problem of binding together activity in different regions of the cerebral cortex has been studied more extensively for vision than for touch. Those studies of the visual system indicate that the brain may bind together the various stimulus features by synchronizing firing in different cortical areas.

The Behavioral Relevance of a Tactile Stimulus Modifies Cortical Responses

Selective attention can modify firing patterns at the higher stages of cortical processing. Although neurons in S-II are activated by embossed letters scanned across their receptive fields, they do not signal the spatial properties of the letters as do neurons in area 3b. Instead, neuronal responses in S-II depend on behavioral context or motivational state. For example, the firing rates can be altered by varying the letters that are reinforced with rewards or by distracting the monkey with an unrelated visual or auditory discrimination task. These same changes in circumstance have little effect on the spatial information conveyed by neurons in S-I.

The S-II cortex provides the gateway to the temporal lobe via the insular cortex. We shall learn in a later chapter that regions of the medial temporal lobe, particularly the hippocampus, are vital to the formation of memories. We do not store in memory every scintilla of tactile information that enters the nervous system, only information that has some behavioral significance. The demonstration that the firing patterns of S-II neurons are modified by selective attention suggests that S-II serves as a decision point for determining whether a particular bit of tactile information is remembered.

Lesions in Somatosensory Areas of the Brain Produce Specific Sensory Deficits

The earliest information about the function of the somatic sensory system came from the analysis of disease states and traumatic injuries of the spinal cord. For example, one of the late consequences of syphilitic infection in the nervous system is a syndrome called *tabes dorsalis*, which destroys the large-diameter neurons in the dorsal root ganglia, causing degeneration of myelinated afferent fibers in the dorsal columns. Patients who have this degeneration as a result of tabes dorsalis have severe deficits in touch and position sense but often little loss of temperature perception and of nociception.

Additional information about the somatic afferent system has come from studies of the behavioral defects produced by transection of the dorsal columns of the spinal cord in experimental animals or by trauma in humans. Injury to the afferent somatosensory pathways in the dorsal columns results in a chronic deficit in certain tactile discriminations, such as detecting the direction of movement across the skin, the frequency of vibration, the relative position of two cutaneous stimuli, and two-point discrimination. The deficit is ipsilateral to the lesion and occurs at levels below the lesion. Interestingly, some simple spatial discriminations, such as differentiating the size of probes pressed on the skin, can be recovered after extensive retraining and rehabilitative therapy. However, perception of stimuli with complex spatio-temporal patterns, such as distinguishing letters drawn on the skin (*graphesthesia*), is permanently impaired.

In addition to sensory deficits, lesions of the dorsal columns distort natural hand movements. For example, macaque monkeys with a lesion of the cuneate fascicle show major deficits in the control of fine finger movements during grooming, scratching, and manipulation of objects. A similar but reversible deficit in the execution of skilled movements can be produced experimentally in monkeys by pharmacological inhibition of neural activity in area 2 of the cortex. When muscimol (a GABA agonist that inhibits cortical cells) is applied to the hand representation of area 2, the monkey is unable to assume normal functional postures of the hand or coordinate the fingers for picking up small objects (Figure 23-15).

Experimental lesions of the various somatic areas of the cortex have also provided valuable information about the function of different Brodmann's areas concerned with somatic sensibility. Total removal of S-I (areas 3b, 3a, 1, and 2) produces deficits in position sense and the ability to discriminate size, texture, and shape. Thermal and pain sensibilities usually are not abolished, but are altered. In addition, serious motor deficits in hand function occur following major lesions in S-I.

Small lesions in the cortical representation of the hand in Brodmann's area 3b produce deficits in the discrimination of the texture of objects as well as their size and shape. Lesions in area 1 produce a defect in the assessment of the texture of objects, whereas lesions in area 2 alter the ability to differentiate the size and shape of objects. This is consistent with the idea that area 3b receives information about texture as well as size and shape (area 3b, together with 3a, is the principal target for the afferent projections from the ventral posterior lateral nucleus of the thalamus). Area 3b projects to both areas 1 and 2. The projection to area 1 is concerned pri-

Ipsilateral hand

Contralateral hand

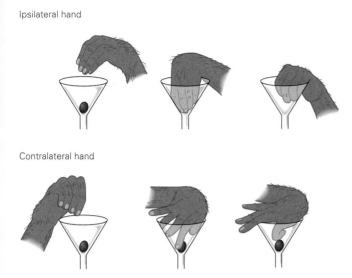

Figure 23-15 A monkey's finger coordination is disrupted when synaptic transmission in the somatic sensory cortex is inhibited. Muscimol, a GABA agonist, was injected into Brodmann's area 2 on the left side of a monkey brain. Within minutes after injection of muscimol, the finger coordination of the right hand (contralateral) is severely disorganized. The monkey is unable to remove a grape piece from a funnel. The injection effects are known to be specific to the injected hemisphere because the left hand (ipsilateral) continues to perform normally. (Adapted from Hikosaka et al. 1985.)

marily with texture, whereas the projection to area 2 is concerned with size and shape.

Because S-II receives inputs from all areas of S-I, removal of S-II causes severe impairment in the discrimination of both shape and texture and prevents monkeys from learning new tactile discriminations based on the shape of an object.

Finally, as we saw in Chapter 20, damage to the posterior parietal cortex produces complex sensorimotor abnormalities. These include the inability to accurately process stimuli in the contralateral visual field or contralateral half of the body. Poor motor coordination and poor eye-hand coordination during reaching, grasping, and hand orientation lead to neglect in usage of the hand.

An Overall View

To perceive how the world impinges on our bodies, the brain is organized to represent the tactile sensory system of the skin. The receptive fields of cortical neurons become progressively more complex with each stage of

information processing, thus extracting more cohesive features of a stimulus at each stage. Cortical receptive fields are larger than those of peripheral receptors due to convergence of inputs from simultaneously stimulated areas of skin.

Cortical neurons are functionally organized in columns, so that all six layers of the cortex in any column receive information representing the same location and modality. The columns are arranged topographically, projecting a precise representation of the external body surface onto the cortical surface. Somatotopy, the orderly projection of the sensory sheet in the brain, permits orderly intracortical connections. However, the somatosensory map or homunculus is not an exact representation of the body surface but is distorted. The finger tips, for example, are represented by a much greater cortical area than are regions like the back. The cortical map represents the density of innervation, hence the functional importance of different areas of the skin.

The body surface has at least eight distinct neural maps in the parietal cortex, four in S-I, two in S-II, and two in the posterior parietal cortex. Each of the four subregions in S-I contains its own map of the body surface, specific to a particular somatic sensory modality. Area 3a receives input primarily from muscle stretch receptors; area 3b receives cutaneous receptor input; area 1 receives input from rapidly adapting receptors; and area 2 contains a map of both cutaneous and deep receptors. As a result, these different regions are responsible for different aspects of somatic sensation. Areas 3b and 1 are involved in sensing surface texture, while area 2 is responsible for sensing the size and shape of objects.

Neurons in areas 2, 5, and 7 are involved in the later stages of somatosensory processing, have more complex feature-detecting properties, receive convergent input from several submodalities, and have larger receptive fields than first-order cortical neurons. At least four types of higher-order somatosensory cells have been found: direction-sensitive, orientation-sensitive, texture-sensitive, and shape-sensitive neurons. Even more complicated processing seems to be carried out by neurons activated when the hand is manipulating an object; these neurons project to the motor cortex for sensory-motor integration. Finally, the S-I cortex sends outputs to the posterior parietal cortex, where integration with other senses and the opposite limb occurs and where an overall picture of the body is formed.

Why are there so many representations of the body surface? Somatic sensation involves the parallel analysis of different stimulus attributes in different cortical areas. Parallel processing in the brain is a form of processing that we shall encounter repeatedly in the sensory systems. It is designed not to achieve multiplication of identical circuitry but to allow different neuronal pathways and brain relays to deal with sensory information in slightly different ways.

Esther P. Gardner
Eric R. Kandel

Selected Readings

Felleman DJ, Van Essen DC. 1991. Distributed hierarchical processing in the primate cerebral cortex. Cereb Cortex 1:1–47.

Gardner EP. 1988. Somatosensory cortical mechanisms of feature detection in tactile and kinesthetic discrimination. Can J Physiol Pharmacol 66:439–454.

Hyvärinen J. 1982. *The Parietal Cortex of Monkey and Man.* Berlin: Springer-Verlag.

Jeannerod M, Arbib MA, Rizzolatti G, Sakata H. 1995. Grasping objects: the cortical mechanisms of visuomotor transformation. Trends Neurosci 18:314–320.

Jones EG. 1986. Connectivity of the primate sensory-motor cortex. In: A Peters, EG Jones (eds). *Cerebral Cortex.* Vol. 5, *Sensory-Motor Areas and Aspects of Cortical Connectivity,* pp. 113–183. New York: Plenum.

Kaas JH, Nelson RJ, Sur M, Merzenich MM. 1981. Organization of somatosensory cortex in primates. In: FO Schmitt, FG Worden, G Adelman, SG Dennis (eds). *The Organization of the Cerebral Cortex: Proceedings of a Neurosciences Research Program Colloquium,* pp. 237–261. Cambridge, MA: MIT Press.

Mountcastle VB. 1995. The parietal system and some higher brain functions. Cereb Cortex 5:377–390.

Mountcastle VB. 1997. The columnar organization of the neocortex. Brain 120:701–722.

References

Bennett-Clarke CA, Chiaia NL, Rhoades RW. 1997. Contributions of raphe-cortical and thalamocortical axons to the transient somatotopic pattern of serotonin immunoreactivity in rat cortex. Somatosens Mot Res 14:27–33.

Burton H, Sinclair RJ. 1994. Representation of tactile roughness in thalamus and somatosensory cortex. Can J Physiol Pharmacol 72:546–557.

Carlson M. 1980. Characteristics of sensory deficits following lesions of Brodmann's areas 1 and 2 in the postcentral gyrus of *Macaca mulatta.* Brain Res 204:424–430.

Carlson M. 1984. Development of tactile discrimination capacity in *Macaca mulatta.* III. Effects of total removal of primary somatic sensory cortex (SmI) in infants and juveniles. Brain Res 318:103–117.

Costanzo RM, Gardner EP. 1980. A quantitative analysis of responses of direction-sensitive neurons in somatosensory cortex of awake monkeys. J Neurophysiol 43: 1319–1341.

Darian-Smith I, Goodwin A, Sugitani M, Heywood J. 1984. The tangible features of textured surfaces: their representation in the monkey's somatosensory cortex. In: G Edelman, WE Gall, WM Cowan (eds). *Dynamic Aspects of Neocortical Function,* pp. 475–500. New York: Wiley.

DiCarlo JJ, Johnson KO, Hsaio SS. 1998. Structure of receptive fields in area 3b of primary somatosensory cortex in the alert monkey. J Neurosci 18:2626–2645.

Favorov O, Kelly DG. 1994. Minicolumnar organization within somatosensory cortical segregates. I. Development of afferent connections. Cereb Cortex 4:408–427.

Favorov O, Kelly DG. 1994. Minicolumnar organization within somatosensory cortical segregates. II. Emergent functional properties. Cereb Cortex 4:428–442.

Favorov O, Whitsel BL. 1988. Spatial organization of the peripheral input to area 1 cell columns. I. The detection of "segregates." Brain Res Rev 472:25–42.

Freund H-J. 1996. Disturbances of motor behavior after parietal lobe lesions in the human. In: O Franzen, R Johansson and L Terenius (eds). *Somesthesis and the Neurobiology of the Somatosensory Cortex,* pp. 331–338. Basel: Birkauser Verlag.

Gardner EP, Hämäläinen HA, Palmer CI, Warren S. 1989. Touching the outside world: representation of motion and direction within primary somatosensory cortex. In: JS Lund (ed). *Sensory Processing in the Mammalian Brain: Neural Substrates and Experimental Strategies,* pp. 49–66. New York: Oxford Univ. Press.

Gardner EP, Ro JY, Debowy D, Ghosh S, 1999. Facilitation of neuronal activity in somatosensory and posterior parietal cortex during prehension. Exp Brain Res 127:(In press).

Hikosaka O, Tanaka M, Sakamoto M, Iwamura Y. 1985. Deficits in manipulative behaviors induced by local injections of muscimol in the first somatosensory cortex of the conscious monkey. Brain Res 325:375–380.

Hsiao SS, O'Shaunessy DM, Johnson KO. 1993. Effects of selective attention on spatial form processing in monkey primary and secondary somatosensory cortex. J Neurophysiol 70:444–447.

Hyvärinen J, Poranen A. 1978. Movement-sensitive and direction and orientation-selective cutaneous receptive fields in the hand area of the post-central gyrus in monkeys. J Physiol (Lond) 283:523–537.

Iwamura Y, Iriki A, Tanaka M. 1994. Bilateral hand representation in the postcentral somatosensory cortex. Nature 369:554–556.

Iwamura Y, Tanaka M. 1991. Organization of the first somatosensory cortex for manipulation of objects: an analysis of behavioral changes induced by muscimol injection into identified cortical loci of awake monkeys. In: O Franzen, J Westman (eds). *Information Processing in the Somatosensory System,* pp. 371–380. London: Macmillan.

Iwamura Y, Tanaka M, Sakamoto M, Hikosaka O. 1985. Comparison of the hand and finger representation in areas 3, 1, and 2 of the monkey somatosensory cortex. In: M Rowe, WD Willis Jr. (eds). *Development, Organization, and Processing in Somatosensory Pathways,* pp. 239–245. New York: Liss.

Johansson RS, Edin BB. 1993. Predictive feed-forward sensory control during grasping and manipulation in man. Biomed Res 14 (Suppl. 4):95–106.

Johnson KO, Hsiao SS, Twombly IA. 1995. Neural mechanisms of tactile form recognition. In: MS Gazzaniga (ed). *The Cognitive Neurosciences,* pp. 253–267. Cambridge: MIT Press.

Jones EG. 1981. Anatomy of cerebral cortex: columnar input-output relations. In: FO Schmitt, FG Worden, G Adelman, SG Dennis (eds). *The Organization of the Cerebral Cortex,* pp. 199–235. Cambridge, MA: MIT Press.

Jones EG, Friedman DP. 1982. Projection pattern of functional components of thalamic ventrobasal complex on monkey somatosensory cortex. J Neurophysiol 48:521–544.

Juliano SL, Hand PJ, Whitsel BL. 1981. Patterns of increased metabolic activity in somatosensory cortex of monkeys, *Macaca fascicularis,* subjected to controlled cutaneous stimulation: a 2-deoxyglucose study. J Neurophysiol 46:1260–1284.

Leinonen L, Hyvärinen J, Nyman G, Linnankowski I. 1979. Functional properties of neurons in lateral part of associative area 7 in awake monkeys. Exp Brain Res 34:299–320.

Leonard CM, Glendinning DS, Wilfong T, Cooper BY, Vierck CJ Jr. 1992. Alterations of natural hand movements after interruption of fasciculus cuneatus in the macaque. Somatosen Motor Res 9:75–89.

Milner AD, Goodale MA. 1995. *The Visual Brain in Action.* Oxford: Oxford Univ. Press.

Mountcastle VB. 1978. An organizing principle for cerebral function: the unit module and the distributed system. In: GM Edelman, VB Mountcastle (eds). *The Mindful Brain,* pp. 7–50. Cambridge, MA: MIT Press.

Mountcastle VB, Powell TPS. 1959. Neural mechanisms subserving cutaneous sensibility, with special reference to the role of afferent inhibition in sensory perception and discrimination. Bull Johns Hopkins Hosp 105:201–232.

Mountcastle VB, Darian-Smith I. 1968. Neural mechanisms in somesthesia. In: VB Mountcastle (ed). *Medical Physiology,* 12th ed., 2:1372–1423. St. Louis: Mosby.

Murray EA, Mishkin M. 1984. Relative contributions of SII and area 5 to tactile discrimination in monkeys. Behav Brain Res 11:67–83.

Nelson RJ, Sur M, Felleman DJ, Kaas JH. 1980. Representations of the body surface in postcentral parietal cortex of *Macaca fascicularis.* J Comp Neurol 192:611–643.

Nicolelis MA, Baccala LA, Lin RC, Chapin JK. 1995. Sensorimotor encoding by synchronous neural ensemble activity at multiple levels of the somatosensory system. Science 268:1353–1358.

Phillips JR, Johnson KO, Hsiao SS. 1988. Spatial pattern representation and transformation in monkey somatosensory cortex. Proc Natl Acad Sci U S A 85:1317–1321.

Pons TP. 1991. A cortical pathway important for tactual object recognition in macaques. In: O Franzen, J Westman (eds). *Information Processing in the Somatosensory System,* pp. 233–244. London: Macmillan.

Pons TP, Garraghty PE, Mishkin M. 1992. Serial and parallel processing of tactual information in somatosensory cortex of rhesus monkeys. J Neurophysiol 68:518–527.

Recanzone GH, Merzenich MM, Jenkins WM, Grajski KA, Dinse HR. 1992. Topographic reorganization of the hand representation in cortical area 3b of owl monkeys trained in a frequency discrimination task. J Neurophysiol 67:1031–1056.

Roland PE. 1993. *Brain Activation.* New York: Wiley-Liss.

Sakata H, Taira M, Murata A, Mine S. 1995. Neural mechanisms of visual guidance of hand action in the parietal cortex of the monkey. Cereb Cortex 5:429–438.

Sur M, Merzenich M, Kaas JH. 1980. Magnification, receptive-field area, and "hypercolumn" size in areas 3b and 1 of somatosensory cortex in owl monkeys. J Neurophysiol 44:295–311.

Sur M, Wall JT, Kaas JH. 1984. Modular distribution of neurons with slowly adapting and rapidly adapting responses in area 3b of somatosensory cortex in monkeys. J Neurophysiol 51:724–744.

Warren S, Hämäläinen HA, Gardner EP. 1986. Objective classification of motion- and direction-sensitive neurons in primary somatosensory cortex of awake monkeys. J Neurophysiol 56:598–622.

Welker E, Van der Loos H. 1986. Quantitative correlation between barrel-field size and the sensory innervation of the whiskerpad: a comparative study in six strains of mice bred for different patterns of mystacial vibrissae. J Neurosci 6:3355–3373.

Woolsey TA, Van der Loos H. 1970. The structural organization of layer IV in the somatosensory region (SI) of mouse cerebral cortex. The description of a cortical field composed of discrete cytoarchitectonic units. Brain Res 17:205–242.

24

The Perception of Pain

T HE SENSATIONS WE CALL PAIN—pricking, burning, aching, stinging, and soreness—are the most distinctive of all the sensory modalities. Pain is, of course, a submodality of somatic sensation like touch, pressure, and position sense and serves an important protective function: It warns of injury that should be avoided or treated. When children with congenital insensitivity to pain injure themselves severely, the injury may go unnoticed and result in permanent damage. Unlike other somatic submodalities, and unlike vision, hearing, and smell, pain has an urgent and primitive quality, a quality responsible for the affective and emotional aspect of pain perception. Moreover, the intensity with which pain is felt is affected by surrounding conditions, and the same stimulus can produce different responses in different individuals under similar conditions.

Pain is a percept; it is an unpleasant sensory and emotional experience associated with actual or potential tissue damage. Although pain is mediated by the nervous system, a distinction between pain and the neural mechanisms of nociception—the response to perceived or actual tissue damage—is important both clinically and experimentally. Certain tissues have specialized sensory receptors, called *nociceptors*, that are activated by noxious insults to peripheral tissues. Nociception, however, does not necessarily lead to the experience of pain. Thus, the relationship between nociception and the perception of pain provides another example of the principle we have encountered in earlier chapters: Perception is a product of the brain's abstraction and elaboration of sensory input.

The highly individual and subjective nature of pain is one of the factors that makes it difficult to define and to treat clinically. There are no "painful stimuli"—stimuli that invariably elicit the perception of pain in all individuals. For example, many wounded soldiers do not feel pain until they are safely removed from battle. Similarly, athletes often do not detect their injuries until their game is over.

Pain can be persistent or chronic. Persistent pain characterizes many clinical conditions and is the major reason why patients seek medical attention, whereas chronic pain appears to serve no useful purpose; it only makes patients miserable. Persistent pains can be subdivided into two broad classes, nociceptive and neuropathic. *Nociceptive pains* result from the direct activation of nociceptors in the skin or soft tissue in response to tissue injury and usually arise from accompanying inflammation. Sprains and strains produce mild forms of nociceptive pain, whereas the pain of arthritis or a tumor that invades soft tissue is much more severe.

Neuropathic pains result from direct injury to nerves in the peripheral or central nervous systems and often have a burning or electric sensation. Neuropathic pains include the syndromes of reflex sympathetic dystrophy and postherpetic neuralgia, a severe pain that occurs in some patients after a bout of shingles. Phantom limb pain can occur after traumatic or surgical limb amputation (see Chapter 20). Anesthesia dolorosa, literally pain in the absence of sensation, sometimes follows therapeutic transection of sensory nerves (eg, the dorsal root nerves) performed in an attempt to block chronic pain.

In this chapter we discuss the basic neural events that underlie the perception of pain as well as abnormal pain states that are clinically important.

Noxious Insults Activate Nociceptors

Harmful stimuli to the skin or subcutaneous tissue, such as joints or muscle, activate several classes of nociceptor terminals, the peripheral endings of primary sensory neurons whose cell bodies are located in the dorsal root ganglia and trigeminal ganglia. We consider here three major classes of nociceptors—thermal, mechanical, and polymodal—as well as a class termed silent nociceptors.

Thermal nociceptors are activated by extreme temperatures (> 45°C or < 5°C). They have small-diameter, thinly myelinated Aδ fibers that conduct signals at about 5–30 m/s. *Mechanical nociceptors* are activated by intensive pressure applied to the skin. They also have

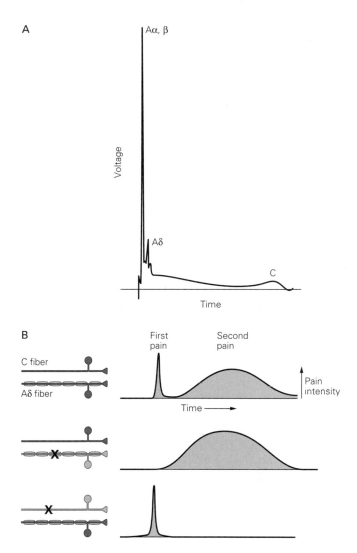

Figure 24-1 Propagation of action potentials in sensory fibers results in the perception of pain. (Modified from Fields 1987.)

A. This electrical recording from a whole nerve shows a compound action potential representing the summated action potentials of all the component axons in the nerve. Even though the nerve contains mostly nonmyelinated axons, the major voltage deflections are produced by the relatively small number of myelinated axons. This is because action potentials in the population of more slowly conducting axons are dispersed in time, and the extracellular current generated by an action potential in a nonmyelinated axon is smaller than the current generated in myelinated axons.

B. First and second pain are carried by two different primary afferent axons. First pain is abolished by selective blockade of Aδ myelinated axons (**middle**) and second pain by blocking C fibers (**bottom**).

Figure 24-2 Nociceptive afferent fibers terminate on projection neurons in the dorsal horn of the spinal cord. Projection neurons in lamina I receive direct input from myelinated (Aδ) nociceptive afferent fibers and indirect input from unmyelinated (C) nociceptive afferent fibers via stalk cell interneurons in lamina II. Lamina V neurons are predominately of the wide dynamic-range type. They receive low-threshold input from the large-diameter myelinated fibers (Aβ) of mechanoreceptors as well as both direct and indirect input from nociceptive afferent fibers (Aδ and C). In this figure the lamina V neuron sends a dendrite up through lamina IV, where it is contacted by the terminal of an Aβ primary afferent. A dendrite in lamina III arising from a cell in lamina V is contacted by the axon terminal of a lamina II interneuron. (Adapted from Fields 1987.)

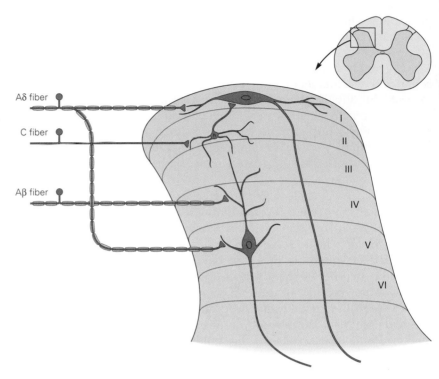

Aδ fiber

C fiber

Aβ fiber

I
II
III
IV
V
VI

thinly myelinated Aδ fibers conducting at 5–30 m/s. *Polymodal nociceptors* are activated by high-intensity mechanical, chemical, or thermal (both hot and cold) stimuli. These nociceptors have small-diameter, nonmyelinated C fibers that conduct slowly, generally at velocities of less than 1.0 m/s (Figure 24-1A).

These three classes of nociceptors are widely distributed in skin and deep tissues and often work together. For example, when you hit your thumb with a hammer, a sharp "first" pain is felt immediately, followed later by a more prolonged aching, sometimes burning "second" pain (Figure 24-1B). The fast sharp pain is transmitted by Aδ fibers that carry information from thermal and mechanical nociceptors. The slow dull pain is transmitted by C fibers that are activated by polymodal nociceptors.

The viscera contain *silent nociceptors*. Normally these receptors are not activated by noxious stimulation yet their firing threshold is dramatically reduced by inflammation and by various chemical insults. Thus, the activation of silent nociceptors may contribute to the development of secondary hyperalgesia and central sensitization, two syndromes discussed later in the chapter.

Unlike the specialized somatosensory receptors for touch and pressure, most nociceptors are free nerve endings. The mechanism by which noxious stimuli depolarize free sensory endings and generate action po-

tentials is not known. The membrane of the nociceptor is thought to contain proteins that convert the thermal, mechanical, or chemical energy of noxious stimuli into a depolarizing electrical potential. One such protein is the receptor for capsaicin, the active ingredient in hot peppers. The capsaicin, or vanilloid, receptor is found exclusively in primary afferent nociceptors and mediates the pain-producing actions of capsaicin. Importantly, the receptor also responds to noxious heat stimuli, which suggests that it also is a transducer of painful heat stimuli.

Many factors in addition to the level of activity of Aδ and C fibers determine the location, intensity, and quality of the pain. Whereas the perception of touch or pressure is consistent when touch-pressure receptors are electrically stimulated, activation of the same nociceptor can lead to different reported sensations. This can be illustrated with a simple experiment in which a blood pressure cuff is placed around the arm and inflated above systolic pressure for about 30 minutes. This procedure produces temporary anoxia and blocks conduction in large-diameter Aα and Aβ fibers; C fibers are still able to conduct action potentials and respond to noxious stimulation. The blockage of conduction occurs because these fibers have a higher metabolic demand than C fibers and, as a result, large motor axons no longer conduct impulses and the arm is paralyzed. In

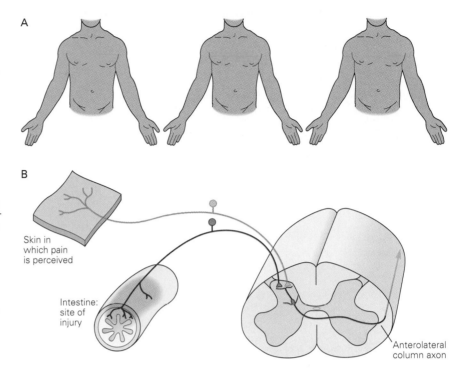

Figure 24-3 Signals from nociceptors in the viscera can be felt as pain elsewhere in the body. The source of the pain can be readily predicted from the site of referred pain.

A. Myocardial infarction and angina can be experienced as deep referred pain in the chest and left arm. (From Teodori and Galletti 1962.)

B. Convergence of visceral and somatic afferent fibers may account for referred pain. According to this hypothesis nociceptive afferent fibers from the viscera and afferents from specific somatic areas of the periphery converge on the same projection neurons in the dorsal horn. The brain has no way of knowing the actual source of the noxious stimulus and mistakenly identifies the sensation with the peripheral structure. (Adapted from Fields 1987.)

addition, there is no touch, vibration, or joint sensation because conduction along Aβ sensory fibers that project into the dorsal column–medial lemniscal system is blocked. In the absence of conduction by the Aα and Aβ fibers, the perception of pain is not normal. For example, a pin prick, a pinch, or ice cannot be distinguished from each other. Rather, each of these normally distinct stimuli now produces burning pain.

This experiment shows that large-diameter Aβ fibers do contribute to the normal perception of stimulus quality, even though they do not respond directly to noxious stimuli. Activity in the large-diameter fiber systems not only modifies the perception of pain but also attenuates it. Thus the reflexive shaking of the hand in response to a burn effectively stimulates large-diameter afferents that can attenuate the pain.

Although the perception of pain normally varies among individuals and in different contexts, abnormal pain states can be diagnosed reliably. In pathological situations activation of nociceptors can lead to two types of abnormal pain states: allodynia and hyperalgesia. In *allodynia*, pain results from stimuli that normally are innocuous: a light stroking of sunburned skin, the movement of joints in patients with rheumatoid arthritis, even getting out of bed the morning after a vigorous workout (particularly when one is not in shape). Pa-

tients with allodynia do not feel constant pain; in the absence of a stimulus there is no pain. In contrast, patients with *hyperalgesia,* an excessive response to noxious stimuli, often perceive pain spontaneously.

Nociceptive Afferent Fibers Terminate on Neurons in the Dorsal Horn of the Spinal Cord

Nociceptive afferent fibers terminate predominantly in the dorsal horn of the spinal cord. The dorsal horn can be subdivided into six distinct layers (laminae) on the basis of the cytological features of its resident neurons (Figure 24-2). Classes of primary afferent neurons that convey distinct modalities terminate in distinct laminae of the dorsal horn. Thus there is a close correspondence between the functional and anatomical organization of neurons in the dorsal horn of the spinal cord.

Nociceptive neurons are located in the superficial dorsal horn, in the marginal layer (also called lamina I) and the substantia gelatinosa (lamina II). The majority of these neurons receive direct synaptic input from Aδ and C fibers. Many of the neurons in the marginal layer (lamina I) respond exclusively to noxious stimulation (and thus are called *nociceptive-specific neurons*) and project to higher brain centers. Some neurons in this layer, called *wide-dynamic-range neurons,* respond in a graded fashion

A

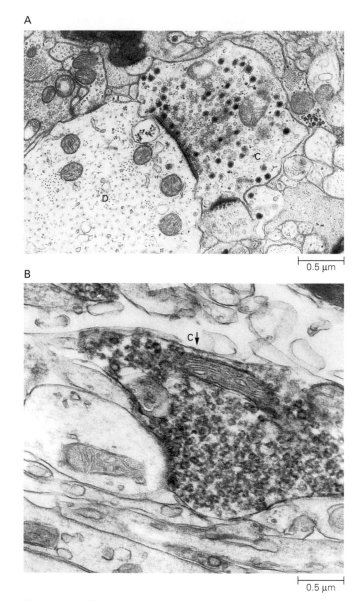

0.5 μm

B

0.5 μm

C

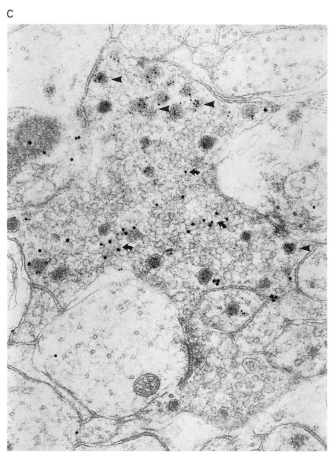

Figure 24-4 Electron micrographs of synapses formed by primary nociceptive neurons with neurons of the substantia gelatinosa in the dorsal horn of the spinal cord.

A. Synapse of an afferent C fiber terminal on the dendrite (**D**) of a dorsal horn neuron. Two classes of synaptic vesicles in the

primary afferent terminal contain different transmitters. Small electron-translucent vesicles contain glutamate, while large dense-core vesicles contain neuropeptides. (Courtesy of H. J. Ralston, III.)

B. Localization of substance P in the terminal of a C fiber afferent (**arrow**) in the dorsal horn. The electron-dense immunoreaction product is confined to large dense-core vesicles. (Courtesy of S. P. Hunt.)

C. Dark scalloped terminals in lamina II of the dorsal horn double-labeled by antisera to glutamate (large gold particles) and to substance P (small gold particles). Glutamate immunoreactivity is scattered in the axoplasm. Substance P immunoreactivity is mostly over large granular vesicles (**arrows**), but not all LGV are labeled (**arrowheads**). (Courtesy of A. Rustioni.)

to both nonnoxious and noxious mechanical stimulation. The substantia gelatinosa (lamina II) is made up almost exclusively of interneurons (both excitatory and inhibitory), some of which respond only to nociceptive inputs while others respond also to nonnoxious stimuli.

Laminae III and IV are located ventral to the substantia gelatinosa and contain neurons that receive monosynaptic input from Aβ fibers. These neurons respond predominantly to nonnoxious stimuli and have quite restricted receptive fields that are organized

topographically. Lamina V contains primarily wide-dynamic-range neurons that project to the brain stem and to regions of the thalamus. These neurons receive monosynaptic input from Aβ and Aδ fibers (Figure 24-2). They also receive input from C fibers, either directly on their dendrites, which extend dorsally into the superficial dorsal horn, or indirectly via excitatory interneurons that themselves receive input directly from C fibers. Many neurons in lamina V also receive nociceptive input from visceral structures.

The convergence of somatic and visceral nociceptive input to lamina V neurons may explain "referred pain," a condition in which pain from injury to a visceral structure is predictably displaced to other areas of the body surface. For example, patients with myocardial infarction frequently report pain not only from the chest but also from the left arm. One explanation for this phenomenon is that a single projection neuron receives input from both regions (Figure 24-3). As a consequence, higher centers cannot discriminate the source of the input and incorrectly attribute the pain to the skin, possibly because the cutaneous input predominates normally. An alternative basis for referred pain is the branching of the axons of peripheral sensory neurons, but this is likely to contribute only to a minority of cases since single afferent fibers rarely innervate both a visceral and a remote cutaneous site.

Neurons in lamina VI receive inputs from large-diameter afferents from muscles and joints and respond to nonnoxious manipulation of joints. These neurons are thought not to contribute to the transmission of nociceptive messages. Finally, neurons in ventral horn laminae VII and VIII, many of which respond to noxious stimuli, have more complex response properties because the nociceptive inputs to lamina VII neurons are polysynaptic. Furthermore, although most dorsal horn neurons receive input from only one side of the body, many neurons in lamina VII respond to stimulation of either side. Thus, neurons of lamina VII, through their connections with the brain stem reticular formation, may contribute to the diffuse nature of many pain conditions.

Nociceptive Afferent Fibers Use Glutamate and Neuropeptides As Neurotransmitters

Synaptic transmission between nociceptors and dorsal horn neurons is mediated by chemical neurotransmitters released from central sensory nerve endings. The major excitatory neurotransmitter released by Aδ and C fibers as well as by nonnociceptive afferents is the amino acid glutamate. The release of glutamate from sensory terminals evokes fast synaptic potentials in dorsal horn neurons by activating the AMPA-type glutamate receptors (see Chapter 12).

The primary afferent fibers of nociceptive neurons also elicit slow excitatory postsynaptic potentials in dorsal horn neurons by releasing peptide transmitters. Small-diameter primary afferent terminals in the dorsal horn contain *both* small electron-translucent synaptic vesicles that store glutamate and large dense-core vesicles that store neuropeptides (Figures 24-4 and 24-5). Of the many neuropeptides present in nociceptive sensory neurons, substance P has been studied in most detail.

Substance P is released from C fibers in response to tissue injury or to intense stimulation of peripheral nerves.

Glutamate and neuropeptides are released together from primary afferent terminals and have distinct physiological actions on postsynaptic neurons, but they act coordinately to regulate the firing properties of postsynaptic neurons. Neuropeptides, including substance P, appear to enhance and prolong the actions of glutamate.

The range of action of the two classes of transmitters may also differ. The actions of glutamate released from sensory terminals are confined to postsynaptic neurons in the immediate vicinity of the synaptic terminal as a result of the efficient reuptake of amino acids into glial cells or nerve terminals. In contrast, neuropeptides released from sensory terminals can diffuse considerable distances from their site of release because there is no specific reuptake mechanism. Thus, the release of neuropeptides from a single afferent fiber is likely to influence many postsynaptic dorsal horn neurons. This feature, together with the fact that peptide levels are significantly increased in persistent pain conditions, suggests that peptide actions contribute both to the excitability of dorsal horn neurons and to the unlocalized character of many pain conditions.

Hyperalgesia Has Both Peripheral and Central Origins

Changes in Nociceptor Sensitivity Underlie Primary Hyperalgesia

Upon repeated application of noxious mechanical stimuli, nearby nociceptors that were previously unresponsive to mechanical stimuli now become responsive, a phenomenon called *sensitization* (Figure 24-6). This mechanism is thought to be mediated by an *axon reflex*, similar to the spread of vasodilation in the vicinity of a localized region of cutaneous injury (discussed below).

The sensitization of nociceptors after injury or inflammation results from the release of a variety of chemicals by the damaged cells and tissues in the vicinity of the injury. These substances include bradykinin, histamine, prostaglandins, leukotrienes, acetylcholine (ACh), serotonin, and substance P (Table 24-1). Each originates from a different population of cells, but all act to decrease the threshold for activation of nociceptors. Some, however, also activate nociceptors. For example, histamine released from damaged mast cells in response to tissue injury activates polymodal nociceptors (Figure 24-7).

ATP, ACh, and serotonin are released from damaged endothelial cells and platelets and act alone or in

A Substance P

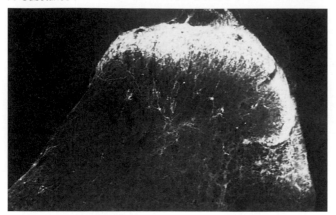

B Enkephalin

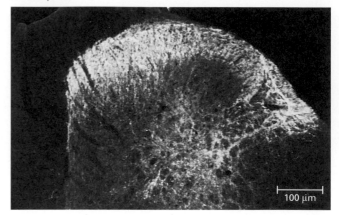

100 µm

C Substance P receptor

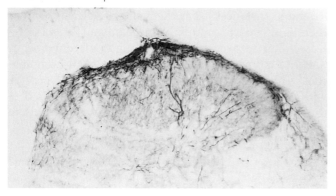

D µ-opioid receptor

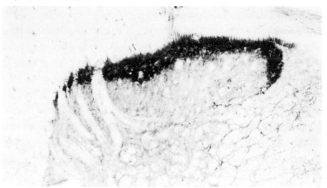

Figure 24-5 Localization of peptides and receptors in the superficial dorsal horn of the spinal cord.

A. Substance P is concentrated in primary afferent terminals located in the superficial dorsal horn.

B. Enkephalin is localized in interneurons concentrated in the superficial dorsal horn, in the same region as afferent terminals

containing substance P. (**A** and **B** courtesy of S.P. Hunt.)

C. Substance P receptor immunoreactivity is localized in the superficial dorsal horn.

D. µ-opioid receptors for enkephalins and other opioids are also localized in the superficial dorsal horn. (**C** and **D** courtesy of A. Basbaum.)

combination to sensitize nociceptors via *other* chemical agents, such as prostaglandins and bradykinin. Prostaglandin E$_2$ is a metabolite of arachidonic acid and is generated by the enzyme cyclooxygenase released from damaged cells. Aspirin and other nonsteroidal anti-inflammatory analgesics are effective in controlling pain because they block the enzyme cyclooxygenase, thereby preventing the synthesis of prostaglandins. The peptide bradykinin is one of the most active pain-producing agents. This high degree of activity is thought to result from its two distinct actions. First, bradykinin activates both Aδ and C nociceptors directly; second, it increases the synthesis and release of prostaglandins from nearby cells.

Primary nociceptive neurons regulate their chemical environment through chemical mediators, which are

synthesized in the cell body (Chapters 4 and 5) and then transported to the peripheral terminal, where they are stored and released upon depolarization of the terminal. For example, injury leads to the release of two neuroactive peptides—substance P and calcitonin gene-related peptide—from nociceptive sensory endings. These two peptides contribute to the spread of edema by acting directly on venules to produce vasodilation. They also contribute to hyperalgesia by leading to the release of histamine from mast cells, which decreases the threshold for activation of nociceptors.

The cardinal signs of inflammation are heat (*calor*), redness (*rubor*), and swelling (*tumor*). Local application of substance P can reproduce all three of these symptoms. Heat and redness are produced by dilation of peripheral blood vessels, whereas swelling results from plasma extravasation, a process in which proteins and cells leak out of postcapillary venules accompanied by fluid. Since this inflammation is mediated by neural activity, it is referred to as *neurogenic inflammation*. Nonpeptide antagonists of substance P can completely block neurogenic inflammation in humans, an example of how the understanding of basic mechanisms of nociception can have clinical applications.

The Hyperexcitability of Dorsal Horn Neurons Underlies Centrally Mediated Hyperalgesia

Under conditions of severe and persistent injury, C fibers fire repetitively and the response of dorsal horn neurons increases progressively. This phenomenon, called "wind-up," is dependent on the release of the excitatory transmitter glutamate from C fibers and consequent opening of postsynaptic ion channels gated by the *N*-methyl-D-aspartate (NMDA)-type glutamate receptor. Thus, blocking NMDA-type receptor activity can block wind-up. Noxious stimulation can therefore produce long-term changes in dorsal horn neurons in a manner similar to long-term potentiation, a process by which long-term changes in synaptic transmission are elicited in the hippocampus and other regions of the brain (see Chapter 63). NMDA-type glutamate receptors also have a role in producing the hyperexcitability of dorsal horn neurons that follows tissue injury. This phenomenon is termed *central sensitization*, to distinguish it from the sensitization that occurs at the peripheral ending of sensory neurons via activation of the arachidonic acid cascade.

These long-term changes in the excitability of dorsal horn neurons constitute a memory of the C fiber input. In response to peripheral noxious stimuli, neurons in the dorsal horn show an induction of immediate early genes that encode transcription factors such as *c-fos*. There is also an upregulation in the expression of neuropeptides and neurotransmitters and their receptors that presumably changes the physiological properties of these neurons.

Alterations in the biochemical properties and excitability of dorsal horn neurons can lead to spontaneous pain and can decrease the threshold for the production of pain. This is evident in the dramatic phenomenon of phantom limb pain, the persistent sensation of pain that appears to originate from the region of an amputated limb. Until recently, limb amputation was performed under general anesthesia in order to eliminate awareness and memory of the procedure. The spinal cord, however, still "experiences" the insult of the surgical procedure because central sensitization still occurs under general anesthesia. To prevent central

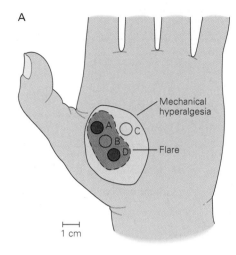

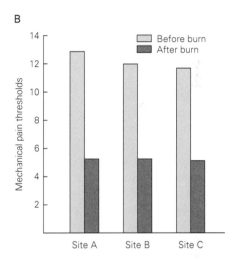

Figure 24-6 Thermal injury can sensitize nociceptors. Burns to the glabrous skin of the hand produce both primary and secondary hyperalgesia to mechanical stimuli, but only primary hyperalgesia to heat stimuli. (Reproduced with permission from Raja et al. 1984.)

A. Mechanical thresholds for pain were recorded at sites A, B, and C before and after burns at sites A and D. The burns consisted of a 53°C stimulus for 30 seconds at both sites. The figure shows the areas of reddening (flare) and mechanical hyperalgesia resulting from the burns in one subject. In all subjects the area of mechanical hyperalgesia was larger than the area of flare. Mechanical hyperalgesia was present even after the flare disappeared.

B. Mean mechanical thresholds for pain before and after burns for seven subjects. The mechanical threshold for pain was significantly decreased after the burn.

sensitization, therefore, general anesthesia is now supplemented with direct spinal administration of an analgesic agent or local infiltration of anesthetics at the injury site.

Table 24-1 Naturally Occurring Agents That Activate or Sensitize Nociceptors[1]

Substance	Source	Enzyme involved in synthesis	Effect on primary afferent fibers
Potassium	Damaged cells		Activation
Serotonin	Platelets	Tryptophan hydroxylase	Activation
Bradykinin	Plasma kininogen	Kallikrein	Activation
Histamine	Mast cells		Activation
Prostaglandins	Arachidonic acid–damaged cells	Cyclooxygenase	Sensitization
Leukotrienes	Arachidonic acid–damaged cells	5-Lipoxygenase	Sensitization
Substance P	Primary afferents		Sensitization

[1]Modified from Fields 1987.

Nociceptive Information Is Transmitted From the Spinal Cord to the Thalamus and Cerebral Cortex Along Five Ascending Pathways

Information about tissue injury is carried from the spinal cord to the brain through five major ascending pathways: the spinothalamic, spinoreticular, spinomesencephalic, cervicothalamic, and spinohypothalamic tracts.

The *spinothalamic tract* is the most prominent ascending nociceptive pathway in the spinal cord. It comprises the axons of nociceptive-specific and wide-dynamic-range neurons in laminae I and V–VII of the dorsal horn (Figure 24-8). These axons project to the contralateral side of the spinal cord and ascend in the anterolateral white matter, terminating in the thalamus. Electrical stimulation of the spinothalamic tract results in pain, whereas lesions of the tract (achieved by a procedure called anterolateral cordotomy) result in marked reductions in pain sensation on the side opposite the spinal cord lesion.

The *spinoreticular tract* comprises the axons of neurons in laminae VII and VIII. It ascends in the anterolateral quadrant of the spinal cord and terminates in both the reticular formation and the thalamus. In contrast to the spinothalamic tract, many of the axons of the spinoreticular tract do not cross the midline.

The *spinomesencephalic tract* comprises the axons of neurons in laminae I and V. It projects in the anterolateral quadrant of the spinal cord to the mesencephalic reticular formation and periaqueductal gray matter, and via the spinoparabrachial tract, it projects to the parabrachial nuclei. In turn, neurons of the parabrachial nuclei project to the amygdala, a major component of the limbic system, the neural system involved in emotion (see Chapter 50). Thus the spinomesencephalic tract is thought to contribute to the affective component of pain. Many of the axons of this pathway project in the dorsal part of the lateral funiculus rather than in the anterolateral quadrant. Thus, if these fibers are spared in surgical procedures designed to relieve pain, such as anterolateral cordotomy, pain may persist or recur.

The *cervicothalamic* tract arises from neurons in the lateral cervical nucleus, located in the lateral white matter of the upper two cervical segments of the spinal cord. The lateral cervical nucleus receives input from nociceptive neurons in laminae III and IV. Most axons in the cervicothalamic cross the midline and ascend in the medial lemniscus of the brain stem to nuclei in the midbrain and to the ventroposterior lateral and posteromedial nuclei of the thalamus. Some axons from laminae III and IV project through the dorsal columns of the spinal cord (together with the axons of large-diameter myelinated primary afferent fibers) and terminate in the cuneate and gracile nuclei of the medulla.

The *spinohypothalamic tract* comprises the axons of neurons in laminae I, V, and VIII. It projects directly to supraspinal autonomic control centers and is thought to activate complex neuroendocrine and cardiovascular responses.

Thalamic Nuclei Relay Afferent Information to the Cerebral Cortex

Several nuclei in the thalamus process nociceptive information. Two are particularly important: the lateral and medial nuclear groups. The *lateral nuclear group* of the thalamus comprises the ventroposterior medial nucleus, the ventroposterior lateral nucleus, and the posterior nucleus. These nuclei receive input via the *spinothalamic tract*, primarily from nociceptive-specific and wide-dynamic-range neurons in laminae I and V of the dorsal horn of the spinal cord. Neurons in these nuclei

Figure 24-7 Chemical mediators can sensitize and sometimes activate nociceptors. Injury or tissue damage releases bradykinin and prostaglandins, which activate or sensitize nociceptors. Activation of nociceptors leads to the release of substance P and CGRP (calcitonin gene related peptide). Substance P acts on mast cells in the vicinity of sensory endings to evoke degranulation and the release of histamine, which directly excites nociceptors. Substance P produces plasma extravasation and CGRP produces dilation of peripheral blood vessels; the resultant edema causes additional liberation of bradykinin. (See Table 24-1 for a list of chemicals that act on nociceptors.) (Adapted from Lembeck and Gamse 1982 and Fields 1987.)

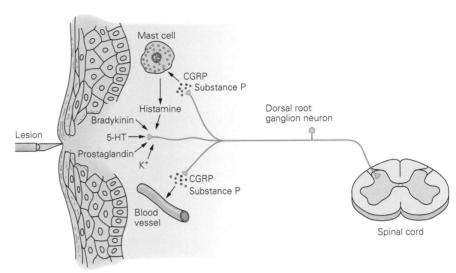

have small receptive fields, as do the spinal neurons that project to them. The lateral thalamus may therefore be mostly concerned with mediating information about the location of an injury, information usually conveyed to consciousness as acute pain.

Injury to the spinothalamic tract and its targets causes a severe pain termed *central pain*. For example, an infarct in a small region of the ventroposterolateral thalamus can produce thalamic (Dejerine-Roussy) syndrome. Patients with this syndrome often experience a spontaneous burning pain and other abnormal sensations (*dysesthesia*) in regions of the body where noxious stimuli normally do not lead to pain. In addition, in certain chronic pain conditions electrical stimulation of the thalamus results in intense pain. In one dramatic case sensations of angina pectoris were rekindled in a patient by electrical stimulation of the thalamus. The report of the patient was so realistic that the anesthesiologist thought the patient was having a heart attack. These observations emphasize that there is a change in thalamic and cortical circuits in chronic pain conditions (Box 24-1). Thus, patients who have experienced persistent pain due to injury have functionally different brains from those who have not experienced such pain.

The *medial nuclear group* of the thalamus comprises the central lateral nucleus of the thalamus and the intralaminar complex. Its major input is from neurons in laminae VII and VIII of the dorsal horn. The pathway to the medial thalamus is the first spinothalamic projection to appear in the evolution of mammals and is therefore known as the *paleospinothalamic tract*. This pathway is also often referred to as the spinoreticulothalamic tract because it includes polysynaptic inputs via the reticular

formation of the brain stem. The projection from the lateral thalamus to the ventroposterior lateral and medial nuclei is most developed in primates and is therefore known also as the *neospinothalamic tract*. Many neurons in the medial thalamus respond optimally to noxious stimuli but also have widespread projections to the basal ganglia and many different cortical areas. They are therefore concerned not only with processing nociceptive information but also with stimuli that activate a nonspecific arousal system.

The Cerebral Cortex Contributes to the Processing of Pain

Until recently most research on the central processing of pain has concentrated on the thalamus. However, pain is a complex perception that is influenced by prior experience and by the context within which the noxious stimulus occurs. Neurons in several regions of the cerebral cortex respond selectively to nociceptive input. Some of these neurons are located in the somatosensory cortex and have small receptive fields. Thus, they may not contribute to the diffuse aches that characterize most clinical pain.

Positron emission tomography (PET) imaging studies of humans also indicate that two other regions of cortex, the cingulate gyrus and the insular cortex, are involved in the response to nociception (Box 24-1). The cingulate gyrus is part of the limbic system and is thought to be involved in processing the emotional component of pain (Chapter 50). The insular cortex receives direct projections from the medial thalamic nuclei and from the ventral and posterior medial thalamic nu-

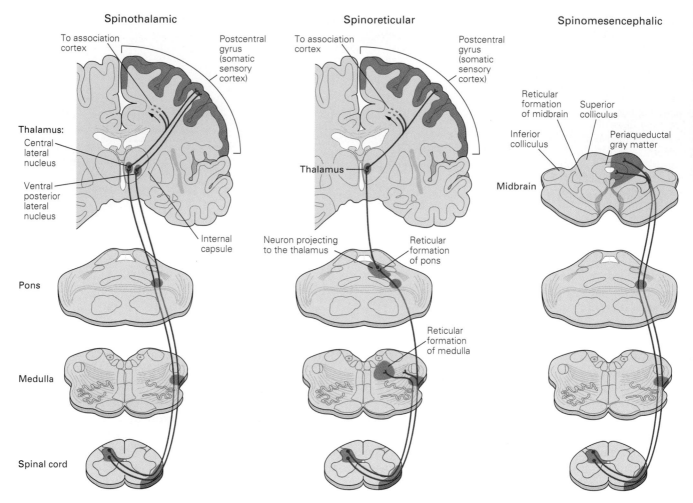

Figure 24-8 Three of the major ascending pathways that transmit nociceptive information from the spinal cord to higher centers. The spinothalamic tract is the most prominent ascending nociceptive pathway in the spinal cord. (Adapted from Willis 1985.)

cleus. The neurons in the insular cortex process information on the internal state of the body, contributing to the autonomic component of the overall pain response. Indeed, lesions of the insular cortex result in an unusual syndrome called *asymbolia for pain*. Patients with this condition perceive noxious stimuli as painful and can distinguish sharp from dull pain but do not display appropriate emotional responses to the pain. The insular cortex may therefore integrate the sensory, affective, and cognitive components, all of which are necessary for normal responses.

Pain Can Be Controlled by Central Mechanisms

One of the most remarkable discoveries in pain research is that the brain has modulatory circuits whose main function is to regulate the perception of pain. Several modulatory systems within the central nervous system affect responses to noxious stimuli. The initial site of modulation is in the spinal cord, where interconnections between nociceptive and nonnociceptive afferent pathways can control the transmission of nociceptive information to higher centers in the brain.

The Balance of Activity in Nociceptive and Nonnociceptive Primary Afferent Fibers Can Modulate Pain: The Gate Control Theory

Pain is not simply a direct product of the activity of nociceptive afferent fibers but is regulated by activity in other myelinated afferents that are not directly concerned with the transmission of nociceptive information. The idea that pain results from the balance of activity in nociceptive and nonnociceptive afferents was formulated in the 1960s and was called the gate control theory (Figure 24-10). This theory incorporates several key observations. First, neurons of lamina V, and possibly lamina I, receive convergent excitatory input from both nonnociceptive Aβ fibers and nociceptive Aδ and C fibers. Second, the large-diameter Aβ fibers inhibit the firing of neurons in lamina V by activating inhibitory interneurons in lamina II. Third, the Aδ and C fibers excite lamina V neurons but also inhibit the firing of the inhibitory interneurons in lamina II, which are activated by the Aβ fibers. Simply put, nonnociceptive afferents "close" and nociceptive afferents "open" a gate to the central transmission of noxious input.

The gate control theory also provides a neurophysiological basis for the observation that a vibratory stimulus that selectively activates large-diameter afferents can reduce pain. The gate control theory is the rationale for the use of transcutaneous electrical stimulation (TENS) and dorsal column stimulation for the relief of pain. In TENS, electrodes are used to activate large-diameter afferent fibers that overlap the area of injury and pain. Stimulation of the dorsal columns via surface electrodes presumably relieves pain because it activates large numbers of Aβ fibers synchronously.

This mechanism of analgesia is topographically specific. The area of the body in which pain is regulated is linked anatomically to the segments of the spinal cord where the nociceptive and nonnociceptive afferents terminate. One does not shake the left leg to relieve pain in the right arm.

Direct Electrical Stimulation of the Brain Produces Analgesia

An even more potent counterbalance to nociception has been found in experimental animals. Here stimulation of the periaqueductal gray region, the gray matter that surrounds the third ventricle and the cerebral aqueduct, produces a profound and selective analgesia. This *stimulation-produced analgesia* is remarkably specific. It is not, for example, associated with a generalized inhibition of afferent inputs. The animal still responds to touch, pressure, and temperature within the body area that is analgesic—it simply feels less pain.

Stimulation of the periaqueductal gray matter also blocks spinally mediated withdrawal reflexes that are normally evoked by noxious stimulation. Blockade occurs because stimulation recruits descending pathways that inhibit nociceptive neurons in the spinal cord. It also inhibits the firing of nociceptive neurons in laminae I and V. Stimulation-produced analgesia has proved to be an effective way of relieving pain in humans under various conditions.

How do the descending pathways recruited by stimulation-produced analgesia relieve pain? Few neurons in the periaqueductal gray matter project directly to the dorsal horn of the spinal cord. Instead they make excitatory connections with neurons of the rostroventral medulla, in particular with serotonergic neurons in the midline of the nucleus raphe magnus. Neurons of this nucleus project to the spinal cord via the dorsal part of the lateral funiculus and make inhibitory connections with neurons in laminae I, II, and V of the dorsal horn (Figure 24-11). Stimulation of the rostroventral medulla inhibits dorsal horn neurons, including neurons of the spinothalamic tract that respond to noxious stimulation.

Other descending inhibitory systems that suppress the activity of nociceptive neurons in the dorsal horn originate in the noradrenergic locus ceruleus and other nuclei of the medulla and pons. These descending projections block the output of neurons in laminae I and V by direct and indirect inhibitory actions. They also interact with endogenous opioid-containing circuits in the dorsal horn (discussed below).

Opiate-Induced Analgesia Involves the Same Pathways as Stimulation-Produced Analgesia

Ever since the discovery of the opium poppy, it has been known that opiates such as morphine and codeine are effective analgesic agents. Are the neural circuits involved in stimulation-produced analgesia and opiate-induced analgesia related?

Microinjection of low doses of morphine or other opiates directly into specific regions of the rat brain produces a powerful analgesia by inhibiting the firing of nociceptive neurons in the dorsal horn. The periaqueductal gray region is among the most sensitive sites for eliciting such analgesia. Morphine-induced analgesia is blocked by injection of the opiate antagonist naloxone into either the periaqueductal gray region or the serotonergic nucleus raphe magnus. Moreover, bilateral transection of the dorsal lateral funiculus in the spinal cord blocks both stimulation-produced and morphine-induced analgesia. These observations indicate that morphine also produces analgesia by activating descending inhibitory pathways.

Opioid Peptides Contribute to the Endogenous Pain Control System

Endogenous Opioid Peptides and Their Receptors Are Located at Key Points in the Pain Modulatory System

The opiate antagonist naloxone blocks stimulation-produced analgesia as well as morphine-induced anal-

Box 24-1 A Sensory Illusion of Pain Localized in the Cerebral Cortex

Thunberg's illusion, first demonstrated in 1896, is a strong, often painful heat felt after touching a grill of alternating warm and cool bars (Figure 24-9A).

This illusory sensation occurs because two classes of neurons in the ascending spinothalamic tract, those that are sensitive to innocuous or noxious cold, respond differently to the grill. This finding has led to a model for the integration of pain perception at the level of the cerebral cortex based on a central disinhibition or unmasking process (Figure 24-9B). The model predicts a quantitative correspondence between grill-evoked pain and cold-evoked pain that has been verified psychophysically. The thalamocortical integration of pain and temperature stimuli can explain the burning sensation felt when nociceptors are activated by cold.

To localize the anatomical site of this unmasking phenomenon in the human brain, positron emission tomography (PET) was used to compare the cortical activation patterns evoked by Thunberg's grill and by cool, warm, noxious cold, and noxious heat stimuli separately. All thermal stimuli activate the insula and somatosensory cortices. Thunberg's grill activates the anterior cingulate cortex (Figure 24-9C). Discrete warm and cool stimuli do not activate this area, whereas noxious heat and cold do.

It appears, therefore, that the anterior cingulate cortex is critical to the perception of thermal pain. Disruption of the integration of thermal and nociceptive stimuli may underlie the central pain syndrome that occurs after damage to neural tissues resulting from a stroke.

A

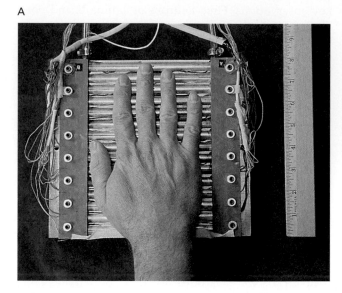

Figure 24-9A The apparatus used to demonstrate Thunberg's illusion. The stimulus surface (20 × 14 cm) was made of 15 sterling silver bars 1 cm wide set about 3 mm apart. Underneath each bar are three longitudinally spaced thermoelectric (Peltier) elements (1 cm²), and on top of each bar is a thermocouple. Alternate (even- and odd-numbered) bars can be controlled independently.

gesia. This finding suggested that the brain contains specific receptors for opiates. Three major classes of opioid receptors have been identified: μ, δ, and κ. The genes encoding each of these receptors have been cloned and found to be members of the G protein-coupled class of receptors (see Chapter 13).

These receptors were originally defined on the basis of their affinity for binding agonists. Opiate alkaloids, such as morphine, are potent agonists at the μ receptor. Indeed, at the μ receptor there is a high correlation between the potency of an analgesic and its affinity for binding to the receptor. Consistent with this idea, mice

in which the gene for the μ opioid receptor has been deleted exhibit an insensitivity to morphine and other μ receptor agonists. Naloxone also binds the μ receptor, but antagonizes the action of morphine by displacing it from the receptor without itself activating the receptor.

The μ-opioid receptors are highly concentrated in periaqueductal gray matter, the ventral medulla, and the superficial dorsal horn of the spinal cord, all of which are important in the regulation of pain. Nevertheless, they are found at many other sites in the central and peripheral nervous systems along with the other opioid receptors. The widespread distribution of these receptors ex-

B

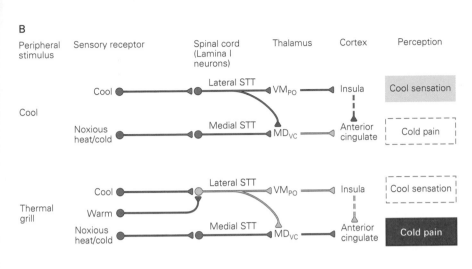

Figure 24-9B Although cool stimuli can excite nociceptive spinothalamic cells, it is hypothesized that they do not produce pain because of the suppressive effect (site of action unknown) of the strongly activated, cool-specific spinothalamic neurons. The grill stimulus has a similar effect, but it is less excitatory to the cool-specific cells so it reduces their suppressive effect on cold pain. Morphine may also activate this pain-suppressive system. "Medial STT" is a conceptual term that refers only to skin temperature test (STT) input to the medial thalamus. In contrast, "lateral STT" is an anatomic term that refers specifically to an ascending bundle (of lamina I axons) in the middle of the lateral funiculus, as opposed to the ventral or anterior STT, which lies in the anterior funiculus. (MD_{VC} = ventral caudal part of medial dorsal nucleus; VM_{PO} = posterior ventral part of medial nucleus.)

C

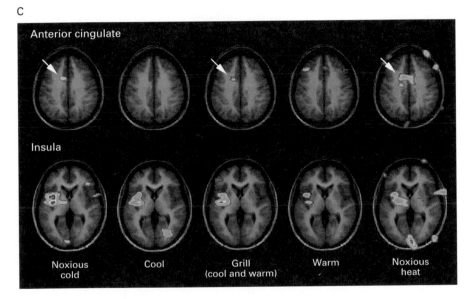

Figure 24-9C The anterior cingulate and insula are activated in human subjects in connection with an intense burning sensation following hand contact with the thermal grill. (Adapted from Craig et al. 1994, 1996.)

plains the finding that systemically administered morphine affects many other physiological processes.

The discovery of endogenous receptors for opiates in the brain raised the question of whether there were corresponding endogenous ligands for these receptors. Three major classes of endogenous opioid peptides that interact with the opioid receptors have now been identified: enkephalins, β-endorphin, and dynorphins (Table 24-2). These three opioid peptides are generated from large polyprotein precursors encoded by three distinct genes: the proenkephalin gene, the proopiomelanocortin gene, and the prodynorphin genes (Figure 24-12).

The two enkephalins—leucine and methionine enkephalin—are both small pentapeptides. β-Endorphin is a product of proopiomelanocortin (POMC), a precursor polypeptide that is expressed primarily in the pituitary and also gives rise to adrenocorticotropic hormone (ACTH). Both β-endorphin and ACTH are released into the bloodstream in response to stress. Dynorphins are derived from the polyprotein product of the *dynorphin* gene. Despite differences in the length of these endogenous opioid peptides, each contains a shared tetrapeptide sequence Tyr-Gly-Gly-Phe (Table 24-2). Enkephalins are active at both μ and δ receptors, and

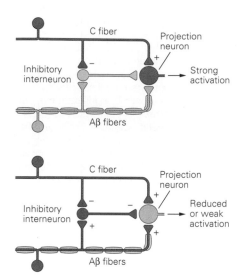

to participate in the regulation of nociception and a broad range of other physiological and behavioral functions.

Activation of Opioid Receptors by Morphine Controls Pain

Opioid receptors are located in regions of the nervous system other than those that mediate pain and thus many of the side effects of using opioids as narcotics can be understood in terms of the distribution of these receptors. For example, receptors are present in the mus-

Figure 24-10 The localized modulation of pain can be explained by the gate control hypothesis. This hypothesis focuses on the interaction of four classes of neurons in the dorsal horn of the spinal cord: (1) nonmyelinated nociceptive afferents (C fibers), (2) myelinated nonnociceptive afferents (Aβ fibers), (3) projection neurons, and (4) inhibitory interneurons. The projection neuron is excited by both nociceptive and nonnociceptive neurons and the balance of these inputs determines the intensity of pain. The inhibitory interneuron is spontaneously active and normally inhibits the projection neuron, thus reducing the intensity of pain. It is excited by the myelinated nonnociceptive afferent but inhibited albeit not directly by the nonmyelinated nociceptor. The nociceptor thus has both direct and indirect effects on the projection neuron.

dynorphin is a relatively selective agonist of the κ receptor.

The peptides encoded by the three opioid genes are distributed differently in the central nervous system, but members of each family are located at sites associated with the processing or modulation of nociception. Neuronal cell bodies and axon terminals containing enkephalin and dynorphin are found in the periaqueductal gray matter, the rostral ventral medulla, and the dorsal horn of the spinal cord, in particular in laminae I and II. β-Endorphin is confined primarily to neurons in the hypothalamus that send projections to the periaqueductal gray region and to noradrenergic nuclei in the brain stem.

In addition to the three classical opioid receptors (the μ, δ, and κ receptors), a novel opioid-like orphan receptor has also been identified. The orphan receptor's endogenous ligand is a 17-amino-acid peptide called orphanin FQ or nociceptin (OFQ/N1-17), which resembles dynorphin. The OFQ/N1-17 receptor is expressed widely in the nervous system, and the peptide appears

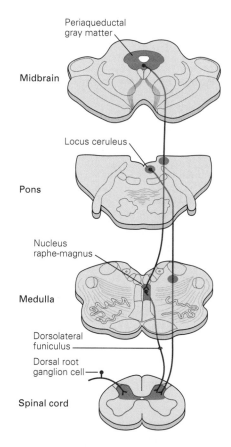

Figure 24-11 A descending pathway regulates nociceptive relay neurons in the spinal cord. The pathway arises in the midbrain periaqueductal gray region and projects to the nucleus raphe magnus and other serotonergic nuclei (not shown), then via the dorsolateral funiculus to the dorsal horn of the spinal cord. Additional spinal projections arise from the noradrenergic cell groups in the pons and medulla and from the nucleus paragigantocellularis, which also receives input from the periaqueductal gray region. In the spinal cord these descending pathways inhibit nociceptive projection neurons through direct connections as well as through interneurons in the superficial layers of the dorsal horn (see Figure 24-10).

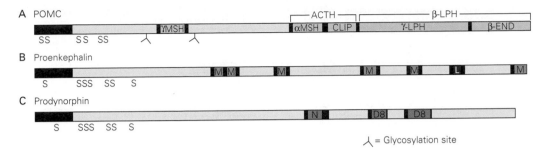

Figure 24-12 The three known families of endogenous opioid peptides arise from three large precursor polyproteins. Each of the precursor molecules gives rise to a variety of biologically active peptide fragments, about half of which are shown in this diagram. (From Fields 1987.)

A. Proopiomelanocortin (POMC) is so named because it gives rise to β-endorphin, melanocyte-stimulating hormone (MSH), adrenocorticotropic hormone (ACTH), and corticotropin-like intermediate lobe peptide (CLIP).

B. Proenkephalin gives rise to multiple copies of metenkephalin (M), a leucine-enkephalin (L), and several extended enkephalins including ME-Arg-Gly-Leu, ME-Arg-Phe, and peptides E, F, and B. Peptide E is further broken down into a family of large enkephalins that appear to be the most potent analgesic fragments derived from proenkephalin.

C. Prodynorphin gives rise to dynorphin (D8), which contains the LE sequence, and neoendorphin (N).

cles of the bowel and the anal sphincter and account for constipation, a common side effect of the action of opiates. Receptors in the cells of the nucleus of the solitary tract in the brain stem account for respiratory depression and cardiovascular changes.

To minimize the side effects of systemic injection, morphine is now also administered locally into the spinal cord. The dorsal horn has a high concentration of opioid receptors, and morphine administration inhibits the firing of dorsal horn neurons responsive to nociceptive stimuli. Indeed, intrathecal or epidural injection of morphine into the cerebrospinal fluid of the spinal cord subarachnoid space produces a profound and prolonged analgesia. These routes of administration are now commonly used in the treatment of postoperative pain, such as the pain that sometimes follows a Caesarean section. In addition to its prolonged effect, the analgesia achieved by intrathecal opiates is associated with minimal side effects because the drug does not diffuse far from the site of injection. Continuous infusion of morphine to the spinal cord has also been used for the treatment of cancer pain.

How does spinal administration of morphine produce its profound analgesic effects? Morphine acts by mimicking the action of the endogenous opioids in this region. The superficial dorsal horn contains a high density

Table 24-2 Amino Acid Sequences of Endogenous Opioid Peptides[1]

Name	Amino acid sequence[2]
Leucine-enkephalin	*Tyr-Gly-Gly-Phe*-Leu-OH
Methionine-enkephalin	*Tyr-Gly-Gly-Phe*-Met-OH
β-Endorphin	*Tyr-Gly-Gly-Phe*-Met-Thr-Ser-Glu-Lys-Ser-Gln-Thr-Pro-Leu-Val-Thr-Leu-Phe-Lys-Asn-Ala-Ile-Val-Lys-Asn-Ala-His-Lys-Gly-Gln-OH
Dynorphin	*Tyr-Gly-Gly-Phe*-Leu-Arg-Arg-Ile-Arg-Pro-Lys-Leu-Lys-Trp-Asp-Asn-Gln-OH
α-Neoendorphin	*Tyr-Gly-Gly-Phe*-Leu-Arg-Lys-Tyr-Pro-Lys

[1]From Fields 1987.
[2]Amino acid sequence in italic is essential for action at opioid receptors.

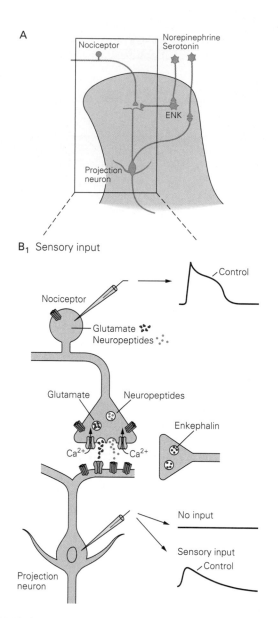

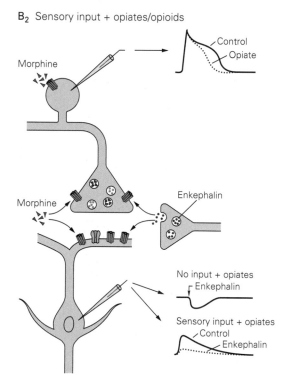

Figure 24-13 Local-circuit interneurons in the superficial dorsal horn of the spinal cord integrate descending and afferent pathways.

A. Possible interactions between nociceptor afferent fibers, local interneurons, and descending fibers in the dorsal horn of the spinal cord. Nociceptive fibers terminate on second-order spinothalamic projection neurons. Local enkephalin-containing interneurons (**ENK**) exert both presynaptic and postsynaptic inhibitory actions at these synapses. Serotonergic and noradrenergic neurons in the brain stem activate the local opioid interneurons and also suppress the activity of spinothalamic projection neurons.

B. 1. Activation of nociceptors leads to the release of glutamate and neuropeptides from sensory terminals in the superficial dorsal horn, thus depolarizing and activating projection neurons. **2.** Opiates decrease the duration of the nociceptor's action potential, probably by decreased Ca^{2+} influx, and thus decrease the release of transmitter from primary afferent terminals. In addition, opiates hyperpolarize the membrane of the dorsal horn neurons by activating a K^+ conductance. Stimulation of the nociceptor normally produces a fast excitatory postsynaptic potential in the dorsal horn neuron; opiates decrease the amplitude of the postsynaptic potential.

of interneurons containing enkephalin and dynorphin, and the terminals of these cells lie close to the synapses between nociceptive afferents and projection neurons (Figure 24-13A). Opioid receptors of all three classes are lo-

cated on the terminals of the nociceptive afferents and on the dendrites of postsynaptic dorsal horn neurons.

Opiates such as morphine and opioid peptides regulate nociceptive transmission with two inhibitory actions: a postsynaptic inhibition, produced partly by increasing K^+ conductance, and presynaptic inhibition of the release of glutamate, substance P, and other transmitters from the terminals of sensory neurons. The opioid-caused decrease in transmitter release from primary afferents results either indirectly from a decrease in Ca^{2+} entry into the sensory terminals (as a result of increased K^+ conductance) or directly from a decrease in Ca^{2+} conductance (Figure 24-13B).

Opioid receptors are not confined to the central terminal of primary afferent fibers but are also located on the peripheral terminals in skin, joints, and muscle. For example, after arthroscopic surgery, prolonged relief of pain results from local injection of morphine into the treated joint at doses that are ineffective when administered systemically. Peripheral administration can significantly reduce side effects. The source of the endogenous opioids that normally activate opioid receptors on peripheral sensory endings is unclear. Two possibilities are the chromaffin cells of the adrenal medulla and various immune cells that migrate to injury sites as part of the inflammatory process and there synthesize endogenous opioids.

Tolerance and Addiction to Opioids Are Distinct Phenomena

As we shall see in Chapter 51, two major problems are associated with the chronic use of morphine: tolerance and addiction. Repeated use of morphine to relieve pain can cause patients to develop increasing resistance to the effects of the drug, so that progressively higher doses are required to achieve the same analgesic effect. Such acquired tolerance is different from addiction, which refers to a psychological craving. Psychological addiction almost never occurs when morphine is used to treat chronic pain, provided the patient has not previously abused opiates.

The mechanisms underlying the development of tolerance are not clear. It has been proposed that tolerance results from an uncoupling of the opioid receptor from its associated G protein. However, naloxone, which binds to the opioid receptor, can precipitate withdrawal in tolerant subjects, suggesting that the opioid receptor is still functional in the tolerant state. Otherwise, naloxone, a drug with no intrinsic activity, would be without effect. Tolerance may therefore result from a compensatory response to the activation of opioid receptors, a response that counteracts the effects of the opiate and returns the system to normal. When the opiate is removed, or when naloxone is administered so as to block the binding of opiates, the compensatory response is unmasked and withdrawal results.

Stress Induces Analgesia Through Both Opioid and Nonopioid Mechanisms

Under conditions of stress or adaptation to an extreme environmental demand, an animal's normal reaction to pain—reflex withdrawal, escape, rest, and recuperation—could be disadvantageous. During stress these reactions to pain may best be suppressed in favor of more adaptive behavior. For example, when a laboratory animal is exposed to a novel and severe adverse stimulus, such as an electric shock to the foot from which it cannot escape, the animal's sensitivity to other painful stimuli is reduced. The time course of such stress-induced analgesia may range from minutes to hours, depending on the nature and severity of the stimulus.

There is now evidence that stress stimulates both opioid and nonopioid mechanisms of analgesia. Some instances of stress-induced analgesia are sensitive to blockade of opiate receptors by naloxone; others are not. Naloxone given alone does not cause pain but can significantly enhance the perceived intensity of protracted clinical pain, for example in patients recovering from dental surgery.

There is anecdotal evidence for stress-induced analgesia in humans. Soldiers wounded in battle and athletes injured in sports events report that they do not feel pain. Indeed, a century ago David Livingstone, the Scottish missionary and explorer of Africa, reported a particularly dramatic personal example. On an early journey to find the source of the Nile, Livingstone was attacked by a lion that crushed his shoulder.

I heard a shout starting, and looking half round, I saw the lion just in the act of springing upon me. I was upon a little height; he caught my shoulder as he sprang, and we both came to the ground below together. Growling horribly close to my ear, he shook me as a terrier does a rat. The shock produced a stupor similar to that which seems to be felt by a mouse after the first shake of the cat. It caused a sort of dreaminess in which there was no sense of pain nor feeling of terror, though quite conscious of all that was happening. It was like what patients partially under the influence of chloroform describe, who see all the operation, but feel not the knife. . . . The shake annihilated fear, and allowed no sense of horror in looking round at the beast. This peculiar state is probably produced in all animals killed by the carnivora; and if so, is a merciful provision by our benevolent creator for lessening the pain of death.

(David Livingstone, *Missionary Travels*, 1857)

An Overall View

Pain is a complex perception. More than any other sensory modality it is influenced by emotional state and environmental contingencies. Because pain is so dependent on experience, and therefore varies from person to person, it is difficult to treat clinically. Although our current understanding of specific pain circuits is still fragmentary, recent advances in understanding the basic physiology of pain mechanisms have led to some effective pain therapies.

First, the finding that the balance of activity in small- and large-diameter fibers is important in pain transmission has led to the use of dorsal column stimulation and transcutaneous electrical nerve stimulation for controlling certain types of peripheral pain. Second, the experimental finding that stimulation of specific sites in the brain stem produces profound analgesia may eventually lead to better ways of controlling pain by activating endogenous pain modulatory systems. Third, the discovery that opiates applied directly to the spinal cord exert potent analgesic effects has led to the administration of opiates in certain conditions by means of intrathecal and epidural routes. Finally, the unraveling of the neurotransmitter systems underlying endogenous pain control circuits should provide a more rational basis for drug therapies in a variety of pain syndromes.

Allan I. Basbaum
Thomas M. Jessell

Selected Readings

Akil H, Watson SJ, Young E, Lewis ME, Khachaturian H, Walker JM. 1984. Endogenous opioids: biology and function. Annu Rev Neurosci 7:223–255.

Basbaum AI. 1995. Unlocking pain's secrets. In: *Encyclopedia Britannica. Medical Health Annual*, pp. 74–95. Chicago: Encyclopedia Britannica.

Basbaum AI, Besson JM (eds). 1991. *Towards a New Pharmacotherapy of Pain*, pp. 1–457. New York: Wiley.

Basbaum AI, Fields HL. 1984. Endogenous pain control systems: brainstem spinal pathways and endorphin circuitry. Annu Rev Neurosci 7:309–338.

Bonica JJ. 1990. *The Management of Pain*, 2nd ed. Philadelphia: Lea & Febiger.

Bromage PR. 1985. Clinical aspects of intrathecal and epidural opiates. In: HL Fields, R Dubner, F Cervero (eds), *Advances in Pain Research and Therapy*, 9:733–748. New York: Raven.

Campbell JN, Raja SN, Cohen RH, Manning DC, Khan AA,

Mayer RA. 1989. Peripheral neural mechanisms of nociception. In: PD Wall, R Melzack (eds), *Textbook of Pain*, 2nd ed., pp. 22–45. Edinburgh: Churchill Livingstone.

Casey KL. 1992. 1991 Bonica lecture. Central pain syndromes: current views on pathophysiology, diagnosis, and treatment. Reg Anesth 17:59–68.

Darland T, Heinricher MM, Grandy DK. 1988. Orphanin FQ/nociceptin: a role in pain and analgesia, but so much more. Trends Neurosci 21:215–221.

Dubner R, Bennett GJ. 1983. Spinal and trigeminal mechanisms of nociception. Annu Rev Neurosci 6:381–418.

Fields HL. 1987. *Pain*. New York: McGraw-Hill.

Fields HL, Liebeskind JC (eds). 1994. *Pharmacological Approaches to the Treatment of Chronic Pain: New Concepts and Critical Issues. The Bristol-Myers Squibb Symposium on Pain Research*. Seattle: IASP Press.

Kelly D (ed). 1986. Stress-induced analgesia. Ann NY Acad Sci 467:1–449.

Levine JD, Fields HL, Basbaum A. 1993. Peptides and the primary afferent nociceptor. J Neurosci 13:2273–2286.

Light AR, Perl ER. 1984. Peripheral sensory systems. In: PJ Dyck, PK Thomas, EH Lambert, R Bunge (eds). *Peripheral Neuropathy*, 2nd ed., 1:210–230. Philadelphia: Saunders.

Melzack R, Wall PD. 1965. Pain mechanisms: a new theory. Science 150:971–979.

Melzack R, Wall PD. 1983. *The Challenge of Pain*. New York: Basic Books.

Price DD. 1988. Psychological and neural mechanisms of pain. New York: Raven.

Terman GW, Shavit Y, Lewis JW, Cannon JT, Liebeskind JC. 1984. Intrinsic mechanisms of pain inhibition: activation by stress. Science 226:1270–1277.

Wall PD, Melzack R (eds). 1994. *Textbook of Pain*, 3rd ed. Edinburgh: Churchill Livingstone.

Wilcox GL. 1991. Excitatory neurotransmitters and pain. In: MR Bond, JE Charlton, CJ Woolf (eds). *Proceedings of the 6th World Congress on Pain*. New York: Elsevier.

Willis WD (ed). 1992. *Hyperalgesia and Allodynia. The Bristol-Myers Squibb Symposium on Pain Research*. New York: Raven.

Willis WD Jr. 1985. *The Pain System: The Neural Basis of Nociceptive Transmission in the Mammalian Nervous System*. Basel: Karger.

Yaksh TL, Noueihed R. 1985. The physiology and pharmacology of spinal opiates. Annu Rev Pharmacol Toxicol 25:433–462.

References

Akil H, Mayer DJ, Liebeskind JC. 1976. Antagonism of stimulation-produced analgesia by naloxone, a narcotic antagonist. Science 191:961–962.

Baumann TK, Simone DA, Shain CN, LaMotte RH. 1991. Neurogenic hyperalgesia: the search for the primary cutaneous afferent fibers that contribute to capsaicin-induced pain and hyperalgesia. J Neurophysiol 66(1):212–227.

Brown JL, Liu H, Maggio JE, Vigna SR, Mantyh PW, Basbaum AI. 1995. Morphological characterization of substance P receptor immunoreactive neurons in the rat spinal cord and trigeminal nucleus caudalis. J Comp Neurol 356:327–344.

Cao YQ, Mantyh PW, Carlson EJ, Gillespie AM, Epstein CJ, Basbaum AI. 1998. Primary afferent tachykinins are required to experience moderate to intense pain. Nature 392:390–394.

Carlen PL, Wall PD, Nadvorna H, Steinbach R. 1978. Phantom limbs and related phenomena in recent traumatic amputations. Neurology 28:211–217.

Cassinari V, Pagni CA. 1969. *Central Pain: A Neurosurgical Survey.* Cambridge, MA: Harvard University Press.

Caterina MJ, Schumacher MA, Tominaga M, Rosen TA, Levine JD, Julius D. 1997. The capsaicin receptor: a heat-activated ion channel in the pain pathway. Nature 389:816–824.

Cervero F, Iggo A. 1980. The substantia gelatinosa of the spinal cord. A critical review. Brain 103:717–772.

Christensen BN, Perl ER. 1970. Spinal neurons specifically excited by noxious or thermal stimuli: marginal zone of the dorsal horn. J Neurophysiol 33:293–307.

Craig AD, Bushnell MC. 1994. The thermal grill illusion: unmasking the burn of cold pain. Science 265:252–255.

Craig AD, Bushnell MC, Zhang ET, Blomqvist A. 1994. A thalamic nucleus specific for pain and temperature sensation. Nature 372:770–773.

Craig AD, Reiman EM, Evans A, Bushnell MC. 1996. Functional imaging of an illusion of pain. Nature 384:258–260.

De Biasi S, Rustioni A. 1988. Glutamate and substance P coexist in primary afferent terminals in the superficial laminae of spinal cord. Proc Natl Acad Sci U S A 85:7820–7824.

Dejerine J, Roussy G. 1906. Le syndrome thalamique. Rev Neurol 14:521–532.

Dickenson AH. 1990. A cure for wind up: NMDA receptor antagonists as potential analgesics. Trends Pharmacol Sci 11:307–309.

Dubner R, Ruda MA. 1992. Activity-dependent neuronal plasticity following tissue injury and inflammation. Trends Neurosci 15:96–103.

Hökfelt T, Zhang X, Wiesenfeld-Hallin Z. 1994. Messenger plasticity in primary sensory neurons following axotomy and its functional implications. Trends Neurosci 17:22–30.

Hosobuchi Y. 1986. Subcortical electrical stimulation for control of intractable pain in humans: report of 122 cases 1970–1984. J Neurosurg 64:543–553.

Koltzenburg M, McMahon SB. 1991. The enigmatic role of the sympathetic nervous system in chronic pain. Trends Pharmacol Sci 12:399–402.

La Motte RH. 1984. Can the sensitization of nociceptors account for hyperalgesia after skin injury? Human Neurobiol 3:47–52.

Lembeck F, Gamse R. 1982. Substance P in peripheral sensory processes. CIBA Found Symp 91:35–54.

Livingstone D. [1857] 1972. *Missionary Travels and Researches in South Africa.* Freeport, NY: Books for Libraries.

Mansour A, Watson SJ, Akil H. 1995. Opioid receptors: past, present and future. Trends Neurosci 18:69–70.

Matthes HW, Maldonado R, Simonin F, Valverde O, Slowe S, Kitchen I, Befort K, Dierich A, Le Meur M, Dollé P, Tzavara E, Hanoune J, Roques BP, Kieffer BL. 1996. Loss of morphine-induced analgesia, reward effect and withdrawal symptoms in mice lacking the μ-opioid-receptor gene. Nature 383:819–823.

McLachlan EM, Jäng W, Devor M, Michaelis M. 1993. Peripheral nerve injury triggers noradrenergic sprouting within dorsal root ganglia. Nature 363:543–546.

McMahon SB, Koltzenburg M. 1990. Novel classes of nociceptors: beyond Sherrington. Trends Neurosci 13:199–201.

McMahon SB, Lewin GR, Wall PD. 1993. Central hyperexcitability triggered by noxious inputs. Curr Opin Neurobiol 3:602–610.

Milne RJ, Foreman RD, Giesler GJ Jr, Willis WD. 1981. Convergence of cutaneous and pelvic visceral nociceptive inputs onto primate spinothalamic neurons. Pain 11:163–183.

Mogil JS, Sternberg WF, Marek P, Sadowski B, Belknap JK, Liebeskind JC. 1996. The genetics of pain and pain inhibition. Proc Natl Acad Sci U S A 93:3048–3055.

Morgan MM, Heinricher MM, Fields HL. 1992. Circuitry linking opioid-sensitive nociceptive modulatory systems in periaqueductal gray and spinal cord with rostral ventromedial medulla. Neuroscience 47:863–871.

Nashold BS Jr, Ostdahl RH. 1979. Dorsal root entry zone lesions for pain relief. J Neurosurg 51:59–69.

Noordenbos W, Wall PD. 1976. Diverse sensory functions with an almost totally divided spinal cord. A case of spinal cord transection with preservation of part of one anterolateral quadrant. Pain 2:185–195.

Raja SN, Campbell JN, Meyer RA. 1984. Evidence for different mechanisms of primary and secondary hyperalgesia following heat injury to the glabrous skin. Brain 107: 1791–1188.

Roberts WJ. 1986. A hypothesis on the physiological basis for causalgia and related pains. Pain 24:297–311.

Ruda MA, Bennett GJ, Dubner R. 1986. Neurochemistry and neural circuitry in the dorsal horn. Prog Brain Res 66: 219–268.

Talbot JD, Marrett S, Evans AC, Meyer E, Bushnell MC, Duncan GH. 1991. Multiple representations of pain in human cerebral cortex. Science 251:1355–1358.

Teodori U, Galletti R. 1962. *Il Dolore nelle Affezioni degli Organi Interni del Torace.* Rome: Pozzi.

Tominaga M, Caterina MJ, Malmberg AB, Rosen TA, Gilbert H, Skinner K, Raumann BE, Basbaum AL, Julius D. 1998. The cloned capsaicin receptor integrates multiple pain-producing stimuli. Neuron 21:531–543.

White JC, Sweet WH. 1969. *Pain and the Neurosurgeon: A Forty-Year Experience.* Springfield, IL: Thomas.

Willis WD Jr. 1995. Neurobiology: cold, pain and the brain. Nature 373:19–20.

Woolf CJ. 1983. Evidence for a central component of post-injury pain hypersensitivity. Nature 306:686–688.

Yaksh TL, Rudy TA. 1976. Analgesia mediated by a direct spinal action of narcotics. Science 192:1357–1358.

25

Constructing the Visual Image

We are so familiar with seeing, that it takes a leap of imagination to realize that there are problems to be solved. But consider it. We are given tiny distorted upside-down images in the eyes, and we see separate solid objects in surrounding space. From the patterns of stimulation on the retina we perceive the world of objects and this is nothing short of a miracle.

Richard L. Gregory, *Eye and Brain*, 1966

MOST OF OUR IMPRESSIONS about the world and our memories of it are based on sight. Yet the mechanisms that underlie vision are not at all obvious to the perceiver or even to the student of perception. How do we see form? How do we perceive movement? How do we distinguish colors? Studies of artificial intelligence and of pattern recognition by computers have shown that the brain recognizes form, motion, depth, and color using strategies that no computer can achieve. Simply to look out into the world and rec-

ognize a face or enjoy a landscape requires an immense computational achievement more difficult than that required for solving logic problems or playing chess.

How is this processing accomplished? This question, which we shall address in this and the next four chapters, is all the more intriguing because information about form, motion, and color is carried not by a single hierarchical pathway, but by at least two (and possibly more) parallel and interacting pathways in the brain.

The existence of parallel pathways in the visual system raises a serious problem that we have considered before—the binding problem. How is information carried by separate pathways brought together into a coherent visual image? In addressing the binding problem in the visual system we confront one of the central questions of cognition: How does the brain construct a perceived world from sensory information, and how does it bring it into consciousness?

Visual Perception Is a Creative Process

Visual perception has often been compared to the operation of a camera. Like the lens of a camera, the lens of the eye focuses an inverted image onto the retina. This analogy breaks down rapidly, however, because it does not capture what the visual system really does, which is to create a three-dimensional perception of the world that is different from the two-dimensional images projected onto the retina. The analogy also fails to reflect the cognitive function of the visual system, such as our ability to perceive an object as the same under strikingly different visual conditions, conditions that cause the image on the retina to vary widely.

As we move about, or as the ambient illumination changes, the size, shape, and brightness of the image projected onto the retina by a single object changes. Yet under most conditions we do not perceive the object itself to be changing. As a friend walks toward you, you perceive the friend as coming closer; you do not perceive the friend as growing larger, even though the image on your retina does enlarge. As we move from a brightly lit garden into a dimly lit room, the intensity of light reaching the retina may vary a thousandfold. Yet in the dim light of a room, as in the bright light of the sun, we see a white shirt as white and a red tie as red. Our ability to perceive an object's size or color as constant illustrates what is so remarkable about the visual system. It does not simply record images passively like a camera. Instead, the visual system transforms transient light patterns on the retina into a coherent and stable interpretation of a three-dimensional world.

The degree to which this processing is creative and not passive has only recently been fully appreciated. Earlier thinking about sensory perception was greatly influenced by the British empiricist philosophers, notably John Locke and George Berkeley, who thought of perception as an atomistic process whereby simple sensory elements, such as color, shape, and brightness, were assembled in an additive way, component by component. The modern view that perception is not atomistic but holistic, that it is an active and creative process that involves more than just the information provided to the retina by any given stimulus element, was first emphasized in the early twentieth century by the German psychologists Max Wertheimer, Kurt Koffka, and Wolfgang Köhler, who founded the school of Gestalt psychology.

The German term *Gestalt* means configuration or form. The central idea of the Gestalt psychologists is that what we see about a stimulus element—the perceptual interpretation we make of any visual object—depends not just on the properties of *that* element, but also on its *contextual interaction,* on the attributes of other features present in the same image. The Gestalt psychologists argued that the visual system accomplishes the organization of these contextual interactions by processing sensory information about the shape, color, distance, and movement of objects according to computational rules that are inherent in the system. That is, the brain makes certain assumptions about what is to be seen in the world, expectations that seem to derive in part from experience and in part from the built-in neural wiring for vision.

Because the elements of an image are selectively organized by our brain to create a form that is more than simply the sum of its elements, the early Gestalt psychologists liked to compare the perception of visual

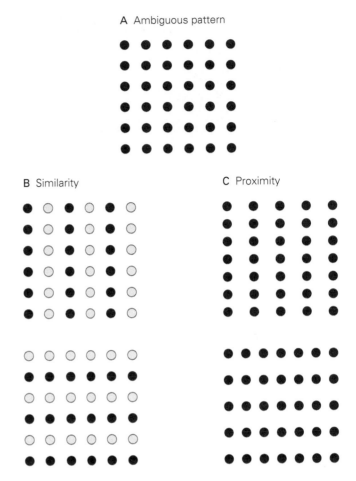

Figure 25-1 Pattern recognition. The array of identical dots in **A** is ambiguous and can be seen alternatively as a pattern of columns or rows. The two lower figures are not ambiguous because of additional cues. In **B** the colors of the dots create a strong pattern of either vertical columns or horizontal rows, while in **C** proximity alone determines whether we see a vertical or horizontal pattern. (From Gleitman 1986.)

form to the hearing of a melody. What we recognize in a melody is not simply the sequence of particular notes but their *interrelationship.* A melody played in different keys will still be recognized as the same melody because the relationship of the notes remains the same. Likewise, we are able to recognize different images under a variety of visual conditions, including differences in illumination, because the relationships between the components of the image are maintained by the brain.

Gestalt psychologists identified specific principles of perceptual organization and illustrated these with examples of visual illusions and perceptual constancies. More recent psychophysical and neurophysiological work has lent further support to a number of these prin-

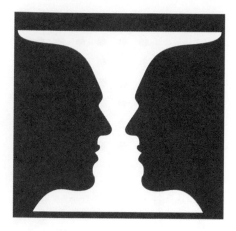

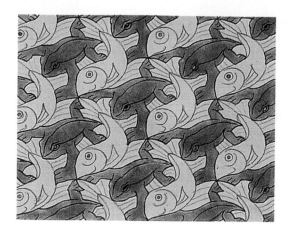

Figure 25-2 Figure-ground recognition.

Left: In this famous illustration of figure and ground by the Danish psychologist Edgar Rubin we sometimes see a pair of faces, sometimes a white vase. If it seems you are seeing both at the same time it is because your perception rapidly alternates between the two figures. The perceptual distinction between figure (or object) and ground is similar to the communication engineer's distinction between signal and noise. As we

focus on one signal, other information is relegated to background noise.

Right: In this repeating pattern by Maurits Escher, both frogs and fishes are formed by the same contours. Normally, contours serve to distinguish an object from an indeterminate background. (M.C. Escher's "Symmetry Drawing E50" © 2000 Cordon Art B.V., Baarn-Holland. All rights reserved.)

ciples. We see a uniform array of 36 undifferentiated dots as *either* rows or columns because of the brain's tendency to impose a pattern on the dots (Figure 25-1A). The specific pattern perceived can be strongly influenced by *similarity or proximity* in the dots. Thus, if the dots in each column are similar, we are more likely to see a pattern of columns (Figure 25-1B). Likewise, if the dots in each column are closer together than those in the rows, we are more disposed to see a pattern of columns. (Figure 25-1C).

The Gestalt psychologists also emphasized the importance of the brain's association of certain parts of a scene to form a recognizable object while relegating other parts to the background. Such separation of *figure* and *ground* can be continuous and dynamic, as is evident in the well-known example of figure-ground reversal (Figure 25-2). This organizational ability of the visual system is creatively exploited by graphic artists. The artist Maurits Escher writes: "Our eyes are accustomed to fixing on specific objects. The moment this happens everything around is reduced to background. . . . The human eye and mind cannot be busy with two things at the same moment, so there must be a quick and continual jumping from one side to the other." The figure-ground dichotomy thus illustrates one principle of visual perception—a winner-take-all perceptual strategy. Like the singleness of action in the motor system described by Charles Sherrington (Chapter 33), in the visual system only part of an image can be selected as the

focus of attention; the rest becomes, at least momentarily, background.

Because contours in the visual field are cues to the edges of objects and thus help us perceive distinct ob-

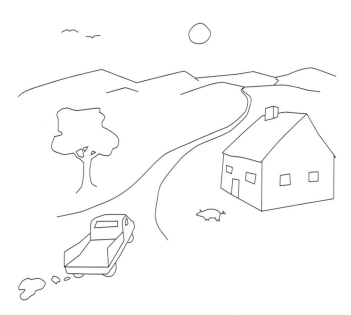

Figure 25-3 Object recognition. An outline drawing, typical of children's drawings, has clearly recognizable objects because edges are powerful cues in the perceptual organization of the visual field.

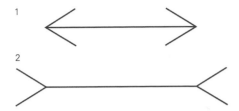

Figure 25-4 Perceived length can differ from measured length. In the classic Müller-Lyer illusion two horizontal lines identical in length appear to have different lengths; line 1 appears shorter than line 2.

jects, we recognize objects in simple line drawings without shading or color (Figure 25-3).

Illusions, which are "misreadings" of visual information by the brain, also illustrate how the brain applies certain assumptions about the visual world to the sensory information it receives. In particular, they demonstrate certain organizational mechanisms of visual perception—selection, distortion, filling in of omissions. In the classic Müller-Lyer illusion two lines of equal length look unequal (Figure 25-4). As is characteristic of many illusions, knowing that the lines are equal does not prevent us from being fooled by this illusion time and again. We perceive the lines to be unequal because the brain uses shape as an indicator of size.

Filling-in is nicely illustrated by the famous Kanizsa triangle (Figure 25-5). The image of the triangle emerges

from contours supplied by the brain—contours that do not actually exist on the page!

The spatial relationships of objects also help us interpret an image. For example, we judge the size of an object by comparing it to its immediate surroundings. When we see two people at different distances, we do not judge the size of each person by comparing them to each other, but by comparing each person to objects immediately around them. In this comparison we also rely on our familiarity with objects in the visual field (Figure 25-6).

The integration of distinctive objects into a coherent visual scene is aided by another central fact of vision: closer structures cover those that are more distant. In Figure 25-7 we "see" a pattern in otherwise unrelated shapes only when the shapes are seen as fragments of an occluded background. Without the assumption of occlusion, our brain would not have enough information to infer a relationship between the assorted shapes.

Perception also is based on inferences about the nature of our world that are built into the wiring of the brain by genetic and developmental processes. A striking example is the perception of shape from shadows. When a round shape is lit from above, it appears to be convex like the exterior of a sphere, whereas when it is lit from below it appears to be concave like the inside of a bowl (Figure 25-8).

This perception seems to be based on the assumption by our visual system that there is only one source of light. When subjects are shown two columns of objects

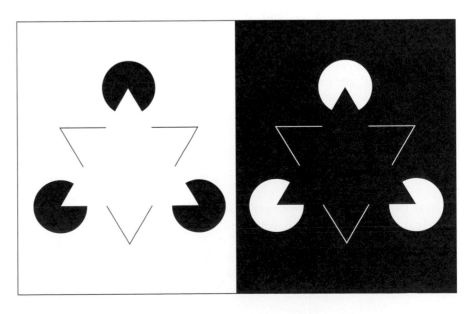

Figure 25-5 The Kanizsa triangle. A triangle is readily perceived in the center of each drawing even though the outline of the triangle does not exist in the drawing and must be inferred from fragments of other objects in the drawing. What is remarkable is that a white triangle emerges from a white background and a black triangle from a black background.

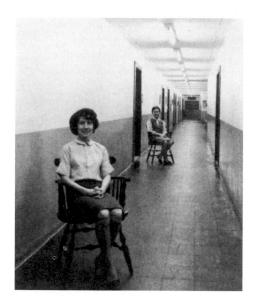 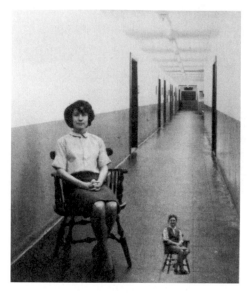

Figure 25-6 The perceived size of an object depends on other objects in the visual field.

Left: The woman in the foreground is nine feet from the camera while the second woman is 27 feet away. Both appear to be the same size.

Right: The photograph was taken with the woman in the foreground only; the photograph of the second woman was pasted into the picture. In the doctored photo the second woman seems small, not far away, because the corridor and tiles around her are not proportional, as they are in the photo at left. To convince yourself that she is the same size as in the photo at left, you will probably need to measure her. (From Brown and Herrnstein 1975.)

that are mirror images, they see one column of objects as concave and the other as convex (Figure 25-8B). Thus the brain must assume that both columns of objects are illuminated by one source of light. Subjects would not perceive both convexity and concavity in different objects if the brain assumed each column had a different light source. The assumption of a single light source may have evolved because our natural environment has only one source of light, the sun, and we assume that the source of light is always above.

As a result of the influence of Gestalt theorists, most perceptual psychologists no longer ask the empiricist's question, "What are the basic components of this perception?" Rather, they—and we—are interested in the question, "How does the brain produce this perception?" This question provides a common framework for the current attempts to merge psychological and neurobiological investigations of vision.

Visual Information Is Processed in Multiple Cortical Areas

In vision, as in other mental operations, various otherwise unrelated attributes—motion, depth, form, and color—are all coordinated in a single percept. This unity

is achieved not by one hierarchical neural system but by multiple visual areas in the brain that are fed by at least two major, interacting neural pathways. Distributed processing has become one of the main tenets of today's neurobiological study of vision. Thus, before we can consider the visual system in cell-physiological terms in later chapters, we must first have an understanding of some of the anatomical features of its pathways.

The photoreceptors of the retina project onto bipolar cells, which in turn have synapses on retinal ganglion cells, the output cells of the retina. The axons of ganglion cells of the retina form the optic nerve, which projects to the lateral geniculate nucleus in the thalamus. The lateral geniculate in turn projects to the primary visual cortex (Brodmann's area 17 or V1, also called the striate cortex). Because the projections are orderly, the striate cortex contains a complete neural map of the retina. Beyond the striate cortex lie the extrastriate areas, a set of higher-order visual areas also containing representations of the retina. The preservation of the spatial arrangement of inputs from the retina is called retinotopy, and the map of the visual field is called a retinotopic map or a retinotopic frame of reference (Box 25-1).

At the beginning of the twentieth century the British neurologist Gordon Holmes concluded that the

Figure 25-7 When one object appears to cover another, we assume the occluded object is in the background and construct our visual image accordingly. (Redrawn from Nakayama and Shimajo 1990, after Bregman 1981.)

Left: Assorted shapes do not appear to be related in any meaningful way. They appear as a jumble of fragments.

Right: When the same shapes are "covered" by an ink blob, we are able to connect the background fragments into the letter B.

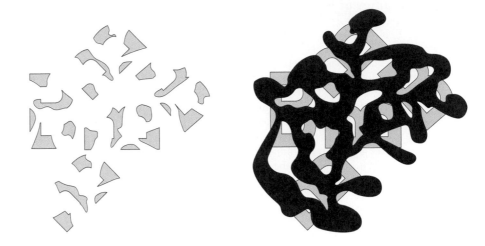

spatial relationship of the photoreceptors in the retina was preserved in the striate cortex, a conclusion based on clinical examination of patients with cortical lesions. This clinical impression was confirmed experimentally in 1941 when Wade Marshall and Samuel Talbot demonstrated that the striate cortex contains a complete retinotopic map.

John Allman and Jon Kaas, as well as Semir Zeki, then identified multiple representations of the retina in the areas outside the striate cortex in monkeys, whose visual capacities are very similar to those of humans. More recently David Van Essen and his collaborators collated information showing at least 32 representations of the retina in the extrastriate areas (Figure 25-9). The amount of the neocortex comprising these visual areas is remarkable. Over 50% of the neocortex of the macaque monkey is devoted to processing visual information, while only 11% is somatosensory cortex and 3% is auditory cortex. Individual visual cortical areas differ enormously in size: The two largest areas (V1 and V2) each occupy over 1100 mm^2 while one of the smallest areas (the middle temporal or MT) occupies only about 55 mm^2.

After identifying multiple areas on anatomical grounds, Zeki went on to investigate the activity of single cells in several of the extrastriate areas. He found that the response properties differed between areas. In the middle temporal area (Figure 25-9) a preponderance of neurons were selective for the direction of stimulus motion but were relatively unselective for color and form. In contrast, in area V4 many of the neurons responded to the color of the stimulus but few were selective for the direction of motion. On the basis of these and other observations, Zeki proposed that each extrastriate area might be specialized for processing a different type of visual information, such as motion, form,

and color. As we shall see in Chapter 28, subsequent studies in these and other extrastriate visual areas have confirmed that cells in different areas have different properties.

Different Cortical Areas Make Different Contributions to the Processing of Motion, Depth, Form, and Color

Can one experimentally relate distinct aspects of what is normally perceived as a unified whole to specific areas

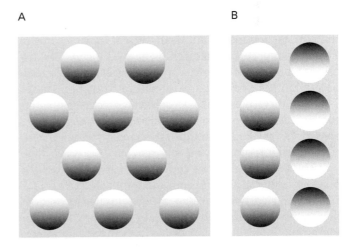

Figure 25-8 Spheres or cavities? The decision depends on where you assume the light source is.

A. You can reverse the depth of these objects by imagining a shift in the light source from the top of the figure to the bottom.

B. In this array, once you see one column as convex the other column will appear concave. It is almost impossible to see both rows as simultaneously convex or concave. (From Ramachandran 1988.)

Box 25-1 Frames of Reference

A major task for the brain is to construct three successive frames of reference for visual perception and the control of movement: a retinotopic frame of reference, a head-centered frame of reference, and a body-centered frame of reference.

Visual information leaving the retina is organized into a two-dimensional map of the visual field. We refer to this map as a *retinotopic map* or a *retinotopic frame of reference*. Each time the eye moves the retinotopic frame of reference moves as well. Anything that is anchored to the frame of reference, such as the afterimage produced by a flash of light, moves with it.

Now suppose we consider the same visual field with respect to the head. In this frame of reference anything in the visual field that moves with the head remains stable. The brain constructs this *head-centered frame of reference* by combining the retinotopic frame of reference with added information about the eye position.

Likewise, a *body-centered frame of reference* can be constructed by combining information about eye movement and head movement with information about posture. Thus one frame of reference is built upon another.

How are these frames of reference established? Some neurons in the parietal cortex that are selectively responsive to visual information have retinal receptive fields that are modulated depending upon the position of the eye in the orbit. These neurons are therefore combining input from the retina with information about eye position—exactly what would be required to move from a retinotopic frame of reference to a head-centered frame of reference. Each time the eye moves, the head-centered frame of reference must be updated. Other neurons in the parietal cortex contribute to this updating by shifting the retinal location of their receptive fields in association with each saccadic eye movement. They could use information from both the retina and the system controlling the eye movements to maintain a stable head-centered representation of the visual field. Similar computations using head-position information may be performed in the ventral premotor cortex and together with the computations from the parietal cortex, they serve to establish a body-centered frame of reference.

---

of the cerebral cortex? How separable is processing of motion from that of form, and either of these from processing of color?

As we have seen in Chapter 20, clinical observations have shown that visual orientation is disrupted in humans with lesions in the parietal cortex. In particular, some patients demonstrate a visual neglect: while they do not have a blind spot or scotoma, as would result from damage to the striate cortex, they do not respond to objects presented in the visual field contralateral to the parietal lesions. In contrast, patients with lesions in the temporal cortex frequently have difficulty in discriminating different forms and have poor visual memory for forms, including an inability to identify faces. These clinical observations suggested to neurologists that the parietal cortex is specialized for spatial representation, whereas the temporal cortex is specialized for object recognition.

The spatial functions of the parietal cortex and the object recognition function of the temporal cortex have been more clearly delineated in behavioral tests of monkeys with lesions in the posterior parietal or inferior temporal cortex. Ablation of the posterior parietal cortex altered the monkey's ability to locate objects visually, including the ability to guide hand movements to reach them, but did not affect the ability of the monkey to identify objects. In contrast, lesions of the inferior temporal cortex impaired the monkey's ability to identify objects when the discriminations required use of color, orientation, pattern, or shape but did not affect the monkey's ability to locate objects in space.

Further evidence that the posterior parietal and inferior temporal cortices have different functions comes from measurements of changes of blood flow using PET scanning. One study compared the responses in the same subjects while locating a point of light and matching faces. During both tasks a lateral occipital extrastriate region was prominent on the scan. However, an area of parietal cortex was active primarily during the object *location* task and an area of occipital temporal cortex was active during the object *recognition* task (Figure 25-10). Similarly, when subjects were asked to attend to the speed or to the color and shape of moving colored bars, attention to speed led to activation in the parietal cortex, whereas attention to color and shape activated areas closer to the temporal area. Thus in normal human subjects there is evidence for a segregation of visual function between areas, with the parietal region being more concerned with spatial relationships and the temporal region with object recognition.

The idea that different aspects of visual perception may be handled in separate areas of the brain dates to the end of the nineteenth century, when Sigmund Freud concluded that the inability of certain patients to recognize specific features of the visual world was due not to a sensory deficit but to cortical defects that affect the ability to combine components of visual impressions into a meaningful pattern. These defects, which Freud called *agnosias* (loss of knowledge), can be quite specific depending on the area of the cortex damaged (Table 25-1). For example, a patient may have a selective defect for the perception of depth as a result of a specific lesion

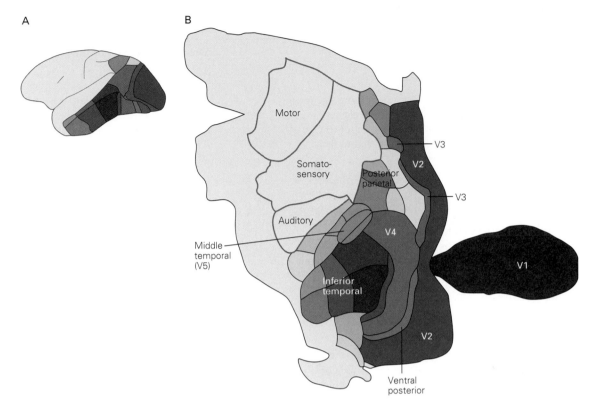

Figure 25-9 Several areas in the cerebral cortex of the monkey are dedicated to processing visual information.

A. Side view of the brain of the macaque monkey.

B. Many areas not visible on the surface of the cortex (because they are buried in the sulci) become visible if the sulci are opened up and spread out on a flattened map. Separate visual areas are outlined on this flattened map. V1, V2, V3, V4 = visual areas 1–4. Areas in **dark purple** are the occipital cortical areas V1, V2, V3, and ventral posterior. Those in shades of **blue** fall primarily in the dorsal visual path. Those in shades of **red-purple** fall primarily in the ventral visual path. (Based on Felleman and Van Essen 1991.)

in the visual cortex. One patient with such a *depth agnosia* had an "inability to appreciate depth or thickness of objects seen. . . . The most corpulent individual might be a moving cardboard figure; everything is perfectly flat." Similarly, a *motion agnosia* can occur after bilateral damage to the middle temporal areas of the cortex (see Chapter 28) and is manifested by an inability to perceive motion without such striking loss of any other perceptual capabilities.

Still other patients lose color vision *(achromatopsia)* because of localized damage to the temporal cortex, while retaining reasonably good perception of form. This color-processing area in the brain can be identified in normal living human subjects using PET scanning. In addition to motion agnosia and achromatopsia, there is an agnosia for form, which can be selective for inanimate or animate objects.

Indeed, there is striking evidence for a discrete cortical region for face recognition from studies of patients who, after a stroke, are unable to recognize particular

faces *(prosopagnosia)*. These patients can identify a face as a face, its parts, and even specific emotions expressed on the face, but they are unable to identify a particular face as belonging to a specific person. Patients with prosopagnosia often cannot recognize their close relatives and may not even recognize their *own* faces in the mirror, even though they will recognize that they are looking at a face. It is not the patient's knowledge of people's identities that has been lost, but the connection between a particular face and a particular identity. To recognize even a close friend, patients must rely on the friend's voice or other nonvisual clues. In the purest form of prosopagnosia, only recognition of faces is impaired; recognition of other objects is not affected. In other cases the failure of recognition extends beyond faces: Stamp collectors do not recognize individual stamps; bird watchers cannot recognize different birds.

Lesions that cause prosopagnosia are always bilateral and are located on the inferior surface of both occipital lobes and extend forward to the inner surface of

Table 25-1 The Visual Agnosias

Type	Deficit	Most probable site of the lesion
Agnosia for form and pattern		
Object agnosia	Naming, using, recognition of real objects	Areas 18, 20, 21 on left and corpus callosum
Agnosia for drawings	Recognition of drawn objects	Areas 18, 20, 21 on right
Prosopagnosia	Recognition of faces	Areas 20, 21 bilaterally
Agnosia for color		
Color agnosia	Association of colors with objects	Area 18 on right
Color anomia	Naming colors	Speech zones or connections from areas 18, 37
Achromtopsia	Distinguishing hues	Areas 18, 37
Agnosia for depth and movement		
Visuospatial agnosia	Stereoscopic vision	Areas 18, 37 on right
Movement agnosia	Discerning movement of object	Medial-temporal area bilaterally (junction of occipital and temporal cortex)

Modified from Kolb and Whishaw 1980.

the temporal lobes. Norman Geschwind suggested that this region must be a critical part of the neural network specialized for the rapid and reliable recognition of faces. Studies of monkeys support this idea and show that the inferior temporal cortex is necessary for normal visual learning and perception. Removal of the inferior

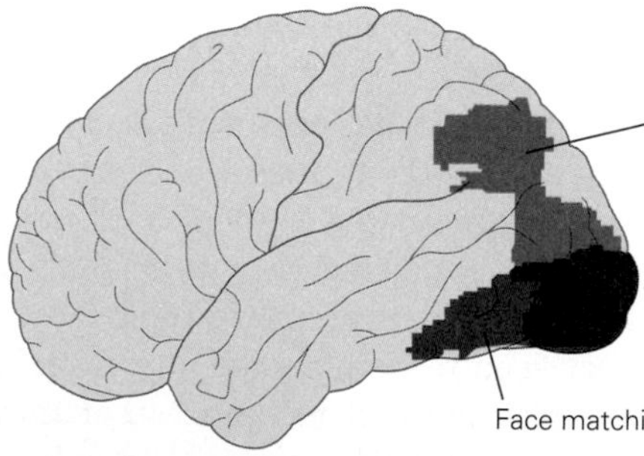

Figure 25-10 Extrastriate cortical areas active in human subjects during visual perception tests. The areas indicated are composites of the cortical regions activated in three or more subjects. Activation was detected in PET scans measuring changes in cerebral blood flow. The location-matching task required the subjects to indicate which of two patterns had a dot in the same position seen in a previously presented pattern. The face-matching task required the subjects to determine which pictures of human faces matched a face they had previously seen. The findings suggest that the lateral occipital extrastriate region is involved in both tasks, the superior parietal area in the location-matching task, and the occipitotemporal region in the face-matching task. (Adapted from Haxby et al. 1994.)

temporal cortex impairs visual recognition of shapes and patterns without in any way disturbing other basic functions of visual perception, such as acuity or recognition of color and movement.

These visual agnosias rarely occur in a pure form. A combination of deficits is not surprising because lesions of the brain due to vascular accidents or tumors are not normally restricted to functionally discrete regions. In animal experiments, on the other hand, a single region can be selectively removed without damage to adjacent areas. Although the clinical evidence for localization of visual agnosias to specific brain regions is not always as precise, it is nevertheless consistent with experiments that show different aspects of vision are mediated by different regions of cerebral cortex.

Parallel Pathways Convey Information From the Retina to Parietal and Temporal Cortical Areas

Since different regions of extrastriate visual cortex appear to have different functions, do these different areas also receive different inputs from the pathways emanating from the retina? Leslie Ungerleider and Mortimer Mishkin addressed this question and argued, based on both the anatomical and functional evidence, that these extrastriate visual areas are organized into two pathways: a *dorsal pathway* from V1 to the posterior parietal cortex, including the middle temporal area, and a *ventral pathway* extending from V1 to the inferior temporal cortex, including area V4 (Figure 25-11). Because of the nature of the deficits resulting from lesions in the targets of these pathways, Ungerleider and Mishkin suggested that the posterior parietal pathway is concerned with localizing *where* objects are and the inferior temporal pathway with identifying *what* the objects are.

How does different information about the visual image reach these cortical pathways? As we shall learn in Chapters 26 and 27, visual information is conveyed from the retina to the cortex in at least two major pathways: the P and the M pathways. This segregation of visual information begins with two types of retinal ganglion cells—large cells (M cells) and small cells (P cells). Each of these cells transmits somewhat different information to different layers in the lateral geniculate nucleus of the thalamus. The axons of the M cells project to the magnocellular layers of the lateral geniculate nucleus (the M pathway), whereas the axons of the P cells project to the parvocellular layers (the P pathway). These two pathways then continue from these separate layers of the lateral geniculate nucleus to separate layers in the primary visual cortex (the M pathway to layer 4Cα and the P pathway to 4Cβ).

Within V1 and V2 there are two important subdivisions, the blobs and stripes respectively, both of which stain intensely for the mitochondrial enzyme cytochrome oxidase. In V1 the heavily staining regions form a repeating polka dot-like pattern of blobs (peg-like structures about 0.2 mm in diameter) separated by unstained regions (the interblobs). In V2 the heavily staining regions form two types of dark stripes, thick and thin, separated by pale interstripe regions. Figure 25-12 outlines these areas and the pathways through them and suggests some of the functions they perform—functions we shall consider in more detail in Chapters 28 and 29.

The P pathway reaches both the blobs and interblobs of the superficial layers of V1. From the blob regions of V1 this pathway goes to the thin stripes of V2, while from the interblob regions it projects to the interstripe regions of V2. Both the thin stripe and interstripe regions of V2 project to V4, forming the ventral pathway, which reaches the inferior temporal cortex (Figure 25-12). The M pathway also contributes to this ventral pathway, which is concerned with the perception of form and color. Because a great deal of information about shape and form is derived from edges and borders (see Figure 25-3), neurons throughout the ventral pathway are sensitive to the outline of images, their orientation, and their boundaries. This system is capable of high resolution, which is important for seeing stationary objects in detail. Thus, this cortical system is more concerned with *what* is seen. In fact, as we have discussed, lesions in the inferior temporal lobe produce deficits related to the recognition of complex objects including the recognition of faces.

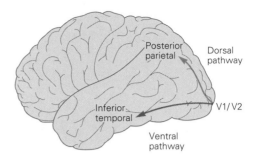

Figure 25-11 Visual processing centers in the cerebral cortex are organized in two pathways. The dorsal processing pathway to the posterior parietal cortex and the ventral pathway to the inferior temporal cortex are shown on a side view of the brain. Although these pathways are depicted on the human brain, the identified areas and their sequence are from research on the monkey. Only forward projections are shown.

The M pathway extends from the magnocellular layers of the lateral geniculate nucleus, through V1, to the thick stripes of V2. Both V1 and V2 project to the middle temporal area to form the dorsal pathway, which extends to the posterior parietal cortex. The middle temporal area (also referred to as V5) is concerned with motion and depth, and the areas in the posterior parietal cortex are concerned with visuospatial function. The neurons in this system are relatively insensitive to color and poor at analyzing stationary objects. The dorsal pathway, therefore, is more concerned with seeing *where* objects are rather than what they are. Lesions in this cortical pathway result in a selective deficit in motion perception and in eye movements directed toward moving targets. The dorsal *where* pathway and the ventral *what* pathway continue rostrally to end in different regions of the prefrontal cortex that specialize, respectively, in visual spatial working memory and object recognition working memory.

Thus the visual system is organized into well-defined pathways extending from the retina into the parietal and temporal lobes. Sequential organization of the sort seen in each pathway is referred to as hierarchical processing.

Visual Attention May Facilitate Coordination Between Separate Visual Pathways

How is information about color, motion, depth, and form, which are carried by separate neuronal pathways, organized into cohesive perceptions? When we see a square purple box we combine into one perception the properties of color (purple), form (square), and dimensions in depth (box). We can equally well combine purple with a round box, a hat, or a coat. Clearly, the possi-

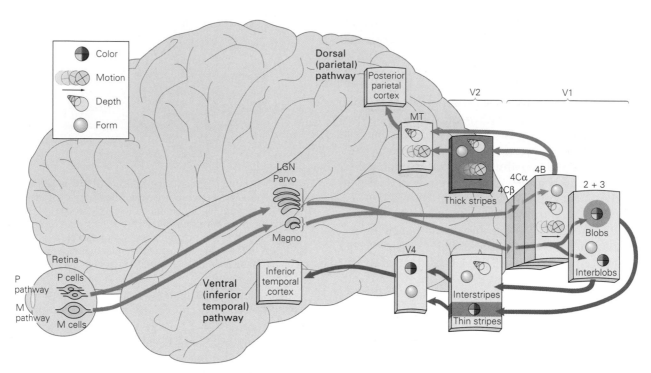

Figure 25-12 Possible functions mediated by the two pathways connecting visual processing centers in the cerebral cortex. The icons represent salient physiological properties of cells in these areas. On the top is the pathway extending to the posterior parietal cortex, which is thought to be particularly involved in processing motion, depth, and spatial information.

On the bottom is the pathway to the inferior temporal cortex, which is more concerned with form and color. Feeding into those two cortical pathways are the P and M pathways from the retina. (**MT** = middle temporal; **LGN** = lateral geniculate nucleus.) (Adapted from Van Essen and Gallant 1994.)

ble combinations are so many that the existence of distinct feature-detecting cells, each responsive to only one set of combinations, is improbable.

Instead, as we have seen in this chapter, visual images typically are built up from the inputs of parallel pathways that process different features—movement, depth, form, and color. To express the specific combination of properties in the visual field at any given moment, independent groups of cells with different functions must temporarily be brought into *association*. As a result, there must be a mechanism by which the brain momentarily associates the information being processed independently by different cell populations in different cortical regions. This mechanism, as yet unspecified, is called the *binding mechanism*.

Anne Treisman and her colleagues and Bela Julesz have independently shown in psychophysical studies that such associations require focused *attention* on elements in the visual field. They began by trying to understand one of the problems addressed by the early Gestalt psychologists: How is attention focused on one object in the visual field? What features of the object make that object stand out from the background?

Treisman and Julesz found that distinctive elementary properties such as brightness, color, and orientation of lines create distinctive boundaries. For example a rectangular area composed of small xs creates distinctive boundaries that allow it easily to stand out within a field of L shapes (Figure 25-13A). In contrast, a rectangular area composed of Ts can be found only after carefully searching the figure because the T shapes are only subtly different from the background of L shapes (Figure 25-13B). In experimental displays such as these, the time required to find a unique item increases with the number of unique items in the display.

On the basis of these observations, Treisman and Julesz suggest two distinct sequential processes are involved in visual perception. A *preattentive process* is concerned only with the detection of objects. This process rapidly scans an object's global texture or features and focuses on the distinction between figure and ground by encoding in parallel the useful elementary properties of the scene: color, orientation, size, or direction of movement. At this point variation in a simple property may be discerned as a border or contour, but complex differences in combinations of properties are not de-

A

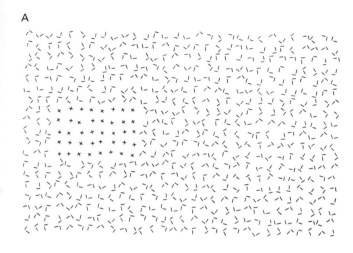

B

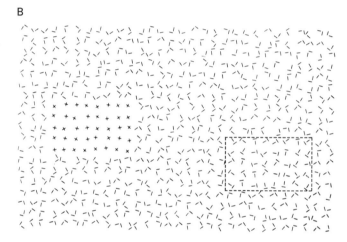

Figure 25-13 Some perceptions are produced by preattentive scanning; others require focal attention. A small subarea composed of x's is easy to pick out from the surrounding area by simply looking at the figure (**A**). The figure also includes a subarea composed of T-shapes. Can you find it? To do so, you must focus on each region of the figure. The less obvious subarea is composed of T-shapes and is outlined in **B**. (From Julesz and Bergen 1983.)

A Color search

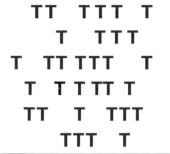

B Conjunction search

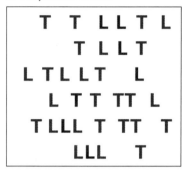

C

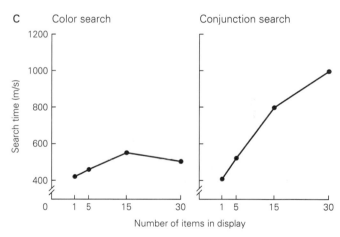

tected (Figure 25-14). Preattentive processing is also referred to as bottom-up processing since it is focused on the properties of individual elements in the scene and emphasizes grouping together the *items* in visual perception that are required to distinguish between figure and ground.

This initial grouping of *items* is followed by an *attentive process* that selects and highlights the still segregated features of an object. In contrast to the parallel processing of the preattentive system, the attentive system processes serially. This attentive system is top-down processing since what is selected must be identified independently of the individual elements of the scene.

Figure 25-14 The search time for a unique item is faster when all items differ by only one attribute than if all items differ by two or more attributes. The subject is instructed to identify whether an item is present or not. The unique stimulus in **A** "pops out," and, as illustrated in the color search in **C**, subjects take about the same time to find the stimulus regardless of how many items are present in the display (**C**). This is consistent with a preattentive process in which all attributes are scanned at once. The unique item in **B** differs by two attributes and does not pop out. In this case of conjunctive search, the more items present, the longer the search takes (**C**). This is consistent with a serial search and successive shifts of attention. Most visual searches probably use a combination of these two processes. (Modified from Treisman et al. 1977 and Treisman 1986.)

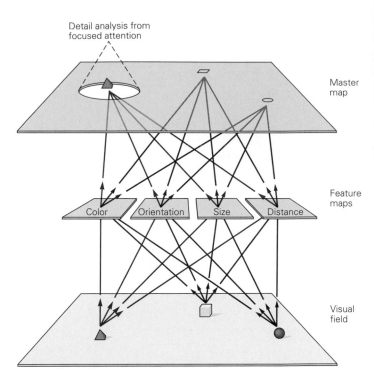

Figure 25-15 A hypothetical model of how different types of visual information processed separately are combined into a coherent image. The elementary properties of objects in the visual field (such as color, orientation, size, and distance) are encoded in separate parallel pathways, each of which generates a feature map. Selected features from these maps are then integrated into a master map, which is a representation of those features that distinguish objects from the background. Focused attention can occur only after features have been associated in a small region of the master map. (After Treisman 1986.)

Treisman has proposed that different properties are encoded in different *feature maps* in different brain regions. To solve the binding problem, Treisman has postulated that there may be a *master map* that codes for conjunctions of features in the image (Figure 25-15). This master map receives input from all feature maps but retains only those features that distinguish the object of attention from its surround. Once these salient features have been represented in the master map, the detailed information associated with each feature can be retrieved by referring back to the individual feature maps. In this way the master map can combine details from the feature maps that are essential for recognition, and Treisman has referred to attention as the glue that binds features together. We will consider other solutions to the binding problem in Chapter 28.

In the examples so far considered, attention is directed at an object or group of objects in a scene. Michael Posner and his collaborators have found that attention is not only directed to the object but to the spatial location as well. Posner conceives of this form of attention as moving from one part of the visual field to another, highlighting objects or places for selective visual processing. An alternative view is that attention is simply the result of competition for the limited visual processing capacity at all stages of the visual system.

How is attention achieved in the visual system? Treisman speaks metaphorically of the spotlight of attention. What might be the switch for this spotlight? What turns it on? As may be appreciated from the evidence presented in this and earlier chapters (such as Chapter

20), the neuronal mechanisms of attention and conscious awareness are one of the great unresolved problems in perception and indeed in all of neurobiology.

The Analysis of Visual Attention May Provide Important Clues About Conscious Awareness

As we saw in Chapter 20, the problem of selective attention was first adressed by William James in 1890. In his essay "The Stream of Thought" he writes:

We see that the mind is at every stage a theatre of simultaneous possibilities. Consciousness consists in the comparison of these with each other, the selection of some, and the suppression of the rest by the reinforcing and inhibiting agency of attention. The highest and most elaborated mental products are filtered from the data chosen by the faculty next beneath, out of the mass offered by the faculty below that, which mass in turn was sifted from a still larger amount of yet simpler material, and so on. The mind, in sort, works on the data it receives very much as a sculptor works on his block of stone.

Much of the sensory information received by the peripheral receptors in our body must eventually be filtered out and eliminated within the brain, much as we disregard the ground when we focus on the figure. Although the visual system contains extensive parallel pathways for simultaneously processing different types of information, selective attention acts to limit the amount of this information that reaches the highest centers of processing in the brain. As we can see in the figure-ground dichotomy, selective attention both filters out some features and sharpens our perception of others. In this winner-take-all strategy, some stimuli stand out in consciousness while others recede into dim awareness.

It is attractive to think that exploration of visual attention will lead us to define the neural mechanisms of a specific instance of consciousness. Despite its central importance in mental processes, the problem of consciousness has so far eluded reductionist approaches. But as this and later chapters illustrate, biological insights into any component of consciousness are likely to give us at least a glimmer of understanding of some of the most complex components: volition, intention, and self-awareness. If there is a common set of neural mechanisms underlying consciousness, then the study of visual attention could put us on the path to a new level of self-understanding.

An Overall View

David Marr began his important book on the computational tasks of vision with the question: "What does it mean, to see?" His answer is that vision is the process of discovering from images what is present in the visual world and where it is.

We now know that the visual system of the brain accomplishes these tasks by distributed processing in many cortical areas. Clinical studies and animal experiments both lead to the conclusion that each area is responsible for a particular aspect of vision, such as depth, form, motion, or color.

Only recently has it become clear that these features are processed in parallel rather than serially. Two pathways (P and M) originate in the retina and continue in two cortical processing pathways leading to the posterior parietal and inferior temporal cortices. The inferior temporal pathway is more involved in determining the *what* of vision, the posterior parietal pathway more with the *where* of vision.

The discovery of these parallel pathways has posed a new problem for the study of visual perception. Integration in a serial pathway is achieved progressively, by the transformation of information carried from one area to the next. In a system of parallel pathways, each with its own function, integration can be achieved only interactively.

How and where does this interaction occur in the visual system? In *A Vision of the Brain,* Semir Zeki puts this issue succinctly:

At first glance, the problem of integration may seem quite simple. Logically it demands nothing more than that all the signals from the specialized visual areas be brought together, to "report" the results of their operations to a single master corti-

cal area. This master area would then synthesize the information coming from all these diverse sources and provide us with the final image, or so one might think. But the brain has its own logic. . . . If all the visual areas report to a single master cortical area, who or what does that single area report to?

Put more visually, what part of the brain is looking at the visual image provided by a master area? The problem is not unique to visual perception. What, for example, listens to the music provided by a master auditory area, or smells the odor provided by the master olfactory cortex? It is in fact pointless pursuing this *grand synthesis* design. For here one comes across an important anatomical fact: There is no single cortical area to which all other cortical areas report exclusively, either in the visual or in any other system. In sum, the cortex must be using a different strategy for generating the integrated visual image.

There are in fact extensive interactions between the visual pathways at almost all cortical levels, as well as reciprocal connections from higher to lower levels both within and between pathways. Cross talk is simply not deferred until late stages of visual processing. This again argues against a grand synthesis and suggests that synthesis occurs all along the pathway and between the pathways. Perceptual integration is therefore likely to be a multi-stage process. Other brain centers that make connections with the visual system and that are known to affect visual attention, such as the prefrontal cortex, the claustrum, or the pulvinar, may allow attention mechanisms to correlate the streams of visual information in a coherent perception.

We have here focused on how we see. Obviously, vision is important not only in gaining information about our environment but also in guiding body movement. It is likely that much visual processing, particularly in the magnocellular pathway and posterior parietal pathway concerned with motion and spatial relationships, is essential for the control of movement. Simply moving about in the world requires complex analyses of visual stimuli. We shall return to the visual guidance of movement later in this book when considering the motor system.

Eric R. Kandel
Robert H. Wurtz

Selected Readings

Albright TD, Jessell TM, Kandel ER, Posner MI. 2000. A century of progress and the mysteries that remain. Cell/Neuron 25:s1–s55.

Desimone R, Duncan J. 1995. Neural mechanisms of selective visual attention. Annu Rev Neurosci 18:193–222.

Felleman DJ, Van Essen DC. 1991. Distributed hierarchical processing in the primate cerebral cortex. Cerebral Cortex 1:1–47.

Gregory RL. 1978. *Eye and Brain: The Psychology of Seeing*, 3rd ed. New York: McGraw-Hill.

Hochberg JE. 1978. *Perception*, 2nd ed. Englewood Cliffs, NJ: Prentice-Hall.

Hubel DH. 1988. *Eye, Brain and Vision*. New York: Scientific American Library.

Marr D. 1982. *Vision: A Computational Investigation Into the Human Representation and Processing of Visual Information*. San Francisco: Freeman.

Posner MI, Petersen SE. 1990. The attention system of the human brain. Annu Rev Neurosci 13:25–42.

Posner MI, Raichle ME. 1994. *Images of Mind*. New York: Scientific American Library.

Rock I, Palmer S. 1990. The legacy of Gestalt psychology. Sci Am 263(6):84–90.

Teuber ML. 1974. Sources of ambiguity in the prints of Maurits C. Escher. Sci Am 231(1):90–104.

Treisman A. 1986. Features and objects in visual processing. Sci Am 255(5):114–125.

Zeki S. 1993. *A Vision of the Brain*. Oxford: Blackwell Scientific.

References

Allman JM, Kaas JH. 1971. Representation of the visual field in striate and adjoining cortex of the owl monkey (*Aotus trivirgatus*). Brain Res 35:89–106.

Andersen RA, Snyder LH, Bradley DC, Xing J. 1997. Multimodal representation of space in the posterior parietal cortex and its use in planning movements. Annu Rev Neurosci 20:303–330.

Bergen JR, Julesz B. 1983. Rapid discrimination of visual patterns. IEEE Trans Syst Man Cybern SMC-13:857–863.

Bregman, AL. 1981. Asking the "what for" question in auditory perception. In: M Kubovy and JR Pomerantz, (eds). *Perceptual Organization*, p. 99. Hillsdale, NJ: Lawrence Erlbaum.

Brown R, Herrnstein RJ. 1975. *Psychology*. Boston: Little, Brown.

Colby CL, Duhamel J-R, Goldberg ME. 1995. Oculocentric spatial representation in parietal cortex. Cereb Cortex 5:470–481.

Corbetta M, Miezin FM, Dobmeyer S, Shulman GL, Petersen SE. 1991. Selective and divided attention during visual discriminations of shape, color, and speed: functional anatomy by positron emission tomography. J Neurosci 11:2383–2402.

Desimone R, Ungerleider LG. 1989. Neural mechanisms of visual processing in monkeys. In: F Boller, J Grafman (eds). *Handbook of Neuropsychology*, pp. 267–299. Amsterdam: Elsevier.

DeYoe EA, Van Essen DC. 1988. Concurrent processing streams in monkey visual cortex. Trends Neurosci 11:219–226.

Escher MC. 1971. *The Graphic Work of M. C. Escher*. New ed., rev. and exp. New York: Ballantine Books.

Farah MJ. 1990. *Visual Agnosias*. Cambridge, MA: MIT Press.

Geschwind N. 1979. Specializations of the human brain. Sci Am 241(3):180–199.

Gleitman H. 1986. *Psychology: The Psychology of Seeing*, 3rd ed. New York: Norton.

Goodale MA, Meenan JP, Bülthoff HH, Nicolle DA, Murphy KJ, Racicot CI. 1994. Separate neural pathways for the visual analysis of object shape in perception and prehension. Curr Biol 4:604–610.

Haxby JV, Horwitz B, Ungerleider LG, Maisog JM, Pietrini P, Grady CL. 1994. The functional organization of human extrastriate cortex: a PET-rCBF study of selective attention to faces and locations. J Neurosci 14(11):6336–6353.

James W. [1890] 1981. *The Principles of Psychology: The Works of William James*, Vol. 1. Cambridge, MA: Harvard University Press.

Julesz B. 1984. Toward an axiomatic theory of preattentive vision. In: GM Edelman, WE Gall, WM Cowan (eds). *Dynamic Aspects of Neocortical Function*, pp. 585–612. New York: Wiley.

Kaas JH. 1989. Changing concepts of visual cortex organization in primates. In: JW Brown (ed). *Neuropsychology of Visual Perception*, pp. 3–32. Hillsdale, NJ: Erlbaum

Kolb B, Whishaw IQ. 1985. *Fundamentals of Human Neuropsychology*, 2nd ed. New York: Freeman.

Livingstone MS. 1988. Art, illusion and the visual system. Sci Am 258(1):78–85.

Marshall WH, Talbot SA. 1942. Recent evidence for neural mechanisms in vision leading to a general theory of sensory acuity. In: H Kluver (ed). *Visual Mechanisms*, pp. 117–164. Lancaster, PA: Cattell.

Nakayama K, Shimojo S. 1990. Toward a neural understanding of visual surface representation. Cold Spring Harb Symp Quant Biol 55:911–924.

Posner MI (ed). 1989. *Foundations of Cognitive Science*. Cambridge, MA: MIT Press.

Ramachandran VS. 1987. Interaction between colour and motion in human vision. Nature 328:645–647.

Ramachandran VS. 1988. Perceiving shape from shading. Sci Am 259(2):76–83.

Rock I. 1984. *Perception*. New York: Scientific American Library.

Talbot SA, Marshall WH. 1941. Physiological studies on neural mechanisms of visual localization and discrimination. Am J Ophthalmol 24:1255–1264.

Treisman A, Gormican S. 1988. Feature analysis in early vision: evidence from search asymmetries. Psychol Rev 95:15–48.

Treisman A, Sykes M, Gelade G. 1977. Selective attention stimulus integration. In S Dornie (ed). *Attention and performance VI*, pp. 333–361. Hilldale, NJ: Lawrence Erlbaum.

Ungerleider LG, Mishkin M. 1982. Two cortical visual systems. In: DJ Ingle, MA Goodale, RJW Mansfield (eds). *Analysis of Visual Behavior*, pp. 549–586. Cambridge, MA: MIT Press.

Van Essen DC, Gallant JL. 1994. Neural mechanisms of form and motion processing in the primate visual system. Neuron 13:1–10.

Zeki S, Shipp S. 1988. The functional logic of cortical connections. Nature 355:311–317.

26

Visual Processing by the Retina

VISUAL PERCEPTION BEGINS in the retina and occurs in two stages. Light entering the cornea is projected onto the back of the eye, where it is converted into an electrical signal by a specialized sensory organ, the retina. These signals are then sent through the optic nerve to higher centers in the brain for further processing necessary for perception. In this chapter we describe the neural processing of visual signals in the retina. The next three chapters explain, in cell-physiological terms, how processing in higher centers underlies the perception of form, motion, and color.

The retina bears careful examination for several reasons. First, it is useful for understanding sensory transduction in general because photoreceptors in the retina are perhaps the best understood of all sensory cells. Second, unlike other sensory structures, such as the cochlea or somatic receptors in the skin, the retina is not a peripheral organ but part of the central nervous system, and its synaptic organization is similar to that of other central neural structures. At the same time, the retina is relatively simple compared with other brain regions. It contains only five major classes of neurons, linked in an intricate pattern of connections but with an orderly, layered anatomical arrangement. This combination of physiological diversity and relatively simple structural organization makes the retina useful for understanding how information is processed by complex neural circuits in the brain.

For these reasons we describe neural processing in the retina in considerable detail. This chapter is divided into two parts. In the first part we describe how photoreceptors transduce light into an electrical signal. In the second we consider how these signals are shaped by other retinal neurons before being sent to the brain and

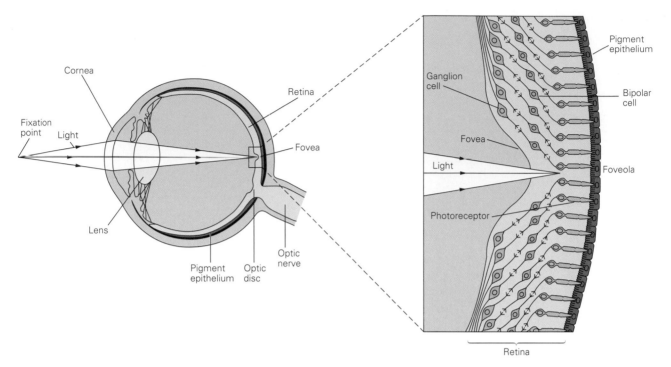

Figure 26-1 Photoreceptors are located in the retina. The location of the retina within the eye is shown at **left**. Detail of the retina at the fovea is shown on the **right** (the diagram has been simplified by eliminating lateral connections mediated by interneurons; see Figure 26-6). In most of the retina light must pass through layers of nerve cells and their processes before it reaches the photoreceptors. In the center of the fovea, or foveola, these proximal neurons are shifted to the side so that light has a direct pathway to the photoreceptors. As a result, the visual image received at the foveola is the least distorted.

how synaptic connections among the retinal neurons are organized to accomplish this processing. Before discussing phototransduction, however, we shall review the organization of the retina and the basic physiological properties of the photoreceptor cells.

The Retina Contains the Eye's Receptor Sheet

The eye is designed to focus the visual image on the retina with minimal optical distortion. Light is focused by the cornea and the lens, then traverses the vitreous humor that fills the eye cavity before reaching photoreceptors in the retina (Figure 26-1). The retina lies in front of the pigment epithelium that lines the back of the eye. Cells in the pigment epithelium are filled with the black pigment melanin, which absorbs any light not captured by the retina. This prevents light from being reflected off the back of the eye to the retina again (which would degrade the visual image).

Because the photoreceptors lie in the back of the eye, immediately in front of the pigment epithelium, all other retinal cells lie in front of the photoreceptors, closer to the lens. Therefore, light must travel through layers of other

retinal neurons before striking the photoreceptors. To allow light to reach the photoreceptors without being absorbed or greatly scattered (which would distort the visual image), the axons of neurons in the proximal layers of the retina are unmyelinated so that these layers of cells are relatively transparent. Moreover, in one region of the retina, the *fovea*, the cell bodies of the proximal retinal neurons are shifted to the side, enabling the photoreceptors there to receive the visual image in its least distorted form (Figure 26-1). This shifting is most pronounced at the center of the fovea, the *foveola*. Humans therefore constantly move their eyes so that scenes of interest are projected onto the fovea. The retina also contains a region called the optic disc, where the optic nerve fibers leave the retina. This region has no photoreceptors and therefore is a blind spot in the visual field (see Figure 27-2). The projection of the visual field onto the two retinas is described in Chapter 27.

There Are Two Types of Photoreceptors: Rods and Cones

The human retina contains two types of photoreceptors, rods and cones. Cones are responsible for day vision;

Table 26-1 Differences Between Rods and Cones and Their Neural Systems

Rods	Cones
High sensitivity to light, specialized for night vision	Lower sensitivity, specialized for day vision
More photopigment, capture more light	Less photopigment
High amplification, single photon detection	Lower amplification
Low temporal resolution: slow response, long integration time	High temporal resolution: fast response, short integration time
More sensitive to scattered light	Most sensitive to direct axial rays
Rod system	**Cone system**
Low acuity: not present in central fovea, highly convergent retinal pathways	High acuity: concentrated in fovea, dispersed retinal pathways
Achromatic: one type of rod pigment	Chromatic: three types of cones, each with a distinct pigment that is most sensitive to a different part of the visible light spectrum

people who lose functioning in the cones are legally blind. Rods mediate night vision; total loss of rods produces only night blindness. Rods are exquisitely sensitive to light and therefore function well in the dim light that is present at dusk or at night, when most stimuli are too weak to excite the cones.

Cones perform better than rods in all visual tasks except the detection of dim stimuli. Cone-mediated vision is of higher acuity than rod-mediated vision and provides better resolution of rapid changes in the visual image (ie, better temporal resolution). Cones also mediate color vision. Although the rod system is more light-sensitive than the cone system, it is achromatic. These differences in performance are due partly to properties of the rods and cones themselves and partly to the connections they make with other neurons in the retina (the rod and cone systems).

The most important factors that contribute to these differences are summarized in Table 26-1 and discussed next.

Rods Detect Dim Light

Rods contain more photosensitive visual pigment than cones, enabling them to capture more light. Even more important, rods amplify light signals more than cones do. A single photon can evoke a detectable electrical response in a rod; in contrast, tens or hundreds of photons must be absorbed by a cone to evoke a similar response. In addition, the rod system is highly convergent: Many rods have synapses on the same target interneuron, known as the bipolar cell (see below). Thus, signals

from the rods are pooled in the bipolar cell and reinforce one another, strengthening the signals evoked by light in individual receptors and increasing the ability of the brain to detect dim lights. In contrast, fewer cones converge on each bipolar cell. In fact, cones in the foveola have small diameters, are closely spaced, and do not converge at all; each bipolar cell receives input from a single cone.

Cones Mediate Color Vision

There are three types of cones, each containing a visual pigment that is sensitive to a different part of the light spectrum (see below). As we shall see in Chapter 29, the brain obtains information about color by comparing the responses of the three types of cones. In contrast, rods contain only one type of pigment and therefore respond in the same way to different wavelengths.

Although rods outnumber cones by roughly 20 to 1, the cone system has better spatial resolution for two reasons. First, because many neighboring rods converge onto a single bipolar cell, differences in the responses of the rods are averaged out in the interneuron. Second, cones are concentrated in the fovea, where the visual image is least distorted.

Like some other sensory receptors, rods and cones do not fire action potentials. Instead, they respond to light with graded changes in membrane potential. Rods respond slowly, so that the effects of all the photons absorbed during a 100 ms interval are summed together. This helps rods detect small amounts of light, but prevents them from resolving light that is flickering faster

A Morphology of photoreceptors

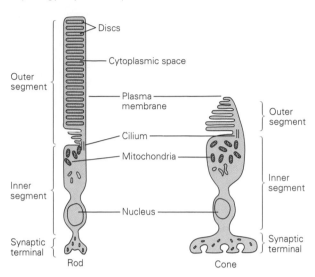

B Outer segments of photoreceptors

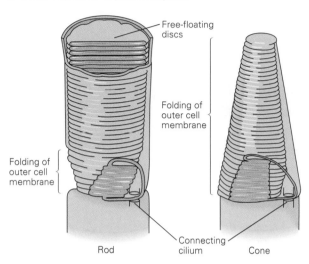

Figure 26-2 The two types of photoreceptors, rods and cones, have similar structures. (Adapted from O'Brien 1982 and Young 1970.)

A. Both rod and cone cells have inner and outer segments connected by a cilium. The inner segment contains the cell's nucleus and most of its biosynthetic machinery. The outer segment contains the light-transducing apparatus.

B. The outer segment consists of a stack of membranous discs, which contain the light-absorbing photopigments. In both types of cells these discs are formed by infolding of the plasma membrane. In rods, however, the folds pinch off from the membrane so that the discs are free-floating within the outer segment, whereas in cones the discs remain part of the plasma membrane.

than about 12 Hz. The response of cones is much faster; they can detect flicker up to at least 55 Hz.

Light Is Absorbed by Visual Pigments in the Photoreceptors

Both rods and cones have three major functional regions (Figure 26-2):

1. The *outer segment*, located at the outer or distal surface of the retina, is specialized for phototransduction.
2. The *inner segment*, located more proximally within the retina, contains the cell's nucleus and most of its biosynthetic machinery.
3. A *synaptic terminal* makes contact with the photoreceptor's target cells.

The outer segments of rods and cones are filled with light-absorbing visual pigments. Each pigment molecule comprises a small light-absorbing molecule attached to a large membrane-spanning protein. Rods and cones can contain a remarkably large number of these membrane proteins (as many as 10^8 in each cell), because they have evolved an elaborate system of stacked membranous discs in their outer segments that dramat-

ically increase the surface area of the membrane in these cells (Figure 26-2B). These discs develop as a series of invaginations of the cell's plasma membrane, ultimately arranging themselves like a roll of pennies in a bank wrapper. In cones the discs are continuous with the plasma membrane, while in rods they pinch off from the plasma membrane and become intracellular organelles.

Like other neurons, photoreceptors do not divide, but their outer segments are constantly renewed. New discs are formed at a rapid rate; in rods about three discs are synthesized every hour. Old discs are discarded at the tips of photoreceptors and removed by the phagocytotic activity of the pigment epithelial cells.

Phototransduction Results From a Three-Stage Cascade of Biochemical Events in the Photoreceptors

The absorption of light by visual pigments in rods and cones triggers a cascade of events that leads to a change in ionic fluxes across the plasma membrane of these cells, and consequently a change in membrane potential. A key molecule in the cascade is the nucleotide cyclic guanosine 3'-5' monophosphate (cGMP). In rods the (cGMP) molecule acts as a second messenger, carry-

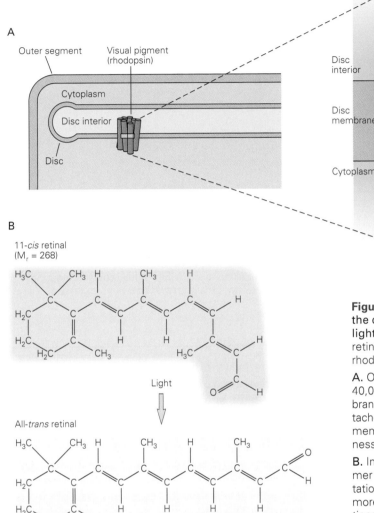

A

Outer segment   Visual pigment (rhodopsin)

Cytoplasm

Disc interior

Disc

NH₂

Residue 296 (attachment site for retinal)

Disc interior

Disc membrane

Cytoplasm

COOH

B

11-*cis* retinal
(M$_r$ = 268)

Light

All-*trans* retinal

Figure 26-3 Rhodopsin, the visual pigment in rod cells, is the covalent complex of a large protein, opsin, and a small light-absorbing compound, retinal. The absorption of light by retinal causes a change in the three-dimensional structure of rhodopsin.

A. Opsin has 348 amino acids and a molecular weight of about 40,000. It loops back and forth seven times across the membrane of the rod disc. Retinal (**green rectangle**) is covalently attached to a side chain of lysine 296 in the protein's seventh membrane-spanning region. (Adapted from Nathans and Hogness 1984.)

B. In its nonactivated form rhodopsin contains the 11-*cis* isomer of retinal. Absorption of light by 11-*cis* retinal causes a rotation around the 11-*cis* double bond. As retinal returns to its more stable all-*trans* configuration, it brings about a conformational change in the opsin portion of rhodopsin, which triggers the other events of visual transduction.

ing information through the cytoplasm connecting the freely floating discs, where light is absorbed, to the cell's plasma membrane, where ionic fluxes are altered. In cones, since the discs are continuous with the plasma membrane, a cytoplasmic messenger is not necessary; nonetheless, cGMP is used in these cells in the same way as in rods. Cyclic GMP controls ionic fluxes by opening a specialized species of ion channels, the cGMP-gated ion channels, which allow an inward current carried largely by Na$^+$ ions to flow into the cell.

In the dark the concentration of cGMP is relatively high, thus maintaining the cGMP-gated channels in an open state and allowing the inward current they carry to maintain the cell in a relatively depolarized state.

Phototransduction then occurs in three stages: (1) Light activates visual pigments; (2) these activated molecules stimulate cGMP phosphodiesterase, an enzyme that reduces the concentration of cGMP in the cytoplasm; and (3) the reduction in cGMP concentration closes the cGMP-gated channels, thus hyperpolarizing the photoreceptor. We shall now examine these events step by step.

Stage 1: Light Activates Pigment Molecules in the Photoreceptors

In rod cells the visual pigment, rhodopsin, has two parts. The protein portion, *opsin*, is embedded in the

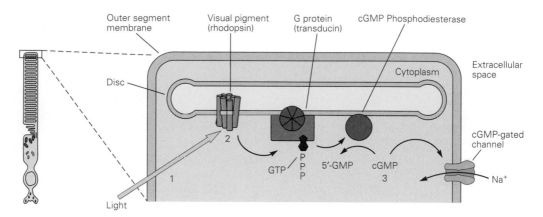

Figure 26-4 Phototransduction involves the closing of cation channels in the outer segment of the photoreceptor membrane. In the absence of light these cation channels are kept open by intracellular cGMP and conduct an inward current, carried largely by Na+.

When light strikes the photoreceptor (illustrated here by a rod cell) the cGMP-gated channels are closed by a three-step process. (**1**) Light is absorbed by and activates pigment mole-cules (rhodopsin in rods) in the disc membrane (the **green rectangle** in the rhodopsin molecule represents the light-absorbing portion, retinal). (**2**) The activated pigment stimulates a G protein (transducin in rods), which in turn activates cGMP phosphodiesterase. This enzyme catalyzes the breakdown of cGMP to 5'-GMP. (**3**) As the cGMP concentration is lowered, the cGMP-gated channels close, thereby reducing the inward current and causing the photoreceptor to hyperpolarize.

disc membrane and does not by itself absorb light. The light-absorbing portion, *retinal,* is a derivative of vita-min A. Retinal can assume several different isomeric conformations, two of which are important in different phases of the visual cycle. In its nonactivated form rhodopsin contains the 11-*cis* isomer of retinal, which fits snugly into a binding site in the opsin molecule (Fig-ure 26-3A).

Activation of rhodopsin starts with the absorption of light, which causes retinal to change from the 11-*cis* to the all-*trans* configuration (Figure 26-3B). This reaction is the only light-dependent step in vision. As a result of this conformational change, retinal no longer fits into the binding site in opsin. The opsin, therefore, under-goes a conformational change to a semistable conforma-tion called metarhodopsin II, which triggers the second step of phototransduction discussed below.

Metarhodopsin II is unstable and splits within min-utes, yielding opsin and all-*trans* retinal. The all-*trans* retinal is then transported from the rods to pigment epithelial cells, where it is reduced to all-*trans* retinol (vitamin A), the precursor in the synthesis of 11-*cis* reti-nal, which is transported back to the rods. All-*trans* retinol is thus a crucial compound in the visual system and, because it cannot be synthesized by humans, must be supplied in the diet. Deficiencies of vitamin A can lead to night blindness and, if untreated, to a deteriora-tion of receptor outer segments and eventually total blindness.

In the retina of primates each of the three types of cone cells contains a different pigment optimized for ab-sorption of light in a different part of the visible light spectrum. As in rods, the visual pigments in cones are composed of two parts: a protein called cone opsin and a light-absorbing portion, 11-*cis* retinal. Each type of cone pigment contains a different isoform of cone opsin that interacts with 11-*cis* retinal in a distinct way, caus-ing it to be most sensitive to a particular part of the visi-ble spectrum. The existence of three types of cones with different absorption characteristics underlies trivariant color vision in humans (see Chapter 29).

Stage 2: Activation of Pigment Molecules Reduces the Cytoplasmic Concentration of Cyclic GMP

The activation of pigment molecules by light leads to a reduction in the cytoplasmic concentration of the sec-ond messenger cGMP. The concentration of cGMP is controlled by two enzymes. It is synthesized from GTP by guanylyl cyclase, and it is broken down to 5'-GMP by cGMP phosphodiesterase, a protein peripherally as-sociated with the disc membrane (see Figure 26-4). The concentration of cGMP is affected by light because cGMP phosphodiesterase is itself controlled by the vi-sual pigments. In darkness cGMP phosphodiesterase is only weakly active, and the concentration of cGMP is therefore relatively high. Activation of pigment mole-cules by light leads to the activation of the phosphodi-

Box 26-1 The Dark Current

In darkness two currents predominate in a photoreceptor. An inward current flows through cGMP-gated channels, which are confined to the photoreceptor's outer segment, while an outward K^+ current flows through nongated K^+-selective channels, which are like those of other neurons and are confined to the inner segment. The outward current carried by the K^+ channels tends to hyperpolarize the photoreceptor toward the equilibrium potential for K^+ (around -70 mV). The inward current tends to depolarize the photoreceptor. The photoreceptor is able to maintain steady intracellular concentrations of Na^+ and K^+ in the face of these large fluxes because its

inner segment has a high density of Na^+-K^+ pumps, which pump out Na^+ and pump in K^+ (Figure 26-5A).

In darkness the cytoplasmic concentration of cGMP is high, thus maintaining the cGMP-gated channels in an open state and allowing a steady inward current, called the dark current (Figure 26-5B). As a result, in darkness the photoreceptor's membrane potential is around -40 mV, significantly more depolarized than that of most neurons. When light reduces the level of cGMP, thus closing cGMP-gated channels, the inward current that flows through these channels is reduced and the cell becomes hyperpolarized (Figure 26-5C).

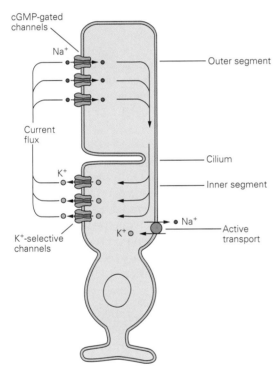

Figure 26-5A. An inward current flows into a photoreceptor through cGMP-gated channels and out of the cell, through nongated K^+ channels. Active transport (Na^+-K^+) pumps maintain the cell's Na^+ and K^+ concentrations at steady levels.

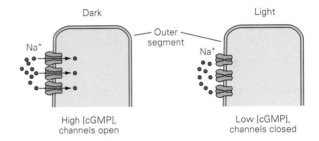

Figure 26-5B. A reduction in the cytoplasmic concentration of cGMP closes the cGMP-gated channels.

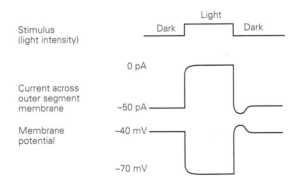

Figure 26-5C. An inward current of -50 pA is suppressed by a bright light, hyperpolarizing the cell to -70 mV, the equilibrium potential for K^+. A light of intermediate intensity would hyperpolarize the cell to potentials between -40 and -70 mV.

Box 26-2 Calcium and Light Adaptation

Calcium modulates the function of several proteins of the phototransduction pathway. The recovery of the cone membrane potential and the desensitization of the cone that underlie light adaptation are mediated by a slow decrease in Ca^{2+} concentration in the cone outer segment during prolonged illumination (the opposite changes occur during dark adaptation).

In darkness Ca^{2+} constantly flows into the outer segment of the cone through the cGMP-gated channels. (Calcium accounts for about one-seventh of the current that flows through these channels). The Ca^{2+} that enters is extruded by a specialized Ca^{2+} carrier in the outer segment membrane, and this process maintains a constant Ca^{2+} concentration in the outer segment. During prolonged illumination the cGMP-gated channels close, thus reducing the influx of Ca^{2+}. This reduction in influx leads to a slow decrease in the intracellular Ca^{2+} concentration because the extrusion of Ca^{2+} continues.

The slow decrease in Ca^{2+} concentration allows the cone membrane potential to recover from its initial hyperpolarizing response to bright illumination because Ca^{2+} inhibits guanylyl cyclase, the enzyme that synthesizes cGMP from GTP. Thus, in darkness, when the Ca^{2+} level is relatively high, guanylyl cyclase is maintained in a partially inhibited state. The slow decrease in Ca^{2+} concentration during illumination relieves the inhibitory effect of Ca^{2+} on guanylyl cyclase. As a result, more cGMP is synthesized, and the concentration of cGMP slowly increases. This results in the reopening of cGMP-gated channels and, consequently, slow depolarization of the cone.

The slow decrease in Ca^{2+} concentration also causes the desensitization of the cone during light adaptation, at least partly through effects on the visual pigments and the cGMP-gated channels. Lowering the Ca^{2+} concentration is believed to speed up the inactivation of the visual pigments, so that the effectiveness of a given light flash in activating cGMP phosphodiesterase is reduced. A lower concentration of Ca^{2+} also decreases the sensitivity of the cGMP-gated channels to changes in cGMP. Because of these effects of Ca^{2+}, a more intense light stimulus is required to close the same number of cGMP-gated channels. Whether these effects entirely account for the desensitization is unknown.

---

esterase, which breaks down cGMP and lowers its concentration.

Photoactivation of a single rhodopsin molecule can lead to the hydrolysis of more than 10^5 molecules of cGMP per second. An activated rhodopsin molecule diffuses within the disc membrane and activates hundreds of molecules of the regulatory protein transducin, each of which stimulates a phosphodiesterase molecule. Each phosphodiesterase molecule in turn is capable of hydrolyzing over 10^3 molecules of cGMP per second.

The biochemical cascade initiated by the photoactivation of rhodopsin resembles the cascades triggered by the binding of many hormones and neurotransmitters to their receptors. Indeed, the rod and cone opsins show a high degree of structural similarity with the family of hormone and transmitter receptors that couple to G proteins (see Chapter 13). Moreover, transducin is a member of the trimeric G protein family. As with other G proteins, the activation of transducin involves a characteristic interaction with guanine nucleotides (see Figure 13-3). Inactive transducin binds a molecule of GDP tightly; upon interaction with activated rhodopsin in the disc membrane, however, transducin exchanges GDP for GTP and itself becomes active. Transducin becomes inactivated because it also has GTPase activity, which breaks down the bound GTP molecule into GDP (see Figure 13-4).

Two mechanisms terminate the light response. As described, transducin inactivates itself by hydrolyzing bound GTP. Also, once activated, rhodopsin becomes a target for phosphorylation by a specific protein kinase, opsin kinase; the phosphorylated rhodopsin then interacts with a specific regulatory protein called arrestin, leading to its rapid inactivation.

Stage 3: The Reduction in Cyclic GMP Concentration Closes cGMP-Gated Ion Channels, Thus Hyperpolarizing the Photoreceptor

The light-evoked decrease in cGMP results in the closure of cGMP-gated ion channels in the photoreceptor (Figure 26-4). Cyclic GMP gates these channels by binding directly to the cytoplasmic face of the channel; the channel is activated by the cooperative binding of at least three molecules of cGMP. The cGMP-gated channel in photoreceptors was the first known example of an ion channel regulated by a cyclic nucleotide acting directly on the channel rather than through a protein kinase. Similar channels are also present in some retinal bipolar cells (see below) and in olfactory neurons (see Chapter 32).

In the absence of a light stimulus the cGMP-gated channels conduct an inward current that tends to depolarize the photoreceptor. The light-evoked closing of

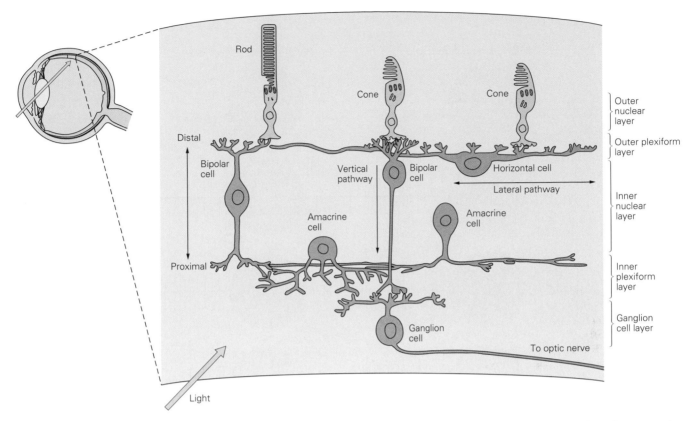

Figure 26-6 The retina has three major functional classes of neurons. Photoreceptors (rods and cones) lie in the outer nuclear layer, interneurons (bipolar, horizontal, and amacrine cells) in the inner nuclear layer, and ganglion cells in the ganglion cell layer. Photoreceptors, bipolar cells, and horizontal cells make synaptic connections with each other in the outer plexiform layer. The bipolar, amacrine, and ganglion cells make contact in the inner plexiform layer. Information flows vertically from photoreceptors to bipolar cells to ganglion cells, as well as laterally via horizontal cells in the outer plexiform layer and amacrine cells in the inner plexiform layer. (Adapted from Dowling 1979.)

these channels reduces this current and therefore hyperpolarizes the cell (Box 26-1).

Photoreceptors Slowly Adapt to Changes in Light Intensity

Whenever we step from a dark environment into bright daylight the light is blinding at first, but over a period of several seconds the eyes adapt. Likewise when we step into a dark movie theater our eyes must adapt before we are able to see our way around. Light or dark adaptation involves many changes in the retina and eye (such as a contraction or expansion of the pupil to reduce or increase the amount of light reaching the retina), but the two most important changes occur in cone photoreceptors. (We describe the events occurring during light adaptation; the opposite events occur during dark adaptation.)

The first change in cones during light adaptation is the slow recovery of the membrane potential. A very bright light closes all cGMP-gated channels, hyperpolarizing the cones to −70 mV, the equilibrium potential for K⁺. In this state the cones cannot respond to further increases in light intensity. If this illumination is maintained, the cones slowly depolarize to a membrane potential between −70 and −40 mV (the resting potential), and are once again capable of hyperpolarizing in response to further increases in light intensity—the bright light is no longer blinding. The second change in cones during light adaption is the desensitization of the receptor. During prolonged illumination by a background light, the smallest increment in light intensity capable of evoking a detectable change in membrane potential increases in proportion to the background intensity, in accordance with Weber's law (Chapter 21). Both changes in the responses of cones—slow recovery of the membrane potential and desensitization—are due to a slow

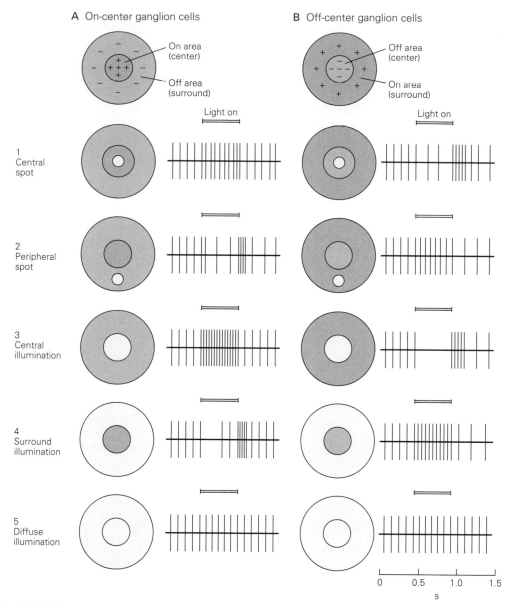

A On-center ganglion cells

On area (center)
Off area (surround)

Light on

1 Central spot

2 Peripheral spot

3 Central illumination

4 Surround illumination

5 Diffuse illumination

B Off-center ganglion cells

Off area (center)
On area (surround)

Light on

0   0.5   1.0   1.5
s

Figure 26-7 Retinal ganglion cells respond optimally to contrast in their receptive fields. Ganglion cells have circular receptive fields, with specialized center (**pink**) and surround (**gray**) regions. On-center cells are excited when stimulated by light in the center and inhibited when stimulated in the surround; off-center cells have the opposite responses. The figure shows the responses of both types of cells to five different light stimuli (the stimulated portion of the receptive field is shown in **yellow**). The pattern of action potentials fired by the ganglion cell in response to each stimulus is also shown in extracellular recordings. Duration of illumination is indicated by a bar above each record. (Adapted from Kuffler 1953.)

A. On-center cells respond best when the entire central part of

the receptive field is stimulated (**3**). These cells also respond well, but less vigorously, when only a portion of the central field is stimulated by a spot of light (**1**). Illumination of the surround with a spot of light (**2**) or ring of light (**4**) reduces or suppresses the cell firing, which resumes more vigorously for a short period after the light is turned off. Diffuse illumination of the entire receptive field (**5**) elicits a relatively weak discharge because the center and surround oppose each other's effects.

B. The spontaneous firing of off-center cells is suppressed when the central area of the receptive field is illuminated (**1, 3**) but accelerates for a short period after the stimulus is turned off. Light shone onto the surround of the receptive field excites the cell (**2, 4**).

decrease in Ca^{2+} concentration, a decrease that affects the function of several proteins in the phototransduction pathway (Box 26-2).

The Output of the Retina Is Conveyed by the Ganglion Cells

We now turn to the second topic of this chapter: How does the retina modify and process the signals evoked by light in photoreceptors before sending them to higher centers? The output of the retina is conveyed by the ganglion cells. Unlike photoreceptors, which respond to light with graded changes in membrane potential, ganglion cells transmit information as trains of action potentials. The axons of these cells form the optic nerve, which projects to the lateral geniculate nucleus of the thalamus and the superior colliculus as well as to the pretectum and other targets (see Chapter 27).

Between the photoreceptors and the ganglion cells are three classes of interneurons: bipolar, horizontal, and amacrine cells (Figure 26-6). These cells do not simply transmit signals from the photoreceptors to the ganglion cells; they also combine signals from several photoreceptors in such a way that the electrical responses evoked in ganglion cells depend critically on the precise spatial and temporal patterns of the light that stimulates the retina. In this section we examine the responses of ganglion cells to different patterns of light. In the final section of this chapter we discuss how the synaptic connections among the photoreceptors, interneurons, and ganglion cells are organized for carrying out the processing of the visual image.

The Receptive Field of the Ganglion Cell Has a Center and an Antagonistic Surround

Individual ganglion cells are never silent, even in the dark, but this spontaneous activity is modulated by the input from retinal interneurons. The inputs to a ganglion cell originate from neighboring photoreceptors in a circumscribed area of the retina, the *receptive field* for that cell. In effect, the ganglion cell's receptive field is the area of retina that the ganglion cell monitors. The receptive fields of ganglion cells have two important features.

First, when small spots of light on the retina are used to probe the properties of ganglion cell receptive fields, the receptive fields prove to be roughly circular.

Second, in most ganglion cells the receptive field is divided into two parts: a circular zone at the center, called the *receptive field center,* and the remaining area of the field, called the *surround.* Ganglion cells respond op-

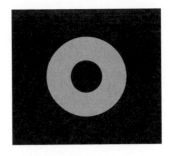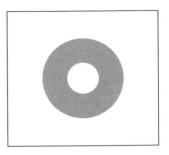

Figure 26-8 The appearance of an object depends principally on the contrast between the object and its background, not on the intensity of the light source. The two gray rings in the figures are identical in hue, but they appear to have different brightness because the different backgrounds produce different contrasts.

timally to differential illumination of the receptive field center and surround.

Two classes of ganglion cells can be distinguished by their responses to a small spot of light applied to the center of their receptive field (Figure 26-7). *On-center ganglion cells* are excited when light is directed to the center of their receptive field. Light applied to the surround inhibits the cell; the most effective inhibitory stimulus is a ring of light on the entire surround. *Off-center ganglion cells* are inhibited by light applied to the center of their receptive field. However, their firing rate increases for a short period of time after the light is removed; that is, they are excited when the spot of light on the center is turned *off.* Light excites an off-center ganglion cell when it is directed to the surround of the receptive field. In both types of cells the response evoked by a ring of light on the entire surround cancels the response evoked by light directed to the center almost completely. For this reason, diffuse illumination of the entire receptive field evokes only a small response in either type of cell (Figure 26-7). Not all ganglion cells have a center-surround receptive field organization. For example, a few ganglion cells respond to changes in the overall luminance of the visual field and are important in controlling pupillary reflexes (see Chapter 27).

On-center and off-center ganglion cells are present in roughly equal numbers, and every photoreceptor sends output to both types. Thus, ganglion cells provide two parallel pathways for the processing of visual information. In addition, their receptive fields vary in size across the retina. In the foveal region of the primate retina, where visual acuity is greatest, the receptive fields are small, with centers that are only a few minutes of arc (60 min = 1 degree). At the periphery of the retina, where acuity is low, the fields are larger, with centers of 3°–5° (1° on the retina is equal to about 0.25 mm).

Box 26-3 The Center-Surround Receptive Field of Bipolar Cells

Cone cells in the center of the receptive field of a bipolar cell synapse directly on the bipolar cell. Each cone cell synapses on both on-center and off-center bipolar cells. Cone cells release a single neurotransmitter, glutamate, which inhibits (hyperpolarizes) on-center bipolar cells and excites (depolarizes) off-center cells.

In the dark the cones are depolarized (around -40 mV), so that voltage-gated Ca^{2+} channels in their synaptic terminals are open, allowing Ca^{2+} to enter the terminals and trigger the release of glutamate. This constant release of glutamate in the dark maintains the on-center bipolar cells in a hyperpolarized state. When illuminated, however, the cones become hyperpolarized, and the voltage-gated Ca^{2+} channels close, reducing the Ca^{2+} influx and therefore the amount of glutamate the cells release; as a result, the on-center bipolar cells depolarize.

Conversely, cone cells maintain off-center bipolar cells in a depolarized state in the dark. When glutamate release is reduced by light the off-center bipolar cells hyperpolarize (Figure 26-9).

Glutamate produces different responses in the two classes of bipolar cells by gating different cation channels. In off-center bipolar cells glutamate opens a type of cation channel that carries an inward (depolarizing) Na^+ current into the cells. In on-center bipolar cells the mechanism by which glutamate hyperpolarizes the cell is unusual and may be different for rods and cones. At some synapses the transmitter appears to act by opening K^+-selective ion channels. At others it closes a cGMP-gated channel that carries an inward Na^+ current. In the absence of transmitter this type of channel is kept open by a high intracellular concentration of cGMP. Glutamate appears to cause the closure of these channels in precisely the same way that light causes the closure of cGMP-gated channels in photoreceptors—by activating a specific glutamate receptor that activates a G protein, which in turn activates cGMP phosphodiesterase and lowers the cytoplasmic concentration of cGMP.

Cones in the surround of a bipolar cell's receptive field synapse on horizontal cells. Horizontal cells do not make direct synaptic contact with the bipolar cells, however. Instead, they have synapses on cones in the center of the bipolar cell's receptive field. When the surround is illuminated, the horizontal cells depolarize the cones in the center, the opposite effect of light absorption by these cones (Figure 26-10). Whether this mechanism alone accounts for the antagonism between center and surround in bipolar cells is not yet known.

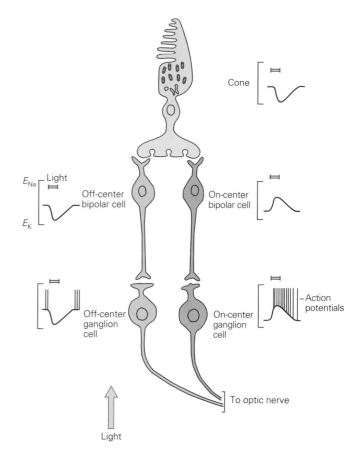

Figure 26-9 On-center and off-center bipolar cells establish parallel pathways for the signal of a single cone. Each bipolar cell makes an excitatory connection with a ganglion cell of the same type. When the cone is hyperpolarized by light, the on-center bipolar cell is excited and the off-center bipolar cell is inhibited. These opposite and simultaneous actions are initiated by the transmitter glutamate. In the dark the cone releases large amounts of transmitter because it is depolarized. Light, by hyperpolarizing the cone, causes a reduction in transmitter release. The same transmitter has different actions because the two types of bipolar cells have different postsynaptic receptors that gate different types of ion channels. The responses of the ganglion cells are largely determined by the inputs from the bipolar cells. The on-center bipolar cell, which becomes depolarized by illumination of its receptive field center, will depolarize the on-center ganglion cells; the off-center cell shows the opposite response.

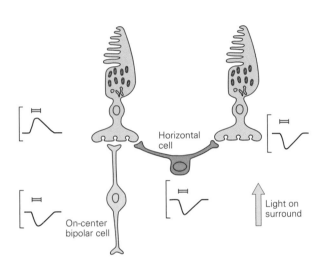

Figure 26-10 Signals from cones in the surround of a bipolar cell's receptive field are mediated by horizontal cells. Center-surround antagonism is illustrated here for an on-center bipolar cell. The horizontal cell receives input from a cone in the surround of the on-center bipolar cell and also has a connection with a postsynaptic cone in the center of the bipolar cell's receptive field. In the dark, horizontal cells release an inhibitory transmitter that maintains postsynaptic cones in the receptive field center in a slightly hyperpolarized state. Illumination of cones in the bipolar cell's surround hyperpolarizes those cones, which in turn hyperpolarize the postsynaptic horizontal cell. (In the dark the cones in the surround are maintained in a depolarized state and thus excite those horizontal cells.) This hyperpolarization of the horizontal cell reduces the amount of inhibitory transmitter released by the horizontal cell onto postsynaptic cones in the receptive field center, and as a result these cones become depolarized (the opposite effect of light absorption by these cones). This in turn allows the on-center bipolar cell to become hyperpolarized, the opposite effect of illumination in the receptive field center.

Ganglion Cells Are Specialized for the Detection of Contrasts and Rapid Changes in the Visual Image

Why do ganglion cells have a center-surround receptive field organization, and why are there parallel on-center and off-center pathways?

As we have just seen, ganglion cells respond only weakly to uniform illumination because of the center-surround structure of their receptive fields. They respond best when the light intensities in the center and surround are quite different. They therefore report principally the contrasts in light, rather than its absolute intensity.

Most of the useful information in a visual scene is, however, contained in the pattern of contrasts. The absolute amount of light reflected by objects is relatively uninformative because it is largely determined by the intensity of the light source. Doubling the ambient light intensity will double the amount of light reflected by objects but does not alter contrasts between the objects. The center-surround organization of the receptive field of ganglion cells is therefore an adaptation for detecting useful information in the visual scene.

As we shall see in Chapters 28 and 29, perception of the brightness and color of objects relies mainly on information about contrast rather than the absolute amount of light and can therefore be influenced by the contrast between an object and its surroundings. For example, the same gray ring looks much lighter against a black background than against a white one (Figure 26-8).

Why does the detection of contrast start in the retina? In principle the information from photoreceptors could be sent directly to higher centers for this processing. However, signals transmitted through several relay steps to the cortex inevitably become slightly distorted. One way of minimizing the effect of transmission errors is for the retina itself to measure the difference and to transmit that information. This, in effect, is what the ganglion cell does. The firing rate of a ganglion cell provides a measure of the difference in the intensities of light illuminating the center and surround. In this way information about small differences in intensities is directly transmitted to higher centers.

Parallel on-center and off-center pathways also enhance the performance of the visual system because each type of ganglion cell responds best to either rapid increases or decreases in illumination. On-center ganglion cells have a low rate of firing under dim illumination; rapid increases in firing thus signal rapid *increases* in light intensity in their receptive field center. In contrast, off-center ganglion cells discharge at a low rate in the light; rapid increases in firing in these cells therefore signal rapid *decreases* in light intensity in their receptive field center. This specialization has been demonstrated by experiments in which the function of on-center ganglion cells in awake monkeys was blocked using a pharmacological agent, aminophosphorobutyrate (APB), which selectively antagonizes transmission from photoreceptors to on-center bipolar cells. Detection of rapid increases, but not decreases, in illumination was severely impaired in these animals.

Specialized Ganglion Cells Process Different Aspects of the Visual Image

In addition to contrast and rapid changes in illumination, the visual system also analyzes several other aspects of the visual image, such as color, form, and movement. As we discussed briefly in the preceding chapter and will discuss again in more detail in subsequent chapters, these features are processed in the visual cortex in parallel pathways. This parallel processing begins in the retina with parallel networks of ganglion cells.

Each region of the retina has several functionally distinct subsets of ganglion cells that convey, in parallel pathways, signals from the same photoreceptors. Most ganglion cells in the primate retina fall into two functional classes, M (for *magni*, or large) and P (for *parvi*, or small). Each class includes both on-center and off-center cells.

M cells have large receptive fields (reflected in their large dendritic arbors) and respond relatively transiently to sustained illumination. They respond optimally to large objects and are able to follow rapid changes in the stimulus. As we shall see in Chapter 27, they appear therefore to be concerned with the analysis of the gross features of a stimulus and its movement. The smaller P cells, which are more numerous, have small receptive fields, respond selectively to specific wavelengths, and are therefore involved in the perception of form and color. P cells are thought to be responsible for the analysis of fine detail in the visual image, although some M cells may also be involved in this function.

The primate retina also contains ganglion cells that do not fall into the P or M classes. The functions of these cells are largely unknown, although one type is known to report on the overall ambient light intensity.

Signals From Photoreceptors Are Relayed to Ganglion Cells Through a Network of Interneurons

How do the relatively simple signals provided by photoreceptors give rise to the complex responses of the ganglion cells? Although the circuitry connecting these cells appears complicated, on close examination it is relatively simple. Each type of retinal interneuron (horizontal, bipolar, and amacrine) plays a specific role in shaping photoreceptor signals transmitted through the retina. The role of retinal interneurons is best illustrated by focusing on the bipolar cells, as they represent the most direct pathway between receptors and ganglion cells. As a further simplification, we restrict our attention to the circuitry for cones, the circuitry that mediates vision in normal daylight.

Bipolar Cells Convey Cone Signals to Ganglion Cells Through Direct or Indirect Pathways

Visual information is transferred from cones to ganglion cells along two types of pathways in the retina. Cones in the *center* of a ganglion cell's receptive field make direct synaptic contact with bipolar cells that in turn directly contact the ganglion cells; these connections are known as direct or vertical pathways. Signals from cones in the *surround* of the ganglion cell's receptive field are also conveyed to the ganglion cell through bipolar cells but only indirectly by means of horizontal and some amacrine cells; these indirect connections are called lateral pathways. Horizontal cells, which have large dendritic trees, transfer information from distant cones to bipolar cells. (Horizontal cells are also electrically coupled to each other by gap junctions and thus are able to respond to inputs from even more distant cones that contact neighboring horizontal cells.) Curiously, the horizontal cells do not appear to convey information to the bipolar cells directly, but rather by feeding back onto cones in the center of the bipolar cell's receptive field (see Figure 26-10). Some types of amacrine cells transfer information from distant bipolar cells to ganglion cells (see Figure 26-6).

Most synaptic contacts in the retina are grouped in two plexiform (network-like) layers. The outer plexiform layer contains the processes of receptor, bipolar, and horizontal cells, while the inner plexiform layer contains the processes of bipolar, amacrine, and ganglion cells (see Figure 26-6). Thus the bipolar cells bridge the two plexiform layers by having processes in both.

We have seen that photoreceptors respond to light with graded changes in membrane potential rather than by firing action potentials. The same is true of horizontal and bipolar cells. These cells lack voltage-gated Na^+ channels capable of generating action potentials; instead they transmit signals passively (see Chapter 8). Because these cells are small and have short processes, the signals spread to their synaptic terminals without significant reduction. (Passive signal spread in cells with short processes occurs in many different parts of the brain.) In contrast, the axons of ganglion cells project considerable distances to their targets in the brain and transfer information in the form of trains of action potentials. Many types of amacrine cells also fire action potentials.

The Receptive Fields of Bipolar Cells Have a Center-Surround Organization

Like ganglion cells, the bipolar cells have receptive fields with an antagonistic center-surround organization, and the cells are either on-center or off-center. When cones in the center of the receptive field are active, on-center bipolar cells depolarize, while off-center bipolar cells hyperpolarize. When cones in the surround are active, the response of the bipolar cell is opposite that evoked by illumination of the center (Box 26-3).

Different Classes of Bipolar Cells Have Excitatory Connections With Corresponding Classes of Ganglion Cells

The receptive field properties of a ganglion cell largely reflect those of the bipolar cells connected to it, because each type of bipolar cell (on-center or off-center) makes excitatory synaptic connections with the corresponding type of ganglion cell. When on-center bipolar cells are depolarized by light, they depolarize on-center ganglion cells (see Figure 26-9 in Box 26-3).

Although the responses of ganglion cells are largely determined by these direct inputs from bipolar cells, they are also shaped by amacrine cells, a group of interneurons with processes in the inner plexiform layer (see Figure 26-6). There are over 20 morphologically distinct types of amacrine cells that use at least 8 different neurotransmitters. Some amacrine cells function like horizontal cells: They mediate antagonistic inputs from bipolar cells in the ganglion cell's surround. Others have been implicated in shaping the complex receptive field properties of specific classes of ganglion cells, such as the M-type ganglion cells that process orientation information (see Chapter 28).

An Overall View

The absorption of light and its transduction into electrical signals is carried out by the photoreceptors. Visual information is then transferred from the receptors to the ganglion cells via the bipolar cells. The ganglion cells in turn project to the brain; their axons form the optic nerve. Two types of interneurons (horizontal cells and amacrine cells) provide lateral inputs to bipolar cells and ganglion cells.

The cyclic nucleotide cGMP plays a central role in phototransduction. Absorption of light by the photosensitive visual pigments in the photoreceptor triggers a second-messenger cascade. The activated pigment molecules stimulate a G protein, transducin, which in turn activates a phosphodiesterase that catalyzes the hydrolysis of cGMP. Light absorption therefore causes a reduction in the cytoplasmic concentration of cGMP. In darkness cGMP opens specialized ion channels that carry a depolarizing current into the cell, so that the reduction in the level of cGMP makes the photoreceptor hyperpolarize.

Signals from photoreceptors to ganglion cells are conveyed in parallel on-center and off-center pathways. An on-center ganglion cell is excited when light stimulates the center of its receptive field and inhibited when light stimulates its surround. An off-center ganglion cell exhibits the opposite responses; it is inhibited when light stimulates its center and excited by light on its surround. These transformations of the visual signal assist higher centers in detecting weak contrasts and rapid changes in light intensity. In addition, ganglion cells are specialized for processing different aspects of the visual image such as movement, fine spatial detail, or color.

The pattern of synaptic connections in the retina explains how the various responses of ganglion cells arise. Interposed between the photoreceptors and ganglion cells are interneurons, the bipolar cells. Bipolar cells, like ganglion cells, fall into two classes, on-center and off-center. The transmitter released by cones excites bipolar cells of one class and inhibits the others. Each cone makes contact with both types of bipolar cells. Cones in the receptive-field center of a ganglion cell synapse onto bipolar cells that make direct contact with the ganglion cell. Inputs from cones in the receptive-field surround are relayed along lateral pathways by horizontal and amacrine cells.

As we shall see in subsequent chapters, the segregation of information into parallel processing pathways and the shaping of response properties by inhibitory lateral connections are pervasive organizational principles in the visual system.

Marc Tessier-Lavigne

Selected Readings

DeVries SH, Baylor DA. 1993. Synaptic circuitry of the retina and olfactory bulb. Cell 72(Suppl):139–149.

Dowling JE. 1987. *The Retina: An Approachable Part of the Brain.* Cambridge, MA: Belknap.

Hurley JB. 1994. Termination of photoreceptor responses. Curr Opin Neurobiol 4(4):481–487.

Lagnado L, Baylor D. 1992. Signal flow in visual transduction. Neuron 8:955–1002.

Nakanishi S. 1995. Second-order neurones and receptor mechanisms in visual- and olfactory-information processing. Trends Neurosci 18(8):359–364.

Schiller PH. 1992. The ON and OFF channels of the visual system. Trends Neurosci 15(3):86–92.

Stryer L. 1987. The molecules of visual excitation. Sci Am 257(1):42–50.

References

Dowling JE. 1979. Information processing by local circuits: the vertebrate retina as a model system. In: FO Schmitt, FG Worden (eds). *The Neurosciences: Fourth Study Program,* pp. 163–181. Cambridge, MA: MIT Press.

Hecht S, Shlaer S, Pirenne MH. 1942. Energy, quanta and vision. J Gen Physiol 25:819–840.

Kuffler SW. 1953. Discharge patterns and functional organization of mammalian retina. J Neurophysiol 16:37–68.

Nathans J, Hogness DS. 1984. Isolation and nucleotide sequence of the gene encoding human rhodopsin. Proc Natl Acad Sci U S A 81:4851–4855.

O'Brien DF. 1982. The chemistry of vision. Science 218: 961–966.

Young RW. 1970. Visual cells. Sci Am 223:80–91.

27

Central Visual Pathways

T HE VISUAL SYSTEM HAS THE most complex neural circuitry of all the sensory systems. The auditory nerve contains about 30,000 fibers, but the optic nerve contains over one million! Most of what we know about the functional organization of the visual system is derived from experiments similar to those used to investigate the somatic sensory system. The similarities of these systems allow us to identify general principles governing the transformation of sensory information in the brain as well as the organization and functioning of the cerebral cortex.

In this chapter we describe the flow of visual information in two stages: first from the retina to the midbrain and thalamus, then from the thalamus to the primary visual cortex. We shall begin by considering how the world is projected on the retina and describe the projection of the retina to three subcortical brain areas: the pretectal region, the superior colliculus of the midbrain, and the lateral geniculate nucleus of the thalamus. We shall then examine the pathways from the lateral geniculate nucleus to the cortex, focusing on the different information conveyed by the magno- and parvocellular divisions of the visual pathways. Finally, we consider the structure and function of the initial cortical relay in the primary visual cortex in order to elucidate the first steps in the cortical processing of visual information necessary for perception. Chapter 28 then follows this visual processing from the primary visual cortex into two pathways to the parietal and temporal cortex.

In examining the flow of visual information we shall see how the architecture of the cortex—specifically its modular organization—is adapted to the analysis of information for vision.

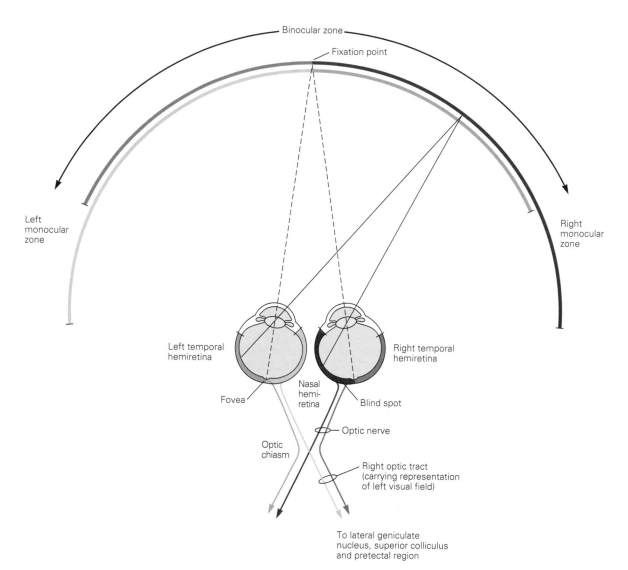

Figure 27-1 The visual field has both binocular and monocular zones. Light from the binocular zone strikes the retina in both eyes, whereas light from the monocular zone strikes the retina only in the eye on the same side. For example, light from a left monocular zone (temporal crescent) falls on only the ipsilateral nasal hemiretina and does not project upon the contralateral retina. The temporal and nasal hemiretinas are defined with respect to the fovea, the region in the center of the retina with highest acuity. The optic disc, the region where the ganglion cell axons leave the retina, is free of photoreceptors and therefore creates a gap, or blind spot, in the visual field for each eye (see Figure 27-2). While each optic nerve carries all the visual information from one eye, each optic tract carries a complete representation of one half of the binocular zone in the visual field. Fibers from the nasal hemiretina of each eye cross to the opposite side at the optic chiasm, whereas fibers from the temporal hemiretina do not cross. In the illustration, light from the right half of the binocular zone falls on the left temporal hemiretina and right nasal hemiretina. Axons from these hemiretinas thus contain a complete representation of the right hemifield of vision (see Figure 27-6).

The Retinal Image Is an Inversion of the Visual Field

For both clinical and experimental purposes it is important to distinguish between the retinal image and the visual field. The surface of the retina is divided with respect to the midline: the *nasal hemiretina* lies medial to the fovea, the *temporal hemiretina* lateral to the fovea. Each half of the retina is further divided into dorsal (or superior) and ventral (or inferior) quadrants.

The visual field is the view seen by the two eyes without movement of the head. Left and right halves of

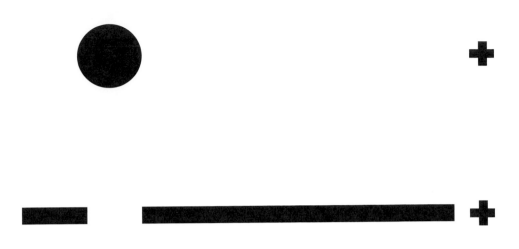

Figure 27-2 Locate the blind spot in your left eye by shutting the right eye and fixating the upper cross with the left eye. Hold the book about 15 inches from the eye and move it slightly nearer and farther from the eye until the circle on the left disappears. At this point the circle occupies the blind spot in the left eye. If you fixate the left eye on the lower cross, the gap in the black line falls on the blind spot and the black line is seen as continuous. (Adapted from Hurvich 1981.)

the visual field can be defined when the foveas of both eyes are fixed on a single point in space. The *left visual hemifield* projects onto the nasal hemiretina of the left eye and the temporal hemiretina of the right eye. The *right visual hemifield* projects onto the nasal hemiretina of the right eye and the temporal hemiretina of the left eye (Figure 27-1). Light originating in the central region of the visual field, called the *binocular zone,* enters both eyes. In each half of the visual field there is also a *monocular zone:* light from the temporal portion of the visual hemifield projects onto only the nasal hemiretina of the eye on the same side (the ipsilateral nasal hemiretina). This monocular portion of the visual field is also called the *temporal crescent* because it constitutes the crescent-shaped temporal extreme of each visual field. Since there is no binocular overlap in this region, vision is lost in the entire temporal crescent if the nasal hemiretina is severely damaged.

The region of the retina from which the ganglion cell axons exit, the optic disc, contains no photoreceptors and therefore is insensitive to light—a *blind spot* in the retina. Since the disc is nasal to the fovea in each eye (Figure 27-1), light coming from a single point in the binocular zone never falls on both blind spots simultaneously so that in normal vision we are unaware of them. We can experience the blind spot only by using one eye (Figure 27-2). The blind spot demonstrates what blind people experience—not blackness, but simply nothing. It also explains why damage to large regions of the peripheral retina goes unnoticed. In these instances no large dark zone appears in the periphery, and it is usually through accidents, such as bumping into an unnoticed object, or through clinical testing of the visual fields, that this absence of sight is noticed.

In tracing the flow of visual information to the brain we should keep in mind the correspondence between regions of the visual field and the retinal image. This relationship can be particularly difficult to follow for two reasons. First, the lens of the eye inverts the visual image (Figure 27-3). The upper half of the visual field projects onto the inferior (ventral) half of the retina, while the lower half of the visual field projects onto the superior (dorsal) half of the retina. Thus, damage to the inferior half of the retina of one eye causes a monocular deficit in the upper half of the visual field. Second, a single point in the binocular portion of one visual hemifield projects onto different regions of the two retinas. For example, a point of light in the binocular half of the right visual hemifield falls upon the temporal hemiretina of the left eye and the nasal hemiretina of the right eye (see Figure 27-1).

Axons from the ganglion cells in the retina extend through the optic disc and, at the optic chiasm, the fibers from the *nasal* half of each retina cross to the opposite side of the brain. The axons from ganglion cells in the temporal hemiretinas do not cross. Thus, the optic chiasm fibers from both retinas are bundled in the left and right optic tracts. In this arrangement the axons from the *left half of each retina* (the temporal hemiretina of the left eye and the nasal hemiretina of the right eye) project in the left optic tract, which thus carries a complete representation of the *right hemifield of vision* (Figure 27-1). Fibers from the *right half of each retina* (the nasal hemiretina of the left eye and the temporal hemiretina of the right eye) project in the right optic tract, which carries a complete representation of the *left hemifield of vision.* This separation of the right visual hemifield into the left optic tract and the left visual hemifield into the right optic tract is maintained in all the projections to the subcortical visual nuclei, which we consider next.

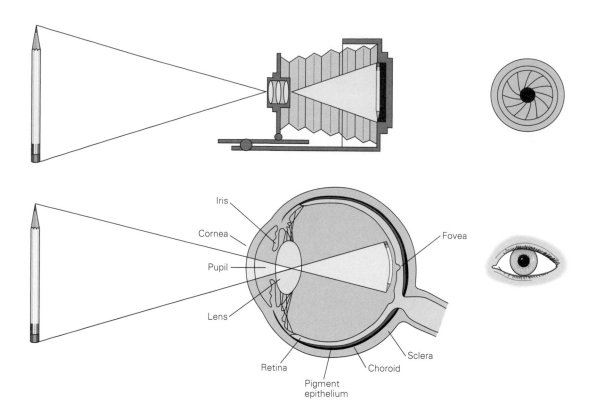

Figure 27-3 The lens of the eye projects an inverted image on the retina in the same way as a camera. (Adapted from Groves and Schlesinger 1979.)

The Retina Projects to Subcortical Regions in the Brain

The axons of all retinal ganglion cells stream toward the optic disc, where they become myelinated and together form the bilateral optic nerves. The optic nerves from each eye project to the optic chiasm, where fibers from each eye destined for one or the other side of the brain are sorted out and rebundled in the bilateral optic tracts, which project to three major subcortical targets: the pretectum, the superior colliculus, and the lateral geniculate nucleus (Figure 27-4). The following discussion of the details of these projections, and particularly our description of cellular activity along these pathways, is based on research in monkeys whose visual systems are similar to those of humans.

The Superior Colliculus Controls Saccadic Eye Movements

The superior colliculus is a structure of alternating gray cellular and white (axonal) layers lying on the roof of the midbrain. Retinal ganglion cells project directly to the superficial layers and form a map of the contralateral visual field. Cells in the superficial layers in turn project through the pulvinar nucleus of the thalamus to a broad area of the cerebral cortex, thus forming an indirect pathway from the retina to the cerebral cortex.

The superior colliculus also receives extensive cortical inputs. The superficial layers receive input from the visual cortex, while deeper layers receive projections from many other areas of the cerebral cortex. These deep layers have the same map of the visual field found in the superficial layers, but the cells also respond to auditory and somatosensory stimuli as well. The locations in space represented by these multisensory inputs are aligned with one another. For example, neurons that respond to a bird flying within the contralateral visual field also will respond to its singing when it is in that same part of the field. In this way, different types of sensory information about an object are conveyed to a common region of the superior colliculus. The auditory and somatosensory inputs are adjusted to fit with the visual map in situations where the maps of these other modalities might diverge. An example of such divergence occurs when our eyes are directed to one side but our head

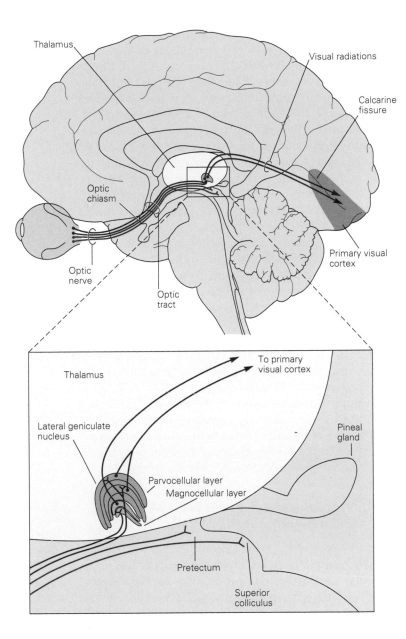

Figure 27-4 A simplified diagram of the projections from the retina to the visual areas of the thalamus (lateral geniculate nucleus) and midbrain (pretectum and superior colliculus). The retinal projection to the pretectal area is important for pupillary reflexes, and the projection to the superior colliculus contributes to visually guided eye movements. The projection to the lateral geniculate nucleus, and from there to the visual cortex, processes visual information for perception.

is directed straight ahead (with respect to the body); a bird sitting where we are looking will fall in the center of the visual field but its song will locate it to one side of the auditory field.

Many cells lying in the deeper layers of the colliculus also discharge vigorously before the onset of saccadic eye movements, those movements that shift the gaze rapidly from one point in the visual scene to another. These cells form a movement map in the intermediate layers of the colliculus, and this map is in register with the visual map: Cells responding to stimuli in the left visual field will discharge vigorously before a leftward-directed saccade. Although the superior colliculus receives direct retinal input, the control of these

saccadic eye movements is thought to be determined more by the inputs from the cerebral cortex that reach the intermediate layers. The organization within the brain of this system for generating saccadic eye movements is considered in Chapter 39.

The Pretectum of the Midbrain Controls Pupillary Reflexes

Light shining in one eye causes constriction of the pupil in that eye (the direct response) as well as in the other eye (the consensual response). Pupillary light reflexes are mediated by retinal ganglion cells that project to the pretectal area of the midbrain, just rostral to the superior colliculus where the midbrain fuses with the thalamus. The cells in the pretectal area project bilaterally to preganglionic parasympathetic neurons in the Edinger-Westphal (or accessory oculomotor) nucleus, which lies immediately adjacent to the neurons of the oculomotor (cranial nerve III) nucleus (Figure 27-5). Preganglionic neurons in the Edinger-Westphal nucleus send axons out of the brain stem in the oculomotor nerve to innervate the ciliary ganglion. This ganglion contains the postganglionic neurons that innervate the smooth muscle of the pupillary sphincter that constricts the pupil. A sympathetic pathway innervates the pupillary radial iris muscles that dilate the pupils.

Pupillary reflexes are clinically important because they indicate the functional state of the afferent and efferent pathways mediating them. As an example, if light directed to the left eye of a patient elicits a consensual response in the right eye but not a direct one in the left eye, then the afferent limb of the reflex, the optic nerve, is intact but the efferent limb to the left eye is damaged, possibly by a lesion of the oculomotor nerve. In contrast, if the afferent optic nerve is lesioned unilaterally, illumination of the affected eye will cause no change in either pupil, but illumination of the *normal* eye will elicit both direct and consensual responses in the two eyes. The absence of pupillary reflexes in an unconscious patient is a symptom of damage to the midbrain, the region from which the oculomotor nerves originate.

The Lateral Geniculate Nucleus Is the Main Terminus for Input to the Visual Cortex

Ninety percent of the retinal axons terminate in the lateral geniculate nucleus, the principal subcortical structure that carries visual information to the cerebral cortex. Without this pathway visual perception is lost, although some very limited stimulus detection and movement toward objects in the visual field still is possible. This residual vision, possibly mediated by the visual pathway passing through the superior colliculus, has been called *blindsight*.

Ganglion cells in the retina project in an orderly manner to points in the lateral geniculate nucleus, so that in each lateral geniculate nucleus there is a retinotopic representation of the contralateral half of the visual field. As in the somatosensory system, all areas of the retina are not represented equally in the nucleus. The fovea, the area of the retina with the highest density of ganglion cells, has a relatively larger representation than does the periphery of the retina. About half of the neural mass in the lateral geniculate nucleus (and in the primary visual cortex) represents the fovea and the region just around it. The much larger peripheral portions

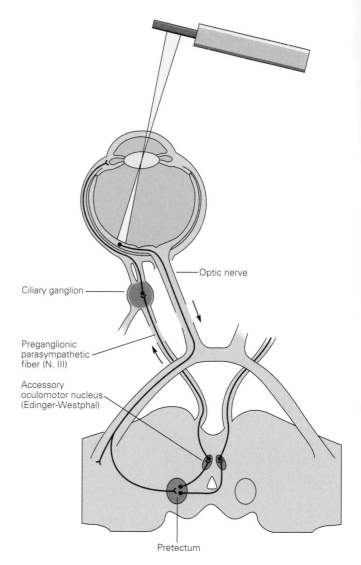

Figure 27-5 The reflex pathway mediating pupillary constriction. Light signals are relayed through the midbrain pretectum, to preganglionic parasympathetic neurons in the Edinger-Westphal nucleus, and out through the parasympathetic outflow of the oculomotor nerve to the ciliary ganglion. Postganglionic neurons then innervate the smooth muscle of the pupillary sphincter.

of the retina, with the lowest density of ganglion cells, are less well represented.

The retinal ganglion cells in and near the centrally located fovea are densely packed to compensate for the fact that the retina's central area is less than its periphery (due to the concavity of the retina). Since this physical limitation does not exist beyond the retina, neurons in the lateral geniculate nucleus and primary visual cortex are fairly evenly distributed—connections from the more numerous neurons in the fovea are distributed over a wide area. The ratio of the area in the lateral geniculate nucleus (or in the primary visual cortex) to the area in the retina representing one degree of the visual field is called the *magnification factor.*

In primates, including humans, the lateral geniculate nucleus contains six layers of cell bodies separated by intralaminar layers of axons and dendrites. The layers are numbered from 1 to 6, ventral to dorsal (Figure 27-6). Axons of the M and P retinal ganglion cells described in Chapter 26 remain segregated in the lateral geniculate nucleus. The two most ventral layers of the nucleus contain relatively large cells and are known as the *magnocellular layers;* their main retinal input is from M ganglion cells. The four dorsal layers are known as *parvocellular layers* and receive input from P ganglion cells. Both the magnocellular and parvocellular layers include on- and off-center cells, just as there are on- and off-center ganglion cells in the retina.

An individual layer in the nucleus receives input from one eye only: fibers from the contralateral nasal hemiretina contact layers 1, 4, and 6; fibers from the ipsilateral temporal hemiretina contact layers 2, 3, and 5 (Figure 27-6). Thus, although one lateral geniculate nucleus carries complete information about the contralateral visual field, the inputs from each eye remain segregated. The inputs from the nasal hemiretina of the contralateral eye represent the complete contralateral visual hemifield, whereas the inputs from the temporal hemiretina of the ipsilateral eye represent only 90% of the hemifield because they do not include the temporal crescent (see Figure 27-1).

Retinal ganglion cells have concentric receptive fields, with an antagonistic center-surround organization that allows them to measure the contrast in light intensity between their receptive field center and the surround (see Chapter 26). Do the receptive fields of lateral geniculate neurons have a similar organization? David Hubel and Torsten Wiesel, who first addressed this question in the early 1960s, found that they did. They directed light onto the retina of cats and monkeys by projecting patterns of light onto a screen in front of the animal. They found that receptive fields of neurons in the lateral geniculate nucleus are similar to those in the retina: small concentric fields about one degree in diameter. As in the retina, the cells are either on-center or off-center. Like the retinal ganglion cells, cells in the lateral geniculate nucleus respond best to small spots of light in the center of their receptive field. Diffuse illumination of the whole receptive field produces only weak responses. This similarity in the receptive properties of cells in the lateral geniculate nucleus and retinal ganglion cells derives in part from the fact that each geniculate neuron receives its main retinal input from only a very few ganglion cell axons.

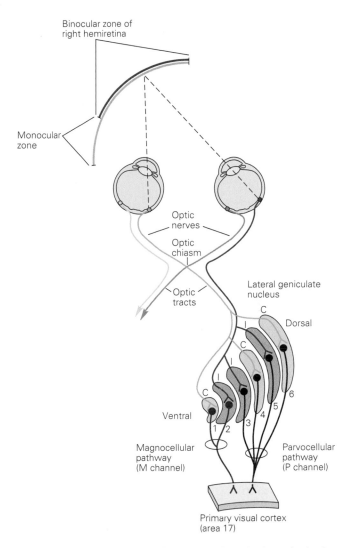

Figure 27-6 The lateral geniculate nucleus is the principal subcortical site for processing visual information. Inputs from the right hemiretina of each eye project to different layers of the right lateral geniculate nucleus to create a complete representation of the left visual hemifield. Similarly, fibers from the left hemiretina of each eye project to the left lateral geniculate nucleus (not shown). The temporal crescent is not represented in contralateral inputs (see Figure 27-1). Layers 1 and 2 comprise the magnocellular layers; layers 3 through 6 comprise the parvocellular layers. All of these project to area 17, the primary visual cortex. (**C** = contralateral input; **I** = ipsilateral input.)

Magnocellular and Parvocellular Pathways Convey Different Information to the Visual Cortex

We have already seen that the M ganglion cells of the retina project to the magnocellular layers of the lateral geniculate nucleus and that the P ganglion cells pro-

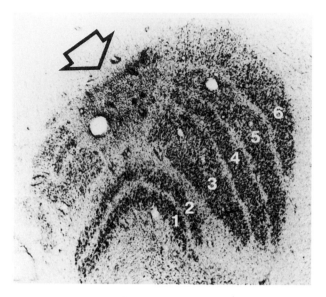

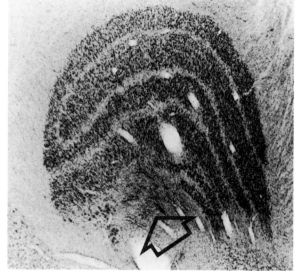

Parvocellular lesion   0.5 mm   Magnocellular lesion

Figure 27-7 Samples of lesions (arrows) in the lateral geniculate nucleus of the monkey that selectively alter visual function. In the photograph on the left the geniculate layers are numbered. Lesions were made with an excitotoxin (ibotenic acid). Coronal sections were stained with cresyl violet. (From Schiller et al. 1990.)

ject to the parvocellular layers. The parvocellular and magnocellular layers in turn project to separate layers of the primary visual cortex as we shall see later in this chapter. This striking anatomical segregation has led to the view that these separate sequences of retinal ganglion, lateral geniculate, and visual cortical cells can be regarded as two parallel pathways, referred to as the M and P pathways.

As indicated in Table 27-1, there are striking differences between cells in the M and P pathways. The most prominent difference between the cells in the lateral geniculate nucleus is their sensitivity to *color contrast.*

Table 27-1 Differences in the Sensitivity of M and P Cells to Stimulus Features

Stimulus feature	Sensitivity	
	M cells	P cells
Color contrast	No	Yes
Luminance contrast	Higher	Lower
Spatial frequency	Lower	Higher
Temporal frequency	Higher	Lower

The P cells respond to changes in color (red/green and blue/yellow) regardless of the relative brightness of the colors, whereas M cells respond weakly to changes of color when the brightness of the color is matched.

Luminance contrast is a measure of the difference between the brightest and darkest parts of the stimulus— M cells respond when contrast is as low as 2%, whereas P cells rarely respond to contrasts less than 10%. The M and P cells also differ in their response to spatial and temporal frequency. *Spatial frequency* is the number of repetitions of a pattern over a given distance. For example, alternating light and dark bars each occurring 10 times over a visual angle of one degree have a spatial frequency of 10 cycles per degree. *Temporal frequency* is how rapidly the pattern changes over time; turning the bars of a grating on and off 10 times per second would produce a temporal frequency of 10 Hz. The M cells tend to have lower spatial resolution and higher temporal resolution than P cells.

One way to explore further the contribution of the M and P pathways is by selectively removing one or the other in a monkey and then measuring the monkey's ability to perform a task that is thought to depend on the ablated pathway. Because the M and P cells are in different layers in the lateral geniculate nucleus, removal of a pathway is possible through localized chemical lesions (Figure 27-7).

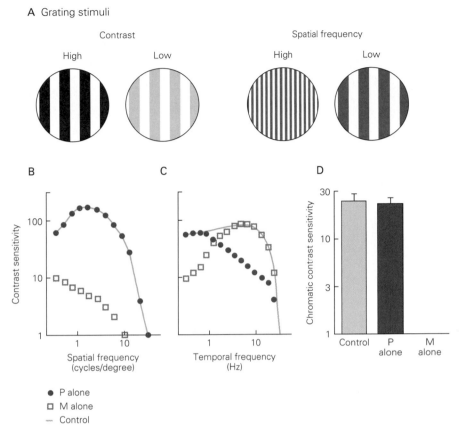

A Grating stimuli

Figure 27-8 Visual losses after selective lesioning of the magnocellular and parvocellular layers of the lateral geniculate nucleus in monkeys. The monkeys were trained to look at a fixation spot on a TV monitor and then grating stimuli were presented at one location in the visual field. The location was selected to coincide with the part of the visual field affected by a lesion in the lateral geniculate nucleus (such as those shown in Figure 27-7). Each lesion was centered on one layer that received information from one eye, so in the test the eye unaffected by the lesion was covered. On each presentation the monkeys indicated whether the gratings were vertical or horizontal, and this distinction became more difficult as the luminance contrast of the gratings became very low or the spatial frequency became very high.

A. Luminance contrast is the difference between the brightest and darkest parts of the grating. Spatial frequency is the number of light and dark bars (cycles) in the grating per degree of visual angle. Temporal frequency (not shown) is how fast the

stationary grating is turned on and off per second (Hz).

B. Contrast sensitivity is the inverse of the lowest stimulus contrast that can be detected. Contrast sensitivity for all spatial frequencies is reduced when only the magnocellular (M) pathway remains after parvocellular (P) lesion. The solid blue line in B and C shows sensitivity of the normal monkey; **filled circles** show the contribution of the P pathway (after M lesions) and **open squares** the contribution of the M pathway (after P lesions).

C. Contrast sensitivity to a grating with low spatial frequency is reduced at lower temporal frequencies when only M cells remain and at higher frequencies when only P cells remain.

D. Color contrast is measured the same way as luminance contrast except that bars of different colors were used instead of light and dark bars. Color contrast sensitivity is lost when only the M cells remain. (Adapted from Merigan and Maunsell 1993.)

The effects of these focal lesions on color vision are striking. Removal of P cells (leaving M cells alone) leads to a complete loss of color vision (Figure 27-8D), a result explained by the color sensitivity of these cells. Lesions in the M cell layers (leaving P cells alone) do not produce such deficits, consistent with the lack of color sensitivity in these cells. Selective lesions of M cells make it difficult for monkeys to perceive a pattern of bright and dark bars that have both low spatial frequency (more

widely spaced bars) and high temporal frequency (bars turned on and off at higher rates). To make the discriminations, the luminance contrast of the bright and dark bars must be higher than for normal monkeys (Figure 27-8B, C). Lesions in the P cell layers produce the opposite effect—they make it difficult for the monkey to discriminate between stimuli that have both high spatial frequency (more closely spaced bars) and low temporal frequency (bars turned on and off at lower rates).

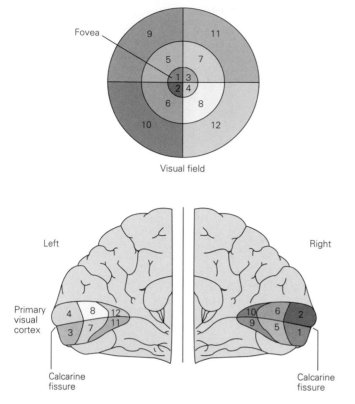

Figure 27-9 Each half of the visual field is represented in the contralateral primary visual cortex. In humans the primary visual cortex is located at the posterior pole of the cerebral hemisphere and lies almost exclusively on the medial surface. (In some individuals it is shifted so that part of it extends onto the lateral surface.) Areas in the primary visual cortex are devoted to specific parts of the visual field, as indicated by the corresponding numbers. The upper fields are mapped below the calcarine fissure, and the lower fields above it. The striking aspect of this map is that about half of the neural mass is devoted to representation of the fovea and the region just around it. This area has the greatest visual acuity.

Thus both the response properties of single cells and the behavioral consequence of removing the cells show that the M and P cells make different contributions to perception. The P cells are critical for color vision and are most important for vision that requires high spatial and low temporal resolution vision. The M cells contribute most to vision requiring low spatial and high temporal resolution. Such specialization of processing is critical for the elemental properties of vision such as spatial and temporal resolution and color vision.

Although we know a great deal about the cell types and circuitry of the lateral geniculate nucleus, and about the information conveyed by the P and M cells, the function of the nucleus is not yet clear. In fact, only 10–20% of the presynaptic connections onto geniculate relay

cells come from the retina! The majority of inputs come from other regions, and many of these, particularly those from the reticular formation in the brain stem and from the cortex, are feedback inputs. This input to the lateral geniculate nucleus may control the flow of information from the retina to the cortex.

The Primary Visual Cortex Organizes Simple Retinal Inputs Into the Building Blocks of Visual Images

The first point in the visual pathway where the receptive fields of cells are significantly different from those of cells in the retina is the primary visual cortex, also called visual area 1 (abbreviated V1). This region of cortex, Brodmann's area 17, is also called the *striate cortex* because it contains a prominent stripe of white matter in layer 4, the *stria of Gennari,* consisting of myelinated axons. Like the lateral geniculate nucleus and superior colliculus, the primary visual cortex in each cerebral hemisphere receives information exclusively from the contralateral half of the visual field (Figure 27-9).

The primary visual cortex in humans is about 2 mm thick and consists of six layers of cells (layers 1–6) between the pial surface and the underlying white matter. The principal layer for inputs from the lateral geniculate nucleus is layer 4, which is further subdivided into four sublayers (sublaminae): 4A, 4B, 4Cα, and 4Cβ. Tracings of resident cells and axonal inputs in the monkey have shown that the M and P cells of the lateral geniculate nucleus terminate in different layers and even in different sublayers. The axons of M cells terminate principally in sublamina 4Cα; the axons of most P cells terminate principally in sublamina 4Cβ (Figure 27-10A). Thus, the segregation of the parvocellular and magnocellular pathways continues to be maintained at this level of processing.

Axons from a third group of cells, located in the intralaminar region of the lateral geniculate nucleus, terminate in layers 2 and 3, where they innervate patches of cells called *blobs,* a functional grouping that we shall discuss below. These intralaminar cells probably receive their retinal inputs primarily from ganglion cells other than those providing inputs to the M and P cells. These cells might therefore represent another pathway in parallel to the P and M pathways from the retina to the visual cortex, but little is now known about their function.

As we have seen in Chapter 17, the cortex contains two basic classes of cells. *Pyramidal cells* are large and have long spiny dendrites; they are projection neurons whose axons project to other brain regions as well as

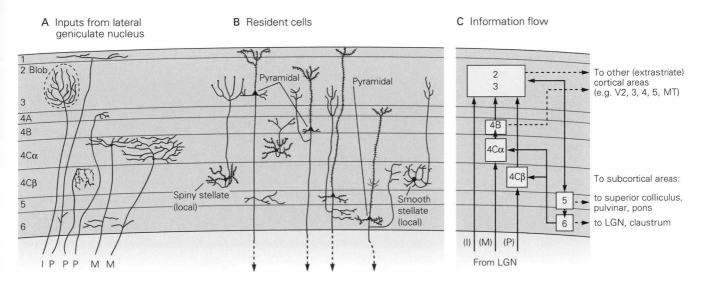

A Inputs from lateral geniculate nucleus

B Resident cells

C Information flow

Figure 27-10 The primary visual cortex has distinct anatomical layers, each with characteristic synaptic connections. (Adapted from Lund 1988.)

A. Most afferent fibers from the lateral geniculate nucleus terminate in layer 4. The axons of cells in the parvocellular layers (P) terminate primarily in layer 4Cβ, with minor inputs to 4A and 1, while the axons of cells in the magnocellular layers (M) terminate primarily in layer 4Cα. Collaterals of both types of cells also terminate in layer 6. Cells of the intralaminar regions (I) of the lateral geniculate nucleus terminate in the blob regions of layers 2 and 3.

B. Several types of neurons make up the primary visual cortex. Spiny stellate and pyramidal cells, both of which have spiny dendrites, are excitatory. Smooth stellate cells are inhibitory. Pyramidal cells project out of the cortex, whereas both types of stellate cells are local neurons.

C. Conception of information flow based on anatomical connec-

tions. (LGN = lateral geniculate nucleus; MT = middle temporal area.)

Inputs. Axons from M and P cells in the lateral geniculate nucleus end on spiny stellate cells in the sublayers of 4C, and these cells project axons to layer 4B or the upper layers 2 and 3. Axons from cells in the intralaminar zones of the lateral geniculate nucleus project directly to layers 2 and 3.

Intracortical connections. Axon collaterals of pyramidal cells in layers 2 and 3 project to layer 5 pyramidal cells, whose axon collaterals project both to layer 6 pyramidal cells and back to cells in layers 2 and 3. Axon collaterals of layer 6 pyramidal cells then make a loop back to layer 4C onto smooth stellate cells.

Output. Each layer, except for 4C, has outputs for V1 and each is different. The cells in layers 2, 3, and 4B project to extrastriate visual cortical areas. Cells in layer 5 project to the superior colliculus, the pons, and the pulvinar. Cells in layer 6 project back to the lateral geniculate nucleus and the claustrum.

interconnecting neurons in local areas. *Nonpyramidal cells* are small and stellate in shape and have dendrites that are either spiny (spiny stellate cells) or smooth (smooth stellates). They are local interneurons whose axons are confined to the primary visual cortex (Figure 27-10B). The pyramidal and spiny stellate cells are excitatory and many use glutamate or aspartate as their transmitters; the smooth stellate cells are inhibitory and many contain γ-aminobutyric acid (GABA).

Once afferents from the lateral geniculate nucleus enter the primary visual cortex, information flows systematically from one cortical layer to another, starting with the spiny stellate cells, which predominate in layer 4. The spiny stellate cells distribute the input from the lateral geniculate nucleus to the cortex and the pyramidal cells feed axon collaterals upward and downward to integrate activity within the layers of V1 (Figure 27-10C).

Simple and Complex Cells Decompose the Outlines of a Visual Image Into Short Line Segments of Various Orientations

How is the complexity of the circuitry in the cerebral cortex reflected in the response properties of cortical cells? Hubel, Wiesel, and their colleagues found that most cells above and below layer 4 respond optimally to stimuli that are substantially more complex than those that excite cells in the retina and lateral geniculate nucleus. Their most unexpected finding was that small spots of light—which are so effective in the retina, lateral geniculate nucleus, and in the input layer of the cortex 4C—are much less effective in all other layers of the visual cortex except possibly the blob regions in the superficial layers. Instead, cells respond best to stimuli that have linear properties, such as a line or bar. These cells belong to two major groups, simple and complex.

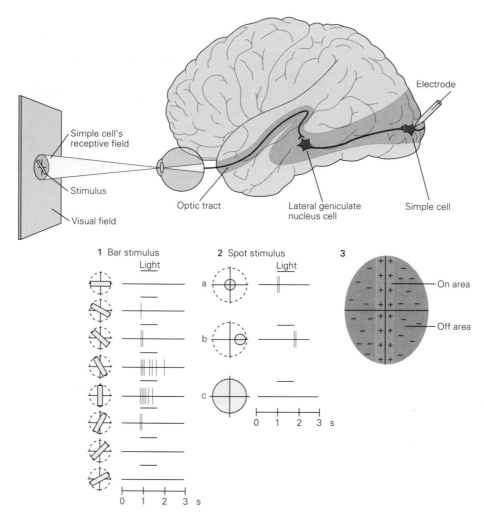

Figure 27-11 Receptive field of a simple cell in the primary visual cortex. The receptive field of a cell in the visual system is determined by recording activity in the cell while spots and bars of light are projected onto the visual field at an appropriate distance from the fovea. The records shown here are for a single cell. Duration of illumination is indicated by a line above each record of action potentials. (Adapted from Hubel and Wiesel 1959 and Zeki 1993.)

1. The cell's response to a bar of light is strongest if the bar of light is vertically oriented in the center of its receptive field.

2. Spots of light consistently elicit weak responses or no response. A small spot in the excitatory center of the field elicits only a weak excitatory response (**a**). A small spot in the inhibitory area elicits a weak inhibitory response (**b**). Diffuse light produces no response (**c**).

3. By using spots of light, the excitatory or "on" areas (+) and inhibitory or "off" areas (−) can be mapped. The map of the responses reveals an elongated "on" area and a surrounding "off" area, consistent with the optimal response of the cell to a vertical bar of light.

The *simple* cells respond best to a bar of light with a specific orientation. For example, a cell that responds best to a vertical bar will not respond, or respond only weakly, to a bar that is horizontal or even oblique (Figure 27-11). Thus, an array of cells in the cortex, all receiving impulses from the same point on the retina but with rectilinear receptive fields with different axes of orientation, is able to represent every axis of rotation for that point on the retina.

Simple cells also have excitatory and inhibitory zones in their receptive fields, although these zones are slightly larger than those for lateral geniculate cells (Figure 27-12A, B). For example, a cell may have a rectilinear excitatory zone (with its long axis running from 12 to 6 o'clock such as in Figure 27-12B upper right). For a cell with such a field, an effective stimulus must excite the specific segment of the retina innervated by receptors in the excitatory zone *and* have the correct linear properties (in this case an edge) *and* have a specific axis of orientation (in this case vertical, running from 12 to 6 o'clock).

Rectilinear receptive fields could be built up from many circular fields if the presynaptic connections from

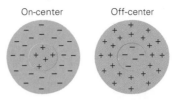

A Receptive fields of concentric cells of retina and lateral geniculate nucleus

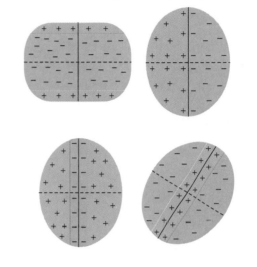

Figure 27-12 The receptive fields of simple cells in the primary visual cortex are different and more varied than those of the neurons in the retina and lateral geniculate nucleus.

A. Cells of the retina and lateral geniculate nucleus fall into two classes: on-center and off-center. The receptive fields of these neurons have a center-surround organization due to antagonistic excitatory (+) and inhibitory (−) regions.

B. The receptive fields of simple cells in the primary visual cortex have narrow elongated zones with either excitatory (+) or inhibitory (−) flanking areas. Despite the variety, the receptive fields of simple cells share three features: (1) specific retinal position, (2) discrete excitatory and inhibitory zones, and (3) a specific axis of orientation.

C. Model of the organization of inputs in the receptive field of simple cells proposed by Hubel and Wiesel. According to this model, a simple cortical neuron in the primary visual cortex receives convergent excitatory connections from three or more on-center cells that together represent light falling along a straight line in the retina. As a result, the receptive field of the simple cortical cell has an elongated excitatory region, indicated by the colored outline in the receptive field diagram. The inhibitory surround of the simple cortical cells is probably provided by off-center cells whose receptive fields (not shown) are adjacent to those of the on-center cells. (Adapted from Hubel and Wiesel 1962).

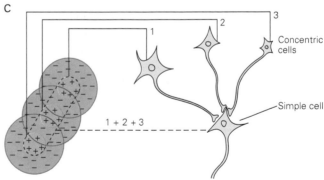

the lateral geniculate nucleus were appropriately arrayed on the simple cell (Figure 27-12C). Indeed, experiments have indicated that the excitatory ("on") regions in the receptive field of simple cells largely represent the input from on-center lateral geniculate cells while the inhibitory ("off") regions represent inputs from off-center lateral geniculate cells.

The receptive fields of *complex cells* in the cortex are usually larger than those of simple cells. These fields also have a critical axis of orientation, but the precise position of the stimulus within the receptive field is less crucial because there are no clearly defined on or off zones (Figure 27-13A). Thus, movement across the re-

ceptive field is a particularly effective stimulus for certain complex cells. Although some complex cells have direct connections with cells of layer 4C, Hubel and Wiesel proposed that a significant input to complex cells comes from a group of simple cortical cells with the same axis of orientation but with slightly offset receptive field positions (Figure 27-13B).

Some Feature Abstraction Is Accomplished by Progressive Convergence

The pattern of convergence of inputs throughout the pathway that leads to the complex cells suggests that

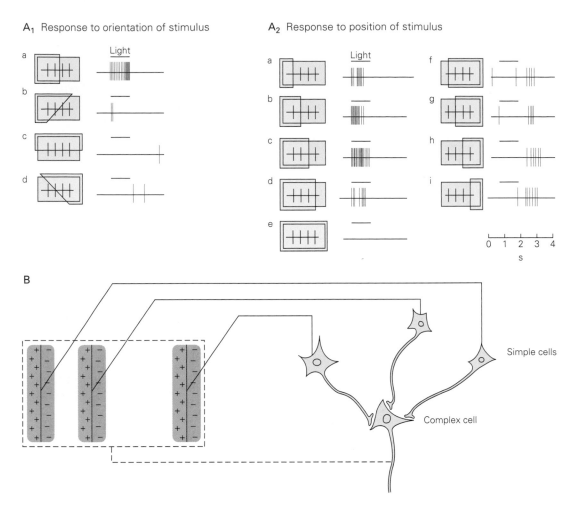

Figure 27-13 The receptive field of a complex cell in the primary visual cortex has no clearly excitatory or inhibitory zones. Orientation of the light stimulus is important, but position within the receptive field is not. (Adapted from Hubel and Wiesel 1962).

A. In this example the cell responds best to a vertical edge moving across the receptive field from left to right. This figure shows the patterns of action potentials fired by the cell in response to two types of variation in the stimulus: differences in orientation and differences in position. The line above each record indicates the period of illumination. **1.** Different orientations of the light stimulus produce different rates of firing in the cell. A vertical bar of light on the left of the receptive field produces a strong excitatory response **(a)**. Orientations other than vertical are less effective **(b–d)**. **2.** The position of the border of

the light within the receptive field affects the type of response in the cell. If the edge of the light comes from any point on the right within the receptive field, the stimulus produces an excitatory response **(a–d)**. If the edge comes from the left, the stimulus produces an inhibitory response **(f–i)**. Illumination of the entire receptive field produces no response **(e)**.

B. According to Hubel and Wiesel, the receptive fields of complex cells are determined by the pattern of inputs. Each complex cell receives convergent excitatory input from several simple cortical cells, each of which has a receptive field with the same organization: a central rectilinear excitation zone (+) and flanking inhibitory regions (−). In this way the receptive field of a complex cell is built up from the individual fields of the presynaptic cells.

each complex cell surveys the activity of a group of simple cells, each simple cell surveys the activity of a group of geniculate cells, and each geniculate cell surveys the activity of a group of retinal ganglion cells. The ganglion cells survey the activity of bipolar cells that, in turn, survey an array of receptors. At each level each cell

has a greater capacity for abstraction than cells at lower levels.

At each level of the afferent pathway the stimulus properties that activate a cell become more specific. Retinal ganglion and geniculate neurons respond primarily to contrast. This elementary information is transformed in the simple and complex cells of the cortex, through the pattern of excitation in their rectilinear fields, into relatively precise line segments and boundaries. Hubel and Wiesel suggest that this processing is an important step in analyzing the contours of objects.

In fact, contour information may be sufficient to recognize an object. Monotonous interior or background surfaces contain no critical visual information! David Hubel describes this unexpected feature of perception:

Many people, including myself, still have trouble accepting the idea that the interior of a form . . . does not itself excite cells in our brain, . . . that our awareness of the interior as black or white . . . depends only on cells' sensitivity to the borders. The intellectual argument is that perception of an evenly lit interior depends on the activation of cells having fields at the borders and on the absence of activation of cells whose fields are within the borders, since such activation would indicate that the interior is not evenly lit. So our perception of the interior as black, white, gray or green has nothing to do with cells whose fields are in the interior—hard as that may be to swallow. . . . What happens at the borders is the only information you need to know: the interior is boring.

It is the information carried by edges that allows us to recognize objects in a picture readily even when the objects are sketched only in rough outline (see Figure 25-3).

Since simple and complex cells in V1 receive input from both the M and P pathways, both pathways could contribute to what the theoretical biologist David Marr called the *primal sketch,* the initial two-dimensional approximation of the shape of a stimulus. We will return in Chapter 28 to the fate of the P and M pathways.

The Primary Visual Cortex Is Organized Into Functional Modules

We have seen how the organization of the receptive fields of neurons in the visual pathway changes from concentric to simple to complex. Do these local transformations reflect a larger organization within the visual cortex? We shall see that the neurons in the visual cortex have a columnar organization, like the somatic sensory cortex, and that sets of columns can be regarded as functional modules, each of which processes visual information from a specific region of the visual field.

Neurons With Similar Receptive Fields Are Organized in Columns

Like the somatic sensory cortex, the primary visual cortex is organized into narrow columns of cells, running from the pial surface to the white matter. Each column is about 30 to 100 μm wide and 2 mm deep, and each contains cells in layer 4C with concentric receptive fields. Above and below are simple cells whose receptive fields monitor almost identical retinal positions and have identical axes of orientation. For this reason these groupings are called *orientation columns.* Each orientation column also contains complex cells. The properties of these complex cells can most easily be explained by postulating that each complex cell receives direct connections from the simple cells in the column. Thus, columns in the visual system seem to be organized to allow local interconnection of cells, from which the cells are able to generate a new level of abstraction of visual information. For instance, the columns allow cortical cells to generate linear receptive field properties from the inputs of several cells in the lateral geniculate nucleus that respond best to small spots of light.

The discovery of columns in the various sensory systems was one of the most important advances in cortical physiology in the past several decades and immediately raised questions that have led to a family of new discoveries. For example, given that cells with the same axis of orientation tend to be grouped into columns, how are columns of cells with *different* axes of orientation organized in relation to one another? Detailed mapping of adjacent columns by Hubel and Wiesel, using tangential penetrations with microelectrodes, revealed a precise organization with an orderly shift in axis of orientation from one column to the next. About every three-quarters of a millimeter contained a complete cycle of orientation changes.

The anatomical layout of the orientation columns was first demonstrated in electrophysiological experiments in which marks were made in the cortex near the cells that are activated by stimuli at a given orientation. Later, this anatomical arrangement was delineated by injecting 2-deoxyglucose, a glucose analog that can be radiolabeled and injected into the brain. Cells that are metabolically active take up the label and can then be detected when sections of cortex are overlaid with x-ray film. Thus, when a stimulus of lines with a given orientation is presented, an orderly array of active and inactive stripes of cells is revealed. A remarkable advance now allows the different orientation columns to be visualized directly in the living cortex. Using either a voltage-sensitive dye or inherent differences in the light scattering of active and inactive cells, a highly sensitive camera can detect the pattern of active and inactive orientation columns during presentation of a bar of light with a specific axis of orientation (Figure 27-14).

The systematic shifts in axis of orientation from one column to another is occasionally interrupted by *blobs,* the peg-shaped regions of cells prominent in layers

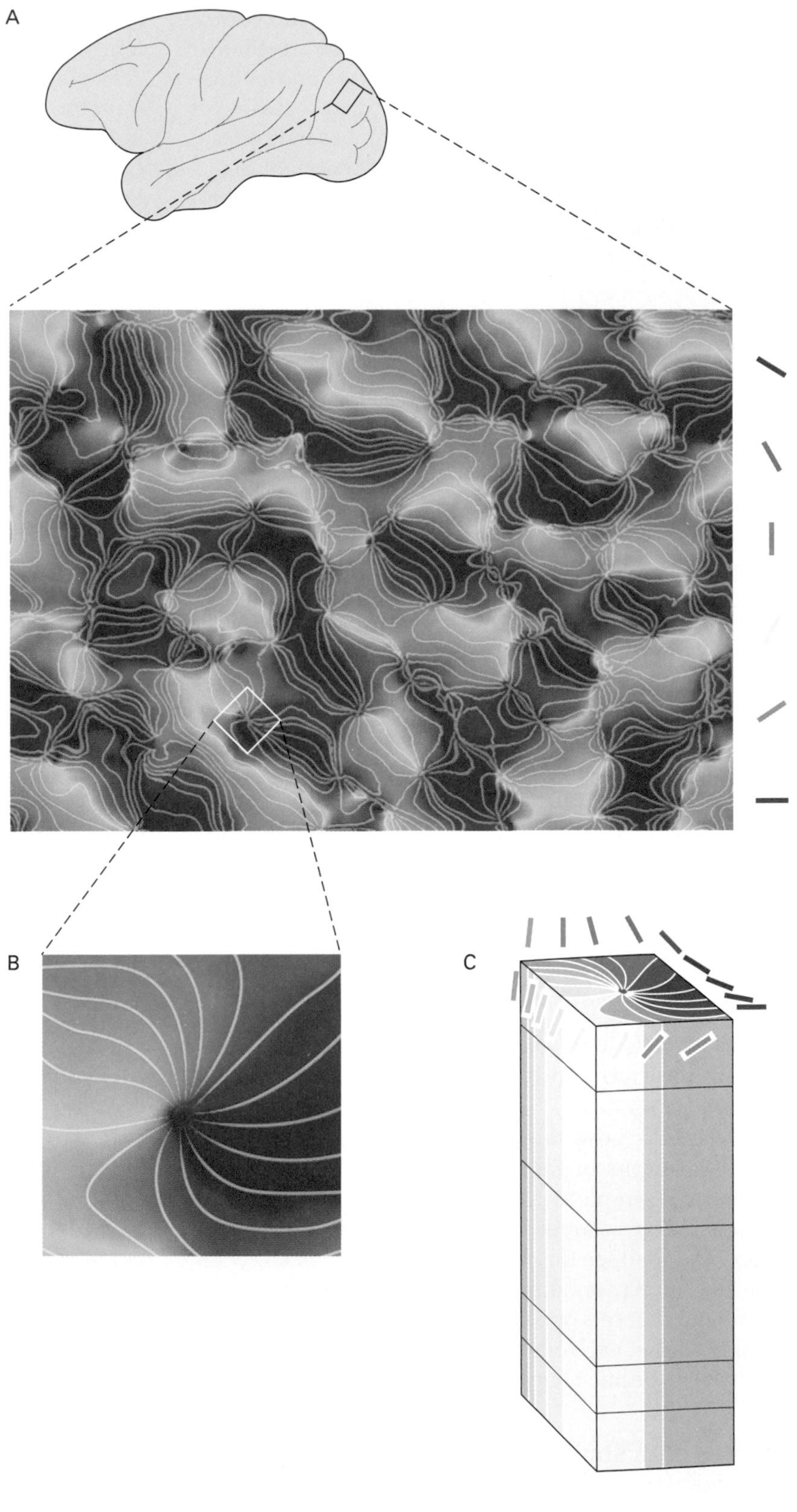

Figure 27-14 Orientation columns in the visual cortex of the monkey. (Courtesy of Gary Blasdel.)

A. Image of a 9 by 12 mm rectangle of cortical surface taken while the monkey viewed contours of different orientations (indicated on the right). This image was obtained through optical imaging and by comparing local changes in reflectance, which indicate activity. Areas that were most active during the presentation of a particular orientation are indicated by the color chosen to represent that orientation (bars on the right). Complementary colors were chosen to represent orthogonal orientations. Hence, red and green indicate maximal activities in response to horizontal and vertical, while blue and yellow indicate greatest activation by left and right oblique.

B. Enlargement of a pinwheel-like area in A. Orientations producing the greatest activity remain constant along radials, extending outward from a center, but change continuously (through ± 180°).

C. Three-dimensional organization of orientation columns in a 1 mm × 1 mm × 2 mm slab of primary visual cortex underlying the square surface region depicted in B.

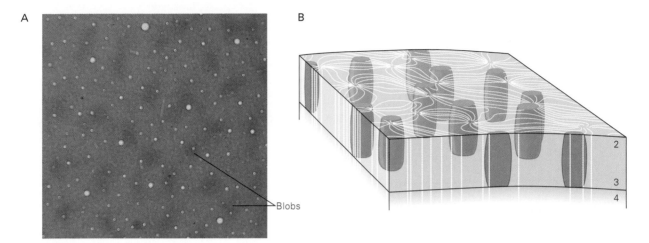

Figure 27-15 Organization of blobs in the visual cortex.

A. Blobs are visible as dark patches in this photograph of a single 40 μm thick layer of upper cortex that has been processed histochemically to reveal the density of cytochrome oxidase, a mitochondrial enzyme involved in energy production. The heightened enzymatic activity in the blobs is thought to represent heightened neural activity. The cortex was sectioned tangentially. (Courtesy of D. Ts'o, C. Gilbert, and T. Wiesel.)

B. Organization of the blobs in relation to the orientation columns. Only the upper layers of the cortex are shown with the blobs extending though these layers. The blobs interrupt the pattern of the orientation columns.

2 and 3 of V1 (Figure 27-15). The cells in the blobs frequently respond to different color stimuli, and their receptive fields, like those of cells in the lateral geniculate nucleus, have no specific orientation.

In addition to columns of cells responsive to axis of orientation and blobs related to color processing, a third system of alternating columns processes separate inputs from each eye. These *ocular dominance* columns, which we shall consider again in Chapter 56, represent an orderly arrangement of cells that receive inputs only from the left or right eye and are important for binocular interaction. The ocular dominance columns have been visualized using transsynaptic transport of radiolabeled amino acids injected into one eye. In autoradiographs of sections of cortex cut perpendicular to the layers, patches in layer 4 that receive input from the injected eye are heavily labeled, and they alternate with unlabeled patches that mediate input from the uninjected eye (Figure 27-16).

A Hypercolumn Represents the Visual Properties of One Region of the Visual Field

Hubel and Wiesel introduced the term *hypercolumn* to refer to a set of columns responsive to lines of all orientations from a particular region in space. The relationship between the orientation columns, the independent ocular dominance columns, and the blobs within a module is illustrated in Figure 27-17. A complete sequence of ocular dominance columns and orientation columns is repeated regularly and precisely over the surface of the primary visual cortex, each occupying a region of about 1 mm². This repeating organization is a striking illustration of the modular organization characteristic of the cerebral cortex. Each module acts as a window on the visual field and each window represents only a tiny part of the visual field, but the whole field is covered by many such windows. Within the processing module all information about that part of the visual world is processed. From what we know now, that includes orientation, binocular interaction, color, and motion.

Each module has a variety of outputs originating in different cortical layers. The organization of the output connections from the primary visual cortex is similar to that of the somatic sensory cortex in that there are outputs from all layers except 4C, and in each layer the principal output cells are the pyramidal cells (see Figure 27-10C). The axons of cells above layer 4C project to other cortical areas; those of cells below 4C project to subcortical areas. The cells in layers 2 and 3 send their output to other higher visual cortical regions, such as Brodmann's area 18 (V2, V3, and V4). They also make connections via the corpus callosum to anatomically symmetrical cortical areas on the other side of the brain. Cells in layer 4B project to the middle temporal area (V5 or MT). Cells in layer 5 project to the superior colliculus, the pons, and the pulvinar. Cells in layer 6 project back to the lateral geniculate nucleus and to the claustrum.

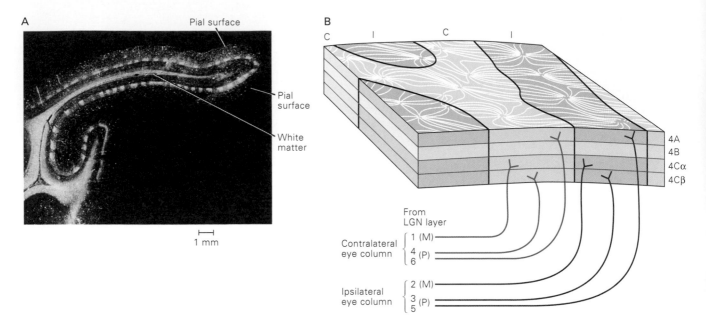

Figure 27-16 The ocular dominance columns.

A. This autoradiograph of the primary visual cortex of an adult monkey shows the ocular dominance columns as alternating white and dark (labeled and unlabeled) patches in layer 4 of the cortex, below the pial surface. One eye of the monkey was injected with a cell label, which over the course of 2 weeks was transported to the lateral geniculate nucleus and then across synapses to the geniculocortical relay cells, whose axons terminate in layer 4 of the visual cortex. Areas of layer 4 that receive input from the injected eye are heavily labeled and appear white; the alternating unlabeled patches receive input from the uninjected eye. In all, some 56 columns can be counted in layer 4C. The underlying white matter appears white because it contains the labeled axons of geniculate cells. (From Hubel and Wiesel 1979.)

B. The scheme of inputs to the alternating ocular dominance columns in layer 4 of the primary visual cortex. Inputs from the contralateral (**C**) and ipsilateral (**I**) eyes arise in different layers in the lateral geniculate nucleus (**LGN**), identified in Figure 27-5, and project to different subdivisions of layer 4.

Since cells in each layer of the visual cortex probably perform a different task, the laminar position of a cell determines its functional properties.

Columnar Units Are Linked by Horizontal Connections

As we have seen, three major vertically oriented systems crossing the layers of primary visual cortex have been delineated: (1) orientation columns, which contain the neurons that respond selectively to light bars with specific axes of orientation; (2) blobs, peg-shaped patches in upper layers (but not layer 4) that contain cells that are more concerned with color than orientation; and (3) ocular dominance columns, which receive inputs from one or the other eye. These units are organized into hypercolumns that monitor small areas of the visual field.

These vertically oriented systems communicate with one another by means of horizontal connections that link cells within a layer. Axon collaterals of individual pyramidal cells in layers 3 and 5 run long distances, parallel with the layers, and give rise to clusters of axon terminals at regular intervals that approximate the width of a hypercolumn (Figure 27-18A). Horseradish peroxidase injected into focal regions within superficial cortical layers (2, 3) reveals an elaborate lattice of labeled cells and axons that encloses unlabeled patches about 500 μm in diameter. Similarly, tracers injected into sites corresponding to blobs label other blobs, producing a honeycomb image. A honeycomb array also appears after labeling the nonblob cortex.

To examine these horizontal connections, recordings were made from pairs of cells in blob regions; each pair was separated by about 1 mm, the distance that typically separates the lattice arrays described above (Figure 27-18B). Many cell pairs were found to fire simultaneously in response to stimuli with a specific orientation and direction of movement. Thus, color-selective cells in one blob are linked to cells with similar responses in other blobs.

Additional evidence that horizontal connections tie together cells with similar response properties in different columns comes from injection of radiolabeled 2-deoxyglucose and fluorescently labeled microbeads

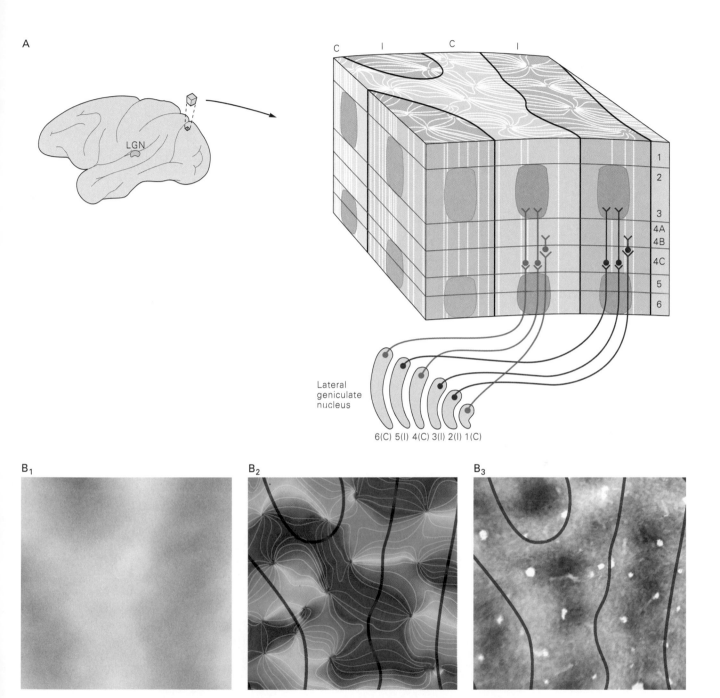

Figure 27-17 Organization of orientation columns, ocular dominance columns, and blobs in primary visual cortex.

A. An array of functional columns of cells in the visual cortex contains the neural machinery necessary to analyze a discrete region of the visual field and can be thought of as a functional *module.* Each module contains one complete set of orientation columns, one set of ocular dominance columns (right and left eye), and several blobs (regions of the cortex associated with color processing). The entire visual field can be represented in the visual cortex by a regular array of such modules.

B. Images depicting ocular dominance columns, orientation columns, and blobs from the same region of primary visual cortex. (Courtesy of Gary Blasdel.) **1.** Images of ocular dominance

columns were obtained using optical imaging and independently stimulating the left and right ocular dominance columns in a particular region. Because neural activity decreases cortical reflectance, the subtraction of one left eye image from one right eye image produces the characteristic pattern of dark and light bands, representing the right and left eyes respectively. **2.** In this image the borders of the ocular dominance columns shown in 1 appear as **black lines** superimposed on the pattern of orientation-specific columns depicted in Figure 27-14. **3.** The borders of the ocular dominance columns shown in 1 are superimposed on tissue reacted for cytochrome oxidase, which visualizes the blobs. The blobs are thus seen localized in the centers of the ocular dominance columns.

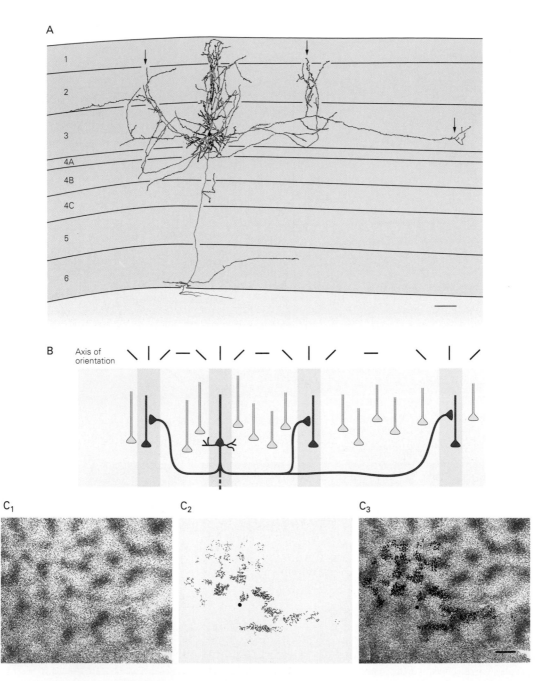

Figure 27-18 Columns of cells in the visual cortex with similar function are linked through horizontal connections.

A. A camera lucida reconstruction of a pyramidal cell injected with horseradish peroxidase in layers 2 and 3 in a monkey. Several axon collaterals branch off the descending axon near the dendritic tree and in three other clusters **(arrows).** The clustered collaterals project vertically into several layers at regular intervals, consistent with the sequence of functional columns of cells. (From McGuire et al. 1991.)

B. The horizontal connections of a pyramidal cell, such as that shown in A, are functionally specific. The axon of the pyramidal cell forms synapses on other pyramidal cells in the immediate vicinity as well as pyramidal cells some distance away. Record-

ings of cell activity demonstrate that the axon makes connections only with cells that have the same functional specificity (in this case, responsiveness to a vertical line). (Adapted from Ts'o et al. 1986.)

C. 1. A section of cortex labeled with 2-deoxyglucose shows a pattern of stripes representing columns of cells that respond to a stimulus with a particular orientation. **2.** Microbeads injected into the same site as in 1 are taken up by the terminals of neurons and transported to the cell bodies. **3.** Superimposition of the images in 1 and 2. The clusters of bead-labeled cells lie directly over the 2-deoxyglucose-labeled areas, showing that groups of cells in different columns with the same axis of orientation are connected. (From Gilbert and Wiesel 1989.)

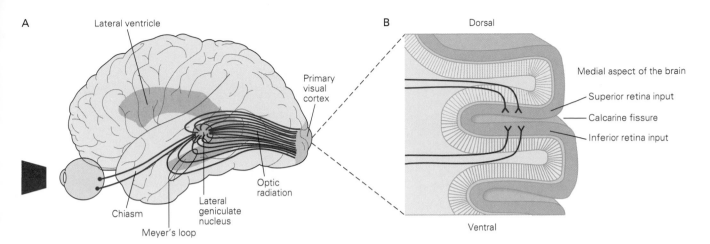

Figure 27-19 Projection of input from the retina to the visual cortex.

A. Fibers from the lateral geniculate nucleus sweep around the lateral ventricle in the *optic radiation* to reach the primary visual cortex. Fibers that relay inputs from the inferior half of the retina loop rostrally around the temporal horn of the lateral ventricle, forming Meyer's loop. (Adapted from Brodal 1981.)

B. A cross section through the primary visual cortex in the occipital lobe. Fibers that relay input from the inferior half of the retina terminate in the inferior bank of the visual cortex, below the calcarine fissure. Those that relay input from the superior half of the retina terminate in the superior bank.

into a column containing cells that respond to a specific orientation. The beads are taken up by axon terminals at the injection site and transported back to the cell bodies. In sections tangential to the pia the overall pattern of cells labeled with the microbeads closely resembles the lattice described above. In fact, the pattern labeled with 2-deoxyglucose is congruent with the pattern obtained with the microbeads (Figure 27-18C). Thus, both anatomical and metabolic studies establish that cortical cells having receptive fields with the same orientation are connected by means of a horizontal network.

The visual cortex, then, is organized functionally into two sets of intersecting connections, one vertical, consisting of functional columns spanning the different cortical layers, and the other horizontal, connecting functional columns with the same response properties. What is the functional importance of the horizontal connections? Recent studies indicate that these connections integrate information over many millimeters of cortex. As a result, a cell can be influenced by stimuli *outside* its normal receptive field. Indeed, a cell's axis of orientation is not completely invariant but is dependent on the context on which the feature is embedded. The psychophysical principle of *contextual effect*, whereby we evaluate objects in the context in which we see them, is thought to be mediated by the horizontal connections between the functional columns of the visual cortex.

Lesions in the Retino-Geniculate-Cortical Pathway Are Associated With Specific Gaps in the Visual Field

As we have seen in Chapter 20, the fact that the connections between neurons in the brain are precise and relate to behavior in an orderly way allows one to infer the site of anatomical lesions from a clinical examination of a patient. Lesions along the visual pathway produce characteristic gaps in the visual field.

The axons in the optic tract form synapses on the principal cells of the lateral geniculate nucleus. In turn, the axons of the principal cells sweep around the lateral ventricle in the optic radiation to the primary visual cortex, radiating on the lateral surface of both the temporal and occipital horns of the lateral ventricle (Figure 27-19A). Fibers representing the inferior parts of the retina swing rostrally in a broad arc over the temporal horn of the ventricle and loop into the temporal lobe before turning caudally to reach the occipital pole. This group of fibers, called *Meyer's loop*, relays input from the inferior half of the retina terminate in the inferior bank of the cortex lining the calcarine fissure. The fibers relaying input from the superior half of the retina terminate in the superior bank (Figure 27-19B). Consequently, unilateral lesions in the temporal lobe affect vision in the superior quadrant of the contralateral visual hemifield

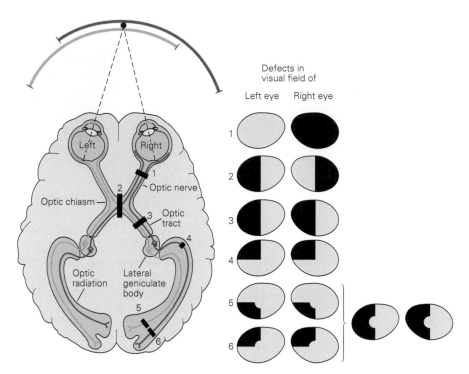

Figure 27-20 Deficits in the visual field produced by lesions at various points in the visual pathway. The level of a lesion can be determined by the specific deficit in the visual field. In the diagram of the cortex the numbers along the visual pathway indicate the sites of lesions. The deficits that result from lesions at each site are shown in the visual field maps on the right as **black areas.** Deficits in the visual field of the left eye represent what an individual would *not* see with the right eye closed rather than deficits of the left visual hemifield.

1. A lesion of the right optic nerve causes a total loss of vision in the right eye.

2. A lesion of the optic chiasm causes a loss of vision in the temporal halves of both visual fields (bitemporal hemianopsia). Because the chiasm carries crossing fibers from both eyes, this is the only lesion in the visual system that causes a *nonhomonymous* deficit in vision, ie, a deficit in two different parts of the visual field resulting from a single lesion.

3. A lesion of the optic tract causes a complete loss of vision in the opposite half of the visual field (contralateral hemianopsia). In this case, because the lesion is on the right side, vision loss occurs on the left side.

4. After leaving the lateral geniculate nucleus the fibers representing both retinas mix in the optic radiation (see Figure 27-19). A lesion of the optic radiation fibers that curve into the temporal lobe (Meyer's loop) causes a loss of vision in the upper quadrant of the opposite half of the visual field of both eyes (upper contralateral quadrantic anopsia).

5, 6. Partial lesions of the visual cortex lead to partial field deficits on the opposite side. A lesion in the upper bank of the calcarine sulcus (5) causes a partial deficit in the inferior quadrant of the visual field on the opposite side. A lesion in the lower bank of the calcarine sulcus (6) causes a partial deficit in the superior quadrant of the visual field on the opposite side. A more extensive lesion of the visual cortex, including parts of both banks of the calcarine cortex, would cause a more extensive loss of vision in the contralateral hemifield. The central area of the visual field is unaffected by cortical lesions (5 and 6), probably because the representation of the foveal region of the retina is so extensive that a single lesion is unlikely to destroy the entire representation. The representation of the periphery of the visual field is smaller and hence more easily destroyed by a single lesion.

because they disrupt Meyer's loop. A lesion in the inferior bank of the calcarine cortex causes a gap in the superior half of the contralateral visual field.

This arrangement illustrates a key principle: At the initial stages of visual processing each half of the brain is concerned with the contralateral hemifield of vision. This pattern of organization begins with the segregation of axons in the optic chiasm, where fibers from the two eyes dealing with the same part of the visual field are brought together (see Figure 27-1). In essence, this is

similar to the somatic sensory system, in which each hemisphere mediates sensation on the contralateral side of the body.

We can understand better the projection of the visual world onto the primary visual cortex by considering the gaps in the visual field produced by lesions at various levels leading up to the cortex. These deficits are summarized in Figure 27-20.

After sectioning one optic nerve the visual field is seen monocularly by the eye on the intact side (Figure

27-20, 1). The temporal crescent is normally seen only by the nasal hemiretina on the same side. A person whose optic nerve is cut would therefore be blind in the temporal crescent on the lesioned side. Removal of binocular input in this way also affects the perception of spatial depth (stereopsis).

Destruction of the fibers crossing in the optic chiasm removes input from the temporal portions of both halves of the visual field. The deficit produced by this lesion is called *bitemporal hemianopsia* and occurs because fibers arising from the nasal half of each retina have been destroyed (Figure 27-20, 2). This kind of damage is most commonly caused by a tumor of the pituitary gland that compresses the chiasm.

Destruction of one optic tract produces *homonymous hemianopsia,* a loss of vision in the entire contralateral visual hemifield (Figure 27-20, 3). For example, destruction of the right tract causes left homonymous hemianopsia, ie, loss of vision in the left nasal and right temporal hemiretinas (Figure 27-20, 4). Finally, a lesion of the optic radiation or of the visual cortex, where the fibers are more spread out, produces an *incomplete* or *quadrantic field defect,* a loss of vision in part of the contralateral visual hemifield (Figure 27-20, 5, 6).

An Overall View

Visual information important for perception flows from the retina to the lateral geniculate nucleus. In both structures cells have small circular receptive fields. The primary visual cortex elaborates the elemental information from these cells in at least three ways. (1) Each part of the visual field is decomposed into short line segments of different orientation, through orientation columns. This is an early step in the process thought to be necessary for discrimination of form. (2) Color processing occurs in cells that lack orientation selectivity in regions called blobs. (3) The input from the two eyes is combined through the ocular dominance columns, a step necessary for perception of depth.

This parallel processing in the visual system is achieved by means of central connections that are remarkably specific. The ganglion cells in the retina project to the lateral geniculate nucleus in the thalamus in an orderly way that creates a complete retinotopic map of the visual field for each eye in the nucleus. Furthermore, the M and P ganglion cells of the retina project to different layers of the lateral geniculate nucleus: the M cells to the magnocellular layers and the P cells to the parvocellular layers. Cells in these layers project to different sublayers in 4C of striate cortex ($4C\alpha$ and $4C\beta$). Thus, two separate pathways (the M and P pathways)

extend from the retina to the primary visual cortex. The functional contribution of the M and P pathways are different. The P pathway is essential for color vision and is particularly sensitive to stimuli with higher spatial and lower temporal frequencies. The M pathway is more sensitive to stimuli with lower spatial and higher temporal frequencies.

Within the striate cortex each geniculate axon terminates primarily in layer 4, from which information is distributed to other layers, each of which has its own pattern of connections with other cortical or subcortical regions. In addition to the circuitry of the layers, cells in the visual cortex are arranged into vertically oriented functional systems: orientation-specific columns, ocular dominance columns, and blobs. Neurons with similar response properties in different vertically oriented systems are linked by horizontal connections. Information thus flows in two directions: between layers and horizontally throughout each layer. This pattern of interconnection links several columnar systems together; for example, a set of linked orientation-specific columns would represent all directions of movement in a specific region of the visual field. Such "hypercolumns" seem to function as elementary computational modules—they receive varied inputs, transform them, and send their output to a number of different regions of the brain.

Robert H. Wurtz
Eric R. Kandel

Selected Readings

Casagrande VA. 1994. A third parallel visual pathway to primate area V1. Trends Neurosci 17:305–310.

Gilbert CD. 1992. Horizontal integration and cortical dynamics. Neuron 9:1–13.

Hubel DH. 1988. *Eye, Brain, and Vision.* New York: Scientific American Library.

Hubel DH, Wiesel TN. 1959. Receptive fields of single neurones in the cat's striate cortex. J Physiol (Lond) 148:574–591.

Hubel DH, Wiesel TN. 1962. Receptive fields, binocular interaction and functional architecture in the cat's visual cortex. J Physiol (Lond) 160:106–154.

Hubel DH, Wiesel TN. 1979. Brain mechanisms of vision. Sci Am 241(3):150–162.

Lund JS. 1988. Anatomical organization of macaque monkey striate visual cortex. Annu Rev Neurosci 11:253–288.

Merigan WH, Maunsell JH. 1993. How parallel are the primate visual pathways? Annu Rev Neurosci 16:369–402.

Schiller PH, Logothetis NK, Charles ER. 1990. Role of the color-opponent and broad-band channels in vision. Vis Neurosci 5:321–346.

Shapley R. 1990. Visual sensitivity and parallel retinocortical channels. Annu Rev Psychol 41:635–658.

Shapley R, Perry VH. 1986. Cat and monkey retinal ganglion cells and their visual functional roles. Trends Neurosci 9:229–235.

References

Blasdel GG. 1992a. Differential imaging of ocular dominance and orientation selectivity in monkey striate cortex. J Neurosci 12:3115–3138.

Blasdel GG. 1992b. Orientation selectivity, preference and continuity in monkey striate cortex. J Neurosci 12:3139–3161.

Brodal A. 1981. The optic system. In: *Neurological Anatomy in Relation to Clinical Medicine,* 3rd ed. New York: Oxford Univ. Press.

Bunt AH, Hendrickson AE, Lund JS, Lund RD, Fuchs AF. 1975. Monkey retinal ganglion cells: morphometric analysis and tracing of axonal projections, with a consideration of the peroxidase technique. J Comp Neurol 164:265–285.

Ferster D. 1992. The synaptic inputs to simple cells of the cat visual cortex. Prog Brain Res 90:423–441.

Gilbert CD, Wiesel TN. 1979. Morphology and intracortical projections of functionally characterised neurones in the cat visual cortex. Nature 280:120–125.

Gilbert CD, Wiesel TN. 1989. Columnar specificity of intrinsic horizontal and corticocortical connections in cat visual cortex. J Neurosci 9:2432–2442.

Groves P, Schlesinger K. 1979. *Introduction to Biological Psychology.* Dubuque, IA: W.C. Brown.

Guillery RW. 1982. The optic chiasm of the vertebrate brain. Contrib Sens Physiol 7:39–73.

Horton JC, Hubel DH. 1981. Regular patchy distribution of cytochrome oxidase staining in primary visual cortex of macaque monkey. Nature 292:762–764.

Hubel DH, Wiesel TN. 1965. Binocular interaction in striate cortex of kittens reared with artificial squint. J Neurophysiol 28:1041–1059.

Hubel DH, Wiesel TN. 1972. Laminar and columnar distribution of geniculo-cortical fibers in the macaque monkey. J Comp Neurol 146:421–450.

Hubel DH, Wiesel TN, Stryker MP. 1978. Anatomical demonstration of orientation columns in macaque monkey. J Comp Neurol 177:361–379.

Hurvich LM. 1981. *Color Vision.* Sunderland, MA: Sinauer.

Kaas JH, Guillery RW, Allman JM. 1972. Some principles of organization of the lateral geniculate nucleus. Brain Behav Evol 6:253–299.

Kisvarday ZF, Cowey A, Smith AD, Somogyi P. 1989. Interlaminar and lateral excitatory amino acid connections in the striate cortex of monkey. J Neurosci 9:667–682.

Livingstone MS, Hubel DH. 1984. Anatomy and physiology of a color system in the primate visual cortex. J Neurosci 4:309–356.

Livingstone MS, Hubel DH. 1984. Specificity of intrinsic connections in primate primary visual cortex. J Neurosci 4:2830–2835.

Marr D. 1982. *Vision: A Computational Investigation Into the Human Representation and Processing of Visual Information.* San Francisco: Freeman.

Marshall WH, Woolsey CN, Bard P. 1941. Observations on cortical somatic sensory mechanisms of cat and monkey. J Neurophysiol 4:1–24.

Martin KAC. 1988. The lateral geniculate nucleus strikes back. Trends Neurosci 11:192–194.

McGuire BA, Gilbert CD, Rivlin PK, Wiesel TN. 1991. Targets of horizontal connections in macaque primary visual cortex. J Comp Neurol 305:370–392.

McGuire BA, Hornung J-P, Gilbert CD, Wiesel TN. 1984. Patterns of synaptic input to layer 4 of cat striate cortex. J Neurosci 4:3021–3033.

Merigan WH. 1989. Chromatic and achromatic vision of macaques: role of the P pathway. J Neurosci 9:776–783.

Merigan WH, Byrne CE, Maunsell JH. 1991. Does primate motion perception depend on the magnocellular pathway? J Neurosci 11:3422–3429.

Merigan WH, Katz LM, Maunsell JH. 1991. The effects of parvocellular geniculate lesions on the acuity and contrast sensitivity of macaque monkeys. J Neurosci 11:994–1001.

Merigan WH, Maunsell JHR. 1993. Macaque vision after magnocellular lateral geniculate lesions. Vis Neurosci 5:347–352.

Rockland KS, Lund JS. 1983. Intrinsic laminar lattice connections in primate visual cortex. J Comp Neurol 216:303–318.

Schiller PH. 1984. The connections of the retinal on and off pathways to the lateral geniculate nucleus of the monkey. Vision Res 24:923–932.

Sclar G, Maunsell JH, Lennie P. 1990. Coding of image contrast in central visual pathways of the macaque monkey. Vision Res 30:1–10.

Shapley R, Kaplan E, Soodak R. 1981. Spatial summation and contrast sensitivity of X and Y cells in the lateral geniculate nucleus of the macaque. Nature 292:543–545.

Shapley R, Lennie P. 1985. Spatial frequency analysis in the visual system. Annu Rev Neurosci 8:547–583.

Sherman SM. 1988. Functional organization of the cat's lateral geniculate nucleus. In: M Bentivoglio, R Spreafico (eds). *Cellular Thalamic Mechanisms,* pp. 163–183. New York: Excerpta Medica.

Stone J, Dreher B, Leventhal A. 1979. Hierarchical and parallel mechanisms in the organization of visual cortex. Brain Res Rev 1:345–394.

Stryker MP, Chapman B, Miller KD, Zahs KR. 1990. Experimental and theoretical studies of the organization of afferents to single-orientation columns in visual cortex. Cold Spring Harbor Symp Quant Biol 55:515–527.

Ts'o DY, Frostig RD, Lieke EE, Grinvald A. 1990. Functional organization of primate visual cortex revealed by high resolution optical imaging. Science 249:417–420.

Ts'o DY, Gilbert CD, Wiesel TN. 1986. Relationships between horizontal interactions and functional architecture in cat striate cortex as revealed by cross-correlation analysis. J Neurosci 6:1160–1170.

Walls GL. 1953. *The Lateral Geniculate Nucleus and Visual Histophysiology.* Berkeley: Univ. California Press.

Wiesel TN, Hubel DH, Lam DMK. 1974. Autoradiographic demonstration of ocular-dominance columns in the monkey striate cortex by means of transneuronal transport. Brain Res 79:273–279.

Weiskrantz L, Harlow A, Barbur JL. 1991. Factors affecting visual sensitivity in a hemianopic subject. Brain 114:2269–2282.

Wong-Riley M. 1979. Changes in the visual system of monocularly sutured or enucleated cats demonstrable with cytochrome oxidase histochemistry. Brain Res 171:11–28.

Yoshioka T, Levitt JB, Lund JS. 1994. Independence and merger of thalamocortical channels within macaque monkey primary visual cortex: anatomy of interlaminar projections. Vis Neurosci 11:467–489.

Zeki S. 1993. *A Vision of the Brain.* Oxford: Blackwell Scientific.

28

Perception of Motion, Depth, and Form

IN VISION, AS IN OTHER mental operations, we experience the world as a whole. Independent attributes—motion, depth, form, and color—are coordinated into a single visual image. In the two previous chapters we began to consider how two parallel pathways—the magnocellular and parvocellular pathways, that extend from the retina through the lateral geniculate nucleus of the thalamus to the primary visual (striate) cortex—might produce a coherent visual image. In this chapter we examine how the information from these two pathways feeds into multiple higher-order centers of visual processing in the extrastriate cortex. How do these pathways contribute to our perception of motion, depth, form, and color?

The magnocellular (M) and parvocellular (P) pathways feed into two extrastriate cortical pathways: a dorsal pathway and a ventral pathway. In this chapter we examine, in cell-biological terms, the information processing in each of these pathways.

We shall first consider the perception of motion and depth, mediated in large part by the dorsal pathway to the posterior parietal cortex. We then consider the perception of contrast and contours, mediated largely by the ventral pathway extending to the inferior temporal cortex. This pathway also is concerned with the assessment of color, which we will consider in Chapter 29. Finally, we shall consider the binding problem in the visual system: how information conveyed in parallel but separate pathways is brought together into a coherent perception.

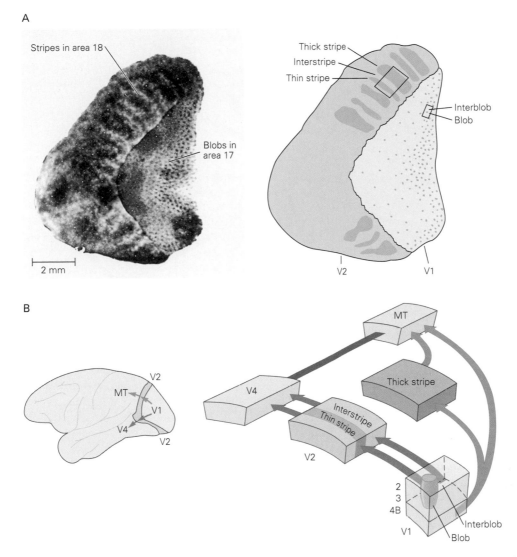

Figure 28-1 Organization of V1 and V2.

A. Subregions in V1 (area 17) and V2 (area 18). This section from the occipital lobe of a squirrel monkey at the border of areas 17 and 18 was reacted with cytochrome oxidase. The cytochrome oxidase stains the blobs in V1 and the thick and thin stripes in V2. (Courtesy of M. Livingstone.)

B. Connections between V1 and V2. The blobs in V1 connect primarily to the thin stripes in V2, while the interblobs in V1 connect to interstripes in V2. Layer 4B projects to the thick stripes in V2 and to the middle temporal area (**MT**). Both thin and interstripes project to V4. Thick stripes in V2 also project to MT.

The Parvocellular and Magnocellular Pathways Feed Into Two Processing Pathways in Extrastriate Cortex

In Chapter 27 we saw that the parallel parvocellular and magnocellular pathways remain segregated even in the striate cortex. What happens to these P and M pathways beyond the striate cortex? Early research on these pathways indicated that the P pathway continues in the ventral cortical pathway that extends to the inferior temporal cortex, and that the M pathway becomes the dorsal pathway that extends to the posterior parietal cortex. However, the actual relationships are probably not so exclusive.

The evidence for separation of function of the dorsal and ventral pathways begins in the primary visual, or striate, cortex (V1). Staining for the mitochondrial enzyme cytochrome oxidase reveals a precise and repeating pattern of dark, peg-like regions about 0.2 mm in diameter called blobs. The blobs are especially prominent in the superficial layers 2 and 3, where they are separated by intervening regions that stain lighter, the in-

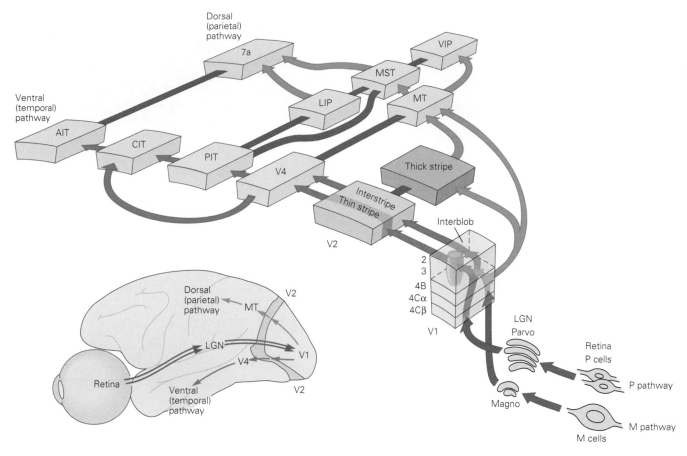

Figure 28-2 The magnocellular (M) and parvocellular (P) pathways from the retina project through the lateral geniculate nucleus (LGN) to V1. Separate pathways to the temporal and parietal cortices course through the extrastriate cortex beginning in V2. The connections shown in the figure are based on established anatomical connections, but only selected connections are shown and many cortical areas are omitted (compare Figure 25-9). Note the cross connections between the two pathways in several cortical areas. The parietal pathway re-

ceives input from the M pathway but only the temporal pathway receives input from both the M and P pathways. (Abbreviations: **AIT** = anterior inferior temporal area; **CIT** = central inferior temporal area; **LIP** = lateral intraparietal area; **Magno** = magnocellular layers of the lateral geniculate nucleus; **MST** = medial superior temporal area; **MT** = middle temporal area; **Parvo** = parvocellular layers of the lateral geniculate nucleus; **PIT** = posterior inferior temporal area; **VIP** = ventral intraparietal area.) (Based on Merigan and Maunsell 1993.)

terblob regions. The same stain also reveals alternating thick and thin stripes separated by interstripes of little activity (Figure 28-1 in the secondary visual cortex, or V2).

Margaret Livingstone and David Hubel identified the anatomical connections between labeled regions in V1 and V2 (Figure 28-1B). They found that the P and M pathways remain partially segregated through V2. The M pathway projects from the magnocellular layers of the lateral geniculate nucleus to the striate cortex, first to layer 4Cα and then to layer 4B. Cells in layer 4B project directly to the middle temporal area (MT) and also to the thick stripes in V2, from which cells also project to MT.

Thus, a clear anatomical pathway exists from the magnocellular layers in the lateral geniculate nucleus to MT and from there to the posterior parietal cortex (Figure 28-2).

Cells in the parvocellular layers of the lateral geniculate nucleus project to layer 4Cβ in the striate cortex, from which cells project to the blobs and interblobs of V1. The blobs send a strong projection to the thin stripes in V2, whereas interblobs send a strong projection to the interstripes in V2. The thin stripe and interstripe areas of V2 may in turn project to discrete subregions of V4, thus maintaining this separation in the P pathway into V4 and possibly on into the inferior temporal cortex. A pathway from the P cells in the lateral geniculate nu-

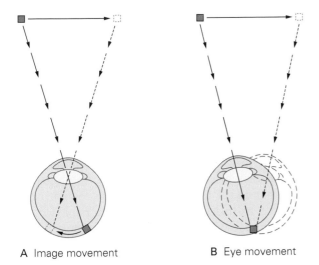

A Image movement   B Eye movement

Figure 28-3 Motion in the visual field can be perceived in two ways.

A. When the eyes are held still, the image of a moving object traverses the retina. Information about movement depends upon sequential firing of receptors in the retina.

B. When the eyes follow an object, the image of the moving object falls on one place on the retina and the information is conveyed by movement of the eyes or the head.

cleus to the inferior temporal cortex can therefore also be identified (Figure 28-2).

But are these pathways exclusive of each other? Several anatomical observations suggest that they are not. In V1 both the magnocellular and parvocellular pathways have inputs in the blobs, and local neurons make extensive connections between the blob and interblob compartments. In V2 cross connections exist between the stripe compartments. Thus, the separation is not absolute, but whether there is an intermixing of the M and P contributions or whether the cross connections allow one cortical pathway to modulate activity in the other is not clear.

Results of experiments that selectively inactivate the P and M pathways as they pass through the lateral geniculate nucleus (described in Chapter 27) also erode the notion of strict segregation between the pathways in V1. Blocking of either pathway affects the responses of fewer than half the neurons in V1, which indicates that most V1 neurons receive physiologically effective inputs from both pathways. Further work has shown that the responses of neurons both within and outside of the blobs in the superficial layers of V1 are altered by blocking only the M pathway. Both observations suggest that there is incomplete segregation of the M and P pathways in V1.

This selective blocking of the P and M pathways also reveals the relative contributions of the pathways to

the parietal and inferior temporal cortices. Blocking the magnocellular layers of the lateral geniculate nucleus eliminates the responses of many cells in MT and always reduces the responses of the remaining cells; blocking the parvocellular layers produces a much weaker effect on cells in MT. In contrast, blocking the activity of either the parvocellular or magnocellular layers in the lateral geniculate nucleus reduces the activity of neurons in V4. Thus, the dorsal pathway to MT seems primarily to include input from the M pathway, whereas the ventral pathway to the inferior temporal cortex appears to include input from both the M and P pathways. We can now see that there is substantial segregation of the P and M pathways up to V1, probably

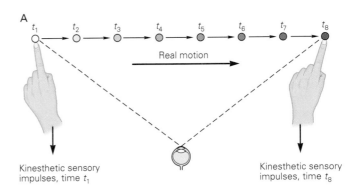

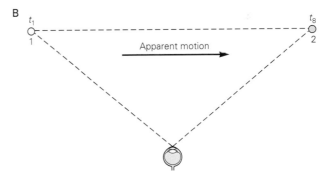

Figure 28-4 The illusion of apparent motion is evidence that the visual system analyzes motion in a separate pathway.

A. Actual motion is experienced as a sequence of visual sensations, each resulting from the image falling on a different position in the retina.

B. Apparent motion may actually be more convincing than actual motion, and is the perceptual basis for motion pictures. Thus, when two lights at positions **1** and **2** are turned on and off at suitable intervals, we perceive a single light moving between the two points. This perceptual illusion cannot be explained by processing of information based on different retinal positions and is therefore evidence for the existence of a special visual system for the detection of motion. (From Hochberg 1978.)

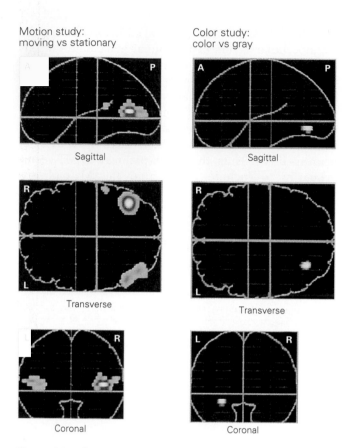

Motion study:
moving vs stationary

Sagittal

Transverse

Coronal

Color study:
color vs gray

Sagittal

Transverse

Coronal

Figure 28-5 Separate human brain areas are activated by motion and color.

Motion studies. Six subjects viewed a black and white random-dot pattern that moved in one of eight directions or remained stationary. The figure shows the effect of motion because the PET scans taken while the pattern was stationary were subtracted from those taken while the pattern was moving. The **white** and **red areas** show the high end of activity (increased blood flow). The areas are located on the convexity of the prestriate cortex at the junction of Brodmann's areas 19 and 37.

Color studies. The subjects viewed a collage of 15 squares and rectangles of different colors or, alternatively, the same patterns in gray shades only. The figure shows the difference in blood flow while viewing the color and gray patterns. The area showing increased flow, subserving the perception of color, is located inferiorly and medially in the occipital cortex. (From Zeki et al. 1991).

separation into V2, a likely predominance of the M input to the dorsal pathway to MT and the parietal cortex, and a mixture of P and M input into the pathway leading to the inferior temporal lobe (as indicated by the lines crossing between the pathways in Figure 28-2).

What should we conclude about the organization of visual processing throughout the multiple areas of the visual cortex? First, we know that there are specific serial pathways through the multiple visual areas, not just

a random assortment of equally connected areas. There is substantial evidence for two major processing pathways, a dorsal one to the posterior parietal cortex and a ventral one to the inferior temporal cortex, but other pathways may also exist. Second, there is strong evidence that the processing in these two cortical pathways is hierarchical. Each level has strong projections to the next level (and projections back), and the type of visual processing changes systematically from one level to the next. Third, the functions of cortical areas in the two cortical pathways are strikingly different, as judged both by the anatomical connections and the cellular activity considered in this chapter and by the behavioral and brain imaging evidence discussed in Chapter 25.

Our examination of the functional organization within these vast regions of extrastriate visual cortex begins with the dorsal cortical pathway and the most intensively studied visual attribute, motion. We then examine the processing of depth information in the dorsal pathway. Finally, we turn to the ventral cortical pathway and consider the processing of information related to form. Color vision is the subject of the next chapter.

Motion Is Analyzed Primarily in the Dorsal Pathway to the Parietal Cortex

We usually think of motion as an object moving in the visual field, a car or a tennis ball, and we easily distinguish these moving objects from the stationary background. However, we often see objects in motion not because they move on our retina, but because we track them with eye movements; the image remains stationary on the retina but we perceive movement because our eyes move (Figure 28-3).

Motion in the visual field is detected by comparing the position of images recorded at different times. Since most cells in the visual system are exquisitely sensitive to retinal position and can resolve events separated in time by 10 to 20 milliseconds, most cells in the visual system should, in principle, be able to extract information about motion from the position of the image on the retina by comparing the previous location of an object with its current location. What then is the evidence for a special neural subsystem specialized for motion?

The initial evidence for a special mechanism designed to detect motion independent of retinal position came from psychophysical observations on *apparent motion,* an illusion of motion that occurs when lights separated in space are turned on and off at appropriate intervals (Figure 28-4). The perception of motion of objects that in fact have not changed position suggests that position and motion are signaled by separate pathways.

Box 28-1 Optic Flow

Optic flow refers to the perceived motion of the visual field that results from an individual's own movement through the environment. With optic flow the entire visual field moves, in contrast to the local motion of objects. Optic flow provides two types of cues: information about the organization of the environment (near objects will move faster than more distant objects) and information about the control of posture (side-to-side patterns induce body sway). Particularly influential in the development of ideas about optic flow was the demonstration by the experimental psychologist James J. Gibson that optic flow is critical for indicating the direction of observer movement ("heading"). For example, when an individual moves forward with eyes and head directed straight ahead, optic flow expands outward from a point straight ahead in the visual field, a pattern that is frequently used in movies to show space ship flight.

Where is optic flow represented in the brain? Neurons in one region of the medial superior temporal area of the parietal cortex in monkeys respond in ways that would make these cells ideal candidates to analyze optic flow. These neurons respond selectively to motion, have receptive fields that cover large parts of the visual field, and respond preferentially to large-field motion in the visual field. Additionally, the neurons are sensitive to shifts in the origin of full-field motion and to differences in speed between the center and periphery of the field. The neurons also receive input related to eye movement, which is particularly significant because forward movement is typically accompanied by eye and head movement. Finally, electrical stimulation of this area alters the ability of the monkey to locate the point of origin of field motion, providing further evidence that the superior temporal area of the parietal cortex is important for optic flow.

Motion Is Represented in the Middle Temporal Area

Experiments on monkeys show that neurons in the retina and lateral geniculate nucleus, as well as many areas in the striate and extrastriate cortex, respond very well to a spot of light moving across their receptive fields. In area V1, however, cells respond to motion in *one* direction, while motion in the opposite direction has little or no effect on them. This *directional selectivity* is prominent among cells in layer 4B of the striate cortex. Thus, cells in the M pathway provide input to cells in 4B, but these input cells themselves do not show directional selectivity. They simply provide the raw input for the directionally selective cortical cells.

In monkeys one area at the edge of the parietal cortex, the middle temporal area (MT), appears to be devoted to motion processing because almost all of the cells are directionally selective and the activity of only a small fraction of these cells is substantially altered by the shape or the color of the moving stimulus. Like V1, MT has a retinotopic map of the contralateral visual field, but the receptive fields of cells within this map are about 10 times wider than those of cells in the striate cortex. Cells with similar directional specificity are organized into vertical columns running from the surface of the cortex to the white matter. Each part of the visual field is represented by a set of columns in which cells respond to different directions of motion in that part of the visual field. This columnar organization is similar to that seen in V1.

Cells in MT respond to motion of spots or bars of light by detecting contrasts in luminance. Some cells in MT also respond to moving forms that are not defined by differences in luminance but by differences only in texture or color. While these cells are not selective for color itself, they nonetheless detect motion by responding to an edge defined by color. Thus, even though MT and the dorsal pathway to the parietal cortex may be devoted to the analysis of motion, the cells are sensitive to stimuli (color) that were thought to be analyzed primarily by cells in the ventral pathway. Stimulus information on motion, form, and color therefore is not processed exclusively in separate functional pathways.

This description of motion processing is based on research on the MT area in monkeys. In the human brain an area devoted to motion has been identified at the junction of the parietal, temporal, and occipital cortices. Figure 28-5 shows changes in blood flow in this area in PET scans made while the subject viewed a pattern of dots in motion.

A cortical area adjacent to MT, the medial superior temporal area (MST), also has neurons that are responsive to visual motion and these neurons may process a type of global motion in the visual field called optic flow, which is important for a person's own movements through an environment (Box 28-1).

Cells in MT Solve the Aperture Problem

We have considered the response of MT neurons to the motion of simple stimulus like an edge or a line. How-

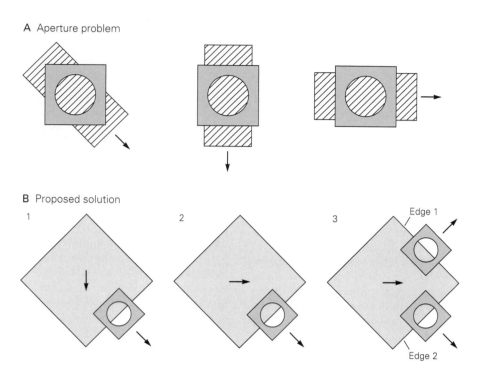

A Aperture problem

B Proposed solution

1   2   3

Edge 1

Edge 2

Figure 28-6 The aperture problem.

A. Three patterns moving in three different directions produce the same physical stimulus if only part of the pattern is within view, and thus all three patterns are perceived as moving in the same direction. Three patterns are shown moving in three directions. When seen through a small aperture the three gratings appear to move in the same direction, downward and to the right. This failure to accurately detect the true direction of motion is called the aperture problem. (Adapted from Movshon et al. 1985.)

B. A formal solution to the aperture problem. When motion in different directions, downward (**1**) or rightward (**2**), is seen through a small aperture, the motion of the edge seen through the aperture does not indicate the true direction of the entire pattern. Assume now that the aperture represents the receptive field of a neuron, and that there are two apertures rather than one (**3**). This represents the situation in which two or more cells that respond to specific directions perpendicular to their axis of orientation are activated by different edges moving in different directions. A higher-order cell that integrates the signals from the lower-order cells could encode the motion of the entire object. (Adapted from Movshon 1990.)

ever, in the everyday world complex two- and three-dimensional patterns often give rise to ambiguous or illusory perception. Consider the example in Figure 28-6A, which shows three gratings moving in three directions. When viewed through a small circular aperture, all three gratings appear to move in the same direction. The observer only reports the component of motion that is perpendicular to the orientation of the bars in the gratings. This phenomenon, known as the *aperture problem*, applies to the study of neurons as well as perception. Since most neurons in V1 and MT have relatively small receptive fields, they confront the aperture problem when an object larger than their receptive field moves across the visual field.

To solve the aperture problem, neurons may extract information about motion in the visual field in two stages. In the initial stage neurons that respond to a specific axis of orientation signal motion of components

perpendicular to their axis of orientation. The second stage is concerned with establishing the direction of motion of the entire pattern. In this stage higher-order neurons integrate the local components of motion analyzed by neurons in the initial stage.

The hypothesis that motion information in the visual system is processed in two stages was tested by Tony Movshon and his colleagues, who recorded the responses of cells in V1 and MT to a moving plaid pattern. The neurons of V1 as well as the majority of neurons in MT responded only to the components of the plaid. Each cell responded best when the lines in the plaid moved in the direction preferred by the cell. Cells did not respond to the direction of motion of the entire plaid. Movshon therefore called these neurons *component direction-selective neurons*. In contrast, about 20% of the neurons in MT responded only to motion of the plaid pattern. These cells, called *pattern direction-*

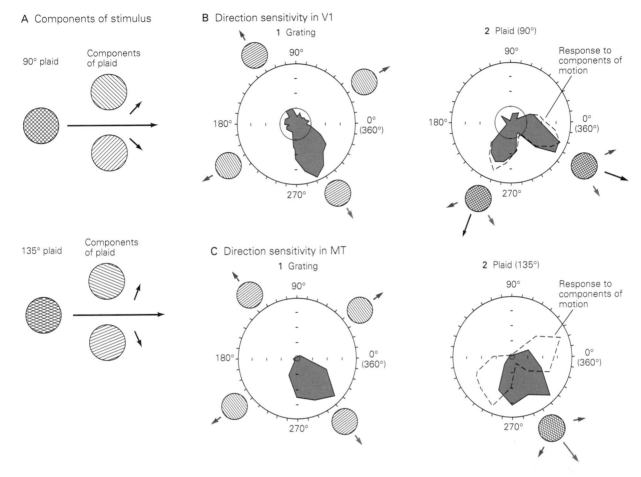

Figure 28-7 Neurons in the middle temporal area of cortex in monkeys are sensitive to the motion of an entire object in the visual field.

A. Stimuli used to activate cells in V1 and MT. Pairs of gratings are oriented at a 90° angle (top) or 135° angle (bottom) to each other. When each pair is superimposed during movement, the resulting plaid pattern appears to move directly to the right. The motion of each component grating is perpendicular to the orientation of its bars. The movement of either component alone should stimulate first-stage neurons that prefer the direction of motion of the one grating. When the two gratings are superimposed to form a moving plaid, other (second-stage) neurons should be activated.

B. Polar plots illustrate the motion signaled by first-stage neurons in V1. The plots show the response of a neuron to the direction (0 to 360°) of motion of individual gratings (**1**) and the plaid (**2**). The response of the neuron to motion in each direction is indicated by the distance of the point from the center of the plot. The circle at the center indicates the neuron's activity when no stimulus is presented.

1. This neuron responds best when the motion of a grating is downward and to the right (**blue arrow**).

2. When presented with the moving plaid, the neuron responds to the motion of each component grating (**solid color**) rather than to the rightward motion of the plaid. The response of the cell to the grating components is expected to have the two-lobed configuration indicated by the **dashed lines**. Neurons that respond only to the motion of the components of the plaid are referred to as component direction-selective neurons.

C. These polar plots illustrate the motion signaled by a higher-order neuron in the middle temporal area (MT).

1. As with the lower-order cell in V1, this cell in MT responds to motion downward and to the right.

2. When presented with the plaid, the neuron responds to the direction of motion of the plaid (**solid color**), not to the directions of the component gratings (**dashed line**). This indicates that the neuron has processed the component signals of V1 into a more accurate perception of the movement of the object, and the neuron is referred to as a pattern direction-sensitive neuron. (Modified from Movshon et al. 1985.)

A

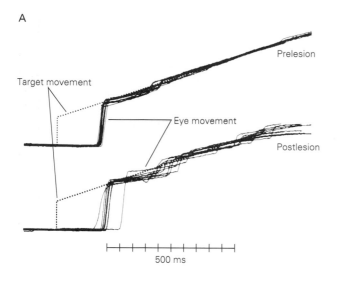

Target movement

Prelesion

Eye movement

Postlesion

500 ms

B

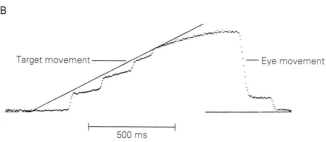

Target movement —————   —— Eye movement

500 ms

Figure 28-8 Cortical lesions in monkeys and humans produce similar deficits in smooth-pursuit eye movement.

A. Smooth-pursuit eye movements of a monkey before a lesion in the foveal region medial superior temporal area (MST) in the right hemisphere (**prelesion**) and 24 h after the lesion (**postlesion**). The monkey's task is to to keep the moving target on the fovea by making smooth-pursuit eye movement. The **dotted line** shows the position of the target over time. The stimulus is turned off where the monkey is fixating and then turned on again as it moves smoothly at 15° per second to the right. The **solid lines** show superimposed eye movements as the monkey pursues the target on 10 separate trials. Note that before the lesion the monkey nearly matches the target motion with smooth-pursuit eye movement, but after the lesion it fails to do so. Instead it makes frequent saccadic eye movements (the series of small steps in the eye movement record) to catch up with the target. (From Dursteler et al. 1987.)

B. Smooth-pursuit eye movements in a human subject with a right occipital-parietal lesion. The patient attempts to follow a target moving 20° per second to the right, but the eye movements do not keep up with the target motion. As with the monkey, the subject uses a series of catch-up saccades to compensate for the slow pursuit. In both humans and monkeys the pursuit deficit is most prominent when the target is moving toward the side of the brain containing the lesion (in these cases, right brain lesions and deficits with rightward pursuit). The human subject, with a large lesion that must include multiple brain areas, has a deficit in smooth-pursuit eye movements very similar to the deficit seen in the monkey with a lesion limited to small and identified visual areas. (From Morrow and Sharpe 1993.)

sensitive neurons, receive input from the component direction-selective cells (Figure 28-7). Thus, as suggested by the two-stage hypothesis, the *global motion* of an object is computed by pattern-selective neurons in MT based on the inputs of the component direction-selective neurons in V1 and MT.

Control of Movement Is Selectively Impaired by Lesions of MT

These correlations of neuronal activity and visual perception raise the question, Is the activity of direction-selective cells in MT causally related to the visual perception of motion and the control of motion-dependent movement? The question whether direction-selective cells in MT directly affect the control of movement was first addressed in an experiment that examined the relationship of these cells to smooth-pursuit eye movements, the movements that keep a moving target in the fovea (see Figure 28-3). When discrete focal chemical lesions were made within different regions of the retinotopic map in MT of a monkey, the speed of the moving target could no longer be estimated correctly in the region of the visual field monitored by the damaged MT area. In contrast, the lesions did not affect pursuit of targets in other regions of the visual field nor did they affect eye movements to stationary targets. Thus, visual processing in MT is selective for motion of the visual stimulus; lesions produce a blind spot, or a scotoma, for motion.

Human patients with lesions of parietal cortex also sometimes have these deficits in smooth-pursuit eye movements, but the most frequent behavioral deficit is quite different from that seen after lesions of MT. The neurologist Gordon Holmes originally reported that these patients were unable to follow a target when it was moving toward the side of the brain that had the lesion. For example, a patient with a lesioned right hemisphere has difficulty pursuing a target moving toward the right (Figure 28-8B). Later experiments on monkeys showed that lesions centered on the medial superior temporal area (MST), the next level of processing for visual motion, produced just such a deficit (Figure 28-8A).

Perception of Motion Is Altered by Lesions and Microstimulation of MT

The question whether MT cells contribute to the perception of visual motion was addressed in an experiment in which monkeys were trained to report the direction of motion in a display of moving dots. The experimenter varied the proportion of dots that moved in the same direction. At zero correlation the motion of all dots was

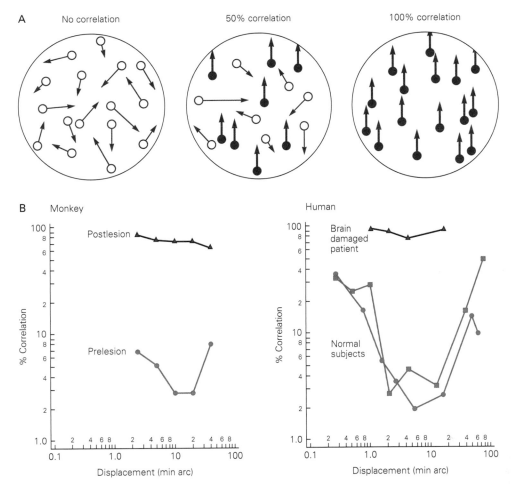

Figure 28-9 A monkey with an MT lesion and a human patient with damage to extrastriate visual cortex have similar deficits in motion perception.

A. Displays used to study the perception of motion. In the display on the left there is no correlation between the directions of movement of several dots, and thus no net motion in the display. In the display on the right all the dots move in the same direction (100% correlation). An intermediate case is in the center; 50% of the dots move in the same direction while the other 50% move in random directions (essentially noise added to the signal). (From Newsome and Pare 1988.)

B. The performance of a monkey before and after an MT lesion (left). The performance of a human subject with bilateral brain damage is compared to two normal subjects (right). The ordinate of the graph shows the percent correlation in the directions of all moving dots (as in part A) required for the monkey to pick out the one common direction. The abscissa indicates the size of the displacement of the dot and thus the degree of apparent motion. Note the general similarity between the performance of the humans and that of the monkey and the devastation to this performance after the cortical lesions. (From Newsome and Pare 1988, Baker et al. 1991.)

random and at 100% correlation the motion of all dots was in one direction (Figure 28-9A). While normal monkeys could perform the task with less than 10% of the dots moving in the same direction, monkeys with a lesion in MT required nearly 100% coherence to perform as well (Figure 28-9B). A human patient with bilateral brain damage also lost the perception of motion when tested on the same task (Figure 28-9B). In both the monkeys and the human subject, visual acuity for stationary stimuli was not affected by the brain damage.

Thus damage to MT reduces the ability of monkeys to detect motion in the visual field, as indicated by disruptions in the pursuit of moving objects and perception of the direction of motion. However, monkeys with MT lesions quickly recover these functions. Directionally selective cells in other areas of cerebral cortex, such as MST, apparently can take over the function performed by MT. Recovery of function is greatly slowed when the lesion affects not only MT but also MST and other extrastriate areas.

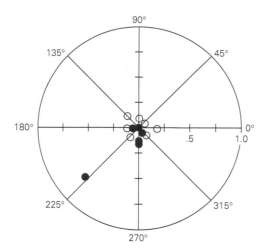

Figure 28-10 Alteration of perceived direction of motion by stimulation of MT neurons. A monkey was shown a display of moving dots with a relatively low correlation of 25.6% (see Figure 28-9A) and instructed to indicate in which of eight directions the dots appeared to be moving. The **open circles** show the proportion of decisions made for each direction of motion—about equal choice for all directions. Electric current was passed through a microelectrode positioned among cells that responded best to stimulus motion in one direction, 225° on the polar plot. The microstimulation was applied for 1 s, beginning and ending with the onset and offset of the visual stimulus. **Filled circles** show the response of the monkey when the MT cells were stimulated at the same time the visual stimulus was presented. Stimulation increased the likelihood that the monkey would indicate seeing motion in the direction preferred by the stimulated MT cells (225°). (Adapted from Salzman and Newsome 1994.)

If cells in MT are directly involved in the analysis of motion, the firing patterns of these neurons should affect perceptual judgments about motion. How well does the firing pattern of these neurons actually correlate with behavior? To address this question, William Newsome and Movshon recorded the activity of direction-selective neurons in MT while the monkeys reported the direction of motion in a random-dot display. Firing of the neurons correlated extremely well with performance. Thus the directional information encoded by the neurons of MT cells is sufficient to account for the monkey's judgment of motion.

If this inference is correct, then modifying the firing rates of the MT neurons should alter the monkey's perception of motion. In fact, Newsome found that stimulating clusters of neurons in a single column of cells sensitive to one direction of motion biases the monkey's judgment toward that direction of motion. The electrical stimulation acts as if a constant visual motion signal were added to the signal conveyed by the

whole population of MT neurons (Figure 28-10). Thus, the firing of a relatively small population of motion-sensitive neurons in MT directly contributes to perception.

Depth Vision Depends on Monocular Cues and Binocular Disparity

One of the major tasks of the visual system is to convert a two-dimensional retinal image into three dimensions. How is this transformation achieved? How do we tell how far one thing is from another? How do we estimate the relative depth of a three-dimensional object in the visual field? Psychophysical studies indicate that the shift from two to three dimensions relies on two types of clues: monocular cues for depth and stereoscopic cues for binocular disparity.

Monocular Cues Create Far-Field Depth Perception

At distances greater than about 100 feet the retinal images seen by each eye are almost identical, so that looking at a distance we are essentially one-eyed. Nevertheless we can perceive depth with one eye by relying on a variety of tricks called monocular depth cues. Several of these monocular cues were appreciated by the artists of antiquity, rediscovered during the Renaissance, and codified early in the sixteenth century by Leonardo da Vinci.

1. *Familiar size.* If we know from experience something about the size of a person, we can judge the person's distance (Figure 28-11A).
2. *Occlusion.* If one person is partly hiding another person, we assume the person in front is closer (Figure 28-11A).
3. *Linear perspective.* Parallel lines, such as those of a railroad track, appear to converge with distance. The greater the convergence of lines, the greater is the impression of distance. The visual system interprets the convergence as depth by assuming that parallel lines remain parallel (Figure 28-11A).
4. *Size perspective.* If two similar objects appear different in size, the smaller is assumed to be more distant (Figure 28-11A).
5. *Distribution of shadows and illumination.* Patterns of light and dark can give the impression of depth. For example, brighter shades of colors tend to be seen as nearer. In painting this distribution of light and shadow is called *chiaroscuro.*

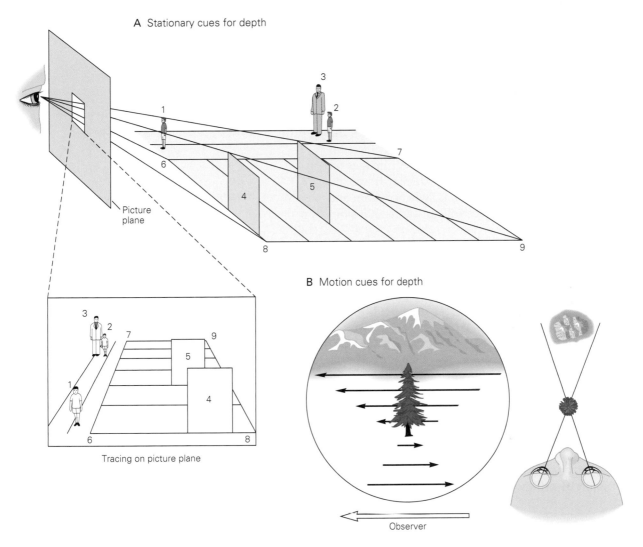

Figure 28-11 Monocular depth cues provide information on the relative distance of objects and have been used by painters since antiquity.

A. The upper drawing shows the side view of a scene. When the scene is traced on a plane of glass held between the eye and the scene (lower drawing) the resulting two-dimensional tracing reveals the cues needed to perceive depth. **Occlusion:** The fact that rectangle 4 interrupts the outline of 5 indicates which object is in front, but not how much distance there is between them. **Linear perspective:** Although lines 6-7 and 8-9 are parallel in reality, they converge in the picture plane. **Size perspective:** Because the two boys are similiar figures, the smaller boy (2) is assumed to be more distant than the larger

boy (1) in the picture plane. **Familiar size:** The man (3) and the nearest boy are drawn to nearly the same size in the picture. If we know that the man is taller than the boy, we deduce on the basis of their sizes in the picture that the man is more distant than the boy. This type of cue is weaker than the others. (Adapted from Hochberg 1968.)

B. Motion of the observer or sideways movement of head and eyes produces depth cues. If the observer moves to the left while looking at the tree, objects closer than the tree move to the right; those farther away move to the left. The full-field motion that results from the observer's own movement is referred to as optic flow. (See Box 28-1.) (Adapted from Busettini et al. 1996).

6. *Motion* (or monocular movement) *parallax.* Perhaps the most important of the monocular cues, this is not a static pictorial cue and therefore does not come to us from the study of painting. As we move our heads or bodies from side to side, the images projected by an object in the visual field move across the retina. Objects closer than the object we are looking at seem to move quickly and in the direction opposite to our own movement, whereas more distant objects move more slowly and in the same direction as our movement (Figure 28-11B).

Stereoscopic Cues Create Near-Field Depth Perception

The perception of depth at distances less than 100 feet also depends on monocular cues but in addition is mediated by stereoscopic vision. Stereoscopic vision is possible because the two eyes are horizontally separated (by about 6 cm in humans) so that each eye views the world from a slightly different position. Thus, objects at different distances produce slightly different images on the two retinas. This can be clearly demonstrated by closing each eye in turn. As vision is switched from one to the other eye, any near object will appear to shift sideways.

Understanding stereopsis begins with an understanding of the simple geometry of the images falling on the retina. When we fixate on a point, the image of this point falls upon corresponding points on the center of the retina in each eye (Figure 28-12). The point of focus is called the *fixation point;* the parallel (vertical) plane of points on which it lies is called the *fixation plane.* The distance of an image from the center of the two eyes allows the visual system to calculate the distance of the object relative to the fixation point. Any point on the object that is nearer or farther than the fixation point will project an image at some distance from the center of the retina. Parts of the object that are closer to us will be farther apart on the two retinas in a horizontal direction. Parts of the object that are farther from us will project closer together on the two retinas.

Clearly, the difference in position, called *binocular disparity,* depends on the distance of the object from the fixation plane. Thus points on a three-dimensional object just outside the fixation plane stimulate different points on each eye, and the multiple disparities provide cues for stereopsis, the perception of solid objects.

Surprisingly, not one of the great early students of optics—Euclid, Archimedes, Leonardo da Vinci, Newton, nor Goethe—understood stereopsis, although each could readily have discovered it with the methods available to them. Stereoscopic vision was not discovered until 1838, when the physicist Charles Wheatstone invented the stereoscope. Two photographs of a scene 60–65 mm apart, one taken from the position of each eye, are mounted into a binocular-like device such that the right eye sees only the picture taken from one position and the left eye sees only the other picture. Remarkably, this presentation produces a three-dimensional scene.

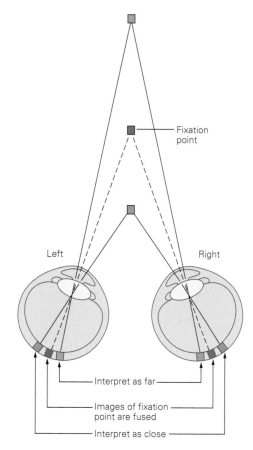

Figure 28-12 When we fix our eyes on a point the convergence of the eyes causes that point (the fixation point) to fall on identical portions of each retina. Cues for depth are provided by points just proximal or distal to the fixation point. These points produce binocular disparity by stimulating slightly different parts of the retina of each eye. When the lack of correspondence is in the horizontal direction only and is not greater than about 0.6 mm or 2° of arc, the disparity is perceived as a single, solid (three-dimensional) spot.

Information From the Two Eyes Is First Combined in the Primary Visual Cortex

How is stereopsis accomplished? Clearly the brain must somehow calculate the disparity between the images seen by the two eyes and then estimate distance based on simple geometric relations. However, this cannot occur before information from the two eyes comes together, and cells in the primary visual cortex (V1) are the first in the visual system to receive input from the two eyes (Chapter 27). Stereopsis, however, requires that the inputs from the two eyes be slightly *different*—there must be a horizontal disparity in the two retinal images (Figure 28-13). The important finding that certain neurons in V1 are actually selective for horizontal disparity was

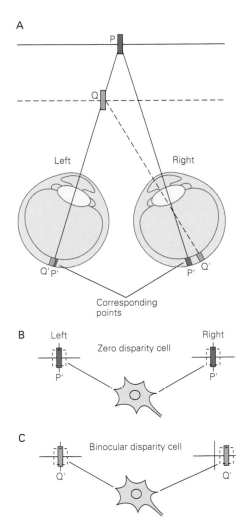

Figure 28-13 Neuronal basis of stereoscopic vision.
(Adapted from Ohzawa et al. 1996.)

A. When an observer looks at point P the image P′ falls on corresponding points on the retina of each eye. These images completely overlap and therefore have zero binocular disparity. When looking at a point to the left and closer, point Q, the image Q′ in the left eye falls on the same point as P′, but the image in the right eye is laterally displaced. These images have binocular disparity.

B. A cortical neuron receiving binocular inputs is maximally activated when the inputs from the two eyes have zero disparity as at P′.

C. Another cortical neuron receiving binocular inputs responds best when the inputs from the two eyes are spatially disparate on the two retinas (Q′); it is most sensitive to near stimuli.

made in 1968 by Horace Barlow, Colin Blakemore, Peter Bishop, and Jack Pettigrew. They found that a neuron that prefers an oriented bar of light at one place in the visual field responds better when that stimulus appears in front of the screen (referred to as a near stimulus)

or when the stimulus is beyond the screen (a far stimulus). There is thus an additional level of organization of information in the ocular dominance columns in V1.

Cells sensitive to binocular disparity are found in several cortical visual areas. In addition to V1, some cells in the extrastriate areas V2 and V3 respond to disparity, and many direction-selective cells in MT respond best to stimuli at specific distances, either at the plane of fixation or nearer or farther than the plane. Some cells in MST, the next step in the parietal pathway, fire in response to combinations of disparity and direction of motion. That is, the direction of motion preferred by the cell varies with the disparity of the stimulus. For example, a cell that responds to leftward-moving far stimuli might also respond to rightward-moving near stimuli. These cells can convey information not only about the direction of motion but about the direction of motion at different depths within the visual field (as in Figure 28-11B).

Studies of cells in the striate and extrastriate cortex that respond selectively to binocular disparity fall into several broad categories. Among these, tuned cells respond best to stimuli at a specific disparity, frequently on the plane of fixation. Other cells respond best to stimuli at a range of disparities either in front of the fixation plane ("near cells") or beyond the plane ("far cells") (Figure 28-14).

Just as the motion information processed in MT is used both for the visual guidance of movement and for visual perception, disparity-sensitive cells in different regions of visual cortex may use disparity information for different purposes. One use is the perception of depth, which we have already considered. Another is in aligning the eyes to focus at a particular depth in the field. The eyes rotate toward each other (convergence) to focus on near objects and rotate apart (divergence) to focus on more distant objects. The ability to align the eyes develops in the first few months of life and disparity information may play a key role in establishing this alignment.

Random Dot Stereograms Separate Stereopsis From Object Vision

Must the brain recognize an object before it can match the corresponding points of the object in the two eyes? Until 1960 this was generally thought to be so, and stereopsis therefore was thought to be a late stage in visual processing. In 1960 Bela Julesz proved that this idea was wrong when he found that stereoscopic fusion and depth perception do not require monocular identification of form. The only clue necessary for stereopsis is retinal disparity.

To demonstrate this remarkable fact, Julesz created a pattern of randomly distributed dots in the middle of which is a square area of dots. He made two copies of

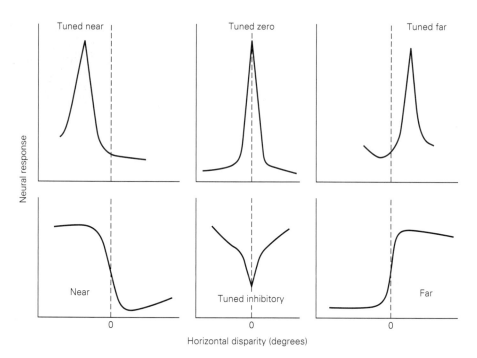

Figure 28-14 Different disparity profiles are found in neurons in cortical visual areas of the monkey. The curves show the responses of six different neurons to bright bars of optimal orientation moving in the preferred direction across the receptive fields at a series of horizontal disparities. These different disparity profiles have been observed in many areas of the monkey visual cortex. The tuned cells are more common in areas V1 and V2, especially in the region of foveal representation, and the "near" and "far" cells are more common in MST. (After Poggio 1995.)

the pattern but in one copy the inner square of dots is positioned slightly differently from the other copy. The inner square of dots is visible only when the identical copies of the pattern are viewed in a stereoscope. If one inner square is displaced so the two squares are closer together, in binocular view the square appears to lie in front of the pattern. If one inner square is shifted so the two squares are further apart, the perceived square appears to lie behind the surrounding dots (Figure 28-15). By itself, each random-dot pattern will not produce any depth clues. Only with stereoscopic vision can one see the square within the pattern. With this method, Julesz demonstrated that humans can detect form based strictly on binocular disparity.

Are there, among the disparity-sensitive neurons in the visual cortex, individual neurons that respond to a stereogram that contains no depth clues except retinal disparity? To answer this question, Gian Poggio first located responsive cells using a bar of light as a stimulus. He then replaced the bar with a random-dot pattern stereogram. Many of the neurons that responded to the solid figure also responded to the random-dot stereogram.

Object Vision Depends on the Ventral Pathway to the Inferior Temporal Lobe

The ventral cortical pathway extends from V1 through V2 to V4 and then to the inferior temporal cortex. We have already noted that V2 has subregions referred to as thick stripes, thin stripes, and interstripes and that the thin and interstripe regions project to V4. As we have indicated, the ventral pathway appears to be concerned with analysis of form and color. Here we will concentrate on the processing of form in V2, V4, and the inferior temporal cortex.

Cells in V2 Respond to Both Illusory and Actual Contours

As in V1, cells in V2 are sensitive to the orientation of stimuli, to their color, and to their horizontal disparity, and they continue the analysis of contour begun by cells in V1. Their response to contours was explored in experiments in which cells were tested for their sensitivity to certain illusory contours of the sort we considered in

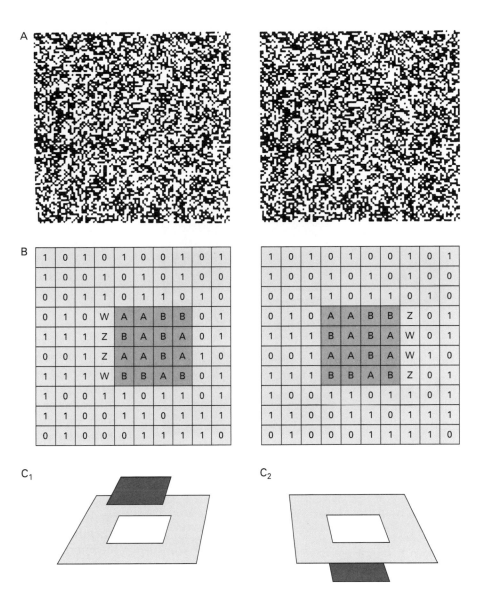

Figure 28-15 Stereopsis does not depend on perception of form.

A. A square form inside these identical random-dot displays cannot be seen by looking at either display alone. It can be seen only when the two identical images are viewed in a stereoscope, or by training the eyes to focus outside the image plane.

B. The square areas in the two random-dot patterns have different positions. The square becomes visible only because of the ocular disparity of the two dot patterns, not because either eye recognizes the form of the square.

C. In the stereoscope the random-dot images are placed behind a rectangular opening. If one inner square of dots is displaced so the left and right inner squares are closer together (**1**), the square is perceived in front of the larger pattern. If the inner squares are shifted so that the two squares are further apart (**2**), the square is perceived behind the larger pattern. (Adapted from Julesz 1971.)

Chapter 25. Many cells in V2 responded to the illusory contours just as they responded to edges (Figure 28-16). In contrast, few cells in V1 responded to the same illusory contours (although other experiments have shown responses of V1 cells to more limited illusory contours). These results suggest that V2 carries out an analysis of contours at a level beyond that of V1, and they are further evidence of the progressive abstraction that occurs in each of the two pathways of the visual system.

Cells in V4 Respond to Form

Initial observations on cells in V4 indicated that the cells were selective for color, and it was thought that they were devoted exclusively to color vision. However, many of these same cells are also sensitive to the orientation of bars of light and are more responsive to finer-grained than to coarse-grained stimuli. Thus, some V4 cells are responsive to combinations of color and form.

Does removal of V4 alter a monkey's responses to color more than to form? Experiments show that ablation of V4 impairs a monkey's ability to discriminate patterns and shapes but only minimally affects its ability to distinguish colors with different hues and saturation. In other experiments ablation of V4 altered only subtle color discriminations, such as the ability to identify colors under different illumination conditions (*color constancy*).

We have noted that some humans lose color vision (achromatopsia) after localized damage to the ventral occipital cortex. PET scans of normal human subjects re-

A

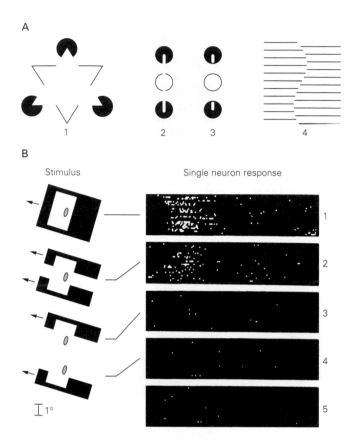

B

Stimulus   Single neuron response

I 1°

Figure 28-16 Illusions of edges used to study the higher level information processing in V2 cells of the monkey.

A. Examples of illusory contours. **1.** A white triangle is clearly seen, although it is not defined in the picture by a continuous border. **2.** A vertical bar is seen, although again there is no continuous border. **3.** Slight alterations obliterate the perception of the bar seen in 2. **4.** The curved contour is not represented by any edges or lines. (From Von der Heydt et al. 1984.)

B. A neuron in V2 responds to illusory contours. The cell's receptive field is represented by an ellipse in the drawings on the left. **1.** A cell responds to a bar of light moving across its receptive field. Each dot in the record on the right indicates a cell discharge and successive lines indicate the cell's response to successive movements of the bar. **2.** The neuron also responds when an illusory contour passes over its receptive field. **3, 4.** When only half of the stimulus moves across the cell's receptive field, the response resembles spontaneous activity (**5**). (Adapted from Von der Heydt et al. 1984.)

veal an increase in activity in the lingual and fusiform gyri when colored stimuli are presented (see Figure 28-5). The deficits in patients with achromatopsia differ from those in monkeys with lesions of V4. The human patients cannot discriminate hues but can discriminate shape and texture, whereas the monkeys' ability to differentiate shapes is markedly diminished while hue discrimination is only minimally affected. It therefore seems unlikely that the area identified in the human brain is directly comparable to the V4 region in the monkey, but instead includes more extended regions, including the inferior temporal cortex, the area we consider next.

Recognition of Faces and Other Complex Forms Depends Upon the Inferior Temporal Cortex

We are capable of recognizing and remembering an almost infinite variety of shapes independent of their size or position on the retina. Clinical work in humans and experimental studies in monkeys suggest that form recognition is closely related to processes that occur in the inferior temporal cortex.

The response properties of cells in the inferior temporal cortex are those we might expect from an area involved in a later stage of pattern recognition. For example, the receptive field of virtually every cell includes the foveal region, where fine discriminations are made. Unlike cells in the striate cortex and many other extrastriate visual areas, the cells in the inferior temporal area do not have a clear retinotopic organization, and the receptive fields are very large and occasionally may include the entire visual field (both visual hemifields). Such large fields may be related to *position invariance*, the ability to recognize the same feature anywhere in the visual field. For example, even a small eye movement can easily move an edge stimulus from the receptive field of one V1 neuron to another. In contrast, such a movement would simply move the edge within the receptive field of one inferior temporal neuron. The larger receptive field of many extrastriate regions, including the inferior temporal, may be important in the ability to recognize the same object regardless of its location.

The most prominent visual input to the inferior temporal cortex is from V4, so it would not be surprising to see a continuation of the visual processing observed in V4. Inferior temporal cortex appears to have functional subregions and, like V4, may have separate pathways to these regions. Also like V4, inferior temporal cells are sensitive to both shape and color. Many cells in inferior temporal cortex respond to a variety of shapes and colors, although the strength of the response varies for different combinations of shape and color (Figure 28-17). Other cells are selective only for shape or color.

Most interesting is the finding that some inferotemporal cells respond only to specific types of complex stimuli, such as the hand or face. For cells that respond to a hand, the individual fingers are a particularly critical visual feature; these cells do not respond when there are no spaces separating the fingers. However, all orientations of the hand elicit similar responses. Among

Figure 28-17 Many inferior temporal neurons respond both to form and color.

A. Average responses for a single neuron to stimuli with different shapes. The height of each bar indicates the average discharge rate during presentation of the stimulus. The **dashed line** indicates the background discharge rate.

B. Responses of the same neuron to colored stimuli. Discharge rates are indicated by the size of each circle. The **open circle** represents a discharge rate of 30 spikes/s. The responses are plotted on a color map with the relative location of colors, red, green, and blue given for reference. The axes are relative amounts of primary colors. (Adapted from Komatsu and Ideura 1993.)

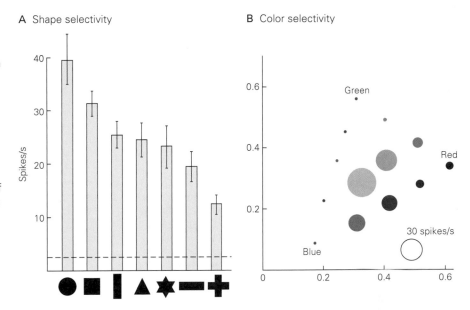

A Shape selectivity

B Color selectivity

neurons selective for faces, the frontal view of the face is the most effective stimulus for some, while for others it is the side view. Moreover, whereas some neurons respond preferentially to faces, others respond preferentially to specific facial expressions. Although the proportion of cells in the inferior temporal cortex responsive to hands or faces is small, their existence, together with the fact that lesions of this region lead to specific deficits in face recognition (Chapter 25), indicates that the inferior temporal cortex is responsible for face recognition.

One of the major issues in understanding the brain's analysis of complex objects is the degree to which individual cells respond to the simpler components of these objects. Certain critical elements of faces are sufficient to activate some inferior temporal neurons. For example, instead of a face, two dots and a line appropriately positioned might activate the cell (Figure 28-18). Other experiments suggest that some cells respond to facial dimensions (distance between the eyes) and others to the familiarity of the face. There is also evidence that cells responding to similar features are organized in columns.

Visual Attention Facilitates Coordination Between Separate Visual Pathways

The limited capacity of the visual system means that at any given time only a fraction of the information available from the visual scene falling on the two retinas can be processed. Thus some information is used to produce perception and movement while other information is lost or discarded. This selective filtering of visual information is achieved by visual attention. As may be appreciated from the evidence presented in this and earlier chapters, understanding the neuronal mechanisms of attention and conscious awareness is one of the great unresolved problems in perception. Can we resolve these mechanisms and understand their contribution to behavior? How does attention alter the processing of visual information?

Investigation of spatial attention at the neuronal level began in the 1970s with exploration of the cellular basis of visual attention in the superior colliculus, the striate cortex (V1), and the posterior parietal cortex of awake primates (see Figure 20-15). Michael Goldberg and Robert Wurtz examined the response of cells to a spot of light under two conditions: (1) when the monkey looked elsewhere and did not attend to the location of the spot, and (2) when the animal was required to fix its gaze on the spot of light by making rapid or saccadic eye movements to the spot. When the animal attended to the spot, cells in the superior colliculus responded more intensely, while the response of cells in V1 showed little modulation. However, the enhanced response of the cells in the superior colliculus did not result from selective attention per se but was dependent upon the initiation of eye movement. In similar tests of the responsiveness of cells in the posterior parietal cortex, a region known from clinical studies to be involved in attention (Chapter 20), the cells' responses were enhanced whether the monkey made an eye movement to the visual target or reached for it (Box 28-2).

The effects of attention on cells in V4 and inferior temporal cortex were next determined by Robert

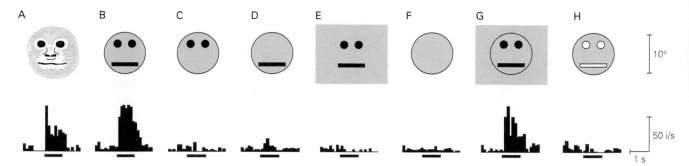

Figure 28-18 Response of a neuron in the inferior temporal cortex to complex stimuli. The cell responds strongly to the face of a toy monkey (**A**). The critical features producing the response are revealed in a configuration of two black spots and one horizontal black bar arranged on a gray disk (**B**). The bar, spots, and circular outline together were essential, as can be seen by the cell's responses to images missing one or more of these features (**C, D, E, F**). The contrast between the inside and outside of the circular contour was not critical (**G**). However, the spots and bar had to be darker than the background within the outline (**H**). (i = spikes.) (Modified from Kobatake and Tanaka 1994.)

Desimone and his colleagues by presenting two stimuli, both falling in the receptive field of one cell. The experimenters found that they could turn a neuron on or off depending on whether they required the monkey to attend to one of the stimuli. The stimulus remained the same between trials; only the monkey's attention shifted.

Since attention is the selection of one stimulus from among many, it would be reasonable to expect that the effect of attention on cell responsiveness would increase with the number of stimuli presented. In one experiment a monkey was required to focus attention on one stimulus in a group of six to eight identical stimuli. The responses of one-third of the neurons in V4 were altered when the monkey's attention shifted to one stimulus. Activity in most of these same neurons was not altered as much when the monkey had to choose from only two identical stimuli. Furthermore, increasing the number of stimuli also enhanced the responses of neurons in earlier stages of the visual pathways, in V2 and V1. As the demands for selection among visual targets increases, so does the relative effect of attention.

Changes in cellular activity also occur when the focus of attention is a specific object rather than a location. In one set of experiments a monkey was cued to select an object, or the color or shape of an object, and then required to select a similar object from among a set of objects presented either simultaneously or in series. Remarkably, presentation of the matching object can have a greater effect on a neuron's response than the sample stimulus that is present. In one of these experiments the cells in V4 responded more vigorously when the color of the matching object was the same as the cue (Figure 28-19). During the search for matching stimuli the activity of neurons in the ventral pathway and inferior temporal cortex is modified. In the dorsal pathway the activity of cells in area 7A, MST, and MT is also modified, particularly when multiple stimuli fall within the receptive field of a cell.

The Binding Problem in the Visual System

We have seen that information about motion, depth, form, and color is processed in many different visual areas and organized into at least two cortical pathways. How can such distributed processing lead to cohesive perceptions? When we see a red ball we combine into one perception the sensations of color (red), form (round), and solidity (ball). We can equally well combine red with a square box, a pot, or a shirt. The possible combination of elements is so great that the existence of an individual feature-detecting cell for each set of combinations is improbable.

Instead, as we have seen in this chapter, the evidence is strongly in favor of a constructive process by which complex visual images are built up at successively higher processing centers. Is there a "final common pathway" where all the elements of a complex percept are brought together? Or do the distributed afferent pathways interact in some continuous fashion to produce coherent percepts? There is as yet no satisfactory solution to the *binding problem,* the problem of how consciousness of an ongoing, coherent experience emerges from the information processing being conducted independently in different cortical areas.

As described in Chapter 25, Anne Treisman and Bela Julesz independently showed that the associative process by which multiple features of one object are

Box 28-2 Parietal Cortex and Movement

The dorsal visual path extends to the posterior parietal cortex, which, based on clinical observations of patients with parietal damage, is known to be involved in the representation of the visual world and the planning of movement. Recent studies of neurons in the parietal cortex of monkeys have revealed several functionally distinct areas, which may account for the varied deficits following damage to the parietal cortex. The activity in most of these areas is related to the transition from sensory processing to the generation of movement.

Neurons in one of these subregions, the lateral intraparietal area, fire in connection with saccadic eye movements (Chapter 39). These neurons fire in response to a visual target, before a saccade to the target, and increase their activity just before the beginning of the saccade, indicating that the activity in these neurons is related both to the visual input and to the motor output of the brain. Between the sensory and motor events, continuing activity in these neurons depends on the condition under which the saccade is made, such as whether the saccade is made to a visual stimulus or the location of a remembered stimulus. Thus, although activity in these neurons is closely associated with the transition from sensory perception to motor movement, it is not exclusively related to one or the other.

These neurons also clearly receive information more complex than either pure sensory and pure motor information. Many neurons respond differently to the same visual stimulus, depending upon where in space the eyes and head are oriented, indicating that they receive input about eye position as well as the visual stimulus. Such neurons might be involved in shifting the frame of reference in which sensory information is processed (from eye to head to body; see Box 25-1) a shift that is necessary to control movements such as reaching. We therefore have strong evidence that parietal neurons are involved in putting visual information in the service of the motor systems and for compensating for the disruption to vision that results from such movement.

---

brought together in a coherent percept requires attention. They suggested that different properties are encoded in different feature maps during a preattentive stage of perception and that attention selects specific features in these different maps and ties them together (as illustrated in Figure 25-15).

A related view of the effect of attention on the binding problem recently was advanced by John Reynolds and Robert Desimone. They based their interpretation on two observations already described in this chapter: neurons have larger and larger receptive fields at higher levels in the cortical visual pathways and attention to one of several stimuli falling in one of these large receptive fields increases the response to that stimulus. They assume that attention acts to increase the competitive advantage of the attended stimulus so that the effect of attention is to shrink the effective size of the field around the attended stimulus. Now instead of many stimuli with different characteristics such as color and form, only the one stimulus is functionally present in the receptive field. Because the effective receptive field now just includes that one stimulus, all the characteristics of the stimulus are effectively bound together.

Another approach to the binding problem has been emphasized by Charles Gray and Wolfgang Singer and Reinhold Eckhorn and their colleagues. They found that when an object activates a population of neurons in the visual cortex, the neurons tend to oscillate and fire in unison. They suggest that these oscillations are indicative of a synchrony among cells and that this synchrony of firing would bind together the activity of cells responding to different features of the same object. To combine the visual features (color, form, motion) of the same object, the synchrony between neurons would, according to this view, extend across neurons in different cortical areas.

Quite a different solution to the binding problem was proposed by Lance Optican, Barry Richmond, and their colleagues. They found that neurons extending from the lateral geniculate nucleus to the inferior temporal cortex convey more information if the temporal pattern of their discharge is considered. Instead of measuring the total number of spikes in a time period, they measured the distribution of the spikes in that time period and found that different stimulus features (eg, form, contrast, color) tended to be represented by different response patterns of the same cell. They propose that the pattern of discharge in each cell carries information about different features so that the problem of binding across cells, each representing a different feature, is eliminated. Cells in different areas would all convey some information about a number of stimulus features, but different cells would carry comparatively more or less about each feature.

Thus, while several solutions to the binding problem have been proposed, it still remains one of the central unsolved puzzles in our understanding of the neurobiological bases of perception.

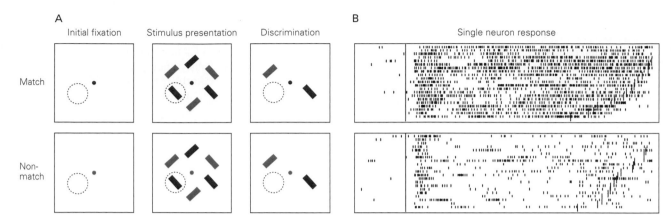

Figure 28-19 The response of V4 neurons to an effective visual stimulus is modified by selective attention.

A. A monkey was trained to shift its attention to one set of stimuli as opposed to another. At the start of each trial (**initial fixation**) the monkey was trained to look at a fixation point on a screen (the dot in the square). At this point in the experiment the receptive field of a V4 cell has been located (**dotted circle**). On any given trial the fixation point was either red (**upper row**) or green (**bottom row**). Then six other stimuli came on, one of which fell into the receptive field of the cell (**stimulus presentation**). The monkey knew from prior training that it would be required to discriminate only those stimuli that were the same color as the fixation point—the three red stimuli in the top row or the three green in the bottom row. The assumption in the experiment is that this requires the monkey to attend to the appropriate three stimuli. If one of those stimuli is in the receptive field of the cell, as in the match trials (top row), the monkey presumably is paying attention to that stimulus in the receptive field. If those stimuli with the same color as the fixation point

lie outside the receptive field, as in the nonmatch trials (bottom row), the monkey presumably is attending to the stimuli outside the receptive field. The responses of the V4 neuron to these match and nonmatch trials were compared. Note that the stimulus falling on the receptive field of the cell is the same in the match and nonmatch trials, only its significance for the monkey has changed. In the last phase of a trial (**discrimination**) only two stimuli remain on, and the monkey, in order to obtain a reward, must indicate whether the matched stimulus is tilted to the right or to the left.

B. Increased response to the same visual stimulus falling on the receptive field of a V4 cell during the match (upper record) as opposed to the nonmatch (lower record) trials. Each line represents a successive trial, and each dot indicates the discharge of the neuron. The vertical tick marks indicate the monkey's behavioral response. While the match and nonmatch trials are shown separately, they were interleaved during the experiment. (After Motter 1994.)

An Overall View

Much like the somatic sensory system the visual system consists of several parallel pathways not a single serial pathway. The M and P pathways pass from the retina, through the parvocellular and magnocellular layers of the lateral geniculate nucleus, to layer 4C of the primary visual cortex (V1), where they feed into parallel pathways extending through the cerebral cortex. A dorsal pathway extends from V1, through areas MT and MST, to the posterior parietal cortex. A ventral pathway extends from V1, through V4, to the inferior temporal cortex. The parietal pathway appears to be dominated by the M input, but the inferior temporal pathway depends upon both the P and the M input.

Several factors lead to the conclusion that these pathways serve different functions much as do the submodalities for somaesthesis: The anatomical connections along these two pathways, differences in neuronal activity, the behavioral deficits occurring after damage

to the terminal areas of the pathways in both humans and monkeys, and the activity detected in the human brain during tasks that should differentially activate the two pathways. One view is that the dorsal or posterior parietal pathway is concerned with determining where an object is, whereas the ventral or inferior temporal pathway is involved in recognizing what the object is. Another view is that the dorsal pathway leads to action, the ventral to perception. But all agree that the function of the two pathways is different.

We have concentrated on the neuronal mechanisms mediating motion and depth information in the dorsal posterior parietal pathway and on form perception in the ventral inferior temporal pathway. Both pathways represent hierarchies for visual processing that lead to greater abstraction at successive levels. Neurons in MT respond to the motion of a patterned stimulus, whereas cells in V1 respond only to motion of the elements of a pattern. Neurons in inferior temporal cortex respond to a given shape at any position in large areas of the visual field, whereas simple cells in V1 respond only when an edge is positioned at one location in the field. In addition, cellular responses along the pathways tend to become increasingly dependent on the stimulus characteristic selected for attention. The effect of the remembered object in a visual search can have more effect on the response of neurons in V4 and the inferior temporal cortex than the stimulus that is present.

While we have considered separately the visual processing for motion, depth, and form, these parallel pathways may not be mutually exclusive pathways. Some processing combines the activity of the pathways. For example, form can be seen when the only cue is the coherent motion of components of the scene (which is regarded as the purview of the parietal pathway). Likewise, some MT cells respond to the motion of an edge defined only by color (a property that should be conveyed by the inferior temporal pathway). Thus, at both a perceptual and a physiological level, cross talk between the posterior parietal and inferior temporal pathways must occur as is also indicated by the anatomical evidence for cross connections.

We know the outline of the steps the brain takes in constructing complex visual images from the pattern of light and dark falling on the retina—the early processing along the M and P pathways and the later, more abstract processing in the dorsal posterior parietal and ventral inferior temporal pathways. But these steps remain only an outline. Many cortical areas must still be explored, and critical details of visual processing are only beginning to be understood.

Robert H. Wurtz
Eric R. Kandel

Selected Readings

Andersen RA, Snyder LH, Bradley DC, Xing J. 1997. Multiple representations of space in the posterior parietal cortex and its use in planning movement. Ann Rev Neurosci 20:303–330.

Felleman DJ, Van Essen DC. 1991. Distributed hierarchical processing in primate cerebral cortex. Cereb Cortex 1:1–47.

Ferrera VP, Nealey TA, Maunsell JH. 1994. Responses in macaque visual area V4 following inactivation of the parvocellular and magnocellular LGN pathways. J Neurosci 14:2080–2088.

Hubel DH. 1988. *Eye, Brain, and Vision*. New York: Scientific American Library.

Julesz B. 1971. *Foundations of Cyclopean Perception*. Chicago: University of Chicago Press.

Livingstone MS, Hubel DH. 1987. Psychophysical evidence for separate channels for the perception of form, color, movement, and depth. J Neurosci 7:3416–3468.

Maunsell JH, Newsome WT. 1987. Visual processing in monkey extrastriate cortex. Annu Rev Neurosci 10:363–401.

Merigan WH, Maunsell JH. 1993. How parallel are the primate visual pathways? Annu Rev Neurosci 16:369–402.

Miyashita Y. 1993. Inferior temporal cortex: where visual perception meets memory. Annu Rev Neurosci 16:245–263.

Poggio GF. 1995. Mechanisms of stereopsis in monkey visual cortex. Cereb Cortex 3:193–204.

Salzman CD, Britten KH, Newsome WT. 1990. Cortical microstimulation influences perceptual judgements of motion direction. Nature 346:174–177.

Singer W, Gray CM. 1995. Visual feature integration and the temporal correlation hypothesis. Annu Rev Neurosci 18:555–586.

Stoner GR, Albright TD. 1993. Image segmentation cues in motion processing: implications for modularity in vision. J Cogn Neurosci 5:129–149.

Tanaka K. 1996. Inferotemporal cortex and object vision. Annu Rev Neurosci 19:109–139.

References

Albright TD, Desimone R, Gross CG. 1984. Columnar organization of directionally selective cells in visual area MT of the macaque. J Neurophysiol 51:16–31.

Baizer JS, Ungerleider LG, Desimone R. 1991. Organization of visual inputs to the inferior temporal and posterior parietal cortex in macaques. J Neurosci 11:168–190.

Baker CL, Hess RF, Zihl J. 1991. Residual motion perception in a "motion-blind" patient, assessed with limited-lifetime random dot stimuli. J Neurosci 11:454–461.

Barlow HB, Blakemore C, Pettigrew JD. 1967. The neural mechanism of binocular depth discrimination. J Physiol (Lond) 193:327–342.

Brewster D. 1856. *The Stereoscope, Its History, Theory and Construction*. London: John Murray.

Bishop PO, Pettigrew JD. 1986. Neural mechanisms of binocular vision. Vision Res 26:1587–1600.

Britten KH, Shadlen MN, Newsome WT, Movshon JA. 1992. The analysis of visual motion: a comparison of neuronal and psychophysical performance. J Neurosci 12:4745–4765.

Busettini C, Masson GS, Miles FA. 1996. A role for stereoscopic depth cues in the rapid visual stabilization of the eyes. Nature 380:342–345.

Desimone R, Wessinger M, Thomas L, Schneider W. 1990. Attentional control of visual perception: cortical and subcortical mechanisms. Cold Spring Harbor Symp Quant Biol 55:963–971.

DeYoe EA, Felleman DJ, Van Essen DC, McClendon E. 1994. Multiple processing streams in occipitotemporal visual cortex. Nature 371:151–154.

Duffy CJ, Wurtz RH. 1995. Response of monkey MST neurons to optic flow stimuli with shifted centers of motion. J Neurosci 15:5192–5208.

Duhamel J-R, Colby CL, Golberg ME. 1992. The updating of the represention of visual space in parietal cortex by intended eye movements. Science 255:90–92.

Dürsteler MR, Wurtz RH, Newsome WT. 1987. Directional pursuit deficit following lesions of the foveal representation within the superior temporal sulcus of the macaque monkey. J Neurophysiol 57:1262–1287.

Eckhorn R, Bauer R, Jordan W, Brosch M, Kruse W, Munk M, Reitboeck HJ. 1988. Coherent oscillations: a mechanism for feature linking in the visual cortex. Biol Cybern 60:121–130.

Escher MC. 1971. *The Graphic Work of M. C. Escher.* New rev. and exp. ed. New York: Ballantine Books.

Fox JC, Holmes G. 1926. Optic nystagmus and its value in the localization of cerebral lesions. Brain 49:333–371.

Gibson JJ. 1950. *The Perception of the Visual World.* Boston: Houghton Mifflin.

Graziano M, Andersen R, Snowden R. 1994. Tuning of MST neurons to spiral motions. J Neurosci 14:54–56.

Haenny PE, Maunsell JH, Schiller PH. 1988. State dependent activity in monkey visual cortex II. Retinal and extraretinal factors in V4. Exp Brain Res 69:245–259.

Hasselmo ME, Rolls ET, Baylis GC. 1989. The role of expression and identity in face-selective response of neurons in the temporal visual cortex of the monkey. Behav Brain Res 32:203–218.

Heywood CA, Cowey A, Newcombe F. 1994. On the role of parvocellular (P) and magnocellular (M) pathways in cerebral achromatopsia. Brain 117:245–254.

Heywood CA, Gadotti A, Cowey A. 1992. Cortical area V4 and its role in the perception of color. J Neurosci 12:4056–4065.

Hochberg JE. 1978. *Perception,* 2nd ed. Englewood Cliffs, NJ: Prentice-Hall.

Horton JC. 1984. Cytochrome oxidase patches: a new cytoarchitectonic feature of monkey visual cortex. Philos Trans R Soc Lond B 304:199–253.

Julesz B. 1986. Stereoscopic vision. Vision Res 26:1601–1612.

Kobatake E, Tanaka K. 1994. Neuronal selectivities to complex object features in the ventral visual pathway of the macaque cerebral cortex. J Neurophys 71:856–867.

Komatsu H, Ideura Y. 1993. Relationships between color, shape, and pattern selectivities of neurons in the inferior temporal cortex of the monkey. J Neurophysiol 70:677–694.

Lueschow A, Miller EK, Desimone R. 1994. Inferior temporal mechanisms for invariant object recognition. Cereb Cortex 4:523–531.

Malpeli JG, Schiller PH, Colby CL. 1981. Response properties of single cells in monkey striate cortex during reversible inactivation of individual lateral geniculate laminae. J Neurophysiol 46:1102–1119.

Maunsell JH, Nealey TA, DePriest DD. 1990. Magnocellular and parvocellular contributions to responses in the middle temporal visual area (MT) of the macaque monkey. J Neurosci 10:3323–3334.

Maunsell JH, Sclar G, Nealey TA, DePriest DD. 1991. Extraretinal representations in area V4 in the macaque monkey. Vis Neurosci 7:561–573.

McClurkin JW, Zarbock JA, Optican LM. 1994. Temporal codes for colors, patterns, and memories. In: A Peters, KS Rockland (eds). *Cerebral Cortex.* Vol. 10, *Primary Visual Cortex in Primates,* pp. 443–467. New York: Plenum.

Moran J, Desimone R. 1985. Selective attention gates visual processing in the extra striate cortex. Science 229:782–784.

Morrow MJ, Sharpe JA. 1993. Retinotopic and directional deficits of smooth pursuit initiation after posterior cerebral hemispheric lesions. Neurology 43:595–603.

Motter BC. 1993. Focal attention produces spatially selective processing in visual cortical areas V1, V2, and V4 in the presence of competing stimuli. J Neurophys 70:909–919.

Motter BC. 1994. Neural correlates of attentive selection for color or luminance in extrastriate area V4. J Neurosci 14:2178–2189.

Movshon JA. 1990. Visual processing of moving images. In: H Barlow, C Blakemore, M Weston-Smith (eds). *Images and Understanding: Thoughts About Images; Ideas About Understanding,* pp. 122–137. New York: Cambridge Univ. Press.

Movshon JA, Adelson EH, Gizzi MS, Newsome WT. 1985. The analysis of moving visual patterns. In: C Chagas, R Gattass, C Gross (eds). *Pattern Recognition Mechanisms,* pp. 117–151. New York: Springer-Verlag.

Nealey TA, Maunsell JH. 1994. Magnocellular and parvocellular contributions to the responses of neurons in macaque striate cortex. J Neurosci 14:2069–2079.

Newsome WT, Pare EB. 1988. A selective impairment of motion perception following lesions of the middle temporal visual area (MT). J Neurosci 8:2201–2211.

Ohzawa I, DeAngelis GC, Freeman RD. 1996. Encoding of binocular disparity by simple cells in the cat's visual cortex. J Neurophysiol 75:1779–1805.

Optican LM, Richmond BJ. 1987. Temporal encoding of two-dimensional patterns by single units in primate inferior temporal cortex. III. Information theoretic analysis. J Neurophysiol 57:162–178.

Perrett DI, Mistlin AJ, Chitty AJ. 1987. Visual neurones responsive to faces. Trends Neurosci 10:358–364.

Poggio GF. 1989. Neural responses serving stereopsis in the visual cortex of the alert macaque monkey: position-disparity and image-correlation. In: JS Lund (ed). *Sensory Processing in the Mammalian Brain: Neural Substrates and Experimental Strategies,* pp. 226–241. New York: Oxford Univ. Press.

Reynolds JH, Desimone R. 1999. The role of neural mechanisms of attention in solving the binding problem. Neuron: In press.

Roy J-P, Komatsu H, Wurtz RH. 1992. Disparity sensitivity of neurons in monkey extrastriate area MST. J Neurosci 12:2478–2492.

Salzman CD, Murasugi CM, Britten KH, Newsome WT. 1992. Microstimulation in visual area MT: effects on direction discrimination performance. J Neurosci 12:2331–2355.

Salzman CD, Newsome WT. 1994. Neural mechanisms for forming a perceptual decision. Science 264:231–237.

Tootell RB, Hamilton SL. 1989. Functional anatomy of the second visual area (V2) in the macaque. J Neurosci 9:2620–2644.

Treisman A. 1986. Features and objects in visual processing. Sci Am 255(5):114B–125.

Treue S, Maunsell JH. 1996. Attentional modulation of visual motion processing in cortical areas MT and MST. Nature 382:539–541.

Ullman S. 1986. Artificial intelligence and the brain: computational studies of the visual system. Annu Rev Neurosci 9:1–26.

Von der Heydt R, Peterhans E. 1989. Mechanisms of contour perception in monkey visual cortex. I. Lines of pattern discontinuity. J Neurosci 9:1731–1748.

Von der Heydt R, Peterhans E, Baumgartner G. 1984. Illusory contours and cortical neuron responses. Science 224:1260–1262.

Wong-Riley MTT, Carrol EW. 1984. Quantitative light and electron microscopic analysis of cytochrome oxidase-rich zones in VII prestriate cortex of the squirrel monkey. J Comp Neurol 222:18–37.

Wurtz RH, Goldberg ME, Robinson DL. 1982. Brain mechanisms of visual attention. Sci Am 246(6):124–135.

Yoshioka AT, Levitt JB, Lund JS. 1994. Independence and merger of thalamocortical channels within macaque monkey primary visual cortex: anatomy of interlaminar projections. Vis Neurosci 11:467–489.

Zeki SM. 1976. The functional organization of projections from striate to prestriate visual cortex in the rhesus monkey. Cold Spring Harbor Symp Quant Biol 40:591–600.

Zeki S, Shipp S. 1988. The functional logic of cortical connections. Nature 355:311–317.

Zeki S, Watson JD, Lueck CJ, Friston KJ, Kennard C, Frackowiak RS. 1991. A direct demonstration of functional specialization in human visual cortex. J Neurosci 11:641–649.

Zihl J, von Cramon D, Mai N, Schmid C. 1991. Disturbance of movement vision after bilateral posterior brain damage. Further evidence and follow-up observations. Brain 114:2235–2252.

29

Color Vision

COLOR ENRICHES OUR VISUAL experience and enables us to discern objects and patterns that would otherwise not be seen. To appreciate this enrichment we need only compare a color photograph with a black-and-white photograph of the same scene (Figure 29-1). In a black-and-white image, details are represented by differences in light and dark. The details are easily made out, but the image lacks the overall richness and structure of a full-color image.

Color vision adds something distinctive and important to simple brightness perception, which we considered in Chapters 26 and 27. Nevertheless, color vision is a poor substitute for brightness vision. We can appreciate this by considering a picture in which variations in brightness have been eliminated, leaving only variations in color (Figure 29-1C). Here the objects are poorly defined and the structure of the scene is obscure. To make sense of variations in color we need information about variations in brightness, and to understand color vision we need to consider it in the broader context of perceiving objects.

Color is a subjective experience tied to the spectral composition of the light reaching the eye. Light visible to the human eye occupies a small part of the electromagnetic spectrum, spanning wavelengths between about 400 nm and 700 nm. (The eye is much more sensitive in the middle of this range than at its limits, so lights of very short wavelength or very long wavelength appear dim.) Light of a single wavelength has a characteristic color (Figure 29-2); mixtures of lights of different wavelengths are seen as a rich range of colors. For example, purple results from mixing short and long wavelengths; white results when all wavelengths are mixed.

But the color of an object does not depend strictly on the spectral composition of the light in its retinal image. The context is important, so an object's appearance might change simply because of a change in the spectral composition of the background against which it is seen. Figure 29-3 demonstrates this. At the same time, an object may retain its color despite large variations in the composition of the light it reflects. For example, a lemon seems yellow whether viewed in sunlight (which is whitish), under the light of a tungsten filament bulb (which is reddish), or by fluorescent (bluish) light.

In this chapter we first describe how light is reflected from surfaces and how the visual system ana-

A Full color image

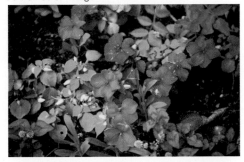

B Black and white only

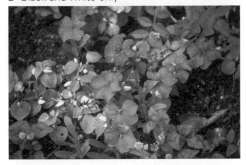

C Color only

Figure 29-1 Color vision enriches visual perception but alone it is a poor detector of spatial detail. (Images courtesy of K. R. Gegenfurtner.)

A. A normal full-color image contains information about variations in brightness and color.

B. An achromatic image captures brightness variations in the scene and is formed by weighting the energy of the reflected light by the overall spectral sensitivity of the eye. Spatial detail is easily discerned in this kind of image.

C. A purely chromatic image contains no information about variations in brightness in the scene; rather it contains only information about hue and saturation. Spatial detail is hard to discern.

lyzes the spectral composition of this light using three different cone systems. We then examine how the nervous system processes this information in the retina and the visual cortex.

Color Vision Captures Properties of Surfaces

Most of the color we see comes from light reflected by the surfaces of objects. Surfaces reflect light in several ways: for example, the shiny skin of an apple contains a pigment that gives it a distinctive reddish or greenish color. It also displays bright highlights that reveal the color of the light falling on it. These highlights, or *specular reflections,* depend on the smoothness of the surface and, although characteristic of some objects, are usually less distinctive than the reflection from surface pigmentation. It is the latter type of reflection we shall be concerned with here.

Surfaces can differ in the *proportion* of incident light they reflect (dark ones reflect less than light ones) and in the *spectral composition* of the light they reflect. These properties can be described by a *reflectance function,* which specifies the fraction of the incident light the surface reflects at each wavelength (Figure 29-4). The reflectance function is a stable and distinctive attribute—it does not change with the spectral composition or the intensity of the light falling on the surface—and can provide a physical signature of an object. To distinguish surfaces reliably, the visual system must distinguish their reflectance functions.

To capture the reflectance function is not a trivial task, as we shall see, and it is potentially greatly complicated by the circumstances under which we normally view objects. The information available to us about the surface reflectance function is contained in the spectral distribution of the light the surface reflects, but that spectral distribution depends on both the surface reflectance function and the spectral distribution of energy in the light that illuminates the surface. Figure 29-5 illustrates just how troublesome this problem might be. Nevertheless, the visual system manages this complexity so well that we are often unaware of large variations in the composition of the light reflected by an object under different conditions of illumination—the color of the object appears constant.

Color Vision Requires at Least Two Types of Photoreceptors With Different Spectral Sensitivities

Color vision depends on the cone photoreceptors. Each cone contains retinal, a photosensitive pigment that, like rhodopsin in rods, is composed of the protein opsin and the light-sensitive compound 11-*cis* retinal.

Light absorption triggers the isomerization of the light-absorbing portion of retinal from the 11-*cis* to the all-*trans* form (see Chapter 26). This results ultimately in

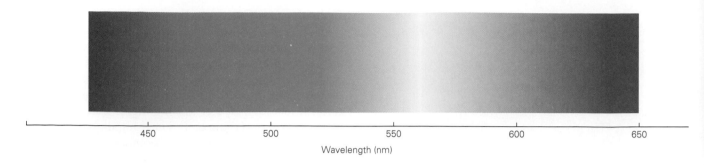

Figure 29-2 The visible spectrum. This is a small part of the electromagnetic spectrum, spanning wavelengths between about 400 and 700 nm. Lights of different wavelengths have characteristic colors. Light drawn from a narrow band of wavelengths is called *monochromatic*. Monochromatic lights are rarely seen in nature.

Figure 29-3 Context influences the appearance of color. The crosses in the two parts of the figure are printed in the same ink (confirm this by looking at where they are joined at the left, yet they look different because they are surrounded by different backgrounds. The perceived color in the cross tends toward the complement of the background color. (From Albers 1975.)

a hyperpolarization of the cell membrane. The absorption of a photon always results in the same electrical response, whatever the wavelength of the photon, so individual cones do not transmit information about the wavelength of a light stimulus. Cones do, however, respond preferentially to particular wavelengths: What varies with wavelength is not the form of the electrical response but the *probability* that a photon will be absorbed.

The nervous system cannot determine from the response of a particular cone whether the cone is illuminated with a weak light at a wavelength to which it is sensitive or a more intense light at a wavelength to which it is less sensitive, or even a combination of lights of several wavelengths. If we had only one type of cone (as some rare individuals do), we would not be able to experience color. Color vision therefore requires at least two sets of photoreceptors with different spectral sensitivities.

A two-receptor, or *dichromatic*, system would generate two different signals for each wavelength. By comparing the two signals the brain could distinguish lights of different wavelengths. For example, if an object reflected primarily long-wavelength light, the response of the cone system sensitive to longer wavelengths would be stronger than the response of the other system, and higher processing centers would interpret the object as being red or yellow. If the object reflected primarily shorter wavelengths, it would evoke a stronger response in the short-wavelength system and the object would be seen as blue. Objects that reflect all wavelengths equally are perceived as colorless (black, gray, or white, depending on the brightness of the background against which they are seen).

A two-cone system will never confuse light of one wavelength with light of any other single wavelength. However, the light reflected from real surfaces in the world rarely contains just one wavelength; rather, it is usually characterized by a continuous distribution of wavelengths (Figure 29-4). A dichromatic visual system must represent this mixture with just two signals that arise from the photon catches in the two classes of cones. Many physically different mixtures of wavelengths could give rise to the same two signals, so sur-

A Flowers

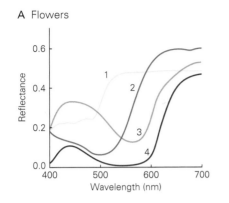

B Human skin

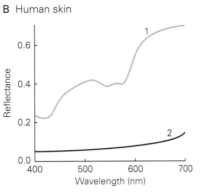

C Paint

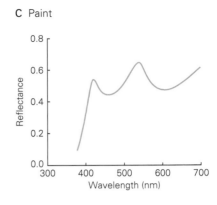

Figure 29-4 An object's surface reflectance function describes the fraction of incident light that its surface reflects at each wavelength. A reflectance of 1 means that all the incident light is reflected. The pigments in natural surfaces generally have reflectance functions that vary slowly and smoothly across the visible spectrum, while synthetic pigments often have a more complex structure.

A. Surface reflectance functions of flowers. (**1**) Pale yellow gladiolus reflects little light at short wavelengths but quite uniformly reflects light at wavelengths greater than about 520 nm. (**2**) Bright orange gladiolus reflects light mostly at wavelengths greater than 580 nm. (**3**) Pale violet rose of Sharon reflects light at long wavelengths and short wavelengths, but not at middle wavelengths (the yellowish-green part of the spectrum). (**4**) Wine-colored gladiolus reflects light at long wavelengths and a little at short wavelengths. (From Evans 1948.)

B. Surface reflectance functions of human skin: (**1**) white skin; (**2**) black skin. (From Evans 1948, after Edwards and Duntley 1939.)

C. Surface reflectance function of light green enamel paint. The surface reflectance functions of synthetic pigments often vary less smoothly with wavelength than do those of natural surfaces. (From Wyszecki and Stiles 1982.)

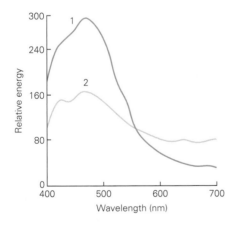

Figure 29-5 The light reflected from a surface depends both upon the object's surface reflectance function and the spectral composition of the illuminant. The plot shows the spectral composition of light reflected from the surface of a blue vase illuminated by direct sunlight (1) and by a uniformly overcast sky (2). The different phases of daylight bring about a substantial change in the distribution of light reflected from the surface of an object. (From Evans 1948.)

faces that reflect light quite differently might appear to be the same color.

A system that used more than two types of cones would generate more signals to describe surfaces and would encounter fewer physically different surfaces that appeared the same color. The normal human visual system uses *three* cone systems to represent the spectral properties of surfaces. As we shall see later, some people have fewer kinds of cones, and they often confuse surfaces that are easily distinguished by people with three types.

Three-Cone Systems of the Human Retina Respond to Different Parts of the Visible Spectrum

The idea that human color vision depends on three mechanisms with broad spectral sensitivities, each most responsive to a different part of the visible spectrum, was made explicit at the beginning of the nineteenth century by Thomas Young. We now know that these mechanisms are three different classes of cones, each containing a different photopigment (Box 29-1) that gives it a distinctive spectral sensitivity. One kind of

Box 29-1 The Cone Pigments

The three cone pigments each contain a different opsin. All three opsins are transmembrane proteins with seven membrane-spanning regions. Thus the cone pigments belong to the family of genes that encode rhodopsin, bacterio-rhodopsins, the invertebrate photopigments, and the oderant receptors, as well as a variety of transmitter receptors that also interact with G proteins (see Chapter 13).

Genes for the three types of cone opsins resemble each other and the rhodopsin gene, suggesting that all four evolved from a common precursor by duplication and divergence. A comparison of amino acid sequences (Figure 29-6) suggests that the gene for the S (short wavelength) cone pigment arose first from the rod gene. This gene then seems to have given rise to a single gene for a long-wavelength cone pigment, an arrangement still found in contemporary New World monkeys, many of which often have only two color pigments.

The long wavelength pigment gene is thought to have duplicated and diverged to give rise to distinct genes for L (long wave length) and M (middle wavelength) pigments only about 30 million years ago, when Old World monkeys (which have three pigments) separated from New World monkeys (which often have only two). The L and M gene products are indeed closely related, with 90% identity in their amino acid sequences (see Figure 29-13).

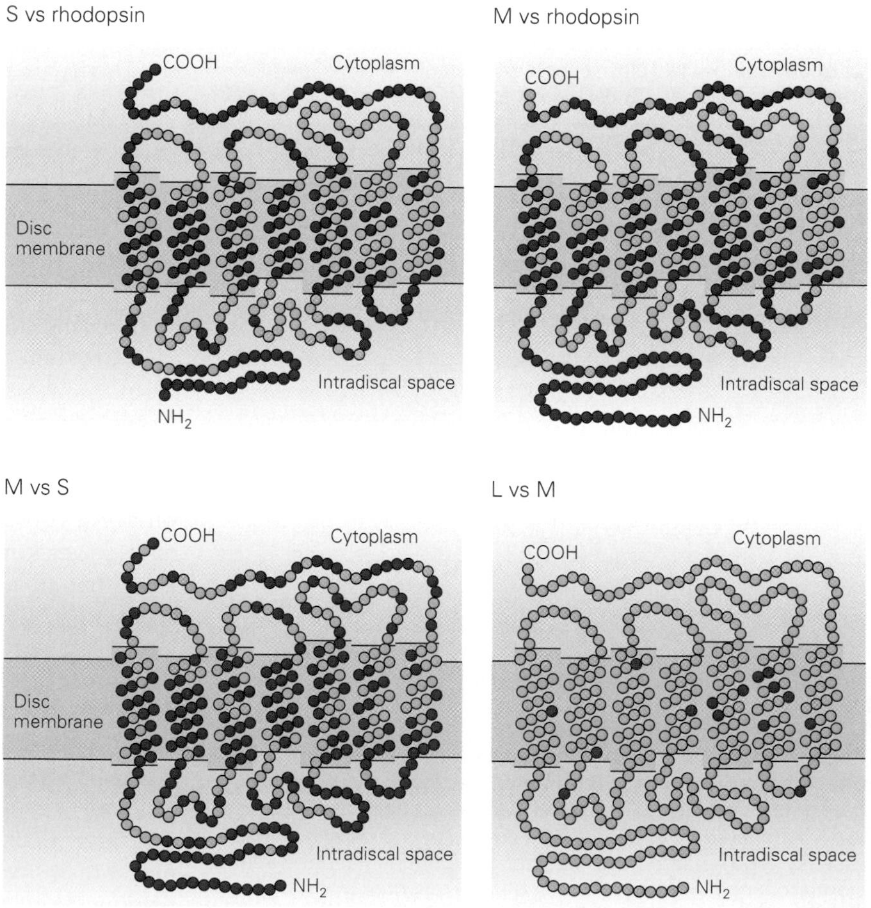

Figure 29-6 Comparisons of the amino acid sequences of selected pairs of photopigments from rods and the L, M, and S cones. Blue circles denote the same amino acid; black circles denote different ones.

cone, the S cone, contains a pigment most sensitive to *short* wavelengths in the visible spectrum. Another, the M cone, is selective for *middle* wavelengths. The third, L cone, responds best to slightly *longer* wavelengths. Recent measurements show that the S pigment absorbs most strongly near 420 nm, the M pigment near 530 nm, and the L pigment near 560 nm (Figure 29-7).

We have seen that using just two values to represent a continuous spectral reflectance function can lead to ambiguous descriptions. How much is the difficulty eased by using three values? The answer depends on the particulars of the surfaces and the particulars of the cone systems that do the sampling.

The reflectance functions of most natural surfaces vary relatively smoothly and slowly with wavelength (see Figure 29-4A, B). The curve that describes surface reflectance can actually be assembled from a small number of even simpler underlying curves that can be thought of as elementary constituents common to all reflectance functions. Figure 29-8 shows a set of three such curves. By adding these three fundamental curves together in appropriate proportions, we can synthesize a real surface reflectance function rather well; by adding yet more fundamental curves we could do better still, though each additional curve would contribute progressively less information about the structure of the full reflectance function.

Thus a visual system with a few sensing mechanisms (perhaps two or three) and spectral sensitivities that allowed the system to represent the *underlying* curves faithfully could do a good job of representing the range of spectral reflectance functions found among natural surfaces. Lawrence Maloney has shown that three mechanisms with the spectral sensitivities of human cones can in fact do the job well. The spectral sensing capabilities of the human eye therefore seem to be reasonably well-matched to the demands of distinguishing natural surfaces.

Although the human visual system will not generally confuse light distributions reflected from different *natural* surfaces, a three-valued representation leaves the system open to confusion by artificial means. We exploit this in color reproduction systems to render a range of colors with only a small number of primary sources. For example, in color television a wide range of colors and lightnesses is synthesized at each point in the image by varying the intensities that excite three phosphors on the surface of the tube: one phosphor that emits long-wavelength light, one that emits middle-wavelength light, and one that emits short-wavelength light (Figure 29-9).

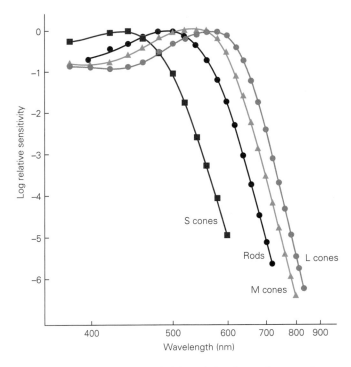

Figure 29-7 Spectral sensitivities of the three classes of cones and the rods. Sensitivity varies over a large range and thus is shown on a logarithmic scale. The different classes of photoreceptors are sensitive to broad and overlapping ranges of wavelengths. The rods normally do not contribute to vision in daylight. (From Schnapf et al. 1988.)

Signals From Cones Are Transformed Early in the Visual Pathway

Although the three kinds of cones can capture and represent the reflectances of natural surfaces, information would not be conveyed efficiently in a system in which each type of cone was connected to its own distinct neural pathway. This is easy to see if we consider the signals that arise in the L and M cones exposed to the kinds of spectral distributions that characterize the samples of flowers and skin in Figure 29-4. Because the reflectance functions vary slowly across the spectrum, and the spectral sensitivities of the L and M cones are similar over a broad spectral region, these classes of cones will generate highly correlated signals when they absorb light from natural surfaces. The correlation between these signals and the signals from the S cones is lower, but still substantial.

The visual pathway could transmit information more efficiently by first removing from the cone signals

Figure 29-8 The reflectance function of a natural surface has component functions.

A. Three component functions, when added together in suitable proportions, provide the best three-variable description of the surface reflectance functions of a large sample of natural objects. One curve can be loosely considered to represent the brightness dimension of the image; two other curves can be loosely thought of as representing dimensions of red-green variation and yellow-blue variation. These three component functions account for over 99% of the variance in the reflectance functions of the natural surfaces that have been studied. The fit can be made almost perfect by using three additional component functions (making six altogether). (From Cohen 1964 and Maloney 1986.)

B. The surface reflectance of an apple was measured at the point marked by the cross.

C. The apple's actual surface reflectance function is closely approximated by the best-fitting curve (dashed line) that could be synthesized by adding together, in appropriate proportions, the three fixed curves from A.

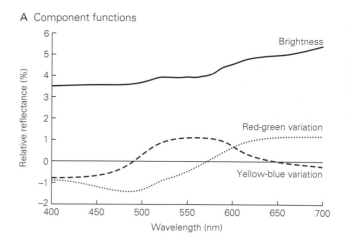

A Component functions

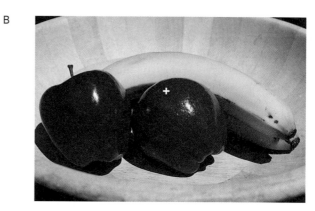

B

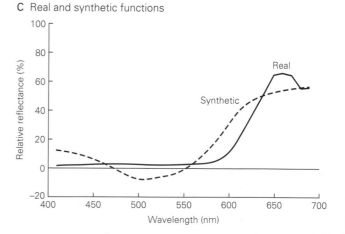

C Real and synthetic functions

those parts that are shared. The simplest way to do this is to transmit the differences among signals. The best transformation would be one that yielded, for the kinds of visual stimuli the eye normally encounters, the smallest correlation among signals in three pathways. Given the spectral composition of the light entering the eye, and the spectral sensitivities of the cone photoreceptors, the best transformations are the following:

The sum of the signals from the three classes of cones (L+M+S).

The difference between the signals from L and M cones (L − M).

The difference between the signal from S cones and some combined signal from the L and M cones (S − LM).

Mechanisms that transformed cone signals in these ways would have spectral sensitivities broadly like those shown in Figure 29-10. This result is very important, for it provides evidence for a transformation of cone signals that had long been suspected from perceptual observations and that has more recently been explored in physiological experiments.

In the late nineteenth century Ewald Hering first drew attention to the fact that the hues red, yellow, green, and blue have special properties: They are fundamental in the sense that other hues can readily be described as mixtures of them, and they seem to be related in mutually exclusive pairs (red vs green and blue vs

yellow), so that a reddish-green color for example is impossible. These observations led Hering to postulate that vision depended on three distinct *opponent mechanisms*. One captured red-green variation in the image, so that it might be excited by red light and inhibited by green light (or vice-versa); another captured blue-yellow variation in the image, being perhaps excited by blue light and inhibited by yellow light. A third captured the light-dark, or *achromatic*, variation in the image, being excited by light and inhibited by dark.

For a considerable time this account was seen as an alternative to the one that postulated three sensing systems of the kind represented by cones, but it eventually came to be seen as a description of mechanisms that receive and transform cone signals. It gained widespread acceptance in the 1950s when Leo Hurvich and Dorothea Jameson marshaled substantial evidence from psychophysical experiments and several other investigators found direct physiological evidence for the existence of mechanisms that combined cone signals in different ways.

The first electrophysiological evidence for opponent mechanisms came from recordings made from horizontal cells in the fish retina. These cells become hyperpolarized in response to lights of certain wavelengths and are depolarized in response to lights of other wavelengths. Recordings in the primate retina by Dennis Dacey and colleagues show that the horizontal cells behave differently, giving responses of the same polarity to lights of all wavelengths. Opponent inputs are clearly evident in extracellular recordings made from primate ganglion cells by Peter Gouras and from lateral geniculate nucleus cells by Russell DeValois and colleagues and by Wiesel and Hubel. The properties of neurons in the lateral geniculate nucleus apparently reflect those of ganglion cells, which in turn probably reflect transformations of cone signals occurring at an earlier stage in the retina. Anatomical considerations suggest these happen in bipolar cells, though this has not yet been established physiologically.

How do ganglion cells convey the red-green, blue-yellow, and achromatic dimensions of variation in the image? There are several kinds of retinal ganglion cells that differ in their anatomical and physiological characteristics. As we have seen in Chapter 26, there are two major classes of ganglion cells, now most often called M cells and P cells for their separate projections to the *magnocellular* (large-cell) and *parvocellular* (small-cell) layers of the lateral geniculate nucleus. These account for about 90% of all ganglion cells. Table 29-1 summarizes some of their properties, and Figure 29-11 shows schematically the organization of receptive fields.

Modern physiological recordings from ganglion cells, and from the neurons to which they project in the lateral geniculate nucleus, have firmly established the chromatic properties of both M and P cells. The receptive fields of M cells have a simple antagonistic center-surround organization. Some cells have on-center receptive fields, others off-center receptive fields, but in both types the center and surround have similar, broad spec-

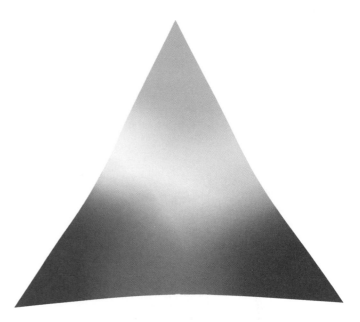

Figure 29-9 A wide range of colors can be synthesized by mixing three primary lights in varying proportions. In this figure the red, green, and blue primaries within the central patch vary only in intensity. Each has a gradient from bright to dark.

tral sensitivities. Information about color is carried almost exclusively in the P cell system.

P cells fall into two subtypes: neurons that receive opposed signals from L and M cones and neurons that receive signals from S cones opposed to some combined signal from L and M cones. These two subtypes of P cells are well suited to provide the red-green and blue-yellow channels postulated by Hering, while M cells appear well equipped to convey the achromatic/brightness signals. However, this scheme looks less satisfactory when we consider how the different kinds of neurons deal with the spatial structure of the image.

Most of the information about the detailed structure of the visual world is conveyed by variations of brightness in the image rather than by variations in color (see Figure 29-1). We might therefore expect much of the visual system's capacity to be devoted to analyzing the brightness variations rather than the color variations. Perceptual experiments confirm this expectation: our capacity to resolve fine spatial variations in brightness exceeds our capacity to resolve spatial variations in hue. Since we know how M cells and P cells are distributed on the retina, we can calculate what kind of image detail each class of cell is capable of conveying.

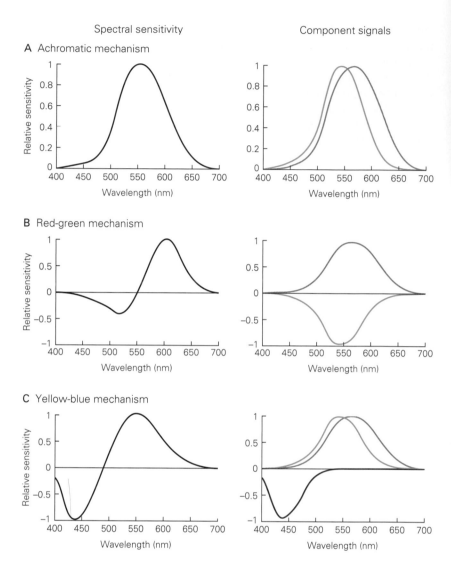

Figure 29-10 Spectral sensitivities of three "second-stage" mechanisms that can transform signals from the three classes of cones.

A. The spectral sensitivity of the achromatic mechanism (**left**) is formed by adding signals from L and M cones (**right**), and possibly a very small contribution from S cones. The spectral sensitivity curves for the components (**right**) are the same as those shown in Figure 29-7 but are drawn on a linear rather than logarithmic sensitivity axis.

B. The spectral sensitivity of the red-green mechanism results from the subtraction of M cone signals from L cone signals. Some psychophysical observations suggest that S cones contribute to this mechanism, with the same sign as L cones, although this has not been found in studies of neurons in the lateral geniculate nucleus.

C. The spectral sensitivity of the yellow-blue mechanism results from the subtraction of L cone and M cone signals from S cone signals.

M cells are arranged much too sparsely to account for our capacity to resolve detail. They are important in the analysis of image movement (see Chapter 28), but they cannot convey information about detailed spatial variations in brightness. P cells, on the other hand, are very densely distributed—in and around the fovea there are two P cells for every cone—and could easily represent the detail that we can resolve in an image. The problem is that P cells appear superficially to be better suited to conveying information about color than to conveying information about the lightness variations that define structure. In fact, however, the spatial organization of the P cell's receptive field allows the cell to convey both brightness and color information in a complex signal.

When the light falling on a P cell's receptive field covers both center and surround, the cell will respond well to variations in color, being excited by some hues and inhibited by others. However, when the light is either very small and confined to the center or distributed over the whole receptive field in a way that does not disturb the average light level on the surround (for example a fine grating pattern), only the central part of the receptive field generates a signal. Because this signal arises from a single type of cone, the cell responds to light over a broad range of wavelengths—it loses its color opponency. Thus a P cell responds well to brightness variations in the fine structure of the image, and it responds well to color variations in the coarse structure of the image.

Not all P cells contribute to this encoding of spatial variations in lightness. The cornea and lens of the eye, when imaging a surface, cannot focus light of all wavelengths in the same plane in the retina. This *chromatic aber-*

Table 29-1 M and P Pathways in the Visual System

Attribute	M Cells	P Cells
Percentage of all ganglion cells	~10	~80
Distribution on retina	Densest in fovea?	Densest in fovea
Conduction velocity	~15 m/s	~6 m/s
Central projection 　Ganglion cells 　LGN[1] cells	LGN, magnocellular V1, layer 4Cα	LGN, parvocellular V1, layer 4Cβ
Chromatic opponency	Almost none	Well-developed (two types: L vs M; S vs L,M)
Rod input	Yes	Sometimes
Contrast sensitivity	High (>60)	Low (<20)
Spatial resolution	Lower	Higher (single-cone center in fovea)
Temporal resolution	Higher (>60 Hz)	High (>30 Hz)
Periphery effects	Some	None?

[1]LGN = lateral geniculate nucleus.

ration prevents all wavelengths from being in focus at the same time, so the visual system opts for a sharp image at middle and long wavelengths at the expense of a blurred image at short wavelengths. The S cones constitute less than 10% of the total (they are actually entirely absent from the center of the fovea). The ganglion cells that receive their inputs probably constitute a similar fraction of P cells and are sparsely distributed on the retina.

P cells that receive inputs from only L and M cones seem to be the ones that can carry both a color-opponent signal and a brightness signal. These signals are conveyed through the ongoing discharge of action potentials and, as far as we know, are confounded in the discharge of a single cell. That is, just as individual cones confuse variations in wavelength and intensity, so too do individual P cells. The ambiguity in the discharge of any one P cell must be resolved by mechanisms in the cortex.

Signals Are Transformed Again in the Primary Visual Cortex

Psychophysical observations suggest that information about color is encoded in the cortex in ways more complex than in the retina and lateral geniculate nucleus.

The Cortex Contains More Than Three Chromatic Channels

Although the idea that there are three "second-stage" mechanisms of color vision is now widely accepted, several lines of evidence suggest that this is a simplification and that, at least at higher levels in the visual pathway, many mechanisms exist, each selectively sensitive to its own small domain of color and lightness. The strongest evidence for this kind of organization comes from psychophysical experiments that show that sensitivity to particular hues is diminished after prolonged viewing of similar and complementary hues and that the loss of sensitivity is confined to spectral regions so narrow as to implicate more than three spectrally selective mechanisms. These experiments do not give a precise indication of how many higher-level mechanisms might exist, but they point firmly to more than three.

Color is not an isolated attribute detached from other properties of an object, such as shape and movement. It is inextricably bound up with other object attributes, a point emphasized by perceptual tests that show how spatial context affects the appearance of colored regions (see Figure 29-3). When we consider the spatial complexities of natural scenes, the color of surfaces can no longer be treated simply as a three-variable problem. We know only a little about how the spatial at-

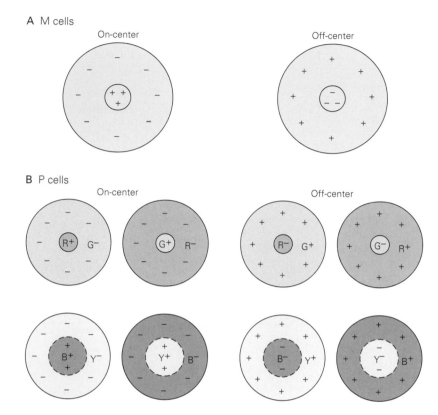

Figure 29-11 The receptive fields of primate retinal ganglion cells have two concentrically organized regions, a center and an antagonistic surround. This fundamental organization is expressed in two basic forms: In an on-center cell, light falling on the center excites the cell while light falling on the surround inhibits it. In an off-center cell, light falling on the center inhibits the cell while light falling on the surround excites it. Different types of ganglion cells are distinguished by the sizes of their receptive fields and by the ways in which their centers and surrounds integrate signals from the different classes of cones.

A. M cells constitute about 8% of all ganglion cells. Even the smallest center receives inputs from several cones. The spectral sensitivities of center and surround differ little, if at all.

B. P cells constitute about 80% of all ganglion cells. Two subtypes are defined by the organization of cone inputs. The "red-green" opponent type receives inputs only from L and M cones, whereas the "yellow-blue" type receives input from all three classes of cones. Within the red-green class different connections to cones give rise to multiple cell subtypes: on- or off-center cells, and centers with L or M cone inputs. The cone inputs to the surround are less firmly established, but are generally thought to arise from the class that does not feed the center. In cells in and near the fovea the center of the receptive field receives input from a single cone; in more peripheral regions of retina several cones provide input to the center. Less is known about the structure of the receptive fields of the blue-yellow type of P cell. The antagonistic mechanisms seem to overlap more, possibly because chromatic aberration defocuses short-wavelength light, and center and surround are harder to distinguish. Cells in which S cones contribute the "off" signal are rare.

tributes of objects influence their color, but it seems likely, given the simple behavior of P cells, that the mechanisms responsible for the influence of context reside in the cortex.

Neurons in Primary Visual Cortex Do Not Fall Into Distinct Color Classes

The P cells project from the lateral geniculate nucleus to neurons in layers 4Cβ and 4A of the primary visual cor-

tex. Most of these neurons respond well to achromatic stimuli and poorly to colored ones. Some cells in layer 4Cβ, however, have receptive fields that resemble those of P cells: They have a concentrically organized color-opponent structure, though in some the antagonistic mechanisms are spatially coextensive. As a result, these cells in layer 4Cβ are most sensitive to changes in the color of a uniform region of light that covers the whole receptive field. They are relatively insensitive to brightness changes in either finely structured or coarsely structured stimuli. Layer 4A also contains a small proportion of cells with similarly organized color-opponent receptive fields. Thus, even in the input layers of the cortex there is substantial transformation of the signals arriving from the lateral geniculate nucleus, and there are probably cells (unlike those in the lateral geniculate nucleus) whose chromatic properties do not depend upon the spatial configuration of the visual stimulus.

Neurons in the upper layers of striate cortex, to which layer 4 cells project heavily and which provide the principal output to higher visual areas, generally have receptive fields with a more elaborate structure. Most simple and complex cells (see Chapters 27 and 28) respond best to achromatic stimuli. Few cells respond well to color variations, even if these variations are configured to match the spatial characteristics of the cell's receptive field. We should not think this surprising, given the relatively small amount of information carried by color variation in images. Some of the cells that respond well to colored stimuli are simple, some are complex. Still other, rare ones have distinctive receptive fields consisting of concentrically organized regions. In the central region certain colors excite the cell while other colors inhibit it. Surrounding the central region is a much larger zone in which light of broad spectral composition will reduce the response (either excitatory or inhibitory) to light in the center. Neurons with fields like this are sometimes called *double-opponent* cells.

Unlike the tight clustering of P cells in the lateral geniculate nucleus into clear "red-green" and "blue-yellow" groups, cells in the primary visual cortex that respond well to changes in color do not fall into distinct groups and are widely scattered, as if each cell is selective for a particular combination of brightness and color contrast.

The code the brain uses to convey information about color is profoundly changed in the primary visual cortex. The general picture emerging from studies of striate cortex is that color is just one of several dimensions of image variation to which an individual neuron is selective; information about color is encoded along with information about other attributes of the image. However, this picture is complicated by the possibility that color-opponent cells are clustered in the striate cortex. Some investigators have found relatively high concentrations of double-opponent cells in the conspicuous "blobs" that regularly punctuate the striate cortex. Because blobs send specific projections to higher visual areas (Chapter 27), any clustering of color-opponent cells in blobs implies the existence of cortical pathways that analyze color.

Signals About Color Are Conveyed to the Temporal Lobe

The secondary visual area, V2, is the principal destination of output from the primary visual cortex. When stained for cytochrome oxidase, V2 in the monkey shows a pattern of stripes, and some of these (the "thin" stripes) receive inputs preferentially from the blobs in striate cortex (see Chapter 28). The thin stripes in turn send projections to area V4, a region that Semir Zeki first showed contained many cells that are selective for the color of visual stimuli. As a result of Zeki's observations, V4 is regarded as an area whose principal role is to analyze and represent the color information in the image.

As discussed in Chapter 28, Zeki's discoveries, in both V4 and MT (the middle temporal area), indicate that different visual cortical areas are specialized for the analysis of different attributes of the image: color, motion, depth, etc. To the extent that color opponent neurons in V1 are associated with the blobs, this evidence points to a pathway specialized for the analysis of color.

Thus, information about the chromatic attributes of objects is confined mainly to pathways that convey information from striate cortex, through areas V2 and V4, to the temporal lobe. Experimental studies of animals with lesions of these pathways, and studies of people who have suffered localized brain damage, usually as a result of stroke, sometimes show impairments of color vision, often in association with other disruptions of object vision.

Recordings made from single neurons at different stages in the pathway connecting the primary visual cortex to the temporal lobe show that their chromatic characteristics are generally like those of neurons in the primary cortex. Some studies of neurons in area V4 have found that a cell's response to a colored stimulus falling on its receptive field is influenced by the color of light falling in a large region surrounding the receptive field. This work implicates V4 in color-contrast phenomena of the kind illustrated in Figure 29-3.

Color Blindness Can Be Congenital or Acquired

Few people are truly color-blind, in the sense of being wholly unable to distinguish a change in the color of a light from a change in its intensity, but many people have severely impaired color vision. Most abnormalities of color vision are congenital and have been reliably characterized; some other abnormalities result from injury or disease of the visual pathway.

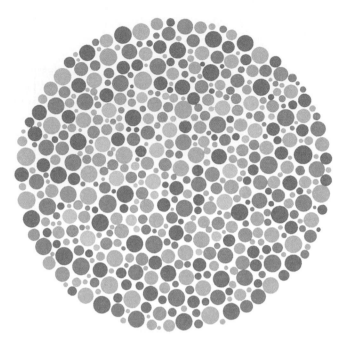

Figure 29-12 Numerals embedded in this color pattern can be distinguished by people with trichromatic vision but not usually by dichromats who are weak in red-green discriminations. (From Ishihara 1993.)

Congenital Abnormalities Take Several Forms

The study of congenital abnormalities has contributed enormously to our understanding of the mechanisms of color vision. The first major insight, well-understood in the nineteenth century, is that some people, instead of having the three classes of receptors that characterize normal trichromatic vision, have only two. These people, called *dichromats*, find it hard or impossible to distinguish some surfaces whose colors appear different to trichromats. The dichromat's problem is that every surface reflectance function is represented by a two-value description rather than a three-value one, and this reduced description causes dichromats to confuse many more surfaces than do trichromats. Simple tests for color-blindness exploit this fact. Figure 29-12 shows an example from the Ishihara test, in which the numerals defined by colored dots are seen by normal trichromats, but not by most dichromats.

If a person with normal color vision fails to distinguish between two physically different surface reflectance functions, a dichromat will also fail to distinguish them. The failure means that each class of cone gives rise to the same signal when absorbing light reflected by either surface, so the fact that the dichromat is confused by the same surfaces that confuse a trichro-

mat proves that the cones in the dichromat have normal pigments.

In principle, there could be three forms of dichromacy, corresponding to the loss of each of the three types of cones. This is in fact the case, though two kinds of dichromacy are much more common than the third. The common forms correspond to the loss of the L cones, or the loss of the M cones, and are called *protanopia* and *deuteranopia,* respectively. Protanopia and deuteranopia almost always occur in males, each with a frequency of about 1%. The third form of dichromacy, *tritanopia,* corresponds to the loss of the S cone. It is rare (affecting about 1 in 10,000 people), afflicts women and men equally, and has a gene on chromosome 7.

Since the L and M cones exist in large numbers, one might think that the loss of one or other type would impair vision generally rather than just weakening color vision. In fact, this does not happen, which suggests that, rather than having lost large numbers of L or M cones, the dichromat possesses the normal number but all are L or M.

In addition to the relatively severe forms of color blindness, such as dichromacy, there are milder forms, again affecting mostly males, that result in a slightly impaired capacity to distinguish reflectance functions that are readily distinguished by normal trichromats. People with these milder impairments are trichromats—their cones provide three-value descriptions of the lights reflected by surfaces—but apparently the spectral sensitivities of their cones differ from those of normal cones. Such *anomalous trichromacy* occurs in different forms, depending on which normal cone pigment is replaced by another pigment with a different spectral sensitivity. In two common forms the normal L or M cone pigment is replaced by one that has some intermediate spectral sensitivity. These forms, called *protoanomaly* and *deuteranomaly* respectively, together affect about 7-8% of males.

The existence of sex-linked inherited defects of the L and M cones points to the X chromosome as the locus of genes that encode the visual pigments of these cones. These genes, and the amino acid sequences of the pigments they encode, have been identified, largely through the work of Jeremy Nathans and colleagues. Their discovery reveals some interesting complexities in the genetic organization underlying color vision. Molecular cloning of the genes for the L and M pigments shows the genes to be very similar and arranged head-to-tail on the X chromosome (Figure 29-13). (The pigments also have very similar structures, differing in only 4% of their amino acids.) People with normal color vision have a single copy of the gene for the L pigment and from one to three (occasionally as many as five) almost identical copies of the gene for the M pigment.

The proximity and similarity of the genes is thought to predispose them to varied forms of recombination, leading either to the loss of a gene or to the formation of hybrid genes that account for the common forms of red-green defect (see Chapter 3). Examination of the genes from color-blind males shows that replacement of the L pigment gene by a hybrid can lead to either protanopia or protanomaly; replacement of an M pigment gene by a hybrid results in either deuteranopia or deuteranomaly (always the latter if there are additional M pigment genes).

Acquired Defects Arise Through Disease or Injury

Disease of the retina can affect color vision, though rarely is color vision the only perceptual capability disturbed. Disturbances of color vision are common in people suffering from diseases of the eye, including retinitis pigmentosa and glaucoma, suggesting that cones are more vulnerable to damage than are rods. One interesting aspect of these disorders is that they affect principally, or initially, the blue-yellow dimension of color appearance. This selectivity seems to reflect the particular vulnerability of S cones, which are more readily damaged than the L and M cones. This vulnerability is exploited by histological methods that selectively label the S cones, revealing their well-defined and almost regular arrangement on the retina (Figure 29-14).

One of the most interesting and puzzling disturbances of color vision results from damage to the visual cortex, usually after stroke. Cases in which weakened color vision is one of a constellation of visual abnormalities do not tell us much about the organization of the underlying neural mechanisms. In some cases, however, weakness or loss of color vision *achromatopsia* is the only or most prominent consequence of the lesion (Box 29-2). The fact that color vision can be selectively damaged suggests that some region of the cortex is specialized for the analysis of information about color. However, the idea of cortical specialization for color processing has proven to be controversial. Although many patients with achromatopsia show a striking defect in color vision, when studied carefully they usually also show other perceptual deficits.

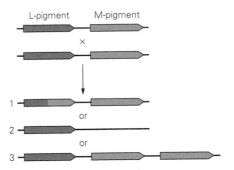

Figure 29-13 The arrangement of L and M pigment genes on the X chromosome might explain variations in these genes observed in both normal and color-blind individuals. Because they are next to each other on a normal X chromosome, recombination between these genes can lead to the generation of a hybrid gene (**1**) or the loss of a gene (**2**), the patterns observed in color-blind men. It can also lead to the duplication of a gene (**3**), a pattern observed in some people with normal color vision. (Adapted from Stryer 1988.)

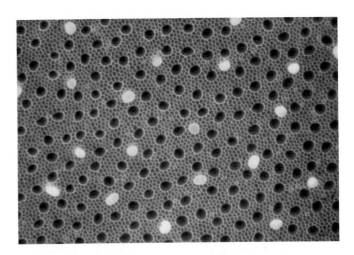

Figure 29-14 The mosaic of cones in the macaque retina, stained with the dye procion yellow to identify the S cones. The S cones are visible as a quasi-regular array of bright yellow spots. The more numerous dark spots are the inner segments of the L and M cones, also arranged quasi-regularly. No anatomical method yet devised can distinguish L and M cones. The small pale spots filling in the spaces between the cones are the rods. (Photograph courtesy of S. Schein and F. M. deMonasterio).

Box 29-2 A Life Without Color Vision: The Case of the Colorblind Painter

Mr. I. had seen normally all his life, had been born with a full complement of cones, or color receptors. . . . He had become colorblind, after sixty-five years of seeing colors normally. And he did not just confuse some colors or see them as gray, as is usually the case with the congenitally colorblind. He had become totally colorblind—as if "viewing a black and white television screen." All this came on suddenly when he had an accident. The suddenness of the event was incompatible with any of the slow deteriorations that can befall the retinal cone cells, and suggested, instead, a mishap at a higher level, in those parts of the brain specialized in perceiving color.

[Some time after the car accident] he decided to go to work again. It seemed to him as if he were driving in a fog, even though he knew it to be a bright and sunny morning. Everything seemed misty, bleached, grayish, indistinct. His bewilderment and fear now became a feeling of horror. . . .

Mr. I arrived at his studio with relief, expecting that the horrible mist would be gone, that everything would be clear again. But as soon as he entered, he found his entire studio, which was hung with brilliantly colored paintings . . . now utterly gray and void of color. His canvases, the abstract color paintings which he was known for, all were grayish or black and white, unintelligible. Now to horror there was added despair: even his art was without meaning, and he could no longer imagine how to go on. . . .

Mr. I. could hardly bear the changed appearances of people ("like animated gray statues") any more than he could bear his own changed appearance in the mirror; he shunned social intercourse and found sexual intercourse impossible. He saw people's flesh, his wife's flesh, his own flesh, as an abhorrent gray; "flesh-colored" now appeared "rat-colored" to him. This was so even when he closed his eyes, for his preternaturally vivid ("eidetic") visual imagery was preserved but now without color, and forced on him images, forced him to "see" but see internally with the wrongness of his achromatopsia. He found foods disgusting in their grayish, dead appearance and had to close his eyes to eat. But this did not help very much, for the mental image of a tomato was as black as its appearance. . . .

Thus reds were seen (or not seen) as black. Yellows and blues, in contrast, were almost white. Further, there was an excessive tonal contrast, with loss of delicate tonal gradations. . . . Objects stood out, if they stood out at all, with inordinate contrast and clarity, like silhouettes. But if the contrast were normal, or low, they might disappear from sight altogether. . . .

His despair of conveying what the world looked like, and the uselessness of the usual black-and-white analogies, finally drove him, some weeks later, to create an entire "gray room," a

gray universe, in his studio, in which tables, chairs, and an elaborate dinner ready for serving were all painted in a range of grays. The effect of this, in three dimensions and in a different tonal scale from the "black and white" we are all accustomed to, was indeed macabre, and wholly unlike that of a black-and-white photograph. As Mr. I. pointed out, "we accept drawings, films, television—small, flat images in black and white you can look at, or away from, when you want. It is only an image, it is not *supposed* to be real. But imagine black and white all around you, 360 degrees, all solid and three-dimensional, and there all the time—a total black and white world. . . . You can't imagine it: the only way I can express it is to make a complete gray room, with everything in it gray—and you yourselves would have to be painted gray, so you'd be part of the world, not just observing it." It was, he once said, like living in a world "molded in lead.". . .

Music, curiously, was impaired for him too, because he had previously (like the Russian composer Scriabin and others) had an extremely intense synesthesia, so that different tones had immediately been translated into color, and he experienced all music simultaneously as a rich tumult of inner colors. With the loss of his ability to generate colors, he lost this ability as well—his internal "color-organ" was out of action, and now he heard music with no visual accompaniment; this, for him, was music with its essential chromatic counterpart missing, music now radically impoverished.

When we asked Mr. I. to examine and paint a copy of a colored spectrum . . . he could see only black and white and varying shades of gray, and painted it as such. Intriguingly, his perception of the spectrum bore no resemblance to that of the retinally color-blind (which has a single peak of luminosity in the green around 500 nanometers) but did resemble that of people with normal ("photopic") vision, whose perception of luminosity reaches a peak in the yellow-green (around 560 nanometers). This showed that his cone mechanisms and discrimination of wavelengths were intact, and only color "perception" (or "construction") was deficient. . . .

Testing up to this point—other forms of visual testing, and a general neurological examination, were entirely negative—had shown an isolated but total achromatopsia or color-blindness. . . .

Efforts had . . . been made to delineate the brain damage in Mr. I.'s case (by the use of special scan techniques: CAT scan, NMR scan), and to measure the physiological reactions of visual cortex (with evoked potential tests), but these tests were all negative. With more sophisticated brain imaging we might well be able to identify the minute brain areas affected; but Mr. I. was getting tired of "all those tests," and for the present it seemed best to return to perceptual testing, but in a more elaborate form.

"Higher" forms of color perception have engaged the interest of Edwin Land in this country and S. Zeki in England, who have both devised a number of experimental and clinical tests. These use complex, subtly juxtaposed blocks of different colors, with a vague resemblance to some paintings of Mondrian (and hence sometimes called "Mondrians"). The colored shapes are projected on a screen through filters that can quickly be changed. In January 1987, with the patient, we met with Professor Zeki, and performed more elaborate testing. A "Mondrian" of great complexity was used as a test object, and this was projected with white light and with extremely narrow-range gel filters allowing the passage of only red, green, and blue light. . . .

Mr. I., it was evident, could distinguish most of the geometric shapes, though only as consisting of differing shades of gray, and he instantly ranked them on a one-to-four gray scale, although he could not distinguish some color boundaries (for example, between red and green, which both appeared to him, in white light, as "black"). With rapid, random switching of the filters, the gray-scale value of all the shapes dramatically changed, some shades previously indistinguishable now becoming very different, and all shades (except actual black) changed, either grossly or subtly, with the wavelength of the illuminating beam. (Thus a green area would be seen by him as "white" in green [medium-wavelength] light, but as "black" in white or red [long-wavelength] light.)

All Mr. I.'s responses were consistent and immediate. . . . Such a response was utterly unlike that which would be made by someone with retinal colorblindness—ie, an absence of receptors sensitive to wavelengths in the eye. Mr. I., it was clear, could discriminate wavelengths—but he could not *go on* from this to "translate" the discriminated wavelengths into color, could not generate the cerebral or mental construct of color. . . .

This showed us with great clarity how his ability to discriminate different wavelengths was preserved, while his color perception was obliterated, how there was a clear dissociation of the two. Such a dissociation could not occur unless there were separate processes for wavelength discrimination and color construction. Thus, Mr. I.'s situation only becomes intelligible with a theory of multistage processing such as Land's or Zeki's; and such a theory can only be grounded, finally and elegantly, in such a patient.

Postscript (October 1987)

It is almost two years since Mr. I. lost his color vision. The intense sorrow that was so characteristic at first, as he sat for hours before his (to him) black lawn, desperately trying to perceive or imagine it as green, has disappeared, as has the revulsion (he no longer sees his wife, or himself, as having "rat-colored" flesh).

There has, we think, been in his case a real "forgetting" color—a forgetting at once psychological and physiological, at once strategic and structural. Perhaps this has to occur in someone who is no longer able to imagine or remember, or in any physiologically based way generate, a lost mode of perception. . . .

In the past few months Mr. I has been changing his habits and behavior—"becoming a night-person"; in his own words he drives, at random, to Boston, Baltimore, or small towns and villages, arriving at dusk, and then wandering about the streets for half the night, occasionally talking to a fellow walker, occasionally going into little diners: "Everything in diners is different at night, at least if it has windows. The darkness comes into the place, and no amount of light can change it. They are transformed into night places. I love the nighttime," Mr. I. says. . . .

Richard Gregory, speaking of those who have never had color vision (owing to absence of cones, or normal cone function, in their eyes) said, "They live in a scotopic world, in a world of bright moonlight," and this now seems to be the only world that Mr. I. can bear. Our world—our "photopic" world, dazzlingly bright and colored—must appear discordant and painful to an achromatope (whether he has been born colorblind, like Gregory's subjects, or become colorblind, like Mr. I.); given this, along with an enhanced, compensatory sensitivity to the nocturnal and scotopic, it is not surprising, it is perhaps inevitable, that achromatopes should be drawn to the only world in which they feel at ease and at home—and that they should, like the loris and the potto, the big-eyed primates that only emerge and hunt at night, turn wholly, or as much as they can, to becoming night creatures in a night world.

Abridged, with permission, from O Sacks, R Wasserman, The case of the colorblind painter, *New York Review of Books*, 19 November 1987, 25–34.

An Overall View

Color vision is a powerful aide to distinguishing and identifying objects. The mechanisms underlying it—three classes of cone photoreceptors with different but overlapping spectral sensitivities—result in the visual system representing every spectral distribution by three values. Although three values seem sufficient to represent, with little ambiguity, surface reflectance functions that have the simple structure typical of natural objects, there remains a vast range of physically different spectral distributions of light that the visual system cannot distinguish. This weakness is exploited in color television, which synthesizes a wide range of colors by mixing three lights of fixed spectral composition in different proportions.

Mechanisms in the retina transform the signals generated by cones to give rise to color-opponent signals. These signals can be thought of as a providing a more efficient code to represent the spectral characteristics of surfaces. The signals for color are conveyed to the cortex by the class of neurons (P cells) that also carries information about the spatial structure of the image.

An important question is whether or not the cortex analyzes color signals in isolation or in conjunction with signals about other image attributes. If color is analyzed in a special pathway, we might expect to see in some higher cortical area a region containing a preponderance of cells that respond well to variations in image color but are relatively unselective for other attributes of visual stimuli. On the other hand, if every neuron is tuned to multiple dimensions along which images vary—movement, color, surface depth, orientation, etc—the analysis of color information will be inextricably bound up with the analysis of information about other attributes of the image. Physiological observations on the extrastriate cortex have not altogether resolved the issue. We have seen that, after a stroke, people can be left with weakness or loss of color vision without corresponding impairment of other visual capabilities. This selective loss, together with the results of recent studies using positron emission tomography (PET) to highlight regions of the visual cortex that are especially active when subjects view colored as opposed to achromatic patterns, suggests that there is a region specialized for the analysis of color within the human cortex. Moreover, experimental studies on monkeys have shown color-opponent neurons to be especially conspicuous in area V4.

Despite these indications of a pathway or region specially concerned with color, other evidence suggests that any specialization must be modest. Some of the best evidence comes from perceptual experiments that show how prolonged viewing of a pattern of particular color, shape, and orientation makes the viewer less sensitive to that pattern but not to others that differ from it in color, shape, or orientation (we know from physiological experiments that such perceptual aftereffects arise in the cortex and not earlier). This evidence implies the existence of fatigable mechanisms, each of which is sensitive not just to one but to *several* dimensions of variation in the image. Other lines of evidence, too, suggest that V4 must have a broader and more complex visual function than just the analysis of color. First, color-selective cells are only a small fraction of those that project from V2 to V4. Second, studies that have examined the visual capabilities of monkeys with lesions in V4 show that the monkeys perform satisfactorily on simple visual discrimination tasks but are grossly impaired in making more complex form discriminations. But perhaps the strongest argument against V4 being an area specialized for color is that it is the gateway to the temporal lobe and the principal conduit of information to higher visual centers known to be important for many aspects of visual perception (see Chapter 28).

On balance, physiological evidence favors the view that information about color is analyzed not in a specialized pathway and module, but is everywhere inextricably bound up with the analysis of other object attributes, at least in the major pathway connecting V1 to the temporal lobe. According to this view, color is just one of several aspects of an image to which a cortical neuron is selective.

Peter Lennie

Selected Readings

Kaiser PK, Boynton RM. 1996. *Human Color Vision,* 2nd ed. Washington, DC: Optical Society of America.

Gouras P (ed). 1991. *The Perception of Colour.* Boca Raton, FL: CRC Press.

Lennie P, D'Zmura M. 1988. Mechanisms of color vision. CRC Crit Rev Neurobiol 3:333–400.

Plant GT. 1991. Disorders of colour vision in diseases of the nervous system. In: DH Foster (ed). *Inherited and Acquired Colour Vision Deficiencies: Fundamental Aspects and Clinical Studies,* pp. 173–198. Boca Raton, FL: CRC Press.

Nathans J, Merbs SL, Sung CH, Weitz CJ, Wang Y. 1992. Molecular genetics of human visual pigments. Annu Rev Genet 26:403–424.

Neitz J, Neitz M. 1994. Color vision defects. In: AF Wright, B Jay (eds). *Molecular Genetics of Inherited Eye Disorders,* pp. 218–257. Chur, Switzerland: Harwood Academic.

Zeki S. 1993. *A Vision of the Brain.* Oxford: Blackwell Scientific.

References

Albers J. 1975. *Interaction of Color.* New Haven, Yale Univ. Press.

Baylor DA, Nunn BJ, Schnapf JL. 1984. The photocurrent, noise, and spectral sensitivity of rods of the monkey *Macaca fascicularis.* J Physiol (Lond) 357:575–607.

Buchsbaum G, Gottschalk A. 1983. Trichromacy, opponent colours coding and optimum colour information transmission in the retina. Proc R Soc Lond B Biol Sci 220:89–113.

Cohen J. 1964. Dependency of the spectral reflectance curves of the Munsell color chips. Psychonom Sci 1:369–370.

Dacey DM, Lee BB, Stafford DK, Pokorny J, Smith VC. 1996. Horizontal cells of the primate retina: cone specificity without spectral opponency. Science 271:656–659.

Dartnall HJ, Bowmaker JK, Mollon JD. 1983. Human visual pigments: microspectrophotometric results from the eyes of seven persons. Proc R Soc Lond B Biol Sci 220:115–130.

DeValois RL, Abramov I, Jacobs GH. 1966. Analysis of response patterns of LGN cells. J Opt Soc Am 56:966–977.

Edwards EA, Duntley SQ. 1939. The pigments and color of living human skin. Am J Anat 65:1–33.

Evans RM. 1948. *An Introduction to Color.* New York: Wiley.

Gouras P. 1968. Identification of cone mechanisms in monkey ganglion cells. J Physiol (Lond) 199:533–547.

Hering E. 1964. *Outlines of a Theory of the Light Sense.* LM Herrick, D Jameson (transl). Cambridge, MA: Harvard Univ. Press.

Hubel DH, Wiesel TN. 1968. Receptive fields and functional architecture of monkey striate cortex. J Physiol (Lond) 195:215–243.

Hurvich LM, Jameson D. 1957. An opponent-process theory of color vision. Psychol Rev 64:384–404.

Ishihara S. 1993. *Tests for Colour-Blindness.* Tokyo: Kanehara.

Krauskopf J, Williams DR, Heeley DW. 1982. Cardinal directions of color space. Vision Res 22:1123–1131.

Lennie P, Krauskopf J, Sclar G. 1990. Chromatic mechanisms in striate cortex of macaque. J Neurosci 10:649–669.

Levitt JB, Kiper DC, Movshon JA. 1994. Receptive fields and functional architecture of macaque V2. J Neurophysiol 71:2517–2542.

Maloney LT. 1986. Evaluation of linear models of surface spectral reflectance with small numbers of parameters. J Opt Soc Am [A] 3:1673–1683.

Nathans J. 1989. The genes for color vision. Sci Am 260:42–49.

Schnapf JL, Kraft TW, Nunn BJ, Baylor DA. 1988. Spectral sensitivity of primate photoreceptors. Vis Neurosci 1:255–261.

Smith VC, Pokorny J. 1975. Spectral sensitivity of the foveal cone photopigments between 400 and 500 nm. Vision Res 15:161–171.

Stryer L. 1988. *Biochemistry,* 3rd ed. New York: Freeman.

Vos JJ, Walraven PL. 1971. On the derivation of the foveal receptor primaries. Vision Res 11:799–818.

Webster MA, Mollon JD. 1991. Changes in colour appearance following post-receptoral adaptation. Nature 349:235–238.

Wiesel TN, Hubel DH. 1966. Spatial and chromatic interactions in the lateral geniculate body of the rhesus monkey. J Neurophysiol 29:1115–1156.

Wyszecki G, Stiles WS. 1982. *Color Science—Concepts and Methods, Quantitative Data and Formulae,* 2nd ed. New York: John Wiley & Sons.

Young T. 1802. The Bakerian lecture. On the theory of light and colours. Philos Trans R Soc Lond 92:12–48.

Zeki SM. 1973. Colour coding in rhesus monkey prestriate cortex. Brain Res 53:422–427.

30

Hearing

HUMAN EXPERIENCE IS enriched by our ability to distinguish a remarkable range of sounds—from the complexity of a symphony, to the warmth of a conversation, to the dull roar of the stadium. This ability depends upon the almost miraculous feats of hair cells, the receptors of the internal ear. Similar hair cells are also responsible for our sense of equilibrium. Human hearing commences when the cochlea, the snail-shaped receptor organ of the inner ear, transduces sound energy into electrical signals and forwards them to the brain. The cochlea, however, is not simply a passive detector. Our ability to recognize small differences in sounds stems from the auditory system's capacity to distinguish among frequency components and to inform us of both the tones present and their amplitudes. The cochlea also contains cellular amplifiers that augment our auditory sensitivity and are responsible for the first stages of frequency analysis.

The paired cochleas contain slightly more than 30,000 receptor cells. These hair cells carry out the process of auditory transduction: They receive mechanical inputs that correspond to sounds and transduce these signals into electrical responses that can be forwarded to the brain for interpretation. Hair cells can measure motions of atomic dimensions and transduce stimuli ranging from static inputs to those at frequencies of tens of kilohertz. Damage to or deterioration of hair cells accounts for most of the hearing loss in the nearly 30 million Americans who are afflicted with significant deafness.

Information flows from the cochlea to the cochlear nuclei, from which signals ascend the brain stem through a richly interconnected series of relay nuclei. The brain stem components are essential for localizing

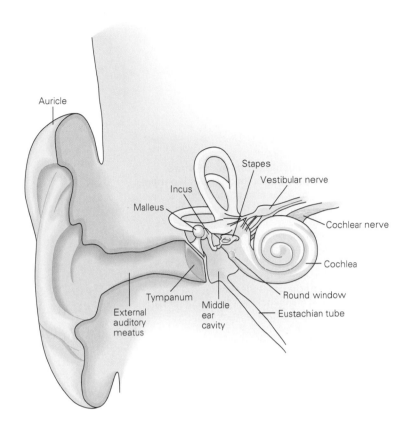

Figure 30-1 **The structure of the human ear.** The external ear, especially the prominent auricle, focuses sound into the external auditory meatus. Alternating increases and decreases in air pressure vibrate the tympanum. These vibrations are conveyed across the air-filled middle ear by three tiny, linked bones: the malleus, the incus, and the stapes. Vibration of the stapes stimulates the cochlea, the hearing organ of the inner ear. (Adapted from Noback 1967.)

sound sources and suppressing the effects of echoes. The auditory regions of the cerebral cortex further analyze auditory information and deconstruct complex sound patterns such as human speech. This chapter considers the cochlea and how it achieves its remarkable performance, examines the central nervous system pathways of the auditory system, describes how humans analyze sounds, and outlines various therapeutic possibilities for the treatment of deafness.

The Ear Has Three Functional Parts

Sound consists of alternating compressions and rarefactions propagating through an elastic medium, air. As we are reminded upon making the effort to shout, producing these pressure changes requires that work be done on the air by our vocal apparatus or some other sound source. Sound carries energy through the air at a speed of about 340 m/s. To hear, our ears must capture this mechanical energy, transmit it to the ear's receptive organ, and transduce it into electrical signals suitable for analysis by the nervous system. These three tasks are the functions of the external ear, the middle ear, and the inner ear (Figure 30-1).

External Ear

The most obvious component of the human external ear is the auricle, a prominent fold of cartilage-supported skin. Much as a parabolic antenna collects electromagnetic radiation, the auricle acts as a reflector to capture sound efficiently and to focus it into the external auditory meatus, or ear canal. The external ear is not uniformly effective for capturing sound from any direction; the auricle's corrugated surface collects sounds of differing frequencies best when they originate at different, but specific, positions with respect to the head. Our capacity to localize sounds in space, especially along the vertical axis, depends critically upon the sound-gathering properties of the external ear. The external auditory meatus ends at the tympanum or eardrum, a thin diaphragm about 9 mm in diameter.

Middle Ear

The middle ear is an air-filled pouch extending from the pharynx, to which it is connected by the Eustachian tube. Mechanical energy derived from airborne sound progresses across the middle ear as motions of three tiny ossicles, or bones: the malleus, or hammer; the incus, or anvil; and the stapes, or stirrup. The base of the malleus

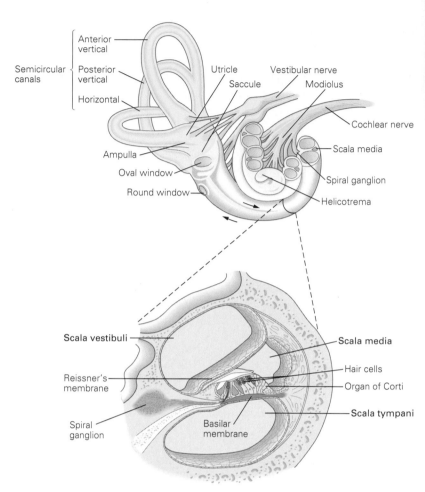

Figure 30-2 The cochlea consists of three fluid-filled compartments throughout its entire length of 33 mm. A cross section of the cochlea shows the arrangement of the three ducts. The oval window, against which the stapes pushes in response to sound, communicates with the **scala vestibuli.** The **scala tympani** is closed at its base by the round window, a thin, flexible membrane. Between these two compartments lies the **scala media,** an endolymph-filled tube whose epithelial lining includes the 16,000 hair cells surmounting the basilar membrane. (Adapted from Noback 1967.)

is attached to the tympanic membrane; its other extreme makes a ligamentous connection to the incus, which is similarly connected to the stapes. The flattened termination of the stapes, the footplate, inserts in an opening—the oval window—in the bony covering of the cochlea. The first two ossicles are relics of evolution, for their antecedents served as components of the jaw in reptilian ancestors.

Inner Ear

The cochlea derives its name from the Greek *cochlos,* the word for snail. A human cochlea consists of slightly less than three coils of progressively diminishing diameter, stacked in a conical structure like a snail's shell. Each cochlea is about 9 mm across, or roughly the size of a chickpea. Covered with a thin layer of laminar bone, the entire cochlea is embedded within the dense structure of the temporal bone. The inner and outer aspects of the cochlea's bony surface are lined with connective-tissue layers, the endosteum and periosteum.

The interior of the cochlea, unlike that of a snail, does not consist of a single cavity. Instead, it contains three fluid-filled tubes, wound helically around a conical bony core, the modiolus (Figure 30-2). If the cochlea is examined in cross-section at any position along its spiral course, the uppermost fluid-filled compartment is the *scala vestibuli.* At the base of this chamber is the oval window, which is sealed by the footplate of the stapes. The lowermost of the three chambers is the *scala tympani;* it, too, has a basal aperture, the round window, which is closed by an elastic diaphragm. The *scala media,* or cochlear duct, separates the other two compartments along most of their length; the scala vestibuli and scala tympani communicate with one another at the helicotrema, an interruption of the cochlear duct at the cochlear apex. The scala media is bounded by a pair of elastic partitions. The thin vestibular membrane (Reissner's membrane) separates the scala media from the scala vestibuli. The basilar membrane, which forms the partition between the scala media and the subjacent scala tympani, is a complex structure upon which auditory transduction occurs.

Hearing Commences With the Capture of Sound Energy by the Ear

Psychophysical experiments have established that we perceive an approximately equal increment in loudness for each 10-fold increase in the amplitude of a sound stimulus. This type of relation is characteristic of many of our senses and is the basis of the Weber-Fechner law (see Chapter 21). To represent sound intensity in a way that corresponds with perceived loudness, it is useful to employ a logarithmic scale. The level, L, of any sound may then be expressed (in units of decibels sound-pressure level, or dB SPL) as

$$L = 20 \times \log_{10}\left(\frac{P}{P_{\text{ref}}}\right),$$

where P, the magnitude of the stimulus, is given as the root mean square of the sound pressure (in units of pascals, or Pa). For a sinusoidal stimulus, the peak amplitude exceeds the root mean square by a factor of the square root of 2. As the reference level on this scale, 0 dB SPL is defined as the sound pressure whose root mean square value is 20 μPa. This intensity corresponds to the approximate threshold of human hearing at 4 kHz, the frequency at which our ears are most sensitive.

That sound consists of alternating compressions and expansions of the air is evident when a loud noise rattles a window. The loudest sound tolerable to humans, with an intensity of about 120 dB SPL, transiently alters the local atmospheric pressure (about 10^5 Pa) by much less than 0.1%. This change nonetheless exerts an oscillatory force of ±28 Pa on a window 1 m on each side. Experience tells us that to rattle the same window by pushing upon it, we would in fact need to exert a comparable force, about ±60 pounds. A faint but clearly audible tone at an intensity of 10 dB SPL produces a periodic pressure change of only ±90 μPa within the ear canal; in this instance the fractional change in the local pressure is less than $\pm 10^{-9}$.

Despite their small magnitude, sound-induced increases and decreases in air pressure push and pull effectively upon the tympanum, moving it inward or outward. Movements of the tympanum displace the malleus, which is fixed to the inner surface of the eardrum. The subsequent motions of the ossicles are complex, depending upon both the frequency and the intensity of sound. In simple terms, however, the actions of these bones may be understood as those of two interconnected levers, the malleus and incus, and a piston, the stapes. The thrust of the incus alternatingly drives the stapes deeper into the oval window and retracts it. The stapes's footplate thus serves as a piston that pushes and pulls cyclically upon the fluid in the scala vestibuli.

Because the energy associated with acoustical signals is generally quite small, compromise of the middle ear's normal structure may lead to *conductive* hearing loss, of which two forms are especially common. First, scar tissue due to middle-ear infection (otitis media) can immobilize the tympanum or ossicles. Second, a proliferation of bone in the ligamentous attachments of the ossicles (otosclerosis) can deprive the ossicles of their normal freedom of motion; this chronic condition of unknown origin can lead to severe deafness.

A clinician may test for conductive hearing loss using the simple Rinné test. A patient is asked to compare the loudness of sound from a vibrating tuning fork held in the air near an affected ear with that perceived when the base of the tuning fork is placed against the patient's head, for example just behind the auricle. If the latter stimulus is perceived as the louder, the patient's conductive pathway may be damaged, but the internal ear may be intact. In contrast, if bone conduction is not more efficient than airborne stimulation, the patient may have inner ear damage, that is, sensorineural hearing loss. The diagnosis of conductive hearing loss is important because surgical intervention is highly effective: removal of scar tissue or reconstitution of the conductive pathway with an inert prosthesis can restore excellent hearing in many instances.

The action of the stapes at the oval window produces pressure changes that propagate throughout the fluid of the scala vestibuli at the speed of sound. Because the aqueous perilymph is virtually incompressible, however, the primary effect of the stapes's motion is to displace the fluid in the scala vestibuli in the one direction not restricted by a firm boundary: toward the elastic cochlear partition. When the fluid deflects the cochlear partition downward, this motion in turn increases the pressure in the scala tympani. This enhanced pressure displaces a fluid mass that causes outward bowing of the round window. Each cycle of a sound stimulus thus evokes a complete cycle of up-and-down movement of a minuscule volume of fluid in each of the inner ear's three chambers. This motion is then sensed from the deflection of the basilar membrane.

Functional Anatomy of the Cochlea

The Basilar Membrane Is a Mechanical Analyzer of Sound Frequency

The mechanical properties of the basilar membrane are key to the cochlea's operation. To appreciate this, suppose that the basilar membrane had uniform dimensions and mechanical properties along its entire length, about 33 mm. Under these conditions a fluctuating pressure difference between the scala vestibuli and the scala tympani, caused by sound waves, would move the entire basilar membrane up and down with similar excursions at all points (Figure 30-3C). This would occur regardless of the frequency of stimulation; any pressure differences between the scala vestibuli and the scala tympani would propagate throughout those chambers within microseconds, and the basilar membrane would therefore be subjected to similar forces at any position along its length. This simple form of basilar-membrane motion occurs in the auditory organs of some reptiles and birds.

The critical characteristic of the basilar membrane in the mammalian cochlea is that it is not uniform. Instead, the basilar membrane's mechanical properties vary continuously along the cochlea's length. At its apical extreme the human basilar membrane is more than fivefold as broad as at the cochlear base. That is, as the cochlear chambers become progressively larger from the organ's apex toward its base, the basilar membrane *decreases* in width. Moreover, the basilar membrane is relatively thin and floppy at the apex of the cochlea but thicker and more taut toward the base. Because its properties vary along its length, the basilar membrane is not like a single string on a musical instrument; instead, it is more like a panoply of strings that vary from the coarsest string on a bass viol to the finest string on a violin.

Because of the systematic variation in mechanical properties along the basilar membrane, stimulation with a pure tone evokes a complex and elegant movement of the membrane. At any instant the partition displays a pattern of up-and-down motion along its length, with the amplitude greatest at a particular position. Over one complete cycle of the sound, each segment along the basilar membrane also undergoes a single cycle of vibration (Figure 30-3D). The various parts of the membrane do not, however, oscillate in phase with one another. As a consequence, some portions of the membrane are moving upward while others move downward. As first demonstrated under stroboscopic illumination by Georg von Békésy, the overall pattern of motion of the membrane is a traveling wave. Each wave reaches its maximal amplitude at the position appropriate for the frequency of stimulation, then rapidly declines in size as it advances toward the cochlear apex. A traveling wave ascending the basilar membrane resembles an ocean wave rolling toward the shore: As the wave nears the beach, its crest grows to a maximal height, then breaks and rapidly fades away.

Although the analogy of an ocean wave gives some sense of the appearance of the basilar membrane's motion, the connection between the traveling wave of the partition's motion and the movement of a wave is wholly metaphorical—the physical bases of the phenomena are quite distinct. The energy carried by an ocean wave resides in the momentum of a wind-blown mass of water. In contrast, most of the energy that evokes movement of each segment of the basilar membrane comes from motion of the fluid masses above and below the membrane. These fluids, in turn, are continuously driven up and down by the energy supplied by the stapes's piston-like movements at the oval window.

The variation in mechanical properties also accounts for the fact that the mammalian basilar membrane is tuned to a progression of frequencies along its length. At the apex of the human cochlea the partition responds best to the lowest frequencies that we can hear, down to approximately 20 Hz. At the opposite extreme, the basilar membrane at the cochlear base responds to frequencies as great as 20 kHz. The intervening frequencies are represented along the basilar membrane in a continuous array (Figure 30-3E). Hermann Helmholtz first appreciated that the basilar membrane's operation is essentially the inverse of a piano's. The piano *synthesizes* a complex sound by combining the pure tones produced by numerous vibrating strings; the cochlea *deconstructs* sounds by confining the action of each component tone to a discrete segment of the basilar membrane.

The arrangement of vibration frequencies in the basilar membrane is an example of a *tonotopic map*. The relation between characteristic frequency and position upon the basilar membrane varies smoothly and monotonically but is not linear. Instead, the *logarithm* of the best frequency is roughly proportional to the distance from the cochlea's apex. The frequencies from 20 Hz to 200 Hz, those between 200 Hz and 2 kHz, and those spanning 2 kHz to 20 kHz are thus each apportioned about one-third of the basilar membrane's extent.

Analysis of the partition's response to a complex sound illustrates how the basilar membrane works. For example, a vowel sound in human speech ordinarily comprises, at any instant, three dominant frequency components. Measurements of the sound pressure outside an ear exposed to such a sound would reveal a complex, seemingly chaotic signal. Likewise, the motions of the tympanum and ossicles in response to a vowel sound appear very complicated. The motion of the basilar membrane, though, is far simpler. Each frequency component of the stimulus establishes a traveling wave that, to a first approximation, is independent of the waves evoked by the others (Figure 30-3F). The amplitude of each traveling wave is proportional, albeit in a complex way, to the intensity of the corresponding

Figure 30-3 Motion of the basilar membrane.

A. A conceptual drawing of an uncoiled cochlea displays the flow of stimulus energy. Sound vibrates the tympanum, which sets the three ossicles of the middle ear in motion. The stapes, a piston-like bone set in the elastic oval window, produces oscillatory pressure differences that rapidly propagate along the scala vestibuli and scala tympani. Low-frequency pressure differences are shunted through the helicotrema.

B. A further simplification of the cochlea converts the spiral organ into a linear structure and reduces the three fluid-filled compartments to two, separated by the elastic basilar membrane.

C. If the basilar membrane had uniform mechanical properties along its full extent, a compression would drive the tympanum and ossicles inward, increasing the pressure in the scala vestibuli and forcing the basilar membrane downward (**top**). Note that the increased pressure in the scala tympani is relieved by outward bowing of the round-window membrane. Under similar circumstances, opposite movements would occur during a rarefaction (**bottom**). Movement of the ossicles is greatly exaggerated here and in **D**.

D. Because the basilar membrane's mechanical properties in fact vary continuously along its length, oscillatory stimulation by sound causes a traveling wave on the basilar membrane. Such a wave is shown, along with the envelope of maximal displacement over an entire cycle. The magnitude of movement is grossly exaggerated in the vertical direction; the loudest tolerable sounds move the basilar membrane by only ±150 nm, a scaled distance less than one hundredth the width of the lines representing the basilar membrane in these figures.

E. Each frequency of stimulation excites maximal motion at a particular position along the basilar membrane. Low-frequency sounds, such as a 100 Hz stimulus, excite basilar-membrane motion near the apex where the membrane is relatively broad and flaccid (**top**). Mid-frequency sounds excite the membrane in its middle (**middle**). The highest frequencies that we can hear excite the basilar membrane at its base (**bottom**). The mapping of sound frequency onto the basilar membrane is approximately logarithmic.

F. The basilar membrane performs spectral analysis of complex sounds. In this example a sound with three prominent frequencies (such as the three dominant components of human speech) excites basilar-membrane motion in three regions, each of which represents a particular frequency. Hair cells in the corresponding positions transduce the basilar-membrane oscillations into receptor potentials, which in turn excite the nerve fibers that innervate these particular regions.

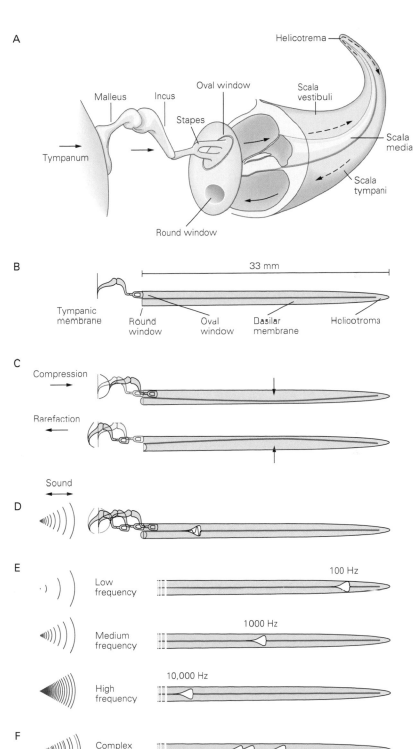

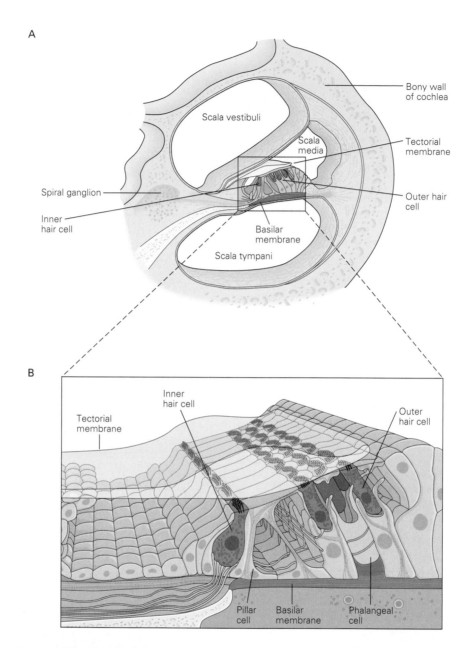

Figure 30-4 Cellular architecture of the organ of Corti in the human cochlea. Although there are differences among species, the basic plan is similar for all mammals.

A. The inner ear's receptor organ is the organ of Corti, an epithelial strip that surmounts the elastic basilar membrane along its 33 mm spiraling course. The organ contains some 16,000 hair cells arrayed in four rows: a single row of inner hair cells and three of outer hair cells. The mechanically sensitive hair bundles of these receptor cells protrude into endolymph, the fluid contents of the scala media. The hair bundles of outer hair cells are attached at their tops to the lower surface of the tectorial membrane, a gelatinous shelf that extends the full length of the basilar membrane.

B. Detailed structure of the organ of Corti. The hair bundle of each inner cell is a linear arrangement of the cell's stereocilia, while the hair bundle of each outer hair cell is a more elaborate, V-shaped palisade of stereocilia. The hair cells are separated and supported by phalangeal and pillar cells (see Figure 30-5A). One hair cell has been removed from the middle row of outer hair cells so that three-dimensional aspects of the relationship between supporting cells and hair cells can be seen. The diameter of an outer hair cell is approximately 7 μm. Empty spaces at the bases of outer hair cells are occupied by efferent nerve endings that have been omitted from the drawing.

A

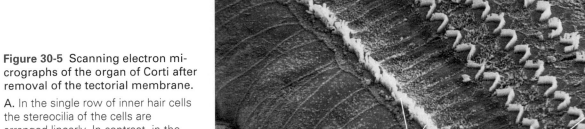

B

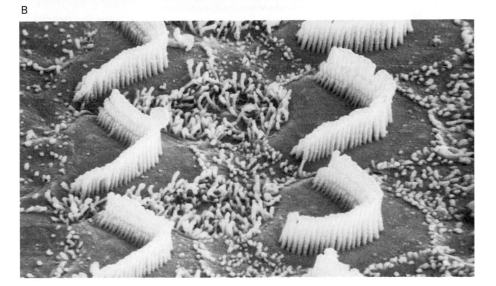

Figure 30-5 Scanning electron micrographs of the organ of Corti after removal of the tectorial membrane.

A. In the single row of inner hair cells the stereocilia of the cells are arranged linearly. In contrast, in the three rows of outer hair cells the stereocilia of each cell are arranged in a V configuration. The surfaces of a number of other cells are visible: the inner spiral sulcus cells, the heads of the inner pillar cells, the phalangeal processes of Deiters' cells, and the surfaces of Hensen's cells.

B. The V-shaped configuration of the stereocilia of the outer hair cells is shown at higher magnification. The apical surfaces of the hair cells surrounding the stereocilia appear smooth, whereas the surfaces of supporting cells are endowed with microvilli.

frequency component. Moreover, each traveling wave reaches its peak excursion at the basilar-membrane position appropriate for the relevant frequency component. The basilar membrane thus acts as a mechanical frequency analyzer by distributing stimulus energy to the hair cells arrayed along its length according to the various pure tones that make up the stimulus. In doing so, the basilar membrane's pattern of motion begins the encoding of the frequencies and intensities in a sound.

The Organ of Corti Is the Site of Mechanoelectrical Transduction in the Cochlea

The organ of Corti is the receptor organ of the inner ear, containing the hair cells and a variety of supporting cells. It appears as an epithelial ridge extending along

the length of the basilar membrane (Figure 30-4). The approximately 16,000 hair cells in each cochlea are innervated by about 30,000 afferent nerve fibers, which carry information into the brain along the eighth cranial nerve. Like the basilar membrane itself, both the hair cells and the auditory nerve fibers are tonotopically organized: At any position along the basilar membrane they are optimally sensitive to a particular frequency, and these frequencies are logarithmically mapped in ascending order from the cochlea's apex to its base.

The organ of Corti includes a wealth of cell types, most of obscure function, but four types have obvious importance. First, there are two varieties of hair cells. The *inner hair cells* form a single row of approximately 3500 cells (Figure 30-5). Farther from the helical axis of the cochlear spiral lie three (or occasionally four) rows

A

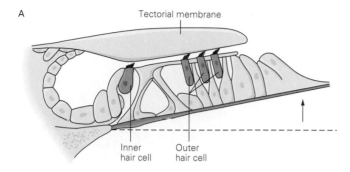

Tectorial membrane

Inner hair cell   Outer hair cell

B

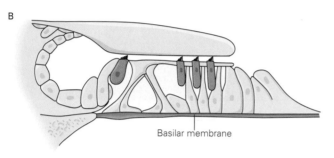

Basilar membrane

C

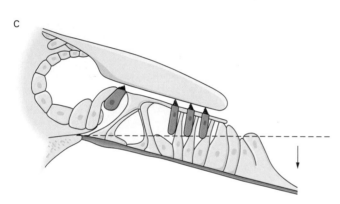

Figure 30-6 Hair cells in the cochlea are stimulated when the basilar membrane is driven up and down by differences in the fluid pressure between the scala vestibuli and scala tympani. Because this motion is accompanied by shearing motion between the tectorial membrane and organ of Corti, the hair bundles that link the two are deflected. This deflection initiates mechanoelectrical transduction of the stimulus. (Adapted from Miller and Towe 1979.)

A. When the basilar membrane is driven upward, shear between the hair cells and the tectorial membrane deflects hair bundles in the excitatory direction, toward their tall edge.

B. At the midpoint of an oscillation the hair bundles resume their resting position.

C. When the basilar membrane moves downward, the hair bundles are driven in the inhibitory direction.

of *outer hair cells,* which total about 12,000 cells. The outer hair cells are supported at their bases by the phalangeal (Deiters') cells; the space between the inner and outer hair cells is delimited and mechanically supported by the pillar cells (Figures 30-4 and 30-5).

A second epithelial ridge adjacent to, but just inside, the organ of Corti gives rise to the tectorial membrane, a cantilevered gelatinous shelf that lies over the organ of Corti (Figure 30-4). The tectorial membrane is anchored at its base by the interdental cells, which are also responsible, at least in part, for producing the structure. The tectorial membrane's tapered distal edge forms a fragile connection with the organ of Corti. More importantly, the longest stereocilia of the outer hair cells are tightly attached to the tectorial membrane's lower surface. In fact, the coupling of hair bundles to the tectorial membrane is so strong that the stereociliary tips are pulled free from the hair cells when the tectorial membrane is lifted from the organ of Corti.

Experimental techniques do not as yet permit detailed examination of how the organ of Corti moves during exposure to sound. From the geometrical arrangement of the organ upon the basilar membrane and from the basilar membrane's measured movements, however, it is possible to infer how stimulation reaches the hair cells. When the basilar membrane vibrates in response to a sound, the organ of Corti and the overlying tectorial membrane are carried with it. However, because the basilar and tectorial membranes pivot about different lines of insertion, their oscillating displacements are accompanied by back-and-forth shearing motions between the upper surface of the organ of Corti and the lower surface of the tectorial membrane. Hair bundles bridge that gap, so they too are deflected (Figure 30-6).

The mechanical deflection of the hair bundle is the proximate stimulus that excites each hair cell of the cochlea—and the appropriate stimulus for hair cells of the vestibular organs as well. This deflection is transduced into a receptor potential (see Chapter 31). The receptor potentials of inner hair cells can be as great as 25 mV in amplitude. As expected from the cells' directional sensitivity, from their geometrical orientation in the organ of Corti, and from the hypothesized motion of the organ of Corti, an upward movement of the basilar membrane leads to depolarization of the cells, whereas a downward deflection elicits hyperpolarization (Figure 30-6).

As a result of the tonotopic arrangement of the basilar membrane, every hair cell is most sensitive to stimulation at a specific frequency. On average, successive inner hair cells differ in characteristic frequency by about 0.2%; adjacent piano strings, in comparison, are tuned to frequencies some 6% apart. A cochlear hair cell is also sensitive to a limited range of frequencies both higher and lower than its characteristic frequency. This follows from the fact that the traveling wave evoked even by a pure sinusoidal stimulus spreads appreciably along the basilar membrane. When a stimulus tone is presented at a pitch lower than the characteristic frequency of a specific cell, the traveling wave passes that cell and peaks somewhat farther up the cochlear spiral. A higher-pitched tone, on the other hand, causes a traveling wave that crests below the cell. Nevertheless, in either instance, the basilar membrane undergoes some motion at the cell's site, so that the cell responds to the stimulus.

The frequency sensitivity of a hair cell may be displayed as a tuning curve. To construct a tuning curve, a cell is stimulated repeatedly with pure-tone stimuli at numerous frequencies below, at, and above its characteristic frequency. For each frequency, the intensity of stimulation is adjusted until the response reaches a predefined criterion level. An investigator might, for example, ask what stimulus intensity is necessary at each frequency to produce a receptor potential 1 mV in peak-to-peak magnitude. The tuning curve is then a graph of sound intensity, presented logarithmically in decibels of sound-pressure level, against stimulus frequency.

The tuning curve for an inner hair cell is characteristically V-shaped (Figure 30-7). The curve's tip, which represents the frequency at which the criterion response is achieved with the stimulus of lowest intensity, corresponds to the cell's characteristic frequency. Sounds of greater or lesser frequency require higher intensity to excite the cell to the criterion response. As a consequence of the traveling wave's shape, the slope of a tuning curve is steeper on its high-frequency flank than on its low-frequency flank.

Sound Energy Is Mechanically Amplified in the Cochlea

Although the task is complex, the hydrodynamic and mechanical properties of the cochlea can be represented in a mathematical model of basilar-membrane motion. Modeling studies show that the inner ear faces an obstacle to efficient operation: A large portion of the energy in an acoustical stimulus must go into overcoming the damping effects of cochlear fluids on basilar-membrane motion, rather than into excitation of hair cells, which would be more efficient. The cochlea nevertheless works extraordinarily well. Most investigators agree that the sensitivity of the cochlea is too great, and auditory frequency selectivity too sharp, to result solely from the inner ear's passive mechanical properties. Thus the cochlea must have some active means of amplifying sound energy.

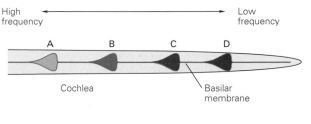

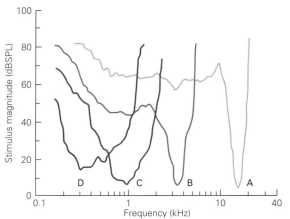

Figure 30-7 Tuning curves for cochlear hair cells. To construct a curve, the experimenter presents sound at each frequency at increasing amplitudes until the cell produces a criterion response, here 1 mV. The curve thus reflects the threshold of the cell for stimulation at a range of frequencies. Each cell is most sensitive to a specific frequency, its characteristic (or best) frequency. The threshold rises briskly (sensitivity falls abruptly) as the stimulus frequency is raised or lowered. (From Pickles 1988.)

One indication that amplification occurs in the cochlea comes from measurements with sensitive laser interferometers of the basilar membrane's movements. When a preparation is stimulated with low-intensity sound, the motion of the membrane is found to be highly frequency-selective. As the sound intensity is increased, however, the membrane's sensitivity declines precipitously and its tuning becomes less sharp: the sensitivity of basilar-membrane motion to 80 dB stimulation is less than 1% that for 10 dB excitation. Interestingly, the sensitivity expected on the basis of modeling studies corresponds to that observed with high-intensity stimuli. These results suggest that the motion of the basilar membrane is augmented over 100-fold during low-intensity stimulation but that this effect diminishes progressively as the stimulus grows in strength.

In addition to the circumstantial evidence that the inner ear's performance requires amplification, two observations support the idea that the cochlea contains a

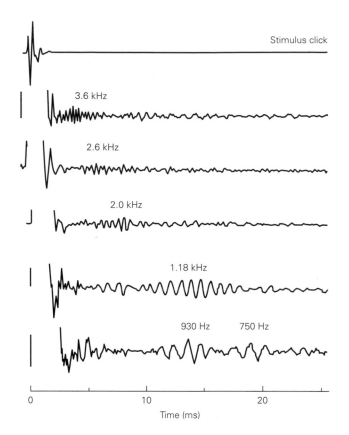

Figure 30-8 Evoked otoacoustical emissions are evidence for a cochlear amplifier. Mechanical amplification of vibrations within the cochlea is an active process that enhances the sensitivity of hearing (see Figure 30-9). The records here show the otoacoustical emissions in the ears of five subjects. For each subject, a brief click was played into an ear through a miniature speaker. A few milliseconds later a tiny microphone in the external auditory meatus detected one or more bursts of sound emission from the ear. (From Wilson 1980.)

tinuously emit one or more pure tones. Although these sounds are generally too faint to be directly audible by others, the phenomenon has been reported by physicians who noted sounds emanating from the ears of newborns! There is no reason to believe that spontaneous otoacoustical emissions are a necessary part of the transduction process. Instead, it is probable that an amplificatory process of the cochlea ordinarily serves to counter the viscous damping effects of cochlear fluids upon the basilar membrane. Just as a public address system howls when its gain is excessive, the ear emits sound when the cochlear amplifier is overly active.

What is the source of evoked and spontaneous otoacoustical emissions, and presumably of cochlear amplification as well? Several lines of evidence implicate outer hair cells as the elements that enhance cochlear sensitivity and frequency selectivity and hence as the energy sources for amplification. The outer hair cells make only token projections via afferent fibers to the central nervous system. However, they receive extensive efferent innervation, whose activation decreases cochlear sensitivity and frequency discrimination. Pharmacological ablation of outer hair cells with selectively ototoxic drugs degrades the ear's responsiveness still more profoundly.

When stimulated electrically, an isolated outer hair cell displays motility: The cell body shortens when depolarized and elongates when hyperpolarized (Figure 30-9). The energy for these movements is drawn from the experimentally imposed electrical field, rather than from hydrolysis of an energy-rich substrate such as ATP. It therefore seems possible that cochlear amplification results when outer hair cells transduce mechanical stimulation of their hair bundles into receptor potentials. Motion of the cell body in response to changes in cell membrane potential may augment basilar-membrane motion.

Although an outer hair cell can flinch under the influence of electrical stimulation in vitro, whether this motion constitutes the only motor for cochlear tuning and otoacoustical emissions remains uncertain. Because sharp tuning, high sensitivity, and otoacoustical emissions are also observed in animals that lack outer hair cells, another active process must complement motion of the outer hair cells. It is possible that hair bundles, in addition to receiving stimuli, are also mechanically active. Hair bundles have been shown to make back-and-forth movements and to exert pulsatile forces against stimulus probes; these bundles contain a form of myosin that might serve as a motor molecule for active movement. It is unknown, however, whether hair bundles can generate forces at the very high frequencies at which sharp frequency selectivity and otoacoustical emissions are observed in the mammalian cochlea.

mechanical amplifier. First, after stimulating a normal human ear with a click, an experimenter can measure the subsequent emission of one to several pulses of sound from that ear. Each pulse includes sound in a restricted frequency band. High-frequency sounds are emitted with the smallest latency, about 5 ms, while low-frequency emissions occur after a delay as great as 20 ms (Figure 30-8). These so-called *evoked otoacoustical emissions* are not simply acoustical echoes; they represent the emission of mechanical energy by the cochlea, triggered by acoustical stimulation.

A second, more compelling manifestation of the cochlea's active amplification is spontaneous otoacoustical emission. If a suitably sensitive microphone is used to measure sound pressure in the ear canals of subjects in a quiet environment, most human ears con-

Neural Processing of Auditory Information

Ganglion Cells Innervate Cochlear Hair Cells

Information flows from cochlear hair cells to neurons whose cell bodies lie in the cochlear ganglion. Because this ganglion follows a spiral course within the bony core (*modiolus*) of the cochlear spiral, it is also called the *spiral ganglion*. About 30,000 ganglion cells innervate the hair cells of each inner ear. The morphological specialization at the hair cell's afferent synaptic contact indicates that transmission between inner hair cells and neurons is chemical (see Chapter 31). In species that have been examined experimentally, the synaptic transmitter glutamate is released in a quantal manner.

The pattern of afferent innervation in the human cochlea emphasizes the functional distinction between inner and outer hair cells. At least 90% of the cochlear ganglion cells terminate on inner hair cells (Figure 30-10). Each axon innervates only a single hair cell, but each inner hair cell directs its output to several nerve fibers, on average nearly 10. This arrangement has three important consequences. First, the neural information from which hearing arises originates almost entirely at inner hair cells, which dominate the input to cochlear ganglion cells. Second, the output of each inner hair cell is sampled by many nerve fibers, which independently encode information about the frequency and intensity of sound. Each hair cell therefore forwards information of somewhat differing nature to the brain along separate axons. Finally, at any point along the cochlear spiral, or at any position within the spiral ganglion, neurons respond best to stimulation at the characteristic frequency of the contiguous hair cells. The tonotopic organization of the auditory neural pathways thus begins at the earliest possible site, immediately postsynaptic to inner hair cells.

Relatively few cochlear ganglion cells innervate the outer hair cells, and each such ganglion cell extends branching terminals to numerous outer hair cells. Although the ganglion cells that innervate outer hair cells are known to extend axons into the central nervous system, these neurons are so few that it is not certain whether their projections contribute significantly to the analysis of sound.

The pattern of efferent innervation of cochlear hair cells is complementary to that of afferent innervation. Inner hair cells receive sparse efferent innervation; just beneath inner hair cells, however, are extensive synaptic contacts between efferent axonal terminals and the endings of afferent nerve fibers. Outer hair cells, by contrast, have extensive connections with efferent nerves on their basolateral surfaces. Each outer hair cell bears

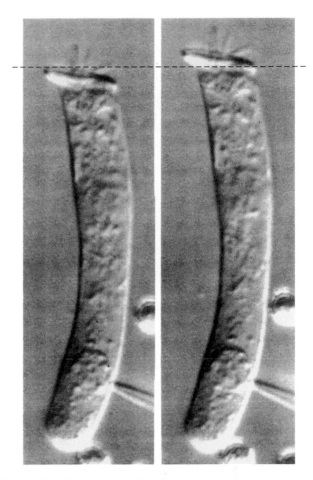

Figure 30-9 Cochlear amplification is mediated by movement of hair cells. When this isolated outer hair cell is depolarized by the electrode at its base, its cell body shortens (**left**). Hyperpolarization, on the other hand, causes the cell to lengthen (**right**). The oscillatory motions of outer hair cells may provide the mechanical energy that amplifies basilar-membrane motion and thus enhances the sensitivity of human hearing. (From Holley and Ashmore 1988.)

several efferent terminals, which largely fill the space between the cell's base and the phalangeal cell.

Cochlear Nerve Fibers Encode Stimulus Frequency and Intensity

The acoustical sensitivity of axons in the cochlear nerve mirrors the innervation pattern of spiral ganglion cells. Each axon is most responsive to stimulation at a particular frequency of sound, its characteristic frequency. Stimuli of lower or higher frequency also evoke responses, but only when presented at greater intensities. An axon's responsiveness may be characterized by a

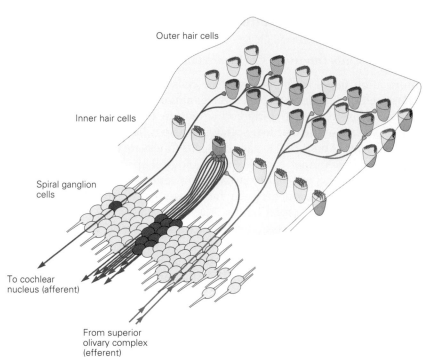

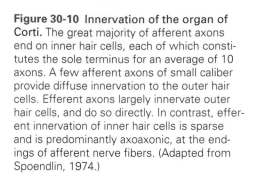

Figure 30-10 Innervation of the organ of Corti. The great majority of afferent axons end on inner hair cells, each of which constitutes the sole terminus for an average of 10 axons. A few afferent axons of small caliber provide diffuse innervation to the outer hair cells. Efferent axons largely innervate outer hair cells, and do so directly. In contrast, efferent innervation of inner hair cells is sparse and is predominantly axoaxonic, at the endings of afferent nerve fibers. (Adapted from Spoendlin, 1974.)

tuning curve, which, like the curves for basilar-membrane motion or hair-cell sensitivity, is a V-shaped relation. The tuning curves for nerve fibers of various characteristic frequencies resemble one another but are shifted along the abscissa so that their characteristic frequencies occur at a range of positions corresponding to the variety of frequencies that we can hear.

The relation between sound-pressure level and firing rate in each fiber of the cochlear nerve is approximately linear. Because of the relation between level and sound pressure, this relation implies that sound pressure is logarithmically encoded by neuronal activity. Very loud sounds saturate a neuron's response; because an action potential and the subsequent refractory period last about 1 ms, the greatest sustainable firing rate is near 500 spikes per second. Even among nerve fibers of the same characteristic frequency, the threshold of responsiveness varies from axon to axon.

The most sensitive nerve fibers, those whose response thresholds extend down to approximately 0 dB SPL, characteristically have high rates of spontaneous activity and produce saturating responses for stimulation at moderate intensities, about 40 dB SPL. At the opposite extreme, some afferent fibers display less spontaneous activity and much higher thresholds but give graded responses to intensities of stimulation in excess of 100 dB SPL. Activity patterns of most fibers range between these extremes.

Differences in neuronal responsiveness originate at the synapses between inner hair cells and afferent nerve fibers. Nerve terminals on the surface of a hair cell nearest the axis of the cochlear spiral belong to the afferent neurons of lowest sensitivity and spontaneous activity. The terminals on a hair cell's opposite side, by contrast, belong to the most sensitive afferent neurons. The multiple innervation of each inner hair cell is therefore not completely redundant. Instead, because of systematic differences in the rate of transmitter release or in postsynaptic responsiveness (or both), the output from a given hair cell is directed into several parallel channels of differing sensitivity and dynamic range.

The firing pattern of fibers in the eighth cranial nerve has both phasic and tonic components. If a tone is presented for a few seconds, brisk firing occurs at the onset of the stimulus. As adaptation occurs, however, the firing rate declines to a plateau level over a few tens of milliseconds. When stimulation ceases, there is usually a transitory cessation of activity, with a similar time course before resumption of the spontaneous firing rate (Figure 30-11).

When a periodic stimulus such as a pure tone is presented, the firing pattern of an eighth-nerve fiber encodes information about the periodicity of the stimulus. If a relatively low-frequency tone is sounded at a moderate intensity, for example, a given nerve fiber might fire one spike during each cycle of stimulation. The phase of firing is also stereotyped: Each action potential might occur, for example, during the compressive phase of the stimulus. As the stimulus frequency rises, stimuli eventually become too rapid for the nerve fiber, whose action potentials can no longer follow the stimulus on a cycle-by-cycle basis. Up to a frequency in excess of 4 kHz, however, phase-locking nonetheless persists; a fiber may fire only every few cycles of the stimulus, but its firing continues to occur at a particular phase in the stimulus cycle.

Periodicity in neuronal firing enhances the transmission of information about the stimulus frequency. Any specific, pure-tone stimulus of sufficient intensity will evoke firing in numerous auditory-nerve fibers. Those fibers whose characteristic frequency coincides with the frequency of the stimulus will begin to respond at the lowest stimulus intensity and will respond most briskly for stimuli of moderate intensity. Other nerve fibers of nearby characteristic frequencies will also respond, although somewhat less vigorously. Regardless of their characteristic frequencies, however, all the responsive fibers will display phase locking; each will tend to fire during a particular part of the stimulus cycle.

The central nervous system can therefore gain information about stimulus frequency in two ways. First, there is a *place code;* the fibers are arrayed in a tonotopic map such that position is related to characteristic frequency. Second, there is a *frequency code;* the fibers fire at a rate reflecting the frequency of the stimulus. Frequency coding is of particular importance when sound is loud enough to saturate the neuronal firing rate. Although fibers of many characteristic frequencies respond to such a stimulus, each will provide information about the stimulus frequency in its temporal firing pattern.

Sound Processing Begins in the Cochlear Nuclei

Axons in the cochlear component of the eighth cranial nerve terminate in the cochlear nuclear complex, which lies at the medullo-pontine junction, medial to the inferior cerebellar peduncle (Figure 30-12). There are three major components to this structure: the dorsal cochlear nucleus and the anteroventral and posteroventral cochlear nuclei. Each auditory nerve fiber branches as it enters the brain stem. The ascending branch terminates in the anteroventral cochlear nucleus, while the descending branch innervates both the posteroventral and dorsal cochlear nuclei. Each of the three cochlear nuclei is tonotopically organized; cells with progressively higher characteristic frequencies are arrayed in an orderly progression along one axis of the structure (Figure 30-13).

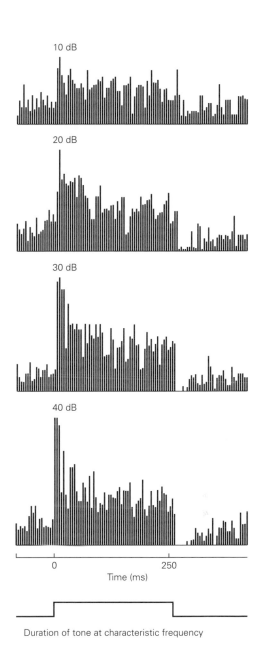

Figure 30-11 The firing pattern in auditory nerve fibers has phasic and tonic components. An auditory nerve fiber was stimulated with tone bursts at about 5000 kHz (the characteristic frequency of the cell) lasting approximately 250 ms. The stimulus was followed by a quiet period, then was repeated, over a period of 2 min. Histograms show the average response patterns of the fiber to tone bursts as a function of stimulus level. The entire sample period is divided into a number of small time units, or bins, and the number of spikes occurring in each bin is displayed. There is an initial, phasic increase in firing correlated with the onset of the stimulus. Following adaptation, discharge continues during the remainder of the stimulus; a decrease in activity follows termination. This pattern is evident when the stimulus is more than 20 dB above threshold. There is a gradual return to baseline activity during the interstimulus interval. (Adapted from Kiang 1965.)

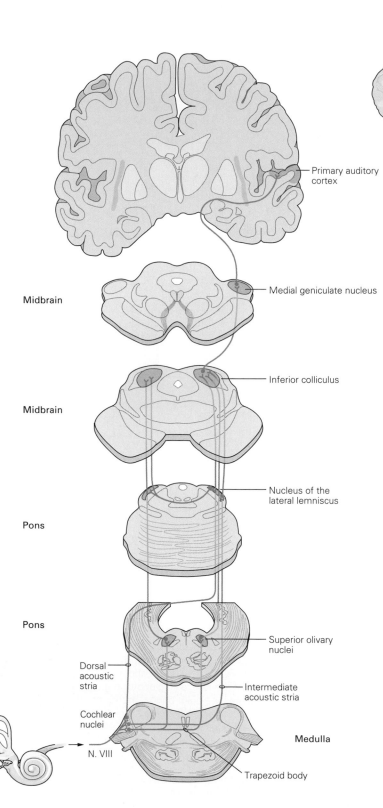

Midbrain

Primary auditory cortex

Medial geniculate nucleus

Inferior colliculus

Midbrain

Nucleus of the lateral lemniscus

Pons

Pons

Superior olivary nuclei

Dorsal acoustic stria

Intermediate acoustic stria

Cochlear nuclei

Medulla

N. VIII

Trapezoid body

Figure 30-12 The central auditory pathways extend from the cochlear nucleus to the auditory cortex. Postsynaptic neurons in the cochlear nucleus send their axons to other centers in the brain via three main pathways: the dorsal acoustic stria, the intermediate acoustic stria, and the trapezoid body. The first binaural interactions occur in the superior olivary nucleus, which receives input via the trapezoid body. In particular, the medial and lateral divisions of the superior olivary nucleus are involved in the localization of sounds in space. Postsynaptic axons from the superior olivary nucleus, along with axons from the cochlear nuclei, project to the inferior colliculus in the midbrain via the lateral lemniscus. Each lateral lemniscus contains axons relaying input from both ears. Cells in the colliculus send their axons to the medial geniculate nucleus of the thalamus. The geniculate axons terminate in the primary auditory cortex (Brodmann's areas 41 and 42), a part of the superior temporal gyrus. (Adapted from Brodal 1981.)

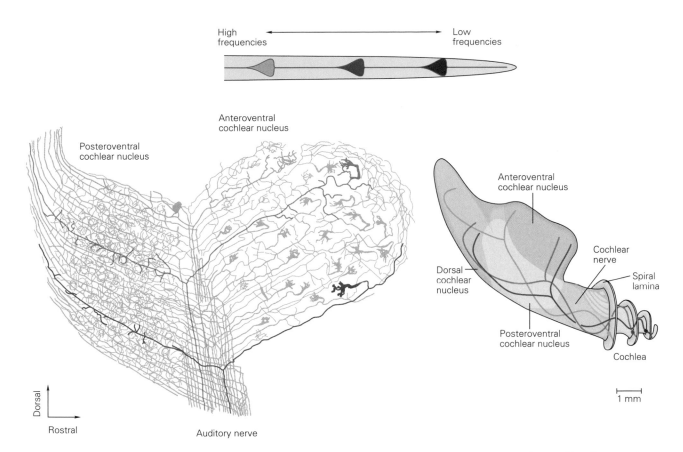

Figure 30-13 The representation of stimulus frequency in the three divisions of the cochlear nucleus. Stimulation with three frequencies of sound vibrates the basilar membrane at three positions (**top**), exciting distinct populations of afferent nerve fibers (**right**, showing three fibers). The fibers project to the components of the cochlear nucleus in an orderly pattern (**left**, showing three fibers).

The cochlear nuclei contain neurons of several types identified by their dendritic configurations. By injecting cells with dyes after characterization of their electrical properties, investigators can correlate particular cell types with specific functions. The ventral cochlear nuclei, for example, contain two major neuronal types. The *stellate cell*, which has several relatively symmetrical dendrites, responds to the injection of depolarizing current with a train of regularly spaced action potentials (Figure 30-14). This behavior identifies stellate cells as the origin of *chopper* responses to auditory inputs. Chopper cells fire at very regular rates despite noise and slight variations in stimulus frequency. Because each cell responds at a characteristic frequency, the ensemble of stellate cells encodes the frequencies present in a given auditory input.

Bushy cells of the ventral cochlear nuclei are so named because each has a single, stout, modestly branched primary dendrite that is adorned with numer-

ous fine branchlets (Figure 30-14). A bushy cell receives one or a few massive axonal terminals, the end-bulbs, whose finger-like branches encircle the entire soma. Electrical stimulation of a bushy cell characteristically elicits only one action potential. Consistent with this pattern of response, bushy cells are thought to respond to auditory stimulation by firing only at a sound's onset. Such cells provide accurate information about the timing of acoustical stimuli, which is valuable for locating sound sources along the azimuthal (horizontal) axis.

The dorsal cochlear nucleus is organized in layers, much like the cerebellar cortex. This similarity is not coincidental, for the neurons of this nucleus originate from the same primordia as cerebellar cells. Fusiform cells in the dorsal nucleus exhibit excitatory or inhibitory responses to a broad range of stimulus frequencies. Through their spatial firing pattern, these cells are thought to participate in locating of sound sources along the elevational (vertical) axis. Another type of

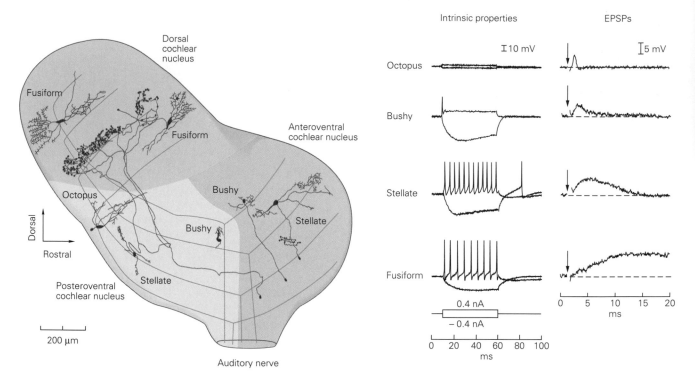

Figure 30-14 Types of cells in the cochlear nuclei and their responses to brief current pulses. A stellate cell has several dendrites that receive numerous small synaptic terminals. The responses of a stellate cell to brief depolarizing and hyperpolarizing current pulses are shown. Depolarizing pulses cause the cell to fire repetitively at a fixed frequency, the so-called *chopper response.* A bushy cell has a single dendritic trunk that re-

ceives a few very large synaptic terminals called end bulbs that surround the cell. Bushy cells respond to a depolarizing current pulse with a single action potential and are therefore thought to signal the onset or timing of a sound. Bushy cells respond like stellate cells to hyperpolarizing currents. (Adapted from Oertel et al. 1988.)

neuron, the tuberculoventral cell, provides a delayed inhibitory output that suppresses the responses of neurons in the ventral cochlear nuclei to echoes.

Relay Nuclei in the Brain Stem Mediate Localization of Sound Sources

The axons of the various cell types in the cochlear nuclei project to several nuclei at more rostral levels of the brain stem. Because of the complexity of the auditory connections in the brain stem, however, we shall restrict our attention to a few major pathways. Three important general principles emerge from considering these connections. First, acoustical information is processed in parallel pathways, each of which is dedicated to the analysis of a particular feature of auditory information. Second, the various cell types of the cochlear nuclei project to specific relay nuclei, so that the separation of information streams commences within the cochlear nuclei. Finally, there is extensive interaction between

auditory structures on the two sides of the brain stem. Accordingly, for optimal excitation many neurons respond to stimulation of either ear, and some require particular patterns of stimulation through both ears. As a consequence, unilateral lesions along the auditory pathways infrequently produce hearing deficits confined to one ear.

The anteroventral cochlear nucleus contributes to the most prominent output, the *trapezoid body* (or ventral acoustical stria), which extends at the level of the pons to three nuclei of the *superior olivary complex:* the lateral and medial superior olives and the nucleus of the trapezoid body (see Figure 30-12). The posteroventral cochlear nucleus also contributes axons to the trapezoid body and provides outflow to the lateral superior olive via the intermediate acoustical stria. Neurons in the dorsal cochlear nucleus do not project to the pontine level; we shall describe the projections of these cells later.

The *medial superior olive* performs a specific function in a readily intelligible way. The ability to localize sound sources along the azimuthal axis stems in part from the processing of information about auditory delays. The sound from a source directly to one side of the head reaches the nearer ear before the farther. Sound travels somewhat slower across a surface, such as the human head, than through free space; as a consequence, the maximal delay in the arrival of sound at the two ears is about 700 µs. The closer a sound source is to the mid-sagittal plane, the shorter the interaural delay; a source in the midplane excites the two ears at the same time.

Thanks to the activity of the medial superior olive, humans can distinguish interaural delays as small as 10 µs and hence locate sound sources with an accuracy of a few degrees. This temporal discrimination does not depend upon a complex computation but makes use of the delay inherent in signaling by means of action potentials. A sound arriving at one ear is transduced by hair cells, elicits firing by fibers of cranial nerve VIII, and evokes spikes in the axons that project from the cochlear nuclei to the medial superior olive. The same sound initiates a similar series of events when it then reaches the opposite ear. In the medial superior olive the axonal terminals from neurons in the contralateral anteroventral cochlear nucleus extend across one surface of the olive. As the action potentials evoked by acoustical stimulation progress across this target nucleus, they evoke excitatory synaptic potentials in successive cells. Excitation from either ear alone is insufficient to bring a neuron in the medial superior olive to threshold. For neurons at some particular position in this nucleus, a given delay in sound stimulation of one ear is exactly counterbalanced by the delay in conduction of an action potential from the opposite side. Those cells will therefore receive simultaneous excitatory inputs from both ears and will be excited to threshold (Figure 30-15). The array of cells in the medial superior olive therefore represents a continuous gradation of interaural time differences: The nucleus contains a map of sound-source location along the azimuth.

The *lateral superior olive* is also involved in the localization of sound sources but employs intensity cues to calculate where a sound originated. Because of the head's sound-absorptive properties, a sound reaching the ear nearer its source is somewhat louder than that traveling to the opposite ear. The lateral superior olive receives inputs from both cochlear nuclei; ipsilateral projections are received directly, whereas contralateral inputs are relayed through the nucleus of the trapezoid body. The two inputs are generally antagonistic in effect. A given neuron in the lateral superior olive responds best when the intensity of a stimulus sound reaching one side of the body exceeds that on the opposite side by a particular amount. The nucleus is tono-

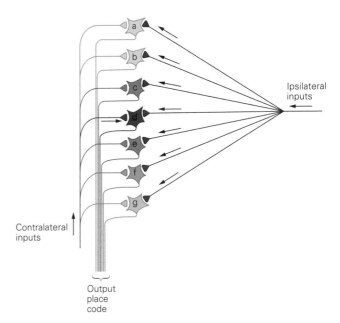

Figure 30-15 Model of neural circuits for measuring and encoding interaural time differences. Any of the binaural neurons (a–g) fires maximally when its ipsilateral and contralateral inputs arrive simultaneously. Each neuron thus serves as a coincidence detector. In the model, delays in signal transmission are a function of the variable lengths of the incoming axons from the contralateral cochlear nucleus. The length of the axonal path from the contralateral nucleus to the binaural neurons increases systematically along the array. Only the place of a neuron in the array determines the interaural time difference to which the neuron responds maximally. If sound were to arrive at the two ears simultaneously, neuron d in the array would be excited by coincident inputs. If sound to the contralateral ear were delayed, neurons e, f, or g would be excited depending on the extent of the delay. The output axons project to higher centers in the brain. (Adapted from Carr and Konishi 1988.)

topically organized as well, so the pattern of neuronal activity represents the intensity differences between the two ears throughout the range of audible frequencies.

Thus, two types of information are used to localize sounds in space. In a sense the two are complementary. Interaural time differences are most striking for relatively low-frequency sounds. Interaural intensity cues are most important for high-frequency stimuli, because the head absorbs short-wavelength sounds better than long-wavelength sounds. The frequency responses of the superior olivary nuclei reflect these differences. The medial superior olive includes many neurons responsive to low-frequency inputs, while the cells of the lateral superior olive are most sensitive to high-frequency stimuli.

The axons from the superior olivary complex constitute the principal component of the *lateral lemniscus*, a

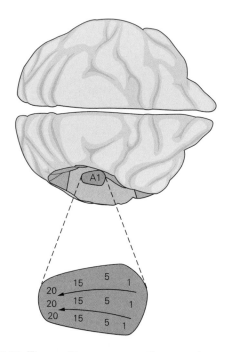

Figure 30-16 The auditory areas on the superior surface of the temporal cortex of the monkey. Neurons in the primary auditory area (A1) are arrayed in a tonotopic map according to their characteristic frequencies, which are expressed in kilohertz (κHz). This area is girdled by higher-order auditory areas whose specific functions have not yet been elucidated; many of these areas are also organized tonotopically. (From Merzenich and Brugge 1973.)

prominent tract that extends to the midbrain. The lateral lemniscus also includes the axons of cells in the contralateral dorsal cochlear nucleus which exit the nucleus as the dorsal accoustical stria. Some axons in the lateral lemniscus terminate in the nucleus of the lateral lemniscus but most extend more rostrally to the inferior colliculus in the midbrain (see Figure 30-12).

The *inferior colliculus* is divisible into two major components. The dorsal part has four prominent layers of neurons, which receive both auditory and somatosensory inputs. The functional significance of this region remains uncertain. Beneath the dorsal layers lies the central nucleus, surrounded by several additional clusters of neurons, the paracentral nuclei. The cell bodies in the central nucleus are arrayed in numerous layers. Cells within each layer exhibit similar characteristic frequencies, so the tonotopic map in this nucleus extends orthogonal to the layers. Both the projections to the central nucleus and the physiological properties of its neurons indicate that this structure is of extraordinary complex-

ity. Each layer of neurons receives inputs from each of the various nuclei whose projections constitute the lateral lemniscus. The inputs from each nucleus are not distributed uniformly throughout the layers but form several patches in each layer.

Because it contains many neurons sensitive to interaural timing or intensity differences, the inferior colliculus is apparently involved in sound localization. This role is well established in the barn owl, in which the homolog of the inferior colliculus (the lateral dorsal mesencephalic nucleus) has been extensively investigated. Barn owls are nocturnal predators whose capacity to localize sounds is so acute as to permit successful hunting in total darkness. Cells in the mesencephalic nucleus are organized in a two-dimensional map of sound sources in space. Differences in interaural sound intensity and especially interaural time delays are interpreted such that each point upon the nuclear surface represents a specific sound-source location in both azimuth and elevation.

The *medial geniculate nucleus* constitutes the thalamic relay of the auditory system (see Figure 30-12). This nuclear complex comprises at least three subdivisions, of which the principal (ventral or lateral) nucleus is the best understood. Neurons in the central nucleus of the inferior colliculus project to the principal nucleus of the medial geniculate nucleus by way of the brachium of the inferior colliculus. The remaining components of the medial geniculate nucleus are multimodal, receiving somatosensory and visual inputs in addition to auditory projections.

Like the earlier stages in auditory processing, the principal nucleus of the medial geniculate nucleus is organized tonotopically. Here neurons with the same characteristic frequency are arrayed in one layer, so that the nucleus consists of a stack of neuronal laminae that represent successive stimulus frequencies. The physiological properties of neurons within the principal nucleus also resemble those in antecedent stages of processing. Most cells are sharply tuned to specific stimulus frequencies, and most are responsive to stimulation through either ear. Sensitivity to interaural time or intensity difference, a property first elaborated in the inferior colliculus, is retained by many neurons in the principal nucleus.

Auditory Information Is Processed in Multiple Areas of the Cerebral Cortex

The ascending auditory pathway terminates in the cerebral cortex, where several distinct auditory areas occur on the dorsal surface of the temporal lobe. The most prominent projection, from the principal nucleus of the medial geniculate nucleus, extends to the primary auditory cortex (area A1, or Brodmann's areas 41 and 42) on the transverse gyrus of Heschl (see Figure 30-16). This cytoarchitectonically distinct region contains a tonotopic representation of characteristic frequencies; neurons tuned to low frequencies occur at the rostral end of the area, while the caudal region includes cells responsive to high frequencies. In its use of parallel processing and conformal mapping, the auditory cortex thus resembles the somatosensory and visual cortices.

Although most neurons in the primary auditory cortex are responsive to stimulation through either ear, their sensitivities are not identical. Instead, the cortex is divided into alternating zones of two types. In half of these strips, known as *summation columns*, neurons are excited by stimulation of either ear (EE cells), though the contralateral input is usually stronger than the ipsilateral contribution. The alternating cortical bands, or *suppression columns*, contain neurons that are excited by a unilateral input but inhibited by stimulation of the opposite ear (EI cells). Because the summation and suppression columns extend at right angles to the axis of tonotopic mapping, the primary auditory cortex is partitioned into columns responsive to every audible frequency and to each type of interaural interaction.

The primary auditory area is surrounded by several distinct regions involved with the elaboration of particular types of auditory information. Some mammals have at least nine such regions, most of which are organized in tonotopic maps of stimulus frequency. It is highly probable that the human auditory cortex itself is subdivided into numerous functional areas, but the positions and roles of such areas remain to be determined.

For humans, the most important aspect of hearing is its role in processing language. Although we know much about the neural processing of sound in general, we know relatively little about how speech sounds are processed: There are no experimental animals in which language processing can be investigated at the neural level. Recently developed techniques for imaging of neural activity, especially positron emission tomography (PET) and functional magnetic resonance imaging (fMRI), are now providing a growing understanding of the localization of cortical areas concerned with language (see Chapter 59). For the most part, however, our limited appreciation of speech processing rests upon analogies to the mechanisms studied in the brains of animals that employ complex auditory signals.

Insectivorous bats provide the best experimental system for investigating the cortical analysis of sound. These animals find their prey almost entirely through echolocation, by emitting sounds that are then reflected

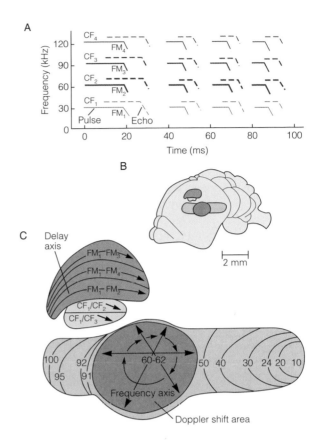

Figure 30-17 Processing of auditory information in the bat's cerebral cortex.

A. Schematized sonogram of the mustached bat's orientation sounds (**solid**) and the Doppler-shifted echoes (**dashed**). Each orientation sound is also called a pulse. The four harmonics of both the orientation sound and the echo each contain a long constant-frequency component (**CF**) and a short frequency modulated component (**FM**). The amplitudes of the four harmonics in the orientation sound differ. The second harmonic is most intense as indicated by the darker lines.

B. This view of the cerebral hemisphere of the mustached bat shows the two functional areas within the auditory cortex: the frequency modulation area, where the range of a target is computed (**brown**), and the constant frequency area, where the velocity of a target is computed (**gold**).

C. Representation of auditory modalities in the bat's cerebral cortex. Although the primary auditory cortex processes information about the full range of frequencies to which a bat can respond, a large portion (Doppler shift area) represents the narrow range of 60–62 kHz that encompasses the frequencies of Doppler-shifted sounds reflected from prey. In the FM-FM area comparison of the delays between emitted sonar pulses and their reflections permits the calculation of target range. This area makes use of information about the frequency-modulated component of a bat's chirp. In the CF/CF area analysis of the Doppler shifts associated with the constant-frequency component of sonar emission leads to an estimate of target velocity.

by flying insects. Most bats emit two types of sounds, and the bat's auditory cortex possesses distinct areas devoted to the processing of echoes elicited by the two emission components. *Constant-frequency emissions* are analogous to human vowel sounds, whose frequency components are relatively stable for tens to hundreds of milliseconds. *Frequency-modulated emissions,* on the other hand, resemble human consonant sounds in their rapid changes of frequency (Figure 30-17A).

Constant-frequency emissions are used to determine an animal's speed with respect to its prey. When a flying bat approaches an insect, the sounds reflected from the target are Doppler-shifted to a frequency higher than that at which they were emitted. A receding insect, on the other hand, yields reflections of lowered frequency. To process these signals, neurons in the constant-frequency region of the cortex are sharply tuned to a narrow range of frequencies near the emission frequency. The cortical surface bears a tonotopic map of the cells' characteristic frequencies and hence of target speed; the orthogonal coordinate represents sound intensity (Figure 30-17C).

Frequency-modulated emissions are used to determine the distance to a target. A bat ascertains target range by measuring the interval between sound emission and the capture of reflected sound; it then calculates the distance neurally on the basis of the relatively constant speed of sound. The cortical area dedicated to target ranging is divided into columns, each of which is responsive to a particular combination of stimulus frequencies and delays. Each neuron in this area responds to a particular combination of frequency-modulated sounds separated by a specific temporal delay (Figure 30-17C).

Sensorineural Hearing Loss Is Common But Can Often Be Overcome

Most deafness, whether mild or profound, falls into the category of *sensorineural hearing loss,* often mistermed nerve deafness. This distinction is of considerable importance; although hearing loss can result from damage to the eighth cranial nerve, for example from an acoustic neuroma (Chapter 44), deafness primarily stems from the loss of cochlear hair cells. Like neurons, the 16,000 hair cells in each human cochlea must last a lifetime; they are not replaced by cell division. Experiments on amphibians and birds have recently demonstrated that supporting cells can be induced to divide and their progeny to produce new hair cells; efforts are now being made to replenish mammalian hair cells as well. Until we understand how hair cells can be restored to the or-

gan of Corti, however, we must cope with hearing losses, the prevalence of which is growing in our aging population and increasingly noisy environment.

Deafness can be devastating. Children who lack hearing as a result of genetic conditions and pre- or perinatal infections are often deprived of the normal avenue to the development of speech, and of reading and writing as well. It is for this reason that a modern pediatric examination must include an assessment of hearing; many children thought to be cognitively impaired are found instead to be hard of hearing, and their intellectual development resumes its normal course when this problem is corrected. For the elderly, hearing loss can result in a painful and protracted estrangement from family, friends, and colleagues.

For those of intermediate years, acute hearing loss exacts an enormous price for two principal reasons. First, hearing plays an important, but often overlooked, role in our psychological well-being. Our daily verbal exchanges with family and colleagues, including even the less pleasant interactions, help to situate us in a social context. Abrupt loss of such intercourse leaves a person distressingly lonely and may lead to depression and even suicide. Hearing serves us in another, subtle way. Our auditory system is a remarkably efficient early-warning system. We are constantly but subconsciously informed about our environment by our hearing, which tells us, for example, when other people approach us or leave the room. Still more obviously, our aural awareness of fire alarms and the sirens of emergency vehicles can be life-saving. Deafness often leaves a person with an ominous sense of vulnerability to unheard changes in the environment.

The last few decades have brought remarkable advances in our ability to treat deafness. For the majority of patients who have significant residual hearing, hearing aids can amplify sounds to a level sufficient to activate the surviving hair cells. A modern aid is custom-tailored to compensate for each individual's hearing loss, so that the device most amplifies sounds at frequencies to which the wearer is least sensitive, while providing little or no enhancement to those that can still be heard well. To the credit of our society, the stigma formerly associated with wearing a hearing aid is gradually dissipating; using such an aid will soon be regarded as no more remarkable than wearing eyeglasses.

When most or all of a person's cochlear hair cells have degenerated, no amount of amplification can restore hearing. Through the use of a cochlear prosthesis, however, it is nonetheless possible to restore hearing by bypassing the damaged cochlea. Such a prosthesis includes an array of tiny electrodes that, when surgically implanted in the scala tympani, can electrically stimu-

A

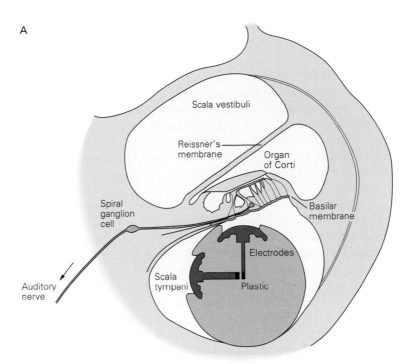

Figure 30-18 A cochlear prosthesis.

A. This cross section of the cochlear spiral shows the placement of the prosthetic electrode array. A portion of the extracellular current passed between an electrode pair is intercepted by nearby auditory nerve fibers, which are thus excited and send action potentials to the brain. (From Loeb et al. 1983.)

B. The inputs to an intracochlear electrode array form a fine cable that passes to a set of receiving antennas implanted subdermally behind the auricle. Complementary broadcasting antennas receive electrical signals from a sound processor, located for example in the subject's breast pocket, and forward them across the skin to the receiving antennas and thence to the electrode array. (From Loeb 1983.)

B

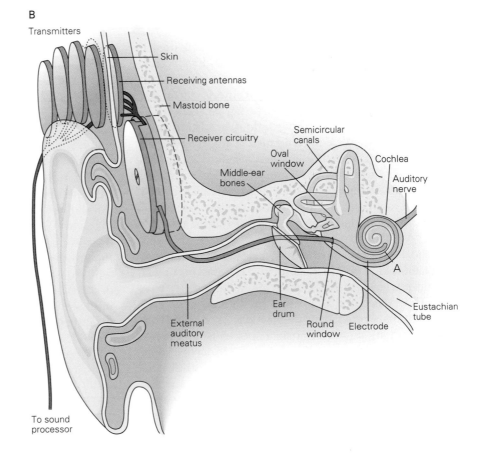

late nerve fibers at various positions along the spiral course of the cochlea (Figure 30-18). A patient wears a pocket-sized unit that picks up sounds, decomposes them into their frequency components, and forwards electronic signals representing these constituents along separate wires. These signals propagate to small antennas, usually worn on eyeglass frames, that transmit the signals transdermally to receiving antennas implanted just behind the auricle. Fine wires then bear the signals to the appropriate electrodes in the intracochlear array, whose activation excites action potentials in nearby axons.

The cochlear prosthesis takes advantage of the tonotopic representation of stimulus frequency along the cochlear spiral. Because axons innervating each segment of the cochlea are concerned with a specific, narrow range of frequencies, each electrode in a prosthesis can excite a cluster of nerve fibers of similar frequency sensitivity. The stimulated neurons then forward their outputs along the eighth cranial nerve to the central nervous system, where these signals are interpreted as a sound of the frequency represented at that position along the basilar membrane. An array of electrodes, as many as 20, can mimic a complex sound by appropriately stimulating several clusters of neurons.

Cochlear prostheses have now been implanted in about 15,000 patients worldwide. Their effectiveness varies widely from person to person. In the best instances an individual wearing a prosthesis can understand speech nearly as well as a hearing person and can even conduct telephone conversations. At the other extreme, some patients derive no benefit from prostheses, presumably because of complete degeneration of the nerve fibers near the electrode array. Most patients, however, find their prostheses of great value; even if hearing is not completely restored, the devices help in lip reading and alert patients to noises in the environment.

The other way to overcoming deafness rests not on high technology but on the efforts of generations of deaf individuals and their teachers. Sign languages have probably existed for as long as humans have spoken, and perhaps even longer. Most such languages have represented attempts to translate spoken language into a system of hand signs. Signed English, for example, provides an effective means of communication that largely obeys the rules of English speech. To the surprise of many, however, sign languages that diverge more radically from spoken languages are far more effective.

Freed from the constraint of mirroring English, American Sign Language, or ASL, has become an elegant and eloquent language in its own right. Linguists now recognize ASL as a distinct language whose range of expressiveness generally matches—and sometimes exceeds—that of spoken English.

An Overall View

Hearing, a key sense in human communication, commences with the ear's capture of sound. Mechanical energy flows through the middle ear to the cochlea, where it makes the elastic basilar membrane vibrate. An array of 16,000 hair cells detects each frequency component of a stimulus, transduces it into receptor potentials, and encodes it in the firing pattern of eighth-nerve fibers. The complex auditory pathways of the brain stem mediate certain functions, such as the localization of sound sources, and forward auditory information to the cerebral cortex. Here, several distinct areas analyze sound to detect the complex patterns characteristic of speech.

As our population ages and as our society becomes more concerned about hearing loss, physicians will increasingly confront patients and families who are experiencing the social difficulties associated with deafness. This subject is at present politically charged. On the one hand, the rapid technical improvement in cochlear prostheses leads their developers to advocate use of the devices whenever practical, including for young children. Many members of the deaf community, on the other hand, believe that widespread implantation of cochlear prostheses, particularly in children, will foster a generation of individuals whose ability to communicate is dependent upon technological support of as yet unproved durability. The extensive application of prostheses might also diminish the use of ASL and thus reverse the deaf community's remarkable recent advances. Although this debate will not soon subside, it is worthwhile to note the most positive aspect of the issue. A few decades ago there were no widely effective ways of coping with profound deafness; now there are two. Moreover, these solutions are not mutually exclusive; a deaf individual can benefit from bilinguality in spoken English, mediated through a cochlear prosthesis, and ASL.

A. J. Hudspeth

Selected Readings

Loeb GE. 1985. The functional replacement of the ear. Sci Am 252(2):104–111.

Pickles JO. 1988. *An Introduction to the Physiology of Hearing*, 2nd ed. New York: Academic.

References

Ashmore JF. 1987. A fast motile response in guinea-pig outer hair cells: the cellular basis of the cochlear amplifier. J Physiol (Lond) 388:323–347.

Brodal A. 1981. The auditory system. In *Neurological Anatomy in Relation to Clinical Medicine*, 3rd ed. New York: Oxford Univ. Press.

Carr CE, Konishi M. 1988. Axonal delay lines for time measurement in the owl's brainstem. Proc Natl Acad Sci U S A 85:8311–8315.

Griffin DR. 1958. *Listening in the Dark; The Acoustic Orientation of Bats and Men*. New Haven: Yale Univ. Press

Helmholtz HLF. [1877] 1954. *On the Sensations of Tone as a Physiological Basis for the Theory of Music*. New York: Dover.

Holley MC, Ashmore JF. 1988. On the mechanism of a high-frequency force generator in outer hair cells isolated from the guinea pig cochlea. Proc R Soc Lond B Biol Sci 232:413–429.

Kiang NY-S. 1965. *Discharge Patterns of Single Fibers in the Cat's Auditory Nerve*. Cambridge, Mass: MIT Press.

Kiang NY. 1980. Processing of speech by the auditory nervous system. J Acoust Soc Am 68:830–835.

Knudsen EI, Konishi M. 1978. A neural map of auditory space in the owl. Science 200:795–797.

Liberman MC. 1982. Single-neuron labeling in the cat auditory nerve. Science 216:1239–1241.

Loeb GE, Byers CL, Rebscher SJ, Casey DE, Fong MM, Schindler RA, Gray RF, Merzenich MM. 1983. Design and fabrication of an experimental cochlear prosthesis.

Med Biol Eng Comput 21:241–254.

Merzenich MM, Brugge JF. 1973. Representation of the cochlear partition on the superior temporal plane of the macaque monkey. Brain Res 50:275–296.

Miller JM, Towe AL. 1979. Audition: structural and acoustical properties. In T Ruch, HD Patton (eds.), *Physiology and Biophysics, Vol 1. The Brain and Neural Function*, 20th ed. pp. 339–375. Philadelphia: Saunders.

Noback CR. 1967. *The Human Nervous System: Basic Elements of Structure and Function*. New York: McGraw-Hill.

Oertel D, Wu SH, Hirsh JA. 1988. Electrical characteristics of cells and neuronal circuitry in the cochlear nuclei studied with intracellular recordings from brain slices. In GM Edelman, WE Gall, WM Cowan (eds). *Auditory Function: Neurobiological Bases of Hearing*, pp. 313–336. New York: Wiley.

Oertel D. 1991. The role of intrinsic neuronal properties in the encoding of auditory information in the cochlear nuclei. Curr Opin Neurobiol 1:221–228.

Ruggero MA. 1992. Responses to sound of the basilar membrane of the mammalian cochlea. Curr Opin Neurobiol 2:449–456.

Spoendlin H. 1974. Neuroanatomy of the cochlea. In: E Zwicker, E Terhardt (eds). *Facts and Models in Hearing*, pp. 18–32. New York: Springer-Verlag.

Suga N. 1990. Biosonar and neural computation in bats. Sci Am 262(6):60–68.

von Békésy G. 1960. *Experiments in Hearing*. EG Wever (ed, transl). New York: McGraw-Hill.

Wilson JP. 1980. Evidence for a cochlear origin for acoustic re-emissions, threshold fine structure and tonal tinnitus. Hearing Res 2:233–252.

Young ED, Sachs MB. 1979. Representation of steady-state vowels in the temporal aspects of the discharge patterns of populations of auditory-nerve fibers. J Acoust Soc Am 66:1381–1403.

31

Sensory Transduction in the Ear

FROM THE COMPLEXITY OF music to the warmth of conversation to the hubbub of adventitious noise, the richness of our aural experience depends on hair cells, the receptors of the internal ear. Similar hair cells are also responsible for our sense of equilibrium. In both contexts hair cells perform almost miraculous feats: They can measure motions of atomic dimensions and transduce stimuli ranging from static inputs to those with frequencies in the tens of kilohertz. Regardless of the type of stimulus to which it responds, a hair cell is a biological strain gauge. Mechanical stimulation opens ion channels in the cell's plasma membrane; the current flowing through these channels alters the cell's membrane potential, which in turn modulates the release of synaptic transmitter. Excited by this chemical transmitter, an af-

ferent nerve fiber contacting the hair cell fires a pattern of action potentials that encodes such features of the stimulus as its intensity, time course, and frequency.

The hair cells of the six receptor organs in the human internal ear are of similar form and function. In this chapter we describe the hair cell's structure and how the cell transduces mechanical energy into electrical signals. In the previous chapter we examined the function of the hair cells in the cochlea, the receptor organ of the auditory system. In Chapter 40 we examine the function of the hair cells in the vestibular labyrinth, the complex of five receptor organs mediating the sense of equilibrium.

Hair cells originate from surface ectoderm and retain an epithelial character. A hair cell is columnar or flask-shaped, lacking both dendrites and axons (Figure 31-1). Around its apex the hair cell is connected to nonsensory supporting cells. A special saline solution (endolymph) bathes the cell's apical aspect; this fluid is kept entirely separate from the ordinary extracellular fluid at the basolateral surface of the cell by a tight junction. Immediately below the tight junction, an intermediate junction, or *belt desmosome*, provides a strong mechanical attachment for the hair cell.

The cell's hair bundle, which serves as a receptor apparatus for mechanical stimuli, projects from the flattened apical surface of the cell (Figure 31-1). Depending upon the organ in which it occurs, a hair bundle may range in height from less than 1 μm to over 100 μm. This organelle is a cluster of 20–300 cylindrical processes, the *stereocilia*, which are arranged in a hexagonal array. Because the stereocilia vary in length continuously across the cell's surface, a hair bundle appears as a beveled

Figure 31-1 Structure of a vertebrate hair cell.

A. The epithelial character of the hair cell is evident in this drawing of the sensory epithelium from a frog's internal ear. The cylindrical hair cell is joined to the adjacent supporting cells by a junctional complex around its apical perimeter. From the cell's apical surface extends the hair bundle, the mechanically sensitive organelle. Afferent and efferent synapses occur upon the basolateral surface of the plasma membrane.

B. This scanning electron micrograph of a hair cell's apical surface reveals the hair bundle protruding about 8 μm into the endolymph. The bundle comprises some 60 stereocilia, each a cylinder with a tapered base, arranged in stepped rows of varying length. At the bundle's tall edge stands the single kinocilium, an axonemal structure with a bulbous swelling at its tip. Deflection of the hair bundle to the right, the positive stimulus direction, depolarizes the hair cell; movement in the opposite direction elicits a hyperpolarization. The hair cell is surrounded by supporting cells, whose apical aspects bear a stubble of microvilli.

A

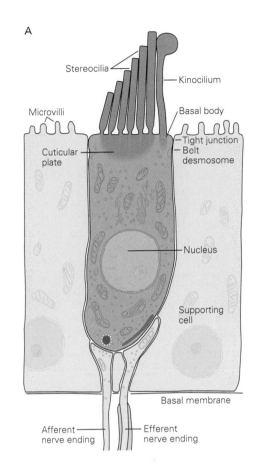

B

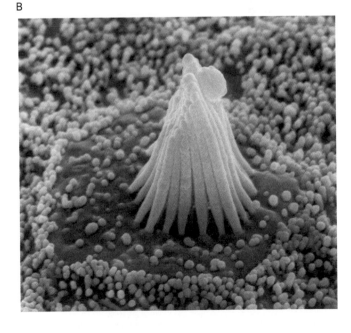

structure, like the tip of a hypodermic needle. Each stereocilium is a rigid cylinder whose cytoskeleton consists of a fascicle of actin filaments cross-linked by the protein fibrin. Cross-linking renders a stereocilium much more rigid than would be expected for a bundle of unconnected actin filaments. The core of the stereocilium is covered by a tubular sheath of plasma membrane.

Although an individual stereocilium is of constant diameter along most of its length, it tapers over the micrometer or so just above its basal insertion. As the stereocilium narrows from about 0.5 μm to roughly one-quarter that diameter, the actin filaments diminish from nearly a thousand to only a few dozen. This attenuated cluster of microfilaments constitutes a rootlet that anchors the stereocilium in the cuticular plate, a thick mesh of interlinked actin filaments lying beneath the apical membrane surface. Because the cytoskeleton of the stereocilium is thinnest at the process's base, application of a mechanical force at the stereocilium's tip causes the process to pivot around its basal insertion.

During its development every hair bundle includes at its tall edge a single true cilium, the *kinocilium*. This structure possesses at its core an axoneme, or array of nine paired microtubules, and sometimes an additional, central pair of microtubules. In organs of the vestibular labyrinth the kinocilium acts as a lever that transmits stimulus forces to the mechanically receptive stereocilia in a hair bundle. The kinocilium is not essential for mechanoelectrical transduction; transduction persists in vitro after its removal from vestibular hair cells, and kinocilia normally degenerate in the hair bundles of the cochlea.

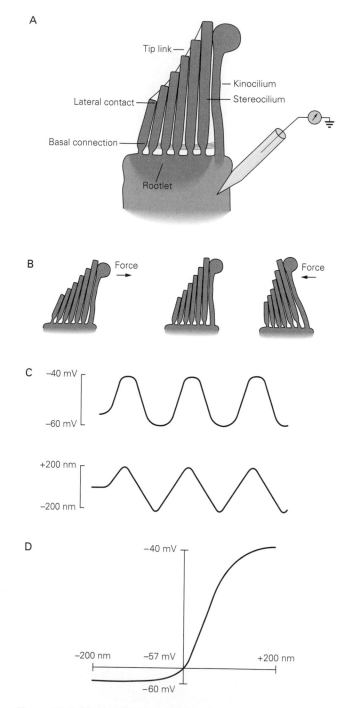

Figure 31-2 Mechanical sensitivity of a hair cell.

A. A schematic drawing of a hair cell with a recording electrode inserted into its cytoplasm.

B. Application of a mechanical force to the hair bundle deflects this elastic structure.

C. When the top of a hair bundle is displaced back and forth by a stimulus probe (**lower trace**), the opening and closing of mechanically sensitive channels produces an oscillatory receptor potential (**upper trace**).

D. The sigmoidal relation between hair-bundle deflection (abscissa) and receptor potential (ordinate) is a stimulated hair cell

Hair Cells Transform Mechanical Energy Into Neural Signals

Deflection of the Hair Bundle Initiates Mechanoelectrical Transduction

Application of a mechanical stimulus to a hair bundle elicits an electrical response, the receptor potential, by gating mechanically sensitive ion channels. In vitro, when a bundle is deflected by a probe attached at its tip, the hair cell's response depends on the direction and magnitude of the stimulus. In an unstimulated cell approximately 15% of the transduction channels are open. As a result, the cell's resting potential, about −60 mV, is determined in part by the inward flow of transduction current. A positive stimulus, which displaces the bundle toward its tall edge, opens additional channels; the resulting influx of cations depolarizes the cell by as much as tens of millivolts (Figure 31-2). In contrast, a negative stimulus, which displaces the bundle toward its short edge, shuts those transduction channels that are open at rest and hyperpolarizes the cell. Stimuli at right angles to the bundle's axis of mirror symmetry are neutral and produce no change from the resting potential. Hair cells respond only to stimulus components parallel to the hair bundle's axis of morphological symmetry; an oblique stimulus accordingly elicits a response proportional to its vectorial projection along that axis.

A hair cell's receptor potential is graded. As the stimulus amplitude increases, the receptor potential grows progressively larger, up to a maximal point of saturation. The relation between a bundle's deflection and the resulting electrical response is sigmoidal (Figure 31-2D). Consistent with the hair cell's sensitivity to very small stimuli, a displacement of only 100 nm represents 90% of the response range. During normal stimulation, a hair bundle therefore moves through an angle of only ±1° or so, that is, by less than the diameter of one stereocilium. Hair cells are so sensitive that the response thresholds of both auditory and vestibular receptor organs are probably set by Brownian motion; weaker stimuli are lost in the thermal clatter of the ear's components. When observed in vitro, a hair bundle exhibits a Brownian motion of about 3 nm. However, because the auditory system averages responses over several cycles to improve its signal-to-noise ratio, the threshold of hearing corresponds to a hair-bundle deflection of only ±0.3 nm. A stimulus of this magnitude evokes a receptor potential of about 100 μV.

The mechanoelectrical transduction channels of hair cells are relatively nonselective, cation-passing pores with a conductance near 100 pS. Because small organic cations can support measurable current, the transduction channel's pore must be at least 0.7 nm in diameter. Most of the transduction current is carried by K^+, the cation with the highest concentration in the endolymph bathing the hair bundle. The poor selectivity of these channels permits them to be blocked by aminoglycoside antibiotics, such as streptomycin, gentamicin, and tobramycin. When used in large amounts against bacterial infections, these drugs have a toxic effect on hair cells; the antibiotics damage hair bundles and eventually kill hair cells. These drugs may insinuate themselves through transduction channels at a low rate and thus cause long-term ototoxic effects by interfering with protein synthesis on the mitochondrial ribosomes, which resemble prokaryotic ribosomes. Consistent with this hypothesis, human sensitivity to aminoglycosides is inherited as a mitochondrial trait.

Single-channel recordings and noise analysis suggest that each hair cell possesses only about 100 transduction channels. Because there is a comparable number of stereocilia in the hair bundle, and because the magnitude of the receptor potential is roughly proportional to the number of stereocilia remaining in a microdissected bundle, there may be only one or a few active transduction channels per stereocilium. The paucity of mechanoelectrical transduction channels in hair cells, along with the lack of high-affinity ligands with which to label them, explains why the biochemical nature of these channels has not yet been described.

Mechanical Force Directly Opens and Closes Transduction Channels

Mechanoelectrical transduction in hair cells involves a mechanism for gating of ion channels that is fundamentally different from those employed in such electrical signals as the action potential or postsynaptic potential. Instead of responding to membrane potential or to ligand binding, the channels in the hair cell are affected by mechanical strain.

Two lines of evidence suggest that the opening and closing of transduction channels is regulated by the tension in elastic structures within the hair bundle. First, it is possible to measure a component of hair-bundle stiffness associated with mechanoelectrical transduction. A bundle is stiffer along its axis of morphological symmetry, and hence of mechanical sensitivity, than at a right angle. This observation suggests that a portion of the work done in deflecting a bundle goes into elastic elements, termed *gating springs,* that pull upon the molecular gates of transduction channels (Figure 31-3). Because the gating springs contribute over half of a hair bundle's stiffness, the transduction channels efficiently capture the energy supplied when a bundle is deflected. In addi-

tion, hair-bundle stiffness decreases during channel gating, a phenomenon expected if channels are directly gated through a mechanical linkage to the hair bundle.

A second line of evidence that the channels involved in mechanoelectrical transduction are directly controlled by gating springs is the rapidity with which hair cells respond. The response latency is so brief, only a few microseconds, that gating is more likely to be direct than indirect, by means of a second messenger (see Chapter 13). Moreover, the electrical responses of hair cells to a series of step stimuli of increasing magnitude not only are progressively larger, but also rise faster. This behavior favors a kinetic scheme in which mechanical force controls the rate constants for channel gating. If the mechanical energy from a stimulus is stored in a spring attached to the channel's gate, the rates of channel opening and closing are determined by the probability that the energy content of the spring exceeds the transition-state energy for channel opening or closing.

The site of mechanoelectrical transduction has been established at the tips of the stereocilia by three experimental techniques. First, the region where cations flow into a hair cell was inferred by measuring small differences in the extracellular potential around a stimulated hair bundle. The voltage signal is strongest at the bundle's top; cations flowing toward transduction channels converge near the stereociliary tips. Second, aminoglycoside antibiotics, which block these channels, have their greatest effect on the top of the hair bundle. Finally, Ca^{2+}-sensitive fluorescent indicators first signal Ca^{2+} entry near the tip of the deflected hair bundles. Transduction current entering channels near the stereociliary tips must flow axially down the stereocilia before it changes the cell's membrane potential and thus influences the rate at which synaptic transmitter is released. Although stereocilia are quite narrow, they are also short, so their cable properties are unlikely to attenuate electrical signals significantly.

The gating spring has been identified as a *tip link,* a filamentous connection between two stereocilia (Figure 31-3B). Each tip link is a fine fiber, possibly a pair of molecular strands, obliquely joining the distal end of one stereocilium to the side of the longest adjacent process. It is thought that each link is attached, at one end or at both, to the molecular gates of one or a few transduction channels. Under this arrangement, pushing a bundle in the positive direction would elongate the tip link and promote channel opening; an oppositely directed stimulus would slacken the link and allow the associated channel to close (Figure 31-3A).

Three lines of evidence suggest that tip links are gating springs. First, the links occur universally in hair bundles, where they are situated at the site of transduc-

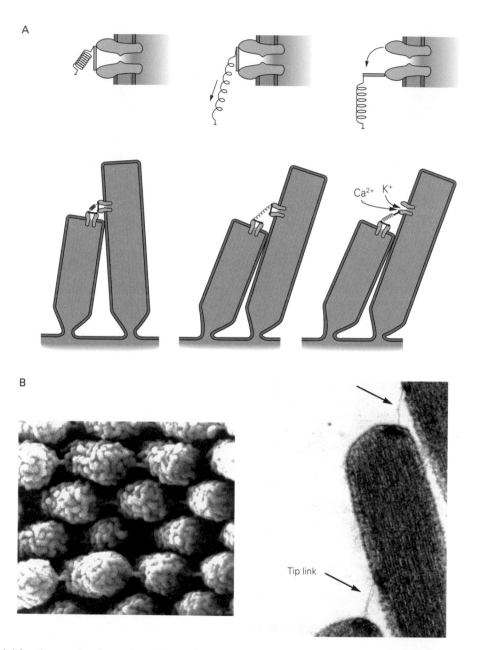

Figure 31-3 A model for the mechanism of mechano-electrical transduction by hair cells.

A. Top: The ion channels that participate in mechanoelectrical transduction in hair cells are gated by elastic structures in the hair bundle. The channel is assumed to be a membrane-spanning protein with a cation-selective pore. Ion permeation through this channel is regulated by a molecular gate, whose opening and closing is controlled by the tension in an elastic element, the gating spring, that senses hair-bundle displacement. (Adapted from Howard and Hudspeth 1988.)

Bottom: When the hair bundle is at rest each transduction channel clatters between closed and open states, spending most of its time shut (**left**). Displacement of the bundle in the positive direction increases the tension in the gating spring, here assumed to be a tip link, attached to each channel's molecular gate (**middle**). The enhanced tension promotes channel opening and the influx of cations, thereby producing a depolarizing receptor potential (**right**). (Adapted from Hudspeth 1989.)

B. The links that connect each stereociliary tip to the side of the longest adjacent stereocilium are visible in this scanning electron micrograph of a hair bundle's top surface (**left**) and transmission electron micrograph (**right**). Although each tip link is only 3 nm in diameter, the links appear stouter in the illustration on the left because of metallic coating during specimen preparation. (From Assad et al. 1991 and Hudspeth and Gillespie 1944.)

tion inferred in biophysical experiments. Second, when tip links are destroyed by exposing hair cells to Ca^{2+} chelators, transduction vanishes. Finally, the orientation of the links is consistent with the vectorial sensitivity of transduction. The links invariably interconnect stereocilia in a direction parallel with the hair bundle's plane of mirror symmetry. Stimulation at a right angle to the bundle's plane of symmetry, which would not be expected to alter the length of the links, elicits little or no response from a hair cell.

Direct Mechanoelectrical Transduction Is Rapid

In contrast to hair cells, many other sensory receptors, such as photoreceptors and olfactory neurons, employ cyclic nucleotides or other second messengers in transduction. As we have seen (Chapter 13), this strategy is advantageous in that the enzymatic apparatus that generates a second messenger provides amplification, and feedback within the metabolic pathway readily permits sensory receptors to have such controls as adaptation or desensitization.

What is the selective advantage of transduction without the intervention of a second messenger? The answer probably lies in the speed of response; hair cells operate much more quickly than do other sensory-receptor cells of the vertebrate nervous system, and indeed more quickly than neurons themselves. To deal with the frequencies of biologically relevant stimuli, transduction by hair cells must be rapid. The behavior of sound in air and the dimensions of sound-emitting and sound-absorbing organs such as vocal cords and eardrums mean that optimal auditory communication occurs in the frequency range of 0.1–100 kHz. Much higher frequencies propagate poorly through air; much lower frequencies are inefficiently produced and captured by animals of moderate size.

The localization of sound sources, one of the most important functions of hearing, sets even more stringent limits on the speed of transduction. If a sound source lies directly to one side of an animal, an emitted sound will reach the nearer ear somewhat sooner than the farther. For a human, this delay is at most 700 μs. Both humans and owls can locate sound sources on the basis of much smaller temporal delays, about 10 μs. For this to occur, hair cells must be capable of detecting acoustical waveforms with microsecond-level resolution. The responsiveness of hair cells to high frequencies of stimulation implies that transduction channels are gated very rapidly. Even in animals sensitive to relatively low frequencies, the response to a stimulus of moderate intensity has a time constant of only 80 μs at 24°C. For mammals to be able to respond to frequencies greater than

100 kHz, the hair cells presumably have gating rates that are an order of magnitude faster.

The Temporal Responsiveness of Hair Cells Determines Their Sensitivity to Stimuli

The responsiveness of hair cells is not constant; mechanical sensitivity varies in such a way that a given cell responds best to behaviorally relevant stimuli. When it is appropriate that low-frequency inputs be disregarded, hair cells possess a unique means of adapting to sustained stimulation. Many hair cells that detect oscillatory stimuli display electrical resonance that tunes each cell to a specific frequency.

Hair Cells Adapt to Sustained Stimuli

Despite the precision with which it grows, a hair bundle is unlikely to develop in such a way that the sensitive transduction apparatus is perfectly poised at its position of greatest mechanosensitivity. Some mechanism must compensate for developmental irregularities, as well as for environmental changes, by resetting the gating springs to correspond with the bundle's resting position. An adaptation process that continuously adjusts the hair bundle's range of mechanical sensitivity does just that; it can maintain a high sensitivity to transient stimuli while rejecting static inputs a million times as large.

Adaptation manifests itself as a progressive decrease in the receptor potential during protracted hair-bundle deflection (Figure 31-4). The process differs from desensitization in that the sensitivity of the receptor persists. However, with prolonged stimulation the hair bundle's range of mechanical sensitivity migrates from that of the bundle's resting position to that of the deflected position maintained by the stimulus. Adaptation occurs on a time scale three orders of magnitude slower than mechanoelectrical transduction: The time constant of adaptation is approximately 25 ms when endolymph bathes the hair bundle. Both the rate and the extent of adaptation increase with increasing concentration of Ca^{2+} in the fluid contacting the apical cellular surface.

How does adaptation occur? Because the stiffness of the hair bundle changes as adaptation proceeds, the process evidently involves an adjustment in the tension borne by the gating springs. It appears likely that the structure anchoring the upper end of each tip link, the *insertional plaque*, is repositioned during adaptation by an active molecular motor. Hair bundles contain several candidates for this role—various forms of myosin, the motor molecules generally associated with motility

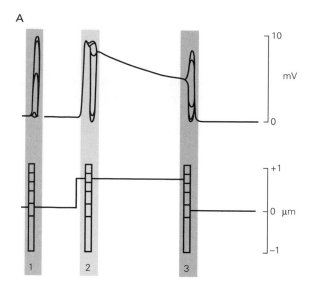

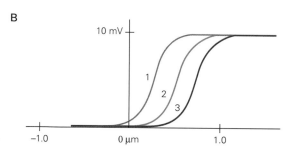

Figure 31-4 Adaptation of mechanoelectrical transduction in hair cells.

A. The hair bundle is subjected to a family of deflections in a series of tests. Test stimuli of various sizes are applied before (**1**) and at two times during a bundle deflection maintained for 100 ms (**2–3**). The family of receptor potentials reveals a rapid depolarization at the outset, followed by gradual decline toward a plateau during maintained stimulation.

B. The relation between displacement and the electrical response of the hair bundle before and during the maintained displacement. As adaptation proceeds, the sigmoidal relation between bundle displacement and receptor potential shifts along the abscissa without substantial changes in the curve's shape or amplitude. This result implies that, during adaptation to a protracted stimulus, a hair bundle's range of mechanical sensitivity migrates toward the position at which the bundle is held.

along actin filaments. For example, immunohistochemical studies indicate that myosin Iβ clusters near the stereociliary tips, possibly at insertional plaques. Myosin VI and myosin VIIa are also found in hair bundles. These isozymes, whose ATPase activity is regulated by several associated calmodulin molecules, are of unknown function. Several such myosin molecules may maintain tension in each tip link by ascending cyto-

skeletal actin filaments, pulling the link's insertion with them (Figure 31-5).

When a stimulus step increases the tension in the gating spring, the associated transduction channel opens, permitting an influx of cations. As Ca^{2+} ions accumulate in the stereociliary cytoplasm, they interact with calmodulin molecules and cause the associated myosin Iβ molecules to produce less upward force. The gating spring is thus able to pull down the myosin molecules and, as a result, it shortens. When the spring reaches its resting tension, closure of the channel reduces the Ca^{2+} influx to its original level, restoring a balance between the upward force produced by myosin and the downward tension in the spring.

Hair Cells Are Tuned to Specific Stimulus Frequencies

Hair cells must contend with acoustical stimuli that have very low energy content. If the stimulus consists of a periodic signal, such as the sinusoidal pressure of a pure tone, a detection system can increase its signal-to-noise ratio by amplifying the response to a relevant frequency selectively. At least two cellular mechanisms are known to accomplish this task.

First, the mechanical properties of the hair bundle act to tune the bundle to a particular frequency. The natural frequency of a hair bundle depends upon its mechanical properties in the same way a tuning fork's resonant frequency depends upon the flexibility and mass of its tines. The flexible elements that restore a bundle to its resting upright position include both gating springs and the actin rootlets at the stereociliary bases. Because the bundle moves through a viscous medium, the relevant mass in the bundle's tuning includes that of a volume of water dragged along by the moving bundle. Viscosity also heavily dampens the motion: Although a bundle responds optimally at a particular frequency, it differs from a tuning fork in being incapable of sustained oscillation after stimulation has ceased.

In many auditory organs the lengths of hair bundles vary systematically along the frequency axis of the organ. Hair cells that respond to low-frequency acoustical, vibrational, and accelerational stimuli have the longest bundles, while receptors for the highest-frequency acoustical signals have the shortest bundles. In the human cochlea, for example, an inner hair cell responsive to frequencies as great as 20 kHz bears a 4 μm hair bundle. At the opposite extreme a cell sensitive to a 20 Hz stimuli has a bundle over 7 μm high. The systematic relation between anatomical position and the frequency to which cells are most sensitive is termed *tonotopic mapping*. This phenomenon is widespread in the auditory system, as we have seen in Chapter 30.

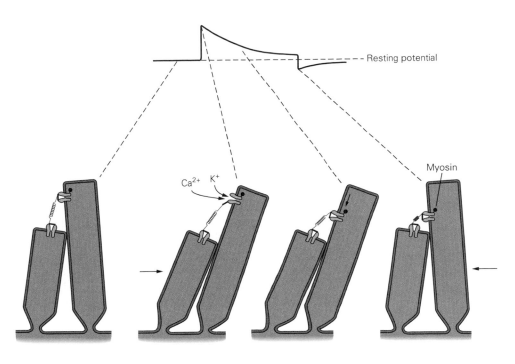

Figure 31-5 A model of adaptation by hair cells. A hair bundle may be subjected to prolonged deflection in the positive or negative direction. The electrical response to a positive stimulus displays an initial depolarization, followed by a decline to a plateau and an undershoot at the cessation of the stimulus. Negative stimulation elicits a complementary response: The receptor potential largely abates during stimulation but shows a rebound at the end. Bundle movement in response to positive stimulation increases tip link tension and opens transduction channels. As stimulation continues, however, the tip link's upper attachment moves down the stereocilium, allowing each channel to close during adaptation. During negative stimulation tension is restored to the initially slack tip link by active ascent of the link's upper insertion.

Computer modeling shows that the tuning-fork mechanism tunes hair cells with free-standing hair bundles, those that are not attached to a tectorial membrane. These cells include the inner hair cells of the human cochlea, the receptors that provide most information conveyed by the cochlear nerve. The length of the stereocilia may also affect the tuning of cells whose hair bundles are inserted into a tectorial membrane, for in these cells, too, there is an inverse relation between bundle length and characteristic frequency.

The second mechanism that tunes individual hair cells to specific frequencies is electrical in nature and occurs after mechanoelectrical transduction. In fishes, amphibians, reptiles, and birds the membrane potential of hair cells resonates at a particular frequency. Whether electrical resonance contributes to frequency tuning in the ears of mammals, including humans, is uncertain. Electrical resonance is demonstrated experimentally by injecting a pulse of current into a hair cell, whereupon the membrane potential undergoes an exponentially damped, sinusoidal oscillation (Figure 31-6A). When the cell is stimulated with mechanical stimuli of constant amplitude, its transduction apparatus responds over a broad range of frequencies. Stimulation at the particular frequency at which a cell's membrane potential resonates when current is injected, however, evokes the greatest receptor potential.

In these species the cells responsive to specific frequencies are generally distributed in a tonotopic map. For example, in the basilar papilla, the auditory receptor organ of reptiles and birds, there is a continuous progression along the organ in the frequencies to which hair cells are tuned. Because the release of synaptic transmitter at the cell's basolateral surface is controlled by membrane potential, the postsynaptic nerve fibers innervating each cell are most responsive to stimuli of a specific frequency.

The origin of electrical resonance has been determined by recording from isolated hair cells using the voltage-clamp technique (see Box 9-1). The depolarizing phase of an oscillation is driven by current carried into a hair cell through voltage-sensitive Ca^{2+} channels, while the repolarizing component results from outward current through Ca^{2+}-sensitive K^+ channels (Figure 31-6B). Several factors establish the frequency and damping of the resonance: the membrane capacitance; the numbers and kinetic properties of the Ca^{2+} and K^+ channels; and the time course of Ca^{2+} removal by diffusion, sequestration, and extrusion.

How hair cells become tuned to their appropriate frequencies during development remains to be determined. It has recently been found, however, that alternative splicing of the mRNA encoding cochlear K^+ channels generates channel isoforms that differ in their

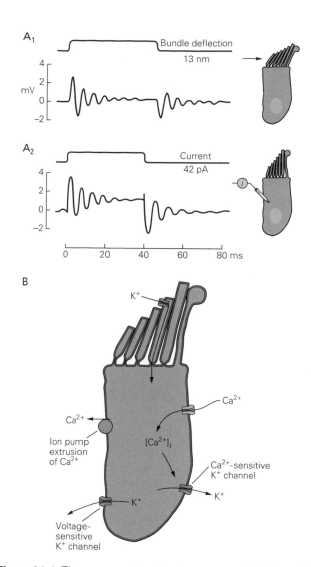

Figure 31-6 The resonant electrical response of a hair cell from the internal ear of a turtle. (From Crawford and Fettiplace 1985.)

A.1. When the hair bundle is deflected the hair cell's receptor potential displays sinusoidal oscillation, or ringing, at a frequency of about 180 Hz. **2.** Passing electrical current into the same hair cell through a microelectrode evokes oscillation of the membrane potential at a similar frequency, an indication that the cell is tuned to a specific stimulus frequency by an electrical resonator.

B. A model of electrical resonance in a hair cell. Positive deflection of the hair bundle or injection of current with a microelectrode allows K^+ influx that depolarizes the cell. The depolarization opens voltage-sensitive Ca^{2+} channels, which augment the depolarization by permitting Ca^{2+} entry. As Ca^{2+} accumulates in the cytoplasm, however, it activates Ca^{2+}-sensitive K^+ channels, which, along with voltage-sensitive K^+ channels, allow K^+ efflux that repolarizes the cell. To maintain an appropriate cytoplasmic Ca^{2+} concentration, the Ca^{2+} must be sequestered and eventually pumped from the cell.

Ca^{2+} and voltage sensitivity. Such variations may underlie differences in the frequency selectivity of the hair cells in which the channels are expressed.

Synaptic Transmission from Hair Cells Is Triggered at Low-Amplitude Receptor Potentials

In addition to being sensory receptors, hair cells are also presynaptic terminals. The basolateral membrane of each cell contains several presynaptic active zones, where chemical neurotransmitter is released. Each active zone is characterized by four prominent morphological features (Figure 31-7). In the cytoplasm adjacent to the release site sits a presynaptic dense body, a spherical or ovoidal, fibrillar, osmiophilic structure about 400 nm in diameter. Although its biochemical constitution is unknown, the dense body resembles the synaptic ribbon of a photoreceptor cell and may be an elaboration of the smaller presynaptic densities found at the neuromuscular junction and at central nervous system synapses. The presynaptic dense body is surrounded by clear-core synaptic vesicles, each 35 nm in diameter, which are sometimes attached to the dense body by tenuous filaments. Between the dense body and the presynaptic plasma membrane lies a striking presynaptic density, which usually comprises several short rows of fuzzy material. Within the plasmalemma, rows of large intramembrane particles occur in register with the strips of presynaptic density. These particles are thought to include the Ca^{2+} channels involved in the release of transmitter as well as the K^+ channels that participate in electrical resonance.

Few physiological studies of the afferent synapses of mammalian hair cells have been performed. Nevertheless, these mammalian synapses are structurally similar to those of other vertebrates, so that conclusions drawn from model systems probably apply to mammalian synapses as well. Studies of nonmammalian vertebrate hair cells show that, as with most other synapses (Chapter 10), the release of transmitter by hair cells is evoked by presynaptic depolarization and requires the presence of Ca^{2+} in the extracellular medium. Postsynaptic recordings indicate that the release of the hair cell's synaptic transmitter is quantal in nature; the statistical behavior of these synapses resembles that of neuromuscular junctions (Chapter 11). The identity of the afferent neurotransmitter is controversial. Glutamate appears to be the transmitter in some instances, but there is evidence for other, as yet unidentified, substances as well.

The afferent synapses of hair cells have several un-

Another unusual feature of the hair cell's synapses is that, like photoreceptors, they must be able to release neurotransmitter reliably in response to a threshold receptor potential of only 100 μV or so. This feature, too, may result from the fact that the presynaptic Ca^{2+} channels are activated at the resting potential.

Finally, hair cells that respond to high-frequency stimuli, especially those of the mammalian cochlea, must be capable of mustering synaptic vesicles at a rate high enough to ensure reliable signaling. Although the function of the presynaptic dense body is unknown, the structure's prominence in hair cells, as well as its close association with the apparatus of vesicle release, suggests that it is involved in the unusually rapid release of neurotransmitter in response to minimal stimulation.

Most hair cells receive efferent synaptic inputs from neurons in the brain stem. Unlike the specialized afferent terminals discussed above, the efferent terminals are of a form typical of peripheral synapses. Efferent axons terminate in relatively large boutons on the hair-cell surface. The presynaptic cytoplasm contains numerous clear synaptic vesicles about 50 nm in diameter, as well as a smaller number of larger, dense-core vesicles. The principal efferent transmitter is acetylcholine (ACh). Calcitonin gene-related peptide (CGRP), however, also occurs in efferent terminals and may be coreleased with ACh. Just beneath each efferent terminal the postsynaptic cytoplasm of a hair cell holds a single cisterna of smooth endoplasmic reticulum. This structure may be involved in the release and reuptake of Ca^{2+} in response to efferent stimulation.

Efferent stimulation has different effects in different hair cells. In the vestibular apparatus it may decrease or increase neural activity in afferent fibers connected to the target hair cells. The role of efferent innervation is best understood in the instance of hair cells that employ electrical resonance for frequency tuning. When the efferent nerve supply is stimulated, the efferent transmitter hyperpolarizes the target hair cells. More importantly, the transmitter-induced increase in membrane conductance perturbs the critically tuned resonant circuit in the hair cell's membrane, thus decreasing both the sharpness of frequency selectivity and the gain of electrical amplification. The complex and unusual role of efferent innervation in the mammalian cochlea is considered in Chapter 30.

An Overall View

As the receptors for the auditory and vestibular systems, hair cells have three major functions. By means of their mechanically sensitive hair bundles, they trans-

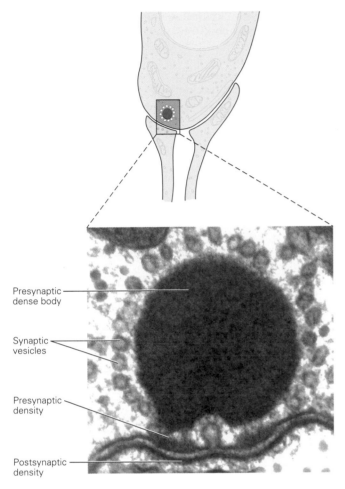

Presynaptic
dense body

Synaptic
vesicles

Presynaptic
density

Postsynaptic
density

Figure 31-7 The afferent synapse of a hair cell. The cytoplasm of a hair cell occupies most of this transmission electron micrograph; an afferent terminal is shown at the bottom of the image. The active zone is characterized by a spherical presynaptic dense body surrounded by a halo of clear-core synaptic vesicles. Beneath the dense body lies a presynaptic density, in the middle of which one vesicle is undergoing exocytosis. The inner aspect of the plasmalemma of the afferent terminal displays a modest postsynaptic density. (From Jacobs and Hudspeth 1990.)

usual features that underlie the specialized signaling abilities of these cells. Many hair cells release transmitter at rest. During synaptic transmission the amount of transmitter released and the consequent activity in the afferent nerve fibers is modulated upward or downward, depending on whether the hair cell is respectively depolarized or hyperpolarized from its resting potential. Consistent with this observation, the Ca^{2+} channels of hair cells are activated at the resting potential, providing a steady leak of Ca^{2+} that causes transmitter release from unstimulated cells.

duce sounds and accelerations into electrical responses. In many instances, hair cells make a mechanical or electrical contribution to a receptor organ's frequency selectivity. Finally, each hair cell is in effect a synaptic terminal whose release of a chemical neurotransmitter excites a response in fibers of the eighth cranial nerve.

A. J. Hudspeth

Selected Readings

Hudspeth AJ. 1989. How the ear's works work. Nature 341:397–404.

Hudspeth AJ, Gillespie PG. 1994. Pulling springs to tune transduction: adaptation by hair cells. Neuron 12:1–9.

References

Art JJ, Crawford AC, Fettiplace R, Fuchs PA. 1985. Efferent modulation of hair cell tuning in the cochlea of the turtle. J Physiol 360:397–421.

Assad JA, Shepherd GM, Corey DP. 1991. Tip-link integrity and mechanical transduction in vertebrate hair cells. Neuron 7:985–994.

Crawford AC, Fettiplace R. 1985. The mechanical properties of ciliary bundles of turtle cochlear hair cells. J Physiol (Lond) 364:359–379.

Fettiplace R. 1987. Electrical tuning of hair cells in the inner ear. Trends Neurosci 10:421–425.

Freeman DM, Weiss TF. 1988. The role of fluid inertia in mechanical stimulation of hair cells. Hearing Res 35:201–207.

Holton T, Hudspeth AJ. 1983. A micromechanical contribution to cochlear tuning and tonotopic organization. Science 222:508–510.

Howard J, Hudspeth AJ. 1988. Compliance of the hair bundle associated with gating of mechanoelectrical transduction channels in the bullfrog's saccular hair cell. Neuron 1:189–199.

Hudspeth AJ. 1982. Extracellular current flow and the site of transduction by vertebrate hair cells. J Neurosci 2:1–10.

Hudspeth AJ, Lewis RS. 1988. A model for electrical resonance and frequency tuning in saccular hair cells of the bull-frog, *Rana catesbeiana*. J Physiol (Lond) 400:275–297.

Jacobs RA, Hudspeth AJ. 1990. Ultrastructural correlates of mechanoelectrical transduction in hair cells of the bullfrog's internal ear. Cold Spring Harb Symp Quant Biol 55:547–561.

Lumpkin EA, Hudspeth AJ. 1998. Regulation of free Ca^{2+} concentration in hair-cell stereocilia. J Neurosci 18:6300–6318.

Rosenblatt KP, Sun Z-P, Heller S, Hudspeth AJ. 1997. Distribution of Ca^{2+}-activated K^+ channel isoforms along the tonotopic gradient of the chicken's cochlea. Neuron 19:1061–1075.

Tilney LG, Tilney MS, Saunders JS, DeRosier DJ. 1986. Actin filaments, stereocilia, and hair cells of the bird cochlea. III. The development and differentiation of hair cells and stereocilia. Dev Biol 116:100–118.

Wright A. 1984. Dimensions of the cochlear stereocilia in man and the guinea pig. Hear Res 13:89–98.

32

Smell and Taste: The Chemical Senses

W E ARE CONTINUOUSLY bombarded by molecules released into our environment. Through the senses of smell and taste these molecules provide us with important information that we use constantly in our daily lives. They inform us about the availability of foods and the potential pleasure or danger to be derived from them. They also initiate physiological changes required for the digestion and utilization of ingested foodstuffs. In many mammals the sense of smell plays an additional role, eliciting physiological and behavioral responses to members of the same species.

Humans and other mammals are capable of discriminating a great variety of odors and flavors. Although the olfactory capability of humans is somewhat limited compared with that of some other mammals, we are nevertheless able to perceive thousands of different odorous molecules (*odorants*). Perfumers, who are highly trained to discriminate odorants, say that they can distinguish as many as 5000 different types of odorants, and wine tasters report that they can distinguish more than 100 different components of taste based on combinations of flavor and aroma.

Molecules that are smelled or tasted are sensed by specialized sensory cells in the nose or mouth that relay information to the brain. In the olfactory system the sensory cells are olfactory sensory neurons that lie within a specialized neuroepithelium in the back of the nasal cavity. The sensory cells of the mouth that sense taste

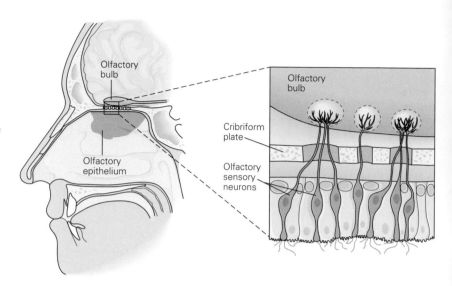

Figure 32-1 Olfactory sensory neurons are embedded in a small area of specialized epithelium in the dorsal posterior recess of the nasal cavity. These neurons project axons to the olfactory bulb of the brain, a small ovoid structure that rests on the cribriform plate of the ethmoid bone.

stimuli (*tastants*) are specialized epithelial cells, called taste cells, that are clustered together in the taste buds. Taste cells are capable of sensing four basic types of taste stimuli: bitter, sweet, salty, and sour. The large variety of flavors that we associate with taste are generated by complex mixtures of molecules that fall into these four categories, together with volatile molecules that reach the olfactory system from the back of the nasal cavity during chewing and swallowing. The somatosensory system also plays a role in taste. It senses the textures of foods and localizes to the mouth sensations of flavors contributed by the olfactory system.

In this chapter we consider how odor and taste stimuli are detected and how they are encoded in patterns of neural signals transmitted to the brain. In recent years much has been learned about the mechanisms of signal detection and transduction in olfactory sensory neurons and taste cells. We shall see that the strategies employed by these cells to sense and transmit information involve specific receptors, signal transduction molecules, and ion channels similar to those of other neural and nonneural systems. We also consider the neural pathways through which olfactory and gustatory information is transmitted, and the organizational strategies used by the olfactory and gustatory systems to discriminate a large variety of chemical stimuli in the environment.

Odors Are Detected by Nasal Olfactory Sensory Neurons

The initial events in olfactory perception occur in olfactory sensory neurons in the nose. These neurons are embedded in the olfactory epithelium, a small patch of spe-

cialized epithelium that in humans covers a region in the back of the nasal cavity about 5 cm² in size (Figure 32-1). The human olfactory epithelium contains several million olfactory sensory neurons interspersed with glia-like supporting cells, both of which lie above a basal layer of stem cells (Figure 32-2). Olfactory neurons are distinctive among neurons in that they are short-lived, with an average life span of only 30–60 days, and are continuously replaced from the basal stem cell population.

The olfactory sensory neuron is a bipolar nerve cell (Figure 32-2). From its apical pole each neuron extends a single dendrite to the epithelial surface, where the dendrite expands into a large knob. From this knob 5–20 thin cilia protrude into the layer of mucus that coats the epithelium. From its basal pole each neuron projects a single axon through the bony cribriform plate above the nasal cavity to the olfactory bulb, where the axon forms synapses with olfactory bulb neurons that relay signals to the olfactory cortex.

The cilia of the olfactory neuron are specialized for odor detection. They have specific receptors for odorants as well as the transduction machinery needed to amplify sensory signals and generate action potentials in the neuron's axon. The mucus that bathes the cilia is secreted by the supporting cells of the olfactory epithelium and by Bowman's glands, which lie under the epithelium and have ducts that open onto the epithelial surface. The mucus is thought to provide the appropriate molecular and ionic environment for odor detection. It also contains soluble odorant-binding proteins, produced by a gland that empties into the nasal cavity. While they are not themselves the olfactory receptors, these soluble odorant-binding proteins could contribute to odorant concentration or removal.

A

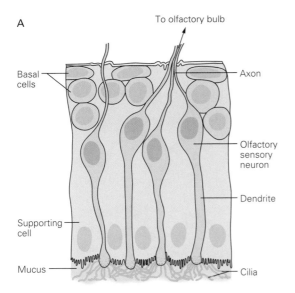

To olfactory bulb

Basal cells

Axon

Olfactory sensory neuron

Dendrite

Supporting cell

Mucus

Cilia

B

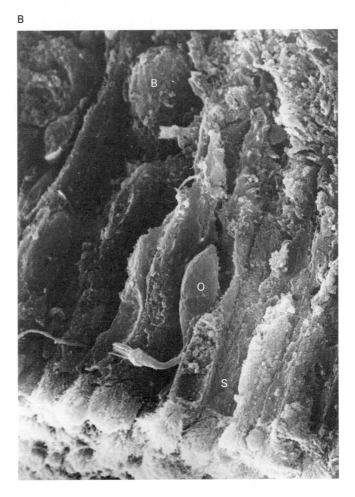

Figure 32-2 Structure of the olfactory epithelium.

A. The olfactory epithelium contains three major cell types: olfactory sensory neurons, supporting cells, and basal stem cells at the base of the epithelium. Each olfactory sensory neuron extends a single dendrite to the epithelial surface. From the dendritic terminus numerous cilia protrude into the layer of mucus lining the nasal lumen. From its basal pole each neuron projects a single axon to the olfactory bulb. Odorants bind to specific odorant receptors on olfactory cilia and initiate a cascade of signal transduction events that lead to the production of action potentials in the sensory axon.

B. This scanning electron micrograph illustrates the structure of the olfactory epithelium and the dense mat of receptive olfactory cilia at the epithelial surface (bottom of image). Supporting cells (**S**) are columnar cells that have apical microvilli and thin

extensions attached to the base of the epithelium. An olfactory sensory neuron (**O**) with its dendrite and cilia and a basal stem cell (**B**) can be seen among the supporting cells (**S**). (From Morrison and Costanzo 1990.)

Different Odorants Stimulate Different Olfactory Sensory Neurons

To be discriminated, an odorant must cause a distinct signal to be transmitted from the nose to the brain. This is accomplished primarily by the differing sensitivities of individual olfactory sensory neurons to different odorants (Figure 32-3). The usual response of the neuron to an odorant consists of depolarization and the production of action potentials. The number of neurons that respond to an odorant varies with odorant concentration; higher concentrations of an odorant stimulate a

larger number of neurons. This may explain why odorants presented to human subjects at different concentrations can be perceived as being different.

A Large Family of Odorant Receptors Permits Discrimination of a Wide Variety of Odorants

Volatile odorants that enter the nasal cavity and dissolve in the nasal mucus are detected by odorant receptors on the cilia of olfactory sensory neurons. A large multigene family, first identified in the rat, appears to

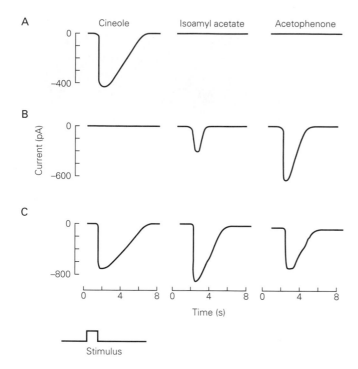

Figure 32-3 Individual olfactory sensory neurons respond to different odorants. The records are from patch clamp recordings of the responses of three neurons (A, B, C) to three odorants, each at a concentration of 5×10^{-4} M. One cell responded only to one of the odorants while another responded to two odorants; the third cell was stimulated by all three odorants. (Adapted from Firestein et al. 1993.)

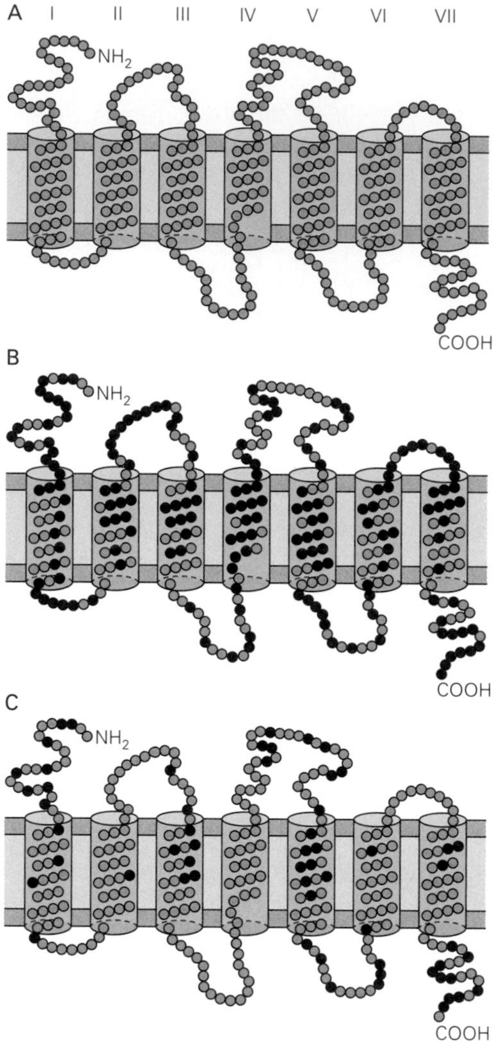

code for as many as 1000 different types of odorant receptors. This gene family, which is also present in humans, is extremely diverse. Although odorant receptors all have the same general structure and have some amino acid sequence motifs in common, each is unique (Figure 32-4). The unprecedented size and diversity of this receptor family are likely to allow for the discrimination of a wide variety of odorants having different sizes, shapes, and functional groups.

The odorant receptors belong to a large superfamily of structurally related receptor proteins that transduce signals by interactions with heterotrimeric GTP-binding proteins (G proteins). Like other G protein-coupled receptors (see Chapters 5 and 13), the odorant receptors have seven hydrophobic regions that are likely to serve as transmembrane domains (Figure 32-4). Detailed studies of some other G protein-coupled receptors (eg, the β-adrenergic receptor) suggest that in many of these receptors the interaction with the ligand occurs in a

Figure 32-4 The amino acid sequences of odorant receptors are extremely diverse.

A. A typical odorant receptor (I15) is shown in its presumed configuration in the membrane, with seven hydrophobic membrane-spanning domains. Each amino acid is represented by a ball.

B. Odorant receptors are extremely diverse in amino acid sequence. The **black balls** indicate amino acids that are different in two odorant receptors (I15 and F6). The extreme diversity in the amino acid sequences of several of the transmembrane domains is consistent with the possibility that a ligand binding pocket is formed in the plane of the membrane by a combination of the transmembrane domains.

C. Although odorant receptors, and the genes that encode them, are extremely variable in sequence, some are closely related. Groups of receptor genes that are more than 80% identical in nucleotide sequence are considered to belong to the same subfamily. The receptors they encode are similar in amino acid sequence and therefore might interact with similar odorants. The **black balls** indicate amino acids that are different in two receptors (I15 and I9) that belong to the same subfamily.

ligand-binding pocket that is formed by a combination of the transmembrane regions. Interestingly, the amino acid sequences of odorant receptors are especially variable in several transmembrane domains, providing a possible mechanism for the recognition of a variety of structurally diverse ligands.

The Interaction Between Odorant and Receptor Activates a Second-Messenger System That Leads to Depolarization of the Sensory Neuron

Odorants induce increases in adenylyl cyclase activity and cAMP in preparations of olfactory cilia. This effect is GTP dependent, suggesting that olfactory transduction, like visual transduction, proceeds via a G protein-coupled mechanism. The existence of an ionic conductance in olfactory cilia that is gated by cyclic nucleotides further suggests a mechanism by which odorant-induced elevations in cAMP could be translated into changes in membrane potential.

Our current understanding of the molecular events underlying olfactory signal transduction is illustrated in Figure 32-5. In this model the interaction of an odorant with its receptor induces an interaction between the receptor and a heterotrimeric G protein. This interaction causes release of the G protein's GTP-coupled α-subunit, $G_{\alpha olf}$, which then stimulates adenylyl cyclase to produce cAMP. The increased cAMP leads to the opening of cyclic nucleotide-gated cation channels in the cilia membrane, causing a depolarization that leads to the generation of action potentials in the sensory axon and the transmission of signals to the olfactory bulb. Additional signal transduction cascades involving inositol 1,4,5-trisphosphate (IP_3), cyclic GMP, and carbon monoxide are also activated after odorant binding, but their roles in transduction are not currently understood.

When we are continuously exposed to a disagreeable odor we cease to notice it after a short time. However, a brief exposure to fresh air allows us to smell the unpleasant odor again. This *adaptation* to odorants is thought to derive from at least two different physiological mechanisms. First, the interaction of an odorant receptor with its ligand may be followed by inactivation, or *desensitization*, of the receptor due to phosphorylation of the receptor by a protein kinase. Second, the olfactory neuron may adapt to different concentrations of an odorant by adjusting the sensitivity of its cyclic nucleotide-gated ion channels to cAMP, an effect conceptually analogous to light adaptation in the visual system, where light sensitivity is adjusted to match the intensity of light in the environment (see Box 26-2).

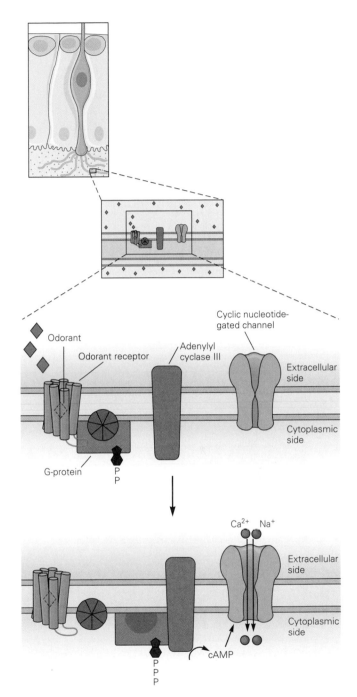

Figure 32-5 Olfactory signal transduction. In this model binding of an odorant to an odorant receptor causes the receptor to interact with a G protein whose GTP-coupled α-subunit ($G_{\alpha olf}$) then stimulates adenylyl cyclase type III. The resultant increase in cAMP opens cyclic nucleotide-gated cation channels, leading to cation influx and a change in membrane potential in the cilium membrane.

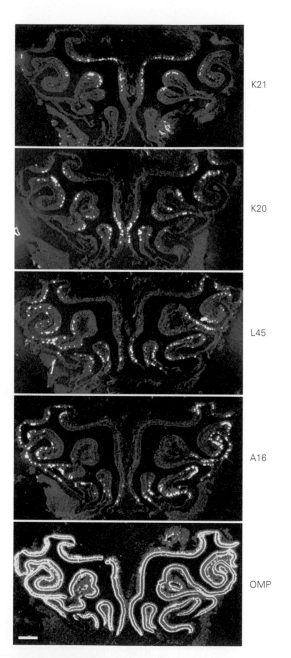

K21

K20

L45

A16

OMP

Figure 32-6 Each odorant receptor type is localized in one of four zones in the olfactory epithelium of the mouse. Sections of mouse olfactory epithelium were hybridized to ^{35}S-labeled probes prepared from genes encoding four different odorant receptors (K21, K20, L45, and A16) or olfactory marker protein (OMP), which is expressed in all olfactory sensory neurons. The nasal septum is in the center of each section, with the two nasal cavities on either side. The pattern of OMP mRNA expression indicates that most of the nasal cavity in this part of the nose is lined by olfactory epithelium. Each receptor probe labeled a small percentage of olfactory sensory neurons. These neurons are confined to one of four zones but are randomly scattered throughout that zone. Each of the receptor probes used here hybridized to neurons in a different zone. Note that the zones are bilaterally symmetrical in the two nasal cavities. Scale bar = 400 μm. (From Sullivan et al. 1996.)

Different Olfactory Neurons Express Different Odorant Receptors

How is the information provided by 1000 different types of odorant receptors organized in the olfactory system? In situ hybridization studies indicate that each odorant receptor gene is expressed in only about 0.1% of olfactory sensory neurons, suggesting that each neuron expresses only one type of odorant receptor. Analysis of receptor expression in single neurons using the polymerase chain reaction also supports this conclusion. Thus each neuron is likely to transmit to the brain information that is derived from only one receptor type.

In rodents different sets of odorant receptor genes are expressed in four zones of the olfactory epithelium (Figure 32-6). Neurons with the same receptors are all located in one zone but are scattered throughout that zone along with neurons expressing other receptors. This arrangement suggests that sensory information is broadly organized into four large sets prior to transmission to the brain. The purpose served by this segregation is unknown. However, the different epithelial zones project axons to different domains in the olfactory bulb, indicating that the organization of epithelial inputs is preserved at the next level in the olfactory pathway.

The highly distributed nature of information coding implied by this arrangement is likely to maximize the information-collecting function of the olfactory epithelium. Since any odorant can be recognized by receptors in many regions of the nasal cavity, responsiveness to an odorant is assured, even if part of the epithelium is damaged, as can occur during respiratory infection or with aging.

Odorant Information Is Encoded Spatially in the Olfactory Bulb

Sensory information from the nose is transmitted to the olfactory bulbs of the brain, paired structures that lie just above and behind the nasal cavities. In the olfactory bulb, incoming sensory axons synapse on the dendrites of olfactory bulb neurons within anatomically discrete synaptic units called glomeruli, of which there are about 2000 per bulb in the mouse (Figure 32-7). In the glomerulus the sensory axon makes synaptic connections with three types of neurons: mitral and tufted relay neurons, which project axons to the olfactory cortex, and periglomerular interneurons, which encircle the glomerulus. The axon of each olfactory sensory neuron synapses in only one glomerulus. Similarly, the primary dendrite of each mitral and tufted relay neuron is confined to a single glomerulus. In each glomerulus the axons of several thousand sensory neurons converge on

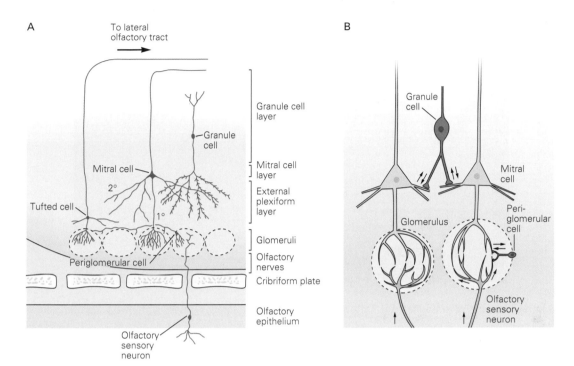

Figure 32-7 The olfactory bulb receives signals from olfactory sensory neurons. (Adapted from Shepherd and Greer 1990.)

A. Each sensory axon terminates in a single glomerulus, forming synapses with the dendrites of periglomerular interneurons and mitral and tufted relay neurons. The primary dendrite of each mitral and tufted cell enters a single glomerulus, where it arborizes extensively. Mitral and tufted cells also extend secondary dendrites into the external plexiform layer, where granule cell interneurons make reciprocal synapses with these secondary dendrites. The output of the bulb is carried by the mitral cells and the tufted cells, whose axons project in the lateral olfactory tract.

B. Within each glomerulus periglomerular cells form inhibitory dendrodendritic synapses with mitral cell dendrites. The periglomerular cells also sometimes make inhibitory contacts with mitral cells that receive input in nearby glomeruli. The secondary dendrites of mitral and tufted cells form excitatory synapses on the dendrites of granule cell interneurons, which form inhibitory synapses on numerous secondary dendrites. These inhibitory connections may provide a curtain of inhibition that must be penetrated by the peaks of excitation generated by odorant stimuli. They may also serve to sharpen or refine sensory information prior to transmission to the olfactory cortex.

the dendrites of about 20–50 relay neurons, resulting in an approximately 100-fold decrease in the number of neurons transmitting olfactory sensory signals.

How is olfactory sensory information organized in the olfactory bulb? Insight into this question has come from experiments that took advantage of the fact that the survival of the olfactory sensory neurons in the nose depends on the integrity of the olfactory bulb. Relatively small lesions in the olfactory bulb lead to the degeneration of individual neurons that are widely dispersed in the olfactory epithelium, suggesting that the axons of sensory neurons in many areas of the epithelium converge on glomeruli in one region of the bulb. Further evidence for this convergence is provided by the observation that a single mitral relay neuron can be stimulated by odorants applied to many different areas of the olfactory epithelium.

The presence of anatomically discrete synaptic units (glomeruli) in the olfactory bulb led early researchers to suggest that the glomeruli might serve as functional units and that information about different odorants might be mapped onto different glomeruli. Evidence for this hypothesis is provided by exposing an animal to different odorants while recording the activity of a single mitral cell. Each mitral cell responds to multiple odorants, but mitral cells connected to different glomeruli generally respond to different sets of odorants. Labeling techniques that monitor neural activity over the entire olfactory bulb also show that each odorant typically stimulates many different glomeruli (Figure 32-8).

What characteristics of the afferent connections explain these observations? Analysis of the patterns of synapses formed in the bulb by sensory neurons ex-

A   B

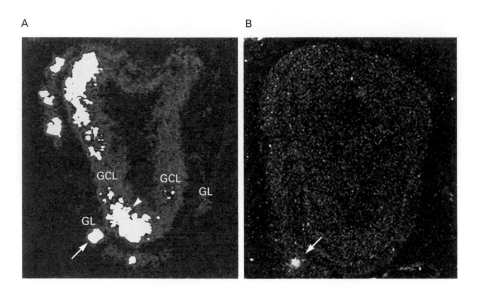

Figure 32-8 Spatial mapping of sensory information in the olfactory bulb of rodents.

A. The pattern of labeling of a ^{35}S-labeled *c-fos* probe in a section through the olfactory bulb of a rat exposed to peppermint odor. Intense hybridization to the probe is observed at several foci in the glomerular layer (**GL; arrow**) as well as in regions of the granule cell layer (**GCL; arrowhead**) deep to those foci. The intense signal in one or more glomeruli at several locations in this section illustrates the finding of numerous studies that a

single odorant typically stimulates multiple glomeruli. Elevated neural activity is reflected here by increases in *c-fos* RNA. (From Guthrie et al. 1993.)

B. A section through the olfactory bulb of a mouse shows intense hybridization of a ^{35}S-labeled odorant receptor gene (*M50*) probe to sensory axons in a single glomerulus (**arrow**). The axons of olfactory sensory neurons that express the *M50* odorant receptor gene are concentrated in only a few glomeruli. (From Ressler et al. 1994.)

pressing different odorant receptors shows that the axons of neurons that express the same receptor all converge on a few glomeruli (Figure 32-8). It appears that each glomerulus may receive input from only one type of receptor. Remarkably, glomeruli that receive input from a specific type of receptor have the same locations in the olfactory bulbs of different animals. Thus, at the level of input to the olfactory bulb, a stereotyped spatial map of sensory information is formed by sensory neurons expressing different odorant receptors projecting to different glomeruli.

This arrangement suggests that an odorant that stimulates many glomeruli is recognized by many different receptors. It also implies that different odorants that activate the same glomerulus are all recognized by the same receptor. Thus, the identity of an odorant may be encoded by a combination of receptors that recognize different structural features of that odorant. That is, each receptor may serve as one component of the code for many odorants, thus allowing for the discrimination of a large number of different odorants. In this model the information map in the olfactory bulb might not be based on different odors but rather on different molecular features, each of which might be shared by a variety

of odorants, including those with very different perceived qualities.

Sensory information is likely to be extensively processed, and perhaps refined, in the olfactory bulb before it is sent to the olfactory cortex. Periglomerular interneurons encircling a glomerulus appear to make inhibitory dendrodendritic synapses with mitral cell dendrites in that glomerulus, and sometimes in adjacent glomeruli (see Figure 32-7). In addition, granule cell interneurons deep in the bulb provide negative feedback circuits. These interneurons are excited by the basal dendrites (secondary dendrites) of mitral cells and also inhibit those mitral cells and others with which they are connected (see Figure 32-7).

Another potential source of signal refinement, or adjustment, is the multiple inputs to the olfactory bulb from olfactory areas of the cortex as well as the basal forebrain (horizontal limb of the diagonal band) and midbrain (locus ceruleus and raphe). These connections may provide a way of modulating olfactory bulb function, so that odors might have different behavioral significance depending on the physiological state of the animal. For example, some centrifugal projections might heighten the perception of the aroma of foods when the animal is hungry.

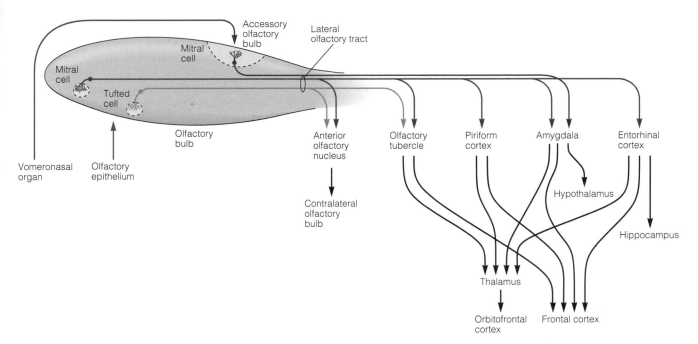

Figure 32-9 Olfactory information is processed in several regions of the cerebral cortex. Information is transmitted from the olfactory bulb by the axons of mitral and tufted relay neurons, which travel in the lateral olfactory tract. Mitral cells project to the five different regions of olfactory cortex: the anterior olfactory nucleus, which innervates the contralateral olfactory bulb; the olfactory tubercle; the piriform cortex; and parts of the amygdala and entorhinal cortex. Tufted cells appear to project primarily to the anterior olfactory nucleus and the olfactory tubercle, while mitral cells in the accessory olfactory bulb project only to the amygdala. The conscious discrimination of odors is thought to depend on the neocortex (orbitofrontal cortex and frontal cortex), which may receive olfactory information via two separate projections: one through the thalamus and one directly to the neocortex. The emotive aspects of olfactory sensation are thought to derive from limbic projections involving the amygdala and hypothalamus. The effects of pheromones are also thought to be mediated by signals from the main and accessory olfactory bulbs to the amygdala and hypothalamus.

Odorant Information Is Transmitted From the Olfactory Bulb to the Neocortex Directly and via the Thalamus

The axons of the mitral and tufted relay neurons of the olfactory bulb project through the lateral olfactory tract to the olfactory cortex (Figure 32-9). The olfactory cortex, defined roughly as that portion of the cortex that receives a direct projection from the olfactory bulb, is divided into five main areas: (1) the anterior olfactory nucleus, which connects the two olfactory bulbs through a portion of the anterior commissure; (2) the piriform cortex; (3) parts of the amygdala; (4) the olfactory tubercle; and (5) part of the entorhinal cortex. From the latter four areas, information is relayed to the orbitofrontal cortex via the thalamus; however, the olfactory cortex also makes direct contacts with the frontal cortex (Figure 32-9). In addition, olfactory information is transmitted from the amygdala to the hypothalamus and from the entorhinal area to the hippocampus.

The afferent pathways through the thalamus to the orbitofrontal cortex are thought to be responsible for the perception and discrimination of odors, because people with lesions of the orbitofrontal cortex are unable to discriminate odors. In contrast, the olfactory pathways leading to the amygdala and hypothalamus are thought to mediate the emotional and motivational aspects of smell as well as many of the behavioral and physiological effects of odors.

Pheromones Are Species-Specific Chemical Messengers

Some species release chemical substances into their surroundings to influence the behavior or physiology of members of the same species. Pheromones play an important role in sexual and social behaviors and reproductive physiology in many animals. Pheromones can influence estrus cycles, regulate the age of onset of puberty, prevent implantation of fertilized embryos, and signal receptivity of females for mating in many species, including mice, rats, cattle, and pigs. The source of pheromones is typically urine or glandular secretions. However, very few pheromones have been chemically defined.

The Vomeronasal Organ Transmits Information About Pheromones

Two separate olfactory systems appear to be involved in sensing pheromones: the main olfactory system, which we have already discussed, and the *accessory olfactory system* or *vomeronasal system*. The accessory system includes the paired vomeronasal organs, which are located at the base of the nasal septum; the vomeronasal nerves; and the accessory olfactory bulbs.

The vomeronasal organ is a fluid-filled, tubular structure that opens into the nasal cavity via a duct at its anterior end. It is lined, in part, with a sensory epithelium that resembles the olfactory epithelium of the nasal cavity. Molecules that dissolve in the mucus of the nasal cavity are pumped into the vomeronasal organ by changes in local blood volume, which change the size of its lumen. The axons of neurons in the vomeronasal organ are bundled in the vomeronasal nerve and project to the accessory olfactory bulb, an anatomically distinct region of the olfactory bulb.

The accessory olfactory bulb differs from the main olfactory bulb in its pattern of projections (Figure 32-9). Mitral cells in the accessory olfactory bulb project almost exclusively to regions of the amygdala that project to the hypothalamus. The anatomical layout of this pathway suggests that molecules sensed by the accessory olfactory system stimulate regions of the hypothalamus that are involved in reproductive physiology and behavior but are not consciously perceived. Consistent with this idea, male hamsters whose vomeronasal nerves have been cut exhibit a severe dysfunction in mating. Similar studies have implicated the vomeronasal system in a variety of behavioral and physiological responses to pheromones.

There has been considerable speculation as to whether humans communicate via body odors. There has also been debate as to whether humans have an accessory olfactory system, although evidence is accumulating that we do not.

Sensory Transduction in the Vomeronasal Organ Differs From That in the Nose

Although sensory neurons in the vomeronasal organ resemble those in the nasal olfactory epithelium, they use different molecules to transduce sensory stimuli. Vomeronasal neurons completely lack several major components of the olfactory sensory transduction cascade ($G_{\alpha olf}$, adenylyl cyclase type III, and one subunit of the olfactory cyclic nucleotide-gated cation channel). In addition, only a rare vomeronasal neuron expresses "classical" odorant receptors. The vomeronasal neurons appear to use two entirely different families, of approximately 100 different receptor types each, to detect sensory ligands.

Although the members of both candidate pheromone receptor families are unrelated in sequence to odorant receptors, they resemble odorant receptors in that they have seven potential transmembrane domains, a feature characteristic of G protein-coupled receptors. The vomeronasal receptor families resemble the odorant receptor family in other ways as well. First, members of these families are diverse, suggesting that they recognize different ligands. Second, it appears that each vomeronasal neuron may express only one type of vomeronasal receptor. And third, neurons that express different receptor types are interspersed in the vomeronasal neuroepithelium (Figure 32-10).

The two families of vomeronasal receptors are expressed in two different spatial zones. In contrast to the spatial zones of odorant receptor expression, the vomeronasal zones consist of two parallel layers of neurons that extend throughout the neuroepithelium. Interestingly, neurons in the upper layer express high levels of the G protein $G_{\alpha i2}$, while those in the lower layer express high levels of $G_{\alpha o}$, suggesting that the two receptor families might couple to different G proteins. An important question still to be answered is what ligands are recognized by the vomeronasal receptors. Another is whether information provided by the two receptor families is transmitted to different areas of the amygdala or hypothalamus that mediate different behavioral or physiological effects of pheromones.

Olfactory Acuity Varies in Humans

Olfactory acuity varies considerably among humans. Sensitivity may vary as much as a thousandfold, even among people with no obvious abnormality. The most common olfactory aberration is *specific anosmia*. An individual with a specific anosmia has lowered sensitivity to a specific odorant even though sensitivity to other odorants appears normal. Specific anosmias to some odorants are common, a few occurring in 1–20% of people. For example, 12% of individuals tested in one study exhibited a specific anosmia for musk. Lack of a specific odorant receptor may explain specific anosmias.

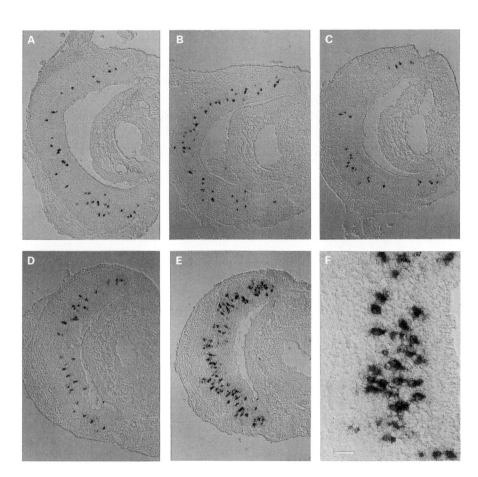

Figure 32-10 The pattern of expression of candidate pheromone receptors in the vomeronasal organ. The expression of one family of vomeronasal receptor genes in the rat was examined by hybridizing digoxigenin-labeled probes to sections through the vomeronasal organ. Probes were prepared from different receptor genes (A–D) or a mix of six such probes (E and F). Each receptor probe hybridized to a small percentage of vomeronasal neurons scattered throughout the upper region of the vomeronasal neuroepithelium. With the mixed probe a much larger percentage of hybridized neurons is seen, indicating that the different receptor genes are expressed in different cells. Although the vomeronasal receptors are likely to recognize pheromones, no differences in hybridization were observed in male versus female rats (A vs B). Scale bar = 120 μm. (From Dulac and Axel 1995.)

Far rarer abnormalities of olfaction, such as *general anosmia* (complete lack of olfactory sensation) or *hyposmia* (diminished sense of smell), can derive from respiratory infections and are often transient. Chronic anosmia or hyposmia can result from damage to the olfactory epithelium caused by infections; from head trauma that severs the olfactory nerves passing through holes in the cribriform plate, which then become blocked by scar tissue; or from particular diseases, such as Parkinson disease. Olfactory hallucinations of repugnant smells (*cacosmia*) can occur as a consequence of epileptic seizures.

Invertebrates and Vertebrates Use Different Strategies to Process Chemosensory Information

Chemosensory mechanisms have been studied in both vertebrates and invertebrates. Certain features are highly conserved in evolution, including the use of chemosensory cells with specialized cilia or microvilli exposed to the external environment. Explorations into the molecular mechanisms underlying chemoreception in several invertebrate species suggest that, like vertebrates, they use G protein-coupled receptors to detect chemosensory stimuli. However, recent studies indicate that the strategies used by the nematode worm *Caenorhabditis elegans* to sort out the complexity of chemical information in its environment are different from those of vertebrates.

The nervous system of *C. elegans* is composed of only 302 neurons, each of which has a characteristic location in the animal. Thirty-two of these cells are chemosensory neurons, which have cilia in contact with the external milieu. *C. elegans* can discriminate between a variety of volatile and nonvolatile chemicals. By killing individual cells with a laser beam, investigators can determine which cells respond to a given chemical. Such studies indicate that responses to volatile and nonvolatile chemicals are generally mediated by different chemosensory neurons. Different neurons respond to different chemicals, but each neuron can recognize a variety of chemicals. The worm moves toward some chemicals but moves away from others, and different chemosensory neurons mediate these attraction and repulsion responses.

Molecular genetic studies have begun to provide insight into the mechanism by which *C. elegans* discriminates among different chemicals. A receptor for a volatile chemical, diacetyl, was identified by cloning genes that are mutated in worms that cannot sense diacetyl (Figure 32-11). Although the diacetyl receptor is unrelated to vertebrate odorant receptors, its structure suggests that it may also transduce signals by interacting with G proteins. The diacetyl receptor belongs to a family of receptors, members of which are expressed by different chemosensory neurons. These receptors are expressed in chemosensory neurons that detect both volatile and nonvolatile chemicals. In striking contrast to vertebrate olfactory systems, a single chemosensory neuron in *C. elegans* expresses several different receptors that belong to the diacetyl receptor family. Each neuron also appears to express several receptors that belong to other families of G protein-coupled receptors, suggesting that each neuron employs a variety of receptor types to detect chemicals in the external environment.

Functional studies indicate that a worm with only one functional chemosensory neuron can distinguish some chemicals. The expression of different classes of receptors in a single cell suggests the intriguing possibility that this discrimination derives from the existence of multiple signaling cascades, each of which is activated by a different receptor type.

Taste Stimuli Are Detected by Taste Cells in the Mouth

Taste Cells Are Clustered in Taste Buds

Molecules that can be tasted are detected by taste cells clustered in taste buds on the tongue, palate, pharynx, epiglottis, and upper third of the esophagus. On the tongue, taste buds are located primarily in the papillae, which are embedded in the epithelium.

In humans three morphological types of papillae are found in different regions of the tongue (Figure 32-12). Several hundred fungiform papillae, which have a peg-like structure, are located on the anterior two-thirds of the tongue. On the posterior third are the large circumvallate papillae, each of which is surrounded by a groove. The foliate papillae, situated on the posterior edge of the tongue, are leaf-like structures, each of which is also surrounded by a groove. Each fungiform papilla contains one to five taste buds, while each circumvallate or foliate papilla contains hundreds of taste buds.

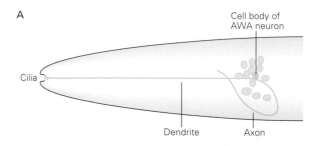

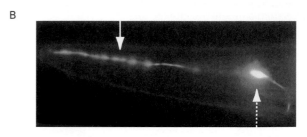

Figure 32-11 The receptor for diacetyl is expressed in a specific chemosensory neuron in the nematode worm *Caenorhabditis elegans.*

A. Diagram of a lateral view of the anterior end of the nematode *C. elegans* showing the cell body and processes of the AWA chemosensory neuron. The dendritic process of the AWA neuron terminates in cilia that are exposed to environmental chemicals. The AWA neuron detects the volatile chemical diacetyl; animals with a mutation in the *odr-10* gene are unable to sense diacetyl.

B. The pattern of expression of the *odr-10* gene was examined by preparing transgenic animals carrying a fusion gene consisting of part of the *odr-10* gene fused to a gene encoding a fluorescent protein (green fluorescent protein). In this lateral view of a transgenic animal, fluorescence is seen only in the AWA neuron, indicating that the *odr-10* gene is normally expressed in this neuron. This is consistent with the conclusion that the *odr-10* gene encodes the diacetyl receptor. **Arrows** indicate the AWA dendrite and cell body. (From Sengupta et al. 1996.)

Four morphologically distinguishable types of cells are found in each taste bud: basal cells, dark cells, light cells, and intermediate cells (Figure 32-13). Basal cells, small round cells at the base of the taste bud, are thought to be the stem cells from which the other cells are derived. Taste cells are very short-lived and are continuously regenerated. The three nonbasal cell types may represent various stages of differentiation of the developing taste cell, with the light cells being the most mature. Alternatively, the light, intermediate, and dark cells could represent different cell lineages. All three types are referred to as taste cells; all have an elongate, bipolar shape and extend from the epithelial opening of the taste bud to its base.

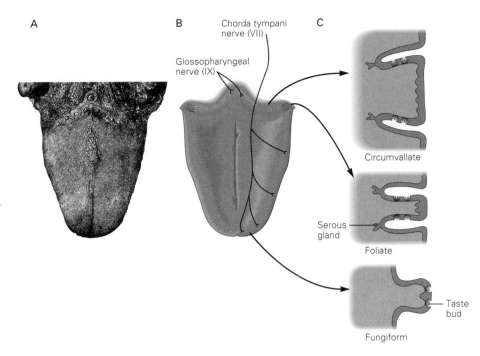

Figure 32-12 Taste buds are located in three types of papillae found in different regions of the human tongue.

A. Surface of the dorsum and root of the human tongue. (From Bloom and Fawcett 1975.)

B. The taste buds of the anterior two-thirds of the tongue are innervated by the gustatory fibers that travel in a branch of the facial nerve (VII) called the chorda tympani. The taste buds of the posterior third of the tongue are innervated by gustatory fibers that travel in the lingual branch of the glossopharyngeal nerve (IX). (Adapted from Shepherd 1983.)

C. The main types of taste papillae are shown in schematic cross sections. Each type predominates in specific areas of the tongue, as indicated by the arrows from **B.**

Each taste bud has a small opening at the surface of the epithelium called a taste pore. The hundred or so taste cells in each bud extend microvilli into the taste pore (Figure 32-13). The microvilli, where sensory transduction takes place, are the only parts of the taste cell that are exposed to the oral cavity. The taste cell is innervated by sensory neurons (primary gustatory afferent fibers) at its basal pole. Although taste cells are nonneuronal epithelial cells, the contacts between taste cells and sensory fibers have the morphological characteristics of chemical synapses. In addition, taste cells, like neurons, are electrically excitable cells with voltage-gated Na^+, K^+, and Ca^{2+} channels capable of generating action potentials.

The Four Different Taste Qualities Are Meditated by a Variety of Mechanisms

The gustatory system distinguishes four basic stimulus qualities: bitter, salty, sour, and sweet. Monosodium glutamate may represent a fifth stimulus category, called *umami*. The molecular mechanisms by which taste stimuli are transduced have been explored in studies using a variety of experimental techniques, including electrophysiology, biochemistry, and molecular biology. These studies have shown that each type of taste stimulus is transduced by a different mechanism (Figure 32-14). In addition, two stimuli may elicit the same taste sensation by different mechanisms. Furthermore,

the molecular mechanisms used by different vertebrate species to sense the same tastant may differ.

In general, tastants interact with either ion channels or specific receptors in the apical membrane of the taste cell. These interactions typically depolarize the cell, either directly or via the action of second messengers. The resulting receptor potential generates action potentials in the taste cell, which, in turn, lead to Ca^{2+} influx through voltage-dependent Ca^{2+} channels and the release of neurotransmitter at synapses formed with sensory fibers. Another alternative mechanism may involve the release of Ca^{2+} from intracellular stores. As discussed below, salty and sour tastes involve permeation, or blockade, of ion channels by Na^+ ions (salty taste) or H^+ ions (sour taste), while sweet and bitter tastes appear to be mediated in some cases by specific G protein-coupled receptors, but in other cases they may result from direct effects on ion channels.

Sweet

Sweet taste is thought to be mediated by the binding of sweet tastants to specific receptors on the apical membrane of the taste cell (Figure 32-14). There may be two different mechanisms for the transduction of sweet tastants. In rodents, one appears to involve a cAMP-dependent closure of basolateral K^+ channels. Since these channels are normally open at the resting membrane potential, their closure leads to depolarization of the cell. The binding of sweet tastants to G protein-

A

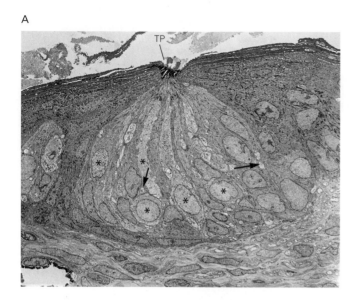

B

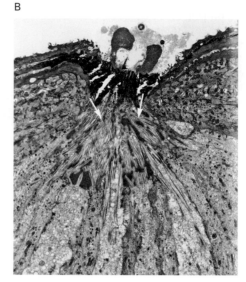

C

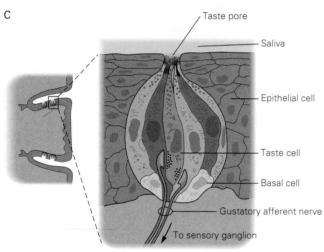

Taste pore

Saliva

Epithelial cell

Taste cell

Basal cell

Gustatory afferent nerve

To sensory ganglion

Figure 32-13 Each taste bud contains many taste cells.

A, B. Transmission electron micrographs of longitudinal sections through a rabbit foliate taste bud show microvilli (**arrows in B**) projecting into the taste pore (**TP**). Also seen are the nuclei and apical processes of the taste cells (**asterisks in A**). Afferent nerve fibers are indicated by **arrows in A**. Magnification approximately × 860. (**A**, from Royer and Kinnamon 1991; **B**, courtesy of Royer and Kinnamon.)

C. Each taste bud contains 50–150 taste cells that extend from the base of the taste bud to the taste pore, where the apical microvilli of taste cells have contact with tastants dissolved in saliva and taste pore mucus. Access of tastants to the basolateral regions of these cells is generally prevented by tight junctions between taste cells. Taste cells are short-lived cells that are replaced from stem cells at the base of the taste bud. Three types of taste cells in each taste bud (light cells, dark cells, and intermediate cells) may represent different stages of differentiation or different cell lineages. Taste stimuli, detected at the apical end of the taste cell, induce action potentials that cause the release of neurotransmitter at synapses formed at the base of the taste cell with gustatory fibers that transmit signals to the brain.

coupled sweet receptors induces an increase in intracellular cAMP, activating a cAMP-dependent kinase that phosphorylates K^+ channels, thereby inactivating them. Evidence for this pathway is provided by studies showing that mouse taste cells depolarize in response to sucrose and that this response can be mimicked by the intracellular injection of cyclic nucleotides or a chemical that specifically blocks K^+ channels. In addition, sucrose causes a dose-dependent rise in cAMP in intact circumvallate taste buds. The observation that increases

in cAMP that are induced by sweet tastants require the presence of GTP further suggests the existence of G protein-coupled receptors for sweet molecules.

A second mechanism of sweet taste transduction in rodents is suggested by the finding that some artificial sweeteners stimulate increases in IP_3. By analogy with signal transduction cascades involving IP_3 induction in some other cell types, some sweet taste receptors may transduce signals via interactions with one or more G proteins that change intracellular concentra-

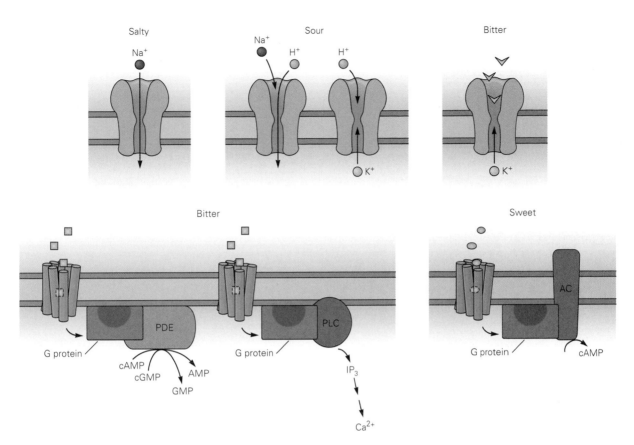

Figure 32-14 Four basic taste stimuli are transduced into electrical signals by different mechanisms.

Salty. Salty taste is mediated by Na⁺ influx through amiloride-sensitive Na⁺ channels. **Sour.** Sour taste can result from either the passage of H⁺ ions through amiloride-sensitive Na⁺ channels or from the blockade of K⁺ channels, which are normally open at resting potential. **Bitter.** Although at least one bitter stimulus, quinine, may depolarize taste cells by blocking apical K⁺ channels, most bitter stimuli are thought to bind to G protein-coupled receptors. There is evidence for two different pathways of bitter taste transduction that involve G proteins. In

one the G protein stimulates phospholipase C (**PLC**) to increase production of inositol 1,4,5-trisphosphate (**IP₃**), which then causes the release of Ca²⁺ from intracellular stores. In the other pathway the G protein gustducin activates a phosphodiesterase (**PDE**) that may reduce intracellular levels of both cAMP and cGMP. **Sweet.** Some sweet tastants are also thought to bind to receptors that couple to gustducin or a G protein that stimulates IP₃ production. However, other sweet receptors may couple to a G protein that interacts with adenylyl cyclase, causing an increase in cAMP that leads to the phosphorylation of K⁺ channels by protein kinase A.

tions of IP₃ rather than cAMP. Such increases in IP₃ are likely to cause the release of Ca²⁺ from intracellular stores.

Yet another possibility has been raised by the observation that mice mutant for the G protein gustducin have defective responses to some sweet substances. Gustducin is similar to transducin, which causes cyclic nucleotide degradation in the visual system. The relative contributions of cAMP production and degradation and IP₃ turnover in sweet taste transduction are currently unclear.

Bitter

Bitter taste is often associated with toxic compounds and is thought to have evolved as a means of preventing ingestion of these molecules. Bitter taste sensations are elicited by a variety of compounds, including divalent cations, some amino acids, alkaloids, and denatonium, the most bitter compound known. The molecular heterogeneity of these bitter-tasting substances and the fact that some are membrane-permeable (eg, quinine) while others are not (eg, denatonium) suggest that bitter taste

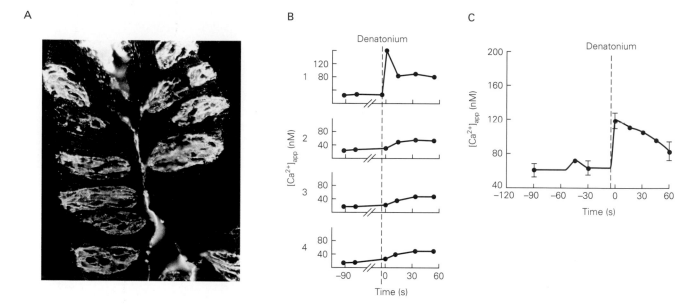

Figure 32-15 Responses of single taste cells to a bitter tastant. (From Akabas et al. 1988.)

A. Taste buds in a circumvallate papilla of the rat tongue labeled with a monoclonal antibody. Many taste cells are clustered in buds lining the wall of the papilla.

B. Intracellular Ca^{2+} concentration increases in a taste cell responsive to a bitter stimulus, denatonium chloride (1). Three

adjacent nonreceptive cells (2, 3, 4) showed no change in intracellular Ca^{2+} concentration. The Ca^{2+} concentration was calculated using a Ca^{2+}-sensitive dye, Fura-2.

C. Increases in intracellular Ca^{2+} concentration in the taste cell are caused by a release of Ca^{2+} from intracellular stores. When taste cells isolated in culture were bathed in a Ca^{2+}-free medium, denatonium remained an effective stimulus.

might be transduced by more than one mechanism. Current evidence supports this idea.

The transduction of many bitter tastes may involve specific G protein-coupled membrane receptors that bind to bitter-tasting compounds (Figure 32-14). This mechanism was suggested by the observation, in optically imaged taste cells impregnated with a calcium-sensitive dye, that intracellular Ca^{2+} changes after exposure to denatonium. Denatonium, as well as some other bitter stimuli, has been found to cause increases in intracellular IP_3 and the release of Ca^{2+} from intracellular stores (Figure 32-15), which are changes elicited by G protein-coupled receptors in many other cell types.

Receptors for some bitter substances, like those for some sweet tastants, may be coupled to the taste cell-specific G protein gustducin. As already mentioned, gustducin is related to transducin, the G protein α-subunit that stimulates cGMP phosphodiesterase in response to visual stimuli in photoreceptor cells. Recent studies suggest that gustducin similarly stimulates a taste cell phosphodiesterase, which then lowers intracellular levels of both cAMP and cGMP. Mice in which the gustducin gene has been deleted are defective in their ability to perceive some bitter compounds as well as some sweet ones.

Some bitter compounds that are membrane-permeable may be sensed by mechanisms that do not involve G proteins (see Figure 32-14). For example, quinine is able to block apically located K^+ channels. This mechanism of bitter taste transduction may explain why a number of different chemicals that block K^+ channels have a bitter taste.

Salty

Salty stimuli, such as NaCl, are transduced at least in part by a diffusion of Na^+ ions down an electrochemical gradient through apical amiloride-sensitive Na^+ channels. This Na^+ influx directly alters the membrane potential of the taste cell (see Figure 32-14). Evidence for this mechanism is provided by studies showing that amiloride interferes with the ability of human subjects to taste Na^+ salts and that it blocks the response of the chorda tympani nerve to NaCl placed on the tongue. The transduction of K^+ salts may similarly involve influx of K^+ ions through apical K^+ channels. Differences in the perceived qualities of various Na^+ salts may be the consequence of differences in the ability of different Na^+ salt anions to penetrate the tight junctions between taste cells and affect ion channels on the basolateral membranes of taste cells.

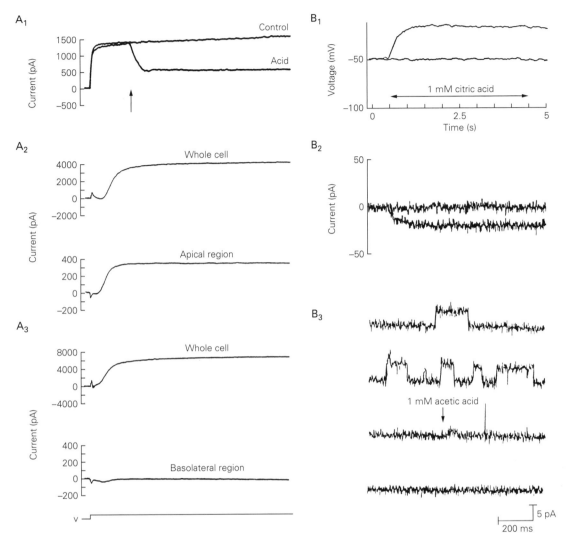

Figure 32-16 Signal transduction of sour tastants can result from a blockade of apical K$^+$ channels.

A. Recordings from isolated mudpuppy taste cells. **1.** Focal application of citric acid to the taste cell reduces the whole-cell K$^+$ current. **2-3.** Approximately 10% of the whole-cell K$^+$ current was recorded near the apical region (**2**), but less than 0.5% near the basolateral region (**3**). Potassium current was recorded in response to a 20 mV depolarization from −100 mV. (From Kinnamon et al. 1988.)

B. Responses of isolated salamander taste cells and cell-free patches to acids. **1.** Citric acid elicited a slow depolarization of the taste cell, which was associated with an increase in membrane resistance (not shown). **2.** Under voltage clamp the acid-induced response was observed as a sustained inward current. **3.** Continuous recording of single K$^+$ channels in outside-out patches of taste cell membrane showed that the channels were rapidly (and reversibly) blocked by acetic acid. (From Teeter et al. 1989.)

Sour

Transduction of sour tastants appears to involve the permeation or blockade of apical ion channels by protons. In the mudpuppy sour taste is mediated by a blockade of apical K$^+$ channels by H$^+$ ions (Figures 32-14 and 32-16). Since the K$^+$ channels are generally open at resting potential, their blockade produces membrane depolarization. In the hamster a different mechanism seems to operate. In this species sour taste results from an influx of H$^+$ ions through amiloride-sensitive Na$^+$ channels (see Figure 32-14). These channels are thought to be permeable to protons when salivary Na$^+$ concentration is low; when Na$^+$ concentrations are high, protons block Na$^+$ flux through the channels and inhibit the response to NaCl. Consistent with this idea, acids reduce the perceived intensity of salts in humans.

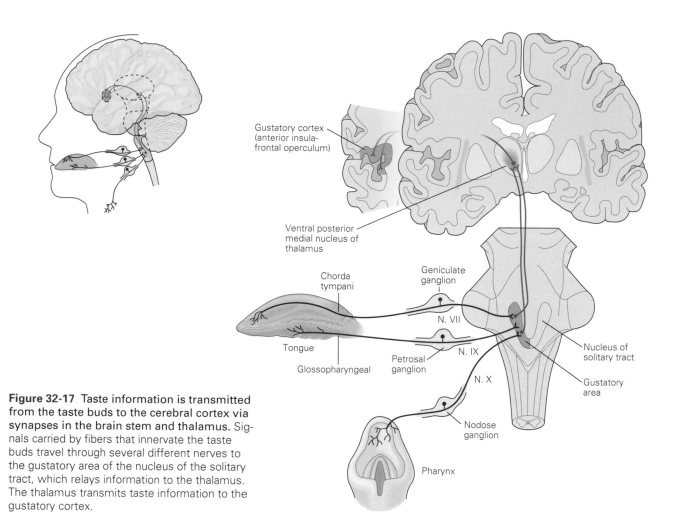

Figure 32-17 Taste information is transmitted from the taste buds to the cerebral cortex via synapses in the brain stem and thalamus. Signals carried by fibers that innervate the taste buds travel through several different nerves to the gustatory area of the nucleus of the solitary tract, which relays information to the thalamus. The thalamus transmits taste information to the gustatory cortex.

Umami

Some consider the taste of monosodium glutamate to represent a fifth category of taste stimuli, umami. Umami taste may be transduced by a specific type of metabotropic glutamate receptor, which is also expressed in certain regions of the brain.

It is clear that a variety of mechanisms serve to transduce sensory stimuli in taste cells and that these mechanisms fall into two general categories: those involving specific membrane receptors and second messengers and those based on the direct permeation or blockade of ion channels. Proteins in the saliva may further contribute to taste sensation by binding taste stimuli and delivering them to the taste cell or, alternatively, by removing taste stimuli.

Information About Taste Is Relayed to the Cortex via the Thalamus

There is some evidence that different taste cells respond to different taste stimuli. However, it is not known whether each cell responds to one tastant or a combination of tastants. Each taste cell is innervated at its base by the peripheral branches of primary gustatory fibers (see Figure 32-13C). Each sensory fiber branches many times, innervating numerous taste buds and, within each taste bud, several taste cells. Thus, the electrical activity recorded from a single sensory fiber represents the input of many taste cells. As already discussed, the release of neurotransmitter from taste cells onto the sensory fibers induces action potentials in the fibers and the transmission of signals to the brain.

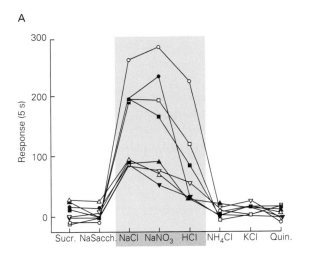

Figure 32-18 Response profiles of chorda tympani fibers of the hamster. (From Frank 1985.)

A. Response profiles for eight fibers that responded more to two sodium salts than to HCl. (**Sucr.** = sucrose; **NaSacch.** = sodium saccharide; **NaCl** = sodium chloride; **NaNO₃** = sodium nitrate; **HCl** = hydrogen chloride; **NH₄Cl** = ammonium chloride; **KCl** = potassium chloride; **Quin.** = quinine.)

B. Profiles for six fibers that responded to HCl, NaCl, and NH₄Cl. (**D-Phe** = D-phenylalanine.)

C. Profiles for six fibers that responded rather specifically to sucrose and D-phenylalanine, which are both sweet.

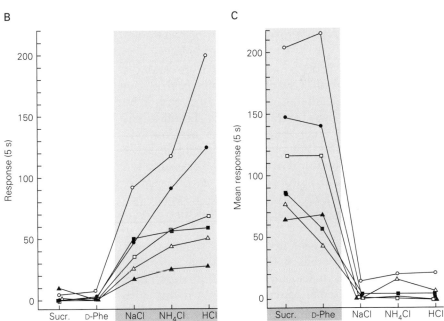

The taste buds in the anterior two-thirds of the tongue (those in the fungiform papillae) are innervated by sensory neurons of the geniculate ganglion whose peripheral branches travel in the chorda tympani, a branch of the facial nerve (cranial nerve VII) (Figures 32-12 and 32-17). Taste buds in the posterior third of the tongue are innervated by sensory neurons of the petrosal ganglion, whose peripheral branches travel in the lingual branch of the glossopharyngeal nerve (cranial nerve IX). The taste buds on the palate are innervated by the greater superficial petrosal branch of cranial nerve VII, and the buds on the epiglottis and esophagus by the superior laryngeal branch of cranial nerve X. Some of these nerves also carry somatosensory afferents that innervate regions of the tongue surrounding the taste buds.

The sensory fibers that receive input from the taste cells and run in cranial nerves VII, IX, and X enter the solitary tract in the medulla (Figure 32-17) and then form synapses on a thin column of cells in the gustatory area of the rostral and lateral part of the nucleus of the solitary tract.

Neurons in the gustatory area project to the thalamus, where they terminate in the small-cell (parvocellular) region of the ventral posterior medial nucleus. There the cells serving taste are grouped separately from neurons concerned with other sensory modalities of the tongue.

Neurons in the parvocellular region of the thalamus that receive taste input project to neurons along the border between the anterior insula and the frontal operculum in the ipsilateral cerebral cortex (Figure 32-17). This region is rostral to the somatosensory (ie, touch, pain, and temperature) representation of the tongue. This projection is believed to provide for the conscious perception and discrimination of taste stimuli.

It was once believed that taste cells responsive to each of the four basic categories of taste stimuli were concentrated exclusively in different areas of the tongue. This is not the case; taste buds responsive to sweet, salty, bitter, and sour tastes are found in all regions of the tongue. However, information derived from different areas of the tongue is spatially segregated in the nucleus of the solitary tract, thalamus, and cortex.

Different Taste Sensations Derive From Variations in Patterns of Activity in the Afferent Fiber Population

How does the gustatory system discriminate among a variety of taste stimuli? One clue has come from studying activity in single afferent gustatory fibers caused by exposure of an animal to different taste stimuli. It has been found that a single gustatory fiber may respond best to one stimulus but may also respond to other types of taste stimuli to varying degrees. For example, a fiber that responds vigorously to salt might also respond to acid (sour taste) and a fiber that responds primarily to acid might also respond to bitter stimuli (Figure 32-18).

This implies that each fiber receives signals from a population of taste cells with a distinctive set of response specificities. It also suggests that different tastes are encoded by different patterns of activity in the entire fiber population or by activation of different, but overlapping, sets of fibers. In this respect, taste coding may resemble sensory information coding in other systems, including the visual and auditory systems, where late steps in the processing of information involve a comparison of the activity of different cells that respond preferentially, but not exclusively, to certain features of sensory stimuli.

The Sensation of Flavors Results From a Combination of Gustatory, Olfactory, and Somatosensory Inputs

Much of what we think of as the flavor of foods derives from information provided by the olfactory system. Volatile molecules released from foods or beverages in the mouth are pumped into the back of the nasal cavity (retronasally) by the tongue, cheek, and throat move-

ments that accompany chewing and swallowing. Although the olfactory epithelium of the nose clearly makes a major contribution to sensations of taste, we experience taste as being in the mouth, not in the nose. It is thought that the somatosensory system is involved in this localization and that the coincidence between somatosensory stimulation of the tongue and retronasal passage of odorants into the nose causes the odorants to be perceived as flavors in the mouth.

Sensations of taste also frequently have a somatosensory component. This component includes the texture of food as well as sensations evoked by spicy and minty foods and by carbonation.

An Overall View

The senses of smell and taste provide us with a means to evaluate volatile molecules in our environment and both volatile and nonvolatile components of foodstuffs. The basic design and functional capacities of these systems are highly conserved across vertebrate species. In addition to providing a means of distinguishing between appropriate and potentially harmful substances prior to ingesting them, in many species these senses, particularly the sense of smell, play an important role in predator-prey relationships as well as in the regulation of social relationships critical to the production and rearing of offspring.

In the olfactory system, chemical stimuli are detected by olfactory sensory neurons that transmit signals to the olfactory bulb of the brain. From the olfactory bulb, olfactory information is relayed through the olfactory cortex to a variety of brain regions that allow for both the conscious discrimination of odors and their various effects on our emotions and behavior. The detection of odorants is accomplished by specific odorant receptors, of which there are as many as 1000 different types. There are millions of olfactory sensory neurons in the nose. Each receptor type is expressed by several thousand neurons, each of which expresses only one type of receptor.

Neurons that express the same type of odorant receptor are restricted to one zone in the nose, but in that zone they are interspersed with neurons expressing other receptor types. In the olfactory bulb the axons of those neurons converge on only a few glomeruli at fixed locations. The olfactory bulb appears to contain a highly organized sensory map in which information provided by different odorant receptors is focused onto different glomeruli. Each odorant may be recognized by several odorant receptors, and each receptor may recognize many odorants. The identity of an odorant is therefore likely to be encoded in the olfactory bulb not by unique odor-specific glomeruli but by unique sets of glomeruli, each of which serves as one component of the multicomponent codes for a variety of odorants. Olfactory information may be processed, or refined, by local circuits within the olfactory bulb prior to transmission to the olfactory cortex. The means by which olfactory information is encoded in the cortex is not yet known.

Taste stimuli are detected in the mouth by taste cells, specialized epithelial cells that are clustered in structures called taste buds. The taste cells are innervated by sensory fibers that transmit signals to the gustatory area of the nucleus of the solitary tract. From there, gustatory information is transmitted to the cortex (through a relay in the thalamus). Four basic categories of taste stimuli—bitter, sweet, salty, and sour—are detected by taste cells. Sweet and some bitter tastants may be detected by specific G protein-coupled receptors on taste cells, while other bitter tastants may stimulate taste cells via direct interactions with ion channels. The detection of salty taste stimuli is mediated by Na^+ ion influx through Na^+ channels, whereas sour tastes can result either from the permeation of Na^+ channels by protons or by proton blockade of apical K^+ channels.

The detection of tastants is transduced into a receptor potential that induces action potentials in the taste cell and the release of neurotransmitter at synapses formed between the taste cell and sensory fibers. Each sensory fiber contacts a number of taste cells and each taste cell synapses with numerous sensory fibers. Each sensory fiber carries information derived from a variety of taste stimuli but is generally dominated by one of these stimuli. Thus, the identity of a taste stimulus appears to be encoded by a unique pattern of inputs from many separate fibers that provide components of the patterns for different stimuli. The multitude of different flavors that one can experience derives from a combination of gustatory, olfactory, and somatosensory components.

Linda B. Buck

Selected Readings

Axel R. 1995. The molecular logic of smell. Sci Am 273:154–159.

Bartoshuk LM, Beauchamp GK. 1994. Chemical senses. Annu Rev Psychol 45:419–449.

Breer H, Boekhoff I, Krieger J, Raming K, Strotmann J, Tareilus E. 1992. Molecular mechanisms of olfactory signal transduction. In: DP Corey, SD Roper (eds). *Society of General Physiologists Series*, 47:93–108. New York: Rockefeller Univ. Press.

Buck LB. 1995. Unraveling chemosensory diversity. Cell 83:349–352.

Buck LB. 1996. Information coding in the vertebrate olfactory system. Annu Rev Neurosci 19:517–544.

Firestein S. 1992. Electrical signals in olfactory transduction. Curr Opin Neurobiol 2:444–448.

Gilbertson TA. 1993. The physiology of vertebrate taste reception. Curr Opin Neurobiol 3:532–539.

Kauer JS. 1987. Coding in the olfactory system. In: TE Finger, WL Silver (eds). *Neurobiology of Taste and Smell*, pp. 205–231. New York: Wiley.

Kauer JS, Cinelli AR. 1993. Are there structural and functional modules in the vertebrate olfactory bulb? Microsc Res Tech 24:157–167.

Margolskee RF. 1993. The biochemistry and molecular biology of taste transduction. Curr Opin Neurobiol 3:526–531.

Pfaff DW, ed. 1985. *Taste, Olfaction, and the Central Nervous System*. New York: Rockefeller Univ. Press.

Reed RR. 1992. Signaling pathways in odorant detection. Neuron 8:205–209.

Roper SD. 1989. The cell biology of vertebrate taste receptors. Annu Rev Neurosci 12:329–353.

Schiffmann SS. 1983. Taste and smell in disease. N Engl J Med 308:1337–1343.

Scott JW, Wellis DP, Riggott MJ, Buonviso N. 1993. Functional organization of the main olfactory bulb. Microsc Res Tech 24:142–156.

Shepherd GM. 1994. Discrimination of molecular signals by the olfactory receptor neuron. Neuron 13:771–790.

Shepherd GM, Greer CA. 1990. Olfactory bulb. In: GM Shepherd (ed). *The Synaptic Organization of the Brain*, 3rd ed., pp. 133–169. New York: Oxford Univ. Press.

Sullivan SL, Ressler KJ, Buck LB. 1995. Spatial patterning and information coding in the olfactory system. Curr Opin Genet Dev 5:516–523.

References

Akabas MH, Dodd J, Al-Awqati Q. 1988. A bitter substance induces a rise in intracellular calcium in a subpopulation of rat taste cells. Science 242:1047–1050.

Amoore JE. 1977. Specific anosmia and the concept of primary odors. Chem Senses Flavor 2:267–281.

Avenet P, Hoffman F, Lindemann B. 1988. Transduction in taste receptor cells requires cAMP-dependent protein kinase. Nature 331:351–354.

Bakalyar HA, Reed RR. 1990. Identification of a specialized adenylyl cyclase that may mediate odorant detection. Science 250:1403–1406.

Behe P, DeSimone JA, Avenet P, Lindemann B. 1990. Membrane currents in taste cells of the rat fungiform papilla: evidence for two types of Ca^{2+} currents and inhibition of K^+ currents by saccharin. J Gen Physiol 96:1061–1084.

Berghard A, Buck LB. 1996. Sensory transduction in vomeronasal neurons: evidence for Gαo, Gαi2, and adenylyl cyclase II as major components of a pheromone signaling cascade. J Neurosci 16:909–918.

Berghard A, Buck LB, Liman ER. 1996. Evidence for distinct signaling mechanisms in two mammalian olfactory sense organs. Proc Natl Acad Sci U S A 93:2365–2369.

Bloom W, Fawcett DW. 1975. *A Textbook of Histology*, 10th ed, pp. 392–410. Philadelphia: Saunders.

Bruch RC, Teeter JH. 1990. Cyclic AMP links amino acid chemoreceptors to ion channels in olfactory cilia. Chem Senses 15:419–430.

Buck L, Axel R. 1991. A novel multigene family may encode odorant receptors: a molecular basis for odor recognition. Cell 65:175–187.

Chaudhari N, Yang H, Lamp C, Delay E, Cartford C, Than T, Roper S. 1996. The taste of monosodium glutamate: membrane receptors in taste cells. J Neurosci 16:3817–3826.

Dawson TM, Arriza JL, Jaworksy DE, Borisy FF, Attramadal H, Lefkowitz RJ, Ronnett GV. 1993. Beta-adrenergic receptor kinase-2 and beta-arrestin-2 as mediators of odorant-induced desensitization. Science 259:825–829.

Dhallan RS, Yau KW, Schrader KA, Reed RR. 1990. Primary structure and functional expression of a cyclic nucleotide-activated channel from olfactory neurons. Nature 347:184–187.

Dulac C, Axel R. 1995. A novel family of genes encoding putative pheromone receptors in mammals. Cell 83:195–206.

Firestein S, Picco C, Menini A. 1993. The relation between stimulus and response in olfactory receptor cells of the tiger salamander. J Physiol 468:1–10.

Gilbertson TA, Avenet P, Kinnamon SC, Roper SD. 1992. Proton currents through amiloride-sensitive Na$^+$ channels in hamster taste cells: role in acid transduction. J Gen Physiol 100:803–824.

Guthrie KM, Anderson AJ, Leon M, Gall C. 1993. Odor-induced increases in c-*fos* mRNA expression reveal an anatomical "unit" for odor processing in olfactory bulb. Proc Natl Acad Sci U S A 90:3329–3333.

Heck GL, Mierson S, DeSimione JA. 1984. Salt taste transduction occurs through an amiloride-sensitive sodium transport pathway. Science 223:403–405.

Jones DT, Reed RR. 1989. G$_{olf}$: an olfactory neuron-specific G protein involved in odorant signal transduction. Science 244:790–795.

Jourdan F, Duveau A, Astic L, Holley A. 1980. Spatial distribution of [^{14}C]2-deoxyglucose uptake in the olfactory bulbs of rats stimulated with two different odors. Brain Res 188:139–154.

Kinnamon SC, Dionne VE, Beam KG. 1988. Apical localization of K$^+$ channels in taste cells provides the basis for sour taste transduction. Proc Natl Acad Sci U S A 85:7023–7027.

McLaughlin SK, McKinnon PJ, Margolskee RF. 1992. Gustducin is a taste-cell-specific G protein closely related to the transducins. Nature 357:563–569.

Mori K, Mataga N, Imamura K. 1992. Differential specifici-
ties of single mitral cells in rabbit olfactory bulb for a homologous series of fatty acid odor molecules. J Neurophysiol 67:786–789.

Morrison EE, Costanzo RM. 1990. Morphology of the human olfactory epithelium. J Comp Neurol 297:1–13.

Nakamura T, Gold GH. 1987. A cyclic nucleotide-gated conductance in olfactory receptor cilia. Nature 325:442–444.

Pace U, Hanski E, Salomon Y, Lancet D. 1985. Odorant-sensitive adenylate cyclase may mediate olfactory reception. Nature 316:255–258.

Pevsner J, Reed RR, Feinstein PG, Snyder SH. 1988. Molecular cloning of odorant-binding protein: member of a ligand carrier family. Science 241:336–339.

Pfaffmann C. 1955. Gustatory nerve impulses in rat, cat and rabbit. J Neurophysiol 18:429–440.

Raming K, Krieger J, Strotmann J, Boekhoff I, Kubick S, Baumstark C, Breer H. 1993. Cloning and expression of odorant receptors. Nature 361:353–356.

Ressler KJ, Sullivan SL, Buck LB. 1993. A zonal organization of odorant receptor gene expression in the olfactory epithelium. Cell 73:597–609.

Ressler KJ, Sullivan SL, Buck LB. 1994. Information coding in the olfactory system: evidence for a stereotyped and highly organized epitope map in the olfactory bulb. Cell 79:1245–1255.

Royer SM, Kinnamon JC. 1991. HVEM Serial-section analysis of rabbit foliate taste buds. I. Type III cells and their synapses. J Comp Neurol 306:49–72.

Ruiz-Avila L, McLaughlin SK, Wildman D, McKinnon PJ, Robicon A, Spickofsky N, Margolskee RF. 1995. Coupling of bitter receptor to phosphodiesterase through transducin in taste receptor cells. Nature 376:80–85.

Saucier D, Astic L. 1986. Analysis of the topographical organization of olfactory epithelium projections in the rat. Brain Res Bull 16:455–462.

Schiffman SS, Lockhead E, Maes FW. 1983. Amiloride reduces the taste intensity of Na$^+$ and Li$^+$ salts and sweeteners. Proc Natl Acad Sci U S A 80:6136–6140.

Sengupta P, Chou JH, Bargmann CI. 1996. *odr-10* encodes a seven transmembrane olfactory receptor required for responses to the odorant diacetyl. Cell 84:899–909.

Sengupta P, Colbert HA, Kimmel BE, Dwyer N, Bargmann CI. 1993. The cellular and genetic basis of olfactory responses in *Caenorhabditis elegans*. Ciba Found Symp 179:235–244.

Shepherd GM. 1994. Discrimination of molecular signals by the olfactory receptor neuron. Neuron 13:771–790.

Stewart WB, Kauer JS, Shepherd GM. 1979. Functional organization of rat olfactory bulb analyzed by the 2-deoxyglucose method. J Comp Neurol 185:715–734.

Sullivan SL, Adamson MC, Ressler KJ, Kozak CA, Buck LB. 1996. The chromosomal distribution of mouse odorant receptor genes. Proc Natl Acad Sci U S A 93:884–888.

Teeter JH, Sugimoto K, Brand JG. 1989. Ionic currents in taste cells and reconstituted taste epithelial membranes. In: JG Brand, JH Teeter, RH Cagan, MR Kare (eds). *Chemical Senses*. Vol. 1, *Receptor Events and Transduction in Taste and*

Olfaction, pp. 151–170. New York: Marcel Dekker.

Tonosaki K, Funakoshi M. 1988. Cyclic nucleotides may mediate taste transduction. Nature 331:354–356.

Troemel ER, Chou JH, Dwyer ND, Colbert HA, Bargmann CI. 1995. Divergent seven transmembrane receptors are candidate chemosensory receptors in *C. elegans*. Cell 83:207–218.

Vassar R, Ngai J, Axel R. 1993. Spatial segregation of odorant receptor expression in the mammalian olfactory epithelium. Cell 74:309–318.

Vassar R, Chao SK, Sitcheran R, Nunez JM, Vosshall LB, Axel R. 1994. Topographic organization of sensory projections to the olfactory bulb. Cell 79:981–991.

Wong GT, Gannon KS, Margolskee RF. 1996. Transduction of bitter and sweet taste by gustducin. Nature 381:796–800.

Part VI

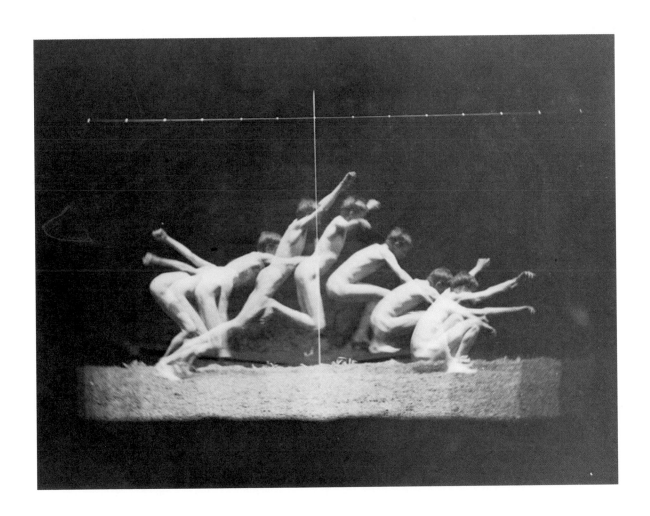

VI Movement

O UR SENSORY SYSTEMS FORM internal representations of our bodies and the external world. One of the principal functions of these internal representations is to guide movement. Even a simple task such as reaching for a glass of water requires visual information to establish an internal representation of the location of the glass in space. It also requires proprioceptive information to form an internal representation of the body so that appropriate motor commands can be sent to the arm. Purposeful action is possible only because the parts of the brain that control movement have access to the ongoing stream of sensory information in the brain. The integrative action of the nervous system—the decision to execute one movement and not another—depends therefore on the interaction between the motor and sensory systems.

The motor systems are organized in a functional hierarchy, with each of these levels concerned with different decisions. The highest, most abstract level, is concerned with the question: What is the purpose of the movement? This level is represented by the dorsolateral frontal cortex. The next level is concerned with the formation of a motor plan. This is accomplished through interactions between posterior parietal and premotor areas. In this interaction, the premotor cortex specifies the spatial characteristics of a movement based on sensory information from the posterior parietal cortex about the environment and about the position of the body in space. The lowest level of the hierarchy coordinates the spatiotemporal details of the muscle contractions needed to execute the planned movement. This coordination is executed by the motor circuits in the spinal cord.

Several anatomically distinct pathways project in parallel to the spinal cord from higher motor centers. Above the spinal cord is the brain stem, and above the brain stem are the cerebellum and the basal ganglia, structures that modulate the actions of brain stem systems. Overseeing these supraspinal structures are the motor centers in the cerebral cortex. As in the sensory systems, most of the motor areas of the brain stem and cerebral cortex are organized somatotypically— movements of adjacent body parts are controlled by contiguous areas of the brain at each level of the motor hierarchy.

Some functions of the motor systems and their disturbance by disease have now been described at the level of the biochemistry of specific transmitter systems. In fact, the discovery that neurons of the basal ganglia in parkinsonian patients lack functional amounts of dopamine was the first important clue that neurological and psychiatric disorders can result from altered chemical transmitter systems. As more of the genes and proteins important for motor functions are identified, we may understand the molecular events essential for the integrative action of the nervous system. Likewise, imaging techniques that can reveal the areas of the brain concerned with the cognitive aspects of motor control may help us understand how attention, intention, and motor learning are integrated to produce a meaningful motor act.

Part VI

33

The Organization of Movement

IN THE PRECEDING PART of this book we considered how the brain constructs internal representations of the world by integrating information from the different sensory systems. These sensory representations are the framework in which the motor systems plan, coordinate, and execute the motor programs responsible for purposeful movement. In this part of the book we shall learn how the motor systems of the brain and spinal cord allow us to maintain balance and posture, to move our body, limbs, and eyes, and to communicate through speech and gesture. In contrast to sensory systems, which transform physical energy into neural signals, motor systems produce movement by translating neural signals into contractile force in muscles.

Just as our perceptual skills reflect the capabilities of the sensory systems to detect, analyze, and estimate the significance of physical stimuli, our motor agility and dexterity reflect the capabilities of the motor systems to plan, coordinate, and execute movements. The accomplished pirouette of a ballet dancer, the powered backhand of a tennis player, the fingering technique of a pianist, and the coordinated eye movements of a reader all require a remarkable degree of motor skill that no robot approaches. Yet, once trained, the motor systems execute the motor programs for each of these skills with ease, for the most part automatically.

The ability of humans to carry out skilled movements while still performing cognitive tasks—such as thinking while using tools or speaking while walking—requires flexibility and skills no other animal has. A striking aspect of motor function is the effortlessness with which we carry out the most complicated motor tasks without a thought given to the actual joint motions or muscle contractions required. Although we are consciously aware of the intent to perform a task, such as driving a car, and planning certain sequences of actions, and at times we are aware of deciding to move at a particular moment, the details of our movements generally seem to occur automatically. The tennis player need not consciously decide which muscles to contract to return a serve with a backhand or which head motions and body parts must be moved to intercept the ball. In fact, thinking about each body movement before it takes place would disrupt the player's performance. Thus, conscious processes are not necessary for the moment-to-moment control of movement.

The graceful and effortless quality of normal movement carried out automatically depends on a continuous flow of visual, somatosensory and postural information to the motor systems. The "effortless" quality of normal motor control is frequently lost if the motor systems are deprived of a continuous flow of sensory information, from vision, somatic sensation, and vestibular inputs. Vision is particularly important to guiding movement and provides critical cognitive information about the location and shape of objects. The blind must explore space using tactile and kinesthetic cues, a more lengthy process, and they need to rely more on memorized representations of the locations of objects than do sighted persons. Similarly, movements become inaccurate and posture unstable when somatic sensation is lost from the limbs. Loss of vestibular input also impairs ability to maintain balance and orientation.

Successively higher levels of the motor hierarchy specify increasingly more complex aspects of a motor task. This hierarchy of motor representations depends on a parallel hierarchy of sensory input; more complex sensory information is extracted, at each level, from the spinal cord to the motor cortex. The crucial insight that the components of the motor systems are organized hierarchically was first obtained in the eighteenth century in studies that showed the spinal cord severed from the brain stem and forebrain is capable of organized behaviors. Relatively automatic behaviors include rhythmic behaviors, such as breathing or running as well as reflexes, such as the knee jerk or coughing. Patterned responses to sensory stimuli differ according to the level at which the neuraxis is transected. These differences therefore provide useful clinical indicators of the level of a lesion and of the integrity of afferent and efferent pathways.

Because reflexes and automatic rhythmic movements are so stereotyped, in contrast to the endless variety of voluntary movements, reflex and voluntary movements were originally thought to be controlled by

qualitatively different neuronal mechanisms. At the beginning of the twentieth century, however, Charles Sherrington in England proposed that voluntary movements represent chains of reflex responses linked together by the brain. Although this is not correct, the spinal cord does contain local circuits that coordinate reflexes, and these same circuits participate in more complex voluntary movements governed by higher brain centers.

In this chapter we first review the principles that govern various classes of movement and action. We shall learn how motor psychophysical studies of movement describe the relationships between intended actions and performance, just as sensory psychophysical studies relate physical stimuli to sensory experience in a quantitative way (Chapter 2). The lawful relationships emerging from these studies provide critical insights into how motor systems operate. Finally, we review the overall anatomical organization of the motor systems, from local spinal reflex circuits to the systems of the brain stem and the cerebral cortex that coordinate simple muscle contractions into elaborate purposeful actions.

The Motor Systems Generate Reflexive, Rhythmic, and Voluntary Movements

Just as there are distinct modalities of sensation, there are three distinct categories of movement: reflexive, rhythmic, and voluntary.

Reflexive and Rhythmic Movements Are Produced by Stereotyped Patterns of Muscle Contraction

Reflexes are *involuntary* coordinated patterns of muscle contraction and relaxation elicited by peripheral stimuli. They are typically isolated in animals in which motor pathways from higher brain centers to the spinal cord have been cut (such animals are called *decerebrate* or *spinal* animals depending on the level of the cut). The spatial and temporal patterns of muscle contraction vary in different reflexes, depending on the type of sensory receptors that are stimulated. Receptors in muscles produce stretch reflexes whereas cutaneous receptors produce withdrawal reflexes. In reflexes the particular muscles that contract in response to a stimulus vary with the site of stimulation, a phenomenon termed *local sign*. If external conditions remain the same, a given stimulus will elicit the same response time after time. However, both the intensity of the response and the local sign of reflexes can be modulated by mechanisms that switch the patterns of connections of afferent fibers to spinal in-

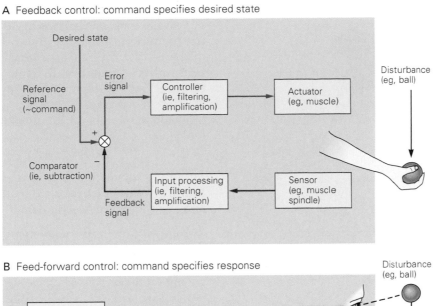

A Feedback control: command specifies desired state

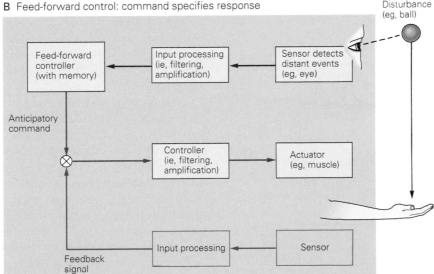

B Feed-forward control: command specifies response

Figure 33-1 Feed-forward and feedback control circuits.

A. In a feedback system a signal from a sensor is compared with a reference signal by a comparator. The difference, the error signal, is sent to a controller and causes a proportional change in output to the actuator. For example, if the task is to maintain the elbow at a given angle, the muscles are the actuators and the controlled system is the elbow. The reference signal specifies the muscle contraction required to maintain the joint at the required angle. Proprioceptive or visual information about the current elbow angle provides the feedback signal. The difference between the current and the reference angle determines the degree to which extensor and flexor muscles are activated.

B. Feed-forward control relies on information acquired before the feedback sensor is activated; this mechanism is essential for rapid movements. For example, a person catching a ball uses visual information about the ball's initial direction to anticipate the path of the ball in order to initiate the correct response to intercept it. Accuracy requires prior knowledge of the trajectories of thrown balls and the factors that might influence trajectory, such as the spin placed on the ball by the thrower. In the diagram a feedback response directly influences the very disturbance picked up by the sensor. This is not always the case with feed-forward control.

terneurons and motor neurons depending on the context of the behavior. We consider reflexes in greater detail in Chapter 36.

Understanding how input connects to output in spinal reflexes is important because the motor systems make use of this circuitry to coordinate muscles in complex purposeful movements. Also, different spinal reflexes are tested clinically to diagnose the integrity of afferent and efferent pathways and to locate the level of a lesion.

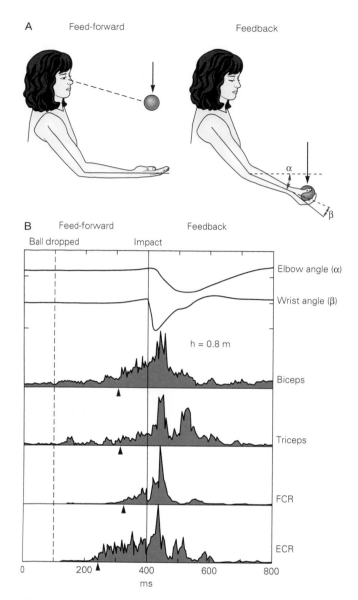

Figure 33-2 Catching a ball requires feed-forward and feedback controls.

A. Setup for ball-catching experiment. The ball can be dropped from any height set by the investigator.

B. The averaged responses of a subject catching a ball falling from a height of 0.8 m. The traces from top to bottom correspond to elbow angle (α), wrist angle (β), and rectified EMG activity of the biceps, triceps, flexor carpi radialis (FCR), and extensor carpi radialis (ECR). The anticipatory responses, before the impact of the ball, consist of coactivation of biceps and triceps muscles (**arrow heads**). After impact there is transient modification of the stretch reflex with further coactivation of flexor and extensors (rather than reciprocal inhibition).

Repetitive rhythmic motor patterns include chewing, swallowing, and scratching, as well as the alternating contractions of flexors and extensors on either side of the body during quadrupedal locomotion. The circuits for these repetitive rhythmic motor patterns lie in the spinal cord and brain stem. Although these patterns may occur spontaneously, they are more commonly triggered by peripheral stimuli that activate the underlying circuits.

Voluntary Movements Are Goal-Directed and Improve With Practice as a Result of Feedback and Feed-Forward Mechanisms

In contrast to reflexes, voluntary movements are initiated to accomplish a specific goal. Voluntary movements may, of course, be triggered by external events—we put on the brakes when we see the traffic light turn red or rush to catch a ball in flight. Voluntary movements improve with practice as one learns to anticipate and correct for environmental obstacles that perturb the body.

The nervous system learns to correct for such external perturbations in two ways. First, it monitors sensory signals and uses this information to act directly on the limb itself. This moment-to-moment control is called *feedback*. Second, the nervous system uses the same or different senses—for example, vision, hearing, and touch—to detect imminent perturbations and initiate proactive strategies based on experience. This anticipatory mode is called *feed-forward* control. Understanding the computations needed for these two forms of control is central to understanding how the motor systems control posture and movement.

In feedback control (also called *servo-control*) signals from sensors are compared with a desired state, represented by a *reference signal*. The difference, or *error signal*, is used to adjust the output (Figure 33-1A). In a negative or proportional feedback system the computed error immediately produces a compensatory change in output. Because the system forms a closed loop, the output of the feedback system itself can be altered by changing the reference signal. For example, in automatic regulation of room temperature a gauge monitors the ambient temperature and compares it with the desired value set on a thermostat. If the temperature is below the value desired, a heater is turned on; if it is too high, the heater is turned off.

Feedback systems are characterized by their *gain*. A high-gain system acts vigorously to minimize deviations from the optimal target state. However, high-gain systems may be unstable if there are large delays across the loop, for example from sensory neurons to interneuron(s) to motor neurons to muscle to a change in contractility. The delay between the input and output of a system is called the *phase lag*. If lags are long and external conditions change rapidly, specific feedback corrections may not be appropriate by the time they are implemented. In many feedback systems the gain is kept relatively low so that corrections do not produce large errors if conditions have changed. In low-gain systems, however, disturbances are corrected slowly, because the small corrections have to be repeated.

Feedback is especially important in maintaining the position of our limbs or the forces we apply to objects that we are holding. Very sensitive mechanoreceptors in muscles (the muscle spindles we shall consider in Chapter 36) and cutaneous afferents in the finger tips provide critical feedback signals for these tasks. Remarkable disorders of posture and movement occur in patients who lack this information. This information is disrupted when the large-diameter fibers that carry the signals from the mechanoreceptors are damaged. Affected patients can neither sense the motions of their joints nor detect objects touching their fingers. They cannot maintain their hand in one position or grasp an object steadily; after a few seconds the force and position of the limb begin to "drift" as fatigue in local groups of muscle fibers goes undetected.

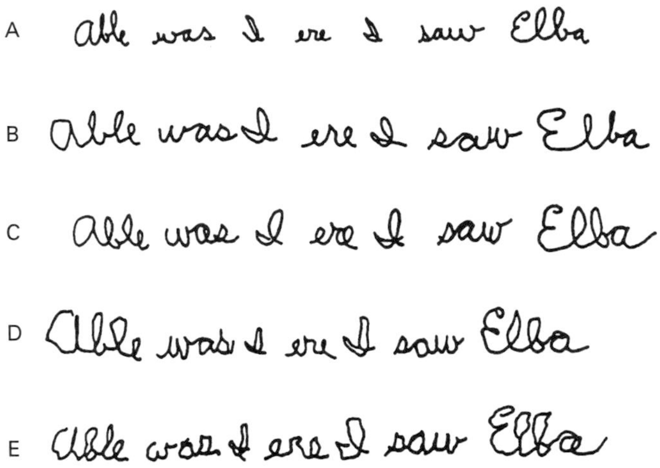

Unlike feedback systems, feed-forward control acts in advance of certain perturbations. When we enter a cold house we can immediately light a fire or close the windows to prevent becoming cold. This form of control is often referred to as *open loop* control to emphasize that feedback sensory signals do not directly affect the timing of the response. The term is somewhat misleading, however, because it suggests that actions controlled in this way are independent of sensory signals. In fact, feed-forward control must rely on a great deal of information—from sensors as well as experience—to operate correctly (Figure 33-1B). *Anticipatory* control is therefore the more appropriate term.

Feed-forward control is widely used by motor systems to control posture and movement. When we lift an arm while standing, we contract the muscles of our legs before those of the arm so that the shift in center of mass will not cause us to fall over. Even without any movement of the limbs, the contraction of our leg muscles is continuously being adjusted to compensate for the changes in center of mass that occur during breathing.

Experience is important in feed-forward control. Catching a ball is a visually triggered feed-forward response. We use visual information about the initial part of the ball's trajectory to predict the ball's path. Only after the ball hits the hand and displaces it can feedback begin to adjust the hand's position. Feed-forward mech-

Figure 33-3 Writing can be performed using **different parts of the body.** The examples here were written with the right (dominant) hand (**A**), with the right arm but with the wrist immobilized (**B**), with the left hand (**C**), with the pen gripped between the teeth (**D**), and with the pen attached to the foot (**E**), The ability of different motor sets to achieve the same behavior is called motor equivalence. (From Raibert 1977.)

anisms allow us to compute the time of the ball's impact and to contract the opposing arm muscles just before the ball reaches the hand (Figure 33-2). Interestingly, this anticipatory contraction always precedes impact by the same amount of time, regardless of the height from which the ball is seen to fall. This demonstrates that catchers use experience (knowledge that the ball is constantly accelerated by gravity) to time their muscle contractions accurately.

What happens after impact? Normally the rapid stretch of a muscle evokes a reflex controlled by spinal circuits: the stretched muscle contracts and its antagonist relaxes. But when people expect to catch a falling ball, the sudden muscle stretch produced by the ball's impact evokes the contraction of *both* the agonist and antagonist muscles. These contractions stiffen the elbow joint and transiently dampen the motions of the joint. Only spinal circuits can mediate such rapid feedback adjustments.

Catching a ball illustrates three key principles in the feed-forward control of movement. First, feed-forward control is essential for rapid action. Second, it depends on the ability of the nervous system to predict the consequences of sensory events, such as where a falling ball will drop. Third, feed-forward mechanisms can modify the operation of feedback mechanisms in the spinal cord.

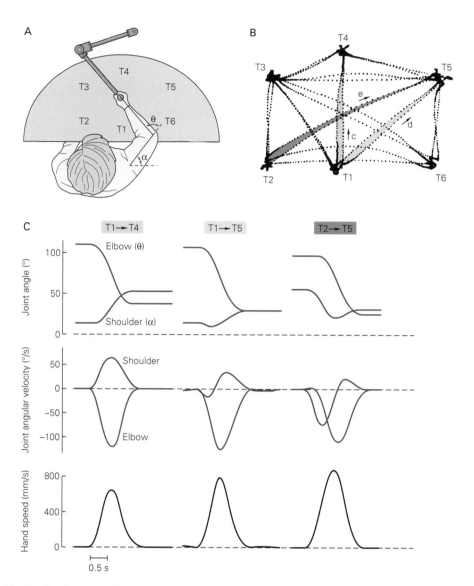

Figure 33-4 The brain plans reaching movements as hand trajectories.

A. Experimental setup. The subject sits in front of a semicircular plate and grasps the handle of a two-jointed apparatus that moves in one plane and records hand position. The subject is instructed to move the hand to various targets (T1–T6).

B. The paths traced by one subject while moving his hand to a series of targets.

C. Kinematic data for hand paths **c, d,** and **e** shown in part B. All paths are roughly straight and all hand speed profiles have the same shape and scale in proportion to the distance covered. In contrast, the profiles for the elbow and shoulder angles for the three hand paths differ. The straight hand paths and common profiles for speed suggest that planning is done with reference to the hand because these parameters can be linearly scaled. Planning with reference to joints would require computing nonlinear combinations of joint angles.

Voluntary Movements Obey Psychophysical Principles

The task of the motor systems is the reverse of the task of the sensory systems. Sensory processing generates an internal representation of the world or the state of the body, but motor processing *begins* with an internal representation, namely the desired result of movement. Nevertheless, just as psychophysical analysis of sensory processing tells us about the capabilities and limitations of the sensory systems, psychophysical analysis of motor performance provides crucial information about how the brain produces voluntary movements.

Psychophysical studies typically involve a subject performing a specific task (pushing a button, pointing, or reaching for an object) on signal. Light or sound cues may be used to instruct the subjects to delay a response or to vary it. The physiological circuits mediating behavior can be understood by combining pychophysical studies with neuroimaging or extracellular recording from single neurons ("single unit") in awake, behaving primates.

Psychophysical studies reveal that voluntary movements are governed by certain laws, which can be modified by learning. Three of these laws have been extensively studied because they have particular, practical significance. First, the brain represents the outcome of motor actions independently of the specific effector used or the specific way the action is achieved. Second, the time taken to respond to a stimulus depends on the amount of information that needs to be processed to accomplish the task. Third, there is a trade-off between the speed of a movement and its accuracy. We shall discuss each of these laws of voluntary movement in turn.

Voluntary Movements Have Certain Invariant Features and Are Governed by Motor Programs

In the early 1950s the psychologist Donald Hebb observed that individual motor actions share important characteristics even when performed in different ways. For example, our handwriting appears about the same regardless of the size of the letters or of the limb or body segment used to produce them (Figure 33-3). Hebb called this *motor equivalence.*

Motor equivalence suggests that a purposeful movement is represented in the brain in some abstract form rather than as a series of joint motions or muscle contractions. The path of the hand on its way to the target is always relatively straight, regardless of its starting or final position. As the target is approached, the speed of the hand at first increases and then declines to zero. In contrast, the motions of the joints in series (shoulder, elbow, and wrist) are complicated and vary greatly with different initial and final positions. Since rotation at a single joint would produce an arc at the hand, both elbow and shoulder joints have to be rotated concurrently to produce a straight path. In some directions the elbow moves more than the shoulder; in others the reverse occurs. When the hand is moved from one side of the body to the other, one or both joints may have to reverse direction in mid course (Figure 33-4).

If the brain forms a representation of a movement before its execution, does it plan the extent of the movement or does it continuously assess the distance between the hand and the target and use visual informa-

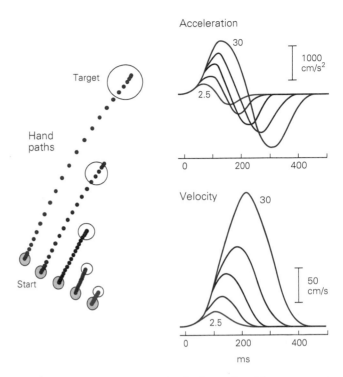

Figure 33-5 Acceleration and velocity scale with movement extent. Hand paths of a subject reaching for targets located 2.5, 5, 10, 20, and 30 cm from the starting position (dots are hand positions at 20 ms intervals) are presented at random. The subject could not see his hand during movement. The average acceleration and velocity profiles are scaled linearly as a function of the extent of movement to the target. The single peaks indicate that the extent of movement is specified prior to actual movement as a scaled impulse of force accelerating the limb.

tion to stop movement once the target is reached? If the brain relied primarily on vision to stop, the initial speed of the hand might be relatively similar in movements of different extents. Instead, both the speed and the acceleration of the hand movement are scaled proportionately to the distance of the target (Figure 33-5). This means that the extent of a movement is planned before the movement is initiated. The representation of this plan for movement is called a *motor program.* The motor program specifies the spatial features of the movement and the angles through which the joints will move. These are collectively known as *movement kinematics.* The program must also specify the forces required to rotate the joints (torques) to produce the desired movement. This is known as *movement dynamics.*

Motor programs not only specify the kinematic and dynamic features of the movement, they also tell the nervous system how to respond to certain patterns of sensory information. In lifting an object between thumb and

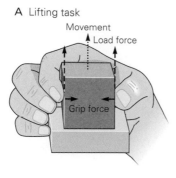

A Lifting task

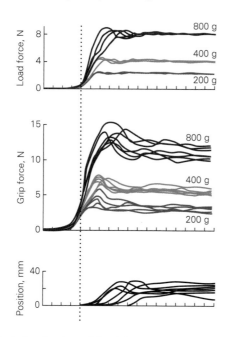

B Correctly anticipated weights

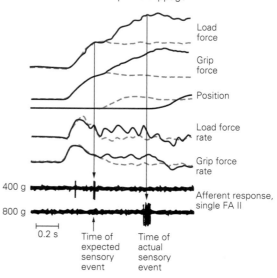

C Correction to unanticipated slippage

Figure 33-6 Both feedback and feed-forward controls are used when lifting a slippery object.

A. The subject lifts a test object from the table. Sensory receptors measure the load force applied to the object to overcome gravity and inertia, the grip force, and vertical motion. The discharge of different sensory receptors is recorded by microelectrodes inserted next to identified sensory axons of the peripheral nerve, a procedure called microneuronography.

B. When the subject knows the weight of the object in advance the applied forces are adequate to lift the object. Three sets of traces (24 trials superimposed) show load force, grip force, and position as subjects lifted three objects of different weights (200, 400, and 800 g). The grip force increases in pro-

portion to the weight of the object. This is done by scaling a preprogrammed force profile. (Notice that the profiles have the same shape but different amplitudes.)

C. When the weight is larger than expected the subject responds to slippage of the object. After being presented with a 400 g object for several trials (**dashed lines**), the subject was given an 800 g object (**solid lines**). On each trial with the 400 g object a burst of action potentials occurs in the afferent axon due to activation of a Pacinian corpuscle, triggering the beginning of the hold phase during which the grip force is constant. When the 800 g object is presented, the absence of burst responses, because of slippage, triggers a slow increase in force that is terminated when movement (the lifting) begins.

index finger we set our grip force and the acceleration of our hand in accordance with the expected slipperiness of the object and its weight using feed-forward control. The absence of the expected activation of cutaneous receptors indicates slippage and our grip force is increased immediately through rapid feedback control via a spinal cord

circuit. This circuit is said to be "gated" during lifting as no such response occurs if the same receptors are stimulated when the hand is at rest (Figure 33-6).

The nervous system deconstructs complex actions into elemental movements that have highly stereotyped spatial and temporal characteristics. For example, the

Figure 33-7 Complex movements are made up of discrete segments. (From Lacquaniti, Terzuolo, and Viviani, 1983.)

A. Figure eight drawn by a subject.

B. The continuous motion of drawing a figure eight consists of regular increases and decreases in the angular motion of the hand. These changes in angular motion occur at regular intervals during which the hand describes approximately equal angles, a feature termed *isogony.* The duration of each hand movement is the same regardless of the length of the hand path, a feature termed *isochrony.* Studies of more complex movements, such as those made during random continuous scribbling, show a similar segmentation. Such studies also reveal a consistent relationship between the speed of hand motion and the degree of curvature of the hand path: Velocity varies as a continuous function of the curvature raised to the 2/3 power. This two-thirds power law governs virtually all movements and expresses an obligatory slowing of the hand during movement segments that are more curved and a speeding up during segments that are straight.

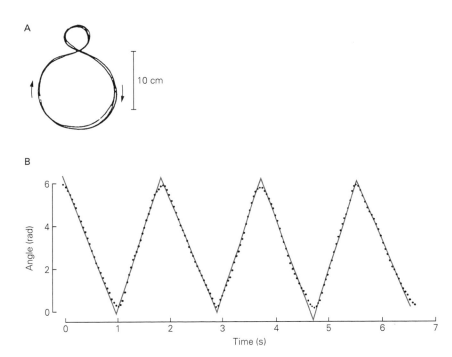

seemingly continuous motion of drawing a figure eight actually consists of discrete movement segments that are constant in duration, regardless of their size (Figure 33-7). The simple spatiotemporal elements of a movement are called *movement primitives* or *movement schemas.* Like the simple lines, ovals, or squares in computer graphics programs, movement primitives can be scaled in size or in time. The neural representations of complex actions, such as prehension, writing, typing, or drawing, are thought to be stored sets of these simple spatiotemporal elements.

Reaction Time Varies With the Amount of Information Processed

Reaction time, the time between the presentation of a stimulus and the initiation of a voluntary response, is an indication of the amount of neural processing taking place between a stimulus and the response. Reaction times also vary with several factors, including the neural conduction distance and the modality of the stimulus.

Voluntary reaction times are significantly longer than the latencies of reflex responses elicited by comparable stimuli. For example, the reaction times for voluntary responses to proprioceptive stimuli range from 80 to 120 ms. In contrast, the shortest latency for a monosynaptic reflex response to comparable muscle stretches is only around 40 ms. The longer time for the voluntary response results from the additional synapses interposed between afferent input and motor output. Thus, reactions to visual stimuli require still more time (150–180 ms) because of the larger number of synaptic relays in the retina. Unfortunately, one cannot compute the number of synapses involved in triggering a movement from the reaction time because the summation time of synapses is highly variable.

Reaction time is shortest if subjects know which response they will have to make when a stimulus is presented. It is prolonged when they must choose among different responses, for example, if a subject is presented with one of several cues signifying different movements. The added time needed to select a particular response is called the *choice effect.* Reaction time increases systematically with the number of choices available (Figure 33-8A). For complex tasks, reaction times are half a second to a second. Analyses of the effect of choice on reaction time gave rise to the idea that voluntary responses are processed in stages, including a step in which an appropriate response is selected from among alternatives (Figure 36-8B). Efforts at quantifying the rate of information processing have yielded delays of 100–150 ms per information bit, a rate much slower than that of even small personal computers.

However, it is now known that multiple stimuli and responses can be processed in parallel pathways (Box 33-1). Parallel processing overcomes the slowness of serial neural processing. Learning continually improves the efficiency of this parallel processing.

Voluntary Movements Trade Speed for Accuracy

In the 1890s the psychologist Robert Woodworth showed that fast movements are less accurate than slow ones. This is in part because fast movements leave less time for feedback corrections. In fact, the fastest movements are shorter than the reaction time itself. But lack of time for correction does not explain fully why fast movements are less accurate and more variable than slow ones; faster movements made without visual feedback are also more variable in both extent and speed.

Several factors contribute to the increase in variability with speed. One of these is the recruitment of additional motor neurons to produce rapid increases in force, since the excitability of motor neurons is subject to random variations. We shall see in the next chapter that a constant incremental increase in force is produced by progressively smaller numbers of motor neurons. Therefore, as force increases, fluctuations in the number of motor neurons lead to proportionately greater fluctuations in force and speed. This proportional relationship is maintained over most of the range of contractile force and corresponds to the proportional increase in variability with the speed of movement (Figure 33-10) and the distance of the target. The slope of the speed-accuracy trade-off is seen in Figure 33-10 and is analogous to the Weber-Fechner law, which characterizes sensory discriminations.

Variability also arises because subjects may be uncertain about the forces and loads that are needed to oppose movement. This uncertainty decreases with practice, however, so that both the accuracy and the speed of movement increase. For example, a monkey that is trained to grasp a handle and move it to a series of targets learns to anticipate opposing forces and to program its movements accurately before initiating a movement. With time, movement paths to each target become straighter and less variable (Figure 33-11).

In competitive sports and other tasks requiring skill the brain eventually learns to take account of even subtle changes in posture and external loads that might influence the trajectory of movement. This

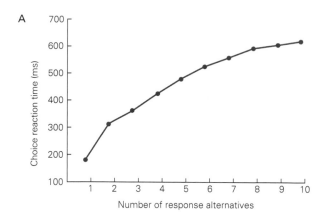

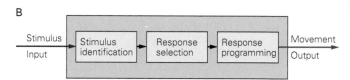

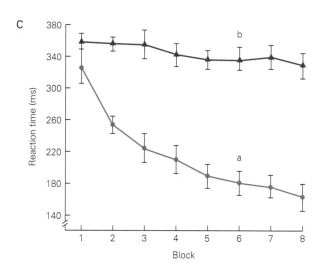

Figure 33-8 Reaction time increases with choice and decreases with learning.

A. Reaction time increases nonlinearly with the number of response alternatives available to the subject (From Woodworth 1938.)

B. In this outdated but still useful model of information processing three stages intervene between stimulus presentation and the motor response: stimulus identification, choice of response to the stimulus, and programming of the chosen response.

C. Reaction time decreases with learning as stimuli become predictable. In the plot each block represents 10 repetitions of a 10-trial sequence. On each trial a light appeared at one of four locations and subjects were instructed to press a key under the light. For one group of subjects (**a**) the same 10-trial sequence was repeated in a single block; the reaction time of this group decreased dramatically. For the other group (**b**) the position of the light in each trial was random; there was no significant decrease in reaction time for this group. (From Nissen and Bullemer 1987.)

principle is beautifully illustrated by expert pistol shooters, who achieve accuracy by synchronizing trigger actions with their involuntary tremors. Only beginners seek to immobilize themselves when pulling the trigger.

The Motor Systems Are Organized Hierarchically

The Spinal Cord, Brain Stem, and Forebrain Contain Successively More Complex Motor Circuits

The motor systems can perform so many different motor tasks—reflex, rhythmic, and voluntary—with speed and accuracy because of two features of their functional organization. First, the processing of sensory inputs and commands to motor neurons and muscles is distributed in hierarchically interconnected areas of the spinal cord, brain stem, and forebrain. Each level has circuits that can, through their input and output connections, organize or regulate complex motor responses. Second, sensory information relating to movement is processed in different systems that operate in parallel. The hierarchical organization of the motor systems is illustrated in Figure 33-12.

The spinal cord is the lowest level of this hierarchical organization. It contains the neuronal circuits that mediate a variety of reflexes and rhythmic automatisms such as locomotion and scratching. Similar circuits governing reflex movements of the face and mouth are located in the brain stem. The simplest neural circuit is monosynaptic; it includes only the primary sensory neuron and the motor neuron. However, most reflexes are mediated by polysynaptic circuits, where one or more interneurons are interposed between the primary sensory neuron and the motor neuron.

Interneurons and motor neurons also receive input from axons descending from higher centers. These supraspinal signals can modify reflex responses to peripheral stimuli by facilitating or inhibiting different populations of interneurons. They also coordinate motor actions through these interneurons. For example, when we flex a joint the descending commands that drive the flexor muscle also inhibit the opposing extensor muscle through the same inhibitory interneuron that is activated during the stretch reflex. Nevertheless, all motor commands eventually converge on motor neurons, whose axons exit the spinal cord or brain stem to innervate skeletal muscles. Thus in Sherrington's words, motor neurons are the "final common pathway" for all motor action.

The next level of the motor hierarchy is in the brain stem. Two systems of brain stem neurons, the medial and lateral, receive input from the cerebral cortex and subcortical nuclei and project to the spinal cord. The *medial descending systems* of the brain stem contribute to the control of posture by integrating visual, vestibular, and somatosensory information. The *lateral descending systems* control more distal limb muscles and are thus important for goal-directed movements, especially of the arm and hand. Other brain stem circuits control movements of the eyes and head.

The cortex is the highest level of motor control. The primary motor cortex and several premotor areas project directly to the spinal cord through the corticospinal tract and also regulate motor tracts that originate in the brain stem. The premotor areas are important for coordinating and planning complex sequences of movement. They receive information from the posterior parietal and prefrontal association cortices (see Chapter 19) and project to the primary motor cortex as well as to the spinal cord.

The variety of reflex circuits in the spinal cord and brain stem simplifies the instructions the cortex must send to lower levels. By facilitating some circuits and inhibiting others, higher levels can let sensory inputs at lower levels govern the temporal details of an evolving movement. The timing of activation of agonists and antagonist muscles is intrinsic to the spinal circuit and thus the descending signals themselves need not be timed as precisely. The patterns of coordination in spinal circuits are relatively stereotyped. A cat with its cervical cord transected can, if provided with body support, walk on a moving treadmill and bring its paw around an obstacle after hitting it. But the spinal cat cannot lift its forelimb *before* impact with an obstacle, as an intact animal does, because this movement requires control of the limbs using visual information. This anticipatory control, in turn, requires intervention by the motor cortex to suppress the oscillatory circuit that coordinates normal stepping.

The Cerebellum and Basal Ganglia Influence Cortical and Brain Stem Motor Systems

In addition to the three hierarchical levels—spinal cord, brain stem, and cortex—two other parts of the brain also regulate the planning and execution of movement. The cerebellum and basal ganglia provide feedback circuits that regulate cortical and brain stem motor areas: They receive inputs from various areas of cortex and project to motor areas of the cortex via the thalamus. The loop circuits of these two structures flow through separate regions of the thalamus and to different cortical areas.

Box 33-1 Parallel Processing in Movement

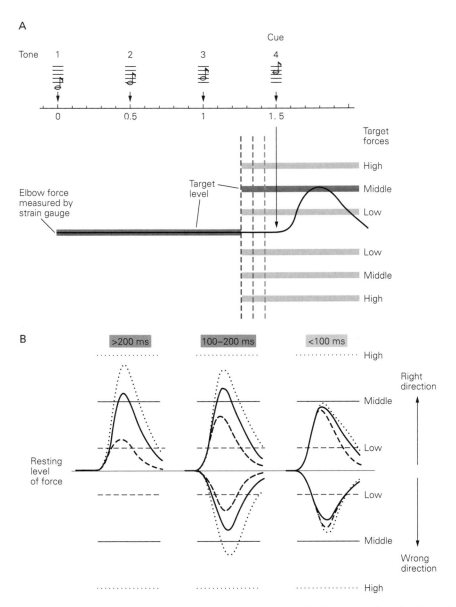

Figure 33-9

A. The timed response paradigm. In each trial four successive tones of increasing pitch are presented to a subject at 0.5-s intervals. The subject, whose arm is immobilized, is instructed to produce a pulse of elbow force (a brief isometric elbow flexion or extension) in synchrony with the fourth tone. The subject is also instructed to attempt to match the peak of the force pulse to a level specified at an unpredictable time between the third and fourth tone but not to correct their response if they were unable to match the target level. There were six possible target levels: three up (flexion) and three down (extension).

B. Average force trajectories of responses. The traces on the **left** are for responses initiated 200 ms or more after the target force was specified. Such responses were fully preprogrammed before execution. The shapes of the trajectories are highly stereotyped and match the target amplitude, and none of the

responses is in the wrong direction (up rather than down). The traces on the right are for responses initiated 0–100 ms after the target was presented, ie, before information about the extent or direction of the movement could be processed. Half are in the right direction and half are wrong. Nevertheless, the shapes of these "default" trajectories are similar to those of fully preprogrammed responses, and their amplitudes are all clustered at the center of the range. The traces in the center are for responses initiated 100–200 ms after the target was presented. Responses in the correct direction begin to show some degree of scaling: Responses to small- and large-amplitude target forces are smaller or larger than responses to the middle target. A second point of interest, however, is that this scaling is equally evident for responses in the wrong direction. This demonstrates that amplitude and direction are specified independently. (From Favilla et al. 1989.)

How long does it take for a motor program (eg, direction or extent) to be fully specified? The answer depends on whether individual parameters are specified in successive stages of processing or in parallel pathways. This issue was first addressed by David Rosenbaum in an experiment to determine whether the delay in choice reaction time can be shortened by providing subjects with partial information about an expected response.

In this experiment the choices available to subjects were which hand to move, the direction to move in, and the distance to move. As expected, reaction time is longest when subjects have no advance information and becomes progressively shorter as more information is provided. This indicates that the brain can program individual features of a movement before executing the movement.

Such experiments do not, however, address the question of whether individual features of a movement can be programmed in separate but parallel pathways while the action is underway. Can subjects initiate a response before its features are fully specified, ie, can they adopt different strategies when one or another parameter is uncertain? To determine whether the extent and direction of a movement can be programmed in separate but parallel pathways and how long it takes to program these features, it is necessary to examine how responses change as a function of the time available to specify a given feature. This was done using the *timed response paradigm* (Figure 33-9A). Subjects were trained to initiate a simple response in synchrony with a predictable auditory cue (as occurs in dancing). They were also given visual cues about the amplitude and direction of each response. Training the subjects to begin their response with the auditory cue ensured that the visual cue did not initiate the response but only provided information about amplitude and direction.

The influence of processing time on the characteristics of the trajectory of a movement was assessed by systematically varying the time between presentation of the information on the expected amplitude and direction of movement and the onset of movement. When subjects have to act before knowing which response to make, they set *default values* for amplitude and direction based on their expectation. When two directions are equally probable, responses are equally distributed in both directions. After the visual cues are presented and information on the extent and direction of movement can be processed, specification occurs over about 200 ms. Interestingly, amplitude is specified progressively for movements in both the correct and wrong directions. Thus, specifications of the extent and direction of movement are processed in parallel. Since the bell-shaped speed profiles, straightness, and movement time are the same for default responses, partially specified responses, and fully specified responses (Figure 33-9B), these movements are not substantially adjusted during execution. Similar results have been obtained for hand movements in space.

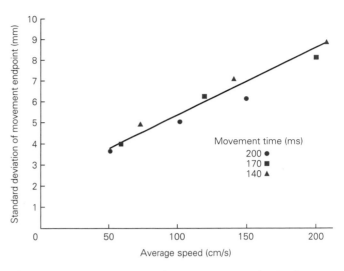

Figure 33-10 The accuracy of a movement varies in direct proportion to the speed of movement. Subjects held a stylus and had to hit a straight line lying perpendicular to the direction in which they moved the stylus. Subjects could not see their hand and thus were unable to correct their movement. The variability in the motion of the subjects' arm movements is shown here as the standard deviation of the extent of movement plotted against average speed (for three different movement times). The variability in movement increases in proportion to the speed and therefore to the force producing the movement. (From Schmidt et al. 1979.)

Likewise, the inputs to them from the cortex are also separate. The cerebellum and basal ganglia do not send significant output to the spinal cord, but they do act directly on projection neurons in the brain stem.

Although the precise contribution of the cerebellum and basal ganglia to motor action is still not clear, both are necessary for smooth movement and posture. Damage to either structure has significant clinical effects. Degenerative diseases of the basal ganglia, such as Parkinson or Huntington disease, produce involuntary movements, abnormalities in posture, and, as recent studies have shown, major impairment in cognitive processing. Thus the basal ganglia have increasingly been implicated in motivation and the selection of adaptive behavioral plans (Chapter 43). Damage to the cerebellum by vascular lesions and certain familial degenerative conditions produces cerebellar ataxia, a characteristic loss of coordination and accuracy of limb movement. Cerebellar circuits are involved with the timing and coordination of movements in progress and with the learning of motor skills (Chapter 42).

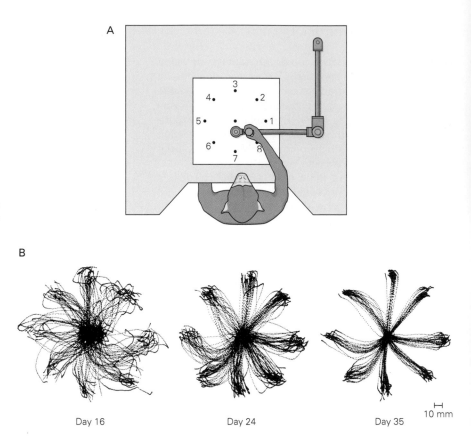

Figure 33-11 Learning improves the accuracy of reaching.

A. A monkey was made to sit at a table and move a handle at the end of a manipulandum (starting from the position shown) over the surface toward targets arranged in a circular array (numbered 1–8). The monkey was required to move the handle from the center of the array to whichever one of the targets lit up, covering the target with a clear plexiglass circle on the end of the manipulandum.

B. Records of movement trajectories for a monkey are shown at successive stages of training. The trajectories become straighter with practice, and increasing accuracy is reflected in the decreased dispersion (variability) of the trajectories. (The persistent curvature of the trajectories to targets 4, 5, and 6 is a result of mechanical constraints of the apparatus.)

Day 16   Day 24   Day 35   10 mm

Lesions of the Motor Pathways Produce Positive and Negative Signs

The nineteenth-century neurologist John Hughlings Jackson, whose clinical insights were so informative for the early understanding of different regions of cortex (Chapter 19), was also the first to recognize that lesions of the nervous system result in both negative and positive signs. Negative signs reflect the loss of particular capacities normally controlled by the damaged system, for example loss of strength. Positive signs, also called *release phenomena,* are abnormal and stereotyped responses that are explained by the withdrawal of tonic inhibition from neuronal circuits mediating a behavior. When cerebral control of the brain stem is disconnected in the cat, ordinary head and neck movements produce postural reflexes that otherwise do not occur in the intact animal.

In humans, lesions that interrupt the descending pathways from the cortex or brain stem produce weakness in voluntary movements (a negative sign) and, at the same time, increase muscle tone, a key feature of the clinical picture of *spasticity.* In this condition, as in decerebrate rigidity, stretch reflexes are abnormally active. Clinicians often must decide if a patient's weakness

arises from a disease that affects systems descending from the cortex and brain stem to motor neurons or from a disease that directly affects the motor neurons or their axons. Although both conditions produce weakness by diminishing neural input to muscle, three important differences distinguish them. First, diseases affecting the descending pathways give rise to spasticity whereas diseases of motor neurons do not. Second, diseases affecting motor neurons directly result in denervation atrophy and reduced muscle volume, whereas this does not occur with damage to the descending pathway. Third, damage to descending systems tends to be distributed more diffusely in limb or face muscles and often affects large groups of muscles, for example the flexors. In contrast, degeneration in local groups of motor neurons tends to affect muscles in a patchy way and may even be limited to single muscles. Nerve lesions result in weakness that reflects the known distribution of individual nerves.

We now consider the organization of the three levels of the motor hierarchy—the spinal cord, brain stem, and cerebral cortex—and how they control proximal and distal muscles.

Spinal Motor Neurons Execute Movement

Primary afferent fibers from cutaneous and deep peripheral receptors (Chapter 22) branch profusely before terminating in the various laminae of the spinal gray matter, where they form connections with four types of neurons: (1) local interneurons, whose axons are confined to the same or adjacent spinal segments; (2) propriospinal neurons, whose axon terminals reach distant spinal segments; (3) projection neurons, whose axons ascend to higher brain centers; and (4) motor neurons, whose axons exit the nervous system to innervate muscles. We first consider the motor neurons and then the interneurons and propriospinal neurons that are important in motor control.

The cell bodies of motor neurons that innervate individual muscles are clustered in motor neuron pools, or *motor nuclei,* which form longitudinal columns extending over one to four spinal segments. The spatial organization of the different motor nuclei follows a *proximal-distal rule.* According to this rule, motor nuclei innervating the most proximal muscles lie most medially within the spinal cord while those innervating more distal muscles are located progressively more laterally. Thus, for the arm, the motor nuclei innervating the axial, shoulder girdle, elbow, wrist, and digit muscles are arrayed from medial to lateral positions (Figure 33-13). The separation of motor neurons innervating axial and proximal muscles from those innervating distal muscles is maintained throughout the spinal cord.

The functional specialization of medial and lateral motor nuclei is also reflected in the organization of the local interneurons of the spinal cord. Interneurons in the most medial parts of the intermediate zone of the spinal cord project to the medial motor nuclei that control axial muscles on both sides of the body. More laterally located interneurons project only to the motor neurons that innervate ipsilateral girdle muscles, while the most lateral ones synapse on motor neurons that innervate the most distal ipsilateral muscles (Figure 33-13).

The axons of propriospinal neurons course up and down the white matter of the spinal cord and terminate on interneurons and motor neurons located several segments away from the cell bodies (Figure 33-13). Axons of medial propriospinal neurons run in the ventral and medial columns. They have long axons that branch extensively; some axons extend through the entire length of the spinal cord to coordinate movements of the neck and pelvis. This organization allows the axial muscles, which are innervated from many spinal segments, to be coordinated easily during postural adjustments.

More laterally placed propriospinal neurons interconnect smaller numbers of segments and have less

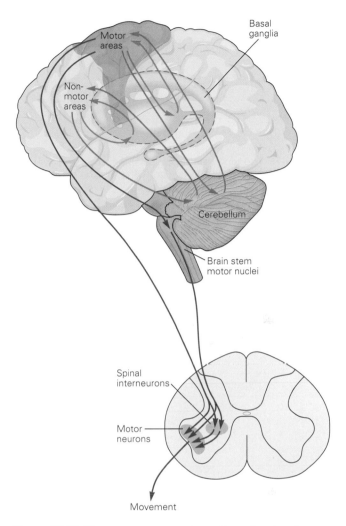

Figure 33-12 The motor systems have three levels of control—the spinal cord, brain stem, and forebrain—organized both serially and in parallel. The motor areas of the cerebral cortex can influence the spinal cord either directly or through the descending systems of the brain stem. All three levels of the motor systems receive sensory inputs and are also under the influence of two independent subcortical systems: the basal ganglia and the cerebellum. (The basal ganglia and cerebellum act on the cerebral cortex through relay nuclei in the thalamus, which are omitted from the diagram for clarity.)

diffuse terminations. This explains the greater independence of action of more distal muscles, allowing a larger variety of muscle activation patterns. Although shoulder and elbow muscles are used to direct the hand in reaching for objects in different directions, shoulder and elbow motions are more stereotyped and less varied than those of the wrist and the elbow. Control of the digits requires the greatest degree of differentiation. Even the movements of a single digit require highly dif-

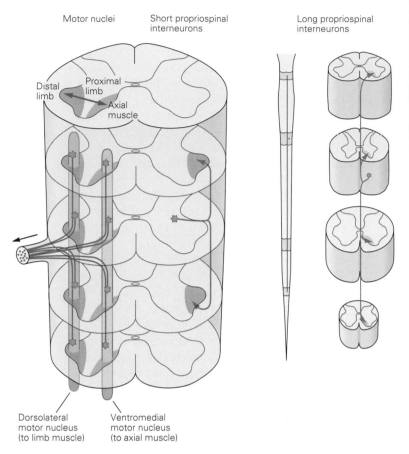

Figure 33-13 The motor nuclei of the spinal cord are arranged along a medial-lateral axis according to function. The medial nuclei contain the motor neurons innervating axial muscles of the neck and back; among the lateral nuclei the most medial motor neurons innervate proximal muscles while the most lateral innervate distal muscles. The medial motor nuclei are interconnected across several segments of the spinal cord by propriospinal neurons with long axons, whereas the lateral nuclei are interconnected across fewer segments by propriospinal neurons with shorter axons.

ferentiated and coordinated contraction of many different muscles (Chapter 38).

The Brain Stem Modulates the Action of Spinal Motor Circuits

The brain stem contains, in addition to the motor nuclei that regulate the facial muscles, many groups of neurons that project to the spinal gray matter. These projections were classified by the Dutch neuroanatomist Hans Kuypers into two main systems: the medial and the lateral brain stem pathways.

The medial pathways provide the basic postural control system upon which the cortical motor areas can organize more highly differentiated movement. They are phylogenetically the oldest component of the descending motor systems and consist of three major tracts: the vestibulospinal (medial and lateral), reticulospinal (medial and lateral), and tectospinal tracts. These pathways descend in the ipsilateral ventral columns of the spinal cord and terminate predominantly on interneurons and long propriospinal neurons in the ventromedial part of the intermediate zone (Figure 33-14A), thus influencing motor neurons that innervate axial and proximal muscles. They also terminate directly on some motor neurons, particularly those of the medial cell group that innervate axial muscles. The wide area of termination of individual axons is important in distributing control to a variety of functionally related motor nuclei.

The lateral brain stem pathways are more concerned with goal-directed limb movements such as reaching and manipulating; they terminate on interneurons in the dorsolateral part of the spinal gray matter and thus influence motor neurons that control distal muscles of the limbs. The main lateral descending pathway from the brain stem is the *rubrospinal tract*, which originates in the magnocellular portion of the red nucleus in the midbrain. Rubrospinal fibers descend through the medulla to the dorsal part of the lateral column of the spinal cord (Figure 33-14B). In

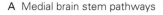

A Medial brain stem pathways

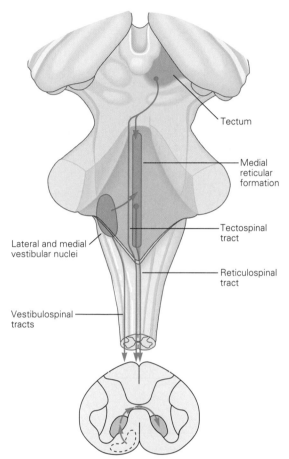

Tectum

Medial
reticular
formation

Tectospinal
tract

Reticulospinal
tract

Lateral and medial
vestibular nuclei

Vestibulospinal
tracts

B Lateral brain stem pathways

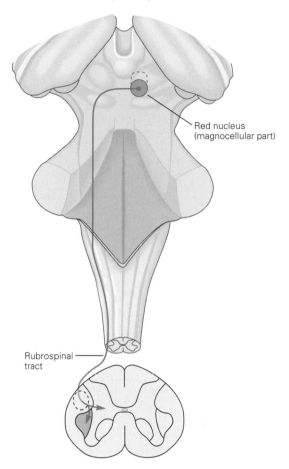

Red nucleus
(magnocellular part)

Rubrospinal
tract

Figure 33-14 Medial and lateral descending pathways from
the brain stem control different groups of neurons and different groups of muscles.

A. The main components of the medial pathways are the reticulospinal, medial and lateral vestibulospinal, and tectospinal
tracts that descend in the ventral column. These tracts termi-

nate in the ventromedial area of the spinal gray matter.

B. The main lateral pathway is the rubrospinal tract, which originates in the magnocellular portion of the red nucleus. The
rubrospinal tract descends in the contralateral dorsolateral column and terminates in the dorsolateral area of the spinal gray
matter.

cats and monkeys the rubrospinal tract is important
in the control of distal limb muscles used for manipulating objects. In anthropoid apes and humans this
function is largely assumed by the corticospinal
system.

The Cerebral Cortex Modulates the Action
of Motor Neurons in the Brain Stem and
Spinal Cord

The ability to organize complex motor acts and execute
fine movements with precision depends on control signals from the motor areas in the cerebral cortex. Cortical

motor commands descend in two tracts. The corticobulbar fibers control the motor nuclei in the brain stem that
move facial muscles, while the corticospinal fibers control the spinal motor neurons that innervate the trunk
and limb muscles. In addition, the cerebral cortex indirectly influences spinal motor activity by acting on the
descending brain stem pathways.

The Cerebral Cortex Acts on Spinal Motor Neurons
Both Directly and Indirectly

At the end of the nineteenth century Gustav Fritsch and
Eduard Hitzig discovered that electrical stimulation of
the cortex produces movements on the contralateral side

A Ventral corticospinal tract

B Lateral corticospinal tract

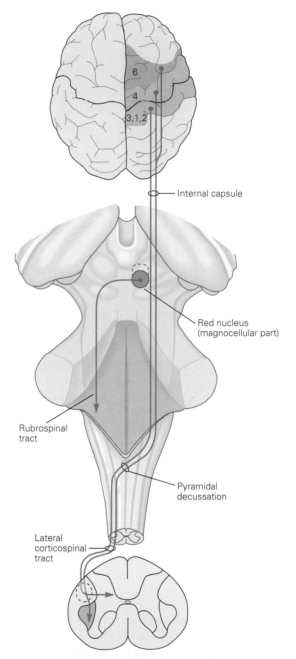

Figure 33-15 The cortex directly controls motor neurons in the spinal cord through two descending pathways.

A. The ventral corticospinal tract originates principally from pre-motor neurons in Brodmann's area 6 and in zones in area 4 controlling the neck and trunk. The descending fibers terminate bilaterally and send collaterals to the medial pathways from the brain stem.

B. The lateral corticospinal tract originates in two motor areas (Brodmann's areas 4 and 6) and three sensory areas (3, 2, and 1). It crosses at the pyramidal decussation, descends in the dorso-lateral column, and terminates in the spinal gray matter. The fibers from the sensory cortex terminate primarily in the medial portion of the dorsal horn. However, collateral fibers project to dorsal column nuclei. These terminations allow the brain to actively modify sensory signals.

of the body. Systematic stimulation of the surface of the cortex in primates revealed somatotopic maps of the body in frontal areas. In addition, lesions of the arm or leg area of motor cortex led to axonal degeneration at cervical and lumbar levels of the spinal cord, respectively. This demonstrated that somatotopic areas project to their expected targets in the spinal cord. The primary motor cortex lies along the precentral gyrus in Brodmann's area 4. Several other motor maps can also be defined in area 6, the premotor cortex. (These maps and their contributions to motor control are described in Chapter 38 in the context of voluntary movement.) The axons of cortical neurons that project to the spinal cord run together in the corticospinal tract, a massive bundle of fibers containing about 1 million axons. About a third of these originate from the precentral gyrus of the frontal lobe. Another third originate from area 6. The rest originate in areas 3, 2, and 1 in the somatic sensory cortex and regulate transmission of afferent input through the dorsal horn.

The corticospinal fibers run together with corticobulbar fibers through the posterior limb of the internal capsule to reach the ventral portion of the midbrain. In the pons they separate into small bundles of fibers that course between the pontine nuclei. They then regroup in the medulla to form the medullary pyramid, a conspicuous landmark on the ventral surface of the medulla. About three-quarters of the corticospinal fibers cross the midline in the pyramidal decussation at the junction of the medulla and spinal cord. The crossed fibers descend in the dorsal part of the lateral columns (dorsolateral column) of the spinal cord, forming the lateral corticospinal tract. The uncrossed fibers descend in the ventral columns as the ventral corticospinal tract (Figure 33-15).

The lateral and ventral divisions of the corticospinal tract terminate in approximately the same regions of spinal gray matter as do the lateral and medial systems from the brain stem. The lateral corticospinal tract projects primarily to motor nuclei in the lateral part of the ventral horn and to interneurons in the intermediate zone. The ventral corticospinal tract projects bilaterally to the ventromedial cell column and to adjoining portions of the intermediate zone that contain the motor neurons that innervate axial muscles.

The Cerebral Cortex Acts on Brain Stem Motor Neurons Through the Corticobulbar Tract

The corticobulbar fibers that control muscles of the head and face terminate in motor and sensory (cranial nerve) nuclei in the brain stem. In humans the corticobulbar fibers form monosynaptic connections with motor neu-

rons in the trigeminal, facial, and hypoglossal nuclei. The trigeminal motor nuclei and facial nuclei receive cortical projections from both hemispheres. The motor neurons innervating muscles of the upper part of the face receive approximately an equal number of axons from both hemispheres, whereas those innervating the lower face receive predominantly contralateral fibers. As a result, damage to corticobulbar fibers on one side produces weakness only of the muscles of the contralateral lower part of the face. Movements of the eyes are controlled by a different system (Chapter 41).

The Motor Cortex Is Influenced by Both Cortical and Subcortical Inputs

The major cortical inputs to the motor areas of cortex are from the prefrontal, parietal, and temporal association areas. These are mainly focused on the premotor cortex and supplementary motor area. There are, however, connections from the primary sensory cortex to the primary motor cortex. Other corticocortical inputs arise from the opposite hemisphere and course through the corpus callosum. Callosal fibers interconnect homologous areas in the two hemispheres. The left and right finger representations, however, do not receive callosal fibers and are thus functionally independent of one another. As we shall see in Chapters 41, 42, and 43, the major subcortical input to the motor cortical areas comes from the thalamus, where separate nuclei convey inputs from the basal ganglia and the cerebellum.

An Overall View

The primary purpose of the elaborate information processing and storage that takes place in the brain is to enable us to interact with our environment. Our infinitely varied and purposeful motor behaviors are governed by the integrated actions of the brain's several motor systems. Nevertheless, the first insight into the neural mechanisms of motor action came from analyses of the motor capabilities remaining when the spinal cord or brain stem is disconnected from the brain or after local damage. The discovery of spinal reflexes showed that the spinal cord contains the neural circuits for generating simple and coordinated movements.

Reflexes do not differ from voluntary movements as fundamentally as was once thought. Reflexes are organized by specific sensory inputs such that the locus and magnitude of the response are appropriate for the site and the intensity of the stimulus. These sensorimotor relationships are not, however, immutable and, as we will see in Chapter 36, the reflex patterns produced through spinal circuits can be converted from one set of movements to another by signals from higher levels of the nervous system. While voluntary movements are strikingly adaptable, they too are governed by well-defined rules.

Motor commands are organized hierarchically. The brain stem integrates spinal reflexes into a variety of automated movements that control posture and locomotion. Several interconnected areas of cortex that project to the descending systems of the brain stem and to the spinal cord itself initiate and control our more complex voluntary movements. Unlike motor systems at lower levels, cortical motor areas are not influenced only by peripheral sensory input; they also receive crucial information from sensory association and prefrontal areas that integrate current sensory information with stored knowledge. In addition, motor areas in the cortex are modulated by two subcortical structures, the basal ganglia and cerebellum.

The corticospinal and corticobulbar pathways are the most direct and powerful route by which the cerebral cortex can control the motor neurons that innervate muscles. The cortex also regulates spinal motor neurons indirectly through its influence on the brain's various descending systems. This redundancy allows for significant recovery of function in cases of injury. In contrast, the only route by which the cortex can control the muscles of our hands and fingers is through the direct projection from the primary motor cortex to distal motor neurons. Therefore, injury to these fibers results in permanent loss of all the skilled movements that we use to manipulate small objects.

Three features of the motor hierarchy are particularly important. First, the inputs to each component create a rough somatotopic map of the body, and this somatotopic organization is preserved in the outputs of each component. For example, regions of primary motor cortex that control the hand receive input from hand control areas in the premotor cortex and influence fibers of the descending brain stem pathways that affect hand movement. Second, each level of motor control receives peripheral sensory information that is used to modify the motor output at that level. At the same time, each level contains distinct populations of neurons that project in parallel to sensory relay nuclei and other structures, including the thalamus and cerebellum. These recurrent pathways provide the sensory systems and other processing systems with information about ongoing motor commands and allow higher motor centers to control the information that reaches them, conveying only such information as may be relevant to a given task.

Third, motor programs are refined continuously by learning. Functional imaging and physiological studies have shown that there are changes and shifts in the anatomical location of representations of motor programs as a motor behavior progresses, through learning, from being novel to being automatic. Even though motor learning is acquired primarily through practice, skilled performers are often unable to express what it is they have learned. Motor learning is thus referred to as "implicit" learning, in contrast to the "explicit" acquisition of knowledge that can be expressed verbally in statements about the world.

Claude Ghez
John Krakauer

Selected Readings

Bernstein N. 1967. *The Co-ordination and Regulation of Movements.* Oxford: Pergamon Press.

Dunn RP, Strick PL. 1996. The corticospinal system: a structural framework for the central control of movement. In: LB Rowell, JT Sheperd (eds). *Handbook of Physiology.* Section 12, *Exercise: Regulation and Integration of Multiple Systems,* pp. 217–254. New York: Oxford University Press.

Jackson JH. 1932. *Selected Writings of John Hughlings Jackson,* Vol. 2, J Taylor (ed). London: Hodder and Stoughton.

Johansson RS. 1996. Sensory control of dexterous manipulation in humans. In: AM Wing, P Haggard, JR Flanagan (eds). *Hand and Brain: The Neurophysiology and Psychology of Hand Movements,* pp. 381–414. San Diego: Academic Press.

Kuypers HGJM. 1981. Anatomy of the descending pathways. In: VB Brooks (ed). *Handbook of Physiology.* Section 1, *The Nervous System.* Vol. 2, *Motor Control,* Part 1, pp. 597–666. Bethesda, MD: American Physiological Society.

Kuypers HGJM. 1985. *The Anatomical and Functional Organization of the Motor System.* In: M Swash, C Kennard (eds). *Scientific Basis of Clinical Neurology,* pp. 3–18. New York: Churchill Livingstone.

Lacquaniti F. 1989. Central representations of human limb movement as revealed by studies of drawing and handwriting. Trends Neurosci 12:287–291.

Lundberg A. 1979. Integration in a propriospinal motor centre controlling the forelimb in the cat. In: H Asanuma, VJ Wilson (eds). *Integration in the Nervous System,* pp. 47–64. Tokyo: Igaku-Shoin.

Marsden CDR, Rothwell JC, Day BL. 1985. The use of peripheral feedback in the control of movement. In: EV Evorts, SP Wise, D Bousfield (eds). *The Motor System in Neurobiology,* pp. 215–222. New York: Elsevier Biomedical Press.

Rosenbaum DA, Host Krist H. 1996. Antecedents of action. In: H Heuer, SW Keefe (eds). *Handbook of Perception and Action*. Vol. 2, *Motor Skills*. San Diego: Academic Press.

Sherrington C. 1947. *The Integrative Action of the Nervous System*, 2nd ed. New Haven: Yale University Press.

References

Brown LL, Schneider JS, Lidsky TI. 1997. Sensory and cognitive functions of the basal ganglia. Curr Opin Neurobiol 7:157–163.

Favilla M, Hening W, Chez C. 1989. Trajectory control in targeted force impulses. VI Independent specification of response amplitude and direction. Exp Brain Res 75(2): 280–294.

Georgopoulos AP, Kalaska JF, Massey JT. 1981. Spatial trajectories and reaction times of aimed movements: effects of practice, uncertainty, and change in target location. J Neurophysiol 46:725–743.

Gordon J, Ghilardi MF, Cooper SE, Ghez C. 1994. Accuracy of planar reaching movements. II. Systematic extent errors resulting from inertial anisotropy. Exp Brain Res 99:112–130.

Hebb DO. 1949. *The Organization of Behavior: A Neuropsychological Theory*. New York: John Wiley.

Hening W, Favilla M, Ghez C. 1988. Trajectory control in targeted force impulses. V. Gradual specification of response amplitude. Exp Brain Res 71:116–128.

Johansson RS, Westling G. 1991. Afferent signals during manipulative tasks in man. In: O Franzen, J Westman (eds). *Somatosensory Mechanisms*, pp. 25–48. London: Macmillan.

Johansson BS, Westling G. 1987. Signals in tactile afferents from the fingers eliciting adaptive motor responses during precision grip. Exp Brain Res 66:141–154.

Lacquaniti F, Maioli C. 1989. The role of preparation in tuning anticipatory and reflex responses during catching. J Neurosci 9:134–148.

Lacquaniti F, Terzuolo C, Viviani P. 1983. The law relating the kinematic and figural aspects of drawing movements. Acta Psycholog 54:115–130.

Morasso P. 1981. Spatial control of arm movements. Exp Brain Res 42:223–227.

Nissen MJ, Bullemer P. 1987. Attentional requirements of learning: evidence from performance measures. Cogn Psychol 19:1–32.

Raibert MH. 1977. *Motor Control and Learning by the State-Space Model*. Cambridge, MA: Artificial Intelligence Laboratory, MIT.

Rothwell JC, Traub MM, Day BL, Obeso JA, Thomas PK, Marsden CD. 1982. Manual motor performance in a de-afferented man. Brain 105:515–542.

Sanes JN, Mauritz KH, Dalakas MC, Evarts EV. 1985. Motor control in humans with large-fiber sensory neuropathy. Human Neurobiol 4:101–114.

Schmidt RA. 1988. *Motor Control and Learning*, 2nd ed. Champaign, IL: Human Kinetics Publishers.

Woodworth RS. 1899. The accuracy of voluntary movement. Psychol Rev 3(Suppl 13):1–114.

Woodworth RS. 1938. *Experimental Psychology*. New York: Holt.

34

The Motor Unit and Muscle Action

. . . to move things is all that mankind can do, for such the sole executant is muscle, whether in whispering a syllable or in felling a forest.

Charles Sherrington, 1924

THE MAJOR CONSEQUENCE of the elaborate information processing that takes place in the brain is the contraction of skeletal muscles. Indeed, animals are distinguishable from plants by their ability to make precise, goal-directed movements of their body parts. The problem of deciding when and how to move is, to a large degree, the driving force behind the evolution of the nervous system. In this chapter we examine how the electrical and chemical signals used to convey information in the nervous system are ultimately converted into the forces and displacements that make up movement.

In all but the most primitive animals movement is generated by specialized muscle cells. There are three general types of muscles: smooth muscle, used primarily for internal actions such as peristalsis and control of blood flow; cardiac muscle, used exclusively for pumping blood; and skeletal muscle, used primarily for moving bones. In this chapter we deal exclusively with the organization and neural control of mammalian skeletal muscles.

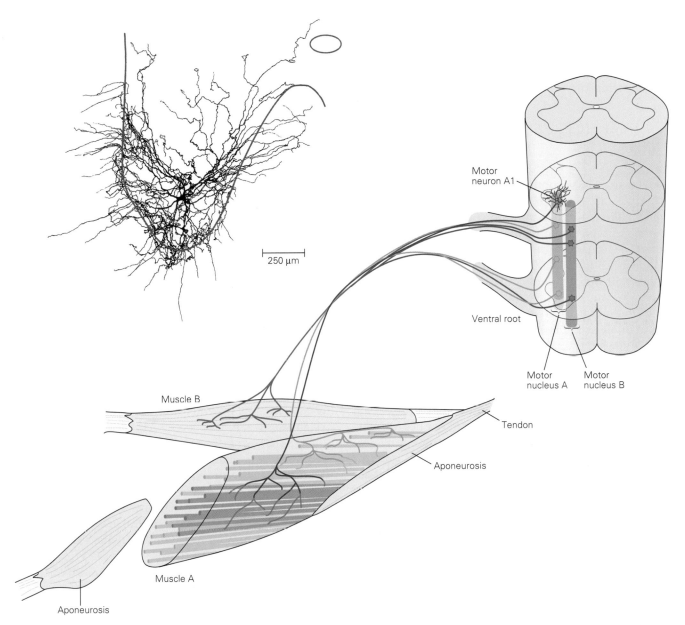

Figure 34-1 A typical muscle consists of many thousands of muscle fibers working in parallel and organized into a smaller number of motor units. A motor unit consists of a motor neuron and the muscle fibers that it innervates. The motor neurons innervating one muscle are usually clustered into an elongated motor nucleus within the ventral spinal cord that may extend over 1–4 segments. In the example shown here the motor neuron A1 plus other motor neurons innervating muscle A form motor nucleus A. Muscle B is innervated by motor neurons lying in a separate motor nucleus B. Note that the extensively branched dendrites of a typical motor neuron (shown for A1 only) tend to intermingle with those from other motor nuclei. The axons from the various motor nuclei are intermingled in the ventral roots and peripheral nerves, but they resegregate to emerge as individual muscle nerves. (Reconstructed motor neuron courtesy of P. K. Rose.)

Much of this chapter concerns the mechanical properties of muscles, tendons, and joints and the laws of physics that govern the motion of limbs. In order to perform a task the brain must solve a control problem that depends on these properties and laws. The difficulty of controlling a system with multiple linked segments can be appreciated by considering that, despite substantial computing power, industrial robots are relatively poor at compensating for unexpected perturbations that would pose no problem even for a simple animal. At least a part of the solution to the control problem resides in the muscles themselves. Our skeletal muscles are endowed with mechanical properties that contribute importantly to the grace, speed, efficiency, and robustness of our movements.

Motor Neurons Convey Commands to Muscle Fibers

Skeletal muscle is subdivided into parallel bundles of stringlike fascicles, which themselves are bundles of even smaller stringlike multinucleated cells called *muscle fibers*. A typical mammalian muscle fiber has a diameter of 50–100 μm and a length of 2–6 cm. Thus a typical muscle is composed of hundreds of thousands, even millions, of independent contractile elements arranged in parallel and, in longer muscles, in series. The main job of the motor nervous system is to control these elements in all of the muscles simultaneously so that the correct tension is applied to the skeleton to produce the desired movement.

A typical muscle is controlled by about a hundred large motor neurons whose cell bodies lie in a distinct cluster called a motor nucleus in the spinal cord or brain stem (Figure 34-1). The axon of each motor neuron exits the spinal cord through a ventral root (or through a cranial nerve from the brain stem) and traverses progressively smaller branches of peripheral nerves until it enters the muscle it controls. There it branches widely to innervate anywhere from 100 to 1000 muscle fibers scattered over a substantial part of the muscle. Except during development, each muscle fiber is normally innervated by only one motor neuron in only one place, usually near its midpoint. The ensemble of muscle fibers innervated by a single motor neuron is called a *muscle unit*, and that ensemble together with its motor neuron is called a *motor unit*. The number of muscle fibers constituting a single motor unit varies greatly in muscles in different parts of the body (see Chapter 35).

The functional connection between a motor neuron and a target muscle fiber is a chemical synapse called the end-plate (Chapter 11). End-plates are usually clustered into bands that extend across some or all of the muscle. The neuromuscular synapse formed by a motor neuron on a muscle fiber is large and filled with many vesicles containing the neurotransmitter acetylcholine. This synapse is constructed so that each action potential in the motor neuron releases sufficient transmitter to depolarize the postsynaptic membrane of the muscle fiber to its threshold for an action potential. The acetylcholine released from the presynaptic terminals is rapidly hydrolyzed by acetylcholinesterase, leaving the

muscle fiber ready to respond again in an all-or-none manner to the next action potential. All of the muscle fibers innervated by the same motor neuron respond faithfully and synchronously to each action potential of the motor neuron.

Once the postsynaptic membrane of the neuromuscular junction is depolarized to its threshold, an action potential propagates along the membrane of the muscle fiber (the sarcolemma). The action potential propagates relatively slowly (3–5 m/s) in both directions away from the end-plate region. A muscle fiber is electrically similar to a large-diameter, unmyelinated axon in that high transmembrane currents are required to propagate the action potential. These currents give rise to relatively large potential gradients in the extracellular fluid around the muscle fiber.

Because a single action potential in a motor neuron can activate hundreds of muscle fibers in synchrony, the resulting currents sum to generate an electrical signal that is readily detectable outside the muscle itself. Furthermore, when more than minimal force is required, many motor neurons generate an asynchronous barrage of action potentials with overlapping action potentials arising in each muscle unit. The result is a complex pattern of electrical potentials (typically on the order of 100 μV in amplitude) that can be recorded as an *electromyogram* (EMG) using simple electrodes on the surface of the overlying skin. The relative timing and amplitude of these patterns recorded over particular muscles reflect closely the aggregate activity of motor neurons that innervate each muscle. Electromyographic signals are valuable for studying motor control and for diagnosing pathology in the motor systems and in the muscles themselves (see Chapter 35).

The Contractile Machinery of Muscle Fibers Is Organized Into Sarcomeres and Cross Bridges

When viewed through the light microscope a single skeletal muscle fiber can be seen to contain many *myofibrils*, each of which has a longitudinally repeating pattern of dark and light bands called *striations*. The dark bands are constant in length, but the light bands tend to become longer or shorter as the muscle lengthens or shortens, respectively.

Sarcomeres Are Composed of Interdigitated Thick and Thin Filaments

Under the electron microscope individual myofibrils can be seen to consist of longitudinally repeated cylindrical units, called *sarcomeres*. Each sarcomere contains contrac-

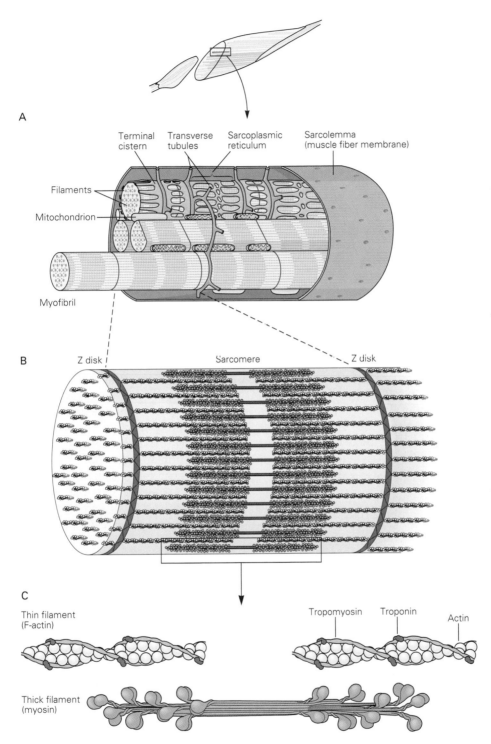

Figure 34-2 A single muscle fiber contains several myofibrils. (Adapted from Bloom and Fawcett, 1975; Loeb and Gans, 1986.)

A. This three-dimensional reconstruction of a section of muscle fiber shows the relationship of the myofibrils to the membrane, transverse tubule system, and sarcoplasmic reticulum.

B. The sarcomere is the functional unit of the muscle. It contains contractile proteins, the thick and thin filaments, bounded by thin Z disks, from which the thin filaments arise. Thick and thin filaments overlap, creating alternating dark bands that give skeletal muscle its characteristic striated appearance. This banded pattern changes as the overlap between the thin and thick filaments changes during shortening or lengthening of the muscle fiber.

C. Detail of the contractile proteins (myofilaments). The thin filaments are composed principally of polymerized actin but also include tropomyosin and troponin. The thick filaments consist of arrays of entwined pairs of myosin molecules; each molecule includes a stem and a double globular head that protrudes from the stem.

tile proteins, organized into a regular interdigitated matrix of thick and thin filaments, and is bounded by Z disks (Figure 34-2). The changing banding pattern with muscle contraction evident in the light microscope results from the changing overlap between these filaments. The sarcomere is the functional unit of length in skeletal muscle. All myofibrils in all muscle fibers of a muscle tend to change length in concert as a result of the various noncontractile components that link them mechanically. The physiological range of length of each sarcomere is 1.5–3.5 μm. A muscle fiber with a 4-cm resting length would have about 20,000 sarcomeres in series.

The thin filaments project in both directions from the Z disks, whereas the thick filaments are discontinuous and float in the middle of the sarcomere. The main constituent of each thin filament is a pair of polymerized actin monomers (F actin) arranged as a helix (Figure 34-2C). The thin filament also contains tropomyosin (a long filamentous protein that lies in the grooves formed by the paired strands of actin) and troponin (small molecular complexes that are attached to the tropomyosin filament at regular intervals).

The thick filament is made up of about 250 myosin molecules entwined together along most of their lengths. The myosin molecules have globular heads on short stems that stick out from the sides of the thick filament in a staggered array, pointing away from a bare region in the middle of the filament where there are no heads (Figure 34-2C).

Contractile Force Is Produced by Cross Bridges

The thick and thin filaments comprise the contractile machinery of the muscle. In a contracting muscle adjacent thick and thin filaments slide past each other, propelled by cyclical interactions between the myosin heads of the thick filaments and binding sites on the actin of the adjacent thin filaments. This is the "sliding filament hypothesis" developed by A.F. Huxley and colleagues starting in the 1950s.

Each globular myosin head contains an ATPase that converts the chemical energy of adenosine triphosphate (ATP) into mechanical energy, resulting in a "cocked" deformation of the myosin head (Figure 34-3). This stored mechanical energy can be released only after the myosin head attaches to a binding site on one of the adjacent thin filaments that has been activated by Ca^{2+} (a process described later). The attached head, or *cross bridge*, then acts like an oar, pulling the thin filament longitudinally in a direction that increases the overlap between the thick and thin filaments and shortening the muscle fiber.

After a sliding motion of about 0.06 μm, the stress in the cross bridge is completely relieved and it can de-

tach. Detachment is accompanied by recocking the head for reattachment to another binding site. The detachment of the myosin head from the actin molecule is an active process that uses energy derived from the hydrolysis of ATP into adenosine diphosphate (ADP) and phosphate in the presence of Ca^{2+}. The process of attachment, rotation, and detachment therefore continues as long as Ca^{2+} and ATP are present in the cell in sufficient amounts. The stiff state of muscles after death known as *rigor mortis* results from cross bridges that cannot detach because ADP is not phosphorylated to replenish the ATP supply.

Noncontractile Components in Muscle Fibers Provide Stability for the Contractile Elements

Muscle fibers contain several structural elements whose mechanical properties ensure stable and efficient production and transmission of the active force generated by the contractile apparatus of the thin and thick filaments. In addition to the contractile myofilaments described above, a set of very thin and highly elastic filaments, the connecting filaments or *connectins,* extend from the ends of the thick filaments and attach on both flanking Z disks (see Figure 34–5 below). These connectins form a continuous elastic structure along the entire length of the muscle fiber, accounting for at least some of the springlike restoring force that can be measured when an inactive muscle is stretched passively (see below). The connecting filaments keep the thick and thin filaments aligned with respect to each other if the muscle is stretched past the overlap of the filaments. The remainder of the passive force is provided by endomysial connective tissue, a loose matrix of collagen that surrounds each muscle fiber and helps to distribute tension and sarcomere length changes evenly. Any active force generated by the contractile mechanism is independent of and additional to the passive force generated by these parallel elastic elements.

At the ends of muscle fibers that insert onto connective tissue the last set of actin filaments attaches to specialized sites on the muscle fiber membrane where the tension is conveyed to invaginated strands of extracellular collagen in the connective tissue. Tendons and aponeuroses (see below) can stretch and store mechanical energy during muscle contraction, particularly if these in-series elastic elements are relatively long compared with the muscle fibers. Some muscles have long fascicles that are staggered bundles of shorter muscle fibers. The intrafascicular ends of these muscle fibers have a long tapered shape that provides a large surface area over which tensile force can be

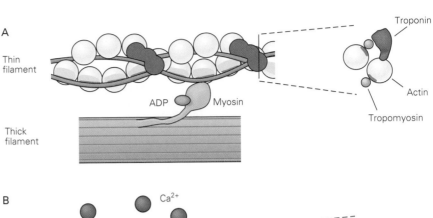

Figure 34-3 Contraction is produced by cyclical attachment and detachment of myosin heads on adjacent thin filaments. (Based on Huxley and Simmons, 1971; Squire, 1983.)

A. In a muscle fiber at rest the myosin heads of the thick filaments are all in a "cocked" position with bound adenosine diphosphate (ADP). The troponin-tropomyosin complexes on the thin filaments have no bound Ca^{2+} and are positioned so as to block the binding sites on the actin (**orange**).

B. When the muscle fiber is activated, Ca^{2+} is released from the cisternae of the sacroplasmic reticulum (see Figure 34-2) and binds to at least some of the tropomyosin sites. This action causes a conformational change in the thin filament that exposes actin-binding sites, allowing the myosin heads to attach and form cross bridges between the thick and thin filaments.

C. Attached myosin heads rotate, exerting longitudinal forces that pull the thick and thin filaments into greater overlap, shortening the muscle fiber.

D. At the end of the cross-bridge power stroke fresh adenosine triphosphate (ATP) binds to the myosin head, which then detaches.

E. Chemical energy released by dephosphorylation of the ATP to bound ADP is used to recock the myosin head for attachment to another binding site and thus another power stroke.

P_i = phosphate.

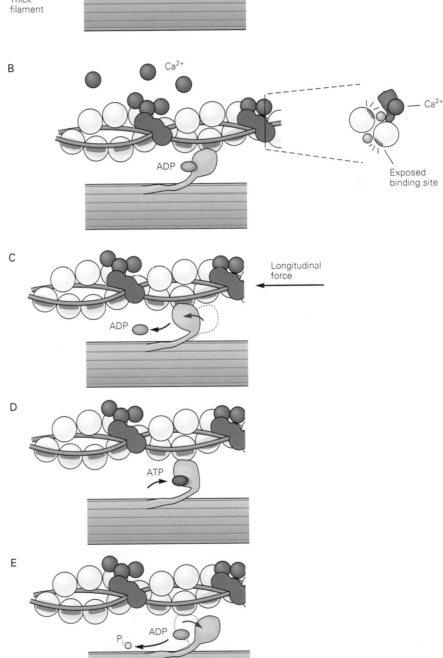

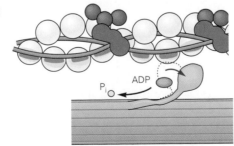

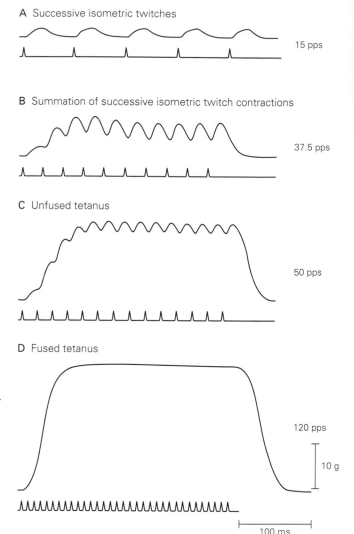

Figure 34-4 The active tension in a muscle varies with the rate of stimulation of the muscle nerve. The muscle nerve is stimulated electrically while the muscle is held at a constant length. The example is from the caudofemoralis, a very fast cat muscle. (All parts are scaled identically to the maximal specific force per unit cross-sectional area shown in D.) The comparable stimulus range for human muscle would be about 5–60 pps. (Courtesy of I. E. Brown and G. E. Loeb).

A. Successive stimuli at a low frequency evoke discrete and separate twitches characterized by a rapid rise in force and a slower decay.

B. If the force produced by a given twitch has not returned to baseline by the time the next is evoked, the contractile force of successive twitches increases at first, but a stable mean level is achieved after a few stimuli, resulting in a ripple of force.

C. Increasing the rate of stimulation produces a higher mean force. However, distinct ripples corresponding to individual stimuli can still be seen.

D. At high rates of stimulation individual stimuli do not produce discrete force fluctuations and the mean force is somewhat greater than during the unfused contraction. Note the delay before force decays back to baseline after the cessation of stimulation. The frequency of action potentials needed to produce a fused tetanic contraction is higher than that occurring during physiological recruitment.

passed as shear force into the surrounding connective tissue. Some of the myopathies described in Chapter 35 may be related to failures of the noncontractile components of muscle.

Contractile Force Depends on the Level of Activation of Each Muscle Fiber and Its Length and Velocity

The total force output that can be measured at the tendon of a muscle reflects the sum of its passive tension plus the instantaneous active tension generated by cross bridges. Three physically independent processes affect active tension: the number of cross bridges formed, the force produced by each cross bridge, and the velocity of cross-bridge motion.

Formation of Cross Bridges Depends on Calcium

The actin-binding sites for the myosin heads are normally covered by troponin-tropomyosin complexes (Figure 34-3A). When a troponin molecule binds with Ca^{2+}, the troponin-tropomyosin complex undergoes a conformational change that exposes local actin-binding sites, permitting a cocked myosin head to attach and exert contractile force as a cross bridge.

Muscle fibers contain an extensive network of longitudinally oriented tubules and chambers called the *sarcoplasmic reticulum* (Figure 34-2) that sequester and release Ca^{2+}. Under resting conditions the amount of intracellular Ca^{2+} is kept very low by active pumping into the sarcoplasmic reticulum. The Ca^{2+} is transported through the tubules to terminal cisternae distributed throughout the cross section of the muscle fiber. These cisternae are tightly bound to the transverse

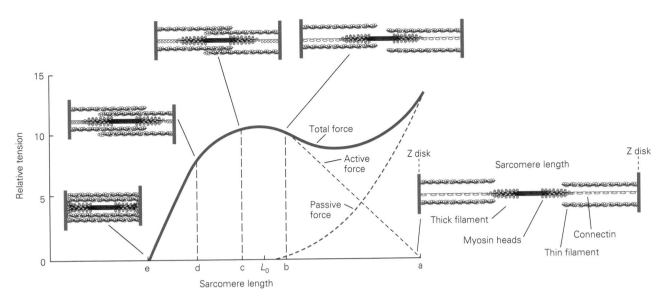

Figure 34-5 The amount of active contractile force developed during contraction depends on the degree of overlap of thick and thin filaments. When the sarcomere is stretched beyond the length at which the thick and thin filaments overlap (length **a**), no active force develops because the myosin heads are not near any binding sites and thus cross bridges cannot form. As the filaments overlap (lengths **a–b**) the force that can develop increases linearly as length decreases because of the progressive increase in the number of binding sites for myosin heads. Around the muscle's optimal length (L_0, between lengths **b–c**) the level of force remains constant because the central portion of the thick filaments is devoid of myosin heads. With further reductions in length (lengths **c–d**) the progressive overlap of thin filaments with each other occludes potential attachment sites and the force begins to fall. Once the thick filaments abut the Z disks (lengths **d–e**), they act like compression springs opposing the active force generated by the cross bridges. Passive force exists in muscle regardless of activation, starting at about L_0 and rising at first exponentially and then linearly as progressive lengthening of the muscle stretches the connectin filaments that tether the thick filaments between the Z disks. Total force is the sum of active and passive force.

tubules, which are actually invaginations of the sarcolemma (Figure 34-2).

When an action potential propagates along the surface of the muscle fiber, it actively depolarizes the transverse tubules within the muscle fiber. Changes in the transmembrane charge in the transverse tubules are coupled to the terminal cisternae by processes that are not yet fully understood. The end result is that Ca^{2+} is released through transmembrane channels in the cisternae, diffuses passively among the myofilaments, and binds reversibly to troponin, thus enabling cross bridges to form (ie, the myosin heads are able to bind to actin).

The release of Ca^{2+} is very rapid, but it may take 20–50 ms to activate the thin filaments fully and for cross bridges to form. Meanwhile, the total amount of free Ca^{2+} is rapidly reduced by reuptake, causing a decrease in cross bridges and a fall in contractile force over a period of 80–200 ms. Activation and calcium reuptake—two competing, time-dependent processes—account for the different time courses of the rise and fall of active tension in a *twitch contraction*, the muscle's response to a single action potential (Figure 34-4A).

The contractile force produced by a single action potential is relatively small because the amount and persistence of released Ca^{2+} is considerably less than that required to activate all of the actin-binding sites (ie, relatively few cross bridges form during a twitch). If another action potential occurs before all the Ca^{2+} released by the first action potential has been resequestered, more cross bridges form, resulting in a greater output of force (Figure 34-4B). The higher the frequency of action potentials, the higher the amount of force up to the point at which all cross bridge binding sites are continuously activated and force output no longer shows any ripples (Figure 34-4D). This smoothly fused contraction is called a *fused tetanus*, or *maximal tetanic contraction*.

The Number of Cross Bridges Depends on the Degree of Overlap Between Actin and Myosin Filaments

Cross bridges can form only in regions of the sarcomere where myosin heads lie adjacent to actin filaments. As

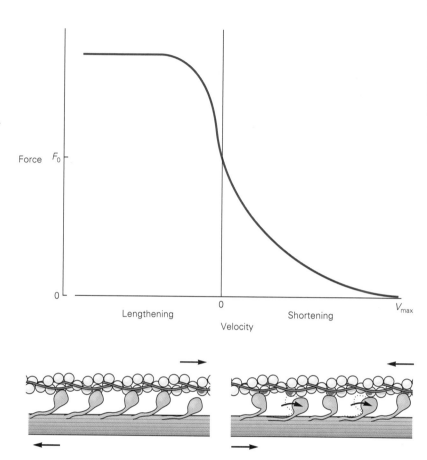

Figure 34-6 The active force produced by muscle depends on the velocity at which it is changing length. Starting from the isometric point (zero velocity), increasing rates of shortening result in decreasing ability to generate force until contractile force drops to zero at V_{max}. As shown in the drawing below, shortening causes the myosin heads to spend more time near the end of their power stroke, when they produce less contractile force, and in detaching, recocking, and reattaching, when they produce no force. When muscle is actively lengthened, contractile force rises rapidly and tends to stay high. The myosin heads spend more time stretched past their angle of attachment and little time in the unattached state because they do not need to be recocked after being pulled away from the actin in this manner (see Figure 34-3).

the muscle fiber and its sarcomeres are stretched, the region of overlap decreases until at zero overlap no active force can be generated (although there is usually considerable passive force at this length). Thus the amount of active force depends on both the frequency of action potentials in the muscle fiber and the fiber's length.

As the sarcomeres shorten, the actin filaments from each end of the sarcomere overlap with a longer portion of the thick filaments (Figure 34-5), thus increasing the ability to generate contractile force. There is a plateau in the force-length relationship, however, because the mid region of the thick filament does not contain myosin heads. With further shortening the actin filaments interdigitate with each other. This interferes with the ability of the myosin heads to find binding sites, decreasing force generation. The thick filaments eventually collide with and crumple against the Z disks, producing a pushing force that increasingly counteracts the contractile force. The force-length relationship thus has an inverted U shape, meaning that the muscle cannot produce active force at either extreme of length and produces maximal force at an intermediate length, usually called L_0 (Figure 34-5).

If the fibers of a muscle extended from the bony origin to the bony insertion of the muscle, the relationship between muscle length and fiber and sarcomere length would be a simple matter, and we could compute the total force output as the sum of the force produced by all active fibers at that length. In many muscles, however, the muscle fibers are arranged obliquely to the long axis of the muscle and are attached to plates of connective tissue that extend over the surface and sometimes into the body of the muscle (see muscle A in Figure 34-1). These *aponeuroses* gather and transmit the force of muscle fibers to a band of connective tissue, the tendon, which typically inserts on the bone. This pennate (feather-like) architecture enhances the total force that can be generated by a given volume of muscle because there are more fibers working in parallel. There is a cost, however, to this mechanical advantage: a change in length of the whole muscle results in a proportionately larger length change in each contractile unit. As we have seen, force generation depends on muscle length; if the muscle fibers start at their optimal length, a large change in length will shift them to a suboptimal point in their force-length relationship (see Figure 34-5).

The Force Produced by Cross Bridges Depends on the Velocity of the Sarcomere

The force-length relationship reflects the ability of cross bridges to produce force when length remains unchanged, that is, when the muscle is isometric. Muscles are rarely isometric, however; they usually work to change the motion of loads. If the load is less than the contractile force, the muscle shortens (sometimes called concentric work). The faster the sarcomeres are shortening and the cross bridges are cycling, the less force they produce (Figure 34-6). The shortening velocity at which active force output goes to zero is called V_{max}. If the load is greater than the contractile force, the muscle will lengthen (active lengthening or eccentric work). In this case, the muscle is absorbing rather than generating mechanical energy, such as is required to decelerate a heavy object when catching it. Lengthening muscles actually produce more force than isometric muscles at the same level of activation.

The rate of energy consumption by the cross bridges is proportional to their velocity, not to the force they produce. During rapid shortening when the muscle produces little force, the rate of energy consumption is very high, because each cross bridge dephosphorylates one ATP molecule in the process of detaching at the end of the power stroke. In contrast, during active lengthening the rate of energy consumption is much lower because the cross bridges are pulled apart without ATP binding. During lengthening, cross bridges that have been ripped away from their actin attachments remain cocked and immediately find another actin-binding site, so they continue to contribute to the force-resisting stretch of the muscle regardless of stretch velocity. The force-velocity relationship modifies force output simultaneously with, and more or less independently of, the force-length relationship (Figure 34-7).

Repeated Activation of Muscle Causes Fatigue

When muscle fibers are repeatedly activated, energy supplies are depleted and the muscles fatigue: they produce less force and the rate of rise of force is reduced. When fatigued, muscle fibers also take longer to relax (ie, to slacken when activation ceases) because relaxation is an active process that requires ATP. This prolongation in relaxation time has the paradoxical effect of allowing the force produced by successive nerve impulses to summate at lower frequencies (longer interspike intervals) than when the muscle is rested. As a result, early during fatigue the summed force produced by unfused tetanic stimulation decreases more slowly than the force of individual twitches. As fatigue develops, the firing frequency of motor neurons is decreased to com-

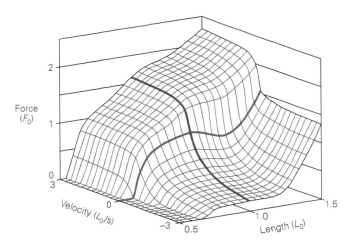

Figure 34-7 The total force (active plus passive) produced by a muscle fiber at a given level of activation depends on both its instantaneous length and velocity, which are independent kinematic variables. Figure 34-5 shows the mechanisms responsible for the effects of length alone and Figure 34-6 the mechanisms responsible for the effects of velocity alone.

This surface plot was generated from a mathematical model that captures the behavior of the slow-twitch soleus muscle of the cat during maximal tetanic activation. It incorporates additional interrelations between length and velocity that occur at nonoptimal lengths. For muscle fibers activated at less than tetanic levels the height of the surface scales downward (lower force), but additional dependencies between activation, length, and velocity change the shape of the surface somewhat. (Adapted from Brown et al. 1996.)

During a natural movement both the length and the velocity of active muscle fibers are likely to change as a result of skeletal motion and stretching of the elastic connective tissues that are in series between the muscle fibers and the bones. Such changes in the kinematic conditions of the muscle fibers alter the force output of the muscle, even if the neural activation of the muscle does not change. In the plot the direction and steepness of the slope of the surface in a particular region represent changes in force output due to small perturbations in the kinematic state of the muscle. Small changes in velocity around zero create particularly large changes in force. These intrinsic changes in force are instantaneous and generally tend to oppose the perturbations, helping to stabilize the muscle in a given kinematic state.

pensate for the summed force. In the next chapter we shall see how receptors in the muscles sense changes in tension and length and can compensate for them through reflex actions on motor neurons.

Three Types of Motor Units Differ in Speed, Strength of Contraction, and Fatigability

Anyone who has carved a roasted chicken knows that its muscles are either light colored ("white" muscle) or

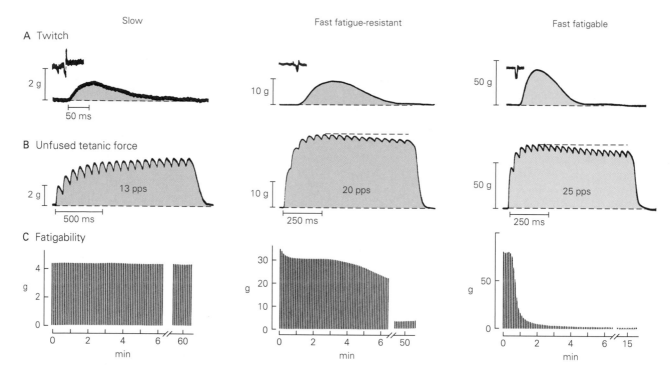

Figure 34-8 Slow, fast fatigue-resistant, and fast fatigable motor units vary in twitch, tetanic force, and fatigability. (From Burke et al. 1973.)

A. Traces show the twitches of the three motor units.

B. Unfused contractions produced by a train of stimuli at a rate typical for each type of motor unit. Fast units produce much larger twitch and tetanic forces than do slow units (vertical scale changed for each).

C. Fatigability can be seen in records of the force produced by

sustained activation. The motor units were activated by stimulus trains (40 pps) lasting 0.33 s and repeated every second. In the records shown here a single vertical line represents the force produced by one contraction, recorded at slow speed. In the slow unit the force remained essentially constant for over an hour of repeated stimulation. In the fast fatigable unit the force dropped abruptly after only a minute. The fast fatigue-resistant unit had substantial resistance to fatigue and the force declined slowly over many minutes; some residual force remained after 50 min.

dark colored ("red") muscle). The red muscles of the legs are specialized for standing and walking, while the white muscles that operate the wings of this flightless bird are used only occasionally in a vigorous escape maneuver. The distinctive appearance and specialized mechanical capabilities of each type of muscle stem from structural specializations and different metabolic properties of the muscle fibers. Most mammalian muscles are composed of a mix of three fiber types: slow-twitch fibers and two types of fast-twitch fibers. All of the muscle fibers innervated by a single motor neuron are of the same type.

Red muscles are composed mostly of slow-twitch fibers, also called type I fibers. The force produced by type I fibers rises and falls relatively slowly in response to an action potential (Figures 34-8A and 34-9). Muscles composed of type I fibers can produce relatively small amounts of tension for long periods without running down their energy stores. This fatigue resistance results

from their reliance on oxidative catabolism, by which glucose and oxygen from the bloodstream can be used almost indefinitely to regenerate the ATP that fuels the contractile apparatus. To support this aerobic metabolism, slow-twitch muscle fibers are surrounded by an extensive network of capillaries. They also are provided with large numbers of mitochondria and oxidative enzymes as well as with myoglobin, a heme protein that helps bind and store oxygen from the blood stream. Individual red muscle fibers produce less contractile force than fast-twitch fibers because they are smaller and have fewer contractile filaments.

White muscles are composed mostly of fast-twitch fibers, also called type II. The force produced by type II fibers rises and falls rapidly (Figure 34-8). These fibers also have a different form of myosin; the cross bridges produce force more effectively at rapid shortening velocities. Fast-twitch fibers are generally categorized into two subtypes depending on their metabolic processes

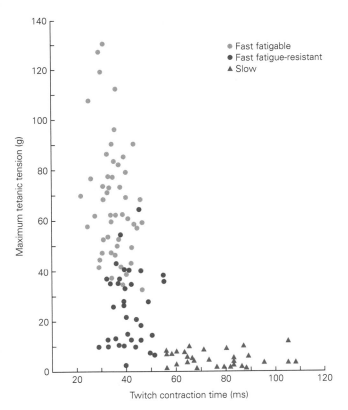

Figure 34-9 This physiological profile of motor units in the gastrocnemius muscle of the cat shows the distinctive actions of slow-twitch and fast-twitch motor units. The fast fatigable units produce larger force than the fast fatigue-resistant units. The slow units have very long twitch-contraction times and generate very low force. (From Burke et al. 1973.)

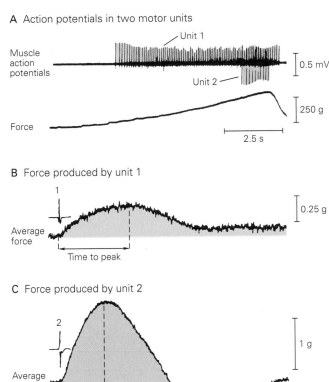

Figure 34-10 Motor units that produce a small amount of force are recruited before motor units that produce larger forces. (Adapted from Desmedt and Godaux, 1977.)

A. Action potentials from two motor units were recorded simultaneously through a single intramuscular microelectrode (**upper trace**) while the subject gradually increased the force produced by the muscle (**lower trace**). The motor neuron labeled unit 1 starts firing near the beginning of the voluntary contraction and increases its firing rate steadily as the force increases. Motor unit 2 starts firing only near the peak of the voluntary contraction and turns off as soon as the force declines.

B-C. Average twitch forces produced by motor units 1 and 2. Because many unrecorded motor units fire asynchronously but more or less at the same time, there is no recognizable deflection in the force trace associated with each of the spikes. To assess the force of a single recorded motor unit, brief segments of the recorded force are aligned with the time of occurrence of each spike and summed. The changes in force that are uncorrelated with a particular action potential, representing noise, will cancel each other out, while the forces that result specifically from this action potential are time locked with it and sum constructively with each added spike. With enough spikes (typically several hundred) the time course of the twitch becomes evident, as in the traces here. Following the size principle of recruitment, the average force produced by unit 1, recruited first, is less than one-quarter that produced by unit 2, while the time from onset to peak force is roughly double.

and fatigue resistance. The *fast fatigable* (type IIB) fibers rely on anaerobic catabolism to sustain force output. They have relatively large stores of glycogen that provide energy to phosphorylate ADP rapidly as the glycogen is converted into lactic acid. However, the rapid depletion of glycogen stores and accumulation of lactic acid limit these fibers to brief bursts of force, after which they take many hours to recover fully. The other fast-twitch subgroup, *fast fatigue-resistant* (type IIA) fibers, combine relatively fast twitch dynamics and contractile velocity with enough aerobic capacity to resist fatigue for several minutes.

The contractile force of a motor unit depends on the force-generating capabilities of its fiber type multiplied by the number of muscle fibers innervated by the motor neuron. The motor neurons that control the fast-twitch (type II) muscle fibers usually innervate many large fibers, thus enhancing their ability to produce large forces rapidly (Figure 34-9). These motor neurons have

Figure 34-11 Two motor neurons of different sizes have the same resting membrane potential (E_m starts at the resting level in both plots) and receive the same excitatory synaptic current (I_{syn}) from a spinal interneuron. Because the small motor neuron has a small surface area, it has fewer parallel ion channels and therefore a higher overall resistance (R_{high}). According to Ohm's Law ($E = IR$) the synaptic current in the small neuron produces a large excitatory postsynaptic potential (**EPSP**) that reaches threshold, resulting in an action potential. The small motor neuron also has a small-diameter axon that conducts the action potential relatively slowly to the few small muscle fibers that comprise its muscle unit. In contrast, the large motor neuron has a larger surface area, resulting in a lower overall transmembrane resistance (R_{low}) and a smaller, subthreshold EPSP in response to I_{syn}. As a result, its many muscle fibers are not recruited.

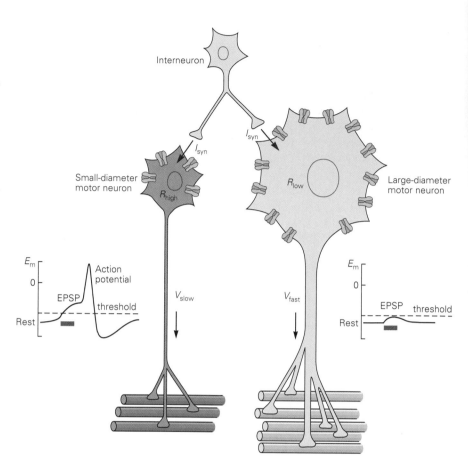

relatively large cell bodies and large-diameter axons that conduct action potentials at high velocities.

The motor neurons that control the slow-twitch (type I) muscle fibers have smaller cell bodies and innervate fewer, thinner fibers, resulting in much smaller force output (as little as 1% of the force produced by fast fatigable units). As might be expected, motor neurons innervating fast fatigue-resistant fibers tend to be intermediate in size and speed.

Motor Units Are Recruited in Fixed Order

In both reflexive and voluntary contractions motor units are recruited in a fixed order from weakest to strongest. Thus when only a small amount of force is required from a muscle innervated by more than one type of motor unit, this force is provided exclusively by the slow-twitch units (Figure 34-10). As more force is required, fast fatigue-resistant and then fast fatigable units are recruited in remarkably precise order according to the magnitude of the force each unit produces. As muscle force is decreased, motor units drop out in the order op-

posite from their recruitment: the largest are the first to cease activity.

The Electrical Properties of Motor Neurons Determine Their Responses to Synaptic Input

The order of recruitment is highly correlated with the diameter and conduction velocity of the axons and the size of the motor neuron cell bodies, as well as the size and strength of their muscle units. A cell's threshold for firing depends on its electrical resistance, which is inversely related to its surface area. The same synaptic input will produce larger changes in membrane potential in small-diameter cells, which have high electrical resistance, than in large-diameter cells (Figure 34-11). Thus, as the net amount of excitatory synaptic input to a motor nucleus increases, individual motor neurons reach threshold levels of depolarization in the order of their size: The smallest fire first and the largest fire last. This is the size principle of motor neuron recruitment.

Size-ordered recruitment serves two important purposes. First, it minimizes the development of fatigue by allowing the most fatigue-resistant muscle fibers to be used most of the time, holding the more fatigable fibers in reserve until needed to achieve higher forces. A cat uses half the motor units in an ankle extensor for standing and walking, activities that require about 20% of the maximal force of the muscle. Only during powerful and rapid movements such as jumping are the rest of the units recruited. Thus, about 80% of the total muscle force is held in reserve for transient use during predatory or escape behaviors. Second, size-ordered recruitment ensures that the increment of force generated by successively activated motor units will be roughly proportional to the level of force at which each individual unit is recruited. In natural conditions spinal motor neurons receive synaptic inputs from many sources (eg, sensory afferents, spinal interneurons, descending projections), causing their membrane potentials to fluctuate somewhat randomly. During a fine motor task requiring only small amounts of force by a few slow-twitch motor units, random recruitment of a fast fatigable motor unit, whose twitch contraction might be larger than all slow-twitch units combined, would seriously disrupt the task.

The Force of Contraction Depends on the Number of Recruited Motor Neurons and Their Individual Firing Rates

When a motor nucleus begins to be activated by peripheral or descending inputs, individual motor neurons begin firing at a slow regular rate (5–10 impulses per second in humans). This results in a partially fused train of contractions in the target muscle fibers. As the net excitatory synaptic input in the nucleus increases, the firing rate of the cells increases and other, slightly larger motor neurons reach their threshold for firing, adding their force as well. In this way the mean level of force produced in the muscle gradually increases (Figure 34-12). The overall force of a contraction depends on both the number and size of active motor units and their individual firing rates (see Figure 34-4D). Because the relative timing of the individual action potentials in the various motor units is asynchronous, the various unfused contractions produced by all active motor units blend together into a smooth contraction.

Movements Are Produced by the Coordinated Work of Many Muscles Acting on Skeletal Joints

The human body has over 250 muscles, each with a distinct mechanical action at one or more joints. The nervous system could, in principle, be wired up to control

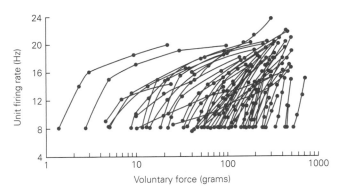

Figure 34-12 For motor tasks that require a slow increase in force, motor units are gradually recruited one at a time and their firing frequency is increased progressively. Units fire at about 8 Hz when first recruited and their firing rate increases as the load on the muscle increases. The record here is from the extensor digitorum communis of a human subject. (Adapted from Monster and Chan 1977.)

each muscle independently, producing any combination of achievable forces in each. However, this would make for a great deal of neural redundancy. In fact, the nervous system must learn which muscles to use to perform a movement, primarily by trial and error exploration of the mechanical advantages of various combinations of muscles. The suitability of particular muscles depends on the distribution of fiber types as well as the mechanical arrangement of fibers (muscle architecture). The choice of a particular combination of muscles influences the efficiency of performance and the ability to recover gracefully from an unexpected perturbation. The spatial and temporal control of different combinations of muscles is mediated by the divergent and convergent patterns of connections of primary afferents, interneurons, and descending axons within the spinal cord.

Muscles Have Different Actions at Individual Joints

The simplest joint is a hinge, like the elbow and interphalangeal joints. These joints allow movement back and forth in only one plane. Because muscles pull but cannot push, hinge joints require at least two muscles pulling in opposite directions, so called *antagonist* muscles. Most joints are not as simple and have at least a limited range of motion in more than one plane. For example, the ankle permits a large range of extension and flexion together with modest amounts of axial rotation and inversion-eversion. Ball joints, such as the shoulder and hip, permit wide ranges of motion in all three possi-

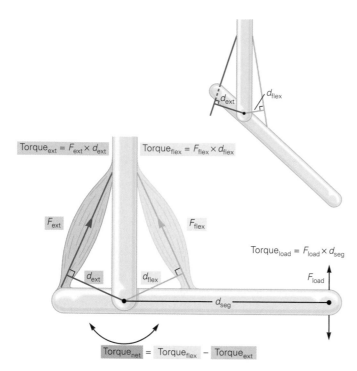

$$\text{Torque}_{ext} = F_{ext} \times d_{ext}$$

$$\text{Torque}_{flex} = F_{flex} \times d_{flex}$$

$$\text{Torque}_{load} = F_{load} \times d_{seg}$$

$$\text{Torque}_{net} = \text{Torque}_{flex} - \text{Torque}_{ext}$$

Figure 34-13 Each muscle produces a torque at a joint that is the product of its contractile force *(F)* and its moment arm at that joint *(d)*. The moment arm of a muscle is defined as the length of a perpendicular from the line of pull of the muscle to the center of rotation of the joint (it may be necessary to extend the line of pull past the end of the muscle to construct such a perpendicular, as done for d_{ext} in the inset). Note that the moment arm changes when the angle of the joint changes if the distance between the tendon and the joint changes (as in the inset). The moment arm at a given angular position is often determined experimentally by measuring the change of length of the muscle produced by a small change in angular position and computing the effective moment arm trigonometrically.

The net torque at a joint is the sum of the torques of all of the muscles crossing the joint. The antagonistic muscles shown here (ext = extensor; flex = flexor) produce torque in opposite directions, so the net torque is the difference between the torques produced by each. If the limb is at rest, the net torque produced by the muscles must be opposed by another equal but opposite torque, such as would be caused by a force from a load at the end of the limb segment. If that external force (F_{load}) is measured perpendicular to the long axis of the limb segment (as depicted here), then this external torque (Torque_{load}) is the product F_{load} times the length of the segment (d_{seg}, which is the moment arm for F_{load}).

ble axes of rotation. A few joints move primarily in translation, rather than rotation, such as the sliding of the scapula on the trunk. The number of different, independently controllable axes of motion possible at a joint is called its degree of freedom and ranges from one, for a simple hinge joint, up to a maximum of six (three rotational and three translational). In a multiarticular limb the degree of freedom is the sum of the degrees of freedom of all of its joints. Thus the arm (not counting the digits) has seven degrees of freedom: three at the shoulder, one at the elbow, and three at the wrist.

The action of a muscle on a simple hinge joint depends on its anatomical orientation with respect to the center of rotation of the joint. The muscle plus any tendon in series acts like a rope pulling on a lever or passing around a pulley, so its action can be described as a *torque* (a force that rotates a joint) according to the laws of physical mechanics. The shortest distance from the muscle's line of pull to the center of the joint is called its *moment arm*, measured in a plane perpendicular to the axis of rotation of the joint (Figure 34-13). This distance can change as the angle of the joint changes; for example, elbow flexor muscles pass closer to the center of rotation when the elbow joint is fully extended rather than in mid position. A muscle with a large moment arm can generate a lot of torque but only at the expense of large changes in length and velocity. The action of a muscle on a joint with several degrees of freedom can be computed for each axis of rotation from the same geometrical principles. In more complex joints the moment arms of muscles often change in complicated ways as a result of shifts in the centers of rotation and the routing of tendons around bony protuberances and through connective tissue sheaths.

Rapid Changes in Joint Torque Involve Sequential Activation of Agonist and Antagonist Muscles

The nervous system controls the torques at joints by varying the frequency of action potentials in motor units. Because the build-up of force at the onset of neural activity and its decay when neural activity ceases are both slow, muscle force cannot follow rapid fluctuations in neural discharge (Figure 34-14A). Yet for many tasks it is necessary to produce rapidly rising and falling torques. The nervous system accomplishes this by activating the agonist muscle more vigorously and then activating an antagonist muscle with a slight delay so that the excess agonist torque is opposed by the antagonist torque (Figure 34-14B).

Muscle Force Is Required to Overcome Inertia

Movement of the body depends on more than just the contractile properties of agonist and antagonist muscles. It also depends on the interplay of external forces such as gravity, the mechanical constraints of joints and ligaments, and the laws of physics governing the movement of mass.

Newton's Laws of mechanics dictate that the velocity of an object will change if and only if acted upon by an external force. For the body to stay motionless in the face of an external force such as gravity, an equal and opposite force must be applied by the muscles. Conversely, muscle force is required to accelerate a limb from rest and then to decelerate it back to rest when the desired new position is attained. This explains why rapid movements are often accompanied by sequences of activity in agonist and antagonist muscles (Figure 34-15).

Muscle Force May Be Used to Create Stiffness at Joints

Movement of any joint crossed by a muscle tends to change the length and velocity of that muscle, whether the movement is caused by the action of the muscle itself, the action of other muscles, or by external forces. Because the force produced by a muscle depends on its length and on the velocity at which its length is changing, joint movement produces an instantaneous change in the muscle's force without any change in its state of activation. At first this might seem like an unfortunate complication, requiring yet more compensatory computations by the nervous system. In fact, the nervous system uses these properties to great advantage in coping with unanticipated perturbations.

When standing still, little or no ankle muscle activity is required to stabilize your body over your ankle joints. But consider the problem of trying to stand on the deck of a small boat pitching back and forth in the water. Now you must apply large forces rapidly in order to pull the center of mass back from any direction. By co-contracting the ankle muscles before these perturbations occur, you increase the stiffness at the joint (ie, the force produced by a given change in length in both directions increases). When the body is rapidly thrown in one direction, the muscles that normally pull in that direction suddenly shorten and their tension drops abruptly, while those that pull one back suddenly lengthen and their force increases. Additionally, because the muscle is active, you can take advantage of the force-velocity relationship of the co-contracting muscles. The resulting changes in force are quite large in precisely the direction required to keep your balance (Figure 34-16). Furthermore, these intrinsic changes in active force are instantaneous. Even the fastest reflex response to the sensory information about the perturbation requires about 50 ms to travel from the sensors to the spinal cord and out along the motor axons, followed by another 50 ms delay for the processes involved in excitation-contraction coupling to change the force output of the muscle. One disadvantage of co-contraction is that

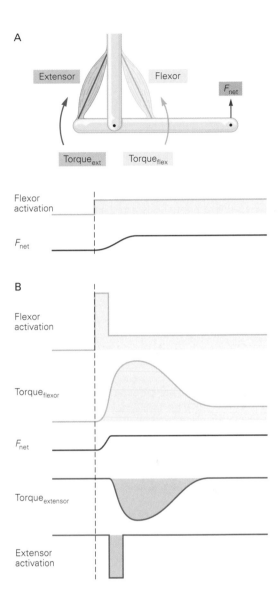

Figure 34-14

A. The ability of a muscle to rapidly exert a force is limited by the relatively slow rate of rise of its contractile force following electrical activation by its motor neurons.

B. The nervous system can increase torque more rapidly by using a larger initial burst of motor neuronal activity, but it must then prevent the net torque from overshooting the desired level. It cannot turn off the agonist muscle quickly enough because the fall time of its contractile force is even slower than the rise time. The nervous system solves this problem by briefly activating the antagonist muscle shortly after activating the agonist, so that the negative torque of the antagonist counteracts the anticipated overshoot from the agonist muscle. In this and the following figures muscle activation and torque are shown as positive for the agonist and negative for the antagonist. In experimental work electrical activation is often estimated by rectifying and smoothing the recorded EMG signal, an amplitude-modulated, broadband AC waveform whose amplitude is highly correlated with the aggregate activation of the muscle fibers in the whole muscle.

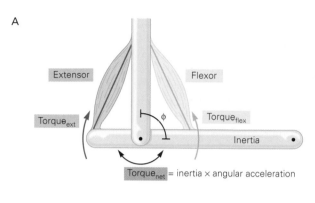

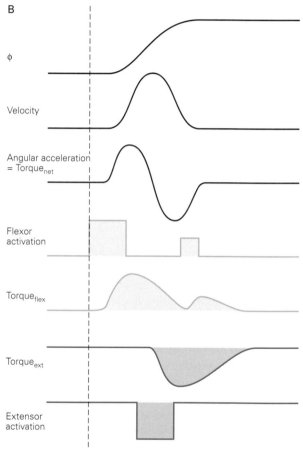

Figure 34-15 Muscle torques are required to overcome inertia when movements are started and stopped.

A. According to Newton's Law, force is required to change the velocity of a mass. The common form of the relationship for linear translation is force = mass × acceleration. Muscles produce torque to rotate the inertial mass of the skeletal segment around a joint. For torque, the equivalent form of Newton's Law is torque = rotational inertia × angular acceleration, where the inertia depends on the mass of the limb segment as well as its distribution over the length of the segment.

B. When humans move their limbs from one position to another they generally change joint angles in a smooth manner, such that angular velocity follows a symmetrical, bell-shaped profile. According to Newton's Law, this requires equal and opposite net torque pulses to produce the corresponding acceleration and deceleration phases. The flexor and extensor muscles are activated in succession, as shown by their activation levels and individual torque contributions. Because the relatively slow fall time of contractile force would tend to cause the decelerating torque from the extensor muscle to overshoot, a small, third phase of activity (from the flexor muscle) is often included to stop the limb exactly on target, particularly for fast movements. (Joint angle ϕ graphed inverted so that flexion is upward.)

it must be initiated and maintained before a perturbation occurs, which increases metabolic cost and risks fatiguing the muscles.

Muscles Act on More Than One Joint

More than half of the muscles of the body cross more than one joint. The ability of a multiarticular muscle to produce force at one joint depends on movement of the other joints that it crosses. For example, the grip strength of the finger flexor muscles in the forearm is greatly reduced when they are shortened by flexion of the wrist joint, because their sarcomere lengths become disadvantageously short (see Figure 34-5).

In physical mechanics work is performed when a force acts over a distance. If the motions at two joints result in offsetting lengthening and shortening effects in a multiarticular muscle, the muscle cannot perform much mechanical work itself because it exerts force over a length change of zero. Nevertheless, it may be useful to activate the muscle so that it acts like a stiff strut in a pantograph (Figure 34-17A). In this case the muscle exerts force over a

Figure 34-16 The intrinsic mechanical properties of muscles restore forces when a limb is perturbed.

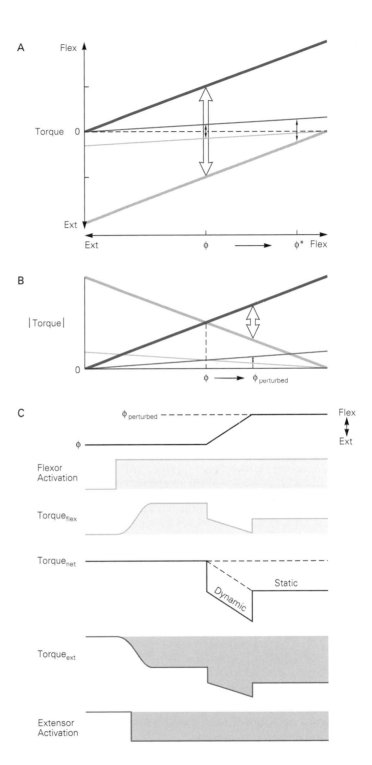

A. Because of the shapes of the active and passive force-length relationships (see Figure 34-5), muscles are springlike, increasing their total force output as they are lengthened. The slope of the relationship (the ratio of force to length) is equivalent to the stiffness of the spring. This ratio can be varied according to the level of activation of the muscle. For an antagonist pair of muscles as shown, the force-length relationships can be graphed as torque versus joint angle (ϕ) relationships with opposite signs. When the torque amplitudes are equal and opposite, the limb will be at rest at an equilibrium position. A given equilibrium position (ϕ) can be achieved with different degrees of coactivation of the antagonist muscles, as long as their torques are equal and opposite. If the relative activation of the two muscles changes, the limb will move to a new equilibrium position, ϕ^*.

B. It is easier to see how the opposing torques interact with each other by inverting one and seeing where they intersect. If the joint is shifted from an equilibrium angle, ϕ, to a new angle, $\phi_{perturbed}$, while the activation levels of the muscles remain constant, there will be a net torque that resists the shift and that is equal to the difference between the two torques at the new angle (**red arrows**). The resisting net torque is much higher when the same joint angles are achieved with higher levels of muscle coactivation (**thick, steep lines**).

C. The nervous system takes advantage of the intrinsic force-length and force-velocity relationships in muscle to produce a resistive force against sudden perturbations. By co-contracting the flexor and extensor muscles as shown in the activation traces, the net torque before the perturbation does not change and the joint angle stays the same but the stiffness increases. When a perturbation in joint angle occurs, the stretch of the extensor muscle and the shortening of the flexor muscle result in a large resisting net torque that occurs before any reflexes could produce a change in muscle activation. This torque has two components: a large dynamic change produced by the force-velocity relationship of the two active muscles and a smaller static force due to the force-length relationship. This intrinsic response is usually supplemented by subsequent reflex effects on muscle activation mediated by stretch receptors in the muscles and their projections onto spinal interneurons and motor neurons (see subsequent chapters).

period of time, which represents momentum in physical mechanics. Such a linkage economically transfers mechanical momentum from one body segment to another. This can greatly improve the overall efficiency of a rhythmic task such as walking, in which individual limb segments must be alternately accelerated and decelerated with each step.

Although a muscle produces torque only at the joint it crosses, this torque may well affect the movement of other joints throughout the body because of mechanical interactions through the skeletal linkage (Figure 34-17B,C). For example, the soleus muscle crosses only the ankle joint and produces only an extensor torque at

A

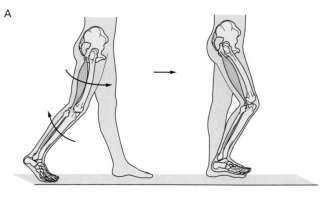

Figure 34-17 A single muscle can affect the motion of many joints.

A. Many muscles cross more than one joint. For example, the hamstring muscles of the leg extend the hip and flex the knee. During the swing phase of walking the knee is flexed, which tends to shorten the hamstrings, while the hip is also flexed, which tends to lengthen the hamstrings (**black arrows**). If the flexion of the knee were accomplished by a monoarticular knee flexor, the muscle would have to work hard and consume much energy to achieve the necessary force while shortening rapidly. The same knee flexion torque is much more easily obtained by the biarticular hamstring muscle, which is working under isometric or even active lengthening conditions. The hip extension torque produced by the hamstrings is also desirable because it helps to decelerate the forward velocity of the leg in preparation for placing the foot on the ground. The stiffened biarticular muscle acts like a strut to convey momentum from one body segment to another without itself doing much mechanical work.

B

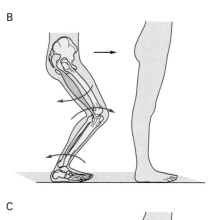

B-C. Muscles produce torques directly on the joints they cross (**red arrows**) but also cause widespread and sometimes counterintuitive accelerations at remote joints (**green arrows**). When standing still, the hip and ankle extensor muscles each cause similar changes in position at three joints (hip, knee, and ankle). The large rotational inertia of the trunk resists tilting backward, so the monoarticular hip extensors tend to pull the thigh into extension (**B**). The weight of the body keeps the foot from sliding backward, so the knee and ankle must extend, even though the hip muscle has no direct action on these joints. The ankle extensors affect acceleration of the knee and hip when the foot is planted on the ground because they can only pull the shank back, not plantarflex the foot down (**C**). If left on indefinitely, the hip, knee, and ankle extensors each would eventually result in different postural results, but the short-term accelerations are similar in their ability to keep the leg extended. When standing quietly, humans naturally rotate the activation of hip, knee, and ankle extensors to minimize fatigue.

C

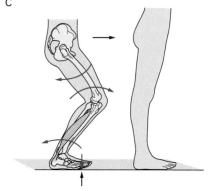

the ankle. However, when standing with the weight of the body on the foot, soleus contraction produces a backward rotation of the shank, which pulls the knee and hip joints into extension.

Contracting a muscle to accelerate one body segment causes mechanical effects that propagate backward and forward through the linkages of the skeleton. For example, if the elbow is flexed with the hand in the prone (palm down) position, the wrist and fingers will tend to lag behind and become flexed unless their extensor muscles are activated at the same time as the elbow flexors. Similarly, the trunk will also be thrown forward unless stiffened by contracting the axial and leg muscles.

While we may describe and plan movements in relatively simple terms (eg, "bend the elbow"), execution of movements by the motor systems must anticipate and correct for these and many other consequences of physical dynamics. In fact, the first muscles recruited when one tries to move the arm as quickly as possible are in the legs, despite their greater distance from the brain. The nervous system normally learns to program its muscle commands in this way through lengthy practice in infancy and early childhood. Nevertheless, changes in body mass and muscle strength throughout life require continuous adjustments in motor programs, and these in turn depend on a steady stream of sensory feedback from muscles that is provided by receptors in muscles and joints (Chapter 36).

An Overall View

The musculoskeletal system is the mechanical apparatus by which our nervous system interacts with the outside world. The mechanical properties of muscles have been largely conserved throughout vertebrate phylogeny and these properties have been a primary determinant in shaping and adapting the neural mechanisms of movement. For an engineer, muscles may appear to be highly imperfect transducers of electrical and chemical energy to mechanical energy. They respond quite slowly to variations in the frequency of action potentials reaching them, and the force they generate in response to neural input varies in a nonlinear fashion with their length, velocity, and activation history. Nevertheless, many of these properties help to make the musculoskeletal system mechanically robust and tolerant of computational noise and delays in the nervous system.

Motor performance improves as we learn to deal appropriately with the many perturbations of the musculoskeletal machinery that occur during skilled movement. These perturbations may be external, such as those produced by unpredictable loads or footing. They may also be internal, due to the nervous system itself; for example, membrane noise affects the recruitment of individual motor units, resulting in some unpredictability in the force produced by the muscles. When the brain decides on a motor program to perform a task it takes into account its stored experience with these various perturbations. It also weighs the importance of speed versus accuracy, the willingness to expend energy, and the ability to tolerate transmission delays in neural circuits.

The brain implements a motor program for limb movement by sending signals to the spinal cord. Some of the signals are transmitted directly to motor neurons, but most are relayed through a variety of interneurons. Most spinal interneurons also receive convergent input from many somatosensory modalities. In turn, they project directly and indirectly to many different motor nuclei. A single motor neuron is thus bombarded with synaptic inputs, and the net result determines whether it reaches threshold and hence whether the muscle fibers it controls will participate in a motor program.

Gerald E. Loeb
Claude Ghez

Selected Readings

Engel AG, Franzini-Armstrong C, eds. 1994. *Myology.* New York: McGraw-Hill.

Freund H-J. 1983. Motor unit and muscle activity in voluntary motor control. Physiol Rev 63:387–436.

Hill AV. 1970. *First and Last Experiments in Muscle Mechanics.* London: Cambridge Univ. Press.

Huxley AF. 1974. Review lecture: muscular contraction. J Physiol (Lond) 243:1–43.

Lieber RL. 1992. *Skeletal Muscle Structure and Function: Implications for Rehabilitation and Sports Medicine.* Baltimore: Williams & Wilkins.

Loeb GE, Gans C. 1986. *Electromyography for Experimentalists.* Chicago: Univ. Chicago Press.

McComas AJ. 1996. *Skeletal Muscle: Form and Function.* Champaign, IL: Human Kinetics.

Needham DM. 1971. *Machina Carnis. The Biochemistry of Muscular Contraction and Its Historical Development.* Cambridge, England: Cambridge Univ. Press.

Vrbova G. 1995. *Nerve-Muscle Interaction,* 2nd ed. New York: Chapman & Hall.

Zajac FE. 1990. Muscle and tendon: properties, models, scaling and application to biomechanics and motor control. CRC Crit Rev Biomed Eng 17:319–411.

References

Alexander RM, Bennet-Clark HC. 1977. Storage of elastic strain energy in muscle and other tissues. Nature 265:114–117.

Bloom W, Fawcett DW. 1975. *A Textbook of Histology,* 10th ed. Philadelphia: Saunders.

Brown IE, Satoda T, Richmond FJR, Loeb GE. 1998. Feline caudofemoralis muscle. Muscle fiber properties, architecture, and motor innervation. Exp Brain Res 121:76–91.

Brown IE, Scott SH, Loeb GE. 1996. Mechanics of feline soleus. II. Design and validation of a mathematical model. J Muscle Res Cell Motil 17:205–218.

Burke RE, Levine DN, Tsairis P, Zajac FE. 1973. Physiological types and histochemical profiles in motor units of the cat gastrocnemius. J Physiol (Lond) 234:723–748.

Burke RE, Rudomin P, Zajac FE III. 1976. The effect of activation history on tension production by individual muscle units. Brain Res 109:515–529.

Calancie B, Bawa P. 1990. Motor unit recruitment in humans. In: MD Binder, L Mendell (eds). *Orderly Recruitment of Motor Units,* pp. 75–95. New York: Oxford Univ. Press.

Catterall WA. 1991. Excitation-contraction coupling in vertebrate skeletal muscle: a tale of two calcium channels. Cell 64:871–874.

Desmedt JE, Godaux E. 1977. Ballistic contractions in man: characteristic recruitment pattern of single motor units of the tibialis anterior muscle. J Physiol (Lond) 264:673–693.

Feldman AG, Adamovich SV, Levin MF. 1995. The relationship between control, kinematic and electromyographic variables in fast single-joint movements in humans. Exp Brain Res 103:440–450.

Gans C, DeVree F. 1987. Functional bases of fiber length and angulation in muscle. J Morphol 192:63–85.

Gielen S, Schenau G, Tax T, Theeuwen M. 1990. The activation of mono- and bi-articular muscles in multi-joint movements. In: J Winters, S Woo (eds). *Multiple Muscle Systems: Biomechanics and Movement,* pp. 303–311. New York: Springer-Verlag.

Gordon AM, Huxley AF, Julian FJ. 1966. The variation in isometric tension with sarcomere length in vertebrate muscle fibres. J Physiol (Lond) 184:170–192.

He J, Levine WS, Loeb GE. 1991. Feedback gains for correcting small perturbations to standing posture. IEEE Trans Automat Contr 36:322–332.

Henneman E, Somjenand G, Carpenter DO. 1965. Functional significance of cell size in spinal motoneurons. J Neurophysiol 28:560–580.

Hill AV. 1938. The heat of shortening and the dynamic constants of muscle. Proc R Soc Lond B Biol Sci 126:136–195.

Hogan N. 1984. Adaptive control of mechanical impedance by coactivation of antagonist muscles. IEEE Trans Automat Contr 29:681–690.

Hogan N. 1985. The mechanics of multi-joint and movement control. Biol Cybern 52:315–331.

Horowits R, Kempnert ES, Bisher ME, Podolsky RJ. 1986. A physiological role for titin and nebulin in skeletal muscle. Nature 323:360–364.

Huxley HE. 1969. The mechanism of muscular contraction. Science 164:1356–1366.

Huxley AF, Simmons RM. 1971. Proposed mechanism of force generation in striated muscle. Nature 233:533–538.

Joyce GC, Rack PMH, Westbury DR. 1969. The mechanical properties of cat soleus muscle during controlled lengthening and shortening movements. J Physiol (Lond) 204:461–474.

Liddell EGT, Sherrington CS. 1925. Recruitment and some other factors of reflex inhibition. Proc R Soc Lond B Biol Sci 97:488–518.

Loeb GE. 1990. The functional organization of muscles, motor units, and tasks. In: MD Binder, LM Mendell (eds). *The Segmental Motor System,* pp. 23–35. New York: Oxford Univ. Press.

Magid A, Law DJ. 1985. Myofibrils bear most of the resting tension in frog skeletal muscle. Science 230:1280–1282.

Monster AW, Chan H. 1977. Isometric force production by motor units of extensor digitorum communis muscle in man. J Neurophysiol 40:1432–1443.

Romanes GJ. 1951. The motor cell columns of the lumbosacral spinal cord of the cat. J Comp Neurol 94:313–363.

Schutte LM, Rodgers M, Zajac FE, Glaser R. 1993. Improving the efficacy of electrical stimulation-induced leg cycle ergometry: an analysis based on a dynamic musculoskeletal model. IEEE Trans Rehab Eng 1:109–125.

Shadmehr R, Mussa-ivaldi FA, Bizzi E. 1993. Postural force fields of the human arm and their role in generating multi-joint movements. J Neurosci 13:45–62.

Sherrington CS. 1979. 1924 Linacre lecture. In: JC Eccles, WC Gibson (eds). *Sherrington: His Life and Thought,* p. 59. New York: Springer-Verlag.

Squire JM. 1983. Molecular mechanisms in muscular contraction. Trends Neurosci 6:409–413.

Trotter JA, Richmond FJR, Purslow PP. 1995. Functional morphology and motor control of series-fibered muscles. Exerc Sport Sci Rev 23:167–213.

Young RP, Scott SH, Loeb GE. 1993. The distal hindlimb musculature of the cat: multiaxis moment arms of the ankle joint. Exp Brain Res 96:141–151.

Zajac FE, Gordon ME. 1989. Determining muscle's force and action in multi-articular movement. Exerc Sport Sci Rev 17:187–230.

35

Diseases of the Motor Unit

I N 1925 CHARLES SHERRINGTON introduced the term *motor unit* to designate the basic unit of motor function—a motor neuron and the group of muscle fibers it innervates (Chapter 34). In this chapter we consider the disorders that affect the motor unit. In addition we describe the impact of molecular genetics in characterizing the genes that underly some muscular dystrophies.

The modern experimental analysis of disorders of the motor unit began in 1929 when Edgar Adrian and Deltev Bronk introduced electromyography, a technique for recording the action potentials from single motor units in human muscles. Electromyography now has a prominent role in the clinical diagnosis of diseases of the motor unit. Today, physiological techniques are combined with molecular genetic analysis to obtain a more detailed understanding of diseases of the motor unit.

Most diseases of the motor unit cause weakness and wasting of skeletal muscles. The distinguishing features of these diseases vary depending on which of the four functional components of the motor unit is primarily affected: the cell body of the motor neuron, its axon, the neuromuscular junction, or the muscle fibers it innervates. As we saw in Chapter 17, diseases were originally classified based on postmortem examination. When pathologists in the nineteenth century studied patients who had died of diseases characterized by progressive weakness and wasting of limb muscles, they found different morphological changes in patients with different symptoms or signs. Some patients had pronounced changes in nerve cell bodies or peripheral nerves but only minor changes in muscle fibers. These neurogenic diseases were then subdivided into those that primarily affect the nerve cell bodies (motor neuron diseases) and those that primarily affect the peripheral axons (peripheral neuropathies). Other patients had advanced degeneration of muscles, with little change in motor neurons or axons; these diseases were called myopathic diseases, or myopathies.

These pathological findings demonstrate two important features of neurological disease. First, some neurological diseases affect only sensory systems, others only motor systems. Second, a neurological disease may affect only one component of the neuron (for example, the axon rather than the cell body). Thus the functional distinctions among the different components of the neuron have important clinical implications.

Neurogenic and Myopathic Diseases Are Distinguished by Clinical and Laboratory Criteria

When a peripheral nerve is cut the muscles innervated by that nerve immediately become paralyzed and then waste progressively; tendon reflexes are lost immediately. Because the nerve carries sensory as well as motor fibers, sensation in the area innervated by the nerve is also lost. In neurogenic diseases the effects of denervation are similar but appear more slowly; that is, the muscles gradually become weak and wasted. The term *atrophy* (literally, lack of nourishment) refers to the wasting away of a once-normal muscle and, by historical usage, "atrophy" appears in the names of several diseases that are now thought to be neurogenic.

The main symptoms of myopathic diseases are due to weakness of skeletal muscle and often include difficulty in walking or lifting. Other, less common symptoms include inability of the muscle to relax *(myotonia)*, cramps, pain *(myalgia)*, or the appearance in the urine of the heme-containing protein that gives muscle its red color *(myoglobinuria)*. The *muscular dystrophies* are myopathies with special characteristics: The diseases are inherited; all symptoms are caused by weakness, the weakness becomes progressively more severe, and signs of degeneration and regeneration are seen histologically, with no evidence of abnormal mitochondria or abnormal accumulations of metabolic products.

Because both neurogenic and myopathic diseases are characterized by weakness of muscle, distinguishing them may be difficult. Classification and differential diagnosis of these diseases involve both clinical and laboratory criteria.

Clinical Criteria Help to Identify Neurogenic and Myopathic Conditions

In general, neurogenic and myopathic disorders tend to cause weakness in different areas: Distal limb weakness most often indicates a neurogenic disorder, and proximal limb weakness a myopathy. Because there are many exceptions to this generalization, however, location of weakness is not a reliable differential sign. Other signs, such as fasciculations, are reliable because they are found only in neurogenic diseases. *Fasciculations* are visible twitches of muscle that can be seen as flickers under the skin. They result from involuntary but synchronous contractions of all muscle fibers in a motor unit. For reasons that are not yet known, fasciculations are characteristic of slowly progressive diseases of the motor neuron itself and are rarely seen in peripheral neuropathies. *Fibrillations*, on the other hand, arise from spontaneous activity within single muscle fibers. They are not visible clinically and can be detected only by electromyography.

For diagnostic purposes, clinicians have found it useful to use the terms lower and upper motor neurons. *Lower motor neurons* are primary motor neurons of the spinal cord and brain stem that directly innervate skeletal muscles. *Upper motor neurons* are neurons that originate in higher regions of the brain, such as the motor cortex, and synapse on the lower motor neurons to convey descending commands for movement. Strictly speaking, upper motor neurons are not motor but *premotor* neurons, and therefore this terminology is no longer used by modern students of the motor system. However, since these premotor neurons affect motor output in such a fundamental way, their functional properties are often considered together with primary motor neurons in the spinal cord. Axons of upper, premotor, and motor neurons make up the corticospinal (pyramidal) tract. The distinction between lower and upper motor neurons is important clinically because diseases involving either class of neurons produce distinctive symptoms. Disorders of lower motor neurons result in atrophy, fasciculations, decreased muscle tone, and loss of tendon reflexes. Disorders of upper motor neurons and their axons result in spasticity, overactive tendon reflexes, and abnormal plantar extensor reflex (the Babinski sign).

Overactive tendon reflexes are evidence of disease of the upper motor neurons, whereas weak, wasted, and twitching muscles are evidence of disease of the lower motor neurons. The concurrence of these apparently incompatible signs in the same limb is virtually diagnostic of *amyotrophic lateral sclerosis* (Lou Gehrig disease), a condition that involves both the upper and lower motor

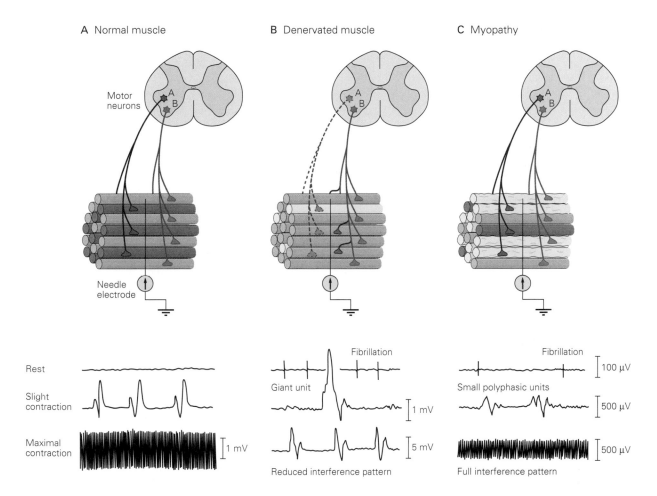

Figure 35-1 Neurogenic and myopathic diseases have different effects on the motor unit.

A. Typical activity in a normal muscle. The muscle fibers innervated by a single motor neuron are not usually adjacent to one another. When a motor unit potential is recorded by a needle electrode inserted into the muscle, the highly effective transmission at the neuromuscular junction ensures that each muscle fiber innervated by the same neuron will contract in response to an action potential.

B. When motor neurons are diseased the number of motor units under voluntary control is reduced. The muscle fibers supplied by the degenerating motor neuron (**cell B**) become denervated and atrophic. However, the surviving neuron (**cell A**) has sprouted an axonal branch that has reinnervated one of the denervated muscle fibers. The electromyogram shows larger

than normal motor unit potentials (**middle trace**) because the surviving motor neuron innervates more than the usual number of muscle fibers (it also innervates formerly denervated fibers). Denervated muscle fibers fire spontaneously even at rest, giving rise to fibrillations (top trace), another characteristic of motor neuron disease. Axons of the surviving motor neurons may also fire spontaneously at rest, giving rise to irregularly occurring motor unit discharges known as fasciculations. Under conditions of maximal contraction the interference pattern is reduced (**lower trace**).

C. When muscle is diseased the number of muscle fibers in each motor unit is reduced. Some muscle fibers innervated by the two motor neurons shrink and become nonfunctional. In the electromyogram the motor unit potentials do not decrease in number but are smaller and of shorter duration than normal.

neurons, as we shall discuss below. When the sole manifestation of a disease is limb weakness (with no fasciculation or upper motor neuron signs), clinical criteria may not be sufficient to distinguish neurogenic and myopathic diseases. To assist in this differentiation, clinicians rely on several laboratory tests: measurement of muscle enzyme activity in serum, electromyography and nerve conduction studies, muscle biopsy, and DNA analysis.

Laboratory Criteria Also Assist in Making the Diagnosis

One test that helps to distinguish myopathic from neurogenic diseases is the measurement of serum enzyme activities. The sarcoplasm of muscle is rich in soluble enzymes that are also found in low concentrations in the serum. In many muscle diseases the concentration of these sarcoplasmic enzymes in serum is elevated, presumably because the diseases affect the integrity of sur-

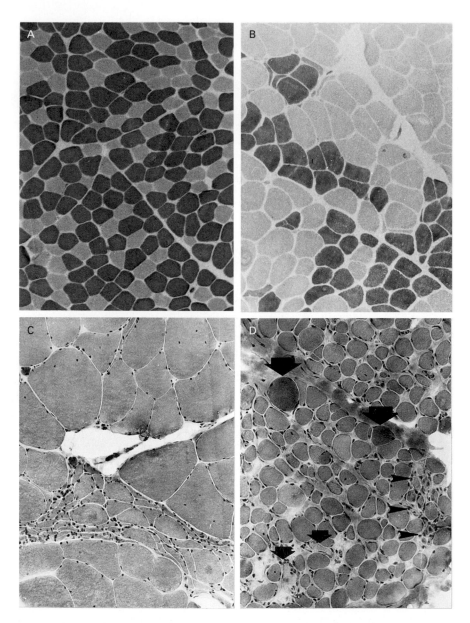

Figure 35-2 Muscle histochemistry helps to distinguish neurogenic and myopathic diseases because the histochemical properties of a muscle are determined by the motor neuron that innervates the muscle. (Courtesy of A. P. Hays.)

A. The two types of muscle fibers (types I and II) are normally roughly equal in number and distributed in a random fashion, as seen in this gastrocnemius muscle from a normal adult. With the myosin ATPase stain at pH 9.4 after incubation, the type I fibers (with predominantly oxidative enzymes) are light and the type II fibers (predominantly glycolytic) are dark. The fiber types are roughly equal in number and are distributed in more or less random fashion, as seen in this gastrocnemius muscle from a normal person. (Stain: myofibrillar [myosin] ATPase, preincubation at pH 9.4, ×100.)

B. In this gastrocnemius muscle from a patient with a chronic sensorimotor polyneuropathy the two types of muscle fibers are no longer distributed randomly but tend to cluster with

other fibers of the same histochemical type (known as fiber-type grouping). Neighboring muscle fibers have assumed uniform histochemical and physiological properties because axon sprouts from surviving motor units have innervated the denervated muscle fibers. (Stain: myofibrillar ATPase, preincubation at pH 9.4, ×100.)

C. In this gastrocnemius muscle from another patient with a chronic sensorimotor polyneuropathy a large concentrated group of muscle fibers has atrophied (middle) and is surrounded by fibers that are normal in size or hypertrophied. This so-called group atrophy is characteristic of disorders of lower motor neurons. (Modified Gomori trichrome, × 60.)

D. In this vastus lateralis muscle from a 4-year-old boy with Duchenne muscular dystrophy the diffuse character of the damage to muscle fibers is evident in the hypercontracted (hyaline) fibers (**large arrows**) and necrotic fibers (**small arrows**). The **arrowheads** indicate muscle fibers with cytological signs of regeneration. (Modified Gomori trichrome, × 60.)

face membranes of the muscle that ordinarily keep soluble enzymes within the sarcoplasm. Slight increases in the serum levels of these enzymes are also found in some denervating diseases, but the level of the increase is usually much less than in a myopathy. The enzyme activity most commonly used for diagnosing myopathy is creatine kinase (CK), an enzyme that phosphorylates creatine and is important in the energy metabolism of muscle. Assays for serum glutamic-oxaloacetictransaminase (SGOT) and lactate dehydrogenase (LDH) are also used.

Some abnormalities can be diagnosed by *electromyography*, a routine clinical procedure in which a small needle is inserted into a muscle to record the electrical activity of several neighboring motor units. Three specific measurements are important: spontaneous activity at rest, the number of motor units under voluntary control, and the duration and amplitude of action potentials in each motor unit. In normal muscle there is usually no activity outside the end-plate in the muscle at rest. During a weak voluntary contraction a series of motor unit potentials is recorded as different motor units become recruited. In fully active normal muscles these potentials overlap in an interference pattern so that it is impossible to identify single potentials (Figure 35-1A). Normal values have been established for the amplitude and duration of motor unit potentials. The amplitude of the motor unit potential is determined by the number of muscle fibers within the motor unit.

In neurogenic disease the denervated muscle is spontaneously active even at rest. The muscle may still contract in response to voluntary motor commands, but because some motor axons have been lost the number of motor units under voluntary control is smaller than normal. The loss of motor units is evident in electromyogram (EMG) records, which show a discrete pattern of motor unit potentials instead of the profuse interference pattern seen in normal muscles (Figure 35-1B). However, the amplitude and duration of individual motor unit potentials may increase, presumably because the remaining axons give off small branches that innervate the muscle fibers denervated by the loss of other axons. Accordingly, surviving motor units contain more than the normal number of muscle fibers.

In myopathic diseases there is no activity in the muscle at rest and no change in the number of motor units firing during a contraction. But because there are fewer surviving muscle fibers in each motor unit, the motor unit potentials are of shorter duration and smaller in amplitude (Figure 35-1C).

The *conduction velocities* of peripheral motor axons can also be measured through electrical stimulation and recording. The conduction velocity of motor axons is slowed in demyelinating neuropathies, as we shall see later, but is normal in neuropathies without demyelination (axonal neuropathies).

In human muscles there are no fast- or slow-twitch fibers; the fibers are identified by histochemical reactions as type I or type II. A muscle biopsy can be examined under the microscope. The predominant metabolic enzymes present in type I are oxidative. In type II the dominant enzymes are anaerobic (glycolytic) (see Chapter 34).

Prolonged stimulation of a single motor axon can deplete the glycogen of type II (glycolytic) muscle fibers. Histochemical stains for glycogen would then show which fibers lacked the substrate and were therefore innervated by that axon and thus define the distribution of muscle fibers within that motor unit. Experiments using this technique indicate that all of the muscle fibers innervated by a single motor neuron are of the same histochemical type. The histochemical type is determined by the neuron; sometimes histochemical types can be reversed by experimental cross-innervation.

The muscle fibers of one motor unit are interspersed among the muscle fibers of other motor units. This is easily seen in a cross-section of normal muscle; when an enzyme stain selective for only one type is used, the stained and unstained fibers alternate in an irregular "checkerboard" pattern (Figure 35-2A).

In chronic neurogenic diseases the muscle innervated by a dying motor neuron becomes atrophic and some muscle fibers disappear. Axons of surviving neurons tend to sprout and innervate some of the remaining muscle fibers that are denervated when neurons die. Because the motor neuron determines the histochemical type, the reinnervated muscle fibers assume the histochemical properties of the innervating neuron. As a result, the fibers of a muscle in neurogenic disease become clustered by type (a pattern called *fiber-type grouping*) (Figure 35-2B). If the disease is progressive and the neurons in the surviving motor units also become affected, atrophy occurs in groups of adjacent muscle fibers belonging to the same histochemical type, a process called *group atrophy* (Figure 35-2C). In contrast, the muscle fibers in myopathic diseases are affected in a more or less random fashion. Sometimes an inflammatory cellular response is evident and sometimes there is prominent infiltration of the muscle by fat and connective tissue (Figure 35-2D).

The main clinical and laboratory features used for the differential diagnosis of diseases of the motor unit are listed in Table 35-1. Some of the major neurogenic and myopathic diseases of the motor unit are listed in Table 35-2. We shall consider in turn diseases that affect motor neurons, peripheral nerves, and skeletal muscle.

Table 35-1 Differential Diagnosis of Neurogenic and Myopathic Diseases of the Motor Unit

Finding	Neurogenic disease[1]	Myopathic disease[2]
Clinical Findings		
Weakness	+ +	+ +
Wasting	+	+
Loss of reflexes	+ (ALS)	0
Fasciculations	+ (PN)	0
Sensory loss	+ (PN)	0
Hyperreflexia, Babinski sign	+ (ALS)	0
Laboratory Findings		
Cerebrospinal fluid protein increased	+ (PN)	0
Slow nerve conduction velocity	+ (PN)	0
Electromyography		
Duration of potentials	Increased	Decreased
Fibrillation, fasciculation	+	0
Number of potentials	Decreased	Normal
Serum enzymes increased	±	+ + + +
Muscle biopsy	Group atrophy, fiber-type grouping	Necrosis and regeneration

[1]ALS = amyotrophic lateral sclerosis; PN = peripheral neuropathy; + + = prominent, + = present; ± = slight change.

[2]+ + = prominent, + = present; 0 = absent; + + + + = marked change.

Diseases of Motor Neurons Are Acute or Chronic

Motor Neuron Diseases Do Not Affect Sensory Neurons

The best-known disorder of motor neurons is amyotrophic lateral sclerosis (Lou Gehrig disease). "Amyotrophy" is another word for neurogenic atrophy of muscle; "lateral sclerosis" refers to the hardness felt when the pathologist examines the spinal cord at autopsy. This hardness results from the proliferation of astrocytes and scarring of the lateral columns of the spinal cord. Scarring is caused by disease of the corticospinal tracts, which carry the axons of premotor cells from the cortex and brain stem to the spinal cord. Although the premotor neurons in the cortex and in the brain stem and spinal cord degenerate progressively, some are spared, notably those supplying ocular muscles and those involved in voluntary control of bladder sphincters.

Symptoms usually start with painless weakness of the arms or legs. Typically the patient, often a man in his 60s, discovers that he has become awkward in executing fine movements of the hands: typing, playing the piano, playing baseball, fingering coins, or working with tools.

This weakness is associated with wasting of the small muscles of the hands and feet and fasciculations of the muscles of the forearm and upper arm. These signs of lower motor neuron disease are often paradoxically associated with *hyperreflexia,* an increase in tendon reflexes that is characteristic of upper motor neuron disease. The cause of amyotrophic lateral sclerosis is not known; it is progressive and may ultimately affect muscles of respiration. There is no effective treatment for this invariably fatal condition.

There are other variants of motor neuron disease—the first symptoms may be restricted to muscles innervated by cranial nerves, with resulting *dysarthria* (difficulty speaking) and *dysphagia* (difficulty swallowing). When cranial symptoms occur alone, the syndrome is called *progressive bulbar palsy* (the term *bulb* is used interchangeably with *medulla,* and *palsy* means weakness). If only lower motor neurons are involved, the syndrome is called progressive *spinal muscular atrophy.*

Spinal muscular atrophy is characterized by weakness, wasting, loss of reflexes, and fasciculation. Although hyperreflexia and other signs of disease of the upper motor neurons are lacking, autopsy usually reveals some degeneration of the myelin sheath of axons in the corticospinal tracts. That is, even though the clinical signs are solely those of the lower motor neuron, the corticospinal tracts are affected in addition to the anterior horn cells. Thus, adult-onset spinal muscular atrophy is probably the same disease as amyotrophic lateral sclerosis. The degeneration of the lower motor neurons in spinal muscular atrophy presumably obscures clinical expression of upper motor neuron signs. (If the extensor of the great toe is paralyzed, it is impossible to elicit the abnormal extensor Babinski sign. Similarly, if tendon reflexes have been lost in spinal muscular atrophy, there cannot be hyperreflexia.)

Amyotrophic lateral sclerosis and its variants are restricted to motor neurons; they do not affect sensory neurons or autonomic neurons. The acute viral disease poliomyelitis is also confined to motor neurons. These diseases illustrate dramatically the individuality of nerve cells and the principle of *selective vulnerability*. The basis of this selectivity is not understood.

Motor Neuron Disease Is Characterized by Fasciculation and Fibrillation

Diseases of the motor neuron lead to two types of spontaneous activity in muscle: fasciculation (visible twitches) and fibrillation (invisible twitches). The cause of fasciculation is not known. The EMG record of a fasciculation is a compound motor unit potential, and these electrical changes may also be seen in disorders of nerve roots or peripheral nerves. In all of these conditions the electrical activity may persist after a nerve has been blocked by injection of a local anesthetic or even after cutting the nerve.

Since nerve block eliminates all activity that originates central to the site of injection (the spinal cord, dorsal and ventral roots, and proximal nerve), continued spontaneous muscle activity must arise distal to the block—in the remote axon just before it branches, in the terminals, or at the neuromuscular junction. Acetyl-

choline (ACh) is thought to be involved in fasciculations because the activity can be abolished by *d*-tubocurarine and because neostigmine (an inhibitor of cholinesterase) can induce fasciculation in a normal mammalian nerve-muscle preparation.

Whereas fasciculations involve activation of an entire motor unit and therefore produce visible twitching of the skin, invisible fibrillations result from the discharge of a single muscle fiber. In some circumstances fibrillations are thought to result from the insertion of new voltage-dependent Na^+ and Ca^{2+} channels into the plasma membranes of denervated muscle fibers. These new channels make the fiber spontaneously active, much like the action of pacemaker cells of the heart. The appearance of new voltage-gated channels cannot be the entire explanation, however, because fibrillations are increased by intra-arterial injection of ACh or epinephrine, suggesting that transmitter-gated channels may also be involved.

Diseases of Peripheral Nerves Are Also Acute or Chronic

Because motor and sensory axons run in the same nerves, disorders of peripheral nerves (neuropathies) usually affect both motor and sensory functions. Some patients with peripheral neuropathy report abnormal, frequently unpleasant, sensory experiences similar to the sensations felt after local anesthesia for dental work; these sensations are variously called numbness, pins-and-needles, or tingling. When these sensations occur spontaneously without an external sensory stimulus, they are called *paresthesias*.

Patients with paresthesias usually have impaired perception of cutaneous sensations (pain and tempera-

Table 35-2 Examples of Neurogenic and Myopathic Diseases of the Motor Unit

Neurogenic diseases		Myopathic diseases	
Motor neuron	Peripheral nerve	Inherited	Acquired
Amyotrophic lateral sclerosis	Guillain-Barré syndrome	Duchenne muscular dystrophy	Dermatomyositis
		Facioscapulohumeral dystrophy	Polymyositis syndrome
	Chronic peripheral neuropathy	Limb-girdle muscular dystrophy	Endocrine myopathies
		Myotonic dystrophy	Myoglobinurias

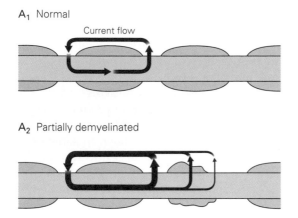

Figure 35-3 In demyelinated nerve fibers conduction is impaired.

A. The demyelinated region of a nerve fiber does not conduct an impulse as well as the normal, myelinated region. Current flow is indicated by the **purple arrow. 1.** In normal, myelinated regions the high resistance and low capacitance of the myelin shunts most of the current from one node of Ranvier to the next. **2.** In a demyelinated region current is lost through the membrane. (Adapted from Waxman 1982.)

B. The densities of Na$^+$ channels and K$^+$ channels differ in the normal (myelinated) and demyelinated regions of the axons. **1.** Sodium channels are dense at the node of Ranvier but sparse or absent in the internodal regions of the axon membrane. The K$^+$ channels are located beneath the myelin sheath in internodal regions. **2.** The conduction properties of the nodal regions of the axon membrane and the internodal regions are therefore different.

ture) because the small myelinated fibers that carry these sensations are selectively affected; the sense of touch may or may not be involved. Proprioceptive sensations (position and vibration) may be lost without loss of cutaneous sensation. Lack of pain perception may lead to injuries. The sensory disorders are always more prominent distally (called a glove-and-stocking pattern), possibly because the distal portions of the nerves are most remote from the cell body and therefore most susceptible to disorders that interfere with axonal transport of essential metabolites and proteins.

The motor disorder of peripheral neuropathy is first manifested by weakness, which may be predominantly proximal in acute cases and is usually distal in chronic disorders. Tendon reflexes are usually depressed or lost. Fasciculation is only rarely seen, and wasting does not ensue unless the weakness has been present for many weeks. The protein content of the cerebrospinal fluid is often increased, presumably because the permeability of the nerve roots within the subarachnoid space of the spinal cord is altered to enhance entry of protein from the blood or to impede absorption of protein from the cerebrospinal fluid.

Neuropathies may be either acute or chronic. The best-known acute neuropathy is the Guillain-Barré syndrome. Most cases follow respiratory infection, but the syndrome may occur without preceding illness. The condition may be mild or so severe that mechanical ven-

tilation is required. Cranial nerves may be affected, leading to paralysis of ocular, facial, and oropharyngeal muscles. The disorder is attributed to an autoimmune attack on peripheral nerves by circulating antibodies. It is therefore treated with plasmapheresis. Even when the condition is so severe as to seem life-threatening, some improvement occurs in all who survive, and no matter how severe the original state, a return to normal function is often possible. Many patients, however, are left with some disability.

The chronic neuropathies also vary from the mildest manifestations to incapacitating or even fatal conditions. There are many varieties, including genetic diseases (acute intermittent porphyria, Charcot-Marie-Tooth disease), metabolic disorders (diabetes, B$_{12}$ deficiency), intoxication (lead), nutritional disorders (alcoholism, thiamine deficiency), carcinomas (especially carcinoma of the lung), and immunological disorders (plasma cell diseases, amyloidosis). Some chronic disorders, such as the neuropathy of B$_{12}$ deficiency in pernicious anemia, are amenable to therapy.

In addition to being acute or chronic, neuropathies may be categorized as *demyelinating* (in which the myelin sheath breaks down) or *axonal* (in which the axon is affected). Demyelinating neuropathies are probably more common. As might be expected from the role of the myelin sheath in saltatory conduction, the velocity of conduction is slow in axons that have lost myelin

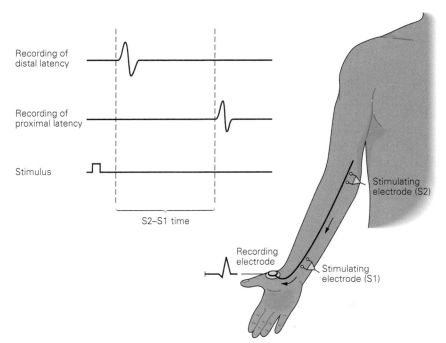

Figure 35-4 Motor nerve conduction velocity can be determined by recording action potentials with two transcutaneous or surface electrodes along the pathway of the motor nerve. The time from S2 to the muscle is the proximal latency; the time from S1 to the muscle is the distal latency. The time from S2 to S1 is divided into the distance between S1 and S2 to give the conduction velocity.

(as discussed below). In axonal neuropathies the myelin sheath is not affected and conduction velocity is normal.

Neuropathies Can Cause Positive or Negative Signs and Symptoms

Axonal and demyelinating neuropathies may lead to positive or negative symptoms. The negative signs consist of weakness or paralysis, loss of tendon reflexes, and impaired sensation, resulting from damage to motor axons. The positive symptoms of peripheral neuropathies consist of paresthesias that arise from abnormal impulse activity in sensory fibers, and either spontaneous activity of injured nerve fibers or electrical interaction (cross-talk) between abnormal axons, a process called *ephaptic transmission* to distinguish it from normal synaptic transmission. For reasons not known, damaged nerves also become hyperexcitable. This is evident in the Tinel sign, named after a French neurologist who studied nerve injuries in World War I. Tinel found that lightly tapping the site of injury evoked a burst of unpleasant sensations in the region over which the nerve is distributed. This sign is useful for both showing peripheral nerve damage and pinpointing the site of the lesion.

Demyelination Leads to a Slowing of Conduction Velocity

Negative symptoms have been studied most thoroughly and can be attributed to three basic mechanisms:

conduction block, slowed conduction, and impaired ability to conduct impulses at higher frequencies.

Conduction block was first recognized in 1876 by the German neurologist Wilhelm Erb, one of the first clinicians to study human nerves with electrical methods. Erb observed that stimulation of an injured peripheral nerve below the site of injury evoked a muscle response, whereas stimulation above the site of injury produced no response. He concluded that the lesion blocked impulses of central origin, even when the segment of the nerve distal to the lesion was still functional. Later experimental studies showed that diphtheria and other toxins produce conduction block by causing demyelination at the site of application.

Why does demyelination produce nerve block and how does it lead to slowing of conduction velocity? As discussed in Chapters 4 and 7, conduction velocity is much more rapid in myelinated fibers than in unmyelinated axons for two reasons. First, there is a direct relationship between conduction velocity and axon diameter, and the axons of myelinated fibers tend to be larger in diameter. Second, although in myelinated axons the action potential undergoes regeneration at regular but short patches of unmyelinated axon (the nodes of Ranvier), propagation along longer stretches of unmyelinated axon attenuates the action potential (Figure 35-3; and see Chapter 38).

When myelination along the axon is disrupted by disease, the action potentials in different axons of the nerve begin to conduct at slightly different velocities, and the nerve loses its normal synchrony of conduction in response to a single stimulus. (Figure 35-4 shows the arrangement for measuring conduction velocities in peripheral nerves.) This slowing and the temporal dispersion are thought to account for some of the early clinical signs of neuropathy. For example, functions that normally depend on the arrival of synchronous bursts of neural activity, such as tendon reflexes and vibratory sensation, are lost soon after the onset of a chronic neuropathy. As demyelination becomes more severe, conduction becomes blocked. This block may be intermittent, occurring only at high frequencies of neural firing, or complete.

Diseases of Skeletal Muscle Can Be Inherited or Acquired

Skeletal muscle diseases are conveniently divided into those that are inherited and those that appear to be acquired.

Muscular Dystrophies Are the Most Common Inherited Myopathies

The best-known inherited diseases are the muscular dystrophies, of which there are four major types based on clinical and genetic patterns (Table 35-3). Two types are characterized by weakness alone: the Duchenne and facioscapulohumeral dystrophies. Duchenne muscular dystrophy starts in the legs, affects males only (because it is transmitted as an X-linked recessive trait), and progresses relatively rapidly, so that patients are in wheelchairs by age 12 and usually die in their third decade. As discussed below, Duchenne muscular dystrophy results from a genetic defect in a membrane-associated muscle protein. Facioscapulohumeral muscular dystrophy is autosomal dominant, affects both sexes equally, starts later (usually in adolescence), affects the shoulder girdle and face early, and may be much milder, resulting in an almost normal life span. These clinical and genetic differences imply different biochemical abnormalities, which have been identified.

The third type of inherited muscular dystrophy also causes weakness but has an additional and characteristic feature, myotonia, and is therefore called myotonic muscular dystrophy. Myotonia is manifest as a delayed relaxation of muscle after vigorous voluntary contraction, percussion, or electrical stimulation. The delayed relaxation is caused by repetitive firing of muscle action potentials and is independent of nerve supply because it persists after nerve block or curarization. In addition to myotonia, the dystrophy has other special characteristics: It involves cranial muscles, and the limb weakness is primarily distal rather than proximal. The symptoms are not confined to muscles; for instance, almost all patients have cataracts and affected men commonly have testicular atrophy and baldness.

Myotonic muscular dystrophy is an example of a group of seven neurodegenerative diseases in which the genetic defect has been identified as an excessive length of repeating units of three nucleotides: CAG, CTG, or CCG. As we have seen in Chapter 3, small tandem repeats of 6–30 triplets do occur normally, but when a disease is present the repeat expands to 35–40 or more. There are two types of triplet repeat diseases. The first is caused by a repeat of CAGs *within* the open reading frame that encodes polyglutamine. An example of this type is Huntington disease (Chapters 3 and 43). Myotonic dystrophy belongs to the second type of triplet repeat disorders, in which CCGs or CTGs are repeated *outside* the open reading frame. Myotonic dystrophy is linked to a gene located in the central region of chromosome 19 that encodes myotonin protein kinase; more than 200 repeated CTGs lie in the 3′-untranslated portion of the mRNA.

A property of these triplet repeats is the formation of a hairpin structure in the DNA that contains them (Chapter 3). The ability to form these rigid structures is thought to be the basis of the expansion of the triplet repeat region from generation to generation, since the longer the repeat domain the more stable is the hairpin structure. This amplification causes the symptoms of the diseases to occur at an earlier age (*anticipation*) and in more severe form (*potentiation*).

Forms of inherited muscular dystrophy that do not fit these three major types are lumped into a fourth group, *limb-girdle muscular dystrophy*. This category certainly includes more than one type because affected families differ in the extent of limb weakness, age at onset, and patterns of inheritance. Some forms of limb-girdle muscular dystrophy have been mapped to specific gene loci, as discussed later. A Tunisian autosomal recessive form maps to chromosome 13q. Another recessive form maps to chromosome 15, and autosomal dominant forms map to chromosomes 2p and 5q.

Dermatomyositis Exemplifies Acquired Myopathy

The prototype of an acquired myopathy is *dermatomyositis*, defined by two clinical features: rash and myopathy. The rash has a predilection for the face, chest, and extensor surfaces of joints, including the fingers. The myopathic weakness primarily affects proximal limb muscles. Both rash and weakness usually appear simultaneously and become worse in a matter of weeks. The

Table 35-3 Four Major Forms of Muscular Dystrophy

	Duchenne	Facioscapulohumeral	Myotonic	Limb-girdle
Sex	Male	Both	Both	Both
Onset	Before age 5	Adolescence	Infancy or adolescence	Adolescence
Initial symptoms	Pelvic	Shoulder girdle	Hands or feet	Either
Face involved	No	Always	Often	No
Pseudohypertrophy	80% of patients	No	No	Rare
Progression	Rapid	Slow	Slow	Slow
Inheritance	X-linked recessive	Autosomal dominant	Autosomal dominant	Autosomal recessive
Serum enzymes	Very high	Normal	Normal	Slight increase
Myotonia	No	No	Yes	No

weakness may be mild or life-threatening, and the disorder affects children or adults. About 10% of adult patients have malignant tumors. Although the pathogenesis is also not known, dermatomyositis is thought to be an autoimmune disorder of small intramuscular blood vessels microvasculopathy.

Another inflammatory myopathy is *polymyositis*, which is also manifest primarily by proximal limb weakness but lacks the characteristic rash. Polymyositis differs from dermatomyositis histologically; it lacks the vascular pathology and shows infiltration of muscle by T and B lymphocytes.

Weakness in Myopathies Need Not Be Due to Loss of Muscle Fibers

The weakness seen in any myopathy is attributed to degeneration of muscle fibers. At first the missing fibers are replaced by regeneration of new fibers. Ultimately, however, renewal cannot keep pace and fibers are lost progressively. This leads to the appearance of compound motor unit potentials of brief duration and reduced amplitude. The decreased number of functioning muscle fibers would then account for the diminished strength.

There may be other contributing factors. For instance, in one form of inherited myopathy, the glycogen storage diseases, large amounts of the polysaccharide accumulate within skeletal muscle cells because breakdown of the complex by glycolysis is blocked due to lack of phosphorylase or phosphofructokinase. Glycogen accumulation disrupts the normal architecture of many muscle fibers; at the ultrastructural level there is major distortion of the myofilaments.

Molecular Genetics Has Illuminated the Physiology and Pathology of Neurogenic and Myopathic Diseases

The first success of the DNA technique called *positional cloning*—now used extensively in mapping gene loci for human diseases—was achieved in the study of two X-linked diseases: *Duchenne muscular dystrophy* and *chronic granulomatous disease*, a disease of polymorphonuclear white blood cells. This advance came from the search for the gene involved in Duchenne muscular dystrophy.

Duchenne muscular dystrophy was recognized to be X-linked because the associated gene is carried by women but symptoms appear only in boys. A myopathy similar to Duchenne muscular dystrophy occurs in young girls; chromosomal translocations of the second band on the short arm of the X chromosome moved the dislocated distal fragment to an autosome. In all cases the breakpoint involved the band called Xp21. That breakpoint pattern implicated Xp21 as a likely site of the gene for Duchenne muscular dystrophy.

As we have seen in Chapter 3 (Box 3-4), it is possible to map the genes responsible for human diseases by mapping DNA polymorphisms called *restriction fragment length polymorphisms*. Kay Davies and her colleagues used this approach to map the gene for Duchenne muscular dystrophy. They found restriction fragment length polymorphisms that were linked to

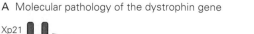

A Molecular pathology of the dystrophin gene

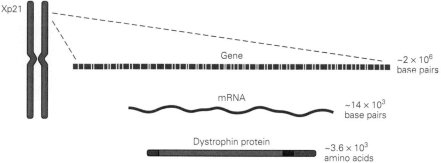

B₁ Deletion resulting in severe (Duchenne) dystrophy

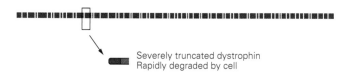

B₂ Deletion resulting in milder (Becker) dystrophy

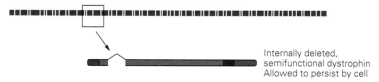

Figure 35-5 A specific deletion mutation in the dystrophin gene can result in different symptoms, depending on its effect on the translational reading frame. (After Hoffman and Kunkel 1989.)

A. The drawing on the left shows the relative position of the dystrophin gene within the Xp21 region of the X chromosome. An enlargement of this locus shows the 65 exons (**white lines**) defining the gene with about 2.0×10^6 base pairs. Transcription of the gene gives rise to mRNA (about 14×10^3 base pairs), and translation of this mRNA gives rise to the protein dystrophin (mol wt 427,000).

B. Two similar deletions can show dramatically different clinical phenotypes. A deletion of genomic DNA encompassing only a single exon results in the clinically severe Duchenne muscular dystrophy. A larger deletion encompassing four exons results in the clinically milder Becker muscular dystrophy. In both cases

the gene is transcribed into mRNA and the exons flanking the deletion are brought together. **1.** If a single exon is deleted and a nonintegral set of codons is missing, the borders of neighboring exons may not match, causing the translational reading frame to shift. As a result, incorrect amino acids are inserted into the growing polypeptide chain until a stop codon is reached, causing premature termination of the protein. The truncated protein may be unstable, may fail to be localized in the membrane, or fail to bind to glycoproteins. Dystrophin is then almost totally absent and the clinical disorder is severe Duchenne muscular dystrophy. **2.** If the deletion is larger but an integral number of codons are deleted, the reading frame can be maintained in the mRNA. This produces a dystrophin molecule with an internal deletion but intact ends. Although the protein is smaller than normal and may be present in less than normal amounts, it would suffice to preserve some muscle function. The resulting myopathy would be Becker muscular dystrophy.

clinical manifestations of the disease and flanked the p21 region of the X chromosome.

A major breakthrough came when a large deletion of the region around Xp21 was identified in a patient with five different X-linked conditions: Duchenne muscular dystrophy, retinitis pigmentosa, mental retardation, an unusual abnormality of blood groups called the McLeod

syndrome, and chronic granulomatous disease. Louis Kunkel and his associates reasoned that the missing area of the X-chromosome must contain the Duchenne gene. By the end of 1987, using specific probes, researchers identified deletions of that area in the DNA of boys with Duchenne muscular dystrophy, and the probes were used to identify and then clone the entire gene.

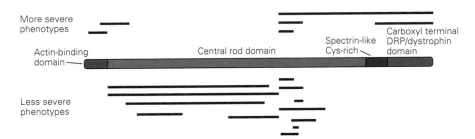

Figure 35-6 The location of a deletion in the dystrophin gene influences the severity of muscular dystrophy. The diagram shows the four domains of the dystrophin protein and the locations of gene deletions (**black bars**) found in patients with Duchenne or Becker muscular dystrophy. The deletions leading to the more severe phenotypes (**above**) were found in both patients with the severe Becker muscular dystrophy (wheelchair-bound before age 20) and those with Duchenne muscular dys-

trophy (wheelchair-bound by age 11). The deletions leading to less severe phenotypes (**below**) were found only in patients with mild to moderate Becker muscular dystrophy (wheelchair-bound after age 20). The deletions at either end of the gene are associated with the more severe forms of muscular dystrophy, while those in the central rod region are associated with less severe symptoms. (From Hoffman 1993.)

The Membrane Protein Dystrophin Is Lacking in Duchenne Muscular Dystrophy

The Duchenne gene is the second largest human gene so far characterized (the largest encodes titin, the protein that spans the length of half a sarcomere). It is about 2.5 million base pairs in length and accounts for 1% of the X chromosome and 0.1% of the total human genome. It contains at least 79 exons that encode a 14 kilobase mRNA. The inferred amino acid sequence of the previously unknown protein, named dystrophin, suggests a rod-like structure and a molecular weight of 427,000, with domains similar to those of two cytoskeletal proteins, α-actinin and spectrin. Antibody studies placed dystrophin on the inner surface of the plasma membrane. The amino terminus of dystrophin is linked to cytoskeletal actin, while the carboxy terminal is linked to the sarcolemma.

Boys with Duchenne muscular dystrophy lack dystrophin (or have less than 5% of the normal amount). In Becker muscular dystrophy the protein is present but is either shorter than normal or present in less than the normal amount. About 70% of all boys with Duchenne muscular dystrophy have a deletion that can be detected with cDNA probes. The specificity of these deletions has been used to practical advantage. In the cases with deletions prenatal diagnosis is relatively simple and rapid. In the cases with no detectable deletion indirect diagnosis is possible using a series of probes for the Xp21 region, defining a consistent pattern called a *haplotype*. The haplotype can be used to identify carriers of the gene and determine whether a fetus is affected.

Alteration of the same gene can result in different diseases. Seemingly identical deletions are seen in some patients with Duchenne muscular dystrophy and others

with the Becker form. Thus, the difference in symptoms depends on the effect of the deletion on the reading frame. If the deletion removes a multiple of three coding nucleotides, the deletion is "in-frame" and the smaller-than-normal mRNA is translated to form a protein lacking only the amino acids encoded by the missing nucleotides (Figure 35-5). The resulting gene product will therefore be shorter than normal but may still be functional; this condition produces the milder Becker form of muscular dystrophy. If the missing peptides are required for full function, that would explain why there are any symptoms at all.

The location of the deletion within the gene also influences the severity of the muscular dystrophy. In general, the more severe forms of Becker muscular dystrophy are associated with mutations at either end of the dystrophin gene, while less severe symptoms occur when the central rod region is affected (Figure 35-6).

Dystrophin-Normal Muscular Dystrophy and Limb-Girdle Muscular Dystrophy Are Associated With Mutations of Genes for Sarcoglycans

The discovery of the affected gene product in Duchenne muscular dystrophy was rapidly followed by advances in the cell biology of muscle and, simultaneously, in the analysis of other muscular dystrophies. As a result of this dual approach, Kevin Campbell and others discovered new proteins that helped to explain the role of dystrophin in normal muscle and, in the process, elucidated the molecular structure of muscle.

The information was gained in large part by mapping the genes responsible for dystrophin-normal mus-

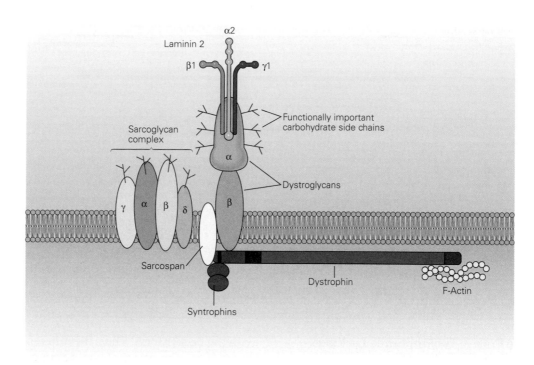

Figure 35-7 Proteins of the cytoskeleton of the muscle surface membrane. Dystrophin is anchored to actin on the cytoplasmic side of the plasma membrane of the muscle cell. Syntrophin links dystrophin to the extracellular dystroglycans, which in turn connect to merosin. The four sarcoglycans are transmembrane proteins. It is thought that the sarcoglycan complex functions as a unit. Hereditary progressive myopathies have been attributed to mutations in each of the sarcoglycans, and merosin is missing in a congenital muscular dystrophy. No patients have yet been identified with an abnormality of dystroglycan or syntrophin. This diagram was adapted from diagrams by Justin Fallon and Kevin Campbell.

cular dystrophies and then identifying the gene products that are altered. These diseases resemble the Duchenne form clinically but differ because dystrophin is normal and because inheritance is autosomal dominant or autosomal recessive instead of X-linked. The international gene-mapping effort started in Tunisia and extended to many other countries. The new information gave evidence of the power of molecular genetics to elucidate diseases and, in turn, to provide new insights into the biology of normal cells.

The dystrophin-associated glycoproteins include some that are extracellular (merosin, formerly called laminin, and dystroglycans), some that are located on the cytoplasmic side of the muscle plasma membrane (dystrophin, syntrophin, and utrophin), and some that span the surface membrane (sarcoglycans) (Figure 35-7).

The importance of the glycoproteins (sarcoglycans and dystroglycans) is emphasized in the dystrophin-normal dystrophies. In these conditions one of the sarcoglycans is missing (Table 35-4). All but one of these newly recognized disease-associated proteins is part of the muscle cytoskeleton; the exception is calpain, a muscle-specific, calcium-activated protease. However, some families show no linkage to any of these loci; identified mutations account for about 10% of all myopathies with normal dystrophin. As a group, these limb-girdle muscular dystrophies exemplify locus heterogeneity, whereby different mutant gene products are encoded on different chromosomes but give rise to clinically similar syndromes.

The "sarcoglycanopathies" teach us that dystrophin is needed to anchor the sarcoglycans, but the glycoproteins are important themselves and seem to function as a complex. If a key sarcoglycan is missing, dystrophin does not function properly. Moreover, mutation of one sarcoglycan leads to secondary loss of the other components of the complex.

Table 35-4 Classification of Limb-Girdle Muscular Dystrophies

Type	Inheritance	Map position	Gene product	Popular name*
LGMD1A	Autosomal dominant	5q	Not known	
	Autosomal dominant	Not 5q	Not known	
LGMD2A	Autosomal recessive	Unlinked	Calpain 3	
LGMD2B	Autosomal recessive	2p	Not known	
LGMD2C	Autosomal recessive	13q12	γ-sarcoglycan	SCARMD
LGMD2D	Autosomal recessive	17q12	α-sarcoglycan (adhalin)	DMD-like
LGMD2E	Autosomal recessive	4q12	β-sarcoglycan	DMD-like

*SCARMD, severe childhood autosomal recessive muscular dystrophy; DMD, Duchenne muscular dystrophy.

Myelin Proteins Are Affected in Some Hereditary Peripheral Neuropathies

Charcot-Marie-Tooth disease is an inherited sensorimotor peripheral neuropathy. As in other peripheral neuropathies, the condition is characterized by muscle weakness and wasting, loss of reflexes, and loss of sensation in the distal parts of the limbs. These symptoms appear in childhood or adolescence and are slowly progressive. The introduction of methods for measuring conduction velocity led to the discovery that one form (type 1) has the features of a demyelinating neuropathy. Conduction in peripheral nerves is slow, with histological evidence of demyelination and remyelination. Sometimes the reactive remyelination leads to gross hypertrophy of the nerves. Type 1 disorders are inexorably progressive, without remissions or exacerbations.

In type 2 Charcot-Marie-Tooth disease nerve conduction velocity is normal. This form is considered an axonal neuropathy without demyelination. Both types 1 and 2 are inherited as autosomal dominant diseases. Type 3 Charcot-Marie-Tooth disease, or Dejerine-Sottas disease, appeared as a very severe condition in children and was originally considered autosomal recessive.

In the 1990s the genetic defects in these conditions began to be localized. The type 1 disease was attributed to mutations on two different chromosomes (locus heterogeneity). A more common form (type 1A) was linked to chromosome 17, while a less common form (1B) was localized to chromosome 1. The genes encoded two myelin proteins: Type 1A involved a defect in peripheral myelin protein 22, and type 1B the myelin protein P_0.

Further study of the syndrome has revealed that mutations in different alleles of the same gene (allelic heterogeneity) give rise to different clinical syndromes. For example, a disorder of intermittent and reversible symptoms (now called *hereditary neuropathy with liability to pressure palsies*) has intermittent and focal characteristics that may affect only one arm; these traits are totally different from the symptoms of Charcot-Marie-Tooth disease, which are permanent and progressive and usually affect both legs. Nevertheless, both hereditary neuropathy with lability to pressure palsies and type 1A Charcot-Marie-Tooth disease map to the same locus on chromosome 17 and involve the same protein, peripheral myelin protein 22 (PMP22) (see Chapter 4). The severe childhood form of Charcot-Marie-Tooth disease (type 3) has also been attributed to mutations of the same gene and gene product. Why the clinical manifestations of these three variants of one disease differ is not known. A modifying gene could be responsible.

Analysis of the PMP22 mutations has led to a new principle in human genetics because gene dosage seems to explain the clinical differences. Normal individuals have two alleles, a "double dose." In Charcot-Marie-Tooth disease type 1 the gene on one chromosome is duplicated. This duplication and the single unaltered gene on the other chromosome add up to a triple dose of the gene. If, however, the gene is altered by a mutation on one chromosome and that allele is absent, then there is only a single dose (the one normal allele on the other chromosome), and the resulting syndrome is hereditary neuropathy with lability to pressure palsies. If there are mutations of both alleles (zero dosage), the resulting syndrome is Charcot-Marie-Tooth disease type 3, the severe childhood form.

An Overall View

The creative interplay of clinical observation and molecular neural science has nowhere been more fruitful than in the analysis of diseases of the motor unit. Molecular genetic analysis of Duchenne muscular dystrophy has provided information that bears importantly on the organization of the human genome, the nature of inherited deletions, and the physiological function of normal muscle.

The severe Duchenne muscular dystrophy and the milder Becker muscular dystrophy are most often due to deletions in the same gene. In the severe form there is a virtual absence of the gene product, dystrophin, while in the milder form the protein is present but in less than normal amounts and with abnormal structure. Identification of dystrophin led to the discovery of related proteins that are essential in maintaining the integrity of the normal muscle surface membrane. When the genes for these dystrophin-associated proteins are mutated, different clinical disorders result.

Other genetic diseases of nerve and muscle have been related to different kinds of mutations. Trinucleotide amplification occurs in myotonic muscular dystrophy, and gene-dosage effects are seen in the Charcot-Marie-Tooth forms of inherited peripheral nerve disease. Different clinical syndromes may result from abnormalities in one gene product; the clinical differences presumably result from the ameliorating or damaging consequence of the actions of a second, modifying gene or from environmental effects. If we are to develop rational therapies, the complete pathogenesis of these diseases has to be unraveled. We will need to understand how the mutation results in the symptoms and signs of disease.

Lewis P. Rowland

Selected Readings

Culp WJ, Ochoa J (eds). 1982. *Abnormal Nerves and Muscles as Impulse Generators.* New York: Oxford Univ. Press.

Dyck PJ, Thomas PK, Griffin JW, Low PA, Poduslo JF (eds). 1993. *Peripheral Neuropathy,* 3rd ed. Philadelphia: Saunders.

Engel AG, Franzini-Armstrong C (eds). 1994. *Myology,* 2nd ed. New York: McGraw-Hill.

Hoffman EP, Kunkel LM. 1989. Dystrophin in Duchenne/

Becker muscular dystrophy. Neuron 2:1019–1029.

Paulson HL, Fischbeck KH. 1996. Trinucleotide repeats in neurogenetic disorders. Annu Rev Neurosci 19:79–107.

Roberts RG. 1995. Dystrophin, its gene, and the dystrophinopathies. Adv Genet 33:177–232.

Rowland LP. 1988. Clinical concepts of Duchenne muscular dystrophy: the impact of molecular genetics. Brain 111:479–495.

Walton JM. 1994. *Diseases of Voluntary Muscle,* 6th ed. Edinburgh: Churchill Livingstone.

References

Adrian ED, Bronk DW. 1929. The discharge of impulses in motor nerve fibres. 2. The frequency of discharge in reflex and voluntary contractions. J Physiol (Lond) 67:119–145.

Ahn AH, Kunkel LM. 1993. The structural and functional diversity of dystrophin. Nat Genet 3:283–291.

Angelini C, Fanin M, Freda MP, Duggan MJ, Siciliano G, Hoffman EP. 1999. The clinical spectrum of sarcoglycanopathies. Neurology 52:176–179.

Azibi K, Bachner L, Beckmann JS, Matsumura K, Hamouda E, Chaouch M, Chaouch A, Ait-Ouarab R, Vignal A, Weissenbach J, et al. 1993. Severe childhood autosomal recessive muscular dystrophy with the deficiency of the 50 kDa dystrophin-associated glycoprotein maps to chromosome 13q12. Hum Mol Genet 2:1423–1428.

Barohn RJ, Amato AA, Griggs RC. 1998. Overview of distal myopathies: from the clinical to the molecular. Neuromuscul Disord 8:309–316.

Beckmann JS, Richard I, Hillaire D, Broux O, Antignac C, Bois E, Cann H, Cottingham RW Jr., Feingold N, Feingold J, et al. 1991. A gene for limb-girdle muscular dystrophy maps to chromosome 15. C R Acad Sci Paris 312:141–148.

Ben Olthame K, Hamida MB, Pericak-Vance MA, et al. 1992. Linkage of Tunisian autosomal recessive Duchenne-like muscular dystrophy to the pericentromeric region of chromosome 1eq. Nat Genet 2:315–317.

Biros I, Forest S. 1999. Spinal muscular atrophy; untangling the knot? J Med Genet 36:1–8.

Bonnemann CG, Modi R, Boguchi S, Mizumo Y, Yoshida M, Gussoni E, McNally EM, Duggan DJ, Angelini C, Hoffman EP, Ozawa E, Kunkel LM. 1995. β-Sarcoglycan (A3b) mutations cause autosomal recessive muscular dystrophy with loss of the sarcoglycan complex. Nat Genet 11:266–273.

Borchelt DR, Wong PC, Sisodia SS, Price DL. 1998. Transgenic mouse models of Alzheimer's disease and amyotrophic lateral sclerosis. Brain Pathol 8:735–757.

Brook JD, McCurrach ME, Harley HG, Buckler AJ, Church D, Aburatani H, Hunter K, Stanton VP, Thirion JP, Hudson T, et al. 1992. Molecular basis of myotonic muscular dystrophy; expansion of a trinucleotide (CTG) repeat at the 3' end of a transcript encoding a protein kinase family member. Cell 68:799–808.

Brown RH Jr. 1997. Dystrophin-associated proteins and the muscular dystrophies. Annu Rev Med 48:456–466.

Bushby KMD, Beckmann JS. 1995. Workshop report: the

limb-girdle muscular dystrophies—proposal for a new nomenclature. Neuromuscul Disord 5:337–343.

Bushby KMD, Gardner-Medwin S. 1993. The clinical, genetic and dystrophin characteristics of Becker muscular dystrophy. 1. Natural history. J Neurol 240:98–104.

Bushby KM, Gardner-Medwin S, Nicholson LV, Johnson MA, Haggerty ID, Cleghorn NJ, Harris JB, Bhattacharya SS. 1993. The clinical, genetic and dystrophin characteristics of Becker muscular dystrophy. II. Correlation of phenotype with genetic and protein abnormalities. J Neurol 240:105–112.

Campbell KP. 1995. Adhalin gene mutation and autosomal recessive limb-girdle muscular dystrophy. Ann Neurol 38:353–354.

Campbell KP. 1995. Three muscular dystrophies: loss of cytoskeleton-extracellular matrix linkage. Cell 80:675–679.

Chance PF, Alderson MK, Lepig KA, et al. 1993. DNA deletion associated with hereditary neuropathy with liability to pressure palsies. Cell 72:143–152.

Chance PF, Bird TD, Matsunami N, et al. 1992. Trisomy 17p associated with Charcot-Marie-Tooth neuropathy type 1A phenotype: evidence for gene dosage as a mechanism in CMT1A. Neurology 42:2295–2299.

Davies KE. 1988. Further studies of gene deletions that cause Duchenne and Becker muscular dystrophies. Genomics 2:109–114.

Duggan DJ, Gorospe JR, Fanin M, Hoffman EP, Angelini C. 1997. Mutations in the sarcoglycan genes in patients with myopathy. N Engl J Med 336:618–624.

Fallon JR, Hall ZW. 1994. Building synapses: agrin and dystroglycan stick together. Trends Neurosci 17:469–473.

Fu YH, Pizzuti A, Fenwick R, et al. 1992. Unstable triplet repeat in a gene related to myotonic muscular dystrophy, myotonin protein kinase. Science 255:1256–1258.

Harper PS. 1989. *Myotonic Dystrophy*. London: Saunders.

Hayasaka T, Takada G, Ionasescu VV. 1993. Mutation of the myelin Po gene in Charcot neuropathy type 1B. Hum Mol Genet 2:1369–1372.

Hayashi YK, Mizuno Y, Yoshida M, Nonaka I, Ozawa E, Arahata K. 1995. The frequency of patients with 50 kd dystrophin-associated glycoprotein (50 DAG or adhalin) deficiency in a muscular dystrophy patient population in Japan: immunocytochemical analysis of 50DAG, 43DAG, dystrophin and utrotrophin. Neurology 45:551–554.

Hoffman EP. 1993. Genotype/phenotype correlations in Duchenne/Becker dystrophy. In: T Partridge (ed). *Molecular and Cell Biology of Muscular Dystrophy*, pp. 12–36. London: Chapman & Hall.

Hoffman EP, Brown RH, Kunkel LM. 1987. Dystrophin: the protein product of the Duchenne muscular dystrophy locus. Cell 51:919–928.

Hoffman EP, Fischbeck KH, Brown RH, Johnson M, Medori R, Loike JD, Harris JB, Waterston R, Brooke M, Specht L, Kupsky W, Chamberlain J, Caskey CT, Shapiro F, Kunkel LM. 1988. Characterization of dystrophin in muscle-biopsy specimens from patients with Duchenne's or Becker's muscular dystrophy. N Engl J Med 318: 1363–1368.

Ince PG, Lowe J, Shaw PJ. 1998. Amyotrophic sclerosis: current issues in classification, pathogenesis, and molecular pathology. Neuropath Appl Neurobiol 24:104–117.

Ionasescu VV, Ionasescu R, Searby C. 1993. Screening of dominantly inherited Charcot neuropathies. Muscle Nerve 176:1232–1238.

Karpati G, Ajdukovic D, Arnold D, et al. 1993. Myoblast transfer in Duchenne muscular dystrophy. Ann Neurol 34:8–17.

Kubisch C, Schnmidt-Rose T, Fontaine B, Bretqag AH, Jentsch T. 1998. CIC-1 chloride channel mutations in myotonia congenita: variable penetrance of mutations shifting the voltage dependence. Hum Molec Genet 7:1753– 1760.

Lim LE, Duclos F, Broux O, Bourg N, Sunada Y, Allamand V, Meyer J, Richard I, Moomaw C, Slaughter C, Tome FMS, Fardeau M, Jackson CE, Beckmann JS, Campbell KP. 1995. β-Sarcoglycan: characterization and role in limb-girdle muscular dystrophy linked to 4q12. Nat Genet 11:257–264.

Lim LE, Campbell KP. 1998. The sarcoglycan complex in limb-girdle muscular dystrophy. Curr Op Neurol 11:443–452.

Ljunggren A, Duggan D, McNally, et al. 1995. Primary adhalin deficiency as a cause of muscular dystrophy in patients with normal dystrophin. Ann Neurol 38:376–372.

Matsumara K, Campbell KP. 1993. Deficiency of dystrophin-associated proteins: a common mechanism leading to muscle cell necrosis in severe childhood muscular dystrophies. Neuromuscul Disord 3:109–118.

Matsumara K, Campbell KP. 1994. Dystrophin-glycoprotein complex: its role in the molecular pathogenesis of muscular dystrophies. Muscle Nerve 17:2–15.

Mendell JB, Sahenk A, Prior TW. 1995. The childhood muscular dystrophies: diseases sharing a common pathogenesis of membrane instability. J Child Neurol 10:150–159.

Minetti C, Beltrame F, Marcenaro G, Bonilla E. 1992. Dystrophin at the plasma membrane of human muscle fibers shows a costameric localization. Neuromuscul Disord 2:99–109.

Monaco AP, Bertelson CJ, Liechti-Gallati S, Moser H, Kunkel LM. 1988. An explanation for the phenotypic differences between patients bearing partial deletions of the DMD locus. Genomics 2:90–95.

Moxley RT III. 1992. Myotonic muscular dystrophy. Handbook Clin Neurol 62:209–261.

Ozawa E, Nogouchi S, Mizuno Y, Hagiwara Y, Yoshida M. 1998. From dystrophenopathy to sarcoglycanopathy: evolution of a concept of muscular dystrophy. Muscle Nerve 21:421–438.

Patel PI, Lupski JR. 1994. Charcot-Marie-Tooth disease: a new paradigm for the mechanism of inherited disease. Trends Genet 10:128–133.

Piccolo F, Roberds SL, Jeanpierre M, Leuturcq F, Azibi K, Beldjord C, Carrie A, Recan D, Chaouch M, Righis A, el Kerch F, Sefiani A, Voit T, Merlini L, Collin H, Eymard B, Beckmann JS, Romero NB, Tome FMS, Fardeau M,

Campbell KP, Kaplan, J-C. 1995. Primary adhalinopathy: a common cause of autosomal recessive muscular dystrophy of variable severity. Nat Genet 10:243–245.

Pizzuti A, Friedman DL, Caskey CT. 1993. The myotonic dystrophy gene. Arch Neurol 50:1173–1179.

Plassart-Schiess E, Gervais A, Eymaard B. 1998. Novel muscle chloride channel (CLCN1) mutations in myotonia congenita with various modes of inheritance including incomplete dominance and penetrance. Neurology 50: 1176–1179.

Richard I, Broux O, Allamand V, Passos-Bueno M-R, Zatz M, Tischfield JA, Fardeau M, Jackson CE, Cohen D, Beckmann JS. 1995. Mutations in the proteolytic enzyme calpain 3 cause limb-girdle muscular dystrophy type 2A. Cell 81:27–40.

Roa BB, Dyck PJ, Marks HG, Chance PF, Lupski JR. 1993. Dejerine-Sottas syndrome associated with point mutation in the peripheral myelin protein 22 (PMP22) gene. Nat Genet 5:269–273.

Rowland LP. 1998. Diagnosis of amyotrophic lateral sclerosis. J Neurol Sci 160(suppl 1):S6–S24.

Sherrington CS. 1929. Some functional properties attaching to convergence. Proc R Soc Lond B Biol Sci 105:332–362.

Suter U, Patel PI. 1994. Genetic basis of inherited peripheral neuropathies. Hum Mutat 3:95–102.

Tinsley JM, Blake DJ, Zuellig RA, Davies KE. 1994. Increasing complexity of the dystrophin-associated protein complex. Proc Natl Acad Sci U S A 91:8307–8313.

Tinsley JM, Davies KE. 1993. Utrophin: a potential replacement for dystrophin. Neuromuscul Disord 3:537–539.

Waxman S. 1982. Membranes, myelin, and the pathophysiology of multiple sclerosis. N Engl J Med 306:1529–1533.

Worton R. 1995. Muscular dystrophies: diseases of the dystrophin-glycoprotein complex. Science 270:755–756.

36

Spinal Reflexes

DURING NORMAL MOVEMENTS the central nervous system uses information from a vast array of sensory receptors to ensure the generation of the correct pattern of muscle activity. Sensory information from muscles, joints, and skin, for example, is essential for regulating movement. Without this somatosensory input, gross movements tend to be imprecise, while tasks requiring fine coordination in the hands, such as fastening buttons, are impossible (see Chapter 33).

Charles Sherrington was among the first to recognize the importance of sensory information in regulating movements. In an influential monograph published in 1906 he proposed that simple reflexes, stereotyped movements elicited by the activation of receptors in skin or muscle, are the basic units for movement. He further proposed that complex sequences of movements can be produced by combining simple reflexes. This view has been the guiding principle in motor physiology for much of this century. Only relatively recently has it been modified by the recognition that many coordinated movements can be produced in the absence of sensory information. For example, in a variety of species locomotor patterns can be initiated and maintained in the absence of patterned sensory input (Chapter 37). Nevertheless, the notion that reflexes play an important role in the patterning of motor activity is beyond doubt. The contemporary view is that reflexes are integrated with centrally generated motor commands to produce adaptive movements.

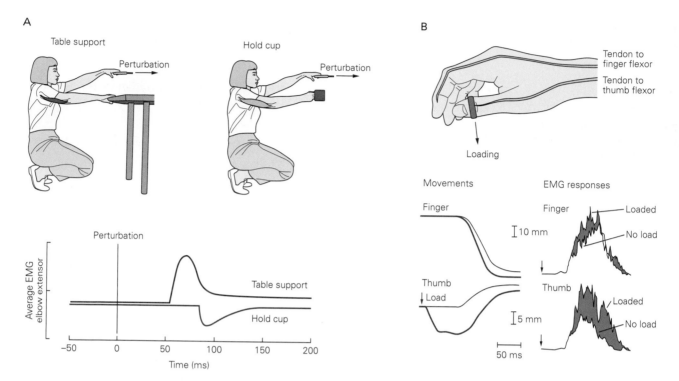

Figure 36-1 Reflex responses are often complex and can change depending on the task.

A. Perturbation of one arm causes an excitatory reflex response in the contralateral elbow extensor muscle when the contralateral limb is used to prevent the body from moving forward, but the same stimulus produces an inhibitory response in the muscle (reduced EMG) when the contralateral hand holds a filled cup. (Adapted from Marsden et al. 1981.)

B. Loading the thumb during a rhythmic sequence of finger-to-thumb movements produces a reflex response (shaded blue area) in the muscle moving the finger as well as the loaded thumb muscle. The additional movement of the finger ensures that the pinching movement remains accurate. (Adapted from Cole et al. 1984.)

In this chapter we consider the principles underlying the organization and function of reflexes, focusing on spinal reflexes. The sensory stimuli for spinal reflexes arise from receptors in muscles, joints, and skin and the neural circuitry responsible for the motor response is entirely contained within the spinal cord. Reflexes have been viewed traditionally as automatic, stereotyped movements in response to stimulation of peripheral receptors. This view arose primarily from early studies on reduced animal preparations in which reflexes were examined under a set of standard conditions. However, as investigators extended their studies to measure reflexes during normal behavior, our concept of reflexes changed substantially. We now know that under normal conditions reflexes can be modified to adapt to the task. This flexibility allows reflexes to be smoothly incorporated into complex movements initiated by central commands.

Reflexes Are Highly Adaptable and Control Movements in a Purposeful Manner

A good example of the adaptability of reflexes is seen when the muscles of the wrist of one arm are stretched while a subject is kneeling or standing. The muscles that are stretched contract, but muscles in other limbs also contract to prevent a loss of balance. Interestingly, the reflex response of the elbow extensor of the *opposite* arm depends on the task being performed by that arm. If the arm is used to stabilize the body (by holding the edge of a table), a large excitatory response is evoked in the elbow extensor muscles to resist the forward sway of the body. If the arm is holding an unsteady object, such as a cup of tea, a reflex inhibition of the elbow extensors prevents movement of the cup (Figure 36-1A).

Another example of adaptability in reflexes is the reflex of finger and thumb flexor muscles in response to stretching the thumb muscles. If flexion of the thumb is resisted while a subject is attempting to touch the tip of the finger rhythmically to the tip of the thumb, a short-latency reflex response is produced in *both* the finger and thumb flexor muscles. The reflex in the finger flexor muscle produces a larger flexion movement of the finger to compensate for the reduced flexion of the thumb, thus ensuring the performance of the intended task (Figure 36-1B). If the subject is simply making rhythmic thumb movements, a reflex response is produced only in the thumb flexor muscle.

A third example of the adaptable nature of reflexes involves a conditioned flexion-withdrawal reflex. Flexion withdrawal can be associated with an auditory tone by classical conditioning techniques (Chapter 62). Subjects are asked to place an index finger, palmar surface down, on an electrode. A mild electrical shock is then paired with the auditory tone. As one might expect, after only a very few such pairings the auditory tone alone will elicit the withdrawal reflex. What exactly has been conditioned? Is it the contraction of a fixed group of muscles or a behavioral *act* that withdraws the finger from the noxious stimulus? This question can be answered by having the subjects turn their hands over after conditioning is complete, so that now the dorsal surface of the finger is in contact with the electrode. Most subjects will withdraw their fingers from the electrode when the tone is played, even though this means that the opposite muscles now contract. Thus, the conditioned reflex in response to the tone is not only a stereotyped set of muscle contractions but also an appropriate behavior.

Three important principles are illustrated by these examples. First, transmission in reflex pathways is set according to the motor task. The state of the reflex pathways for any task is referred to as *functional set*. Exactly how functional set is established for most motor tasks is largely unknown (the unraveling of the underlying mechanisms constitutes one of the challenging and exciting areas of contemporary research on motor systems). Second, sensory input from a localized source generally produces reflex responses in many muscles, some of which may be distant from the stimulus. These multiple responses are coordinated to achieve an intended goal. Third, supraspinal centers play an important role in modulating and adapting spinal reflexes, even to the extent of reversing movements when appropriate.

In order to understand the neural basis for reflexes and how they are modified for a particular task, we must first have a thorough knowledge of the organization of reflex pathways in the spinal cord. The spinal cord is a major site for integrating reflexes with central commands, and many qualitative features of reflexes are maintained after transection of the spinal cord.

Spinal Reflexes Produce Coordinated Patterns of Muscle Contraction

Cutaneous Reflexes Produce Complex Movements That Serve Protective and Postural Functions

A familiar example of a spinal reflex is the flexion-withdrawal reflex, in which the limb is quickly withdrawn from a painful stimulus, usually by simultaneous contraction of all the flexor muscles in the limb. We know that this is a spinal reflex because it persists after complete transection of the spinal cord, a condition that isolates the spinal circuits from the brain. Flexion withdrawal is a protective reflex in which a discrete stimulus causes muscles to contract in a coordinated fashion at multiple joints. Through divergent polysynaptic reflex pathways the sensory signal both excites motor neurons that innervate flexor muscles of the stimulated limb and inhibits motor neurons that innervate extensor muscles of the limb (Figure 36-2A).

Excitation of one group of muscles and inhibition of their antagonists is what Sherrington first called *reciprocal innervation*. (Antagonist muscles are those that act in the opposite direction of a given muscle; for example, knee extensors are the antagonists of knee flexors.) Reciprocal innervation is a key principle of motor organization and is discussed later in this chapter.

Along with flexion of the stimulated limb, the reflex can produce an opposite effect in the contralateral limb, that is, excitation of extensor motor neurons and inhibition of flexor motor neurons. This *crossed-extension reflex* serves to enhance postural support during withdrawal of a foot from a painful stimulus. Contraction of the extensor muscles in the opposite leg counteracts the increased load caused by lifting the stimulated limb. Thus, flexion withdrawal is a complete, albeit simple, motor act.

While flexion reflexes are relatively stereotyped in form, both the spatial extent and the force of muscle contraction depend on stimulus intensity (Chapter 33). Touching a stove that is only slightly hot may produce moderately fast withdrawal only at the wrist and elbow, while touching a stove that is very hot invariably leads to a forceful contraction at all joints, leading to a rapid withdrawal of the entire limb. The duration of the reflex usually increases with stimulus intensity, and the contractions produced in a flexion reflex always outlast the stimulus. Thus, reflexes are not simply repetitions of a stereotyped movement pattern; they are modulated by properties of the stimulus.

A Flexion and crossed-extension reflex

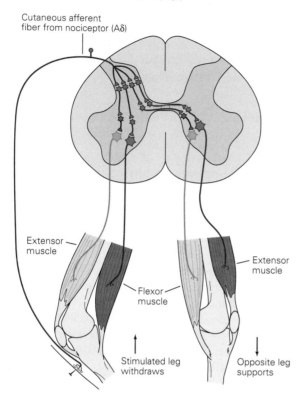

Cutaneous afferent
fiber from nociceptor (Aδ)

Extensor
muscle

Extensor
muscle

Flexor
muscle

Stimulated leg
withdraws

Opposite leg
supports

Figure 36-2 Spinal reflexes involve coordinated contractions of numerous muscles in the limbs.

A. Flexion and crossed-extension reflexes are mediated via polysynaptic pathways in the spinal cord. An excitatory pathway activates motor neurons supplying ipsilateral flexor muscles, which withdraw the limb from noxious stimuli. At the same time, motor neurons supplying contralateral extensor muscles are excited to provide support during withdrawal of the limb. Inhibitory interneurons (gray) ensure that the motor neurons supplying antagonist muscles are inactive during the reflex response. (Adapted from Schmidt 1983.)

B.1. Stretch reflexes are mediated by monosynaptic pathways. Ia afferent fibers from muscle spindles make excitatory connections on two sets of motor neurons: alpha motor neurons that innervate the same (homonymous) muscle from which they arise and motor neurons that innervate synergist muscles. They also act through inhibitory interneurons to inhibit the motor neurons that innervate antagonist muscles. When a muscle is stretched the Ia afferents increase their firing rate. This leads to contraction of the same muscle and its synergists and relaxation of the antagonist. The reflex therefore tends to counteract the stretch, enhancing the spring-like properties of the muscles. **2.** The reflex nature of contractions produced by muscle stretch is revealed by the large contraction of an extensor muscle when it is stretched compared with the small force increase after cutting the sensory afferents in the dorsal roots. (Adapted from Liddell and Sherrington 1924.)

B₁ Stretch reflex

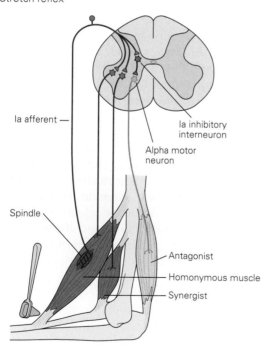

Ia afferent

Ia inhibitory
interneuron

Alpha motor
neuron

Spindle

Antagonist

Homonymous muscle

Synergist

B₂

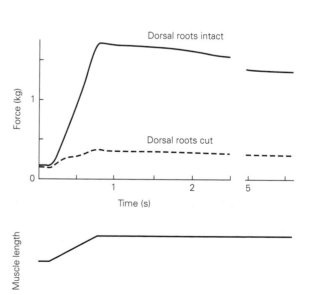

Dorsal roots intact

Dorsal roots cut

Force (kg)

Time (s)

Muscle length

Because of the similarity of the flexion-withdrawal reflex to stepping, it was once thought that walking might be generated merely as a series of flexion reflexes. We now know that a major component of the neural control system for walking is a set of intrinsic spinal circuits that do not require sensory stimuli to produce the basic walking pattern (see Chapter 37). Nevertheless, in mammals the intrinsic spinal circuits that control walking share many of the same interneurons that are involved in flexion reflexes.

The Stretch Reflex Acts to Resist the Lengthening of a Muscle

Perhaps the most important and certainly the most studied spinal reflex is the *stretch reflex*, a contraction of muscle that occurs when the muscle is lengthened. Stretch reflexes were originally thought to be an intrinsic property of muscles. However, Sherrington showed at the turn of the century that they could be abolished by cutting either the dorsal or the ventral roots, thus establishing that they require sensory input from the muscle to the spinal cord and a return path to the muscles. We now know that the receptor that senses the change of length is the muscle spindle (see Box 36-1) and that the afferent axons from this receptor make direct excitatory connections to motor neurons (Figure 36-2B).

In his investigation of reflexes, Sherrington developed a valuable experimental model for investigating spinal circuitry. He carried out his experiments with cats whose brain stems had been surgically transected at the level of the midbrain, between the superior and inferior colliculi. This is referred to as a *decerebrate preparation*. The effect of this procedure is to disconnect the rest of the brain from the spinal cord, thus blocking sensations of pain as well as interrupting normal modulation of reflexes by higher brain centers.

When Sherrington attempted to flex passively the rigidly extended hindlimb of a decerebrate cat, he felt increased contraction of the muscles being stretched (Figure 36-2 B2). He called this the stretch reflex. Sherrington also discovered that stretching a muscle caused the antagonist muscles to relax. He concluded that the stretch stimulus caused excitation of certain motor neurons and inhibition of others (reciprocal innervation).

Decerebrate animals have stereotyped and usually heightened spinal reflexes, making it is easier to examine the factors controlling their expression. They also show a dramatic increase in extensor muscle tone, sometimes sufficient to support the animal in the standing position. Muscle tone is increased because, in the absence of control by higher brain centers, descending pathways from the brain stem powerfully facilitate the neuronal circuits involved in the stretch reflexes of extensor muscles.

In normal animals spinal reflexes are weaker and considerably more variable in strength than those in decerebrate animals because there is a balance between facilitation and inhibition. Descending pathways from the cerebral cortex and other higher centers of the brain continuously modulate the strength of stretch reflexes.

Neuronal Networks in the Spinal Cord Contribute to the Purposeful Integration of Reflex Responses

The Stretch Reflex Involves a Monosynaptic Pathway

The neural circuit responsible for the stretch reflex was one of the first reflex pathways to be examined in detail (see Chapter 4). The physiological basis of this reflex was elucidated by measuring the latency of the response evoked in ventral roots when the dorsal roots were stimulated electrically. When the large Ia afferent fibers from the primary spindle endings are selectively activated, the reflex latency through the spinal cord is less than 1 ms. (The classification of sensory fibers from muscle is discussed in Box 36-2.) Since the delay introduced by a single synapse is between 0.5 and 0.9 ms, it can be inferred that the Ia fibers make direct connections on the alpha motor neurons, creating a *monosynaptic pathway* (Figure 36-4).

Ia fibers from a muscle excite not only the motor neurons innervating that muscle (*homonymous connections*) but also those innervating muscles having a similar mechanical action (*heteronymous connections*). The pattern of connections of Ia fibers to motor neurons can be shown directly by intracellular recording techniques. Intracellular recording has also shown that alpha motor neurons innervating antagonistic muscles receive inhibition from Ia fibers via a specific class of inhibitory interneurons, the *Ia inhibitory interneurons*. This disynaptic inhibitory pathway is the basis for reciprocal innervation; when a muscle is stretched, the antagonists relax.

Inhibitory Interneurons Coordinate the Muscles Surrounding a Joint

Reciprocal innervation is useful not just in stretch reflexes but also in voluntary movements. Relaxation of the antagonist muscle during movements enhances speed and efficiency because the muscles that act as prime movers are not working against the contraction of opposing muscles. The Ia inhibitory interneurons

Box 36-1 Muscle Spindles

Muscle spindles are small encapsulated sensory receptors that have a spindle-like or fusiform shape and are located within the fleshy part of the muscle. Their main function is to signal changes in the length of the muscle within which they reside. Changes in the length of muscles are closely associated with changes in the angles of the joints that the muscles cross. Thus, muscle spindles can be used by the central nervous system to sense relative positions of the body segments.

Each spindle has three main components: (1) a group of specialized *intrafusal* muscle fibers whose central regions are noncontractile; (2) large-diameter myelinated sensory endings that originate from the central regions of the intrafusal fibers; and (3) small-diameter myelinated motor endings that innervate the polar contractile regions of the intrafusal fibers (Figure 36-3A). When the intrafusal fibers are stretched, often referred to as "loading the spindle," the sensory endings are also stretched and increase their firing rate. Because muscle spindles are arranged in parallel with the extrafusal muscle fibers that make up the main body of the muscle, the intrafusal fibers change in length as the whole muscle changes. Thus, when a muscle is stretched, the activity in the sensory endings of muscle spindles is increased. When a muscle shortens, the spindle is unloaded and the activity decreases.

The motor innervation of the intrafusal muscle fibers comes from small-diameter motor neurons, called *gamma* motor neurons to distinguish them from the large-diameter *alpha* motor neurons that innervate the extrafusal muscle fibers. Contraction of the intrafusal muscle fibers does not contribute to the force of muscle contraction. Rather, activation of gamma motor neurons causes shortening of the polar regions of the intrafusal fibers. This in turn stretches the noncontractile central region from both ends, leading to an increase in firing rate of the sensory endings or to a greater likelihood that stretch of the muscle will cause the sensory ending to fire. Thus, the gamma motor neurons provide a mechanism for adjusting the sensitivity of the muscle spindles.

The structure and functional behavior of muscle spindles is considerably more complicated than this simple description implies. When a muscle is stretched, there are two phases of the change in length: a dynamic phase, the period during which length is changing, and a static or steady-state phase, when the muscle has stabilized at a new length. Structural specializations within each component of the muscle spindles allow spindle afferents to signal aspects of each phase separately.

There are two types of intrafusal muscle fibers: nuclear bag fibers and nuclear chain fibers. The bag fibers can be divided into two groups, dynamic and static. A typical spindle has 2 or 3 bag fibers and a variable number of chain fibers, usually about 5. Furthermore, there are two types of sensory fiber endings: a single primary ending and a variable number of secondary endings (up to 8). The primary (Ia fiber) ending spirals around the central region of all the intrafusal muscle fibers (Figure 36-3B). The secondary (group II fiber) endings are located adjacent to the central regions of the static bag and chain fibers. The gamma motor neurons can also be divided into two classes, dynamic and static. Dynamic gamma motor neurons innervate the dynamic bag fibers, while the static gamma motor neurons innervate the static bag and the chain fibers.

This duality of structure is reflected in a duality of function. The steady-state or tonic discharge of both primary and secondary sensory endings signals the steady-state length of the muscle. The primary endings are, in addition, highly sensitive to the velocity of stretch, allowing them to provide information about the speed of movements. Because they are highly sensitive to small changes, primary endings provide quick information about unexpected changes in length, useful for generating quick corrective reactions.

Increases in activity of *dynamic* gamma motor neurons increase the dynamic sensitivity of the primary endings but have no influence on the secondary endings. Increases in activity of *static* gamma motor neurons increase the tonic level of activity in both primary and secondary endings, decrease the dynamic sensitivity of primary endings, and can prevent the silencing of primary activity when a muscle is released from stretch (Figure 36-3C). Thus, the central nervous system can independently adjust the dynamic and static sensitivity of the sensory fibers from muscle spindles.

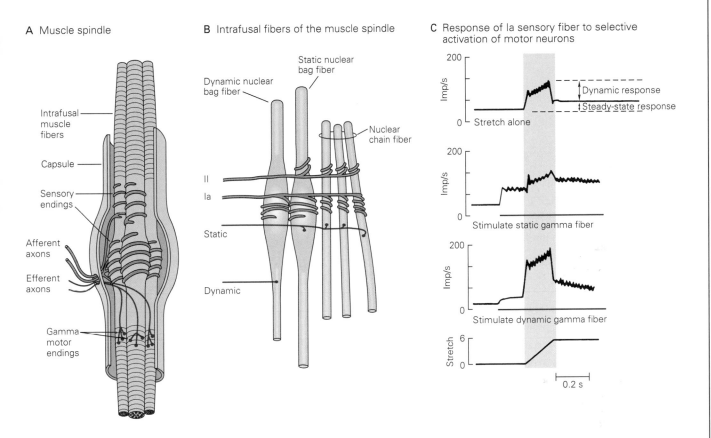

A Muscle spindle

Intrafusal muscle fibers

Capsule

Sensory endings

Afferent axons

Efferent axons

Gamma motor endings

B Intrafusal fibers of the muscle spindle

Static nuclear bag fiber

Dynamic nuclear bag fiber

Nuclear chain fiber

II

Ia

Static

Dynamic

C Response of Ia sensory fiber to selective activation of motor neurons

Dynamic response

Steady-state response

Stretch alone

Stimulate static gamma fiber

Stimulate dynamic gamma fiber

0.2 s

Figure 36-3

A. The main components of the muscle spindle are intrafusal muscle fibers, afferent sensory fiber endings, and efferent motor fiber endings. The intrafusal fibers are specialized muscle fibers; their central regions are not contractile. The sensory fiber endings spiral around the central regions of the intrafusal fibers and are responsive to stretch of these fibers. Gamma motor neurons innervate the contractile polar regions of the intrafusal fibers. Contraction of the intrafusal fibers pulls on the central regions from both ends and changes the sensitivity of the sensory fiber endings to stretch. (Adapted from Hulliger 1984.)

B. The muscle spindle contains three types of intrafusal fibers: dynamic nuclear bag, static nuclear bag, and nuclear chain fibers. A single Ia sensory fiber innervates all three types of fibers, forming a primary sensory ending. A group II sensory fiber innervates nuclear chain fibers and static bag fibers, form-

ing a secondary sensory ending. Two types of motor neurons innervate different intrafusal fibers. Dynamic gamma motor neurons innervate only dynamic bag fibers; static gamma motor neurons innervate various combinations of chain and static bag fibers. (Adapted from Boyd 1980.)

C. Selective stimulation of the two types of gamma motor neurons has different effects on the firing of the primary sensory endings in the spindle (the Ia fibers). Without gamma stimulation the Ia fiber shows a small dynamic response to muscle stretch and a modest increase in steady-state firing. When a static gamma motor neuron is stimulated the steady-state response of the Ia fiber increases but there is a decrease in the dynamic response. When a dynamic gamma motor neuron is stimulated the dynamic response of the Ia fiber is markedly enhanced but the steady-state response gradually returns to its original level. (Adapted from Brown and Matthews 1966.)

Box 36-2 Selective Activation of Sensory Fibers from Muscle

Sensory fibers are classified according to their diameter. Axons with larger diameters conduct action potentials more rapidly. Because each class of receptors gives rise to afferent fibers with diameters within a restricted range, this method of classification distinguishes to some extent the fibers that arise from the different groups of sensory receptors. The main groups of sensory fibers from muscle are listed in Table 36-1 (see Chapter 22 for the classification of sensory fibers from skin and joints).

The organization of reflex pathways in the spinal cord has been established primarily by electrically stimulating the sensory fibers and recording evoked responses in different classes of neurons in the spinal cord. This method of activation has three advantages over natural stimulation. The timing of afferent input can be precisely established, the central responses evoked by different classes of sensory fibers can be assessed by grading the strength of the electrical stimulus, and certain classes of receptors can be activated in isolation (impossible in natural conditions).

The strength of electrical stimuli required to activate a sensory fiber is measured relative to the strength required to activate the largest afferent fibers since the largest fibers have the lowest threshold for electrical activation. Thus group I fibers are usually activated over the range of one to two times the threshold of the largest afferents (with Ia fibers having, on average, a slightly lower threshold than Ib fibers). Most group II fibers are activated over the range of 2–5 times the threshold, while the small group III and IV fibers require stimulus strengths in the range of 10–50 times the threshold for activation.

Table 36-1 Classification of Sensory Fibers from Muscle

Type	Receptor	Axon	Sensitive to
Ia	Primary spindle endings	12–20 μm myelinated	Muscle length and rate of change of length
Ib	Golgi tendon organs	12–20 μm myelinated	Muscle tension
II	Secondary spindle endings	6–12 μm myelinated	Muscle length (little rate sensitivity)
II	Nonspindle endings	6–12 μm myelinated	Deep pressure
III	Free nerve endings	2–6 μm myelinated	Pain, chemical stimuli, and temperature (important for physiological response to exercise)
IV	Free nerve endings	0.5–2 μm nonmyelinated	Pain, chemical stimuli, and temperature

involved in the stretch reflex are also used to coordinate muscle contraction during voluntary movements. The interneurons receive inputs from collateral fibers of axons descending from neurons in the motor cortex, which make direct excitatory connections to spinal motor neurons (Figure 36-5A). This organizational feature simplifies the control of voluntary movements since higher centers do not have to send separate commands to the opposing muscles.

Reciprocal innervation of opposing muscles is not the only useful mode of coordination. Sometimes it is advantageous to contract the prime mover and the antagonist at the same time. Such *co-contraction* has the effect of stiffening the joint and is most useful when precision and joint stabilization are critical. An example of this phenomenon is the co-contraction of flexor and extensor muscles of the elbow immediately before catching a ball (see Chapter 33). The Ia inhibitory interneurons receive both excitatory and inhibitory signals from all of the major descending pathways (Figure 36-5A). By changing the balance of excitatory and inhibitory inputs onto these interneurons, supraspinal centers can reduce reciprocal inhibition and enable co-contraction, thus controlling the relative amount of joint stiffness to meet the requirements of the motor act.

The activity of spinal motor neurons is also regulated by another important class of inhibitory interneurons, the *Renshaw cells* (Figure 36-5B). Renshaw cells are excited by collaterals of the axons of motor neurons, and they make inhibitory synaptic connections to several populations of motor neurons, including the same motor neurons that excite them, and to the Ia inhibitory interneurons. The connections of Renshaw cells to motor neurons form a negative feedback system that may help stabilize the firing rate of the motor neurons, while the connections to the Ia inhibitory interneurons may regulate the strength of reciprocal inhibition to antagonistic motor neurons. In addition, Renshaw cells receive significant synaptic input from descending pathways and distribute inhibition to task-related groups of motor neurons and Ia interneurons. Thus, it is likely that they contribute to establishing the pattern of transmission in divergent group Ia pathways according to the motor task.

Divergence in Reflex Pathways Amplifies Sensory Inputs and Coordinates Muscle Contractions

In all reflex pathways in the spinal cord the afferent neurons form divergent connections with a large number of target neurons through branching of the central component of the axon. The flexion-withdrawal reflex, for example, involves extensive divergence within the spinal cord. Stimulation of a small number of sensory afferents from a localized area of skin is sufficient to cause contractions of widely distributed muscles and thus to produce a coordinated motor pattern.

Lorne Mendell and Elwood Henneman used computer enhancement techniques to determine the extent to which action potentials in single Ia afferent fibers are distributed among spinal motor neurons. Examining the medial gastrocnemius motor neurons of the cat, they found that individual Ia axons make excitatory synapses with all homonymous motor neurons. This widespread divergence effectively amplifies the effect of the signals in individual Ia fibers, producing a strong excitatory drive to the muscle within which they originate (*autogenic excitation*).

Group Ia axons also provide excitatory inputs to many of the motor neurons innervating synergist muscles (up to 60% of the motor neurons for some synergists). These connections, though widespread, are not quite as strong as the connections to homonymous motor neurons. The strength of these connections varies from muscle to muscle in a complex way according to the similarity of the mechanical actions of the synergists. We have already noted that, in the control of voluntary movements, descending pathways make use of reciprocal inhibition of antagonists in the stretch reflex. A similar principle holds for synergist muscles. Thus, stretch reflex pathways provide a principal mechanism by which the contractions of different muscles can be linked together in voluntary as well as reflex actions.

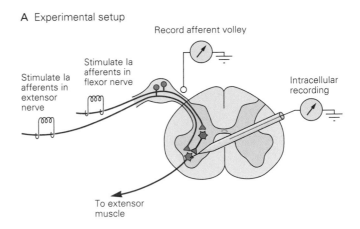

A Experimental setup

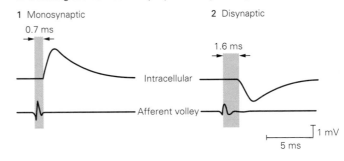

B Inferring the number of synapses in a pathway

Figure 36-4 Intracellular recording can be used to infer the number of synapses in a reflex pathway.

A. An intracellular recording electrode is inserted into the cell body of a motor neuron in the spinal cord that innervates an extensor muscle. Afferent axons (Ia fibers) in the nerves of flexor and extensor muscles are stimulated and the volley of action potentials that results is recorded at the dorsal root.

B.1. When Ia fibers in the nerve to the extensor muscle are stimulated, the latency between the recording of the afferent volley and the excitatory postsynaptic potential in the motor neuron is 0.7 ms. Since this is approximately equal to the duration of signal transmission across a single synapse, it can be inferred that the excitatory action of the stretch reflex pathway is monosynaptic. **2.** When Ia fibers in the nerve of an antagonist flexor muscle are stimulated, the latency between the recording of the afferent volley and the inhibitory postsynaptic potential in the motor neuron is 1.6 ms. Since this is approximately twice the duration of signal transmission across a single synapse, it can be inferred that the inhibitory action of the stretch reflex pathway is disynaptic.

Convergence of Inputs on Interneurons Increases the Flexibility of Reflex Responses

Thus far we have considered reflex pathways as though each was specialized for transmitting information from one type of sensory fiber. However, an enormous amount of sensory information from many different

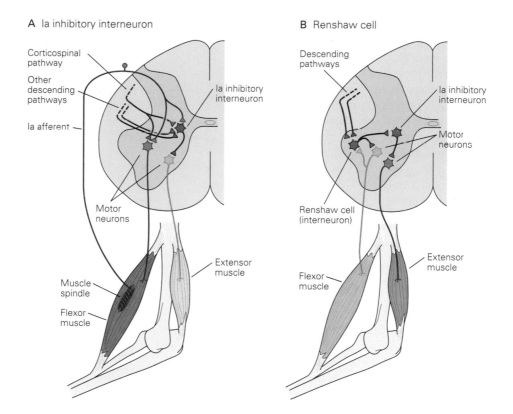

A Ia inhibitory interneuron

Corticospinal pathway
Other descending pathways
Ia afferent

Ia inhibitory interneuron

Motor neurons

Muscle spindle
Flexor muscle

Extensor muscle

B Renshaw cell

Descending pathways

Ia inhibitory interneuron
Motor neurons

Renshaw cell (interneuron)

Flexor muscle

Extensor muscle

Figure 36-5 Inhibitory interneurons play special roles in coordination of reflex actions.

A. The Ia inhibitory interneuron allows higher centers to coordinate opposing muscles at a joint through a single command. This inhibitory interneuron mediates reciprocal innervation in stretch reflex circuits. In addition, it receives inputs from corticospinal descending axons, so that a descending signal that activates one set of muscles automatically leads to relaxation of the antagonists. Other descending pathways make excitatory and inhibitory connections to this interneuron. When the balance of input is shifted to greater inhibition of the Ia inhibitory

interneuron, reciprocal inhibition will be decreased and cocontraction of opposing muscles may occur.

B. Renshaw cells produce recurrent inhibition of motor neurons. These spinal interneurons are excited by collaterals from motor neurons and then inhibit those same motor neurons. This negative feedback system regulates motor neuron excitability and stabilizes firing rates. Renshaw cells also send collaterals to synergist motor neurons (not shown) and Ia inhibitory interneurons. Thus, descending inputs that modulate the excitability of the Renshaw cell adjust the excitability of all the motor neurons around a joint.

sources converges on interneurons in the spinal cord. The *Ib inhibitory interneurons* are one of the most intensively studied groups of interneurons that receive extensive convergent input. These interneurons receive their principal input from Golgi tendon organs, sensory receptors that signal the tension in a muscle (Box 36-3).

Stimulation of tendon organ afferent fibers produces disynaptic or trisynaptic inhibition of homonymous motor neurons (*autogenic inhibition*). The action of Ib fibers is complex because the interneurons mediating these effects also receive input from the Ia fibers from

muscle spindles, low-threshold afferent fibers from cutaneous receptors, and afferent fibers from joints, as well as both excitatory and inhibitory input from various descending pathways (Figure 36-7A). Moreover, Ib fibers form widespread connections with motor neurons innervating muscles acting at different joints. Therefore, the spinal cord connections of the afferent fibers from tendon organs are thought to be part of spinal reflex networks that regulate whole limb movements.

Golgi tendon organs were originally thought to have a protective function, preventing damage to muscle, since

Box 36-3 Golgi Tendon Organs

Golgi tendon organs are sensory receptors located at the junction between muscle fibers and tendon; they are therefore connected in series to a group of skeletal muscle fibers. These receptors are slender, encapsulated structures about 1 mm long and 0.1 mm in diameter. Each tendon organ is innervated by a single (group Ib) axon that loses its myelination after it enters the capsule and branches into many fine endings, each of which intertwines among the braided collagen fascicles. Stretching of the tendon organ straightens the collagen fibers, thus compressing the nerve endings and causing them to fire (Figure 36-6A). Because the free nerve endings intertwine among the collagen fiber bundles, even very small stretches of the tendon organs can deform the nerve endings.

Whereas muscle spindles are most sensitive to changes in length of a muscle, tendon organs are most sensitive to changes in muscle tension. A particularly potent stimulus for activating a tendon organ is a contraction of the muscle fibers connected to the collagen fiber bundle containing the receptor. The tendon organs are thus readily activated during normal movements. This has been demonstrated by recordings from single Ib axons in humans making voluntary finger movements and in cats walking normally.

Studies in more restricted situations have shown that the average level of activity in the population of tendon organs in a muscle gives a fairly good measure of the total force in a contracting muscle (Figure 36-6B). This close agreement between firing frequency and force is consistent with the view that the tendon organs continuously measure the force in a contracting muscle.

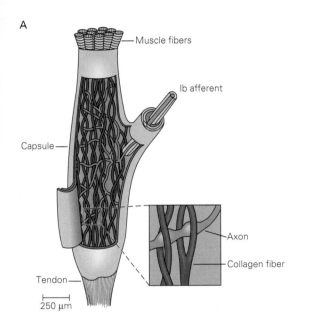

A

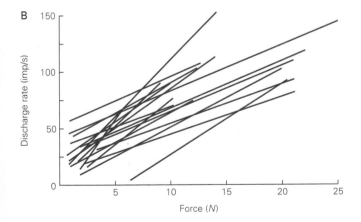

B

Figure 36-6A When the Golgi tendon organ is stretched (usually because of contraction of the muscle), the afferent axon is compressed by the collagen fibers (see inset) and its rate of firing increases. (Adapted from Schmidt 1983; inset adapted from Swett and Schoultz 1975.)

Figure 36-6B The discharge rate of a population of Golgi tendon organs signals the force in a muscle. Linear regression lines show the relationship between discharge rate and force for Golgi tendon organs of the soleus muscle of the cat. (Adapted from Crago et al 1982.)

it was assumed that they fired only when high tensions were achieved. But we now know that they also signal minute changes in muscle tension, thus providing the nervous system with precise information about the state of contraction of the muscle. The convergence of afferent input from tendon organs, cutaneous receptors, and joint receptors onto interneurons that inhibit motor neurons may allow for precise spinal control of muscle tension in activities such as grasping a delicate object. Combined input from these receptors excites the Ib inhibitory interneurons

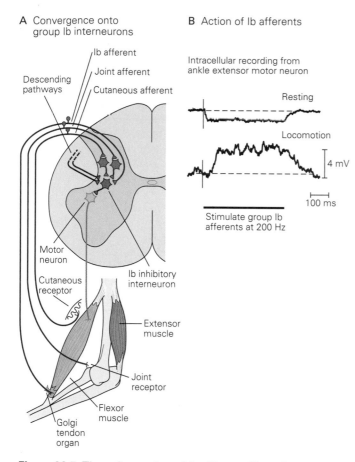

A Convergence onto group Ib interneurons

Descending pathways

Ib afferent

Joint afferent

Cutaneous afferent

Motor neuron

Cutaneous receptor

Ib inhibitory interneuron

Extensor muscle

Joint receptor

Flexor muscle

Golgi tendon organ

B Action of Ib afferents

Intracellular recording from ankle extensor motor neuron

Resting

Locomotion

4 mV

100 ms

Stimulate group Ib afferents at 200 Hz

Figure 36-7 The reflex action of Ib afferent fibers from Golgi tendon organs is modulated by multiple inputs to Ib inhibitory interneurons and depends on the behavioral state of an animal.

A. The Ib inhibitory interneurons receive convergent input from tendon organs, muscle spindles (not shown), joint and cutaneous receptors, and descending pathways.

B. When an animal is resting (quiescent), stimulation of Ib afferent fibers from the ankle extensor muscle (plantaris) *inhibits* ankle extensor motor neurons via Ib inhibitory interneurons, as shown by the intracellular recording from a motor neuron (top trace). During locomotion the same stimulus *excites* the motor neurons via polysynaptic excitatory pathways (bottom trace).

when the limb contacts the object and so reduces the level of muscle contraction to permit an appropriate soft grasp.

Centrally Generated Motor Commands Can Alter Transmission in Spinal Reflex Pathways

Both the strength and sign of synaptic transmission in spinal reflex pathways can be altered during behavioral acts. An interesting example is the change in sign in the responses evoked by stimulation of group Ib axons during

walking. As we have seen, the Ib afferent fibers from extensor muscles have an inhibitory effect on extensor motor neurons in the absence of locomotor activity. However, during locomotion the same Ib fibers produce an excitatory effect on extensor motor neurons, and transmission in the disynaptic Ib inhibitory pathway is depressed (Figure 36-7B). This phenomenon is referred to as *state-dependent reflex reversal*. Another example is the progressive decline in the strength of the monosynaptic reflex in leg extensor muscles of humans in going from standing to walking to running. In both these examples descending signals associated with the central motor command for walking modify the properties of transmission in spinal reflex pathways.

Tonic and Dynamic Mechanisms Regulate the Strength of Spinal Reflexes

Earlier we noted that the force of a reflex can vary even though the sensory stimulus stays constant. This variability in reflex strength depends on the flexibility of synaptic transmission in reflex pathways. There are three possible sites in the spinal cord for modulating the strength of a spinal reflex: the alpha motor neurons, interneurons in all reflex circuits except those having monosynaptic pathways with group Ia afferent fibers, and the presynaptic terminals of the afferent fibers (Figure 36-8A).

Descending neurons from higher centers of the nervous system, as well as from other regions of the spinal cord, make synaptic connections at these sites. These neurons can thus regulate the strength of reflexes by changing the background (tonic) level of activity at any of these sites. For example, an increase in the tonic excitatory input to the alpha motor neurons moves the membrane potential of these cells closer to threshold so that even the slightest reflex input will more easily activate the motor neurons (Figure 36-8B).

In addition to the modulatory effect of changes in the level of tonic activity, we have seen that reflex strength can be dynamically modulated depending on the task and the behavioral state. The mechanisms for this dynamic modulation are thought to be similar to those for tonic modulation. However, intracellular recording experiments have suggested that presynaptic inhibition of the primary (Ia) afferent fibers is particularly important. During locomotor activity the level of presynaptic inhibition is rhythmically modulated; this action presumably modulates the strength of reflexes during walking.

Gamma Motor Neurons Provide a Mechanism for Adjusting the Sensitivity of Muscle Spindles

Reflexes that are initiated by stimulation of muscle spindles can also be modulated by changing the level of activity in the gamma motor neurons, which innervate the intrafusal muscle fibers (see Box 36-1). During large muscle contractions the spindle slackens and therefore is unable to signal further changes in muscle length. One role of the gamma motor neurons is to maintain tension in the muscle spindle during active contraction, thereby ensuring its responsiveness at different lengths. When alpha motor neurons are selectively stimulated under experimental conditions, the firing of the spindle sensory fiber shows a characteristic pause during the contraction because the muscle is shortening and therefore unloading (slackening) the spindle. If, however, gamma motor neurons are activated at the same time as alpha motor neurons, the pause becomes filled in because contraction of the intrafusal fibers keeps the central region of the spindle loaded, or under tension (Figure 36-9). Thus, an essential role of intrafusal fiber innervation by gamma motor neurons is to prevent the spindle sensory fiber from falling silent when the muscle shortens as a result of active contraction, therefore enabling it to signal length changes over the full range of muscle lengths.

This mechanism maintains the spindle firing rate within an optimal range for signaling length changes, whatever the actual length of the muscle. In many voluntary movements alpha motor neurons are normally activated more or less in parallel with gamma motor neurons, a pattern referred to as *alpha-gamma coactivation*. This results in an automatic maintenance of sensitivity.

In addition to the axons of the gamma motor neurons, collaterals from alpha motor neurons also innervate the intrafusal fibers. These are referred to as *skeletofusimotor*, or *beta*, efferents. A significant, though still unquantified, amount of skeletofusimotor innervation has been found in spindles in both cats and humans. These efferents provide the equivalent of alpha-gamma coactivation; when skeletofusimotor neurons are activated, unloading of the spindle by contraction of extrafusal fibers is at least partially compensated by loading due to intrafusal contraction.

Nevertheless, the existence of a skeletofusimotor system, with its forced linkage of extrafusal and intrafusal contraction, serves to highlight the importance of the independent fusimotor system made up of the gamma motor neurons. Apparently, mammals have evolved a mechanism that allows for uncoupling the control of muscle spindles from the control of their parent muscles. In principle, this uncoupling would allow greater flexibility in controlling the spindle output for different types of motor tasks.

This conclusion is supported by recordings in primary spindle afferents during a variety of natural movements in cats. The amount and type of activity in

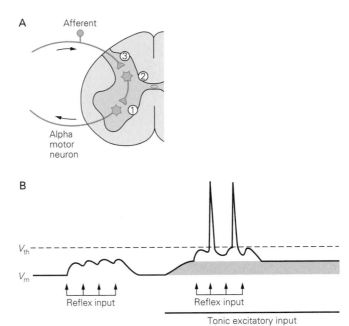

Figure 36-8 The strength of a spinal reflex can be modulated by changes in transmission in the reflex pathway.

A. A reflex pathway can be modified at three sites: (**1**) alpha motor neurons, (**2**) interneurons in polysynaptic pathways, and (**3**) afferent axon terminals. Transmitter release from the primary afferent fibers is regulated by presynaptic inhibition (see Chapter 14).

B. An increase in tonic excitatory input maintains depolarization in the neuron (**shaded**) and enables an otherwise ineffective input to initiate action potentials in the neurons (V_{th} = threshold voltage; V_m = membrane potential).

gamma motor neurons (static or dynamic) are preset at a fairly steady level but vary according to the specific task or context. In general, both static and dynamic gamma motor neurons are set at higher levels as the speed and difficulty of the movement increase. Unpredictable conditions, as when a cat is picked up or handled, lead to marked increases in dynamic gamma activity reflected in increased spindle responsiveness when muscles are stretched. When an animal is performing a difficult task, such as walking across a narrow beam, high levels of both static and dynamic gamma activation are present (Figure 36-10).

Thus, the nervous system uses the fusimotor system—adjusting the level of activation and the balance between activation of static and dynamic gamma motor neurons—to fine-tune the spindles so that the ensemble output of the muscle spindles provides information most appropriate for a task. The task conditions under which independent activation of alpha and gamma motor neurons occurs in humans have not yet been established.

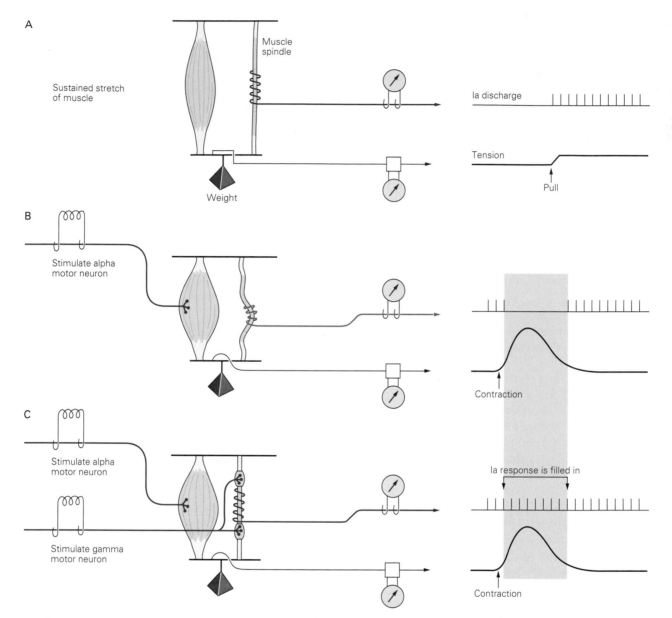

Figure 36-9 Activation of gamma motor neurons during active muscle contraction enables the muscle spindles to continue sensing changes in muscle length. (Adapted from Hunt and Kuffler 1951.)

A. Sustained tension elicits steady firing in the Ia sensory fiber.

B. A characteristic pause occurs in the ongoing discharge of the Ia fiber when the alpha motor neuron alone is stimulated. The Ia fiber stops firing because the spindle is unloaded by the resulting contraction.

C. If a gamma motor neuron to the spindle is also stimulated, the spindle is not unloaded during the contraction and the pause in discharge of the Ia fiber is filled in.

Proprioceptive Reflexes Play an Important Role in the Regulation of Both Voluntary and Automatic Movements

All movements activate receptors in the muscles, joints, and skin. These sensory signals generated by the body's own movements were referred to as *proprioceptive* by Sherrington, who proposed that they control important aspects of normal movements. A good example is the Hering-Breuer reflex, which regulates the amplitude of inspiration. Stretch receptors in the lungs are activated during inspiration, and the Hering-Breuer reflex even-

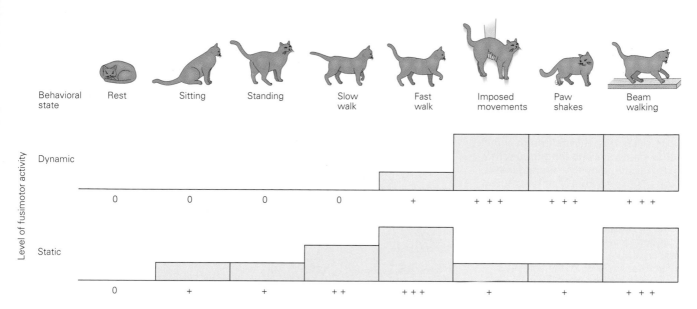

Figure 36-10 Activity in the fusiform system (dynamic and static gamma motor neurons) is set at different levels for different types of behavior. During activities in which muscle length changes slowly and predictably only static gamma motor neurons are active. Dynamic gamma motor neurons are activated during behaviors in which muscle length may change rapidly and unpredictably. (Adapted from Prochazka et al. 1988.)

tually triggers the transition from inspiration to expiration when the lungs are expanded. A similar situation exists in the walking systems of many animals; sensory signals generated near the end of the stance phase initiate the onset of the swing phase (see Chapter 37 for details).

Proprioceptive signals can also contribute to the generation of motor activity during ongoing movements. This has been demonstrated in recent studies on individuals with sensory neuropathy of the arms. These patients have abnormal reaching movements and have difficulty in accurately positioning the limb because the lack of proprioception results in a failure to compensate for the complex inertial properties of the human arm.

The primary function of proprioceptive reflexes in regulating voluntary movements is to adjust the motor output according to the biomechanical state of the body and limbs. This ensures a coordinated pattern of motor activity during an evolving movement, and it provides a mechanism for compensating for the intrinsic variability of motor output.

Reflexes Involving Limb Muscles Are Mediated Through Spinal and Supraspinal Pathways

Reflexes involving the limbs are mediated by multiple pathways acting in parallel via spinal and supraspinal pathways (Figure 36-11A). Consider the response evoked by a sudden stretch of a flexor muscle of the thumb. This response has two discrete components. The first, the M1 response, is generated via the monosynaptic connection of muscle spindle afferents to the spinal motor neurons. The second response, the M2 response, is also a reflex response since its latency is shorter than the voluntary reaction time.

The M2 response has been observed in virtually all limb muscles. In the distal muscles M2 responses are evoked via pathways that include the motor cortex, as shown in studies of patients with Klippel-Feil syndrome (Figure 36-11B). In this unusual condition neurons descending from the motor cortex bifurcate and make connections to homologous motor neurons on both sides of the body. One consequence is that when the individual voluntarily moves the fingers of one hand, these movements are mirrored by movements of the fingers of the other hand. Similarly, when the M2 component is evoked by stretching muscles of one hand, a response with the same latency is evoked in the corresponding muscle of the other hand even though there is no M1 response in the other hand. Thus, the reflex pathway responsible for the M2 response must have traversed the motor cortex.

Reflex responses mediated via the motor cortex and other supraspinal structures are termed *long-loop reflexes*. Long-loop reflexes have been investigated in numerous muscles in humans and other animals. The gen-

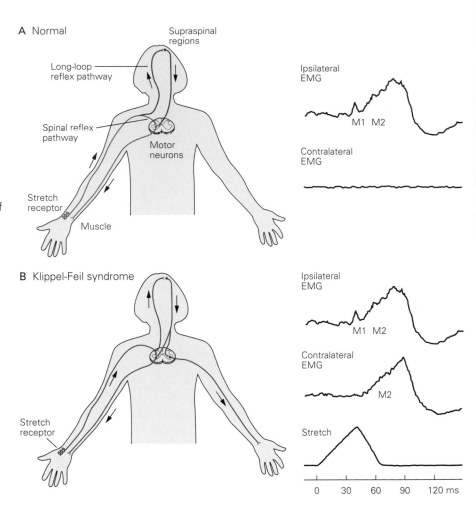

Figure 36-11 Sensory signals produce reflex responses through spinal reflex pathways and long-loop reflex pathways that involve supraspinal regions. (Adapted from Matthews 1991.)

A. In normal individuals a brief stretch of a thumb muscle produces a short-latency M1 response in the stretched muscle followed by a long-latency M2 response. The M2 response is the result of transmission of the sensory signal via the motor cortex.

B. In individuals with Klippel-Feil syndrome M2 response is also evoked in the corresponding thumb muscle of the opposite hand because neurons in the motor cortex activate motor neurons bilaterally. **EMG** = electromyogram.

eral conclusion is that the cortical route for long-loop reflexes may be of primary importance in regulating contractions in distal muscles, while subcortical reflex pathways may be largely responsible for the afferent regulation of proximal muscles. This type of organization is related to functional demands. Many tasks involving distal muscles require precise regulation by voluntary commands. Presumably, the transmission of afferent signals to regions of the cortex most involved in controlling voluntary movements allows the commands to be quickly adapted to the evolving needs of the task. On the other hand, more automatic motor functions, such as maintaining balance and producing gross bodily movements, can be efficiently executed largely via subcortical and spinal pathways.

Stretch Reflexes Reinforce Central Commands for Movements

Proprioceptive reflexes can modulate motor output during voluntary movements because they function not only as discrete reflexes but also as closed feedback loops (Figure 36-12A). For example, stretch of a muscle produces an increase in spindle discharge, leading to muscle contraction and a consequent shortening of the muscle. But this muscle shortening leads to a decrease in spindle discharge, a reduction of muscle contraction, and a lengthening of the muscle. Thus, the stretch reflex loop acts continuously, tending to keep muscle length close to a desired or reference value. This is referred to as feedback because the output of the system (a change in muscle length) is "fed back" and becomes the input. The stretch reflex is a negative feedback system because it tends to counteract or reduce deviations from the reference value of the regulated variable.

In 1963 Ragnar Granit proposed that, in voluntary movements, the reference value is set by descending signals that act on both the alpha and gamma motor neurons. The rate of firing of alpha motor neurons is set to produce the desired shortening of the muscle, while the rate of firing of gamma motor neurons is set to produce an equivalent shortening of the intrafusal fibers of the muscle spindle. If shortening of the whole muscle is less than what is required by a task, as when a load is greater than predicted, spindle afferent fibers increase their firing rate since the contracting intrafusal fibers are stretched (loaded) by the relatively longer length of the whole muscle. If shortening is more than is necessary, spindle afferents decrease their firing rate since the intrafusal fibers are relatively slackened (unloaded).

Thus, one function of the monosynaptic excitatory pathway may be to provide a compensatory mechanism for unexpected alterations in load encountered by the muscles. Although direct evidence for this role of proprioceptive reflexes is lacking, there is strong evidence that alpha and gamma motor neurons are coactivated during voluntary movements by human subjects. In the late 1960s Åke Vallbo and Karl-Erik Hagbarth developed a technique known as microneurography to record from the largest afferents in peripheral nerves. Vallbo later showed that during slow movements of the fingers the primary spindle afferents (group Ia fibers) from the contracting muscles increase their rate of firing even when the muscle shortens as it contracts (Figure 36-12B). The only explanation for this finding is that the gamma motor neurons are active in synchrony with alpha motor neurons.

Further, when subjects attempted to make slow movements at a constant velocity, the trajectory of the movements showed small deviations from a constant velocity—at times the muscle shortened quickly and at others times more slowly. The firing of the Ia sensory fiber mirrored the irregularities in the trajectory. When the velocity of flexion increased transiently, the rate of firing in the Ia fibers decreased because the muscle was shortening more rapidly and therefore exerted less tension on the intrafusal fibers. When the velocity decreased, Ia fiber firing increased because the muscle was shortening more slowly and therefore relative tension on the intrafusal fibers increased. This information can be used by the nervous system to compensate for irregularities in the movement trajectory by exciting the alpha motor neurons.

Thus the stretch reflex may function as a *servomechanism*, that is, a feedback loop in which the output variable (actual muscle length) automatically follows a changing reference value (intended muscle length). In theory this mechanism could permit the nervous system to produce a movement of a given distance without having to know in advance the actual load or weight being moved. In practice, however, the stretch reflex pathways do not exert sufficient influence over motor neurons to overcome large unexpected loads. This is immediately obvious if we consider what happens when we attempt to lift a heavy suitcase that we thought was empty. We have to pause briefly and make a new movement with much greater muscle activation.

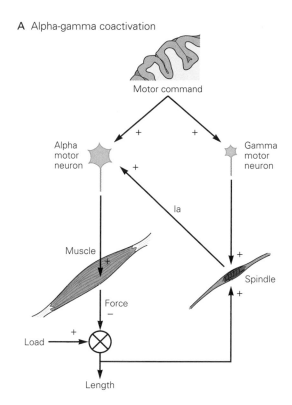

A Alpha-gamma coactivation

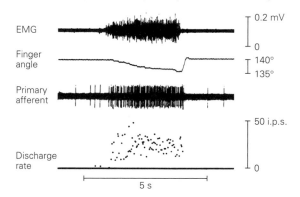

B Increased spindle activity during muscle shortening

Figure 36-12 Alpha and gamma motor neurons are coactivated during voluntary movements.

A. Coactivation of alpha and gamma motor neurons by a motor command allows feedback from muscle spindles to reinforce the activation of the alpha motor neurons. Since any disturbance during the movement alters the length of the muscle and changes the activity in the muscle spindles, altering the spindle input to the alpha motor neuron compensates for the disturbance.

B. Recordings from the primary sensory fiber of a spindle during slow flexion of a finger show the spindle's discharge increasing. This increase in discharge rate depends on alpha-gamma coactivation. If the gamma motor neurons were not active the spindle would slacken and its discharge rate would decrease as the muscle shortened. (Adapted from Vallbo 1981.)

Stretch reflex pathways therefore provide a mechanism for compensating for small changes in load and intrinsic irregularities in the muscle contraction. This action is mediated by both monosynaptic and long-loop pathways, with the relative contribution of each pathway dependent on the muscle and the task.

Damage to the Central Nervous System Produces Characteristic Alterations in Reflex Responses and Muscle Tone

Stretch reflexes can be evoked in many muscles throughout the body and are routinely used in clinical examinations of patients with neurological disorders. These are typically elicited by sharply tapping the tendon of a muscle with a reflex hammer. Hence, they are often referred to as *tendon reflexes* or *tendon jerks*, although the receptor that is stimulated, the muscle spindle, is in the muscle belly, not the tendon. Only the primary sensory fibers in the spindle participate in the tendon reflex since these are selectively activated by the rapid stretch of the muscle produced by the tendon tap. An electrical analog for the tendon jerk reflex is the Hoffmann reflex (Box 36-4).

Measuring alterations in the strength of the stretch reflex can assist in the diagnosis of certain conditions and in the localization of injury or disease in the central nervous system. Absent or weak stretch reflexes often indicate a disorder of one or more of the components of the reflex arc: sensory or motor axons, the cell bodies of motor neurons, or the muscle itself. However, because the excitability of motor neurons is dependent on both excitatory and inhibitory descending influences, either hyperactive or hypoactive stretch reflexes can result from lesions of the central nervous system.

Interruption of Descending Pathways to the Spinal Cord Frequently Produces Spasticity

Muscle tone, the force with which a muscle resists being lengthened, depends on the intrinsic elasticity, or stiffness, of the muscles. Because muscle has elastic elements in series and parallel that resist lengthening, it behaves like a spring. In addition to this intrinsic stiffness, however, there is a neural contribution to muscle tone; the stretch reflex feedback loop also acts to resist lengthening of the muscle. The neural circuits responsible for stretch reflexes provide the higher centers of the nervous system with a mechanism for adjusting muscle tone under different circumstances.

Disorders of muscle tone are frequently associated with lesions of the motor system, especially those that interfere with descending motor pathways, because the strength of stretch reflexes is controlled by higher brain centers. These may involve both abnormal increases in tone (*hypertonus*) and decreases (*hypotonus*). The most common form of hypertonus is spasticity, which is characterized by hyperactive tendon jerks and an increase in resistance to rapid muscle stretch. Slowly applied stretch of a muscle in a patient with spasticity may elicit little resistance. As the speed of the stretch is progressively increased, resistance to the stretch also increases progressively. Thus spasticity is primarily a phasic phenomenon. An active reflex contraction occurs only during a rapid stretch; when the muscle is held in a lengthened position the reflex contraction subsides. In some patients, however, the hypertonus also has a tonic component; that is, the reflex contraction continues even after the muscle is no longer being lengthened.

The pathophysiology of spasticity is still unclear. It was long thought that the increased gain of stretch reflexes in spasticity resulted from hyperactivity of the gamma motor neurons. Recent experiments, however, have cast doubt on this explanation. While gamma overactivity may be present in some cases, changes in the background activity of alpha motor neurons and interneurons are probably a more important factor.

Whatever the precise mechanism that produces spasticity, the effect is a strong facilitation of transmission in the monosynaptic reflex pathway from Ia sensory fibers to alpha motor neurons. Indeed, this has been the basis for therapeutic treatment. A common procedure today is to mimic presynaptic inhibition in the terminals of the Ia fibers. This is done by intrathecally administering the drug baclofen to the spinal cord. This drug is an agonist of the γ-aminobutyric acid $(GABA)_B$ receptors; binding of GABA to these receptors decreases the influx of calcium into the presynaptic terminals and hence reduces the amount of transmitter released.

Transection of the Spinal Cord in Humans Leads to a Period of Spinal Shock Followed by Hyperreflexia

Damage to the spinal cord can cause large changes in the strength of spinal reflexes. Each year about 10,000 individuals in the United States have spinal cord injuries in which the cord is effectively damaged. More than half of these injuries produce permanent disability, including impairment of motor and sensory functions (Box 36-5) and disruption of voluntary control of bowel and bladder function.

When transection is complete there is usually a period immediately after the accident when all spinal reflexes below the level of the transection are reduced or completely suppressed. This condition is known as

Box 36-4 The Hoffmann Reflex

An important technique, based on early work by P. Hoffmann, was introduced in the 1950s to examine the characteristics of the monosynaptic connections from Ia sensory fibers to spinal motor neurons in humans. This technique involves electrically stimulating the Ia fibers in a peripheral nerve and recording the reflex response in the homonymous muscle. This is known as the *Hoffmann reflex*, or *H-reflex* (Figure 36-13A).

The H-reflex is readily measured in the soleus muscle (an ankle extensor). The Ia fibers from the soleus and its synergists are excited by an electrode placed above the tibial nerve behind the knee. The response recorded from the soleus muscle depends on stimulus strength. At low stimulus strengths a pure H-reflex is evoked, since the threshold for activation of the Ia fibers is lower than the threshold for motor axons. As the stimulus strength is increased, motor axons supplying the soleus are excited and two distinct responses are recorded. The first results from direct activation of the motor axons, and the second is the H-reflex evoked by stimulation of the Ia fibers (Figure 36-13B). These two components of the evoked electromyogram are called the *M-wave* and the *H-wave*, respectively. The H-wave occurs later because it results from signals that travel to the spinal cord, across a synapse, and back again to the muscle. The M-wave, in contrast, results from direct stimulation of the muscle.

As the stimulus strength is increased still further, the M-wave continues to become larger and the H-wave progressively declines (Figure 36-13C). The decline in the H-wave amplitude occurs because action potentials in the motor axons propagate toward the cell body (antidromic conduction) and cancel reflexively evoked action potentials in the same motor axons. At very high stimulus strengths only the M-wave is evoked.

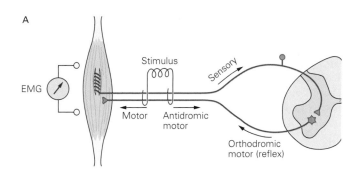

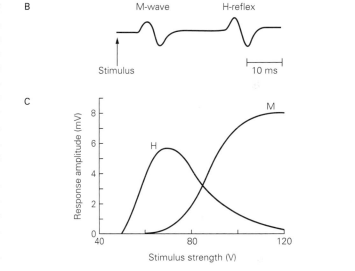

Figure 36-13

A. The H-reflex is evoked by direct electrical stimulation of afferent sensory fibers from primary spindle endings in mixed nerves. The evoked volley in the sensory fibers monosynaptically excites alpha motor neurons, which in turn activate the muscle. Muscle activation is detected by recording the electromyogram (**EMG**) from the muscles. At very low stimulus strengths a pure H-reflex can be evoked because the axons from the primary spindle endings have a lower threshold for activation than all other axons.

B. As the stimulus strength is increased, motor axons are excited and spindle afferents are activated. The former produces the M-wave that precedes the H-reflex in the EMG.

C. The magnitude of the H-reflex declines at high stimulus strengths because the signals generated reflexively in the motor axon are cancelled by action potentials initiated by the electrical stimulus in the same motor axons. At very high stimulus strengths only an M-wave is evoked. (Adapted from Schieppati 1987.)

---

spinal shock. During the course of weeks and months spinal reflexes gradually return, often greatly exaggerated compared with normal. For example, a light touch to the skin of one foot may elicit a strong flexion withdrawal reflex of the leg.

The mechanisms underlying spinal shock and recovery are poorly understood. The initial shock is considered to be due to the sudden withdrawal of tonic facilitatory influence from the brain. Several different mechanisms may contribute to the recovery: denervation supersensitivity, increased numbers of postsynaptic receptors, and sprouting of afferent terminals. Interestingly, the period of recov-

Box 36-5 Sensory and Motor Signs of Spinal Cord Lesions

Lesions of the spinal cord give rise to motor or sensory symptoms that are often related to a particular sensory or motor segmental level of the spinal cord. Identification of the level of sensory or motor loss is crucial for recognizing focal lesions within the spinal cord or external compressive lesions that interrupt function below the level of the damage. Key landmarks for locating sensory and motor lesions are listed in Tables 36-2 and 36-3.

Table 36-2 Indicators of Motor Level Lesions

Root	Major muscles affected	Reflex loss
C3-5	Diaphragm	—
C5	Deltoid, biceps	Biceps
C7	Triceps, extensors of wrist and fingers	Triceps
C8	Interossei, abductor of fifth finger	—
L2-4	Quadriceps	Knee jerk
L5	Long extensor of great toe, anterior tibial	—
S1	Plantar flexors, gastrocnemius	Ankle jerk

Motor Signs

When motor roots are injured, or when motor neurons are affected focally, symptoms in the affected muscles include weakness, wasting, fasciculation, and loss of tendon reflexes. When descending motor tracts are injured, symptoms in the muscles innervated below the level of the lesions include weakness, increased tendon reflexes, and spasticity. For unilateral lesions of the spinal cord motor signs will almost always be ipsilateral, since the main motor tracts, and especially the corticospinal tract, cross in the brain stem and descend on the same side of the spinal cord as the motor neurons they innervate.

Sensory Signs

The characteristic pattern of sensory loss is loss of cutaneous sensation below the level of the lesion. For unilateral lesions, however, the pattern may be complex. The pathway carrying pain and temperature information *(the anterolateral system)* ascends on the opposite side of the cord, while the pathway responsible for discriminative touch, vibration sense, and position sense ascends on the same side of the cord. In addition, it is necessary to distinguish between sensory loss resulting from spinal lesions and sensory loss caused by lesions of peripheral nerves or isolated nerve roots.

When multiple peripheral nerves are affected by disease *(polyneuropathy)*, cutaneous sensation loss occurs in the hands and feet (Figure 36-14A). This predominantly distal pattern is attributed to impaired axonal transport, or *dying back* (Chapter 16). The parts most affected are those most distant from the sensory neuron cell bodies in the dorsal root ganglia. When single peripheral nerves or sensory roots are injured, the distribution of sensory loss is more restricted and can be recognized by reference to sensory charts (Figure 36-15).

Complete Transection of the Spinal Cord

Complete transection of the spinal cord leads to loss of all sensation and all voluntary movement below the level of the lesion (Figure 36-14B). Bladder and bowel control are also lost. If the lesion is above C3, breathing may be affected. It is important to remember that the spinal cord ends at the level of the base of the second lumbar vertebra. Below this level the spinal

Table 36-3 Indicators of Sensory Level Lesions

Root	Major sensory areas affected
C4	Clavicle
C8	Fifth finger
T4	Nipples
T10	Umbilicus
L1	Inguinal ligament
L3	Anterior surface of the thigh
L5	Great toe
S1	Lateral aspect of the foot
S3-5	Perineum

canal is occupied by the lower nerve roots. Therefore, injuries to the spinal canal below vertebral level L2 cause sensory loss in the regions of the body innervated by the lower lumbar and sacral nerve roots as well as weakness and decreased tendon reflexes in certain leg muscles (Figure 36-14C).

Partial Transection

With partial transection of the spinal cord some ascending or descending tracts may be spared. Partial function is retained but specific motor and sensory signs are evident. Hemisection of the spinal cord, also called Brown-Séquard syndrome, causes a characteristic and easily recognized pattern (Figure 36-14D). If one side of the cord is transected, there are ipsilateral weakness and spasticity in certain muscle groups (corticospinal tract), ipsilateral loss of discriminative touch, vibration, and position sense (dorsal column), and contralateral loss of pain and temperature (anterolateral system). While a precise hemisection is quite rare, this syndrome is fairly common since many traumatic lesions predominately affect one side of the cord or the other.

Another example of a lesion that causes an incomplete transection is *syringomyelia*, a condition in which cysts form within the central portion of the spinal cord and progressively worsen. Because the lesions start centrally, the first fibers to be affected are those carrying pain and temperature fibers, since they decussate in the anterior commissure. This usually causes bilateral loss of pain and temperature sensation, restricted to the segments involved (Figure 36-14E). Unless and until the cysts significantly enlarge, discriminative touch and position sense are usually spared.

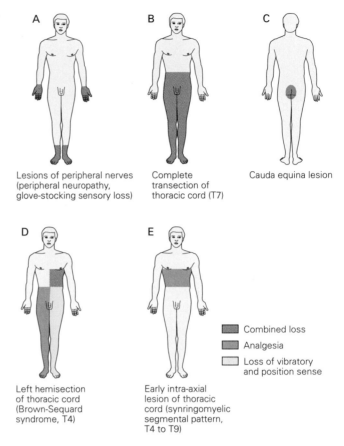

A Lesions of peripheral nerves (peripheral neuropathy, glove-stocking sensory loss)

B Complete transection of thoracic cord (T7)

C Cauda equina lesion

D Left hemisection of thoracic cord (Brown-Sequard syndrome, T4)

E Early intra-axial lesion of thoracic cord (synringomyelic segmental pattern, T4 to T9)

■ Combined loss
■ Analgesia
□ Loss of vibratory and position sense

Figure 36-14 Sensory deficits resulting from damage to the spinal cord or nerve roots (segmental) and deficits resulting from damage to peripheral nerves.

(Continued)

Box 36-5 Sensory and Motor Signs of Spinal Cord Lesions (continued)

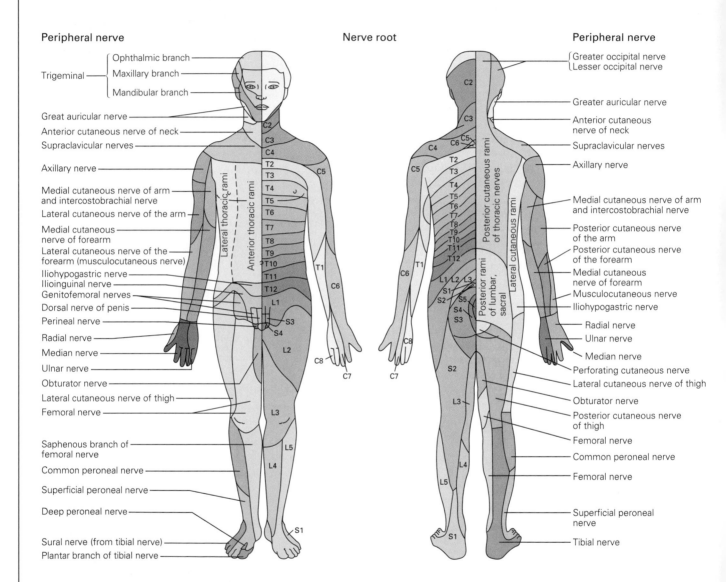

Peripheral nerve

Trigeminal
- Ophthalmic branch
- Maxillary branch
- Mandibular branch

Great auricular nerve
Anterior cutaneous nerve of neck
Supraclavicular nerves
Axillary nerve
Medial cutaneous nerve of arm and intercostobrachial nerve
Lateral cutaneous nerve of the arm
Medial cutaneous nerve of forearm
Lateral cutaneous nerve of the forearm (musculocutaneous nerve)
Iliohypogastric nerve
Ilioinguinal nerve
Genitofemoral nerves
Dorsal nerve of penis
Perineal nerve
Radial nerve
Median nerve
Ulnar nerve
Obturator nerve
Lateral cutaneous nerve of thigh
Femoral nerve
Saphenous branch of femoral nerve
Common peroneal nerve
Superficial peroneal nerve
Deep peroneal nerve
Sural nerve (from tibial nerve)
Plantar branch of tibial nerve

Nerve root

Peripheral nerve

Greater occipital nerve
Lesser occipital nerve
Greater auricular nerve
Anterior cutaneous nerve of neck
Supraclavicular nerves
Axillary nerve
Medial cutaneous nerve of arm and intercostobrachial nerve
Posterior cutaneous nerve of the arm
Posterior cutaneous nerve of the forearm
Medial cutaneous nerve of forearm
Musculocutaneous nerve
Iliohypogastric nerve
Radial nerve
Ulnar nerve
Median nerve
Perforating cutaneous nerve
Lateral cutaneous nerve of thigh
Obturator nerve
Posterior cutaneous nerve of thigh
Femoral nerve
Common peroneal nerve
Femoral nerve
Superficial peroneal nerve
Tibial nerve

Figure 36-15 Maps of cutaneous innervation of the body differ depending on whether one is looking at the areas of skin innervated by nerve roots (center) or peripheral nerves (right and left). By carefully mapping the area of sensory loss, therefore, one can determine the locus of damage (nerve root or peripheral nerve) and the specific nerves or roots involved. Note that the area of skin innervated by a single nerve root is often referred to as a dermatome.

ery from spinal shock is much shorter in animals than in humans. In nonhuman primates the recovery period is rarely more than a week; in cats and dogs it is only a few hours. The longer recovery period for humans presumably reflects the greater influence of descending input on spinal reflex circuits. This may in turn reflect the increased complexity of upright bipedal locomotion. Indeed, as we shall see in the next chapter, in humans with spinal cord injury recovery of automatic locomotor patterns is slight when compared with that of quadrupedal mammals.

An Overall View

Reflexes are coordinated, involuntary motor responses initiated by a stimulus applied to peripheral receptors. Some reflexes initiate movements to avoid potentially hazardous situations, whereas others automatically adapt motor patterns to maintain, or to achieve, a behavioral goal. The purposeful responses evoked by reflexes depend on mechanisms that set the strength and pattern of responses according to the task and behavioral state (known as functional set). Currently we know little about the details of these mechanisms, except for the fact that modification of transmission in spinal reflex pathways by descending signals from the brain is thought to be an important factor.

Many groups of interneurons in the reflex pathways of the spinal cord are also involved in producing complex movements such as walking and transmitting voluntary commands from the brain. In addition, some components of reflex responses, particularly components of reflexes involving the limbs, are mediated via supraspinal centers (brain stem nuclei, cerebellum, and motor cortex). The convergence of afferent signals onto spinal and supraspinal interneuronal systems involved in initiating movements provides the basis for the smooth integration of reflexes into centrally generated motor commands. Establishing details of these integrative events is one of the major challenges of contemporary research on reflex regulation of movement.

Because descending pathways from the brain continuously modulate transmission in spinal reflex pathways, damage or disease of the central nervous system often results in significant alterations in the strength of spinal reflexes. The pattern of changes is an important aid to diagnosis of patients with neurological disorders.

Keir Pearson
James Gordon

Selected Readings

Baldissera F, Hultborn H, Illert M. 1981. Integration in spinal neuronal systems. In: JM Brookhart, VB Mountcastle, VB Brooks, SR Geiger (eds). *Handbook of Physiology: The Nervous System,* pp. 509–595. Bethesda, MD: American Physiological Society.

Boyd IA. 1980. The isolated mammalian muscle spindle. Trends Neurosci 3:258–265.

Dietz V. 1992. Human neuronal control of automatic functional movements: interaction between central programs and afferent input. Physiol Rev 72:33–61.

Jankowska E. 1992. Interneuronal relay in spinal pathways from proprioceptors. Prog Neurobiol 38:335–378.

Matthews PBC. 1991. The human stretch reflex and the motor cortex. Trends Neurosci 14:87–90.

Prochazka A. 1996. Proprioceptive feedback and movement regulation. In: L Rowell, JT Sheperd (eds). *Handbook of Physiology: Regulation and Integration of Multiple Systems,* pp. 89–127. New York: American Physiological Society.

References

Appenteng K, Prochazka A. 1984. Tendon organ firing during active muscle lengthening in normal cats. J Physiol (Lond) 353:81–92.

Brown MC, Matthews PBC. 1966. On the sub-division of the efferent fibres to muscle spindles into static and dynamic fusimotor fibres. In: BL Andrew (ed). *Control and Innervation of Skeletal Muscle,* pp. 18–31. Dundee, Scotland: University of St. Andrews.

Cole KJ, Gracco VL, Abbs JH. 1984. Autogenetic and nonautogenetic sensorimotor actions in the control of multiarticulate hand movements. Exp Brain Res 56:582–585.

Crago A, Houk JC, Rymer WZ. 1982. Sampling of total muscle force by tendon organs. J Neurophysiol 47:1069–1083.

Gossard JP, Brownstone RM, Barajon I, Hultborn H. 1994. Transmission in a locomotor-related group Ib pathway from hindlimb extensor muscles in the cat. Exp Brain Res 98:213–228.

Granit R. 1970. *Basis of Motor Control.* London: Academic.

Hagbarth KE, Kunesch EJ, Nordin M, Schmidt R, Wallin EU. 1986. Gamma loop contributing to maximal voluntary contractions in man. J Physiol (Lond) 380:575–591.

Hoffman P. 1922. *Untersuchungen über die Eigenreflexe (Sehuenreflexe) menschlicher Muskeln.* Berlin: Springer.

Hulliger M. 1984. The mammalian muscle spindle and its central control. Rev Physiol Biochem Pharmacol 101:1–110.

Hunt CC, Kuffler SW. 1951. Stretch receptor discharges during muscle contraction. J Physiol (Lond) 113:298–315.

Liddell EGT, Sherrington C. 1924. Reflexes in response to stretch (myotatic reflexes). Proc R Soc Lond B Biol Sci 96:212–242.

Marsden CD, Merton PA, Morton HB. 1981. Human postural responses. Brain 104:513–534.

Matthews PBC. 1972. *Muscle Receptors.* London: Edward Arnold.

Mendell LM, Henneman E. 1971. Terminals of single Ia

fibers: location, density, and distribution within a pool of 300 homonymous motoneurons. J Neurophysiol 34:171–187.

Pearson KG, Collins DF. 1993. Reversal of the influence of group Ib afferents from plantaris on activity in model gastrocnemius activity during locomotor activity. J Neurophysiol 70:1009–1017.

Prochazka A, Hulliger M, Trend P, Dürmüller N. 1988. Dynamic and static fusimotor set in various behavioural contexts. In: P Hnik, T Soukup, R Vejsada, J Zelena (eds). *Mechanoreceptors: Development, Structure and Function*, pp. 417–430. New York: Plenum.

Schieppati M. 1987. The Hoffman reflex: a means of assessing spinal reflex excitability and its descending control in man. Prog Neurobiol 28:345–376.

Schmidt RF. 1983. Motor systems. In: RF Schmidt and G Thews (eds), MA Biederman-Thorson (transl). *Human Physiology*, pp. 81–110. Berlin: Springer.

Sherrington CS. 1906. *Integrative Actions of the Nervous System*. New Haven, CT: Yale Univ. Press.

Swett JE, Schoultz TW. 1975. Mechanical transduction in the Golgi tendon organ: a hypothesis. Arch Italian Biol 113:374–382.

Vallbo ÅB. 1981. Basic patterns of muscle spindle discharge in man. In: A Taylor and A Prochazka (eds). *Muscle Receptors and Movement*, pp. 263–275. London: Macmillan.

Vallbo ÅB, Hagbarth KE, Torebjörk HE, Wallin BG. 1979. Somatosensory, proprioceptive, and sympathetic activity in human peripheral nerves. Physiol Rev 59:919–957.

37

Locomotion

A N ESSENTIAL FEATURE OF animal life is the ability to move from one place to another. Although many different forms of locomotion have evolved, including swimming, crawling, flying, and walking, a common feature is rhythmic and alternating movements of the body or appendages. Its rhythmicity makes locomotion appear to be a stereotyped action involving repetitions of the same movements. Indeed, we shall see that this repetitive quality allows locomotion to be controlled automatically at relatively low levels of the nervous system without intervention by higher centers. Nevertheless, locomotion usually takes place in unpredictable environments. Therefore locomotor movements must be continually modified, usually in a subtle fashion, to adapt otherwise stereotyped movement patterns to the immediate surroundings.

Thus, in the study of the neural control of locomotion neurobiologists must address two fundamental questions. First, how do systems of nerve cells generate the rhythmic motor patterns associated with locomotor movements? Second, how does sensory information modify these patterns to adjust the locomotor movements to both anticipated and unexpected events in the environment? In this chapter we address both these questions by examining the mammalian neural mechanisms controlling walking. Most of our information on walking has come from studying the control of the cat's stepping movements. However, important insights have come from other animals, as well as from studies on rhythmic behaviors other than locomotion. Therefore, we shall also consider the more general issue of how rhythmic motor activity can be generated and sustained by networks of neurons.

Several critical insights into the mammalian neural mechanisms controlling stepping were made nearly a

Box 37-1 Preparations Used to Study the Neural Control of Stepping

The literature on the neural control of stepping can be confusing because different experimental preparations are used in different studies. In addition to intact animals, two reduced preparations, spinal and decerebrate cats, are commonly used in studies of the neural mechanisms of locomotor rhythmicity. Two additional experimental strategies, deafferentation and immobilization, are used with each of these preparations, depending on what is being investigated. Finally, a neonatal rat preparation has recently been introduced that promises to be useful for analyzing the cellular properties of neurons generating the locomotor rhythm.

Spinal Preparations

In spinal preparations the spinal cord is transected at the lower thoracic level (Figure 37-1A), thus isolating the spinal segments that control the hind limb musculature from the rest of the central nervous system. This allows investigations on the role of spinal circuits in generating rhythmic locomotor patterns.

In *acute* spinal preparations adrenergic drugs such as L-DOPA and nialamide are administered immediately after the transection. These drugs elevate the level of norepinephrine in the spinal cord and lead to the spontaneous generation of locomotor activity about 30 minutes after administration. Clonidine, another adrenergic drug, enables locomotor activity to be generated in acute spinal preparations but only if the skin of the perineal region is also stimulated.

In *chronic* spinal preparations animals are studied for weeks or months after transection. Locomotor activity without drug treatment can return within a few weeks of cord transection. Locomotor function returns spontaneously in kittens, but in adult cats daily training sessions are usually required.

Decerebrate Preparations

In decerebrate preparations the brain stem is completely transected at the level of the midbrain, preventing more rostral brain centers, especially the cerebral cortex, from influencing the locomotor pattern. These preparations allow investigation of the role of the cerebellum and structures in the brain stem in controlling locomotion.

Two decerebrate preparations are commonly used. In one the locomotor rhythm is generated spontaneously, while in the other it is evoked by electrical stimulation of the mesencephalic locomotor region. This difference depends on the level of decerebration. Spontaneous walking occurs in *premammillary preparations,* in which the brain stem is transected from the anterior margin of the superior colliculi to a point immediately rostral to the mammillary bodies. When the transection is made caudal to the mammillary bodies, spontaneous stepping does not occur; rather, electrical stimulation of the mesencephalic locomotor region is required to evoke walking (Figure 37-1B). When supported on a motorized treadmill both preparations walk with a coordinated stepping pattern in all

four limbs, and the rate of stepping is matched to the treadmill speed. The motor activity can be recorded during stepping, and sensory nerves can be stimulated via implanted electrodes to examine reflex mechanisms regulating stepping.

Deafferented Preparations

An early view of the neural control of locomotion was that it involved a "chaining" of proprioceptive reflexes; successive stretch reflexes in flexor and extensor muscles were thought to produce the basic rhythm of walking. This view was disproved by Graham Brown, who showed that rhythmic locomotor patterns were generated even after complete removal of all sensory input from the moving limbs.

Deafferentation is accomplished by transection of all the dorsal roots that innervate the limbs. Since the dorsal roots carry only sensory axons, motor innervation of the muscles remains intact. Deafferented preparations were once useful for demonstrating the capabilities of isolated spinal cord but are rarely used today, principally because the loss of all tonic sensory input drastically reduces the excitability of interneurons and motor neurons in the spinal cord. Thus, changes in the locomotor pattern after deafferentation might result from the artificial reduction in excitability of neurons rather than from the loss of specific sensory inputs.

Immobilized Preparations

The role of specific sensory input from the limbs can be more systematically investigated by preventing the motor neurons from actually causing any movement. This is typically accomplished by paralyzing the muscles with *d*-tubocurare, a competitive inhibitor of acetylcholine that blocks synaptic transmission at the neuromuscular junction. When locomotion is initiated in such an immobilized preparation, often referred to as *fictive locomotion,* the motor nerves to flexor and extensor muscles fire alternately but no actual movement takes place. Thus, the effect of proprioceptive reflexes is removed while tonic sensory input is preserved. Because immobilized preparations allow intracellular and extracellular recording from neurons in the spinal cord, they are used to examine the synaptic events associated with locomotor activity and the organization of central and reflex pathways controlling locomotion.

Neonatal Rat Preparation

When the spinal cord is removed from neonatal rats (0–5 days after birth) and placed in a saline bath, it will generate coordinated bursts of activity in leg motor neurons when exposed to NMDA and serotonin (Figure 37-1C). This promising new preparation allows more detailed analysis of the locations and roles of the specific neurons involved in rhythm generation, as well as pharmacological studies on the rhythm-generating network.

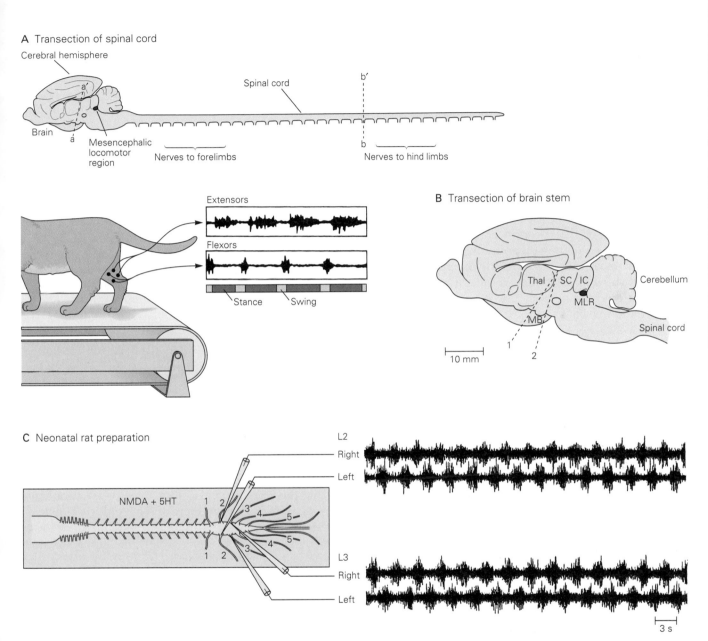

Figure 37-1

A. Transection of the spinal cord of a cat at the level of **b–b'** isolates the hind limb segments of the cord, but the hind limbs are still able to step on a treadmill (either immediately after recovery from surgery if adrenergic drugs are administered or a few weeks after surgery if the animal is exercised regularly on the treadmill). Locomotor patterns can also be evoked in spinal animals after eliminating all phasic sensory feedback, either by cutting the dorsal roots or immobilizing the animal with curare. Transection of the brain stem at the level a–a' isolates the spinal cord and lower brain stem from the cerebral hemispheres.

B. Depending on the exact level of the transection of the brain stem, locomotion either occurs spontaneously (**cut 1**) or can be

initiated by electrical stimulation of the mesencephalic locomotor region (**MLR**) after a more caudal transection (**cut 2**). The MLR is a small region of the brain stem close to the cuneiform nucleus about 6 mm below the surface of the inferior colliculus (**IC**). **Thal** = thalamus; **SC** = superior colliculus; **MB** = mammillary body.

C. The spinal cord is removed from a neonatal animal (0–5 days of age) and placed in a saline bath. Addition of *N*-methyl-D-aspartate (NMDA) and serotonin (5-hydroxytryptamine, or 5-HT) to the bath elicits rhythmic bursting in the motor neurons supplying leg muscles. Intracellular or patch clamp recordings can be made from lumbar neurons during periods of rhythmic activity. (Adapted from Cazalets et al. 1995.)

century ago when it was found that removing the cerebral hemispheres in dogs did not abolish walking. These animals walked spontaneously, and one was observed to rear itself in order to rest its forepaws on a gate at feeding time. It was soon discovered that stepping of the hind legs could be induced in cats and dogs after complete transection of the spinal cord. The stepping movements in these *spinal preparations* (Box 37-1) were similar to normal stepping. Nonrhythmic electrical stimulation of the cut cord elicited stepping, with the rate of stepping related to the intensity of the stimulating current. Another important early observation was that passive movement of a limb by the experimenter could initiate stepping movements in spinal cats and dogs, suggesting that proprioceptive reflexes have a crucial role in regulating stepping movements. Finally, in 1911 Thomas Graham Brown discovered that rhythmic, alternating contractions could be evoked in deafferented hind leg muscles immediately after transection of the spinal cord.

Four conclusions can drawn from these early studies:

1. Supraspinal structures are not necessary for producing the basic motor pattern for stepping.
2. The basic rhythmicity of stepping is produced by neuronal circuits contained entirely within the spinal cord.
3. The spinal circuits can be activated by tonic descending signals from the brain.
4. The spinal pattern-generating networks do not require sensory input but nevertheless are strongly regulated by input from limb proprioceptors.

For almost half a century after these early studies few investigations were aimed at establishing the neural mechanisms for walking. During this period research on the motor systems focused on establishing the organization of reflex pathways and the mechanisms of synaptic integration within the spinal cord (see Chapter 36). Contemporary research on the neural control of locomotion dates from the 1960s and two major experimental successes. First, rhythmic patterns of motor activity were evoked in spinal preparations by the application of adrenergic drugs (Box 37-1). Second, walking on a treadmill was evoked in decerebrate cats by electrical stimulation of a small region in the brain stem. At about the same time the first electromyographic recordings were made from numerous hind leg muscles during unrestrained walking in intact cats. These recordings revealed the complexity of the locomotor pattern and brought to prominence the question of how spinal reflexes are integrated into intrinsic spinal circuits to produce the locomotor pattern.

A Complex Sequence of Muscle Contractions Is Required for Stepping

For the purpose of examining the patterns of muscle contraction during locomotion the step cycle in cats and humans can be divided into four distinct phases: flexion (F), first extension (E_1), second extension (E_2), and third extension (E_3) (Figure 37-2A). The F and E_1 phases occur during the time the foot is off the ground (*swing*), while E_2 and E_3 occur when the foot is in contact with the ground (*stance*).

Swing commences with flexion at the hip, knee, and ankle (the F phase). Approximately midway through swing the knee and ankle begin to extend while the hip continues to flex (the E_1 phase). Extension at the knee and ankle during E_1 moves the foot ahead of the body and prepares the leg to accept weight, in anticipation of foot contact at the onset of stance. During early stance (the E_2 phase) the knee and ankle joints flex, even though extensor muscles are contracting strongly. The lengthening of the contracting ankle and knee extensor muscles is due to weight being transferred to the leg. The yielding of these muscles as weight is accepted allows the body to move smoothly over the foot and is essential for establishing an efficient gait. During late stance (the E_3 phase) the hip, knee, and ankle all extend to provide a propulsive force to move the body forward.

The rhythmic movements of the legs during stepping are produced by contractions of a large number of muscles. In general, contractions of flexor muscles occur during the F phase, and contractions of extensor muscles occur during one or more of the E phases. However, the timing and level of activity in different muscles vary widely (Figure 37-2B). For example, the hip flexor muscle (iliopsoas) contracts continuously during the F and E_1 phases, while the knee flexor muscle (semitendinosus) contracts briefly at the beginning of each of these phases. An additional complexity is that some muscles contract during both swing and stance. The complex sequence of muscle contractions is the *motor pattern for stepping*.

The Motor Pattern for Stepping in Mammals Is Produced at the Spinal Level

Transection of the spinal cord of quadrupeds initially causes complete paralysis of the hind legs. However, this operation does not permanently abolish the capacity of hind legs to make stepping movements; hind leg stepping often recovers spontaneously over a period of a few weeks, particularly if the transection is made in young animals. Recovery of stepping in adult cats can

A Four phases of the step cycle

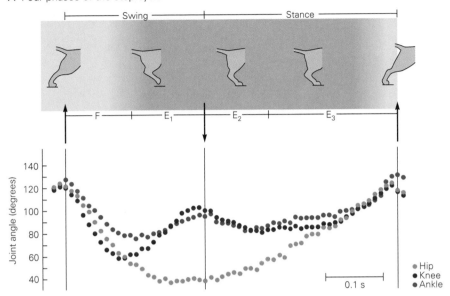

B Activity in hind leg muscles during the step cycle

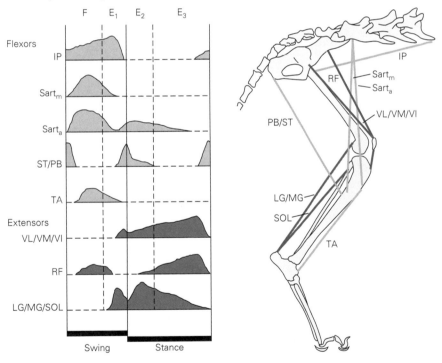

Figure 37-2 Stepping is produced by complex patterns of contractions in leg muscles.

A. The step cycle is divided into four phases: flexion (F) and first extension (E₁) occur during swing, and second extension (E₂) and third extension (E₃) occur during stance. Second extension is characterized by flexion at the knee and the ankle resulting from the animal's weight. The contracting knee and ankle extensor muscles lengthen during this phase. (Adapted from Engberg and Lundberg 1969.)

B. Profiles of electrical activity in some of the hind leg flexor

and extensor muscles in the cat during stepping. Although activity of flexor and extensor muscles generally occurs during swing and stance, respectively, the overall pattern of activity is complex in both timing and amplitude. The positions of the muscles are illustrated on the right. **IP** = iliopsoas; **LG** and **MG** = lateral and medial gastrocnemius; **PB** = posterior biceps; **RF** = rectus femorus; **Sart_m** and **Sart_a** = medial and anterior sartorius; **SOL** = soleus; **ST** = semitendinosus; **TA** = tibialis anterior; **VL, VM,** and **VI** = vastus lateralis, medialis, and intermedialis.

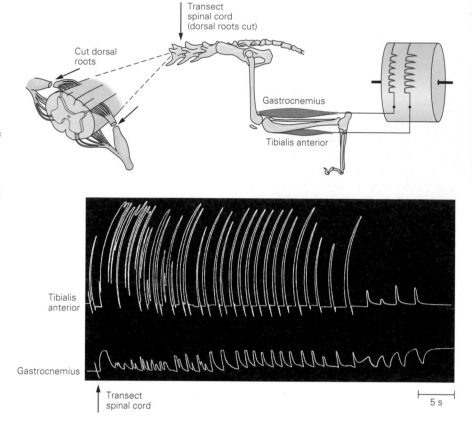

Figure 37-3 Rhythmic activity for walking is generated by networks of neurons in the spinal cord. The existence of such spinal networks was first demonstrated by Thomas Graham Brown in 1911. Graham Brown developed an experimental animal system in which dorsal root nerves were cut so that sensory information from the limbs could not reach the spinal cord. An original record from Graham Brown's study shows that rhythmic alternating contractions of ankle flexor (tibialis anterior) and extensor (gastrocnemius) muscles begin very soon after transection of the spinal cord.

be facilitated by daily training on a treadmill combined with nonspecific cutaneous stimulation of the perineal region. In chronic spinal cats electromyographic records from hind leg muscles during stepping are very similar to those from normal walking animals. Many of the reflex responses occurring in normal animals can be evoked in spinal animals.

Neuronal Networks Within the Spinal Cord Generate Rhythmic Alternating Activity in Flexor and Extensor Muscles

From the studies by Graham Brown early in the twentieth century we know that the isolated spinal cord can generate rhythmic bursts of reciprocal activity in flexor and extensor motor neurons of the hind legs even in the absence of sensory input (Figure 37-3). Graham Brown proposed that contractions in the flexor and extensor muscles were controlled by two systems of neurons, which he termed *half-centers*, that mutually inhibit each other. He suggested that the switching of activity from one half-center to the other depended on fatigue in the inhibitory connections.

The half-center hypothesis was supported by studies in the 1960s of the effects of the drug L-dihydroxyphenylalanine (L-DOPA, a precursor for the monoamine transmitters dopamine and norepinephrine) in spinal cats. After the cats were treated with L-DOPA, brief trains of electrical stimuli were applied to small-diameter cutaneous and muscle afferents. These evoked long-lasting bursts of activity in either flexor or extensor motor neurons depending on whether ipsilateral or contralateral nerves were stimulated. Collectively the group of small-diameter afferents producing these effects are referred to as *flexor reflex afferents* (FRA). Additional administration of nialamide (a drug prolonging the action of released norepinephrine in the spinal cord) often resulted in short sequences of rhythmic reciprocal activity in flexor and extensor motor neurons (Figure 37-4A).

The system of interneurons generating the flexor bursts was found to inhibit the system of interneurons generating the extensor bursts, and vice versa (Figure 37-4B). This organizational feature is consistent with Graham Brown's notion that mutually inhibiting half-centers produce the alternating burst activity in flexor

Figure 37-4 Elements of the central pattern generator are revealed by electrical stimulation of high-threshold cutaneous and muscle afferents (flexor reflex afferents, FRA) in spinal cats treated with L-DOPA (L-dihydroxyphenylalanine) and nialamide.

A. Brief stimulation of ipsilateral FRA evokes a short sequence of rhythmic activity in flexor and extensor motor neurons. (Adapted from Jankowska et al. 1967a.)

B. Reciprocal inhibition between interneurons in the pathways mediating long-latency reflexes from the ipsilateral and contralateral FRA. This half-center organization of the flexor and extensor interneurons is likely the basis for central rhythm generation for stepping. **MN** = motor neuron.

C. Interneurons in the half-centers are located in the intermediate region of the gray matter. Delayed, long-duration bursts of activity are evoked in these interneurons by stimulation of the ipsilateral FRA. (Adapted from Jankowska et al. 1967b.)

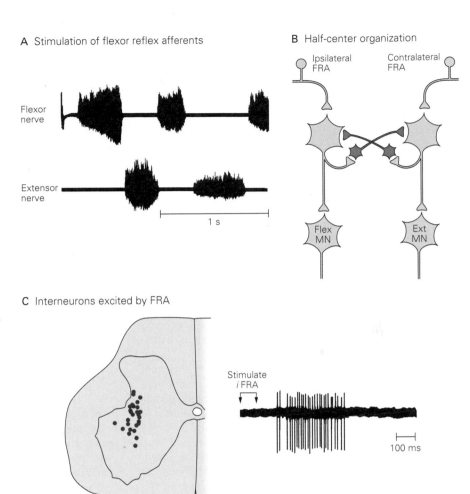

A Stimulation of flexor reflex afferents

Flexor nerve

Extensor nerve

1 s

B Half-center organization

Ipsilateral FRA   Contralateral FRA

Flex MN   Ext MN

C Interneurons excited by FRA

Stimulate *i* FRA

100 ms

and extensor motor neurons. The interneurons mediating the reflexes from the flexor reflex afferents have not yet been fully identified, but they may include interneurons in the intermediate region of the gray matter in the sixth lumbar segment. Interneurons in this region of the cord produce prolonged bursts of activity in response to brief stimuli to either ipsilateral or contralateral FRA in spinal cats treated with L-DOPA (Figure 37-4C).

Very little is known about the interneuronal network generating the locomotor rhythm in mammals. Although rhythmically active interneurons are widely distributed in the gray matter of lumbar and sacral segments, there is no information on the interconnections between these interneurons or whether any of them are members of the rhythm-generating network. Recent studies on rhythm generation in the spinal cord of neonatal rats have revealed that some rhythmically active interneurons can sustain depolarizations *(plateau potentials)* in response to weak synaptic input. Because this active membrane property is known to be impor-

tant for rhythm generation in invertebrate systems, it is likely that it also contributes to rhythm generation in the mammalian spinal cord.

We lack detailed information on the neuronal circuitry and mechanisms of rhythm generation in the mammalian spinal cord largely because the mammalian nervous system is so complex. In contrast, we have much more detailed knowledge about the mechanisms of rhythm generation in invertebrates and lower vertebrates, which have relatively less complex nervous systems. The neuronal networks capable of generating rhythmic motor activity in the absence of sensory feedback are termed *central pattern generators* (Box 37-2).

The Rhythm-Generating System in the Spinal Cord Can Generate Complex Motor Patterns

In general, the locomotor patterns generated in deafferented or immobilized spinal preparations are much simpler than normal stepping patterns; they usually consist

Box 37-2 Central Pattern Generators

A central pattern generator (CPG) is a neuronal network capable of generating a rhythmic pattern of motor activity in the absence of phasic sensory input from peripheral receptors. CPGs have been identified and analyzed in more than 50 rhythmic motor systems, including those controlling such diverse behaviors as walking, swimming, feeding, respiration, and flying. Although the centrally generated pattern is sometimes very similar to the normal motor pattern, as in lamprey swimming, there are often significant differences. The basic pattern produced by a CPG is usually modified by sensory information from peripheral receptors and signals from other regions of the central nervous system.

The generation of rhythmic motor activity by CPGs depends on three factors: (1) the cellular properties of individual nerve cells within the network, (2) the properties of the synaptic junctions between neurons, and (3) the pattern of interconnections between neurons (Table 37-1). Modulatory substances, usually amines or peptides, can alter cellular and synaptic properties, thereby enabling a CPG to generate a variety of motor patterns.

The simplest CPGs contain neurons that are able to burst spontaneously. Such *endogenous bursters* can drive motor neurons, and some motor neurons are themselves endogenous bursters. Bursters are common in CPGs producing continuous rhythms such as those for respiration. They are also found in locomotor systems. Locomotion, however, is an episodic behavior, so bursters in locomotor systems must be regulated. Bursting is often induced by neuromodulators. Neuromodulators can also alter the cellular properties of neurons so that brief depolarizations lead to maintained depolarizations (*plateau potentials*) that far outlast the initial depolarization. Neurons with the capacity to generate plateau potentials have been found in a large number of CPGs, and in some cases the ability of neurons to generate plateau potentials is essential for rhythm generation.

Rhythmicity in CPGs does not always depend on bursting or plateau potential properties of neurons in the network. A simple network can generate rhythmic activity if it includes some time-dependent process that enhances or reduces activity within some of the neurons. One process is postinhibitory rebound, a transient increase in excitability of a neuron after the termination of inhibitory input. Two neurons that mutually inhibit each other can oscillate in an alternating fashion if each neuron has the property of postinhibitory rebound. Other time-dependent processes include synaptic depression, delayed onset of activity after a depolarization (delayed excitation), and differences in the time course of synaptic actions via parallel pathways connecting two neurons.

Most CPGs produce a complex temporal pattern of activation of different groups of motor neurons. Sometimes the pattern can be divided into a number of distinct phases; even within a phase the timing of activity can vary in different motor neurons. The sequencing of motor patterns is regulated by a number of mechanisms. Perhaps the simplest mechanism is mutual inhibition; interneurons that fire out of phase with each other are usually reciprocally coupled by inhibitory connections. Another mechanism is the rate of recovery from inhibition, which can influence the relative time of onset of activity in two neurons simultaneously released from inhibition. Finally, mutual excitation is an important mechanism for establishing the more or less synchronous firing of a group of neurons. Electrical junctions often mediate mutual excitation, particularly when it is important to rapidly generate a high-intensity burst within a group of neurons.

One of the best-analyzed CPGs is the one for lamprey swimming. Lampreys swim by alternating activation of motor neurons on the two sides of each body segment (Figure 37-5). Each segment contains a network capable of generating the rhythmic, alternating activity in motor neurons on the two sides (Figure 37-6).

Table 37-1 Building Blocks of Rhythm-Generating Networks

Cellular properties	Synaptic properties	Patterns of connection
Threshold	Sign	Reciprocal inhibition
Frequency-current relationship	Strength	Recurrent inhibition
Spike frequency adaptation	Time course	Parallel excitation and inhibition
Postburst hyperpolarization	Transmission:	Mutual excitation
Delayed excitation	Electrical	
Postinhibitory rebound	Chemical	
Plateau potentials	Release mechanisms:	
Bursting:	Spike	
Endogenous	Graded	
Conditional	Multicomponent postsynaptic potentials	
	Facilitation/depression:	
	Short term	
	Long term	

A number of cellular and synaptic mechanisms are involved in the initiation and termination of activity on one side of the network. One important mechanism in the initiation of activity is the opening of NMDA receptor-channels to produce plateau potentials. Once the inhibition from the contralateral I interneuron is terminated, NMDA receptor-channels in all ipsilateral neurons are opened by a depolarization resulting from postinhibitory rebound. The voltage-dependency of the NMDA receptor-channels then leads to the generation of plateau potentials. Activation of low-voltage Ca^{2+} channels further strengthens the depolarization. The influx of Ca^{2+} through these channels and the NMDA receptor-channels activates calcium-dependent K^+ channels. The resultant increase in K^+ conductance terminates the plateau potentials and so contributes to the termination of activity.

Two additional mechanisms contribute to the termination of activity in each half of the network. One is a progressive decline in the discharge rate of the neurons resulting from the summation of slow after-hyperpolarizations. The other is delayed excitation of the L interneurons, which inhibit the I interneurons (Figure 37-6) and thereby remove inhibition from the contralateral half of the network, enabling it to become active.

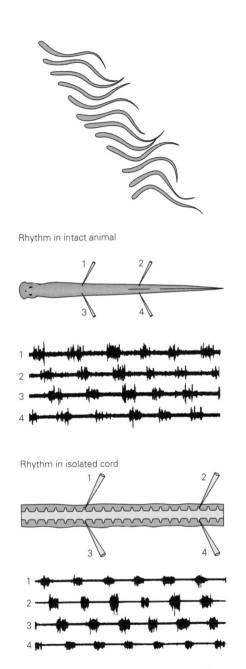

Rhythm in intact animal

Rhythm in isolated cord

Figure 37-5 The lamprey swims by means of a wave of muscle contractions traveling down one side of the body 180° out-of-phase with a similar traveling wave on the opposite side. This pattern can be detected by recording from different sites along the animal during normal swimming. Electromyogram recordings from four sites on the intact body are shown in the middle. The central origin of this pattern is revealed when a similar pattern is recorded from four spinal roots in an isolated cord (bottom). (Adapted from Grillner et al. 1987.)

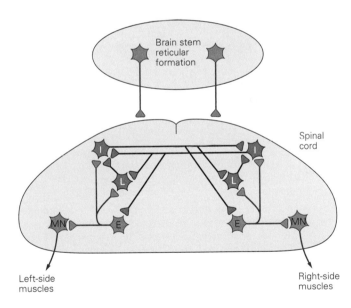

Brain stem reticular formation

Spinal cord

Left-side muscles

Right-side muscles

Figure 37-6 Some of the main features of the neuronal network in each body segment of the lamprey responsible for the rhythmic locomotor pattern for swimming. Activity in each segmental network is initiated by activity in glutaminergic axons descending from the reticular formation. The reticulospinal neurons increase the excitability of all neurons in the segmental networks by activation of both NMDA and non-NMDA receptors.

On each side of the network excitatory interneurons (**E**) drive the motor neurons (**MN**) and two classes of inhibitory interneurons (**I** and **L**). The axons of the I interneurons cross the midline and inhibit all neurons in the contralateral half of the network, ensuring that when muscles on one side of the network are active, muscles on the other side are silent. The L interneurons inhibit the I interneurons on the same side. (Adapted from Grillner et al. 1995.)

A Spinal cat immobilized

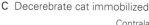

G

Q

ST

|— 1 s —|

B Decerebrate cat walking

LG

EDB

IP

ST

|————— 1 s —————|

C Decerebrate cat immobilized

Contralateral stimulus

Sart

RF

ST

Ipsilateral stimulus

Sart

RF

ST

|— 1 s —|

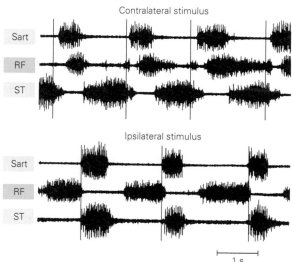

D Locomotor pattern generator

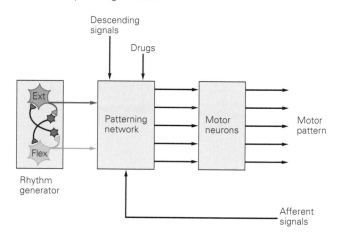

Descending
signals

Drugs

Ext

Flex

Patterning
network

Motor
neurons

Motor
pattern

Rhythm
generator

Afferent
signals

Figure 37-7 A variety of motor patterns can be generated in the absence of phasic sensory signals input to the spinal cord.

A. Reciprocal pattern of activity recorded from flexor and extensor nerves in an immobilized spinal cat treated with L-DOPA and nialamide. **G** = gastrocnemius; **Q** = quadriceps; **ST** = semitendinosus. (Adapted from Edgerton et al. 1976.)

B. Complex motor pattern recorded from a walking decerebrate cat with deafferented hind-leg muscles. **LG** = lateral gastrocnemius; **EDB** = extensor digitorum brevis; **IP** = iliopsoas; **ST** = semitendinosus. (Adapted from Grillner and Zangger 1984.)

C. Fictive motor patterns recorded in an immobilized decorticate cat when the ipsilateral and contralateral paw is squeezed.

The pattern is radically altered by changing the site of the sensory stimulus. **SART** = sartorius; **RF** = rectus femoris; **ST** = semitendinosus. (Adapted from Perret and Cabelguen 1980.)

D. In this hypothetical locomotor pattern generator the basic rhythmic pattern is produced by mutually inhibiting flexor and extensor half-centers (see Figure 37–4B). The output from the interneurons of these half-centers drives the motor neurons via an intermediate system of interneurons (patterning network) that control the timing of activation of different classes of motor neurons. Descending signals, drugs, or afferent signals could modify the temporal motor activity pattern by altering the functioning of interneurons in the patterning network.

of alternating bursts of activity in flexor and extensor motor neurons (Figure 37-7A). However, more complex locomotor patterns can be generated in immobilized spinal animals with the application of additional drugs (such as 4-aminopyridine) or after a period of training. Moreover, in decerebrate preparations elaborate locomotor patterns can be generated in hind limb motor neurons after deafferentation (Figure 37-7B); these patterns resemble those recorded in the same animals be-

fore deafferentation. Finally, a variety of patterns can be generated in immobilized decerebrate preparations, and these patterns can be altered significantly by changing the level of tonic sensory input (Figure 37-7C).

From these observations it is clear that the spinal pattern-generating network can generate a variety of motor patterns. Which pattern is generated depends on multiple factors, such as the supraspinal and tonic sensory inputs to the spinal pattern generators as well as the drugs used to initiate rhythmicity. This functional flexibility in the spinal pattern generator may be explained by a scheme in which mutually inhibiting half-centers produce the basic rhythmicity and establish a general pattern of reciprocity in the activity of flexor and extensor motor neurons while the details of the temporal pattern are established by the organization and properties of an interneuronal network between the half-centers and the motor neurons (Figure 37–7D).

Sensory Input From Moving Limbs Regulates Stepping Patterns

Although normal walking is automatic, it is not necessarily stereotyped. Outside the laboratory mammals constantly use sensory input to adjust their stepping patterns to variations in the terrain and to unexpected events. Three important types of sensory information are used to regulate stepping: somatosensory input from the receptors of muscle and skin, input from the vestibular apparatus (for controlling balance), and visual input.

In considering the role of somatosensory input in stepping, Charles Sherrington made the distinction between proprioceptors and exteroceptors. *Proprioceptors* are located in muscles and joints and are excited by body movements; input from proprioceptors is involved in the automatic regulation of stepping. *Exteroceptors* are located in the skin; their main function is to adjust stepping to external stimuli. This distinction is still considered valid, although it is now recognized that skin afferents can provide important feedback about body movements.

Proprioception Regulates the Timing and Amplitude of the Stepping Patterns

One of the clearest indications that somatosensory afferents from the limbs regulate the step cycle is that the rate of stepping in spinal and decerebrate cats matches the speed of the motorized treadmill belt on which they are stepping. Specifically, afferent input regulates the duration of the stance phase. As the stepping rate increases, stance duration decreases, while the duration of the swing phase remains relatively constant. This observation suggests that some form of sensory input signals the end of stance and thus leads to the initiation of swing.

Sherrington was the first to propose that proprioceptors in muscles acting at the hip were primarily responsible. He noticed that rapid extension at the hip joint, but not at the knee and ankle joints, led to contrac-

tions in the flexor muscles of chronic spinal cats and dogs. More recent studies have shown that preventing hip extension in a limb suppresses stepping in that limb, whereas rhythmically moving the hip can entrain locomotor rhythm. During entrainment, a burst activity in flexor motor neurons is initiated in synchrony with hip extension (Figure 37-8A). The afferents responsible for signaling hip angle for swing initiation arise from the muscle spindles in hip flexor muscles. Stretching hip flexor muscles in decerebrate animals to mimic the lengthening that occurs at the end of the stance phase inhibits the extensor half-center and thus facilitates the initiation of burst activity in flexor motor neurons during walking (Figure 37-8B).

Other important signals for regulating the step cycle arise from the Golgi tendon organs and muscle spindles of extensor muscles. Electrical stimulation of the afferents from these receptors prolongs the stance phase, often delaying the onset of swing until the stimulus has terminated (Figure 37-9A). Both groups of afferents are active during stance, with the Golgi tendon organs providing a measure of the load carried by the leg. The excitatory action of the Golgi tendon organs on extensor motor neurons during walking is opposite to their inhibitory action when locomotor activity is not being generated (see Chapter 36). The functional consequence of this reflex reversal is that the swing phase will not be initiated until the leg is unloaded and the forces exerted by extensor muscles are low (signaled by a decrease in activity from Golgi tendon organs). Limb unloading normally occurs near the end of leg extension, when the animal's weight is being borne by the other legs and the extensor muscles are shortened and thus unable to produce optimal forces.

In addition to regulating the transition from stance to swing, proprioceptive feedback from muscle spindles and Golgi tendon organs contributes significantly to the generation of burst activity in extensor motor neurons. Reducing feedback from these afferents in cats reduces the level of extensor activity by more than 50%, while in humans up to 30% of the excitatory input to the ankle extensor motor neurons arises from Ia afferents of extensor muscles.

At least three excitatory pathways transmit information from extensor sensory fibers to extensor motor neurons: (1) a monosynaptic pathway from Ia fibers, (2) a disynaptic pathway from Ia and Ib fibers, and (3) a polysynaptic pathway from Ia and Ib fibers (Figure 37-9B). The polysynaptic pathway includes the extensor half-center of the central rhythm generator, so in addition to regulating the level of extensor activity this pathway also controls the stance duration. The disynaptic excitatory pathway is active only during the extension

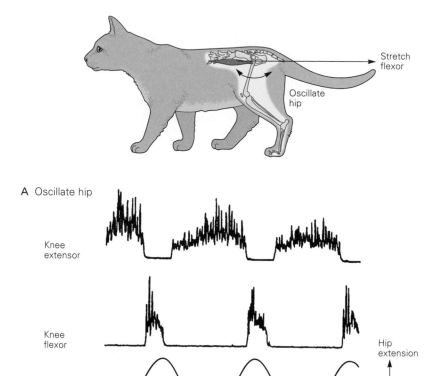

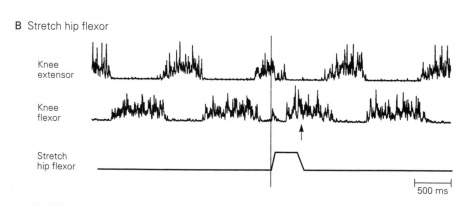

Figure 37-8 Information on hip extension controls the transition from stance to swing.

A. Oscillating movements around the hip joint in an immobilized decerebrate cat entrains the fictive locomotor pattern in extensor and flexor motor neurons. Note that the flexor bursts, corresponding to the swing phase, are generated when the hip is extended. (Adapted from Kriellaars et al. 1994.)

B. Stretching the detached hip flexor muscle (iliopsoas) in a walking decerebrate cat causes inhibition of extensor activity and an earlier onset of flexor activity. The **arrow** indicates the expected time of the onset of flexor activity had the flexor muscle not been stretched. Activation of sensory fibers from muscle spindles is responsible for this effect. (Adapted from Hiebert et al. 1996.)

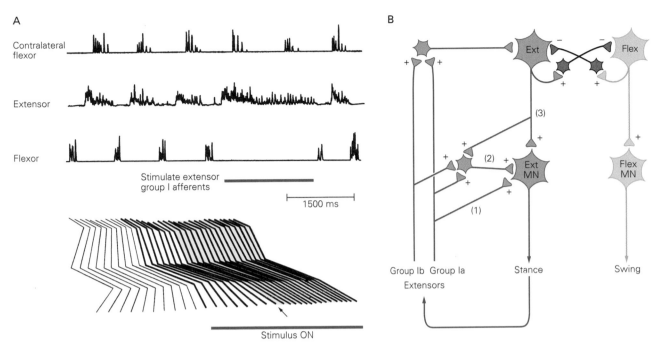

Figure 37-9 Initiation of the swing phase of walking is controlled by feedback from Golgi tendon organs and muscle spindles in extensor muscles.

A. Electrical stimulation of the group Ib sensory fibers from ankle extensor muscles inhibits bursting in ipsilateral flexors and prolongs the burst in the ipsilateral extensors during walking in a decerebrate cat. The timing of flexor activity in the contralateral leg is not altered. Stimulating group Ib afferents from the extensors prevents the initiation of the swing phase, as can be seen in the position of the leg during a stimulated trial (**bottom**). The **arrow** shows the point at which the swing phase would normally have occurred had the extensor afferents not been stimulated. (Adapted from Whelan et al. 1995.)

B. Afferent pathway from extensor muscles regulating stance. The central pattern generator is represented by mutually inhibiting groups of interneurons (**Ext** and **Flex**). Feedback from Ia and Ib afferent fibers from extensor muscles influences extensor activity via three excitatory (**+**) pathways: (**1**) monosynaptic connections from Ia fibers to extensor motor neurons (**MN**); (**2**) disynaptic connections from Ia and Ib fibers that are functional during the extension phase; and (**3**) a polysynaptic excitatory pathway via the extensor interneurons of the central pattern generator. These pathways increase the level of activity in extensor motor neurons during stance and maintain extensor activity when the extensor muscles are loaded.

(possibly by excitatory input to the interneurons in this pathway from the extensor half-center). The continuous regulation of the level of extensor activity by proprioceptive feedback presumably allows automatic adjustment of force and length in extensor muscles to unexpected unloading and loading of the leg.

Sensory Input From the Skin Allows Stepping to Adjust to Unexpected Obstacles

Exteroceptors in the skin have a powerful influence on the central pattern generator for walking. One important function for these receptors is to detect external obstacles and adjust the stepping movements to avoid them. A well-studied example is the stumbling-corrective reaction in cats. A mild mechanical stimulus applied to the dorsal part of the paw during the swing

phase produces excitation of flexor motor neurons and inhibition of extensor motor neurons, leading to rapid flexion of the paw away from the stimulus and elevation of the leg in an attempt to step over the object. Because this corrective response is readily observed in spinal cats, it must be produced to a large extent by circuits entirely contained within the spinal cord.

One of the interesting features of the stumbling-corrective reaction is that corrective flexion movements are produced only when the paw is stimulated during the swing phase. An identical stimulus applied during the stance phase produces an opposite response: excitation of extensor muscles that reinforces the ongoing extensor activity. This extensor action is appropriate; if a flexion reflex were produced, the animal might collapse because its weight is being supported by the limb. This is an example of a phase-dependent reflex reversal: the

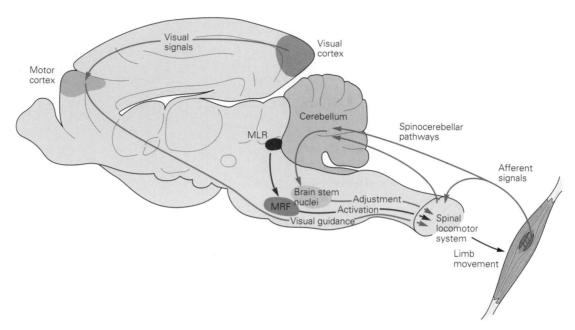

Figure 37-10 Descending signals from the brain stem and motor cortex initiate locomotion and adjust stepping movements to the immediate needs of the animal. The spinal locomotor system is activated by signals from the mesencephalic locomotor region (**MLR**) relayed via neurons in the medial reticular formation (**MRF**) (see Figure 37–11). The cerebellum receives signals via spinocerebellar pathways from both peripheral receptors and the spinal central pattern generators and adjusts the locomotor pattern via brain stem nuclei. Modification of stepping by visual signals is mediated via the motor cortex.

same stimulus will excite one group of motor neurons during one phase of locomotion and excite the antagonist motor neurons during another phase.

Descending Pathways Are Necessary for Initiation and Adaptive Control of Walking

Although the basic motor pattern for stepping is generated in the spinal cord, fine control of stepping movements involves numerous regions of the brain, including the motor cortex, cerebellum, and various sites within the brain stem. Recordings from neurons in all these regions have shown that many are rhythmically active during locomotor activity and hence involved in some way with the production of the normal motor pattern. Each region, however, appears to play a different role in the regulation of locomotor function.

Supraspinal regulation of stepping can, in broad terms, be divided into three functional systems. One activates the spinal locomotor system and controls the overall speed of locomotion, another refines the motor pattern in response to feedback from the limbs, and the third guides limb movement in response to visual input (Figure 37-10).

Descending Pathways From the Brain Stem Initiate Walking and Control Its Speed

In their seminal studies of decerebrate cats, Mark Shik, Fidor Severin, and Grigori Orlovsky found that tonic electrical stimulation of the mesencephalic locomotor region initiates stepping when animals are placed on a freely moving treadmill. The rhythm of the locomotor pattern is not related to the pattern of electrical stimulation but depends only on its intensity. Weak stimulation produces a walking gait that increases in speed as the intensity increases; progressively stronger stimulation produces trotting and finally galloping (Figure 37-11A). Thus, a relatively simple control signal from the brain stem, modulated only in intensity, not only initiates locomotion but also controls the overall speed of walking.

It is especially interesting to note that the changes in gait are associated with changes in the coordination between legs: an out-of-phase relationship between left and right legs in walking changes to an in-phase relationship in galloping. These shifts in interlimb coordination are most likely implemented by local circuits in the spinal cord, since they are also observed in spinal cats walking on a motorized treadmill as the treadmill speed is increased.

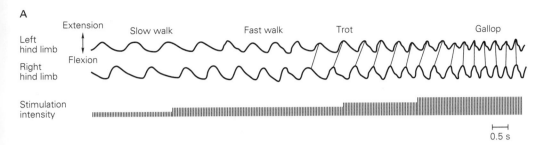

A

Extension

Left hind limb

Flexion

Right hind limb

Slow walk   Fast walk   Trot   Gallop

Stimulation intensity

0.5 s

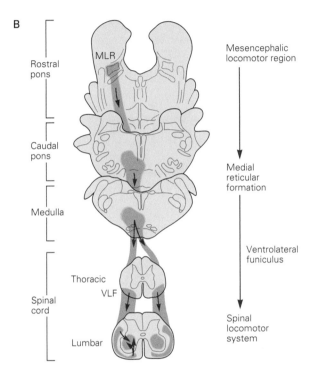

B

Rostral pons

MLR

Mesencephalic locomotor region

Caudal pons

Medulla

Medial reticular formation

Ventrolateral funiculus

Thoracic

VLF

Spinal cord

Lumbar

Spinal locomotor system

Figure 37-11 Locomotor responses to electrical stimulation of the mesencephalic locomotor region.

A. Increasing the strength of stimulation to the mesencephalic locomotor region (MLR) in a decerebrate cat walking on a treadmill progressively changes the gait and rate of stepping from slow walking to trotting and finally to galloping. As the cat progresses from trotting to galloping the hind limbs shift from alternating to simultaneous flexion and extension.

B. Efferent projection from the MLR. Stimulation of the MLR excites interneurons in the medial reticular formation whose axons descend to the spinal locomotor system via the ventrolateral funiculus (VLF). (Adapted from Mori et al. 1992.)

In addition to the mesencephalic locomotor region several other motor regions of the brain, including a subthalamic motor region and a pontine locomotor region, can produce locomotion when stimulated experimentally. How these different brain stem regions interact in normal control of locomotion is not yet known.

The Descending Signals That Initiate Locomotion Are Transmitted via the Reticulospinal Pathway

How are signals from brain stem locomotor regions transmitted to pattern-generating networks in the spinal cord? Because application of adrenergic drugs is often sufficient to initiate stepping in acute spinal animals, an early hypothesis was that the initiation and maintenance of locomotor activity depends on activity in the descending noradrenergic pathway from the locus ceruleus or the descending serotonergic pathway from the raphe nucleus.

However, neither of these two aminergic pathways is essential for locomotion, since locomotor activity can be evoked after depletion of these amines. The current view is that biogenic amines regulate the magnitude and timing of motor neuron activity in the locomotor networks in the spinal cord. Thus, while adrenergic drugs can initiate stepping movements in the spinal preparation, aminergic systems may not serve this function in intact animals.

If aminergic systems do not initiate locomotion, what descending signals are necessary for the initiation of locomotor activity? Clues to the answer to this question have come from studies on the initiation of locomotor activity in the neonatal rat and lamprey. In both animals administration of glutamate receptor agonists initiates locomotor activity. Recently a similar phenomenon has been observed in the cat. In decerebrate cats intrathecal administration of agonists that bind to NMDA-type glutamate receptors in the spinal cord ini-

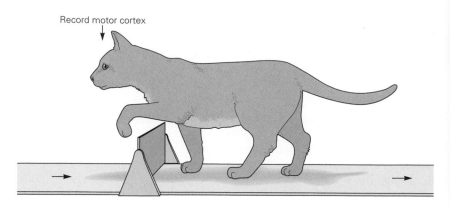

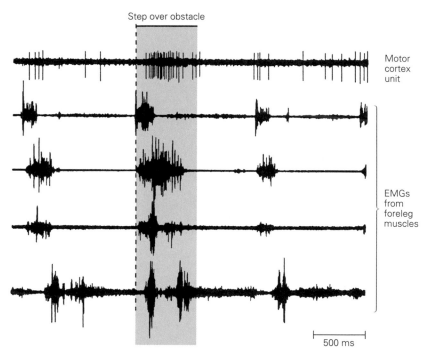

Figure 37-12 Activity in neurons in the motor cortex is modulated by visual system inputs to adapt stepping movements. When a normal cat steps over objects fixed to the belt of a treadmill, neurons in the motor cortex increase in activity. This increase in cortical activity is associated with enhanced activity on electromyograms (EMGs) in foreleg muscles. (Adapted from Drew 1988.)

tiates locomotion, while application of glutamate receptor antagonists prevents initiation of locomotor activity when the mesencephalic locomotor region is stimulated. These observations suggest that descending glutaminergic pathways are involved in initiating locomotor activity.

Considerable research has focused on identifying the origin and location of the pathways involved in initiating locomotor activity. The axons of neurons in the nuclei near the mesencephalic locomotor region do not descend directly to the cord and therefore do not directly activate central pattern generators. Instead, neurons in the medullary reticular formation, whose axons descend in the ventrolateral region of the spinal cord, are considered important elements in initiating locomotor activity (Figure 37-11B). These neurons are excited by stimulation of the mesencephalic locomotor region,

and transection of their axons in the ventrolateral funiculus of the spinal cord prevents stimulation of the mesencephalic locomotor region from initiating locomotor activity. Thus, the current evidence indicates that the signals that activate locomotion and control its speed are transmitted to the spinal cord by glutaminergic neurons whose axons travel in the reticulospinal pathway.

The Motor Cortex Is Involved in the Control of Precise Stepping Movements in Visually Guided Walking

During normal walking we often must guide our walking using visual cues. The motor cortex is essential in such visuomotor coordination. Experimental lesions of the motor cortex do not prevent animals from walking on a smooth floor or even on smooth inclines. However, they do severely impair tasks requiring a high degree of visuomotor coordination, such as walking on the rungs of horizontal ladders, stepping over a series of barriers, and stepping over single objects placed on a treadmill belt. Such "skilled walking" is associated with considerable modulation in the activity of a large number of neurons in the motor cortex (Figure 37-12). Since many of these neurons project directly into the spinal cord, they may regulate the activity of interneurons that form part of, or are influenced by, the central pattern generator for locomotion.

The Cerebellum Fine-Tunes the Locomotor Pattern by Regulating the Timing and Intensity of Descending Signals

Damage to the cerebellum results in marked abnormalities in locomotor movements, including abnormal variations in the speed and range of movements at different joints in single limbs and abnormal coupling between stepping in different limbs. These symptoms are collectively referred to as ataxia (see Chapter 42). Ataxic walking resembles a drunken gait. Since ataxic gait is apparent in patients with cerebellar lesions even when they are walking on a flat, smooth surface, we can conclude that the cerebellum is involved in the regulation of all stepping movements.

The cerebellum receives information about both the actual stepping movements and the state of the spinal rhythm-generating network via two ascending pathways. For the hind legs of the cat these are the dorsal and ventral spinocerebellar tracts. Neurons in the dorsal tract are strongly activated by numerous leg proprioceptors and thus provide the cerebellum with detailed information about the biomechanical state of the hind legs. In contrast, neurons in the ventral tract are activated primarily by interneurons in the central pattern generator, thus providing the cerebellum with information about the state of the spinal locomotor network.

It is thought that the cerebellum compares the *actual* movements of the legs (proprioceptive signals in the dorsal spinocerebellar tract) with the *intended* movements (information on the central pattern generator carried by the ventral spinocerebellar tract) and computes corrective signals that are then sent to various brain stem nuclei (see Figure 37-10). Thus the cerebellum may adjust the locomotor pattern when stepping movements unexpectedly deviate from the intended movements. The brain stem nuclei influenced by the cerebellum during walking include the vestibular nuclei, red nucleus, and nuclei in the medullary reticular formation. Cerebellar output to the vestibular nuclei may be involved in integrating proprioceptive information from the legs with vestibular signals for the control of balance.

Human Walking May Involve Spinal Pattern Generators

Unlike spinal cats and other quadrupeds, humans with spinal lesions that effectively transect the spinal cord generally are not able to walk spontaneously. Nevertheless, some observations of patients with spinal cord injury parallel the findings from studies of spinal cats.

In one striking case, only recently reported, an individual with near complete transection of the spinal cord showed spontaneous uncontrollable rhythmic movements of the legs when the hips were extended. This closely parallels the finding that rhythmic stepping movements can often be evoked in chronic spinal cats by hip extension. In another study a drug influencing the biogenic amines (clonidine) was found to improve stepping on a treadmill in a few patients with severe spinal cord injury, as it does in spinal cats.

Compelling evidence for the existence of spinal rhythm-generating networks in humans comes from studies of development. Human infants produce rhythmic stepping movements immediately after birth if held erect and moved over a horizontal surface. This strongly suggests that some of the basic neuronal circuits for locomotion are established genetically. These circuits must be located at or below the brain stem (possibly entirely within the spinal cord) since stepping can occur in anencephalic infants.

These basic circuits are thought to be brought under supraspinal control in two ways during the first year of life, as automatic stepping is transformed into functional walking. First, the infant develops the ability to control locomotion voluntarily. From what we know about the neuronal mechanisms in the cat, this ability could depend on the development of reticulospinal pathways and regions activating reticulospinal neurons (such as the mesencephalic locomotor region). Second, the stepping pattern gradually develops from a primitive flexion-extension pattern that generates little effective propulsion to the complex mature pattern. Again, based on studies of cats, it is plausible that this adaptation is a result of maturation of descending systems originating from the motor cortex and brain stem nuclei modulated by the cerebellum.

We can conclude, therefore, that human walking relies on the same general principles of neuronal organization as walking in other mammals: Intrinsic oscillatory networks are activated and modulated by other brain structures and by afferent input. Nevertheless, human locomotion differs from most animal locomotion in that it is bipedal, placing significantly greater demands on descending systems that control balance during walking. Indeed, some investigators believe that what allows the infant to begin to walk independently at the end of the first year is not necessarily maturation of the stepping pattern, but instead maturation of the system that enables successful balance control. Contrast this with horses, which can stand and walk within hours after birth. It is likely, therefore, that the spinal networks that contribute to human locomotion are more dependent on supraspinal centers than those in quadrupedal animals. This dependence may in part explain the relatively few observations of spontaneous stepping movements in humans with spinal cord injury.

An Overall View

Locomotion in mammals typically involves rhythmic movements of the body and one or more appendages. These movements depend on the precise regulation of the timing and the strength of contractions in numerous muscles. Centrally located neuronal circuits, known as central pattern generators, can generate the basic motor pattern for locomotion even without afferent feedback from peripheral receptors. Numerous central pattern generators have now been analyzed at the cellular level, and it is clear that a wide variety of cellular, synaptic, and network properties are involved in these local networks. Central pattern generators are extremely flexible. Their cellular and synaptic properties can be modified by chemical signals, and their functioning depends on how they are activated and the pattern of afferent input they receive.

Contemporary research on mammalian locomotion dates from the 1960s, when two important experimental animal preparations were introduced. In the decerebrate animal stepping can be initiated by electrical stimulation of a site in the brain stem (the mesencephalic locomotor region). In the spinal preparation centrally generated locomotor activity can be evoked after the administration of L-DOPA and nialamide. Investigations using these preparations have confirmed and extended fundamental observations made near the turn of the century, namely that the basic rhythm for locomotion is generated centrally in spinal networks, that the transition from stance to swing is regulated by afferent signals from leg flexor and extensor muscles, and that descending signals from the brain regulate the intensity of locomotion and modify stepping movements according to the terrain on which the animal is walking.

Recent studies of humans with spinal cord injury and normal infants indicate that many of the basic features of the neural control of human bipedal walking are similar to those in quadrupedal locomotion.

Keir Pearson
James Gordon

Selected Readings

Getting PA. 1989. Emerging principles governing the operation of neural circuits. Annu Rev Neurosci 12:185–204.

Grillner S. 1981. Control of locomotion in bipeds, tetrapods and fish. In: VB Brooks (ed). *Handbook of Physiology*. Sect. 1, *The Nervous System*. Vol. 2, *Motor Control*, pp. 1179–1236. Bethesda, MD: American Physiological Society.

Marder E, Calabrese R. 1996. Principles of rhythmic motor pattern generation. Physiol Rev 76:687–717.

Pearson KG. 1993. Common principles of motor control in vertebrates and invertebrates. Annu Rev Neurosci 16:265–297.

Pearson KG. 1995. Proprioceptive regulation of locomotion. Curr Opin Neurobiol 5:786–791.

References

Belanger M, Drew T, Provencher J, Rossignol S. 1996. A comparison of treadmill locomotion in adult cats before and after spinal transection. J Neurophysiol 76:471–491.

Calancie B, Needham-Shropshire B, Jacobs P, Willer K, Zych G, Green BA. 1994. Involuntary stepping after chronic spinal cord injury: evidence for a central rhythm generator for locomotion in man. Brain 117:1143–1159.

Cazalets J-R, Borde M, Clarac F. 1995. Localization and organization of the central pattern generator for hindlimb locomotion in newborn rat. J Neurosci 15:4943–4951.

Douglas JR, Noga BR, Dai X, Jordan LM. 1993. The effects of intrathecal administration of excitatory amino acid agonists and antagonists on the initiation of locomotion in the adult cat. J Neurosci 13:990–1000.

Drew T. 1988. Motor cortical cell discharge during voluntary gait modification. Brain Res 457:181–187.

Edgerton VR, Grillner S, Sjöström A, Zangger P. 1976. Central generation of locomotion in vertebrates. In: RM Herman, S Grillner, PSG Stein, DG Stuart (eds). *Neural Control of Locomotion*, pp. 439–467. New York: Plenum.

Engberg I, Lundberg A. 1969. An electromyographic analysis of muscular activity in the hindlimb of the cat during unrestrained locomotion. Acta Physiol Scand 75:614–630.

Forssberg H. 1985. Ontogeny of human locomotor control. I. Infant stepping, supported locomotion and transition to independent locomotion. Exp Brain Res 57:480–493.

Forssberg H. 1979. Stumbling corrective reaction: a phase dependent compensatory reaction during locomotion. J Neurophysiol 42:936–953.

Graham Brown T. 1911. The intrinsic factors in the act of progression in the mammal. Proc R Soc Lond B Biol Sci 84:308–319.

Graham Brown T. 1914. On the nature of the fundamental activity of the nervous centres; together with an analysis of the conditioning of rhythmic activity in progression, and a theory of the evolution of function in the nervous system. J Physiol (Lond) 48:18–46.

Grillner S, Deliagina T, Ekebuerg Ö, El Manira A, Hill RH, Lansner A, Orlovsky GN, Wallen P. 1995. Neural networks that co-ordinate locomotion and body orientation in lamprey. Trends Neurosci 18:270–280.

Grillner S, Wallén P, Dale N, Brodin L, Buchanan J, Hill R. 1987. Transmitters, membrane properties and network circuitry in the control of locomotion in the lamprey. Trends Neurosci 10:34–41.

Grillner S, Zangger P. 1984. The effect of dorsal root transection on the efferent motor pattern in the cat's hindlimb during locomotion. Acta Physiol Scand 120:393–405.

Hiebert GW, Whelan PJ, Prochazka A, Pearson KG. 1996. Contribution of hindlimb flexor muscle afferents to the timing of phase transitions in the cat step cycle. J Neurophysiol 75:1126–1137.

Jankowska E, Jukes MGM, Lund S, Lundberg A. 1967a. The effect of DOPA on the spinal cord. 5. Reciprocal organization of pathways transmitting excitatory action to alpha motoneurones of flexors and extensors. Acta Physiol Scand 70:369–388.

Jankowska E, Jukes MGM, Lund S, Lundberg A. 1967b. The effect of DOPA on the spinal cord. VI. Half-centre organization of interneurons transmitting effects from flexor reflex afferents. Acta Physiol Scand 70:389–402.

Kriellaars DJ, Brownstone RM, Noga BR, Jordan LM. 1994. Mechanical entrainment of fictive locomotion in the decerebrate cat. J Neurophysiol 71:2074–2086.

Mori S, Matsuyama K, Kohyama J, Kobayashi Y, Takakusaki K. 1992. Neuronal constituents of postural and locomotor control systems and their interactions in cats. Brain Dev 14:S109–S120.

Noga BR, Kriellaars DJ, Jordan LM. 1991. The effect of selective brain stem or spinal cord lesions on treadmill locomotion evoked by stimulation of the mesencephalic or pontomedullary locomotor region. J Neurosci 11:1691–1700.

Perret C, Cabelguen JM. 1980. Main characteristics of the hindlimb locomotor cycle in the decorticate cat with special reference to bifunctional muscles. Brain Res 187:333–352.

Sherrington CS. 1910. Flexor-reflex of the limb, crossed extension reflex, and reflex stepping and standing (cat and dog). J Physiol (Lond) 40:28–121.

Shik ML, Severin FV, Orlovsky GN. 1966. Control of walking and running by means of electrical stimulation of the mid-brain. Biophysics 11:756–765.

Thelen E. 1985. Developmental origins of motor coordination: leg movements in human infants. Dev Psychobiol 18:1–22.

Whelan PJ, Hiebert GW, Pearson KG. 1995. Stimulation of the group I extensor afferents prolongs the stance phase in walking cats. Exp Brain Res 103:20–30.

38

Voluntary Movement

IN PREVIOUS CHAPTERS WE saw how spinal and brain stem circuits can organize elementary movement patterns in response to somatosensory, vestibular, and other stimuli. However such reflex actions are relatively stereotyped and the repertory of movements is limited. In this chapter we shall see how the motor areas of the cerebral cortex integrate visual, proprioceptive, and other information to produce the more elaborate voluntary movements that require planning.

Voluntary movements differ from reflexes in several important ways. First, voluntary movements are organized around the performance of a purposeful task. Thus the selection of which joints and body segments will be used for a movement depends on the goal of the movement, whether it is designed to reach for and lift a glass of water or to return a tennis serve. In contrast to the stereotyped relation between response and stimulus, characteristic of reflexes, voluntary movements vary in response to the same stimulus depending on the behavioral task. Second, the effectiveness of voluntary movements improves with experience and learning. Finally, unlike reflexes, voluntary movements are not mere responses to environmental stimuli but can be generated internally. The higher levels of our motor systems can therefore dissociate two aspects of a stimulus—its informational content and its capacity to trigger a movement. In the cortex the information content of a stimulus signals where to move or what to do, but the occurrence of the stimulus may or may not actually initiate the appropriate movement. In reflexes these aspects of the stimulus are linked.

The motor areas of the cerebral cortex are subdivided into a primary motor area and several premotor areas. Each area contains populations of neurons that

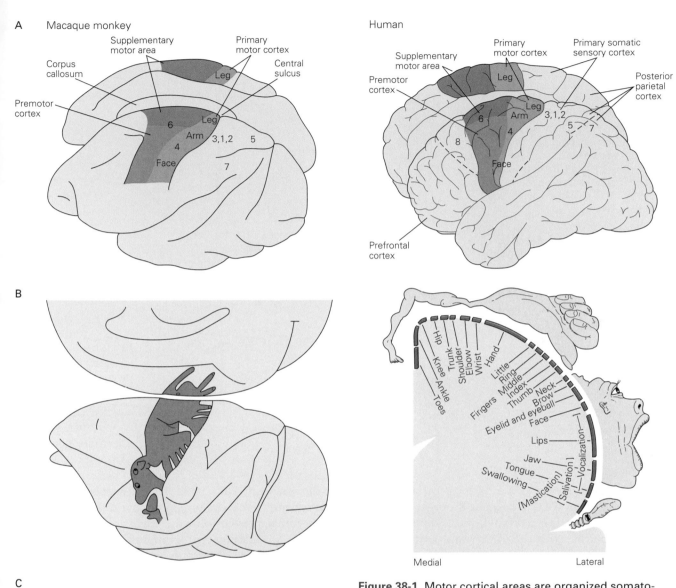

Figure 38-1 Motor cortical areas are organized somatotopically.

A. Brodmann's cytoarchitectural areas in monkeys and humans.

B. Comparison of the somatotopic organization of the primary motor cortex in monkeys and humans. The sequence of representation of body parts is similar. The ankle control area is medial while the face, mouth, and mastication control areas are lateral. The face and fingers in the human motor cortex have much larger representations because of the greater degree of cortical control of these areas. (Left: from Woolsey 1958; right: adapted from Penfield and Rasmussen 1950.)

C. Somatotopic organization of the medial and lateral motor cortex in the monkey, showing the arm and leg representations. (**ArSi,** arcuate sulcus, inferior limb; **ArSs**=arcuate sulcus, superior limb; **CS**=central sulcus; **M1**=primary motor cortex; **PMd**=dorsal premotor area; **PMv**=ventral premotor area; **PS**=precentral sulcus; **SGm**=superior frontal gyrus, medial wall; **SMA**=supplementary motor area; **pre-SMA**=presupplementary motor area; **SPcS**=superior precentral sulcus.) (From Dum and Strick 1996.)

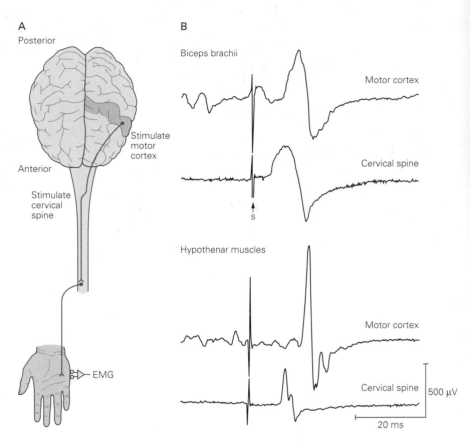

Figure 38-2 The motor cortex can be stimulated directly in awake humans.

A. Magnetic stimulation of the motor cortex or cervical spine produces muscle contraction painlessly. Stimulation of the motor cortex activates the corticospinal fibers and produces a short-latency electromyographic (EMG) response in contralateral muscles.

B. The traces show activation of arm and hand muscles (biceps brachii and hypothenar) when stimulation is applied over the cortex or the cervical spine. The peaks occur earlier from cervical stimulation because the corticospinal impulse has less distance to travel. The point marked **s** is a stimulus artifact, reflecting the application of the magnetic field pulse. (From Rothwell 1994.)

project from the cortex to the brain stem and spinal cord. In this chapter we first describe the organization of the motor areas of the cerebral cortex, showing how they communicate with each other and with primary sensory and association areas. We then examine how these different motor areas control simple and complex aspects of movement.

Voluntary Movement Is Organized in the Cortex

The Primary Motor Cortex Controls Simple Features of Movement

The discovery in 1870 that electrical stimulation of different parts of the frontal lobe produces movements of muscles on the opposite side of the body had a major impact on neurological thinking. In the early twentieth century electrical stimulation was used to identify the specific motor effects of discrete sites in the frontal lobe in different species—including primates and humans—and the resulting *motor maps* were correlated with anatomical and clinical observations on the effects of

local lesions. The contralateral precentral gyrus (Brodmann's area 4), the region now called the *primary motor cortex,* proved to be the area in which the lowest-intensity stimulation elicited movements. At low intensities the effects of stimuli can be attributed to the activation of neurons near the electrode that are connected to the spinal cord either directly or via only a small number of synapses.

The motor maps produced by these experiments show an orderly arrangement along the gyrus of control areas for the face, digits, hand, arm, trunk, leg, and foot. However, the fingers, hands, and face—which are used in tasks requiring the greatest precision and finest control—have disproportionately large representations in the motor areas of cortex (Figure 38-1), much as the inputs from regions of the body that have important roles in perception predominate in the sensory areas of the cortex. Consistent with the overall somatotopic organization, lesions in the arm representation lead to degeneration of myelinated fibers in the cevical cord, while lesions in the leg representation produce degeneration extending all the way to the lumbar spinal cord. These axons arise from specialized large pyramidal neurons in lamina V named Betz cells after their discoverer.

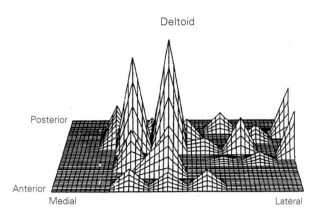

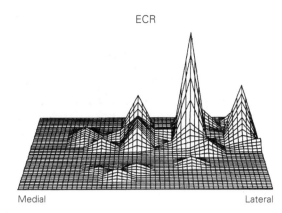

Figure 38-3 Sites controlling an individual muscle are not located together but are distributed over a wide area of motor cortex. Intracortical microstimulation was used to identify sites in monkey primary motor cortex at which low-threshold stimulation evoked electromyographic activity (indicating monosynaptic connections) in a shoulder abduction muscle (middle head of deltoid muscle) and a wrist extensor muscle (extensor carpi radialis; **ECR**). Topographic maps of the identified sites, reveal overlap between shoulder and wrist representations. The maps were constructed based on the inverse of the threshold (1/threshold) in microamperes, with the peaks representing approximately 1/3 µA and the valleys 1/40 µA. (From Humphrey DR, Tanji J. 1991. In: DR Humphrey, HJ Freund (eds.). *Motor Control: Concepts and Issues*, pp 413–443. New York: Wiley.)

The results of animal experiments done in the early 1900s helped explain the clinical signs in patients produced by traumatic, vascular, and other forms of local damage to the contralateral frontal lobe. They also explained focal epilepsy, which can develop as a result of traumatic injury or tumors. The abrupt rhythmic flexion-extension movements seen in focal seizures resemble the movements produced by electrical stimulation of the primary motor cortex. Indeed, in the nineteenth century, before electroencephalographic recordings were available, John Hughlings Jackson had already proposed that seizure activity resulted from paroxysmal increases in local neuronal activity in a limited area of cerebral cortex that corresponds to the primary motor cortex. Focal seizures often start in the fingers and spread proximally down the limb as the focus of discharges spreads from the hand area to adjacent sites controlling more proximal muscles. Clinically this is known as the *Jacksonian march*.

In the past decade it has become possible to stimulate motor cortical areas in alert humans by inducing electrical fields in the brain using rapidly alternating magnetic fields produced by wire coils applied to the scalp. The responses in muscles (eg, of the hand) are recorded with surface electrodes. The motor action potentials are large and have a short latency, consistent with the fact that they are conducted by corticospinal fibers (Figure 38-2). Magnetic stimulation can be used to map the body representation in the primary motor cortex or to perturb processing in local cortical areas.

The early mapping experiments stimulating the cortical surface electrically (and more recently magnetically) initially led to the simplistic idea that the primary motor cortex acts as a massive switchboard with individual switches controlling individual muscles or small groups of adjacent muscles. More detailed studies, however, using microelectrodes inserted into the depths of the cortex (intracortical microstimulation or ICMS) to stimulate small groups of output neurons indicate that this simple view is incorrect. Whereas the weakest stimuli may evoke the contraction of individual muscles, the same muscles are invariably activated from several separate sites as well, indicating that neurons in several cortical sites project axons to the same target (Figure 38-3).

In addition, most stimuli activate several muscles, with muscles rarely being activated individually. This is corroborated by recent anatomical and physiological experiments showing that the terminal distributions of individual corticospinal axons diverge to motor neurons innervating more than one muscle. Instead of a simple switchboard of muscle representations, detailed maps of monkey motor cortex suggest a concentric organization: sites influencing distal muscles are contained at the center of a wider area containing sites that also influence more proximal muscles, while sites in the peripheral ring around this central area influence proximal muscles alone. An implication of the redundancy in muscle representation is that inputs to motor cortex from other cortical areas can combine proximal and distal muscles in different ways in different tasks.

A Inputs to primary motor cortex

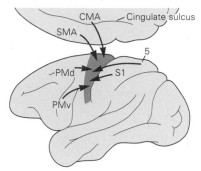

B Inputs to premotor areas

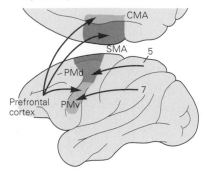

Figure 38-4 The major inputs to the motor cortex in monkeys.

A. The major inputs to the primary motor cortex. (**PMd**=dorsal premotor area; **PMv**=ventral premotor area; **S1**=primary sen-

sory cortex; **SMA**=supplementary motor area; **CMA** = cingulate motor area.)

B. The major inputs to the premotor areas. Dense interconnections between the premotor areas are not shown here.

Premotor Cortical Areas Project to the Primary Motor Cortex and Spinal Cord

In the late 1930s it was discovered that movements can also be elicited by direct electrical stimulation of the *premotor areas,* Brodmann's area 6, although the intensity of stimulation necessary to produce movement is greater here than in the primary motor cortex. Brodmann's area 6 lies anterior to the precentral gyrus, on the lateral and medial surfaces of the cortex. Like the primary motor cortex, the premotor areas contain pyramidal (output) neurons in layer V that project to the spinal cord, although the cell bodies are smaller than those in the primary motor cortex.

Recent anatomical studies indicate there are four main premotor areas in primates—two on the lateral convexity and two on the medial convexity. The two on the lateral convexity are the *lateral ventral* and *lateral dorsal premotor areas.* The two in the medial wall of the hemisphere are the *supplementary motor area* and the *cingulate motor areas,* located in the banks of the cingulate sulcus. Similar premotor areas exist in humans, but differences in size and sulcal patterns make it difficult to identify homologous areas with precision.

Motor maps of the face and extremities can be delineated in each premotor area (Figure 38-1C). However, unlike the primary motor cortex, where stimulation typically evokes simple movements of single joints, stimulation of the premotor areas often evokes more complex movements involving multiple joints and resembling natural coordinated hand shaping or reaching movements. Stimulation of the medial parts of area 6, the supplementary motor area, can give rise to

bilateral movements, suggesting that this area has a role in coordinating movements on the two sides of the body.

All the premotor areas project to both the primary motor cortex and the spinal cord, although there are fewer projections from the premotor areas to the spinal cord than from the primary motor cortex. In the spinal cord the areas of termination of the premotor and primary motor projections overlap. For example, the corticospinal axons of neurons in the supplementary motor area terminate in motor nuclei innervating digit and hand muscles, as do those of neurons in the hand area in the primary motor cortex. The corticospinal projections from the dorsal premotor area terminate mainly in motor nuclei innervating proximal limb musculature. The existence of these direct monosynaptic connections suggests that the premotor neurons can control hand movements independently of the primary motor cortex.

Each Cortical Motor Area Receives Unique Cortical and Subcortical Inputs

The primary motor cortex receives somatotopically organized inputs directly from two sources. First, it receives inputs from the primary somatosensory cortex (areas 1, 2, and 3). This means that, like neurons in somatosensory cortex, neurons in the motor cortex have receptive fields in the periphery. For example, some neurons in the motor cortex receive proprioceptive input from the muscles to which they project and many neurons in the hand region of the motor map respond to

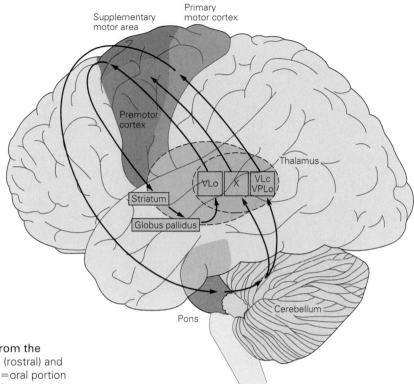

Figure 38-5 The motor cortex receives inputs from the cerebellum via the thalamus. **VLo** and **VLc**=oral (rostral) and caudal portions of the ventrolateral nucleus; **VPLo**=oral portion of the ventral posterolateral nucleus; **X**=nucleus X.

tactile stimuli applied to specific regions of the digits and palms. These so-called *transcortical* circuits are discussed later. Second, the primary motor cortex receives inputs from posterior parietal area 5. Posterior parietal areas 5 and 7 are involved in integrating multiple sensory modalities for motor planning (Figure 38-4A).

The premotor areas receive major inputs from areas 5 and 7 as well as from area 46 in the prefrontal cortex (Figure 38-4B). Each premotor area has its own pattern of inputs from distinct locations in areas 5 and 7. Area 46 projects mainly to the ventral premotor area and is important in working memory; it is thought to store information about the location of objects in space only long enough to guide a movement. There are also dense connections between the premotor areas themselves. These connections are thought to allow working memory to influence specific aspects of motor planning that are mediated by the different premotor subregions.

The premotor areas and primary motor cortex also receive input from the basal ganglia and cerebellum via different sets of nuclei in the ventrolateral thalamus (Figure 38-5). The basal ganglia and cerebellum do not project directly to the spinal cord.

An important feature of the relationship between cortical areas and subcortical structures is the reciprocal nature of their connections. Each cortical motor area appears to have a unique pattern of cortical and subcortical input. Thus there are many cortico-subcortical loops, each one making a different contribution to a motor behavior (Chapter 43).

The Somatotopic Organization of the Motor Cortex Is Plastic

The somatotopic organization of the motor cortex is not fixed but can be altered during motor learning and following injury. This plasticity has been demonstrated in many experiments and clinical studies. In one study using mature rats the representation of the whiskers in the primary motor cortex was first mapped using intracortical microstimulation. The whiskers were then denervated. Electrical stimulation of the cortical region that had caused whisker movement subsequently produced forelimb movement (Figure 38-6). This shift in functionality may be due to facilitation of preexisting circuits in the whisker region that are connected to the forelimb. The change can take place in just a few hours. The loss of sensory inputs from the whiskers into the motor area is thought to trigger the reorganization. This indicates that neurons influencing facial musculature are more widely distributed than is revealed by local electrical stimulation at any given point in time.

The idea that the organization of at least some ma-

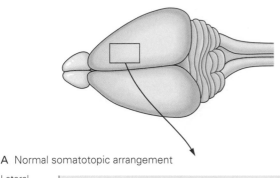

Figure 38-6 The functional organization of the primary motor cortex of a rat changes after transection of the facial nerve. (From Sanes et al. 1991.)

A. Surface view of the rat frontal cortex shows the normal somatotopic arrangement of areas representing forelimb, whisker, and periocular muscles.

B. Same view after transection of branches of the facial nerve. Areas of cortex devoted to forelimb and periocular control have increased, extending into the area previously devoted to whisker control.

A Normal somatotopic arrangement

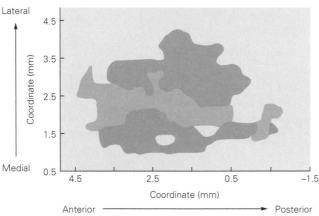

B Somatotopic arrangement after 7th nerve transection

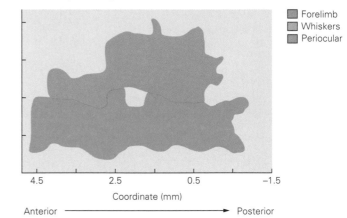

ture motor circuits in the cortex can change depending on sensory or motor activity holds important promise for the rehabilitation of patients who have had strokes and other forms of brain injury. Evidence in favor of this possibility has recently been obtained in animal experiments. In one such experiment, a small cortical artery was occluded in squirrel monkeys to destroy a portion of the population of cells in the primary motor cortex controlling the hand and digits. The animals lost the ability to retrieve food pellets from the smallest of a series of wells, and with time the area of hand representation around the lesion shrank.

Some animals were retrained and others not. The changes in the cortical maps of hand and forearm representation were strikingly different in the two groups. In animals that had not practiced using the hand and relied only on proximal muscle control, all areas of hand and forearm representation were lost. The neurons outside the lesion did not die but elbow and shoulder areas expanded into the remaining (undamaged) hand area. In animals that practiced using their hand daily, the undamaged cortex controlling the hand and digit expanded into adjacent undamaged cortex previously occupied by neurons controlling the elbow and shoulder. These animals fully recovered the ability to retrieve pel-

lets after 3 or 4 weeks. This result emphasizes the importance of practice in sensorimotor tasks for rehabilitation following stroke and other focal brain damage.

As noted in the introduction, a characteristic feature of voluntary movements is that they improve with practice. This may be associated with cortical reorganization. In one study striking changes were found in the motor cortex in human subjects after practice of a single motor task. Subjects were asked to practice a finger opposition task for about 20 minutes every day, touching the thumb to the tip of each finger in a specific repeating sequence. As one can readily appreciate, at first this task was performed slowly and hesitatingly. However, as with typing or playing the piano, speed and accuracy increased with each successive day of practice until the performance learning curve reached asymptote in about 3 weeks. Functional magnetic resonance imaging (MRI) scans revealed that the area of cortex activated during performance of the trained sequence was larger than that activated during a novel untrained sequence (Figure 38-7).

It is important to emphasize that subjects performed both the novel and learned sequences at the same rate. This is crucial in order to exclude the possibility that the differences in activation are simply due to differences in the speed of finger movements. Moreover,

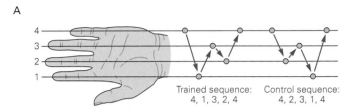

Figure 38-7 As a movement becomes more practiced, it is represented more extensively in primary motor cortex.

A. Human subjects performed two finger-opposition tasks, touching the thumb to each fingertip in the sequences shown. Digits are numbered 1 through 4. Both the practiced and the novel sequence were performed at a fixed, slow rate of two component movements per second.

B. Functional MRI scans show the area in the primary motor cortex activated during the performance of a finger-opposition sequence that had been practiced daily for 3 weeks (**left**) followed by a novel sequence (**right**). The area of activation is larger when the practiced sequence is performed. The experimenters interpret the increased area of metabolic activity as indicating that long-term practice results in a specific and more extensive representation of the trained sequence of movements in the primary motor cortex.

C. In another trial the practiced sequence followed the novel sequence, yet the area of activation in the primary motor cortex during the learned sequence is still larger. Thus the extent of activation is not merely an effect of the order in which the tasks were performed. (From Karni et al 1995.)

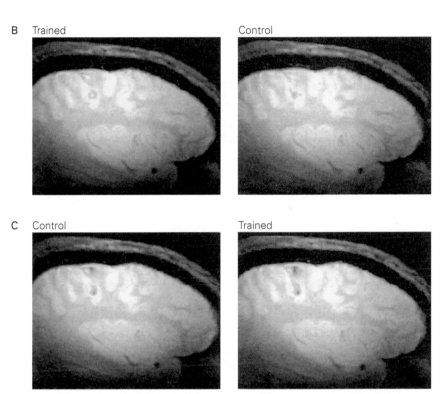

practice with one finger sequence did not facilitate performance of a new sequence nor did it transfer to the untrained hand. (Hand areas are unique in that they are not connected across the corpus callosum.) Such experience-dependent change in the primary motor cortex is likely to be important for the acquisition and retention of other motor skills.

Corticospinal Axons Influence Spinal Motor Neurons Through Direct and Indirect Connections

Corticospinal neurons make powerful and direct excitatory connections with alpha motor neurons in the spinal cord. A unique feature of the corticospinal synapse is that successive cortical stimuli produce progressively larger excitatory postsynaptic potentials in spinal motor neurons. This potentiating connection is one of the mechanisms that permit monkeys to perform individual movements of the digits, including the grasping of small objects (Figure 38-8A) and to isolate movement of proximal joints. This ability is lost permanently after sectioning the pyramidal tracts in the medulla (Figure 38-8B) or after ablating the hand-control area of the motor cortex. Corticospinal fibers also terminate on interneurons in the spinal cord, which in turn project to alpha motor neurons. These indirect connections with motor neurons regulate a larger number of muscles than do the direct connections and so may contribute to the organization of multijointed movements such as reaching and walking.

Sectioning the medullary pyramidal tracts, which interrupts the projection of corticospinal axons from the primary motor cortex and premotor areas, produces contralateral weakness in monkeys. But the animals recover after a period of months, leaving only deficits in speed of movement and in the rate of force development. These deficits can be attributed to interruption of the projections from the primary motor cortex because

A Normal

B After sectioning of
   corticospinal fibers

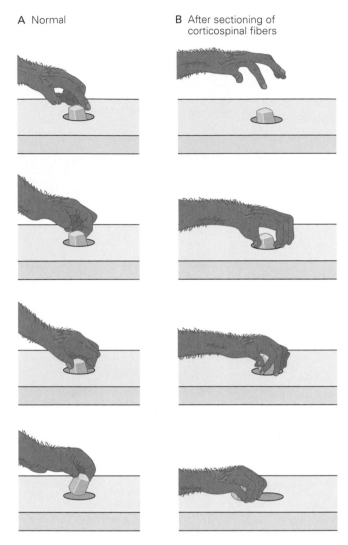

Figure 38-8 Direct corticospinal control of motor neurons is necessary for fine control of the digits.

A. A monkey is able to pick up a food morsel from a small well using the index finger and thumb.

B. After bilateral sectioning of the pyramidal tract the monkey can only remove food from the well by grabbing with the whole hand. (From Lawrence DG, Kuypers HGJM. 1968. The functional organization of the motor system in the monkey. Brain XCI.)

similar deficits arise from lesions in primary motor cortex but not from lesions in premotor areas. Animals with pyramidal tract lesions climb, jump, and appear generally normal. Their partial recovery is possible because cortical commands have indirect access to spinal motor neurons through the descending systems of the brain stem (Chapter 33). Nevertheless, individuated movements of the digits are lost permanently, and the wrist, elbow, and shoulder become linked in extensor or flexor synergies.

Corticospinal projections also have inhibitory effects on spinal motor neurons. Direct recordings in monkeys and indirect evidence from reflex testing in humans indicate that corticospinal inhibition is mediated by the Ia inhibitory interneuron, the same interneuron responsible for the reciprocal inhibition of stretch reflexes (Figure 38-9). Because these spinal interneurons receive peripheral inputs and are able to respond directly to ongoing changes in somatic sensory input, the higher centers of the brain are freed from the need to manage all the details of movements and instead can use the spinal circuits as components of more complex behaviors, much like the subroutines of a computer program.

The Primary Motor Cortex Executes Movements and Adapts Them to New Conditions

Activity in Individual Neurons of the Primary Motor Cortex Is Related to Muscle Force

To understand how cortical motor areas contribute to movement it is necessary to study how individual neurons are modulated in natural motor behaviors. This became possible in the 1960s when Edward Evarts succeeded in correlating the activity of single neurons with specific motor behaviors in active monkeys. Evarts found that activity in individual neurons in the primary motor cortex is modulated when monkeys either flex or extend the individual joints of their contralateral limbs. Individual neurons are maximally activated during movement of a particular joint and particular direction of movement. The changes in neuronal activity begin some 100 ms or more before the onset of movement.

In a classic experiment Evarts showed that, during wrist flexion, the firing of primary motor cortex neurons varied with the amount of force the animal had to exert to move its hand, not with the amplitude of the hand's displacement (Figure 38-10). The activity of these cortical neurons therefore appears to signal the direction and amplitude of muscle force required to produce a movement rather than the actual displacement of the joint.

Jun Tanji and Evarts found another, more surprising property of some primary motor cortex neurons. In these cells the baseline discharge changed while the animal waited for a signal to move in a predetermined direction. For example, a cell would change its level of baseline activity when a green light instructed the animal that an extension movement was to be made at a later signal (an instructed delay task). This pattern of activity was termed *set related* because it reflected the animal's preparation—or *preparatory set*—to respond to a later stimulus. These discharges demonstrated that the intent to perform a movement alters the firing pattern of neurons in the primary motor cortex hundreds of milliseconds before the movement takes place.

Simple correlations of neuronal activity and behavior do not prove causality. Movement or set-related neurons might be concerned with early changes in postural muscle activity or some other process, rather than with the voluntary movement. The most common (and often the only possible) approach to relating neuronal activity to a specific behavior is to exclude confounding sources of correlation. However, in the case of primary motor cortex neurons, what is really needed is a way to know for sure whether activity that precedes a voluntary movement directly influences the muscles used in the movement. Only after a direct influence has been established can the relationship of these cells' activity to specific aspects of the movement be addressed meaningfully.

A major advance in this direction was made in the mid-1970s by Eberhard Fetz and co-workers, who used the spike-triggered averaging technique (Box 38-1) to identify neurons in the primary motor cortex that project directly to motor neurons, called *corticomotoneuronal (CM) cells*. They found that individual CM cells project monosynaptically to more than one motor nucleus and sometimes to muscles controlling different joints. Thus, muscles are not mapped one-to-one in cortical output neurons. Most of the neurons recorded by Fetz have phasic-tonic patterns of activity, firing most briskly during the dynamic phase of movement and settling down to a lower tonic rate when a steady force is reached (Figure 38–12A). For almost all neurons there is a range over which force is related linearly to firing rate. Often, however, this range is quite small, and maximal firing is achieved for relatively small forces.

Direction of Movement Is Encoded by Populations of Cortical Neurons

Most movements involve rotating multiple joints and require sequential and temporally precise activation of many muscles. This raises the question of whether cells in motor cortex directly control the specific spatiotemporal patterns of muscle activation or do they encode more global features of the movement such as its direction, extent, or joint angle changes?

This was examined by Apostolos Georgopoulos, who trained monkeys to move a joystick toward visual targets located in different directions and recorded the associated changes in activity in the primary motor cortex. All neurons fired briskly before and during movements in a broad range of directions (Figure 38-13A).

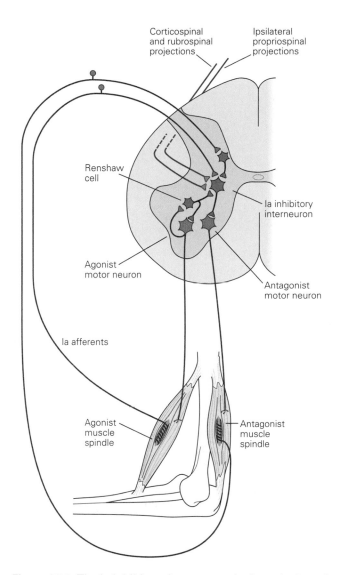

Figure 38-9 The Ia inhibitory interneuron in the spinal cord sends inhibitory signals to antagonist motor neurons when muscle spindles in the agonist muscle are activated. The interneuron receives complex excitatory and inhibitory inputs, including direct input from the motor cortex. These direct cortical connections allow the motor cortex to use reflex circuits as components of complex movements, thereby simplifying the motor cortical program. (Based on Lundberg 1979.)

How can movement direction be coded precisely by neurons that are so broadly tuned? Georgopoulos proposed that movement in a particular direction is determined not by the action of single neurons but by the net action of a large population of neurons. He suggested that the contribution of each neuron to movement in a particular direction be represented as a vector whose length indicates the level of activity during movement

Experimental setup

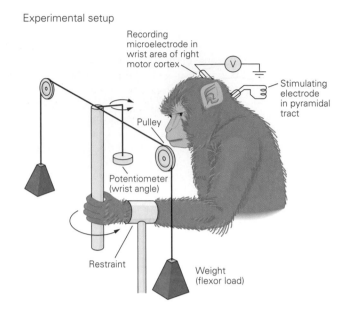

Records of behavior and cell activity

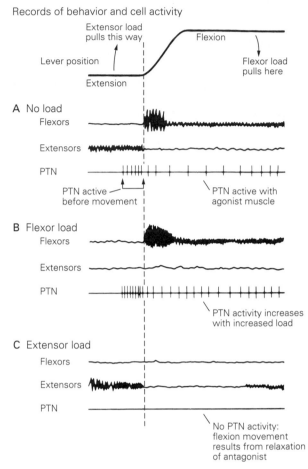

Figure 38-10 Activity in a corticospinal axon correlates with the direction and amplitude of muscle force rather than the direction of displacement. Records shown here were made while a monkey flexed its wrist under three load conditions. In each set of traces the **top trace** indicates the activity in a corticospinal neuron and the **bottom trace** wrist position, with upward deviation being flexion. When no load was applied (**A**) the neuron fired before and during flexion. When a load-opposing flexion was applied, activity in the neuron increased (**B**). When a load-assisting flexion was applied, the neuron fell silent (**C**). In all three conditions the wrist displacement was the same but the neuronal activity changed as the load changed. Thus the firing of the corticospinal neuron in this experiment is related to the force exerted during a movement and not to the displacement of the wrist. (From Evarts 1968.)

in that direction. The contributions of individual cells could then be added vectorially to produce a *population vector*. In fact, the directions of such computed population vectors closely match the directions of movement (Figure 38-13B).

The directionally tuned neurons described by Georgopoulos are modulated strongly by the presence of external loads during reaching movements in a given direction, and this modulation depends on the force required to displace the limb. A cell's firing rate increases if a load opposes movement of the arm in the cell's preferred direction; it decreases if the load pulls the arm in the cell's

preferred direction (Figure 38-14). This dependence of firing rate on load shows that the activity of neurons in the primary motor cortex varies with the direction of forces as well as with movement direction during reaching with the whole arm. This force coding is similar to that for single-joint movements, discussed earlier.

Together these various studies show that motor cortex activity signals not only "lower level" movement parameters, such as muscle forces, but also "higher level" parameters related to the trajectory of the hand during reaching. This feature of motor cortex neurons distinguishes them from alpha motor neurons.

Box 38-1 Postspike Facilitation of Muscle Activity

Recording from cortical neurons in awake animals and relating the neuronal activity to movement parameters has led to significant insights about cortical control of movement. However, studies of this type are limited by their inability to identify functional connections between cortical neurons and the motor neurons of target muscles. This becomes possible with a technique developed by Ebehard Fetz and his colleagues called spike-triggered averaging (STA).

Cortical motor neurons with direct excitatory synaptic connections to motor neurons produce individual EPSPs with a fixed latency. Any one EPSP is unlikely to fully depolarize a motor neuron but it transiently increases the probability the motor neuron will fire by bringing it closer to threshold. The EMG profile is the sum of spike trains of a population of motor units within a muscle and is a reliable indicator of the firing of spinal motor neurons. By averaging the EMG profile over thousands of discharges of one cortical neuron, the effect of a single cortical neuron on an EMG profile can be ascertained. This averaging cancels out random associations of cortical neuronal firing and motor unit discharge; the signal-to-noise ratio improves with the square root of the number of discharges used to compile the average.

Figure 38-11 shows the relation of the discharge of a single cortical neuron to an extension movement of the wrist. A cumulative average over 2000 discharges of the cortical neuron reveals a clear peak in the EMG profile beginning at a latency of 6 ms. This transient increase is called *postspike facilitation* and its short latency is interpreted as evidence of an underlying synaptic connection between the cortical neuron and the motor neurons.

Figure 38-11 Spike-triggered averaging can detect the effects of a single cortical neuron on motor units. The records on the left show discharges of a cortical cell and normal and rectified EMG activity of one agonist muscle associated with wrist extension. From these records 30 μs segments of EMG activity associated with each cortical spike were averaged. The cumulative average of EMG segments associated with the first five spikes are shown on the right. No clear effect can be seen after averaging over only five spikes, but at 2000 spikes postspike facilitation can clearly be seen. (From Fetz and Cheney 1980.)

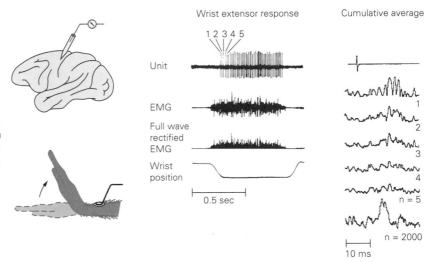

Neurons in the Primary Motor Cortex Are Activated Directly by Peripheral Stimulation Under Particular Conditions

The simplest behaviors controlled by the primary motor cortex are those elicited directly by sensory stimuli. Motor cortical neurons receive strong sensory inputs from the limb whose muscles they control. When a standing human subject pulls on a handle, the sudden postural perturbation elicits a rapid counter-response in the stretched muscle at a latency shorter than a simple reaction time but longer than for a spinal reflex. However, this counter-response happens only when the person is told to resist. Such rapid motor adjustments are mediated mainly by relatively simple transcortical pathways through which somatosensory inputs reach the primary motor cortex directly via projections from the thalamus or primary sensory cortex. This transcortical pathway provides a degree of flexibility to rapid responses that is unavailable in spinal reflexes. These long-loop or transcortical responses are selectively increased in several movement disorders, such as Parkinson disease and myoclonus, while spinal reflexes remain normal.

Individual Movement of Digits Is Controlled by Patterns of Activity in a Population of Cortical Neurons

As noted earlier, anatomical studies and lesion experiments have suggested that the primary motor cortex

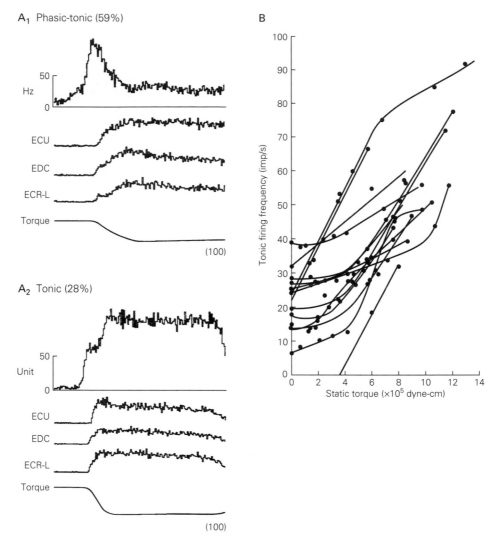

A₁ Phasic-tonic (59%)

A₂ Tonic (28%)

B

Figure 38-12 There is a direct relationship between the firing rate of motor cortical cells and force generation. (From Fetz EE and Cheney 1980.)

A. Two types of motor cortical neurons, phasic-tonic and tonic, are predominant in the primary motor cortex. Each has a characteristic response pattern during isometric wrist torques in which the torque level is reached and held. (Similar patterns are seen for torques accompanied by wrist displacement.)

1. Phasic-tonic cell activity begins with a dynamic burst during the initial increase in torque and then decreases to a steady level when torque is maintained. **2.** Tonic cell activity follows the rise in torque and remains at a high level.

B. In both cell types activity increases with torque. The plot shows the relation between tonic firing rate, (impulses per second) and static torque during wrist extension.

plays a special role in producing individuated movement of the digits in primates.

Although individual neurons fire maximally when a particular finger is moved, digit neurons are dispersed throughout the hand control area of primary motor cortex (Figure 35-15). The manner in which such activity is coordinated to produce a finger movement is analogous to the population coding that underlies reaching movements.

This observation is not surprising, since the digits are biomechanically coupled by common tendons and thus are not anatomically independent of each other. Moving a single digit alone requires activating and inhibiting muscles acting on all the digits. Current evidence indicates that each corticomotoneuronal (CM) cell influences activity in a small group of target muscles. Very few of these cells have been found that control only a single muscle. Even CM cells involved in individuated

A

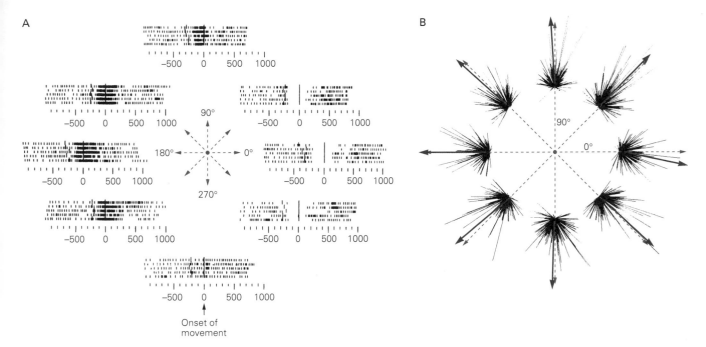

B

Figure 38-13 Direction of movement is encoded in the motor cortex by the pattern of activity in an entire population of cells. (From Georgopoulos et al. 1982.)

A. Motor cortical neurons are broadly tuned to the direction of movement, but individual cells fire preferentially in connection with movement in certain directions. Raster plots of the firing pattern of a single neuron during movement in eight directions show the cell firing at relatively higher rates during movements in the range from 90 degrees to 225 degrees. Different cells have different preferred movement directions. For these recordings a monkey was trained to move a handle to eight locations arranged radially in one plane around a central starting

position. Each row of tics in each raster plot represents activity in a single trial; the rows are aligned at zero time (the onset of movement).

B. Cortical neurons with different preferred directions are all active during movement in a particular direction. The entirety of this activity results in a population vector that closely matches that of the direction of movement. The eight clusters shown here represent the activity of the same population of neurons during reaching movements in eight different directions. **Solid arrows** are the population vectors; **dashed arrows** are the direction of movement of the limb.

finger movements have axons that diverge to more than one motor nucleus in the spinal cord. In addition, as noted earlier, the same target muscle may be influenced by CM cells that are dispersed throughout the hand representation. The cells activated will depend on the task in which the muscle is used.

Roger Lemon and R. B. Muir demonstrated how different tasks determine which of the neurons in the primary motor cortex will be used to control a particular muscle. They examined the activity of individual CM cells in monkeys during two different finger tasks, a power grip and a precision grip, both of which involve contraction of the intrinsic hand muscles controlled by the identified CM cells. Cells that are active during the precision grip remain silent during the power grip, even though the contraction of the target muscle is stronger

for the power grip than for the precision grip (Figure 38-16).

The observation that activity in a CM cell is not invariably coupled with activation of its target muscle fundamentally distinguishes CM cells from spinal motor neurons. The finding that a distinct population of cells in the primary motor cortex is active only during the precision grip is further evidence of the special role of the primary motor cortex in controlling individuated movements of the fingers. The power grip, which does not require individual finger movements, can be controlled by descending pathways, arising either within or outside of the primary motor cortex, that diverge extensively in the spinal cord and therefore can recruit a large number of muscles in a less differentiated synergy.

A Unloaded   B Loaded

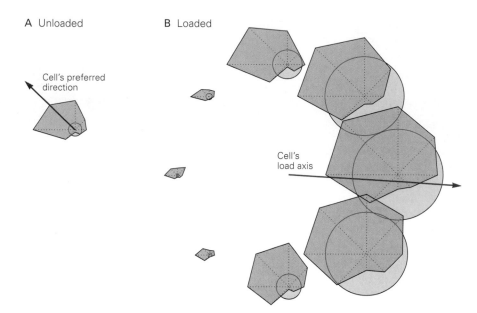

Cell's preferred
direction

Cell's
load axis

Figure 38-14 Motor cortical cells can code for the force required to maintain a trajectory. A monkey was trained to
reach in eight directions while external loads pulled the arm in
one of these directions. Polar plots represent the activity of a
single cell in the primary motor cortex while the arm moved
with external loads. The magnitude of the cell's discharge is
plotted as the length of a vector extending in the direction of
the executed movement (**dotted line**). The tips of all vectors
are joined by a **solid line**. The radius of the circle indicates the
magnitude of cell activity while holding the arm at the central
starting position before movement.

A. Plot showing the preference of the cell for movement to the

upper left during movements in eight directions without an external load applied to the arm.

B. Polar plots for the same cell when loads are applied in eight
directions. The position of each polar plot corresponds to the
direction in which the load pulled the arm. The cell's firing rate
increases in all directions when the arm is pulled right. This
rightward direction is the load axis of the cell, which is approximately opposite to its preferred movement direction. Thus the
cell's firing rate is related to the amount of force required to
maintain an arm trajectory in a given direction, not just to the
direction itself. (From Kalaska et al. 1989.)

Certain motor cortical cells fire less and less often as
muscle force increases. That is, their activity is correlated negatively with force. However, like neurons with
positive correlations (see Figure 38-12), these cells also
facilitate their target muscles. They discharge only during tasks that require precise control of force and
smooth changes in force. Thus their function may be to
provide more precise derecruiting of motor units than
would be afforded simply by inhibiting the so-called
positive cortical neurons. This would be helpful, for example, in releasing delicate objects carefully.

In conclusion, the primary cortex has two levels of
functional organization. First, a low-level control system, the CM cells, controls groups of muscles that can be
brought together into task-specific combinations. Second, a higher-level control system encodes more global
features of the movement. Practice and learning adjust
the relation between these two levels of organization.

Each Premotor Area Contributes to Different
Aspects of Motor Planning

Although the outputs of the premotor areas and the primary motor cortex overlap in the spinal cord, the inputs
to the premotor areas are quite different from those to
the primary motor cortex (see Figure 38-4). Moreover,
damage to premotor areas causes more complex motor
impairments than does damage to primary motor cortex. When a monkey with a large lesion of the premotor
area is presented with food behind a transparent shield
it will reach directly for the food and bump into the
shield. Unlike a normal animal it is unable to incorporate visuospatial information about the shield into the
kinematic plan for moving its hand.

The idea that premotor areas are involved in planning movement has received crucial support during the
past 20 years from physiological and imaging studies of

humans and monkeys performing a variety of special tasks. In monkeys distinct populations of cells are active in connection with ipsilateral movements, bilateral movements, or specific combinations of movements. Set-related and preparatory activity predominates, and cell activity is often associated primarily with specific tasks as we will see below.

Studies of the premotor areas have identified several basic features of the neural organization of motor preparation. First, movements that are initiated internally by the subject—such as the sequencing of finger movements when manipulating an object—involve primarily the supplementary motor area. Second, movements triggered by external sensory events involve primarily the lateral premotor areas. More specifically, separate populations of lateral premotor neurons map the often arbitrary relationship between stimulus and response. The lateral dorsal premotor area is also concerned with delayed action (executed later on cue), whereas the lateral ventral premotor area is concerned with conforming the hand to the shape of objects.

Third, mental rehearsal of a movement—that is, the use of visual imagery to plan a movement—invokes the same patterns of activity in the premotor and posterior parietal cortical areas as those that occur during performance of the movement. Psychophysical studies have shown that mental rehearsal of movement has a similar time course and closely simulates task performance. This observation helps explain the importance of mental rehearsal to athletes and skilled performers. Fourth, the motor and premotor neurons activated during a particular task are not the same over time but change progressively as performance becomes automatic.

The Supplementary and Presupplementary Motor Areas Play an Important Role in Learning Sequences of Discrete Movements

Motor actions are often self-initiated without an environmental cue. Nearly a full second before a self-initiated voluntary movement begins, a characteristic negative shift in cortical potentials is seen in the electroencephalogram (EEG) record of medial premotor regions, where the supplementary motor area is situated. This negative potential, referred to as the *preparatory potential* or Bereitschaft potential, signals the planning that occurs before movement is executed.

The region responsible for this negative potential was localized more precisely in a study comparing increases in regional cerebral blood flow (a measure of increases in neuronal activity) during simple, complex,

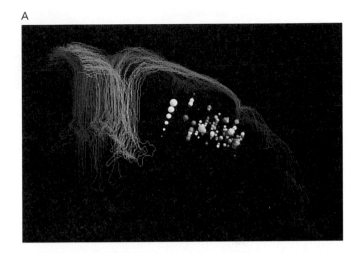

A

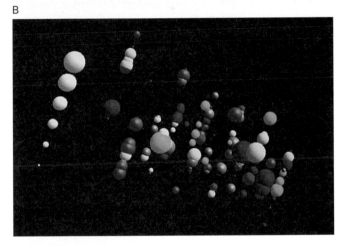

B

Figure 38-15 Cortical neurons that govern finger movements are distributed throughout the hand-control area of the primary motor cortex. (From Schieber and Hibbard 1993.)

A. View of the frontal pole of the monkey cortex, showing the interhemispheric fissure and the lateral convexity. The **colored dots** and **spheres** represent sites of single neurons in the hand-control region of the primary motor cortex from which recordings were made.

B. A plot of each neuron's maximal activity shows that neurons that are maximally active for a particular digit or for the wrist are not grouped together but instead are distributed throughout the hand-control area of the primary motor cortex. Each digit and the wrist are represented by a different color. The diameter of the sphere is proportional to the neuron's activity (the radii of the white spheres represent changes in firing frequency of 0, 40, 80, 120, 160, and 200 spikes per second.)

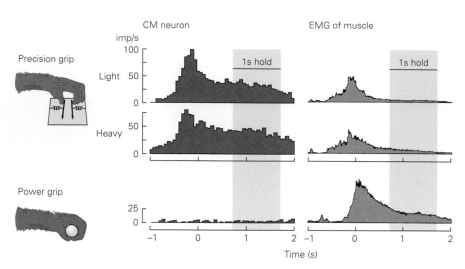

Figure 38-16 Whether an individual corticomotoneuronal (CM) cell is active depends on the motor task. The activity of a CM cell and the activity in its target muscle are not directly related. Cumulative histograms show the activity of a single neuron during a precision grip and a power grip. During the precision grip the neuron's activity is the same whether overall force is light or heavy and the level of electromyographic (EMG) activity in the target muscle is similar for both forces. During the power grip there is almost no activity in the neuron despite a greater amount of EMG activity in the muscle. Thus, even if a given motor neuron is monosynaptically connected to a given CM cell, their firing patterns do not have to parallel each other because the multiplicity of connections to motor neurons allows task flexibility. (**imp/s** = impulses per second.) (From Muir RB, Lemon RN. 1983. Corticospinal neurons with a special role in precision grip. Brain Res 261:312–316.)

and imagined sequences of finger movements. Complex movement sequences require more planning than do simple repetitive movements. Imagining complex movements might require the same amount of planning as real movements. As expected, during forceful repetitive finger flexions against a spring-loaded movable cylinder, increases in regional cerebral blood flow were largely confined to the contralateral primary sensorimotor hand-control region. A complex sequence of finger movements was accompanied by regional cerebral blood flow increases within the supplementary motor area. Remarkably, when the complex sequence of finger movements was simply imagined, regional cerebral blood flow increased in an area anterior to the supplementary motor area on both sides (Figure 38-17). This area, the presupplementary motor area, provides the main input to the supplementary motor area and is discussed in detail below.

The specific role of the supplementary motor area in the internal representation of sequences of movements was examined in another experiment, in which recordings were made from neurons in the primary motor cortex, supplementary motor area, and lateral premotor areas of monkeys while the animals performed two variations of an *instructed-delay task*. In this type of task

subjects are taught which movements to make and later given a cue telling them when to make the movements. The monkeys in this experiment were instructed to touch three panels in a specific sequence. In one variation the instruction was visual: Three panels were lit up in a sequence that the monkeys had to follow. In the other variation the monkeys were instructed to perform a previously memorized sequence. As expected, neurons in the primary motor cortex generally discharged before and during movements to the same degree for visually guided and memorized sequences. In contrast, many supplementary motor area neurons fired only before and during performance of a memorized sequence. The reverse was true for the lateral premotor neurons (Figure 38-18). In addition, the movement-related discharge of some supplementary motor area neurons is specific to a particular sequence of movements such as pushing followed by turning a handle. The cells do not fire in connection with other combinations of the same movements. Thus the supplementary motor area seems to be involved in preparing movement sequences from memory in the absence of visual cues.

The main cortical input to the supplementary motor area arises from the presupplementary motor area (see Figure 38-4). This region projects only to the supple-

A Simple finger flexion

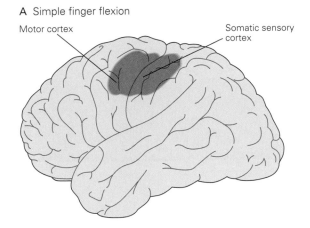

B Sequential finger movements (performance)

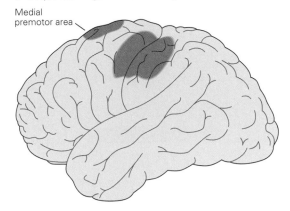

Figure 38-17 Different areas of cortex are activated during simple, complex, and imagined sequences of finger movements. Local increases in cerebral blood flow during a behavior indicate which areas of motor cortex are involved in the behavior. In the experiment illustrated here blood flow was measured by intravenously injecting radioactive xenon dissolved in a saline solution and measuring the radioactivity over different parts of cortex using arrays of detectors placed over the scalp. Because local tissue perfusion varies with neural activity, the measured radioactivity provides a good index of regional activity in the surface of the brain. (Adapted from Roland et al. 1980.)

A. When a finger is pressed repeatedly against a spring, increased blood flow is detected in the hand-control areas of the primary motor and sensory cortices. The increase in the motor area is related to the execution of the response, whereas the increase in the sensory area reflects the activation of peripheral receptors.

B. During a complex sequence of finger movements the increase in blood flow extends to the medial premotor area,

C Mental rehearsal of finger movements

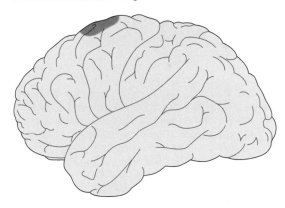

which includes the supplementary motor area (SMA) and presupplementary motor area (preSMA).

C. During mental rehearsal of the same sequence illustrated in part B, blood flow increases only in the medial motor area.

mentary motor area and has no clear somatotopy. Whereas the supplementary motor area is involved in setting the motor programs for learned sequences, the presupplementary motor area is thought to be involved in learning these sequences. For example, in one study the presupplementary motor area was preferentially activated while subjects learned a new sequence of button presses; the supplementary motor area became active only during the performance of the movements once they were learned. This motor learning likely involves a continuous interchange of information with the prefrontal cortex (area 46) and other areas of cortex.

When proficiency and skill are gained, the neural control of task performance can also shift from the sup-

plementary motor area to the primary motor cortex. In one recent study with monkeys, premovement activity in the supplementary motor area during the performance of a key-pressing task disappeared after 12 months of overtraining. Subsequently, an experimental lesion in the right primary motor cortex of these overtrained monkeys caused weakness in the left digits, thereby greatly compromising the monkeys' ability to perform the task. After 21 days the monkeys had recovered sufficiently to press the keys with the same skill as before they received the lesion. Twenty-two days after the monkeys received the lesion recordings from the supplementary motor area showed that neurons were again very active before movement.

Much as extended practice influences the extent of

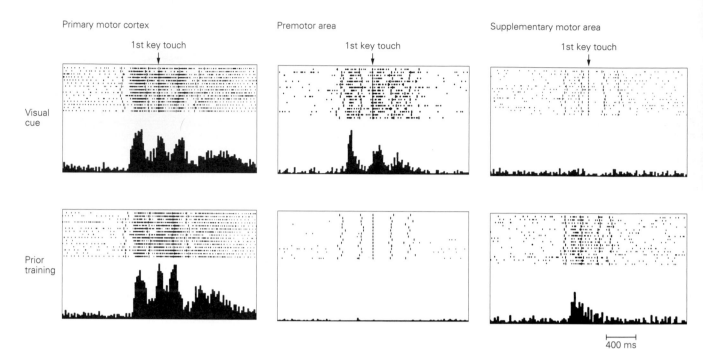

Figure 38-18 Cell activity in the motor cortex depends on whether a sequence of movements is guided by visual cues or by prior training. Monkeys were required to press three buttons either in a sequence presented by lighting three panels in turn or in a sequence they had learned previously. After being instructed to perform the observed sequence or the trained sequence, there was a delay before the animal was given a signal to initiate the movement. Raster plots represent cell discharge before and during movement on 16 trials, and the his-togram shows the summed activity over all trials. Data are aligned to the onset of the first key touch. The cell in the primary cortex fired whether the sequence performed was the one learned in prior training or the one cued by lighted panels. The cell in the lateral premotor area fired only when the visually cued sequence was used, whereas the cell in the supplementary motor area fired only when the trained sequence was used. (From Mushiake et al.1991.)

motor representation in the primary motor cortex, a shift in representation occurs in the supplementary motor cortex as a task goes from being novel to automatic. Conversely, recovery of function following damage to the primary motor cortex represents a new learning challenge in which the supplementary and perhaps pre-supplementary motor areas participate anew.

The Lateral Premotor Areas Contribute to the Selection of Action and to Sensorimotor Transformations

Selection of appropriate action can be the result of internal reflection, which may involve evocation of mental imagery. More often, however, actions are responses to visual or auditory cues. Such cues may signify that a particular action is required immediately (eg, a red light telling us to stop) or that some type of situation is imminent in which action will be required (eg, a yellow light

signaling an imminent change to red). The ability to learn new, adaptive responses to particular environmental stimuli is crucial to effective and accurate movement.

We have seen that set-related activity occurs in the primary motor cortex and supplementary motor area before movement is executed. In the primary motor cortex this activity represents specific parameters of a particular movement; in the supplementary motor area it represents a specific order of responses. In the lateral premotor areas it represents how visual or other sensory stimuli are to be used to direct the movement. Characteristically, set-related activity in the premotor area persists during the entire interval between an anticipatory cue and the signal to move (Figure 38-19).

Set-related activity in the lateral dorsal premotor area is related predominantly to sensory stimuli that do not convey spatial cues to direct movement. For example, the stimulus could be a light in a location that is not

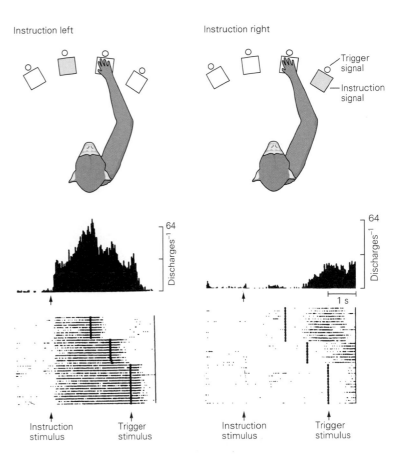

Figure 38-19 A set-related neuron in the dorsal premotor area becomes active while the monkey prepares to make a movement to the left. An instruction signal (illumination of one of four panels) tells the monkey which panel it will have to depress when a trigger signal (illumination of a nearby light-emitting diode) is presented. In the raster plots each dot on each line represents a spike in the recorded neuron. Each line is one trial, and successive trials are aligned on the onset of the instruction signal. The delay between the instruction and trigger signals varied randomly among three values. In the raster plots and histograms the responses made with each delay time are grouped to show that the discharge of the neuron coincides with the instruction signal and lasts until the response is made after the trigger signal. (From Weinrich and Wise 1982.)

Figure 38-20 The visuomotor transformations required for reaching and grasping involve two different pathways from the primary visual cortex to the premotor areas.

Reaching. A path connects the parieto-occipital extrastriate area (**PO**) and the dorsal premotor area (**PMd**). Some of these connections reach PMd directly, and some relay via areas in the intraparietal sulcus: the medial dorsal parietal (**MDP**) and medial intraparietal (**MIP**) areas. This system is responsible for transforming visual information about the location of objects in extrapersonal space into the direction of a reaching movement.

Grasping. A path connects the dorsal extrastriate (**ES**) cortex and the ventral premotor area (**PMv**) via the anterior intraparietal area (**AIP**). This system is responsible for transforming visual information about the properties of objects, such as shape and size, into commands for effective grasping.

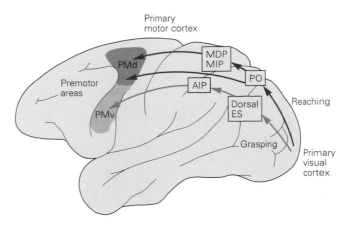

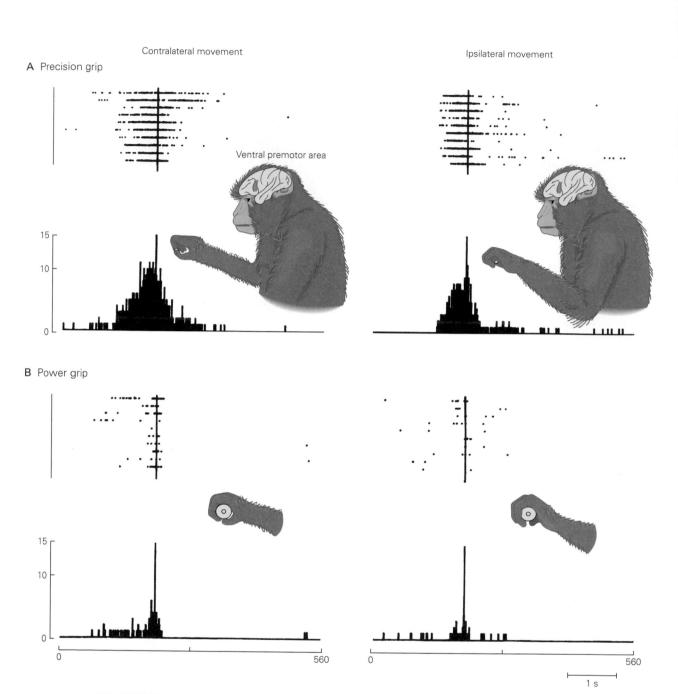

Figure 38-21 Individual neurons in the ventral premotor area fire during specific hand actions only. Raster plots and cumulative histograms show the discharge of a single neuron in the lateral ventral premotor area of a monkey during a precision grip and a power grip involving all the fingers. The cell is active during the precision grip by either arm but not during the power grip by either arm. Thus its activity is specific to the grip type employed by either hand. The fact that the neuron is active during movement of both arms excludes the possibility that this difference is due solely to the different patterns of corticospinal activation required by the two grips; if this were the case, only contralateral activation would occur. (From Rizzolatti et al. 1996.)

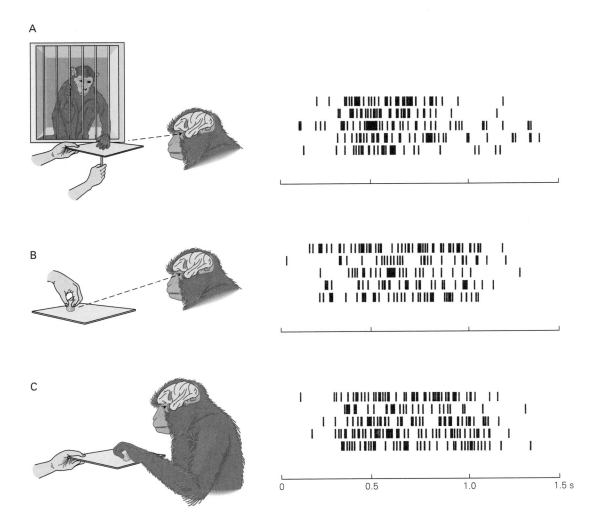

Figure 38-22 An individual cell in the ventral premotor area is active whether the monkey performs a task or observes someone else perform the task. The fact that the same cell is active during action or observation suggests that it is involved in the abstract representation of the motor task.

A. Activity in the neuron as the monkey observes another mon-

key make a precision group.

B. Activity in the same neuron as the monkey observes the human experimenter make the precision grip.

C. Activity in the same neuron as the monkey itself performs a precision grip. (From Rizzolotti et al 1996.)

related to the direction in which the movement is to be executed. Thus the lateral dorsal premotor area is involved in learning to associate a particular sensory event with a specific movement (associative learning). Consistent with this, monkeys with lesions in the lateral dorsal premotor area have difficulty with associative learning. In one study monkeys were taught to associate pulling or pushing a joystick with a particular background light (red or blue). The lateral premotor cortex was then removed from both hemispheres and the animals were retrained two weeks after surgery. Although

the monkeys were able to execute the required movements without impairment, none was able to relearn the association between the background color and whether to push or pull.

Reaching and Grasping Are Mediated by Separate Parieto-Premotor Channels

Goal-directed movements require transformation of sensory representations of the environment into muscle-control signals, a process termed *sensorimotor transformation*. Reaching, a goal-directed movement, requires that visual information about target location and the position of the upper limb be used to specify critical features of the upcoming arm movement. In addition, reaching is commonly coupled with grasping an object.

The parameters for reaching movement, notably direction and extent, depend on the location of the target relative to the body, shoulder, or hand. Grasping, in contrast, is governed mainly by the shape and dimensions of the object. Grasping involves first a separation of the fingers sufficient to enclose the object and then closure as the object is gripped between the pads. Separation of the fingers occurs during transport of the hand toward the object. The kinematics of grasping thus depend on the object itself and not on its location. Thus reaching and grasping are interesting behaviors to study in order to better understand the process of visuomotor transformation.

Anatomical evidence and single-cell recordings have shown that separate but parallel parieto-premotor channels mediate visuomotor transformations required for reaching and grasping (Figure 38-20). During reaching, neurons in parietal area 5 code for direction of the movement but discharge later than dorsal premotor neurons to which they are connected. These neurons could monitor ongoing movements and improve the planning and execution of subsequent reaches by premotor areas.

During grasping, different neurons in the lateral ventral premotor area of monkeys fire in connection with different hand actions and object shapes. These neurons are active throughout reach, well before the fingers begin to grasp. Moreover, different cells fire during different patterns of hand shaping. Some neurons are active only when the action is a precision grip; others are active only when the action is a swiping movement to retrieve food; still others are active only if the action is a power grip (Figure 38-21A). The cells in the lateral ventral premotor area thus seem to direct motor acts that can be guided by visual information about object shape received from the posterior parietal cortex. Another set of neurons discharges whether an object is grasped or bitten.

A unique type of neuron has been discovered in the lateral ventral premotor area. Like others, these neurons discharge when the monkey performs a specific grasping movement, but they also discharge when the monkey observes the same movement being made by another monkey or even by the experimenter. These neurons have been called *mirror neurons* (Figure 38-22).

These different neurons all share the characteristic of encoding a vocabulary of goal-directed behaviors rather than how these behaviors will be carried out.

The ventral premotor area receives its main input from neurons with similar task related properties in the anterior intraparietal region, a region buried in the intraparietal sulcus. Recordings of these neurons were made while a monkey performed a series of tasks involving several different switches and knobs. Cells fired selectively when particular switches were grasped and also fired when the monkey visually fixated the same switch without grasping it. These cells may have a role in transforming the dimensions of an object in visual space into motor signals.

An Overall View

Our understanding of the functional organization of the motor areas of the cerebral cortex has undergone substantial change in recent years, as a new picture of the cortical control of movement has emerged. The primary motor cortex can no longer be seen as a simple motor map of the body, in which adjacent muscles or joints are represented in adjacent cortical sites. Instead, individual muscles and joints are represented repeatedly in a complex mosaic that makes it possible for the cortex to organize combinations of movements suitable to specific tasks. Each muscle and joint is represented by columnar arrays of neurons whose axons branch and make connections with several functionally related motor nuclei. This branching is more modest for cells that control distal muscles, providing these muscles with more independent control.

In addition to terminating on spinal motor neurons, corticospinal neurons also terminate on interneurons in the spinal cord. These connections can gate reflex circuits, allowing voluntary movements to take advantage of spinal circuits, as these circuits can link local sensory input to output.

Distinct populations of motor cortical neurons appear to have specialized roles in determining specific features of motor performance. The characteristics of these different populations and their distribution within the motor areas of cortex point to a hierarchical organization of motor tasks. Thus most neurons in the primary motor cortex become active only shortly before and during movement. Neurons of the primary motor cortex differ from spinal motor neurons in that the former fire only in connection with certain tasks and spatial patterns of muscle activation (eg, precision grip versus power grip), they encode a more restricted range of contractile force than do spinal motor neurons, and some even encode decrements in force. The kinematic details of movement are determined by population codes, the summed activity of entire populations of neurons.

In contrast to neurons in the primary motor cortex, movement-related neurons in the premotor areas may fire during movements that are related to specific tasks and not others to encode a more global feature. Set-related neurons, which are relatively rare in the primary motor cortex, are more common in premotor areas. These cells are active in the absence of any overt behavior, such as during a delay between task instructions and execution of the task. Some encode a response to be made after a delay; others encode a global sensorimotor transformation (eg, "always move at 180 degrees from the visual stimulus"). Thus, just as there is a hierarchy of spinal and supraspinal motor control, there is a hierarchy of neuronal representations of task features within the different cortical areas.

The planning and execution of voluntary movement relies on sensorimotor transformations in which representations of the external environment are integrated into motor programs. This integration is the product of premotor and primary motor areas operating in conjunction with sensory and association areas. We have seen an example of this in the communication between parietal and motor areas during visually guided reaching.

In contrast to reflex movements, voluntary movements are highly adaptable—they improve in speed and accuracy with repeated trials of practice. This adaptability may reflect an optimization process in which the minimal circuits needed to accomplish a behavior are, with training, selected from redundant sensorimotor connections. Such an optimization process could be responsible for the observed shift in the encoding of particular parameters of movement from one group of cells to another, or from one area of cortex to another, as proficiency develops.

A novel behavior initially requires processing in multiple motor and parietal areas as it is continuously monitored for errors and subsequently modified. As the behavior becomes more accurate, the need for sampling of the sensory inflow and updating of the motor program decreases and the need for the computational power of large networks lessens. For example, the pre-supplementary motor area is active during the learning of a behavior but becomes less active as learning progresses. After long periods of practice, when the behavior becomes automatic, activity in the supplementary motor area ceases.

John Krakauer
Claude Ghez

Selected Readings

Dum R, Strick PL. 1996. The corticospinal system: a structural framework for the central control of movement. In: LB Rowell, JT Sheperd (eds). *Handbook of Physiology.* Section 12, *Exercise: Regulation and Integration of Multiple Systems.* Oxford: Oxford Univ. Press (for the American Physiological Society).

Jeannerod M. 1997. *The Cognitive Neuroscience of Action.* Cambridge, MA: Oxford.

Picard N, Strick PL. 1996. Motor areas of the medial wall: a review of their location and functional activation. Cerebral Cortex 6:342–353.

Porter R, Lemon R. 1993. *Corticospinal Function and Voluntary Movement.* Oxford: Clarendon.

Rothwell J. 1994. *Control of Human Voluntary Movement,* 2nd ed. London: Chapman & Hill.

References

Aizawa H, Inase M, Mushiake H, Shima K, Tanji J. 1991. Reorganization of activity in the supplementary motor area associated with motor learning and functional recovery. Exp Brain Res 84:668–671.

Asanuma H, Rosen I. 1972. Topographical organization of cortical efferent zones projecting to distal forelimb muscles in the monkey. Exp Brain Res 14:243–256.

Betz V. 1874. Anatomischer Nachweis zweier Gehimcentra. Centralbl Med Wiss 12:578–580, 595–599.

Brinkman C. 1984. Supplementary motor area of the monkey's cerebral cortex: short- and long-term deficits after unilateral ablation and the effects of subsequent callosal section. J Neurosci 4:918–929.

Cheney PD, Fetz EE. 1980. Functional classes of primate corticomotoneuronal cells and their relation to active force. J Neurophysiol 44:773–791.

Deecke L, Kornhuber HH. 1969. Distribution of readiness potential, pre-motion positivity, and motor potential of the human cerebral cortex preceding voluntary finger movements. Exp Brain Res 7:158–168.

Evarts EV. 1966. Pyramidal tract activity associated with a conditioned hand movement in the monkey. J Neurophysiol 29:1011–1027.

Evarts EV. 1968. Relation of pyramidal tract activity to force exerted during voluntary movement. J Neurophysiol 31:14–27.

Evarts EV, Tanji J. 1976. Reflex and intended responses in motor cortex pyramidal tract neurons of monkey. J Neurophysiol 39:1069–1080.

Fetz EE, Cheney PD. 1980. Postspike facilitation of forelimb muscle activity by primate corticomotoneuronal cells. J Neurophysiol 44:751–772.

Fetz EE, Cheney PD, German DC. 1976. Corticomotoneuronal connections of precentral cells detected by postspike averages of EMG activity in behaving monkeys. Brain Res 114:501–510.

Fritsch G, Hitzig E. 1870. Ueber die elektrische Erregbarkeit des Grosshirns. Arch Anat Physiol Wiss Med, pp. 300–332.

Georgopoulos AP, Kalaska JF, Caminiti R, Massey JT. 1982. On the relations between the direction of two-dimensional arm movements and cell discharge in primate motor cortex. J Neurosci 2:1527–1537.

Goldberger ME. 1972. Restitution of function in the CNS: the pathologic grasp in *Macaca mulatta*. Exp Brain Res 15:79–96.

Halsband U, Freund HJ. 1990. Premotor cortex and conditional motor learning in man. Brain 113:207–222.

He SQ, Dum RP, Strick PL. 1995. Topographic organization of corticospinal projections from the frontal lobe: motor areas on the medial surface of the hemisphere. J Neurosci 15:3284–3306.

Hebb DO, Donderi DC. 1987. *Textbook of Psychology*, 4th ed. Hillsdale, NJ: Lawrence Erlbaum.

Hepp-Reymond MC, Trouche E, Wiesendanger M. 1974. Effects of unilateral and bilateral pyramidotomy on a conditioned rapid precision grip in monkeys (*Macaca fascicularis*). Exp Brain Res 21:519–527.

Jackson JH. 1931. *Selected Writing of John Hughlings Jackson*, Vol. 1. J. Taylor (ed). London: Hodder & Stoughton.

Jankowska E, Padel Y, Tanaka R. 1976. Disynaptic inhibition of spinal motoneurons from the motor cortex in the monkey. J Physiol 258:467–487.

Jeannerod M, Arbib MA, Rizzolatti G, Sakata H. 1995. Grasping objects: the cortical mechanisms of visuomotor transformation. Trends Neurosci 18:314–320.

Jeannerod M, Decety J. 1995. Mental motor imagery: a window into the representational stages of action. Curr Opin Neurobiol 5:727–732.

Kalaska JF. 1996. Parietal cortex area 5 and visuomotor behavior. Can J Physiol Pharmacol 74:483–498.

Kalaska JF, Cohen DA, Hyde ML, Prud'homme M. 1989. A comparison of movement direction-related versus load direction-related activity in primate motor cortex using a two-dimensional reaching task. J Neurosci 9:2080–2102.

Kalaska JF, Crammond DJ. 1995. Deciding not to go: neuronal correlates of response selection in a GO/NOGO task in primate premotor and parietal cortex. Cerebral Cortex 5:410–428.

Karni A, Meyer G, Jezzard P, Adams MM, Turner R, Ungerlieder LG. 1995. Functional MRI evidence for adult motor cortex plasticity during motor skill learning. Nature 377:155–158.

Leyton ASF, Sherrington ES. 1917. Observations on the excitable cortex of the chimpanzee, orangutan, and gorilla. Q J Exp Physiol 11:135–222.

Lundberg A. 1979. Multisensory control of spinal reflex pathways. Prog Brain Res 50:11–28

Lynch JC, Mountcastle VB, Talbot WH, Yin TCT. 1977. Parietal lobe mechanisms for directed visual attention. J Neurophysiol 40:362–389.

Maier MA, Bennett KMB, Hepp-Reymond MC, Lemon RN. 1993. Contribution of the monkey corticomotoneuronal system to the control of force in precision grip. J Neurophysiol 69:772–785.

Moll L, Kuypers HGJM. 1977. Premotor cortical ablations in monkeys: contralateral changes in visually guided reaching behavior. Science 198:317–319.

Mountcastle VB, Lynch JC, Georgopoulos A, Sakata H, Acuna C. 1975. Posterior parietal association cortex of the monkey: command functions for operations with extrapersonal space. J Neurophysiol 38:871–908.

Mushiake H, Inase M, Tanji J. 1991. Neuronal activity in the primate premotor, supplementary, and precentral motor cortex during visually guided and internally determined sequential movements. J Neurophysiol 66:705–718.

Nudo RJ, Wise BM, SiFuentes F, Milliken GW. 1996. Neural substrates for the effects of rehabilitative training on motor recovery after ischemic infarct. Science 272: 1791–1794.

Passingham RE. 1985. Premotor cortex: sensory cues and movement. Behav Brain Res 18:175–186.

Passingham RE, Perry VH, Wilkinson F. 1983. The long term effects of removal of sensory motor cortex in adult and rhesus monkey. Brain 106:675–705.

Penfield W, Rasmussen T. 1950. *The Cerebral Cortex of Man. A Clinical Study of Localization of Function*. New York: Macmillan.

Rizzolatti G, Camarda R, Fogassi L, Gentilucci M, Luppino G, Matelli M. 1988. Functional organization of inferior area 6 in the macaque monkey. II. Area F5 and the control of distal movement. Exp Brain Res 71:491–507.

Rizzolatti G, Fadiga L, Gallesi V, Fogassi L. 1996. Premotor cortex and the recognition of motor actions. Brain Res Cogn Brain Res 3:131–141.

Roland PE, Larsen B, Lassen NA, Skinhoj E. 1980. Supplementary motor area and other cortical areas in organization of voluntary movements in man. J Neurophysiol 43:118–136.

Sanes JN, Suner S, Donoghue JP. 1990. Dynamic organization of primary motor cortex output to target muscles in adult rats. I. Long-term patterns of reorganization following motor or mixed peripheral nerve lesions. Exp Brain Res 79:479–491.

Schell GR, Strick PL. 1984. The origin of thalamic inputs to the arcuate premotor and supplementary motor areas. J Neurosci 4:539–560.

Schieber MH, Hibbard LS. 1993. How somatotopic is the motor cortex hand area? Science 261:489–492.

Shima K, Aya K, Mushiake H, Inase M, Aizawa H, Tanji J. 1991. Two movement-related foci in the primate cingulate cortex observed in signal-triggered and self-paced fore-limb movements. J Neurophysiol 65:188–202.

Smith AM, Hepp-Reymond MC, Wyss UR. 1975. Relation of activity in precentral cortical neurons to force and rate of force change during isometric contractions of finger muscles. Exp Brain Res 23:315–332.

Stephan KM, Fink GR, Passingham RE, Silbersweig D, Ceballos-Haumann RA, Frith CD, Frackowiak R. 1995. Functional anatomy of the mental representation of upper extremity movements in healthy subjects. J Neurophysiol 73:373–386

Weinrich M, Wise SP. 1982. The premotor cortex of the monkey. J Neurosci 2:1329–1345.

Woolsey CN. 1958. Organization of somatic sensory and motor areas of the cerebral cortex. In: HF Harlow, CN Woolsey (eds). *Biological and Biochemical Bases of Behavior*, pp. 63–81. Madison: Univ. Wisc. Press.

39

The Control of Gaze

In the last several chapters we learned about the motor systems that control the movements of the body in space. In this and the next two chapters we consider the motor systems concerned with gaze, balance, and posture. As we explore the world around us these motor systems act to stabilize our body, particularly our eyes, in space. In examining these motor systems we shall be concerned with the following questions: How do we know where we are in space? How do we compensate for planned and unplanned movements of the head? How do we stay upright?

In this chapter we describe the organization of the ocular motor system and how visual information guides eye movements. In the next chapter we discuss the vestibular system and how vestibular reflexes adjust the eyes when the head moves. In the third chapter of this sequence (Chapter 41) we examine how vestibular and proprioceptive information is used by the skeletomotor system to maintain upright posture, including stabilizing the head.

The importance of the gaze system arises from the anatomy of the eye. Although the eye can detect objects anywhere in front of us, we see best with the *fovea*, the specialized area at the center of the retina that is less than 1 mm in diameter and detects a tiny fraction of the visual field, less than the diameter of a full moon. When we want to examine an object in the world, we have to move the fovea to it. The *gaze system* performs this function through two components: the *oculomotor system*, which moves the eyes in the orbit, and the *head movement system*, which moves the orbits in space. The gaze system also prevents the image of an object from moving on the retina. It keeps the eye still when the image is still and stabilizes the image when the object moves in the world or when the head itself moves.

Stabilizing the fovea when the head moves requires information about head motion. This information can be supplied by the visual system—because the image moves on the retina when the eyes move with the head—but this visual processing is relatively slow. Instead, the nervous system relies on sensors in the inner ear that detect head motion directly. Information on movements of the head and the position of the head relative to gravity is processed by the vestibular system. This information is used by the vestibulo-ocular reflex to move the eyes directly without relying on visual information to control the movement.

Six Neuronal Control Systems Keep the Fovea on Target

Hermann Helmholtz and other nineteenth century psychophysicists who studied vision were also interested in eye movement. They appreciated that an analysis of these movements was essential for understanding visual perception but they did not realize that there is more than one kind of eye movement. However, in 1890 Edwin Landott discovered that, when we read, the eyes do not move smoothly along a line of text but make little jerky movements—saccades—each followed by a short pause. By 1902 Raymond Dodge was able to outline five separate movement systems that put the fovea on a target and keep it there. Each of these movement systems shares the same effector pathway—the three bilateral groups of oculomotor neurons in the brain stem.

These five systems include three that keep the fovea on a visual target in the environment and two that stabilize the eye during head movement. *Saccadic eye movements* shift the fovea rapidly to a visual target in the periphery. *Smooth pursuit movements* keep the image of a moving target on the fovea. *Vergence movements* move the eyes in opposite directions so that the image is posi-

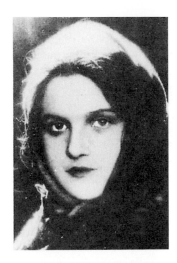

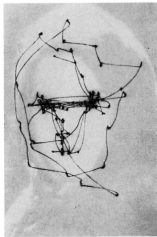

Figure 39-1 Saccadic eye movements are used to explore the visual environment. Alfred Yarbus discovered that the pattern of an observer's eye movements can describe the objects of attention in the environment. In Yarbus's experiment an observer looks at a picture of a woman for 1 min. The resulting eye positions are shown superimposed on the picture of the woman as **dark lines.** Note that the eye movements concentrate on certain features of the face. The eye lingers over the woman's eyes and mouth *(fixations)* and spends less time over intermediate positions. The rapid movements between fixation points are *saccades.* (From Yarbus 1967.)

tioned on both foveae. *Vestibulo-ocular movements* hold images still on the retina during brief head movements and are driven by signals from the vestibular system. *Optokinetic movements* hold images during sustained head rotation and are driven by visual stimuli.

All eye movements but vergence movements are conjugate: Each eye moves the same amount in the same direction. Vergence movements are disconjugate: The eyes move in different directions and sometimes by different amounts. Finally, there are times that the eye must stay still in the orbit so that it can examine a stationary object. Thus, a sixth system, the *fixation system,* holds the eye still during intent gaze. This requires active suppression of eye movement. The vestibular and optokinetic systems are discussed in Chapters 40 and 41. We discuss the remaining four here.

An Active Fixation System Keeps the Eyes on a Stationary Target

Vision is most accurate when the eyes are still. When we look at an object of interest a neural system of fixation actively prevents the eyes from moving. The fixation system is not as active when we are doing something that does not require vision, for example, mental arithmetic. Some patients with disorders of the fixation system—for example, those with congenital nystagmus—have poor vision not because their eyes are abnormal but because they cannot hold their eyes still enough for the visual system to work accurately.

The Saccadic System Points the Fovea Toward Objects of Interest

Our eyes explore the world in a series of active fixations connected by saccades (Figure 39-1). The purpose of the saccade is to move the eyes as quickly as possible. Sac-

cades are highly stereotyped; they have a standard waveform with a single smooth increase and decrease of eye velocity. Saccades are extremely fast, occurring within a fraction of a second, at speeds up to 900°/s (Figure 39-2). Only the distance of the target from the fovea determines the velocity of a saccadic eye movement. We can change the amplitude and direction of our saccades voluntarily but we cannot change their velocities.

Ordinarily there is no time for visual feedback to modify the course of the saccade; corrections to the direction of movement are made in successive saccades. Only fatigue, drugs, or pathological states can slow saccades. Accurate saccades can be made not only to visual targets but also to sounds, tactile stimuli, memories of locations in space, and even verbal commands ("look left").

The Smooth Pursuit System Keeps Moving Targets on the Fovea

The smooth pursuit system keeps the image of a moving target on the fovea by calculating how fast the target is moving and moving the eyes accordingly. The system requires a moving stimulus in order to calculate the proper eye velocity. Thus, a verbal command or an imagined stimulus cannot produce smooth pursuit. Smooth pursuit movements have a maximum velocity of about 100°/s, much slower than saccades. Drugs, fa-

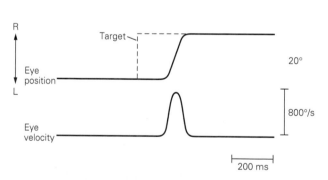

Figure 39-2 The human saccade. Eye position, target position, and eye velocity are shown plotted against time. At the beginning of the plot the eye is on the target—the traces representing eye and target positions are superimposed. Suddenly the target jumps to the right (**dotted line**). Almost immediately, 200 ms later, the eye moves to bring the target back to the fovea. Note the smooth symmetric velocity profile. Because eye movements are rotations of the eye in the orbit they are described in terms of the angle of rotation. Similarly, objects in the visual world are described by the angle of arc they subtend at the eye. A thumb, viewed at arm's length subtends an angle of about 1°. A saccade from one side of the thumb to the other traverses 1° of arc.

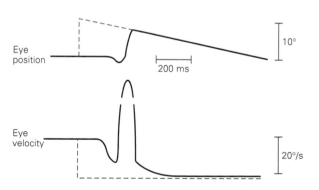

Figure 39-3 Human smooth pursuit. Eye position plotted over time with the target position superimposed (dotted line). Eye and target velocity are plotted beneath. In this example the subject was asked to make a saccade to a target that jumps away from the center of gaze and then moves back. Note that the very first movement seen in the position and velocity traces is a smooth pursuit movement with the same velocity as the target. As can be seen from the eye position trace, the eye briefly moves *away* from the target. The saccade enables the eye to adjust its position to catch the target, and from then on the smooth pursuit keeps the eye on the target. The saccade velocity trace is clipped so that the movement can be shown on the scale of the pursuit movement, an order of magnitude slower than the saccade.

tigue, alcohol, and even distraction degrade the quality of these movements.

The saccadic and smooth pursuit systems have very different central control systems. This is best seen when a target jumps away from the center of gaze and then moves slowly back toward it. The eye begins smooth pursuit movement first and then, paradoxically, moves *away* from the target with a velocity briefly equal to that of the target (Figure 39-3).

The Vergence Movement System Aligns the Eyes to Look at Targets at Different Depths

The smooth pursuit and saccadic systems produce conjugate movements of both eyes. In contrast, the vergence system produces disconjugate movements of the eyes. When we look at an object that is close to us our eyes rotate toward each other, or *converge;* and when we look at an object further away they rotate away from each other, or *diverge* (Figure 39-4). These disconjugate movements ensure that the object of interest is on the same place in both retinas, since objects ordinarily occupy slightly different places on the two retinas. The visual system uses slight differences of retinal position, or *retinal disparity,* to create a sense of depth. The vergence system uses retinal disparity to drive disconjugate movements.

At any given time the entire visual world is not in focus on the retina. When we look at something close by, distant objects are blurred. When we look at something far away, near objects are blurred. When the eyes shift gaze in depth, the new object of interest must be brought into focus. The ciliary muscle adjusts the curvature of the crystalline lens in the eye that focuses the world on the retina. To bring the object into focus the oculomotor system contracts the ciliary muscle, thereby changing the radius of curvature of the lens to focus the world on the retina. This process is called *accommodation.*

Accommodation and vergence are linked. Blur is the stimulus that induces accommodation; whenever accommodation occurs, the eyes also converge. Similarly, retinal disparity induces vergence; whenever the eyes converge, accommodation also takes place. At the same time the pupils transiently constrict to increase the depth of field of the focus. The linked systems of accommodation, vergence, and pupillary constriction comprise the *near response.*

The Eye Is Moved by Six Muscles

Eye Movements Rotate the Eye in the Orbit

To understand how the eyes move it is necessary to understand the geometry of the eye and the extraocular

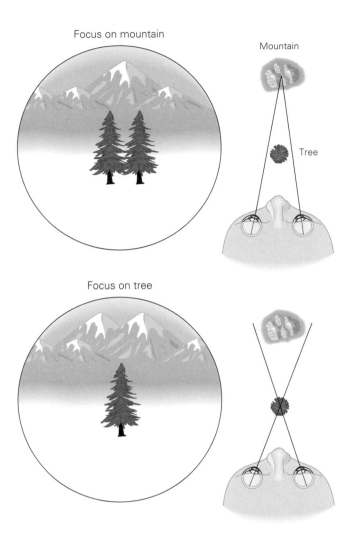

Focus on mountain

Focus on tree

Figure 39-4 Vergence movements. When the eyes focus on a distant mountain, the nearer tree occupies relatively different retinal positions in the two eyes and is seen as a double image. When the viewer wishes to look at the tree, the vergence system must rotate each eye inward. Now the tree image occupies the same position on both retinas and is seen as one object, but the mountain occupies different locations on the retinas and appears double. (From Dr. F. A. Miles.)

muscles. To a good approximation, eye movements are the rotation of the globe of the eye in the socket of the orbit. The eye's orientation can be defined by three axes of rotation—horizontal, vertical, and torsional—that intersect at the center of the eyeball, and eye movements are described as rotations around these axes.

Abduction rotates the eye away from the nose and *adduction* rotates the eye toward the nose. *Elevation* rotates the eye vertically up; *depression* rotates it down.

A Lateral view

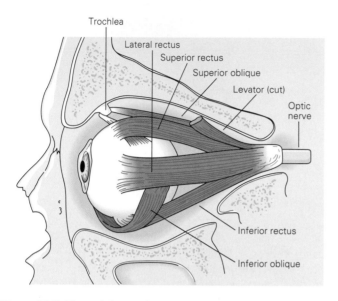

B Superior view

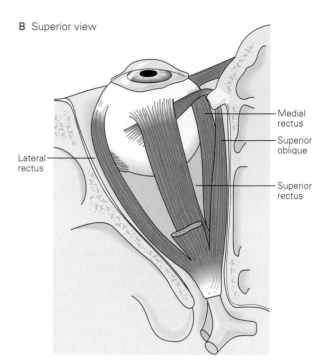

Figure 39-5 The origins and insertions of the extraocular muscles.

A. Lateral view of a left eye with the orbital wall cut away. The recti insert in front of the equator of the globe, so that contraction rotates the cornea toward the muscle. The obliques insert behind the equator, and contraction rotates the cornea away

from the insertion. The superior oblique muscle passes through a pulley of bone, the trochlea, before it inserts.

B. Superior view of the left eye with the roof of the orbit cut away. The superior rectus passes over the superior oblique and inserts in front of it.

Torsional movements do not change the line of sight, but rotate the eye around it: *Intorsion* rotates the top of the cornea toward the nose and *extorsion* rotates it away from the nose. Torsional movements maintain the perceptual stability of vertical lines. The eye must maintain the same amount of torsion in all positions in the orbit, or else lines perceived as vertical in some positions of gaze would be perceived to tilt in others. Torsional movements become apparent only when they are exaggerated by pathological processes.

The Six Extraocular Muscles Form Three Complementary Pairs

Six muscles attach to each eye: four rectus muscles (superior, inferior, medial, and lateral) and two oblique (superior and inferior). The recti originate at the apex of the orbit and insert on the *sclera,* the outer coat of the eyeball, anterior to the equator of the eye (Figure 39-5).

The obliques approach the eye from the anteromedial aspect and insert behind the equator. Because the obliques attach behind the equator, they pull the

back of the eye toward their insertions, tilting the pupil away. Thus the superior oblique depresses the eye and the inferior oblique elevates it. The superior oblique muscle travels first through a pulley *(trochlea)* of bone and then to the eye.

The medial rectus adducts the eye; the lateral rectus abducts it. The actions of the four remaining muscles are complicated because they do not perform purely vertical or torsional rotations but a combination of the two. The proportion of torsional and vertical rotation performed by each muscle depends on the horizontal position of the eye in the orbit (Table 39-1 and Figure 39-6).

For all but vergence movements the two eyes are yoked together: To follow a target moving upward to the left, the left eye moves upward and away from the nose while the right eye moves upward and toward the nose. This requires that each pair of muscles in one orbit have a functional complement in the other so that the eye can rotate in the same plane, but in the opposite direction. The horizontal recti complement each other, but the vertical muscles do not. The superior oblique muscle of one eye has roughly the same pulling plane as

A   Left superior rectus

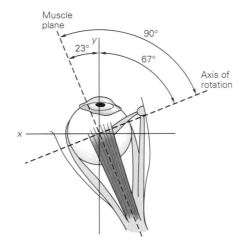

B   Left superior oblique

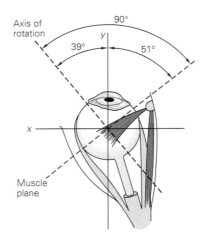

Figure 39-6 Each superior rectus and oblique muscle has torsional and elevational components to its actions. How much each muscle elevates and provides torsion depends on the position of the eye. (Adapted from von Noorden 1980.)

A. When the eye is in the primary visual axis (the *y* axis in the diagram) or lateral to it *(abduction)* the superior rectus rotates the eye vertically upward and all of the intorsion comes from the superior oblique muscle. When the eye is completely medial to the visual axis *(adduction)* the superior rectus predomi-

nantly intorts the eye and the inferior oblique provides most of the elevation.

B. When the eye is 16° or more lateral from the primary visual axis the superior oblique intorts the eye and depression comes from the inferior rectus. When the eye is completely medial to the visual axis the superior oblique rotates the eye vertically downward and all of the intorsion comes from the superior rectus.

the inferior rectus of the other, and the inferior oblique of one eye has the same pulling plane as the superior rectus of the other.

Extraocular Muscles Are Controlled by Three Cranial Nerves

Extraocular muscles are innervated by three groups of motor neurons whose cell bodies form nuclei in the brain stem (Figure 39-7). The lateral rectus is innervated by the *abducens nerve* (cranial nerve VI), whose nucleus lies in the pons in the floor of the fourth ventricle. The superior oblique muscle is innervated by the *trochlear nerve* (cranial nerve IV) located in the midbrain at the level of the inferior colliculus. The trochlear nerve gets its name from the bony pulley through which the superior oblique muscle travels. The medial, inferior, and superior recti and the inferior oblique muscles are all innervated by the *oculomotor nerve* (cranial nerve III), located in the midbrain at the level of the superior colliculus. The levator palpebrae that raises the eyelid and the ciliary muscles that constrict the pupil and adjust the curvature of the lens are also innervated by parasympathetic fibers traveling in the oculomotor nerve.

The pupil and levator palpebrae also have sympathetic innervation. The sympathetic innervation of the pupil dilates the eye. The sympathetic fibers reach the

eye via a circuitous route that is clinically important. Preganglionic fibers have their nuclei in the intermediolateral column of the upper thoracic spinal cord. They leave the spinal cord in the first thoracic root, traverse the apex of the pleura, and synapse in the superior cervical ganglion. The postganglionic fibers travel with the carotid artery and join the ophthalmic branch of the trigeminal nerve near its entrance into the orbit.

Patients with lesions of the extraocular muscles or their nerves complain of double vision *(diplopia)*, because the image of the object of gaze no longer lies on the same retinal location in each eye. Lesions of each nerve have a characteristic syndrome.

An isolated lesion of the abducens nerve (VI) results in loss of abduction beyond the midline, causing

Table 39-1 Vertical Muscle Action in Adduction and Abduction

Muscle	Adduction	Abduction
Superior rectus	Intorsion	Elevation
Inferior rectus	Extorsion	Depression
Superior oblique	Depression	Intorsion
Inferior oblique	Elevation	Extorsion

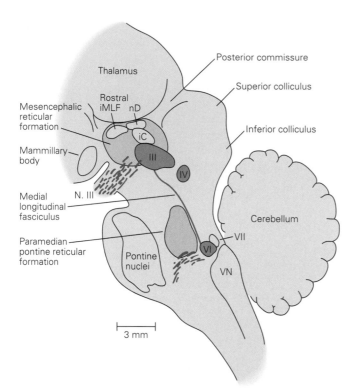

Figure 39-7 The ocular motor nuclei in the brain stem (parasagittal section through the thalamus, pons, midbrain, and cerebellum of a rhesus monkey). The oculomotor nucleus (cranial nerve III) is in the midbrain at the level of the mesencephalic reticular formation. The trochlear nucleus (nerve IV) is slightly caudal, and the abducens nucleus (nerve VI) lies in the pons at the level of the paramedian pontine reticular formation, adjacent to the fasciculus of the facial nerve (VII). iC = interstitial nucleus of Cajal; iMLF = interstitial nucleus of the medial longitudinal fasciculus; nD = nucleus of Darkshevich; VN = vestibular nuclei. (Adapted from Henn et al. 1984.)

diplopia when patients attempt to look in the direction of the paralyzed lateral rectus muscle. Because convergence adducts each eye, patients with a partial paralysis of the abducens nerve will have less diplopia when they look at a near object than when they look at a far object.

An isolated lesion of the trochlear nerve results in deficits in extorsion and depression that vary with the position of the eye in the orbit. This results in a *skew deviation* (eyes at different vertical positions in the orbit) and a torsional deficit. Patients with damage of the trochlear nerve frequently keep their heads tilted toward the side of the weak muscle to minimize diplopia (Figure 39-8).

A lesion of the oculomotor nerve results in loss of eye movement medially or upward from the mid position. Downward movement is partial because the superior oblique muscle (trochlear nerve) function is intact but the torsional function of the superior oblique is not balanced by that of the inferior rectus muscle, so the eye intorts as it moves downward.

Since fibers that control lid elevation, accommodation, and pupillary constriction travel in the oculomotor nerve, damage to this nerve also results in drooping of the eyelid *(ptosis)*, blurred vision for near objects, and pupillary dilatation *(mydriasis)*. The ptosis is not complete because the sympathetic innervation is still intact. Lesions anywhere along the course of the sympathetic fibers result in ptosis and a relative pupillary constriction *(meiosis)*. For example, many patients with lesions at the apex of a lung show ptosis and meiosis of the ipsilateral eye.

Extraocular Motor Neurons Signal Eye Position and Velocity

To understand how the brain generates eye movements it is necessary to understand the motor signals sent to the extraocular muscles. The best way to understand these motor signals is to examine the activity of an extraocular motor neuron during a saccade. The discharge frequency of an extraocular motor neuron is directly proportional to the position and velocity of the eye (Figure 39-9A). As the eye velocity goes from 0°/s to 900°/s the firing rate of the neuron increases rapidly, described as a *pulse* of activity. This rapid rise of neuronal activity drives the eyes as quickly as possible and overcomes the viscous drag of the eye in the orbit. Once the eyes have reached their new position they are held there by steady contraction of the extraocular muscles. The difference between the initial and final discharge levels is described as a *step* in activity.

Thus the saccade signal of an ocular motor neuron has the form of a pulse-step (Figure 39-9B). The height of the step determines the amplitude of the saccade, while the height of the pulse determines the speed of the saccade. The duration of the pulse determines the duration of the saccade. Inputs from different neural pathways determine the pulse and the step of the motor signal.

Ocular motor units differ from skeletal motor units in several ways. There are no ocular stretch reflexes, although the extraocular muscles are rich in muscle spindles. Recurrent inhibition does not occur on oculomotor neurons, nor are there special fast-twitch and slow-twitch muscles. All eye motor neurons participate equally in all types of eye movements; no motor neurons are specialized for saccades or smooth pursuit. However, like skeletal motor units, eye motor units have a fixed sequence of recruitment. Regardless of the type of eye movement, eye motor neurons are recruited according to the position of the eye in the orbit. For example, the further the eye moves laterally, the more abducens neurons discharge, causing more lateral rectus muscle fibers to contract.

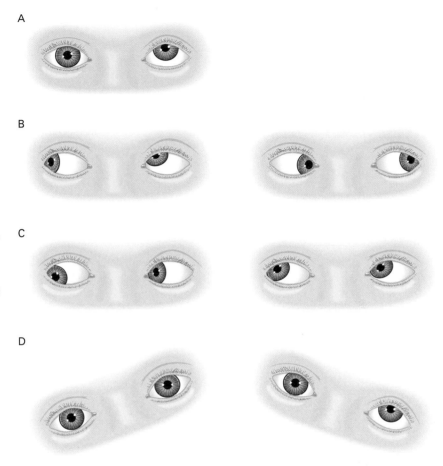

Figure 39-8 A patient with a deficit of the left superior oblique muscle. When the patient looks straight ahead, the left eye is mildly elevated relative to the right (**A**). This elevation occurs because there is no superior oblique tension to counteract the left superior oblique. When the patient looks to the right, the eye becomes even more elevated as more of the superior oblique force is dedicated to elevation (**B**). When the patient attempts to look down, the left eye cannot be depressed below the midline (**C**). When the head tilts to the right, the vertical deviation is lessened (**D**). Patients with a lesion of the trochlear nerve frequently adopt this posture to eliminate diplopia. (Adapted from Leigh and Zee 1991.)

The Motor Circuits for Saccades Lie in the Brain Stem

Ocular motor signals describe the velocity and the position of the eye at any given time. How are these parameters of movement determined? The higher centers that control gaze (discussed in the next section) specify only a desired change in eye position. This signal is then transformed by interneurons in the brain stem reticular formation into the necessary velocity and position instructions to the motor neurons. The horizontal component of this movement, the signals going to the horizontal recti muscles, is organized in the paramedian pontine reticular formation and the rostral medulla. The vertical component is organized in the mesencephalic reticular formation. In each of these circuits different neurons are responsible for the step and the pulse components of the motor signal.

Horizontal Saccades Are Generated in the Pontine Reticular Formation

Patients with brain stem lesions cannot make conjugate horizontal eye movements to the side with the lesion. Electrical stimulation of the paramedian pontine reticular formation drives the eyes in the ipsilateral direction, and chemical lesions destroying the cells in this region eliminate saccades without affecting the vestibulo-ocular reflex or smooth pursuit. When the lesions are limited to the pons, the effect may be limited to ipsilateral saccades only.

Recall that a saccade motor signal has both pulse and step components. The neurons that give rise to the pulse component are called *burst cells*. The burst neurons for horizontal saccades lie within the paramedian pontine reticular formation. These cells fire at a high frequency just before and during ipsilateral saccades, and

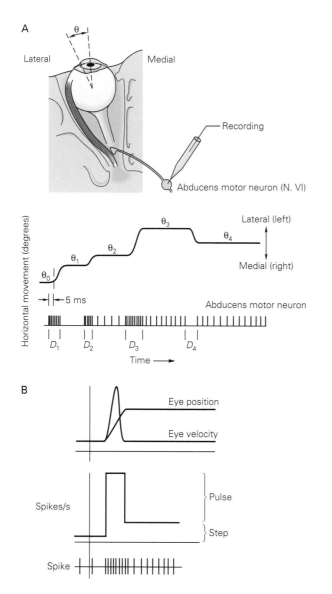

Figure 39-9 Motor neurons signal eye position and velocity.

A. Relation of the discharge rate of a right abducens neuron in the monkey to eye position and velocity. When the eye is positioned in the left side of the orbit the cell is silent (position θ_0). As the monkey makes a rightward saccade there is a burst (D_1), but in the new position (θ_1) the eye is still too far to the left for the cell to discharge. During the next saccade there is a burst (D_2), and at the new position (θ_2) there is a tonic position-related discharge. Before and during the next saccade (D_3) there is again a pulse of activity and a higher baseline discharge when the eye is at the new position (θ_4). When the eye makes a leftward movement there is a period of silence during the saccade (D_4) even though the eye ends up at a position associated with a tonic discharge. (Adapted from Dr. A. Fuchs.)

B. Saccades are associated with a step of activity, which signals the change in eye position, and a pulse of activity, which signals eye velocity. The neural activity (**below**) corresponding to eye position and velocity (**above**) is illustrated here both as a train of individual spikes and as an estimate of the instantaneous firing rate (spikes per second).

their activity resembles the pulse component of motor neuron discharge (Figure 39-10).

There are a variety of burst cells. *Medium-lead burst cells* make direct excitatory connections to motor neurons and interneurons in the ipsilateral abducens nucleus. *Long-lead burst neurons* drive the medium-lead burst cells and receive excitatory input from higher centers. *Inhibitory burst neurons* located more caudally suppress contralateral abducens neurons and excitatory burst neurons and are excited by medium-lead burst neurons.

A second class of pontine cells, *omnipause cells*, fire continuously except around the time of a saccade; firing ceases shortly before and during all saccades. Omnipause cells are located in the nucleus of the dorsal raphe on the midline just behind and below the abducens nucleus (Figure 39-10A). They project to contralateral pontine and mesencephalic burst neurons. Electrical stimulation of omnipause neurons during a saccade stops the saccade, which resumes when the stimulation stops. The omnipause neurons are GABA-ergic neurons that inhibit the burst neurons. By pausing in their firing they allow burst cells to initiate a saccade. Because a saccade requires both the excitation of burst cells and inhibition of omnipause cells, the system is stable, and unwanted saccades are made only infrequently.

If the motor neurons received a signal only from the burst cells, the eyes would drift back to the starting position because there would be no new position signal to hold the eyes in place after they have been moved by the pulse. David A. Robinson pointed out that this signal can be generated from the velocity burst signal by the neural equivalent of the mathematical process of integration. (Velocity can be computed by differentiating position with respect to time. Position can be computed by integrating velocity with respect to time.)

Neural integration of the velocity signal requires the cerebellar flocculus and two brain stem nuclei, the medial vestibular nucleus and the nucleus prepositus hypoglossi. Neurons in these areas are *tonic* neurons that maintain a steady signal related to eye position; they do not generate any saccadic burst signal. A monkey with a lesion of these areas makes normal saccades, but after a saccade the eyes drift back toward the mid position because the cells responsible for the integrated step signal that keeps the eyes at the new position are destroyed. Integration of the burst requires coordination of the nuclei prepositi hypoglossi and the medial vestibular nuclei on both sides of the brain stem. A simple midline disconnection causes a failure of eye position. Tonic cells are also found in the paramedian pontine reticular formation.

The lateral rectus motor neurons in the pons are driven directly by medium-lead burst neurons, which

A

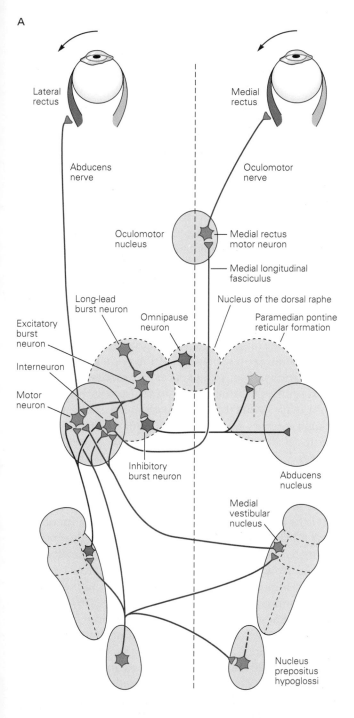

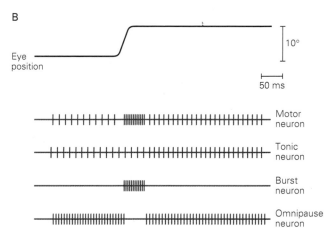

Figure 39-10 The motor circuit for horizontal saccades in the brain stem. Excitatory neurons are **orange** and inhibitory neurons are **gray**. The **dotted line** represents the midline of the brain stem.

A. Long-lead burst neurons relay signals from higher centers to the excitatory burst neurons. The eye velocity component of the motor signal arises from excitatory burst neurons in the paramedian pontine reticular formation that synapse on motor neurons and interneurons in the abducens nucleus. The abducens motor neurons project to the ipsilateral lateral rectus muscles while the interneurons project to the contralateral medial rectus muscle via fibers that cross the midline and ascend in the medial longitudinal fasciculus. Excitatory burst neurons also drive ipsilateral inhibitory burst neurons that inhibit contralateral abducens and excitatory burst neurons. The medial vestibular nucleus also inhibits contralateral abducens neurons. Omnipause neurons inhibit excitatory burst neurons and abducens neurons, preventing unwanted eye movements. The eye position component of the motor signal arises from a "neural integrator" comprised of neurons distributed throughout the medial vestibular nuclei and nucleus prepositus hypoglossi on both sides of the brain stem. These neurons receive velocity signals from excitatory burst neurons and integrate this velocity signal to a position signal. The position signal is transmitted to the ipsilateral abducens neurons.

B. Different neurons provide different information for a horizontal saccade (**above**). The motor neuron has both position and velocity signals. The tonic neuron in the nucleus prepositus hypoglossi has only an eye position signal. The excitatory burst neuron in the paramedian pontine reticular neuron has only eye velocity information. The omnipause neuron discharges at a high rate except before, during, and after the saccade.

supply the burst, and the vestibular and prepositus nuclei neurons, which supply the tonic signal. The medial rectus motor neurons in the midbrain are not directly excited by these burst and tonic neurons. Instead, the burst and tonic signals for the medial recti are first sent to a population of interneurons in the abducens nucleus,

which in turn project to motor neurons in the contralateral oculomotor nucleus through a tract that crosses the midline and ascends in the *medial longitudinal fasciculus* (Figure 39-10A). This tract is critical for coordinating the medial lateral recti for all lateral gaze processes, and its length and vulnerability make it clinically important.

Vertical Saccades Are Generated in the Mesencephalic Reticular Formation

Only horizontal saccades are organized in the paramedian pontine reticular formation. The burst and tonic neurons for vertical saccades lie in the *rostral* interstitial nucleus of the medial longitudinal fasciculus in the mesencephalic reticular formation. The pontine omnipause cells control both pontine and mesencephalic burst neurons. Both the pontine and mesencephalic systems participate in the generation of oblique saccades, which have both horizontal and vertical components. Purely vertical saccades require activity on both sides of the mesencephalic reticular formation, and communication between the two sides traverses the posterior commissure.

Patients With Brain Stem Lesions Have Characteristic Deficits in Eye Movements

We can now understand how different brain stem lesions can cause characteristic syndromes. Lesions that include the pontine gaze centers result in paralysis of ipsilateral horizontal gaze but can leave pure vertical gaze intact. Conversely, lesions that include the midbrain gaze centers cause paralysis of vertical gaze. Lesions of the medial longitudinal fasciculus disconnect the medial rectus motor neurons from the abducens interneurons. As a result, the medial rectus is unable to contract during horizontal saccades or smooth pursuit but functions perfectly well in vergence because the upper motor neurons for vergence all lie in the midbrain, as will be discussed later. This combination of medial rectus dysfunction in lateral gaze and normal medial rectus function in vergence is called *internuclear ophthalmoplegia* and is often seen in patients with multiple sclerosis.

Saccades Are Controlled by the Cerebral Cortex

The pontine and mesencephalic burst circuits provide the necessary motor signals to drive the muscles for saccades. However, eye movements are a component of the cognitive behavior of higher mammals and the decision when and where to make a saccade is usually made in the cerebral cortex when that saccade is important to visual behavior. The cortex ordinarily controls the saccadic system through the *superior colliculus* (Figure 39-11).

The Superior Colliculus Integrates Visual and Motor Information Into Oculomotor Signals to the Brain Stem

The superior colliculus is a major visuomotor integration region. It is a multilayered structure in the midbrain and is the mammalian homolog of the optic tectum in lower vertebrates. The superior colliculus can be divided into two functional regions: the superficial layers and the intermediate and deep layers.

The three superficial layers of the superior colliculus receive both direct input from the retina and a projection from striate cortex for the entire contralateral visual hemifield. Neurons in the superficial layers respond to visual stimuli. In monkeys the responses of half of these vision-related neurons are quantitatively enhanced when the animal is going to make a saccade to a stimulus in the cell's receptive field. This enhancement is specific for saccades. If the monkey attends to the stimulus without making a saccade to it—for example, by making a hand movement in response to a brightness change—the neuron's response is not enhanced.

In the two intermediate and deep layers cell activity is primarily related to oculomotor actions. These movement-related cells receive visual information from prestriate, middle temporal, and parietal cortices and motor information from the frontal eye field. These layers also contain representations of the body surface and of the locations of sound in space. As described in Chapter 29, these neural "maps" are in register with the visuotopic maps. Thus if the image of a bird excites a vision-related neuron, the bird's chirp will excite an adjacent audition-related neuron, and both will excite a bimodal neuron.

Much of the early work describing the sensory responsiveness of neurons in the intermediate layer was done in anesthetized animals. However, to understand how the brain generates movement, the activity of neurons must be studied in alert animals while they behave normally, a technique pioneered for the skeletomotor system by Edward Evarts. One of the earliest cellular studies of active animals revealed that the majority of neurons in the intermediate layers fire before contralateral saccades of specific size and direction. These neurons drive the long-lead burst cells of the paramedian pontine reticular formation.

Individual movement-related neurons in the superior colliculus discharge before saccades of specific amplitudes and directions, just as individual vision-related neurons in the superior colliculus respond to stimuli at specific distances and direction from the fovea. The movement-related neurons form a map of potential eye movements that is in register with visual and auditory receptive maps, so that the neurons that control eye movements to a certain target are found in the same region as the cells excited by the sounds and image of that target. The region of the visual field that contains the targets for the saccades controlled by a given movement-related neuron in the superior colliculus is called the *movement field* of that neuron. Electrical stimulation of the intermediate layers of the superior colliculus evokes saccades into the movement fields of the neurons at the site of the stimulating electrode.

Movement fields are large, so each cell fires before a wide range of saccades, although each cell fires most intensely before saccades of a specific direction and amplitude. Therefore a large population of cells is active before each saccade. The actual eye movement is encoded by the entire ensemble of these broadly tuned cells. Since each cell makes only a small contribution to the direction and amplitude of the movement, any variability or noise in the discharge of a given cell is minimized. Similar population coding is found in the olfactory system (Chapter 32) and skeletal motor system (Chapter 38).

Activity in the superficial and intermediate layers of the superior colliculus can occur independently. Thus sensory activity in the superficial layers need not lead to motor output, and motor output can occur without sensory activity in the superficial layers. In fact, the neurons in the superficial layers do not have a large, direct projection to the intermediate layers. Instead, their axons terminate on neurons in the pulvinar and lateral posterior nuclei of the thalamus, from which their signals are relayed to cortical regions that project back to the intermediate layers. Lesions of a small part of the colliculus affect the latency, accuracy, and velocity of saccades; lesions of the entire colliculus render a monkey unable to make any contralateral saccades, although with time the ability to make contralateral saccades is recovered.

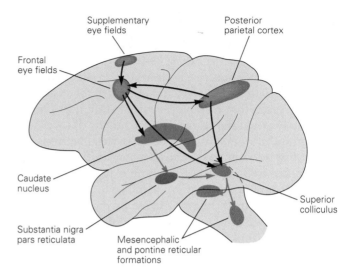

Figure 39-11 Cortical pathways for saccadic eye movements in the monkey. The brain stem saccade generator receives a command from the superior colliculus. The colliculus receives direct excitatory projections from the frontal eye field and the lateral intraparietal area and an inhibitory projection from the substantia nigra. The substantia nigra is suppressed by the caudate nucleus, which in turn is excited by the frontal eye field. Thus the frontal eye field directly excites the colliculus and indirectly releases it from suppression by the substantia nigra by exciting the caudate nucleus, which inhibits the substantia nigra. Cortical areas controlling saccades are in **purple,** the intermediate supranuclear structures in **blue,** and the brain stem reticular formation in **brown.** (Courtesy of Dr. R. J. Krausliz.)

The Rostral Superior Colliculus Facilitates Visual Fixation

The most rostral portion of the superior colliculus has a representation of the fovea. Neurons in the intermediate layers in this region discharge strongly during active visual fixation and before small contralateral saccades. Because the neurons are active during visual fixation, the most rostral part of the superior colliculus is often called the "fixation zone." Neurons here inhibit the movement-related neurons in the more caudal parts of the colliculus and also project directly to the nucleus of the dorsal raphe, where they inhibit saccade generation by exciting the omnipause neurons, which themselves inhibit saccades. With lesions in the fixation zone an animal is more likely to make saccades to distracting stimuli.

The Basal Ganglia Inhibit the Superior Colliculus

The substantia nigra pars reticulata sends a powerful GABA-ergic inhibitory projection to the superior col-

liculus. Neurons in the substantia nigra are spontaneously active with high frequency, and this discharge is suppressed at the time of voluntary eye movements to the contralateral visual field. These cells control the superior colliculus in the same way the omnipause cells control the pontine burst neurons: The inhibitory activity of the substantia nigra must be suppressed before the superior colliculus can drive a saccade. This suppression is mediated by inhibitory input from neurons in the caudate nucleus, which fire before saccades to the contralateral visual field.

The superior colliculus is controlled by two regions of the cerebral cortex that have overlapping but different functions in the generation of saccades. The lateral intraparietal area of the posterior parietal cortex (part of Brodmann's area 7) modulates visual attention and the frontal eye field (part of Brodmann's area 8) provides motor commands.

The Parietal Cortex Controls Visual Attention

Saccadic eye movements and visual attention are closely intertwined. As seen in Figure 39-1, the content of a subject's visual attention can be traced from the course of that person's saccades. Certain neurons in the posterior parietal cortex that respond to visual stimuli fire more vigorously when the stimuli are the targets of saccades. In contrast, in monkeys these same parietal neurons increase firing when the animal attends to the stimulus but without looking at it (for example, when the animal uses the dimming of the peripheral cue to signal a hand movement). Thus the signal carried by these neurons is best interpreted as an attentional signal, not dependent on either a visual stimulus or eye movement but relevant to both. This is in distinction to the superior colliculus, where enhanced activity is associated only with saccades, not with saccade-free attentive behavior.

In monkeys, lesions of the posterior parietal cortex result in increases in the latency of saccades and some inaccuracy in targeting. They also result in selective neglect. Monkeys with unilateral parietal lesions preferentially attend to stimuli in the contralateral visual hemifield. In humans as well, parietal lesions, especially right parietal lesions, initially cause dramatic attentional deficits (Chapter 19). Patients act as if the objects in the neglected field do not exist, and they have difficulty making eye movements into that field. Patients with Balint's syndrome, which is usually the result of bilateral lesions of posterior parietal and prestriate cortex, tend to see and describe only one object in their visual environment at a time. These patients make few saccades, as if they are unable to shift the focus of their attention from the fovea, and thus can only describe the foveal target. Even after these patients have recovered from most of their deficits, their contralateral saccades are inaccurate and they take more time to initiate contralateral saccades.

The Frontal Eye Field Sends a Specific Movement Signal to the Superior Colliculus

Compared to the neurons in the parietal cortex, neurons in the frontal eye field are more closely associated with saccades. Three different types of neurons in the frontal eye field discharge before saccades. *Visual neurons* respond to visual stimuli, and half of these neurons respond more vigorously to stimuli that will be the targets of saccades. Unlike neurons in the parietal cortex, activity in these cells is not enhanced when the animal attends to the stimulus without making a saccade to it. Monkeys can be trained to make saccades of specific direction and amplitude in total darkness, but the visual

neurons of the frontal eye field do not discharge before saccades that are made without visual targets.

Movement-related neurons fire before and during all saccades, whether or not they are made to a visual target, and do not respond to visual stimuli that are not the targets of saccades. Unlike the movement-related cells in the superior colliculus that fire before all saccades, these cells fire only before saccades that are relevant to the monkey's behavior. This class, and not the visual neurons, projects to the superior colliculus. *Visuomovement neurons* have both visual and movement-related activity and discharge best before visually guided saccades. Electrical stimulation of the frontal eye field evokes saccades to the movement fields of the stimulated cells. Bilateral stimulation of the frontal eye field evokes vertical saccades.

The frontal eye field controls the superior colliculus in two ways. First, the movement-related neurons project directly to the intermediate layers of the superior colliculus, exciting movement-related neurons there. Second, movement-related neurons from the same layer of the frontal eye field form excitatory synapses on neurons in the caudate nucleus that inhibit the substantia nigra. Thus, activity of movement-related cells in the frontal eye field simultaneously excites the superior colliculus and releases it from the inhibitory signals of the substantia nigra. The frontal eye field also projects to the pontine and mesencephalic reticular formations, although not directly to the burst cells.

Two other cortical regions with inputs to the frontal eye field are thought to be important in the control of saccades, particularly more cognitive aspects of saccades. The *supplementary eye field* at the most rostral part of the supplementary motor area has neurons that describe saccades to a part of a target rather than an absolute saccade direction. Thus a neuron in the left supplementary eye field that ordinarily fires before rightward eye movements will fire before a leftward saccade if that saccade is to the right side of a target. The *dorsolateral lateral prefrontal cortex* has neurons that discharge when a monkey makes a saccade to a remembered target. The activity starts at the stimulus appearance and continues throughout the interval through which the monkey must remember the location of the target.

We can now understand the effects of lesions of these regions on the generation of saccades. In monkeys lesions of the superior colliculus produce only transient damage to the saccadic system because the projection from the frontal eye field to the brain stem is intact. Similarly, animals can recover from cortical lesions because the superior colliculus is intact. Lesions of the frontal eye field and the colliculus together permanently damage the ability to make saccades. The predominant effect of a parietal lesion is an attentional deficit. When the attentional deficit recovers, the system can function normally because the frontal signals are sufficient to suppress the substantia nigra and stimulate the colliculus.

Damage to the frontal eye field causes more subtle deficits. In monkeys lesions of the frontal eye field cause a transient contralateral neglect and paresis of contralateral gaze that rapidly recover. This paralysis may be related to the fact that, in the absence of inputs from the frontal eye field, there is no adequate control on the substantia nigra, which then will not permit the colliculus to generate any saccades. Eventually the system adapts so that the colliculus can respond to the remaining parietal signal. After recovery the animals have no trouble making visually guided saccades but have great difficulty learning to make memory-guided saccades. As compared with these subtle deficits, bilateral lesions of both the frontal eye fields and the superior colliculus render monkeys unable to make saccades at all.

Humans with lesions of the frontal cortex have difficulty suppressing unwanted saccades to attended stimuli. This is easily shown by asking subjects to make an eye movement away from a stimulus. When the stimulus appears the subject must attend to it, without turning the eyes toward it, and use its location to calculate the desired saccade. Patients with frontal lesions who can make normal saccades to visual targets have difficulty with this task. They cannot suppress the saccade to the stimulus. As we have seen, in monkeys neurons in the lateral intraparietal area are active when the animal attends to a visual stimulus whether or not the animal makes a saccade to the stimulus. In the absence of a frontal eye field this undifferentiated attention signal is the only one to arrive at the superior colliculus. Thus the human patient's failure to suppress a saccade is to be expected if the superior colliculus responds to a parietal signal that generates attention to the stimulus, without the frontal-nigral control that normally prevents saccades in response to parietal signals.

The Control of Saccades Can Be Modified by Experience

The quantitative study of the neural control of movement is possible because the discharge rate of a motor neuron has a predictable effect on a movement. For example, a certain frequency of firing in the abducens motor neuron has a predictable effect on eye position and velocity. Sometimes, however, this relationship can change, for example, if the muscle becomes weak through disease. The brain can compensate to some degree for such changes.

With the saccadic system, moving the eyes a certain distance may require a much stronger signal for a weak muscle than for a stronger one. *Gain* is the relationship between the input to a system and its output. The gain of the saccadic system can be modulated by experience. Adaptation to partial paralysis occurs through two mechanisms: (1) change in the duration of the innervation pulse, and (2) change in the height of the step relative to the pulse size (see Figure 39-9B).

Patients are occasionally forced to use an eye with weak muscles because they have poor vision in the eye with normal muscles. If the eye with normal muscles is patched to prevent diplopia, the gain of the system increases so that the weak eye makes adequate saccades. This results in an excess of innervation to the normal eye, which thus makes more powerful movements. Because this eye is behind the patch, no visual information tells the system that the saccades are inaccurate. Because the burst is too large for the step, the integrated signal is too small and the eye drifts backward *(post-saccadic drift)*.

Damage to the cerebellum prevents both of these adaptive changes. Lesions of the dorsal cerebellar vermis and fastigial nuclei prevent changes in the pulse size while lesions of the flocculus prevent the matching of step size and pulse size. Thus the flocculus maintains the pulse-step match and the dorsal vermis and fastigial nuclei maintain pulse size.

Smooth Pursuit, Vergence, and Gaze Are Controlled by Distinct Systems

Smooth Pursuit Involves the Cerebral Cortex, the Cerebellum, and the Pons

The task of the smooth pursuit system is different from that of the saccadic system. Instead of driving the eyes as rapidly as possible to a point in space, it must match the velocity of the eye to that of a target in space. Neurons that signal eye velocity for smooth pursuit are found in the medial vestibular nucleus and the nucleus prepositus hypoglossi. They project to the abducens nucleus as well as the ocular motor nuclei in the midbrain (Figure 39-12) and receive projections from the flocculus of the cerebellum. Neurons in the paramedian pontine reticular formation also carry smooth pursuit signals and receive signals from the vermis of the cerebellum. Neurons in both the vermis and flocculus transmit an eye velocity signal that correlates with smooth pursuit. These areas receive signals from the cerebral cortex relayed by the dorsolateral pontine nucleus. Lesions in the dorsolateral pons disrupt ipsilateral smooth pursuit.

There are two major cortical inputs to the smooth pursuit system in monkeys. One arises from motion-sensitive regions in the superior temporal sulcus and

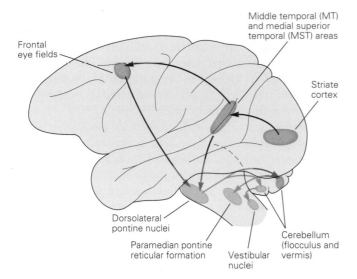

Frontal
eye fields

Middle temporal (MT)
and medial superior
temporal (MST) areas

Striate
cortex

Dorsolateral
pontine nuclei

Paramedian pontine
reticular formation

Vestibular
nuclei

Cerebellum
(flocculus and
vermis)

Figure 39-12 Pathways for smooth pursuit eye movements in the monkey. The cerebral cortex processes information about motion in the visual field and sends it to the motor neurons via the dorsolateral pons, the vermis and flocculus of the cerebellum, the vestibular nuclei, and the paramedian pontine reticular formation. The initiation signal for smooth pursuit may come in part from the frontal eye field. (Courtesy of Dr. R. J. Krausliz.)

the middle temporal (MT) and medial superior temporal (MST) areas (Chapter 28). The other arises from the frontal eye field.

Neurons in both MT and MST calculate the velocity of the target. When the eye speeds up to match target speed, the relative speed of the target's motion on the retina decreases. Neurons in MT, which describe retinal image motion, stop firing as the speed of the retinal image decreases, even though the target continues to move in space. Neurons in MST continue to fire and fire even if the target disappears briefly. These neurons have access to a process that adds the speeds of both the moving eye and the target motion on the retina to compute the speed of the target in space. Lesions of either MT or MST disrupt the ability of a subject to respond to targets moving in regions of the visual field represented in the damaged cortical area. Lesions of MST also diminish smooth pursuit movements toward the side of the lesion, no matter where the target is on the retina.

The temporal cortex provides the sensory information to guide pursuit movements but may not be able to initiate them. Electrical stimulation of MT and MST does not initiate smooth pursuit but can affect ongoing pursuit movement, speeding up ipsilateral pursuit and slowing down contralateral pursuit. The frontal eye field may be more important for initiating pursuit. This

area has neurons that fire in association with ipsilateral smooth pursuit. Electrical stimulation of the frontal eye field initiates ipsilateral pursuit, and lesions of the frontal eye field diminish, but do not eliminate, smooth pursuit.

In humans disruption anywhere along the pursuit pathway, including cortical, cerebellar, and brain stem areas, prevents patients from making adequate smooth pursuit eye movements. Instead, they track moving targets using a combination of defective smooth pursuit movements, whose velocity is less than that of the target, and small saccades. Patients with brain stem and cerebellar lesions cannot pursue targets moving toward the side of the lesion. Patients with parietal deficits have two different sorts of deficits. The first is a directional deficit that resembles that of monkeys with MST lesions: They cannot pursue targets moving toward the side of the lesion. The second is a retinotopic deficit that resembles the deficit of monkeys with MT lesions. As shown in Figure 39-3, normal subjects can generate smooth pursuit eye velocity to match the velocity of a stimulus in the periphery. Most patients cannot generate smooth pursuit to a stimulus limited to the visual hemifield opposite the lesion, regardless of the direction of motion.

Vergence Is Organized in the Midbrain

Vergence is a function of the horizontal rectus muscles only. Near-field viewing is accomplished by simultaneously increasing the tone of both medial recti and decreasing the tone of the lateral recti. Distance viewing is accomplished by relaxing medial rectus tone and increasing lateral rectus tone. Accommodation and vergence are controlled by neurons in the midbrain in the region of the oculomotor nucleus. Neurons in this region discharge with vergence, accommodation, or both.

Gaze Involves Combined Head and Eye Movements

So far we have described how the eyes are moved when the head is still. When we look around, however, our head is usually moving. The coordination of head and eye movements to direct the fovea is called *gaze*. Because the head has a much higher inertia, during small *gaze movements* the fovea reaches its target before the head begins to move. Therefore a small gaze movement consists of saccade followed by head movement and then a compensatory vestibulo-ocular reflex (Chapter 40) that moves the eyes back to the center of the orbit in the new position (Figure 39-13A). For larger gaze movements the eyes and the head move simultaneously in the same direction (Figure 39-13B). Since the vestibulo-ocular reflex ordinarily moves the eyes in the direction

A Small gaze shift

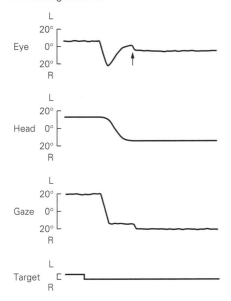

B Large gaze shift

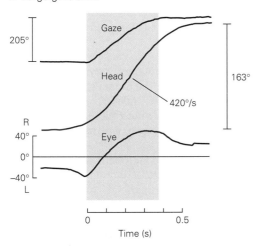

Figure 39-13 Directing the fovea to an object when the head is moving requires coordinated head and eye movements.

A. For a small gaze shift the eye and head move in sequence. The eye begins to move 300 ms after the target appears. Near the end of the eye movement the head begins to move. The eye then rotates back to the center of the orbit to compensate for the head movement. The gaze tracing is the sum of eye and head movements, only it looks like a saccade. (From Zee 1977.)

B. For a large gaze shift the eye and head move in the same direction simultaneously. Near the end of the gaze shift the eye remains still while the head continues to move. (From Laurutis and Robinson 1986.)

opposite that of the head, the reflex must be temporarily suppressed in order for the eyes and the head to move simultaneously.

Many of the same centers that control simple saccades also control gaze movements. For example, electrical stimulation of the superior colliculus evokes eye saccades in a monkey with its head fixed. The same stimulation in an animal whose head can move freely results in saccades combined with head movement. Neurons in the superior colliculus that carry eye movement signals also project to the reticular formation neurons that drive the neck muscles, presumably enabling a combined head and eye movement to bring the fovea to an object of interest.

An Overall View

The oculomotor system provides a spectacular window into the nervous system for both clinician and scientist. Patients with oculomotor deficits experience diplopia, and this alarming symptom sends them quickly to seek medical help. A physician with a thorough knowledge of the oculomotor system can describe and diagnose most oculomotor deficits at the bedside and localize the site of the lesion within the brain based on the neuroanatomy and neurophysiology of eye movements. Much of our understanding of neural processes arises from our knowledge of the oculomotor system as a microcosm of human behavior.

The oculomotor system is the simplest motor control system, requiring the coordination of only 12 muscles that move the two eyes. In humans and primates the main job of the oculomotor system is to control the position of the fovea, the most sensitive part of the retina. Six different systems control the eye. *Fixation* keeps the fovea still on a target; *saccades* move the fovea from one object of interest to another; *smooth pursuit* keeps the fovea on a moving target; *vestibular* and *optokinetic movements* keep the eye still in space when the head moves; and *vergence* adjusts the individual angles of each eye to keep objects at a certain depth focused on equivalent retinal positions. In addition, movements of the head help position the fovea on a target in the visual field. Combined eye and head movements are called gaze movements.

The cerebral cortex chooses significant objects in the environment as targets for eye movements. Cortical signals are relayed to motor circuits in the brain stem by the superior colliculus. The cortical and collicular signals do not specify the contribution of each muscle to the movement. Instead, the motor programming for eye movements is performed in the brain stem, which translates the signals from higher centers into signals appropriate for each muscle.

The neural signal sent to each muscle has two components, one related to eye position and the other to eye velocity. Velocity and position signals are generated by different neural systems, which converge on the motor neuron. Horizontal and vertical eye movements are specified independently; vertical movements are generated in the mesencephalic reticular formation and horizontal movements in the pontine reticular formation.

Inhibitory neurons prevent unwanted eye movements. Omnipause neurons in the pontine reticular formation prevent excitatory neurons in the brain stem from stimulating the motor neurons. Fixation neurons in the rostral superior colliculus inhibit movement-related neurons in the colliculus while exciting omnipause neurons in the pons. Inhibitory neurons in the substantia nigra inhibit these same movement-related neurons from firing except during saccades.

Michael E. Goldberg

Selected Readings

Becker W. 1989. Metrics. In: RH Wurtz, ME Goldberg (eds). *The Neurobiology of Saccadic Eye Movements.* Vol. 3, *Reviews of Oculomotor Research.* Amsterdam: Elsevier.

Colby CL, Duhamel J-R, Goldberg ME. 1995. Oculocentric spatial representation in parietal cortex. Cerebr Cortex 5:470–481.

Hepp K, Henn V, Vilis T, Cohen B. 1989. Brainstem regions related to saccade generation. In: RH Wurtz, ME Goldberg (eds). *The Neurobiology of Saccadic Eye Movements.* Vol. 3, *Reviews of Oculomotor Research*, pp. 105–212. Amsterdam: Elsevier.

Hikosaka O, Wurtz RH. 1989. The basal ganglia. In: RH Wurtz, ME Goldberg (eds). *The Neurobiology of Saccadic Eye Movements.* Vol. 3, *Reviews of Oculomotor Research*, pp. 257–284. Amsterdam: Elsevier.

Leigh RJ, Zee DS. 1999. *The Neurology of Eye Movements*, 3rd ed. Philadelphia: FA Davis.

Schall JD. 1995. Neural basis of saccade target selection. Rev Neurosci 6:63–85.

Sparks DL, Mays LE. 1990. Signal transformations required for the generation of saccadic eye movements. Annu Rev Neurosci 13:309–336.

Wurtz RH, Komatsu H, Dürsteler MR, Yamasaki DSG. 1990. Motion to movement: cerebral cortical visual processing for pursuit eye movements. In: G Edelman, WE Gall, WM Cowan (eds). *Signal and Sense: Local and Global Order in Perceptual Maps*, pp. 233–260. New York: Wiley.

Yarbus AL. 1967. In: (ed). *Eye Movements and Vision.* New York: Plenum.

References

Andersen RA, Asanuma C, Essick G, Siegel RM. 1990. Corticocortical connections of anatomically and physiologically defined subdivisions within the inferior parietal lobule. J Comp Neurol 296:65–113.

Baker R, Highstein SM. 1975. Physiological identification of interneurons and motoneurons in the abducens nucleus. Brain Res 91:292–298.

Bruce CJ, Goldberg ME. 1985. Primate frontal eye fields. I. Single neurons discharging before saccades. J Neurophysiol 53:603–635.

Bruce CJ, Goldberg ME, Stanton GB, Bushnell MC. 1985. Primate frontal eye fields. II. Physiological and anatomical correlates of electrically evoked eye movements. J Neurophysiol 54:714–734.

Bushnell MC, Goldberg ME, Robinson DL. 1981. Behavioral enhancement of visual responses in monkey cerebral cortex. I. Modulation in posterior parietal cortex related to selective visual attention. J Neurophysiol 46:755–772.

Büttner-Ennever JA, Büttner U, Cohen B, Baumgartner G. 1982. Vertical gaze paralysis and the rostral interstitial nucleus of the medial longitudinal fasciculus. Brain 105:125–149.

Büttner-Ennever JA, Cohen B, Pause M, Fries W. 1988. Raphe nucleus of the pons containing omnipause neurons of the oculomotor system in the monkey, and its homologue in man. J Comp Neurol 267:307–321.

Cohen B, Henn V. 1972. Unit activity in the pontine reticular formation associated with eye movements. Brain Res 46:403–410.

Colby CL, Duhamel J-R, Goldberg ME. 1996. Visual, presaccadic and cognitive activation of single neurons in monkey lateral intraparietal area. J Neurophysiol 76:2841–2852.

Cumming BG, Judge SJ. 1986. Disparity-induced and blur-induced convergence eye movement and accommodation in the monkey. J Neurophysiol 55:896–914.

Deng S-Y, Goldberg ME, Segraves MA, Ungerleider LG, Mishkin M. 1986. The effect of unilateral ablation of the frontal eye fields on saccadic performance in the monkey. In: E Keller, DS Zee (eds). *Adaptive Processes in the Visual and Oculomotor Systems*, pp. 201–208. Oxford: Pergamon.

Duhamel J-R, Colby CL, Goldberg ME. 1992. The updating of the representation of visual space in parietal cortex by intended eye movements. Science 255:90–92.

Dürsteler MR, Wurtz RH, Newsome WT. 1987. Directional pursuit deficits following lesions of the foveal representation within the superior temporal sulcus of the macaque monkey. J Neurophysiol 57:1262–1287.

Evarts EV. 1966. Methods for recording activity of individual neurons in moving animals. In: RF Rushmer (ed). *Methods in Medical Research*, pp. 241–250. Chicago: Year Book.

Fuchs AF, Luschei ES. 1970. Firing patterns of abducens neurons of alert monkeys in relationship to horizontal eye movement. J Neurophysiol 33:382–392.

Funahashi S, Bruce CJ, Goldman-Rakic PS. 1993. Dorsolateral prefrontal lesions and oculomotor delayed-response performance: evidence for mnemonic "scotomas." J Neurosci 13:1479–1497.

Funahashi S, Bruce CJ, Goldman-Rakic PS. 1989. Mnemonic coding of visual space in the monkey's dorsolateral prefrontal cortex. J Neurophysiol 61:331–349.

Goldberg ME, Bushnell MC. 1981. Behavioral enhancement of visual responses in monkey cerebral cortex. II. Modulation in frontal eye fields specifically related to saccades. J Neurophysiol 46:773–787.

Goldberg ME, Wurtz RH. 1972a. Activity of superior colliculus in behaving monkey. I. Visual receptive fields of single neurons. J Neurophysiol 35:542–559.

Goldberg ME, Wurtz RH. 1972b. Activity of superior colliculus in behaving monkeys. II. Effect of attention on neuronal responses. J Neurophysiol 35:560–574.

Gottlieb JP, MacAvoy MG, Bruce CJ. 1994. Neural responses related to smooth-pursuit eye movements and their correspondence with electrically elicited smooth eye movements in the primate frontal eye field. J Neurophysiol 74:1634–1653.

Hecaen J, Ajuriguerra JD. 1954. Balint's syndrome (psychic paralysis of visual fixation). Brain 77:373.

Henn V, Hepp K, Büttner-Ennever JA. 1984. The primate oculomotor system. II. Premotor system. Hum Neurobiol 1:87–95.

Henn V, Lang W, Hepp K, Resine H. 1984. Experimental gaze palsies in monkeys and their relation to human pathology. Brain 107:619–636.

Highstein SM, Baker R. 1978. Excitatory termination of abducens internuclear neurons on medial rectus motoneurons: relationship to syndrome of internuclear ophthalmoplegia. J Neurophysiol 41:1647–1661.

Hikosaka O, Sakamoto M, Usui S. 1989. Functional properties of monkey caudate neurons. I. Activities related to saccadic eye movements. J Neurophysiol 61:780–798.

Horn AK, Büttner-Ennever JA, PW, Reichenberger I. 1994. Neurotransmitter profile of saccadic omnipause neurons in nucleus raphe interpositus. J Neurosci 4:2032–2046.

Judge SJ, Cumming BG. 1986. Neurons in the monkey midbrain with activity related to vergence eye movement and accommodation. J Neurophysiol 55:915–930.

Kanaseki T, Sprague JM. 1974. Anatomical organization of pretectal and tectal laminae in the cat. J Comp Neurol 158:319–337.

Keller EL. 1974. Participation of medial pontine reticular formation in eye movement generation in monkey. J Neurophysiol 37:316–332.

Komatsu H, Wurtz RH. 1989. Modulation of pursuit eye movements by stimulation of cortical areas MT and MST. J Neurophysiol 62:31–47.

Laurutis VP, Robinson DA. 1986. The vestibular reflex during human saccadic eye movements. J Physiol (Lond) 373:209–233.

Lee C, Rohrer WH, Sparks DL. 1988. Population coding of saccadic eye movements by neurons in the superior colliculus. Nature 332:357–360.

Luschei ES, Fuchs AF. 1972. Activity of brain stem neurons during eye movements of alert monkeys. J Neurophysiol 35:445–461.

Lynch JC, Graybiel AM, Lobeck LJ. 1985. The differential projection of two cytoarchitectonic subregions of the inferior parietal lobule of macaque upon the deep layers of the superior colliculus. J Comp Neurol 235:241–254.

Lynch JC, McLaren JW. 1989. Deficits of visual attention and saccadic eye movements after lesions of parieto-occipital cortex in monkeys. J Neurophysiol 61:74–90.

Lynch JC, Mountcastle VB, Talbot WH, Yin TCT. 1977. Parietal lobe mechanisms for directed visual attention. J Neurophysiol 40:362–389.

May JG, Keller EL, Suzuki DA. 1988. Smooth-pursuit eye movement deficits with chemical lesions in the dorsolateral pontine nucleus of the monkey. J Neurophysiol 59:952–977.

McFarland JL, Fuchs AF. 1992. Discharge patterns in nucleus prepositus hypoglossi and adjacent medial vestibular nucleus during horizontal eye movement in behaving macaques. J Neurophysiol 68:319–332.

Morrow MJ, Sharpe JA. 1993. Retinotopic and directional deficits of smooth pursuit initiation after posterior cerebral hemispheric lesions. J Neurol 43:595–603.

Munoz DP, Wurtz RH. 1993a. Fixation cells in monkey superior colliculus. I. Characteristics of cell discharge. J Neurophysiol 70:559–575.

Munoz DP, Wurtz RH. 1993b. Fixation cells in monkey superior colliculus. II. Reversible activation and deactivation. J Neurophysiol 70:576–589.

Mustari MJ, Fuchs AF, Wallman J. 1988. Response properties of dorsolateral pontine units during smooth pursuit in the rhesus macaque. J Neurophysiol 60:664–686.

Newsome WT, Wurtz RH, Dürsteler MR, Mikami A. 1985. Deficits in visual motion processing following ibotenic acid lesions of the middle temporal visual area of the macaque monkey. J Neurosci 5:825–840.

Newsome WT, Wurtz RH, Komatsu H. 1988. Relation of cortical areas MT and MST to pursuit eye movements. II. Differentiation of retinal from extraretinal inputs. J Neurophysiol 60:604–620.

Olson CR, Gettner SN. 1995. Object-centered direction selectivity in the macaque supplementary eye field. Science 269:985–988.

Raybourn MS, Keller EL. 1977. Colliculo-reticular organization in primate oculomotor system. J Neurophysiol 269:985–988.

Robinson DA. 1975. Oculomotor control signals. In: G Lennerstrand, P Bach–y-Rita. *Basic Mechanisms of Ocular Motility and Their Clinical Implications*, pp. 337–374. Oxford: Pergamon.

Robinson DA. 1970. Oculomotor unit behavior in the monkey. J Neurophysiol 33:393–404.

Schiller PH, Koerner F. 1971. Discharge characteristics of single units in superior colliculus of the alert rhesus monkey. J Neurophysiol 34:920–936.

Schiller PH, True SD, Conway JL. 1980. Deficits in eye movements following frontal eye field and superior colliculus ablations. J Neurophysiol 44:1175–1189.

Segraves MA, Goldberg ME. 1987. Functional properties of corticotectal neurons in the monkey's frontal eye field. J Neurophysiol 58:1387–1419.

Suzuki DA, Keller EL. 1984. Visual signals in the dorsolateral pontine nucleus of the alert monkey: their relationship to smooth-pursuit eye movements. Exp Brain Res 53:473–478.

Suzuki DA, May J, Keller EL. 1984. Smooth-pursuit eye movement deficits with pharmacological lesions in monkey dorsolateral pontine nucleus. Soc Neurosci Abst 10:58.

Tyler HR. 1968. Abnormalities of perception with defective eye movements (Balint's syndrome). Cortex 4:154–171.

von Noorden GK. 1980. *Burian-Von Noorden's Binocular Vision and Ocular Motility.* St. Louis: Mosby.

Wurtz RH, Goldberg ME. 1972. Activity of superior colliculus in behaving monkey. III. Cells discharging before eye movements. J Neurophysiol 35:575–586.

Zee DS. 1977. Disorders of eye-head coordination. In: BA Brooks, FJ Bajandas. *Eye Movements,* pp. 9–39. New York: Plenum.

40

The Vestibular System

AIRPLANES AND SUBMARINES navigate in three dimensions using sophisticated guidance systems that register every acceleration and turn. Laser gyroscopes and computers have afforded such navigational aids unprecedented precision. Yet the principles of inertial guidance are ancient—vertebrates have used analogous systems for 500 million years, and invertebrates for still longer.

The vestibular system is designed to answer two of the questions basic to human life: "Which way is up?" and "Where am I going?" It does so by measuring linear and angular acceleration of the head through an ensemble of five sensory organs in the inner ear (the membranous or vestibular labyrinth). Acceleration of the head deflects hair bundles attached to hair cells in the vestibular labyrinth. This distortion changes membrane potential and transmitter release patterns in these cells, thereby affecting the discharge patterns of the vestibular neurons that innervate them. In turn, the vestibular neurons carry head velocity and acceleration signals to the vestibular nuclei in the brain stem. This information helps us maintain balance and influences how we perceive space. In this chapter we consider how the hair cells of the vestibular apparatus generate the primary signals for head acceleration and how the brain integrates these signals.

The early origin of the vestibular system is seen in the outputs of the labyrinthine receptors, which flow to vestibular nuclei that occupy a prominent position in the brain stem. As we shall learn in the next chapter, various components of the vestibular system subserve a variety of postural reflexes, including those that make possible upright, bipedal posture. Finally, through pathways involving the ocular motor nuclei and cerebellum,

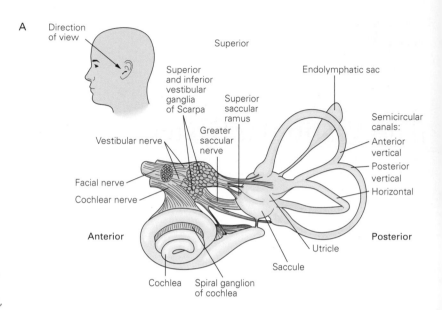

Figure 40-1 The vestibular labyrinth.

A. Location of vestibular and cochlear divisions of the inner ear with respect to the head.

B. The inner ear is divided into bony and membranous labyrinths. The bony labyrinth is bounded by the petrous portion of the temporal bone. Lying within this structure is the membranous labyrinth, which contains the organs of hearing (the cochlea) and equilibrium (the utricle, saccule, and semicircular ducts). The space between bone and membrane is filled with perilymph, while the membranous labyrinth is filled with endolymph. Sensory cells in the utricle, saccule, and the ampullae of the semicircular ducts respond to motion of the head. (Adapted from Iurato 1967.)

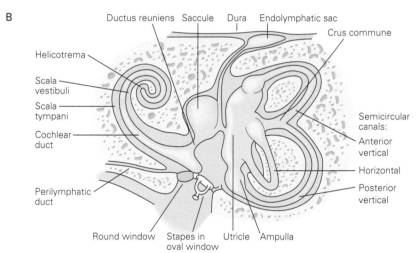

the vestibular system also controls reflex eye movements that stabilize retinal images despite head and body motions.

The Vestibular Labyrinth Houses Five Receptor Organs

Hair Cells Transduce Mechanical Stimuli into Receptor Potentials

The two vestibular labyrinths are mirror-symmetric structures within the inner ears (Figure 40-1). Each vestibular labyrinth comprises five receptor organs that, complemented by those of the contralateral ear, can measure linear acceleration along any axis and angular acceleration about any axis. Linear accelerations, in-

cluding those produced by gravity and those resulting from body motions are detected by the *utricle* and the *saccule*. Angular accelerations caused by rotation of the head or the body are measured by the semicircular canals. The receptive organs are ensheathed by the connective tissue that delineates the *membranous labyrinth;* a layer of laminar bone, the *bony labyrinth*, invests the membranous labyrinth and separates it from the cancellous bone of the skull.

Although the labyrinth's very name betokens its geometric complexity, the fundamental organization of the five constituent receptors is not dauntingly complicated. In keeping with its origin from the embryonal surface ectoderm, each organ is lined with a continuous sheet of epithelial cells. By the action of ion pumps, certain cells in this epithelium produce the *endolymph*, a special extracellular fluid that bathes the apical cellular

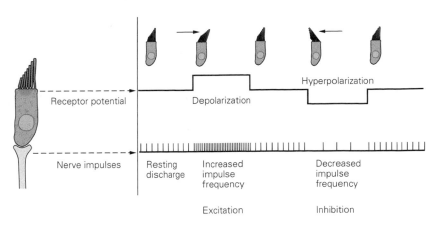

Figure 40-2 Hair cells in the vestibular labyrinth transduce mechanical stimuli into neural signals. At the apex of each cell is a hair bundle in which a number of stereocilia taper in length toward a single kinocilium. The membrane potential of the receptor cell depends on the direction in which the hair bundle is bent. Deflection toward the kinocilium causes the cell to depolarize and thus increases the rate of firing in the afferent fiber. Bending away from the kinocilium causes the cell to hyperpolarize, thus decreasing the afferent firing rate. (Adapted from Flock 1965.)

surfaces. Like cochlear endolymph, this fluid is rich in K^+ but relatively poor in Na^+ and Ca^{2+}. A junctional complex girdling the apex of each cell includes tight junctions that separate the endolymph from the ordinary extracellular fluid, the *perilymph*, that surrounds the membranous labyrinth and bathes the basolateral epithelial surfaces.

During its development the labyrinth progresses from a simple sac to a complex of interconnected organs. However, its fundamental topological organization persists: Each organ originates as an epithelium-lined pouch that buds from the otic cyst, and the endolymphatic spaces within the several organs remain continuous in the adult. The endolymphatic spaces of the vestibular labyrinth are also connected to the scala media of the cochlea through the ductus reuniens.

Among the epithelial cells lining the membranous labyrinth are five clusters of hair cells, one cluster in each receptor organ. Like the hair cells that mediate hearing in the cochlea, the hair cells of the vestibular labyrinth are endowed with hair bundles that transduce mechanical stimuli into receptor potentials. The general principles of mechanoelectrical transduction by hair cells (Chapter 31) also apply to these cells. Deflection of a hair bundle toward the kinocilium elicits a depolarization, which in turn enhances the release of synaptic transmitter. Deflection away from the kinocilium hyperpolarizes the hair cell and reduces neurotransmitter release (Figure 40-2).

The Vestibular Nerve Transmits Sensory Information From the Vestibular Organs

The hair cells of the vestibular labyrinth send their outputs to the vestibular nuclei of the brain stem by 20,000 myelinated axons, which constitute the vestibular component of the eighth cranial nerve. The cell bodies of the vestibular neurons are clustered in the *vestibular ganglion*, which lies in a swelling of the vestibular nerve within the internal auditory meatus (Figure 40-1). Most vestibular afferent fibers fire both tonically and phasically; in some cells firing persists indefinitely, but in other cells the firing adapts during protracted stimulation. Vestibular afferents thus provide information about sustained stimulation, such as the acceleration from gravity, and about abrupt changes in bodily accelerations. The time-dependent decrease in vestibular-afferent firing is likely to stem from adaptation at several levels, including that of mechanoelectrical transduction by hair cells and accommodation by the nerve fibers.

Like most other hair cells, those of the human vestibular system receive efferent inputs from the brain stem. Although the effect of these inputs has not been extensively studied by recording from hair cells in situ, stimulation of the fibers from the brain stem has dramatic effects on the sensitivity of the afferent axons from the hair cells. Stimulation decreases the excitability of some hair cells, as would be expected if activation of the efferent fibers elicited inhibitory postsynaptic potentials in hair cells. In other hair cells, however, activation of the efferent fibers leads to increased excitability, the cause of which is unknown.

Given that hair cells are essentially strain gauges, explained in Chapter 31, the key to understanding how each vestibular organ operates lies in grasping how mechanical stimuli are delivered to the constituent hair cells. Distinctive mechanical linkages account for the contrasting sensitivities of the utricle and saccule, on the one hand, and the three semicircular canals, on the other.

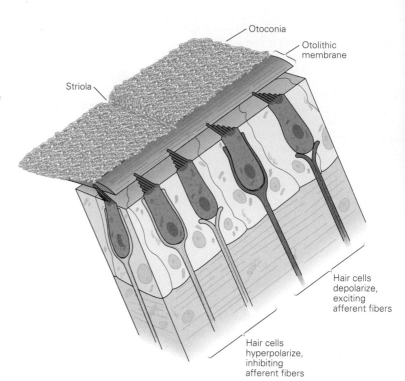

Figure 40-3 The utricle is organized to detect tilt of the head. The hair cells in the epithelium of the utricle have apical hair bundles that project into the otolithic membrane, a gelatinous material embedded with calcium carbonate stones (otoconia). The hair bundles are polarized, but not all cells are oriented in the same direction. The response of an individual hair cell in the utricle to a tilt of the head depends on the direction in which its hairs are bent by the gravitational force of the otoliths. When the head is tilted in the direction of the axis of polarity for a particular hair cell, that cell depolarizes and excites the afferent fiber. When the head is tilted in the opposite direction, the hair cell hyperpolarizes and inhibits the afferent fiber (see Figure 40-2). (Adapted from Iurato 1967.)

The Utricle and the Saccule Detect Linear Accelerations

The simplest labyrinthine organs are the utricle (or *utriculus*) and the saccule (or *sacculus*), each of which consists of an ovoidal sac of membranous labyrinth about 3 mm in the longest dimension. The complement of hair cells in each organ is localized to a roughly elliptical patch, called the *macula*. The human utricle contains about 30,000 hair cells, while the saccule contains some 16,000.

The hair bundle at the apex of each hair cell extends into the endolymphatic space of the utricle or saccule, where the bundle's top is attached to a gelatinous sheet, the *otolithic membrane*, that covers the entire sensory macula (Figure 40-3). Embedded within and lying on the otolithic membrane are fine, dense particles, the *otoconia* ("ear dust"); consisting of calcium carbonate in the form of the mineral calcite. Otoconia are typically 0.5–10 μm long and millions of these particles fill the endolymphatic cavities of the utricle and the saccule. Because of the prominence of otoconia, the utricle and saccule are named the *otolithic organs*.

When the head undergoes linear acceleration the membranous labyrinth moves along as well because it is fixed to the skull. The otoconial mass, however, is free to shift within the receptor organ. Because of its inertia this mass lags behind movement of the head. The motion of the otoconia is communicated to the gelatinous otolithic

membrane, which thus shifts with respect to the underlying epithelium. This motion in turn deflects the hair bundles that link the otolithic membrane to the macula, thus exciting an electrical response in the hair cells.

Although a linear acceleration may be of any magnitude and may be oriented in any direction, the otolithic organs are arranged to provide the central nervous system with a unique pattern of signals for any acceleration within the physiological range. With the head in its normal position, the macula in each utricle is approximately horizontal. Any substantial acceleration in the horizontal plane therefore deflects at least some hair bundles. Any particular horizontal acceleration maximally depolarizes one group of hair cells and maximally inhibits a complementary set because the various hair cells are so oriented that their axes of greatest mechanosensitivity (Chapter 31) lie in all possible directions (Figure 40-4). Other hair cells, whose axes of sensitivity lie at various angles to the acceleration, are excited or inhibited according to their orientations. The afferent nerve fibers from each utricle therefore provide a rich and redundant representation of the magnitude and orientation of any acceleration in the horizontal plane. Because the utricles are bilateral, the brain receives additional information from the contralateral labyrinth.

The operation of the paired saccules resembles that of the utricles. The hair cells represent all possible orientations within the plane of each macula, but the maculas are oriented vertically in nearly parasagittal planes. The saccules are therefore especially sensitive to vertical accelerations, of which gravity is the most ubiquitous and the most important. Certain saccular hair cells also respond to accelerations in the horizontal plane; in particular, a saccule is sensitive to motions along the anterior-posterior axis.

The Semicircular Canals Detect Angular Accelerations

Angular acceleration occurs whenever an object alters its rate of rotation about an axis. Our head therefore undergoes angular acceleration during turning or tilting motions of the head, rotatory body movements, and turning movements during active or passive locomotion. The three semicircular canals of each vestibular labyrinth detect these angular accelerations and report their magnitudes and orientations to the brain.

The name of the semicircular canal aptly reflects its gross structure, which is a roughly semicircular tube of membranous labyrinth extending from the utricle (Figure 40-1). The term "canal" is misleading, however, as the organ is actually a closed tube, nearly 8 mm in overall diameter, and filled with endolymph.

Like the otolithic organs, the semicircular canals detect accelerations by means of the inertia of their internal contents. Here, however, it is the mass of endolymph itself that responds to accelerations. Consider the simplest instance of a smoothly increasing rotatory motion, and hence a constant angular acceleration, about an axis passing perpendicularly through the center of a semicircular canal. As the head rotates faster and faster it carries the bony and membranous labyrinths with it. Because of its inertia, however, the endolymph tends to lag behind and therefore rotates within the semicircular canal in a direction opposite that of the head.

A cup of coffee can demonstrate the motion of endolymph in a semicircular canal. While gently twisting the cup about its vertical axis, one can observe a particular bubble near the fluid's outer boundary. As the cup begins to turn, the coffee tends to maintain its original orientation in space and thus counterrotates in the vessel. At the conclusion of the turning motion, when the cup decelerates, the coffee moves in the opposite direction.

Fluid cannot freely move around the whole of a semicircular canal. Instead, the endolymphatic space of each canal is interrupted by a gelatinous diaphragm, the *cupula*, that extends across the canal in its widest region, a dilatation termed the *ampulla* (Figure 40-5). Around most of its perimeter the cupula is attached to the epi-

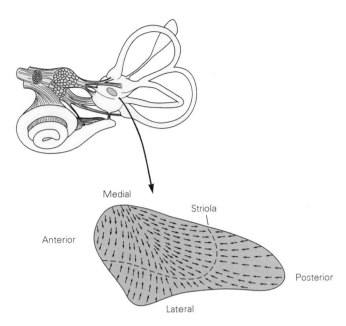

Figure 40-4 The axis of mechanical sensitivity of each hair cell in the utricle is oriented toward the striola, a curved border running across the surface of the macula. The drawing shows the resulting variation in axes (**arrows**) in the population of hair cells. Because of this arrangement, tilt in any direction depolarizes some cells and hyperpolarizes others, while having no effect on a third group. (Adapted from Spoendlin 1966.)

thelium lining the canal. The portion of the cupula contacting the ampullary crista, however, is less firmly anchored; there the cupula is penetrated by hair bundles extending from a patch of nearly 7000 hair cells.

When endolymph begins to move as the result of an acceleration, this fluid presses against one surface of the cupula. Because of its flexibility the cupula bows; the margin into which the hair bundles insert also flexes, thus stimulating the associated hair cells. Because all the hair bundles in each semicircular canal share a common orientation, angular acceleration in one direction depolarizes hair cells and excites afferent axons, while acceleration in the opposite direction hyperpolarizes the receptor cells and diminishes spontaneous neural activity. As with the other receptor organs of the internal ear, the magnitude of the response of the hair cells, as well as that of the afferent axons, is graded with the amplitude of stimulation.

In each labyrinth the three canals are almost precisely perpendicular to one another, so that the canals represent accelerations about three mutually orthogonal axes (Figure 40-6). The planes in which the semicircular canals lie do not, however, correspond with the head's major anatomical planes. As its name indicates, the hor-

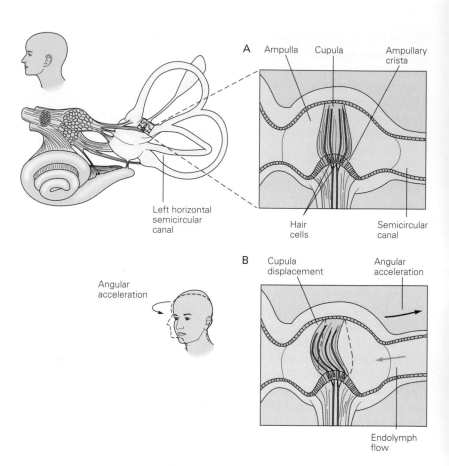

Figure 40-5 The organization of the ampulla of a semicircular canal.

A. A thickened zone of epithelium, the ampullary crista, contains the hair cells. The hair bundles of the hair cells extend into a gelatinous diaphragm called the cupula, which stretches from the crista to the roof of the ampulla.

B. The cupula is displaced by the flow of endolymph when the head moves. As a result, the hair bundles extending into the cupula are also displaced.

izontal semicircular canal of each ear lies nearly horizontally with the head in its ordinary, upright position. This canal is accordingly sensitive to rotations about a *vertical* axis, for example to twisting the neck. The plane in which each anterior vertical semicircular canal lies is slanted about 45° with respect to the coronal plane, so that the lateral extreme of each canal lies rostrally to the medial edge. The planes of the two posterior vertical canals are canted approximately 45° in the opposite direction.

The vestibular labyrinths on the two sides of the head are systematically arranged with respect to one another. The two horizontal canals thus lie in a common plane and hence function together (Figure 40-7). Each anterior vertical canal, in contrast, lies in the same plane as the contralateral *posterior* vertical canal.

Most Movements Elicit Complex Patterns of Vestibular Stimulation

Although the actions of the vestibular organs may be separated conceptually and experimentally, as may be the operation of the right and left vestibular labyrinths, actual human movements generally elicit a complex pattern of excitation and inhibition in several receptor organs on both sides of the body. Consider, for example, the act of rising from the driver's seat of an automobile. As one begins to swivel toward the door, both horizontal semicircular canals are strongly stimulated. The simultaneous lateral movement out the car's door stimulates hair cells in both utricles in a pattern that changes continuously as the orientation of the turning head changes with respect to the direction of bodily movement. An appropriately oriented complement of hair cells in each of the saccules is excited, and an oppositely oriented group inhibited, by the vertical acceleration that accompanies rising to a standing position. Finally, the maneuver's conclusion involves linear and angular accelerations opposite to those at the inception.

The coffee cup example again confirms the complex pattern of accelerations involved in even a simple movement. One may, for example, examine the result of extending the cup from a position immediately in front of the body to one laterally and at arm's length—the movements involved in serving another person. The angular component of acceleration causes the coffee to rotate within the cup, while the linear component causes the liquid to slosh toward the cup's rim. The conclusion

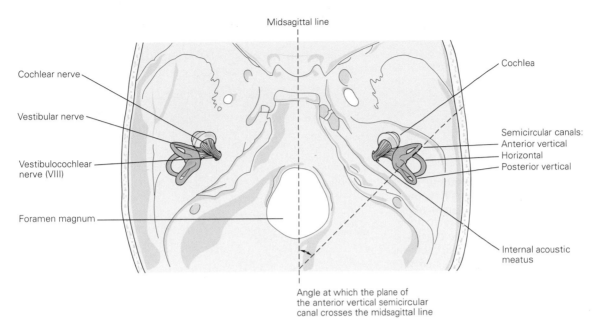

Midsagittal line

Cochlear nerve

Vestibular nerve

Vestibulocochlear
nerve (VIII)

Foramen magnum

Cochlea

Semicircular canals:
Anterior vertical
Horizontal
Posterior vertical

Internal acoustic
meatus

Angle at which the plane of
the anterior vertical semicircular
canal crosses the midsagittal line

Figure 40-6 The bilateral symmetry of the semicircular canals. The horizontal canals on both sides lie in the same plane and therefore are functional pairs. In contrast, the anterior vertical canal on one side and the posterior vertical canal on the opposite side lie in the same plane and are therefore functional pairs.

of the movement evokes contrary fluid motions that reflect linear and angular accelerations in the opposite direction.

In view of the complexity of the sensory stimuli associated with seemingly simple everyday acts, one may better appreciate why infants need many months of training to support bipedal locomotion. Even as adults we must work diligently to incorporate into reflexes the new patterns of vestibular stimulation associated with new experiences, for example, piloting an airplane. It also seems likely that the need for continual practice by athletes results from constant fine-tuning of vestibular pathways and the associated motor outflows.

The complementary and redundant pattern of stimulation of various receptor organs, both within one vestibular labyrinth and between the two internal ears, explains why lesions of the vestibular receptors and pathways can cause disorientation and vertigo. The central nervous system associates a particular pattern of neuronal activity with each motor action in our repertory of behavior. If a component of the vestibular system is excessively active or abnormally silent, the brain receives inappropriate information on acceleration and the reflexes driven by vestibular inputs understandably falter. Only then do we become consciously aware of the vestibular system at work. In the most severe cases a diseased labyrinth must be surgically destroyed in or-

der to relieve the brain of erratic and disabling vestibular signals.

Menière Disease Affects the Vestibular Labyrinth

In addition to problems that affect hair cells in general, the receptor cells of the vestibular labyrinth are vulnerable to a poorly understood, spontaneous condition called *Menière disease*. This syndrome is characterized by intermittent, relapsing vertigo, with attacks lasting from tens of minutes to tens of hours and varying in severity from mild to debilitating. The vestibular symptoms are often accompanied by noise in the ears (*tinnitus*) and distorted hearing, which indicate that the cochleas are also involved.

The condition usually afflicts middle-aged individuals and is generally unilateral. In certain patients attacks are precipitated or exacerbated by high salt intake or anxiety. Although some people find relief from diuretics, sedatives, or steroids, there is no consistently effective therapy for the condition. In extreme cases of Menière disease it is necessary to destroy vestibular hair cells with the antibiotic streptomycin or to remove the affected labyrinth surgically in order to relieve severe vertigo.

The cause of Menière disease is unknown. Histological examination of an affected ear reveals endolymphatic hydrops, or edema of the endolymphatic spaces,

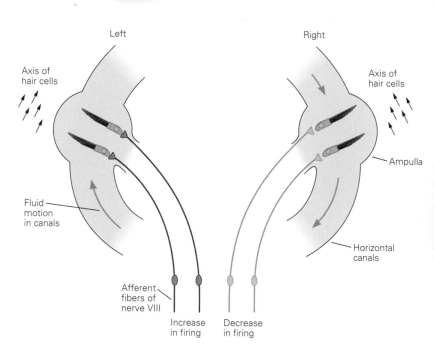

Figure 40-7 This view of the horizontal semicircular canals from above shows how the paired canals work together to signal head movement. Because of inertia, rotation of the head in a counterclockwise direction causes endolymph to move clockwise with respect to the canals. This reflects the stereocilia in the left canal in the excitatory direction, thereby exciting the afferent fibers on this side. In the right canal the hair cells are hyperpolarized and afferent firing there decreases.

associated with damage to epithelial cells, especially the hair cells. The histopathology suggests that attacks ensue from poor drainage of endolymph, which normally exits the labyrinth through the endolymphatic duct and is resorbed into the cerebrospinal fluid in the endolymphatic sac. Patients are sometimes treated by surgical insertion of a shunt that diverts excess endolymph directly to the cerebrospinal fluid, a procedure that is not always effective.

Vestibular Reflexes Stabilize the Eyes and the Body When the Head Moves

The vestibular nerve transmits information about head acceleration to the vestibular nuclei in the medulla, which then distribute it to higher centers. This central network of vestibular connections is responsible for the various reflexes that the body uses to compensate for head movement and the perception of motion in space. These reflexes include the *vestibulo-ocular reflexes*

that keep the eyes still when the head moves and the *vestibulospinal reflexes* that enable the skeletomotor system to compensate for head movement.

The Vestibulo-Ocular Reflexes Compensate for Head Movement

We perceive stable images on the retina better than moving ones. When the head moves the eyes are kept still by the vestibulo-ocular reflexes of the eye muscles. If a person were to shake her head while reading this paragraph she would still be able to read it because of the vestibulo-ocular reflexes. If she moved the book at the same speed, however, she would no longer be able to read it because vision would be the only cue the brain had to stabilize the image of the moving book on the retina. Visual processing is much slower and less efficient than vestibular processing for image stabilization.

The vestibular apparatus signals how fast the head is rotating, and the oculomotor system uses this information to stabilize the eyes in order to keep visual images motionless on the retina (Chapter 39). Loss of this reflex is devastating. A physician who lost his vestibular hair cells because of a toxic reaction to streptomycin wrote a dramatic account of this loss. Immediately after the onset of streptomycin toxicity he could not read in bed without steadying his head to keep it motionless. Even after partial recovery he still could not read street signs or recognize friends while walking in the street; he had to stop to see clearly.

Three different vestibulo-ocular reflexes arise from the three major components of the labyrinth:

1. The *rotational vestibulo-ocular reflex* compensates for head rotation and receives its input predominantly from the semicircular canals.
2. The *translational vestibulo-ocular reflex* compensates for linear head movement.
3. The *ocular counter-rolling response* compensates for head tilt in the vertical.

The second and third reflexes receive their input predominantly from the otolith organs and thus are sometimes called the *otolith reflexes*. Although most head movement is a complex combination of rotation and translation, the reflexes have properties that enable the components to be analyzed independently.

Vestibular Nystagmus Resets Eye Position During Sustained Rotation of the Head

Of the three vestibulo-ocular reflexes the rotational reflex is the simplest. When the semicircular canals sense head rotation in one direction, the eyes slowly rotate in the opposite direction. As a result the eyes remain still and vision is clear. One would think that sustained rotation in any direction would drive the eyes to the edge of the orbit and keep them there. This does not occur because the eyes make a rapid resetting movement back across the center of the gaze (Figure 40-8). The combination of slow and quick phases of eye movement results in a repetitive pattern, *nystagmus* (Greek, "nod"), so called because a nod has a slow phase as the head drops and a quick phase as the head snaps back to an erect position. The vestibular signal drives the slow phase of nystagmus and brain stem circuits generate the quick phase.

The Otolith Reflexes Compensate for Linear Motion and Head Deviations Relative to Gravity

The semicircular canals signal head rotation only. They are silent during linear, sideways motion, which is sensed by the otolith organs. Linear movement provides

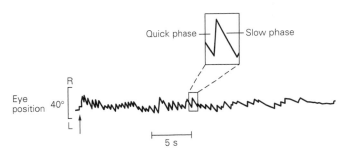

Figure 40-8 Vestibular nystagmus. The trace shows the eye position of a subject in a chair rotated counterclockwise at a constant rate in the dark. At the beginning of the trace the eye moves slowly at the same speed as the chair (slow phase) and occasionally makes rapid resetting movements (quick phase). The speed of the slow phase gradually decreases until the eye no longer moves regularly. (From Leigh and Zee 1991.)

a more complex geometric problem for the vestibular system to solve than does rotation. When the head rotates, images move with the same velocity on the retina. When the head moves sideways, however, the image of a close object moves more rapidly on the retina than an image of a distant one. This can be easily understood by considering what happens when a person looks out of the side window of a moving car: Objects near the side of the road move out of view almost with the speed of the car, but distant objects move more slowly.

To compensate for linear head movement the translational vestibulo-ocular reflex must take into account the distance to the object being viewed. The more distant the object, the smaller the eye movement. Such graded modification is not necessary for the rotational vestibulo-ocular reflex because the reflex is independent of viewing distance.

Since gravity exerts a constant linear acceleration on the head, the otolith organs also sense the orientation of the head relative to gravity. When the head tilts out of its vertical position along an axis running from the occiput to the nose, the otolith organs estimate the deviation from the vertical and initiate the counter-rolling response of the eyes to compensate.

The Optokinetic System Supplements the Vestibulo-Ocular Reflexes

The vestibular apparatus is not a perfect transducer of head movement. It has two serious problems. First, it habituates. In the dark nystagmus does not continue as long as the head moves, but gradually slows and stops (see Figure 40-8). It stops because the semicircular canals habituate exponentially with a time constant of

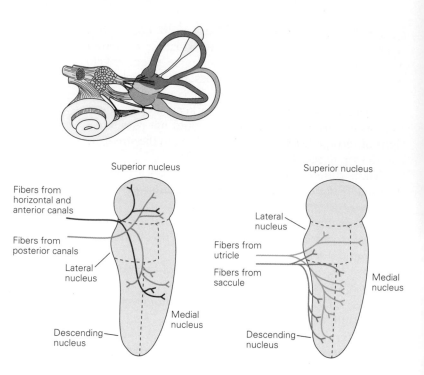

Figure 40-9 The afferent inputs to the vestibular nuclei. The superior and medial nuclei receive input predominantly from the semicircular canals, but also from the otolith organs, and send efferent fibers in the medial longitudinal fasciculus. The lateral nucleus (Deiters' nucleus) receives input from the canals and otolith organs and projects mostly in the lateral vestibulospinal tract. This nucleus is concerned predominantly with postural reflexes. The descending nucleus receives input predominantly from the otolith organs and projects to the cerebellum and reticular formation as well as the contralateral vestibular nuclei and spinal cord. (Adapted from Gacek and Lyon 1974.)

5 s (ie, the signal at 5 s is $1/e$ of its original value). Brain stem circuitry extends the time constant of vestibular nystagmus to 15 s, but during sustained rotation the vestibular signal ultimately fails and the eyes begin to move in space. Second, the canals do not respond well to very slow head movement. To compensate for such deficiencies in the vestibular apparatus the *optokinetic system* provides the central vestibular system with visual information that is used to stabilize the eyes.

When the eyes move in space, fixed objects in the environment—for example, trees and buildings—seem to move in a direction opposite to that of the head. The optokinetic system drives the eyes in the direction of this image motion, an eye movement which, if it were perfect, would stabilize the image on the retina. The optokinetic reflex has the properties needed to complement the vestibulo-ocular reflex: It responds to very slow visual image motion and it builds up slowly, so as to provide a motion signal that can take over as the vestibular signal decays. The combination of vestibular and optokinetic reflexes enables rotatory nystagmus to continue in a lit environment for as long as the head moves.

Vestibulospinal Reflexes Are Important in Maintaining Vertical Posture

How do people know when they are falling? One way is visual—they see the world move. They also know be-

cause the head moves, developing both an angular velocity and a deviation from its normal position relative to the force of gravity. Because the vestibular system responds much faster than the visual system and provides an early warning for derangements of posture, signals from the vestibular nuclei to the spinal cord are a major factor in the maintenance of posture. Vestibular control of posture is discussed in Chapter 41.

Central Connections of the Vestibular Apparatus Integrate Vestibular, Visual, and Motor Signals

The Vestibular Nerve Signals Head Velocity to the Vestibular Nuclei

As we have seen, vestibular neurons fire tonically in the steady state and phasically in response to head movement. Some neurons innervating the otoliths respond tonically to the acceleration provided by gravity. These neurons signal the degree of tilt of the head. The phasic response of neurons innervating the semicircular canals and otolith organs correlates with the velocity of head movement. Head movement to the contralateral side increases neuronal discharge, and head movement to the ipsilateral side decreases it.

The vestibular nerve projects from the vestibular ganglion (Figure 40-1) to the ipsilateral vestibular com-

A Excitatory connections

B Inhibitory connections

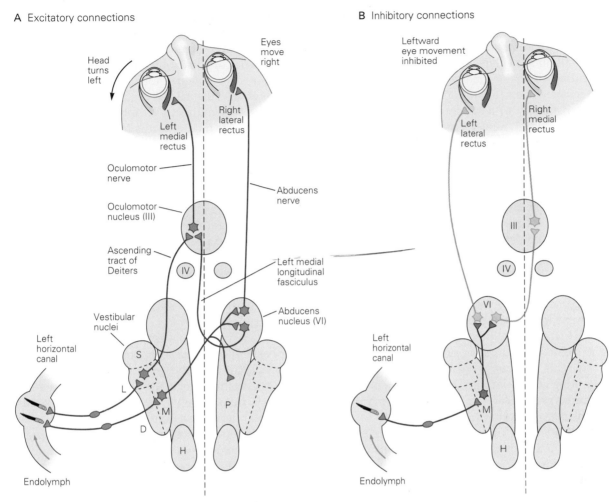

Figure 40-10 Horizontal vestibulo-ocular reflex.

A. Counterclockwise head rotation excites the left horizontal canal, which then excites neurons that evoke rightward eye movement. One population of first-order neurons lies in the medial vestibular nucleus (**M**): Its axons cross the midline and excite neurons in the right abducens nucleus (**VI**) and nucleus prepositus hypoglossi (**P**). The other population is in the lateral vestibular nucleus (**L**). Its axons ascend ipsilaterally in the ascending tract of Deiters and excite neurons in the left oculomotor nucleus (**III**), which project in the oculomotor nerve to the left medial rectus muscle. There are two populations of neurons in the right abducens nucleus (**VI**): motor neurons that project in the abducens nerve and excite the right lateral rectus muscle and interneurons whose axons cross the midline and ascend in the left medial longitudinal fasciculus to the oculomotor nucleus, where they excite the neurons that project to

the left medial rectus muscle. These connections facilitate the rightward horizontal eye movement that compensates for counterclockwise head movement. The illustration also shows the superior (**S**) and descending (**D**) vestibular nuclei, the trochlear nucleus (**IV**), and the nucleus prepositus hypoglossi (**H**).

B. During counterclockwise head movement leftward eye movement is inhibited by sensory fibers from the left horizontal canal. These afferent fibers excite neurons in the medial vestibular nucleus that inhibit left abducens neurons and interneurons. This action reduces the excitation of the motor neurons for the left lateral and right medial rectus muscles. The same head movement results in a decreased signal in the right horizontal canal (not shown), which has similar connections. This movement results in decreased inhibition of the right lateral and left medial rectus muscles and decreased excitation of the left lateral and right medial rectus muscles.

plex of four major nuclei in the dorsal part of the pons and medulla, in the floor of the fourth ventricle (Figure 40-9). The vestibular nuclei integrate signals from the vestibular organs with those from the spinal cord, cere-

bellum, and visual system and project to several central targets: the oculomotor nuclei, reticular and spinal centers occupied with skeletal movement, the vestibular regions of the cerebellum (flocculus, nodulus, ventral paraflocculus, and ventral uvula), and the thalamus. In addition, each vestibular nucleus projects to other ipsilateral and contralateral vestibular nuclei.

The vestibular nuclei—medial, lateral, superior, and descending—were originally distinguished by their cytoarchitecture. Their anatomical differences correspond approximately to a functional segregation. The superior and medial nuclei receive fibers predominantly from the semicircular canals. They send fibers through the medial longitudinal fasciculus rostrally to oculomotor centers and caudally to the spinal cord. Neurons in the medial nucleus are predominantly excitatory, and those in the superior nucleus are predominantly inhibitory. These nuclei are concerned primarily with reflexes that control gaze.

The lateral nucleus (Deiters' nucleus) receives fibers from the semicircular canals and otolith organs and projects mostly into the lateral vestibulospinal tract; this nucleus is concerned mainly with postural reflexes. The descending nucleus receives predominantly otolith input and projects to the cerebellum and reticular formation, as well as to the contralateral vestibular nuclei and the spinal cord. This nucleus is probably most concerned with integrating vestibular signals and central motor signals. Vestibular projections to the spinal systems are discussed in the next chapter, which is on posture.

As we have seen, the three pairs of semicircular canals are organized roughly in three mutually perpendicular planes (Figure 40-6). Each of these planes lies approximately in the pulling direction of each of two pairs of complementary extraocular muscles: the left and right horizontal canals in the plane of the medial and lateral recti; the left anterior and right posterior canals in a plane close to that of the left superior and inferior recti and right superior and inferior obliques; and the right anterior and left posterior canals near that of the right vertical recti and the left obliques. (See Figure 39-5 for the anatomical relationships of the extraocular muscles.)

The anatomical connections of the vestibular nerves mirror the geometric arrangement. Signals from each canal thus project to the motor nuclei in such a way that each canal excites the pair of muscles whose direction of action opposes the direction of head rotation that stimulates the canal and inhibits the pair whose action is in the same direction.

This reciprocity can be seen easily in the horizontal vestibulo-ocular reflex. Leftward head rotation, for example, excites the left horizontal canal, increasing the discharge level in the left vestibular nerve and decreasing the discharge level in the right vestibular nerve in an amount proportional to head velocity. These changes in input result in excitation of the right lateral and left medial rectus muscles and inhibition of the left lateral rec-

tus and right medial rectus muscles. The change in activity is proportional to head velocity.

The motor signals for the horizontal vestibulo-ocular reflex are distributed to the muscles by a network of interneurons (Figure 40-10). As in the saccade system (Chapter 39), the lateral rectus motor neurons in the pons are driven directly by interneurons in the vestibular nuclei. The medial rectus motor neurons in the midbrain are driven by abducens interneurons as well as by a direct projection from the vestibular nuclei. The abducens interneurons receive the same signal as the motor neurons but project to the midbrain via the contralateral medial longitudinal fasciculus rather than to the muscle. This pathway is critical for coordinating the medial and lateral rectus muscles for all lateral gaze processes.

Recall that the ocular motor signal has two components: a velocity signal and a position signal (see Figure 39-9B). If the motor signal from the vestibular nuclei were the only one to reach the eye muscle as a result of head movement, the eyes would drift back to their starting position once the head stopped because no new position signal would be generated. As in the saccade system, the vestibulo-ocular system obtains the necessary position information from the velocity signal in the vestibular nerve by a neural equivalent of mathematical integration (see Chapter 39). This processing is performed by neurons in the nucleus prepositus hypoglossi and medial vestibular nucleus for the horizontal vestibulo-ocular reflex.

As described earlier the eyes remain still when the head is still because the tonic discharges from all canals to all of the extraocular motor neurons are in balance. Disease in a canal usually causes a decrease of this tonic signal. The resulting imbalance in vestibular signals causes pathological nystagmus: The imbalance drives both eyes in one direction and the quick-phase mechanism jerks them back in the other. Nystagmus when the head is still resembles the normal nystagmus that occurs with head rotation and is the hallmark of disease of the vestibular labyrinth and its central connections.

Subcortical and Cortical Structures Contribute to the Optokinetic Reflex

Movement of images on the retina or head movement can induce nystagmus and the perception of self-motion. This perception occurs because vision-related neurons project to the vestibular nuclei: Retinal neurons project to the nucleus of the optic tract in the pretectum, which projects to the same medial vestibular nucleus that receives signals from vestibular afferents. Neurons that receive input from this nucleus cannot distinguish

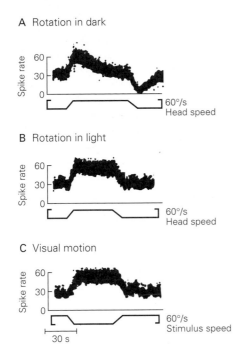

A Rotation in dark

B Rotation in light

C Visual motion

Figure 40-11 Convergence of visual and vestibular signals on a neuron in the medial vestibular nucleus. Each panel shows the neuronal spike rate as a function of time.

A. Rotation of animal in the dark. The **lower trace** shows the angular velocity of the turntable used to rotate the animal subject. The activity of the neuron falls to the baseline even while the animal is still rotating.

B. Rotation of animal in the light. The discharge is maintained throughout rotation.

C. The animal is still but the visual environment rotates around it. At the steady state the neuron responds as if the animal were rotating in the light, although it takes somewhat longer for the neuron to reach the steady state. The similarity of response between body rotation in the light and rotation of the environment in the light may explain why people sometimes feel that they are moving when the visual environment moves. For example, people often feel they are moving backward when they are stopped at a red light and the car next to them moves forward. (Adapted from Waespe and Henn 1977.)

between visual and vestibular signals (Figure 40-11). In principle, they respond identically to head movement and movement of an image on the retina, and presumably that is why people sometimes cannot distinguish between the two.

The cells in the nucleus of the optic tract respond preferentially to stimuli moving across the retina in a temporal-to-nasal direction and stimuli moving with low velocity. In rabbits this nucleus provides the major visual input to the vestibular system, so that the optokinetic reflex in these animals is most responsive to stimuli moving slowly in a temporal-to-nasal direction.

In primates the optokinetic reflex is supplemented by a cortical system that responds to stimuli moving with higher velocities or in a nasal-to-temporal direction. This cortical system includes the visual motion pathway: the magnocellular layers of the lateral geniculate nucleus, the striate cortex, the middle temporal area, and the medial superior temporal area (Chapter 28).

Patients with lesions of this pathway have defective optokinetic nystagmus to visual stimuli moving toward the side with the lesion. Humans with a hereditary lack of color vision (*achromatopsia*) have an optokinetic reflex similar to that of rabbits, with a sensitivity to visual stimuli moving slowly in a temporal-to-nasal direction.

The Vestibular Projection to the Cerebral Cortex Allows Perception of Rotation and Vertical Orientation

All vestibular nuclei project to the ventral posterior and ventral lateral nuclei of the thalamus, which then project to two cortical areas, 2V and 3a. These areas form parts of the primary somatosensory cortex. Vernon Mountcastle first showed that electrical stimulation of the vestibular nerve in the cat evoked activity in the primary somatosensory cortex and in a parietal association cortex. Otto-Joachim Grüsser described neurons in areas 2V and 3a in the monkey that respond to head rotation. Vestibular activity has also been found in the monkey in the parietovestibular insular cortex, which is near the secondary somatosensory area (S-II), and also in parietal association area 7.

Although the vestibular apparatus measures how one accelerates and tilts, the cortex uses this information to generate a subjective measure of self-movement and the external world. Patients with lesions in this area perceive vertical objects to be tilted toward the side of the lesion.

An Overall View

When the head moves the oculomotor system knows how much to move the eyes to compensate for the head movement in order to maintain clear vision. It is possible to derive the velocity of head motion from visual information because when the head moves the image of the world also moves on the retina. It is also possible to derive head velocity from the tactile sensation of the air moving across one's face. If head movement is associated with neck or body movement, then the velocity of head movement can be derived from proprioceptive systems of the neck and body. However, these sensory mechanisms are slow and cumbersome. In contrast, the hair cells of the vestibular system sense head acceleration directly, and this sensing in turn allows those reflexes that require information about head motion to act efficiently and quickly.

Projections from the vestibular nuclei to the oculomotor system allow eye muscles to compensate for head movement by moving in such a way as to hold the image of the external world motionless on the retina. Rotatory vestibulo-ocular reflexes compensate for angular movement and depend on the semicircular canals. Translational vestibulo-ocular reflexes compensate for linear movement and depend on the otolith organs.

Sustained rotation results in a pattern of alternating slow and fast eye movements called nystagmus. The slow eye movement is equal and opposite to the head movement while the fast eye movement is a resetting movement in the opposite direction. Nystagmus in the absence of sustained head rotation is a sign of disease of the vestibular apparatus or its central connections. Vestibular signals habituate during sustained rotation and are relatively insensitive to very slow head movements.

Head movement evokes motion of the visual image on the retina as the moving eyes sweep across a stable visual field. This visual signal is used by the brain to supplement the vestibular signal and compensate for the tendency of the vestibular signal to adapt during prolonged rotation. The optokinetic system provides the visual input to the central vestibular system. The retinal image motion induced by head movement enables the optokinetic system to induce eye movements and perceptions that are equivalent to those induced by actual head movement.

Michael E. Goldberg
A. J. Hudspeth

Selected Readings

Baloh RW, Honrubia V. 1990. *Clinical Neurology of the Vestibular System*. Philadelphia: FA Davis.

Highstein SM, McCrea RA. 1988. The anatomy of the vestibular nuclei. Rev Oculomot Res 2:177–202.

Leigh RJ, Zee DS. 1991. *The Neurology of Eye Movements*, 2nd ed. Philadelphia: FA Davis.

References

Benser ME, Issa NP, Hudspeth AJ. 1993. Hair bundle stiffness dominates the elastic reactance to otolithic-membrane shear. Hear Res 68:243–252.

Bergström B. 1973. Morphology of the vestibular nerve. II. The number of myelinated vestibular nerve fibers in man at various ages. Acta Otolaryngol (Stockh) 76:173–179.

Brandt T, Dieterich M. 1994. Vestibular syndromes in the roll plane: topographic diagnosis from brainstem to cortex. Ann Neurol 36:337–347.

Dieterich M, Brandt T. 1995. Vestibulo-ocular reflex. Curr Opin Neurol 8:83–88.

Fernandez C, Goldberg JM. 1976a. Physiology of peripheral neurons innervating otolith organs of the squirrel monkey. I. Response to static tilts and to long-duration centrifugal force. J Neurophysiol 39:970–984.

Fernandez C, Goldberg JM. 1976b. Physiology of peripheral neurons innervating otolith organs of the squirrel monkey. II. Directional selectivity and force-response relations. J Neurophysiol 39:985–995.

Fernandez C, Goldberg JM. 1971. Physiology of peripheral neurons innervating semicircular canals of the squirrel monkey. II. Response to sinusoidal stimulation and dynamics of peripheral vestibular system. J Neurophysiol 34:661–675.

Fernandez C, Goldberg JM, Abend WK. 1972. Response to static tilts of peripheral neurons innervating otolith organs of the squirrel monkey. J Neurophysiol 35:978–997.

Flock Å. 1965. Transducing mechanisms in the lateral line canal organ receptors. Cold Spring Harbor Symp Quant Biol 30:133-145.

Fukushima K. 1997. Corticovestibular interactions: anatomy, electrophysiology, and functional considerations. Exp Brain Res 117:1–16.

Gacek RR, Lyon M. 1974. The localization of vestibular efferent neurons in the kitten with horseradish peroxidase. Acta Otolaryngol (Stockh) 77:92–101.

Goldberg JM, Fernández C. 1971. Physiology of peripheral neurons innervating semicircular canals of the squirrel monkey. I. Resting discharge and response to constant angular accelerations. J Neurophysiol 34:635–660.

Grüsser OJ, Pause M, Schreiter U. 1990. Localization and responses of neurons in the parieto-insular vestibular cortex of awake monkeys (*Macaca fascicularis*). J Physiol (Lond) 430:537–557.

Hillman DE, McLaren JW. 1979. Displacement configuration of semicircular canal cupulae. Neuroscience 4:1989–2000.

Iurato S. 1967. Submicroscopic Structure of the Inner Ear. Oxford: Pergamon Press.

Mustari MJ, Fuchs AF. 1990. Discharge patterns of neurons in the pretectal nucleus of the optic tract (NOT) in the behaving primate. J Neurophysiol 64:77–90.

Mustari MJ, Fuchs AF, Kaneko CRS, Robinson F. 1994. Anatomical connections of the primate pretectal nucleus of the optic tract. J Comp Neurol 349:111–128.

Spoendlin H. 1966. Ultrastructure of the vestibular sense organ. In: RJ Wolfson (ed). *The Vestibular System and Its Diseases,* pp. 39–68. Philadelphia: University of Pennsylvania Press.

Waespe W, Henn V. 1977. Neuronal activity in the vestibular nuclei of the alert monkey during vestibular and optokinetic stimulation. Exp Brain Res 27:523–538.

Watanuki K, Schuknecht HF. 1976. A morphological study of human vestibular sensory epithelia. Arch Otolaryngol Head Neck Surg 102:583–588.

Yee RD, Baloh RW, Honrubia V. 1981. Eye movement abnormalities in rod monochromacy. Ophthalmology 88:1010–1018.

41

Posture

WHEN WE MOVE WE ARE usually unaware of the complex neuromuscular processes that control our posture. But postural control is obvious enough when we accidentally fall or when disease damages parts of the postural system. The mechanical problem of maintaining posture is particularly challeng-ing for erect bipeds. Even with the more stable four-legged animals successful postural control is no mean achievement. Imagine a predator chasing its prey at full gallop and then suddenly changing direction. Before doing so it must first throw its center of gravity into the curve, correctly predicting the new gravito-inertial force vector introduced by centrifugal force.

Humans also make this kind of postural adjustment, usually without thinking. In fact, conscious control can be disastrous. One might think that to make a rightward turn on a bicycle the rider simply rotates the handlebars to the right. Wrong! Rotation to the right would move the center of gravity to the left, and the cyclist would quickly crash to the ground. Instead, without realizing it, the cyclist first turns the handlebars briefly leftward to generate a centrifugal force that moves the body rightward into the intended curve. Only then does he steer the bicycle to the right until the new force vector properly lines up with wheel contact on the ground. Children must learn this postural adjustment when switching from a tricycle (in which the handlebars must first be turned in the direction the rider wants to go) to a bicycle.

The postural system must therefore meet three main challenges. It must maintain a *steady stance* (balance) in the presence of gravity, it must generate responses that *anticipate* volitional goal-directed movements, and it must be *adaptive.*

Systematic investigation of posture began with experiments on four-legged animals, notably the decerebrate cat, in which cerebral control of the brain stem is disconnected by a transection at a midbrain level (see Box 37-1). This preparation was devised by Charles Sherrington at the beginning of the twentieth century to study spinal reflexes isolated from higher levels of motor control. In a series of classic experiments on decerebrate cats and dogs early in the twentieth century, Sherrington, Rudolf Magnus, and other physiologists uncovered a variety of stretch reflexes because these reflexes are exaggerated in the decerebrate animal (Chapter 36). When the cut is between the superior and inferior colliculi, contraction of extensor and other antigravity muscles is intensified, producing what is called *decerebrate rigidity*. The rigidity may be great enough to allow the animal to stand unsupported. When the sensory nerves from the limbs of decerebrate animals are cut, the enhanced tone of antigravity muscles collapses dramatically, revealing that afferent signals from muscle are crucial to efferent motor control.

Sherrington went so far as to suggest that rigidity of extensor muscles in the face of gravity represents the foundation of postural control expressed in "grotesque form," although he knew that there was more to postural control than this. When Magnus and his colleagues transected the brain at higher levels they observed a hierarchy of automated responses to postural disturbance—ranging from head and neck reflexes to the so-called righting reflexes—that are not possible in the midbrain decerebrate preparation. Magnus concluded that postural control could be explained by the simple summation of these reflexes.

Postural reflexes do not fully account for postural control during skilled, purposeful movements, however. For example, the simple act of reaching out to grasp an object can destabilize balance unless precisely timed compensatory action is initiated before the arm is extended. Thus a system is needed to generate anticipatory responses. In addition, a wide range of automatic response patterns must be available to cope with any unexpected disturbances. Finally, because postural control must be integrated with voluntary movement, postural control systems must be capable of adaptive learning. Thus the current view is that postural control involves the behaviorally meaningful integration of many different neural systems, including those associated with cognition.

Posture and Equilibrium

How should posture be defined? What are its behavioral goals? Posture is essentially the relative position of the various parts of the body with respect to one another (the *egocentric coordinate system*) and to the environment (the *exocentric coordinate system*). A third frame of reference is that of the gravitational field (the *geocentric coordinate system*). The orientation of a body part can

be described in terms of each of these frameworks, depending on the behavioral context. For example, knowing the position of the head relative to the environment is important in stabilizing vision, while knowing its position relative to the rest of the body is important in maintaining erect posture. Regulation of posture with respect to gravity is obviously important in maintaining *postural equilibrium*, which may be defined as the state in which all forces acting on the body are balanced so that the body rests in an intended position (*static equilibrium*) or is able to progress through an intended movement without losing balance (*dynamic equilibrium*).

Postural control may have different goals under different circumstances, such as longitudinal alignment of the whole body to maintain a steady, erect stance; remodeling of stance in preparation for a voluntary movement; shaping of the body for display purposes, as in dance; maintenance of balance, as on the gymnast's beam; or conservation of energy in a demanding task.

Different animals may use quite different postural strategies to achieve a steady stance in the face of gravity. Thus, as a result of size-dependent mechanics (*allometry*), the elephant mechanically locks its legs in line with the gravity vector to minimize the muscle forces supporting its heavy body. In contrast, small quadrupeds tense the muscles around flexed limb joints, thus permitting rapid responses to danger. (Tensing the muscles around flexed joints enhances muscle stiffness; since stiff muscle pairs mechanically resist change virtually instantaneously and hence well ahead of any active reflex response, opposition to unexpected perturbations is optimal.)

Posture and Movement

Both of these strategies are used by humans. We stand like elephants. Instead of flexing the knees as if to spring forward, we lock the knee joints so that the legs become static and structural, thus off-loading antigravity muscles until they are needed for movement. On the other hand, like smaller animals we flex the weight-supporting limbs in preparation for intended movement, as at the start of a sprint.

Postural Readjustment Must Be Preceded by Anticipatory Motor Action

Now consider what happens when one leg is actively lifted sideways while a subject maintains balance on the other. Since the center of gravity's force vector is initially projected midway between the two feet, the body would fall to the side of the lifted leg if no *anticipatory* action were

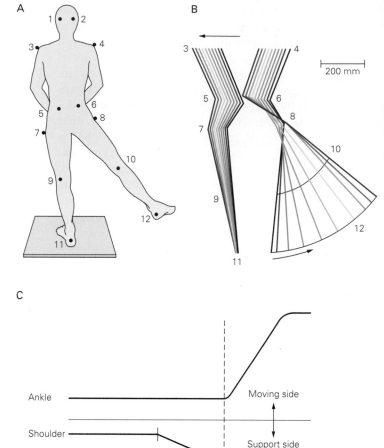

Figure 41-1 Postural adjustments require anticipatory motor actions. (Adapted from Lee et al. 1995.)

A. Rear view of a subject standing on a force-transducing platform and lifting the right leg sideways to the right. The **numbered points** identify points on the body from which the image in part B is constructed.

B. A record of trunk and limb movements during this maneuver. The **black lines** represent the subject with both feet resting symmetrically on the ground. The **colored lines,** separated by 50 ms intervals and moving in the direction of the **arrows,** show the moment-to-moment pattern of postural adjustment employed to reestablish static equilibrium on the left leg without falling.

C. Kinematic records show the hip and the shoulders beginning to move long before the ankle starts to rise. The center of pressure registered by the force-transducing platform first moves outward toward the leg that is to be lifted in order to move the center of gravity over the supporting leg. Then, as the shoulders and the hip begin to move, it moves back under the supporting leg to maintain the new posture.

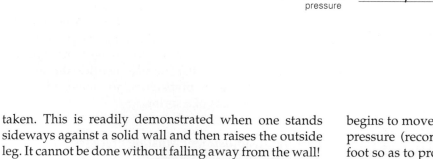

taken. This is readily demonstrated when one stands sideways against a solid wall and then raises the outside leg. It cannot be done without falling away from the wall!

To maintain balance, the voluntary movement must be preceded by a counterbalancing movement that shifts the center of gravity over the leg on which the person intends to remain standing. This apparently simple procedure invokes a complex set of interactive responses, however. Some 600 ms before the rising ankle

begins to move, a subject will briefly move the center of pressure (recorded on a platform) toward the outside foot so as to provide the necessary force for transferring the body's center of mass over the inside foot. Since shoulder and hip movements are driven by the changing center of pressure, they too are initiated before the ankle begins to move. As the shoulders and the hips begin to move, the center of pressure returns to the support leg (Figure 41-1).

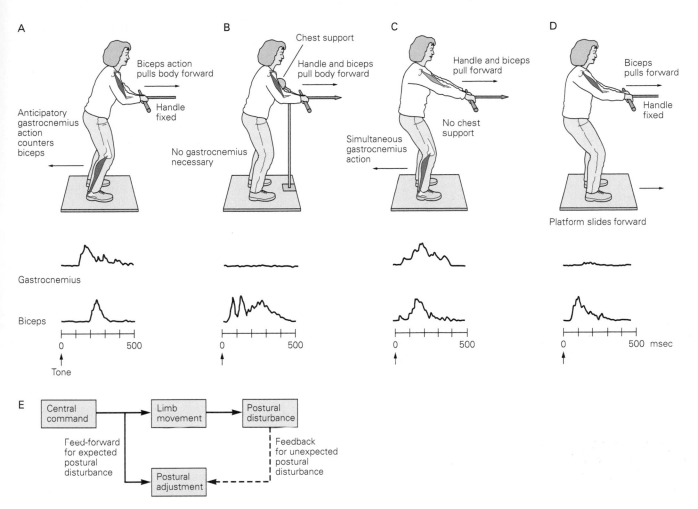

Figure 41-2 Anticipatory motor action in response to postural disturbance adapts to the behavioral context. The illustrations show the postural activity of the gastrocnemius muscle in four behavioral contexts. (Adapted from Cordo and Nashner 1982.)

A. The subject stands on a firm platform and pulls on a fixed handle as soon as possible after an auditory cue. To maintain posture, backward-acting contraction of the leg muscle (gastrocnemius) starts before the biceps begin pulling the handle.

B. When the chest is supported and the handle is suddenly pulled forward, there is a very early reflex response in the bi-

ceps and the gastrocnemius remains silent.

C. When the handle suddenly pulls the unsupported subject forward, the early biceps reflex is suppressed so that counterbalancing arm and leg muscles can act simultaneously.

D. Finally, when the foot support unexpectedly slides forward, tilting the subject backward, the gastrocnemius is silent (otherwise it would tilt the subject further back) and an early biceps response is brought into play.

E. The feed-forward and feedback components of postural control. (Adapted from Gahéry and Massion 1981.)

Postural Control Can Be Adapted to Suit Specific Behaviors

Anticipatory action is remarkably adaptable and varies according to behavioral demand (Figure 41-2). One can easily demonstrate the dependence of postural control on behavioral context, or *postural set*. First, place the right upper arm beside the body with the forearm horizontal so that the elbow of the arm is at a right angle. Then, while actively maintaining this posture with the

eyes closed, try to press that forearm down with the left hand. If one suddenly releases the downward pressure of the left hand, there is little or no movement of the right forearm. Anticipatory suppression of the right forearm flexors is synchronized with the predicted removal of the left hand. Next, again with the eyes shut, have a colleague apply downward pressure on the right forearm, and then ask that it be suddenly removed without warning. Now the right forearm flies upward.

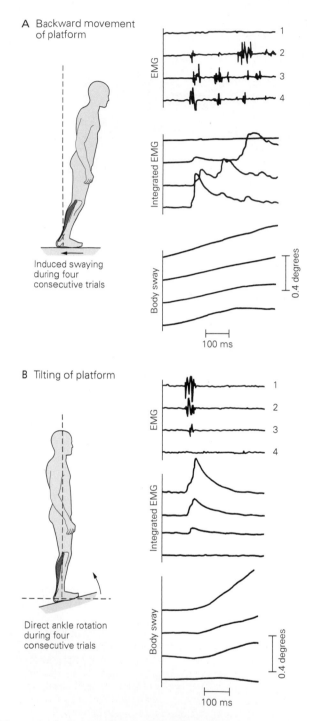

A Backward movement
of platform

EMG

1
2
3
4

Integrated EMG

Body sway

0.4 degrees

100 ms

Induced swaying
during four
consecutive trials

B Tilting of platform

EMG

1
2
3
4

Integrated EMG

Body sway

0.4 degrees

100 ms

Direct ankle rotation
during four
consecutive trials

Figure 41-3 Appropriate anticipatory responses to postural disturbances can be learned. (Adapted from Nashner 1976.)

A. Backward movement of the sliding platform tilts the body forward, calling for countervailing action in the stretched gastrocnemius to maintain balance. In successive trials the muscular response is enhanced and its latency reduced.

B. When the platform is tilted up, action by the gastrocnemius would worsen the backward body tilt. Accordingly, in successive trials the muscle's response is decreased, with a corresponding decrease of backward sway.

Anticipatory responses depend on feed-forward control. The central command for a voluntary limb movement is associated with a simultaneous feed-forward command anticipating an expected postural perturbation. Postural adjustments to unexpected disturbances depend on feedback, however. These adjustments may be relatively simple and fast, as in the biceps stretch reflex (Figure 41-2B), but usually they are the product of complex motor reactions that are learned and released as a whole (Figure 41-2C). The interaction of feed-forward and feedback control of posture is summarized in Figure 41-2E.

While the basic elements of postural control are innate, they nevertheless can be greatly modified by learning. The rigid stance of the decerebrate quadruped is innate, as is the stereotyped response of a standing quadruped when it loses the support of one or more limbs. If support from diagonally opposite legs is unexpectedly withdrawn, the decerebrate animal actively reacts by supporting itself on the other pair of legs. The advantage of this strategy is that the center of gravity need not be moved, although it does create a problem with stabilization. If an intact animal is trained to *expect* loss of support from one paw, it adopts a quite different strategy at the time of unloading: The center of gravity is actively moved within the triangular support of the other three limbs. This action provides support *and* ensures subsequent postural equilibrium.

Russian investigators in the early twentieth century used classical Pavlovian conditioning to show that animals can learn anticipatory feed-forward patterns of response. They trained animals with deafferented limbs to remove the support of one limb by actively lifting one paw in response to an auditory cue. Recordings of postural muscle activity showed that the trained animals always appropriately activated the antigravity muscles of the other three limbs *before* raising the paw.

Later, Lew Nashner devised an ingenious way to demonstrate adaptive learning of postural control in humans. The subject stands erect on a platform, which can be made to slide backward without tilting or to tilt toe-up without sliding. Both maneuvers stretch the gastrocnemius. But while forward sway calls for contraction of the muscle, backward sway calls for its relaxation. In both conditions there is clear evidence that the subject learns the appropriate response (Figure 41-3).

Adaptive Postural Control Requires an Intact Cerebellum

Nashner also observed that patients with cerebellar lesions were largely unable to make adaptive changes in postural control, suggesting an important role for the cerebellum in this form of motor learning. Fay Horak and Hans Diener studied adaptation of postural control in patients with anterior cerebellar lobe lesions. As in Nashner's experiments, the subjects stood erect on a platform that could suddenly be moved backward. The platform was moved under two different conditions. In one series of trials the platform was displaced at different distances in an unpredictable order. In the second series it was moved the same distance in all trials.

Recordings of ankle torque and integrated electromyograms were made during the first 75 ms of the stimulus—before there could have been sensory-motor feedback from the event. Neither the patients nor the control subjects could scale their response to the random displacement trials. When the platform was displaced the same distance in successive trials, normal subjects systematically learned to scale their responses appropriately; patients with cerebellar lesions failed to do so (Figure 41-4).

Adaptive Postural Control Is Learned During Locomotion

A normal blindfolded person can walk straight ahead quite well. This task requires precise neuromuscular control of horizontal trunk rotation relative to the stance foot on the ground in order to prevent curvature in the trajectory of locomotion. This neuromuscular control must be learned.

In a recent series of experiments subjects were required to walk on the perimeter of a rotating disc without moving in space, much like walking on a treadmill. After an hour or so of this unusual experience, blindfolded subjects could no longer walk straight ahead on firm ground. Instead, they unknowingly walked in curved trajectories, even though the rate of rotation relative to space was then well above the threshold of vestibular sensation. In contrast, the same subjects were able to propel themselves manually in a wheelchair along a straight path, demonstrating that the learning was restricted to the postural components exposed to the adaptive stimulus, namely, those of the lower limb locomotor system (Figure 41-5). That is, the adaptive learning took place within a "bottom-up" flow of postural information. In contrast, control of spatial relations between the head and the trunk by the vestibular-neck postural system involves "top-down" information flow.

Vestibular and Neck Contributions

When subjects are rotated in one direction for a minute or so and then try to stand up while suddenly tilting the head relative to the trunk, they throw themselves to the

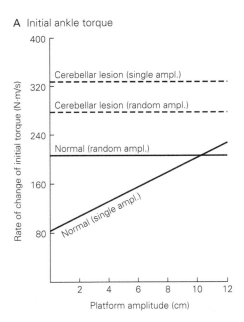

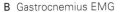

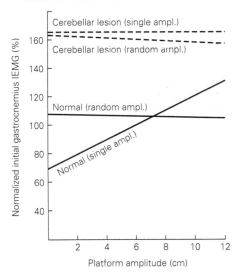

Figure 41-4 Atrophy of the anterior cerebellar lobe prevents appropriate scaling of an anticipatory postural response. Subjects stood on a platform that could be moved backward over controlled distances suddenly and unexpectedly. The two plots represent average regressions of initial ankle torque (**A**) and the gastrocnemius electromyogram (**B**) for a variety of displacement distances (amplitudes) in two sets of trials. The data are for 10 patients with anterior cerebellar lobe lesions and 10 normal subjects. Each individual was exposed to two series of 10 trials. In the first series the platform was moved at different amplitudes in a random, unpredictable sequence. In the second series displacement amplitude was the same in all trials. The normal subjects learned to scale their responses to the predictable displacements of constant amplitude, but the patients with cerebellar lesions could not do so. (Adapted from Horak and Diener 1994.)

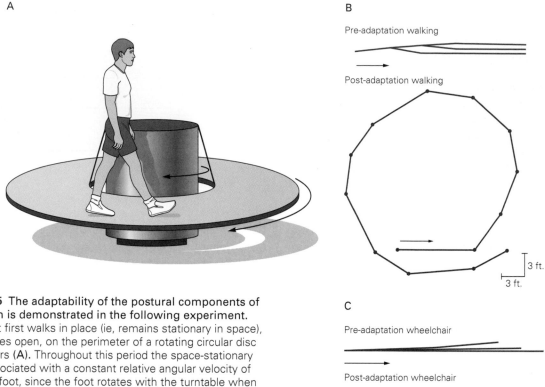

Figure 41-5 The adaptability of the postural components of locomotion is demonstrated in the following experiment. The subject first walks in place (ie, remains stationary in space), with the eyes open, on the perimeter of a rotating circular disc for 1–2 hours (**A**). Throughout this period the space-stationary trunk is associated with a constant relative angular velocity of the stance foot, since the foot rotates with the turntable when planted on it. Before adaptation to the rotating treadmill a blindfolded subject can walk straight ahead on firm ground quite well. After adaptation the blindfolded subject can no longer walk straight ahead. When trying to do so he *unknowingly* walks in a circular path on the ground by steadily rotating the trunk relative to the stance foot (**B**), even when the resulting body angular velocity is well above the vestibular threshold of rotational sensation. In contrast, after adaptation the blind-

folded subject can readily propel a wheelchair straight ahead with the hands (**C**), demonstrating that the motor learning is localized in the podokinetic system for sensory-motor control of trunk rotation relative to the stance foot. (Adapted from Gordon et al. 1995.)

ground because of powerful but inappropriate vestibulospinal postural reflexes (don't try this without restraint—it's dangerous!). Why are these reflexes so inappropriate in these circumstances? The grossly misleading vestibulospinal response that occurs after prolonged rotation becomes mismatched to the concurrent but normal afferent stimulation of neck afferents introduced by head tilt.

In normal circumstances we can sharply rotate the head relative to the trunk without any disturbance of equilibrium, but only because of the precisely calibrated offset of vestibulospinal reflexes by neck afferent signals. With the trunk stationary, the two separate but powerful influences normally cancel one another perfectly so that their presence in the central nervous system goes unnoticed by the subject. When the trunk moves relative to space, the separate roles of the two pathways that project to the spinal cord become apparent.

Vestibular and Neck Reflexes Are Subject to Volitional Control

Many now-classical behavioral studies done early in the twentieth century identified a series of vestibular-neck (vestibulocollic), vestibulospinal, neck-neck (cervicocollic), and cervicospinal reflexes, all of which appear to be innate.

Since the vestibular sensory signal relays a message of head movement relative to inertial space (Chapter 40), it is not surprising that the vestibulocollic reflex plays an important role in stabilizing the head relative to space. Significantly, however, the vestibulocollic reflex acts in a fundamentally different way from the more familiar vestibulo-ocular reflexes that stabilize the eyes (Chapter 39). When the vestibulocollic reflex acts on neck muscles to stabilize the head relative to space, the motor response, by opposing the perturbing head movement, necessarily tends to null the vestibular signal at its source. In other words, this reflex functions as an error-activated negative feedback system.

In contrast, the cervicocollic reflex responds to neck muscle stretch and joint afferents and therefore stabilizes the head relative to the trunk (rather than to space). Consequently, when the trunk is stationary the vestibulocollic and cervicocollic reflexes collaborate in head stabilization. But when the trunk turns relative to the head, as when one looks at a fixed object while turning a corner, the cervicocollic reflex must be suppressed so that the vestibulocollic reflex alone stabilizes the head. Thus, even though innate, these reflexes can be brought under higher control to suit the intended pattern of voluntary movement.

Vestibulospinal and Cervicospinal Reflexes Collaborate in Maintaining Postural Stability

The innate vestibulospinal and cervicospinal reflexes automatically maintain postural stability. For example, if the head and trunk of a quadruped are both passively tilted to the left, vestibulospinal responses extend the left limbs and flex the right ones to oppose the perturbation. If the trunk alone is passively tilted left while the head is held stationary, the cervicospinal response produces opposition to the tilt. However, if the head is rotated while the trunk remains stationary, these two reflexes oppose one another, so that the animal's stance is not disturbed (Figure 41-6). Again, even though these reflexes are innate, they can be altered or superseded by higher brain centers to suit the behavioral context.

Another innate vestibulospinal response occurs during sudden falls. Humans dropped unexpectedly exhibit a stereotyped extensor response in the antigravity muscles of the lower limbs that serves to break the fall. Due to the fixed latency of this response (less than 100 ms), it is useful only for falls from heights sufficiently great (5″–6″) to allow the response to come into play. Here, too, there is a need for flexibility in an innate reflex response, which must be integrated with volitional control based on the subject's assessment of the distance to the ground.

When a cat with clear vision is suddenly dropped, the short-latency vestibulospinal response is superimposed upon by context-dependent muscle activity, which is nicely timed within a millisecond or two of the anticipated moment of landing. Spinal stretch reflexes alone would not serve to resist the landing from any height because the latency of such a reaction, which includes the electromechanical coupling time, would be far too long to permit muscular deceleration even by the monosynaptic stretch reflex. This long latency creates a problem when, for example, one descends a step of unanticipated depth. If the time of fall is less than the latency of the vestibulospinal response, muscular deceler-

A Normal position

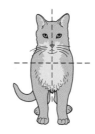

B Head and trunk together (vestibular stimulation)

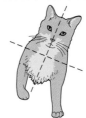

C Trunk alone (cervical stimulation)

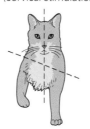

D Head alone (vestibular–neck stimulation)

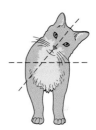

Figure 41-6 The vestibulospinal and cervicospinal reflexes act synergistically to maintain body posture whether the head and trunk move together or independently.

A. The head and the trunk are in the normal standing position with both forelegs extended.

B. Passive rotation of both the head and the trunk to the left leads to left leg extension and right leg flexion. This pattern of reflex response is a purely vestibulospinal one since there is no relative movement between the head and the trunk.

C. Tilting the trunk left-side down while keeping the head stationary in space produces the same behavior as in B. Here, however, the reflex response is purely cervicospinal.

D. When the head is rotated relative to both gravity and the trunk, the two reflexes oppose one another and limb extension remains balanced, thus allowing the head to rotate relative to the trunk without postural disturbance.

ation is not possible, and a dangerous skeletal impact is bound to occur.

The vestibular contribution to postural control depends on the kind of perturbation imposed. For example, if the platform on which a subject stands is suddenly and unexpectedly moved backward, patients with defective vestibular labyrinths make normal postural muscle reactions to the forward-induced fall. If the head rather than the foot position is perturbed, the same patients cannot make normal short-latency corrective responses (Figure 41-7).

A primary function of the vestibular response is to stabilize the head in space. When a normal subject balances on a small support surface, a so-called hip balanc-

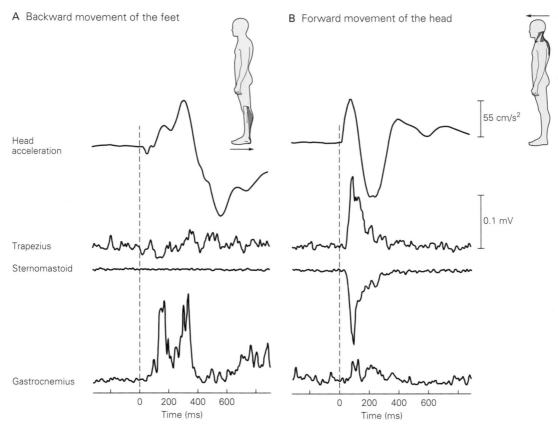

A Backward movement of the feet

Head
acceleration

Trapezius

Sternomastoid

Gastrocnemius

0   200   400   600
Time (ms)

B Forward movement of the head

55 cm/s^2

0.1 mV

0   200   400   600
Time (ms)

Figure 41-7 The vestibular contribution to postural adjustment depends on whether the primary perturbation is to the feet or the head. (Adapted from Horak et al. 1994.)

A. Sudden backward movement of the feet leads to a large and early response in the gastrocnemius muscle but no relevant action in the trapezius or sternomastoid neck muscles. Although the head does move when the feet are displaced, the resulting

vestibular activity cannot be responsible for the gastrocnemius response since the latency of the response is too brief. In fact, the latency is that of the stretch reflex.

B. In contrast, sudden forced acceleration of the head produces the opposite effects: a strong, short-latency response in the neck muscle and little or no response in the gastrocnemius.

ing strategy is brought into play. With the head held steady, one maintains balance by continually shifting the pelvic girdle back and forth. Under conditions in which a normal subject copes quite well, the patient with a labyrinth defect quickly loses balance because the vestibular components of head stabilization are lacking. Furthermore, when cats who have just been labyrinthectomized turn their heads relative to both trunk and space, they immediately lose their balance and fall because the cervicospinal reflexes are no longer balanced by matching vestibular input.

Perhaps a similar rationale explains why, while a normal cat readily learns to walk along a rotating beam without falling, an animal with bilateral labyrinthectomy never recovers this remarkable ability. In contrast, the unilaterally defective animal can relearn this demanding postural motor task through adaptive mechanisms of the kind discussed in the next section. Signifi-

cantly, the potential for long-term recovery is highly dependent on postoperative management. Animals normally recover completely within about 7 weeks. But if the animal is artificially constrained for 1 week during the first 10 days after surgical lesioning, the *ultimate* degree of recovery is severely impaired; no more than about 40% of the possible extent of recovery is achieved. Constraint in the middle of the recovery period severely prejudices the potential achievement, but constraint after full recovery has no effect since the motor learning is then complete (Figure 41-8).

Motor Learning in Vestibulo-Ocular Control

Adaptive motor learning has been extensively studied in the vestibulo-ocular system. Here we summarize current views on the central mechanisms involved.

Figure 41-8 After unilateral removal of a cat's vestibular labyrinth, the ultimate degree of recovery of the animal's ability to maintain dynamic equilibrium is highly dependent on postoperative management. The **curves** show recovery patterns in the ability to walk along a beam that can be rotated at various speeds. (The curves begin 12 days after surgery because before that time none of the cats could perform the task even on a static beam.) The unrestrained cat achieved full postoperative recovery after about 7 weeks of practice. A period of 1 week's physical restraint after full recovery had no effect **(A)**. Restraint in the middle of the recovery period seriously reduced the otherwise attainable degree of recovery **(B)**. One week of restraint immediately after operation reduced the *ultimate* level of recovery to only 40% of the potential level **(C)**. (Adapted from Xerri and Lacour 1980.)

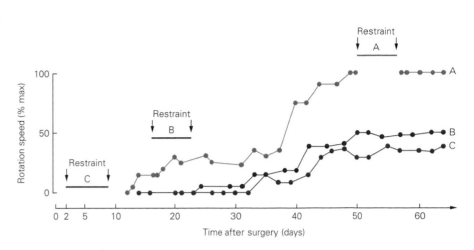

When a subject wears magnifying lenses the retinal image of the outside world is magnified, as is the velocity of the retinal image relative to that of the head. The normal vestibulo-ocular reflex rotates the eyes in a compensatory direction at the same speed as that of the head relative to space, ie, with a gain of approximately unity. The magnifying lenses initially make this response inappropriate. After the lenses have been worn continually for a week the vestibulo-ocular reflex is again effective in stabilizing the retinal image because the gain of the reflex has been augmented appropriately. This change is due to adaptive adjustment of synaptic efficacy (*neural gain*) in the reflex path, which allows the adjusted response to occur without further feedback. The temporal pattern of increase (or decrease) of the gain of the vestibulo-ocular reflex in monkeys fitted with magnifying (or minifying) lenses is shown in Figure 41-9.

The reflex is said to be *adaptive* because it tends to meet the new behavioral demand of automatic image stabilization during head rotation with modified optics. It is *plastic* because it retains its adapted state: If at any time during the adaptive sequence the animal is placed in darkness or the head is fixed in space with clear vision, the gain stays put at the value then attained, since both these conditions remove the driving force of visual-vestibular conflict. Thus, once a change of gain has been established, the normal condition can be restored only by active readaptation. When a patient acquires new prescription spectacles that magnify or reduce the retinal image, time is required for an adaptive change of vestibulo-ocular gain to recover automatic image stabilization. During this adaptive period patients may be frustrated with the resulting disturbance of visual postural control as well as visual blurring during head movements.

The Cerebellum Plays a Key Role in Adapting Vestibulo-Ocular Control

As discussed earlier, the cerebellum is a necessary component of adaptation of postural control. It is also necessary in adaptation of the vestibulo-ocular reflex, although how the cerebellum participates in this adaptation remains controversial. Masao Ito proposed a likely hypothesis based on experimental studies of rabbits. In addition to direct excitatory input to the vestibular nuclei in the brain stem, the sensory neurons of the vestibular labyrinth also provide input to Purkinje cells in the flocculo-nodular lobes of the cerebellum via a pathway of mossy and parallel fibers. In turn, the Purkinje cells project an *inhibitory* influence back onto the vestibular nuclei (Figure 41-10A). Ito argued that the gain of the vestibulo-ocular reflex can be adaptively modulated by altering the relative strengths of the direct excitatory and indirect inhibitory pathways.

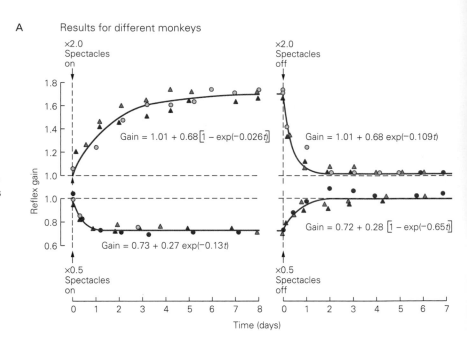

A   Results for different monkeys

$Gain = 1.01 + 0.68[1 - exp(-0.026t)]$

$Gain = 1.01 + 0.68\,exp(-0.109t)$

$Gain = 0.73 + 0.27\,exp(-0.13t)$

$Gain = 0.72 + 0.28[1 - exp(-0.65t)]$

Figure 41-9 Monkeys wearing magnifying (× 2) or minifying (× 0.5) spectacles gradually augment (or diminish) the intrinsic gain of the vestibulo-ocular reflex. (Adapted from Miles and Eighmy 1980.)

A. The results for *different* animals indicate consistency of the phenomenon between different animals.

B. The results for the *same* animal on different occasions indicate that adaptation does not depend on previous adaptation experience. In the fitted equations time (t) is expressed in hours. There are no obvious effects of one learning cycle on the next.

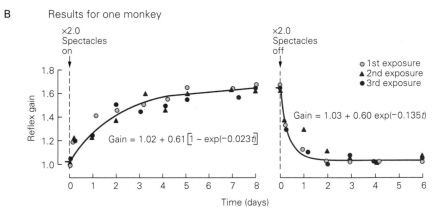

B   Results for one monkey

○ 1st exposure
▲ 2nd exposure
● 3rd exposure

$Gain = 1.02 + 0.61[1 - exp(-0.023t)]$

$Gain = 1.03 + 0.60\,exp(-0.135t)$

Figure 41-10 (Opposite) Two hypotheses of adaptive adjustment in the vestibulo-ocular reflex.

A. Ito's original hypothesis proposed that the "teaching line" is represented by the climbing fiber pathway from the inferior olivary nucleus to Purkinje cells of the cerebellar cortex, while the site of adaptative "learning" is in the cerebellar cortex at the synapses of vestibular parallel fibers onto the Purkinje cells. (Adapted from Ito 1984.)

B. The Miles-Lisberger hypothesis proposes that the "teaching line" is represented by the Purkinje cell *output*, while the site of "learning" is at Purkinje cell target neurons in the vestibular nuclei of the brain stem. If the direction of gaze is properly stabilized in space by the vestibulo-ocular reflex during head rotation, the vestibular signal of head rotation relative to space and that of the motor copy of eye motion relative to the head (conveyed in mossy fiber projections to cerebellar cortex) should normally be equal and opposite. That is, during normal head movement the two signals cancel one another by summation at the Purkinje cell level. Thus there would appropriately be no "teaching" signal discharged by the Purkinje cell output from the cerebellar cortex.

However, if the vestibulo-oculomotor output is too low for retinal image stabilization (as when first donning magnifying spectacles or in the early stages of clinical oculomotor paresis), visual pursuit will force increased eye movement and thus increase the motor copy signal fed into the cerebellar cortex relative to that of the opposing vestibular input. As a result the Purkinje cells now carry a difference signal that represents the relevant underperformance of the vestibulo-ocular reflex. This error signal then "teaches" relays in the vestibular nuclei to augment the vestibulo-oculomotor drive and hence recover automatic vestibulo-ocular stabilization of the retinal image during head rotation.

Note that in the *general* case it is the sum of eye movement relative to the head and spatial image movement relative to the retina that properly represents the visual system's "estimate" of head movement relative to space. This sum accounts for the discrete parallel pathways for "eye velocity" and "retinal image slip" (right) in mossy fiber projections to the cerebellar cortex. In both figures the stars indicate the proposed site of synaptic learning. (Adapted from Lisberger 1988.)

A Ito hypothesis

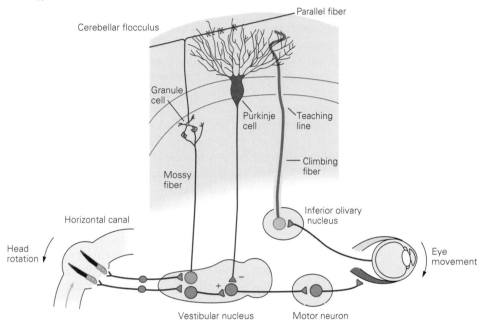

B Miles-Lisberger hypothesis

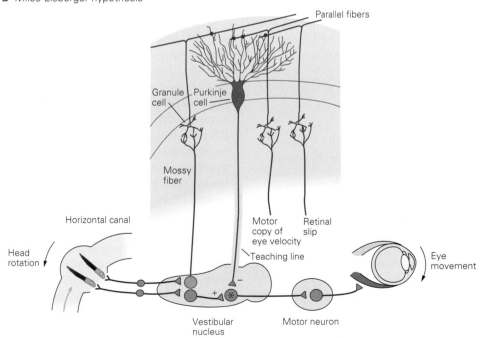

The question remained, how could this modulation be achieved in a controlled manner? David Marr had suggested earlier that the synaptic efficacy of parallel fiber input to a specific Purkinje cell could be modified by the concurrent action of a climbing fiber input. Thus, Ito argued, a message of retinal image slip (the "error" signal) carried by the climbing fiber could be the modulating influence. In fact, Ito and his colleagues showed that such a signal is conveyed in the accessory optic pathway from the retina to the inferior olivary nucleus and from the nucleus into climbing fiber pathways that project to the vestibular cerebellum.

The latter pathway thus could represent a "teaching" line that establishes the parameters for adaptation at the parallel fiber–Purkinje cell synapse (Figure 41-10A). Consistent with this idea is that cerebellar lesions abolish the learning potential. Moreover, simultaneous electrical stimulation of related mossy and climbing fiber projections produces long-term changes in the efficacy of the synapse of the parallel fiber and the Purkinje cell through the mechanism of long-term depression.

Later experiments with monkeys by Frederick Miles and Stephen Lisberger questioned this interpretation. In these experiments Purkinje cell output was modulated only *during* the process of adaptive learning; the output returned to its original state after completion of the adaptation, apparently leaving no "memory trace" in the cerebellar cortex. This work suggests that the Purkinje cell output, rather than the climbing fiber input, is the "teaching" line. Accordingly, Miles and Lisberger concluded that the brain stem neurons targeted by the Purkinje cells are the site of adaptive learning and that the cerebellum constructs the signal that drives this adaptation (Figure 41-10B).

The Memory of Adaptive Learning in the Vestibulo-Ocular Reflex Probably Occurs in the Brain Stem Under Cerebellar Control

Anne Luebke and David Robinson devised a method of reversibly "shutting down" the floccular cortex in the cerebellum of alert cats using unnaturally strong electrophysiological stimulation of its climbing fiber input. This enabled them to test two fundamental questions. First, would cortical shutdown prevent behaviorally induced adaptive learning in the alert cat? It did, as was expected from previous lesion studies. Second, and more important, would the memory of an adaptive change in vestibulo-ocular reflex gain disappear during the shutdown period (as predicted by Ito's model, Figure 41-10A), or would it remain intact (as predicted by Miles and Lisberger's model, Figure 41-10B)? It remained, thus demonstrating that the cerebellar cortex is

not the primary site of adaptive change in the reflex even though it has a necessary role in the change.

Vision

Vestibular stabilization of the eye relative to space allows unequivocal determination of which objects in the visual scene are fixed in space and which are moving. The contribution of the visual system to spatial orientation can be misleading when the whole visual scene moves steadily relative to a stationary subject, as in the familiar impression of backward movement caused by the forward motion of an adjacent train pulling out of the station. This form of *optokinetic* stimulation can have a dramatic destabilizing effect on posture in the newly walking infant or an adult performing a difficult balancing task.

In a well-researched form of visually generated illusion a subject is seated at the center of a concentric "optokinetic" cylinder that is rotated about the stationary subject at constant speed in the light. At first the subject correctly perceives that the cylinder is turning relative to himself. Gradually the subject perceives himself rotating in the opposite direction while the rotating cylinder appears to slow down. After about 30 s the subject feels as though he is rotating at constant speed relative to a stationary cylinder. This illusion, known as *circular vection,* is very compelling and feels just like the normal vestibular sensation of real body rotation relative to space.

Circular vection led to experiments with alert head-fixed monkeys in which neural activity was recorded in the brain stem vestibular nuclei during pure optokinetic stimulation. This stimulation generates a response in the nuclei even though there is no concurrent peripheral vestibular stimulation, thus accounting for the human vestibular-like illusion of circular vection described earlier. Further experiments suggested that optokinetic and vestibular peripheral inputs converged on the vestibular nuclei, as would occur during *natural* rotation of the whole body relative to a *stationary* visual scene.

David Robinson first pointed out another important advantage of converging vestibular and optokinetic signals during natural rotational movement. If one suddenly starts rotating relative to space at a constant speed with clear vision of the space-stationary surrounding scene, the vestibular nuclei initially receive an accurate peripheral vestibular input, but with continued rotation the input decays exponentially to zero, resulting in high-pass filtering of the vestibular signal (Figure 41-11). Meanwhile, the optokinetic pathway simultaneously feeds an exponentially *rising* signal of similar time

Figure 41-11 Integration of vestibular and optokinetic signals in the vestibular nuclei of the brain stem. The vestibular signal is fed in through its inherent high-pass (*first-order lead*) transfer function (1). The optokinetic signal is fed back through the low-pass (*first-order lag*) transfer function as a summed signal of eye movement relative to the head and image slip relative to the retina. This sum represents the visual "estimate" of head movement relative to space (2), closing a positive feedback loop at the vestibular nuclei (**VN**). Ideally the vestibular and optokinetic signals will cancel out their individual "errors" to reconstruct a veridical central representation of actual rotation that is independent of stimulus duration and quite different from either of the original sensory inputs, as indicated by the inset diagram at the bottom right of the figure. (Adapted from Wilson and Melvill Jones 1979.)

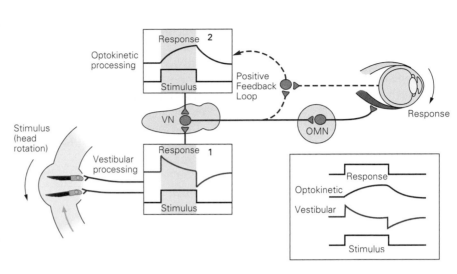

constant into the vestibular nuclei, resulting in low-pass filtering of the signal (Figure 41-11). In these *normal* circumstances the summed output of these two different responses to the same rotational stimulus emerges as a single constant neural signal, resulting in broad band-pass filtering of the signal (see bottom right of Figure 41-11) that represents the actual constant rotation of the subject relative to space. In the *abnormal* situation of purely optokinetic stimulation the subject experiences a false, exponentially rising, vestibular-like sensation of self-rotation.

Circular vection can also have a powerful destabilizing effect relative to the geocentric framework. If one stands in front of a large-diameter circular disc that is rotating in a frontal plane about a horizontal fore-aft axis, circular vection gradually leads to a sensation of body rotation (tilt) in the direction opposite to that of the turning disc. In time, postural correction for this illusion leads one to tilt the whole body in the same direction as the turning disc, even to the point of losing one's balance and falling in that direction.

Perceptual Correlates

The powerful effects of illusory self-motion indicate that cognitive perception plays an important role in postural control. To study this matter Thomas Mergner and his colleagues assembled a device that allows the human head, trunk, and feet to be independently turned relative to space and one another. The subject's perception in the dark of the relative movement of these body parts and their place in space were quantitatively recorded while turning first the whole body relative to space, then the trunk relative to the stationary head, and finally the feet relative to the stationary trunk.

As expected, rotation of the whole body relative to space showed the normal high-pass response typical of the vestibular system, with a sensation threshold of around 2°/s and an associated sensation "decay" time constant of 10–15 s. However, perception of the relative movement of the head, trunk, and feet was found to depend on which body parts were moved and the nature of the perceptual task. For example, when the trunk was turned at various sinusoidal frequencies relative to the stationary head, the subject's estimate of trunk rotation relative to *space* reflected the high-pass dynamics of vestibular sensation, even though rotational vestibular stimulation was completely lacking in this situation. On the other hand, the subject's estimate of head rotation relative to the trunk had no vestibular-like dynamics, and the sensation threshold was decreased by an order of magnitude to around 0.2°/s. Similarly, when the foot and the trunk were turned relative to one another, the perception of foot rotation relative to the trunk reflected vestibular-like high-pass dynamics, while that of trunk rotation relative to the feet reflected the same low-pass characteristics and low threshold as those of head sensation relative to the trunk.

Thus there appear to be two discrete modes of perceiving these postural relations. One, stemming from the vestibular system, takes the head as a reference and projects information in a "top-down" manner from head to trunk to feet. The other takes the stable ground as a reference and projects in a "bottom-up" manner from feet to trunk to head. The top-down pathway faithfully registers high-frequency components of movement, such as those that occur during jogging, for which the high-pass filtering of the vestibular system is well adapted. The bottom-up pathway serves the complementary role of registering low-frequency and low-amplitude angular movements, such as those encountered during a change of direction while walking.

Our conscious ideas about postural changes have physiological consequences. This is demonstrated by an experiment in which the whole body is passively rotated while the subject tries to visually fixate an imagined stationary target in the dark. If gaze direction drifts away from the target because of underperformance of the compensatory vestibulo-ocular reflex, the intended goal tends nevertheless to be achieved by *internally generated* corrective saccadic eye movements (termed *vestibular memory-contingent saccades*). These corrective oculomotor saccades are presumably activated when there is a difference between a valid vestibular perceptual estimate of rotation relative to the target and a calibrated motor copy of the total angle of compensatory eye movement relative to the head. The corrective saccades occur only if the subject consciously tries to maintain target fixation, however. As observed by the Russian physiologist Viktor Gurfinkel, "The system of internal (perceptual) representation plays a dominant role in postural control."

An Overall View

The goal of postural control is to orient body parts relative to one another and the external world without loss of balance. Posture must be controlled both while the body is still (static equilibrium) and during movement (dynamic equilibrium). In the dynamic states of natural behavior voluntary movement can perturb postural equilibrium, but knowledge of these potential perturbations is built into the motor program and used to offset their adverse effects *ahead* of the event by anticipatory (feed-forward) motor action. These anticipatory responses tend to be complex, involving many synergistic muscle groups. Anticipatory responses must be learned, but eventually they operate automatically, being triggered by specific intended movements.

The postural system is also equipped with stereotyped response patterns that are rapidly corrected for *unexpected* perturbations. Some of these responses are innate, while others have to be acquired by motor learning that involves the cerebellum. These responses are characteristically driven by immediate feedback from visual, vestibular, and somatosensory information.

In the past, posture might have been explained by the parallel action of involuntary reflexes controlled at relatively low levels of the nervous system. Today we recognize that postural control is complex and context-dependent and that all levels of the nervous system must be examined to account for this complexity.

Geoffrey Melvill Jones

Selected Readings

Berthoz A, Melvill Jones G. 1985. *Adaptive Mechanisms in Gaze Control.* Amsterdam: Elsevier.

du Lac S, Raymond JL, Sejnowski TJ, Lisberger SG. 1995. Learning and memory in the vestibulo-ocular reflex. Annu Rev Neurosci 18:409–441.

Gahéry Y, Massion J. 1981. Coordination between posture and movement. Trends Neurosci 4:199–202.

Horak FB, Macpherson JM. 1996. Postural orientation and equilibrium. In: LB Rowell, JT Shepherd (eds). *Handbook of Physiology.* Sect. 12, *Exercise: Regulation and Integration of Multiple Systems,* pp. 255–292. New York: Oxford Univ. Press.

Lisberger SG. 1988. The neural basis for motor learning in the vestibulo-ocular reflex in monkeys. Trends Neurosci 11:147–152.

Massion J. 1992. Movement, posture and equilibrium: interaction and coordination. Prog Neurobiol 38:35–56.

Mergner T, Huber W, Becker W. 1997. Vestibular-neck interaction and transformation of sensory coordinates. J Vestib Res 7:347–367.

Miles FA, Lisberger SG. 1981. Plasticity in the vestibulo-ocular reflex: a new hypothesis. Annu Rev Neurosci 4:273–299.

Roberts TDM. 1978. *Neurophysiology of Postural Mechanisms,* 2nd ed. London: Butterworths.

Thach WT, Goodkin HG, Keating JG. 1992. Cerebellum and the adaptive coordination of movement. Annu Rev Neurosci 15:403–442.

Wilson VJ, Melvill Jones G. 1979. *Mammalian Vestibular Physiology.* New York, London: Plenum.

References

Allum JH, Honegger F. 1992. A postural model of balance-correcting movement strategies. J Vestib Res 2:323–347.

Berthoz A, Pozzo T. 1988. Intermittent head stabilization

during postural and locomotory tasks in humans. In: B Amblard, A Berthoz, F Clarac (eds). *Posture and Gait: Development, Adaptation and Modulation*, pp. 189–198. Amsterdam: Elsevier.

Bloomberg J, Melvill Jones G, Segal B. 1991. Adaptive modification of vestibularly perceived self-rotation. Exp Brain Res 84:47–56.

Cordo PJ, Nashner LM. 1982. Properties of postural adjustments associated with rapid arm movements. J Neurophysiol 47:287–302.

Forget R, Lamarre Y. 1990. Anticipatory postural adjustments associated with rapid voluntary arm movements. I. Electromyographic data. J Neurol Neurosurg Psychiatry 47:611–622.

Glasauer S, Amorim M-A, Vitte E, Berthoz A. 1994. Goal-directed linear locomotion in normal and labyrinthine-defective subjects. Exp Brain Res 98:323–335.

Gordon CR, Fletcher WA, Melvill-Jones G, Block E. 1995. Adaptive plasticity in the control of locomotor trajectory. Exp Brain Res 102:539–545.

Greenwood R, Hopkins A. 1976. Muscle responses during sudden falls in man. J Physiol (Lond) 254:507–518.

Grillner S. 1975. Locomotion in vertebrates: central mechanisms and reflex interaction. Physiol Rev 55:247–304.

Gurfinkel VS. 1994. The mechanisms of postural regulation in man. In: T Turpaev (ed). *Physiology and General Biology Reviews*, Vol. 7, pp. 59–89. Yverdon, Switzerland: Harwood Academic. (Also obtainable from Box 786, Cooper Station, New York, NY 10276.)

Henn V, Young LR, Finley C. 1974. Vestibular nucleus units in alert monkeys are also influenced by moving visual fields. Brain Res 71:144–149.

Horak FB, Diener HC. 1994. Cerebellar control of postural scaling and central set in stance. J Neurophysiol 72:479–493.

Horak FB, Shupert CL, Dietz V, Horstmann G. 1994. Vestibular and somatosensory contributions to responses to head and body displacements in stance. Exp Brain Res 100:93–106.

Ito M. 1984. *The Cerebellum and Neural Control*. New York: Raven.

Lee RG, Tonolli E, Viallet F, Aurenty R, Massion J. 1995. Preparatory postural adjustments in Parkinsonian patients with postural instability. Can J Neurol Sci 22:126–135.

Luebke AE, Robinson DA. 1994. Gain changes of the cat's vestibulo-ocular reflex after flocculus deactivation. Exp Brain Res 98:379–390.

Magnus R. 1926. Some results of studies in the physiology of posture. I. Lancet 221:531–536.

Marr D. 1969. A theory for cerebellar cortex. J Physiol (Lond) 202:437–470.

Martin TA, Keating JG, Goodkin HP, Bastian AJ, Thach WT. 1996. Throwing while looking through prisms. II. Specificity and storage of multiple gaze-throw calibrations. Brain 119:1183–1198.

Melvill Jones G. 1992. On the role of perception in oculomotor control. In: H Shimazu, Y Shinoda (eds). *Vestibular and Brainstem Control of Eye, Head and Body Movements*, pp. 365–378. Tokyo: Springer-Verlag.

Melvill Jones G, Watt DGD. 1971. Muscular control of landing from unexpected falls in man. J Physiol (Lond) 219:729–737.

Mergner T, Hlavacka F, Schweigart G. 1993. Interaction of vestibular and proprioceptive inputs. J Vestib Res 3:41–57.

Miles F, Eighmy BB. 1980. Long-term adaptive changes in primate vestibuloocular reflex. I. Behavioral observations. J Neurophysiol 43:1406–1425.

Nashner LM. 1976. Adapting reflexes controlling the human posture. Exp Brain Res 26:49–72.

Robinson DA. 1977. Linear addition of optokinetic and vestibular signals in the vestibular nucleus. Exp Brain Res 30:447–450.

Schor RH, Kearney RE, Dieringer N. 1988. Reflex stabilization of the head. In: BW Peterson, FJ Richmond (eds). *Control of Head Movement*, pp. 141-166. New York: Oxford Univ. Press.

Sherrington C. 1961. *The Integrative Action of the Nervous System*, 2nd ed. New Haven, CT: Yale Univ. Press. (1st ed., 1906, London: Constable.)

Thach WT. 1996. On the specific role of the cerebellum in motor learning and cognition: clues from PET activation and lesion studies in humans. Behav Brain Sci 19:411–431.

von Holst E, Mittelstaedt H. 1950. Das Reafferenzprinzip. Wechselwirkung zwischen Zentralnervensystem und Peripherie. Naturwissenschaften 37:464–476.

Watt DGW. 1976. Responses of cats to sudden falls: an otolith-origin reflex assisting landing. J Neurophysiol 39:257–265.

Xerri C, Lacour M. 1980. Compensation des déficits posturaux et cinétiques après neurectomie vestibulaire unilatérale chez le chat. Rôle de l'activité sensori-motrice. Acta Otolaryngol (Stockh) 90:414–424.

42

The Cerebellum

T HE CEREBELLUM (Latin, little brain) constitutes only 10% of the total volume of the brain but contains more than half of all its neurons. These neurons are arranged in a highly regular manner as repeating units, each of which is a basic circuit module. Despite its structural regularity the cerebellum is divided into several distinct regions, each of which receives projections from different portions of the brain and spinal cord and projects to different motor systems. These features suggest that regions of the cerebellum perform similar computational operations but on different inputs.

The cerebellum influences the motor systems by evaluating disparities between intention and action and by adjusting the operation of motor centers in the cortex and brain stem while a movement is in progress as well as during repetitions of the same movement. Three aspects of the cerebellum's organization underlie this function. First, the cerebellum is provided with extensive information about the goals, commands, and feedback signals associated with the programming and execution of movement. The importance of this input is evident in the fact that 40 times more axons project into the cerebellum than exit from it. Second, the output projections of the cerebellum are focused mainly on the premotor and motor systems of the cerebral cortex and brain stem, systems that control spinal interneurons and motor neurons directly. Third, synaptic transmission in

A

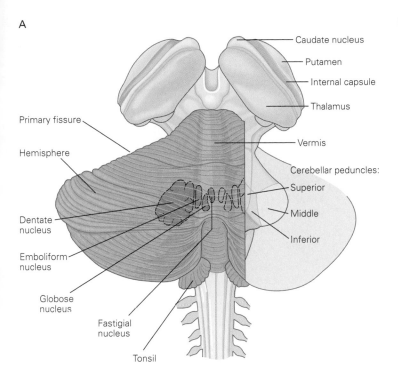

Caudate nucleus

Putamen

Internal capsule

Thalamus

Primary fissure

Vermis

Hemisphere

Cerebellar peduncles:

Superior

Middle

Dentate
nucleus

Inferior

Emboliform
nucleus

Globose
nucleus

Fastigial
nucleus

Tonsil

B

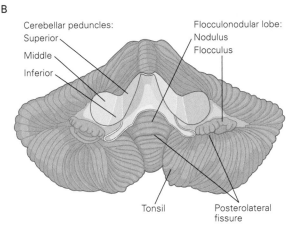

Cerebellar peduncles:
Superior
Middle
Inferior

Flocculonodular lobe:
Nodulus
Flocculus

Tonsil

Posterolateral
fissure

C

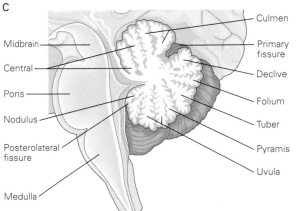

Midbrain

Central

Pons

Nodulus

Posterolateral
fissure

Medulla

Culmen

Primary
fissure

Declive

Folium

Tuber

Pyramis

Uvula

Figure 42-1 Gross features of the cerebellum, including the nuclei, cerebellar peduncles, lobes, folia, and fissures. (Adapted from Nieuwenhuys et al. 1988.)

A. Dorsal view. Part of the right hemisphere has been cut out to show the underlying cerebellar peduncles.

B. Ventral view of the cerebellum detached from the brain stem.

C. Midsagittal section through the brain stem and cerebellum, showing the branching structures of the cerebellum.

the circuit modules can be modified, a feature that is crucial for motor adaptation and learning.

Removal of the cerebellum does not alter sensory thresholds or the strength of muscle contraction. Thus the cerebellum is not necessary to basic elements of perception or movement. Rather, damage to the cerebellum disrupts the spatial accuracy and temporal coordination of movement. It impairs balance and reduces muscle tone. It also markedly impairs motor learning and certain cognitive functions.

In this chapter we first consider briefly the functional organization of the cerebellum into regions with different inputs and outputs. We then examine how these regions are connected to see how information is processed within the cerebellum. Finally, we describe in detail the contributions of each region to sensorimotor processing and the disorders that result from damage to each region.

The Cerebellum Has Three Functionally Distinct Regions

The cerebellum occupies most of the posterior cranial fossa. It is composed of an outer mantle of gray matter (the *cerebellar cortex*), internal white matter, and three pairs of deep nuclei: the *fastigial,* the *interposed* (itself composed of two nuclei, the *globose* and *emboliform*), and the *dentate* (Figure 42-1). The cerebellum is connected to the dorsal aspect of the brain stem by three symmetrical pairs of tracts: the *inferior cerebellar peduncle* (also called the *restiform body*), the *middle cerebellar peduncle* (or *brachium pontis*), and the *superior cerebellar peduncle* (or *brachium conjunctivum*). The superior cerebellar peduncle contains most of the efferent projections. With one exception, cerebellar output originates from cell bodies in the deep nuclei. The exception is a relatively small portion of cerebellar cortex—the *flocculonodular*

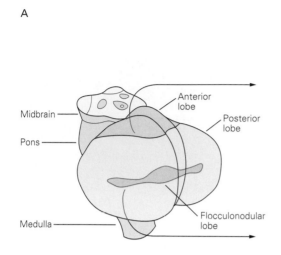

A

B

Figure 42-2 The cerebellum is divided into anatomically distinct lobes.

A. The cerebellum is unfolded to reveal the lobes normally hidden from view.

B. The main body of cerebellum has three functional regions: the central vermis and the lateral and intermediate zones in

each hemisphere. It is divided by the primary fissure into anterior and posterior lobes. The posterolateral fissure separates the flocculonodular lobe. Shallower fissures divide the anterior and posterior lobes into nine lobules (anatomists consider the flocculonodular lobe as the tenth lobule).

lobe—whose cells project to the lateral and medial vestibular nuclei in the brain stem.

A striking feature of the surface of the cerebellum is the presence of many parallel convolutions called *folia* (Latin, leaves) that run from side to side (Figure 42-1). Two deep transverse fissures divide the cerebellum into three lobes. The primary fissure on the dorsal surface separates the anterior and posterior lobes, which together form the body of the cerebellum. The posterolateral fissure on the ventral surface separates the body from the much smaller flocculonodular lobe (Figure 42-2). Sagittal section through the midline shows that shallower fissures further subdivide each lobe into several lobules comprising a variable number of folia.

Two longitudinal furrows, which are most prominent ventrally, distinguish three mediolateral regions that are important functionally. The furrows define an elevated ridge in the midline known as the *vermis* (Latin, worm). On either side of the vermis are the *cerebellar hemispheres,* each of which is divided into intermediate and lateral regions (Figure 42-2). The three mediolateral regions of the body of the cerebellum (the vermis and intermediate and lateral parts of the hemispheres) and the flocculonodular lobe receive different afferent inputs, project to different parts of the motor systems, and represent distinct functional subdivisions.

The flocculonodular lobe is the most primitive part of the cerebellum, appearing first in fishes. Its cor-

tex receives input directly from primary vestibular afferents and projects to the lateral vestibular nuclei (Figure 42-3). In higher vertebrates its function is limited to controlling balance and eye movements and is thus called the *vestibulocerebellum.*

The vermis and hemispheres develop later in phylogeny. The vermis receives visual, auditory, and vestibular input as well as somatic sensory input from the head and proximal parts of the body. It projects by way of the fastigial nucleus to cortical and brain stem regions that give rise to the medial descending systems that control proximal muscles of the body and limbs. The vermis governs posture and locomotion as well as gaze. The adjacent intermediate part of the hemisphere also receives somatosensory input from the limbs. This region projects via the interposed nucleus to lateral corticospinal and rubrospinal systems and thus controls the more distal muscles of the limbs and digits. Because the vermis and intermediate hemispheres are the only regions to receive somatosensory inputs from the spinal cord, they are often called the *spinocerebellum.*

The lateral parts of the hemispheres, which are phylogenetically most recent, are much larger in humans and apes than in monkeys or cats. This region receives input exclusively from the cerebral cortex and is thus called the *cerebrocerebellum.* Its output is mediated by the dentate nucleus, which projects to motor, premotor, and prefrontal cortices. Recent imaging data indicate that

A Inputs

B Outputs

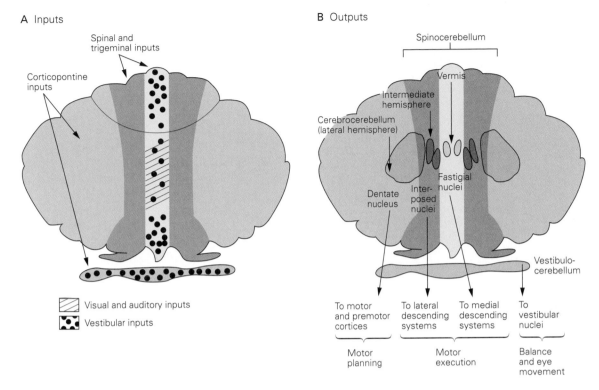

Figure 42-3 The three functional regions of the cerebellum have different inputs and outputs.

the cerebrocerebellum is intimately involved in planning and mental rehearsal of complex motor actions and in the conscious assessment of movement errors.

Cerebellar Circuits Consist of a Main Excitatory Loop and an Inhibitory Side-Loop

The cerebellar cortex is a simple three-layered structure consisting of only five types of neurons: the inhibitory stellate, basket, Purkinje, and Golgi neurons; and the excitatory granule cells.

Neurons in the Cerebellar Cortex Are Organized into Three Layers

The outermost or *molecular layer* of the cerebellar cortex contains the cell bodies of two types of inhibitory interneurons, the stellate and basket cells, dispersed among the excitatory axons of granule cells and the dendrites of inhibitory Purkinje cells, whose cell bodies lie in deeper layers (Figure 42-4). The axons of the granule cells in this layer run parallel to the long axis of the folia and therefore are called *parallel fibers*. The dendrites of Purkinje neurons are oriented perpendicular to these axons.

Beneath the molecular layer is the *Purkinje cell layer,* consisting of a single layer of Purkinje cell bodies. Purkinje neurons have large cell bodies (50–80 μm) and fan-like dendritic arborizations that extend upward into the molecular layer. Their axons project into the underlying white matter to the deep cerebellar or vestibular nuclei and provide the output of the cerebellar cortex. This output is entirely inhibitory and mediated by the neurotransmitter γ-aminobutyric acid (GABA).

The innermost or *granular layer* contains a vast number (estimated at 10^{11}) of granule cells (so called because they appear as small and densely packed darkly stained nuclei in histological sections) and a few larger Golgi interneurons. The mossy fibers, the major source of afferent input to the cerebellum (see below), terminate in this layer. The bulbous terminals of the mossy fibers contact granule cells and Golgi neurons in synaptic complexes called *cerebellar glomeruli* (Figure 42-4).

The Purkinje Cells Receive Excitatory Input From Two Afferent Fiber Systems and Are Inhibited by Three Local Interneurons

The cerebellum receives two main types of afferent inputs, mossy fibers and climbing fibers. Both groups of

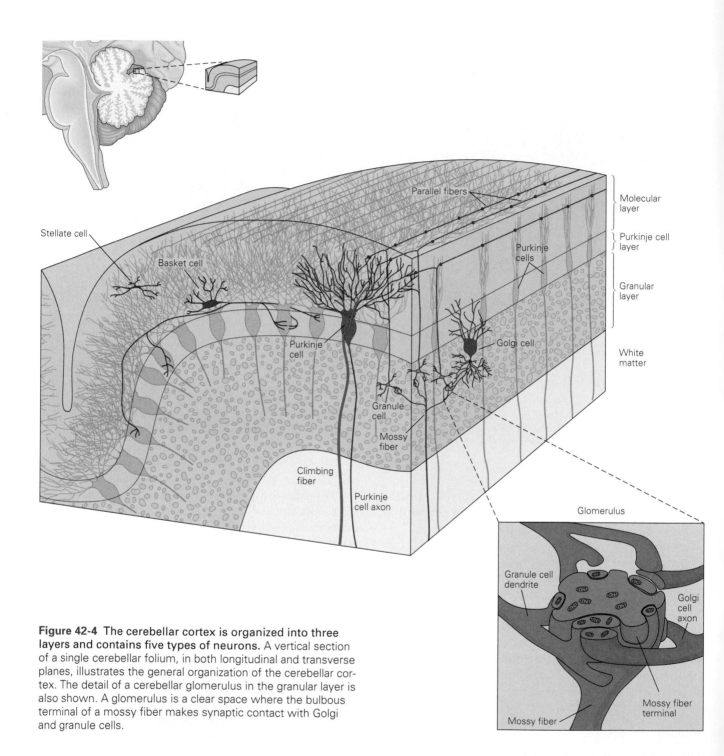

Figure 42-4 The cerebellar cortex is organized into three layers and contains five types of neurons. A vertical section of a single cerebellar folium, in both longitudinal and transverse planes, illustrates the general organization of the cerebellar cortex. The detail of a cerebellar glomerulus in the granular layer is also shown. A glomerulus is a clear space where the bulbous terminal of a mossy fiber makes synaptic contact with Golgi and granule cells.

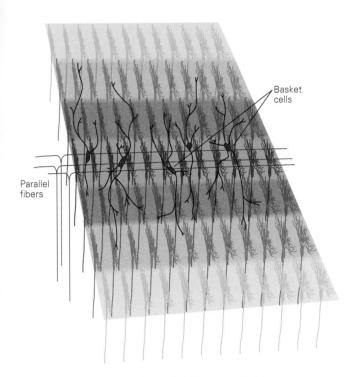

Figure 42-5 Bundles of parallel fibers, called beams, run transversely and excite the dendrites of Purkinje cells and basket cells. The basket cells then inhibit the Purkinje cells flanking the parallel fiber beam.

fibers form excitatory synapses with cerebellar neurons, but the two groups terminate differently in the cerebellar cortex and produce different patterns of firing in the Purkinje neurons.

Mossy fibers originate from nuclei in the spinal cord and brain stem and carry sensory information from the periphery as well as information from the cerebral cortex. They terminate as excitatory synapses on the dendrites of granule cells in the granular layer (Figure 42-4). The axons of the granule cells (the parallel fibers) travel long distances (up to one-third of the width of the cerebellar hemisphere) along the long axis of the cerebellar folia in the molecular layer, thus exciting large numbers of Purkinje neurons in the same transverse plane (Figure 42-5). In humans each Purkinje cell receives input from as many as one million granule cells, each of which collects input from many mossy fibers.

Climbing fibers originate from the inferior olivary nucleus and convey somatosensory, visual, or cerebral cortical information. The climbing fibers are so named because they wrap around the cell bodies and proximal dendrites of Purkinje neurons like a vine on a tree, making numerous synaptic contacts. Individual Purkinje neurons receive synaptic input from only a single climbing fiber, whereas each climbing fiber contacts 1–10

Purkinje neurons. The terminals of the climbing fibers in the cerebellar cortex are arranged topographically; the axons of clusters of olivary neurons terminate in thin parasagittal strips that extend across several folia. In turn, the Purkinje neurons within each strip project to common groups of deep nuclear neurons. This highly specific connectivity of the climbing fiber system contrasts markedly with the massive convergence and divergence of the mossy and parallel fibers.

The basic circuit of the cerebellum is illustrated in Figure 42-6, which shows the excitatory and inhibitory connections between different cell types. The geometry of the principal connections—the mossy, parallel, and climbing fiber systems—is shown in Figure 42-7.

Climbing fibers have unusually powerful synaptic effects on Purkinje neurons. Each action potential in a

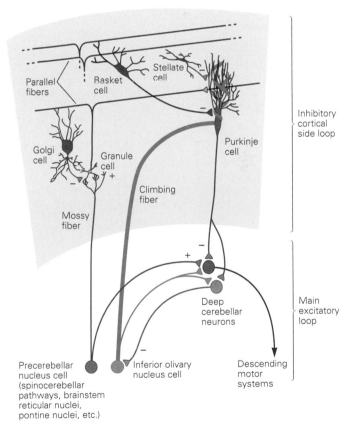

Figure 42-6 Synaptic organization of the basic cerebellar circuit module. Mossy and climbing fibers convey output from the cerebellum via a main excitatory loop through the deep nuclei. This loop is modulated by an inhibitory side-loop passing through the cerebellar cortex. This figure shows the excitatory (+) and inhibitory (−) connections among the cell types. Figures 42-4, 42-5, and 42-7 show the geometry of the divergence and convergence of these basic connections.

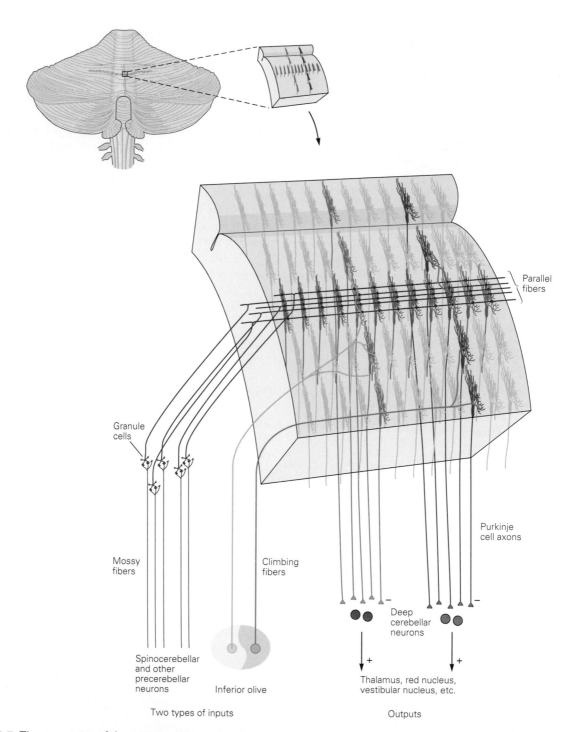

Parallel fibers

Granule cells

Purkinje cell axons

Mossy fibers

Climbing fibers

Deep cerebellar neurons

Spinocerebellar and other precerebellar neurons

Inferior olive

Thalamus, red nucleus, vestibular nucleus, etc.

Two types of inputs

Outputs

Figure 42-7 The geometry of the mossy and parallel fiber system contrasts with that of the climbing fiber system. Mossy fibers excite granule cells whose parallel fibers branch transversely to excite hundreds of Purkinje cells several millimeters from the branch point, both medially and laterally. By contrast, climbing fibers branch in the sagittal dimension to excite 10 or so Purkinje cells anterior and posterior to the branch point. The transverse connections of the parallel fibers and the sagittal connections of the climbing fibers thus form an orthogonal matrix.

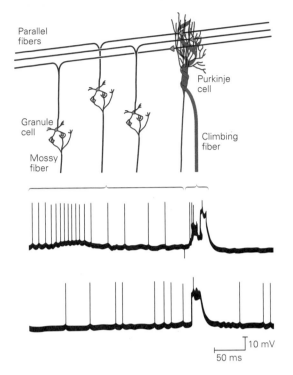

Figure 42-8 Simple and complex spikes recorded intracellularly from cerebellar Purkinje cells. Complex spikes (right bracket) are evoked by climbing fiber synapses, while simple spikes (left bracket) are produced by mossy fiber input. (From Martinez et al. 1971.)

center-surround antagonism in visual and somatosensory pathways.

The Golgi cell has an elaborate dendritic tree in the overlying molecular layer. The GABA-ergic terminals of Golgi cells form axodendritic synapses with the granule cells in the glomeruli (Figure 42-4). Golgi cell firing, initiated by firing in the parallel fibers, suppresses mossy fiber excitation of the granule cells and thus tends to shorten the duration of bursts in the parallel fibers.

Mossy and Climbing Fibers Encode Peripheral and Descending Information Differently

Mossy and climbing fibers respond very differently to sensory stimulation and during motor activity. Spontaneous activity in mossy fibers produces a steady stream of simple spikes in Purkinje cells. Somatosensory, vestibular, or other sensory stimuli change the frequency of the simple spikes, which may reach several

A

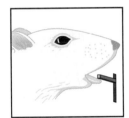

B

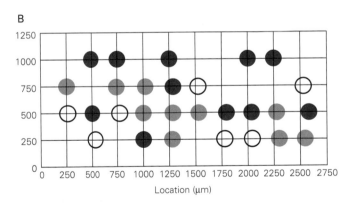

Figure 42-9 Synchronization of complex spikes in the Purkinje neurons. (From Welsh et al 1995. Nature 374:453–457.)

A. A rat performing trained licking.

B. The grid represents the spatial locations of 29 Purkinje cells from which complex spikes were recorded while the rat was licking. The cells in **red** fired synchronously at one time; those in **blue** fired synchronously at another time; cells represented by open circles were not synchronized. Synchronous complex spikes occurred in neighboring Purkinje cells even after the peripheral nerves from the face had been sectioned, suggesting that the synchronized firing was central in origin.

climbing fiber generates a prolonged voltage-gated calcium conductance in the soma and dendrites of the postsynaptic Purkinje cell. This results in prolonged depolarization that produces a *complex spike*: an initial large-amplitude spike followed by a high-frequency burst of smaller-amplitude action potentials. In contrast, parallel fibers produce a brief excitatory postsynaptic potential that generates a single action potential or *simple spike* (Figure 42-8). Consequently, spatial and temporal summation of inputs from several parallel fibers are needed before the Purkinje cell will fire.

The activity of the Purkinje neurons is inhibited by the stellate, basket, and Golgi interneurons. The short axons of stellate cells contact the nearby dendrites of Purkinje cells, and the long axons of basket cells run perpendicular to the parallel fibers and form synapses with Purkinje neurons anterior and posterior to the parallel fiber beam (Figure 42-4). Stellate and basket cells are facilitated by parallel fibers. This arrangement—facilitation of a central array of neurons and inhibition of surrounding cells by local input—resembles the

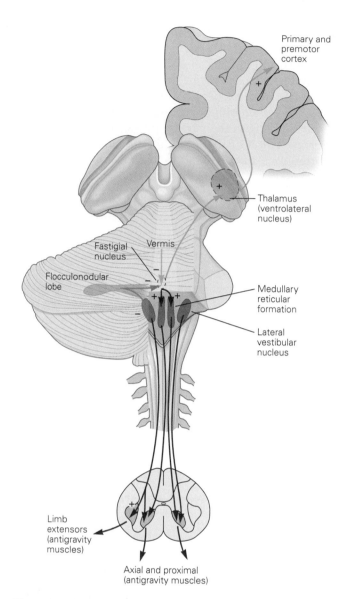

Figure 42-10 The flocculonodular lobe and the vermis control proximal muscles and limb extensors. The vestibulo-cerebellum (flocculonodular lobe) receives input from the vestibular labyrinth and projects directly to the vestibular nuclei. (Oculomotor connections of the vestibular nuclei are omitted for clarity.) The vermis receives input from the neck and trunk, the vestibular labyrinth, and the retinal and extraocular muscles. Its output is focused on the ventromedial descending systems of both the brain stem (mainly the reticulospinal and vestibulospinal tracts) and cortex (corticospinal fibers acting on medial motor neurons).

hundred spikes per second. Voluntary eye or limb movements are also associated with a marked change in frequency. Thus the frequency of simple spikes can readily encode the magnitude and duration of peripheral stimuli or centrally generated behaviors.

In contrast, climbing fibers fire spontaneously at very low rates, and these spontaneous rates are changed only modestly by sensory stimuli or during active movement. The frequency of complex spikes in Purkinje cells is rarely more than 1–3 per second. Such low frequencies cannot by themselves carry substantial information about the magnitude of natural stimuli or behavior.

What could be encoded by the complex spikes? One possibility is that complex spikes might signal the timing of peripheral events or act as triggers for behavior. Rodolfo Llinás has suggested that a form of timing signal might be provided by the synchronous firing of multiple Purkinje cells. Neurons in the inferior olivary nucleus are often electrotonically connected to one another through dendrodendritic synapses and therefore can fire in synchrony. The synchronous inputs of olivary neurons in climbing fibers produces complex spikes in many Purkinje cells at almost the same time.

Interestingly, the electrotonic coupling of olivary neurons is under efferent control by GABA-ergic fibers from the cerebellar nuclei terminating in the olivary nucleus (Figure 42-6). By functionally disconnecting certain olivary neurons through inhibition the nervous system could be selecting a specific array of Purkinje neurons for synchronous activation. This idea is supported by cell recordings in which different patterns of synchronous discharge in different sets of Purkinje neurons are correlated with different phases of a natural behavior (Figure 42-9). Thus, although there is little divergence of climbing fibers, synchronization of inputs may allow populations of postsynaptic neurons with different inputs to act cooperatively.

Climbing Fiber Activity Produces Long-Lasting Effects on the Synaptic Efficacy of Parallel Fibers

Despite the low frequency of their discharge, climbing fibers may alter cerebellar output by modulating the synaptic effect of parallel fiber input to Purkinje cells in two ways. First, climbing fiber action potentials slightly reduce the strength of the parallel fiber input to the Purkinje cell. Thus, experimental lesions or localized cooling of the inferior olivary nucleus produce a large increase in the frequency of simple spikes generated in the Purkinje cells by the parallel fibers.

Second, activity in climbing fibers can induce selective *long-term depression* in the synaptic strength of parallel fibers that are active concurrently. Long-term depression has been analyzed in slices of cerebellum in which Purkinje cell responses to concurrent stimulation of climbing fibers and parallel fibers can be recorded intracellularly. Masao Ito and co-workers found that concurrent stimulation of climbing fibers and one set of parallel fibers depresses the effect of later stimulation of the same parallel fibers but has no effect on the stimulation of another set of parallel fibers. For this depression to occur, however, the parallel fiber's simple spike must occur within some 100–200 ms of the climbing fiber's complex spike.

The resulting depression can last minutes to hours and depends critically on the prolonged depolarization and large influx of calcium produced by the climbing fiber in Purkinje cell dendrites. This long-term effect of the climbing fiber on the transmission of signals from the mossy fiber, granule cell, and parallel fiber through to the Purkinje cell may be important in the cerebellar role in motor learning.

The Vestibulocerebellum Regulates Balance and Eye Movements

The vestibulocerebellum (flocculonodular lobe) receives information from the semicircular canals and the otolith organs, which sense motion of the head and its position relative to gravity (Chapter 40). Mossy fibers that terminate in the vestibulocerebellar cortex arise from neurons in the vestibular nuclei. The vestibulocerebellar cortex also receives visual input via mossy fibers from the superior colliculi and from the striate cortex, the latter relayed through the pontine nuclei.

Purkinje neurons in the vestibulocerebellum inhibit neurons in the medial and lateral vestibular nuclei. Through the lateral nucleus they modulate the lateral and medial vestibulospinal tracts, which predominantly control axial muscles and limb extensors, assuring balance during stance and gait (Figure 42-10). The inhibitory projection to the medial vestibular nucleus controls eye movements and coordinates movements of the head and eyes via the medial longitudinal fasciculus (Chapter 41).

Disruption of these projections through lesions or disease impairs an individual's ability to use vestibular information to control eye movements during head rotations and movements of the limbs and body during standing and walking. Patients have difficulty maintaining balance; they attempt to compensate by separating their feet widely while standing or walking, thus increasing their base of support. They move their legs irregularly and often fall, whether their eyes are open or closed. In contrast, patients have no difficulty moving their arms or legs accurately while lying down or when their body and head are supported. This test indicates that the primary difficulty is in using vestibular cues for standing and walking, not in controlling the limbs for all movements.

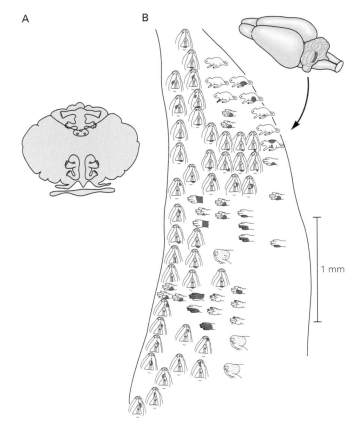

Figure 42-11 The spinocerebellum contains two somatotopic neural maps of the body.

A. Two regions of the cerebellar surface contain somatotopic maps of the entire body. In both maps the head and trunk are located in the vermis, which also receives input from vestibular, visual, and auditory receptors. The limb representations are located on either side of the midline, in the intermediate part of the cerebellar hemispheres.

B. Recordings of the receptive fields of granule cells in the rat cerebellar cortex reveal multiple representations of the same body parts in different locations, an arrangement referred to as *fractured somatotopy*. The receptive fields of individual granule cells are indicated by the **red areas** on body parts. (Adapted from Shambes et al. 1978.)

The Spinocerebellum Regulates Body and Limb Movements

Somatosensory Information Reaches the Spinocerebellum Through Direct and Indirect Mossy Fiber Pathways

Cerebellar afferents from the spinal cord—mainly from somatosensory receptors—are distributed exclusively to the spinocerebellum (see Figure 42-3). Somatosensory information is conveyed to the spinocerebellum through several direct and indirect pathways.

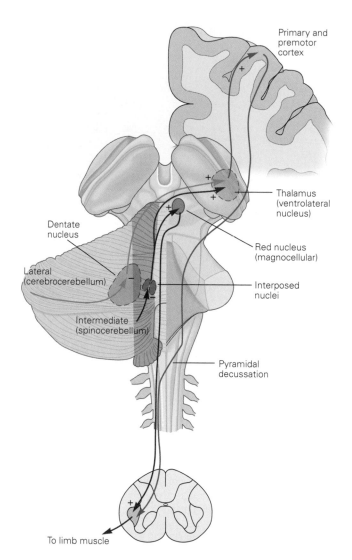

Figure 42-12 Neurons in the intermediate and lateral parts of the cerebellar hemisphere project to the contralateral red nucleus and motor cortex. The intermediate zone (spinocerebellum) receives sensory information from the limbs and controls the dorsolateral descending systems (rubrospinal and corticospinal tracts) acting on the ipsilateral limbs. The lateral zone (cerebrocerebellum) receives cortical input via the pontine nuclei and influences the motor and premotor cortices via the ventrolateral nucleus of the thalamus.

Direct pathways originate from interneurons in the spinal gray matter and terminate as mossy fibers in the vermis or intermediate cortex. Two important pathways are the ventral and dorsal spinocerebellar tracts. These pathways from spinal interneurons provide the cerebellum with somatic sensory information from the legs—notably from muscle and joint proprioceptors—and with information about descending commands reaching the interneurons.

Recordings from neurons in the dorsal and ventral spinocerebellar tracts of decerebrate cats walking on a treadmill show that both systems are modulated rhythmically and in phase with the step cycle. However, when the dorsal roots are cut, preventing spinal neurons from receiving phase-dependent peripheral excitation, dorsal spinocerebellar neurons fall silent while ventral spinocerebellar neurons continue to be modulated. This finding demonstrates that the ventral tract carries internally generated information about the central locomotor rhythm as well as the rhythmic discharge of somatic sensory receptors, while the dorsal tract provides the cerebellum with sensory feedback only during evolving movements. Other direct pathways provide comparable information from the upper extremities.

Direct pathways from the spinal cord to the cerebellum synapse first with neurons in one of several so-called *precerebellar nuclei* in the brain stem reticular formation (the lateral reticular nucleus, reticularis tegmenti pontis, and paramedian reticular nucleus). These inputs provide the cerebellum with different versions of the changing state of the organism and its environment and permit comparisons between such signals. Similar monitoring of outgoing commands is as crucial for perception as for movement, since the internal sensory signals resulting from movement must be distinguished from the external sensory signals in the environment.

The Spinocerebellum Contains Sensory Maps

The initial mapping studies of the spinocerebellum by Edgar Adrian and Ray Snider in the 1940s revealed two inverted somatotopic maps. In both maps the head is represented in the posterior vermis, and the representations of the neck and trunk extend on either side along the dorsal and ventral portions of the vermis. Arms and legs are represented adjacent to the vermis over the intermediate cortex of the hemispheres (Figure 42-11A). Visual input from the superior colliculi and visual cortex is distributed to both vermal and paravermal portions of the posterior lobe (Figure 42-3).

This early mapping was based on recordings of surface potentials, which reflect the predominant input and provide only a coarse representation of somatotopic connections. More refined mapping studies of the cerebellar cortex based on single-cell recordings reveal that input from a given peripheral site, such as a local area of skin, diverges to multiple discrete patches of granule cells, an arrangement called a *fractured somatotopy* (Figure 42-11B).

Recent anatomical studies of primates show that the deep cerebellar nuclei are also organized somatotopically. They are arranged to receive projections from the two maps on the dorsal and ventral surfaces of the intermediate and lateral zones of the cerebellar cortex and project to the magnocellular red nucleus and primary motor cortex via the thalamus (Figure 42-12).

The Spinocerebellum Modulates the Descending Motor Systems in the Brain Stem and Cerebral Cortex

Purkinje neurons in the spinocerebellum project somatotopically to different deep nuclei that control various components of the descending motor pathways. Neurons in the vermis in both the anterior and posterior lobes send projections to the fastigial nucleus, which in turn projects bilaterally to the brain stem reticular formation and lateral vestibular nuclei. The latter areas project directly to the spinal cord (Figure 42-10). Axons of the fastigial nucleus also cross to the contralateral side and project to the area's primary motor cortex controlling proximal muscles via a synapse in the ventrolateral nucleus of the thalamus (Figure 42-12). Thus the medial region of the cerebellum controls mainly the cortical and brain stem components of the medial descending systems. This control affects primarily the head and neck and proximal parts of the limb, rather than the wrist and digits. It is therefore important for movements of the face, mouth, and neck and for balance and postural control during voluntary motor tasks.

Purkinje neurons in the intermediate part of the cerebellar hemisphere project to the interposed nucleus (Figure 42-12). Some axons of this nucleus exit through the superior cerebellar peduncle and cross to the contralateral side to terminate in the magnocellular portion of the red nucleus, whose axons cross back and descend to the spinal cord. Other axons from the interposed nucleus continue rostrally and terminate in the ventrolateral nucleus of the thalamus. This cerebellar receiving area (in ventral lateral thalamus) is located posterior to the area that receives input from the basal ganglia (the ventral anterior nuclei) and anterior to the area recieving from the lemniscal sensory system (ventral posterior lateral nucleus) (see Figure 18-5).

These thalamic neurons project to the limb control areas of the primary motor cortex. By acting on the neurons that give rise to the rubrospinal and corticospinal systems, the intermediate cerebellum focuses its action on limb muscles and axial musculature. Because the axons of the interposed nucleus cross to the contralateral side and the rubrospinal and corticospinal tracts cross back (Figure 42-12), cerebellar lesions can disrupt movements of ipsilateral limbs.

The Spinocerebellum Uses Feed-Forward Mechanisms to Regulate Movements

Because deep nuclear neurons are tonically active and produce powerful excitatory postsynaptic potentials in their target neurons, damage to the interposed nucleus reduces the activity of rubrospinal and corticospinal neurons through disfacilitation. This in turn reduces the excitability of motor neurons themselves and results in a reduction in muscle tone (cerebellar hypotonia). Experimental lesions of the interposed nucleus also disrupt the accuracy of reaching movements because of increased errors in timing the components of movements and systematic errors in direction and extent, a clinical sign called *dysmetria* (Greek, abnormal measure). Joint motions are poorly coordinated or *ataxic* (Greek, loss of order) so that the path of the hand in reaching is curved rather than straight. Attempts by patients to correct such movements are associated with new errors, and the hand oscillates irregularly around the target, with a characteristic *terminal tremor*. Another deficit is seen in stretch reflexes: Although tendon reflexes may be strong, the limb tends to oscillate as it returns to its initial position (*pendular reflexes*).

Are these abnormalities the result of an impairment in correcting movement errors or in programming the movement itself? This question was addressed by Tutis Vilis and Jonathan Hore, who trained monkeys to hold a motor-driven handle in a fixed position and to resist perturbing forces applied unpredictably to the handle. Once an animal was trained, Vilis and Hore compared its performance in circumstances in which the dentate and interposed nuclei were reversibly inactivated with a cooling probe implanted in the nuclei.

When a normal animal is attempting to keep its arm in a fixed position, the application of a transient force to extend the elbow evokes a short-latency stretch reflex in the biceps; the arm then returns rapidly and precisely to its initial position. The precision of the return movement depends on the contraction of the extensor triceps muscle, which prevents the elbow from overshooting. Activation of the triceps occurs shortly after that of the biceps (Figure 42-13A). At this point the perturbation still extends the elbow and shortens the triceps. This extensor contraction is therefore an anticipatory or *feed-forward* response rather than a stretch reflex.

When the dentate and interposed nuclei are inactivated by cooling, the elbow shows a pronounced oscillation after the perturbation instead of returning

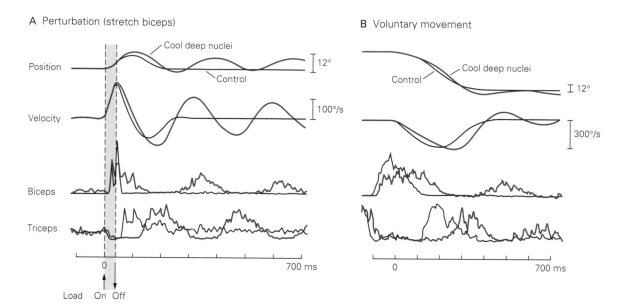

Figure 42-13 Inactivation of the interposed and dentate nuclei disrupts the precisely timed sequence of agonist and antagonist activation that follows external perturbations during normal rapid movements. (Courtesy of Vilis and Hore 1977.)

A. The records show position, velocity, and electromyographic responses in biceps and triceps of a trained monkey after the forearm was suddenly displaced from a held stationary position. Prior to inactivation of the deep nuclei, through local cooling, the limb returns to its original position after the external torque is stopped; only minimal overshooting is evident on the

position trace. While the nuclei are cooled the limb returns with marked overshoot and sequential corrections produce oscillations. (From Vilis and Hore 1977.)

B. With inactivation (cooling) of the nuclei, agonist (biceps) activation becomes slower and more prolonged; activation of the antagonist (triceps), which is needed to stop the movement at the correct location, is delayed and prolonged so that the initial movement overshoots its appropriate extent. Similar delays in successive phases of the movement produce oscillations similar to the terminal tremor seen in patients with cerebellar damage.

precisely to its initial position. The triceps is no longer activated during the initial shortening phase, but only after it has been stretched, when the flexion produced by the biceps contraction overshoots its mark (Figure 42-13A). This delayed contraction of the triceps represents a *feedback* correction to excessive flexion rather than an anticipatory response. Moreover, active triceps force is now superimposed with the elastic recoil of the limb and extends the limb excessively, evoking a new flexor response in the biceps and triggering another cycle of flexion-extension. The same mechanism accounts for the oscillations in the pendular knee jerks observed in humans who have cerebellar diseases.

Vilis and Hore also examined whether the same mechanism might account for the terminal tremor after movement. Rapid single-joint movements are initially accelerated by the contraction of an agonist muscle and decelerated by an appropriately timed contraction of the antagonist (Chapter 33). When the dentate and interposed nuclei are inactivated by cooling, contraction of the antagonist muscle is delayed until the limb has overshot the target (Figure 42-13B). The anticipatory con-

traction has been replaced by a feedback correction. This correction is itself dysmetric and results in another error, necessitating a new adjustment. Thus both the oscillatory response to an external perturbation and the terminal tremor at the end of a voluntary reaching movement result from defective anticipatory control of limb motion.

The failure to decelerate the limb at the correct time reflects defective adaptation of motor commands to the aim of the movement. Specifically, the sequence of muscle commands is not matched correctly to the inertial and viscoelastic properties of the limb. As we saw in Chapter 33, multi-joint movements of a limb are more complicated than single-joint movements because motions at several joints of the limb produce interaction torques that vary with time at each joint. We normally learn to anticipate these forces and continuously recalibrate the internal representation of our limbs. This ability, however, depends on cerebellar processing of proprioceptive information from the limb. The inherent difficulty in controlling the inertial interactions among the multiple segments of a limb accounts for the greater inaccuracy of multi-joint movements in cerebellar ataxia.

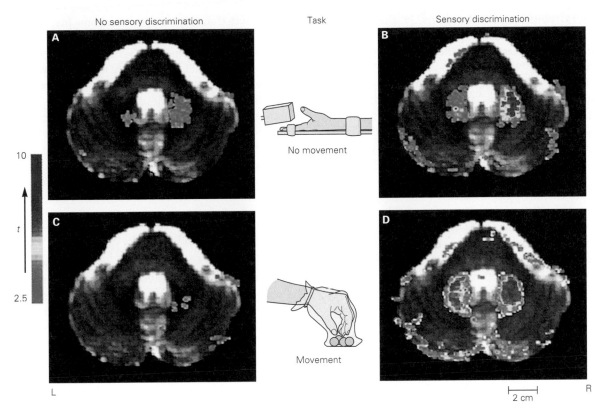

Figure 42-14 Activity in the dentate nucleus is significantly greater when the subject is mentally active during movement. A functional magnetic resonance image (color) overlaid on an anatomical image (gray) shows activation of the dentate nucleus during two pairs of tests. In one pair, subjects first passively experienced sandpaper rubbed across the fingers (A) and then were asked to discriminate the degree of roughness of the sandpaper (B). In the other pair, subjects were asked to lift and drop a series of objects (C) and then had to identify the felt object from a similar group near the other hand (D). (From Gao JH et al. 1996. Science 272:545–547.)

The Cerebrocerebellum Is Involved in Planning Movement and Evaluating Sensory Information for Action

Clinical observations of neurologists and neurosurgeons initially suggested that, like the rest of the cerebellum, the lateral hemispheres were primarily concerned with motor function. However, recent studies of patients with lesions of the lateral hemisphere and experiments using functional brain imaging indicate that the lateral hemispheres, or cerebrocerebellum, also have a variety of perceptual and cognitive functions. In addition, the lateral hemispheres are much larger in humans than in monkeys, consistent with a role in higher cognitive functions.

The Cerebrocerebellum Is Part of a High-Level Internal Feedback Circuit That Regulates Cortical Motor Programs

In contrast to other regions of the cerebellum, which receive sensory information more directly, the lateral hemispheres receive input exclusively from the cerebral cortex. This cortical input originates mainly in the pontine nuclei and projects through the middle cerebellar peduncle to the contralateral dentate nucleus and terminate as mossy fibers in the lateral cerebellar cortex.

Purkinje neurons in the lateral cerebellar cortex project to the dentate nucleus. Most dentate axons exit the cerebellum via the superior cerebellar peduncle and have two main terminations. One termination is in the contralateral ventrolateral thalamus, in the same area receiving input from the interposed nucleus. These thalamic cells project to premotor and primary motor areas of the cerebral cortex (Figure 42-12). The second main termination of dentate neurons is in the contralateral parvocellular red nucleus, a portion of the red nucleus that is distinct from the part receiving input from the interposed nucleus. These neurons project to the inferior olivary nucleus, which in turn projects back to the contralateral cerebellum in the climbing fibers, thus forming a feedback loop. In addition to receiving input from the dentate nucleus, parvocellular neurons also receive input from the lateral premotor areas. The intriguing suggestion has been made, based on brain imaging, that this premotor-cerebello-rubrocerebellar loop is involved in the mental rehearsal of movements and perhaps with motor learning.

Lesions of the Cerebrocerebellum Disrupt Motor Planning and Prolong Reaction Time

In the first half of the twentieth century Gordon Holmes and Jean Babinski identified two characteristic motor disturbances in patients with localized damage in the cerebrocerebellum: variable delays in initiating movements and irregularities in the timing of movement components. The same defect is seen in primates with lesions of the dentate nucleus.

Many motor acts are made up of multiple components, each of which is initiated before the preceding one is completed. An example is *prehension,* in which the shaping of the hand to the object to be grasped begins during the transport phase. During each component of movement the motions at each joint are coordinated precisely one with another (see Chapter 33). Lateral cerebellar lesions disrupt the timing of the various components, which appear to take place sequentially rather than being coordinated smoothly, a defect known as *decomposition of movement.* One of Holmes's patients, who had a lesion of his right cerebellar hemisphere, reported that "movements of my left arm are done subconsciously, but I have to think out each movement of the right arm. I come to a dead stop in turning and have to think before I start again." In humans and primates lesions of the dentate nucleus in particular impair the coordination of distal and proximal components of prehensile movements and the independent use of the digits in manipulatory tasks.

These increases in reaction time and abnormalities in hand paths suggest that the cerebrocerebellum has a role in the planning and programming of hand movements. The activity patterns of single dentate neurons in primates support this idea. Recordings from primates show that dentate nucleus neurons fire some 100 ms before a movement begins. This firing occurs before the discharge of neurons in either the primary motor cortex or interposed nuclei, which are more directly concerned with the execution of movement itself. Hore and his colleagues inactivated the dentate nucleus by localized cooling. Inactivation of the early output from the dentate nucleus delayed the onset of firing in the primary motor cortex, which delayed the onset of movement. Because movement was eventually initiated, the dentate nucleus is not absolutely necessary for initiation.

The Cerebrocerebellum Also Has Purely Cognitive Functions

When patients with cerebellar lesions attempt to make regular tapping movements with their hands or fingers, the rhythm is irregular and the motions are variable in duration and force. Richard Ivry and Steven Keele first sought to determine whether this defect results from a motor deficit or from a more fundamental defect in the timing of serial events. Based on a theoretical model of how such tapping movements are generated, Ivry and Keele found that medial cerebellar lesions interfered only with accurate execution of the response, whereas lateral cerebellar lesions interfered with the timing of serial events. This timing defect was not limited to motor events. It also affected the patient's ability to judge elapsed time in purely mental or cognitive tasks, as in the ability to distinguish whether one tone was longer or shorter than another or whether the speed of one moving object was greater or less than another.

This demonstration that the cerebellum is responsible for a cognitive computation independent of motor execution prompted other researchers to investigate purely cognitive functions of the cerebellum. Steve Petersen, Julie Fiez, and Marcus Raichle used positron emission tomography to image the brain activity of people during silent reading, reading aloud, and speech. As expected, cerebral cortical areas known to be involved in the control of mouth movements were more active when subjects read words aloud than when they read silently. Brain activity during the generation of language was assessed using a verb association task in which subjects had to identify the actions corresponding to certain nouns (eg, a subject might respond with "bark" if he saw the word "dog"). Compared with the brain activity associated with reading aloud, verb generation produced an expected increase in activity in the left frontal lobe, corresponding to Broca's area (see Chapter 59), as well as a pronounced increase within the right lateral cerebellum. Further support of the conclusion that the cerebellum has cognitive functions independent of motor functions comes from the observation that a patient damaged in the right cerebellum (blocked posterior inferior cerebellar artery) could not learn a word association task.

Functional magnetic resonance imaging data have provided evidence for the role of the lateral cerebellum in other cognitive activities. For example, Peter Strick and co-workers showed that solving a pegboard puzzle involves greater activity in the dentate nucleus and lateral cerebellum than does the simple motor task of moving the pegs on the board. Interestingly, the area activated in the dentate nucleus corresponds to the area receiving input from the part of cortex (area 46) involved in working memory (Chapter 62). Another example in which cognitive activity could be isolated from sensory stimulation or movement is shown in Figure 42-14. Activity in the dentate nucleus increased dramatically when subjects were required to evaluate sensory information consciously.

Thus the dentate nucleus appears to be particularly important in acquiring and processing sensory information for tasks requiring complex spatial and temporal judgments, which are essential for programming complex motor actions and sequences of movements. However, the specific contribution of the cerebrocerebellum to sensory discrimination remains to be determined.

The Cerebellum Participates in Motor Learning

On the basis of mathematical modeling of cerebellar function, David Marr and James Albus independently suggested in the early 1970s that cerebellar cortical circuits might be used in learning motor skills. Specifically, they proposed that the climbing fiber input to Purkinje neurons modifies the response of the neurons to mossy fiber inputs and does so for a prolonged period of time. Experimental evidence discussed earlier in the chapter supports this idea: The climbing fiber weakens the parallel fiber–Purkinje cell synapse in a process called long-term depression.

According to the theories of Marr and Albus, altering the strength of certain parallel fiber–Purkinje cell synapses would select specific Purkinje cells to program or correct eye or limb movements. During a movement the climbing fibers would provide an error signal that would depress parallel fibers that are active concurrently and allow "correct" movements (with no error) to emerge. With successive movements the effects of parallel fiber inputs associated with a flawed central command would increasingly be suppressed and a more appropriate pattern of activity would emerge over time. In accordance with this idea, climbing fibers detect differ-ences between expected and actual sensory inputs rather than simply monitoring afferent information. Also, as is reviewed below, motor learning is often impaired following cerebellar damage. It is not yet clear, however, whether climbing fibers can, under natural conditions, also produce the appropriate and specific long-term changes in parallel fiber activation required by the theory.

Initial studies by Masao Ito and his colleagues focused on the vestibulo-ocular reflex, a coordinated response that maintains the eyes on a fixed target when the head is rotated (Chapter 39). In this short-latency reflex motion of the head in one direction is sensed by the vestibular labyrinth, which initiates eye movements in the opposite direction in order to maintain the image in the same position on the retina. When humans and experimental animals wear prism glasses that reverse the left and right visual fields, the vestibulo-ocular reflex is initially maladaptive because the reflex accentuates the motion of the visual field on the retina rather than stabilizing it. After the glasses have been worn continuously for several days the direction of the reflex becomes progressively reduced and eventually reverses direction. This adaptation can be blocked by lesions of the vestibulocerebellum in experimental animals, indicating that the cerebellum has an important role in mediating this form of learning.

Control of limb movements also adapts when subjects wear prisms for an extended period. A striking example is the adjustment of eye-hand coordination in throwing darts. When people throw darts they normally fixate the target visually, and the direction of the throw matches the direction of gaze. When people wear prisms, which bend the light path sideways, the initial throw in the direction of gaze misses the target to the side by an amount proportional to the diopter of the prism (how much the light is bent by the prism). The prisms thus require subjects to shift their gaze to the opposite side, along the bent light path, if they are to fixate the target. With repeated throws aimed at the perceived target, subjects gradually increase the angle between the direction of gaze and the direction of throw, so that the darts land on target within 10–30 throws (Figure 42-15).

At that point the subjects have learned to aim their throw in a direction different from the direction of gaze. When the prisms are removed, gaze is now on target but the widened angle between the direction of gaze and the direction of throw persists: hits miss the target to the side opposite by roughly the same distance as the initial prism-induced error (this is called an *after-effect*).

Patients with a damaged cerebellar cortex or inferior olive (the source of climbing fibers to the cerebellar cortex) are severely impaired or unable to adapt at

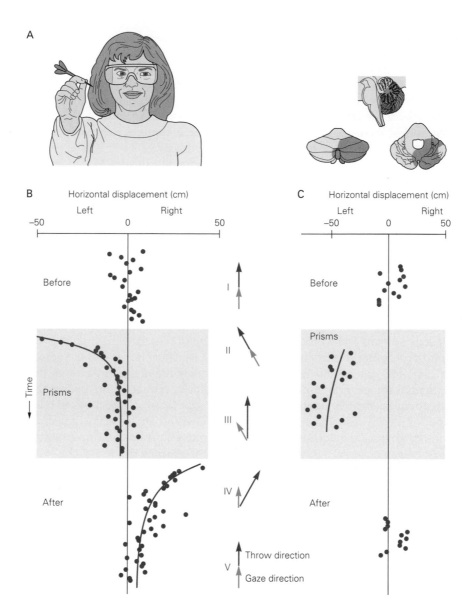

Figure 42-15 Readjustment of eye-hand coordination during adaptation to prism glasses. (Adapted from Martin et al. 1996a and 1996b.)

A. Laterally displacing prisms bend the optic path to the subject's right. The subject looks to the left along the bent light path to see the target directly in front of her. Her hand is held in position ready to throw a dart at the target in front of her.

B. While wearing the prisms (gaze shifted to the left), the first hit is displaced left of center: The hand throws to where the eyes are looking toward the target. Thereafter, hits trend rightward away from where the eyes are looking. After removing the prisms the gaze is centered on the target, and the first throw hits right of center, away from where the eyes are looking. Thereafter hits trend toward the target where the eyes are looking. Data during and after prism use have been fit with exponential curves. Gaze and throw directions are indicated by the **arrows** on the right. Inferred gaze (eye and head) direction assumes the subject is fixating the target. The **roman numer-**

als next to the arrows indicate times during the prism adaptation experiment. **I.** Before donning prisms, when gaze is directed toward the target and the throw is toward the target. **II.** Just after donning prisms, when gaze is directed along the bent light path away from the target and the throw is in the direction of gaze away from the target. **III.** Still wearing prisms and after adapting to them, when gaze is directed along the bent light path away from the target but the throw is directed toward the target. **IV.** Just after doffing the prisms, when the gaze is now directed toward the target and the adapted throw is to the right of the direction of gaze and to the right of the target. **V.** After disadapting the gaze-throw coordination, when gaze is now directed to the target and the throw is in the direction of gaze toward the target as originally.

C. Adaptation fails in a patient with unilateral infarctions in the territory of the posterior inferior cerebellar artery and involves inferior cerebellar peduncle (inferior olivary climbing fibers) and/or inferior lateral posterior cerebellar cortex.

all. Experiments have shown that the kind of motor adaptation and learning with which the cerebellum is concerned requires trial-and-error practice. Once the behavior becomes adapted as learned, it is performed automatically.

The cerebellum's contribution to motor adaptation may occur also in certain forms of associative learning (Chapter 62). Richard Thompson and Christopher Yeo and their colleagues found that lesions of the cerebellum in the rabbit disrupt the acquisition and retention of a classically conditioned eyeblink reflex. After many couplings of an air puff (the unconditioned stimulus) to a sound (the conditioned stimulus), the eye blinked to the sound alone.

Cerebellar Diseases Have Distinctive Symptoms and Signs

Disorders of the human cerebellum result in distinctive symptoms and signs, described originally by Babinski in 1899 and in the 1920s and 1930s by Holmes. Following the plan of Luigi Luciani based on his animal studies, Holmes grouped the abnormalities into three categories.

The first category is hypotonia, a diminished resistance to passive limb displacements. Hypotonia is also thought to explain pendular reflexes. After a knee jerk produced by the tap of a reflex hammer, the leg normally comes to rest after the jerk. In patients who have cerebellar disease the leg may oscillate up to 6 or 8 times before coming to rest.

The second category of symptoms includes a variety of abnormalities in the execution of voluntary movements, collectively referred to as ataxia, or lack of coordination. Examples are a delay in initiating responses with the affected limb, errors in the range of movement (dysmetria), and errors in the rate and regularity of movements (Figure 42-16). This last deficit, discovered by Babinski, is most readily demonstrated when the patient attempts to perform rapid alternating movements, such as tapping one hand with the other, alternating between the back and the palm of the hand. Patients cannot sustain a regular rhythm nor produce an even amount of force, a sign referred to as *dysdiadochokinesia*. Holmes also noted that patients made errors in the relative timing of the components of complex multi-joint movements (decomposition of movement) and frequently failed to brace proximal joints against the forces generated by movement of more distal joints.

The third type of abnormality in movement due to cerebellar disease is a specific form of tremor during movement that is most marked at the end of a move-

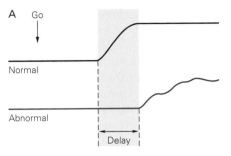

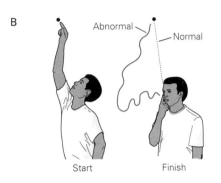

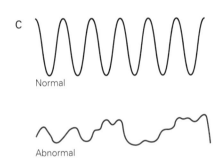

Figure 42-16 Typical defects observed in cerebellar diseases.

A. A lesion in the right cerebellar hemisphere delays the initiation of movement. The patient is told to clench both hands at the same time on a "go" signal. The right hand is clenched later than the left, as evident in the recordings from a pressure bulb transducer squeezed by the patient.

B. A patient moving his arm from a raised position to touch the tip of his nose exhibits dysmetria (inaccuracy in range and direction) and decomposition of movement (moves shoulder first and elbow second). Tremor increases on approaching the nose.

C. Dysdiadochokinesia, an irregular pattern of alternating movements, can be seen in the abnormal position trace of the hand and forearm as cerebellar subjects attempt alternately to pronate and supinate the forearm while flexing and extending at the elbow as rapidly as possible.

ment, when the patient attempts to stop the movement by using antagonist muscles. Such *action* or *intention tremors* represent a series of erroneous corrections in the range of movement due to the failure of adaptive control. Cerebellar action tremor has been duplicated in monkeys by inactivating the interposed and dentate nuclei by cooling.

Sites of damage in the cerebellum can be identified based on a knowledge of the somatotopic organization of the spinocerebellum. Lesions of the vermis and fastigial nuclei produce disturbances principally in the control of axial and trunk muscles during attempted antigravity posture. Thus, when standing or sitting, patients with these lesions spread their feet apart in an attempt to stabilize their balance. Because facial and vocal control is also localized in the vermis, lesions in this area may result in slurring and slowing of speech with a characteristic one-word-at-a-time quality known as *scanning speech*. Degeneration of the anterior lobes (the vermis and the trunk and leg areas) is common in the thiamine deficiency seen in alcoholic or malnourished patients. These patients have ataxia and tremor of the legs and trunk in standing and walking but not of the arms or head.

Lesions of the intermediate cerebellum or the interposed nuclei produce action tremor of the limbs. The disorders produced by lesions of the lateral cerebellar hemispheres consist principally of delays in initiating movement and in decomposition of multi-joint movements—patients cannot move all limb segments together in a coordinated fashion but instead move one joint at a time. This deficit is seen even in movements of the distal joints; patients are unable to combine thumb and index flexion in a precise pinch.

Cases of recovery from atrophy of the cerebellum in childhood have been reported, and many of these patients had large focal lesions in the lateral cerebellar cortex. We now know that lesions of the lateral hemisphere may produce cognitive deficits but little in the way of easily recognized motor abnormality. The misconception has therefore developed that deficits due to cerebellar lesions sustained in youth are well compensated by the functioning of other parts of the nervous system. Deficits due to lesions of the more medial "motor" parts of the cerebellum become permanent disabilities.

An Overall View

Whereas lesions of other motor processing centers produce paralysis or involuntary movements, lesions of the cerebellum result in errors in large numbers of muscles. How do these errors occur?

The organization of inputs to and outputs from the cerebellum indicates that the cerebellum compares internal feedback signals that report the intended movement with external feedback signals that report the ac-

tual movement. When the movement is repeated, the cerebellum is able to generate corrective signals and thus gradually reduce the error. The corrective signals are feed-forward or anticipatory actions that operate on the descending motor systems of the brain stem and cerebral cortex. The oscillations and tremor that follow lesions of the cerebellum are due to the failure of such feed-forward mechanisms.

The cerebellum also plays a role in motor learning. Most motor actions are initiated and executed without immediate feedback and thus have to be well planned. Because there is no opportunity for quick corrections by sensory feedback, planning (feed-forward control) requires calibration and adaptive adjustments of motor programs. The Marr-Albus-Ito model describes how the cerebellum, and specifically the climbing fibers, might participate in motor learning. Because of their low firing frequencies, climbing fibers have a very modest capacity for transmitting moment-to-moment changes in sensory information. Instead, they are thought to be involved in detecting the error in one movement and in changing the program for the next movement.

Finally, the cerebellum seems to have a role in some purely mental operations. In many respects the cerebellum's cognitive functions appear to be similar to its motor functions. For instance, the lateral cerebellum appears to be particularly important for learning both motor and cognitive tasks in which skilled responses are developed through repeated practice. We shall consider the role of the cerebellum in learning again in Chapter 62.

Claude Ghez
W. Thomas Thach

Selected Readings

Adams RD, Victor M. 1989. *Principles of Neurology*, 4th ed. New York: McGraw-Hill.

Brooks VB, Thach WT. 1981. Cerebellar control of posture and movement. In: VB Brooks (ed). *Handbook of Physiology*. Section 1: *The Nervous System*. Vol. 2: *Motor Control*, Part 2, pp. 877–946. Bethesda, MD: American Physiological Society.

Fiez JA, Petersen SE, Cheney MK, Raichle ME. 1992. Impaired non-motor learning and error detection associated with cerebellar damage. Brain 115:155–178.

Gilman S. 1985. The cerebellum: its role in posture and movement. In: M Swah, C Kennard (eds). *Scientific Basis of Clinical Neurology*, pp. 36–55. New York: Churchill Livingston.

Glickstein M, Yeo C. 1990. The cerebellum and motor learning. J Cogn Neurosci 2:69–80.

Holmes G. 1939. The cerebellum of man. Brain 62:1–30.

Ito M. 1984. *The Cerebellum and Neural Control*. New York: Raven.

Keele SW, Ivry R. 1990. Does the cerebellum provide a common computation for diverse tasks? A timing hypothesis. Ann N Y Acad Sci 608:179–211.

Llinás RR. 1981. Electrophysiology of the cerebellar networks. In: VB Brooks (ed). *Handbook of Physiology*. Section 1: *The Nervous System*. Vol. 2: *Motor Control*, Part 2, pp. 831–876. Bethesda, MD: American Physiological Society.

Thach WT. 1996. On the specific role of the cerebellum in motor learning and cognition: clues from PET activation and lesion studies in humans. Behav Brain Sci 19:411–431.

Thach WT, Goodkin HG, Keating JG. 1992. Cerebellum and the adaptive coordination of movement. Annu Rev Neurosci 15:403–442.

References

Adrian ED. 1943. Afferent areas in the cerebellum connected with the limbs. Brain 66:289–315.

Albus JS. 1971. A theory of cerebellar function. Math Biosci 10:25–61.

Allen GI, Tsukahara N. 1974. Cerebrocerebellar communication systems. Physiol Rev 54:957–1006.

Arshavsky YI, Berkenblit MB, Fukson OI, Gelfand IM, Orlovsky GN. 1972. Recordings of neurones of the dorsal spinocerebellar tract during evoked locomotion. Brain Res 43:272–275.

Arshavsky YI, Berkenblit MB, Fukson OI, Gelfand IM, Orlovsky GN. 1972. Origin of modulation in neurones of the ventral spinocerebellar tract during locomotion. Brain Res 43:276–279.

Asanuma C, Thach WT, Jones EG. 1983. Anatomical evidence for segregated focal groupings of efferent cells and their terminal ramifications in the cerebellothalamic pathway of the monkey. Brain Res Rev 5:267–297.

Botterell EH, Fulton JF. 1938. Functional localization in the cerebellum of primates. II. Lesions of midline structures (vermis) and deep nuclei. J Comp Neurol 69:47–62.

Botterell EH, Fulton JF. 1938. Functional localization in the cerebellum of primates. III. Lesions of hemispheres (neocerebellum). J Comp Neurol 69:63–87.

Chan-Palay V, Palay SL. 1984. Cerebellar Purkinje cells have glutamic acid decarboxylase, motilin, and cysteine sulfinic acid decarboxylase immunoreactivity: existence and coexistence of GABA, motilin, and taurine. In: V Chan-Palay and SL Palay (eds). *Coexistence of Neuroactive Substances in Neurons*, pp. 1–22. New York: Wiley.

Eccles JC, Ito M, Szentagothai J. 1967. *The Cerebellum as a Neuronal Machine*. New York: Springer.

Flament D, Hore J. 1986. Movement and electromyographic disorders associated with cerebellar dysmetria. J Neurophysiol 55:1221–1233.

Flament D, Hore J. 1988. Comparison of cerebellar intention tremor under isotonic and isometric conditions. Brain Res 439:179–186.

Flament D, Vilis T, Hore T. 1984. Dependence of cerebellar tremor on proprioceptive but not visual feedback. Exp Neurol 84:314–325.

Gibson AR, Robinson FR, Adam J, Houk JC. 1987. Somatotopic alignment between climbing fiber input and nuclear output of the cat intermediate cerebellum. J Comp Neurol 260:362–377.

Gilbert PFC, Thach WT. 1977. Purkinje cell activity during motor learning. Brain Res 128:309–328.

Gilman S. 1969. The mechanism of cerebellar hypotonia. An experimental study in the monkey. Brain 92:621–638.

Gilman S, Carr D, Hollenberg J. 1976. Kinematic effects of deafferentation and cerebellar ablation. Brain 99:311–330.

Gonshor A, Melvill Jones G. 1976. Short-term adaptive changes in the human vestibulo-ocular reflex arc. J Physiol 256:361–379.

Gravel C, Hawkes R. 1990. Parasagittal organization of the rat cerebellar cortex: direct comparison of Purkinje cell compartments and the organization of the spinocerebellar projection. J Comp Neurol 291:79–102.

Groenewegen HJ, Voogd J. 1977. The parasagittal zonation within the olivocerebellar projection. I. Climbing fiber distribution in the vermis of cat cerebellum. J Comp Neurol 174:417–488.

Groenewegen HJ, Voogd J, Freedman SL. 1979. The parasagittal zonation within the olivocerebellar projection. II. Climbing fiber distribution in the intermediate and hemispheric parts of cat cerebellum. J Comp Neurol 183:551–601.

Hore J, Flament D. 1986. Evidence that a disordered servo-like mechanism contributes to tremor in movements during cerebellar dysfunction. J Neurophysiol 56:123–136.

Hore J, Vilis T. 1984. Loss of set in muscle responses to limb perturbations during cerebellar dysfunction. J Neurophysiol 51:1137–1148.

Ivry RB, Keele SW. 1989. Timing functions of the cerebellum. J Cogn Neurosci 1:136–152.

Ivry RB, Keele SW, Diener HC. 1988. Dissociation of the lateral and medial cerebellum in movement timing and movement execution. Exp Brain Res 73:167–180.

Jansen J, Brodal A (eds). 1954. *Aspects of Cerebellar Anatomy*. Oslo: Grundt Tanum.

Llinás R. 1985. Functional significance of the basic cerebellar circuit in motor coordination. In: JR Bloedel, J Dichgans, W Precht (eds). *Cerebellar Functions*, pp. 170–180. Berlin: Springer.

Lundberg A, Weight F. 1971. Functional organization of connections to the ventral spinocerebellar tract. Exp Brain Res 12:295–316.

Marr D. 1969. A theory of cerebellar cortex. J Physiol 202:437–470.

Martin TA, Keating JG, Goodkin HP, Bastian AJ, Thach WT. 1996a. Throwing while looking through prisms. I. Focal olivocerebellar lesions impair adaptation. Brain 119:1183–1198.

Martin TA, Keating JG, Goodkin HP, Bastian AJ, Thach WT. 1996b. Throwing while looking through prisms. II. Specificity and storage of multiple gaze-throw calibrations. Brain 119:1199–1211.

Martinez FE, Crill WE, Kennedy TT. 1971. Electrogenesis of the cerebellar Purkinje cell response in cats. J Neurophysiol. 34:348–356.

McCormick DA, Thompson RF. 1984. Cerebellum: essential involvement in the classically conditioned eyelid response. Science 223:296–299.

Meyer-Lohmann J, Conrad B, Matsunami K, Brooks VB. 1975. Effects of dentate cooling on precentral unit activity following torque pulse injections into elbow movements. Brain Res 94:237–251.

Meyer-Lohmann J, Hore J, Brooks VB. 1977. Cerebellar participation in generation of prompt arm movements. J Neurophysiol 40:1038–1050.

Miall RC, Weir DJ, Stein JF. 1987. Visuo-motor tracking during reversible inactivation of the cerebellum. Exp Brain Res 65:455–464.

Nieuwenhuys T, Voogd J, van Huijzen C. 1988. *The Human Central Nervous System: A Synopsis and Atlas,* 3rd rev ed. Berlin: Springer.

Oscarsson O. 1973. Functional organization of spinocerebellar paths. In: A Iggo (ed). *Handbook of Sensory Physiology.* Vol. 2: *Somatosensory System,* pp. 339–380. New York: Springer.

Raichle ME, Fiez JA, Videen TO, MacLeod AMK, Pardo JV, Fox PT, Petersen SE. 1994. Practice-related changes in human brain functional anatomy during non-motor learning. Cerebral Cortex 4:8–26.

Robinson DA. 1976. Adaptive gain control of vestibuloocular reflex by the cerebellum. J Neurophysiol 39:954–969.

Shambes GM, Gibson JM, Welker W. 1978. Fractured somatotopy in granule cell tactile areas of rat cerebellar hemispheres revealed by micromapping. Brain Behav Evol 15:94–140.

Snider RS, Stowell A. 1944. Receiving areas of the tactile, auditory, and visual systems in the cerebellum. J Neurophysiol 7:331–357.

Strata P, Montarolo PG. 1982. Functional aspects of the inferior olive. Archieves Italiennes de Biologie 120:321–329.

Strick PL. 1983. The influence of motor preparation on the response of cerebellar neurons to limb displacements. J Neurosci 3:2007–2020.

Thach WT. 1978. Correlation of neural discharge with pattern and force of muscular activity, joint position, and direction of intended next movement in motor cortex and cerebellum. J Neurophysiol 41:654–676.

Thach WT, Perry JG, Kane SA, Goodkin HP. 1993. Cerebellar nuclei: rapid alternating movement, motor somatotopy, and a mechanism for the control of muscle synergy. Rev Neurol 149:607–628.

Vilis T, Hore J. 1977. Effects of changes in mechanical state of limb on cerebellar intention tremor. J Neurophysiol 40:1214–1224.

Vilis T, Hore J. 1980. Central neural mechanisms contributing to cerebellar tremor produced by limb perturbations. J Neurophysiol 43:279–291.

Voogd J, Bigar F. 1980. Topographical distribution of olivary and cortico nuclear fibers in the cerebellum: a review. In: J Courville, C de Montigny, Y Lamarre (eds). *The Inferior Olivary Nucleus: Anatomy and Physiology,* pp. 207–234. New York: Raven.

Yeo CH, Hardiman MJ, Glickstein M. 1984. Discrete lesions of the cerebellar cortex abolish the classically conditioned nictitating membrane response of the rabbit. Behav Brain Res 13:261–266.

43

The Basal Ganglia

THE BASAL GANGLIA CONSIST of four nuclei, portions of which play a major role in normal voluntary movement. Unlike most other components of the motor system, however, they do not have direct input or output connections with the spinal cord. These nuclei receive their primary input from the cerebral cortex and send their output to the brain stem and, via the thalamus, back to the prefrontal, premotor, and motor cortices. The motor functions of the basal ganglia are therefore mediated, in large part, by motor areas of the frontal cortex.

Clinical observations first suggested that the basal ganglia are involved in the control of movement and the production of movement disorders. Postmortem examination of patients with Parkinson disease, Huntington disease, and hemiballismus revealed pathological changes in these subcortical nuclei. These diseases have three characteristic types of motor disturbances: (1) tremor and other involuntary movements; (2) changes in posture and muscle tone; and (3) poverty and slowness of movement without paralysis. Thus, disorders of the basal ganglia may result in either diminished movement (as in Parkinson disease) or excessive movement (as in Huntington disease). In addition to these disorders of movement, damage to the basal ganglia is associated with complex neuropsychiatric cognitive and behavioral disturbances, reflecting the wider role of these nuclei in the diverse functions of the frontal lobes.

Primarily because of the prominence of movement abnormalities associated with damage to the basal ganglia, they were believed to be major components of a motor system, independent of the pyramidal (or corticospinal) motor system, the "extrapyramidal" motor system. Thus, two different motor syndromes were

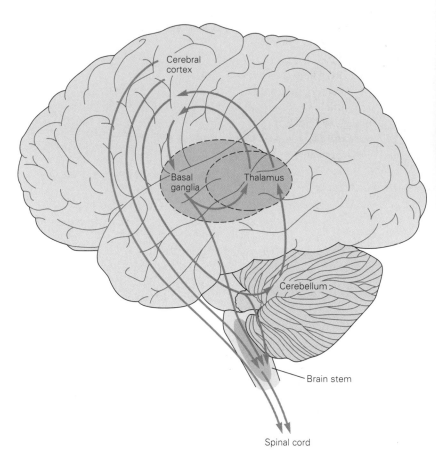

Figure 43-1 The relationships of the basal ganglia to the major components of the motor system. The basal ganglia and the cerebellum may be viewed as key elements in two parallel reentrant systems that receive input from and return their influences to the cerebral cortex through discrete and separate portions of the ventrolateral thalamus. They also influence the brain stem and, ultimately, spinal mechanisms.

distinguished: the *pyramidal tract syndrome,* characterized by spasticity and paralysis, and *the extrapyramidal syndrome,* characterized by involuntary movements, muscular rigidity, and immobility without paralysis.

There are several reasons why this simple classification is no longer satisfactory. First, we now know that, in addition to the basal ganglia and corticospinal systems, other parts of the brain participate in voluntary movement. Thus, disorders of the motor nuclei of the brain stem, red nucleus, and cerebellum also result in disturbances of movement. Second, the extrapyramidal and pyramidal systems are not truly independent but are extensively interconnected and cooperate in the control of movement. Indeed, the motor actions of the basal ganglia are mediated in large part through the supplementary, premotor, and motor cortices via the pyramidal system.

Because they are so common, disorders of the basal ganglia have always been important in clinical neurology. Parkinson disease was the first disease of the nervous system to be identified as a molecular disease caused by a specific defect in transmitter metabolism. Therefore, in addition to providing important informa-

tion about motor control, the study of diseased basal ganglia has provided a paradigm for studying the relationship of transmitters to disorders of mood, cognition, and nonmotor behavior, topics that will be considered in detail in Chapters 60 and 61. The use of a variety of anatomical, molecular, and neural imaging techniques as well as animal models of basal ganglia disorders has led to major advances in understanding the organization and function of the basal ganglia. These insights have, in turn, led to new pharmacologic and neurosurgical approaches to treatment of diseases of the basal ganglia.

The Basal Ganglia Consist of Four Nuclei

The basal ganglia consist of several interconnected subcortical nuclei with major projections to the cerebral cortex, thalamus, and certain brain stem nuclei. They receive major input from the cerebral cortex and thalamus and send their output back to the cortex (via the thalamus) and to the brain stem (Figure 43-1). Thus, the basal ganglia are major components of large cortical-

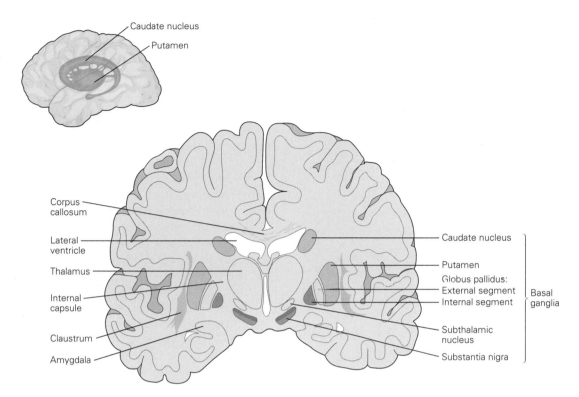

Caudate nucleus

Putamen

Corpus callosum

Lateral ventricle

Thalamus

Internal capsule

Claustrum

Amygdala

Caudate nucleus

Putamen

Globus pallidus:
External segment
Internal segment

Basal ganglia

Subthalamic nucleus

Substantia nigra

Figure 43-2 This coronal section shows the basal ganglia in relation to surrounding structures. (Adapted from Nieuwenhuys et al. 1981.)

subcortical reentrant circuits linking cortex and thalamus.

The four principal nuclei of the basal ganglia are (1) the striatum, (2) the globus pallidus (or pallidum), (3) the substantia nigra (consisting of the pars reticulata and pars compacta), and (4) the subthalamic nucleus (Figure 43-2). The striatum consists of three important subdivisions: the caudate nucleus, the putamen, and the ventral striatum (which includes the nucleus accumbens). Except at its most anterior pole, the striatum is divided into the caudate nucleus and putamen by the *internal capsule,* a major collection of fibers that run between the neocortex and thalamus in both directions. All three subdivisions of the striatum have a common embryological origin.

The striatum is the major recipient of inputs to the basal ganglia from the cerebral cortex, thalamus, and brain stem. Its neurons project to the globus pallidus and substantia nigra. Together these two nuclei, whose cell bodies are morphologically similar, give rise to the major output projections from the basal ganglia. The globus pallidus lies medial to the putamen, just lateral to the internal capsule, and is divided into external and internal segments. The internal pallidal segment is related functionally to the pars reticulata of the substantia

nigra, which lies in the midbrain on the medial side of the internal capsule. The cells of the internal pallidal segment and pars reticulata use γ-aminobutyric acid (GABA) as a neurotransmitter. Just as the caudate nucleus is separated from the putamen by the internal capsule, the internal pallidal segment is separated from the substantia nigra.

In addition to its reticular portion, the substantia nigra also has a compact zone (pars compacta). This zone is a distinct nucleus that lies dorsal to the pars reticulata although some of its neurons lie within the pars reticulata. The cells of the pars compacta are dopaminergic and also contain neuromelanin, a dark pigment derived from oxidized and polymerized dopamine. Neuromelanin, which accumulates with age in large lysosomal granules in cell bodies of dopaminergic neurons, accounts for the dark discoloration of this structure. Dopaminergic cells are also found in the ventral-tegmental area, a medial extension of the pars compacta.

The subthalamic nucleus is closely connected anatomically with both segments of the globus pallidus and the substantia nigra. It lies just below the thalamus and above the anterior portion of the substantia nigra. The glutaminergic cells of this nucleus are the only excitatory projections of the basal ganglia.

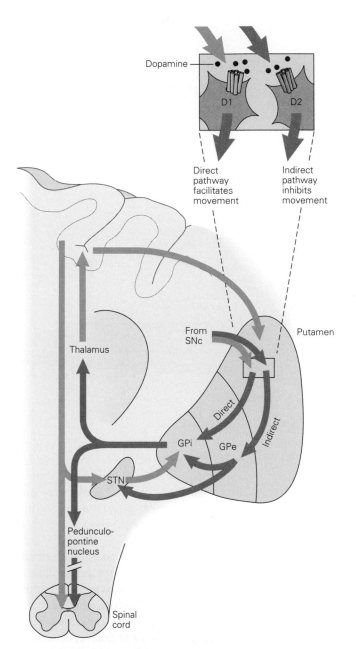

Figure 43-3 The anatomic connections of the basal ganglia–thalamocortical circuitry, indicating the parallel direct and indirect pathways from the striatum to the basal ganglia output nuclei. Two types of dopamine receptors (D1 and D2) are located on different sets of output neurons in the striatum that give rise to the direct and indirect pathways. Inhibitory pathways are shown as **gray arrows;** excitatory pathways, as **pink arrows. GPe** = external segment of the globus pallidus; **GPi** = internal segment of the globus pallidus; **SNc** = substantia nigra pars compacta; **STN** = subthalamic nucleus.

The Striatum, the Input Nucleus to the Basal Ganglia, Is Heterogeneous in Both Its Anatomy and Function

All areas of cortex send excitatory, glutaminergic projections to specific portions of the striatum. The striatum also receives excitatory inputs from the intralaminar nuclei of the thalamus, dopaminergic projections from the midbrain, and serotonergic input from the raphe nuclei.

Although the striatum appears homogeneous on routine staining, it is anatomically and functionally highly heterogeneous. It consists of two separate parts, the *matrix* and *striosome* compartments (the latter also referred to as *patches*). These compartments differ histochemically from one another and have different receptors. The striosome compartment receives its major input from limbic cortex and projects primarily to the substantia nigra pars compacta.

Although the striatum contains several distinct cell types, 90–95% of them are GABA-ergic medium-spiny projection neurons. These cells are both major targets of cortical input and the sole source of output. They are largely quiescent except during movement or in response to peripheral stimuli. In primates the medium-spiny neurons of the striatum can be subdivided into two groups. Those that project to the external pallidal segment express the neuropeptides enkephalin and neurotensin; those that project to the internal pallidal segment or substantia nigra pars reticulata express substance P and dynorphin.

The striatum also contains two types of local inhibitory interneurons: large cholinergic neurons and smaller cells that contain somatostatin, neuropeptide Y, or nitric oxide synthetase. Both classes of inhibitory interneurons have extensive axon collaterals that reduce the activity of the striatal output neurons. Although few in number, they are responsible for most of the tonic activity in the striatum.

The Striatum Projects to the Output Nuclei via Direct and Indirect Pathways

The two output nuclei of the basal ganglia, the internal pallidal segment and the substantia nigra pars reticulata, tonically inhibit their target nuclei in the thalamus and brain stem. This inhibitory output is thought to be modulated by two parallel pathways that run from the striatum to the two output nuclei: one direct and the other indirect. The indirect pathway passes first to the external pallidal segment and from there to the subthalamic nucleus in a purely GABA-ergic pathway, and finally from the subthalamic nucleus to the output nuclei in an excitatory glutaminergic projection (Figure 43-3). The projection from the subthalamic nucleus is the only excitatory intrinsic connection of the basal ganglia; all others are GABA-ergic and inhibitory.

The neurons in the two output nuclei discharge tonically at high frequency. When phasic excitatory inputs transiently activate the *direct* pathway from the striatum to the pallidum, the tonically active neurons in the pallidum are briefly suppressed, thus permitting the thalamus and ultimately the cortex to be activated. In contrast, phasic activation of the *indirect* pathway transiently increases inhibition of the thalamus, as can be determined by considering the polarity of the connections between the striatum and the external pallidal segment, between the external segment and the subthalamic nucleus, and between the subthalamic nucleus and the internal pallidal segment (Figure 43-3).

Thus, the direct pathway can provide *positive* feedback and the indirect pathway *negative* feedback in the circuit between the basal ganglia and the thalamus. These efferent pathways have opposing effects on the basal ganglia output nuclei and thus on the thalamic targets of these nuclei. Activation of the direct pathway disinhibits the thalamus, thereby increasing thalamocortical activity, whereas activation of the indirect pathway further inhibits thalamocortical neurons. As a result, activation of the direct pathway facilitates movement, whereas activation of the indirect pathway inhibits movement.

The two striatal output pathways are affected differently by the dopaminergic projection from the substantia nigra pars compacta to the striatum. Striatal neurons that project directly to the two output nuclei have D1 dopamine receptors that facilitate transmission, while those that project in the indirect pathway have D2 receptors that reduce transmission.

Although their synaptic actions are different, the dopaminergic inputs to the two pathways lead to the same effect—reducing inhibition of the thalamocortical neurons and thus facilitating movements initiated in the cortex. We can now see how depletion of dopamine in the striatum, as occurs in Parkinson disease, may lead to impaired movement. Without the dopaminergic action in the striatum, activity in the output nuclei increases. This increased output in turn increases inhibition of the thalamocortical neurons that otherwise facilitate initiation of movement. Dopaminergic synapses are also found in the pallidum, the subthalamic nucleus, and the substantia nigra. Dopaminergic action at these sites, and in the cortex, could further modulate the actions of the direct and indirect pathways from the striatum.

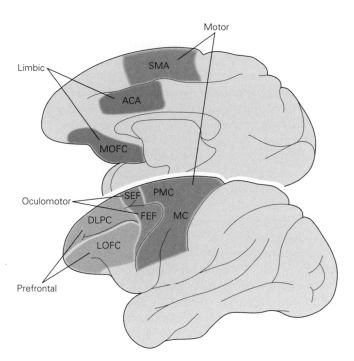

Figure 43-4 The frontal lobe targets of the basal ganglia–thalamocortical circuits. **ACA** = anterior cingulate area; **DLPC** = dorsolateral prefrontal cortex; **FEF** = frontal eye field; **LOFC** = lateral orbitofrontal cortex; **MC** = primary motor cortex; **MOFC** = medial orbitofrontal cortex; **PMC** = premotor cortex; **SEF** = supplementary eye field; **SMA** = supplementary motor area.

The Basal Ganglia Are the Principal Subcortical Components of a Family of Parallel Circuits Linking the Thalamus and Cerebral Cortex

The basal ganglia were traditionally thought to function only in voluntary movement. Indeed, for some time it was believed that the basal ganglia sent their entire output to the motor cortex via the thalamus and thus act as a funnel through which movement is initiated by different cortical areas. It is now widely accepted, however, that through their interaction with the cerebral cortex the basal ganglia also contribute to a variety of behaviors other than voluntary movement, including skeletomotor, oculomotor, cognitive, and even emotional functions.

Several observations point to diversity of function. First, certain experimental and disease-related lesions of the basal ganglia produce adverse emotional and cognitive effects. This was first recognized in patients with Huntington disease. Patients with Parkinson disease also have disturbances of affect, behavior, and cognition. Second, the basal ganglia have extensive and highly organized connections with virtually the entire cerebral cortex, as well as the hippocampus and amygdala. Finally, a wide range of motor and nonmotor behaviors have been correlated with activity in individual basal ganglia neurons in experimental animals and with metabolic activity in the basal ganglia as seen by imaging studies in humans.

The basal ganglia may be viewed as the principal subcortical components of a family of circuits linking the thalamus and cerebral cortex. These circuits are largely segregated, both structurally and functionally. Each circuit originates in a specific area of the cerebral cortex and engages different portions of the basal ganglia and thalamus. The thalamic output of each circuit is directed back to the portions of the frontal lobe from which the circuit originates. Thus, the *skeletomotor circuit* begins and ends in the precentral motor fields (the premotor cortex, the supplementary motor area, and the motor cortex); the *oculomotor circuit,* in the frontal and supplementary eye fields; the *prefrontal circuits,* in the dorsolateral prefrontal and lateral orbitofrontal cortices; and the *limbic circuit,* in the anterior cingulate area and medial orbitofrontal cortex (Figure 43-4). Each area of the neocortex projects to a discrete region of the striatum and does so in a highly topographic manner. Association areas project to the caudate and rostral putamen; sensorimotor areas project to most of the central and caudal putamen; and limbic areas project to the ventral striatum and olfactory tubercle.

The concept of segregated basal ganglia–thalamocortical circuits is a valuable anatomic and physiologic framework for understanding not only the diverse movement disorders associated with basal ganglia dysfunction but also the many-faceted neurologic and psychiatric disturbances resulting from basal ganglia disorders. Structural convergence and functional integration occur *within,* rather than between, the five identified basal ganglia–thalamocortical circuits. For example, the skeletomotor circuit has subcircuits centered on different precentral motor fields, with separate somatotopic pathways for control of leg, arm, and orofacial movements.

Within each of these subunits there may even be discrete pathways responsible for different aspects of motor processing. Injection of transsynaptically transported herpes simplex virus that is transmitted in the retrograde direction into the primary motor cortex, supplementary motor area, and lateral premotor area results in labeling of distinct populations of output neurons in the internal pallidal segment (see Figure 5-9 for technique). Virus transported in the anterograde direction was labeled in distinctly separate regions of the putamen. Given the highly topographic connections between the striatum and the pallidum and between the pallidum and the subthalamic nucleus, it is unlikely that there is significant convergence between neighboring circuits. There is, however, some anatomical evidence that the circuits converge to some degree in the substantia nigra pars reticulata.

The Skeletomotor Circuit Engages Specific Portions of the Cerebral Cortex, Basal Ganglia, and Thalamus

Since movement disorders are prominent in diseases of the basal ganglia, it is appropriate here to focus on the skeletomotor circuit. In primates the skeletomotor circuit originates in the cerebral cortex in precentral motor fields and postcentral somatosensory areas and projects largely to the putamen. The putamen is thus an important site for integration of movement related and sensory feedback information related to movement. The putamen receives topographic projections from the primary motor cortex and premotor areas, including the arcuate premotor area and the supplementary motor area. Somatosensory areas 3a, 1, 2, and 5 project in an overlapping manner to the motor portions of the putamen. Topographically organized projections from each cortical area result in a somatotopic organization of movement-related neurons in the putamen. The leg is represented in a dorsolateral zone, the orofacial region in a ventromedial zone, and the arm in a zone between the two (Figure 43-5). Each of these representations extends along virtually the entire rostrocaudal axis of the putamen. Recent anatomical and physiological data indicate that the skeletomotor circuit is further subdivided into several independent subcircuits, each centered on a specific precentral motor field.

Output neurons in the putamen project topographically to the caudoventral portions of both segments of the pallidum and to the caudolateral portions of the substantia nigra pars reticulata. In turn, the motor portions of the internal pallidal segment and substantia nigra pars reticulata send topographic projections to specific thalamic nuclei, including three ventral nuclei—the ventral lateral nucleus (pars oralis) and the lateral ventral anterior nuclei (pars parvocellularis and pars magnocellularis)—and the centromedian nucleus (see Figure 18-4 for the organization of the thalamic nuclei). The skeletomotor circuit is then closed by projections from the ventral lateral and ventral anterior (pars magnocellularis) nuclei to the supplementary motor area, from the lateral ventral anterior (pars parvocellularis) and the ventral lateral nuclei to the premotor cortex, and from the ventral lateral and centromedian nuclei to the precentral motor fields.

Single Cell Recording Studies Provide Direct Insight into the Role of the Motor Circuits

The contribution of the basal ganglia to movement can be assessed most directly by studying the activity of neurons within the skeletomotor circuit of behaving primates, especially activity in the internal segment of the pallidum, the principal output nucleus. The onset of rapid, stimulus-triggered limb movements is proceeded first by changes in neuronal firing in the motor circuits of the cortex and only later in the basal ganglia. This sequential firing suggests that a *serial* processing occurs within the basal ganglia–thalamocortical circuits and that much of the activity within these circuits is initiated at the cortical level.

During the execution of a specific motor act, such as wrist flexion or extension, the normally high rate of spontaneous discharge in movement-related neurons in the internal pallidal segment becomes even higher in the majority of cells, but in some it decreases. Neurons that exhibit phasic decreases in discharge may play a crucial role in movement by disinhibiting the ventrolateral thalamus and thereby gating or facilitating cortically initiated movements (via excitatory thalamocortical connections). Populations of neurons that show phasic increases in discharge would have the opposite effect, further inhibiting thalamocortical neurons and thus suppressing antagonistic or competing movements.

Little is known about how movement-related signals from the direct and indirect pathways are integrated in the internal pallidal segment to control basal ganglia output. One possibility, of course, is that signals associated with a particular voluntary movement are directed over both pathways to the same population of pallidal neurons. With this arrangement, the inputs from the indirect pathway might assist in braking or possibly smoothing the movement, while those in the direct pathway simultaneously facilitate the movement. This reciprocal regulation would be consistent with the basal ganglia's apparent role in *scaling* the amplitude or velocity of movement. Alternatively, the direct and indirect inputs associated with a particular movement could be directed to separate sets of neurons in the output nuclei of the basal ganglia. In this configuration, the skeletomotor circuit might play a dual role in modulating voluntary movements by both reinforcing the selected pattern (via the direct pathway) and suppressing potentially conflicting patterns (via the indirect pathway). This dual role could result in *focusing* the neural activity

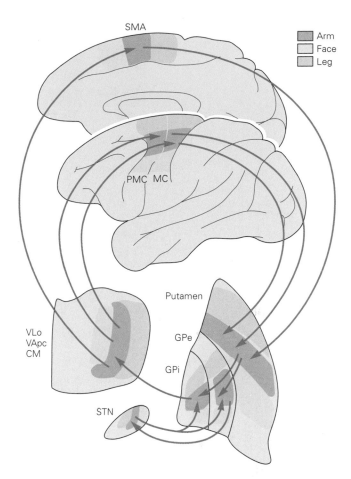

Figure 43-5 The somatotopic organization of the basal ganglia–thalamocortical motor circuit is illustrated in these mesial and lateral views of a monkey brain, as well as the basal ganglia and thalamus. The motor circuit is divided into a "face" representation (**blue**), "arm" representation (**dark green**), and "leg" representation (**light green**). **Arrows** show subcircuits within the portion of the motor circuit concerned with the arm. **CM** = centromedian nucleus of the thalamus; **GPe** = external segment of the globus pallidus; **GPi** = internal segment of the globus pallidus; **MC** = primary motor cortex; **PMC** = prefrontal motor cortex; **SMA** = supplementary motor area; **STN** = subthalamic nucleus; **VApc** = parvocellular portion of the ventral anterior nucleus of the thalamus; **VLo** = pars oralis of the ventrolateral nucleus of the thalamus.

that mediates each voluntary movement in a way similar to the inhibitory surround described for various sensory systems.

Neuronal activity within the skeletemotor circuit has been examined in monkeys performing a variety of motor tasks. At all stages of the circuit (cortical, striatal, and pallidal) the activity of substantial proportions of movement-related neurons depends upon the direction of limb movement, independent of the pattern of mus-

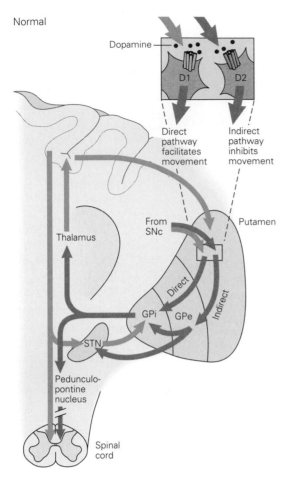

Normal

Dopamine

D1   D2

Direct pathway facilitates movement

Indirect pathway inhibits movement

From SNc

Putamen

Thalamus

Direct

GPi   GPe

Indirect

STN

Pedunculo-pontine nucleus

Spinal cord

Parkinson disease

D1   D2

From SNc

Putamen

Thalamus

Direct

GPi   GPe

Indirect

STN

Pedunculo-pontine nucleus

Spinal cord

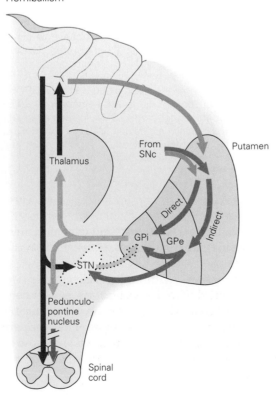

Hemiballism

From SNc

Putamen

Thalamus

Direct

GPi   GPe

Indirect

STN

Pedunculo-pontine nucleus

Spinal cord

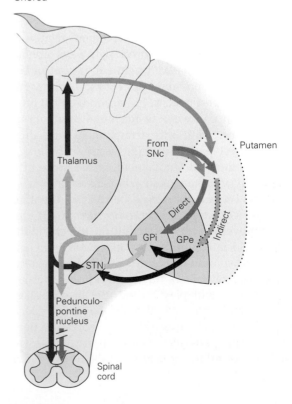

Chorea

From SNc

Putamen

Thalamus

Direct

GPi   GPe

Indirect

STN

Pedunculo-pontine nucleus

Spinal cord

cle activity. These directional cells comprise 30–50% of the movement-related neurons in the supplementary motor area, motor cortex, putamen, and pallidum. All of these neurons are arranged somatotopically. In the motor cortical, but not in the basal ganglia many movement-related cells have been found whose firing does depend on the pattern of muscle activity. In trained primates, the activity in arm-related neurons of the internal pallidal segment also is clearly correlated with amplitude and velocity.

Studies combining behavioral training and single-cell recording indicate that the skeletomotor circuit is involved not only in the execution but also in the preparation for movement. In the precentral motor fields, including the premotor cortex, supplementary motor area, and motor cortex, striking changes in discharge rate occur in some neurons after the presentation of a cue that specifies the direction of limb movement to be executed later. These changes in activity persist until the movement-triggering stimulus is presented. They thus represent a neural correlate of one of the preparatory aspects of motor control referred to as "motor set" (Chapter 38).

Directionally selective activity before movement also occurs within the putamen and the internal segment of the pallidum. Individual neurons within these structures tend to exhibit *either* preparatory (set-related) or movement-related responses, suggesting that the preparation and execution of motor action are mediated by separate subchannels in the skeletomotor circuit. In the internal segment of the pallidum subpopulations of neurons that receive input from the supplementary motor area tend to exhibit set-like preparatory responses. However, neurons receiving inputs from the motor cortex tend to exhibit phasic, movement-related responses. These different response patterns further support the idea that the skeletomotor circuit is composed of distinct subcircuits that connect to different precentral motor fields (motor cortex, supplementary

motor area, and arcuate premotor area). These subcircuits may have distinctive roles in motor control and in the pathogenesis of specific motor signs and symptoms that occur in Parkinson disease and other diseases of the basal ganglia.

Studies of the Oculomotor Circuit Provided Important Insight Into How the Skeletomotor Circuit Operates

The oculomotor circuit is involved in the control of saccadic eye movements. It originates in the frontal and supplementary motor eye fields and projects to the body of the caudate nucleus. The caudate nucleus in turn projects via the direct and indirect pathways to the lateral portions of the substantia nigra pars reticulata, which projects back to the frontal eye fields as well as to the superior colliculus. Inhibition of tonic activity in the substantia nigra pars reticulata disinhibits output neurons in the deep layers of the superior colliculus whose activity is associated with saccades. Inactivation of neurons in the pars reticulata results in involuntary saccades to the contralateral side. These observations provided the critical clue that the skeletomotor circuit might similarly disinhibit thalamocortical neurons phasically during movement, thus facilitating the intended movement.

Some Movement Disorders Result From Imbalances in the Direct and Indirect Pathways in the Basal Ganglia

Considerable progress has been made in understanding the mechanisms underlying the major movement disorders of the basal ganglia. *Hypokinetic disorders* (of which Parkinson disease is the best-known example) are characterized by impaired initiation of movement (*akinesia*) and by a reduced amplitude and velocity of voluntary movement (*bradykinesia*). They are usually accompanied by muscular rigidity (increased resistance to passive displacement) and tremor.

Hyperkinetic disorders (exemplified by Huntington disease and hemiballismus) are characterized by excessive motor activity, the symptoms of which are involuntary movements (*dyskinesias*) and decreased muscle tone (*hypotonia*). The involuntary movements may take several forms—slow, writhing movements of the extremities (athetosis); jerky, random movements of the limbs and orofacial structures (chorea); violent, large-amplitude, proximal limb movements (ballism), and more sustained abnormal postures and slower movements with underlying cocontraction of agonist and

Figure 43-6 (Opposite) The basal ganglia–thalamocortical circuitry under normal conditions and in Parkinson disease, hemiballism, and chorea. Inhibitory connections are shown as **gray and black arrows;** excitatory connections, as **pink and red.** Degeneration of the nigrostriatal dopamine pathway in Parkinson disease leads to differential changes in activity in the two striatopallidal projections, indicated by changes in the darkness of the connecting arrows (**darker arrows** indicate increased neuronal activity and **lighter arrows,** decreased activity). Basal ganglia output to the thalamus is increased in Parkinson disease and decreases in ballism and chorea. **GPe** = external segment of the globus pallidus; **Gpi** = internal segment of the globus pallidus; **SNc** = substantia nigra pars compacta; **STN** = subthalamic nucleus.

antagonist muscles (dystonia). Various types of involuntary movements often occur in combination and some appear to have a common underlying cause. The best example is the similarity between chorea and ballism, which may simply be distal (chorea) or proximal (ballism) forms of the same underlying disorder.

In recent years the development of primate models of both hypo- and hyperkinetic disorders, induced by systemic or local administration of selective neurotoxins, has made it possible to study some of the pathophysiologic mechanisms underlying this diverse symptomatology. Both extremes of the movement disorder spectrum can now be explained as specific disturbances within the basal ganglia–thalamocortical motor circuit. Normal motor behaviors depend on a critical balance between the direct and indirect pathways from the striatum to the pallidum. In the simplest of terms, overactivity in the indirect pathway relative to the direct pathway results in hypokinetic disorders, such as Parkinson disease; underactivity in the indirect pathway results in chorea and ballism (Figure 43-6).

Overactivity in the Indirect Pathway Is a Major Factor in Parkinsonian Signs

Parkinson disease, first described by James Parkinson in 1817, is one of the most common movement disorders, affecting up to one million people in the United States alone. It is also one of the most studied and best understood. Parkinson's description still captures the characteristic posture and movements of the patients with this disease:

. . . involuntary tremulous motion, with lessened muscular power, in parts not in action and even when supported, with a propensity to bend the trunk forwards, and to pass from a walking to a running pace, the senses and intellects being uninjured.

The cardinal symptoms of the disease include a paucity of spontaneous movement, akinesia, bradykinesia, increased muscle tone (rigidity), and a characteristic tremor (4–5 per second) at rest. A shuffling gait as well as flexed posture and impaired balance are also prominent. The appearance of the typical patient with Parkinson disease is instantly recognizable and unforgettable: tremor, mask-like facial expression, flexed posture, and paucity and slowness of movement.

Parkinson disease is the first example of a brain disorder resulting from a deficiency of a single neurotransmitter. In the mid 1950s Arvid Carlson showed that 80% of the brain's dopamine is in the basal ganglia. Next, Oleh Horynekiewicz found that the brains of patients with Parkinson disease are deficient in dopamine, in the striatum, most severely in the putamen. In the early 1960s Parkinson disease was shown to result largely from the degeneration of dopaminergic neurons in the substantia nigra pars compacta. Walter Brikmayer and Horynekiewicz found that intravenous administration of L-dihydroxyphenylalanine (L-DOPA), the precursor of dopamine, provided a dramatic, although brief, reversal of symptoms. The subsequent demonstration by George Cotzias that gradual increases in oral administration of L-DOPA could provide significant and continuous benefit began the modern era of pharmacologic therapy. Even with the development of newer and more effective antiparkinsonian drugs, the benefits of drug therapy usually begin to wane after about five years; and troublesome side effects develop in the form of motor response fluctuations and drug related dyskinesias.

Research in Parkinson disease was recently revitalized by William Langston's discovery that drug addicts exposed to the meperidine derivative 1-methyl-4-phenyl-1,2,3,6-tetrahydropyridine (MPTP) develop a profound Parkinsonian state. This observation led to intense investigation of the role of exogenous toxins in the pathogenesis of Parkinson disease and to the development of a nonhuman primate animal model for experimental study. Primarily on the basis of studies in MPTP-treated primates, a working model of the pathophysiology of Parkinson disease has been developed. According to this model, loss of dopaminergic input from the substantia nigra pars compacta to the striatum leads to increased activity in the indirect pathway and decreased activity in the direct pathway (see Figure 43-6) because of the different actions of dopamine on the two pathways (via D1 and D2 receptors, respectively). Both of these changes lead to increased activity in the internal pallidal segment, which results in increased inhibition of thalamocortical and midbrain tegmental neurons and thus the hypokinetic features of the disease.

Experiments with MPTP-treated monkeys have shown significant changes in neuronal activity along the indirect pathway. For example, microelectrode recording studies have shown that tonic activity is decreased in the external pallidal segment but increased in the subthalamic nucleus and internal pallidal segment. The changes in tonic discharge in the pallidum (and the abnormal motor signs) are reversed by systemic administration of the dopamine receptor agonist apomorphine. The excessive activity in the indirect pathway at the subthalamic nucleus appears to be an important factor in the production of parkinsonian signs, since lesioning of the subthalamic nucleus, which reduces the excessive

Parkinson disease + surgical therapies

STN lesion

GPi lesion

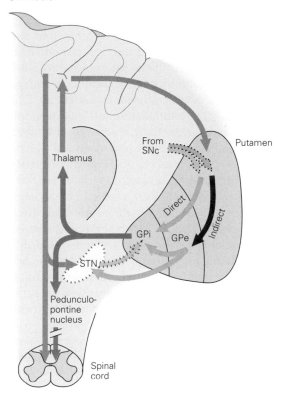

Figure 43-7 Sites of surgical intervention in Parkinson disease. Lesions of the subthalamic nucleus (left) or internal segment of the globus pallidus (right) effectively reduce parkinsonian signs and dyskinesias by respectively normalizing or

eliminating abnormal and excessive output from the internal pallidal segment. **GPe** = external segment of the globus pallidus; **GPi** = internal segment of the globus pallidus; **STN** = subthalmic nucleus; **SNc** = substantia nigra pars compacta.

excitatory drive on the internal pallidal segment, markedly ameliorates parkinsonian signs in MPTP-treated monkeys. Selective inactivation of the *sensorimotor* portion of either the subthalamic nucleus or the internal pallidal segment is sufficient to ameliorate the cardinal parkinsonian motor signs (akinesia, tremor, and rigidity) in MPTP-treated animals (Figure 43-7). Surgical lesions of the posterior (sensorimotor) portion of the internal pallidal segment (pallidotomy) in patients with advanced, medically intractable cases of Parkinson disease is also highly effective in reversing parkinsonian signs. Pallidotomy has undergone a revival in recent years as an effective treatment of patients with advanced disease whose symptoms are poorly controlled by medication alone and who experience drug-induced motor complications (as will be further discussed later).

Thus the hypokinetic features of Parkinson disease appear to result from increased (inhibitory) output from the internal pallidal segment as a result of increased (excitatory) drive from the subthalamic nucleus. Accordingly akinesia and bradykinesia are no longer viewed as negative signs that reflect loss of basal ganglia function, but rather as positive signs that, like rigidity and tremor, result from excessive and abnormal activity in intact structures. This abnormal motor activity can be reversed by reducing or abolishing the pathological output.

In addition to the increase in tonic output of the internal pallidal segment in MPTP-treated monkeys, phasic activity also changes. These changes in the *pattern* of discharge in basal ganglia output are likely to be equally as important as the changes in the rate of discharge. Indeed, recent data suggest that tremor may be due to increased synchronization of oscillatory discharge within the basal ganglia nuclei. Differences in spatial temporal patterns and discharge may account for differences in clinical features among the various hyperkinetic disorders.

The Level of Dopamine in the Basal Ganglia Is Decreased in Parkinson Disease

Measurements of dopamine in the striatum and the metabolic activity of individual basal ganglia nuclei in patients with Parkinson disease are consistent with the pathophysiologic model proposed. Uptake of dopamine in the putamen of these patients is greatly reduced, as assessed earlier by direct biochemical assays and more recently by uptake of the precursor ^{18}F-DOPA measured by positron emission tomography (PET) (see Chapter 19). Imaging of patients with Parkinson disease has shown less synaptic activity (as measured by activated blood flow in the contralateral putamen, the anterior cingulate, the supplementary motor area, and the dorsolateral prefrontal cortex) both when the patients were moving a joystick and when they were resting. Administration of dopamine agonists increased the blood flow to the supplementary motor and anterior cingulate areas during movement tests. Surgical destruction of the pallidum in patients with Parkinson disease has been shown to restore activity in the supplementary motor and premotor areas during this same movement task. These neuroimaging studies lend strong additional support to the importance of the pallidothalamocortical portion of the motor circuit in normal movement and the production of akinesia and bradykinesia.

Underactivity in the Indirect Pathway Is a Major Factor in Hyperkinetic Disorders

Involuntary movements in patients with basal ganglia disorders may result either from clear-cut lesions of these nuclei or from imbalances in neurotransmitter systems. Apart from parkinsonism, the basal ganglia disorder for which the neuropathology is least in doubt is hemiballism. In humans, lesions (usually due to small strokes) restricted to the subthalamic nucleus may result in involuntary, often violent, movements of the contralateral limbs (called "ballism" because of the superficial resemblance of the movements to throwing). In addition to the involuntary movements of the proximal limbs, involuntary movements of more distal limbs may occur in an irregular (choreic) or more continuous writhing form.

Experimental lesions of the subthalamic nucleus in monkeys show that dyskinesias result only when lesions are made selectively in the nucleus, leaving intact the adjacent projections from the internal pallidal segment to the thalamus. More recent studies combining selective lesioning, microelectrode recording, and functional imaging provide new insights into the pathophysiology of ballism and the hyperkinetic disorders in general. The output of the internal pallidal segment is *reduced* in hemiballism, as expected if the projection from the subthalamic nucleus is excitatory. Experimental lesions of the subthalamic nucleus in monkeys significantly reduce the tonic discharge of neurons in the internal pallidal segment and decrease the phasic responses of these neurons to limb displacement. Thus hemiballism may result from disinhibition of the thalamus due to reduction in the tonic (and perhaps phasic) output from the internal pallidal segment. Reduced inhibitory input from the internal pallidal segment might permit thalamocortical neurons to respond in an exaggerated manner to cortical or other inputs, or it might increase the tendency of these neurons to discharge spontaneously, leading to involuntary movements. Alternatively, a changed discharge pattern (rather than lowered rate per se) may play a significant role. Consistent with this idea, pallidotomy relieves hemiballism and other forms of dyskinesia, as well as parkinsonian signs.

Huntington Disease Is a Heritable Hyperkinetic Disorder

The other hyperkinetic disorder most often associated with dysfunction of the basal ganglia is Huntington disease. This disease affects men and women with equal frequency, about 5–10 per 100,000. It is characterized by five features: heritability, chorea, behavioral or psychiatric disturbances, cognitive impairment (dementia), and death 15 or 20 years after onset. In most patients the onset of the disease occurs in the third to fifth decade of life. Many people have already had children by the time the disease is diagnosed.

The Gene for Huntington Disease Has Been Identified

Huntington disease is one of the first complex human disorders to be traced to a single gene, which was identified by mapping genetic polymorphisms (see Box 3-3). The disease is a highly penetrant, autosomal dominant disorder with a gene defect on chromosome 4. This gene encodes a large protein, huntingtin, the function of which has yet to be determined (Chapter 3). The protein normally is located in the cytoplasm. As we have seen in Chapter 3, the first exon of the gene contained repeats of the trinucleotide sequence CAG, which encodes the amino acid glutamine. Whereas normal subjects have less than 40 CAG repeats in the first exon, patients with Huntington disease have more than 40 repeats. Those that have between 70 and 100 repeats develop Huntington disease as juveniles. Once expanded beyond 40 copies, the repeats become unstable and tend to increase from generation to generation, a phenomenon which accounts for genetic "anticipation," the earlier onset of the disease in the offspring than in the parent.

In research aimed at determining why the CAG repeats in the first exon caused disease, the first exon from the mutant human huntingtin protein was expressed in mice and was found to be sufficient to cause a progressive neurological phenotype. Expression of this one exon led to accumulation in the nucleus of multiple inclusions made up of the huntingtin protein. A similar accumulation of huntingtin protein has now been found in the nuclei of brain cells from patients with Huntington disease.

A *Drosophila* model of Huntington disease has been developed by expressing an amino terminal fragment of the human huntingtin protein containing 2, 75, and 120 repeating glutamine residues. By expressing this fragment in photoreceptor neurons of the compound eye of the fly the polyglutamine-expanded huntingtin induced neuronal degeneration much as it does in human neurons. The age on the onset and severity of the neuronal degeneration again correlated with the length of the repeat, and the nuclear localization of huntingtin again presaged neuronal degeneration.

Finally, a cellular model of Huntington disease has been created by transfecting the mutant Huntington's gene into cultured striatal neurons. Here the gene induced neurodegeneration by an apoptotic mechanism, consistent with the idea that the Huntington protein acts in the nucleus to induce apoptosis. Blocking nuclear localization of the mutant huntingtin suppresses its ability to form intranuclear inclusions and to induce apoptosis. However, this apoptotic death did not correlate with the formation of intranuclear inclusions. Full length huntingtin forms inclusions very rarely, raising the possibility that intranuclear inclusions may not play a causal role in mutant huntingtin's induced death. In fact, exposure of transfected striatal neurons to conditions that suppressed the formation of inclusions resulted in an increase in huntingin-induced death. These findings suggests that mutant huntingtin may act within the nucleus to induce neurodegeneration, but that the intranuclear inclusions themselves may reflect a defense mechanism designed to protect against the death induced by huntingtin rather than reflecting a mechanism of cell death.

Although Huntington disease is characterized by widespread loss of neurons in the brain, the pathology is seen earliest in the striatum. A common mechanism appears to underlie both the choreiform movements of Huntington disease and the dyskinetic movements in hemiballism. Striatal neurons that give rise to the indirect pathway are preferentially lost. As a result, the inhibition of neurons in the external pallidum is reduced, causing excessive discharge of these neurons and inhibition of subthalamic nucleus neurons. The resulting *functional* inactivation of the subthalamic nucleus could explain the choreiform symptoms that, in the early stages of the disease, resemble those seen in hemiballism. The rigidity and akinesia in advanced Huntington disease are associated with the loss of the striatal neurons that project to the internal pallidal segment. This loss would reduce inhibition in the internal pallidal segment and thus increase firing in these neurons.

Drug-induced dyskinesias, which closely resemble chorea, are a side effect of dopamine replacement therapy for Parkinson disease. The pathophysiology of these pharmacologically induced dyskinesias may be in part similar to that of chorea in Huntington disease: excessive dopaminergic inhibition of the striatal neurons that project to the external pallidal segment, leading to reduced inhibition of external pallidal neurons and excessive inhibition of the subthalamic nucleus by overactive neurons in the external pallidal segment. The decrease in activity in the subthalamic nucleus would lower the output from the internal pallidal segment in a manner similar to that seen after direct inactivation of the subthalamic nucleus by surgical lesions. This decreased excitatory drive on the internal pallidal segment would be compounded by excessive dopaminergic stimulation of striatal neurons of the direct pathway and the resulting increased inhibitory input to the internal pallidum. Since administration of L-DOPA does not produce dyskinesias in normal individuals or in patients with Parkinson disease early in the course of therapy, the symptoms probably result from receptor upregulation, supersensitivity, and altered gene expression caused by prolonged administration of the drug. Intermittent dosing of L-DOPA appears to be a significant factor in the emergence of drug-induced dyskinesias.

Glutamate-Induced Neuronal Cell Death Contributes to Huntington Disease

Glutamate is the principal excitatory transmitter in the central nervous system. It excites virtually all central neurons and is present in nerve terminals at high concentration (10^{-3} M). In normal synaptic transmission the extracellular glutamate rises transiently, and this rise is restricted to the synaptic cleft. In contrast, sustained and diffuse increases in extracellular glutamate kill neurons. This mechanism of cell death occurs primarily by the persistent action of glutamate on the N-methyl-D-aspartate (NMDA) type of glutamate receptors and the resulting excessive influx of Ca^{2+} (Chapter 12). Excess Ca^{2+} has several damaging consequences that lead to cytotoxicity and death. First, it can activate calcium-dependent proteases (calpains). Second, Ca^{2+} activates phospholipase A_2, which liberates arachidonic acid, leading to the production of eicosanoids, substances that produce inflammation and free radicals that cause tissue damage.

Toxic changes produced by glutamate, called *glutamate excitotoxicity,* are thought to cause cell damage and death after acute brain injury such as stroke or excessive convulsions. In addition, excitotoxicity may contribute to chronic degenerative diseases of the brain, such as Huntington disease. It has been shown that injection of NMDA agonists into the rat striatum reproduces the pattern of neuronal cell loss characteristic of Huntington disease. Thus, it is possible that the altered gene on chromosome 4 produces an abnormality that leads to excessive activation of NMDA receptors or release of glutamate.

The Basal Ganglia Have a Role in Cognition, Mood, and Nonmotor Behavior

Some circuits in the basal ganglia are involved in nonmotor aspects of behavior. These circuits originate in the prefrontal and limbic regions of the cortex and engage specific areas of the striatum, pallidum, and substantia nigra.

The *dorsolateral prefrontal circuit* originates in Brodmann's areas 9 and 10 and projects to the head of the caudate nucleus, which then projects directly and indirectly to the dorsomedial portion of the internal pallidal segment and the rostral substantia nigra pars reticulata. Projections from these regions terminate in the ventral anterior and medial dorsal thalamic nuclei, which in turn project back upon the dorsolateral prefrontal area. The dorsolateral prefrontal circuit has been implicated broadly in so-called "executive functions" (Chapter 19). These include cognitive tasks such as organizing behavioral responses and using verbal skills in problem solving. Damage to the dorsolateral prefrontal cortex or subcortical portions of the circuit is associated with a variety of behavioral abnormalities related to these cognitive functions.

The *lateral orbitofrontal circuit* arises in the lateral prefrontal cortex and projects to the ventromedial cau-

date nucleus. The pathway from the caudate nucleus follows that of the dorsolateral circuit (through the internal pallidal segment and substantia nigra pars reticulata and thence to the thalamus) and returns to the orbitofrontal cortex. The lateral orbitofrontal cortex appears to play a major role in mediating empathetic and socially appropriate responses. Damage to this area is associated with irritability, emotional lability, failure to respond to social cues, and lack of empathy. A neuropsychiatric disorder thought to be associated with disturbances in the lateral orbitofrontal cortex and circuit is obsessive-compulsive disorder (Chapter 61).

The *anterior cingulate* circuit arises in the anterior cingulate gyrus and projects to the ventral striatum. The ventral striatum also receives "limbic" input from the hippocampus, amygdala, and entorhinal cortices. The projections of the ventral striatum are directed to the ventral and rostromedial pallidum and the rostrodorsal substantia nigra pars reticulata. From there the pathway continues to neurons in the paramedian portion of the medial dorsal nucleus of the thalamus, which in turn project back upon the anterior cingulate cortex. The anterior cingulate circuit appears to play an important role in motivated behavior, and it may convey reinforcing stimuli to diffuse areas of the basal ganglia and cortex via inputs through the ventral tegmental areas and the substantia nigra pars compacta. These inputs may play a major role in procedural learning (see Chapter 62). Damage to the anterior cingulate region bilaterally can cause akinetic mutism, a condition characterized by profound impairment of movement initiation.

In general, the disorders associated with dysfunction of the prefrontal cortex and corticobasal ganglia–thalamocortical circuits involve action rather than of perception or sensation. These disturbances are associated both with either intensified action (impulsivity) and flattened action (apathy). Obsessive-compulsive behavior can be viewed as a form of hyperactivity. The disturbances of mood associated with circuit dysfunction are believed to span the extremes of mania and depression. Both dopamine and serotonin, two biogenic amines that modulate neuronal activity within the circuits, are important to depression (Chapter 61).

These observations suggest that the neural mechanisms underlying complex behavioral disorders might be analogous to the dysfunctions of the motor circuits described in this chapter. Thus, schizophrenia might be viewed as a "Parkinson disease of thought." By this analogy, schizophrenic symptoms would arise from disordered modulation of prefrontal circuits. Other cognitive and emotional symptoms may similarly be equivalents of motor disturbances such as tremor, dyskinesia, and rigidity.

An Overall View

In 1949 Linus Pauling revolutionized medical thinking by coining the term "molecular disease." He and his collaborators observed the altered electrophoretic mobility of hemoglobin S and reasoned that sickle cell anemia, a disease known to be genetic, could be explained by a mutation of a gene for a specific protein. A decade later Vernon Ingram showed that this alteration in charge occurs in the amino acid sequence of hemoglobin S, where a glutamic acid residue is replaced by a valine. This change from a single negatively charged residue in normal hemoglobin to a neutral one explains the altered molecular properties of hemoglobin S, and these in turn account for the intermolecular differences and disordered cell stacking observed in sickled red cells. Thus, a single molecular change is fundamental to understanding the patient's pathology, symptoms, and prognosis.

While the explanation for other diseases may not be as simple, it is a fundamental principle of modern medicine that every disorder has a molecular basis. Research in Parkinson disease and myasthenia gravis first made the medical community realize that particular components of chemical synapses can be specific targets for disease. In myasthenia gravis the molecular target is the acetylcholine receptor. In the disorders of the basal ganglia some components of the synthesis, packaging, or turnover of dopamine and serotonin are altered. The causes of the pathological alterations of these loci, whether genetic, infectious, toxic, or degenerative, are not yet known. Although we have identified the mutant gene for Huntington disease, as yet we have no idea about the function of the protein that the wild-type gene encodes. It is clear that rational treatment for diseases of transmitter metabolism requires a good understanding of synaptic transmission in the affected pathways.

Mahlon R. DeLong

Selected Readings

Albin RL. 1995. The pathophysiology of chorea/ballism and parkinsonism. Parkinsonism and Related Disorders 1:3–11.

Brooks DJ. 1995. The role of the basal ganglia in motor control: contributions from PET. J Neurol Sci 128:1–13.

Chesselet MF, Delfs JM. 1996. Basal ganglia and movement disorders: an update. Trends Neurosci 19:417–422.

Graybiel AM. 1995. Building action repertoires: memory and learning functions of the basal ganglia. Curr Opin Neurobiol 5:733–741.

Wichmann T, DeLong MR. 1996. Functional and pathological models of the basal ganglia. Curr Opin Neurobiol 6:751–758.

References

Albin RL, Young AB, Penney JB. 1989. The functional anatomy of basal ganglia disorders. Trends Neurosci 12:366–375.

Alexander GE, Crutcher MD, DeLong MR. 1990. Basal ganglia-thalamocortical circuits: parallel substrates for motor, oculomotor, 'prefrontal' and 'limbic' functions. Prog Brain Res 85:119–146.

Baron MS, Vitek JL, Bakay RAE, Green J, Kaneoke Y, Hashimoto T, Turner RS, Woodard JL, Cole SA, McDonald WM, DeLong MR. 1996. Treatment of advanced Parkinson's disease by GPi pallidotomy: 1 year pilot-study results. Ann Neurol 40:355–366.

Bergman H, Wichmann T, DeLong MR. 1990. Reversal of experimental parkinsonism by lesions of the subthalamic nucleus. Science 249:1436–1438.

Gash DM, Zhang Z, Ovadia A, Cass WA, Yi A, Simmerman L, Russell D, Martin D, Lapchak PA, Collins F, Hoffer BJ, Gerhardt GA. 1996. Functional recovery in parkinsonian monkeys treated with GDNF. Nature 380:252–255.

Gerfen CR. 1995. Dopamine receptor function in the basal ganglia. Clin Neuropharmacol 18:S162–S177.

Hikosaka O, Matsumara M, Kojima J, Gardiner TW. 1993. Role of basal ganglia in initiation and suppression of saccadic eye movements. In: N Mano, I Hamada, M DeLong (eds.). Role of the Cerebellum and Basal Ganglia in Voluntary Movement. Amsterdam: Elsevier.

Hoover JE, Strick PL. 1993. Multiple output channels in the basal ganglia. Science 259:819–821.

Kordower JH, et al. 1995. Neuropathological evidence of graft survival and striatal reinnervation after the transplantation of fetal mesencephalic tissue in a patient with Parkinson's disease. N Engl J Med 332:1118–1124.

Marsden CD, Obeso JA. 1994. The functions of the basal ganglia and the paradox of sterotaxic surgery in Parkinson's disease. Brain 117:877–897.

Nieuwenhuys R, Voogd J, van Huijzen C. 1981. The Human Central Nervous System: A Synopsis and Atlas. 2nd ed. Berlin: Springer.

Part VII

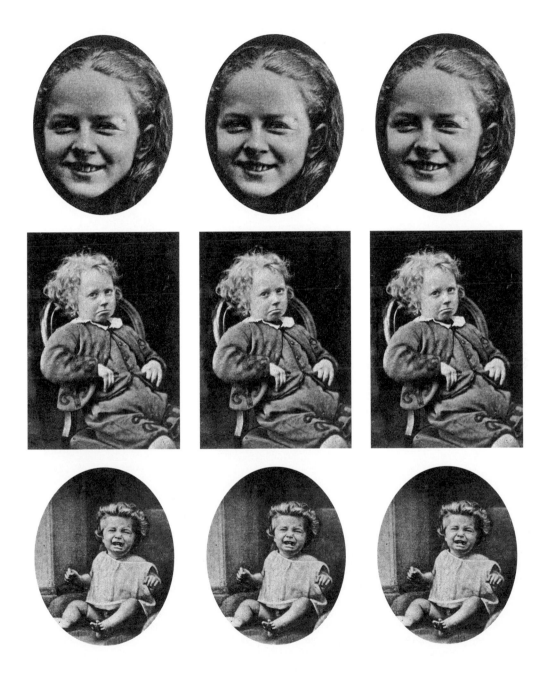

Preceding page

Emotional Facial Expression. Based on observation of his friends and their children, as well as on reports of travelers to various parts of the world, Darwin proposed that emotions have a universal expression—a smile for happiness, a pout for sadness, and crying for misery. He believed not only that all societies express emotions in the same way, but also that animals express emotions similarly. He wrote, "Seeing a dog, horse, and man yawn, makes one feel how all animals are built on only one structure." Some anthropologists question whether Darwin's ideas on emotions are entirely correct. Nevertheless, the expressions shown in these photographs are likely to convey happiness, sadness, and misery to most modern readers. (Reproduced from Darwin's *The Expression of the Emotions in Man and Animals.* 1872.)

VII Arousal, Emotion, and Behavioral Homeostasis

MANY ASPECTS OF BEHAVIOR, ESPECIALLY emotional and homeostatic behaviors, are unconscious and mediated almost reflexively by systems in the brain that are concerned with feeding, drinking, temperature regulation, and sex.

Thus we experience emotional states not only consciously but also unconsciously. The cognitive elements in emotions are mediated by pathways that connect the amygdala to the cerebral cortex. The unconscious autonomic, endocrine, and skeletal motor responses depend on subcortical parts of the nervous system, especially connections between the nuclei of the amygdala, the hypothalamus, and the brain stem. These unconscious responses prepare the body for action and communicate emotional states to other people. A key question in the neurobiology of emotion is whether the somatic responses precede our cognitive awareness of an emotional state or follow from an "emotional idea" that is largely cognitive.

We begin our consideration of these systems with the brain stem. The clinical significance of this small region of the central nervous system—located between the spinal cord and the diencephalon—is disproportionate to its size. Damage to the brain stem can profoundly affect motor and sensory processes because the brain stem contains all of the ascending tracts that bring sensory information from the surface of the body to the cerebral cortex and all the descending tracts from the cerebral cortex that deliver motor commands to the spinal cord. Damage to the brain stem also can affect consciousness because the brain stem contains the locus coeruleus, a center thought to be crucial for attention and therefore for cognitive functions. In fact, fully half of all nonadrenergic neurons of the brain are clustered together in this small nucleus. Finally, the brain stem contains neurons that control respiration and heart beat as well as nuclear groups that give rise to most of the cranial nerves that innervate the head and neck.

One function of the nervous system is to maintain the stability of the internal environment. Homeostatic processes in the nervous system have intrigued some of the founders of modern physiology, including Claude Bernard, Walter B. Cannon, and Walter Hess. Neurons controlling the internal environment are concentrated in the hypothalamus, a small area of the diencephalon that comprises less than 1% of the total volume of the brain. The hypothalamus, with closely linked structures in the brain stem and limbic system, acts directly on the internal environment through its control of the endocrine system and autonomic nervous system. It acts indirectly through its control of emotional and motivational states. In addition to regulating specific motivated behaviors, the hypothalamus, together with the brain stem below and the cerebral cortex above, maintains a general state of arousal, which ranges from excitement and vigilance to drowsiness and stupor.

Six neural systems in the brainstem modulate sensory, motor, and arousal systems. The dopaminergic pathways that connect the midbrain to the limbic system and cortex are particularly important because they are involved in reinforcement of behavior and therefore contribute to motivational state. Addictive drugs such as nicotine, alcohol, opiates, and cocaine are thought to produce their actions by co-opting the same neural pathways that positively reinforce behaviors essential for survival.

Part VII

44

Brain Stem, Reflexive Behavior, and the Cranial Nerves

IN PRIMITIVE VERTEBRATES—reptiles, amphibians, and fish—the forebrain is only a small part of the brain. It is devoted mainly to olfactory processing and integrating autonomic and endocrine function with the basic behaviors necessary for survival: feeding, drinking, sexual reproduction, sleep, and emergency responses. These basic behaviors are organized by the brain stem and consist of relatively simple, stereotypic motor responses. Feeding, for example, involves coordination of chewing, licking, and swallowing, motor responses that are controlled by local ensembles of neurons in the brain stem.

Although we are accustomed to thinking that human behavior originates mainly in the forebrain, many complex human responses, such as feeding, are made up of relatively simple, stereotyped motor responses governed by the brain stem. A striking indicator of this pattern of organization in humans is the rare infant born without a forebrain (hydrencephalus). It is surprisingly difficult to distinguish hydrencephalic infants from normal babies. They also cry, smile, suckle, and move their eyes, face, arms, and legs. As these sad cases illustrate, the brain stem can organize virtually the entire repertory of the newborn's behavior.

In this chapter and the next we shall examine the role of the brain stem in behavior. Here we shall review the cranial nerves and their origin in the brain stem as well as the ensembles of local circuit neurons in the brain stem that organize the simple behaviors involving the face and head. In the next chapter we shall explore how the brain stem acts via long ascending and descending pathways to the forebrain and spinal cord to modulate behavior that is organized at other levels of the nervous system.

The brain stem and the motor and sensory components of the spinal cord are similar in structure. However, the portions of the brain stem concerned with the cranial nerves are much more complex than the corresponding portions of the spinal cord concerned with spinal nerves because the cranial nerves mediate more complex regulatory systems. The core of the brain stem, the *reticular formation*, is homologous to the intermediate gray matter of the spinal cord and is likewise more complex. Nevertheless, like the spinal cord, the reticular formation of the brain stem also contains ensembles of local-circuit interneurons that generate motor patterns and coordinate reflexes and simple stereotyped behaviors.

Table 44-1 Functions of the Cranial Nerves

Cranial nerve	Type of nerve	Functions
(I) Olfactory	Sensory	Smell
(II) Optic	Sensory	Vision
(III) Oculomotor	Motor	Extraocular motor: innervates all extraocular muscles except the superior oblique and lateral rectus muscles (see N. IV and VI), plus striated muscle of the eyelid Autonomic: mediates pupillary constriction and accommodation of the lens for near vision
(IV) Trochlear	Motor	Extraocular motor: innervates superior oblique muscle
(V) Trigeminal	Mixed	Sensory: cutaneous and proprioceptive sensations from skin, muscles, and joints in the face and mouth, and sensory innervation of the teeth and jaws Motor: innervates muscles of mastication, plus tensor tympani, tensor veli palatini, mylohyoid muscle, and anterior belly of digastric muscle
(VI) Abducens	Motor	Extraocular motor: innervates lateral rectus muscle
(VII) Facial	Mixed	Sensory: mediates sensation from the skin of the external ear canal; taste from the anterior two-thirds of the tongue Motor: innervates muscles of facial expression, plus stylohyoid, stapedius, and posterior belly of digastric muscle Autonomic: innervates all salivary glands except parotid as well as lacrimal glands and cerebral vasculature
(VIII) Vestibulocochlear	Sensory	Hearing and sense of motion (angular and linear acceleration)
(IX) Glossopharyngeal	Mixed	Sensory: mediates taste from the posterior third of the tongue and sensation from the posterior palate and tonsillar fossae and carotid sinus Motor: innervates stylopharyngeus muscle Autonomic: innervates parotid gland
(X) Vagus	Mixed	Sensory: mediates sensation from the posterior pharynx, visceral sensation from pharynx, larynx, thoracic and abdominal organs; taste from posterior tongue and oral cavity Motor: innervates striated muscles of larynx and pharynx Autonomic: innervates smooth muscle and glands of gastrointestinal, pulmonary, cardiovascular systems in neck, thorax, and abdomen
(XI) Spinal accessory	Motor	Innervates trapezius and sternocleidomastoid muscles
(XII) Hypoglossal	Motor	Innervates intrinsic muscles of the tongue

Clinical examination	Typical symptoms of dysfunction	Cranial nerve
Various odors applied to each nostril	Loss of sense of smell (anosmia)	I
Visual acuity, map field of vision	Loss of vision (anopsia)	II
Reaction to light, medial and vertical movements of eyes, eyelid movement	Double vision (diplopia); large pupil; uneven dilation of pupils; drooping eyelid (ptosis); deviation of eye outward	III
Downward and inward eye movements	Double vision	IV
Light touch by cotton swab; pain by pinprick; thermal by hot and cold; corneal reflex by touching cornea; jaw reflex by tapping chin; jaw movements	Decreased sensitivity or numbness of face; brief attacks of severe pain (trigeminal neuralgia); weakness and wasting of jaw muscles; asymmetric chewing	V
Lateral movements of eyes	Double vision; inward deviation of the eye	VI
Facial movements and expression; test for taste	Facial paralysis; loss of taste over anterior two-thirds of tongue	VII
Audiogram tests hearing; stimulate by rotating patient or by irrigating the ear with hot or cold water (caloric test)	Deafness; sensation of noise in ear (tinnitus); dysequilibrium, feeling of disorientation in space	VIII
Test for sweet, bitter, and sour tastes on tongue; test pharyngeal or gag reflex by touching walls of pharynx	Spasms of pain in posterior pharynx, sometimes with fall in blood pressure	IX
Observe palate in phonation; palatal reflex by touching palate	Hoarseness, poor swallowing, and loss of gag reflex	X
Movement, strength, and bulk of neck and shoulder muscles	Wasting of neck with weakened rotation; inability to shrug	XI
Tongue movements, tremor, wasting or wrinkling of tongue	Wasting of tongue with deviation to side of lesion on protrusion	XII

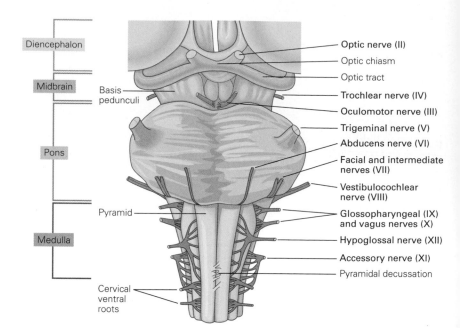

Figure 44-1 The origins of the bilateral cranial nerves seen from the ventral surface of the brain stem. The olfactory nerve (I) is not shown because it terminates in the olfactory bulb in the cerebral hemispheres.

The Cranial Nerves Are Functionally Homologous to the Spinal Nerves

Because the spinal nerves end at the second cervical vertebra, the cranial nerves provide the somatic and visceral sensory and motor innervation for the head. Nerves IX and X also supply visceral sensory and motor innervation of the neck, chest, and most of the abdominal organs with the exception of the pelvis. Unlike the spinal nerves, which supply all sensory and motor functions for a specific body segment, each cranial nerve is associated with a specific function or set of functions and may take in a larger territory (Table 44-1). Assessment of the cranial nerves is an important part of the neurological examination because abnormalities of function can pinpoint the site in the nervous system that has been damaged or injured. Therefore, it is important to know the origins of the cranial nerves, their intracranial course, and where they exit from the skull.

Cranial nerves are traditionally numbered I–XII in rostrocaudal sequence. Each cranial nerve exits the brain stem at a characteristic location (Figures 44-1 and 44-2). Most exit in numerical order from the ventral surface of the brain stem. An exception is the trochlear nerve (IV), which leaves the midbrain from its dorsal surface, just behind the inferior colliculus, and wraps around the lateral surface of the brain stem to join the other cranial nerves concerned with eye movements. The abducens nerve (VI) has the longest intracranial course. As a result, when intracranial pressure increases,

it is often the first cranial nerve to be affected, resulting in inability of the eye on that side to abduct. The cranial nerves with sensory functions (V, VII, IX, and X) each have associated sensory ganglia that operate much as dorsal root ganglia do for spinal nerves. These are located along the course of each nerve, at or just shortly after its entrance into the skull.

The olfactory nerve (I), which is associated with the forebrain, and the optic nerve (II), which is associated with the diencephalon, are described in detail in Chapter 32 (olfaction) and Chapter 26 (vision). The spinal accessory nerve (XI) can be considered a cranial nerve anatomically, but is really a spinal nerve, originating from the higher cervical motor rootlets that innervate the trapezius and sternocleidomastoid muscles in the neck.

The Cranial Nerves Leave the Skull in Groups and Therefore Are Likely to Be Injured Together

In assessing dysfunction of the cranial nerves it is important to determine whether the injury has occurred within the brain or further along the course of the nerve. This task is made simpler because the cranial nerves leave the skull in groups via specific foramena, and hence they are often injured in characteristic combinations by damage at these locations.

The cranial nerves concerned with orbital sensation and movement of the eyes (III, IV, VI, and the oph-

Figure 44-2 A lateral view of the brain stem illustrating the location of the cranial nerves. This view clearly shows the emergence of the trochlear (IV) nerve from the dorsal surface of the midbrain and the facial (VII) and vestibulocochlear (VIII) nerves from the cerebellopontine angle.

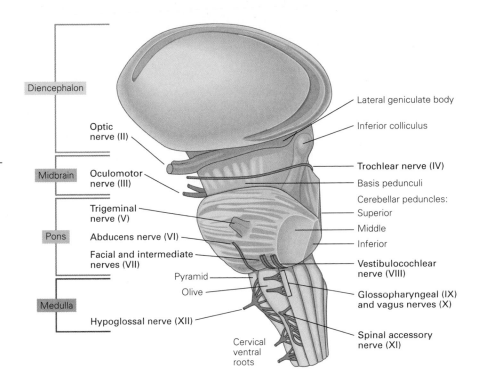

thalmic division of the trigeminal nerve, V₁) are gathered together in the *cavernous sinus*, along the lateral margins of the sella turcica, and then exit the skull through the *superior orbital fissure*, adjacent to the optic foramen through which the optic nerve passes (Figure 44-3). Tumors that occur in this region, such as those arising from the pituitary gland, often first make their presence known by pressure on these nerves or the adjacent optic chiasm.

The cranial nerves that exit the brain stem at the cerebellopontine angle include nerves VII and VIII (Figure 44-4). A common tumor of the cerebellopontine angle is the "acoustic neuroma," which is actually misnamed because it derives from Schwann cells in the vestibular component of nerve VIII. If the tumor is large, it may not only impair the function of nerves VII and VIII but may also press on nerve V near its site of emergence from the middle cerebellar peduncle as well as the cerebellum or its peduncles on the same side, causing ipsilateral clumsiness.

The *lower cranial nerves* (IX, X, and XI) are vulnerable to compression by tumors as they exit through the *jugular foramen* (Figure 44-4B). Nerve XII, which leaves the skull through its own (hypoglossal) foramen, is generally not involved unless the tumor is quite large. If nerve XI is spared, the injury is generally within the substance of the brain stem rather than near the foramen.

The Cranial Nerves Supply the Sensory and Motor Functions of the Face and Head and Autonomic Functions of the Body

The *ocular motor nerves*—the oculomotor (III), trochlear (IV), and abducens (VI)—control movements of the eyes. The abducens nerve has the simplest action, contracting the lateral rectus muscle to move the globe laterally. The trochlear nerve also innervates a single muscle, the superior oblique, but its action both depresses the eye and turns it inward, depending on the eye's position. The oculomotor nerve supplies all of the other muscles of the orbit, including the retractor of the lid. It also provides the parasympathetic innervation responsible for pupillary constriction in response to light and accommodation of the lens for near vision. The ocular motor system is considered in detail in Chapter 41.

The *trigeminal (V) nerve* is a mixed nerve (containing both sensory and motor components) that leaves the brain stem in two roots. The *motor root* innervates the muscles of mastication (the masseter, temporalis, and pterygoids) and a few muscles of the palate (tensor veli palatini), inner ear (tensor tympani), and upper neck (anterior belly of the digastric muscle). The *sensory root* passes into the trigeminal ganglion, located in the floor of the skull in the middle cranial fossa, adjacent to the sella turcica. Three branches emerge from the trigeminal

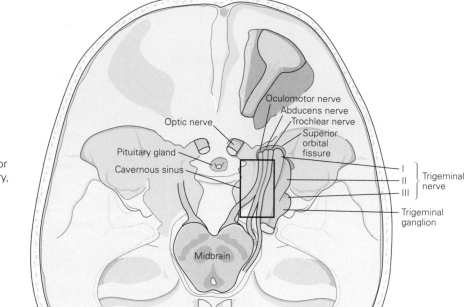

Figure 44-3 The cranial nerves concerned with eye movement exit the skull through the superior orbital fissure. Any enlarging mass in the cavernous sinus, such as a pituitary tumor or an aneurysm of the internal carotid artery, can damage these nerves.

ganglion. The *ophthalmic division* (V₁) runs with the ocular motor nerves through the superior orbital fissure to innervate the structures of the orbit, the nose, and the forehead and scalp back to the vertex of the skull (Figure 44-5). Some fibers from the ophthalmic division also innervate the meninges and blood vessels of the anterior and middle intracranial fossas. The *maxillary division* (V₂) runs through the round foramen of the sphenoid bone to provide sensation from the skin over the cheek, and to the upper portion of the oral cavity. The *mandibular division* (V₃) leaves the skull along with the motor trigeminal branch through the oval foramen of the sphenoid bone. It supplies sensation from the skin over the jaw, the area above the ear, and the lower part of the oral cavity, including the tongue.

A patient with a complete lesion of the trigeminal nerve has numbness that includes not only the entire face but also the inside of the mouth. Patients with psychosomatic complaints rarely know the distribution of the nerve, and so an examination of oral sensation is very important in establishing a trigeminal nerve injury. Trigeminal motor weakness, if one-sided, does not cause much weakness of jaw closure because the muscles of mastication on only one side are sufficient to close the jaw. Nevertheless, the jaw tends to deviate toward the side of the lesion when the mouth is opened. This surprising symptom occurs because the internal pterygoid muscle on the side opposite the lesion is so

powerful that, when unopposed, it pulls the jaw toward the weak side.

The *facial* (VII) *nerve* is also a mixed nerve. Its *motor branch* supplies the muscles of facial expression as well as the stapedius muscle in the inner ear, stylohyoid, and posterior belly of the digastric muscle in the upper neck. The *sensory component* often runs as a separate bundle, the nervus intermedius. Its sensory ganglion, the geniculate, is located near the middle ear. After the geniculate ganglion, the sensory fibers diverge from the motor branch. Some innervate skin of the external auditory meatus, whereas others form the chorda tympani nerve, which joins the lingual nerve and provide taste sensation to the anterior two-thirds of the tongue. The *autonomic component* of the facial nerve includes parasympathetic fibers that innervate lacrimal and salivary glands (except the parotid gland) and the cerebral vasculature.

The facial nerve may suffer isolated injury in *Bell's palsy,* a common complication of certain viral infections. If there is a herpes zoster infection of the geniculate ganglion, small blisters may form in the outer ear canal, the ganglion's cutaneous sensory field; taste sensation may also be lost on the anterior two-thirds of the tongue on that side. Early on the patient may complain mainly of the face pulling toward the unaffected side because of the ipsilateral weakness. Later the entire side of the face becomes weak and the cornea may dry out because the eye does not close during blinking. The patient may com-

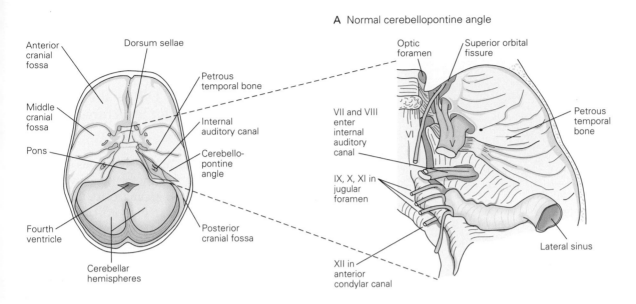

A Normal cerebellopontine angle

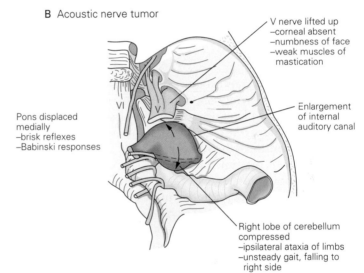

B Acoustic nerve tumor

Figure 44-4 The cranial nerves that exit the brain stem at the cerebellopontine angle. The structures of the cerebellopontine angle are vulnerable to compromise by an enlarging mass, such as a glial tumor of the vestibulocochlear (VIII) nerve (often erroneously called an acoustic neuroma).

A. The relationships of the cranial nerves in the cerebellopontine angle and the jugular foramen are shown in this view of the inner surface of the skull with the brain stem and cerebellum removed.

B. The effects of an enlarging acoustic neuroma on adjacent structures of the cerebellopontine angle. (Adapted from Patten 1977.)

plain that sound has a booming quality in the affected ear, where the stapedius muscle fails to tense the ossicles.

The *vestibulocochlear* (VIII) *nerve* contains two main bundles of sensory axons. The fibers emerging from the vestibular ganglion relay sensation of linear and angular acceleration from the semicircular canals, utricle, and saccule in the inner ear. The auditory fibers from the cochlear ganglion relay information from the cochlea concerning sound. A vestibular schwannoma, one of the most common intracranial tumors, may form along the vestibular component of nerve VIII as it runs within the internal auditory meatus. Patients complain mainly about hearing loss, as the brain is able to adapt to the gradual loss of vestibular information.

The *glossopharyngeal* (IX) and *vagus* (X) *nerves* are mixed but predominantly autonomic nerves. These closely related nerves transmit sensation from the pharynx and upper airway as well as taste in the posterior third of the tongue and oral cavity. The glossopharyngeal nerve transmits visceral information from the neck (for example, information on blood oxygen and pressure from the carotid sinus body), whereas the vagus nerve transmits visceral sensation from the rest of the respiratory, cardiovascular, and gastrointestinal organs (down to the transverse colon). Both nerves include parasympathetic motor fibers; the glossopharyngeal nerve provides parasympathetic control of the parotid salivary gland while the vagus nerve innervates the rest of the internal

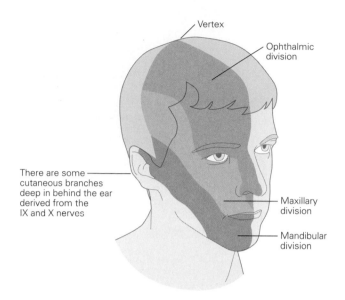

Figure 44-5 The areas of innervation of the three sensory divisions of the trigeminal (V) nerve.

organs of the neck, thorax, and abdomen. The glossopharyngeal nerve innervates only one muscle of the palate, the stylopharyngeus, which raises and dilates the pharynx. The other voluntary muscles of the larynx and pharynx are under the control of the vagus nerve.

Because many of the functions of nerves IX and X are bilateral, unilateral injury may cause relatively minor problems. Patients with unilateral nerve X injury are hoarse, because one vocal cord is paralyzed, and may have some difficulty swallowing. Examination of the oropharynx shows weakness and numbness of the palate on one side.

The *spinal accessory* (XI) *nerve* is a purely motor nerve, which originates from motor neurons in the upper cervical spinal cord. It innervates the trapezius and sternocleidomastoid muscles. The sternocleidomastoid is the only muscle in the body whose action is toward the opposite side of space (it turns the head to the opposite side). Thus an injury of the right XI nerve causes weakness of turning the head to the left. In contrast, a cortical lesion causing weakness of the entire right side of the body will involve the *left* sternocleidomastoid (because the left cerebral cortex is concerned with movement toward the right side of the world). The sternocleidomastoid is the only muscle with this predominantly ipsilateral cortical control.

The *hypoglossal* (XII) *nerve* is also purely motor in function, innervating the muscles of the tongue. When nerve XII is injured, for example, during surgery for head and neck cancer, the tongue atrophies on that side.

The muscle fibers exhibit twitches of muscle fascicles (*fasciculations*), which may be seen clearly through the thin mucosa of the tongue.

The Cranial Nerve Nuclei Follow the Basic Plan for Sensory and Motor Structures in the Spinal Cord

Just as the cranial nerves are homologous to spinal nerves, so are the sensory and motor nuclei within the brain stem similar to those of the spinal cord. Like the sensory and motor laminae of the spinal cord, the neurons of the cranial nerve nuclei are organized into longitudinal columns (Figure 44-6). Although these columns are not always continuous along the longitudinal axis of the brain stem, nuclei with similar functions (sensory or motor, somatic or visceral) tend to be located in characteristic positions at each level of the brain stem. Within individual cranial nerve nuclei neurons are organized in topographically ordered longitudinal columns. For example, motor nuclei consist of elongated clusters of motor neurons that innervate individual muscles. Likewise, longitudinal clusters of neurons in the sensory nuclei tend to be arranged in a topographic map of the body surface they innervate. This pattern of organization can best be understood in light of the basic plan of the spinal cord.

During development the neural tube is divided by the *sulcus limitans,* a longitudinal fissure along the walls of the central canal, into an *alar* (dorsal) and a *basal* (ventral) plate (Figure 44-7). The alar plate differentiates into the sensory structures of the dorsal horn of the spinal cord and the basal plate into the ventral horn motor structures. The intermediate gray matter of the spinal cord contains primarily interneurons that coordinate spinal reflexes and motor responses.

This organizational plan extends to the brain stem. In its rostral extension along the wall of the fourth ventricle through the cerebral aqueduct and into the diencephalon, the sulcus limitans marks the border between sensory (dorsal) and motor (ventral) nuclei. The somatic and visceral, sensory and motor nuclei are further divided into general nuclei that provide functions similar to spinal nerves and special nuclei that provide functions unique to the head (such as hearing, balance, and taste) (Table 44-2).

The Sensory Nuclei

General Somatic Afferent Column

The general somatic afferent column occupies the most lateral portion of the alar plate and includes the trigem-

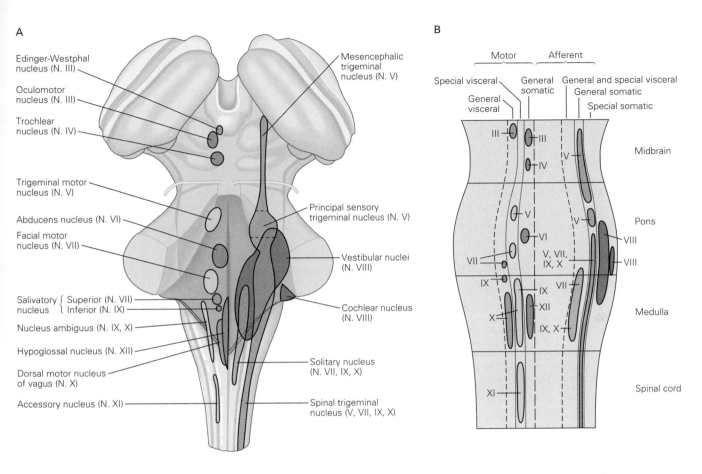

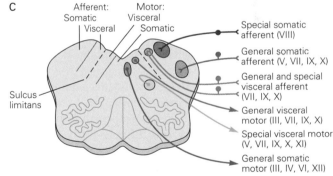

Figure 44-6 Cranial nerve nuclei are organized into functional columns.

A. This dorsal view of the brain stem shows the organization of the cranial nerve sensory columns (**right**) and motor columns (**left**).

B. This simplified schematic view of the same structures as in panel **A** shows more clearly the organization of the motor and sensory columns.

C. The locations of the cranial nuclei with respect to one another and the sulcus limitans (see Figure 44-7) as seen in a cross section at the level of the medulla.

inal sensory nuclei. The *spinal trigeminal nucleus* is essentially a continuation of the superficial laminae of the spinal dorsal horn into the medulla (Figure 44-8). Its outer surface is capped by a superficial fiber tract, the spinal trigeminal tract, which is a direct continuation of Lissauer's tract of the spinal cord (Chapter 23). This arrangement permits trigeminal and upper cervical sensory axons to ascend or descend for several segments. It also allows sensory information from the head and neck carried by the spinal and trigeminal nerves to be knit to-

gether to form an uninterrupted map of the entire body surface.

The spinal trigeminal nucleus also receives sensory axons from all of the cranial nerves concerned with sensation in the head, including axons from the facial nerve that convey information from the external auditory meatus, fibers from the glossopharyngeal nerve that carry input from the posterior part of the palate and tonsillar fossa, and fibers from the vagus nerve that relay sensory information from the posterior wall of the

Table 44-2 Functional Classes of Cranial Nerves

Classification	Functions	Structures innervated	Cranial nerve
Sensory			
General somatic	Touch, pain, and temperature Proprioception	Skin, skeletal muscles of head and neck, mucous membrane of mouth, and teeth	V, VII, IX, X
Special somatic[1]	Hearing, balance	Cochlea, vestibular organ	VIII
General visceral	Mechanical Chemosensory	Pharynx, larynx, neck, gut	V, VII, IX, X
Special visceral	Olfaction, taste	Taste buds, olfactory epithelium	I, VII, IX, X
Motor			
General somatic	Skeletal muscle control (somites)	Extraocular and tongue muscles	III, IV, VI, XII
General visceral	Autonomic control	Tear glands, sweat glands, gut	III, VII, IX, X
Special visceral	Skeletal muscle control (branchiomeric)	Muscles of facial expression, jaw, neck, larynx, and pharynx	V, VII, IX, X, XI

[1]The optic nerve (II) is considered part of the somatic afferent class but is not included here because it does not contain the axons of primary sensory neurons, but rather those of third-order neurons in the visual pathway.

pharynx. The spinal trigeminal nucleus thus contains a map of the entire oral cavity as well as the surface of the face. The nucleus is organized topographically, with the forehead represented ventrally and the oral region dorsally. The tongue representation projects medially from the mouth toward the taste representation in the nucleus of the solitary tract.

The *principal sensory trigeminal nucleus,* which lies in the midpons just lateral to the trigeminal motor nucleus, receives the same type of sensory information from the face that is carried by the dorsal columns from the body. The axons from the principal sensory trigeminal nucleus join those from the dorsal column nuclei in the medial lemniscus through which they ascend to the ventroposterior medial thalamus. An additional component of the trigeminal sensory system, located at the midbrain level in the lateral surface of the periaqueductal gray matter, is the *mesencephalic trigeminal nucleus,* which receives proprioceptive information from the muscles of mastication. The large cells of this nucleus are not central neurons but rather trigeminal ganglion cells that have migrated into the central nervous system. The central branches of the axons from these unipolar cells contact motor neurons in the trigeminal motor nucleus, providing a monosynaptic feedback arc for controlling jaw movement, which is critical for maintaining precise control of biting and chewing.

Special Somatic Afferent Column

The special somatic afferent column is concerned with inputs from the acoustic and vestibular nerves; it develops from the intermediate portion of the alar plate. The *cochlear nuclei,* which hang off the lateral margin of the brain stem at the pontomedullary junction like the floppy ears of a dog, receive the auditory afferents from the spiral ganglion of the cochlea. The cochlear nuclei relay their outputs through the pons to the superior olivary and trapezoid nuclei and on to the inferior colliculus bilaterally (see Chapter 30). The *vestibular nuclei* are more complex. They include four distinct cell groups that relay information from the vestibular ganglion to various motor and oculomotor sites in the brain stem, cerebellum, and spinal cord concerned with maintaining balance and coordination of eye and head movements (see Chapter 41).

Visceral Afferent Column

The visceral afferent column is concerned with special visceral afferent sensation (taste) and general visceral sensation from the facial, glossopharyngeal, and vagus nerves; it derives from the most medial tier of neurons in the alar plate. All of the fibers in this column terminate in a single cell group, the *nucleus of the solitary tract.* The solitary tract is analogous to the spinal trigeminal tract or Lissauer's tract, bundling afferents from different cranial nerves and allowing them to run rostrally or caudally along the length of the nucleus. As a result, visceral sensory information from different afferent nerves interacts in the nucleus of the solitary tract to produce a single visceral sensory map of the body.

Special visceral (taste) afferents from the anterior two-thirds of the tongue reach the nucleus of the solitary tract in the facial nerve, whereas those from the posterior oral cavity arrive via the glossopharyngeal and vagus nerves. These afferents terminate in roughly topographic fashion in the anterior third of the nucleus. General visceral afferents are relayed via the glossopharyngeal and vagus nerves. Those from the rest of the gastrointestinal tract (up to the transverse colon) terminate in the middle portion of the nucleus in topographic order, while those from the cardiovascular and respiratory systems terminate in the posterior portion.

The nucleus of the solitary tract projects directly to parasympathetic and sympathetic preganglionic neurons in the medulla and spinal cord that mediate various autonomic reflexes, as well as to parts of the reticular formation that coordinate autonomic responses. Most ascending visceral outputs to the forebrain are relayed via the parabrachial nucleus in the pons, although some reach the forebrain directly from the nucleus of the solitary tract. Together, the two cell groups supply visceral sensory information to the hypothalamus, basal forebrain, amygdala, thalamus, and cerebral cortex.

The Motor Nuclei

The basal plate of the brain stem gives rise to three motor columns.

General Somatic Motor Column

The general somatic motor column consists of nuclei that develop at the base of the central canal and remain near the midline at the floor of the ventricular system. The *oculomotor* (III) and *trochlear* (IV) *nuclei* lie at the midbrain level just ventral to the cerebral aqueduct (Figure 44-8). The *abducens* (VI) *nucleus* lies beneath the floor of the fourth ventricle at the midpontine level. The *hypoglossal* (XII) *nucleus* is located near the midline beneath the floor of the fourth ventricle and central canal in the medulla.

Special Visceral Motor Column

The special visceral motor column includes motor nuclei that innervate muscles derived from the branchial arches. During development, these cell groups originate

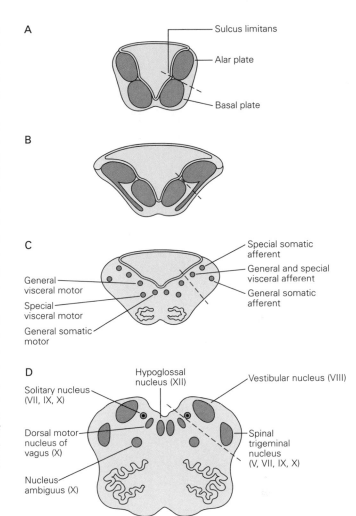

Figure 44-7 The brain stem develops along the same general plan as the spinal cord.

A. The neural tube is divided into a dorsal sensory portion (the alar plate) and a ventral motor portion (the basal plate) by a longitudinal impression along the wall of the neural tube, the sulcus limitans (**dashed line**).

B–D. During development, these structures migrate slightly into their adult positions. In maturity (**D**) the sulcus limitans continues to be recognizable in the walls of the third and fourth ventricles and the cerebral aqueduct, and it still demarcates a border between dorsal sensory structures (**orange**) and ventral motor structures (**green**).

just dorsal to the somatic motor nuclei and migrate ventrolaterally into the tegmentum. The *trigeminal* (V) *motor nucleus*, which innervates the muscles used in chewing, lies ventrolaterally at a midpontine level. Associated with it are the accessory trigeminal nuclei innervating the tensor tympani, tensor veli palatini, and mylohyoid muscles, and the anterior belly of the digastric muscle.

Section through superior colliculus

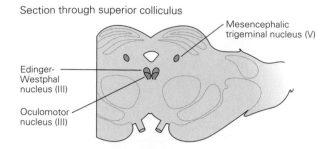

Section through inferior colliculus

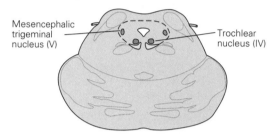

Section through middle cerebellar peduncle

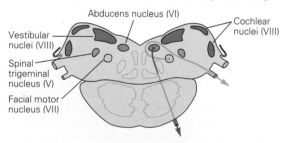

Section through cochlear nuclei and the trapezoid body

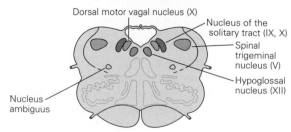

Section through medulla oblongata

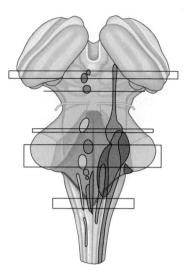

Figure 44-8 The cranial nerve nuclei at various levels of the brain stem.

The facial (VII) *motor nucleus* lies caudal to the trigeminal motor nucleus, at the level of the caudal pons, and contains the motor neurons for the muscles of facial expression. The adjacent accessory facial nucleus innervates the stylohyoid and stapedius muscles and the posterior belly of the digastric muscle.

The motor neurons contributing to the glossopharyngeal and vagus nerves lie in a longitudinal cluster, the *nucleus ambiguus,* that runs the length of the ventrolateral part of the medulla. The nucleus ambiguus is a mixed cell group, containing branchial motor neurons that innervate the striated muscles of the larynx and pharynx as well as preganglionic parasympathetic neurons innervating the thoracic organs (see below).

General Visceral Motor Column

The general visceral motor column begins during development in the most dorsal part of the basal plate just below the sulcus limitans. The neurons of the Edinger-Westphal nucleus and the dorsal motor vagal and inferior salivatory nuclei maintain this position, but during development the preganglionic parasympathetic neurons in the nucleus ambiguus and superior salivatory nucleus follow those of the branchial motor nuclei and migrate into the ventrolateral tegmentum.

The *Edinger-Westphal nucleus* is located at the level of the midbrain along the dorsomedial margin of the oculomotor complex just below the floor of the cerebral aqueduct. It contains the preganglionic neurons that control pupillary constriction and lens accommodation; the axons of these cells run in the oculomotor nerve.

The *superior salivatory nucleus* lies at the level of the pons near the facial nerve. These cells, whose axons exit with the facial nerve, innervate the salivary glands (except for the parotid), the lacrimal glands, and the cerebral vasculature.

Preganglionic neurons associated with the gastrointestinal tract form a column at the level of the medulla just dorsal to the hypoglossal nucleus and ventral to the nucleus of the solitary tract. At the most rostral end of this column is the *inferior salivatory nucleus,* comprising the preganglionic neurons that run through the glossopharyngeal nerve to innervate the parotid gland. The rest of this column is the *dorsal motor vagal nucleus.* Most of the preganglionic neurons in this nucleus innervate the gastrointestinal tract; a few are cardiomotor neurons. The axons of these cells pass through the vagus nerve.

The *nucleus ambiguus,* in the ventrolateral medulla, contains preganglionic neurons that innervate thoracic organs, including the esophagus, heart, and respiratory system. These neurons are organized in a topographic fashion, with the esophagus represented most rostrally, and they are closely associated with the special visceral motor neurons that innervate the larynx and pharynx.

The Brain Stem Deviates From the Organization of the Spinal Cord in Two Important Ways

The first difference between the organization of the brain stem and the spinal cord is that the long ascending and descending sensory tracts, which run along the outside of the spinal cord, are incorporated within the substance of the brain stem. Thus, the ascending sensory lemniscal tracts (the medial lemniscus and spinothalamic tract) run through the reticular formation of the brain stem, as do the auditory, vestibular, and visceral sensory pathways.

A second major difference is that in the brain stem the cerebellum and its associated pathways are superimposed upon the basic plan. Fibers of the cerebellar tracts and nuclei join those of the pyramidal and extrapyramidal motor systems to form a large ventral portion of the brain stem. Thus, from the midbrain to the medulla the brain stem is divided into a dorsal portion, the tegmentum, which follows the basic spinal segmental plan, and a ventral portion, which contains the structures associated with the descending motor systems. At the level of the midbrain the ventral (motor) portion includes the cerebral peduncles, substantia nigra, and red nuclei. At the level of the pons the motor structures oc-

cupying the ventral portion or base of the pons include the pontine nuclei, corticospinal tract, and middle cerebellar peduncle. In the medulla they include the pyramidal tracts and inferior olivary nuclei.

Neuronal Ensembles in the Brain Stem Reticular Formation Coordinate Reflexes and Simple Behaviors Mediated by the Cranial Nerves

The core of the brain stem tegmentum is called the reticular formation. This region is homologous to the intermediate gray matter of the spinal cord, containing interneurons responsible for generating spinal reflexes and simple motor patterns. In early studies the reticular formation was described as poorly organized because its cell clusters lack distinct boundaries and are penetrated by bundles of long ascending and descending fibers that give the entire region a net-like or reticulated appearance. It is now clear, however, that the reticular formation is highly organized and differentiated, consisting of distinct populations of neurons with specific functions.

The reticular formation can be divided functionally into lateral and medial regions (Figure 44-10). Groups of interneurons close to the motor nuclei of the cranial nerves coordinate reflexes and simple stereotyped behaviors mediated by the cranial nerves. As a rule, these local-circuit neurons are located in the *lateral* reticular formation and are relatively small. In contrast, neurons of the *medial* reticular formation tend to be large and have long ascending and descending axons that modulate the actions of neurons involved in movement and posture, pain, autonomic functions, and arousal. Here we briefly describe the actions of the interneurons related to cranial nerve function. The modulatory systems of the brain stem are described in the next chapter.

Neurons in the *ventrolateral medullary reticular formation* are important for coordinating a variety of stereotyped motor patterns and behaviors related to the visceral functions of the vagus nerve. These include gastrointestinal responses (such as swallowing and vomiting), respiratory activities (including the initiation and modulation of respiratory rhythm, coughing, hiccupping and sneezing), and cardiovascular responses (such as baroreceptor reflexes and responses to cerebral ischemia and hypoxia). Many components of these responses require coordination of several organ systems and involve complex patterns of autonomic and somatic motor response that are organized by assemblies of neurons in the reticular formation. Autonomic and respiratory reflex mechanisms are discussed in more detail in Chapter 49.

The *lateral medullary* and *pontine reticular formation*

Box 44-1 Identifying the Site of Lesions in the Brain Stem

The level of the brain stem affected by a lesion is generally determined by assessing which cranial nerves are impaired, whereas the location of the site of injury within that level of the brain stem is inferred by identifying the long tracts that are damaged.

For example, a common clinical syndrome includes (1) dizziness, suggesting impairment of the vestibular component of nerve VIII, (2) hoarseness and difficulty in swallowing, indicating involvement of nerves IX and X, and (3) loss of pain and temperature sensation in the face, implying dysfunction of the spinal trigeminal nucleus. All of the cranial nerve nuclei implicated by these symptoms are located at the level of the medulla.

Patients presenting with this syndrome usually have lost

pain and temperature sensation on the opposite side of the body because of injury to the spinothalamic tract. In addition, clumsiness of the arm and leg on the side of the injury are typical because the inferior cerebellar peduncle is involved. Also, the pupil on the side of the injury may be small, and there may be loss of sweating from injury to the descending hypothalamo-spinal tract.

All of these structures are located in the lateral part of the brain stem. This combination of symptoms, known as *Wallenberg syndrome*, therefore pinpoints the injury to the lateral medulla. Adolph Wallenberg, who first described this syndrome, showed that it can occur when the posterior inferior cerebellar artery is occluded (Figure 44-9).

A Wallenberg's drawing

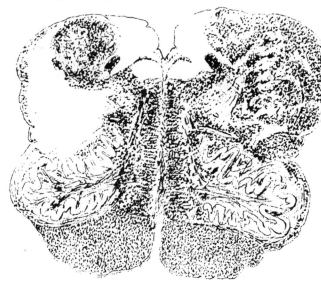

Figure 44-9 Wallenberg syndrome is a combination of symptoms due to damage of cranial nuclei and tracts in the lateral medulla. Part **A** shows Wallenberg's drawing of the affected area. Part **B** illustrates the nuclei and fiber tracts contained in this region. Part **C** shows the pattern of blood supply by the posterior inferior cerebellar artery.

B Areas affected by lateral medullary syndrome

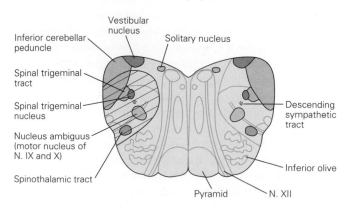

Vestibular nucleus
Inferior cerebellar peduncle
Solitary nucleus
Spinal trigeminal tract
Spinal trigeminal nucleus
Nucleus ambiguus (motor nucleus of N. IX and X)
Descending sympathetic tract
Spinothalamic tract
Inferior olive
Pyramid
N. XII

C Blood supply to medulla

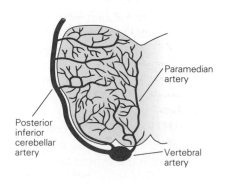

Paramedian artery
Posterior inferior cerebellar artery
Vertebral artery

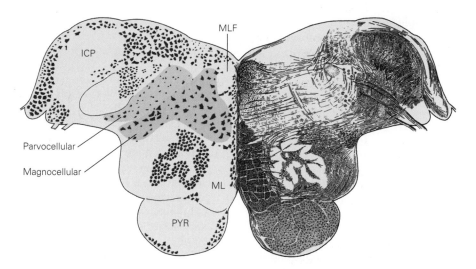

Figure 44-10 The brain stem reticular formation at the level of the medulla. The magnocellular neurons in the medial region give rise to long descending pathways, whereas the parvocellular neurons in the lateral region are mainly involved in modulating reflexes mediated by local cranial nerves IX, X, and XII. **ICP** = inferior cerebellar peduncle; **ML** = medial lemnicus; **MLF** = medial longitudinal fasciculus; **PYR** = pyramid.

extends from the region lateral to the hypoglossal and ambiguus nuclei through the area surrounding the facial nucleus up to and adjacent to the trigeminal motor nucleus. Neurons in this region are involved with the coordination of orofacial motor responses. Most important among these are the motor activities that constitute eating: chewing is coordinated by neurons adjacent to the trigeminal motor nucleus; lip movements are coordinated by neurons near the facial motor nucleus; and movements of the tongue are coordinated by neurons near the hypoglossal nucleus. All of these movements must not only be coordinated with one another (and with respiratory movements) but also highly responsive to sensory feedback from the nucleus of the solitary tract (taste) and the trigeminal sensory nuclei (food texture, temperature, jaw position).

Neurons in the reticular formation surrounding the facial motor nucleus are also important in organizing emotional facial expressions, such as smiling or crying. It is extraordinarily difficult to generate these expressions voluntarily (thus the posed smile in a photograph looks artificial). Actors learn to produce emotion in the face by imagining situations that trigger the motor patterns controlled by the reticular formation. The autonomous control of facial expression is illustrated in patients who have paralysis of voluntary movement on one side of the face because of a stroke. Despite the paralysis they are able to smile *symmetrically* when told a joke. This apparently paradoxical response occurs because the descending input to the reticular formation that triggers emotional facial expression is bilateral and facial expressions can be triggered by either hemisphere.

The *paramedian reticular formation* of the pons adjacent to the abducens nucleus and in the midbrain adjacent to the oculomotor nucleus coordinates eye movements. The pontine paramedian reticular formation on each side of the brain stem controls horizontal eye movements to the ipsilateral side of space. The neurons lateral to the oculomotor nucleus in the midbrain coordinate vertical eye movements as well as the convergence of the eyes necessary to focus at close range.

Diagnosis of a patient with a lesion to the brain stem requires knowledge of the cranial nerves and the anatomy of the long tracts. This is explained in Box 44–1.

An Overall View

Just as the spinal nerves subserve specific sensory or motor functions related to their segmental level, the cranial nerves subserve specific functions for the head, neck, and internal viscera. The organization of the cranial nerve nuclei also follows the basic pattern of the spinal cord, with sensory functions localized dorsally and motor functions ventrally. Finally, like the intermediate gray matter of the spinal cord, the reticular formation of the brain stem contains ensembles of neurons that coordinate reflexes and simple stereotyped motor patterns mediated by the cranial nerves.

These simple motor responses, ranging from facial emotional expressions to the mechanisms for breathing and eating, may be assembled into more complex behaviors under voluntary control by the forebrain. But the precise patterns of motor response are organized locally in the brain stem reticular formation.

Clifford B. Saper

Selected Readings

Carpenter MB, Sutin J. 1983. The medulla, the pons and the mesencephalon. In *Human Neuroanatomy*, 8th ed., pp. 315–453. Baltimore: Williams and Wilkins.

Leigh RJ, Zee DS. 1982. The diagnostic value of abnormal eye movements: a pathophysiological approach. Johns Hopkins Med J 151:122–135.

Martin JH (ed). 1996. General organization of the cranial nerve nuclei and the trigeminal system, and the somatic and visceral motor functions of the cranial nerves. In: *Neuroanatomy, Text and Atlas*, pp. 291–347. New York: Elsevier.

Miller NR. 1985. The autonomic nervous system: Pupillary function, accommodation and lacrimation, and the ocular motor system: Embryology, anatomy, physiology and topographic diagnosis. In: Walsh FB, Hoyt WF. Vol. 2, *Clinical Neuro-Ophthalmology*, 4th ed., pp. 385–995. Baltimore: Williams and Wilkins.

Saper CB. 1995. The central autonomic system. In: G Paxinos (ed). *The Rat Nervous System*, 2nd ed., pp. 107–135. San Diego: Academic.

References

Altschuler SM, Bao XM, Bieger D, Hopkins DA, Miselis RR. 1989. Viscerotopic representation of the upper alimentary tract in the rat: sensory ganglia and nuclei of the solitary and spinal trigeminal tracts. J Comp Neurol 283:248–268.

Berlit P. 1991. Isolated and combined pareses of cranial nerves III, IV, and VI: a retrospective study of 412 patients. J Neurol Sci 103:10–15.

Bieger D, Hopkins DA. 1987. Viscerotopic representation of the upper alimentary tract in the medulla oblongata in the rat: the nucleus ambiguus. J Comp Neurol 262:546–562.

Blessing WW, Li Y-W. 1989. Inhibitory vasomotor neurons in the caudal ventrolateral region of the medulla oblongata. Prog Brain Res 81:83–97.

Braun JP, Tournade A, Adynowski J. 1984. A comparative anatomical CT study of the vascular and nervous structures of the cerebello-pontine angle. Neuroradiology 26:3–7.

Fukushima K. 1991. The interstitial nucleus of Cajal in the midbrain reticular formation and vertical eye movement. Neurosci Res 10:159–187.

Haxhiu MA, Jansen AS, Cherniack NS, Loewy AD. 1993. CNS innervation of airway-related parasympathetic preganglionic neurons: a transneuronal labeling study using pseudorabies virus. Brain Res 618:115–134.

Herbert H, Moga MM, Saper CB. 1990. Connections of the parabrachial nucleus with the nucleus of the solitary tract and the medullary reticular formation in the rat. J Comp Neurol 293:540–580.

Jenny AB, Saper CB. 1987. Organization of the facial nucleus and corticofacial projection in the monkey: a reconsideration of the upper motor neuron facial palsy. Neurology 37:930–939.

Kolb B, Whishaw IQ. 1990 and 1996. *Fundamentals of Human Neuropsychology*, 1990, 3rd ed.; 1996, 4th ed. New York: Freeman.

Kruse MN, Mallory BS, Noto H, Roppolo JR, deGroat WC. 1992. Modulation of the spinobulbospinal micturition reflex pathway in cats. Am J Physiol 262:R478–R484.

Kuypers HGJM. 1958. Corticobulbar connexions to the pons and lower brain stem in man. Brain 81:364–388.

Patten J. 1977. *Neurological Differential Diagnosis*. New York: Springer.

Rinaman L, Card JP, Schwaber JS, Miselis RR. 1989. Ultrastructural demonstration of a gastric monosynaptic vagal circuit in the nucleus of the solitary tract in rat. J Neurosci 9:1985–1996.

Smith JC, Ellenberger HH, Ballanyi K, Richter DW, Feldman JL. 1991. Pre-Bötzinger complex: a brainstem region that may generate respiratory rhythm in mammals. Science 254:726–729.

Spencer SE, Sawyer WB, Wada H, Platt KB, Loewy AD. 1990. CNS projections to the pterygopalatine parasympathetic preganglionic neurons in the rat: a retrograde transneuronal viral cell body labeling study. Brain Res 534:149–169.

Svien HJ, Baker HL, Rivers MH. 1963. Jugular foramen syndrome and allied syndromes. Neurology 13:797–809.

Wallenberg A. 1971. Acute disease of the medulla: Embolus to the posterior inferior cerebellar artery? In: JK Wolf, ed. *The Classical Brain Stem Syndromes*, pp. 119–136. Springfield, IL: Thomas.

Wallin BG, Westerberg CE, Sundlöf G. 1984. Syncope induced by glossopharyngeal neuralgia: sympathetic outflow to muscle. Neurology 34:522–524.

45

Brain Stem Modulation of Sensation, Movement, and Consciousness

IN THE LAST CHAPTER WE examined the groups of interneurons surrounding cranial nerve nuclei in the reticular formation of the brain stem. These reticular interneurons have local projections that mediate reflexes and simple stereotyped behaviors, such as chewing and swallowing. In this chapter we shall explore the *long projection systems* of the reticular formation: the neurons whose axons ascend to the forebrain or descend to the spinal cord. These neurons regulate complex functions of the central nervous system, including the perception of pain and the control of posture and wakefulness. Through these long projection systems the brain stem maintains the level of activity necessary for sensory awareness, motor responses, and arousal related to behavioral states.

Cell Groups in the Brain Stem With Long Projections Can Be Defined by Their Neurotransmitters

Although early neuroanatomists described the reticular formation as being poorly organized, modern methods have demonstrated that it is composed of systems of neurons with specific neurotransmitters and connections. Such systems often extend beyond the borders of the nuclei defined by traditional cell and fiber stains. To overcome this discrepancy, earlier researchers used a combination of letters and numbers to identify clusters of neurotransmitter-specific neurons: letters to identify the neurotransmitter and numbers to indicate the rostrocaudal order of the cell group. Although this nomenclature is convenient and still widely used, it tends to

Box 45-1 The Major Modulatory Systems of the Brain

Noradrenergic Cell Groups

Noradrenergic neurons are located in two columns, one dorsal and one ventral (Figure 45-1). At the level of the medulla the ventral column contains neurons associated with the *nucleus ambiguus* (A1 group); those in the dorsal column are a compo-

nent of the nucleus of the solitary tract and the dorsal motor vagal nucleus (A2 group). Both groups project to the hypothalamus and control cardiovascular and endocrine functions. In the pons the ventral column includes the A5 and A7 cell groups, located in the ventrolateral reticular formation of the pons. These A5 and A7 groups provide mainly projections to

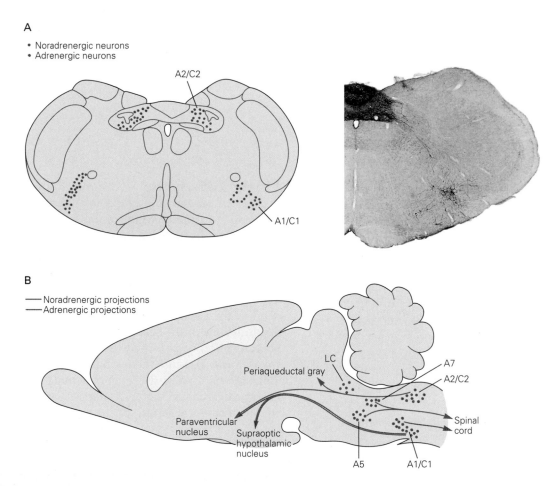

Figure 45-1 Noradrenergic and adrenergic neurons in the medulla and pons.

A. The catecholaminergic neurons in the dorsal medulla (the **A2** noradrenergic and **C2** adrenergic groups) are part of the nucleus of the solitary tract. Those in the ventrolateral medulla (the **A1** noradrenergic and **C1** adrenergic groups) are located near the nucleus ambiguus.

B. The adrenergic projection to the spinal cord arises in the **C1** neurons while the noradrenergic projection to the spinal cord comes from the **A5** and **A7** groups as well as the locus ceruleus (**LC**) (A6 group) in the pons. The ascending noradrenergic input to the hypothalamus stems from both the **A1** and **A2** cell groups while adrenergic input to the hypothalamus comes from the **C1** cell group.

the spinal cord that modulate autonomic reflexes and pain sensation. The A6 cell group, the *locus ceruleus*, sits dorsally and laterally in the periaqueductal and periventricular gray matter (Figure 45-2). The locus ceruleus, which maintains vigilance and responsiveness to unexpected environmental stimuli, has extensive projections to the cerebral cortex and cerebellum, as well as descending projections to the brain stem and spinal cord.

Adrenergic Cell Groups

Some neurons in the two columns of cells in the medulla identified as catecholaminergic were later found to synthesize epinephrine. The C1 adrenergic cell group forms a rostral extension from the A1 column in the rostral ventrolateral medulla (Figure 45-1). Many C1 neurons project to the spinal cord, particularly to the sympathetic preganglionic column, where they

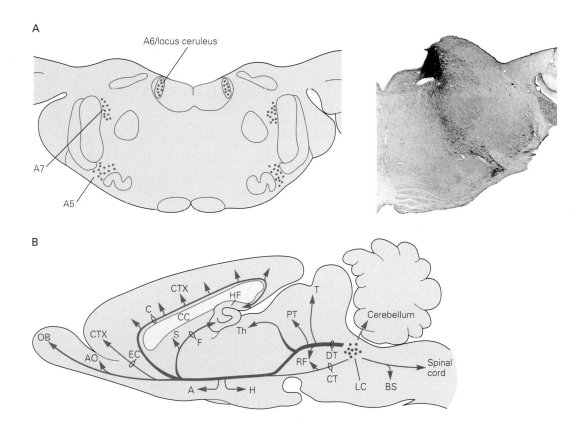

Figure 45-2 Noradrenergic neurons in the pons.

A. Noradrenergic neurons are spread across the pons in three more or less distinct groups: the locus ceruleus (**A6** group) in the periaqueductal gray matter, the **A7** group more ventrolaterally, and the **A5** group along the ventrolateral margin of the pontine tegmentum.

B. The A5 and A7 neurons mainly innervate the brain stem and spinal cord, whereas the **locus ceruleus** provides a major ascending output to the thalamus and cerebral cortex as well as

descending projections to the brain stem, cerebellum, and spinal cord. **A** = amygdala; **AO** = anterior olfactory nucleus; **BS** = brain stem; **C** = cingulate bundle; **CC** = corpus callosum; **CT** = central tegmental tract; **CTX** = cerebral cortex; **DT** = dorsal tegmental bundle; **EC** = external capsule; **F** = fornix; **H** = hypothalamus; **HF** = hippocampal formation; **LC** = locus ceruleus; **OB** = olfactory bulb; **PT** = pretectal nuclei; **RF** = reticular formation; **S** = septum; **T** = tectum; **Th** = thalamus.

(continued)

Box 45-1 The Major Modulatory Systems of the Brain (continued)

are thought to provide tonic excitatory input to vasomotor neurons. Other C1 neurons terminate in the hypothalamus, where they modulate cardiovascular and endocrine responses. The C2 adrenergic neurons, which are a component of the *nucleus of the solitary tract*, contribute to the ascending pathway to the *parabrachial nucleus* (Figure 45-1), which is thought to transmit gastrointestinal information. The C3 adrenergic group is located near the midline at the rostral end of the medulla. Neurons mixed in with the C3 and C1 groups provide a major input to the locus ceruleus, but most of the cells contributing to this pathway are not adrenergic.

Dopaminergic Cell Groups

The dopaminergic cell groups in the midbrain and forebrain were originally numbered as if they were a rostral continuation of the noradrenergic system because identification was based on histofluorescence, which does not distinguish dopamine from norepinephrine very well.

The A8-A10 cell groups include the substantia nigra pars compacta and the adjacent areas of the midbrain tegmentum (Figure 45-3). They send the major ascending dopaminergic inputs to the telencephalon, including the nigrostriatal pathway

Figure 45-3 Dopaminergic neurons in the brain stem and hypothalamus.

A. Dopaminergic neurons in the substantia nigra (**A9** group) and the adjacent retrorubral field (**A8** group) and ventral tegmental area (**A10** group) provide a major ascending pathway that terminates in the striatum, the frontotemporal cortex, and the limbic system, including the central nucleus of the amygdala and the lateral septum.

B. Hypothalamic dopaminergic neurons in the **A11** and **A13** cell groups, in the zona incerta, provide long descending pathways to the autonomic areas of the lower brain stem and the spinal cord. Neurons in the **A12** and **A14** groups, located along the wall of the third ventricle, are involved with endocrine control. Some of them release dopamine as a prolactin release inhibiting factor in the hypophysial portal circulation.

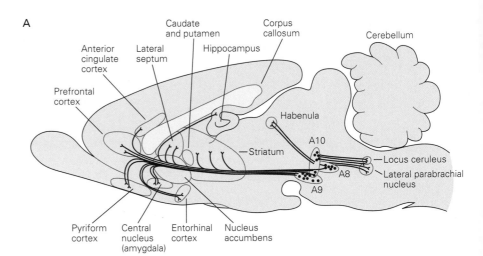

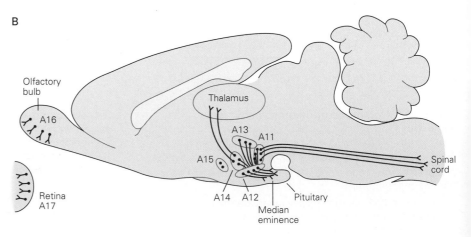

that innervates the striatum and is thought to be involved in initiating motor responses. Mesocortical and mesolimbic dopaminergic pathways arising from the A10 group innervate the frontal and temporal cortices and the limbic structures of the basal forebrain. These pathways have been implicated in emotion, thought, and memory storage. The A11 and A13 cell groups, in the dorsal hypothalamus, send major descending dopaminergic pathways to the spinal cord. These pathways are believed to regulate sympathetic preganglionic neurons. The A12 and A14 cell groups, along the wall of the third ventricle, are components of the tuberoinfundibular hypothalamic neuroendocrine system. Dopaminergic neurons are also found in the olfactory system (A15 cells in the olfactory tubercle and A16 in the olfactory bulb) and in the retina (A17 cells).

Serotonergic Cell Groups

Most serotonergic neurons are located along the midline of the brain stem in the *raphe nuclei* (from *raphé,* French for *seam*). Raphe neurons in the B1-B3 cell groups along the midline of the caudal medulla (Figure 45-4) send descending projections to the motor and autonomic systems in the spinal cord. The raphe magnus nucleus (B3) at the level of the rostral medulla projects to the spinal dorsal horn and is thought to modulate the perception of pain. The serotonergic groups in the pons and midbrain (B4-B9) include the pontine, dorsal, and median raphe nuclei and project to virtually the whole of the forebrain. Serotonergic pathways play important regulatory roles in hypothalamic cardiovascular and thermoregulatory control and modulate the responsiveness of cortical neurons.

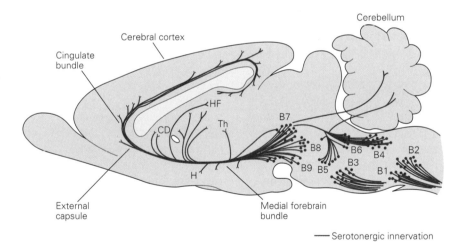

Figure 45-4 Serotonergic neurons along the midline of the brain stem. Neurons in the B1–3 groups, corresponding to the raphe magnus, raphe pallidus, and raphe obscurus nuclei in the medulla, project to the lower brain stem and spinal cord. Neurons in the B4–9 groups, including the raphe pontis, median raphe, and dorsal raphe nuclei, project to the upper brain stem, hypothalamus, thalamus, and cerebral cortex. **CD** = caudate nucleus; **HF** = hippocampal formation; **H** = hypothalamus; **Th** = thalamus.

(continued)

Box 45-1 The Major Modulatory Systems of the Brain (continued)

Cholinergic Cell Groups

Acetylcholine is the transmitter used by both somatic and autonomic motor neurons. Certain populations of cholinergic interneurons are found in the brain stem and forebrain, and large cholinergic neurons in the mesopontine tegmentum and basal forebrain give rise to long ascending projections (Figure 45-5). The mesopontine cholinergic neurons are divided into a ventrolateral column (Ch6 cell group, or the *pedunculopontine nucleus*), close to the lateral margin of the superior cerebellar peduncle, and a dorsomedial column (Ch5 cell group, or the *laterodorsal tegmental nucleus*), a component of the periaqueductal gray matter just rostral to the locus ceruleus. These two cell groups send a major descending projection to the pontine and medullary reticular formation and provide extensive ascending cholinergic innervation of the thalamus. These projections are thought to play an important role in regulating wake-sleep cycles (Chapter 47).

Histaminergic Cell Groups

The histaminergic neurons in the mammalian brain are located in a major cluster in the posterior lateral hypothalamus, the *tuberomammillary nucleus,* and in several minor associated clusters (E1-E5 cell groups) (Figure 45-6). There are roughly as many histaminergic neurons in the tuberomammillary nucleus as there are noradrenergic neurons in the locus ceruleus, and their projections are equally diverse, ranging from the spinal cord to the entire cortical mantle. Histaminergic neurons in the tuberomammillary nucleus may help maintain arousal in the forebrain. Other neurons in the lateral hypothalamic area, containing the peptide neurotransmitters orexin or melanin concentrating hormone also have diffuse cortical, brain stem, and spinal projections (see Figure 45-10) and contribute to arousal responses.

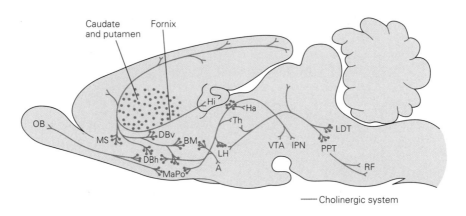

Figure 45-5 Cholinergic neurons in the upper pontine tegmentum and basal forebrain diffusely innervate much of the brain stem and forebrain. The basal forebrain cholinergic groups include the medial septum (**MS**) (Ch1 group), nuclei of the vertical and horizontal limbs of the diagonal band (**DBv** and **DBh**) (Ch2 and Ch3 groups), and the nucleus basalis of Meynert (**BM**) (Ch4 group), which topographically innervate the entire cerebral cortex, including the hippocampus (**Hi**) and the amyg-

dala (**Am**). The pontine cholinergic neurons, in the laterodorsal (**LDT**) (Ch5 group), and pedunculopontine (**PPT**) (Ch6 group), tegmental nuclei, innervate the brain stem reticular formation (**RF**) as well as the thalamus (**Th**). Ha = habenular nucleus; **IPN** = interpeduncular nucleus; **LH** = lateral hypothalamus; **MaPo** = magnocellular preoptic nucleus; **OB** = olfactory bulb; **VTA** = ventral tegmental area.

obscure functional relationships between these cell groups and Nissl-stained nuclei.

The first cell populations in the brain stem to be defined by neurotransmitter substance were identified by histofluorescence, a method that visualizes nerve cells containing norepinephrine, dopamine, and serotonin.

The organization of these monoaminergic systems was later refined by immunocytochemistry, using antisera against specific transmitters or the enzymes that synthesize them. Later studies showed that some of the catecholaminergic neurons in the medulla use epinephrine as neurotransmitter, instead of norepinephrine or

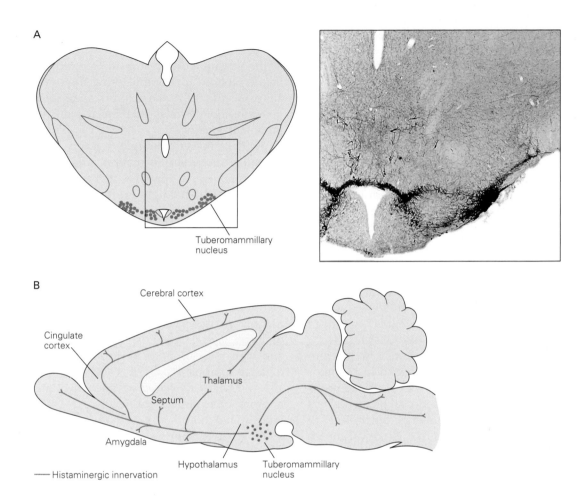

Figure 45-6 All of the histaminergic neurons in the brain are located in the hypothalamus.

A. Histaminergic cells are clustered in the tuberomammillary nucleus in the posterior lateral hypothalamus. There are two main clusters, one located ventrolaterally along the edge of the brain and the other dorsomedially along the edge of the mam-

millary recess of the third ventricle. The photograph on the right shows that some histaminergic cells bridge these two main groups.

B. The histaminergic neurons innervate the entire neuraxis, from the cerebral cortex to the spinal cord.

dopamine, and that a fifth monoaminergic system of neurons in the brain stem uses histamine. Finally, a system of cholinergic neurons was discovered. Each of these six neuronal systems has extensive connections in most areas of the brain and each plays a major role in modulating sensory, motor, and arousal tone. The

major components of these systems are summarized in Box 45-1.

The largest collection of *noradrenergic neurons* is in the pons in the locus ceruleus (Figures 45-1 and 45-2). Remarkably, although the locus ceruleus projects to every major region of the brain and spinal cord, in humans it contains only about 10,000 neurons on each side of the brain. The locus ceruleus maintains vigilance and responsiveness to novel stimuli. It therefore influences both arousal at the level of the forebrain and sensory perception and motor tone in the brain stem and spinal cord.

The largest group of *dopaminergic neurons* in the brain is in the midbrain, including the substantia nigra and the adjacent ventral tegmental area (Figure 45-3). These neurons provide a major ascending input to the cerebral cortex and the basal ganglia that is important in the initiation of behavioral responses. Dopaminergic neurons in the hypothalamus participate in autonomic and endocrine regulation.

Serotonergic neurons are found mainly in the raphe nuclei, located along the midline of the brain stem from the midbrain to the medulla (Figure 45-4). The rostral end of this system projects mainly to the forebrain, where it helps regulate wake-sleep cycles, affective behavior, food intake, thermoregulation, and sexual behavior. In contrast, the neurons of the raphe in the lower pons and medulla project to the brain stem and the spinal cord, where they participate in regulating tone in motor systems and pain perception (see Chapter 24).

The largest groups of *cholinergic neurons* in the brain (aside from the motor neurons) are found in the midbrain and the basal forebrain (Figure 45-5). The neurons in the pedunculopontine and laterodorsal tegmental nuclei of the midbrain provide cholinergic innervation to the brain stem and the thalamus that is critical for inducing a state of cortical arousal, both during wakefulness and dreaming. The cholinergic neurons in the basal forebrain, mainly found in humans in the nucleus basalis of Meynert, also participate in this process. They project largely to the cerebral cortex, where they enhance cortical responses to incoming sensory stimuli.

Histaminergic neurons are found in the tuberomammillary nucleus in the posterior lateral hypothalamus (Figure 45-6). These cells project to all major parts of the nervous system, like the locus ceruleus. They are thought to be important in regulating the level of behavioral arousal.

Descending Projections From the Brain Stem to the Spinal Cord Modulate Sensory and Motor Pathways

Pain Is Modulated by Descending Monoaminergic Projections

Monoaminergic projections to the dorsal horn of the spinal cord descend from the serotoninergic raphe magnus nucleus in the midline of the rostral medulla and from the noradrenergic cell groups in the pons. Activation of either of these monoaminergic pathways can inhibit the

transmission of nociceptive information (see Chapter 24).

The serotonergic neurons in the raphe magnus nucleus receive afferents from enkephalinergic neurons in the periaqueductal gray matter. Electrical stimulation of the periaqueductal gray matter produces analgesia that is blocked by administering the opiate antagonist naloxone into the raphe magnus, suggesting that the endogenous opiates released there activate the descending modulatory pathway.

Other, nonserotonergic neurons in the medial medullary reticular formation adjacent to the raphe magnus have firing patterns that are correlated with reflex responses to painful stimuli. These neurons may also contribute to descending modulation of nociception.

Posture, Gait, and Muscle Tone Are Modulated by Two Reticulospinal Tracts

Two long descending pathways from the reticular formation are associated with control of posture: the medial and lateral reticulospinal tracts. These pathways and their roles in motor control are discussed in more detail in Chapter 41.

The *medial reticulospinal tract* originates from large neurons in the upper pontine reticular formation. It facilitates spinal motor neurons that innervate axial muscles and extensor responses in the legs to maintain postural support. Neurons in the mesopontine reticular formation are also capable of producing patterned, stereotyped movements. For example, stepping movements can be induced by electrically stimulating the midbrain locomotor region, an area adjacent to the cholinergic pedunculopontine nucleus with extensive inputs from the extrapyramidal system (see Chapter 37).

The lateral reticulospinal pathway arises from neurons in the medial medullary reticular formation and inhibits the firing of spinal and cranial motor neurons. Activity of glycinergic neurons in this pathway causes volleys of inhibitory synaptic potentials in motor neurons, producing a loss of motor tone, or *atonia*. Intense volleys of firing of the neurons in the medial medullary reticular formation are associated with the atonia that occurs in rapid eye movement (REM) sleep. These volleys are thought to be under the control of cholinergic neurons in the pedunculopontine nucleus.

Ascending Projections From the Brain Stem Modulate Arousal and Consciousness

The ascending pathways from monoaminergic cell groups in the brain stem and hypothalamus to the cere-

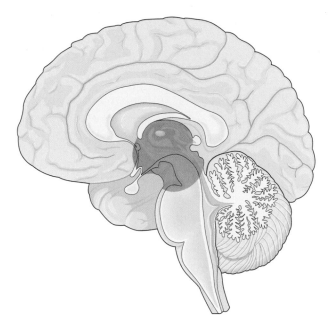

Figure 45-7 Injuries to the ascending arousal system, from the rostral pons through the thalamus and hypothalamus (purple area), can cause loss of consciousness.

bral cortex and thalamus increase wakefulness and vigilance, as well as the responsiveness of cortical and thalamic neurons to sensory stimuli, a state known as *arousal*. These pathways are joined by ascending cholinergic inputs from the pedunculopontine and laterodorsal tegmental nuclei and by other cell groups from the parabrachial nucleus through the paramedian midbrain reticular formation to form an *ascending arousal system.*

The ascending arousal system divides into two major branches at the junction of the midbrain and diencephalon. One branch enters the thalamus, where it activates and modulates thalamic relay nuclei as well as intralaminar and related nuclei with extensive diffuse cortical projections. The other branch travels through the lateral hypothalamic area and is joined by the ascending output from the hypothalamic and basal forebrain cell groups, all of which diffusely innervate the cerebral cortex. Lesions that disrupt either of these two branches impair consciousness (Figure 45-7).

Consciousness Represents the Summated Activity of the Cerebral Cortex

The nature of consciousness has been a subject of intense philosophical concern at least since Plato's *Meno.* However, only within the past 100 years has speculation on the basis of consciousness been informed by scientific understanding of how the brain works. Currently, there is general agreement that consciousness is the property of being aware of oneself and one's place in the environment. Scientifically, this is a very difficult property to measure (see Chapter 20).

As a result, clinicians generally rely on a pragmatic definition based on observation: the ability of the individual to respond appropriately to environmental stimuli. Careful clinical observations show that this ability to orient appropriately to stimuli is dependent upon the summated activity of the two cerebral hemispheres. When parts of the cerebral cortex are damaged a patient may be unable to process certain types of information, and thus the patient is not conscious of certain aspects of the environment. For example, a patient with a lesion in Wernicke's area in the dominant hemisphere may not be aware of the semantic content of speech, and thus would use and interpret language only for emotional gesturing. This type of "fractional" loss of consciousness is discussed in greater detail in Chapter 19. According to this view of conciousness, generalized impairment of consciousness implies diffuse dysfunction in both cerebral hemispheres.

One problem with a definition of consciousness based on responsiveness to stimuli emerged at the beginning of the twentieth century, when clinicians began to report cases of patients with injuries to the brain stem but no injuries to the cerebral hemispheres who were unable to respond to stimuli. Most observers thought that the inability to respond reflected mainly impairment of sensory and motor pathways. In the absence of an independent measure of cortical activity, this view was difficult to disprove.

Fortunately, in the late 1920s Hans Berger, a Swiss psychiatrist, invented the electroencephalogram (EEG) to assess the electrical activity of the cerebral cortex (see Box 46-1). During alert wakefulness the EEG shows a pattern of low-voltage, fast ($\gg$12 Hz) electrical activity called *desynchronized*. During deep sleep the EEG is dominated by high-voltage, slow ($\ll$3 Hz) electrical activity called *synchronized* (Figure 45-8). These patterns are discussed in detail in Chapter 47.

The EEG Reflects Two Modes of Firing of Thalamic Neurons

The EEG is important in assessing wakefulness because electrical activity in the cerebral cortex reflects the firing patterns in the thalamocortical system, a necessary component of maintaining a waking state. As we shall learn in the next two chapters, electrical activity measured from the surface of the skull reflects the summated activity of synaptic potentials in the dendrites of cortical neurons. The specific rhythmic pattern of the EEG waveform thus reflects synchronized waves of

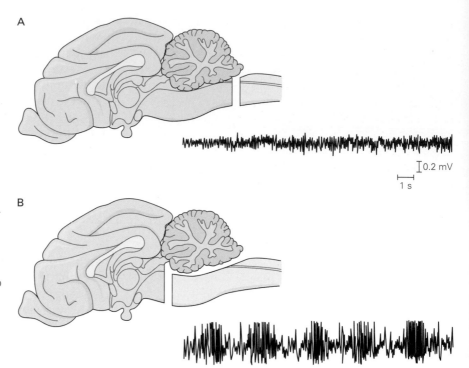

Figure 45-8 The electroencephalogram measures electrical activity in the cerebral cortex.

A. Transection of the lower brain stem at the level shown in the drawing isolates the brain from incoming sensory signals through the spinal cord, a preparation the Belgian neurophysiologist Frederic Bremer called the *encephale isolé*. Animals with this lesion are awake, respond to trigeminal sensory as well as visual and auditory cues, and move their faces and eyes in a normal fashion. The electroencephalogram (EEG) of such animals is typically low voltage and fast, a *desynchronized* pattern typical of waking.

B. When a cut is made at the level indicated in the drawing, between the superior and inferior colliculi, the cat appears to be sleeping, with no eye movement responses to visual stimuli. In animals the EEG pattern is typically high voltage and slow, a *synchronized* pattern consistent with sleep.

excitatory synaptic potentials reaching the cerebral cortex from the thalamus. The rhythmic nature of the thalamic activity is due, in turn, to two important properties of the thalamic relay neurons.

First, the thalamic relay neurons have two distinct physiological states: a transmission mode and a burst mode (Figure 45-9). When the resting membrane potential of the thalamic relay neuron is near the firing threshold, the neuron is in *transmission mode*: incoming excitatory synaptic potentials can drive the neuron to fire in a pattern that reflects the sensory stimulus. When the thalamic neuron is hyperpolarized by inhibitory input, it is in burst mode.

As we shall learn in detail in Chapter 46, the thalamic relay neurons have a special voltage-gated calcium channel that is inactivated when the membrane potential is near threshold. When the relay cell is hyperpolarized incoming excitatory synaptic potentials can trigger transient opening of the calcium channels. These channels produce a calcium current that brings the neuron's membrane potential above threshold for firing action potentials. The cell now fires a burst of action potentials that produce further calcium channel openings,

until sufficient calcium has entered the cell to trigger a calcium-activated potassium current. This potassium current hyperpolarizes the cell, resetting it for another cycle of burst firing.

This raises some questions. How do the thalamic relay cells become hyperpolarized in the first place? What is the nature of the inhibitory input? The thalamic relay neurons have a strong reciprocal interaction with GABA-ergic inhibitory interneurons in the reticular nucleus of the thalamus. The reticular nucleus forms a sheet of GABA-ergic neurons that sits along the outer surface of the thalamus. Their dendrites receive collaterals from both thalamocortical and corticothalamic axons that pass through it. The reticular nucleus is topographically organized, and its neurons project back to relay nuclei from which they receive their inputs. When the reticular nucleus neurons fire, they hyperpolarize thalamic relay neurons, thereby determining whether the thalamic relay neurons will be able to reach firing threshold in response to sensory inputs.

Both the thalamic relay nuclei and the inhibitory neurons of the reticular nucleus enter burst mode when they are hyperpolarized. The input from the reticular neurons produces inhibitory synaptic potentials in the relay neurons that are mediated by GABA$_B$ receptors. This inhibitory input removes inactivation of the calcium channels, and the rebound of the membrane potential sets off a burst of action potentials. In turn, the thalamic relay neurons provide excitatory inputs to the reticular neurons, which trigger another burst of firing in the reticular neurons.

The resulting rhythmic and synchronous firing of thalamic relay neurons produces waves of excitatory postsynaptic potentials in dendrites of cortical neurons. These waves of depolarization show up on the EEG as rhythmic slow waves, a pattern indicating that the thalamus is unable to relay sensory information to the cortex (Figure 45-9). This synchronized pattern of EEG activity is associated with deep sleep (Chapter 47) and is also seen in pathological states in which thalamocortical transmission is blocked, such as coma or during certain types of seizures (see Chapter 46). In contrast, when the thalamus is in transmission mode (eg, during wakefulness), the desynchronized pattern of the EEG reflects ongoing sensory stimuli.

During normal wakefulness the thalamus is kept in the transmission mode by the action of cholinergic inputs from the rostral pons and basal forebrain. The major cholinergic input to the thalamic relay nuclei is from the pedunculopontine and laterodorsal tegmental nuclei in the brain stem. These same nuclei, along with cholinergic neurons in the basal forebrain, innervate the reticular nucleus of the thalamus, reducing its activity and thus preventing it from hyperpolarizing the thalamic relay neurons during wakefulness.

Damage to Either Branch of the Ascending Arousal System May Impair Consciousness

Experimental lesion studies and clinical experience indicate that injury to either branch of the ascending arousal system—the pathway through the thalamus or the pathway through the hypothalamus—can impair consciousness (Figure 45-10). Transection of the brain stem below the level of the rostral pons does not affect the level of consciousness. Acute transections rostral to the level of the inferior colliculus invariably result in coma, a state of profound unarousability. Smaller lesions involving just the paramedian reticular formation of the midbrain are sufficient to produce this result, whereas large lesions of the lateral tegmentum of the upper brain stem do not cause coma. Lesions of the paramedian reticular formation up to the junction of the midbrain and the diencephalon damage axons arising from all components of the ascending arousal system and result in impairment of consciousness.

Lesions of the posterior lateral hypothalamus interrupt the pathway through the hypothalamus. This injury results in profound slowing of the EEG and behav-

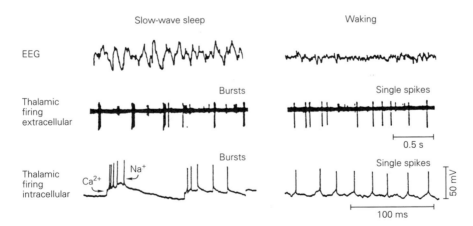

Figure 45-9 Thalamic relay neurons have transmission and burst modes of signaling activity.

Left. Burst mode. When thalamic neurons are hyperpolarized by inhibitory postsynaptic potentials they respond to brief depolarizations with a burst of action potentials (**left**). Each burst of action potentials causes a barrage of synchronized excitatory postsynaptic potentials in the dendrites of cortical neurons, producing an EEG slow-wave pattern known as synchronized activity.

Right. Transmission mode. When thalamic neurons are in a more depolarized state, incoming excitatory potentials produce single action potentials. In this mode the thalamic neuron faithfully transmits sensory impulses to the cerebral cortex but the complex patterning of thalamic firing produces nearly constant, small-scale alterations in the dendritic potentials of cortical neurons. The resulting EEG pattern of fast, low-voltage waves is termed desynchronized.

Figure 45-10 The ascending arousal system consists of the axons of cell populations in the upper brain stem, hypothalamus, and basal forebrain. These pathways diffusely innervate the thalamus and cerebral cortex and keep the thalamus and cortex in a state in which they can respectively transmit and respond appropriately to incoming sensory information. Damage to either the main pathway in the brain stem or its branches in the thalamus or hypothalamus can cause loss of consciousness. **RT** = reticular nucleus of the thalamus; **ILT** = intralaminar thalamic nuclei.

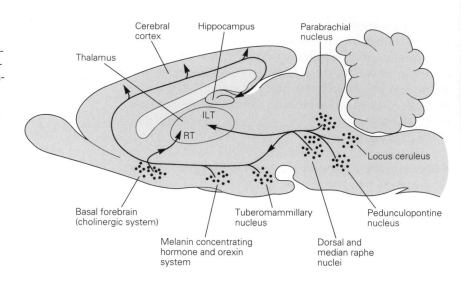

ioral unarousability, even though the branch through the thalamus remains intact. Conversely, injury to the thalamus or its reticular input prevents the brain from achieving a desynchronized or wakeful state. If the injury is sufficiently severe, the EEG rhythm itself is lost.

Bilateral Forebrain Damage May Cause Coma or Persistent Vegetative State or Be Symptomatic of Brain Death

Coma may also be caused by bilateral impairment of the cerebral hemispheres. For example, bilateral subdural hematomas (blood clots in the space between the dura and the arachnoid membranes, usually as a result of head trauma) or multiple (or very large) brain tumors or associated areas of swelling can compress both hemispheres. More often, bilateral forebrain impairment results from a diffuse metabolic process, such as an imbalance of electrolytes or a lack of oxygen. If metabolic imbalance persists, permanent diffuse cortical injury may result.

The large pyramidal neurons in the hippocampal formation and cerebral cortex (particularly laminae III and V) are the cells most severely damaged by inadequate oxygenation (*hypoxia*) or insufficient blood flow (*ischemia*). If many of these neurons are damaged there may not be sufficient numbers of remaining normal neurons to maintain a conscious state. After a period of 1 or 2 weeks of coma these patients enter a contentless wake-sleep cycle called a *persistent vegetative state*. They appear wakeful and may even eat food placed in the mouth, smile or cry, and fixate objects in the environ-

ment, similar to a hydrencephalic infant. Their actions, however, have no cognitive content and bear little relationship to events that surround them.

The persistent vegetative state must be distinguished from *brain death*, in which all brain functions cease. Brain dead patients may have spinal level motor responses, which may include patterned activity such as withdrawal movements or even in rare instances sitting up or moving the arms (the Lazarus syndrome). Even so, there are no purposeful movements of the limbs, face, or eyes; no brain stem reflex responses to sensory stimulation (see below); and no respiratory movements.

An Overall View

The human brain stem is capable of organizing many stereotyped behaviors ranging from eye movements, orofacial responses, and breathing to postural control and even walking. These behaviors are controlled by descending motor pathways from the forebrain. At the same time, the brain stem regulates the overall level of activity of the forebrain itself by controlling wake-sleep cycles and modulating the passage of sensory information, especially pain, to the cerebral cortex.

These regulatory processes are illustrated poignantly in patients who have injury to the lower brain stem. These patients remain awake, but the intact forebrain is unable to interact with the external world, a condition described clinically as *locked-in*. This condition is the exact opposite of patients in a persistent vegetative state, who have extensive forebrain impairment as a result of hypoxia and appear to be awake but lack completely the content of consciousness.

These unfortunate clinical examples underscore the important role of the brain stem in modulating motor and sensory systems through its descending pathways and regulating the wakefulness of the forebrain through its ascending pathways.

Postscript: Examination of the Comatose Patient

More than any other part of the neurological examination the evaluation of a comatose patient must be based on an understanding of the functional anatomy of the brain stem. Two principles of organization are important in pinpointing the cause of coma. First, impairment of consciousness implies dysfunction of the ascending arousal system in the paramedian portion of the upper pons and midbrain, its targets in the thalamus or hypothalamus, or both cerebral hemispheres. Second, dysfunction of cranial nerves indicates injury to the cranial nerves or their nuclei, or the networks of local interneurons that control them. Because the cranial nerves and nuclei are found at specific locations, their dysfunction can indicate the level at which the brain stem has been injured.

States of Consciousness Are Assessed Clinically in Terms of Responsiveness to the Environment

Consciousness is evaluated clinically as the ability of the patient to respond appropriately to environmental stimuli. Loss of this ability is generally judged as an alteration of consciousness. Two major aspects of consciousness must be assessed. First, the *level* of consciousness describes the arousability of the individual. Patients with a mildly depressed level of consciousness are generally classed as *lethargic* and can be easily aroused to full wakefulness. Patients who cannot be fully aroused are *obtunded,* and those who remain in a sleep-like state are *stuporous.* A patient who cannot make a purposeful response to stimulation is *comatose.*

Second, the *content* of consciousness may be assessed in terms of the appropriateness of the patient's responses. We have seen in Chapters 19 and 20 that accurate, purposeful behavioral response depends on the normal function of the higher-order cognitive processes of the forebrain. Impairment of specific cognitive systems may leave the patient unable to appreciate or respond to entire classes of stimuli. For example, the patient with a large right parietal lesion and left-sided neglect is unaware of the left side of his body or the world (Chapter 19). Acute multifocal or diffuse impairment of

Table 45-1 Common Causes of Metabolic Encephalopathy Presenting as Coma

Loss of substrate of cerebral metabolism
   Hypoxia
   Hypoglycemia
   Global ischemia
   Multifocal ischemia resulting from emboli or diffuse
      intravascular coagulation
   Multifocal ischemia resulting from cerebral vasculitis

Derangement of normal physiology
   Hyponatremia or hypernatremia
   Hyperglycemia/hyperosmolar
   Hypercalcemia
   Hypermagnesemia
   Ongoing seizures
   Postseizure state
   Postconcussive state
   Hypothyroidism
   Hypocortisolism

Toxins
   Drugs
   Hypercarbia
   Liver failure
   Renal failure
   Sepsis
   Meningitis/encephalitis
   Subarachnoid blood

the content of consciousness is called *encephalopathy* by neurologists and *acute organic brain syndrome* by psychiatrists, while chronic impairment is *dementia. Delirium* occurs when a patient with diffuse cortical impairment misinterprets sensory information, causing inappropriate excitement or arousal.

Loss of Consciousness May Be Either Structural or Metabolic in Origin

Because the level of arousal of the forebrain is governed by the ascending arousal system, impairment of consciousness reflects either injury to this pathway or diffuse dysfunction of its targets in the forebrain.

Both cerebral hemispheres are most commonly impaired as a result of a metabolic or toxic insult that affects the entire brain. The most common causes of metabolic encephalopathy are listed in Table 45-1. These patients are characterized by normal function of brain stem reflex responses.

In contrast, impairment of the ascending arousal system in the brain stem or diencephalon often results from structural injury. As the ascending arousal system is located

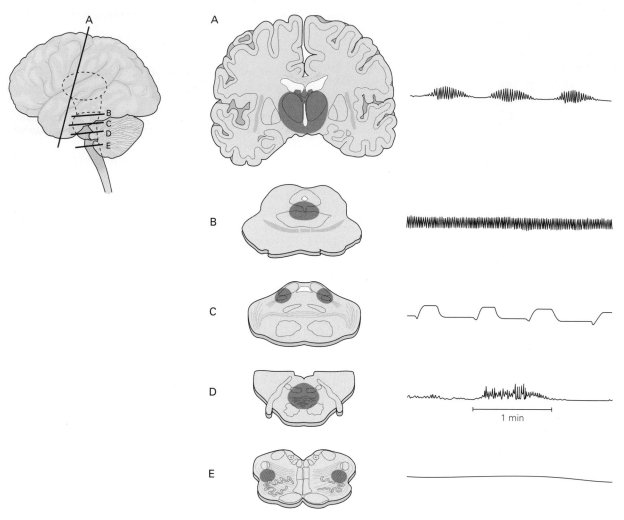

Figure 45-11 The respiratory pattern is a key indicator of level of the brain that is not functioning properly in the comatose patient. When there is diffuse forebrain depression (A), as in a metabolic encephalopathy such as liver failure, the respirations may take on a waxing-and-waning pattern, with variable periods of apnea (no breathing), called *Cheyne-Stokes respiration*. Injury to the midbrain (B) can cause hyperventila-tion. Injury to the rostral pons may produce a peculiar pattern of respiration known as *apneusis* (C), in which the breathing halts briefly at full inspiration. When there is injury to the lower pons or upper medulla, respirations may become irregular and of uneven depth, known as *ataxic* breathing (D). This pattern often heralds a respiratory arrest (E). (Adapted from Plum and Posner 1980.)

close to many cranial nerve nuclei, focal impairment of brain stem reflexes is the hallmark of coma caused by structural damage. Because the critical structures in the brain stem for supporting life are tightly packed within a very small space, even a small progression of an injury can be life-threatening. Hence, it is essential for the physician to recognize focal brain stem impairment and intervene quickly.

Testing Four Functional Systems Gives Important Clues to the Cause of Structural Coma

The examination of the comatose patient is neither diffi-cult nor time-consuming. However, it does require an understanding of how the brain stem is organized. The failure of brain function is important, and all physicians should be able to assess patients with coma and to start immediate lifesaving measures.

Respiratory Patterns

The first systems to be examined in a comatose patient are always cardiovascular and respiratory. In any pa-tient with impaired consciousness, the first step is to make sure that there is adequate perfusion and oxygen supply to the brain. Diffuse forebrain impairment without brain stem injury often induces a pattern of

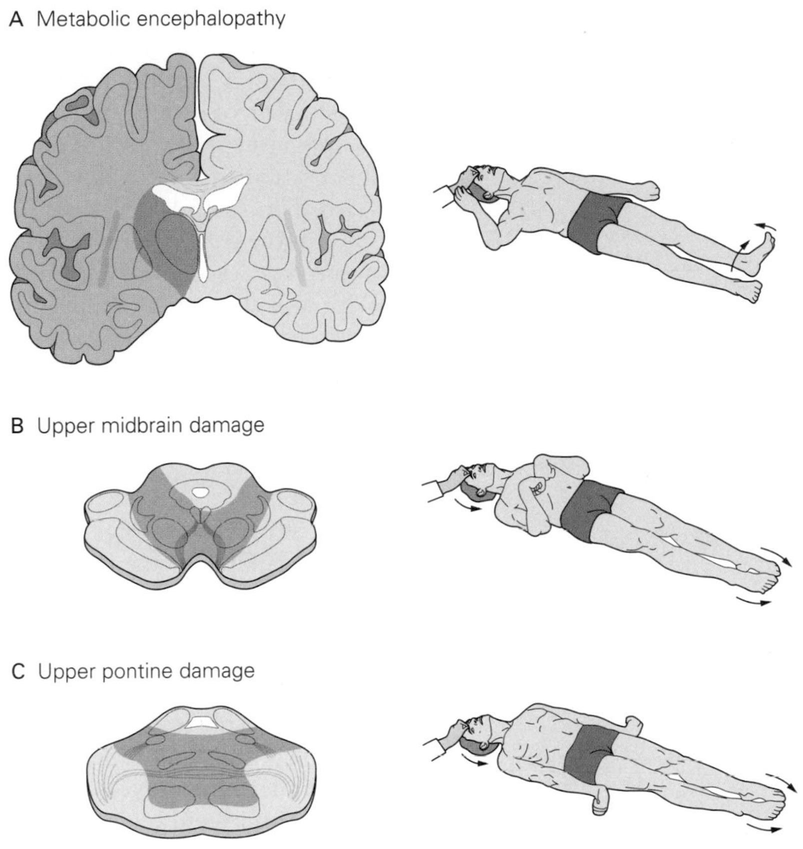

A Metabolic encephalopathy

B Upper midbrain damage

C Upper pontine damage

Figure 45-12 The motor response to painful stimulation is a key indicator of the anatomical site of brain dysfunction causing coma.

A. A patient with a diffuse metabolic encephalopathy may respond to painful stimulation by trying to brush the examiner away (in this case the examiner is pressing on the supraorbital ridge, just above the eye). If one hemisphere is injured more than the other, the motor response may be asymmetric. The contralateral arm may not respond, the leg may be externally rotated, and stimulation of the sole of the foot may cause the big toe to flex upward (the Babinski reflex).

B. Damage to the upper midbrain may cause decorticate posturing: the upper extremities flex, the lower extremities are extended, and the toes extend downward.

C. Damage to the lower midbrain or upper pons causes decerebrate posturing, in which both the upper and lower extremities are extended. Progression from decorticate to decerebrate posturing heralds rostro-caudal deterioration of the brain stem, which may progress in a matter of minutes to failure of the medulla and respiratory arrest. (Adapted from Plum and Posner 1980.)

waxing-and-waning depth of respiration, with interposed apneas, known as Cheyne-Stokes respiration (Figure 45-11). Injury at the pontine level can cause apneusis (inspiratory cramps), while an irregular respiratory cycle suggests involvement of the lower brain stem. Only a bilateral lesion at the level of the ventrolateral medulla or more caudally will cause complete apnea.

Level of Arousability and Motor Responses

The patient should be able to respond to verbal instruction or local painful stimulus (eg, rubbing the sternum, pressing on a nail bed) with appropriate movements of all four limbs (Figure 45-12). Depressed responsiveness

to painful stimuli indicates the depth of the coma. Asymmetric motor responses, eg, failure to move the limbs on one side, are ominous, suggesting a focal injury to the descending motor control systems. Similarly, asymmetry of the muscle stretch reflexes (on tapping the biceps, triceps, knee or ankle tendons) or plantar responses to noxious stimulation of the sole of the foot indicates a focal injury to the descending motor system.

Injury to the upper brain stem can produce posturing of the limbs, either spontaneously or in response to pain. For example, the patient may extend both arms and legs (*decerebrate posturing*), or flex the arms and extend the legs (*decorticate posturing*) bilaterally or unilaterally. This posturing is an ominous sign indicating injury to the upper brain stem reticular formation and

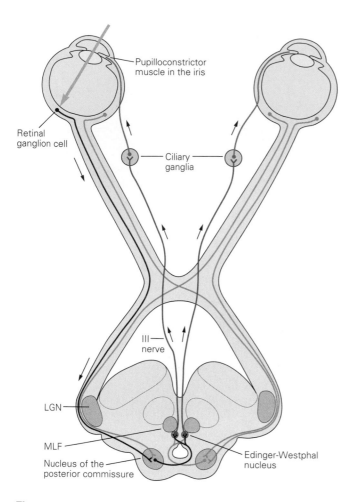

adjacent midbrain. These neurons innervate the parasympathetic ganglion cells in the orbit, which in turn activate the iris constrictor muscle bilaterally, resulting in constriction of both pupils (Figure 45-13).

Dilation of the pupil is provided by the sympathetic innervation of the iris from the superior cervical ganglion (Figure 45-14). The pupillary preganglionic neurons, in the upper thoracic spinal cord, are under tonic excitatory descending control from the hypothalamus. With diffuse forebrain impairment (eg, in metabolic encephalopathy), the pupils are typically small in diameter but react to light (Figure 45-15). Pontine injury may also produce very small but reactive pupils because the pupillodilator pathways are interrupted. Sedative drugs, particularly opiates, may also cause small, reactive pupils.

Loss of pupillary light responses, in contrast, almost always signifies structural injury. Damage to the dorsal midbrain involving the pretectal area causes midposition (or slightly large) pupils that do not react to light. Injury to the midbrain at the level of the third nerve causes complete loss of pupillary responses (because it generally damages the descending sympathetic pupillary dilator system, running through the midbrain lateral to the third nerve nuclei, as well as the pupillary constrictor system).

Unilateral pupillary dilation may result from injury to the oculomotor nerve as it exits the brain stem (the intact sympathetic system causes the pupil with parasympathetic loss to be large). The most common causes of unilateral oculomotor nerve compression in a comatose patient are either an aneurysm of the posterior communicating artery or pressure on the oculomotor nerve when the temporal lobe is pushed through the tentorial opening, for example, by a tumor. Temporal or uncal herniation (the displacement of the uncus, or medial edge of the temporal lobe) may lead to imminent death.

Figure 45-13 The state of the pupil represents a balance between tone in the parasympathetic pupilloconstrictor system (shown here) and the sympathetic pupillodilator pathway (Figure 45-14). Pupillary constriction to light is due to retinal ganglion cells projecting through the optic tract to the pretectal nuclei, at the junction of the thalamus and the midbrain. The pretectal neurons send axons through the posterior commissure to the contralateral parasympathetic preganglionic neurons in the Edinger-Westphal nucleus. These cells, in turn, innervate the ciliary ganglion cells that control the pupilloconstrictor muscle in the iris. **LGN** = lateral geniculate nucleus; **MLF** = medial longitudinal fasciculus. (Adapted from Plum and Posner 1980.)

requires immediate intervention if the patient is to survive.

Pupillary Light Response

The pupillary light response is elicited by shining a bright light in one eye. Retinal ganglion cell axons travel through the optic nerve, optic chiasm, and optic tract to the pretectal area, which then projects to the parasympathetic preganglionic neurons associated with the oculomotor complex, in the Edinger-Westphal nucleus and

Eye Movements

More than any other pathways, those concerned with eye movements run in parallel with the ascending arousal system through the paramedian tegmentum of the upper brain stem. In patients with diffuse forebrain impairment the eyes often rove aimlessly or do not move spontaneously. However, there should be appropriate conjugate eye movement when a vestibular stimulus is provided, by turning the head or by putting cool or warm water in the ear canal (Figure 45-16). Turning the head to the right or left, or up or down, induces eye movement in the opposite direction. Cool water in the ear canal sets up a convection current in the semicircular canals, resulting in conjugate deviation of

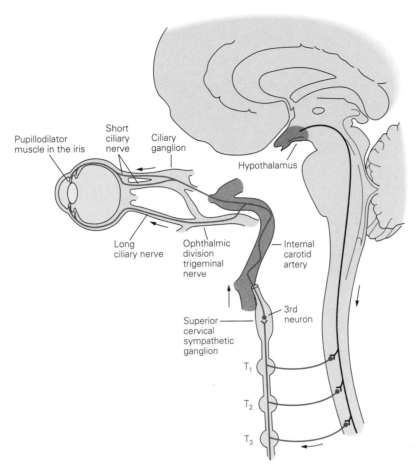

Figure 45-14 Pupillary dilation is regulated by a descending pathway from the hypothalamus. The pathway courses through the lateral part of the brain stem, to the sympathetic preganglionic neurons in the first three segments of the thoracic in-termediolateral cell column. These cells project to the superior cervical ganglion from which sympathetic axons run along the carotid artery to the orbit, where they innervate the pupillodilator muscle in the iris. (Adapted from Plum and Posner 1980.)

the eyes toward that side; warm water has the opposite effect.

Loss of normal reflex eye movements is evidence of brain stem injury. A focal injury of the pons involving the abducens nerve would cause loss only of abduction of the ipsilateral eye. A large lesion of the lateral pontine tegmentum, damaging either the abducens nucleus or the paramedian pontine reticular formation, results in loss of conjugate movements of *both* eyes toward that side. An injury of the medial longitudinal fasciculus, connecting the abducens and oculomotor nuclei, would only prevent adduction of the ipsilateral eye during contralateral gaze.

A lesion at the level of the midbrain, involving the oculomotor nerve either within the brain stem or after it exits, causes loss of elevation, depression, and adduction of the ipsilateral eye, as well as loss of the pupillary light response. Nevertheless, the opposite pupil will still constrict when a light is shined in the paralyzed eye (the consensual pupillary light response). This response indicates that the optic nerve is still intact, as is the dorsal midbrain and opposite third nerve.

Emergency Care of the Comatose Patient Can Be Lifesaving

Although the treatment of the comatose patient is beyond the scope of this book, it is important to understand that a careful examination of a comatose patient, based on the principles in this chapter, is crucial to the outcome of the illness. If the examination demonstrates a depressed level of consciousness but normal function of the brain stem systems that run alongside the ascending arousal system, then the cause of the coma is likely to be diffuse or metabolic impairment of the cerebral hemispheres. These patients require further evaluation with blood tests, scanning of the brain, and often examination of the cerebrospinal fluid during the next few

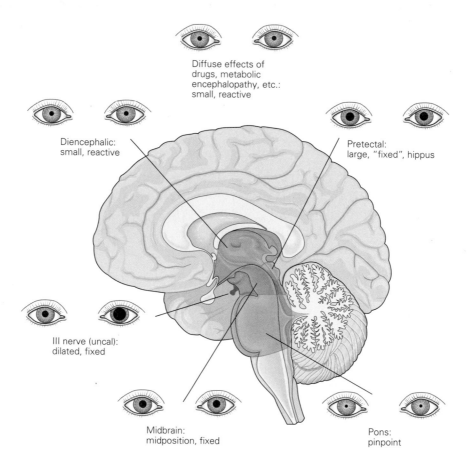

Diffuse effects of drugs, metabolic encephalopathy, etc.: small, reactive

Diencephalic: small, reactive

Pretectal: large, "fixed", hippus

III nerve (uncal): dilated, fixed

Midbrain: midposition, fixed

Pons: pinpoint

Figure 45-15 Pupillary response can help determine the level of the nervous system dysfunction in a comatose patient. In patients with depressed consciousness due to metabolic encephalopathy, drug ingestion, or diffuse pressure on the diencephalon, the pupils are slightly smaller than normal but respond vigorously to light (**top**). Pressure on the pretectal area (eg, from a pineal tumor) prevents visual stimulation from causing pupillary constriction, resulting in large, unreactive pretectal pupils. Injury to the oculomotor (III) nerve itself is usually one-sided, because of swelling in the ipsilateral hemisphere causing the uncus (the medial edge of the temporal lobe) to herniate through the tentorial opening and crush the oculomotor nerve.

A unilateral large, unreactive pupil is an ominous sign that the brain stem is about to be compressed from above. Damage to the midbrain tegmentum itself causes complete loss of pupillary response to light, although the pupils may dilate if a painful stimulus (eg, pinching the neck) is applied, as a purely sympathetic response (the ciliospinal response). Injury to the **pons** may result in pinpoint pupils, which can be seen with a magnifying lens to respond slightly to light. **Pontine** injury not only disrupts the descending hypothalamic pupillodilator pathway but also interrupts ascending inputs to the Edinger-Westphal nucleus that inhibit its tone. (Adapted from Plum and Posner 1980.)

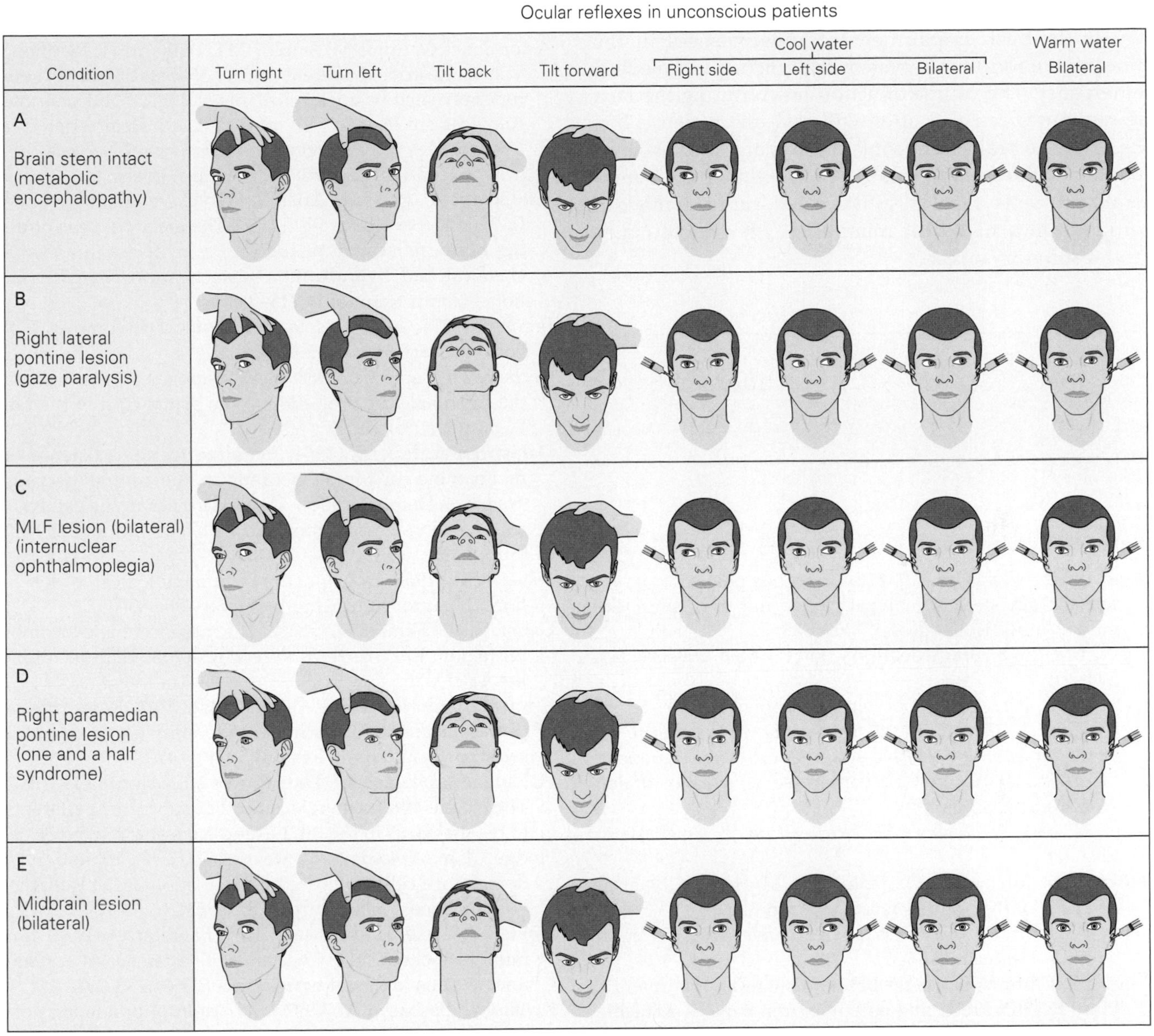

Ocular reflexes in unconscious patients

Figure 45-16 Oculomotor responses provide important information on the level of brain dysfunction in the comatose patient.

A. In patients with metabolic encephalopathy, in whom the brain stem is intact, the eyes rotate counter to the direction of head movement (the *doll's head maneuver*). Placing cold water in the external ear canal (*caloric stimulation*) activates the semicircular canals and causes the eyes to turn to the ipsilateral side, whereas cold water in both ears causes the eyes to look downward and warm water causes the eyes to look upward. In a patient who is feigning unconsciousness, doll's head eye movements are almost impossible to reproduce, and caloric stimulation produces nystagmus.

B. Damage to the lateral pons removes the vestibular input on one side and will block caloric responses in that ear, but the eyes will still show doll's head responses because of input from the other ear. More extensive injury to the pons on one

side will cause loss of movement of either eye to that side (*gaze paralysis*).

C. An injury to the medial longitudinal fasciculus (**MLF**), which connects the oculomotor nuclei with the pontine lateral gaze system, results in loss of adduction of the ipsilateral eye (*internuclear ophthalmoplegia*).

D. The combination of gaze paralysis in one direction and internuclear ophthalmoplegia in the other direction indicates an extensive paramedian pontine lesion. As a result, one eye does not adduct and the other does not abduct or adduct, termed by C. Miller Fisher "the one-and-a-half syndrome."

E. A lesion involving the midbrain oculomotor nuclei allows abduction of the eyes but not adduction or vertical eye movement. (Adapted from Plum and Posner 1980.)

hours to determine the cause of the coma and correct it.

In contrast, impairment of consciousness in the presence of focal brain system dysfunction is a medical emergency. The course of action taken during the next few minutes can and often will save the patient's life. Because the brain stem contains so many vital systems packed within such a small area, pressure on the midbrain or pons that is sufficient to cause coma can progress in a matter of minutes to irreversible injury and respiratory arrest.

Clifford B. Saper

Selected Readings

Basbaum AI, Fields HL. 1984. Endogenous pain control systems: brain stem spinal pathways and endorphin circuitry. Annu Rev Neurosci 7:309–338.

Black PM. 1978. Brain death. N Engl J Med 299:338–344, 393–401.

Celesia GG, Breuer AC, Goldblatt D, Rottenberg DA, Saper CB, Scneck SA, Schutta H, Trauner DA, Whitehouse PJ. 1993. Persistent vegetative state: report of the American Neurological Association committee on ethical affairs. Ann Neurol 33:386–390.

Fisch BJ. 1991. *Spehlmann's EEG Primer,* 2nd ed. Amsterdam: Elsevier.

Hökfelt T, Johansson O, Goldstein M. 1984. Chemical anatomy of the brain. Science 225:1326–1334.

Jennett B, Plum F. 1972. Persistent vegetative state after brain damage. Lancet 1:734–737.

Levy DE, Caronna JJ, Singer BH, Lapinski RH, Frydman H, Plum F. 1985. Predicting outcome from hypoxic-ischemic coma. JAMA 253:1420–1426.

Max MB, Lynch SA, Muir J, Shoaf SE, Smoller B, Dubner R. 1992. Effects of desipramine, amitriptyline, and fluoxetine on pain in diabetic neuropathy. N Engl J Med 326:1250–1256.

Plum F, Posner JB. 1980. *The Diagnosis of Stupor and Coma,* 3rd ed., Philadelphia: Davis.

Saper CB. 1987. Diffuse cortical projection systems: Anatomical organization and role in cortical function. In: F Plum (ed). *Handbook of Physiology.* V, *The Nervous System,* pp. 169–210. Bethesda, MD: American Physiological Society.

Steriade M, Llinás RR. 1988. The functional states of the thalamus and the associated neuronal interplay. Physiol Rev 68:649–742.

Steriade M, McCormick DA, Sejnowski TJ. 1993. Thalamocortical oscillations in the sleeping and aroused brain. Science 262:679–685.

References

Aston-Jones G, Ennis M, Shipley MT, Williams JT, Pieribone V. 1990. Restricted afferent control of locus coeruleus neurones revealed by anatomical, physiological and pharmacological studies. In: CA Marsden, DJ Heal (eds). *The Pharmacology of Noradrenaline in the Central Nervous System,* pp. 187–247. Oxford: Oxford Univ. Press.

Bittencourt JC, Presse F, Arias C, Peto C, Vaughan J, Nahon JL, Vale W, Sawchenko PE. 1992. The melanin-concentrating hormone system of the rat brain: an immunohistochemical and hybridization histochemical characterization. J Comp Neurol 319:218–245.

Bremer F. 1935. Cerveau isolé et physiologie du sommeil. C R Soc Biol (Paris) 118:1235–1242.

Cechetto DF, Saper CB. 1988. Neurochemical organization of the hypothalamic projection to the spinal cord in the rat. J Comp Neurol 272:579–604.

Dahlström A, Fuxe K. 1964. Evidence for the existence of monoamine-containing neurons in the central nervous system. I. Demonstration of monoamines in the cell bodies of brain stem neurons. Acta Physiol Scand 232:1–55 (Suppl. 62).

Fisher CM. 1967. Some neuro-ophthalmological observations. J Neurol Neurosurg Psychiatry 30:383–392.

Garcia-Rill E, Skinner RD. 1987. The mesencephalic locomotor region. II. Projections to reticulospinal neurons. Brain Res 411:13–20.

Grant SJ, Aston-Jones G, Redmond DE Jr. 1988. Responses of primate locus ceruleus neurons to simple and complex sensory stimuli. Brain Res Bull 21:401–410.

Hallanger AE, Levey AI, Lee HJ, Rye DB, Wainer BH. 1987. The origins of cholinergic and other subcortical afferents to the thalamus in the rat. J Comp Neurol 262:105–124.

Hodge CJ Jr., Apkarian AV, Stevens RT. 1986. Inhibition of dorsal-horn cell responses by stimulation of the Kolliker-Fuse nucleus. J Neurosurg 65:825–833.

Hökfelt T, Fuxe K, Goldstein M, Johansson O. 1974. Immunohistochemical evidence for the existence of adrenaline neurons in the rat brain. Brain Res 66:235–251.

Kwiat GC, Basbaum AI. 1992. The origin of brainstem noradrenergic and serotonergic projections to the spinal cord dorsal horn in the rat. Somatosens Mot Res 9:157–173.

Lai YY, Siegel JM. 1990. Cardiovascular and muscle tone changes produced by microinjection of cholinergic and glutamatergic agonists in dorsolateral pons and medial medulla. Brain Res 514:27–36.

Lin JS, Sakai K, Jouvet M. 1988. Evidence for histaminergic arousal mechanisms in the hypothalamus of cat. Neuropharmacology 27:111–122.

Lindvall O, Bjorklund A. 1974. The organization of the ascending catecholamine neuron systems in the rat brain as revealed by the glyoxylic acid fluorescence method. Acta Physiol Scand Suppl 412:1–48.

Loewy AD, McKellar S, Saper CB. 1979. Direct projections from the A5 catecholamine cell group to the intermediolateral cell column. Brain Res 174:309–314.

Magoun HW, Rhines R. 1946. An inhibitory mechanism in

the bulbar reticular formation. J Neurophysiol 9:165–171.

Mason P, Back SA, Fields HL. 1992. A confocal laser microscopic study of enkephalin-immunoreactive appositions onto physiologically identified neurons in the rostral ventromedial medulla. J Neurosci 12:4023–4036.

McCarley RW, Nelson JP, Hobson JA. 1978. Ponto-geniculo-occipital (PGO) burst neurons: correlative evidence for neuronal generators of PGO waves. Science 201:269–272.

Mesulam MM, Mufson EJ, Levey AI, Wainer BH. 1983. Cholinergic innervation of cortex by the basal forebrain: cytochemistry and cortical connections of the septal area, diagonal band nuclei, nucleus basalis (substantia innominata) and hypothalamus in the rhesus monkey. J Comp Neurol 214:170–197.

Moruzzi G, Magoun HW. 1949. Brain stem reticular formation and activation of the EEG. Electroencephalogr Clin Neurophysiol 1:455–473.

Panula P, Airaksinen MS, Pirvola U, Kotilainen E. 1990. A histamine-containing neuronal system in human brain. Neuroscience 34:127–132.

Rye DB, Saper CB, Lee HJ, Wainer BH. 1987. Pedunculopontine tegmental nucleus of the rat: cytoarchitecture, cytochemistry, and some extrapyramidal connections of the mesopontine tegmentum. J Comp Neurol 259:483–528.

Saper CB. 1984. Organization of cerebral cortical afferent systems in the rat. II. Magnocellular basal nucleus. J Comp Neurol 222:313–342.

Saper CB. 1985. Organization of cerebral cortical afferent systems in the rat. II. Hypothalamocortical projections. J Comp Neurol 237:21–46.

Saper CB, Plum F. 1985. Disorders of consciousness. In: JAM Frederiks (ed). Handbook of Clinical Neurology. Vol 45, Clinical Neuropsychology, pp. 107–128. Amsterdam: Elsevier.

Skagerberg G, Lindvall O. 1985. Organization of diencephalic dopamine neurons projecting to the spinal cord in the rat. Brain Res 342:340–351.

Stevens RT, Hodge CJ Jr., Apkarian AV. 1982. Kolliker-Fuse nucleus: the principal source of pontine catecholaminergic cells projecting to the lumbar spinal cord of cat. Brain Res 239:589–594.

Wilson MA, Molliver ME. 1991. The organization of serotonergic projections to cerebral cortex in primates: retrograde transport studies. Neuroscience 44:555–570.

46

Seizures and Epilepsy

UNTIL RECENTLY, ANALYSIS of brain function relied in large part on observations of the behavioral consequences of brain damage caused by strokes or trauma. These natural "experiments" provided early evidence that distinct brain regions subserve specific functions. Also important in this regard has been the analysis of patients with seizures and epilepsy, because the behavioral consequences of a seizure depend on where in the brain a seizure originates. However in ancient times the dramatic, sometimes bizarre, behavioral manifestations of seizures initially created misperceptions of their neurological origins.

Seizures have fascinated and plagued humanity since antiquity. The Greeks in the time of Hippocrates (circa 400 BC) were aware of the relationship between head injuries and seizure activity involving movements of the opposite side of the body. Despite the observed association with physical injury, epilepsy was widely believed to occur in individuals possessed by evil spirits. Seizures were also associated with prescience or special creative powers. For example, many important historical figures in science, politics, and the arts are thought to have been epileptics. However, in earlier times, epilepsy appears to have been defined according to criteria quite different from those used today; other causes of episodic unconsciousness such as syncope, mass hysteria, or psychogenic seizures were almost certainly called epilepsy. Moreover, historical writings typically described generalized convulsive seizures, and it is thus likely that many cases of partial seizures were misdiagnosed or never diagnosed. Even today, it can be difficult for physicians to distinguish between episodic loss of consciousness and the various types of seizures.

The modern neurobiological analysis of epilepsy began with John Hughlings Jackson's work at Queen Square in London in the 1860s. Jackson realized that seizures need not involve loss of consciousness but could be associated with focal symptoms, such as the jerking of an arm. This observation was the first formal recognition of what we now call partial (or focal) seizures. He also observed patients whose seizures began with focal neurological symptoms, then progressed to convulsions with loss of consciousness (a so-called Jacksonian march). Another important early development was the first surgical treatment for epilepsy by Victor Horsley, who in 1886 resected cortex adjacent to a depressed skull fracture and cured a patient with focal motor seizures. The modern surgical treatment for epilepsy, however, dates to the work of Wilder Penfield and Herbert Jasper in Montreal in the early 1950s. Medical innovations include the first use of phenobarbital as an anticonvulsant in 1912 by A. Hauptmann, the development of electroencephalography by Hans Berger in 1929, and the discovery of phenytoin (Dilantin) by Houston Merritt and Tracey Putnam in 1937. The physiological features of seizures are not the only consideration in the care and management of patients with epilepsy. Psychosocial factors are also extremely important. In particular, the diagnosis of epilepsy still carries a social stigma that can affect all aspects of everyday life including driving, employment, and educational opportunities.

Classification of Seizures and the Epilepsies Is Important for Pathogenesis and Treatment

Not all seizures are the same. Thus an understanding of the pathophysiology of seizures must first take into account their clinical features. Seizures and the chronic condition of repetitive seizures (epilepsy) are common clinical problems. Based on epidemiological studies in the United States, about 3% of all people living to the age of 80 will be diagnosed with epilepsy. The highest incidence occurs in young children and the elderly. In many respects, seizures represent a prototypic neurological disease in that the symptoms include both "positive" and "negative" sensory or motor manifestations. Examples of positive signs that can occur during a seizure include the perception of flashing lights or the jerking of an arm. Negative signs can include a slowing of normal brain function resulting in depression of consciousness or even transient blindness or paralysis. These symptoms underscore another general feature of seizures: The symptoms are dependent on the location and extent of brain tissue that is affected. Finally, the manifestations of seizures result in part from the involvement of normal tissue with normal excitability.

Seizures can be classified clinically into two categories: partial and generalized (Table 46-1). This simple classification has proved extremely useful to clinicians because the effectiveness of anticonvulsant medications depends on the type of seizure.

Table 46-1 International Classification of Seizures and Epilepsies

---

Seizures

I. Partial (focal) seizures

    A. Simple partial seizures (with motor, sensory, autonomic, or psychological symptoms)

    B. Complex partial seizures

    C. Complex partial seizures evolving to secondarily generalized seizures

II. Generalized seizures (convulsive or nonconvulsive)

    A. Absence

        1. Typical (petit mal)

        2. Atypical

    B. Myoclonic

    C. Clonic

    D. Tonic

    E. Tonic-clonic (grand mal)

    F. Atonic

III. Unclassified

Epilepsies (abbreviated classification)

1. Localization-related epilepsies and syndromes

    1.1 Idiopathic with age-related onset (eg, benign childhood epilepsy with centrotemporal spikes)

    1.2 Symptomatic (eg, post-traumatic epilepsy)

2. Generalized epilepsies and syndromes

    2.1 Idiopathic with age-related onset (eg, juvenile myoclonic epilepsy)

    2.2 Idiopathic and/or symptomatic (eg, Lennox-Gastaut syndrome)

    2.3 Symptomatic

3. Epilepsies and syndromes undetermined with respect to 1 or 2

    3.1 With both partial and generalized seizures (eg, neonatal seizures)

    3.2 Without unequivocal generalized or partial features

4. Special syndromes (eg, febrile convulsions)

Commission on Classification and Terminology of the International League Against Epilepsy, 1981; Commission on Classification and Terminology of the International League Against Epilepsy, 1985.

Partial seizures originate in a small group of neurons that constitute a seizure focus. Thus the symptomatology depends on the location of the focus within the brain. Partial seizures can be either *simple partial* (with-

A Standard electrode placement

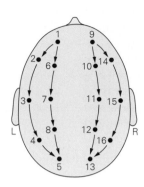

B EEG of awake human

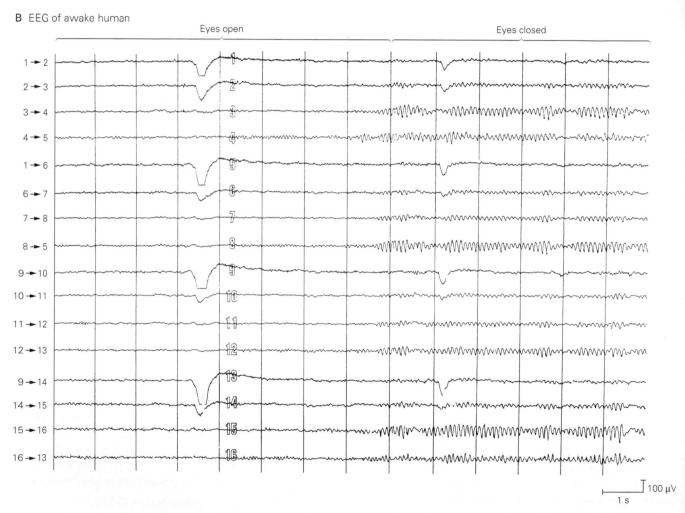

Figure 46-1 The normal electroencephalogram (EEG) in an awake human subject.

A. A standard set of placements for EEG electrodes over the surface of the scalp. The electrical activity between electrode pairs in this bipolar montage is compared.

B. EEG activity of an awake human subject. At the beginning of the recording, the EEG shows low-voltage (circa 20 µV) activity

over the surface of the scalp. The **vertical lines** are placed at 1-s intervals. During the first 8 s the subject rested quietly with eyes open, then closed his eyes. Note the development of larger-amplitude (8–10 Hz) activity over the occipital region (traces 3→4, 4→5, 8→5, 12→13, 15→16, and 16→13). This is the normal alpha rhythm characteristic of the relaxed, wakeful state. Note the slow large-amplitude eye blink artifact at 3.5 s and the artifact on eye closure at 9 s. Calibration 1 s, 100 µV.

out alteration of consciousness) or *complex partial* (with alteration of consciousness). An example of a partial seizure is localized jerking beginning in the right hand and progressing to clonic movements (ie, jerks) of the entire right arm. (Such a seizure formerly was called a focal motor seizure.) If a partial seizure progresses further, the patient may lose consciousness, fall to the ground, rigidly extend all extremities (*tonic phase*), then have jerks in all extremities (*clonic phase*). These symptoms are classified as a secondarily generalized tonic-clonic seizure (formerly called a grand mal seizure).

Symptoms preceding the onset of a partial seizure are called *auras*. Auras commonly include abnormal sensations such as a sense of fear, a rising feeling in the abdomen, or even a specific odor. The aura is due to electrical activity originating from the seizure focus and thus represents the earliest manifestations of a partial seizure. The time after a partial seizure before the patient returns to normal neurological function is called the *postictal period*.

Generalized seizures begin without a preceding aura or focal seizure and involve both hemispheres from the onset. They can be further divided into convulsive or nonconvulsive types, depending on whether the seizure is associated with tonic or clonic movements. The prototypic nonconvulsive generalized seizure is the typical *absence seizure* (formerly called petit mal) found in children. These seizures begin abruptly, usually last less than 10 s, are associated with cessation of all motor activity, and result in loss of consciousness. Unlike a partial seizure, there is no aura or postictal period. Patients may exhibit mild motor manifestations such as eye blinking but do not fall or have tonic-clonic movements. Typical absence seizures have very distinctive electrical characteristics on the electroencephalogram (EEG).

Other generalized seizures can consist only of motor movements (myoclonic, clonic, or tonic) or a sudden loss of motor tone (atonic). However, the most common generalized seizure is the tonic-clonic, or grand mal, seizure. These convulsive seizures also begin abruptly, often with a grunt or cry as tonic contraction of the diaphragm and thorax creates a forced expiration. It is during the tonic phase that the patient may fall to the ground rigid with clenched jaw, lose bladder or bowel control, and become blue *(cyanotic)*. The tonic phase typically lasts 30 s before evolving into clonic jerking of the extremities lasting 1–2 min. This active phase of the generalized tonic-clonic seizure is followed by a postictal phase during which the patient is sleepy and may complain of headache and muscle soreness. Clinically, it can be difficult to distinguish a primary generalized tonic-clonic seizures from a secondarily generalized tonic-clonic seizure with a brief aura. This distinction is not simply academic, as it can be vital to choosing proper treatment as well as pinpointing the underlying cause.

Numerous factors that affect the type and severity of seizures are ignored in the seizure classification shown in Table 46-1. Such factors as the underlying etiology of the seizures, the age of onset, and family history all contribute to the clinical characteristics of the syndrome of recurrent seizures. Recurrent unprovoked seizures constitute the minimal criteria for the diagnosis of *epilepsy*. The factors influencing seizure type and severity can often be recognized in patterns of symptoms resulting in the identification of an *epilepsy syndrome*. Thus a classification of the epilepsies (Table 46-1) continues to evolve, principally based on clinical observation rather than a precise cellular, molecular, or genetic understanding of the underlying pathophysiology. The primary variables are the presence of a focal brain abnormality (localization-related) and whether there is an identifiable cause (symptomatic) or not (idiopathic). The great majority of adult-onset epilepsies are classified as symptomatic, localization-related epilepsy. This category includes such causes as trauma, stroke, tumors, and infections. Understanding the epilepsy syndrome has important implications for prognosis and, for some cases, therapy. Unfortunately many epilepsy syndromes do not fit neatly in this scheme, as indicated by the need for categories 3 and 4 in Table 46-1. One expects that this classification will be greatly refined as the criteria become based on the underlying etiologies rather than clinical observation.

The Electroencephalogram Represents the Collective Behavior of Cortical Neurons

Neurons are excitable cells. Thus it is logical to assume that seizures result either directly or indirectly from a change in the excitability of single neurons or groups of neurons. This view dominated early experimental studies of seizures. Electrical recordings of brain activity can be made with intracellular electrodes that record the electrical activity of individual neurons or with extracellular electrodes that sense action potentials in nearby neurons. Extracellular recording can also detect the synchronized activity of large numbers of cells; such signals are called *field potentials*. At the slow time resolution of extracellular recording (hundreds of milliseconds to seconds), field potentials appear as single electrical transients called *spikes*. These macroscopic events should not be confused with spikes of single neurons, which represent individual action potentials lasting only 1 or 2 ms. The EEG represents a set of field potentials as recorded by multiple electrodes on the surface of the scalp. The set

Box 46-1 The Nature of the EEG

The contribution of single neuron activity to the EEG can be understood by examining a simplified cortical circuit and some basic electrical principles. Pyramidal neurons are the major projection neurons in the cortex. The apical dendrites of pyramidal cells, which are oriented perpendicular to the cell surface, receive a variety of synaptic inputs. Synaptic activity in the pyramidal cells is the principle source of EEG activity.

To understand the contribution of a single neuron to the EEG, consider the flow of current produced by an *excitatory synaptic potential (EPSP)* on the apical dendrite of a cortical pyramidal neuron (Figure 46-2). Current flows into the dendrite at the site of generation of the EPSP, creating a current sink. It then must complete a loop by flowing down the dendrite and back out across the membrane at other sites, creating a current source. The size of the voltage created by the synaptic current is approximately predicted by Ohm's Law ($V = IR$ where V is voltage, I is current, and R is resistance). Because the membrane resistance (R_m) is much larger than that of the salt solution that constitutes the extracellular medium (R_e), the voltage recorded across the membrane with an intracellular

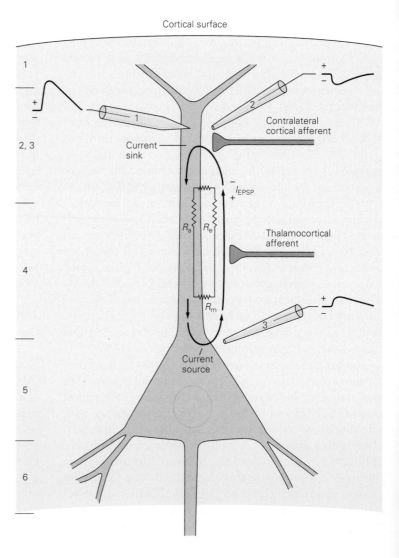

Cortical surface

Figure 46-2 The pattern of electrical current flow for an excitatory postsynaptic potential (EPSP) on the apical dendrite of a pyramidal neuron in the cerebral cortex. The activity is detected by an intracellular electrode (**1**), an extracellular electrode positioned near the site of the EPSP in layer 2 of the cortex (**2**), and an extracellular electrode near the cell body in layer 5 (**3**). At the site of the EPSP (sink), current flows across the cell membrane into the cytoplasm. The current (I_{EPSP}) then flows down the dendritic cytoplasm and completes the loop by exiting through the membrane (source). Note that the polarity of the potentials recorded by extracellular electrodes at the sink and the source are opposite. The intracellular electrode has the same polarity regardless of the site of the input. R_m, R_a, and R_e are the resistances of the membrane, cytoplasm, and extracellular space, respectively.

electrode (electrode 1) is also larger than at an extracellular electrode positioned near the current sink (electrode 2).

At the site of generation of an EPSP the extracellular electrode detects current flowing away from the electrode into the cytoplasm as a downward deflection. However, an extracellular electrode near the source has an opposite polarity (compare electrodes 2 and 3, Figure 46-2). The situation is reversed if the site of the EPSP generation is on a proximal dendrite. In the cortex excitatory inputs from the contralateral hemisphere contact the pyramidal neurons primarily on distal parts of the

dendrite in layers 2 and 3, whereas thalamocortical inputs terminate in layer 4. The activity measured at a surface EEG electrode will have opposite polarities for these two inputs, even though the basic electrical event, membrane depolarization, is the same. EPSPs in superficial layers and *inhibitory postsynaptic potentials (IPSPs)* in deeper layers appear as upward (negative) potentials, whereas EPSPs in deeper layers and IPSPs in superficial layers have downward (positive) potentials (Figure 46-3). Thus cortical synaptic events cannot be unambiguously determined from EEG recordings alone.

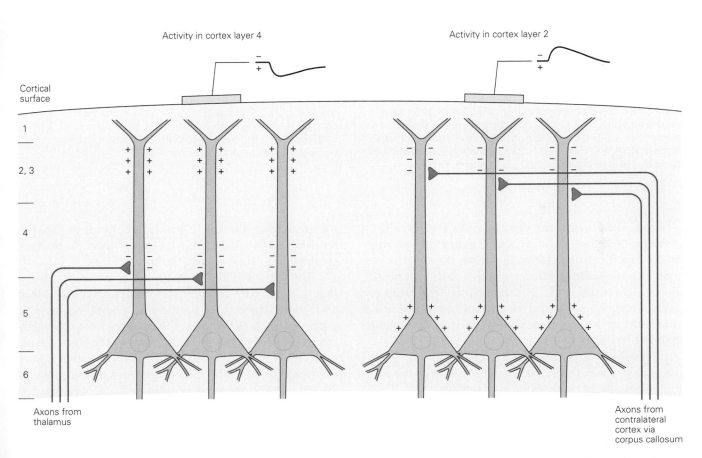

Figure 46-3 The polarity of the surface EEG depends on the location of the synaptic activity within the cortex. A thalamocortical excitatory input in layer 4 (**left**) causes a downward deflection at the surface EEG electrode because the EEG electrode is nearer to the source. In contrast, excitatory input from the contralateral hemisphere in layer 2 (**right**) causes an upward deflection because it is nearer to the sink.

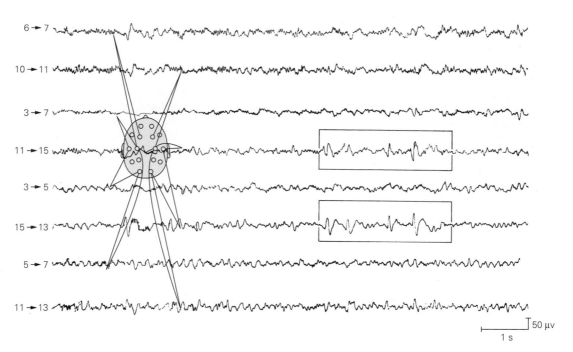

Figure 46-4 Electroencephalogram (EEG) activity in a patient with epilepsy shows focal sharp waves in the EEG electrodes located over the right temporal area (enclosed in boxes). Note that this paroxysmal activity arises suddenly and disrupts the normal background EEG pattern. The focal abnormality suggests that the seizure focus in this patient is in the right temporal lobe. Because the patient had no clinical seizures during the recording, these are interictal spikes. (Adapted from Lothman and Collins 1990.)

of locations for electrodes placed on the skull is called a *montage*. Montages may consist of monopolar arrangements in which each electrode records the electrical activity at a site *(active electrode)* relative to a distant site *(indifferent electrode),* such as the ear lobe. Alternatively, pairs of scalp electrodes can be interconnected and in this case both electrodes are active. A typical bipolar montage is shown in Figure 46-1A.

The electrical activity of the EEG is an attenuated measure of the extracellular current flow from the summated activity of many neurons. However, not all cells contribute equally to the EEG. The surface EEG predominantly reflects the activity of cortical neurons close to the EEG electrode. Thus deep structures such as the hippocampus, thalamus, or brain stem do not contribute directly to the surface EEG. The contributions of individual nerve cells to the EEG as recorded at the cortical surface are schematized in Box 46-1.

Because the electrical activity originates in neurons in the underlying brain tissue, the waveform recorded by the surface electrode depends on the orientation and distance of the electrical source with respect to the electrode. The EEG signal is inevitably distorted by the filtering and attenuation produced by intervening layers of tissue and bone, which act like resistors and capacitors in an electric circuit. Thus the amplitude of EEG potentials (microvolts) is much smaller than the voltage changes in a single neuron (millivolts).

The surface EEG shows typical patterns of activity that can be correlated with various stages of sleep and wakefulness, and with some pathophysiological processes such as seizures. EEG patterns are characterized by the frequency and amplitude of the electrical activity. The normal human EEG shows activity over the range of 1–30 Hz with amplitudes in the range of 20–100 μV. The observed frequencies have been divided into several groups: alpha (8–13 Hz), beta (13–30 Hz), delta (0.5–4 Hz), and theta (4–7 Hz). Alpha waves of moderate amplitude are typical of relaxed wakefulness and are most prominent over parietal and occipital sites. Lower-amplitude beta activity is more prominent in frontal areas and over other regions during intense mental activity. Alerting a relaxed subject results in so-called desynchronization of the EEG, with a reduction in alpha activity and an increase in beta (Figure 46-1B). Theta and delta waves are normal during drowsiness and early slow-wave sleep, but if present during wakefulness represent a sign of brain dysfunction.

As neuronal aggregates become synchronized, the summated currents become larger and can be seen as abrupt changes from the baseline activity. Such "paroxysmal" activity can be normal, eg, the 1–2 s, 7–15 Hz episodes of high-amplitude activity that represent sleep spindles. However, a sharp wave or EEG spike can also represent a clue to the location of a seizure focus in a patient with epilepsy. An example of localized high-amplitude sharp waves is shown in Figure 46-4.

Partial Seizures Originate Within a Small Group of Neurons Known as a Seizure Focus

Despite the range of seizure types that can be distinguished by their clinical features, the generation of seizure activity can be understood by considering two characteristic electrographic patterns: the partial seizure and the (primary) generalized seizure. These two seizure types have different pathophysiological substrates.

The defining feature of partial (and secondarily generalized) seizures is that the abnormal electrical activity originates from a seizure focus. The *seizure focus* is a small collection of neurons that trigger enhanced (epileptiform) excitability. Enhanced excitability may result from many different factors such as altered cellular properties or altered synaptic connections caused by a local scar, blood clot, or tumor. A discrete focus in the primary motor cortex may cause twitching of a finger or jerking of a limb (simple partial seizure), whereas a focus in the limbic system is often associated with unusual behaviors or an alteration of consciousness (complex partial seizure). The phases in the development of a partial seizure can be arbitrarily divided into the interictal period, followed by neuronal synchronization, seizure spread, and finally secondary generalization. Different factors contribute to each of these phases. Most of our knowledge about the pathophysiology of seizures is derived from studies of animal models of partial seizures. In these studies, a seizure is induced by acute injection of a convulsant agent or by focal electrical stimulation. This approach has provided a good understanding of electrical events within the focus during a seizure as well as during the interictal period (Figure 46-5). The development of in vitro tissue slice preparations has also been particularly valuable in the study of seizures (Box 46-2).

Neurons in a Seizure Focus Have Characteristic Activity

Experimental studies of partial seizures have long been directed at how electrical activity in a single neuron or group of neurons leads to the generation of a seizure.

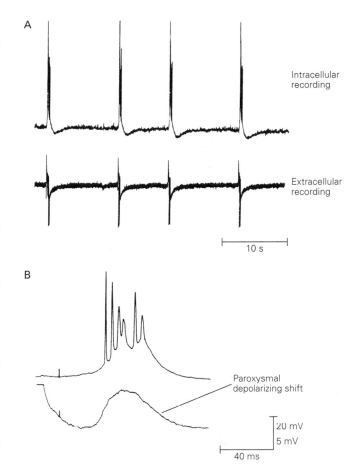

Figure 46-5 Interictal spikes correspond to synchronized discharges of a group of neurons in an in vitro brain slice. (Adapted from Wong et al. 1984.)

A. Rhythmic discharges are present in the intracellular recording from a normal hippocampal pyramidal cell (**top trace**). The discharge of many neurons is manifest as a synchronous interictal spike as recorded by an extracellular electrode (**bottom trace**).

B. The brain slice is perfused with bicuculline, which blocks inhibition mediated by γ-aminobutyric acid (GABA)_A receptors. A hippocampal pyramidal cell is depolarized and fires several superimposed action potentials (**top trace**). Injection of current to hyperpolarize the membrane and prevent action potential firing reveals the large paroxysmal depolarizing shift characteristic of neurons in a seizure focus (**bottom trace**).

Each neuron within a seizure focus has a stereotypic and synchronized electrical response called *the paroxysmal depolarizing shift* (PDS). The PDS consists of a sudden, large (20–40 mV), long-lasting (50–200 ms) depolarization (see Figure 46-5B), which triggers a train of action potentials at the peak of the PDS. The PDS is followed by an afterhyperpolarization. The PDS and the afterhyperpolariza-

Box 46-2 Mammalian Brain Slice Preparation

The tissue slice technique has revolutionized the study of the electrophysiological properties of mammalian neurons. Brain slices, which range from 70–400 μM thick, are prepared by quickly removing the brain and immersing it into chilled saline

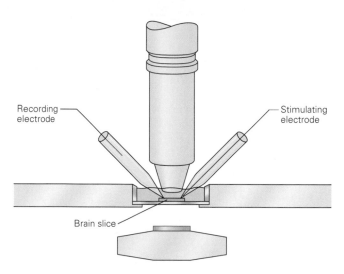

Figure 46-6 Set-up for recording from neurons in a brain slice. The slice is mounted in a chamber to the X-Y stage of a microscope. A water-immersion objective allows visualization of the slice at high power through the saline solution. Separate stimulating and recording electrodes can be placed in the tissue under direct visualization through a microscope. (Adapted from Konnerth 1990.)

and then sectioning the tissue with a special type of microtome. This technique preserves the basic circuitry of neurons in the slice. The slice is placed in a recording chamber (Figure 46-6) through which oxygenated saline solution is circulated.

There are two principal advantages to recording from neurons in tissue slices. First, more stable electrophysiological recordings can be made because there are no mechanical pulsations resulting from respiration or the pumping of blood. This allows recording from very fine neuronal processes, such as dendrites. Second, the tissue is visualized under a microscope. When the microscope is equipped with special optics, for example Nomarski optics, individual neurons actually can be seen (Figure 46-7). Direct visualization of neurons allows them to be identified from their morphology or from their efferent projections, for example, by retrogradely filing a neuron's cell body with a fluorescent compound before the slice is removed from the brain. In addition, direct visualization facilitates patch clamping of individual neurons.

Recording from brain slices has been used to investigate various aspects of the function of mammalian neurons, including the response of neurons to different neurotransmitters and neuromodulators and the properties of single channels. Through the use of tissue slice techniques, cell and molecular biological approaches can be applied to virtually any part of the mammalian brain. Information obtained from recordings made in brain slices has provided important insights into such problems as synaptic plasticity, the mechanisms of epilepsy, and the actions of drugs on the brain.

A

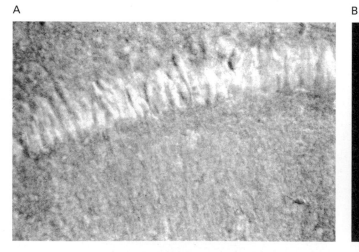

B

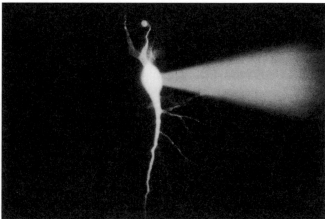

Figure 46-7 Photograph of a rat hippocampal slice. (Courtesy of Dr. A. Konnerth.)

A. Nomarski image from the cut surface of the slice revealing the pyramidal cell layer in the CA1 region of the hippocampus.

B. A single pyramidal cell is filled with the fluorescent dye

Lucifer yellow. The upside-down configuration of the hippocampus results in the large apical dendrite projecting toward the bottom of the photograph, and the basilar dendrites toward the top. The large neuronal cell body can be seen at the tip of the dye-containing pipette.

tion are shaped by the intrinsic membrane properties of the neuron (eg, voltage-gated Na^+, K^+, and Ca^{2+} channels) and synaptic inputs from excitatory (glutamatergic) and inhibitory (GABAergic) neurons, respectively. The depolarizing phase results primarily from activation of excitatory glutamate-mediated channels such as AMPA (α-amino-3-hydroxy- 5-methylisoxazole-4-propionate) and NMDA (N-methyl-D-aspartate) receptor-channels as well as voltage-gated Ca^{2+} channels (Figure 46-8A). The NMDA receptor-channel is particularly suited to enhance excitability because its contribution is increased by membrane depolarization, and it allows Ca^{2+} to enter the neuron.

Although most neurons normally do not exhibit PDS behavior, some (such as hippocampal pyramidal neurons in the CA3 region) do under normal conditions. Likewise, the normal response of a typical cortical pyramidal neuron to excitatory input is an excitatory postsynaptic potential (EPSP) followed by an inhibitory postsynaptic potential (IPSP) (because of the basic circuitry shown in Figure 46-8B). Thus the PDS can be viewed as a gross exaggeration of the normal depolarizing and hyperpolarizing components observed in neurons in a typical cortical circuit.

The afterhyperpolarization limits the duration of the PDS; its gradual disappearance is the most important factor in the onset of a clinical seizure, as discussed later in this chapter. The afterhyperpolarization is generated primarily by calcium- and voltage-dependent K^+ channels as well as GABA-mediated chloride ($GABA_A$) and K^+ ($GABA_B$) conductances (Figure 46-8A). The Ca^{2+} entry through voltage-dependent Ca^{2+} channels and NMDA channels triggers calcium-dependent channels, particularly calcium-dependent K^+ channels. This alternating sequence of depolarization and hyperpolarization is driven by incoming synaptic activity. Thus it is not surprising that many convulsants act by either enhancing excitation or blocking inhibition. Conversely, drugs that block excitation or enhance inhibition are effective anticonvulsants. For example, the benzodiazepines diazepam (Valium) and lorazepam (Ativan) enhance $GABA_A$-mediated inhibition and are the standard emergency treatment for prolonged repetitive seizures. The commonly used anticonvulsants phenytoin (Dilantin) and carbamazepine (Tegretol) cause a use-dependent reduction in voltage-dependent Na^+ channels.

Many other factors also can influence the excitability of neurons within the seizure focus. Examples include the contribution of glia to potassium homeostasis and neurotransmitter uptake, as well as the action of membrane ion pumps to remove ions that accumulate because of the excess electrical activity. The increase in extracellular potassium that accompanies electrical ac-

tivity depolarizes neurons and thus enhances excitability. Under normal circumstances, uptake by glial cells buffers this potassium. Whether glia within seizure foci function normally is not clear. Calcium signaling through glia networks may be a factor in generating seizures. Many factors contribute to PDS and after hyperpolarization; the contribution of each factor may vary considerably in a particular situation.

Synchronization Results From the Breakdown of Surround Inhibition

As long as the abnormal electrical activity is restricted to 1000 or so neurons that constitute the seizure focus, there are no clinical manifestations. The synchronized activity of this small neuronal ensemble can sometimes be detected at the surface of the skull as an interictal spike or a sharp wave on the EEG (see Figure 46-4). During the interictal period the abnormal activity is confined to the seizure focus by the afterhyperpolarization. The afterhyperpolarization is particularly dependent on intact feed-forward and feedback inhibition by GABA-ergic inhibitory interneurons. This circuitry provides a powerful "inhibitory surround" (Figure 46-9). Although this inhibition can be diagrammed simply (see Figure 46-8B), the morphology and connectivity of inhibitory neurons in the cortex is considerably more complex (Box 46-3).

During the development of a focal seizure the surround inhibition is overcome, the afterhyperpolarization gradually disappears in individual neurons, and the seizure begins to spread beyond the original focus (Figure 46-12). In individual neurons the membrane repolarization fails and nearly continuous high-frequency action potentials are generated. What causes the breakdown of surround inhibition?

The most important factor appears to be that GABA-ergic transmission is quite labile; intense discharges result in the failure of the GABA response, although the interneurons remain viable. Whether this labile behavior results from changes in the release of GABA (presynaptic mechanisms) or a change in GABA-ergic receptors (postsynaptic mechanisms) remains unclear. Other factors that may contribute to the loss of surround inhibition include chronic changes in dendritic structure, the density of receptors or channels, or extracellular ions, as mentioned above. Prolonged action potential discharges are also transmitted to distant sites in the brain, which may trigger trains of action potentials in neurons that project back to the neurons in the seizure focus (back-propagation). Reciprocal connections between the neocortex and the thalamus may be particularly important in this regard.

A   Interictal PDS within seizure focus

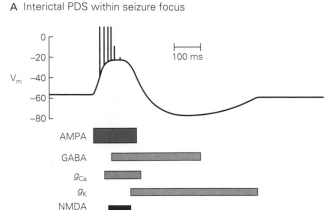

B   Basic cortical circuit

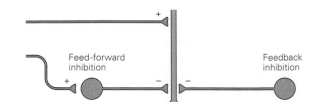

Figure 46-8 The conductances that underlie the paroxysmal depolarizing shift of a neuron in a seizure focus in a simple cortical circuit.

A. The paroxysmal depolarizing shift (**PDS**) consists of a large depolarization that triggers a burst of action potentials. The depolarization is largely dependent on α-amino-3-hydroxy-5-methylisoxazole-4-propionate (**AMPA**) and N-methyl-D-aspartate (**NMDA**) channels activated by the excitatory neurotransmitter glutamate and by voltage-dependent Ca^{2+} channels (g_{Ca}). After the depolarization, the cell is hyperpolarized by activation of

GABA receptors (both GABA$_A$ and GABA$_B$) as well as voltage- and calcium-dependent K$^+$ channels (g_K). (Adapted from Lothman 1993a.)

B. A simplified version of the circuitry impinging on a cortical pyramidal neuron. The **pink** terminals are excitatory, whereas the **gray** terminals are inhibitory. Recurrent axon branches activate inhibitory neurons and cause **feedback inhibition** of the pyramidal neuron. Extrinsic excitatory inputs can also activate feed-forward inhibition.

Despite our understanding of the mechanisms that cause the surround inhibition to break down, we still do not know what causes a seizure to occur at any particular moment. As clinical factors such as stress and sleep deprivation can trigger seizures in some patients, it is possible that diffuse cortical cholinergic, nonadrenergic, or serotonergic projections may play crucial modulatory roles in some cases. In others sensory stimuli such as flashing lights can trigger seizures, suggesting that repeated excitation of some circuits causes a frequency-dependent change in excitability. Both NMDA-receptor activity and labile GABA-ergic inhibition change in a frequency-dependent manner providing one possible cellular mechanism for changing network excitability.

The Spread of Seizure Activity Involves Normal Cortical Circuitry

If activity in the seizure focus is sufficiently intense, the electrical activity begins to spread to other brain regions. The spread of seizure activity from the focus generally follows the same pathways as does normal cortical activity. For example, the primary motor and sensory cortex are organized into vertical columns that run from the pial surface to the underlying white matter. The major input to the sensory cortex comes from

the thalamus and terminates in layer 4, whereas the output cells are in layer 5. The thalamus and cortex are connected by reciprocal thalamocortical pathways. Intracortical connections occur via short U fibers between adjacent sulci and via the corpus callosum, the major interhemispheric connection. Thus thalamocortical, subcortical, and transcallosal pathways can all become involved in seizure spread. Seizure activity can spread via various fiber pathways to involve other areas of the same hemisphere or across the corpus callosum to involve the contralateral hemisphere (Figure 46-13). Once both hemispheres become involved, the seizure has become "secondarily" generalized. At this point, the patient generally loses consciousness. Seizure spread usually occurs rapidly during a few seconds, but can also evolve over many minutes.

As the seizure begins to spread, the patient may experience an aura. If the seizure spreads slowly across the cortex, this may be manifest as a progression of clinical symptoms, called a *Jacksonian march* in the case of a simple partial seizure involving the motor cortex. Alternatively, partial seizures may quickly generalize with little or no warning. Rapid secondary generalization is more characteristic of seizures with a neocortical focus than those originating in the limbic system (in particular, the hippocampus and amygdala). An interesting

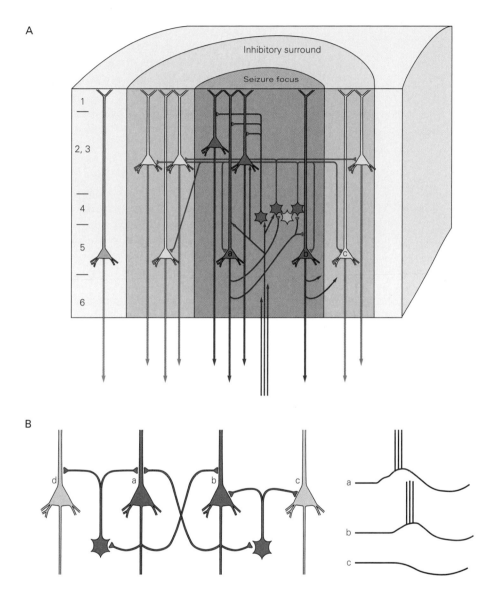

Figure 46-9 The spatial and temporal organization of a seizure focus depends on the interplay between excitation and inhibition in the neural circuits.

A. In this hypothetical neocortical seizure focus the neuron labeled **a** is in the focus and would show characteristic electrical properties such as paroxysmal depolarizing discharges. Activity in cell a can activate another pyramidal cell (b), and when many such cells fire synchronously, a spike can be recorded on the EEG. However, cell a also activates GABA-ergic inhibitory interneurons (**gray**), which through feedback inhibition can reduce the activity of cells a and b (temporal containment) as well

as block the firing of cells outside the focus (cell c). This block is called *surround inhibition* and provides spatial containment of the seizure focus. When extrinsic or intrinsic factors alter this balance of excitation and inhibition, the surround inhibition begins to break down and the spread of the seizure activity begins. (From Lothman and Collins 1990.)

B. The synaptic connections for cells a, b, c, and d are shown at the **left.** The activity at cell a in the focus consists of a paroxysmal depolarizing shift. However, cell c in the surround inhibition region is hyperpolarized because of GABA-ergic inhibition.

Box 46-3 Synaptic Inhibition in the Cerebral Cortex

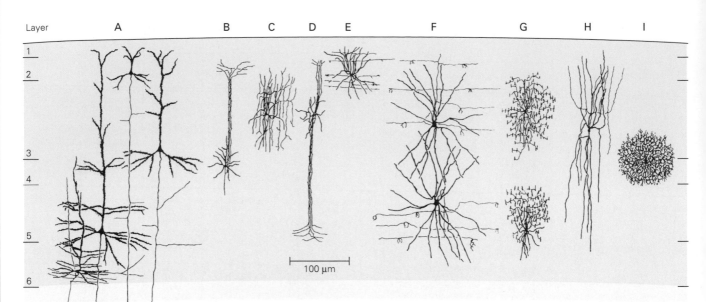

Figure 46-10 Morphological types of cells identifiable in monkey cerebral cortex, based on studies of the primary somatic sensory and motor cortex. Pyramidal cells (**A**) contain dendritic spines and are the only output neurons in the cortex. They are likely to use glutamate as a neurotransmitter and therefore are excitatory neurons, as is the interneuron (**B**).

Most nonpyramidal cells are thought to use GABA, and in some cases neuropeptides, as a transmitter. These neurons do not have dendritic spines. **C** = cell with axonal "arcades"; **D** = double bouquet cell; **E** and **F** = basket cells; **G** = chandelier cells; **H** = long, stringy cells (contain neuropeptides or acetylcholine); **I** = neurogliaform cell. (Adapted from Jones 1987.)

unanswered question is what terminates a seizure. Currently, the only definitive conclusion is that seizures do not stop because of metabolic exhaustion (see below).

During the initial 30 s or so of a typical secondarily generalized tonic-clonic seizure, neurons in the involved areas undergo prolonged depolarization and continuously fire action potentials. This is associated with the loss of afterhyperpolarization that follows a PDS. This period correlates with the tonic phase of muscle contraction, when descending pathways excite motor neurons in the brain stem and spinal cord. As the seizure evolves, the neurons begin to repolarize and the afterhyperpolarization reappears. The cycles of depolarization and repolarization correspond to the clonic phase of the seizure (see Figure 46-12). This phase of the seizure is often followed by a period of decreased electrical activity (the postictal period), which may be accompanied by clinical symptoms of confusion, drowsiness, or even focal neurological deficits such as a hemiparesis *(Todd paralysis)*. A neurological exam in the postictal period can lead to insights about the locus of the seizure focus.

Generalized Seizures Evolve From Thalamocortical Circuits

A generalized seizure shows simultaneous disruption of normal brain activity in both cerebral hemispheres from the onset. Generalized seizures and the associated epilepsies are heterogeneous in terms of their manifestations and underlying etiologies. Furthermore, a partial seizure that rapidly generalizes can be difficult to distinguish from a primary generalized seizure. However, the cellular mechanism of a primary generalized seizure differs in several interesting respects from that of partial or secondarily generalized seizures.

The best-understood type of primary generalized seizure is the childhood absence seizure, whose typical EEG pattern (3-Hz spike-wave pattern, Figure 46-14A) was first recognized by Hans Berger in 1933. F. A. Gibbs saw the relationship of this characteristic EEG pattern to absence seizures (he aptly described the pattern as "dart and dome"), and attributed the mechanism to an unknown generalized cortical disturbance. The distinctive clinical features of absence seizures are clearly corre-

Inhibition in the cerebral cortex is mediated principally by GABA. GABA or its synthesizing enzyme glutamic acid decarboxylase can be found in a variety of nonpyramidal cells using immunological staining techniques. These nonpyramidal cells are largely devoid of dendritic spines and hence are termed *non-spiny neurons* (Figure 46-10). Neurons that contain GABA (or glutamic acid decarboxylase) project locally. (An interesting exception is the Purkinje cell of the cerebral cortex, a GABA-ergic projection neuron.) A large percentage of cortical neurons that are immunoreactive for GABA are also immunoreactive for many of the known neuropeptides (see Chapter 14). Inhibition in the cortex, as well as other supraspinal structures, is powerful and may do more than simply cancel the effect of excitation. In the cortex inhibitory synapses generally are located close to the cell body, whereas excitatory synapses are located primarily on the dendrites. For example, *basket cells* (Figure 46-10) are inhibitory interneurons that synapse on the cell bodies of pyramidal cells. Therefore they have a direct inhibitory influence on action potential generation at the initial axon segment of the pyramidal cell. Inhibitory synapses on cortical neurons not only are strategically placed for influencing signaling, but their action also endures. Cortical inhibitory presynaptic potentials are much larger and last 10–20 times longer than the inhibitory actions exerted on spinal motor neurons (Figure 46-11).

Large cortical inhibitory postsynaptic potentials have a powerful influence on the activity of a population of cells. For example, in normal tissue recurrent inhibition may limit the size of a neuronal population that responds to a stimulus and thereby serve as a mechanism for enhancing the contrast between active and inactive cells in the population (see Chapter 26).

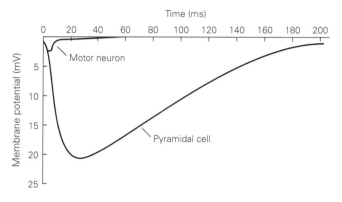

Figure 46-11 The inhibitory postsynaptic potential recorded from a hippocampal pyramidal cell is much greater than that recorded from a spinal motor neuron. (From Spencer and Kandel 1968.)

lated with the EEG activity. The typical absence seizure begins suddenly, lasts 10–30 s, and produces loss of awareness and minor motor manifestations such as blinking or lip smacking. Unlike secondarily generalized seizures, generalized seizures are not preceded by an aura or followed by postictal symptoms. The spike-wave EEG pattern involves all cerebral areas simultaneously and is immediately preceded and followed by normal background activity. Very brief 3-Hz activity without apparent clinical symptoms is common in patients with childhood absence seizures. In contrast to Gibbs's hypothesis of diffuse cortical hyperexcitability, Wilder Penfield and Herbert Jasper noted the similarity of the EEG in absence seizures to rhythmic EEG activity in sleep (so-called sleep spindles). They proposed the "centrencephalic" hypothesis, which suggests that rapid generalization was due to rhythmic activity (*pacing*) by neuronal aggregates in the upper brain stem or thalamus that project diffusely to the cortex.

Research on animal models of generalized seizures suggests that elements of both hypotheses are correct. In cats, parenteral injections of penicillin, a weak $GABA_A$ agonist, produce behavioral unresponsiveness associ-

ated with an EEG pattern of bilateral synchronous slow waves (*generalized penicillin epilepsy*). During this seizure, thalamic and cortical cells become synchronized through the same reciprocal thalamocortical connections that contribute to normal sleep spindles during slow-wave sleep (Chapter 47). Cortical cells become synchronized several cycles before "recruiting" synchronization of thalamic cells, although in primary generalized seizures it is not clear whether activity in the cortex precedes that in the thalamus. Nonetheless, these seizures might represent a form of diffuse cortical hyperexcitability. Recordings from individual cortical neurons show an increase in the number of action potentials during a depolarizing burst, which in turns produces a powerful stimulation of feedback GABA-ergic inhibition that hyperpolarizes the cell for approximately 200 ms after each burst (Figure 46-14C). This cell activity differs fundamentally from the PDS of partial seizures in that the GABA-ergic inhibition is preserved. The summated activity of the bursts produces the spike while the summated inhibition produces the wave of the typical spike-wave EEG pattern of an absence seizure.

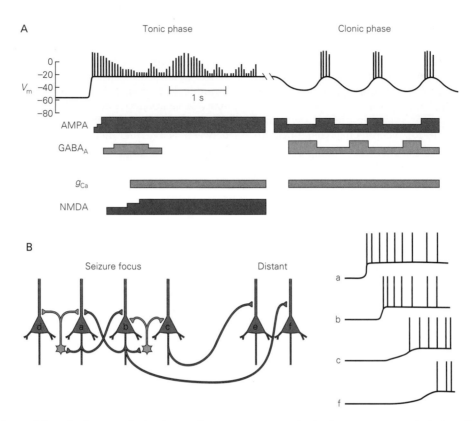

Figure 46-12 The loss of the afterhyperpolarization and surround inhibition accompanies the onset of a partial seizure.

A. With the onset of a seizure, neurons in the focus depolarize as in the first phase of a paroxysmal depolarizing shift. However, unlike the interictal period, the depolarization persists for seconds or minutes. Note that the GABA-mediated inhibition fails, whereas the glutamate-mediated AMPA and NMDA receptor activity is functionally enhanced. This activity occurs during the tonic phase of a secondarily generalized tonic-clonic seizure. As the GABA-mediated inhibition gradually returns, the neurons in the focus enter a period of oscillation, as shown at the **right.** This activity occurs during the clonic phase of a tonic-clonic seizure.

B. As the surround inhibition mediated by GABA-ergic interneurons breaks down, neurons in the focus become synchronously excited and send trains of action potentials to distant neurons, beginning the spread of seizure activity from the focus to distant sites (**left**). Compare the activity in cells a–d (**right**) with their activity during the interictal period shown in Figure 46-9B. (Adapted from Lothman 1993a.)

What are the properties of individual cells that facilitate this generalized and synchronous activity? As we saw in Chapter 45, one clue comes from studies of the intrinsic bursting of thalamic relay neurons. Henrik Jahnsen and Rodolfo Llinàs found that these neurons have a special Ca^{2+} channel that is inactivated at the resting membrane potential but becomes available for activation when the cell is hyperpolarized. Depolarization then transiently opens the channel (thus its name the T channel). Consistent with a contribution of T-type channels to absence seizures, anticonvulsant agents that block absence seizures, such as ethosuximide (Zarontin) and valproic acid (Depakote), also block T-type channels.

The circuitry of the thalamus seems ideally suited to the generation of primary generalized seizures. As we have seen in Chapter 45, the pattern of activity in the thalamic relay neurons during sleep spindles suggests a reciprocal interaction between the thalamic relay neurons and GABA-ergic neurons in thalamic nuclei—the neurons of the reticular nucleus and the perigeniculate nucleus (Figure 46-14B). Recent studies of thalamic brain slices by David McCormick and his colleagues suggest that inhibition of thalamic relay neurons by GABA-ergic interneurons hyperpolarizes the relay neuron, thus removing inactivation of the T-type Ca^{2+} channels. This sequence of events leads to a rebound burst of action potentials after each IPSP. The action potential stimulates the GABA-ergic neurons by a reciprocal excitatory connection. The action potentials in the relay neurons also excite cortical neurons and thus can be manifested in the EEG as a "spindle." Block of $GABA_A$ channels enhances $GABA_B$ IPSPs in relay neurons, resulting in an increase in rebound bursts of action potentials. Thus the T-type Ca^{2+} channel and $GABA_B$ receptors appear to play an important role in generating activity resembling that of human absence seizures.

Several other modulatory influences can alter thalamocortical activity and thus could contribute to the transition from normal spindle activity to the synchronized pattern of primary generalized seizures. Calcium-dependent K^+ conductances could serve to hyperpolarize the neurons and thus remove inactivation of T-type channels. The resulting activation of the hyperpolarization-activated cation current (I_h) in thalamic relay neurons may control rhythmic discharges in this circuit. Diffuse monoamine projections from the locus ceruleus (norepinephrine), raphe magnus (serotonin), and ventral tegmentum (dopamine) may also play a role. The possibility that norepinephrine is a contributing factor is supported by studies of the mouse mutant *tottering* by Jeff Noebels and his colleagues. These animals develop a paroxysmal spike-wave discharge and behavioral arrest seizures in adolescence that are similar to childhood absence seizures. A diffuse hyperinnervation of the cortex by noradrenergic axons and terminals from the locus ceruleus appears to contribute to the seizure phenotype. In addition, a neurotoxin that destroys noradrenergic neurons prevents expression of the seizures. Thus it is possible that β-adrenergic receptor stimulation of cortical neurons is the trigger that leads to enhanced excitability and seizures in the *tottering* mutant.

Locating the Seizure Focus Is Critical to the Surgical Treatment of Epilepsy

The pioneering studies of Penfield in Montreal led to the recognition that removal of the temporal lobe in certain patients with partial seizures of hippocampal origin could reduce or cure epilepsy. As surgical treatment for the partial epilepsies increased, it became clear that the benefit from the surgery is directly related to the adequacy of the resection. Thus precise localization of the seizure focus is essential. Electrical mapping of seizure foci originally relied on the surface EEG, which, as we have seen, is biased toward particular sets of neurons in the cortex immediately adjacent to the skull. However, intractable seizures often begin in deep structures that show little or no abnormality on the surface EEG at the onset of the seizure. Recent developments in magnetic resonance imaging (MRI) have markedly improved the noninvasive anatomical mapping of seizure foci. This technique is now used to evaluate partial epilepsies of the temporal lobe and also shows great promise for extratemporal epilepsies. The scientific basis of anatomical mapping by MRI was the observation that a majority of patients with intractable complex partial seizures have atrophy and cell loss in the mesial portions of the hippocampal formation. There is a dramatic loss of neurons

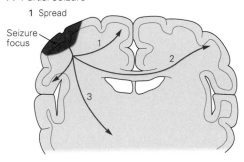

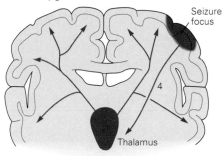

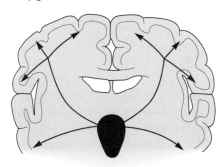

Figure 46-13 The pathways for seizure propagation in partial seizures and primary generalized seizures. (From Lothman 1993b.)

A. Partial seizures. 1. Seizure activity can spread from a **focus** (shown as **red** area of neocortex) and spread via intrahemispheric commissural fibers (**1**) to the homotopic contralateral cortex (**2**) and subcortical centers (**3**). **2.** The secondary generalization of partial seizure activity spreads to subcortical centers via projections to the thalamus (**4**). Widespread thalamocortical interconnections then cause rapid activation of both hemispheres.

B. In a primary generalized seizure, such as a typical absence seizure, diffuse interconnections between the thalamus and cortex (**arrows**) are the primary route of seizure propagation.

A Spike and wave activity in typical absence seizure

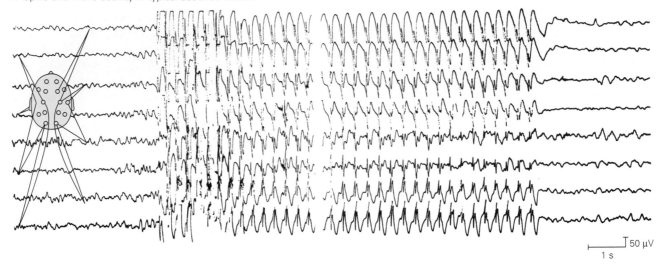

50 µV

1 s

B Thalamocortical projections

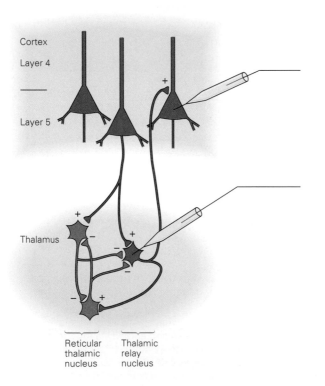

Cortex

Layer 4

Layer 5

Thalamus

Reticular
thalamic
nucleus

Thalamic
relay
nucleus

C Synchrony of neuronal activity in primary generalized (spike-wave) seizure

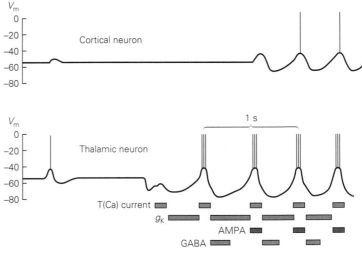

V_m

Cortical neuron

V_m

1 s

Thalamic neuron

T(Ca) current

g_K

AMPA

GABA

Figure 46-14 The generation of primary generalized seizures.

A. This EEG from a 12-year-old patient with typical absence (petit mal) seizures shows the sudden onset of synchronous spike (3/s) and wave activity (approximately 14/s). The seizure was clinically manifest as a staring spell with occasional eye blinks. Note that, unlike a partial seizure, there is no buildup of activity preceding the seizure and that the electrical activity returns abruptly to the normal background level after the seizure.

Discontinuity in the trace is due to removal of a 3s period of recording. (From Lothman and Collins 1990.)

B. The thalamocortical connections that participate in the generation of sleep spindles (Chapter 47) are thought to be essential for the generation of primary generalized seizures. Pyramidal cells in the cortex are reciprocally connected by excitatory synapses with thalamic relay neurons. GABA-ergic neurons in the reticular thalamic nucleus are excited both by pyramidal cells in the cortex and by thalamic relay neurons. In turn the reticular thalamic neurons inhibit the thalamic relay neurons.

C. Neuronal activity of cortical neurons and thalamic relay neurons is synchronized during a primary generalized seizure. The depolarization is dependent on AMPA receptors and T-type Ca^{2+} channels. The repolarization is due to GABA-mediated inhibition as well as voltage- and calcium-dependent K^+ conductances (g_K). (From Lothman 1993a.)

within the hippocampus (mesial temporal sclerosis), changes in dendritic morphology of surviving cells, and collateral sprouting of some axons.

The anatomical resolution of modern MRI scanning has allowed a quantitative, noninvasive assessment of hippocampal size in patients with epilepsy. Loss of volume of the hippocampus has been shown to agree with the localization of seizure foci by electrical criteria. The typical patient with mesial temporal epilepsy has unilateral shrinkage of the hippocampus that can be associated with apparent dilatation of the temporal horn of the lateral ventricle. A typical case is illustrated in Box 46-4. However, in many patients abnormalities cannot be detected using current MRI techniques; thus nonanatomical mapping techniques would be useful.

Metabolic mapping offers an alternative to anatomical methods. This method takes advantage of the changes in cerebral metabolism and blood flow that occur in the seizure focus during the ictal and interictal periods. The electrical activity associated with a seizure places a large metabolic demand on brain tissue. Neurotransmitters are synthesized, released, and transported, ion gradients across membranes are depleted, and ATPases actively work to restore homeostasis. The metabolic demand during a partial seizure results in an approximately 3-fold increase in glucose and oxygen utilization. Increased metabolism in the focus during a seizure can be measured as changes in glucose utilization or cerebral blood flow. In contrast, the focus often has decreased metabolism between seizures. Despite the increased metabolic demands, the brain is able to maintain normal levels of ATP during a partial seizure.

On the other hand, the transient interruption of breathing during a generalized convulsive seizure causes a decrease in oxygen levels in the blood. This results in decreased ATP concentrations and an increased anaerobic metabolism, as indicated by rising lactate levels. This oxygen debt is quickly replenished in the postictal period, and no permanent damage to brain tissue results from a single generalized seizure. A generalized seizure also abolishes the normal autoregulation of cerebral blood flow; thus increases in systemic blood pressure lead to increased cerebral blood flow. The increased cerebral blood flow compensates for the increased demand for glucose and oxygen, necessary for ion pumps to restore the large ion shifts that occur.

Positron emission tomography (PET) scans of patients with complex partial seizures originating in the mesial temporal lobe frequently show interictal hypometabolism, with the extent of the metabolic change extending to the lateral temporal lobe, ipsilateral thalamus, basal ganglia, and frontal cortex (Figure 46-18). PET imaging has been particularly helpful in identify-

ing seizure foci in patients with normal MRI scans and in some early childhood epilepsies.

A related technique, single photon emission computed tomography (SPECT), has shown some promise. SPECT does not have the resolution of PET but can be performed in the nuclear medicine department of many large hospitals. Injection of radioisotopes and SPECT imaging at the time of a seizure has shown a pattern of hypermetabolism followed by hypometabolism in the seizure focus and surrounding tissue.

Prolonged Seizures Can Cause Brain Damage

Repeated Convulsive Seizures (Status Epilepticus) Are a Medical Emergency

As discussed above, brain tissue can compensate for the metabolic stress of a partial seizure or the transient decrease in oxygen delivery during a single generalized tonic-clonic seizure. In a generalized seizure, stimulation of the hypothalamus leads to massive activation of the "stress" response of the sympathetic nervous system. Initially, the increased systemic blood pressure and serum glucose compensate for increased metabolic demand, but these homeostatic mechanisms fail during prolonged seizures. The resulting systemic metabolic derangements, including hypoxia, hypotension, hypoglycemia, and acidemia, lead to a reduction in high-energy phosphates (ATP and phosphocreatine) in the brain and thus can be devastating to brain tissue.

Systemic complications such as cardiac arrhythmias, pulmonary edema, hyperthermia, and muscle breakdown can also occur. Repeated generalized seizures without return to full consciousness between seizures is called *status epilepticus*. This is a true medical emergency requiring aggressive seizure management and general medical support, because 30 or more minutes of continuous convulsive seizures leads to brain injury or even death. Status epilepticus involving nonconvulsive seizures (simple partial, complex partial, or absence seizures) can also occur, but the metabolic consequences are much less severe.

Excitotoxicity Underlies Seizure-Related Brain Damage

Brain damage from repeated seizures can occur independently of cardiopulmonary or systemic metabolic changes, suggesting that local factors in the brain can result in neuronal death. The immature brain appears particularly vulnerable to such damage, perhaps because of factors such as electrotonic coupling between neurons, less effective

Box 46-4 Surgical Treatment of Temporal Lobe Epilepsy

A 27-year-old woman had episodes of decreased responsiveness beginning at age 19. At first she would stare off and appear confused during the episodes. Later she developed a warning (*aura*) consisting of a feeling of fear. This fear was followed by altered consciousness, a wide-eyed stare, tightening of the left arm, and a scream that lasted for 14–20 s (Figure 46-15). These spells were diagnosed as complex partial seizures. The seizures occurred several times per week despite treatment with several antiepileptic drugs. The patient was unable to work or drive because of frequent seizures. She had

a history of meningitis at age 6 months and throughout childhood had experienced brief episodes of altered perception described as being "like someone threw a switch."

Based on the results of the evaluation summarized in Figures 46-16 and 46-17, a right amygdalohippocampectomy was performed. The patient has been seizure free in the 14 months since the operation and has returned to full-time employment. (Courtesy of Dr. Martin Salinsky, Oregon Health Sciences University Epilepsy Center.)

A

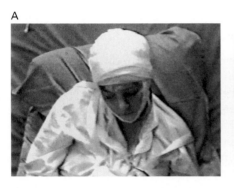

B

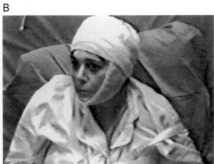

C

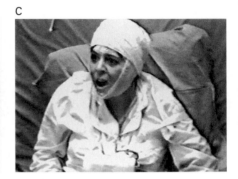

Figure 46-15 The patient was monitored with closed-circuit television simultaneous EEG and telemetry. The monitoring revealed stereotypical complex partial seizures. The patient is shown reading quietly in the period preceding the seizure (A), during the period when she reported a feeling of fear (B), and during the period when there was alteration of consciousness and an audible scream (C). (Courtesy of Dr. Martin Salinsky, Oregon Health Sciences University Epilepsy Center.)

potassium buffering by immature glia, and decreased glucose transport across the blood-brain barrier.

The pattern of brain injury is particularly striking in the hippocampus, with preferential loss of the pyramidal neurons in the CA1 and CA3 regions. The selective vulnerability of the hippocampus was first noted by Sommer in the 1880s and has been produced by electrical stimulation of afferents to the hippocampus or by injection of excitatory amino acid analogs such as kainic acid. Interestingly, the injection of kainic acid into the brain causes local damage but also damage in terminals of afferents that originate at the injection site. These observations suggest that release of the normal excitatory amino acid transmitter, L-glutamate, can itself cause neuronal damage during a seizure. John Olney coined the term *excitotoxicity* for these phenomena. Because it has been difficult to detect increases in extracellular glutamate during sta-

tus epilepticus, it would appear that the trigger is excessive stimulation of glutamate receptors rather than tonic increases in extracellular glutamate per se. The histological appearance of acute excitotoxicity includes massive swelling of neuronal cell bodies and dendrites consistent with the predominant somatodendritic location of glutamate receptors and excitatory synapses (Figure 46-19).

The cellular and molecular mechanisms of excitotoxicity are still not fully understood. However, several features are clear. Excessive stimulation with the release of excitatory amino acid transmitters causes overactivation of glutamate receptors. This leads to an excessive increase in intracellular calcium, which can then activate a self-destructive cellular cascade involving many calcium-dependent enzymes, such as phosphatases (eg, calcineurin), proteases (the calpains), and lipases. Lipid peroxidation can also cause production of free radicals,

Figure 46-16 Simultaneous EEG shows low-amplitude background rhythms at the beginning (left). At the point when the patient reported fear (B) there is a buildup of EEG activity at the onset of a complex partial seizure, but this activity is confined to the EEG electrodes over the right hemisphere (see Figure 46-1 for electrode placement). The seizure activity spreads to the left hemisphere at the point where there is alteration of consciousness (C). EEG spike-waves are particularly prominent in leads 9 → 10 and 9 → 14 over the right anterior temporal region. (Courtesy of Dr. Martin Salinsky.)

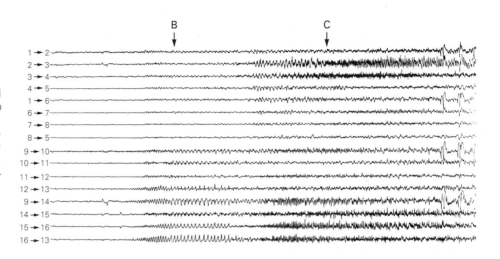

Figure 46-17 Enhanced magnetic resonance imaging of the patient revealed atrophy of the right hippocampus (arrows on right). The left hippocampus is normal (arrows on left). (Courtesy of Dr. Martin Salinsky.)

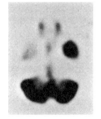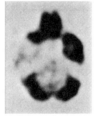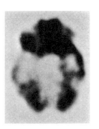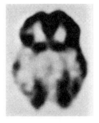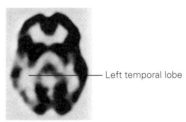

Left temporal lobe

Figure 46-18 Positron emission tomography (PET) scan from a patient with temporal lobe epilepsy. The scan was obtained in the interictal period using ^{18}F-fluorodeoxyglucose as a metabolic tracer. **Dark regions** of the scan reflect higher levels of metabolism. For example, metabolism is higher in the cortex than in the underlying white matter. The left temporal lobe shows an area of hypometabolism. This is most prominent in the first and second scans starting from the left side of the figure. The patient underwent left temporal lobectomy for control of epilepsy and the tissue showed characteristic mesial hippocampal sclerosis. (From Engel et al. 1986.)

which damage vital cellular proteins and lead to cell death. The role of mitochondria in Ca^{2+} homeostasis and in controlling free radicals may also be important. The pattern of cell death was first thought to reflect necrosis from the autolysis of critical cellular proteins. However, recent evidence suggests that activation of "death" genes characteristic of programmed cell death *(apoptosis)* may be involved in excitotoxic damage of neurons.

Within particular brain regions, seizure-related brain damage or excitotoxicity can be specific to certain

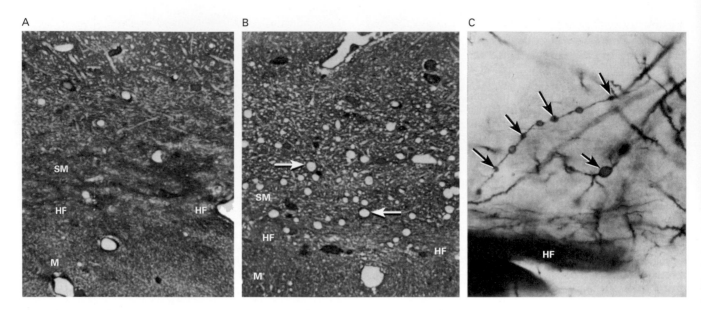

Figure 46-19 Electrical stimulation causes the dendrosomatic swelling characteristic of excitotoxicity.

A, B. Photomicrographs (×260) from the stratum moleculare (**SM**) of the CA1 region in a control rat (**A**) and in a rat after 2 hours of continuous stimulation of the perforant path (**B**). The perforant path forms excitatory synapses on the distal apical dendrites of CA1 pyramidal cells in the stratum moleculare. The spherical swellings (**arrows**) are dendrites of CA1 pyramidal

cells. Presynaptic structures are unaffected by excitotoxic stimuli (not shown). Other labeled structures are the hippocampal fissure (**HF**) and the molecular layer of the dentate gyrus (**M**).

C. A section of the same region as in **A** using the rapid Golgi stain technique that labels occasional neurons. The **arrows** indicate swellings along the distal apical dendrites of a CA1 neuron. (Adapted from Sloviter 1983.)

types of neurons, perhaps because of protective factors such as calcium-binding proteins or sensitizing factors such as the expression of calcium-permeable glutamate receptors. For example, excitotoxicity induced in vitro by activation of AMPA receptors preferentially affects interneurons. These cells show expression of AMPA receptor subtypes that have high Ca^{2+} permeability, providing a possible mechanism for their selective vulnerability.

Recent outbreaks of "amnestic" shellfish poisoning provide a vivid example of the consequences of overactivation of glutamate receptors. Domoic acid, a glutamate analog not present in the brain, is a natural product of certain species of marine algae that flourish during appropriate ocean conditions. Domoic acid can be concentrated by filter feeders such as shellfish. Ingestion of domoic-contaminated shellfish sporadically causes outbreaks of neurological damage, including severe seizures and amnesia. The area most sensitive to damage is the hippocampus, providing further support for the excitotoxicity hypothesis and the role of the hippocampus in learning and memory (Chapter 62).

The Factors Leading to Development of the Epileptic Condition Are an Unsolved Mystery

A single seizure does not warrant a diagnosis of epilepsy. Normal individuals can have a seizure under extenuating circumstances, such as after drug ingestion or extreme sleep deprivation. Our understanding of what factors contribute to a chronic susceptibility to seizures (epilepsy) is still rudimentary. Some forms of epilepsy (mostly with generalized seizures) may be due in part to a genetic predisposition. For example, infants with febrile seizures often have a family history of similar seizures. The role of genetics in epilepsy is supported by the existence of several familial epileptic syndromes in humans as well as seizure-prone animal models with such exotic names as papio papio (a baboon with photosensitive seizures), audiogenic mice (loud sound induces seizures), and *reeler* and *tottering* mice (names alluding to the clinical manifestations of cerebellar mutations in these animals). Recent studies in mice have provided insights into the molecular genetics of epilepsy, with nearly 25 single gene mutations having been linked to an epileptic phenotype. The affected proteins include ion channel subunits, proteins involved in synaptic transmission, synaptic receptors, and molecules involved in calcium signaling. For example, a spontaneous mutation in the α1A voltage-sensitive calcium channel gene is the cause of the *tottering* phenotype. That mutations in these classes of proteins cause epilepsy is perhaps not unexpected given the dependence of seizures on synaptic transmission and neuronal excitability. However, some of the other identified genes, such as genes for Centromere BP-B, a DNA binding protein, or the sodium/hydrogen exchanger, the affected gene in the *slow wave epilepsy* mouse have been more surprising. Regardless of the exact molecular link to the epileptic phenotype, it is clear (at least in mice) that mutations in many different genes may result in epilepsy.

In most cases genetic epilepsy syndromes in humans have complex rather than simple (Mendelian) inheritance patterns, suggesting the involvement of many genes rather than a single one. However, Steinlein and colleagues reported in 1995 that a mutation in the α4 subunit of the neuronal nicotinic acetylcholine receptor is responsible for autosomal dominant nocturnal frontal lobe epilepsy, the first example of an autosomal gene defect in human epilepsy. Subsequently, a novel potassium channel gene was linked to another rare generalized epilepsy syndrome, benign familial neonatal convulsions. The increased resolution of MRI scans has also revealed an unexpectedly large number of cortical malformations and localized areas in patients with epilepsy, suggesting that altered cortical development may be a common cause of epilepsy. This is supported by the recent mapping of two X-linked cortical malformations with epileptic phenotypes, familial periventricular heterotopia, and familial subcortical band heterotopia. The gene responsible for the latter (*doublecortin*) has recently been identified as a putative signal transduction molecule, presumably involved in neuronal migration.

While these studies are promising, genetic studies in epilepsy syndromes with complex inheritance, such as juvenile myoclonic epilepsy, are likely to progress much more slowly, for genetic mapping studies have revealed linkages to several chromosomal loci. In addition, virtually all of the genetic defects are associated with generalized seizures rather than partial or secondarily generalized seizures.

In the more mundane situation, epilepsy often develops after a discrete cortical injury such as a penetrating head wound. Here, the factors leading to the development of epilepsy are less clear. Certain regions of the brain such as the hippocampus are more susceptible to the development of epilepsy. Studies of temporal lobe epilepsy have also indicated an association between an early initial insult (eg, a prolonged febrile convulsion or an episode of encephalitis) and the later development of complex partial seizures. This has led to the idea that the early insult acts as a switch that turns on a set of progressive physiological or anatomical changes leading to the development of chronic seizures. The most promising evidence for this hypothesis has come from studies of tissue removed from patients undergoing temporal lobectomy and models of limbic seizures in rodents.

Chronic stimulation of hippocampal inputs to the dentate gyrus or CA1 leads to hyperexcitability and the loss of neurons in the affected neurons. As discussed above, the death of neurons is thought to result from overexcitation by the release of large amounts of the excitatory neurotransmitter glutamate. Similar pathological changes have been observed in brain tissue removed from the temporal lobe of patients for intractable complex partial seizures. However, the cell loss is selective; certain GABA-ergic interneurons that contain calcium-binding proteins such as parvalbumin and calbindin are spared. These include both basket cells and axoaxonic GABA-ergic neurons.

Despite the morphological preservation of certain types of GABA-ergic interneurons, physiological studies have indicated that GABA-ergic inhibition is reduced in the animal models of temporal lobe epilepsy. This led Robert Sloviter to propose the "dormant inhibition" hypothesis. For example, in mesial temporal sclerosis there is a selective loss of mossy cells in the hilum of the dentate gyrus. The mossy cells provide excitatory feedback to the GABA-ergic interneurons (Chapter 63). Loss of mossy cells functionally removes the surround inhibition in the dentate gyrus, leading to hyperexcitability. The dentate gyrus also provides the main entry point to the hippocampal formation from the neocortex. Thus the dentate gyrus can be thought of as the "gatekeeper" of excitability in the hippocampus. A schema of how reorganization of circuits in the dentate gyrus might lead to the development of temporal lobe epilepsy is diagrammed in Figure 46-20.

One experimental model of hyperexcitability is induced by repeated stimuli of limbic structures, such as the amygdala or hippocampus. The initial stimulus is followed by an electrical response (the *afterdischarge*) that becomes more extensive and prolonged with repeated stimuli until a generalized seizure occurs. This process is called *kindling* and can be induced by both

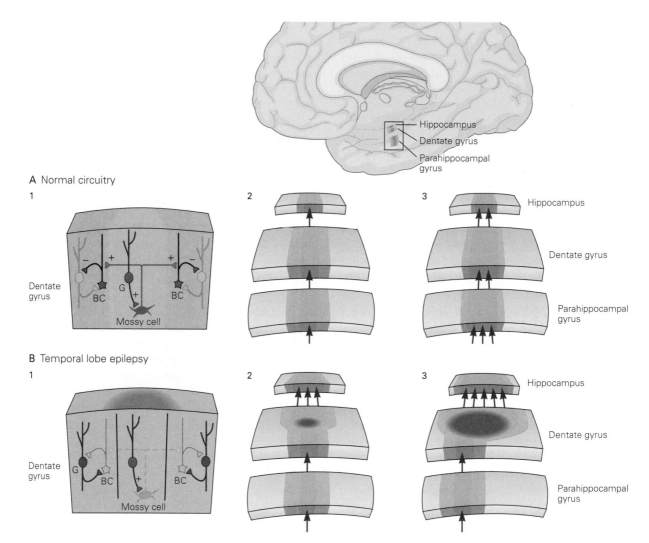

Figure 46-20 Hypothetical role of the dentate gyrus as the "gatekeeper" for seizures involving the hippocampus. (From Sloviter 1994.)

A. Under normal conditions surround inhibition is mediated by GABAergic interneurons activated by mossy cells in the dentate hilus (**1**). This inhibition limits the incoming excitation from the parahippocampal gyrus (red) to a single lamella (**2**). In the presence of a seizure focus in the neocortex (i.e. extrahippocampal), seizure activity spreads to the parahippocampal gyrus, activating multiple lamella (**3**). This strong activation (3 arrows) overcomes the surround inhibition, despite the normal circuitry of the dentate gyrus and thus seizure activity is conveyed to the relatively nor-

mal hippocampus. G = granule cell; BC = GABAergic basket cell.

B. Loss of neurons in the dentate hilus in temporal lobe epilepsy causes erosion of surround inhibition in a confined area (**1**). The resulting enlarged aggregate of hyperexcitable granule cells may then respond to a normal neocortical input to that lamella (single arrow in B2) with excessive discharges, resulting in the onset of seizure in the hippocampus (**2**). With severe mesial temporal sclerosis, loss of large numbers of hilar neurons causes a large area of dentate to become disinhibited. Thus neocortical inputs to any of the surrounding lamella can activate the abnormal tissue and cause the onset of a seizure (**3**)

electrical or chemical stimuli. Many investigators believe that kindling also contributes to the development of human epilepsy.

The synaptic plasticity associated with kindling resembles normal plasticity of synapses, which embraces

both short-term changes in excitability and morphology, including axonal sprouting (Chapter 63). Morphological rearrangements of synaptic connections have been observed in the dentate gyrus of patients with long-standing complex partial seizures as well as after kindling in

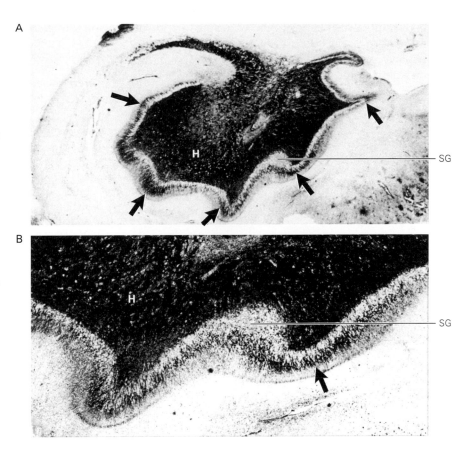

Figure 46-21 Mossy fiber synaptic reorganization (sprouting) in the epileptic human temporal lobe may be one of the changes that causes hyperexcitability. (From Sutula et al. 1989.)

A. Timm stain of a transverse section of hippocampus removed from a patient with epilepsy at the time of temporal lobectomy for control of epilepsy. The stain appears black in the axons of the dentate granule cells (mossy fibers) because of the presence of zinc in these axons. The mossy fibers normally pass through the dentate hilus (**H**) on their way to synapse in the hilus and on CA3 pyramidal cells. In the epileptic tissue shown here, stained fibers appear in the supragranular (**SG**) layer of the dentate gyrus (indicated by **arrows**). This represents aberrant sprouting of mossy fibers that form new recurrent excitatory synapses on dentate granule cells. Similar sprouting of mossy fibers is also seen in experimental animals after kindling.

B. High magnification of a segment of the supragranular layer of the dentate gyrus revealing Timm-stained mossy fibers.

experimental animals (Figure 46-21). The axons of dentate gyrus granule cells proliferate after the death of their target cells in the dentate hilus; they then reinnervate the dendrites of granule cells in the molecular layer of the dentate gyrus. It has been postulated that this sprouting contributes to the hyperexcitability of epileptic brain tissue.

The long-term changes that lead to epilepsy also are likely to involve specific patterns of gene expression. For example, the proto-oncogene *c-fos* and other immediate early genes can be activated by seizures. Because many immediate early genes encode transcription factors that control other genes, the set of gene products that result from epileptiform activity could initiate a cascade of changes leading to the development of epilepsy.

An Overall View

Seizures are one of the most dramatic examples of the collective electrical behavior of the mammalian brain. The distinctive clinical pattern of partial seizures and generalized seizures can be attributed to the distinctly different patterns of activity of cortical neurons. Studies of partial seizures in animals reveal a series of events—from the activity of neurons in the seizure focus to synchronization and subsequent spread of epileptiform activity throughout the cortex. The gradual loss of GABA-ergic surround inhibition is critical to the early steps in this progression. In contrast, generalized seizures are thought to arise from activity in thalamocortical circuits, perhaps combined with a general abnormality in the membrane excitability of all cortical neurons. The recent discovery of several genes associated with epilepsy provides the prospect of a better understanding of the mechanisms of generalized seizures.

The EEG has long provided a window on the electrical activity of the cortex, both in normal phases of arousal and during abnormal activities such as seizures. The EEG can be used to identify certain electrical activity patterns associated with seizures, but it provides limited insight into the pathophysiology of seizures. Several much more powerful and noninvasive approaches are now available to locate the focus of a partial seizure. This has led to the widespread and successful use of epilepsy surgery for selected patients, particularly those with complex partial seizures of hippocampal onset.

Gary L. Westbrook

Selected Readings

Choi DW. 1992. Excitotoxic cell death. J Neurobiol 23:1261–1276.

Dichter MA. 1993. The premise, the promise, and the problems with basic research in epilepsy. Epilepsia 34:791–799.

Dichter MA, Ayala GF. 1987. Cellular mechanisms of epilepsy: a status report. Science 237:157–164.

Engel J. 1989. *Seizures and Epilepsy.* Philadelphia: Davis.

Fisch BJ. 1991. *Spehlmann's EEG Primer,* 2nd ed. Amsterdam: Elsevier.

Fischer RS. 1989. Animal models of the epilepsies. Brain Res Rev 14:245–278.

Gloor P, Fariello RG. 1988. Generalized epilepsy: some of its cellular mechanisms differ from those of focal epilepsy. Trends Neurosci 11:63–68.

Henry TR, Engel J Jr, Mazziotta JC. 1993. Clinical evaluation of interictal fluorine-18-fluorodeoxyglucose PET in partial epilepsy. J Nucl Med 34:1892–1898.

Jahnsen H, Llinás R. 1984. Ionic basis for the electro-responsiveness and oscillatory properties of guinea-pig thalamic neurones in vitro. J Physiol (Lond) 349: 227–247.

Lennox WG, Lennox MA. 1960. *Epilepsy and Related Disorders.* Boston: Little, Brown.

Lothman EW. 1992. Basic mechanisms of the epilepsies. Curr Opin Neurol Neurosurg 5:216–223.

McCormick DA. 1989. Cholinergic and noradrenergic modulation of thalamocortical processing. Trends Neurosci 12:215–221.

McNamara JO, Puranam RS. 1998. Epilepsy genetics: an abundance of riches for biologists. Curr Biol 8:R168–R170.

Noebels JL. 1991. Mutational analysis of spike-wave epilepsy phenotypes. Amsterdam, Elsevier Science Publishers BV Epilepsy Res Suppl 4:201–212.

Noebels JL. 1996. Targeting epilepsy genes. Neuron 16:241–244.

Penfield W, Jasper H. 1954. *Epilepsy and the Functional Anatomy of the Human Brain.* Boston: Little, Brown.

Prince DA, Connors BW. 1986. Mechanisms of interictal epileptogenesis. Adv Neurol 44:275–299.

Snead OC. 1995. Basic mechanisms of generalized absence seizures. Ann Neurol 37:146–157.

von Krosigk M, Bal T, McCormick DA. 1993. Cellular mechanisms of a synchronized oscillation in the thalamus. Science 261:361–364.

References

Berger H. 1929. Über das Elektrenkephalogram des Menchen. Arch Psychiatr Nervenkr 87:527–570.

Biervert C, Schroeder BC, Kubisch C, Berkovic SF, Propping P, Jentsch TJ, Steinlein OK. 1998. A potassium channel mutation in neonatal human epilepsy. Science 279: 403–406.

Commission on Classification and Terminology of the International League Against Epilepsy. 1985. Proposal for classification of epilepsies and epileptic syndromes. Epilepsia 26:268–278.

Commission on Classification and Terminology of the International League Against Epilepsy. 1981. Proposal for revised clinical and electroencephalographic classification of epileptic seizures. Epilepsia 22:489–501.

Engel J Jr, Crandall PH, Rausch R. 1983. The partial epilepsies. In: RN Rosenberg (ed). Vol. 2, *The Clinical Neurosciences,* pp. 1349–1380. New York: Churchill Livingstone.

Hauptmann A. 1912. Luminal bei epilepsie. Munich Med Wochenschr 59:1907–1909.

Horsley V. 1886. Brain surgery. BMJ 2:670–675.

Jones EG. 1987. GABA-peptide neurons of the primate cerebral cortex. J Mind Behav 8:519–536.

Konnerth A. 1990. Patch-clamping in slices of mammalian CNS. Trends Neurosci 13:321–323.

Lothman EW. 1993a. The neurobiology of epileptiform discharges. Am J EEG Technol 33:93–112.

Lothman EW. 1993b. Pathophysiology of seizures and epilepsy in the mature and immature brain: Cells, synapses and circuits. In: WE Dodson, JM Pellock (eds). *Pediatric Epilepsy: Diagnosis and Therapy,* pp. 1–15. New York: Demos Publications.

Lothman EW, Collins RC. 1990. Seizures and epilepsy. In: AL Pearlman, RC Collins (eds). *Neurobiology of Disease,* pp. 276–298. New York: Oxford Univ. Press.

McNamera JO, Bonhaus DW, Shin C. 1992. The kindling model of epilepsy. In: P Schwartzkroin (ed). *Epilepsy: Models, Mechanisms, and Concepts,* pp. 27–47. Cambridge: Cambridge Univ. Press.

Merritt H, Putnam TJ. 1938. A new series of anticonvulsant drugs tested by experiments on animals. Arch Neurol Psychiatry 39:1003–1015.

Morgan JI, Curran T. 1991. Proto-oncogene transcription factors and epilepsy. Trends Pharmacol Sci 12:343–349.

Olney JW, Sharpe LG. 1969. Brain lesions in an infant rhesus monkey treated with monosodium glutamate. Science 166:386–388.

Sloviter RS. 1983. "Epileptic" brain damage in rats induced by sustained electrical stimulation of the perforant path. I. Acute electrophysiological and light microscopic studies. Brain Res Bull 10:675–697.

Sloviter RS. 1994. The functional organization of the hippocampal dentate gyrus and its relevance to the pathogenesis of temporal lobe epilepsy. Ann Neurol 35:640–654.

Sommer W. 1880. Erkrankung des Ammonshorns als Actiologisches Moment der Epilepsie. Arch Psychiatr Nervenkr 10:631–675.

Spencer WA, Kandel ER. 1968. Cellular and integrative properties of the hippocampal pyramidal cell and the comparative electrophysiology of cortical neurons. Int J Neurol 6:266–296.

Steinlein OK, Mulley JC, Propping P, Wallace RH, Phillips HA, Sutherland GR, Scheffer IE, Berkovic SF. 1995. A missense mutation in the neuronal nicotinic adetylcholine receptor alpha 4 subunit is associated with autosomal dominant nocturnal frontal lobe epilepsy. Nat Genet 11:20–203.

Sutula T, Cascino G, Cavazos J, Parada I, Ramirez L. 1989. Mossy fiber synaptic reorganization in the epileptic human temporal lobe. Ann Neurol 26:321–330.

Tyler KL. 1984. Hughlings Jackson: the early development of his ideas on epilepsy. J Hist Med Allied Sci 39:55–64.

Wong RKS, Miles R, Traub RD. 1984. Local circuit interactions in synchronization of cortical neurones. J Exp Biol 112:169–178.

47

Sleep and Dreaming

WHY DO WE SPEND SO much time sleeping? What mechanisms produce this state? What makes us dream? These are some of the central questions confronting the biology of sleep.

The age-old, commonsense explanation for sleep is that it results from reduced brain activity, induced by fatigue. Until 1945 most scientists working on sleep shared this view. They thought that the awake state is actively maintained by sensory stimulation and that the brain falls asleep when fatigue causes a decrease in sen-sory stimulation. In the late 1940s and early 1950s Guiseppi Moruzzi made two startling discoveries that ultimately disproved this idea. First, Moruzzi and Horace Magoun found that transection of the ascending sensory pathways in the brain stem did not interfere with either wakefulness or sleep. In contrast, lesions of the reticular formation of the brain stem produced behavioral stupor and an electroencephalographic pattern resembling sleep even though these lesions did not interfere with the ascending sensory pathways. From these results Moruzzi and Magoun concluded that the tonic activity of the reticular formation, driven by sensory input, keeps the forebrain awake, and that a reduction in the activity of the reticular formation produces sleep.

This new variation on the passive view of sleep dominated sleep research until the late 1950s, when Moruzzi and his colleagues made a second major discovery: transecting the brain stem, including its reticular formation through the pons, greatly *reduced* sleep. This finding suggested that the reticular formation of the brain stem does not act uniformly in regulating sleep. Rather, the rostral portion of the reticular formation—the portion above the pons—contains neurons whose activity contributes to wakefulness. This activity is normally inhibited by neurons in the portion of the reticular formation below the pons.

In the early 1950s Nathaniel Kleitman and two of his graduate students, Eugene Aserinsky and William Dement, made the remarkable discovery that sleep is not a single process but has two distinct phases. One phase is characterized by rapid eye movements (*REM sleep*); while in the other phase there are no rapid eye movements (*non-REM sleep*). These two phases alternate cyclically in a highly structured pattern. The discovery of the two phases of sleep and the subsequent finding by Moruzzi of a zone in the reticular formation that inhibits sleep displaced the old idea that sleep is simply a state of reduced activity. These two studies clearly showed that sleep is an actively induced and highly organized brain state with different phases.

In this chapter we describe the major stages of normal sleep and the neural mechanisms underlying them. In the next chapter we consider the disorders of sleep.

Sleep Follows a Circadian Rhythm

Sleep and wakefulness, like many behaviors and physiological activities, have a circadian periodicity of about 24 hours. Circadian rhythms are endogenous; they can persist without environmental cues. However, under normal circumstances the rhythms are modulated by external timing cues called *zeitgebers* (time givers) that adapt the rhythm to the environment. Sunlight, a powerful timing cue, is linked to the active phase of the circadian rhythm in some animals and the inactive phase in others. Thus, most adult humans sleep at night when it is dark; nocturnal animals such as rats and mice sleep mostly when it is light.

Since circadian rhythms are endogenous, they require a pacemaker or internal clock (see Chapter 3 for a discussion of clock genes). One major internal clock in mammals is the suprachiasmatic nucleus of the anterior hypothalamus. Light entrains this rhythm by means of the *retinohypothalamic tract,* a pathway that runs from the retina to the suprachiasmatic nucleus. Lesions of the suprachiasmatic nucleus dampen the circadian rhythm of sleep, as they dampen other circadian rhythms. When this nucleus is damaged, the rhythm governing sleep can be restored by transplanting a fetal suprachiasmatic nucleus.

The timing of circadian pacemaker neurons can be reset. Familiar examples of resetting are jet lag and the readjustment in daily living required of people who work at night. Resetting is accompanied by considerable discomfort, since, in addition to the sleep-wake cycle, many physiological mechanisms regulated by circadian rhythms are affected.

Even though the pattern of sleep and wakefulness within a day is normally under the influence of circadian regulators, sleep is not simply the result of troughs in circadian activity cycles. Although the suprachiasmatic nucleus regulates the *timing* of sleep, it is not responsible for sleep itself. Rats with lesions of the suprachiasmatic nucleus sleep in both light and dark, whereas normal rats sleep primarily during periods of light. Nevertheless, the lesioned animals sleep the same *total* amount of time in each 24-hour period as do normal animals. Furthermore, lesioned animals show rebounds of increased sleep after sleep deprivation, as do normal rats.

Total sleep time remains fairly stable from day to day even under widely varying conditions, and is only modestly affected by variations in activity and sensory stimulation. Thus, sleep time is not appreciably affected by exercise, eventful days, prolonged bed rest, profound sensory deprivation, or increased visual stimulation. In fact, day-to-day changes in total sleep time are typically not as great as day-to-day variations in food intake, physical or mental work, and mood. The only behavioral factor that reliably and substantially increases sleep is prior sleep loss.

Sleep Is Not Uniform But Is Organized in Cycles of Non-REM and REM Stages

Sleep is defined behaviorally by four criteria: (1) reduced motor activity, (2) decreased response to stimulation, (3) stereotypic postures (in humans, for example, lying down with eyes closed), and (4) relatively easy reversibility (distinguishing it from coma, hibernation, and estivation). Physiological activity during sleep can be conveniently monitored by electrical recordings: Muscle activity is monitored by electromyography, eye movements by electro-oculography, and the collective activity of cortical neurons by electroencephalography.

Humans usually fall asleep by entering non-REM sleep, a phase accompanied by characteristic changes in the electroencephalogram (EEG). The sleeper next moves into REM sleep, which is characterized not only by rapid eye movements but also by a surprisingly complete inhibition of skeletal muscle tone. It is during this phase of sleep that most dreams are thought to occur.

Non-REM Sleep Comprises Four Stages

During non-REM sleep neuronal activity is low, and metabolic rate and brain temperature are at their lowest. In addition, sympathetic outflow decreases and heart rate and blood pressure decline. Conversely, parasympathetic activity increases and then dominates during the non-REM phase, as evidenced by constriction of the pupils. Muscle tone and reflexes are intact. Non-REM sleep is divided into four characteristic stages.

Stage 1 represents the transition from wakefulness to the onset of sleep and lasts several minutes. Awake people show low-voltage EEG activity (10–30 µV and 16–25 Hz). As they relax, they show sinusoidal (alpha)

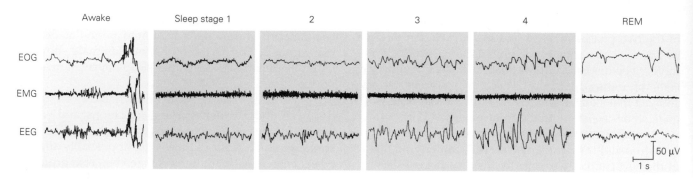

Figure 47-1 Electroencephalogram (EEG) patterns in the stages of human sleep. Non-REM sleep has four stages. Stage 1 is characterized by a slight slowing of the EEG, **stage 2** by high-amplitude K complexes and spindles (low-amplitude clusters). Slow, high-amplitude delta waves characterize **stages 3** and **4.** REM sleep is characterized by eye movements and loss of muscle tone, in conjunction with a stage 1 EEG. The higher-voltage activity in the EOG tracings during stages 3 and 4 reflects high-amplitude EEG activity in prefrontal areas rather than eye movements. **EOG** = electro-oculogram; **EMG** = electromyogram. (From Rechtschaffen and Kales 1968.)

activity of about 20–40 µV and 10 Hz. In the transition to stage 1 slower frequencies emerge and the EEG shows a low-voltage, mixed-frequency pattern. In stage 1 and throughout the non-REM phase there is some activity of skeletal muscle but no rapid eye movements. Rather, the sleeper shows slow, rolling eye movements, and the EEG is characterized by low-voltage activity of mixed frequencies (Figure 47-1).

Stage 2 is characterized by bursts of sinusoidal waves called *sleep spindles* (12–14 Hz) and high-voltage biphasic waves called K complexes, which occur episodically against a background of continuing low-voltage EEG activity.

The EEG in stage 3 shows high-amplitude, slow (0.5–2 Hz) delta waves. In stage 4 the slow-wave activity increases and dominates the EEG record. Stages 3 and 4 in humans are sometimes called *slow-wave sleep.* In some animals all of non-REM sleep is called slow-wave sleep.

REM Sleep Is an Active Form of Sleep

In humans the EEG during REM sleep reverts to a low-voltage, mixed-frequency pattern similar to stage 1 of non-REM sleep. In some animals the EEG patterns of REM sleep and wakefulness are similar. For this reason REM sleep has also been called *paradoxical sleep.* Indeed, during REM sleep the discharge patterns of most neurons resemble those during active wakefulness. Certain neurons—those in the pons, the lateral geniculate nucleus, and the occipital cortex—actually fire in more intense bursts during REM sleep than during wakefulness.

These intense bursts of firing generate high-voltage spike potentials in the EEG called ponto-geniculo-occipital spikes (*PGO spikes*), after the brain structures in which the spikes appear most prominently. PGO spikes originate in the pontine reticular formation and propagate through the lateral geniculate nucleus to the occipital cortex. Waves resembling PGO spikes can be evoked in alert subjects by abrupt stimuli, similar to those that elicit the startle response, suggesting that the spontaneous PGO spikes of REM sleep may be generated by internal activation of the neural circuit for the startle response. PGO spikes are correlated with the bursts of eye movements in REM sleep.

Consistent with the overall increase in neural activity during REM sleep, brain temperature and metabolic rate rise; in some brain regions these levels can be equal to or greater than those during the waking state. In contrast to the waking state, however, almost all skeletal muscle tone is lost (*atonia*); the skeletal muscles that remain active are those controlling the movements of the eyes, middle ear ossicles, and diaphragm. In addition, some small, phasic twitches occur.

During REM sleep penile erections occur regularly in men, and women show clitoral engorgement. In both sexes the pupils become highly constricted (*miosis*), reflecting the high ratio of parasympathetic to sympathetic output to the pupil. Homeostatic mechanisms are attenuated: respiration is relatively unresponsive to changes in blood CO_2, and responses to heat and cold are greatly reduced or even absent. As a result, body temperature drifts toward ambient temperatures.

These observations make it clear that sleep does not easily fit a continuum from "light" to "deep" but consists of distinctive phases. Each phase is behaviorally complex and each is the expression of a distinctive configuration of physiological mechanisms representing a distinctive brain state. By some criteria REM sleep might be considered lighter than non-REM sleep; for example, humans are easier to awaken from REM sleep than from non-REM stages 3 and 4. By other criteria non-REM sleep might be considered lighter than REM sleep; muscle tone, spinal reflexes, and the regulation of body temperature are maintained during non-REM sleep but are reduced during REM sleep.

The non-REM and REM phases alternate cyclically during sleep. Human adults usually begin sleep by progressing from stage 1 through stage 4 of non-REM sleep. This progression is intermittently interrupted by body movements and partial arousals. After about 70–80 minutes the sleeper usually returns briefly to stage 3 or stage 2 and then enters the first REM phase of the night, which lasts about 5–10 minutes. In humans the length of the cycle from the start of non-REM sleep to the end of the first REM phase is about 90–110 minutes. This cycle of non-REM and REM sleep is typically repeated four to six times a night. In successive cycles the duration of non-REM stages 3 and 4 decreases while the length of REM phases increases.

In young adults the largest amount of sleep time (50–60%) is spent in stage 2 non-REM sleep; REM phases constitute 20–25% of total sleep time, stages 3 and 4 non-REM about 15–20%, and stage 1 non-REM about 5% (Figure 47-2).

Different Neural Systems Promote Arousal and Sleep

In their classic study, Moruzzi and Magoun demonstrated that electrical stimulation of the midbrain reticular formation promotes the waking state. Conversely, damage to this region produces a comatose state followed by a long-term reduction in waking. Moruzzi and his colleague also found that the midbrain reticular formation is normally inhibited by a system in the medulla. Disconnecting this medullary inhibitory region, by transecting the brain stem at the level of the pons just behind the midbrain (the midpontine-pretrigeminal transection), produces an animal whose forebrain spends most of its time "awake."

Stimulation of the posterior hypothalamus, rostral to the midbrain, produces an arousal resembling that produced by stimulation of the midbrain. This hypothalamic arousal is partly mediated by histaminergic neurons that connect with cells in the brain stem below and with cells in the forebrain above. Destruction of the histaminergic neurons in the posterior hypothalamus increases sleep. Similarly, blockade of histaminergic outputs with antihistaminic drugs promotes sleep.

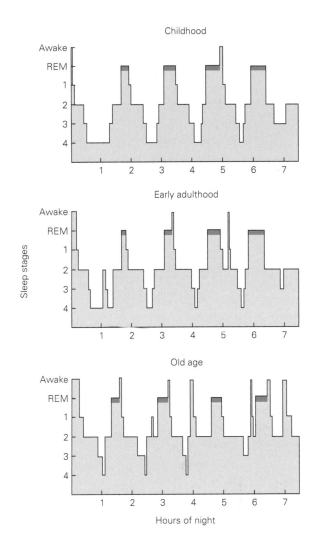

Figure 47-2 The cycling of human sleep stages at different times of life. Childhood is broadly defined to include early adolescence, and "old age" spans the period from the mid 50s to the early 70s. (From Zepelin 1983, by permission.)

Whereas the posterior hypothalamus induces arousal, electrical stimulation of the anterior hypothalamus and the adjacent basal forebrain region rapidly induces sleep, and lesions produce a long-lasting reduction in sleep. The sleep-inducing action of these regions is thought to be mediated by GABA-ergic inhibitory neurons called the *non-REM-on* cells (Figure 47-3). These cells are thought to produce sleep by inhibiting the histaminergic cells in the posterior hypothalamus as well as cells of the nucleus reticularis pontis oralis in the midbrain that mediate arousal. They are maximally active in non-REM sleep and inactive during waking and REM sleep. Many non-REM-on cells are activated by heat and thus may mediate the sleep-inducing effects of elevated temperature.

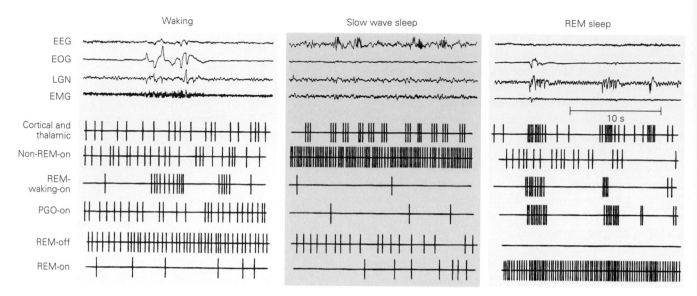

Figure 47-3 The patterns of activity of key cell groups during waking and slow wave and REM sleep are illustrated in these samples of electrode recordings from a cat. Each vertical line represents an action potential. EEG = sensorimotor electroencephalogram; EMG = dorsal neck electromyogram; EOG = eye movement; LGN = lateral geniculate nucleus electrode showing ponto-geniculo-occipital (PGO) spike activity during REM sleep.

Cortical and thalamic cells. The rate of firing of cortical and thalamic cells increases slightly during non-REM sleep and again in REM sleep. These bursts are synchronized with individual waves of the EEG (sleep spindles and slow waves).

Non-REM-on cells. These cells are located in the anterior hypothalamus and the basal forebrain region and participate in the

generation of non-REM sleep.

REM-waking-on cells. These cells predominate in the brain stem reticular formation and are active in both waking and REM sleep. Many excite motor neurons; others control the EEG.

PGO-on cells. These pontine cells fire in high-frequency bursts before PGO waves recorded in the lateral geniculate nucleus.

REM-off cells. These cells include noradrenergic, adrenergic, and serotonergic cells in the brain stem and histaminergic cells in the forebrain. Most skeletal motor neurons have a similar pattern.

REM-on cells. These cells are maximally active in REM sleep and are involved in various aspects of this state.

Non-REM Sleep Is Regulated by Interacting Sleep-Inducing and Arousal Mechanisms

Non-REM sleep is characterized by EEG spindles and slow waves that are produced by synchronized synaptic potentials in cortical neurons. These synchronized synaptic potentials are generated by the rhythmic firing of thalamic relay neurons that project to the cortex. The rhythmic firing of the relay neurons is a result of the actions of GABA-ergic inhibitory neurons in the nucleus reticularis, a nucleus that forms a shell around the thalamus (Chapter 45).

The GABA-ergic neurons of the nucleus reticularis generate a novel type of action potential that is a key event in the sequence of membrane currents generating EEG spindles. Calcium is admitted into the reticularis cells through voltage-sensitive membrane channels that open *only* when the cells are hyperpolarized. During the calcium spike the cells produce a burst of action potentials. After the calcium spike the membrane currents re-

turn the cells to the hyperpolarized state, restarting the process. This cycle of calcium influx followed by hyperpolarization results in rhythmic firing. The GABA released by the reticularis neurons hyperpolarizes thalamocortical neurons, and this hyperpolarization results in a rebound low-threshold calcium spike in the thalamocortical cells. The rhythmic firing of the thalamocortical cells (Figure 47-3) produces synchronized postsynaptic potentials in cortical neurons and it is these potentials that cause the spindle waves seen in the sleep EEG. The rhythmic firing of thalamic and cortical cells occludes the transmission of sensory information through the thalamus and the cortex.

REM Sleep Is Regulated Primarily by Nuclei Located at the Junction of the Midbrain and Pons

During both REM sleep and waking the EEG spindles and slow waves are blocked. During REM sleep there

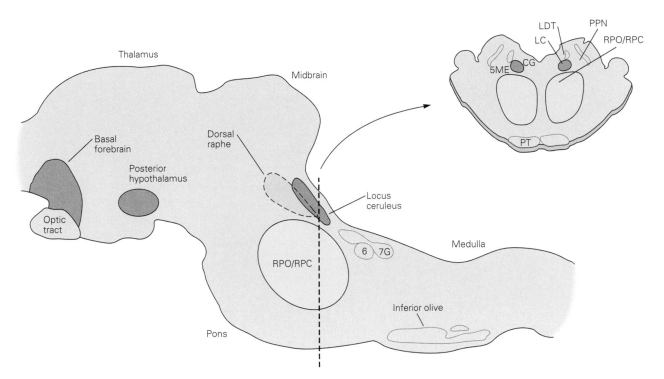

Figure 47-4 The major regions of the brain stem and fore-brain involved in sleep control are shown in this sagittal section. Nuclei in the pontine region critical for triggering REM sleep are shown in a coronal section through the center of the region (**upper right**). Stimulation of neurons in the nucleus reticularis pontis oralis/caudalis (**RPO/RPC**) region produces various characteristics of REM sleep. Depending on their exact size and location, bilateral lesions within this region completely block REM sleep or block components of REM sleep. **CG** = central gray; **LC** = locus ceruleus; **LDT** = lateral-dorsal tegmental nucleus; **PPN** = pedunculopontine nucleus; **PT** = pyramidal tract; **5ME** = mesencephalic nucleus of the trigeminal nerve; **7G** = genu of the seventh cranial nerve; **6** = nucleus of the sixth nerve.

also are PGO waves, muscle atonia, and phasic motor action. How do these events come about?

We first consider EEG voltage reduction, the phenomenon whereby EEG spindles and slow waves are blocked. An important component of the midbrain arousal system arises from cholinergic neurons in the midbrain and the adjacent dorsal pons (Chapter 45). Many of these cholinergic cells and cells adjacent to them are maximally active during waking and REM sleep, and their activity contributes to the blocking of the slow waves of the EEG (Figure 47-3). Acetylcholine (ACh) and other transmitters released by these cells depolarize the GABA-ergic inhibitory neurons in the reticularis nucleus. This depolarization prevents the hyperpolarization that activates the low-threshold Ca^{2+} channels, which in turn initiate the rhythmic firing of the reticular neurons. In the absence of rhythmic firing of the reticular neurons, the thalamocortical relay cells fire only asynchronously, and this asynchronous activity results in the low-voltage EEG characteristic of waking and REM sleep.

Other neuronal machinery important for REM sleep resides in the *nucleus reticularis pontis oralis*, which extends from the rostral pons to the caudal midbrain (Figure 47-4). Bilateral destruction of this nucleus eliminates REM sleep for extended periods. Many of the neurons in the nucleus reticular pontis oralis critical for REM sleep receive input from cholinergic cells located dorsal and lateral to them. Microinjection of the ACh agonist carbachol into the nucleus elicits extended periods of REM sleep.

Three classes of neurons in the nucleus reticularis pontis oralis are of particular interest. The cholinergic *PGO-on cells* fire in bursts to initiate PGO spikes in cells of the lateral geniculate nucleus. Destruction of PGO-on cells blocks the PGO spikes but does not interfere with other aspects of REM sleep. Conversely, stimulation of this area produces PGO spikes even in the absence of REM sleep.

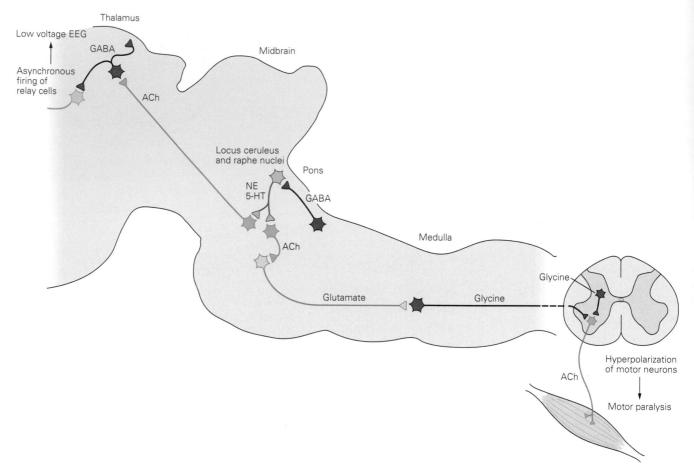

Figure 47-5 A simplified model of the possible connections between the key neuronal groups that control REM sleep. These cell groups are shown on a sagittal section of the brain stem of the cat.

During REM sleep these cell groups cause muscle tone to be turned off and the high-voltage electroencephalogram (EEG) of slow wave sleep to be replaced by the low-voltage EEG of REM sleep. A key event in this process is the activation of GABA-ergic neurons in the pons. The reason for the activation of GABA-ergic cells is not known. The GABA activation causes the inhibition of noradrenergic and serotonergic neurons and the activation (or disinhibition) of cholinergic neurons in the pons. Muscle tone is turned off by a descending system. The cholinergic neurons of the pons excite glutamatergic neurons in the pons. The glutamatergic neurons project to the medulla,

where they terminate on interneurons that release glycine onto motor neurons. This release of glycine hyperpolarizes the motor neurons, producing the motor paralysis of REM sleep. Reduced release of serotonin and norepinephrine may also contribute to muscle tone reduction by disfacilitating motor neurons.

A pontine system with ascending connections causes the reduction in EEG voltage during REM sleep. Some cholinergic cells and adjacent noncholinergic cells activated during REM sleep project to GABA-ergic cells in the thalamus. The release of acetylcholine by these cells blocks the burst firing mode of these neurons. It is the burst firing mode that produces high voltage waves in the EEG. **ACh** = acetylcholine; **NE** = norepinephrine; **5-HT** = serotonin.

The PGO-on cells are regulated by serotonergic *REM-off cells* in the raphe nuclei of the brain stem. The firing of the REM-off cells during waking activity (Figure 47-3) is thought to hyperpolarize and thereby block the burst firing of PGO-on cells. In the transition from non-REM to REM sleep the cessation of activity in the REM-off cells allows the PGO cells to begin discharging in bursts, generating PGO waves. Noradrenergic neu-

rons in the locus ceruleus and histaminergic neurons in the posterior hypothalamus have a pattern of activity that is similar to that of the serotonergic REM-off cells. Cessation of activity in these three cell groups may contribute to changes in autonomic tone, EEG, and muscle tone during REM sleep.

Another class of cells in the nucleus reticularis pontis oralis, the *REM-waking-on cells,* fire during active waking as well as during REM sleep (Figure 47-3) and fire at lower rates during non-REM sleep. Some of these cells project to the motor neurons in the spinal cord, and others project to the motor neurons that drive the extraocular muscles. The burst firing of these cells during waking mediates movements of the head, the neck, the limbs, and the eyes. Their firing during REM sleep produces rapid eye movements and muscle twitches, breaking through the concurrent inhibition of motor neurons.

The third class of cells in the nucleus reticularis pontis oralis, the *REM-on cells*, show little or no activity during waking and non-REM sleep but have high levels of activity in REM sleep (Figure 47-3). Although few in number, these cells play a key role in REM sleep control. One subtype of these cells is GABA-ergic and is responsible for the inhibition of activity in serotonergic and noradrenergic cells during REM sleep; another subtype, possibly glutamatergic, is responsible for the loss of muscle tone in REM sleep.

Muscle tone is lost during REM sleep because motor neurons are actively inhibited. The circuitry mediating inhibition of muscle tone resides in the pons and medulla. A small lesion within a portion of the nucleus reticularis pontis oralis critical for REM sleep releases motor activity during REM sleep. Cats with this lesion have normal non-REM sleep episodes, but when they enter REM sleep they raise their heads, walk, and engage in a variety of vigorous motor activities. A similar syndrome can be produced by lesions of the medial medulla.

The suppression of muscle tone in REM sleep is mediated by interconnections between several types of REM-on neurons. Abnormal activity in these neurons during waking is believed to cause a sudden loss of muscle tone (*cataplexy*), one of the primary symptoms of narcolepsy. Excessive activity in these neurons during sleep may contribute to a collapse of the airway resulting from reduction in muscle tone (*sleep apnea*). Insufficient activity in these neurons during sleep may cause a release of motor activity during REM sleep, during which dreams are acted out (the REM sleep behavior disorder). We shall consider these sleep disorders in greater detail in the next chapter.

The connections thought to mediate the interactions between the key groups of neurons that mediate REM sleep are illustrated in Figure 47-5.

Several Endogenous Substances Affect Sleep

For nearly a century sleep researchers have searched for substances that accumulate during waking and are metabolized in sleep. An understanding of how soluble substances might determine sleepiness would provide an important insight into sleep function, as well as the development of potent "natural" sleeping pills. However, no endogenous substance is yet widely accepted as causing sleep. Among the substances that have been identified as having hypnogenic properties are muramyl peptides (a chemical related to substances found in bacterial cell walls), interleukin-1 (a cytokine that may mediate the effects of muramyl peptides as well as immune responses), adenosine, delta sleep-inducing peptide (a substance isolated from the blood of sleeping rabbits), prostaglandin D_2, and a long-chain fatty acid primary amide, *cis*-9,10-octadecenoamide.

Melatonin, a hormone synthesized in the brain, stimulates wakefulness when given to rats during the daytime and has a powerful hypnotic effect in birds. Human studies have not shown a consistent hypnotic effect, although recent studies have indicated that it can facilitate sleep onset in old people who are deficient in melatonin and may be of value in treating jet lag. It remains unclear whether it is effective as a treatment for insomnia, despite its popular promotion as a safe, natural sleeping pill.

Sleep Periods Change Over the Life Span

In humans daily sleep declines sharply from a peak of 17–18 hours at birth to 10–12 hours at age 4 and then more gradually to a fairly stable duration of 7–8.5 hours by age 20. The initial pattern of infancy, consisting of 3- to 4-hour bouts of sleep alternating with brief feedings, is gradually replaced by more continuous sleep. By age 4 sleep becomes consolidated into a single long nocturnal period and sometimes a daytime nap.

In the newborn, REM phases constitute about 50% of sleep, but these REM phases differ from their adult form. The atonia is very irregular, and rapid eye movements and muscle twitches occur on a background of low muscle tone and a relatively undifferentiated EEG. The proportion of time spent in REM sleep declines rapidly until about 4 years of age, when it stabilizes near the level of young adults (20–25%). With increasing age, REM declines gradually to 15–20% (Figure 47-2).

The high-amplitude, slow EEG waves of the non-REM phase are absent at birth. In humans these slow waves appear during the first year of life and their amplitudes greatly increase, reaching a stable, high plateau between 3–11 years of age. These developmental changes in sleep are accelerated in animals that mature rapidly. For example, in rats a mature sleep pattern is achieved 30 days after birth. In humans slow-wave activity begins to decline during adolescence and continues to decline for the rest of life. Like newborns, many people over age 50 show almost no high-amplitude EEG activity (Figure 47-2). Also, the nocturnal sleep of the elderly tends to be interrupted by many short awakenings.

There Are Phylogenetic Variations in Sleep

All mammals sleep, but the length and form of sleep (the proportion of non-REM and REM phases) vary greatly. Daily sleep ranges from about 4–5 hours in giraffes and elephants to 18 hours or more in bats, opossums, and giant armadillos. Small mammals generally sleep more than larger mammals. REM sleep as a percentage of total sleep ranges from 10.5% in guinea pigs and baboons to 25% or more in opossums, hedgehogs, dogs, and giraffes. Mammals born immature tend to have more REM sleep, both in infancy and adulthood, than precocial mammals. The length of the (non-REM–REM sleep cycle) ranges from 12 min or less in shrews, bats, rats, and mice to 30 min or longer in humans, pigs, cattle, and elephants. Brain weight is positively correlated with the length of the cycle, independent of the relationship of brain weight to body weight.

Specific characteristics of sleep have presumably evolved as adaptations to each animal's way of life. For example, several marine mammals show non-REM sleep patterns in only one cerebral hemisphere at a time, an apparent accommodation to respiration. If a dolphin is awakened when only one hemisphere sleeps, that hemisphere later shows a sleep rebound while the other does not. Like mammals, birds show non-REM and REM sleep but their sleep episodes are much shorter; REM episodes may last only several seconds, muscle atonia during the REM phase is rare, and the occurrences of non-REM sleep patterns in only one hemisphere are more frequent. Lower orders show quiescent periods that resemble sleep behaviorally; whether these periods are ancestral to mammalian sleep or simply species-specific forms of rest is not clear.

Phylogenetic differences suggest that sleep is largely under genetic control. This idea is supported by laboratory studies that show significant correlations of total sleep time and the proportion of REM in monozygotic but not dizygotic twins. Moreover, heritability of sleep patterns has been demonstrated within species. Inbred mice strains show differences in total sleep time, REM sleep, and circadian rhythms, and crossbreeding studies of mice indicate that each of these sleep characteristics is inherited independently.

The Functions of Sleep and Dreaming Are Not Yet Known

Various Theories of the Function of Sleep Have Been Proposed

It is likely that sleep is functionally important because it has persisted throughout the evolution of mammals and birds (and is perhaps present in lower forms as well). Its importance is also indicated by the rebound of sleep after total sleep deprivation and the rebound of slow-wave or REM sleep after selective deprivation of these stages, as well as by the functional impairments after sleep loss. Rats that have been chronically deprived of sleep for 2–3 weeks die. Rats deprived only of REM sleep survive about twice as long. Despite these considerations, there is no agreement on why sleep is important. Several ideas have been advanced, but they all have been challenged by contrary evidence or shown to have limited generality.

Conservation of Metabolic Energy

The idea that sleep conserves energy is supported by the fact that humans and laboratory animals increase their food intake during sleep deprivation. However, the metabolic rate during sleep is only 15% less than during quiet wakefulness; the energy loss of a sleepless night could be compensated by only a small amount of food. The idea that sleep enforces body rest is supported by the fact that small mammals tend to sleep the most. These animals have high energy demands for thermoregulation and locomotion but low energy reserves. However, rest is possible during wakefulness. Why suffer a form of rest with impaired vigilance? Nevertheless, rest without sleep leaves us sleepy. Because we feel refreshed after sleep, the idea that sleep is restitutive is intuitively appealing, but precisely what may get restored during sleep has not been identified.

Cognition

Humans show little or no physiological impairment after several days of sleep deprivation but do show impaired intellectual performance. Thus, it has been proposed that sleep serves higher mental functions. However, the performance deficit could result from a homeostatic pressure to enter sleep rather than from impaired intellectual capacity. Most of the deficits can be reversed by strong motivation or analeptic drugs.

Thermoregulation

There are strong indications that sleep has thermoregulatory functions. Body and brain temperatures are usually reduced during sleep. Heating the hypothalamus induces sleep in animals, and body heating prior to sleep increases subsequent slow wave sleep in humans. Rats that are chronically deprived of sleep show an increase in preferred ambient temperature of 10°C or more. These facts suggest that sleep has cooling functions. On the other hand, rats deprived of sleep for two weeks show a significant drop in body temperature in spite of a doubling of metabolic rate, suggesting that sleep may also have a role in heat retention.

Neural Maturation and Mental Health

The idea that REM sleep aids neural maturation is strongly supported by the association of REM sleep and immaturity at birth both across and within species. But why would REM sleep then persist and rebound after its selective deprivation in adults? Early anecdotal reports of disturbed behavior after REM sleep deprivation suggested that REM sleep is important for mental health, but none of several controlled studies has demonstrated that mental health is impaired as a result of REM deprivation. In fact, severely depressed patients improve after extended REM deprivation.

Some reports indicate that REM sleep facilitates learning or memory, but the effects of REM sleep deprivation on learning and memory have not always been very strong or very consistent. In fact, learning can occur without sleep. The fact that REM sleep follows non-REM sleep suggests that REM sleep compensates for the cerebral inactivation or temperature declines of non-REM sleep. However, even when wakefulness (with its cerebral activation and increased temperature) follows selective REM sleep deprivation, compensatory increases of REM sleep follow later.

In light of the many ideas about the function of sleep, sleep may have many functions. Alternatively, it may serve a single, as yet unidentified, cellular function important to a variety of processes: maturational processes in the young, temperature regulation in small animals, and cognitive processes in adult humans.

Modern Research Has Increased Our Knowledge About Dreaming

When Kleitman, Aserinsky, and Dement studied the REM and non-REM phases of sleep they also studied the relation of each phase to dreaming. They awakened subjects during REM and non-REM sleep and asked them to describe any dreams they were having. Dreams were far more likely to be recalled when subjects were awakened from REM sleep (74% or more of awakenings) than from non-REM sleep (less than 10% of awakenings). The preponderance of reports after REM sleep led to the belief that dreaming occurs exclusively during REM sleep (the non-REM reports were dismissed as recall from earlier REM sleep). It was widely believed that the physiological basis of dreaming would soon be discovered. This expectation has not yet been realized.

Although REM sleep is the phase from which dreams may be most reliably elicited, REM sleep is not necessary for dreaming. In almost all more recent studies the frequency of dream recall after non-REM sleep is higher than in the earliest studies—as high as 70% in some studies. Many dream reports are elicited on awakenings from non-REM sleep that occurs before the first REM phase of the night; these dream reports do not represent recall from REM periods earlier in the night. In fact, dream reports have also been elicited from subjects at the onset of sleep and from subjects lying quietly awake in a darkened room.

Reports of non-REM dreams tend to be shorter, less vivid, less emotional, and more coherent than reports of REM dreams. But there are no qualitative differences between REM and non-REM reports of the same length. Thus, the major difference is that REM dreams tend to be longer than non-REM dreams.

REM sleep is not sufficient for dreaming, which varies with cognitive abilities as well as sleep stages. Even though children have abundant REM sleep, they rarely report thematically organized dreams before ages 7–9 years; appearance of organized dreams is correlated with the development of visuospatial skills. Dreaming may be absent in a variety of patients with neurological damage who nevertheless show REM sleep.

According to Sigmund Freud, dreams are disguised manifestations of strong, unacceptable, unconscious wishes. Much of the impetus for modern dream research was motivated by the interest in the psychoanalytic interpretation of dream content. Although modern dream research has identified the phases of sleep when dreams are likely to occur—and has thus facilitated fresh recall of dreams—it has no special procedures for uncovering hidden meanings and has therefore contributed little to identifying unconscious determinants of dreams. Nor has it had much success in specifying other sources of dream content. However, it has shown that dream content is not greatly influenced by external environmental stimuli during sleep. Even on the relatively infrequent occasions when external stimuli are incorporated into dreams, they usually appear to be incidental to the dream narrative. In one study subjects had their eyelids taped open and had various objects presented to them during REM sleep. None of the objects appeared in any of the subsequently reported REM dreams.

Systemic stimulation of one or another internal homeostatic system also does not have a consistent effect on dream content. For example, restricting fluid intake over a 24-hour period does not routinely lead to the appearance of thirst in REM dream reports, and only one-third of dream reports following fluid restriction contain any references to drinking. Although full or partial penile erections occur in 80–95% of REM periods, only 12% of men's dreams contain manifestly sexual content. Moreover, patients with spinal cord transections that preclude genital sensations report dreams with orgasmic imagery. Even experiences that immediately precede sleep do not appear to affect our dreams consistently. For example, viewing violent films does not reliably produce violent dreams, nor do pornographic films increase sexual dreams substantially.

Although modern dream research has contributed relatively little to uncovering hidden meanings in dreams, it has greatly enlarged the empirical information on the phenomenology and correlates of dreams by systematically collecting detailed dream reports in the laboratory. Dreams are not kaleidoscopic jumbles of visual fragments, but are organized thematically and perceptually. The old view that dreams occur in an instant is not consistent with the correlation between the duration of the REM period, the length of the dream report, and the actual time taken by subjects to reenact a dream experience after they have been awakened. Although threads of specific content or personal concerns may appear in several discrete dreaming periods during a single night, dreams do not appear as successive chapters in a book, but rather as separate short stories.

Dreams and waking mentation are similar in several respects. Most dreams collected over the course of a night are quite ordinary. Dreams have an undeserved reputation for being extremely bizarre because our spontaneous recall of dreams is usually limited to the longer, more exciting dreams that typically occur before morning awakening. In general a person's mood, anxiety, imaginativeness, and expressiveness in dreams are positively correlated with these traits in their waking experience. Except for some decrease in the clarity of background detail and color saturation, visual dream imagery resembles waking visual imagery. Like waking imagery, most dreams are in color; the mystery is why 20–30% of dreams are achromatic.

Perhaps the greatest difference between dreaming and ordinary wakefulness is that we are able to differentiate between real and imagined images only when we are awake. Except for the relatively rare lucid dreams in which we know we are dreaming, *all* dream images seem real at the time. In spite of a lifetime of discriminating between dreams and reality, we can make the discrimination only after awakening. Identifying the neural substrates that are responsible for critical self-reflection during wakefulness, and that fail us while dreaming, is a major challenge for sleep and dream research.

An Overall View

The circadian rhythm of sleep is controlled by the suprachiasmatic nucleus of the hypothalamus. Non-REM sleep is generated by the interaction of neurons in the basal forebrain and medulla with neurons in the midbrain and diencephalon. REM sleep is generated by the interaction of neurons in the caudal midbrain and pons with neurons in the medulla and forebrain. Thus, sleep is actively generated by the interplay of several neuronal populations using different transmitters.

Sleep serves important functions, as is indicated by its ubiquitous persistence in different environments and throughout evolution, by the rebound of sleep after sleep loss, and by the functional impairments (to the point of death) produced by sleep deprivation. No theory of sleep, however, has yet succeeded in explaining the exact function of sleep or providing a unified way of integrating the wealth of data now available on sleep.

The discovery of a relationship between REM sleep and dreaming was a major impetus for modern sleep research. However, we now know that REM sleep is not necessary for dreaming, that dreaming can also occur during non-REM sleep, and that dreamlike experiences can be elicited during quiet wakefulness. REM sleep is also not sufficient for dreaming, since the integrity of certain cognitive skills is also necessary.

Nevertheless, REM sleep is the state from which long vivid dreams are retrieved most reliably. As a result, studies of REM sleep have greatly increased knowledge about the number of dreams per night and their temporal characteristics, perceptual features, stimulus determinants, and cognitive features. The sources of specific dream content and an understanding of why we are usually unaware that we are dreaming while the dream is in progress still remain a mystery.

Allan Rechtschaffen
Jerome Siegel

Selected Readings

Anch AM, Browman CP, Mitler MM, Walsh JK. 1988. *Sleep: A Scientific Perspective.* Englewood Cliffs, NJ: Prentice Hall.

Antrobus JS, Bertini M (eds). 1992. *The Neuropsychology of Sleep and Dreaming.* Hillsdale, NJ: Erlbaum.

Carskadon MA, Rechtschaffen A, Richardson G, Roth T, Siegel J (eds). 1993. *Encyclopedia of Sleep and Dreaming.* New York: Macmillan.

Cavallero C, Foulkes D (eds). 1993. *Dreaming as Cognition.* London: Harvester Wheatsheaf.

Horne J. 1988. *Why We Sleep: The Functions of Sleep in Humans and Other Mammals.* New York: Oxford Univ. Press.

Klein DC, Moore RY, Reppert SM (eds). 1991. *Suprachiasmatic Nucleus: The Mind's Clock.* New York: Oxford Univ. Press.

Kleitman N. 1963. *Sleep and Wakefulness.* Chicago: Univ. Chicago Press.

Kryger MH, Roth T, Dement WC (eds). 1994. *Principles and Practice of Sleep Medicine,* 2nd ed. Philadelphia: Saunders.

Rechtschaffen A. 1973. The psychophysiology of mental activity during sleep. In: FJ McGuigan, RS Schoonover (eds). *The Psychophysiology of Thinking,* pp. 153–205. New York: Academic.

Rechtschaffen A. 1978. The single-mindedness and isolation of dreams. Sleep 1:97–109.

Rechtschaffen A. 1998. Current perspectives on the function of sleep. Perspect Biol Med 41:359-390.

Siegel JM. 1994. Brainstem mechanisms generating REM sleep. In: MH Kryger, T Roth, WC Dement (eds). *Principles and Practice of Sleep Medicine,* 2nd ed., pp. 125–144. Philadelphia: Saunders.

Steriade M, McCarley RW. 1990. *Brainstem Control of Wakefulness and Sleep.* New York: Plenum.

Zepelin H. 1983. A life span perspective on sleep. In: A Mayes (ed). *Sleep Mechanisms and Functions in Humans and Animals: An Evolutionary Perspective,* pp. 126-160. Cambridge: Cambridge Univ. Press.

References

Aserinsky E, Kleitman N. 1953. Regularly occurring periods of eye motility, and concomitant phenomena, during sleep. Science 118:273–274.

Baghdoyan HA, Mallios J, Duckrow RB, Mash DC. 1994. Localization of muscarinic receptor subtypes in brain stem areas regulating sleep. Neuroreport 5:1631–1634.

Bard P, Macht MB. 1958. The behavior of chronically decere-brate cats. In: GEW Wolstenholme, CM O'Conner (eds). *Neurological Basis of Behavior,* pp. 55–75. London: Churchill.

Dement W, Wolpert EA. 1958. The relation of eye movements, body motility, and external stimuli to dream content. J Exper Psychol 55:543–553.

Foulkes WD. 1982. *Children's Dreams: Longitudinal Studies.* New York: Wiley-Interscience.

Freud S. 1953 (1900). *The Interpretation of Dreams.* James Strachey (trans). London: Hogarth.

Haimov I, Lavie P, Laudon M, Herer P, Vigder C, Zisapel N. 1995. Melatonin replacement therapy of elderly insomniacs. Sleep 18:598–603.

Hobson JA, McCarley RW. 1977. The brain as a dream state generator: an activation-synthesis hypothesis of the dream process. Am J Psychiatry 134:1335–1348.

Jouvet M. 1967. Neurophysiology of the states of sleep. Physiol Rev 47:117–177.

Luebke JJ, Greene RW, Semba K, Kamondi A, McCarley RW, Reiner PB. 1992. Serotonin hyperpolarizes cholinergic low-threshold burst neurons in the rat laterodorsal tegmental nucleus in vitro. Proc Natl Acad Sci U S A 89:743–747.

Moruzzi G, Magoun HW. 1949. Brain stem reticular formation and activation of the EEG. Electroencephalogr Clin Neurophysiol 1:455–473.

Nitz D, Siegel JM. 1997. GABA release in the dorsal raphe nucleus: role in the control of REM sleep. Am J Physiol 273:R451–R455.

Ralph MR, Foster RG, Davis FC, Menaker M. 1990. Transplanted suprachiasmatic nucleus determines circadian period. Science 247:975–978.

Rechtschaffen A, Bergmann BM. 1995. Sleep deprivation in the rat by the disk-over-water method. Behav Brain Res 69:55–63.

Rechtschaffen A, Kales A. 1968. *A Manual of Standardized Terminology, Techniques and Scoring System and Sleep Stages of Human Subjects.* Los Angeles: University of California Brain Information Service.

Schenkel E, Siegel JM. 1989. REM sleep without atonia after lesions of the medial medulla. Neurosci Lett 98:159–165.

Shouse MN, Siegel JM. 1992. Pontine regulation of REM sleep components in cats: integrity of the pedunculopontine tegmentum (PPT) is important for phasic events but unnecessary for atonia during REM sleep. Brain Res 571:50–63.

Siegel JM, Nienhuis R, Fahringer HM, Paul R, Shiromani P, Dement WC, Mignot E, Chiu C. 1991. Neuronal activity in narcolepsy: identification of cataplexy related cells in the medial medulla. Science 252:1315–1318.

Solms M. 1996. *The Neuropsychology of Dreams: A Clinico-Anatomical Study.* Mahwah, NJ: Erlbaum.

Steriade M, McCormick DA, Sejnowski TJ. 1993. Thalamo-cortical oscillations in the sleeping and aroused brain. Science 262:679–685.

48

Disorders of Sleep and Wakefulness

A S WE HAVE SEEN IN THE previous chapter, sleep is an actively induced state distinct from wakefulness. Disorders of sleep have a variety of causes. Some represent an exacerbation of a waking medical disorder whereas others are primary disorders of sleep. In this chapter we describe the major disorders of sleep in the context of the neural mechanisms of sleep and wakefulness.

We first discuss the general consequences of sleep disorders and then consider several specific ones. These disorders can be classified according to patients' primary complaints: excessive sleepiness (difficulty maintaining wakefulness), difficulty initiating and maintaining sleep (insomnia), or difficulties with partial arousal from sleep.

There is a surprising difference in the incidence of insomnia as compared with that of excessive sleepiness. A large number of people, about 15%, have chronic insomnia, but only about 2% have excessive sleepiness. Yet more people seek help for excessive sleepiness than for insomnia or any other sleep disorder, because excessive sleepiness is much more disruptive to life than insomnia. Nearly half of the people who seek medical attention for excessive sleepiness have had automobile accidents. More than half have had occupational accidents, some life-threatening. Because of their sleepiness, many have lost jobs, and the impact of sleepiness on family life is very disruptive. Insomnia, however, is by no means innocuous. Among people complaining of chronic insomnia the rate of automobile accidents resulting from daytime sleepiness is twice that of people with occasional or no insomnia.

Both insomnia and excessive sleepiness are complaints—they are symptoms. Like many symptoms, insomnia or daytime sleepiness can be caused by any of a number of different disorders or combination of disorders. Evaluation of sleep disorders starts with an assessment of the patient's sleep habits—the amount and timing of sleep—and drug use, since some drugs can disturb sleep or waking alertness.

Disturbances of sleep are frequently seen in depression, with early morning awakening being most common. Curiously, sleep deprivation transiently alleviates the psychological symptoms. Thus, keeping the depressed patient from sleeping for one or two consecu-

Table 48-1 Electrophysiological Measures Used in Clinical Polysomnograms

Documenting sleep states
  Left electro-oculogram
  Right electro-oculogram
  Electromyogram (submental muscle)
  Electroencephalogram (C3/A2 or C4/A1 placements)

Documenting cardiac arrhythmias
  Electrocardiogram (V5 placement)

Identifying periodic leg movements
  Electromyogram (tibialis muscle)

Documenting apnea and hypopnea with the associated desaturation
  Nasal/oral airflow (thermistor)
  Thoracic movement (strain gauge)
  SaO$_2$ (oxygen desaturation by oximetry)

tive nights (done only in a hospital setting) results in a day without symptoms. The symptoms return, however, when the patient resumes regular sleep patterns.

Electrophysiological methods used to document sleep are described in the previous chapter. Additional physiological monitoring, referred to as *clinical polysomnography*, helps to identify the various sleep pathologies and their consequences (Table 48-1).

A Variety of Medical Disorders Are Associated With Excessive Sleepiness

A variety of medical conditions can be associated with excessive daytime sleepiness. Primary sleep pathologies such as apnea (cessation of breathing for more than 10 s) and periodic limb movements (typically in the legs, lasting 0.5 to 5 s) can lead to excessive daytime sleepiness if they occur frequently. Irregular or insufficient sleep can also result in excessive daytime sleepiness. Obstructive sleep apnea syndrome is the most frequent complaint at sleep disorder centers; the next most frequent disorder is narcolepsy. These two disorders are also the most interesting scientifically.

Persistent Daytime Sleepiness Is the Most Prominent Symptom of Narcolepsy

Narcolepsy is a primary sleep disorder that affects between 20–45 people per 100,000 in the United States. Its most prominent symptom is excessive sleepiness. This

disorder was first identified in 1880 by Jean-Baptiste Gelineau, who described a condition of irresistible, recurring, short episodes of sleep, accompanied by *cataplexy* (an abrupt and reversible loss of muscle tone elicited by strong emotion, commonly anger or laughter).

In the 1950s the *narcoleptic syndrome* was defined as consisting of four symptoms: (1) daytime sleepiness, (2) cataplexy, (3) sleep paralysis, and (4) hypnagogic hallucinations. Shortly after the discovery of rapid eye movement (REM) sleep it was observed that patients with narcolepsy begin sleep with REM sleep, whereas, as we saw in the last chapter, sleep normally begins with non-REM sleep. Onset of sleep with a REM period is now considered to be the pathognomonic sign of narcolepsy (Figure 48-1).

The persistent daytime sleepiness of narcolepsy is debilitating. Sleep intrudes into wakefulness during physical as well as sedentary activities. These unwanted sleep episodes recur throughout the day, lasting from minutes to an hour. Patients report feeling refreshed when they awaken from these brief sleep episodes. Between episodes there is a refractory period lasting several hours. Poor work performance, memory lapses, and behavioral automatisms are typical symptoms reported by patients with narcolepsy. Excessive sleepiness is usually the first symptom that develops in narcolepsy, generally between 15 and 25 years of age.

Whereas the key sign of narcolepsy is the onset of sleep with a REM period, its major symptom is cataplexy, the reversible loss of muscle tone. The cataplectic attack, or *sleep paralysis,* can involve all skeletal musculature or only isolated muscle groups. It can result in total collapse, slight buckling of the knees, or only a sagging jaw. Attacks are usually short-lived and do not impair consciousness and memory. There is some disagreement, however, whether cataplexy is an inherent feature of narcolepsy and whether its presence is essential to make the diagnosis. Cataplexy does not occur in all patients showing the other signs and symptoms of narcolepsy, while other patients with narcolepsy experience cataplexy only.

Sleep paralysis typically occurs as patients with narcolepsy fall asleep or awaken. At these transitions between sleep and wakefulness patients find themselves unable to move or speak, even if they have awakened. They are aware of the paralysis and able to recall the experience later. For some patients sleep paralysis is quite upsetting. *Sleep onset paralysis* is often accompanied by visual hallucinations but is relatively rare in the general population. *Sleep offset paralysis* occurs on awakening from REM sleep and is common. Not all patients with narcolepsy experience sleep paralysis or hypnagogic

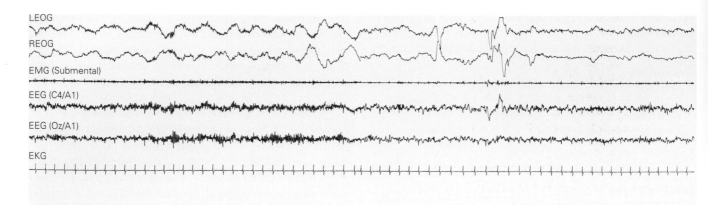

Figure 48-1 A 1-minute sample of a polysomnogram showing a sleep-onset rapid eye movement period (SOREMP). SOREMPs are considered to be the pathognomonic sign of narcolepsy. The **left** side of the traces shows rolling eye movements in the left and right electro-oculograms (**LEOG** and **REOG**), some submental electromyographic (**EMG**) activity, and low-voltage fast electroencephalographic (**EEG**) activity with bursts of alpha waves (8–12 Hz) from the central (**C4/A1**) and occipital (**Oz/A1**) EEG electrode placements. These are the characteristics of eyes-closed, relaxed wakefulness. The **middle** of the traces shows a loss of submental EMG activity (ie, atonia of REM sleep), the appearance of rapid eye movements (REMs) in the LEOG and REOG tracings, and a slowing of EEG activity with sawtooth-like waves. These are the characteristics of REM sleep.

hallucinations. When they do occur, these symptoms usually develop after the onset of the primary symptom, excessive sleepiness.

The clinical symptoms of cataplexy, sleep paralysis, and hypnagogic hallucinations are all pathologic manifestations of REM sleep. In fact, cataplexy appears to be neurophysiologically similar to this atonia of REM sleep without having REM sleep. As we have seen in Chapter 47, the medulla and pons contain a system that actively suppresses skeletal muscle tone during REM sleep. The muscle atonia of REM sleep occurs through inhibition of spinal motor neurons, probably by glycinergic inhibitory interneurons in the spinal cord. Loss of muscle tone without complete induction of REM sleep can be elicited experimentally by local injection of cholinergic and glutamatergic agonists into the brain stem, pons, and medulla of cats. Cataplexy appears to be neurophysiologically similar to this atonia without REM sleep. In patients with narcolepsy, neural systems that normally produce arousal seem to malfunction during wakefulness; instead of producing arousal, they trigger atonia but without the other features of REM sleep.

Other findings for narcolepsy include excessive sleepiness on the *multiple sleep latency test,* a standard test of sleepiness in which latency to sleep onset is repeatedly tested (Figure 48-2). Regardless of time of day, patients with narcolepsy fall asleep in 2–3 minutes whereas healthy normal subjects fall asleep in 10–15 minutes and display a circadian rhythm in their sleep latency. On these latency tests normal people rarely en-

ter sleep with REM sleep, whereas patients with narcolepsy typically do. In healthy normal subjects REM latency is shortened after they take REM-suppressing drugs or are awakened every time REM occurs. Decreased REM latency is an indication of REM pressure. However, in narcolepsy the fact that sleep begins with REM sleep does not indicate the existence of REM pressure since the other typical signs (increased REM percent and more frequent eye movements) do not occur. In fact, when sleep does not begin with REM sleep the REM latency of patients with narcolepsy is normal. Their nocturnal sleep is often disturbed, however, with frequent awakenings and brief arousals associated with apneas and leg movements.

Narcolepsy has long been known to have a familial incidence strongly associated, perhaps up to 90%, with a class II antigen of the major histocompatibility complex on chromosome 6 at the HLA-DR2 or HLA-DQW1 locus.[1] This strong genetic association suggests a genetic basis for the susceptibility to narcolepsy. What environmental factors lead to the expression of narcolepsy, or whether the syndrome is polygenetic in origin, is not known. HLA-DR2 is also associated with autoimmune diseases such as multiple sclerosis and rheumatoid

---

1. The association, originally thought to be 98–100%, may be somewhat lower.

arthritis, raising the possibility that narcolepsy has an immunological basis, possibly a viral infection. However, infectious processes have not yet been clearly implicated.

Some dogs are narcoleptic, and their narcolepsies are similar in most respects to human narcolepsy, except for the mode of genetic transmission. In these dogs abnormalities have been found in cholinergic and monoaminergic synaptic transmission, important components of REM sleep regulation (Chapter 47). Dogs with narcolepsy have more muscarinic M2 receptors in the pons, suggesting a defect in cholinergic sensitivity. Consistent with this, cholinergic antagonists inhibit and agonists exacerbate canine cataplexy. Norepinephrine function also seems abnormal in that the number of α-2 receptors in the locus ceruleus is larger than normal. Moreover, the density of dopamine D2 receptors is greater in both dogs and humans with narcolepsy. Finally, some of the selective serotonin reuptake inhibitors reduce cataplexy in dogs and humans, thereby implicating serotonergic systems, at least in cataplexy.

Given the incomplete understanding of the etiology and pathophysiology of narcolepsy, the treatment focuses on symptoms. Excessive sleepiness is treated with stimulants such as pemoline, methylphenidate, and amphetamine, drugs that enhance noradrenergic function. Cataplexy is treated with tricyclic antidepressants and monoamine oxidase inhibitors, drugs most effective in suppressing REM sleep. The effectiveness of antidepressants against cataplexy and sleep paralysis is probably due to their ability to inhibit norepinephrine reuptake.

Although stimulants and tricyclics are helpful, they do not completely reverse the symptoms. Moreover, tolerance develops to the stimulants. These limitations require careful clinical and behavioral management, including introduction of periods without drugs (drug holidays) and the use of napping strategies for better maintenance of alertness.

Breathing Is Compromised in Obstructive Sleep Apnea Syndrome

Obstructive sleep apnea syndrome is another primary sleep disorder. It is a disorder of physiological functions normally altered by sleep rather than a disorder of sleep-wake cycles. Breathing is compromised because during sleep there is a reduction in skeletal muscle tone. Obstruction of the upper airway produces frequent *apnea* (breathing cessation for more than 10 seconds) and leads to frequent, brief arousals from sleep in order to reestablish upper airway muscle tone to resume breathing (Figure 48-3).

In a recent study in the United States of employed men and women aged 30–60 years, 2% of women and 4% of men had five or more episodes of apnea per hour of sleep (considered to be an abnormal level of apnea) and also complained of excessive sleepiness. In those aged 50–60 years, 4% of women and 9% of men were estimated to have obstructive sleep apnea syndrome.

Snoring is the most common patient complaint, although snorers do not necessarily have apnea. The next most prominent symptoms are excessive daytime sleepiness and nonrefreshing sleep. Unless observed by a bed partner, the frequent apnea is often not known to the patient, and it is the snoring or excessive sleepiness that brings medical attention.

Patients may also report restlessness and choking during sleep, as well as morning headaches. As with narcolepsy, the daytime sleepiness may be accompanied by memory problems or mental confusion. Obstructive sleep apnea syndrome is seen usually in obese, middle-aged men. Twice as many men as women have the disorder. The typical patient with obstructive sleep apnea is in good general health except for obesity. When the patient has had the apnea for longer periods of time, cardiovascular complications, such as cardiac arrhythmias or hypertension, may occur.

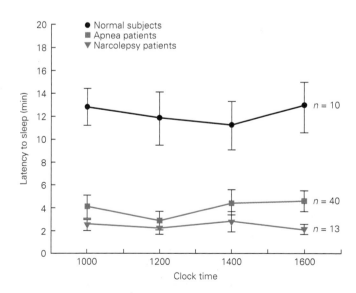

Figure 48-2 Sleep latency is measured by the multiple sleep latency test (MSLT). The data here are for tests conducted at 2-hour intervals across the day on patients with narcolepsy and apnea compared with healthy normal subjects matched for age. Normal subjects fall asleep in 10–15 min, with slight reductions in latency later in the day (at 1400). Patients with narcolepsy or apnea consistently fall asleep in 5 min or less.

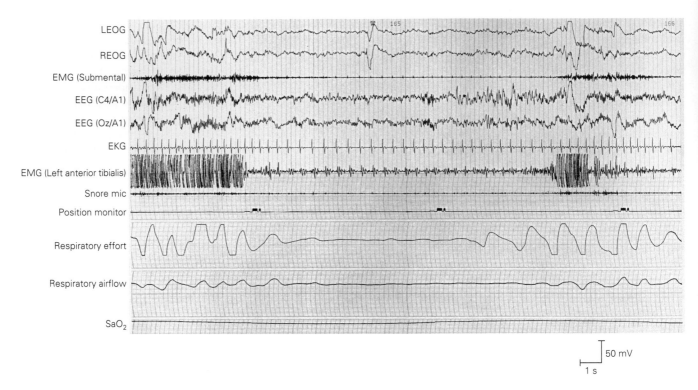

Figure 48-3 This polysomnogram sample illustrates an episode of apnea (mixed type). Starting at the left, the tracings reflect the arousal that terminated the previous apnea episode. After approximately six breaths the respiratory effort (as measured by a strain gauge placed over the rib cage) ceases, as does respiration airflow (recorded by naso-oral thermistors). The EEG from the central (**C4/A1**) and occipital placements (**Oz/A1**) shows a sleep spindle (12–14 Hz) in the middle of the episode, and the C4/A1 tracing shows a K complex toward the end of the episode. Resumption of the respiratory effort leads to arousal, as reflected in the EEG speeding and the increase in submental EMG activity. With arousal the airway opens again and airflow resumes. **EKG** = electrocardiogram; **LEOG** and **REOG** = left and right electro-oculograms; **SaO₂** = oxygen desaturation by oximetry.

Evaluation of a patient suspected of obstructive sleep apnea syndrome typically reveals frequent episodes of apnea, characterized by the absence of airflow and increasing efforts to breathe, which last 20–30 seconds and in some cases as long as 2–3 minutes. During each episode oxygen saturation drops progressively and heart rate slows. At the end of the episode the electroencephalogram (EEG) shows a brief (3–10 seconds) speeding or burst of alpha activity; the electromyogram (EMG) is elevated; and the heart rate is accelerated. Normal breathing resumes and oxygen saturation returns to the level of wakefulness. This pattern recurs repeatedly throughout sleep.

Over the night there is no reduction in sleep time, but rather a fragmentation of sleep. The percentage of stage 1 non-REM sleep, normally 10% or less, can be as great as 30–50%. There usually is very little slow-wave non-REM sleep, and REM sleep can also be somewhat reduced. When tested for sleepiness on the multiple sleep latency test, patients with severe obstructive sleep apnea syndrome fall asleep on average in 2–4 minutes (Figure 48-2). In less severe cases the apnea may be specific to REM sleep (probably because of REM atonia) or may occur only when the patient is sleeping supine (because gravitational forces contribute to collapse of the airway). Less severe cases may also result from *hypopnea* (reduced respiratory airflow) rather than complete obstruction.

The pathophysiology of obstructive sleep apnea syndrome involves two normal events: a reduction in neuromuscular tone at sleep onset and a change in the central nervous system's control of respiration during sleep. The combination of these two events results in anatomical abnormalities in the upper airway, specifically the pharynx.

The first event occurs because the pharynx, which is important in respiration, swallowing, and speech, is collapsible. To serve these multiple functions the pharynx is one of the few collapsible segments of the airway. Several muscle groups control the size and stiffness of the upper airway. Because of the collapsibility of the pharynx, airway patency is normally maintained through a balance between the inward pressures during inspiration and the outward forces of the airway muscles contracting to keep it open.

As noted earlier, obstructive sleep apnea syndrome typically occurs in obese people, and its severity fluctuates as body weight changes. It is assumed that an increase in body weight is reflected in an increase of fatty tissue in the pharynx and other upper-airway structures. The gain in weight leads to a reduction in the size and patency of the pharynx in patients with apnea. Pressures causing pharyngeal collapsibility are enhanced by the excess fatty tissue or other abnormal anatomical features (deviated septum, mandibular retrognathia), and thus muscle activity must increase to counteract the collapsing pressures when the patient is awake. Awake patients with the syndrome show greater electromyographic activity in the airway muscles, particularly the genioglossus, than do normal subjects. This compensatory response is sufficient when the patient is awake; it is during sleep that the problem arises.

At the onset of non-REM sleep, skeletal muscles become hypotonic. Electromyographic activity of some upper-airway muscles decreases, and both the tonic background electromyographic activity and the phasic activity associated with the respiratory cycle are reduced. Animal studies show that the hypotonia of sleep occurs as a result of inhibition of motor neurons. In the transition to REM sleep the motor neurons are even further hyperpolarized, leading to skeletal muscle atonia.

In patients with obstructive sleep apnea syndrome the non-REM hypotonia and REM atonia, coupled with the increased airway resistance resulting from the anatomical abnormalities, lead to collapse of the airway. Brief arousal from sleep occurs, the muscle tonus is restored, and normal respiration returns, thus completing the cycle. This pattern of breathing cessation, arousal, and resumption of breathing can recur up to 400–600 times in an 8-hour sleep period. The brief arousals from sleep compromise the restorative capacity of sleep and lead to the excessive daytime sleepiness.

In healthy normal individuals disruption of sleep by tones, presented through earphones, leads to brief arousals and increased daytime sleepiness. The excessive sleepiness in turn leads to further skeletal muscle hypotonia during sleep. Some studies have shown that sleep deprivation, like central nervous system depressants such as alcohol and the benzodiazepines, reduces tonic genioglossal activity.

The second important event in the pathophysiology of obstructive sleep apnea syndrome is the change in respiratory control with sleep. The respiratory muscles are controlled by a respiratory center in the medulla that receives three types of information: (1) information from chemoreceptors that monitor oxygen and carbon dioxide in the arterial blood, (2) information from mechanical receptors in the lung and the chest wall, and (3) feedback from higher cortical centers. The carotid bodies, located in the bifurcations of the carotid arteries, sense oxygen, carbon dioxide, and pH levels and send impulses via the ninth cranial nerve to the medulla. When oxygen drops (*hypoxia*) and carbon dioxide rises (*hypercapnia*), ventilatory effort is increased. In REM sleep the hypoxic response is reduced and the hypercapnic response is almost nonexistent. These sleep-related respiratory changes in control cause problems for the patient with a compromised airway. In less severe cases episodes of apnea are limited to REM sleep; in most patients with obstructive sleep apnea syndrome the apnea episodes become longer in REM sleep.

The most effective treatment for obstructive sleep apnea syndrome is continuous positive airway pressure delivered through a mask placed over the nose. This positive pressure counteracts the developing negative pressures caused by the narrowing and collapse of the pharynx. When optimal continuous positive airway pressure is achieved, respiratory disturbance is reversed, the hypoxia during sleep is improved, the brief arousals from sleep do not occur, and daytime sleepiness rapidly subsides. Even so, patients find the continuous positive airway pressure mask uncomfortable and claustrophobic, either rejecting it immediately or discontinuing or minimizing its use later.

Chronic Insufficient Sleep Syndrome Reflects a Failure to Obtain Sufficient Sleep

Chronic insufficient sleep syndrome results when a person persistently fails to obtain the amount of sleep necessary to maintain normal alertness throughout the day. The essential feature of this syndrome is that the sleep stages are normally distributed (as described in Chapter 47), but patients spend an unusually high percentage of their bedtime asleep.

Chronic insufficient sleep syndrome typically occurs in adults during the third to sixth decades of life and is more common in men. People at risk might include students, those working two jobs, those with very early morning work report times, or those with unusually extensive work and homecare responsibilities. Patients may consume unusually large amounts of caffeine or resort to the use of over-the-counter stimulants to combat sleepiness. As children and adolescents are given greater latitude in setting bedtimes, chronic insufficient sleep syndrome may become a more widespread problem in pediatric clinics.

Clinical evaluation reveals normal psychological and physical health, no history of a prior medical cause of the sleepiness, and the absence of alcohol or drug abuse. Patients do not have a disease that would interfere with their ability to initiate or maintain biologically necessary sleep—they just don't spend enough time in bed. Insufficient sleep is indicated where the patient reports sleeping more on weekends than on weekdays, often by two hours or more. Excessive daytime sleepiness may become more pronounced in the late afternoon and early evening. Patients report that excessive sleepiness improves while on vacations, without recognizing that this is due to their increased time in bed.

Excessive sleepiness in chronic insufficient sleep syndrome is thus a voluntary restriction of daily sleep time that does not meet the patient's specific biological sleep need. Individual sleep need is genetically determined and varies widely. The average adult sleeps 7–8 hours per night. Reductions from this norm, or adherence to the norm by people who need more sleep, results in an accumulated sleep loss and excessive daytime sleepiness. In healthy normal people a reduction of sleep time by as little as two hours a night increases daytime sleepiness, and this daytime sleepiness intensifies over successive days without adequate sleep. Full recovery of alertness requires at least one week of extended nightly sleep. Patients must be warned of the inevitable consequences of restricted sleep and its cumulative effects.

Insomnia Can Be Transient or Persistent

Insomnia Is the Most Frequent of All Complaints About Sleep and Wakefulness

About one-third of the general population reports at least some difficulty in falling or staying asleep or both. Women are more likely than men to report sleeping troubles, regardless of severity, and the likelihood of insomnia increases with age.

The transient and short-term insomnias, which last days or weeks, are due to disruptions of the sleep schedule, a nonconducive sleep environment, or a stressful life experience. When the insomnia persists for months, it is secondary to various medical and psychiatric disorders. Also, primary sleep pathologies (eg, apnea and periodic limb movements) and behavioral processes (eg, hyperarousal and conditioning) can produce a chronic insomnia. Finally, chronic circadian rhythm disorders have been identified in some people with insomnia.

Disturbed Circadian Rhythm Causes Insomnia

Numerous biological processes are synchronized with sleep-wake behavior and the light-dark cycle, including body temperature, hormone production, and brain metabolism with approximately 24-hour rhythms (Chapter 51). When sleep and wake periods are altered, these biological processes normally readjust to the new cycle. However, without a parallel change in the light-dark cycle, good adjustment never seems to occur and a persistent misalignment results. Persistent circadian rhythm disorders can be contrasted with transient disturbances, such as jet lag or radical changes in work schedule. These transient disturbances disappear when a stable sleep schedule is reestablished.

The pathophysiology of persistent circadian rhythm disorders is not known. An approximately 24-hour rhythm of sleep and wakefulness and associated biological functions have been observed in most mammals; in humans the cycle is 24.1 to 24.7 hours. The rhythm is endogenous and genetically determined (Chapter 51); it persists when all external time cues are removed. Light is the major synchronizing stimulus. The disorder is presumed to be associated with the pacemaker, the coupling mechanisms, or the synchronizing mechanisms.

The *delayed sleep phase syndrome* is an inability to fall asleep and arise at conventional times. Onset of sleep is often delayed until early morning (3–6 AM). When the patient is not attempting to conform to the environment, the usual rise time is 11 AM to 2 PM. Delayed sleep phase can be a transient problem, such as in jet lag and shift work, or a persistent problem. Eastward flights create delayed sleep phases that usually require a day-and-a-half adjustment for every hour of phase delay (Figure 48-4). When delayed sleep phase is a chronic problem in one's home environment (a stable light-dark cycle), attempts to advance bedtime and sleep onset fail and the patient experiences chronic difficulties falling asleep but no problems maintaining sleep. When forced to arise at 6–7 AM for social or occupational requirements, the patient finds it difficult to get up. The early rise time shortens total sleep time; when enforced chronically, daytime sleepiness develops.

The *advanced sleep phase syndrome* is the reciprocal of the delayed sleep phase syndrome: the person falls asleep in early evening (8–9 PM) and awakens in early morning (3–5 AM). In jet lag this phase shift occurs after westward flights (Figure 48-4). Because the phase shift is consistent with the biological free-run of circadian rhythms (a 1-hour phase delay per 24 hours), adaptations to westward shifts are more rapid than in eastward flights. If the advanced sleep phase syndrome is chronic, attempts to delay sleep onset and avoid early awakenings generally fail. If sleep onset is successfully delayed to a later hour, the person still awakens in early morning. There is no disturbance of sleep with the advanced sleep phase syndrome.

The sleep pattern of normal elderly people is thought to have characteristics of the advanced sleep phase syndrome in the young. Elderly people fall asleep in early evening and rise in the early morning. In addition, the circadian rhythms of body temperature and cortisol in elderly people are also phase advanced. Aging animals lose cells from the suprachiasmatic nucleus, suggesting a possible pathophysiology for the age-related phase advance seen in humans. The elderly also tend to sleep for shorter periods and have more disturbed sleep than do younger people. These changes may be due to a weakened circadian rhythm (temperature and cortisol rhythms). Interestingly, partial lesions of the suprachiasmatic nucleus can advance the sleep phase and reduce the strength of circadian rhythms.

The effects of bright light on circadian phase have been well established. In healthy normal people the timing of bright light exposure has a direct effect on the direction and magnitude of phase shifts. Bright light has been used successfully to realign the circadian phase of shift workers. However, therapeutic application of bright light demands total control of light and dark exposure during the whole day. The clinical efficacy of bright light in treating the delayed sleep phase syndrome has not been evaluated systematically.

Periodic Limb Movement Disorder Is a Primary Sleep Pathology

Periodic limb movements during sleep should be differentiated from movement disorders present during wakefulness that also can have an impact on sleep. These include parkinsonian tremor and tics or normal waking movements that occur inappropriately during sleep (sleepwalking, sleeptalking). The periodic limb movements during sleep can be described as stereotypical rhythmic extensions of the big toe and dorsiflexion of the ankle and knee. Less commonly, the upper limbs may also be involved. The movements are slower (0.5–5 s) than myoclonic activity and recur at intervals of 20–40 s. Most patients are unaware of the limb movements, although a bed partner may report restless sleep or even accurately describe the movements. Patients typically complain of insomnia and restless or nonrestorative sleep, and may complain of excessive sleepiness when the movements occur often throughout sleep. The prevalence of periodic limb movement increases in the elderly.

Periodic limb movements are reflected in bursts of electromyographic activity, typically during the first

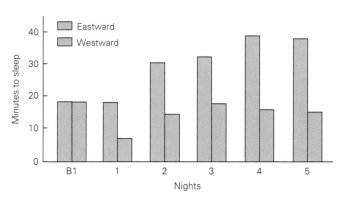

Figure 48-4 The symptoms one experiences after rapid travel through time zones (jet lag) are more severe after eastward flights, and reentrainment of the sleep-wake cycle takes longer. The data here are for subjects who flew from London to Detroit and back (a 5-hour shift in time zones). After eastward travel to London, subjects took longer to fall asleep once in bed. Night B1 is a baseline night's sleep before the flight. Subjects experienced increased sleepiness and reduced performance during waking periods after both eastward and westward flights. (Adapted from Nicholson et al. 1986.)

hours of non-REM sleep. Usually the EMG bursts cease during REM sleep, most likely because of the skeletal atonia of REM. The EMG bursts are often associated with brief EEG signs of arousal, and these recur in cycles that often end with the patient awakening. The duration of stage 1 non-REM sleep, or wakefulness, may increase and the duration of stages 3 and 4 non-REM sleep may be reduced compared with that of age-matched normal individuals. The degree of daytime sleepiness depends on the extent to which sleep is fragmented by limb movements and partial arousals. The most consistently effective treatment for periodic limb movements is the benzodiazepines, which suppress the arousals associated with the periodic limb movements.

Parasomnias Are Disorders of Arousal From Non-REM and REM Sleep

Disorders of arousal from sleep, or *parasomnias*, are a heterogeneous group of disorders that can be classified according to when they occur, either at the transition from wakefulness to sleep during non-REM sleep or during REM sleep. Dysfunctional arousal or partial arousal from sleep is commonly manifested in sleepwalking, sleeptalking, and bed-wetting. These disorders have an estimated prevalence of 2.5%, 5.3%, and 2.1%, respectively. Another parasomnia, the REM behavior disorder, has a dramatic impact on the patient and the patient's spouse but has not been evaluated epidemiologically.

REM Behavior Disorder Gives Rise to Violent Dream Enactment During Sleep

Studies of the neuroanatomy of REM sleep in cats in the early 1960s were predictive of what was identified and described in 1988 as REM behavior disorder in humans. Lesions of the pons that destroy the ventral locus ceruleus in cats produce REM sleep without atonia called *dream enactment* (Chapter 47). Dream enactment in humans can involve complex, vigorous, and even violent movements, with vivid dream recall. The patient or a patient's spouse may report physical injury as a result of dream enactment. Episodes can occur as often as one or two times a night or as infrequently as once every 1 or 2 weeks. REM behavior disorder is more common in men, the elderly, and people with neurological disorders.

The amount and cycling of sleep stages from non-REM to REM is normal. The distinctive finding is the presence of, and even an increase in, a persistent muscular tone during REM sleep (Figure 48-5). Episodes of REM behavior disorder begin with a burst of excessive limb and body movements and progress to more complex movements, which can become vigorous and violent. Prominent muscle twitching and body movement accompany the phasic events of REM sleep, such as the rapid eye movements.

The pathophysiology of REM behavior disorder is not known. It was first thought that the pathology should be similar to that of the experimental lesions in cats that produced REM sleep without atonia. However, a heterogeneous group of neurological and toxic-metabolic conditions has been identified in patients with REM behavior disorder. Moreover, about half of the cases have no associated neuropathological disorders (such cases have been classified as idiopathic). Thus, it is now thought that some subtle dysfunction of the balance between the atonic and phasic mechanisms of REM sleep may be occurring at the spinal cord, brain stem, or even higher cortical regions.

Animal studies have shown that REM atonia can be interrupted at multiple brain sites and that locomotor tracts run parallel with the neural tracts producing atonia. In other words, there may be some dysfunction in the motor-generating system in addition to the atonia. The demographic characteristics of reported cases may provide clues to the pathophysiology. Most notably, the male predominance raises questions about possible hormonal influences. Other characteristics—onset late in life and an association with alcoholism—point to organic brain factors.

Abrupt Arousal From Non-REM Sleep Gives Rise to a Variety of Dysfunctional Behaviors

Confusional arousals—also called sleep drunkenness, sleepwalking, and sleep terrors—are parasomnias that occur as abrupt arousals from non-REM slow-wave sleep in the first hours of the sleep period. These parasomnias are most common in children but can occur at any age. They differ from each other in the extent to which the motor, cognitive, or emotive systems are involved, but can be considered to be on a continuum.

Sleep drunkenness is an episode of marked confusion and disorientation on sudden arousal from deep sleep; no sleepwalking or terror is associated with the confusional state. *Sleepwalking* involves complex automatic behaviors, which may include walking for some distance. The sleepwalker is not awake or conscious during the episode and communication is difficult. *Sleep terror* consists of a sudden awakening in which the patient screams and sits up in bed in an acute state of terror. There is heightened autonomic nervous system arousal with tachypnea, tachycardia, and elevated muscle tone. No cognitive or dream content is associated with sleep terror and no complex motor responses occur beyond sitting up. Patients do not remember confusional arousals.

All three parasomnias typically begin during slow-wave sleep; high-amplitude delta activity is characteristic. Episodes are thought to be induced by abrupt awakening from slow-wave sleep. These parasomnias do not occur during REM sleep and thus should be differentiated from the REM-associated disorders, such as the REM behavior disorder and nightmares. During sleep drunkenness the EEG may indicate some delta-wave activity or stage 1 non-REM sleep with theta activity. The EEG in sleepwalking (recorded via telemetry) shows stage 1 non-REM patterns with a slow alpha rhythm. In sleep terrors there are clear signs of autonomic arousal on the electrocardiogram and the respiratory tracing. In all other aspects the amount and cycling of sleep from non-REM to REM are normal except that stages 3 and 4 non-REM sleep and delta-wave activity are intense.

The pathophysiology of these parasomnias is uncertain, although clear precipitating factors can be identified. Anything that intensifies delta-wave sleep is a precipitant, including sleep deprivation, central nervous system depressants (including alcohol), fever, and young age. In most cases these parasomnias are clearly not nocturnal epileptic seizures. There usually is a family history for one or another of these parasomnias; family members are reported as being "deep sleepers." Also, the presence of one parasomnia in a patient increases the likelihood of that patient experiencing other parasomnias.

A

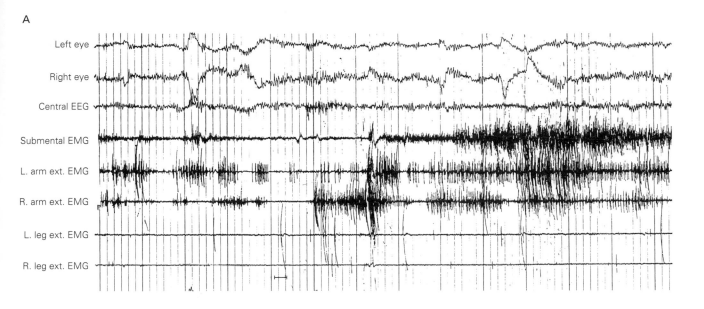

B

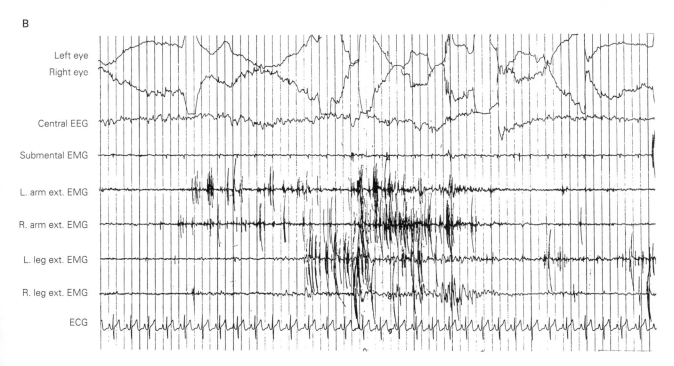

Figure 48-5 Polysomnograms of patients with REM behavior disorder.

A. This polysomnogram shows prominent tonic and phasic EMG activity during REM sleep. Throughout this patient's study REM sleep was almost indistinguishable from wakefulness because of nearly continuous persistence of EMG tone and prominent phasic movement of the limbs. **Ext** = extensor.

B. This polysomnogram shows phasic EMG activity in the limbs during REM sleep. The subject, a 36-year-old male, had a 4- to 5-year history of progressively prominent movements during sleep that progressed to screaming and flying out of bed. During these episodes he sustained multiple fractures, including those of both wrists and the left arm. On one occasion he fell from the bed and sustained a severe head injury requiring prolonged hospitalization for post-traumatic amnesia, fractured right zygoma, fractured clavicle, severe laceration of his ear resulting in significant blood loss, and a chipped tooth. He did not recall any dreams associated with his sleep-related behaviors.

Children usually outgrow parasomnia. Thus, treatment of children is usually not necessary unless the parasomnia is frequent and disruptive. Protection against injury in the case of sleepwalking, or comfort and reassurance in the case of sleep terror, is usually sufficient. In all cases of non-REM parasomnias avoidance of a known precipitant, particularly sleep deprivation, is an important prophylactic. Adults who sleep less than their biological sleep need, as well as young children who are allowed to establish their own bedtimes (and thus do not get enough sleep) accumulate a sleep debt that leads to intensified slow-wave sleep. Just as healthy people who are excessively sleepy because of insufficient sleep can increase their daytime alertness by increasing the amount of sleep over one or two weeks, so too can people with parasomnias lessen the frequency of confusion arousals by getting more sleep each night. Medication can be considered in the more severe cases. The benzodiazepines suppress slow-wave sleep and can reduce the occurrence of parasomniac episodes.

An Overall View

Sleep disorders are common. As much as 20% of the population has some chronic sleep difficulty. These disorders not only are common but also have significant effects on both longevity and quality of life. Patients with sleep disorders typically complain of difficulty sleeping at night, maintaining alertness during the day, or experiencing abnormal behaviors during sleep.

Difficulty sleeping at night, insomnia, is the most common sleep problem. Disorders with daytime sleepiness are less common in the general population but quite common in medical clinics. The reason for the discrepancy is the highly disabling nature of daytime sleepiness. The signs and symptoms of two of the disorders, narcolepsy and sleep apnea, are well understood and hence can be easily diagnosed and treated. Finally, abnormal behaviors during sleep can occur in a variety of populations and are associated with different pathologies. Sleepwalking and sleep terrors are disorders of non-REM sleep occurring mostly in children. In contrast, REM motor dysfunction is an abnormality of muscle control during REM sleep and is seen mostly in elderly patients.

Clear patterns of symptoms are associated with the various disorders. In addition, testing procedures such as all-night sleep studies and the daytime multiple sleep latency test make the identification and diagnosis of sleep disorders relatively easy.

Treatments for the various disorders are effective but they are symptomatic and do not correct the pathophysi-ology of the disorders. For example, the sleepiness of narcolepsy is treated with stimulants, and sleep apnea is treated by mechanically splinting the upper airway with continuous positive airway pressure. A better understanding of basic sleep processes and their pathological variations is needed before treatment can be directed to the primary pathophysiology of sleep disorders.

Thomas Roth
Timothy Roehrs

Selected Readings

Chokroverty S (ed). 1994. *Sleep Disorders Medicine: Basic Science, Technical Considerations, and Clinical Aspects.* Boston: Butterworth-Heinemann.

Dijk DJ, Czeisler CA. 1995. Contribution of the circadian pacemaker and the sleep homeostat to sleep propensity, sleep structure, electroencephalographic slow waves, and sleep spindle activity in humans. J Neurosci 15:3526–3538.

Kleitman N. 1963. *Sleep and Wakefulness.* Chicago: Univ. Chicago Press.

Kryger MH, Roth T, Dement WC (eds). 1994. *Principles and Practice of Sleep Medicine,* 2nd ed. Philadelphia: Saunders.

Thorpy M (ed). 1990. *Handbook of Sleep Disorders.* New York: Marcel Dekker.

References

Aldrich MS. 1990. Narcolepsy. N Engl J Med 323:389–394.

Association of Sleep Disorders Centers and the Association for the Psychophysiological Study of Sleep. 1979. Diagnostic classification of sleep and arousal disorders. Sleep 2:1–137.

Broughton R. 1994. Parasomnias. In: S Chokroverty (ed). *Sleep Disorders Medicine: Basic Science, Technical Considerations, and Clinical Aspects,* pp. 381–399. Boston: Butterworth-Heinemann.

Carskadon MA, Dement WC, Mitler MM, Roth T, Westbrook PR, Keenan S. 1986. Guidelines for the Multiple Sleep Latency Test (MSLT): a standard measure of sleepiness. Sleep 9:519–524.

Coleman RM. 1983. Diagnosis, treatment, and followup of about 8,000 sleep/wake disorder patients. In: C Guilleminault, E Lugaresi (eds). *Sleep/Wake Disorders: Natural History, Epidemiology, and Long-Term Evolution,* pp. 87–98. New York: Raven.

Czeisler CA, Kronauer RE, Allan JS, Duffy JF, Jewett ME, Brown EN, Ronda JM. 1989. Bright light induction of strong (Type 0) resetting of the human circadian pacemaker. Science 244:1328–1333.

Czeisler CA, Weitzman ED, Moore-Ede MC, Zimmerman JC, Knauer RS. 1980. Human sleep: its duration and organization depend on its circadian phase. Science 210:1264–1267.

Diagnostic Classification Steering Committee, Thorpy MJ, chairman. 1990. *The International Classification of Sleep Disorders*. Rochester, MN: American Sleep Disorders Association.

The Gallup Organization. 1991. *Sleep in America: A National Survey of US Adults*. Princeton, NJ: The Gallup Organization.

Gelineau J. 1880. De la narcolepsie. Gozttop (Paris) 53:626–628, 54:635–737.

Guilleminault C. 1994. Clinical features and evaluation of obstructive sleep apnea. In: MH Kryger, T Roth, WC Dement (eds). *Principles and Practice of Sleep Medicine*, 2nd ed., pp. 667–677. Philadelphia: Saunders.

Hening W, Walters A, Chokroverty S. 1994. Motor functions and dysfunctions of sleep. In: S Chokroverty (ed). *Sleep Disorders Medicine: Basic Science, Technical Considerations, and Clinical Aspects*, pp. 255–293. Boston: Butterworth-Heinemann.

Isono S, Remmers J. 1994. Anatomy and physiology of upper airway obstruction. In: MH Kryger, T Roth, WC Dement (eds). *Principles and Practice of Sleep Medicine*, 2nd ed., pp. 642–656. Philadelphia: Saunders.

Mahowald M, Schenck C. 1994. REM sleep behavior disorder. In: MH Kryger, T Roth, WC Dement (eds). *Principles and Practice of Sleep Medicine*, 2nd ed., pp. 574–588. Philadelphia: Saunders.

Mellinger GD, Balter MB, Uhlenhuth EH. 1985. Insomnia and its treatment: prevalance and correlates. Arch Gen Psychiatry 42:225–232.

Nicholson AN, Pascoe PA, Spencer MB, Stone BM, Roehrs T,

Roth T. 1986. Sleep after transmeridian flights. Lancet 2:1205–1208.

Partinen M. 1994. Epidemiology of sleep disorders. In: MH Kryger, T Roth, WC Dement (eds). *Principles and Practice of Sleep Medicine*, 2nd ed., pp. 437–452. Philadelphia: Saunders.

Powell N, Guilleminault C, Riley R. 1994. Surgical therapy for obstructive sleep apnea. In: MH Kryger, T Roth, WC Dement (eds). *Principles and Practice of Sleep Medicine*, 2nd ed., pp. 706–721. Philadelphia: Saunders.

Rechtschaffen A, Wolpert E, Dement WC, Mitchell SA, Fisher C. 1963. Nocturnal sleep of narcolpetic. Electroencephalogr Clin Neurophysiol 15:599–609.

Roehrs T, Zorick F, Sicklesteel J, Wittig R, Roth T. 1983. Excessive daytime sleepiness associated with insufficient sleep. Sleep 6:319–325.

Roth T, Roehrs T, Carskadon M, Dement WC. 1994. Daytime sleepiness and alertness. In: MH Kryger, T Roth, WC Dement (eds). *Principles and Practice of Sleep Medicine*, 2nd ed., pp. 40–49. Philadelphia: Saunders.

Sullivan C, Grunstein R. 1994. Continuous positive airway pressure in sleep-disordered breathing. In: MH Kryger, Roth T, WC Dement (eds). *Principles and Practice of Sleep Medicine*, 2nd ed., pp. 694–705. Philadelphia: Saunders.

Wagner D. 1990. Circadian rhythm sleep disorders. In: M Thorpy (ed). *Handbook of Sleep Disorders*. Vol. 6, *Neurological Disease and Therapy*, pp. 493–527. New York: Marcel Dekker.

Walsh J, Hartman P, Kowall J. 1994. Insomnia. In: S Chokroverty (ed). *Sleep Disorders Medicine: Basic Science, Technical Considerations, and Clinical Aspects*, pp. 219–239. Boston: Butterworth-Heinemann.

Young T, Palta M, Dempsey J, Skatrud J, Weber S, Badr S. 1993. The occurrence of sleep disordered breathing among middle-aged adults. N Engl J Med 328:1230–1235.

49

The Autonomic Nervous System and the Hypothalamus

WHEN WE ARE FRIGHTENED our heart races, our breathing becomes rapid and shallow, our mouth becomes dry, our muscles tense, our palms become sweaty, and we may want to run. These bodily changes are mediated by the *autonomic nervous system*, which controls heart muscle, smooth muscle, and exocrine glands. The autonomic nervous system is distinct from the *somatic nervous system*, which controls skeletal muscle. As we shall learn in the next chapter, even though the neural control of emotion involves several regions, including the amygdala and the limbic association areas of the cerebral cortex, they all work through the hypothalamus to control the autonomic nervous system. The hypothalamus coordinates behavioral response to insure bodily *homeostasis*, the constancy of the internal environment. The hypothalamus, in turn, acts on three major systems: the autonomic nervous system, the endocrine system, and an ill-defined neural system concerned with motivation. In this chapter we shall first examine the autonomic nervous system and then go on to consider the hypothalamus. In the next two chapters, we shall examine emotion and motivation, behavioral states that depend greatly on autonomic and hypothalamic mechanisms.

The Autonomic Nervous System Is a Visceral and Largely Involuntary Sensory and Motor System

In contrast to the somatic sensory and motor systems, which we considered in Parts IV and V of this book, the autonomic nervous system is a *visceral* sensory and motor system. Virtually all visceral reflexes are mediated by local circuits in the brain stem or spinal cord. Although these reflexes are regulated by a network of central autonomic control nuclei in the brain stem, hypothalamus, and forebrain, these visceral reflexes are not under voluntary control, nor do they impinge on consciousness, with few exceptions. The autonomic nervous system is thus also referred to as the *involuntary* motor system, in contrast to the voluntary (somatic) motor system.

The autonomic nervous system has three major divisions: sympathetic, parasympathetic, and enteric. The *sympathetic* and *parasympathetic divisions* innervate cardiac muscle, smooth muscle, and glandular tissues and mediate a variety of visceral reflexes. These two divisions include the sensory neurons associated with spinal and cranial nerves, the preganglionic and postganglionic motor neurons, and the central nervous system circuitry that connects with and modulates the sensory and motor neurons. The *enteric division* has greater autonomy than the other two divisions and comprises a largely self-contained system, with only minimal connections to the rest of the nervous system. It consists of sensory and motor neurons in the gastrointestinal tract that mediate digestive reflexes.

The American physiologist Walter B. Cannon first proposed that the sympathetic and parasympathetic divisions have distinctly different functions. He argued that the parasympathetic nervous system is responsible for *rest and digest*, maintaining basal heart rate, respiration, and metabolism under normal conditions. The sympathetic nervous system, on the other hand, governs the emergency reaction, or *fight-or-flight reaction*. In an emergency the body needs to respond to sudden changes in the external or internal environment, be it emotional stress, combat, athletic competition, severe change in temperature, or blood loss. For a person to respond effectively, the sympathetic nervous system increases output to the heart and other viscera, the peripheral vasculature and sweat glands, and the piloerector and certain ocular muscles. An animal whose sympathetic nervous system has been experimentally eliminated can only survive if sheltered, kept warm, and not exposed to stress or emotional stimuli. Such an animal cannot, however, carry out strenuous work or fend for itself; it cannot mobilize blood sugar from the

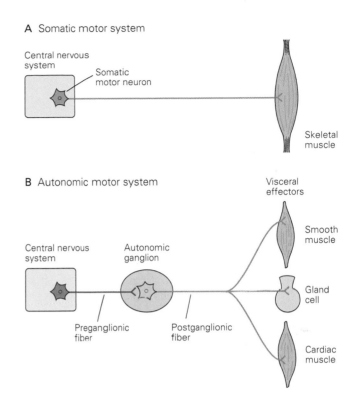

Figure 49-1 Anatomical organization of the somatic and autonomic motor pathways.

A. In the somatic motor system, effector motor neurons in the central nervous system project directly to skeletal muscles.

B. In the autonomic motor system, the effector motor neurons are located in ganglia outside the central nervous system and are controlled by **preganglionic** central neurons.

liver quickly and does not react to cold with normal vasoconstriction or elevation of body heat.

The relationship between the sympathetic and parasympathetic pathways is not as simple and as independent as suggested by Cannon, however. Both divisions are tonically active and operate in conjunction with each other and with the somatic motor system to regulate most behavior, be it normal or emergency. Although several visceral functions are controlled predominantly by one or the other division, and although both the sympathetic and parasympathetic divisions often exert opposing effects on innervated target tissues, it is the balance of activity between the two that helps maintain an internal stable environment in the face of changing external conditions.

The idea of a stable internal environment in the face of changing external conditions was first proposed in the nineteenth century by the French physiologist Claude Bernard. This idea was developed further by Cannon, who put forward the concept of homeostasis as the com-

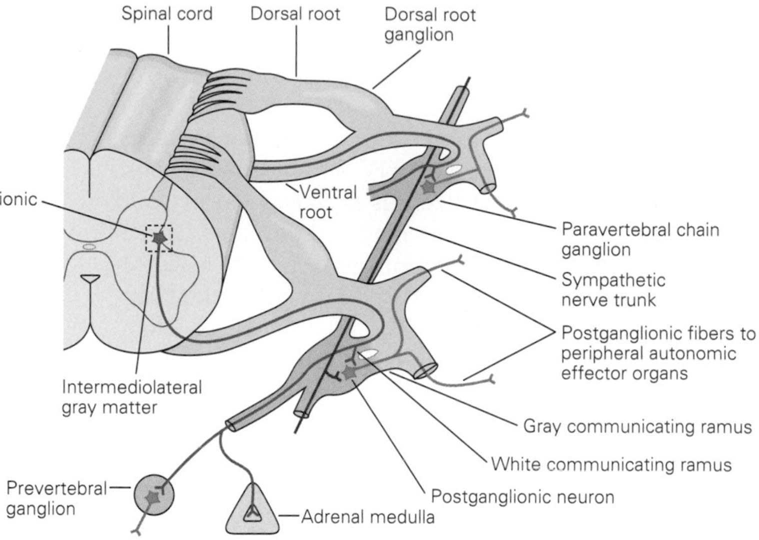

Figure 49-2 Anatomical organization of the sympathetic preganglionic and postganglionic axons. (Adapted from Loewy and Spyer 1990.)

plex physiological mechanisms that maintain the internal milieu. In his classic book *The Wisdom of the Body* published in 1932, Cannon introduced the concept of negative feedback regulation as a key homeostatic mechanism and outlined much of our current understanding of the functions of the autonomic nervous system.

If a state remains steady, it does so because any change is automatically met by increased effectiveness of the factor or factors that resist the change. Consider, for example, thirst when the body lacks water; the discharge of adrenaline, which liberates sugar from the liver when the concentration of sugar in the blood falls below a critical point; and increased breathing, which reduces carbonic acid when the blood tends to shift toward acidity.

Cannon further proposed that the autonomic nervous system, under the control of the hypothalamus, is an important part of this feedback regulation. The hypothalamus regulates many of the neural circuits that mediate the peripheral components of emotional states: changes in heart rate, blood pressure, temperature, and water and food intake. It also controls the pituitary gland and thereby regulates the endocrine system.

Each of the Three Divisions of the Autonomic Nervous System Has a Distinctive Anatomical Organization

The Motor Neurons of the Autonomic Nervous System Lie Outside the Central Nervous System

In the somatic motor system the motor neurons are part of the central nervous system: They are located in the spinal cord and brain stem and project directly to skeletal muscle. In contrast, the motor neurons of the sympathetic and parasympathetic motor systems are located outside the spinal cord in the *autonomic ganglia.* The autonomic motor neurons (also known as *postganglionic neurons*) are activated by the axons of central neurons (the *preganglionic neurons*) whose cell bodies are located in the spinal cord or brain stem, much as are the somatic motor neurons. Thus, in the visceral motor system a synapse (in the autonomic ganglion) is interposed between the efferent neuron in the central nervous system and the peripheral target (Figure 49-1).

The sympathetic and parasympathetic nervous systems have clearly defined sensory components that provide input to the central nervous system and play an important role in autonomic reflexes. In addition, some sensory fibers that project to the spinal cord also send a branch to autonomic ganglia, thus forming reflex circuits that control some visceral autonomic functions.

The innervation of target tissues by autonomic nerves also differs markedly from that of skeletal muscle by somatic motor nerves. Unlike skeletal muscle, which has specialized postsynaptic regions (the endplates; see Chapter 14), target cells of the autonomic nerve fibers have no specialized postsynaptic sites. Nor do the postganglionic nerve endings have presynaptic specializations such as the active zones of somatic motor neurons. Instead, the nerve endings have several swellings (*varicosities*) where vesicles containing transmitter substances accumulate (see Chapter 15).

Synaptic transmission therefore occurs at multiple sites along the highly branched axon terminals of autonomic nerves. The neurotransmitter may diffuse for distances as great as several hundred nanometers to reach its targets. In contrast to the point-to-point contacts made in the somatic motor system, neurons in the autonomic motor system exert a more diffuse control over target tissues, so that a relatively small number of highly branched motor fibers can regulate the function of large masses of smooth muscle or glandular tissue.

Sympathetic Pathways Convey Thoracolumbar Outputs to Ganglia Alongside the Spinal Cord

Preganglionic sympathetic neurons form a column in the intermediolateral horn of the spinal cord extending from the first thoracic spinal segment to rostral lumbar segments. The axons of these neurons leave the spinal cord in the ventral root and initially run together in the spinal nerve. They then separate from the somatic motor axons and project (in small bundles called *white myelinated rami*) to the ganglia of the *sympathetic chains,* which lie along each side of the spinal cord (Figure 49-2).

Axons of preganglionic neurons exit the spinal cord at the level at which their cell bodies are located, but they may innervate sympathetic ganglia situated either more rostrally or more caudally by traveling in the sympathetic nerve trunk that connects the ganglia (Figure 49-2). Most of the preganglionic axons are relatively slow-conducting, small-diameter myelinated fibers. Each preganglionic fiber forms synapses with many postganglionic neurons in different ganglia. Overall, the ratio of preganglionic fibers to postganglionic fibers in the sympathetic nervous system is about 1:10. This divergence permits coordinated activity in sympathetic neurons at several different spinal levels.

The axons of postganglionic neurons are largely unmyelinated and exit the ganglia in the *gray unmyelinated rami.* The postganglionic cells that innervate structures in the head are located in the superior cervical ganglion, which is a rostral extension of the sympathetic chain. The axons of these cells travel along branches of the carotid arteries to their targets in the head. The postganglionic fibers innervating the rest of the body travel in spinal nerves to their targets; in an average spinal nerve about *8%* of the fibers are sympathetic postganglionic axons. Some neurons of the cervical and upper thoracic ganglia innervate cranial blood vessels, sweat glands, and hair follicles; others innervate the glands and visceral organs of the head and chest, including the lacrimal and salivary glands, heart, lungs, and blood vessels. Neurons in the lower thoracic and lumbar paravertebral ganglia innervate peripheral blood vessels, sweat glands, and pilomotor smooth muscle (Figure 49-3).

Some preganglionic fibers pass through the sympathetic ganglia and branches of the splanchnic nerves to synapse on neurons of the *prevertebral ganglia,* which include the coeliac ganglion and the superior and inferior mesenteric ganglia (Figure 49-3). Neurons in these ganglia innervate the gastrointestinal system and the accessory gastrointestinal organs, including the pancreas and liver, and also provide sympathetic innervation of the kidneys, bladder, and genitalia. Another group of preganglionic axons runs in the thoracic splanchnic nerve into the abdomen and innervates the adrenal medulla, which is an endocrine gland, secreting both epinephrine and norepinephrine into circulation. The cells of the adrenal medulla are developmentally and functionally related to postganglionic sympathetic neurons.

Parasympathetic Pathways Convey Outputs From the Brain Stem Nuclei and Sacral Spinal Cord to Widely Dispersed Ganglia

The central, preganglionic cells of the parasympathetic nervous system are located in several brain stem nuclei and in segments S2–S4 of the sacral spinal cord (Figure 49-3). The axons of these cells are quite long because parasympathetic ganglia lie close to or are actually embedded in visceral target organs. In contrast, sympathetic ganglia are located at some distance from their targets.

The preganglionic parasympathetic nuclei in the brain stem include the Edinger-Westphal nucleus (associated with cranial nerve III), the superior and inferior salivary nuclei (associated with cranial nerves VII and IX, respectively), and the dorsal vagal nucleus and the nucleus ambiguus (both associated with cranial nerve X). Preganglionic axons exiting the brain stem through cranial nerves III, VII, and IX and project to postganglionic neurons in the ciliary, pterygopalatine, submandibular, and otic ganglia (Figure 49-3). Parasympathetic preganglionic fibers from the dorsal vagal nucleus project via nerve X to postganglionic neurons embedded in thoracic and abdominal targets—the stomach, liver, gall bladder, pancreas, and upper intestinal tract (Figure 49-3). Neurons of the ventrolateral nucleus ambiguus provide the principal parasympathetic innervation of the cardiac ganglia, which innervate the heart, esophagus, and respiratory airways.

In the sacral spinal cord the parasympathetic preganglionic neurons occupy the intermediolateral column. Axons of spinal parasympathetic neurons leave the spinal cord through the ventral roots and project in the pelvic nerve to the pelvic ganglion plexus. Pelvic ganglion neurons innervate the descending colon, bladder, and external genitalia (Figure 49-3).

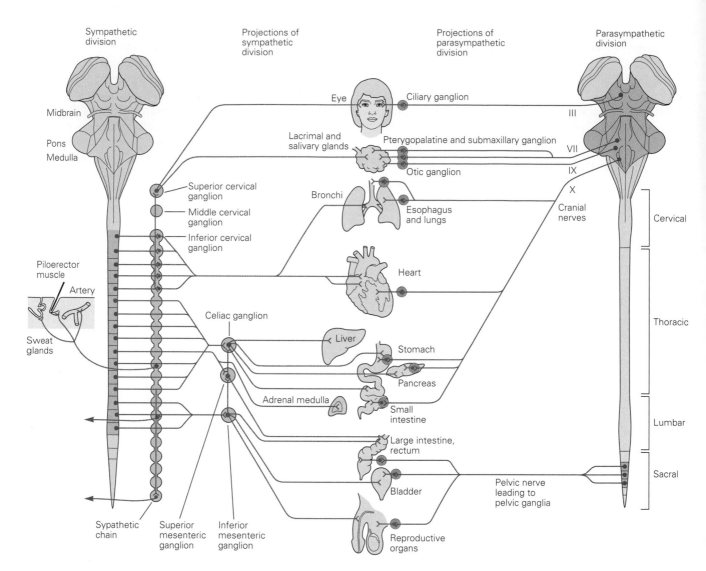

Figure 49-3 Sympathetic and parasympathetic divisions of the autonomic nervous system. Sympathetic preganglionic neurons are clustered in ganglia in the sympathetic chain alongside the spinal cord extending from the first thoracic spinal segment to upper lumbar segments. Parasympathetic preganglionic neurons are located within the brain stem and in segments S2–S4 of the spinal cord. The major targets of autonomic control are shown here.

The sympathetic nervous system innervates tissues throughout the body, but the parasympathetic distribution is more restricted. There is also less divergence, with an average ratio of preganglionic to postganglionic fibers of about 1:3; in some tissues the numbers may be nearly equal.

The Enteric Nervous System Is Largely Autonomous

The enteric nervous system controls the function of the gastrointestinal tract, pancreas, and gallbladder. It contains local sensory neurons and interneurons as well as motor neurons and is responsive to alterations in the tension of gut walls and changes in the chemical environment in the gut. The enteric motor neurons control smooth muscle of the gut, local blood vessels, and secretion by the mucosa. The human enteric nervous system has 80–100 million neurons, approximately as many as are found in the spinal cord.

Two major plexuses of nerve cell bodies and fibers extend continuously along the entire length of the gastrointestinal tract (Figure 49-4). These are the *myenteric (Auerbach's) plexus,* between the outer longitudinal and inner circular smooth muscle layers, and the *submucous (Meissner's) plexus* between the circular muscle layer and the mucosa. In general, the submucous plexus is con-

A

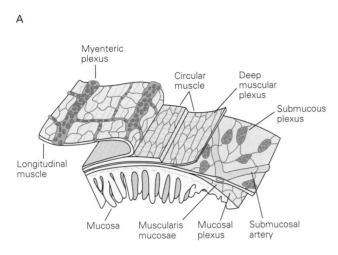

B

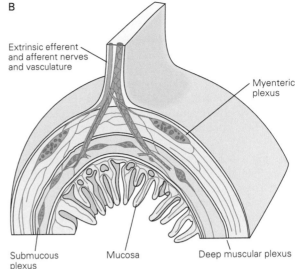

Figure 49-4 The locations of the mucosal, submucous, and myenteric plexuses between the layers of intestinal wall are shown in three dimensions (A) and in cross-section (B). (Adapted from Furness and Costa 1980.)

cerned with control of the secretory functions of the gut, while the myenteric plexus controls gut motility. The two plexuses are interconnected, and they contain motor neurons that innervate both smooth muscle and secretory cells in the mucosa, as well as sensory neurons that respond to stretch, tonicity, and specific chemical signals.

The enteric nervous system is relatively independent of the central nervous system. Although it does have both sympathetic and parasympathetic inputs, these are relatively sparse in relation to the large numbers of enteric neurons. Parasympathetic preganglionic fibers project to enteric ganglia in the stomach, colon, and rectum through the vagus, pelvic, and splanchnic nerves. The sympathetic fibers originate primarily in paravertebral ganglia, although some originate in the prevertebral ganglia, and project mainly to the myenteric and submucous plexuses.

Disruption of enteric connections to the central nervous system results in little or no impairment in function of the small and large bowels; the esophagus and stomach, however, appear to be more dependent on sympathetic and parasympathetic innervation for normal function. The innervation of parts of the gastrointestinal system by the sympathetic and parasympathetic systems may be a way that the other divisions of the autonomic nervous system can override the local nervous control of gut function.

Sensory Inputs Produce a Wide Range of Visceral Reflexes

To maintain homeostasis the autonomic nervous system responds to many different types of sensory inputs. Some of these are somatosensory. For example, a noxious stimulus activates sympathetic neurons that regulate local vasoconstriction (necessary to reduce bleeding when the skin is broken). At the same time, the stimulus activates nociceptive afferents in the spinothalamic tract with axon collaterals to an area in the rostral ventrolateral medulla that coordinates reflexes. These inputs cause widespread sympathetic activation that increases blood pressure and heart rate to protect arterial perfusion pressure and prepares the individual for vigorous defense.

Homeostasis also requires important information about the internal state of the body. Much of this information from the thoracic and abdominal cavities reaches the brain via the vagus nerve. The glossopharyngeal nerve also conveys visceral sensory information from the head and neck. Both of these nerves and the facial nerve relay special visceral sensory information about taste (a visceral chemosensory function) from the oral cavity. All of these visceral sensory afferents synapse in a topographic fashion in the *nucleus of the solitary tract*. Taste information is represented most anteriorly; gastrointestinal information, in an intermediate

Box 49-1 First Isolation of a Chemical Transmitter

The existence of chemical messengers was first postulated by John Langley and Henry Dale and their students on the basis of their pharmacological studies dating from the beginning of the century. However, convincing evidence for a neurotransmitter was not provided until 1920, when Otto Loewi, in a simple but decisive experiment, examined the autonomic innervation of two isolated, beating frog hearts. In his own words:

The night before Easter Sunday of that year I awoke, turned on the light, and jotted down a few notes on a tiny slip of paper. Then I fell asleep again. It occurred to me at six o'clock in the morning that during the night I had written down something most important, but I was unable to decipher the scrawl. The next night, at three o'clock, the idea returned. It was the design of an experiment to determine whether or not the hypothesis of chemical transmission that I had uttered seventeen years ago was correct. I got up immediately, went to the laboratory, and performed a simple experiment on a frog heart according to the nocturnal design. I have to describe briefly this experiment since its results became the foundation of the theory of chemical transmission of the nervous impulse.

The hearts of two frogs were isolated, the first with its nerves, the second without. Both hearts were attached to Straub cannulas filled with a little Ringer solution. The vagus nerve of the first heart was stimulated for a few minutes. Then the Ringer solution that had been in the first heart during the stimulation of the vagus was transferred to the second heart. It slowed and its beat diminished just as if its vagus had been stimulated. Similarly, when the accelerator nerve was stimulated and the Ringer from this period transferred, the second heart speeded up and its beat increased. These results unequivocally proved that the nerves do not influence the heart directly but liberate from their terminals specific chemical substances which, in their turn, cause the well-known modifications of the function of the heart characteristic of the stimulation of its nerves.

Loewi called this substance *Vagusstoff* (vagus substance). Soon after, Vagusstoff was identified chemically as acetylcholine.

---

position; cardiovascular inputs, caudomedially; and respiratory inputs, in the caudolateral part of the nucleus.

The nucleus of the solitary tract distributes visceral sensory information within the brain along three main pathways. Some neurons in the nucleus of the solitary tract directly innervate preganglionic neurons in the medulla and spinal cord, triggering direct autonomic reflexes. For example, there are direct inputs from the nucleus of the solitary tract to vagal motor neurons controlling esophageal and gastric motility, which are important for ingesting food. Also, projections from the nucleus of the solitary tract to the spinal cord are involved in respiratory reflex responses to lung inflation.

Other neurons in the nucleus project to the lateral medullary reticular formation, where they engage populations of premotor neurons that organize more complex, patterned autonomic reflexes. For example, groups of neurons in the rostral ventrolateral medulla control blood pressure by regulating both blood flow to different vascular beds and vagal tone in the heart to modulate heart rate. Other groups of neurons control complex responses such as vomiting and *respiratory rhythm* (a somatic motor response that has an important autonomic component and that depends critically on visceral sensory information).

The third main projection from the nucleus of the solitary tract provides visceral sensory input to a net-work of cell groups that extend from the pons and midbrain up through the hypothalamus, amygdala, and cerebral cortex. This network coordinates autonomic responses and integrates them into ongoing patterns of behavior. These will be described in more detail after we consider more elementary autonomic reflexes.

Discrete Autonomic Reflexes Produce Both Slow and Rapid Visceral Responses

The usual role of the autonomic nervous system is to control a variety of visceral and ocular reflexes. Some of these reflexes are relatively fast, for example, adjustment of pupil size in response to light. Others, such as glandular secretion or gastrointestinal responses to food, are slow. Some bodily functions are under the dual control of the autonomic and somatic motor systems.

Ocular Reflexes

The autonomic nervous system controls two movements of the eye: opening the pupils and focusing the lens. Pupil size determines the amount of light impinging on the retina. Sympathetic fibers from the superior cervical ganglion innervate the muscles of the iris that dilate the pupil, while parasympathetic fibers innervate circular muscle fibers of the iris that constrict the pupil. Ordinarily, the parasympathetic and sympathetic con-

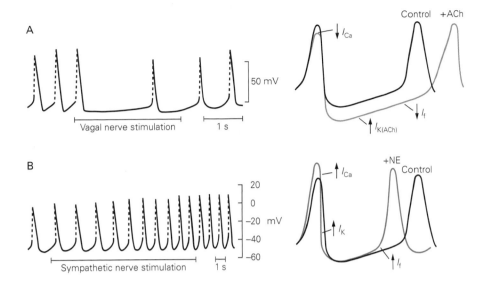

Figure 49-5 Acetylcholine (ACh) and norepinephrine (NE) acting on the same cells produce different firing patterns in cardiocytes in the sinoatrial node.

A. Stimulation of the cholinergic vagal nerve slows firing and shortens the amplitude of the action potential in the target cell. (Adapted from Toda and West 1967.)

B. Stimulation of the adrenergic sympathetic nerve of the frog sinus venosus increases the rate of firing of the cardiac cell. (Adapted from Hutter and Trautwein 1956.)

trols are balanced to achieve the appropriate pupillary opening, although fine-tuning of pupil size may be largely under parasympathetic control. Under conditions of excitement or alarm there is a shift in this balance, inhibiting pupillary constriction and increasing tone in the pupillodilator muscle of the iris. Focusing of the lens is regulated almost entirely by parasympathetic control of ciliary muscles, whereas Muller's muscle, which retracts the eyelids, is under sympathetic control.

Cardiovascular Reflexes

Arterial blood pressure is determined by the rate of output of blood from the heart and the resistance to blood flow through the blood vessels. The sympathetic system increases heart rate and strength of contraction; the parasympathetic slows the heart. Sympathetic stimulation increases blood pressure by increasing cardiac output and peripheral resistance (by constricting small arterioles). Parasympathetic stimulation has a smaller effect on peripheral resistance, although some vasodilatory responses occur, as in blushing. Parasympathetic vasodilation may involve unconventional chemical messengers such as nitric oxide. Under resting conditions almost all systemic arterioles are constricted to approximately half maximal diameter by ongoing sympathetic tonic activity. A decrease in sympathetic output leads to vasodilation; an increase, to further constriction. Without ongoing tonic activity of the sympathetic system, sympathetic output could only increase and thus control only constriction.

Sympathetic vasoconstrictor tone results from continuous firing of mainly adrenergic neurons in the ros-

tral ventrolateral medulla, which innervate sympathetic vasoconstrictor preganglionic neurons. Activation of pressure-sensitive (*baroreceptor*) neurons that innervate the aortic arch and the carotid sinus signal an increase in blood pressure to the nucleus of the solitary tract. Neurons of this nucleus excite interneurons in the caudal ventrolateral medulla, which in turn both inhibit the tonic vasomotor neurons and excite vagal cardiomotor neurons. The result, the *baroreceptor reflex*, is a fall in both arterial blood pressure and heart rate.

The actions of norepinephrine and acetylcholine (ACh) on the heart are worth considering in detail as examples of the complex cellular regulatory systems involved in autonomic control. Norepinephrine acts on cardiac muscle to stimulate heart rate and force of contraction. It increases the force of contraction by acting on β-adrenergic receptors that activate the cyclic adenosine monophosphate (cAMP) second-messenger system, which in turn increases the long-lasting (L-type) Ca^{2+} channel current in the muscle (Chapter 14). Activation of the β-adrenergic receptors also decreases the threshold for firing the cardiac pacemaker cells in the sinoatrial node, thereby increasing heart rate. These effects of norepinephrine can be potently reinforced by circulating epinephrine released from the adrenal medulla.

ACh is released from parasympathetic nerve terminals, as first shown by Otto Loewi in his classic experiment proving the existence of chemical neurotransmitters (Box 49-1). ACh slows the heart by acting on muscarinic receptors in the cardiocytes of the sinoatrial and atrioventricular nodes of cardiac muscle, thus increasing a resting K^+ conductance in these cells. The increase in K^+ conductance hyperpolarizes sinoatrial cells, thus slowing conductance through the atrioventricular node. Hyperpolarization of the sinoatrial cells appears to involve direct gating of a K^+ channel by a G protein activated by the muscarinic receptor. ACh also decreases heart rate by increasing the threshold for firing the pacemaker cells in a manner opposite to that of norepinephrine, thereby slowing the heart rate (Figure 49-5). ACh also reduces the force of contraction by decreasing intracellular cAMP, thus reducing the L-type Ca^{2+} current.

Glandular Reflexes

Nasal, lacrimal, and many gastrointestinal glands are strongly stimulated by parasympathetic inputs. The enteric glands most strongly stimulated by the parasympathetic system are in the upper alimentary tract, particularly in the mouth and stomach. Glandular secretion in lower parts of the alimentary tract is mostly under the autonomous control of the enteric nervous system. Salivary glands respond to both parasympathetic and sympathetic stimulation with secretion. Sympathetic stimulation elicits viscous secretion with a high amylase content, and parasympathetic stimulation elicits a more copious, watery saliva.

Sympathetic activity generally reduces glandular secretion because it causes vasoconstriction, whereas parasympathetic stimulation increases local blood flow, promoting secretion. Sweat glands are an exception to this rule, as sympathetic stimulation increases sweating. Most of the sympathetic fibers are cholinergic rather than adrenergic, but in humans many sympathetic fibers to sweat glands are under {α}-adrenergic control.

Gastrointestinal Reflexes

Gastrointestinal function is controlled by many autonomic reflexes. Some depend on input from the parasympathetic or sympathetic nervous systems (eg, control of gastric acid secretion in the stomach), while others are mainly under local control of the enteric nervous system. For example, intestinal *peristalsis*—the wave of muscle contractions along the length of the intestine that propels intestinal contents toward the anus—is controlled entirely by the enteric nervous system.

As food enters the intestine it pushes the intestinal wall outward, thus stretching sensory neurons in the wall. When sufficiently stretched, these neurons activate interneurons and motor neurons in the myenteric plexus to move the food forward. Peristalsis starts with the activation of excitatory motor neurons whose fibers

project orally, causing the circular muscle at the oral end of the intestinal distention to contract. At the same time, reflex activation of inhibitory motor neurons, whose fibers project anally, relaxes the circular smooth muscle at the anal end of the distention. The waves of contraction and relaxation of the intestinal wall propel the food through the intestines. During peristalsis, parasympathetic nerves excite enteric neurons through nicotinic receptors and contracts smooth muscle through muscarinic receptors. Nitric oxide is thought to mediate smooth muscle relaxation in peristalsis.

Urogenital Reflexes

The control of bladder emptying is unusual because it involves both involuntary autonomic reflexes and some voluntary control. The excitatory input to the bladder wall that causes contraction and promotes emptying is parasympathetic. Activation of parasympathetic postganglionic neurons in the pelvic ganglion plexus near to and within the bladder wall contracts the bladder's smooth muscle. These neurons are quiet when the bladder begins to fill but are activated reflexly by visceral afferents when the bladder is distended.

The sympathetic nervous system relaxes the bladder smooth muscle. Axons of preganglionic sympathetic neurons project from the thoracic and upper lumbar spinal cord to the inferior mesenteric ganglion. From there, postganglionic fibers travel to the bladder in the hypogastric nerve. When the sympathetic system is activated by low-frequency firing in sensory afferents that respond to tension in the bladder wall, the parasympathetic neurons in the pelvic ganglion are inhibited, relaxing bladder smooth muscle and exciting the internal sphincter muscle. Thus, during bladder filling the sympathetic system promotes relaxation of the bladder wall directly while maintaining closure of the internal sphincter.

Somatic motor neurons in the ventral horn of the sacral spinal cord innervate striated muscle fibers in the external urethral sphincter, causing it to contract. These motor neurons are stimulated by visceral afferents that are activated when the bladder is partially full. As the bladder fills, spinal sensory afferents relay this information to a region in the pons that coordinates micturition. This pontine area, sometimes called *Barrington's nucleus* after the British neurophysiologist who first described it, also receives important descending inputs from the forebrain concerning behavioral cues for emptying the bladder. Descending pathways from Barrington's nucleus cause coordinated inhibition of sympathetic and somatic systems, relaxing both sphincters. The onset of urinary flow through the urethra causes reflex contrac-

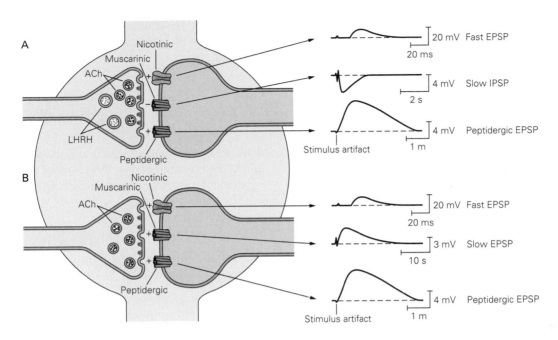

Figure 49-6 Both acetylcholine (ACh) and a luteinizing hormone-releasing hormone (LHRH)-like peptide are released by presynaptic cells at synapses in the sympathetic chain ganglia in the bullfrog. The two transmitters produce different types of postsynaptic potentials in different postganglionic neurons because of their actions on different receptors. (Adapted from Jan and Jan 1983.)

A. In one type of postganglionic neuron a single presynaptic stimulus evokes a fast excitatory postsynaptic potential (fast EPSP) at a nicotinic ACh receptor. Repetitive stimulation

evokes a slow inhibitory postsynaptic potential (slow IPSP) at a muscarinic ACh receptor and a slow EPSP at a peptidergic receptor.

B. In another class of postganglionic neurons a single presynaptic stimulus also evokes a fast EPSP at the nicotinic ACh receptor but repetitive stimulation leads to a slow EPSP at the muscarinic ACh receptor. This class of neurons also evokes the slow peptidergic EPSP, but only in response to stimulation of the preganglionic fibers shown in **A.** The peptide diffuses from these terminals to distant receptors.

tion of the bladder that is under parasympathetic control.

In patients with spinal cord injuries at the cervical or thoracic levels, the spinal reflex control of micturition remains intact, but the connections with the pons are severed. As a result, micturition cannot be voluntarily controlled. When it does occur as a spinal reflex resulting from bladder overfilling, urination is incomplete. As a result, urinary tract infections are common, and it may be necessary to empty the bladder mechanically by catheterization.

Sexual reflexes are organized in a pattern that is analogous to those controlling bladder function. Erectile tissue is controlled largely by the parasympathetic nervous system, involving neurons that produce nitric oxide as their main mediator. Glandular secretion is also parasympathetically mediated. Ejaculation in males is caused by sympathetic control of the seminal vesicles and vas deferens, and emission involves control of striated muscles in the pelvic floor as well. Supraspinal in-

puts play an important role in producing the coordinated pattern of sexual response, although some simple sexual reflexes can be activated even after spinal transection (eg, penile erection can be elicited by local sensory stimuli).

Autonomic Neurons Use a Variety of Chemical Transmitters

Autonomic ganglion cells receive and integrate inputs from both the central nervous system (through preganglionic nerve terminals) and the periphery (through branches of sensory nerves that terminate in the ganglia). Most of the sensory fibers are nonmyelinated and may release neuropeptides, such as substance P and calcitonin gene-related peptide (CGRP), onto ganglion cells. Preganglionic fibers primarily use ACh and norepinephrine as transmitters.

Ganglionic Transmission Involves Both Fast and Slow Synaptic Potentials

Preganglionic activity induces both brief and prolonged responses from postganglionic neurons. ACh released from preganglionic terminals evokes fast excitatory postsynaptic potentials (EPSPs) mediated by nicotinic ACh receptors. The fast EPSP is often large enough to generate an action potential in the postganglionic neuron, and it is thus regarded as the principal synaptic pathway for ganglionic transmission in both the sympathetic and parasympathetic systems.

ACh also evokes slow EPSPs and inhibitory postsynaptic potentials (IPSPs) in postganglionic neurons. These slow potentials can modulate the excitability of these cells. They have been most often studied in sympathetic ganglia but are also known to occur in some parasympathetic ganglia. Slow EPSPs or IPSPs are mediated by muscarinic ACh receptors (Figure 49-6). The slow excitatory potential results when Na^+ and Ca^{2+} channels open and M-type K^+ channels close. The M-type channels are normally active at the resting membrane potential, so their closure leads to membrane depolarization (Chapter 13). The slow inhibitory potential results from the opening of K^+ channels, allowing K^+ ions to flow out of the nerve terminals, resulting in hyperpolarization.

The fast cholinergic EPSP reaches a maximum within 10–20 ms; the slow cholinergic synaptic potentials take up to half a second to reach their maximum and last for a second or more (Figure 49-6). Even slower synaptic potentials, lasting up to a minute, are evoked by neuropeptides, a variety of which are present in the terminals of preganglionic neurons and sensory nerve endings. The actions of one peptide have been studied in detail and reveal important features of peptidergic transmission.

In some, but not all, preganglionic nerve terminals in bullfrog sympathetic ganglia, ACh is colocalized with a luteinizing hormone–releasing hormone (LHRH)-like peptide. High-frequency stimulation of the preganglionic nerves causes the peptide to be released, evoking a slow, long-lasting EPSP in all postganglionic neurons (Figure 49-6), even those not directly innervated by the peptidergic fibers. The peptide must diffuse over considerable distances to influence distant receptive neurons. The slow peptidergic EPSP, like the slow cholinergic excitatory potential, also results from the closure of M-type channels and the opening of Na^+ and Ca^{2+} channels. The peptidergic excitatory potential alters the excitability of autonomic ganglion cells for long periods after intense activation of preganglionic inputs. No mammalian equivalent of the actions of the LHRH-like peptide in amphibians has yet been identified, but the neuropeptide substance P released from sensory afferent terminals in mammals evokes a similar slow, long-lasting EPSP.

Norepinephrine and Acetylcholine Are the Predominant Transmitters in the Autonomic Nervous System

Most postganglionic sympathetic neurons release norepinephrine, which acts on a variety of different adrenergic receptors. There are five major types of adrenergic receptors, and these are the target for several medically important drugs (Table 49-1).

ATP and Adenosine Have Potent Extracellular Actions

Adenosine triphosphate (ATP) is an important cotransmitter with norepinephrine in many postganglionic sympathetic neurons. By acting on ATP-gated ion channels (P_2 purinergic receptors), it is responsible for some of the fast responses seen in target tissues (Table 49-1). The proportion of ATP to norepinephrine varies considerably in different sympathetic nerves. The ATP component is relatively minor in nerves to blood vessels in the rat tail and rabbit ear, while the responses of guinea pig submucosal arterioles to sympathetic stimulation appear to be mediated solely by ATP.

The nucleotide adenosine is formed from the hydrolysis of ATP and is recognized by P_1 purinergic receptors (Table 49-1) located both pre- and postjunctionally. It is thought to play a modulatory role in autonomic transmission, particularly in the sympathetic system. Adenosine may dampen sympathetic function after intense sympathetic activation by activating receptors on sympathetic nerve endings that inhibit further norepinephrine and ATP release. Adenosine also has inhibitory actions in cardiac and smooth muscle that tend to oppose the excitatory actions of norepinephrine.

Many Different Neuropeptides Are Present in Autonomic Neurons

Neuropeptides are colocalized with norepinephrine and ACh in autonomic neurons. Cholinergic preganglionic neurons in the spinal cord and brain stem and their terminals in autonomic ganglia may contain enkephalins, neurotensin, somatostatin, or substance P. Noradrenergic postganglionic sympathetic neurons may also express a variety of neuropeptides. Neuropeptide Y is present in as many as 90% of the cells and modulates sympathetic transmission. In tissues in which the nerve endings are distant from their targets (more than 60 nm,

Table 49-1 Pharmacology of the Autonomic Nervous System

Receptor category	Functional roles[1]	Drugs that act selectively at these receptors	Medical use
Norepinephrine			
Adrenergic α_1	Contractile effects of NE on smooth muscle, especially blood vessels, urogenital, and sphincter muscles	Prazosin (antagonist)	Hypertension
Adrenergic α_2	Presynaptic control (inhibitory) of release of NE, ATP, and ACh from nerve terminals	Yohimbine (antagonist)	Delay ejaculation
Adrenergic β_1	Stimulatory effects of NE and circulating epinephrine on heart	Atenolol (antagonist)	Hypertension
Adrenergic β_2	Relaxant effects of NE on smooth muscle in gastrointestinal tract, urinogenital system, and airways	Salbutamol (agonist)	Bronchodilator for asthma
Adrenergic β_3	Stimulate release of free fatty acids from adipose tissue	None	Potential in obesity
Acetylcholine			
Cholinergic-nicotinic (ganglionic type)	Fast excitation of postganglionic neurons in autonomic ganglia	Hexamethonium (antagonist)	Hypertension (formerly)
Cholinergic-muscarinic M_1	Inhibit ACh and NE release from autonomic nerve terminals	Pirenzepine (antagonist)	Anti-ulcerogenic
Cholinergic-muscarinic M_2	Effects of ACh on heart and smooth muscle	Atropine (nonselective antagonist)	Mydriatic
Cholinergic-muscarinic M_3	ACh-induced secretion from glandular tissues (eg, salivary gland)	Atropine (nonselective antagonist)	Reduced drooling in Parkinson disease
Others			
Purinergic P_1 (Four subtypes)	Modulatory effects of adenosine on autonomic effector tissues	Theophylline (antagonist)	Bronchodilator
Purinergic P_2 (Two subtypes)	Fast and slow responses to ATP in smooth muscle	Few drugs; suramin is P_{2Y} antagonist	None
Nitric oxide (NO)	Relaxant effects on smooth muscle, especially blood vessels	Glyceryl trinitrate and nitroprusside (generate NO)	Coronary vasodilators for angina

[1]ACh = acetylcholine; ATP = adenosine triphosphate; NE = norepinephrine.

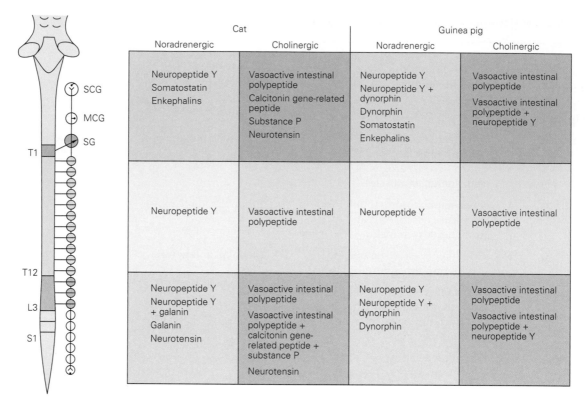

| | Cat | | Guinea pig | |
	Noradrenergic	Cholinergic	Noradrenergic	Cholinergic
	Neuropeptide Y Somatostatin Enkephalins	Vasoactive intestinal polypeptide Calcitonin gene-related peptide Substance P Neurotensin	Neuropeptide Y Neuropeptide Y + dynorphin Dynorphin Somatostatin Enkephalins	Vasoactive intestinal polypeptide Vasoactive intestinal polypeptide + neuropeptide Y
	Neuropeptide Y	Vasoactive intestinal polypeptide	Neuropeptide Y	Vasoactive intestinal polypeptide
	Neuropeptide Y Neuropeptide Y + galanin Galanin Neurotensin	Vasoactive intestinal polypeptide Vasoactive intestinal polypeptide + calcitonin gene-related peptide + substance P Neurotensin	Neuropeptide Y Neuropeptide Y + dynorphin	Vasoactive intestinal polypeptide Vasoactive intestinal polypeptide + neuropeptide Y

Figure 49-7 A variety of neuropeptides coexist with norepinephrine and acetylcholine in neurons of the sympathetic ganglia, as shown here for the cat and the guinea pig. The sympathetic preganglionic nuclei extend from T1 to L3. **MCG** = middle cervical ganglion; **SCG** = superior cervical ganglion; **SG** = stellate ganglion. (Adapted from Elfvin et al. 1993.)

as for the rabbit ear artery), neuropeptide Y potentiates both the purinergic and adrenergic components of the tissue response, probably by acting postsynaptically. In contrast, in tissues with dense sympathetic innervation and where the target is closer (20 nm, such as the vas deferens), neuropeptide Y acts presynaptically to inhibit release of ATP and norepinephrine, thus dampening the tissue response. The peptides galanin and dynorphin are often found with neuropeptide Y in sympathetic neurons, which can contain several neuropeptides. Cholinergic postganglionic sympathetic neurons commonly contain CGRP and vasoactive intestinal polypeptide (VIP) (Figure 49-7).

In postganglionic parasympathetic neurons that express VIP together with ACh, the peptide may contribute to the response of the target tissue because of its powerful vasodilator effects. For example, ACh triggers salivary gland secretion while VIP is responsible for the local increase in blood flow, which is important to the secretory response. Some of the complex modulatory functions that neuropeptides perform are illustrated in Figure 49-8.

A Central Autonomic Network Coordinates Autonomic Function

Autonomic functions ultimately must be coordinated with one another and the ongoing behavioral needs of the individual. This coordination is carried out by a highly interconnected set of structures in the brain stem and forebrain that form a central autonomic network.

A key component of this network is the *nucleus of the solitary tract*. The nucleus receives visceral input from cranial nerves VII, IX, and X and then uses this information to modulate autonomic function in two ways (Figure 49-9).

First, the nucleus of the solitary tract projects to neurons forming brain stem and spinal circuits that control simple autonomic responses. For example, visceral afferents relayed through the nucleus of the solitary tract directly regulate vagal motor control of the stomach and heart rate. Other outputs from the nucleus of the solitary tract innervate neurons in the ventrolateral medullary reticular formation and control blood pressure by regulating the blood flow in different vascular beds (Figure 49–10).

Second, the nucleus of the solitary tract acts to integrate autonomic function with more complex endocrine and behavioral responses, a process in which the hypothalamus, which we will consider below, plays an important role.

The visceral sensory outflow from the nucleus of the solitary tract is relayed to the forebrain by the *parabrachial nucleus,* which is important for the behavioral responses to taste and other visceral sensations. Lesions of the parabrachial nucleus prevent conditioned behavioral responses resulting from gustatory cues. The parabrachial nucleus surrounds the superior cerebellar peduncle in the upper pons and provides inputs to the hypothalamus, the periaqueductal gray matter, the amygdaloid complex, the visceral sensory thalamus, and the cortex. In turn, the parabrachial nucleus receives descending connections from these regions.

The *periaqueductal gray matter* surrounds the cerebral aqueduct in the midbrain. It receives inputs from the nucleus of the solitary tract, the parabrachial nucleus, and the hypothalamus and projects to the medullary reticular formation, where it produces behaviorally coordinated patterns of autonomic response. For example, during a "fight-or-flight" response, the periaqueductal gray matter redirects blood flow from internal organs to the hind limbs to support running behavior.

The *amygdaloid complex* plays a key role in regulation of the autonomic components of conditioned behavioral responses. Inputs to the amygdala from areas of the cortex and the thalamus concerned with behavior enter the lateral and basal nuclei, whereas the central nucleus receives inputs from the central autonomic system. Complex internal circuits allow the amygdala to associate autonomic responses with specific behaviors. For example, as we shall learn in the chapter on emotion (Chapter 50), when a rat learns that an auditory cue is followed by an electric shock, the auditory cue itself eventually produces an elevation of heart rate and behavioral freezing previously associated with the shock. Lesions of the central nucleus of the amygdala, which projects to the hypothalamus and the medulla, prevent this response.

Visceral sensory areas of the thalamus and the *visceral sensory cortex* both receive visceral sensory afferents directly from the parabrachial nucleus. In primates, the taste component of the nucleus of the solitary tract also

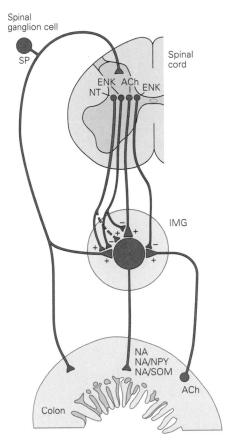

Figure 49-8 Complex modulatory functions of neuropeptides. Sensory neurons in the wall of the **colon** that excite **sympathetic ganglion cells** in the inferior mesenteric ganglion (IMG) use several neuropeptides along with acetylcholine **(ACh)** as transmitters. The neurons that contain cholecystokinin and the vasoactive intestinal polypeptide (VIP) are mechanosensory. Other mechanosensory fibers originate in spinal ganglion cells and contain substance P **(SP)**. They provide excitatory synapses to the sympathetic ganglion cells. Cholinergic fibers originating in the preganglionic spinal cord nuclei contain either enkephalins **(ENK)** or neurotensin **(NT)**. The cholinergic neurons form an excitatory input to the ganglion cells. The enkephalin pathway inhibits release of ACh and SP, whereas the NT pathway facilitates release of SP and gives rise to an excitatory potential in some IMG neurons. Excitatory neurotransmitters and peptides are indicated in **orange;** inhibitory in **gray. NA** = noradrenaline (= norepinephrine); **NPY** = neuropeptide Y; **SOM** = somatostatin. (Adapted from Elfvin et al. 1993.)

projects to the thalamus, thus providing an even more direct relay of taste information to consciousness. The visceral sensory thalamic areas are located in a small-celled nucleus adjacent to the ventroposterior (somatic sensory) complex, the *ventroposterior parvocellular nucleus.* This thalamic nucleus relays taste and other visceral

Figure 49-9 Pathways that distribute visceral sensory information in the brain. Visceral afferent information (**solid line**) enters the brain through the nucleus of the solitary tract. It is distributed to preganglionic neurons, to an area in the ventrolateral medulla that coordinates autonomic and respiratory reflexes, and via an ascending pathway to the forebrain. Less direct inputs (**dotted line**) relayed from the parabrachial nucleus bring visceral sensory information to the hypothalamus, the amygdala, the septum (not shown), the cortex, and the periaqueductal gray matter.

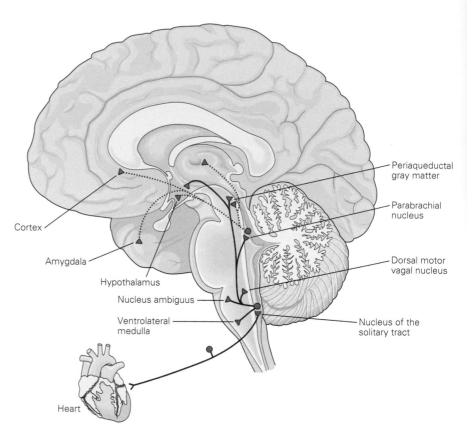

sensations (hunger pangs, abdominal fullness, breath-holding sensations) to the *anterior insular* cortex, where there is a topographic map of the internal organ systems. Taste is located most anteriorly in the insular cortex, with gastrointestinal, then cardiorespiratory sensations, more posteriorly.

The visceral sensory cortex interacts with a portion of the anterior tip of the cingulate cortex, called the *infralimbic area,* which is a visceral motor region. Electrical or chemical stimulation here can cause gastric contractions or changes in blood pressure. Both the anterior insular and infralimbic areas project to the amygdala, hypothalamus, periaqueductal gray matter, parabrachial nucleus, nucleus of the solitary tract, and medullary reticular formation. Lesions of the visceral sensory cortex cause loss of conscious appreciation of visceral sensation such as taste. The visceral motor cortex is part of a region of cingulate cortex in which injury causes abulia, a condition in which patients fail to show emotional reactions to external stimuli.

The Hypothalamus Integrates Autonomic and Endocrine Functions With Behavior

The hypothalamus plays a particularly important role in regulating the autonomic nervous system and was once

referred to as the "head ganglion" of the autonomic nervous system. But recent studies of hypothalamic function have led to a somewhat different view. Whereas early studies found that electrical stimulation or lesions in the hypothalamus can profoundly affect autonomic function, more recent investigations have demonstrated that many of these effects are due to involvement of descending and ascending pathways of the cerebral cortex or the basal forebrain passing through the hypothalamus. Modern studies indicate that the hypothalamus functions to integrate autonomic response and endocrine function with behavior, especially behavior concerned with the basic homeostatic requirements of everyday life.

The hypothalamus serves this integrative function by regulation of five basic physiological needs:

1. It controls blood pressure and electrolyte composition by a set of regulatory mechanisms that range from control of drinking and salt appetite to the maintenance of blood osmolality and vasomotor tone.
2. It regulates body temperature by means of activities ranging from control of metabolic thermogenesis to behaviors such as seeking a warmer or cooler environment.

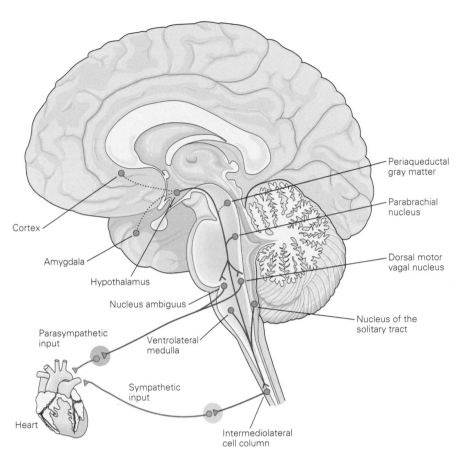

Figure 49-10 Pathways that control autonomic responses. Direct outputs to autonomic preganglionic neurons (**solid line**) arise from the paraventricular and lateral hypothalamus, the parabrachial nucleus, the nucleus of the solitary tract, certain monoamine groups such as the A5 noradrenergic neurons (not shown), serotonergic raphe neurons (not shown), and adrenergic neurons in the ventrolateral medulla. Less direct outputs from the cerebral cortex, amygdala, and periaqueductal gray matter (**dotted lines**) are relayed into the cell groups with direct input to the preganglionic inputs. Nearly all of the cell groups illustrated in these drawings are also connected with one another, forming a central autonomic network.

3. It controls energy metabolism by regulating feeding, digestion, and metabolic rate.
4. It regulates reproduction through hormonal control of mating, pregnancy, and lactation.
5. It controls emergency responses to stress, including physical and immunological responses to stress by regulating blood flow to muscle and other tissues and the secretion of adrenal stress hormones.

The hypothalamus regulates these basic life processes by recourse to three main mechanisms. First, the hypothalamus has access to sensory information from virtually the entire body. It receives direct inputs from the visceral sensory system and the olfactory system, as well as the retina. The visual inputs are used by the suprachiasmatic nucleus to synchronize the internal clock mechanism to the day-night cycle in the external world (Chapter 3). Visceral somatosensory inputs carrying information about pain are relayed to the hypothalamus from the spinal and trigeminal dorsal horn (Chapters 23 and 24). In addition, the hypothalamus has internal sensory neurons that are responsive to changes in local temperature, osmolality, glucose, and sodium,

to name a few examples. Finally, circulating hormones such as angiotensin II and leptin enter the hypothalamus at specialized zones along the margins of the third ventricle called *circumventricular organs,* where they interact directly with hypothalamic neurons.

Second, the hypothalamus compares sensory information with biological set points. It compares, for example, local temperature in the preoptic area to the set point of 37°C and, if the hypothalamus is warm, activates mechanisms for heat dissipation. There are set points for a wide variety of physiological processes, including blood sugar, sodium, osmolality, and hormone levels.

Finally, when the hypothalamus detects a deviation from a set point, it adjusts an array of autonomic, endocrine, and behavioral responses to restore homeostasis. If the body is too warm, the hypothalamus shifts blood flow from deep to cutaneous vascular beds and increases sweating, to increase heat loss through the skin. It increases vasopressin secretion, to conserve water for sweating. Meanwhile, the hypothalamus activates coordinated behaviors, such as seeking to change the local ambient temperature or seeking a cooler environment.

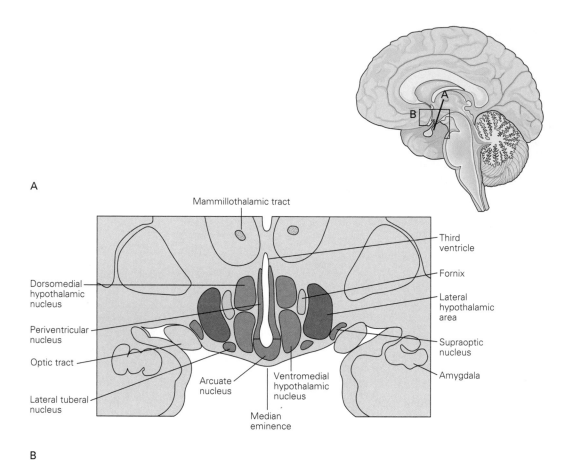

Figure 49-11 The structure of the hypothalamus.

A. Frontal view of the hypothalamus (section along the plane shown in part B).

B. A medial view shows most of the main nuclei. The hypothal-

amus is often divided analytically into three areas in a rosto-caudal direction: the preoptic area, the tuberal level, and the posterior level.

All of these processes must be precisely coordinated. For example, adjustments in blood flow in different vascular beds are important for such diverse activities as thermoregulation, digestion, response to emergency, and sexual intercourse. In order to do this, the hypothalamus contains an array of specialized cell groups with different functional roles.

The Hypothalamus Contains Specialized Groups of Neurons Clustered in Nuclei

Although the hypothalamus is very small, occupying only about 4 grams of the total 1400 grams of adult human brain weight, it is packed with a complex array of cell groups and fiber pathways (Figure 49-11). The hypothalamus can be divided into three regions: anterior, middle, and posterior. The most anterior part of the hypothalamus, overlying the optic chiasm, is the preoptic area. The preoptic nuclei, which include the circadian pacemaker (suprachiasmatic nucleus), are mainly concerned with integration of different kinds of sensory information needed to judge deviation from physiological set point. The preoptic area controls blood pressure and composition; cycles of activity, body temperature, and many hormones; and reproductive activity.

The middle third of the hypothalamus, overlying the pituitary stalk, contains the dorsomedial, ventromedial, paraventricular, supraoptic, and arcuate nuclei. The paraventricular nucleus includes both magnocellular and parvocellular neuroendocrine components controlling the posterior and anterior pituitary gland. In addition, it contains neurons that innervate both the parasympathetic and sympathetic preganglionic neurons in the medulla and the spinal cord, thus playing a major role also in regulating autonomic responses. The arcuate and periventricular nuclei, along the wall of the third ventricle, like the paraventricular nucleus contain parvocellular neuroendocrine neurons, whereas the supraoptic nucleus contains additional magnocellular neuroendocrine cells. The ventromedial and dorsomedial nuclei project mainly locally within the hypothalamus and to the periaqueductal gray matter, to regulate complex integrative functions such as control of growth, feeding, maturation, and reproduction.

Finally, the posterior third of the hypothalamus includes the mammillary body and the overlying posterior hypothalamic area. In addition to the mammillary nuclei, whose function remains enigmatic, this region includes the tuberomammillary nucleus, a histaminergic cell group that is important in regulating wakefulness and arousal.

The major nuclei of the hypothalamus are located for the most part in the medial part of the hypothala-

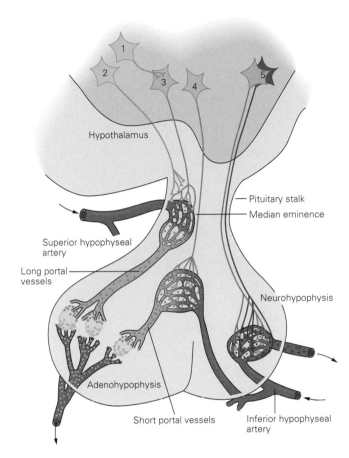

Figure 49-12 The hypothalamus controls the pituitary gland both directly and indirectly through hormone-releasing neurons. Peptidergic neurons (**5**) release oxytocin or vasopressin into the general circulation through the posterior **pituitary**. Two general types of neurons are involved in regulation of the anterior pituitary. Peptidergic neurons (**3, 4**) synthesize and release hormones into the hypophyseal-portal circulation. The second type of neuron is the link between the peptidergic neurons and the rest of the brain. These neurons, some of which are monoaminergic, are believed to form synapses with peptidergic neurons either on the cell body (**1**) or on the axon terminal (**2**).

mus, sandwiched between two major fiber systems. A massive longitudinal fiber pathway, the *medial forebrain bundle,* runs through the lateral hypothalamus. The medial forebrain bundle connects the hypothalamus with the brain stem below, and with the basal forebrain, amygdala, and cerebral cortex above. Large neurons scattered among the fibers of the medial forebrain bundle provide long-ranging hypothalamic outputs that reach from the cerebral cortex to the sacral spinal cord. They are involved in organizing behaviors as well as autonomic responses.

A second, smaller fiber system is located medial to the major hypothalamic nuclei, in the wall of the third

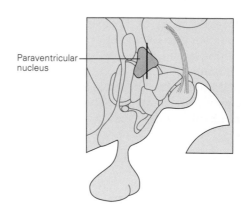

Figure 49-13 The paraventricular nucleus of the hypothalamus is a microcosm of the autonomic and endocrine control systems. Two distinct populations of magnocellular neuroendocrine neurons produce oxytocin or vasopressin, which are secreted into the bloodstream in the posterior pituitary gland. Parvocellular neuroendocrine neurons in the medial paraventricular nucleus (medial parvocellular neuroendocrine neurons) contain hypothalamic releasing hormones, such as corticotropin-releasing hormone and release-inhibiting hormones, such as dopamine and somatostatin. Their axons project to the median eminence, where they release their hormones into the hypophysial portal circulation to control the anterior pituitary gland. Dorsal, ventral, and lateral (not shown) parvocellular neurons project to the preganglionic cell groups in the medulla and the spinal cord, as well as to other autonomic control nuclei in the brain stem. They use mainly oxytocin and vasopressin as neuromodulators. However, this is a completely distinct population from the magnocellular oxytocin and vasopressin neurons, as few if any cells send axons to both the posterior pituitary and the brain stem.

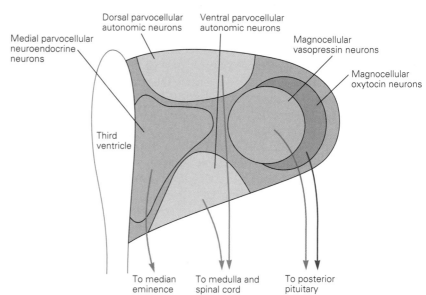

ventricle. This periventricular fiber system contains longitudinal fibers that link the hypothalamus to the periaqueductal gray matter in the midbrain. This pathway is thought to be important in activating simple, stereotyped behavioral patterns, such as posturing during sexual behavior. The periventricular system also conveys the axons of the parvocellular neuroendocrine neurons located in the periventricular region, and including the paraventricular and arcuate nuclei, to the median eminence, for control of the anterior pituitary gland. They are met in the median eminence by the axons from the magnocellular neurons, which continue down the pituitary stalk to the posterior pituitary gland.

The Hypothalamus Controls the Endocrine System

The hypothalamus controls the endocrine system *directly*, by secreting neuroendocrine products into the general circulation from the posterior pituitary gland, and *indirectly*, by secreting regulatory hormones into the local portal circulation, which drains into the blood vessels of the anterior pituitary (Figure 49-12). These regulatory hormones control the synthesis and release of anterior pituitary hormones into the general circulation. The highly fenestrated (perforated) capillaries of the posterior pituitary and median eminence of the hypothalamus facilitate the entry of hormones into the gen-

Table 49-2 Hormones of the Posterior Pituitary Gland

Name	Structure	Function
Vasopressin	H-Cys-Tyr-Phe-Gln-Asn-Cys-Pro-Arg-Gly-NH$_2$ S-S	Vasoconstriction, water resorption by the kidney
Oxytocin	H-Cys-Tyr-Ile-Glu-Asn-Cys-Pro-Leu-Gly-NH$_2$ S-S	Uterine contraction and milk ejection

eral circulation or the portal plexus. Direct and indirect control form the basis of our modern understanding of hypothalamic control of endocrine activity.

Magnocellular Neurons Secrete Oxytocin and Vasopressin Directly From the Posterior Pituitary Gland

Large neurons in the paraventricular and supraoptic nuclei, constituting the magnocellular region of the hypothalamus, project to the posterior pituitary gland (*neurohypophysis*). Some of the magnocellular neuroendocrine neurons in the paraventricular and supraoptic nuclei release the neurohypophyseal hormone oxytocin, while others release vasopressin into the general circulation by way of the posterior pituitary (Figure 49-13). These peptides circulate to target organs of the body that control water balance and milk release.

Oxytocin and vasopressin are peptides that contain nine amino acid residues (Table 49-2). Like other peptide hormones, they are cleaved from larger prohormones (see Chapter 15). The prohormones are synthesized in the cell body and cleaved within transport vesicles as they travel down the axons. The peptide neurophysin is a cleavage product of the processing of vasopressin and oxytocin and is released along with the hormone in the posterior pituitary. The neurophysin formed in neurons that release vasopressin differs somewhat from that produced in neurons that release oxytocin.

Parvocellular Neurons Secrete Peptides That Regulate Release of Anterior Pituitary Hormones

Geoffrey Harris proposed in the 1950s that the anterior pituitary gland is regulated indirectly by the hypothalamus. He demonstrated that the hypophysial portal veins, which carry blood from the hypothalamus to the anterior pituitary gland, convey important signals that control anterior pituitary secretion. In the 1970s the structure of a series of peptide hormones that carry these signals was elucidated. These hormones fall into two classes: releasing hormones and release-inhibiting hormones (Table 49-3). Of all the anterior pituitary hormones, only prolactin is under predominantly inhibitory control. Hence transection of the pituitary stalk causes insufficiency of adrenal cortex, thyroid, gonadal, and growth hormones, but increased prolactin secretion.

Systematic electrical recordings have not been made from neurons that secrete releasing hormones. However, they are believed to fire in bursts because of the pulsatile nature of secretion of the anterior pituitary hormones, which show periodic surges throughout the day. Episodic firing may be particularly effective for causing hormone release and may limit receptor inactivation.

The neurons that make releasing hormones are found mainly along the wall of the third ventricle. The gonadotropin-releasing hormone (GnRH) neurons tend to be located most anteriorly, along the basal part of the third ventricle. Neurons that make somatostatin, corticotropin-releasing hormone (CRH), and dopamine are located more dorsally and are found in the medial part of the paraventricular nucleus. Neurons that make growth hormone–releasing hormone (GRH), thyrotropin-releasing hormone (TRH), GnRH, and dopamine are found in the arcuate nucleus, an expansion of the periventricular gray matter that overlies the median eminence, in the floor of the third ventricle (see Figure 49-10). The median eminence contains a plexus of fine capillary loops. These are fenestrated capillaries, and the terminals of the neurons that contain releasing hormones end on these loops. The blood then flows from the median eminence into a secondary (portal) venous system, which carries it to the anterior pituitary gland (See Figure 49-11).

Table 49-3 Hypothalamic Substances That Release or Inhibit the Release of Anterior Pituitary Hormones

Hypothalamic substance	Anterior pituitary hormone
Releasing	
Thyrotropin-releasing hormone (TRH)	Thyrotropin, prolactin
Corticotropin-releasing hormone (CRH)	Adrenocorticotropin, β-lipotropin
Gonadotropin-releasing hormone (GnRH)	Luteinizing hormone (LH), follicle-stimulating hormone (FSH)
Growth hormone-releasing hormone (GHRH or GRH)	Growth hormone (GH)
Prolactin-releasing factor (PRF)	Prolactin
Melanocyte-stimulating hormone-releasing factor (MRF)	Melanocyte-stimulating hormone (MSH), β-endorphin
Inhibiting	
Prolactin release-inhibiting hormone (PIH), dopamine	Prolactin
Growth hormone release-inhibiting hormone (GIH or GHRIH; somatostatin)	Growth hormone, thyrotropin
Melanocyte-stimulating hormone release-inhibiting factor (MIF)	Melanocyte-stimulating hormone (MSH)

An Overall View

The three divisions of the autonomic nervous system comprise an integrated motor system that acts in parallel with the somatic motor system and is responsible for homeostasis. Essential to the functioning of the motor outflow are the visceral sensory afferents that are relayed from the nucleus of the solitary tract through a network of central autonomic control nuclei. The hypothalamus integrates somatic, visceral, and behavioral information from all of these sources, thus coordinating autonomic and endocrine outflow with behavioral state.

Several features of the autonomic nervous system permit rapid integrated responses to changes in the environment. The activity of effector organs is finely controlled by coordinated and balanced excitatory and inhibitory inputs from tonically active postganglionic neurons. Moreover, the sympathetic system is greatly divergent, permitting the entire body to respond to extreme conditions.

In addition to the small molecule neurotransmitters— ACh and norepinephrine—a wide variety of peptides are thought to be released by autonomic neurons either onto postganglionic cells or their targets. Many of these peptides act to alter the efficacy of cholinergic or adrenergic transmission. The autonomic nervous system uses a rich variety of chemical mediators, several of which may commonly coexist in single autonomic neurons. The release of different combinations of chemical mediators from autonomic neurons may represent a means of "chemical coding" of information transfer in the different branches of the autonomic nervous system, although we are still only beginning to learn how to read the code.

As we shall also see in the following two chapters, the autonomic nervous system is a remarkably adaptable system of homeostatic control. It can function locally through branches of primary sensory fibers that terminate in autonomic ganglia, or intrinsically through the entire nervous system on the functions of the digestive tract. Control centers in the brain stem are involved in several autonomic reflexes. While the hypothalamus integrates behavioral and emotional responses arising from the forebrain with ongoing metabolic need to produce highly coordinated autonomic control and behavior.

Susan Iversen
Leslie Iversen
Clifford B. Saper

Selected Readings

Bacq ZM. 1974. *Chemical Transmission of Nerve Impulses: A Historical Sketch.* New York: Pergamon.

Burnstock G. 1972. Purinergic nerves. Pharmacol Rev 24:509–581.

Burnstock G, Hoyle CHV (eds). 1995. *The Autonomic Nervous System.* Vol. 1, *Autonomic Neuroeffector Mechanisms.* London: Harwood Academic.

Cannon WB. 1932. *The Wisdom of the Body.* New York: Norton.

Costa M, Brookes SJ. 1994. The enteric nervous system. Am J Gastroenterol 89 (Suppl):S129–137.

Furness JB, Bornstein JC, Murphy R, Pompolo S. 1992. Roles of peptides in transmission in the enteric nervous system. Trends Neurosci 15:66–71.

Langley JN. 1921. *The Autonomic Nervous System.* Cambridge: Heffer & Sons.

Milner P, Burnstock G. 1995. Neurotransmitters in the autonomic nervous system. In: AD Korczyn (ed). *Handbook of Autonomic Nervous System Dysfunction*, pp. 5–32. New York: Marcel Dekker.

References

Brown DA, Adams PR. 1980. Muscarinic suppression of a novel voltage-sensitive K^+ current in a vertebrate neurone. Nature 283:673–676.

Elfvin LG, Lindh B, Hokfelt T. 1993. The chemical neuroanatomy of sympathetic ganglia. Annu Rev Neurosci 16:471–507.

Fredholm BB, Abbracchio MP, Burnstock G, Daly JW, Harden TK, Jacobson KA, Leff P, Williams M. 1994. Nomenclature and classification of purinoceptors. Pharmacol Rev 46:143–156.

Furness JB, Costa M. 1980. Types of nerves in the enteric nervous system. Neuroscience 5:1–20.

Gershon M. 1998. *The Second Brain.* New York: Harper Collins.

Guillemin R. 1978. Control of adenohypophysial functions by peptides of the central nervous system. Harvey Lect 71:71–131.

Hugdahl K. 1995. Classical conditioning and implicit learning: The right hemisphere hypothesis. In: RJ Davidson, K Hugdahl (eds). *Brain Asymmetry*, pp. 235–268. Cambridge, MA: MIT Press.

Hugdahl K, Berardi A, Thompson WL, Kosslyn SM, Macy R, Baker DP, Alpert NM, LeDoux JE. 1995. Brain mechanisms in human classical conditioning: a PET blood flow study. Neuroreport 6:1723–1728.

Hutter OF, Trautwein W. 1956. Vagal and sympathetic effects on the pacemaker fibers in the sinus venosus of the heart. J Gen Physiol 39:715–733.

Jan LY, Jan YN. 1983. A LHRH-like peptidergic neurotransmitter capable of action at a distance in autonomic ganglia. Trends Neurosci 6:320–325.

Loewy AD, Spyer KM (eds). 1990. *Central Regulation of Autonomic Function.* New York: Oxford Univ. Press.

Randall WC (ed). 1984. *Nervous Control of Cardiovascular Function.* New York: Oxford Univ. Press.

Reuter H, Scholz H. 1977. The regulation of the calcium conductance of cardiac muscle by adrenaline. J Physiol (Lond) 264:49–62.

Silverman AJ, Zimmerman EA. 1983. Magnocellular neurosecretory system. Annu Rev Neurosci 6:357–380.

Swanson LW, Sawchenko PE. 1983. Hypothalamic integration: organization of the paraventricular and supraoptic nuclei. Annu Rev Neurosci 6:269–324.

Toda N, West T. 1967. Interactions of K, Na and vagal stimulation in the S-A node of the rabbit. Am J Physiol 22:416–423.

Tranel D, Damasio AR. 1985. Knowledge without awareness: an autonomic index of facial recognition by prosopagnosics. Science 228:1453–1454.

Yuan SY, Bornstein JC, Furness JB. 1995. Pharmacological evidence that nitric oxide may be a retrograde messenger in the enteric nervous system. Br J Pharmacol 114:428–432.

50

Emotional States and Feelings

P LEASURE, ELATION, EUPHORIA, ecstasy, sadness, despondency, depression, fear, anxiety, anger, hostility, and calm—these and other emotions color our lives. They contribute to the richness of our experiences and imbue our actions with passion and character. Moreover, as we shall learn in Chapter 61, disorders of emotion contribute importantly to several major psychiatric illnesses. An emotional state has two components, one evident in a characteristic physical sensation and the other as a conscious feeling—we sense our heart pounding *and* we consciously feel afraid. To maintain the distinction between these two components, the term *emotion* sometimes is used to refer only to the bodily state (ie, the emotional state) and the term *feeling* is used to refer to conscious sensation.

Like perception and action, emotional states and feelings are mediated by distinct neuronal circuits within the brain. In fact, many drugs that affect the mind—ranging from addictive street drugs to therapeutic agents—do so by acting on specific neural circuits concerned with emotional states and feelings.

Conscious feeling is mediated by the cerebral cortex, in part by the cingulate cortex and by the frontal lobes. Emotional states are mediated by a family of peripheral, autonomic, endocrine, and skeletomotor responses. These responses involve subcortical structures: the amygdala, the hypothalamus, and the brain stem. When frightened we not only feel afraid but also experience increased heart rate and respiration, dryness of the mouth, tense muscles, and sweaty palms, all of which are regulated by subcortical structures. To understand an emotion such as fear we therefore need to understand the relationship between cognitive feeling represented in the cortex and the

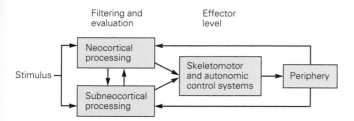

Figure 50-1 Model of the basic neural systems that control emotions. Emotions are typically elicited by a specific stimulus. The stimulus affects both neocortical and subcortical structures, such the amygdala. In turn, cortical structures and the amygdala and other subcortical structures regulate the systems that mediate the peripheral manifestations of emotional behaviors. The particular emotion experienced is a function of cross-talk between neocortical and subcortical structures, as well as feedback from peripheral receptors.

associated physiological signs orchestrated in subcortical structures.

In this chapter we examine how emotion is represented in the brain. A neural analysis of emotion must take into account at least four issues. First, we must understand how stimuli acquire emotional significance and what roles conscious cognitive processes and automatic unconscious processes have in determining whether a particular stimulus at a particular moment will have emotional significance (Figure 50-1). Second, we must understand how certain autonomic and skeletomotor responses are triggered once a stimulus acquires emotional significance. Third, we must identify the circuits in the cerebral cortex responsible for feelings. Finally, we need to understand how somatic emotional states and conscious feeling states interact—how feedback from peripheral, autonomic, and skeletomotor systems to the cerebral cortex shapes emotional experience. As we will see, various theories of emotion largely differ in their emphasis on the importance of this feedback.

The Peripheral Components of Emotion Prepare the Body for Action and Communicate Our Emotional States to Other People

The peripheral, skeletomotor, and autonomic aspects of emotion have preparatory and communicative functions. The preparatory function involves both *general arousal*, which prepares the organism as a whole for action, and *specific arousal*, which prepares the organism for a particular behavior. For example, sexual arousal involves an increase of heart rate, a change that prepares the organism generally for physical exertion. In addi-

tion, it involves more localized changes, such as tumescence, that are specific to sexual behavior. The mechanisms of generalized and specific arousal act synergistically to prepare the periphery (muscles, glands, blood vessels) and the cerebral cortex for ongoing or upcoming events. Unless it is extreme, arousal enhances intellectual and physical performance (Figure 50-2).

The peripheral component of emotion also communicates emotion to others. In humans social communication of emotion is mediated primarily by the skeletomotor system, in particular by the muscles that control facial and postural expressions.

A Theory of Emotion Must Explain the Relationship of Cognitive and Physiological States

Until the late nineteenth century the traditional view of the evocation and expression of emotion consisted of the following sequence. First, an important event is recognized—for example, you see your house on fire. This recognition in turn produces in the cerebral cortex a conscious emotional experience—fear—that triggers signals to peripheral structures including the heart, blood vessels, adrenal glands, and sweat glands. According to this traditional view, a conscious, emotional event initiates reflexive autonomic responses in the body.

In the James-Lange Theory Emotions Are Cognitive Responses to Information From the Periphery

In 1884 the American psychologist William James rejected the traditional view that emotions are initiated by

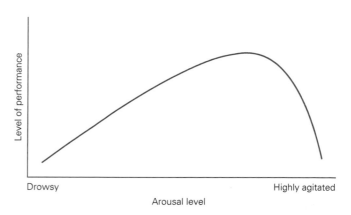

Figure 50-2 Performance is affected by arousal level. An intermediate level of arousal is optimal; performance is less adequate at both very high and very low levels of arousal.

cognitive activity. In an article entitled *What Is Emotion*? James proposed that the cognitive experience of emotion is secondary to the physiological expression of emotion. He suggested that when we encounter a potentially dangerous situation—for example, a bear sitting in the middle of our path—the evaluation of the bear's ferocity does not itself generate a consciously experienced emotional state. We do not experience fear until after we have run away from the bear. That is, we act instinctively by running away and then consciously explain our action and the changes in our body (the increase in heart rate and respiration) as "driven by fear."

Based on this idea, James and the Danish psychologist Carl Lange proposed an alternative hypothesis: The feeling state, the conscious experience of emotion, occurs *after* the cortex receives signals about changes in our physiological state. Feelings are preceded by certain physiological changes—an increase or decrease in blood pressure, heart rate, and muscular tension. Thus, when you see a fire you feel afraid because your cortex has received signals about your racing heart, knocking knees, and sweaty palms. James wrote: "We feel sorry because we cry, angry because we strike, afraid because we tremble and not that we cry, strike or tremble because we are sorry, angry or fearful as the case may be." According to this view, emotions are cognitive responses to information from the periphery.

There is now experimental support for aspects of the James-Lange theory. For example, objectively distinguishable emotions can be correlated with specific patterns of autonomic, endocrine, and voluntary responses. Furthermore, patients in whom the spinal cord has been accidentally severed so that they lack feedback from the autonomic nervous system appear to experience a reduction in the intensity of their emotions.

However, the James-Lange theory fails to explain certain aspects of emotional behavior. For example, one often continues to be emotionally aroused even after the physiological changes have subsided. Were physiological feedback the only controlling factor, the emotions should not outlast the physiological change. Yet a person can sustain a feeling of fear long after a threat has abated. Conversely, some feelings arise faster than the changes in bodily state normally associated with those feelings. Thus there may be more to emotions than just cortical interpretation of feedback information from the periphery.

Perhaps the most serious challenge to the James-Lange theory came in the 1920s from Walter B. Cannon's study of peripheral responses to intense emotion. Cannon's work indicated that intense emotion triggered an emergency reaction—a *fight-or-flight response*—in anticipation of additional behavioral responses and expenditure of energy. Cannon suggested that this flight-or-fight response was mediated by the sympathetic component of the autonomic nervous system and that it acted as a whole, almost in an all-or-none way, independent of the specific emotionally significant stimuli that elicited it. He therefore proposed that the physiological responses to emotionally significant stimuli are too undifferentiated to convey to the cortex specific, detailed information about the nature of an emotional event.

The Cannon-Bard Theory Emphasizes the Role of the Hypothalamus and Other Subcortical Structures in Mediating Both the Cognitive and Peripheral Aspects of Emotion

To deal with the shortcomings of the James-Lange theory, Cannon and Philip Bard suggested that two subcortical structures, the hypothalamus and the thalamus, have a key role in mediating emotions, including regulating the peripheral signs of emotion and providing the cortex with the information required for the cognitive processing of emotion. This idea was based on studies by Cannon and Bard using cats in which the whole cerebral cortex had been removed. Such animals retain fully integrated emotional responses, termed *sham rage* because the responses appear to lack elements of conscious experience that are characteristic of genuine, naturally occurring rage.

Sham rage also differs from genuine rage because responses can be triggered by very mild stimuli, such as a weak touch, or can even occur spontaneously, without provocation. No matter how it is elicited, sham rage subsides very quickly once the stimulus is removed. In addition, sham rage is undirected, and the animals sometimes even bite themselves. When Bard analyzed sham rage by progressive transections he found that the coordinated response disappeared, leaving only isolated elements of the response, when the hypothalamus was included in the ablation (Figure 50-3).

The question whether conscious feeling follows bodily changes (James-Lange) or bodily changes follow feeling continued to dominate modern discussions of emotional states for many years. Emotions are increasingly viewed as the outcome of a dynamic, ongoing interaction, perhaps at the level of the amygdala, of peripheral factors mediated by the hypothalamus and central factors mediated by the cerebral cortex. This synthesis of two theories, which now seems obvious, has emerged only slowly over the past three decades.

According to the Schachter Theory Feelings Are Cognitive Translations of Ambiguous Peripheral Signals

The James-Lange view of emotion has been refined in important ways, first by Stanley Schachter and more recently by Antonio Damasio. In the 1960s Schachter began to emphasize that the cortex actually constructs emotion—much like it does vision—out of often ambiguous signals it receives from the periphery. According to the James-Lange theory emotional experience is the direct consequence of information arriving in the cerebral cortex from the periphery. Instead of this simple relation, Schachter proposed that the cortex actively translates peripheral signals, even nonspecific ones, into specific feelings. He suggested that the cortex creates a cognitive response to peripheral information consistent with the individual's expectations and social context.

In one study Schachter injected volunteers with epinephrine; some subjects were informed of the side effects (eg, pounding heart), others were not. All of the subjects were then exposed either to annoying or amusing conditions. The subjects who had been warned about the side effects of epinephrine exhibited less anger or less pleasurable feelings. Schachter interpreted this finding as indicating that the informed subjects attributed their arousal to the drug, whereas the other group perceived their arousal as an emotional response—as strong anger or pleasant feelings depending on the conditions. More recent experiments have shown that the general arousal produced by exercise can lead to specific arousal, such as sexual arousal.

Schachter's refinement of the James-Lange theory was elaborated even further by Damasio, who argues that the feeling state, the experience of emotion, is essentially a story that the brain constructs to explain bodily reactions. Indeed, recent studies indicate that autonomic responses are not as uniform and stereotyped as Cannon had originally believed. Different emotional states are typically accompanied by different patterns of autonomic responses, such as changes in blood flow or heart rate.

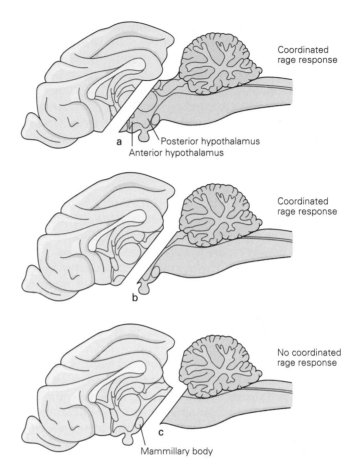

Figure 50-3 This midsagittal section of the cat brain shows the levels of brain transection used to study sham rage. Transection of the forebrain (**level a**) and the disconnection of everything above the transection causes an animal to exhibit sham rage. Transection at the level of the hypothalamus (**level b**) and the disconnection of everything above it also produces sham rage. If, however, the posterior hypothalamus also is disconnected (**level c**), only isolated elements of rage can be elicited.

In the Arnold Theory Autonomic Responses Are Not an Essential Component of Emotion

Magda Arnold has advanced this line of thinking further. She argues that emotion is the product of unconscious evaluation of a situation as potentially harmful or beneficial, while feeling is the conscious reflection of the unconscious appraisal. Feeling is therefore a tendency to respond in a particular way, not the response itself. Emotions differ from one another because they elicit different action tendencies. Thus, unlike the James-Lange theory, Arnold's view does not require that we have an autonomic response to experience emotion.

A consensus is emerging that Arnold's "appraisal" theory provides a good overall description of how emotions are generated: unconscious, implicit evaluation of

a stimulus is followed by action tendencies, then peripheral responses, and finally conscious experience. A key finding supporting this idea is that we can have emotional reactions to subliminal stimuli. An important implication of Arnold's view is that emotions may have their own logic, one that is not derived from either conscious cognitive processes or somantic events associated with emotional states.

To what degree do emotions require conscious and unconscious processes or feedback from peripheral organs? To answer these questions we must ground the study of emotion in neural science. During the past decade the neural pathways for the peripheral (autonomic) and central (evaluative components of emotion) have been identified with some precision. It is now clear from Cannon's work that the peripheral component involves the hypothalamus, while the central, evaluative component, both unconscious and conscious, involves the cerebral cortex, especially the cingulate and the prefrontal cortex. Central to both of these systems is the amygdala, a subcortical nuclear complex thought to coordinate the conscious experience of emotion and the peripheral expressions of emotions, in particular fear.

Neural studies by Joseph LeDoux, by Michael Davis, and by Michael Fanslow indicate that the unconscious evaluation of the emotional significance of a stimulus begins before the conscious processing of the stimulus. Moreover, the neural systems for storing unconscious memories about emotional states (somatic response) are different from those responsible for the memory of conscious feeling. Damage to the amygdala, a system concerned with the experience and memory of fear, disrupts the ability of an emotionally charged stimulus to elicit an unconscious emotional response. In contrast, damage to the hippocampus, the core of the medial temporal lobe system concerned with conscious memory (Chapter 62), interferes with remembering the cognitive features of fear—where the fear-provoking stimulus was and in what context it occurred. Whereas cognitive systems present us with a choice of action, unconscious appraisal systems limit the options to a few adaptively important choices.

An attractive feature of this view is that it brings the study of emotion in line with studies of memory storage, which indicate that memory has two major forms: a conscious (*explicit*) memory for facts and personal events and an unconscious (*implicit*) memory for motor and sensory experience (Chapter 62). Memory of emotional states (autonomic and somatic responses) involves implicit memory storage, whereas memory of feelings involves explicit memory storage.

The Hypothalamus Coordinates the Peripheral Expression of Emotional States

How does the hypothalamus regulate the physiologic expression of emotion? We now appreciate that the hypothalamus acts on the autonomic nervous system by modulating visceral reflex circuitry that is basically organized at the level of the brain stem. This was first shown in 1932 by Stephen Ranson in anesthetized animals, using stereotaxic methods that permit precise and reproducible placement of electrodes in the different regions of the hypothalamus. By stimulating these differ-

ent hypothalamic regions Ranson evoked almost every conceivable autonomic reaction, including alterations in heart rate, blood pressure, and gastrointestinal motility, as well as erection of hairs and bladder contraction.

In the 1940s Walter Hess extended Ranson's approach to awake, unanesthetized cats and found that different parts of the hypothalamus produce characteristic constellations of reactions that appear to be parts of organized responses characteristic of specific emotional states. For example, electrical stimulation in cats of the lateral hypothalamus and the fibers of passage in this area (see Chapter 51) elicits autonomic and somatic responses characteristic of anger: increased blood pressure, raising of the body hair, pupillary constriction, arching of the back, and raising of the tail.

These observations provided the basis for the important conclusion that the hypothalamus is not only a motor nucleus for the autonomic nervous system. Rather, it is a coordinating center that integrates various inputs to ensure a well-organized, coherent, and appropriate set of autonomic and somatic responses. Since many of these responses resemble those seen during various types of emotional states, Hess suggested that the hypothalamus coordinates the peripheral expression of emotional states. This idea is supported by lesion studies that associate different hypothalamic structures with a wide range of emotional states. For example, animals with lesions in the lateral hypothalamus become placid, whereas animals with lesions of the medial hypothalamus are highly excitable and easily become aggressive.

The Search for Cortical Representation of Feeling Has Led to the Limbic System

Emotionally significant stimuli activate sensory pathways that trigger the hypothalamus to modulate heart rate, blood pressure, and respiration. (These observations are consistent with the James-Lange and Schachter-Damasio theories.) In turn, information about emotionally significant stimuli also is conveyed to the cerebral cortex both directly from the peripheral organs whose homeostatic state has been disturbed and indirectly from the hypothalamus, the amygdala, and related structures.

How are feeling and emotion represented in the cortex? In 1937 James Papez proposed that the cortical machinery for feeling involves the *limbic lobe*, a region identified by Paul Broca. The limbic lobe comprises a ring of phylogenetically primitive cortex around the brain stem and includes the cingulate gyrus, the parahippocampal gyrus (which is the anterior and inferior continuation of the cingulate gyrus), and the hippocampal formation, which lies deep in the parahip-

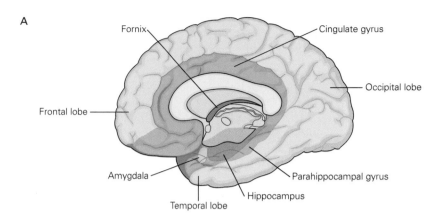

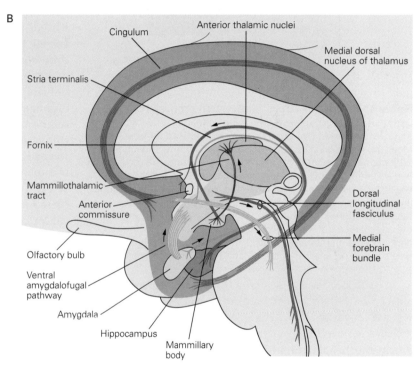

Figure 50-4 The limbic system consists of the limbic lobe and deep-lying structures. (Adapted from Nieuwenhuys et al. 1988.)

A. This medial view of the brain shows the prefrontal limbic cortex and the limbic lobe. The limbic lobe consists of primitive cortical tissue (**blue**) that encircles the upper brain stem as well as underlying cortical structures (hippocampus and amygdala).

B. Interconnections of the deep-lying structures included in the limbic system. The predominant direction of neural activity in each tract is indicated by an **arrow**, although these tracts are typically bidirectional.

pocampal gyrus and is morphologically simpler than the overlying cortex (Figure 50-4). The hippocampal formation includes the hippocampus proper, the dentate gyrus, and the subiculum.

Papez argued that, since the hypothalamus communicates reciprocally with areas of the cerebral cortex, information about the conscious and peripheral aspects of emotion affect each other. Papez proposed that the neocortex influences the hypothalamus by means of connections to the cingulate gyrus and from the cingulate gyrus to the hippocampal formation. According to this idea, the hippocampal formation processes information from the cingulate gyrus and conveys it to the mammillary bodies of the hypothalamus by way of the fornix (a fiber bundle that carries part of the outflow of the hippocampus; see Figure 50-4). In turn, the hypothalamus

provides information to the cingulate gyrus by a pathway from the mammillary bodies to the anterior thalamic nuclei (the mammillothalamic tract) and from there to the cingulate gyrus (Figure 50-5). Consistent with this idea is the clinical observation that patients who have been infected with the rabies virus—which characteristically attacks the hippocampus—show profound changes in emotional state, including bouts of terror and rage.

The concept of the limbic system was later expanded by Paul MacLean to include parts of the hypothalamus, the septal area, the nucleus accumbens (a part of the striatum), neocortical areas such as the orbitofrontal cortex, and most important, the amygdala. Modern anatomical studies have also shown that there are extensive direct connections between neocortical

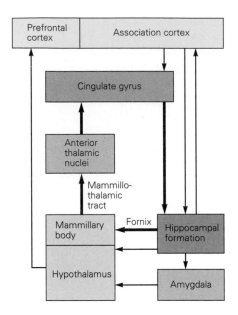

Figure 50-5 A neural circuit for emotion proposed by James Papez and extended by Paul MacLean. The circuit originally proposed by Papez is indicated by **thick lines;** more recently described connections are shown by **fine lines.** Known projections of the fornix to hypothalamic regions (mammillary bodies and other hypothalamic areas) and of the hypothalamus to the prefrontal cortex are indicated. A pathway interconnecting the amygdala to limbic structures is shown. Finally, reciprocal connections between the hippocampal formation and the association cortex are indicated. The hippocampal formation includes the hippocampus proper and surrounding structures, including entorhinal cortex and the subicular complex.

areas, the hippocampal formation, and the amygdala (Figure 50-5).

As we will see below, Papez was correct in attributing an important role to the cingulate cortex and the parahippocampal gyrus in the perception of feeling and emotion. He was incorrect, however, in thinking that the hippocampus coordinates the activity of the hypothalamus with these cortical areas: that coordinating role is carried out by the amygdala.

The first clue to the representation of emotion in the limbic system was found in 1939, when Heinrich Klüver and Paul Bucy showed that bilateral removal of the temporal lobes in monkeys—including the amygdala and the hippocampal formation, as well as the nonlimbic temporal cortex—produced a dramatic behavioral syndrome that included a major change in emotional behavior. After the operation, the monkeys, which had been quite wild before the procedure, became tame and fearless and their emotions flattened. They also exhib-

ited a variety of other behavioral changes not directly related to emotions. They put inedible objects into their mouths and exhibited an enormous increase in sexual behavior, including mounting inappropriate objects and species. Finally, the animals showed a compulsive tendency to observe and react to every visual stimulus but failed to recognize familiar objects.

The Amygdala Is the Part of the Limbic System Most Specifically Involved With Emotional Experience

Because Papez's ideas were so influential, the whole Klüver-Bucy syndrome was for some years ascribed largely to the limbic system. It is now clear that the syndrome can be fractionated and that only some components involve the limbic system. For example, the visual deficits in Klüver-Bucy syndrome are mostly due to damage to the visual association areas of the inferior temporal cortex, the area concerned with, among other things, the recognition of faces and other complex visual forms (Chapter 28). Most important, the hippocampus, the mammillary bodies, and anterior thalamic nuclei, which were central to Papez's thinking about emotion, were found not to be involved in emotion but are critical for cognitive forms of memory storage (Chapter 62). Thus, with the exception of the cingulate and parahippocampal gyri, most parts of the limbic system as originally defined by Papez appear not to play a major role in the emotional components of the Klüver-Bucy syndrome or in emotion in general.

Considerable evidence from both humans and experimental animals now indicates that the amygdala rather than the hippocampus intervenes between the regions concerned with the somatic expression of emotion (the hypothalamus and the brain stem nuclei) and the neocortical areas concerned with conscious feeling, especially fear (the cingulate, parahippocampal, and prefrontal cortices).

For example, electrical stimulation of the amygdala in humans produces feelings of fear and apprehension. Conversely, damage to the amygdala in experimental animals produces tameness. Isolated lesions of the amygdala rarely occur in humans, but lesions of the amygdala occur as part of the widespread Urbach-Wiethe disease, a degenerative condition associated with calcium deposition in the amygdala. If the lesion occurs early in life, patients with bilateral amygdala damage fail to learn the cues that normal subjects use to discern fear in facial expressions and to discriminate fine differences in other facial expressions. Thus Urbach-Wiethe disease disrupts the unconscious pro-

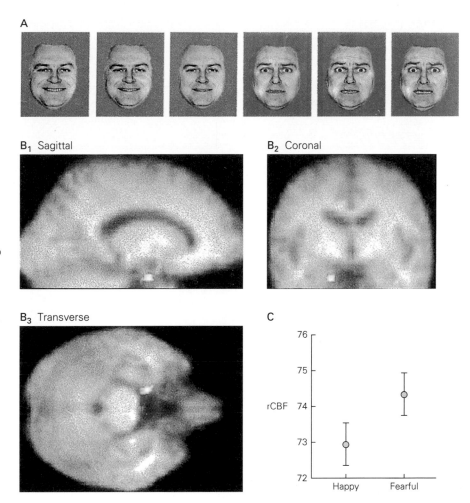

Figure 50-6 Brain imaging studies demonstrate the role of the amygdala in emotional responses. (From Morris et al. 1996.)

A. A series of faces shows a continuum of expression between happiness and fear. Activity in the brain of normal subjects was recorded as they viewed these faces.

B. With the presentation of each of the faces only the left amygdala was found to vary in a systematic fashion. The region with activity that was correlated with the type of face that was shown is indicated in **yellow** and **red**.

C. The mean regional cerebral blood flow (**rCBF**) for the predominantly happy and predominantly fearful expressions. These results are consistent with recording and ablation experiments on animals that suggest the amygdala has a critical role in emotions, particularly in fear.

cessing of cues to fear in both real faces and imagined faces drawn from memory.

The disease does not impair the conscious ability to discriminate complex visual stimuli such as faces. Indeed, patients can accurately identify familiar people from photographs. For example, one patient with degeneration of the amygdala was tested for her ability to rate the intensity of human facial expressions of happiness, surprise, fear, anger, disgust, and sadness. She rated fear, anger, and surprise as less intense than did any of the controls, although she was able to recognize the identity of familiar faces, some of which she had not seen for many years.

These results suggest that there are two anatomically separate neural systems. One, located in the inferotemporal cortex, is involved in the explicit memory of facial identity. The other, located in the amygdala, is concerned with the implicit memory of the appropriate cues that signal emotions expressed by faces. Consistent with this idea, studies using positron emission tomography (PET) and functional magnetic resonance imaging (fMRI) clearly show that recognition of emotional ex-

pression in faces involves the amygdala. When subjects were asked to view photographs of fearful or happy faces, the responses in the amygdala, especially in the amygdala of the left hemisphere, were significantly greater to fearful expressions than to happy expressions. Moreover, the response in the left amygdala increases with increasing fearfulness and decreases with increasing happiness (Figure 50–6).

How does the amygdala participate in forming an emotional response to visual stimuli? Appropriate responses to the sight of emotionally charged signals are coded by the inferior temporal cortex. Neurons in the inferior temporal cortex respond to facial features, including the direction of gaze. Lesions in this area impair the ability to discriminate the direction of gaze in other faces. Since the amygdala receives input from the inferior temporal cortex and has strong connections to the autonomic nervous system, it can mediate emotional responses to complex visual stimuli.

As Charles Darwin first pointed out in 1872, fearful, angry, and happy facial expressions are virtually uni-

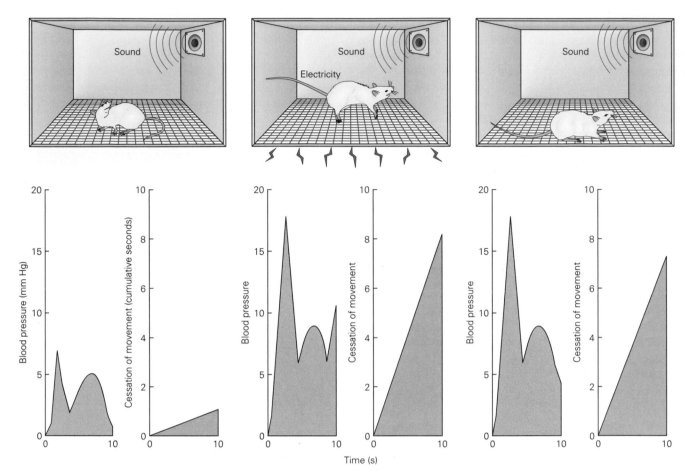

Figure 50-7 Classical fear conditioning can be demonstrated by pairing a sound with a mild electric shock to the foot of a rat. In one set of trials the rat hears a sound (**left panel**), which has relatively little effect on the animal's blood pressure or patterns of movement. Next, the same sound is coupled with a foot shock (**center**). After several pairings the rat's blood pressure rises and the animal freezes; it does not move for an extended period when it hears the sound. The rat has been fear-conditioned. Now, when the sound alone is given, it evokes physiological changes in blood pressure and freezing similar to those evoked by the sound and shock together (**right**). (From LeDoux 1994.)

versal and have not only personal but social significance. Indeed, the recognition of facial expressions is essential for successful social behavior in a complex social environment. Thus, the behavioral impairments resulting from damage to the amygdala suggest that the amygdala may be important for social cognition.

Learned Emotional Responses Are Processed in the Amygdala

The amygdala is a complex structure, consisting of about 10 distinct nuclei. The sensory inflow for various learned emotional states, particularly fear and anxiety, enters the amygdala by means of a particular set of nuclei: the basolateral complex.

The amygdala mediates both inborn and acquired emotional responses. The best studied example of a learned emotional state is the classical conditioning of fear (Chapter 62). Bilateral lesions of the basolateral complex of the amygdala in experimental animals abolish this learned response to fear. In this form of learning an initially neutral stimulus, such as a sound that does not evoke autonomic responses, is paired with an electric shock to the feet, which produces pain, fear, and autonomic responses. After several pairings the sound itself elicits a fearful reaction, such as freezing in place or changes in heart rate or blood pressure (Figure 50-7).

The sensory information about sound is conveyed to the basolateral complex from two sources: directly and rapidly from the auditory sensory nucleus in the

Figure 50-8 Some of the pathways involved in the processing of emotional information. Sensory information is transmitted to the thalamus via lemniscal pathways. The auditory input, for example, arrives in the ventral division of the medial geniculate nucleus. Other extralemniscal pathways deliver auditory information to other parts of the thalamus: the medial division of the medial geniculate nucleus and the posterior intralaminar nucleus. The lemniscal pathway of the ventral division of the medial geniculate nucleus projects only to the primary auditory cortex, but the extralemniscal auditory pathways of the medial geniculate nucleus and posterior intralaminar nucleus project to both the primary auditory cortex and auditory association cortex as well as to the basolateral nuclei of the amygdala. These pathways from the thalamus to the amygdala have been implicated in emotional learning. The anterior nucleus (not shown) projects widely to cortical areas and the central nucleus of the amygdala. The output nucleus of the amygdala, the central nucleus, makes extensive connections with brain stem areas involved in the control of emotional responses. It also projects to the nucleus basalis, which projects widely to cortical areas. The cholinergic projections from the nucleus basalis to the cortex have been implicated in cortical arousal. (Adapted from LeDoux 1992.)

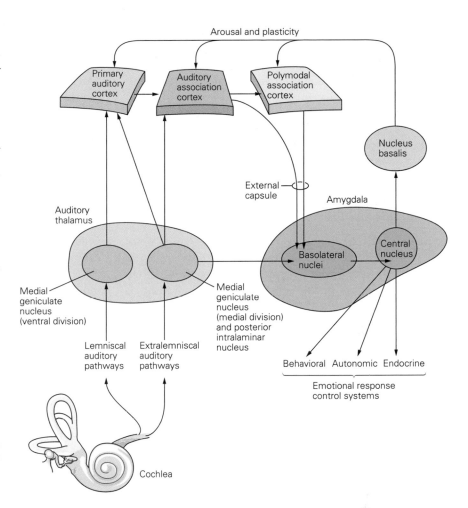

thalamus, and indirectly and more slowly from the primary sensory areas of the cortex. For many types of emotions, particularly fear, information conveyed from the thalamus to the amygdala is especially important because it can initiate short-latency, primitive emotional responses that may be important in situations of immediate danger. This rapidly available information may also prepare the amygdala to receive more highly processed information from cortical centers, which project mainly into the basolateral nuclei but also to the accessory basomedial nuclei (Figure 50-8). Consistent with their role in memory storage, stimulation of either thalamic or cortical pathways produces long-lasting alterations of synaptic efficacy (long-term potentiation; see Chapter 63) in the basolateral complex.

This pattern of responses to a once-neutral sound resembles human anxiety states, as we shall see in Chapter 61. For example, subjects presented repeatedly with a neutral sound together with an offensively loud noise soon show an emotional response—sweating hands, dry mouth, and facial perspiration—to the neutral sound alone. In contrast, patients with damage to the amygdala do not learn to fear the neutral sound even though most were consciously aware that the neutral sound and the offensive noise were paired together.

In addition to simple conditioned fear, both experimental animals and people can also acquire fear-potentiated startle. People and experimental animals will startle more powerfully in response to a loud noise when they are frightened than if they are relaxed. For example, once a rat has learned fear by associating a neutral sound with a foot shock, it will startle much more forcefully to a loud noise heard with the conditioned sound (when the animal is fearful) than it would to the same noise in the absence of the conditioned sound (when the animal is relaxed). Bilateral destruction of the amygdala also eliminates this form of learned fear.

Where is the memory for learned fear stored? One possibility is that emotional memories such as fear are directly stored in the amygdala itself since lesioning of the amygdala abolishes the emotional component of the learned response. Ablation of the amygdala, however, eliminates not only the learned response to fear, but also the innate (unconditioned) response to fear. It eliminates the very ability to express emotion. This leaves open the possibility that emotional memories are not stored in the amygdala directly but are stored in the cingulate and parahippocampal cortices, with which the amygdala is interconnected.

The Amygdala May Be Involved in Both Pleasurable and Fearful Responses to Stimuli

In addition to its role in fear and other negative emotional reactions, the amygdala may also play a role in pleasure or other appetitive, emotional reactions. When a neutral discriminative stimulus such as a tone is paired with a positive reinforcing stimulus such as food, the tone can become associated either with rewarding attributes of the food (its taste) or with nonrewarding attributes (its visual appearance). Lesions of the basolateral nuclei leave intact the learned association between the tone and the nonrewarding aspects of the food, but they disrupt the association of the tone with rewarding attributes of the food. Recall that animals with Klüver-Bucy syndrome frequently take inedible (nonrewarding) objects into their mouths.

Finally, the amygdala is required for a type of learning termed *context conditioning*, (or *place-preference*) by which an animal learns to increase its contact with environments in which it has previously encountered stimuli essential for survival and to minimize contact with environments that are aversive or dangerous. The positive preferences for place can be conditioned not only to food or sexual partners but also to drugs, such as stimulants.

Place preference can be used to measure the rewarding properties of stimuli ranging from simple rewards (sweets) to complex ones (sexual partners). The constellation of stimuli that make up the distinctive environment in which a reward is obtained becomes associated with the reward. As a result, these *place cues* later take on positive values and increase the likelihood that the animal will again seek out this place and maintain contact with it, even in the absence of the primary reward. Presumably, place cues gain positive properties in part by means of classical conditioning (Chapter 62). There is considerable evidence that the amygdala, particularly the basolateral complex, which integrates incoming sensory input, is involved in associating place cues with reward value. Contextual conditioning also involves acquiring and binding together a variety of sensory information about place, a process that requires the hippocampus (Chapter 62).

The Amygdala Mediates Both the Autonomic Expression and the Cognitive Experience of Emotion

The amygdala appears to be involved in mediating both the unconscious emotional state and conscious feeling. Consistent with this dual function of emotion, the amygdala has two projections. Many of the autonomic expressions of emotional states are mediated by the amygdala through its connections to the hypothalamus and the autonomic nervous system. The influence of the amygdala on conscious feeling is mediated by its projections to the cingulate gyrus and prefrontal cortex.

The nuclei of the amygdala are reciprocally connected to the lateral hypothalamus, brain stem, hippocampus, thalamus, and neocortex. The basolateral nucleus of the amygdala receives important afferent information from all sensory modalities and relays this information to the major output region, the central nucleus, both directly and by way of the basolateral and accessory basal nuclei. The central nucleus is reciprocally connected to its target structure by means of two major efferent projections: the *stria terminalis* and the *ventral amygdalofugal pathway* (see Figure 50-4B). As one might expect from its dual role, the output of the amygdala influences both the autonomic and cognitive components of emotion. The stria terminalis projects to the hypothalamus as well as to the bed nucleus of the stria terminalis and the nucleus accumbens. The ventral amygdalofugal pathway projects to the brain stem, the dorsal medial nucleus of the thalamus, and the rostral cingulate gyrus of the cortex and the orbitofrontal cortex.

Electrical stimulation of the central nucleus produces increases in heart rate, blood pressure, and respiration via its two output pathways to the lateral hypothalamic and brain stem regions (Figure 50-9). Conversely, lesions of this nucleus block these autonomic changes. The central nucleus also projects directly and indirectly (via the bed nucleus of the stria terminalis) to the paraventricular nucleus of the hypothalamus, which may be important in mediating neuroendocrine responses to fearful and stressful stimuli.

The central nucleus also plays an important role in arousal and the conscious perception of emotion. It does this by means of its projections to the association areas of the cortex, especially the rostral cingulate gyrus and the orbitofrontal cortex. Projections from the central nucleus are thought to mediate these aspects of arousal, not only by direct projections to various nuclei (Figure 50-9) but also through indirect projections to the nucleus basalis.

In mice and other animals β-adrenergic mechanisms in the limbic system are known to be involved in the storage of emotional events. Lawrence Cahill, James McGaugh, and co-workers investigated the effect of propranolol, a β-adrenergic receptor blocker, on the

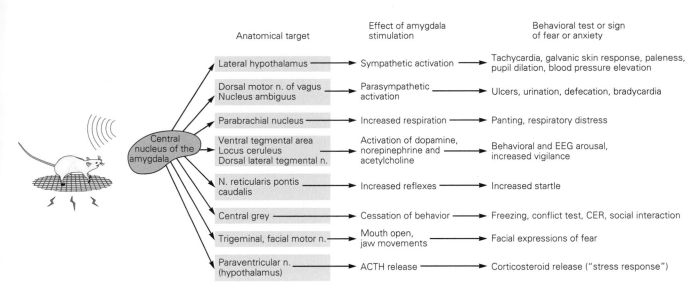

Figure 50-9 The direct connections between the central nucleus of the amygdala and a variety of hypothalamic and brain stem areas that may be involved in different animal tests of fear and anxiety. ACTH = adrenocorticotropin; CER = conditioned emotional response; EEG = electroencephalographic; N = nucleus. (From Davis 1992.)

long-term memory of an emotionally arousing short story or a closely matched, but more emotionally neutral, story. The β-adrenergic blocker selectively impaired the memory for the emotional story, suggesting that nonspecific effects of the drug on arousal or attention could not account for the result. Furthermore, the drug did not block the subjects' initial emotional reaction to the story when it was first presented, but selectively blocked the subjects' memory of it.

The Frontal, Cingulate, and Parahippocampal Cortices Are Involved in Emotion

Electrical stimulation of the orbitofrontal cortex produces many autonomic responses (increases in arterial blood pressure, dilation of the pupils, salivation, and inhibition of gastrointestinal contractions), suggesting that this area is involved in generalized arousal. Lesions of the orbitofrontal cortex reduce the normal aggressiveness and emotional responsiveness of primates, and lesioned animals sometimes fail to show anger when they do not receive expected rewards in a training task. Lesions that include the anterior cingulate cortex also reduce chronic intractable pain, suggesting still another effect of the limbic cortex on emotional behavior.

In 1935 John Fulton and Carlyle Jacobsen first reported that removing the frontal cortex (*lobotomy*) had a calming effect in chimpanzees. Within a few months of Fulton and Jacobsen's report, Egas Moniz, a Portuguese neuropsychiatrist, performed the first prefrontal lobotomy in humans. In an attempt to treat the emotional impairment that often accompanies severe mental illness, Moniz cut the limbic association connections, thereby isolating the orbital frontal cortex.

The early results of frontal lobotomy appeared favorable; many patients seemed less anxious. However, later, more controlled studies led to abandonment of this procedure, in part because lobotomy was associated with a high incidence of complications, including the development of epilepsy and abnormal personality changes, such as a lack of inhibition or a lack of initiative and drive. In addition, the advent of effective psychotherapeutic drugs made radical surgical intervention unnecessary.

The reciprocal connections between the amygdala and the neocortex could permit learning and experience to be incorporated into the cognitive aspects of emotion. Cortical mechanisms provide a means by which memory and imagination, not just external stimuli, can evoke emotional feelings and they enable us to use emotional information generally in cognitive processing. Cortical structures also provide the means by which conscious thought can suppress reflex emotional responses. Once we know that a "bear" is only a shadow that looks like a bear, the fear subsides. The ventromedial frontal cortex is thought to provide one source of cognitive control of emotional responses, but we still understand relatively little of the role of the forebrain in complex feeling states.

Lesions to the ventral sector of the frontal lobe result in disinhibition of inappropriate behavior in social situations. This lack of restraint has frequently been noted in patients after psychosurgery to the frontal lobes. It was a prominent behavioral feature in the historical case of Phineas Gage, who survived a traumatic lesion to the anterior part of his brain when a metal bolt was blown through his skull in a mining accident. Gage made a remarkable recovery from this horrendous accident, but he was a changed person. He could no longer plan for the future, conduct himself according to the social rules he had followed previously, or decide on a course of action that would be most advantageous to his survival. At his death more than a decade later no autopsy was performed, but fortunately his skull, with the bolt hole, was kept in a museum. Medical detective work by Hannah Damasio using modern skull measurements led to the conclusion that the bolt almost certainly destroyed the ventromedial aspect of his frontal lobe (See Figure 19–2C).

Rigorous neuropsychological tests have been used on patients with ventromedial frontal lobe damage to evaluate the influence of affective information on behavior. One such test is a "gambling experiment" in which a player sits in front of four decks of cards, labeled A, B, C, and D. The player is given a loan of $2000 (play money looking like the real thing) and is told that the game is about losing as little as possible and trying to make more money. Play consists of turning one card at a time from any of the four decks until the experimenter says "stop." The player is told that turning every card results in earning more money, but occasionally a card will be turned that results in paying back money to the experimenter. No information is given about the size of the gains or losses or about the cards to be found in the different decks. Only when a card is turned does the player learn its value. No tally of gains and losses is available except in the subject's mind. The undisclosed rules are that A and B cards yield $100 but occasionally require the subject to repay $1250. Cards C and D yield $50 but only require repayment of small sums (less than $100).

Normal people, lured by high rewards, initially play decks A and B, but gradually, usually within 30 of the designated 100 trials of the game, they switch to a preference for decks C and D. Thus normal subjects appear to develop a hunch that decks A and B are more "dangerous" than the others. Patients with frontal lesions behave in quite a different way. After an early general sampling of the card decks they prefer cards from decks A and B and, despite the high penalties and the need to borrow from the bank, they hold to this prefer-

ence throughout the test. They clearly know which decks are riskier but they continue to behave in this inappropriate way even when retested at a later time.

In patients with either amygdala or frontal lobe damage there is a clear dissociation between autonomic responses to emotive stimuli and cognitive evaluation of those stimuli. Lesions of the amygdala do not impair autonomic responses to aversive stimuli, but they do prevent the subject from learning to associate a particular stimulus with a negative consequence. Patients with frontal lesions have normal galvanomic skin responses (sweating measured electrically) to "startle" stimuli, such as unexpected loud noises or bright lights, indicating a normal autonomic response mechanism. However, when patients with frontal lobe lesions were presented with disturbing images interspersed among a series of slides showing bland scenes or abstract patterns, they failed to show the expected autonomic responses to these emotionally charged stimuli. These patients sometimes commented that they knew they should have been disturbed by certain pictures but found themselves unmoved.

Two clinical syndromes dramatically illustrate the dissociation between conscious processing of visual information and unconscious processing of emotional information associated with an image. Patients with prosopagnosia (Chapter 25) cannot consciously identify faces, even those of familiar associates and relatives. Yet they exhibit autonomic responses (eg, skin conductance change) to familiar faces but not to unfamiliar faces. Conversely, patients who suffer from the rare Capgras syndrome can readily recognize familiar faces but apparently do not have emotional responses to them. Remarkably, these patients report that the face shown to them is that of an imposter who looks identical to the person they know.

The Hippocampus Has Only an Indirect Role in Emotion

Early theories of the neural control of emotional states accorded the hippocampus a major role in coordinating the activity of the hypothalamus and cerebral cortex (see Figure 50–5). Subsequent experimental studies on both monkeys and humans showed that the coordinating role is carried out by the amygdala rather than the hippocampus. The hippocampal system is involved in explicit (declarative) memory (Chapter 62).

The distinctive roles of the amygdala and the hippocampus were clearly demonstrated in a study of three patients with selective damage to the amygdala, the hippocampus, or both. These patients were shown monochromatic slides (green, blue, yellow, or red) and their autonomic responses were measured. After some of the colored slides a frightening loud horn was sounded. Patients with the amygdala lesion did not become conditioned to the associated color. Yet when asked how many different colors they observed and how many were followed by the loud horn, the patients responded correctly and had clearly acquired explicit knowledge about the testing situation. Patients with hippocampal damage, on the other hand, became conditioned to colors associated with the loud horn but did not learn how many colors were associated with the sound of the loud horn. Patients with lesions in both the amygdala and hippocampus showed neither autonomic conditioning nor knowledge of the testing situation.

An Overall View

The emotional experiences that we perceive as fear, anger, pleasure, and contentment reflect an interplay between higher brain centers and subcortical regions such as the hypothalamus and amygdala. This is illustrated dramatically in patients in whom the prefrontal cortex or the cingulate gyrus has been removed. These patients are no longer bothered by pain. They experience pain as a sensation and exhibit appropriate autonomic reactions, but the sensation is not felt as a powerful unpleasant experience.

Thus, noxious and pleasurable stimuli have dual effects. First, they trigger autonomic and endocrine responses, integrated by subcortical structures, that immediately alter internal states, thereby preparing the organism for attack, flight, sex, or other adaptive behaviors. These behaviors are relatively simple to execute and require no conscious control. Thereafter a second set of mechanisms come into play, involving the cerebral cortex. Cortical processing of emotionally significant stimuli results in a conscious experience of emotion (feeling) as well as in signals to lower centers that can suppress or enhance the somatic manifestations of emotions.

Many aspects of our primary emotional responses are learned, and during this learning visceral feedback probably has an important role. But with experience we depend increasingly on cognition to evaluate the significance of our environment, and visceral sensations probably play a less important role. The anatomical connections of the amygdala with the temporal (cingulate gyrus) and frontal (prefrontal) association cortices provide the means by which visceral sensations trigger a rich assortment of associations and narratives, the cognitive interpretation of emotional states.

Nevertheless, emotional states may contribute to conscious feeling in a less direct way than originally proposed by William James. Antonio Damasio has suggested that when we think about the potential consequences of a behavior, the memory of our emotional state (visceral experiences) in similar circumstances may provide useful information for evaluating the behavior. The memory may activate ascending noradrenergic and cholinergic projections of the brain stem and basal forebrain, thereby activating the cortex and replicating the conscious sensations of the remembered emotional state, bypassing the feedback of the autonomic nervous system. This may be the basis of what we refer to as "gut feelings."

As discussed in the next chapter, emotions and feelings are closely linked to motivated behaviors such as feeding, drinking, and sexual behaviors. Appropriately motivated animals seek particular stimuli in the environment: food, water, warmth, and novelty. These stimuli are related to survival and consequently are particularly meaningful. Almost by definition they evoke pleasure and pain and generate emotional responses.

Susan Iversen
Irving Kupfermann
Eric R. Kandel

Selected Readings

Cannon WB. 1927. The James-Lange theory of emotions: a critical examination and an alternative theory. Am J Psychol 39:106–124.

Cannon WB. 1932. *The Wisdom of the Body.* New York: Norton.

Damasio AR. 1994. *Descarte's Error: Emotion, Reason and the Human Brain.* New York: Grosset-Putnam.

Damasio AR. 1999. *The Feeling of What Happened.* New York: Harcourt Brace.

Davis M. 1992. The role of the amygdala in fear and anxiety. Annu Rev Neurosci 15:353–375.

Fridlund AJ. 1994. *Human Facial Expression: An Evolutionary View.* New York: Academic.

Gallagher M, Holland PC. 1992. Understanding the function of the central nucleus: Is simple conditioning enough? In: J Aggleton (ed). *The Amygdala: Neurobiological Aspects of Emotion, Memory, and Mental Dysfunction*, pp. 307–321. New York: Wiley-Liss.

Hess WR. 1954. *Diencephalon: Autonomic and Extrapyramidal Functions.* New York: Grune & Stratton.

LeDoux JE. 1996. *The Emotional Brain.* New York: Simon & Schuster.

Loewy AD, Spyer KM (eds). 1990. *Central Regulation of Autonomic Functions.* New York: Oxford Univ. Press.

Papez JW. 1937. A proposed mechanism of emotion. Arch Neurol Psychia 38:725–743.

Ranson SW. 1934. The hypothalamus: its significance for visceral innervation and emotional expression. Trans Coll Physicians Phila Ser 4 2:222–242.

Schachter S. 1964. The interaction of cognitive and physiological determinants of emotional state. In: L Berkowitz (ed). *Advances in Experimental Social Psychology,* 1:49–80. New York: Academic.

Zagonic RB. 1980. Feeling and thinking: preferences need no inferences. Am Psychol 35:151–175.

References

Adolphs R, Tranel D, Damasio H, Damasio AR. 1995. Fear and the human amygdala. J Neurosci 15:5879–5891.

Adolphs R, Tranel D, Damasio H, Damasio AR. 1994. Impaired recognition of emotion in facial expression following bilateral damage to the human amygdala. Nature 372:669–672.

Aggleton JP. 1993. The contribution of the amygdala to normal and abnormal emotional states. Trends Neurosci 16:328–333.

Arnold MB. 1960. *Emotion and Personality.* New York: Columbia University Press.

Bandler R, Shipley MT. 1994. Columnar organisation in the midbrain periaqueductal gray: modules for emotional expression. Trends Neurosci 17:379–389.

Bard P. 1928. A diencephalic mechanism for the expression of rage with special reference to the sympathetic nervous system. Am J Physiol 84:490–515.

Bard P, Mountcastle VB. 1948. Some forebrain mechanisms involved in expression of rage with special reference to suppression of angry behavior. Res Publ Assoc Res Nerv Ment Dis 27:362–404.

Bechara A, Tranel D, Damasio H, Damasio A. 1994. Impaired recognition of emotion in facial expressions following bilateral damage to the human amygdala. Nature 372:669–672.

Bernard C. 1878–1879. *Leçons sur les Phénomènes de la vie Communs aux Animaux et aux Végétaux,* Vols. 1, 2. Paris: Baillière.

Breiter HC, Etcoff NO, Whalen PJ, Kennedy WA, Rauch SL, Buckner RL, Strauss MM, Hyman SE, Rosen BR. 1996. Response and habituation of the human amygdala during visual processing of facial expression. Neuron 17:875–887.

Broca P. 1878. Anatomie comparée de circonvolutions cérébrales. Le grand lobe limbique et al scissure limbique dans la série des mammiféres. Rev Anthropol 1:385–498.

Cahill L, Prins B, Weber M, McGaugh JL. 1994. β-Adrenergic activation and memory for emotional events. Nature 371:702–704.

Cannon WB, Britton SW. 1925. Pseudoaffective meduliadrenal secretion. Am J Physiol 72:283–294.

Damasio AR. 1995. Toward a neurobiology of emotion and feeling: operational concepts and hypotheses. Neuroscientist 1:19–25.

Damasio H, Grabowski T, Frank R, Glaburda AM, Damasio AR. 1994. The return of Phineas Gage: the skull of a famous patient yields clues about the brain. Science 264:1102–1105.

Darwin C. 1872. *The Expression of the Emotions in Man and Animals.* London: John Murray. (Repr 1998. Elkman P, ed. New York: Oxford Univ. Press.)

Davidson RJ, Sutton SK. 1995. Affective neuroscience: the emergence of a discipline. Curr Opin Neurobiol 5:217–224.

Davis M. 1992. The role of the amygdala in fear and anxiety. Ann Rev Neurosci 15:353–375.

Ekman P. 1992. Facial expressions of emotion: new findings, new questions. Psychol Sci 3:34–38.

Ekman P, Levernson RW, Friesers WV. 1983. Autonomic nervous system activity distinguishes among emotions. Science 221:1208–1210.

Gallagher M, Chiba AA. 1996. The amygdala and emotion. Curr Opin Neurobiol 6:221–227.

Giros B, Jaber M, Jones SR, Wightman RM, Caron MG. 1996. Hyperlocomotion and indifference to cocaine and amphetamine in mice lacking the dopamine transporter. Nature 379:606–612.

Hess WR. 1954. *Diencephalon: Autonomic and Extrapyramidal Functions.* New York: Grune & Stratton.

Hirstein W, Ramachandran VS. 1997. Capgras syndrome: a novel probe for understanding the neural representation of the identity and familiarity of persons. Proc R Soc Lond B Biol Sci 264:437–444.

Hohmann GW. 1966. Some effects of spinal cord lesions on experienced emotional feelings. Psychophysiology 3:143–156.

Iversen SD, Iversen LL. 1981. *Behavioural Pharmacology.* New York: Oxford Univ. Press.

Jacobsen CF. 1936. Studies of cerebral function in primates: I. The functions of the frontal association areas in monkeys. Comp Psychol Monogr 13:1–60.

James W. 1884. What is an emotion? Mind 9:188–205. Reprinted in: M Arnold. 1968. *The Nature of Emotion.* Baltimore: Penguin.

Klüver H, Bucy PC. 1939. Preliminary analysis of functions of the temporal lobes in monkeys. Arch Neurol Psych 42:979–1000.

Lange CG. 1985. *Om Sindsbevaegelser et Psyko. Fysiolog. Studie.* Copenhagen: Kromar.

LeDoux JE. 1992. Brain mechanisms of emotion and emotional learning. Curr Biol 2:191–197.

LeDoux JE. 1994. Emotion, memory and the brain. Sci Am 270:50–57.

MacLean PD. 1955. The limbic system ("visceral brain") and emotional behavior. Arch Neurol Psych 73:130–134.

Moniz E. 1936. *Tentatives Opératoires dans le Traitement de Certaines Psychoses.* Paris: Masson.

Morris JS, Frilt CD, Perrett DI, Rowland D, Yong AN, Calder AJ, Dolan RJ. 1996. A different neural response in the human amygdala is fearful and happy facial expressions. Nature 383:812–815.

Nieuwenhuys R, Voogd J, van Huijzen Chr. 1988. *The Human Central Nervous System: A Synopsis and Atlas,* 3rd ed.

Berlin: Springer-Verlag.

Papez JW. 1937. A proposed mechanism of emotion. Arch Neurol Psych 38:725–743.

Phillips RG, Le Doux JE. 1995. Lesions of the fornix but not the entorhinal or perirhinal cortex interfere with contextual fear conditioning. J Neurosci 15:5308–5315.

Ranson SW. 1934. The hypothalamus: its significance for visceral innervation and emotional expression. Trans Coll Physicians Phila Ser 4 2:222–242.

Rolls ET, Hornak J, Wade D, McGrath JMc. 1994. Emotion-related learning in patients with social and emotional changes associated with frontal lobe damage. J Neurol Neurosurg Psychiatry 57:1518–1524.

Woodworth WS, Sherrington CS. 1904. A pseudaffective reflex and its spinal path. J Physiol (Lond) 31:234–243.

Young AW, Aggleton JP, Hanley JR. 1995. Face processing impairments after amygdalectomy. Brain 118:15–24.

51

Motivational and Addictive States

S O FAR IN THIS BOOK OUR discussion of the neural control of behavior has focused on how the brain translates external sensory information about events in the environment into coherent perceptions and motor action. In the final two parts of the book we examine how development and learning profoundly shape the brain's ability to do this. These parts of the book are to a large degree concerned with the cognitive aspects of behavior—what a person knows about the outside world. However, behavior also has noncognitive aspects that reflect not what the individual knows but what he or she needs or wants. Here we are concerned with how individuals respond to *internal* rather than external stimuli. This is the domain of motivation.

Motivation is a catch-all term that refers to a variety of neuronal and physiological factors that initiate, sustain, and direct behavior. These internal factors are thought to explain, in part, variation in the behavior of an individual over time. As discussed earlier in this book, the behaviorists who dominated the study of behavior in the first half of this century largely ignored internal factors in their attempts to explain behavior. With the rise of cognitive psychology a few decades ago the behaviorist paradigm has receded and motivation, with all of its complexity, has become the subject of serious scientific study once again.

The biological study of motivation has until quite recently been confined to studies of simple physiological or homeostatic instances of motivation called drive states. For this reason our discussion here focuses primarily on drive states, which are the outcome of homeostatic processes related to hunger, thirst, and temperature regulation. Drive states are characterized by tension and discomfort due to a physiological need followed by relief when the need is satisfied.

It is important to recognize, however, that drive states are merely one subtype, perhaps the simplest examples, of the motivational states that direct behavior. In general, motivational states may be broadly classified into two types: (1) elementary drive states and more complex physiological regulatory forces brought into play by alterations in internal physical conditions such as hunger, thirst, and temperature, and (2) personal or social aspirations acquired by experience. Freud and contemporary cognitive psychologists have suggested that both forms, but especially personal and social aspirations, represent a complex interplay between physiological and social forces, and between conscious and unconscious mental processes. The neurobiological study of the second type of motivational states is in its infancy.

The issues that surround drive states relate to survival. Activities that enhance immediate survival, such as eating or drinking, or those that ensure long-term survival, such as sexual behavior or caring for offspring, are pleasurable and there is a great natural urge to repeat these behaviors. Drive states steer behavior toward specific positive goals and away from negative ones. In addition, drive states require organization of individual behaviors into a goal-oriented sequence. Attainment of the goal decreases the intensity of the drive state and thus the motivated behavior ceases. A hungry cat is ever alert for the occasional mouse, ready to pounce when it comes into sight. Once satiated, the cat will not pounce again for some time. Finally, drive states have general effects; they increase our general level of arousal and thereby enhance our ability to act.

Drive states therefore serve three functions: they direct behavior toward or away from a specific goal; they organize individual behaviors into a coherent, goal-oriented sequence; and they increase general alertness, energizing the individual to act.

The drive states that neurobiologists have studied most effectively are those related to temperature regulation, hunger, and thirst. Until recently, these drive states were inferred from behavior alone. But as we learn more about the physiological correlates of drive states, we rely less on traditional psychological concepts of motivation and more on concepts derived from servo-control models applied to living organisms. Admittedly, such an approach reduces drive states to a complex homeostatic reflex that is responsive to multiple stimuli. Some of these stimuli are internal in response to tissue deficits; others are external (eg, the sight or smell of food) and are regulated by excitatory and inhibitory systems. Since regulation of internal states involves the autonomic nervous system and the endocrine system, we shall consider the relationship of motivational states to autonomic and neuroendocrine responses.

We first examine how servo-control models have made the study of drive states amenable to biological experimentation. We then examine the regulation of these simple motivational states by factors other than tissue deficits, such as circadian rhythms, ecological constraints, and pleasure. Finally, we discuss the neural systems of the brain concerned with reward or reinforcement, an important component of motivation. These neural systems have been well delineated. Most addictive drugs, such as nicotine, alcohol, opiates, and cocaine, produce their actions by acting on or co-opting the same neural pathways that mediate positively motivated behaviors essential for survival.

Drive States Are Simple Cases of Motivational States That Can Be Modeled as Servo-Control Systems

Drive states can be understood by analogy with control systems, or *servomechanisms*, that regulate machines. While specific physiological servomechanisms have not yet been demonstrated directly, the servomechanism model permits us to organize our thinking about the complex operation of homeostasis, and makes it possible to define experimentally the physiological control of homeostasis.

This approach has been most successfully applied to temperature regulation. Because body temperature can be readily measured, the mechanism regulating temperature has been studied by examining the relationship between the internal stimulus (temperature) and various external stimuli. This control system approach has been less successful when applied to more complex regulatory behaviors, such as feeding, drinking, and sex, in which the relevant internal stimuli are difficult to identify and measure. Nevertheless, at present, the control systems model is probably the best approach to analyzing even these more complex internal states.

Servomechanisms maintain a *controlled variable* within a certain range. One way of regulating the controlled variable is to measure it by means of a feedback detector and compare the measured value with a desired value, or *set point*. The comparison is accomplished by an error detector, or *integrator*, that generates an *error signal* when the value of the controlled variable does not match the set point. The error signal then drives controlling elements that adjust the controlled system in the desired direction. The error signal is controlled not only by internal feedback stimuli but also by external stimuli. All examples of physiological control seem to involve both inhibitory and excitatory effects, which function together to adjust the control system (Figure 51-1).

The control system used to heat a home illustrates these principles. The furnace system is the controlling

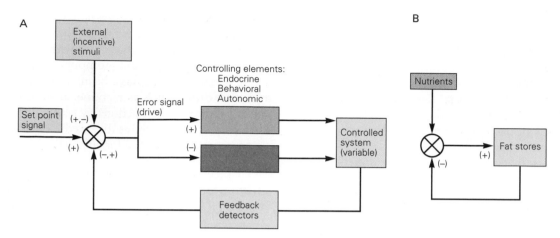

Figure 51-1 Homeostatic processes can be analyzed in terms of control systems.

A. A control system regulates a controlled variable. When a feedback signal indicates the controlled variable is below or above the set point an error signal is generated. This signal turns on (or facilitates) appropriate behaviors and physiological responses, and turns off (or suppresses) incompatible responses. An error signal also can be generated by external (incentive) stimuli.

B. A negative feedback system without a set point controls fat stores. (Based on data of DiGirolamo and Rudman 1968.)

element. The room temperature is the controlled variable. The home thermostat is the error detector. The setting on the thermostat is the set point. Finally, the output of the thermostat is the error signal that turns the control element on or off.

Temperature Regulation Involves Integration of Autonomic, Endocrine, and Skeletomotor Responses

Temperature regulation nicely fits the model of a control system. Normal body temperature is the set point in the system of temperature regulation. The integrator and many controlling elements for temperature regulation appear to be located in the hypothalamus. Because temperature regulation requires integrated autonomic, endocrine, and skeletomotor responses, the anatomical connections of the hypothalamus make this structure well suited for this task. The feedback detectors collect information about body temperature from two main sources: peripheral temperature receptors located throughout the body (in the skin, spinal cord, and viscera) and central receptors located mainly in the hypothalamus. The detectors of temperature, both low and high, are located only in the anterior hypothalamus. The hypothalamic receptors are probably neurons whose firing rate is highly dependent on local temperature, which in turn is importantly affected by the temperature of the blood.

Although the anterior hypothalamic area is involved in temperature sensing, control of body temperature appears to be regulated by separate regions of the hypothalamus. The anterior hypothalamus mediates decreases and the posterior hypothalamus (preoptic area) mediates increases in body temperature. Thus, electrical stimulation of the anterior hypothalamus causes dilation of blood vessels in the skin, panting, and a suppression of shivering, responses that decrease body temperature. In contrast, electrical stimulation of the posterior hypothalamus produces an opposing set of responses that generate or conserve heat (Figure 51-2). As with fear responses, which are evoked by electrical stimulation of the hypothalamus (Chapter 50), temperature regulatory responses evoked by electrical stimulation also include appropriate nonvoluntary responses involving the skeletomotor system. For example, stimulation of the anterior hypothalamus (preoptic area) produces panting, while stimulation of the posterior hypothalamus produces shivering.

Ablation experiments corroborate the critical role of the hypothalamus in regulating temperature. Lesions of the anterior hypothalamus cause chronic hyperthermia and eliminate the major responses that normally dissipate excess heat. Lesions in the posterior hypothalamus have relatively little effect if the animal is kept at room temperature (approximately 22°C). If the animal is exposed to cold, however, it quickly becomes hypothermic because the homeostatic mechanisms fail to generate and conserve heat.

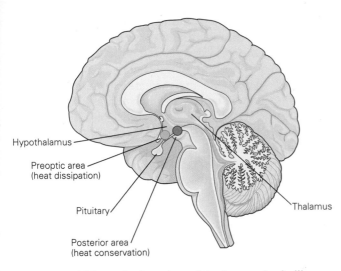

Figure 51-2 This sagittal section of the human brain illustrates the hypothalamic regions concerned with heat conservation and heat dissipation.

Labels on figure:
Hypothalamus
Preoptic area (heat dissipation)
Pituitary
Posterior area (heat conservation)
Thalamus

The hypothalamus also controls endocrine responses to temperature challenges. Thus, long-term exposure to cold can enhance the release of thyroxine, which increases body heat by increasing tissue metabolism. In addition to driving appropriate autonomic, endocrine, and nonvoluntary skeletal responses, the error signal of the temperature control system can also drive voluntary behaviors that minimize the error signal. For example, a rat can be taught to press a button to receive puffs of cool air in a hot environment. After training, when the chamber is at normal room temperature, the rat will not press the button for cool air. If the anterior hypothalamus is locally warmed by perfusing it with warm water through a hollow probe, the rat will run to the cool-air button and press it repeatedly.

Hypothalamic integration of peripheral and central inputs can be demonstrated by heating the environment (and thereby the skin of the animal) and concurrently cooling or heating the hypothalamus. When both the environment and hypothalamus are heated, the rat presses the cool-air button faster than when either one is heated alone. However, even in a hot environment the pressing of the button for cool air can be suppressed completely by cooling the hypothalamus (Figure 51-3).

Recordings from neurons in the preoptic area and the anterior hypothalamus support the idea that the hypothalamus integrates peripheral and central information relevant to temperature regulation. Neurons in this region, called *warm-sensitive neurons*, increase their firing when the local hypothalamic tissue is warmed. Other neurons, called *cold-sensitive neurons*, respond to local cooling. The warm-sensitive neurons, in addition to

responding to local warming of the brain, are usually excited by warming the skin or spinal cord and are inhibited by cooling the skin or spinal cord. The cold-sensitive neurons exhibit the opposite behavior. Thus, these neurons could integrate the thermal information from peripheral receptors with that from neurons within the brain. Furthermore, many temperature-sensitive neurons in the hypothalamus also respond to nonthermal stimuli, such as osmolarity, glucose, sex steroids, and blood pressure.

In humans the set point of the temperature control system is approximately 98.6°F (37°C), although it normally varies somewhat diurnally, decreasing to a minimum during sleep. The set point can be altered by pathological states, for example by the action of pyrogens, which induce fever. Systemic pyrogens, such as the macrophage product interleukin-1, enter the brain at regions in which the blood-brain barrier is incomplete, such as the preoptic area, and act there to increase the set point. The body temperature then rises until the new set point is reached.

When this occurs a part of the brain known as the antipyretic area is activated and limits the magnitude of the fever. The *antipyretic area* includes the septal nuclei,

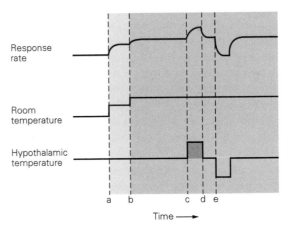

Labels on figure:
Response rate
Room temperature
Hypothalamic temperature
a b   c d e
Time ⟶

Figure 51-3 Peripheral and central information on temperature is summated in the hypothalamus. Changes in either room temperature or local hypothalamic temperature alter the response rate of rats trained to press a button to receive a brief burst of cool air. When the room temperature is increased, thus presumably increasing skin temperature, the response rate increases roughly in proportion to the temperature increase (points **a** and **b**). If the temperature of the hypothalamus is also increased (by perfusing warm water through a hollow probe), the response rate reflects a summation of information on skin temperature and hypothalamic temperature (points **c** and **d**). If the skin temperature remains high enough but the hypothalamus is cooled, the response rate decreases or is suppressed altogether (point **e**). (From data of Corbit 1973 and Satinoff 1964.)

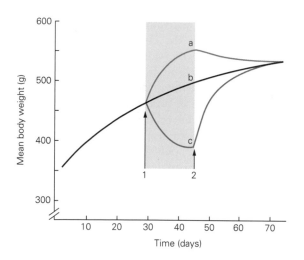

Figure 51-4 Animals tend to adjust their food intake to achieve a normal body weight. The plots show a schematized growth curve for a group of rats. At **arrow 1** one-third of the animals were maintained on their normal diet (**curve b**), one-third were force-fed (**curve a**), and one-third were placed on a restricted diet (**curve c**). At **arrow 2** all rats were placed on a normal (ad libitum) diet. The force-fed animals lost weight and the starved animals gained weight until the mean weight of the two groups approached that of the normal growth curve (**b**). (Adapted from Keesey et al. 1976.)

which are located anterior to the hypothalamic preoptic areas, near the anterior commissure. The antipyretic area is innervated by neurons that use the peptide vasopressin as transmitter. Injection of vasopressin into the septal area counteracts fever in a manner similar to that of antipyretic drugs, such as aspirin and indomethacin, suggesting that some of the effects of these drugs are mediated by the central release of vasopressin. The antipyretic action of aspirin and indomethacin is blocked by injection into the septal nuclei of a vasopressin antagonist. In fact, convulsions brought on by high fevers may in part be evoked by vasopressin released in the brain as part of the antipyretic response.

The control of body temperature is a clear example of the integrative action of the hypothalamus in regulating autonomic, endocrine, and drive-state control. It illustrates how the hypothalamus operates both directly on the internal environment and indirectly, by providing information about the internal environment to higher neural systems.

Feeding Behavior Is Regulated by a Variety of Mechanisms

Like temperature regulation, feeding behavior may also be analyzed as a control system, although at every level

of analysis the understanding of feeding is less complete. One reason for thinking that feeding behavior is subject to a control system is that body weight seems to be regulated by a set point. Humans often maintain the same body weight for many years. Since even a small increase or decrease of daily caloric intake could eventually result in a substantial weight change, the body must be governed by feedback signals that control nutrient intake and metabolism.

Control of nutrient intake is seen most clearly in animals in which body weight is altered from the set point by food deprivation or force-feeding. In both instances the animal will adjust its subsequent food intake (either up or down) until it regains a weight appropriate for its age (Figure 51-4). Animals are thus said to *defend* their body weight against perturbations.

Whereas body temperature is remarkably similar from one individual to another, body weight varies greatly. Furthermore, the apparent set point of an individual can vary with stress, palatability of the food, exercise, and many other environmental and genetic factors. One possible explanation for this difference between regulation of temperature and body weight is that the set point for body weight can itself be changed by a variety of factors. Another possibility is that body weight is regulated by a control system that has no formal set-point mechanism but which nevertheless functions as if there were a set point (Figure 51-1B).

Dual Controlling Elements in the Hypothalamus Contribute to the Control of Food Intake

Food intake is thought to be under the control of two regions in the hypothalamus: a ventromedial region and a lateral region. In 1942 Albert W. Hetherington and Stephen Walter Ranson discovered that destruction of the ventromedial nuclei of the hypothalamus produces overeating (*hyperphagia*) and severe obesity. In contrast, bilateral lesions of the lateral hypothalamus produce severe neglect of eating (*aphagia*) so that the animal dies unless force-fed. Electrical stimulation produces the opposite effects of lesions. Whereas stimulation of the ventromedial region suppresses feeding, stimulation of the lateral hypothalamus elicits feeding.

These observations were originally interpreted to mean that the lateral hypothalamus contains a *feeding center* and the medial hypothalamus a *satiety center.* This conclusion was reinforced by studies showing that chemical stimulation of these parts of the hypothalamus can also alter feeding behavior. This conceptually attractive conclusion proved faulty, however, as it became clear that the brain is not organized into discrete centers that by themselves control specific functions. Rather, as with perception and action, the neural circuits mediating homeostatic functions such as feeding are distributed among several structures in the brain.

The effects of lateral or medial hypothalamic lesions on feeding are thought to be due in part to dysfunctions that result from damage to other structures. Three factors are particularly important: (1) alteration of sensory information, (2) alteration of set point, and (3) interference with behavioral arousal because of damage to dopaminergic fibers of passage.

First, lateral hypothalamic lesions sometimes result in sensory and motor deficits as a result of the destruction of fibers of the trigeminal system and the dopaminergic fibers of the medial forebrain bundle. The sensory loss can contribute to the loss of feeding as well as to the so-called sensory neglect seen after lateral hypothalamic lesions. Thus, a unilateral lesion of the lateral hypothalamus results in loss of orienting responses to visual, olfactory, and somatic sensory stimuli presented contralateral to the lesion. Similarly, feeding responses to food presented contralaterally are also diminished. It is not clear whether this sensory neglect is due to disruption of sensory systems or to interference with motor systems directing responses contralateral to the lesion.

Altered sensory responses are also seen in animals with lesions in the region of the ventromedial nucleus. These animals have heightened responses to the aversive or attractive properties of food and other stimuli. On a normal diet they eat more than do animals without lesions, but if the food is adulterated with a bitter substance, they eat less than normal animals. Since the reduction in eating is similar to that seen in normal animals made obese by force-feeding, the enhanced sensory response to food of animals with ventromedial hypothalamic lesions is partly a consequence rather than a cause of the obesity. This is supported by the finding that some obese humans with no evidence of damage to the region of the ventromedial hypothalamus are also unusually responsive to the taste of food.

Second, hypothalamic lesions may alter the set point for regulating body weight. Rats that were starved to reduce their weight before a small lesion was made in the lateral hypothalamus ate more than normal amounts and gained weight when they resumed eating, whereas the controls (nonstarved) lost weight (Figure 51–5). The starvation apparently brings the weight of these animals below the set point determined by the lateral lesion. Conversely, animals that were force-fed before *ventromedial* hypothalamic lesions did not overeat, which they would have done if they had not been previously force-fed.

Third, lesions of the lateral hypothalamus can damage dopaminergic fibers that course from the substantia

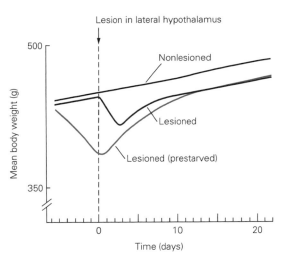

Figure 51-5 The set point for body weight appears to be altered by lesions of the lateral hypothalamus. Three groups of rats were used in this experiment. The control group was maintained on a normal diet. On day 0 the animals of the other two groups received small lesions in the lateral hypothalamus. One of these groups had been maintained on a normal diet; the other group had been starved before the lesion and consequently had lost body weight. After the lesion all animals were given free access to food. The lesioned animals that had not been prestarved initially decreased their food intake and lost body weight, while those that were prestarved rapidly gained weight until they reached the level of the other lesioned animals. (Adapted from Keesey et al. 1976.)

nigra to the striatum via the medial forebrain bundle as well as those that emanate from the ventral tegmental area (the mesolimbic projections) and innervate structures associated with the limbic system (the prefrontal cortex, amygdala, and nucleus accumbens; see Chapter 45). When nigrostriatal dopaminergic fibers are experimentally sectioned bilaterally below or above the level of the hypothalamus or are destroyed by a specific toxin 6-OH dopamine, animals exhibit a hypoarousal state and life-threatening aphagia similar to that observed after lateral hypothalamic lesions.

The loss of dopamine does not account entirely for the lateral hypothalamus syndrome. The physiological profile and recovery of eating patterns are different after lesions of the lateral hypothalamus and depletion of dopamine, demonstrating that both the dopamine system and hypothalamic substrates contribute to the control of feeding.

Lesioning of dopaminergic neurons alone or loss of the neurons of the lateral hypothalamus alone (using the excitotoxins kainic or ibotenic acid) produces less severe behavioral deficits than those seen after the classical lateral hypothalamus lesions. The combined loss of

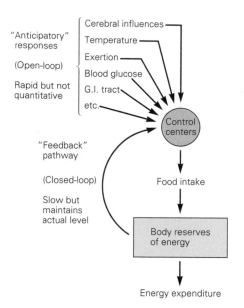

Figure 51-6 Hypothetical model of the mechanisms that regulate energy balance in mammals. (Adapted from Hervey 1969.)

lateral hypothalamic neurons and dopaminergic fibers results in the classical syndrome by impairing both the substrate for monitoring physiological feedback and the neural systems that generate appropriate behavior. In fact, the dopamine agonist apomorphine restores eating and drinking responses to physiological challenges in rats after depletion of dopamine, but not in rats with lateral hypothalamic lesions. Below we shall examine the role of dopamine in food reward and reinforcement more generally when we consider studies of intracranial self-stimulation, the effect of dopamine-blocking drugs on learned behavior to obtain food, and the reinforcing effects of drugs of addiction.

Some of the strongest evidence implicating the hypothalamus in the control of feeding comes from studies showing that a wide spectrum of transmitters produces profound alterations of feeding behavior when injected into the lateral hypothalamus and the area of the paraventricular nuclei. These studies also illustrate that different chemical systems are involved in the control of different classes of nutrients. Application of norepinephrine to the paraventricular nucleus greatly stimulates feeding; but, if given a choice, animals will eat more carbohydrate than protein or fat. In contrast, application of the peptide galanin selectively increases ingestion of fat whereas opiates enhance consumption of protein.

Food Intake Is Controlled by Short-Term and Long-Term Cues

What cues does an organism use to regulate feeding? Two main cues for hunger have been identified: short-term cues that regulate the size of individual meals and long-term cues that regulate overall body weight (Figure 51-6). Short-term cues consist primarily of chemical properties of the food that act in the mouth to stimulate feeding behavior and in the gastrointestinal system and liver to inhibit feeding. The short-term satiety signals impinge on the hypothalamus through visceral afferent pathways, communicating primarily with the lateral hypothalamic regions. The effectiveness of short-term cues is modulated by long-term signals that reflect body weight. As we shall discuss in greater detail below, one such important signal is the peptide leptin, which is secreted from fat storage cells (*adipocytes*). By means of this signal, body weight is kept reasonably constant over a broad range of activity and diet.

Daily energy expenditure is remarkably consistent when expressed as a function of body size (Figure 51-7A). Body weight is also maintained at a set level by self-regulating feedback mechanisms that adjust metabolic rate when the organism drifts away from its characteristic set point (Figure 51-7B). An animal maintained on a reduced-calorie diet eventually needs less food to maintain its weight because its metabolic rate decreases.

Several humoral signals are thought to be important for short-term regulation of feeding behavior. The hypothalamus has glucoreceptors that respond to blood glucose levels. This system probably stimulates feeding behavior (in contrast to autonomic responses to blood glucose) primarily during emergency states in which blood glucose falls drastically. In addition, gut hormones released during a meal may contribute to satiety. Considerable evidence for such a humoral short-term signal comes from studies of the peptide cholecystokinin. Cholecystokinin is released from the duodenum and upper intestine when amino acids and fatty acids are present in the tract. Cholecystokinin released in the gut acts on visceral afferents that affect brain stem and hypothalamic areas, which are themselves sensitive to cholecystokinin. Injection into the ventricles or specifically into the paraventricular nucleus of small quantities of cholecystokinin and several other peptides (including neurotensin, calcitonin, and glucagon) also inhibits feeding. Therefore, cholecystokinin released as a neuropeptide in the brain may also inhibit feeding, independently of its release from the gut.

Cholecystokinin is an example of a hormone or neuromodulator that has independent central and peripheral actions that are functionally related. Other examples include luteinizing hormone–releasing hormone (sexual behavior), adrenocorticotropin (stress and

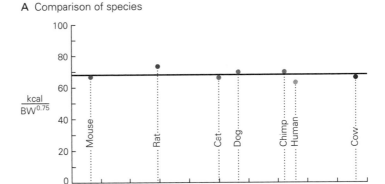

A Comparison of species

$\frac{kcal}{BW^{0.75}}$

Log body weight (kg)

Figure 51-7 Daily energy expenditure (kcal) is relatively constant when expressed per metabolic body size (body weight$^{0.75}$ or BW$^{0.75}$). (Adapted from Keesey 1989, and Kleiber 1947.)

A. Body weight and daily energy expenditure of various species of mammals.

B. Relative constancy of kcal per BW$^{0.75}$ of individual male rats of the same strain and age at the body weight each spontaneously maintains. If rats are forced to increase or decrease their weight they become, respectively, hypermetabolic (**upward-pointed arrow**) or hypometabolic (**downward-pointed arrow**). (Example is for rats normally weighing 410 grams.)

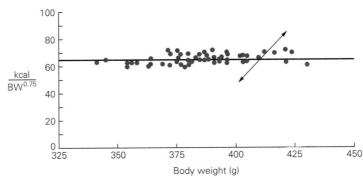

B Comparison of individual male rats

$\frac{kcal}{BW^{0.75}}$

Body weight (g)

avoidance behavior), and angiotensin (responses to hemorrhage). The use of the same chemical signal for related central and peripheral functions is widespread in both vertebrates and invertebrates. Certain invertebrates, such as the sea slug *Aplysia*, have specific serotonergic neurons that both enhance feeding responses (by acting directly on muscles involved in consuming food) and promote arousal (by enhancing the excitability of central motor neurons that innervate these same muscles).

Specific Genes Are Involved in the Control of Food Intake

Selective breeding of mutant mice with chronic disorders of weight control led to the discovery of important genes involved in the long-term regulation of food intake. One of these, is the *ob* gene (Chapter 3). The gene product, leptin, is expressed in fat storage cells and acts as a circulating hormone that enters the brain and informs hypothalamic neurons about the abundance of fat. As a result, feeding behavior, metabolism, and endocrine physiology are coupled to the nutritional state of the organisms. Leptin leads to weight loss both by suppressing appetite and by stimulating metabolic rate. Physiologists have long known of the existence of a

powerful, slow feedback pathway that regulates energy expenditure and controls body fat to within ±1% over a period of years (Figure 51-7). The *ob* gene provides a critical link in this feedback pathway. When functional leptin is absent in homozygous *ob* mutants, obesity and type II (late-onset) diabetes result.

Rats forced to overeat store excess fat, but when offered a normal diet they eat less until the normal weight is regained. Surgical removal of fat mass is followed by increased eating until fat stores are restored. Parabiotic experiments, in which two animals are surgically joined so as to share the same circulatory system, demonstrate the existence of blood-borne factors. Overeating by one joined animal reduces food intake and induces weight loss in the partner. Likewise, when one joined animal becomes obese because of a lesion in the ventromedial hypothalamic nucleus, the other animal reduces its food intake and loses weight, presumably because of enhanced levels of circulating hormones from the obese partner. However, an *ob* mutant animal joined to a normal animal eats less and gains less weight, suggesting that the mutation is associated with a lack of a circulating hormone. Leptin binds to a receptor, so that mutations of the leptin receptor should also result in disturbance of long-term regulation of food intake and fat stores. Indeed, the obesity of mutant *db/db* mice, in which the leptin receptor is defective, is not ameliorated by injection of leptin. In humans, however, the genetic causes of obesity are primarily due to an absence of an appropriate response to leptin, downstream from the leptin receptor, rather than to a deficiency in leptin itself.

How does circulating leptin lead to changes in feeding behavior? There is evidence that leptin produces its action, in part, by regulating the release of neuropeptide Y (NPY). NPY is synthesized by neurons of the arcuate nucleus of the hypothalamus, and these neurons project to other regions of the hypothalamus that control feeding. Release of NPY in the hypothalamus stimulates feeding behavior. Chronic administration of NPY in the brain simulates the phenotype of leptin deficiency and produces hyperphagia, obesity, and inhibition of the production of growth hormone. These findings suggest that leptin acts by inhibiting the actions of NPY. Consistent with this idea, neurons in the arcuate nucleus that express NPY have leptin receptors, and leptin acts on these neurons to inhibit expression of the peptide and its release from the neurons. A critical component of leptin's effect on body weight is its ability to diminish the effects of neurons that secrete NPY and thus decrease the effect of the short-term cues that stimulate feeding. Conversely, low levels of leptin enhance the action of the short-term cues that stimulate feeding.

Drinking Is Regulated by Tissue Osmolality and Vascular Volume

The hypothalamus regulates water balance by its control of hormones, such as antidiuretic hormone. The hypothalamus also regulates aspects of drinking behavior. Unlike feeding, where intake is critical, the amount of water taken in is relatively unimportant as long as the minimum requirement is met. Within broad limits, excess intake is readily eliminated by the kidney. Nevertheless, a set point, or ideal amount of water intake, appears to exist, since too much or too little drinking represents inefficient behavior. If an animal takes in too little liquid at one time, it must soon interrupt other activities and resume its liquid intake to avoid underhydration. Likewise, drinking a large amount at one time results in unneeded time spent drinking as well as urinating to eliminate the excess fluid.

Drinking is controlled by two main variables: tissue osmolality and vascular (fluid) volume. This has led Alan Epstein and James Fitzsimons to propose that the inputs controlling thirst arise when either physiological variables are depleted (*double depletion hypothesis*). Signals related to the variables reach mechanisms in the

brain that control drinking either through afferent fibers from peripheral receptors or by humoral actions on receptors in the brain itself. These inputs control the physiological mechanisms of water conservation in such a way that fluid intake is coordinated with the control of fluid loss so as to maintain water balance.

Thus, the hypothalamus integrates hormonal and osmotic cues sensing cell volume and the state of the extracellular space. The volume of water in the intracellular compartment is normally approximately double that of the extracellular space. This delicate balance is determined by the osmotic equilibrium between the compartments, which in turn is determined by extracellular sodium. The control of sodium is therefore a key element in the homeostatic mechanism regulating thirst. The two drives, thirst and salt appetite, appear to be handled by separate but interrelated mechanisms. Drinking also can be controlled by dryness of the tongue. Hyperthermia, detected at least in part by thermosensitive neurons in the anterior hypothalamus, may also contribute to thirst.

The feedback signals for water regulation derive from many sources. Osmotic stimuli can act directly on osmoreceptor cells (or receptors that sense the level of Na^+), probably neurons, in the hypothalamus. The feedback signals for vascular volume are located in the low-pressure side of the circulation—the right atrium and adjacent walls of the great veins—and large volume changes may also affect arterial baroreceptors in the aortic arch and carotid sinus. Signals from these sources can initiate drinking. Low blood volume, as well as other conditions that decrease body sodium, also results in increased renin secretion from the kidney. Renin, a proteolytic enzyme, cleaves plasma angiotensinogen into angiotensin I, which is then hydrolyzed to the highly active octapeptide angiotensin II. Angiotensin II elicits drinking as well as three other physiological actions that compensate for water loss: vasoconstriction, increased release of aldosterone, and increased release of vasopressin.

For blood-borne angiotensin to affect behavior it must pass through the blood-brain barrier at specialized regions of the brain. The *subfornical organ* is a small neuronal structure that extends into the third ventricle and has fenestrated capillaries that readily permit the passage of blood-borne molecules (see Appendix B on the blood-brain barrier). The subfornical organ is sensitive to low concentrations of angiotensin II in the blood, and this information is conveyed to the hypothalamus by a neural pathway between the subfornical organ and the preoptic area. Neurons in this pathway in turn use an angiotensin-like molecule as a transmitter. Thus the same molecule regulates drinking by functioning as a hormone and a neurotransmitter. The preoptic area also receives information from baroreceptors throughout the body. This information is conveyed to various brain structures that initiate a search for water and drinking. Information from baroreceptors is also sent to the paraventricular nucleus, which mediates the release of vasopressin, which in turn regulates water retention.

The signals that terminate drinking are less well understood than those that initiate drinking. It is clear, however, that the termination signal is not always merely the absence of the initiating signal. This principle holds for many examples of physiological and behavioral regulation, including feeding. Thus, for example, drinking initiated by low vascular fluid volume (eg, after severe hemorrhage) terminates well before the deficit is rectified. This is highly adaptive since it prevents water intoxication from excessive dilution of extracellular fluids and seems to prevent overhydration that could result from absorption of fluid in the alimentary system long after the cessation of drinking.

Motivational States Can Be Regulated by Factors Other Than Tissue Needs

We have so far concentrated on simple forms of motivational states—drive states that minimize or eliminate physiological deficits and are initiated rather directly by feedback systems. Obviously, however, human behavior depends on many factors not related to tissue deficit. Sexual responses and sexual curiosity, for example, do not appear to be controlled by deficits of specific substances in the body. Even homeostatic responses to tissue deficits, such as drinking and feeding, are regulated by innate and learned mechanisms that modulate the direct action of the feedback signals that indicate tissue deficits. Learned habits and subjective feelings of pleasure can override interoceptive feedback signals. For example, people often choose to go hungry rather than eat food they have learned to avoid. Three factors not related to tissue needs are particularly important in regulating motivated behaviors: the particular ecological requirements of the organism, anticipatory mechanisms, and hedonic (pleasure) factors.

Ecological Constraints

The details of particular behaviors, such as the rate of feeding and type of food selection, are determined by evolutionary selection, which shapes responses so that they are appropriate for the ecology of the particular animal. One means of analyzing the ecological value of motivated behaviors is to do cost-benefit analyses similar to those done by economists. For feeding behavior, costs include the time and effort needed to search for and procure food. The benefit consists of nutrient intake that will ultimately support a given level of reproductive success. The spacing and duration of meals can be considered to reflect the operation of brain mechanisms that have evolved to maximize gain and minimize cost.

According to this type of analysis, carnivores may eat very rapidly not because they have exceptionally powerful feedback signals that indicate severe deprivation but because they have evolved mechanisms that help ensure that their kill will not have to be shared with other animals. Ecological considerations need not preclude consideration of homeostatic mechanisms, since homeostatic mechanisms also have evolved to assist the organism in adapting to its particular environmental conditions.

Anticipatory Mechanisms

Homeostatic regulation often is anticipatory. Intrinsic circadian clock mechanisms as well as other timing mechanisms turn physiological behavioral responses on and off before a tissue deficit or need occurs. In the presence of a repeated 24-hour signal (typically light-dark cycles) the circadian rhythm runs exactly 24 hours. However, as we have seen in Chapter 3, circadian rhythms are autogenous—they continue under constant dark, although in periods of somewhat more or less than 24 hours.

There is a circadian rhythm for virtually every homeostatic function. Since many of the rhythms are coordinated, the hypothalamus would be the ideal location for a major clock mechanism that would drive them, or at least coordinate independent clock mechanisms located throughout the brain. Indeed, the suprachiasmatic nucleus has been shown to serve this function.

Animals with lesions of the suprachiasmatic nucleus lose 24-hour rhythmicity of corticosteroid release, feeding, drinking, locomotor activity, and several other responses. Exposure of animals to light pulses just at the phases of the circadian rhythm during which light can shift the rhythm leads to an increase in the products of immediate-early genes, such as *c-fos*, in neurons in the suprachiasmatic nucleus. The immediate-early gene products are thought to affect downstream genes that play a role in regulating the circadian pacemaker (see Chapter 3).

Hedonic Factors

Pleasure is unquestionably a key factor in controlling the motivated behaviors of humans. Humans will

Box 51-1 Cocaine Craving Can Be Elicited by Environmental Cues Reminiscent of Cocaine Usage

Activity in the brain region implicated in several forms of memory—working, episodic and emotional—is directly related to the intensity of craving for cocaine. In a positron emission tomography (PET) scan study both cocaine abusers and normal volunteers were compared in two environments. The volunteers participated in two test sessions separated by at least 1 week. Neutral stimuli were presented during the first session and cocaine-related stimuli were presented during the other session. The neutral stimuli consisted of objects used for arts and crafts (a leather pouch, a paintbrush, paint bottles, etc) and a videotape of a person handling seashells. No drug was present or offered. The cocaine-related stimuli consisted of drug-related paraphernalia: glass pipe, mirror, razor blade, straw, a $10 bill, 40 mg of L-cocaine hydrochloride mixed with an equal mass of lactose, and a videotape showing cocaine self-administration, smoking, and inhalation and handling of white powder crystals. To elicit the likelihood of craving in the abuser group, subjects in the cocaine abusers group were told they would be allowed to partake of the cocaine that had been

in view after all the experimental procedures had been completed.

Cocaine-related cues did not significantly alter blood flow or elicit self-reports of craving in normal volunteers. In contrast, in the cocaine abusers the cues were associated with increases in blood flow in the dorsolateral prefrontal cortex, medial temporal lobe, and cerebellum and the degree of blood-flow changes was correlated with the degree of reported craving (Figure 51–8). Thus, the effects of the stimuli depend on the prior experience with cocaine use.

This study suggests that the mechanisms mediating memory processing are as germane to cocaine craving as are the neural substrates mediating the direct effect of cocaine. Identification of a specific pattern of brain activation correlated with cocaine craving can direct future investigations into the mechanisms of and therapeutic interventions for craving and drug addiction and possibly other repetitive disorders that involve powerful drugs.

A Self-reported craving

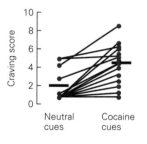

Figure 51-8 Reports by cocaine abusers of craving are correlated with increases in cerebral blood flow.

A. Responses of individual subjects to the question, "Do you have a craving or urge for cocaine?" during exposure to neutral and cocaine-related stimuli. The mean craving score (**horizontal bar**) is significantly higher during exposure to the cocaine-related stimuli than during exposure to the neutral stimuli, and the magnitude of the response across individuals varies considerably.

B. Correlation of change in self-reported craving with the change in regional cerebral metabolic rate for glucose (CMRglc) in two regions of cerebral cortex in the group receiving cocaine-related stimuli. The ordinate represents the difference between the average of the responses to the question, "Do you have a craving or urge for cocaine?" taken at three times during the 30-min presentation of the neutral and cocaine-related stimuli. The abscissa represents the difference in rCMRglc between the two sessions (cocaine cues minus neutral cues).

C. Pseudocolored PET images of metabolic activity in the dorsolateral prefrontal cortex and medial temporal lobe (superimposed on structural magnetic resonance images) illustrate increases of rCMRglc associated with self-reports of craving. Metabolic activity outside these two areas is not shown. **DL** = dorsolateral prefrontal cortex; **Am** = amygdala; **Ph** = parahippocampal gyrus. (Adapted from Grant et al., 1996.)

B Change in metabolic rate
1 Dorsolateral prefrontal cortex

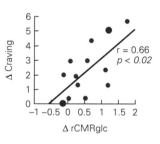

$r = 0.66$
$p < 0.02$

2 Medial temporal lobe

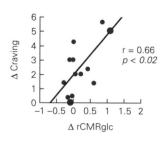

$r = 0.66$
$p < 0.02$

C

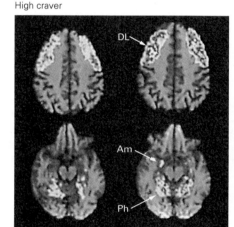

High craver

DL
Am
Ph

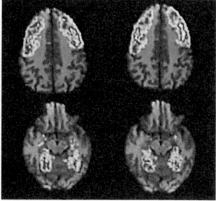

Low craver

Neutral cues   Cocaine cues

sometimes even subject themselves to deprivation to heighten the pleasure obtained when the deprivation is relieved (skipping lunch so as to enjoy dinner more), or to obtain pleasure by satisfying some other need (dieting to look attractive).

Since pleasure is subjective, it is difficult to study experimentally in animals, but there are reasons to believe that a similar variable may control motivated animal behavior. For example, rats given a very palatable diet containing a variety of junk foods (chocolate-chip cookies, salami) eat much more than when they are given a bland and comparably nutritious diet of rat chow.

The neural mechanisms of pleasure are poorly understood, but it seems reasonable to think that they overlap or even coincide with brain mechanisms (including those in the hypothalamus) concerned with reward and the reinforcement of learned behavior (Box 51–1).

The Mesolimbic Dopaminergic Pathways Important for Reinforcement Are Also Recruited by Some Drugs of Abuse

One of the most important discoveries for understanding motivation was the finding in 1954 by James Olds and Peter Milner that intracranial electrical stimulation of the hypothalamus and associated structures can act as a reinforcer of or reward for behavior (see Chapter 62). Brain stimulation acts in many respects like ordinary rewards, but with one important difference. Whereas ordinary rewards are effective only if the animal is in a particular drive state (for example, food serves as a reward only when the animal is hungry), electrical stimulation of the brain works regardless of the drive state of the animal. This observation led to the idea that electrical stimulation of the brain acts as a reward because (1) it evokes a drive state and (2) it recruits neural systems that are ordinarily activated by reinforcing stimuli.

The Limbic Dopaminergic Neurons Are Involved in Behavioral Activation

The human brain has relatively few dopaminergic neurons, and these are equally divided between the substantia nigra, which gives rise to the nigrostriatal pathway, and the ventral tegmental area, which gives rise to the mesocorticolimbic projections (Chapter 45). The neurons of the ventral tegmental area form most of the mesolimbic and mesocortical projections involved in reward. These neurons send their axons to the nucleus ac-

cumbens, the striatum, and the frontal cortex, three structures thought to be involved in motivation.

When animals are trained to stimulate themselves electrically, these stimuli activate dopaminergic neurons in the ventral tegmental area, thereby increasing the output of dopamine at synapses of the mesolimbic and mesocortical projections. Pathways associated with the dopaminergic neurons are also optimal targets for electrical self-stimulation. Rats often choose self-stimulation over food and sex. Receptor blockers such as the antipsychotic drug haloperidol reduce the rewarding effect of food and intracranial self-stimulation. This action is seen as strong evidence that dopamine has a general role in reinforcement mechanisms in limbic areas.

These several arguments implicate midbrain dopaminergic neurons in reward-dependent learning. However, dopamine also is essential for sensory-motor coordination. Selective depletion of dopamine from the ventrolateral sector of the striatum impairs orientation to tactile and olfactory stimuli as well as motor coordination. In experiments with drugs that block dopamine receptors in both the limbic and dorsal striatum, it is difficult to know whether the observed reduction in the hedonic value of reinforcers is due to anhedonia and lack of motivation or an inability to respond to the reinforcement.

The mesolimbic dopamine system is thought to gate signals that regulate biological drives and motivation. Drugs that facilitate dopamine transmission enhance the processes by which otherwise neutral stimuli acquire incentive or reinforcing properties and facilitate further drug-seeking behavior. It is not clear, however, how the dopamine system mediates reinforcement. Brain stimulation is in a sense an unnatural reward, so we may ask: Are the dopamine neurons important for natural rewards such as food, water, and sex? Many experiments support the idea that dopamine is important not only in mediating the immediate pleasurable aspects of natural rewards, but also in mediating the arousal effects that are predictive of impending rewards.

As previously discussed, lesion studies demonstrate that dopamine systems innervating the striatum contribute to feeding, drinking, and other motivated behavior in a crucial way. This view is supported by studies of intracranial self-stimulation and the demonstration that pharmacological blockade of dopamine systems impairs feeding behavior. Additional information comes from recordings by Wolfram Schultz and his colleagues of single dopaminergic neurons in alert monkeys while they receive rewards. When a monkey is presented with various appetitive stimuli (eg, fruit juice), dopaminergic neurons respond with short phasic bursts

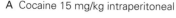

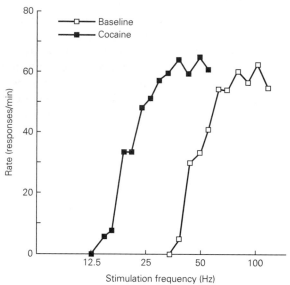

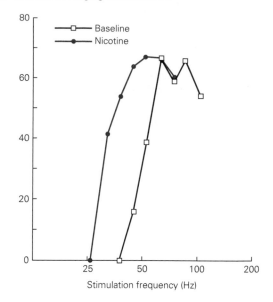

Figure 51-9 Cocaine and nicotine affect the rate of electrical self-stimulation of the brain. As the frequency of the self-stimulation current increases, the rate at which the subject presses a self-stimulation lever increases. In the presence of the drugs animals self-stimulate with a lower-frequency current that was previously ineffective. (Adapted from Wise et al. 1992.)

of activity. Aversive stimuli like air puffs to the hand or drops of saline to the mouth do not cause these transient activations. Thus, dopaminergic neurons are only activated by novel stimuli that elicit reward.

After repeated pairing of visual and auditory cues followed by reward, the time of phasic activation of the dopaminergic neurons changes from firing just after the reward is delivered to firing at the exact time the cue is presented. The changes in dopaminergic activity strongly resemble the transfer of an animal's appetitive behavioral reaction from the unconditional stimulus to the conditional stimulus. These arguments suggest that dopaminergic neurons encode expectations about external rewards.

In one experiment a naive monkey was required to touch a lever before the appearance of a light. Before training, most of the dopaminergic neurons fired a short burst of action potentials after delivery of the reward. After several days of training, the animal learned to reach for the lever as soon as the light was turned on, and this behavioral change correlated with two striking changes in the firing patterns of the dopaminergic neurons. First, the primary reward no longer elicited a phasic response. Second, the onset of the predictive light now caused a phasic activation in the dopaminergic cells' firing. Again, the changes in dopaminergic activity resemble the transfer of the animal's appetitive behavioral reaction from the unconditional to the conditional stimulus.

In trials where the reward is not delivered after the light is turned on, the firing rate of dopaminergic neurons decreases below the basal rate at exactly the time the reward should have occurred. This well-timed decrease in the firing rate of dopaminergic neurons shows that the expected time of reward delivery, based on the occurrence of the light, is also encoded in the fluctuation in dopaminergic activity. In contrast, very few dopaminergic neurons respond to stimuli that predict aversive outcomes.

Drugs of Abuse Increase the Level of Dopamine Released in the Brain

Addictive drugs such as cocaine, amphetamine, opiates, and nicotine act like positive reinforcers. Animals will readily press a lever to give themselves an intravenous infusion of amphetamine, for example. Animals can be conditioned to self-administer addictive drugs directly to certain brain sites through a microcannula. The ability of a drug to act as a positive reinforcer that sustains behavior in experimental animals is highly correlated with the abuse potential of the drug for humans. Drugs of abuse potentiate the reinforcing effects of electrical brain stimulation, reducing the frequency of shock pulses needed to produce a given level of behavioral responses. It is as if the drugs enhance the pleasure produced by electrical brain stimulation (Figure 51-9).

Psychoactive drugs that are reinforcing also increase the levels of dopamine released at terminals of the projections of the ventral tegmental area. Some drugs do so by blocking the dopamine transporter. Thus, cocaine and amphetamine both raise the level of dopamine in the nucleus accumbens by blocking the dopamine transporter (Chapter 15), thereby prolonging the time dopamine remains in the synaptic cleft. The dopamine transporter may be the site of action for both cocaine and amphetamine and as such could be a molecular target for drugs developed to control addiction.

To test this idea, Marc Caron and associates disrupted the gene encoding the dopamine transporter through homologous recombination in a laboratory strain of mice. Homozygotic mice showed no behavioral activation after cocaine or amphetamine were administered systemically, consistent with the notion that the transporter is a critical participant in the mechanism of amphetamine and cocaine action. Study of slices of the striatum in vitro revealed that amphetamine releases dopamine in the wild-type mice but not in the mutant mice.

Although many drugs of abuse modulate dopaminergic transmission, not all of them do so by means of the dopamine transporter. Nicotine, possibly the most addictive and most widely abused drug, increases the level of dopamine in the mesocorticolimbic pathway, as do cocaine and amphetamine. Nicotine enhances release of dopamine by acting on presynaptic cholinergic receptors. This enhancement of dopamine may serve as a constant reinforcement for cigarette smoking. By contrast,

mu opioid agonists appear to be rewarding because they inhibit GABA-ergic neurons that normally suppress dopaminergic neurons in the ventral tegmental area.

The nucleus accumbens, a target for the action of these drugs of addiction, has two functional sectors: the core and the shell. The shell has strong connections to the limbic system and the hypothalamus and is particularly sensitive to addictive drugs. Thus, intravenous injection of cocaine, morphine, and amphetamine results in greater release of dopamine from the shell of the nucleus.

Pathways using other transmitters are also involved in regulating self-stimulation in animals and pleasure in humans. In fact, electrical stimulation of the medial forebrain bundle maintains self-stimulation by activating dopaminergic cells only indirectly. The most effective electrical stimuli activate a group of nondopaminergic neurons in the medial forebrain bundle that project to the midbrain and there activate the ascending dopaminergic neurons (Figure 51-10). Moreover, not all drugs of dependence require the dopamine system. At least some dependence on opiates, alcohol, and benzodiazepines can occur in the absence of dopaminergic mechanisms.

Indeed, addiction involves more than just the positive reinforcement derived from the drug and the resulting anticipation of the euphoria it produces. Two other features characterize addiction: tolerance and dependence. *Tolerance* refers to progressive adaption to the dosage that produces euphoria, so that higher and higher dosages are needed to achieve the same euphoric effect. *Dependence* refers to the negative visceral consequences of withdrawal of the drug, such as nausea. Thus, drug abuse is driven not only by the rewarding ef-

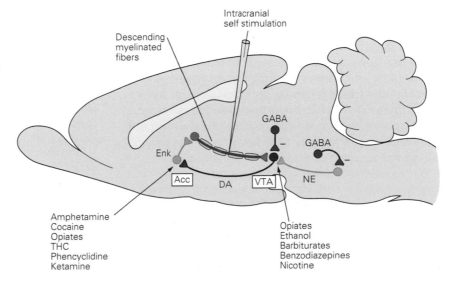

Figure 51-10 Brain-reward circuitry in the rat. Intracranial self-stimulation may act directly on descending myelinated fibers. Suspected sites of drug actions are shown in boxes. **Acc** = nucleus accumbens; **DA** = dopaminergic fibers; **Enk** = enkephalin and other opioid-containing neurons; **GABA** = GABA-ergic inhibitory interneurons; **NE** = norepinephrine-containing fibers; **THC** = tetrahydrocannabinol; **VTA** = ventral tegmental area. (Adapted from Gardner and Lowinson 1993.)

fects of the drug but also by avoidance of the highly aversive effects of withdrawal. Tolerance may be due in part to a drug-induced desensitization of the positive reinforcing system. Likewise, some of the symptoms of withdrawal may be due to a rebound depression of the dopaminergic reinforcing system.

An Overall View

Traditionally, motivational states were inferred internal conditions used to explain variations in behavior that could not be explained by observable learning, damage, or developmental changes. Today we are able to specify the actual physiological bases of at least some of the internal states that affect behavior.

Motivational states involve neural mechanisms that are widely distributed throughout the brain, but hypothalamic mechanisms play a particularly prominent role. The hypothalamus is intimately involved in regulating various behaviors that are directed toward homeostatic goals, such as obtaining food and water and regulating temperature. The hypothalamus contributes to these behaviors by receiving information from both external (incentive) stimuli and internal stimuli that report on the homeostatic status of the animal. The hypothalamus, through its control of hormonal release and the autonomic nervous system, is also involved in the regulation of behavioral states such as stress and anxiety.

Many functions of the hypothalamus can be understood in terms of control systems that respond to specific deficits of physiological needs. However, motivated behaviors are also regulated by factors that do not directly correspond to tissue needs. One such important variable is the pleasurable and reinforcing effects of a stimulus. The neural systems that mediate reward and pleasure use a variety of neurotransmitter agents, and dopamine in particular has been implicated. Dopaminergic pathways important for reinforcement are recruited by some commonly abused drugs that are reinforcing.

We saw in Chapter 24 that the endogenous pain control pathways of the brain provided a useful conceptual framework for understanding the analgesic actions of the opiates. So, too, do the endogenous reward pathways of the brain provide a framework for understanding the mechanisms of action of addictive drugs.

Irving Kupfermann
Eric R. Kandel
Susan Iversen

Selected Readings

Arnold MB. 1960. *Emotion and Personality*. New York: Columbia Univ. Press.

Boulant JA. 1981. Hypothalamic mechanisms in thermoregulation. Fed Proc 40:2843–2850.

Campfield LA, Smith FJ, Burn P. 1996. The OB protein (leptin) pathway: a link between adipose tissue mass and central neural networks. Horm Metab Res 28:619–632.

Friedman MI, Stricker EM. 1976. The physiological psychology of hunger: a physiological perspective. Psychol Rev 83:409–431.

Giros B, Jaber M, Jones SR, Wightman RM, Caron MG. 1996. Hyperlocomotion and indifference to cocaine and amphetamine in mice lacking the dopamine transporter. Nature 379:606–612.

Iversen SD. 1981. Neuropeptides: do they integrate body and brain? Nature 291:454.

Johnson AK, Thunhorst RL. 1995. Sensory mechanisms in the behavioral control of body fluid balance: thirst and salt appetite. Prog Psychobiol Physiol Psychol 16:145–176.

Keesey RE. 1989. Physiological regulation of body weight and the issue of obesity. Med Clin North Am 73:15–27.

Kissileff HR, Van Itallie TB. 1982. Physiology of the control of food intake. Annu Rev Nutr 2:371–418.

Kupfermann I. 1994. Neural control of feeding. Curr Opin Neurobiol 4:869–876.

Kupfermann I, Teyke T, Rosen SC, Weiss KR. 1991. Studies of behavioral state in Aplysia. Biol Bull 180:262–268.

Leibowitz SF, Stanley BG. 1986. Brain peptides and the control of eating behavior. In: TW Moody (ed). *Neural and Endocrine Peptides and Receptors*, pp. 333–352. New York: Plenum.

McEwen BS, Sapolsky RM. 1995. Stress and cognitive function. Curr Opin Neurobiol 5:205–216.

Moore-Ede MC. 1983. The circadian timing system in mammals: two pacemakers preside over many secondary oscillators. Fed Proc 42:2802–2808.

Robbins TW, Everitt BW. 1992. Functions of dopamine in the dorsal and ventral striatum. Sem Neurosci 4:119–127.

Rolls ET. 1981. Central nervous mechanisms related to feeding and appetite. Br Med Bull 37:131–134.

Rolls ET. 1994. Neural processing related to feeding in primates. In: CR Legg, DA Booth (eds). *Appetite: Neural and Behavioral Bases*, 2:11–53. Oxford: Oxford Univ. Press.

Rolls BJ, Rolls ET. 1982. *Thirst*. Cambridge: Cambridge Univ. Press.

Schachter S. 1971. Some extraordinary facts about obese humans and rats. Am Psychol 26:129–144.

Schoener TW. 1971. Theory of feeding strategies. Annu Rev Ecol Syst 2:369–404.

Stellar JR, Stellar E. 1985. *The Neurobiology of Motivation and Reward*. New York: Springer.

Toates F. 1986. *Motivational Systems*. Cambridge: Cambridge Univ. Press.

Vale W, Spiess J, Rivier C, Rivier J. 1981. Characterization of a 41 residue ovine hypothalamic peptide that stimulates secretion of corticotropin and β-endorphin. Science 213:1394–1397.

References

Anand BK, Brobeck JR. 1951. Localization of a "feeding center" in the hypothalamus of the rat. Proc Soc Exp Biol Med 77:323–324.

Bernard C. 1878–1879. *Leçons sur les Phénomènes de la vie Communs aux Animaux et aux Végétaux*, Vols 1, 2. Paris: Ballière.

Bligh J. 1973. *Temperature Regulation in Mammals and Other Vertebrates*. Amsterdam: North-Holland.

Booth DA, Toates FM, Platt SV. 1976. Control system for hunger and its implications in animals and man. In: D Novin, W Wyrwicka, GA Bray (eds). *Hunger: Basic Mechanisms and Clinical Implications*, pp. 127–143. New York: Raven.

Corbit JD. 1973. Voluntary control of hypothalamic temperature. J Comp Physiol Psychol 83:394–411.

DiGirolamo M, Rudman D. 1968. Variations in glucose metabolism and sensitivity to insulin of the rat's adipose tissue, in relation to age and body weight. Endocrinology 82:1133–1141.

Dourish CT, Ruckert AC, Tattersall FD, Iversen SD. 1989. Evidence that decreased feeding induced by systemic injection of cholecystokinin mediated by CCK-A receptors. Eur J Pharmacol 173:233–234.

Epstein AN, Kissileff HR, Stellar E (eds). 1973. *The Neuropsychology of Thirst: New Findings and Advances in Concepts*, p. 357. Washington, DC: V.H. Winston & Sons.

Erikson G, Hollopeter G, Palmiter RD. 1996. Attenuation of obesity syndrome of ob/ob mice by loss of neuropeptide Y. Science 274:1704–1707.

Gardner EL, Lowinson JH. 1993. Drug craving and positive/negative hedonic brain substrates activated by addicting drugs. Sem Neurosci 5:359–368.

Grant S, London ED, Newlin DB, Villemagne VL, Liu X, Contoreggi C, Phillips RL, Kimes AS, Margolin A. 1996. Activation of memory circuits during cue-elicited cocaine craving. Proc Natl Acad Sci USA Oct 15, 93(21): 12040–12045.

Hervey GR. 1969. Regulation of energy balance. Nature 222:629–631.

Hetherington AW, Ranson SW. 1942. The spontaneous activity and food intake of rats with hypothalamic lesions. Am J Physiol 136:609–617.

Hori T, Nakashima T, Koga H, Kiyohara T, Inoue T. 1988. Convergence of thermal, osmotic and cardiovascular signals on preoptic and anterior hypothalamic neurons in the rat. Brain Res Bull 20:879–885.

Kasting NW. 1989. Criteria for establishing a physiological role for brain peptides. A case in point: the role of vasopressin in thermoregulation during fever and antipyresis. Brain Res Rev 14:143–153.

Keesey RE. 1989. Physiological regulation of body weight and the issue of obesity. Med Clin North Am 7:371–418.

Keesey RE, Boyle PC, Kemnitz JW, Mitchel JS. 1976. The role of the lateral hypothalamus in determining the body weight set point. In: D Novin, W Wyrwicka, GA Bray (eds). *Hunger: Basic Mechanisms and Clinical Implications*, pp. 243–255. New York: Raven.

Kleiber M. 1947. Body size and metabolic rate. Physiol Rev 27:511–541.

Koob GF. 1992a. Dopamine, addiction and reward. Sem Neurosci 4:139–148.

Koob GF. 1992b. Drugs of abuse: anatomy, pharmacology and function of reward pathways. Trends Pharmacol Sci 13:177–184.

Mirenowicz J, Schultz W. 1996. Preferential activation of mid brain dopamine neurons by appetitive rather than aversive stimuli. Nature 379:449–451.

Nauta WJH, Feirtag M. 1986. *Fundamental Neuroanatomy*, pp. 120–131. New York: Freeman.

Olds J, Milner P. 1954. Positive reinforcement produced by electrical stimulation of septal area and other regions of rat brain. J Comp Physiol Psychol 47:419–427.

Robbins TW, Everitt BJ. 1996. Neurobehavioural mechanisms of reward and motivation. Curr Opin Neurobiol 6:228–236.

Satinoff E. 1964. Behaviorial thermoregulation in response to local cooling of the rat brain. Am J Physiol 206:1389–1394.

Schultz W, Dayan P, Montague PR. 1997. A neural substrate of prediction and reward. Science 275:1593–1599.

Self DW, Barnhart WJ, Lehman DA, Nestler EJ. 1996. Opposite modulation of cocaine seeking behaviour by D_1 and D_2-like dopamine receptor agonists. Science 271:1586–1589.

Smith GP. 1995. Dopamine and food reward. Prog Psychobiol Physiol Psychol 16:83–144.

Tartaglia LA, Dembski M, Weng X, Deng N, Culpepper J, Devos R, Richards GJ, Campfield LA, Clark FT, Deeds J, Muir C, Sanker S, Moriarty A, Moore KJ, Smutko JS, Mays GG, Woolf EA, Monroe CA, Tepper RI. 1995. Identification and expression cloning of a leptin receptor, OB-R. Cell 83:1263–1271.

Ungerstedt U. 1971. On the anatomy, pharmacology and function of the nigro-striatal dopamine system. Acta Physiol Scand 367(Suppl).

Uno H, Tarara R, Else JG, Suleman MA, Sapolsky RM. 1989. Hippocampal damage associated with prolonged and fatal stress in primates. J Neurosci 9:1705–1711.

Wise RA, Bauco P, Carlezon WA Jr, Trojniar W. 1992. Self-stimulation and drug reward mechanisms. Ann N Y Acad Sci 654:192–198.

Zhang Y, Proenca R, Maffei M, Barone M, Leopold L, Friedman JM. 1994. Positional cloning of the mouse obese gene and its human homologue. Nature 372:425–432.

Part VIII

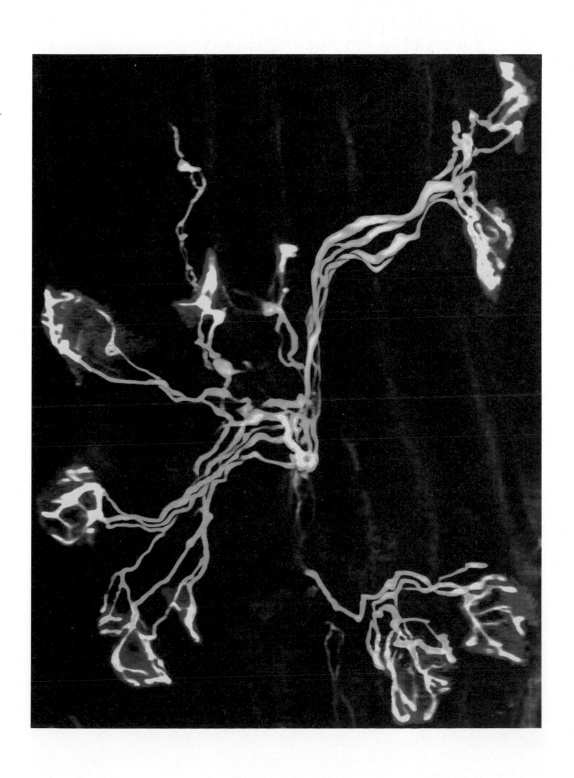

VIII The Development of the Nervous System

ACH OF THE BEHAVIORAL TASKS performed by the mature nervous system—from the perception of sensory input and the control of motor output to cognitive functions such as learning and memory—depends on precise interconnections of many millions of neurons. These connections are made during embryonic and postnatal development.

Over a century ago Santiago Ramón y Cajal undertook a comprehensive and now classical series of anatomical studies that culminated in a clearer appreciation of the structure and organization of the nervous system. Modern studies on the development of the nervous system aim to uncover the cellular and molecular processes underlying the formation of the neural circuits that Ramón y Cajal described. During the past decade in particular there have been many striking advances in understanding the molecular basis of neural development. These advances include the identification of proteins that determine how nerve cells acquire their identities, extend axons to target cells, and form synaptic connections, and have provided insight into how synaptic connections are modified by experience.

Development of the nervous system depends on the expression of particular genes at particular places and times during development. This spatial and temporal pattern of gene expression is regulated by both hard-wired molecular programs and epigenetic processes. The factors that control neuronal differentiation originate both from cellular sources within the embryo and from the external environment. Internal influences include cell surface and secreted molecules that control the fate of neighboring cells, as well as transcription factors that act at the level of DNA to control gene expression. External factors include secreted factors, nutrients, sensory stimuli, and social experience, the effects of which are mediated through patterned changes in the activity of nerve cells. The interaction of these intrinsic and environmental factors is critical for the proper differentiation of each nerve cell.

The recent progress in defining the mechanisms that control the development of the nervous system is due largely to molecular biological studies of neural function. To take but one example, the molecular cloning of genes encoding extrinsic factors (eg, secreted proteins) and intrinsic determinants (eg, transcription factors) has provided unanticipated insight into the differentiation of the nervous system. Moreover, the function of specific genes can now be tested directly in transgenic animals or in animals in which individual genes have been inactivated by mutation.

Other important advances have emerged from the analysis of simple and genetically accessible organisms such as the fruit fly *Drosophila* and the nematode worm *Caenhorabitis elegans*. Indeed, the DNA sequence of the entire genome of *C. elegans* is now known. Most of the key molecules that control the formation of the nervous system are found in organisms separated by millions of years of evolution. Thus, despite the great diversity of animal forms, the developmental programs that govern body plan and neural connectivity are conserved throughout phylogeny.

In this part of the book we examine vertebrate development in a sequential manner. Beginning with the early stages of neural development we concentrate on the factors that control the diversity and survival of nerve cells, guide axons, and regulate the formation of synapses. We then explain how interaction with the environment, both social and physical, modifies or consolidates the neural connections formed during early development. Depriving individuals of their normal environment during the early critical period of development can have profound consequences for the later maturation of the brain and thus for behavior. Finally, we examine factors, such as steroid hormones, that continue to influence the structure of the brain during early postnatal development and the biochemical changes that occur as the brain ages.

It is now clear that mutations in genes that regulate the development of the human nervous system are responsible for many degenerative disorders and cancers. Thus, studies of neural development are beginning to provide practical insight into neurological diseases and to suggest rational strategies for restoring neural connections and function after disease or traumatic injury.

Part VIII

52

The Induction and Patterning of the Nervous System

THE DIVERSE FUNCTIONS OF the vertebrate nervous system, which range from sensory perception and motor coordination to motivation and memory, depend on precise connections formed between distinct types of nerve cells. These connections develop in several steps. First, a uniform population of neural progenitors, the cells of the *neural plate,* are recruited from a large sheet of ectodermal cells that have not yet committed to a specific pathway of differentiation. Once recruited, the cells of the neural plate rapidly begin to acquire differentiated properties, giving rise both to immature neurons and to glial cells. The immature neurons then migrate from zones of cell proliferation to their final positions and extend axons toward their target cells. The formation of contacts between the growing axon and its target cell then initiates a process of selective synapse formation, during which some synaptic contacts are strengthened and others eliminated. Finally, electrical and chemical signals passed across synapses can control patterns of connectivity, as well as the phenotype of the neurons themselves.

This developmental program culminates in a great variety of neural cell types—both neurons and glial cells. There are now thought to be many hundreds of different neuronal types, far more than in any other organ of the body. Nevertheless, the principles underlying the differentiation of neural cells are similar to those governing other developmental processes. Thus the development of the nervous system merely represents a more elaborate version of the most basic problem of developmental biology: How does a single cell, the fertilized egg, give rise to each of the differentiated cell types comprising the mature organism?

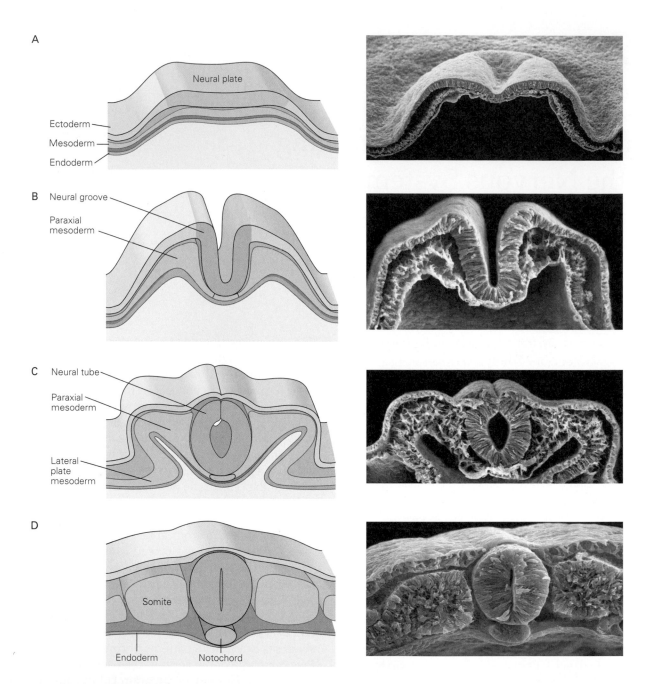

Figure 52-1 The neural plate folds in stages to form the neural tube. (Scanning electron micrographs of chick embryos provided by G. Schoenwolf.)

A. Position of the neural plate in relation to the nonneural ectoderm, the mesoderm, and the endoderm.

B. Folding of the neural plate to form the neural groove.

C. Dorsal closure of the neural folds to form the neural tube.

D. Maturation of the neural tube and its position relative to the axial mesodermal structure, notochord, and somites (derived from the paraxial mesoderm.)

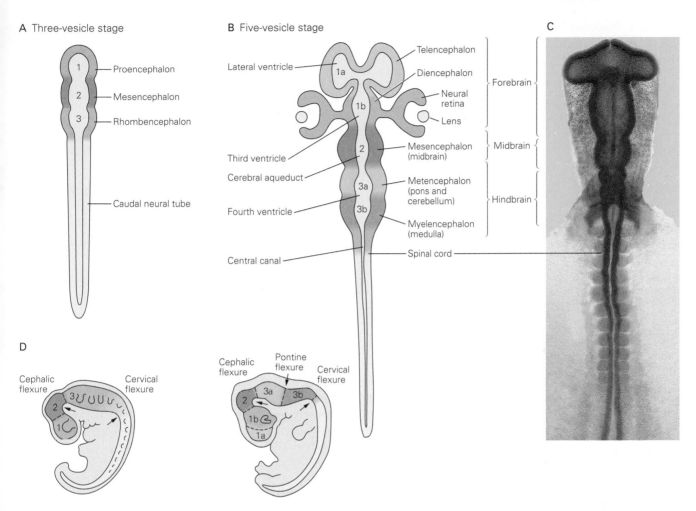

Figure 52-2 Successive stages in the development of the neural tube.

A. Three-vesicle stage. At early stages of development only three brain vesicles are present.

B. Five-vesicle stage. At later stages two additional vesicles form, one in the area of the forebrain (1a and 1b) and the other in the hindbrain (3a and 3b). The relationships between these early structures and the mature nervous system are summarized in Table 52-1.

C. Micrograph showing a dorsal view of the neural tube at an early stage of development. The expansion of the future telencephalic vesicle is apparent. (Micrograph of chick neural tube provided by G. Schoenwolf.)

D. The positions of the cephalic, pontine, and cervical flexures.

Many of the mechanisms governing neural development are conserved in different organisms. Indeed, much of what we have learned about the molecular basis of neural development in vertebrates derives from organisms such as the fruit fly *Drosophila melanogaster* and the nematode worm *Caenorhabditis elegans*, organisms amenable to genetic analysis. Here, however, we shall illustrate the principles of the development of the nervous system primarily with reference to the vertebrate nervous system. In this chapter we shall discuss first the signaling events that establish the early pattern of cell types in the developing nervous system.

The Entire Nervous System Arises From the Ectoderm

The nervous system begins to develop at a relatively late stage in embryogenesis. Prior to its formation, three main cell layers have been generated. The *endoderm*, the innermost layer, gives rise to the gut, lungs, and liver; the *mesoderm*, the middle layer, gives rise to connective tissues, muscle, and the vascular system; and the *ectoderm*, the outermost layer, gives rise to the major tissues of the central and peripheral nervous systems. Neural and glial cells derive from a sheet of ectodermal cells located along the dorsal midline of the embryo at the gas-

Table 52-1 The Main Subdivisions of the Embryonic Central Nervous System and Mature Adult Forms

Three-vesicle stage	Five-vesicle stage	Major mature derivatives	Related cavity
1. Forebrain (prosencephalon)	1a. Telencephalon (endbrain)	1. Cerebral cortex, basal ganglia, hippocampal formation, amygdala, olfactory bulb	Lateral ventricles
	1b. Diencephalon	2. Thalamus, hypothalamus, sub-thalamus, epithalamus, retina, optic nerves and tracts	Third ventricle
2. Midbrain (mesencephalon)	2. Mesencephalon (midbrain)	3. Midbrain	Cerebral aqueduct
3. Hindbrain (rhomb-encephalon)	3a. Metencephalon (afterbrain)	4. Pons and cerebellum	Fourth ventricle
	3b. Myelencephalon (medullary brain)	5. Medulla	Fourth ventricle
4. Caudal part of neural tube	4. Caudal part of neural tube	6. Spinal cord	Central canal

trula stage. As this ectodermal sheet begins to acquire neural properties it forms the neural plate, a columnar epithelium (Figure 52-1). Ectodermal cells that fail to follow the neural program of differentiation give rise instead to the epidermis of the skin.

Soon after the neural plate has formed it begins to fold into a tubular structure, called the *neural tube,* through a process called neurulation (see Figure 52-1). The caudal region of the neural tube gives rise to the spinal cord, and the rostral region becomes the brain. During these early stages of neural development, cells divide rapidly. Moreover, the extent of cell proliferation is not uniform along the length of the neural tube. Individual regions of the neural epithelium expand at different rates and begin to form the various specialized regions of the mature central nervous system. The proliferation of cells in the rostral part of the neural tube initially forms three brain vesicles: the *forebrain* (or prosencephalon), the *midbrain* (or mesencephalon), and the *hindbrain* (or rhombencephalon) (Figure 52-2).

At this early stage of development (the three-vesicle stage) the brain flexes twice: at the junction of the spinal cord and hindbrain, called the *cervical flexure,* and at the junction of the hindbrain and midbrain, the *cephalic flexure.* A third flexure, the *pontine flexure,* forms at a later stage. Both the cervical and the pontine flexures eventually straighten out, but the cephalic flexure remains prominent throughout development. The persistence of this flexure is what causes the longitudinal axis of the forebrain to differ from that of the brain stem and spinal cord. Later in development two of the three primary embryonic vesicles subdivide (Table 52-1). The fore-

brain vesicle gives rise to the telencephalon and diencephalon, and the hindbrain vesicle gives rise to the metencephalon and myelencephalon. These subdivisions, together with the spinal cord, make up the six major regions of the mature central nervous system (see Chapter 17).

Inductive Signals Control Neural Cell Differentiation

What factors determine whether cells embark on the pathway of differentiation that results in the formation of neural tissue? The differentiation of cells in the nervous system, as in other organs, is the consequence of a complex program that directs the expression of specific genes within individual cells. Two major groups of factors determine which genes are expressed in a cell. The first, termed *inducing factors,* are signaling molecules provided by other cells. These factors can be freely diffusible and thus exert their actions over a long range, or they can be tethered to the cell surface and act locally. Because cells in different positions in the embryo are exposed to different inducing factors, the position that a cell occupies early in development is of critical importance in determining its fate.

The second group of factors are the molecules that are activated or induced in cells upon exposure to an inducing factor from another cell. These molecules include surface receptors that mediate the effect of inducing factors. Activation of these receptors then modulates the activity of the transcription factors and regulates expression

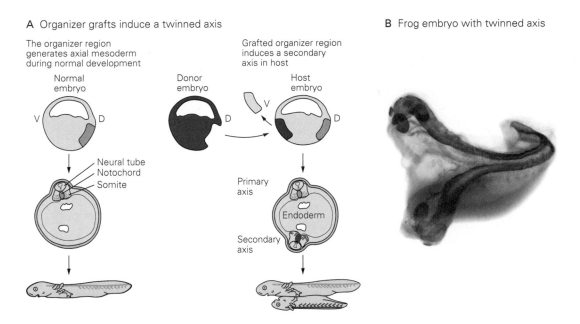

A Organizer grafts induce a twinned axis

The organizer region
generates axial mesoderm
during normal development

Normal
embryo

Grafted organizer region
induces a secondary
axis in host

Donor
embryo

Host
embryo

Neural tube
Notochord
Somite

Primary
axis

Endoderm

Secondary
axis

B Frog embryo with twinned axis

Figure 52-3 Generation of a second neural axis in amphibian embryos.

A. The organizer graft experiment of Spemann and Mangold. The dorsal blastopore lip from an early gastrula is transplanted into the region of a host embryo that normally gives rise to the ventral epidermis. The transplanted tissue induces a second embryonic axis that includes an entire nervous system. Both the pigmented donor tissue (**dark blue**) and the host tissue (**light**) are seen in the induced neural tube, notochord, and

somites. As the embryo matures, the secondary axis becomes fully developed. V = ventral; D = dorsal.

B. Experimental induction of a secondary axis in a *Xenopus* embryo. Secondary axes can be induced by injection of *noggin* or *wnt* RNAs into a normal embryo at the two-cell stage of development. The primary axis is also apparent. The twinned nervous system is revealed by expression of the neural cell adhesion molecule (NCAM) (**brown staining**). (Micrograph provided by P. Eimon, H. Yue, and R. Harland.)

of genes that encode the proteins carrying out the specialized functions of the cell. The ability of the cell to respond to inductive signals, termed its *competence*, depends on the precise repertoire of receptors, transduction molecules, and transcription factors expressed by the cell.

Thus, a cell's fate is determined in part by the signals to which it is exposed—in turn largely a consequence of where it finds itself in the embryo—and in part by the profile of genes it expresses as a consequence of its developmental history. A key to understanding the mechanisms that generate the large number of cell types found in the nervous system has been the identification of the intercellular signals (inducers) that trigger the formation of the neural plate and the intracellular machinery that regulates responsiveness to the inducers.

The Neural Plate Is Induced by Signals From Adjacent Mesoderm

In 1924 Hans Spemann and Hilde Mangold made the fundamental discovery that the differentiation of the neural plate from uncommitted ectoderm in amphibian embryos depends on signals secreted by a specialized

group of cells later called the *organizer region*. Spemann and Mangold originally demonstrated the contribution of the organizer region to the formation of the nervous system by transplanting small pieces of tissue to new locations at the gastrula stage of development. The critical set of experiments involved a region of the embryo called the dorsal lip of the blastopore, which was destined to form the dorsal mesoderm. The dorsal lip was excised from one embryo and transplanted into or underneath the ventral ectoderm of a host embryo, a region that normally gives rise to ventral epidermal tissues. The transplanted cells were removed from a pigmented embryo and grafted into an unpigmented host to facilitate identification of the grafted and host cells.

Spemann and Mangold found that the transplanted cells followed their normal developmental program, generating midline (axial) mesoderm, the notochord. However, the transplanted cells caused a dramatic change in the fate of host ectodermal cells. The host cells formed a duplicate body axis that included a virtually complete second nervous system (Figure 52-3). Only cells from the organizer region had this effect; tissue

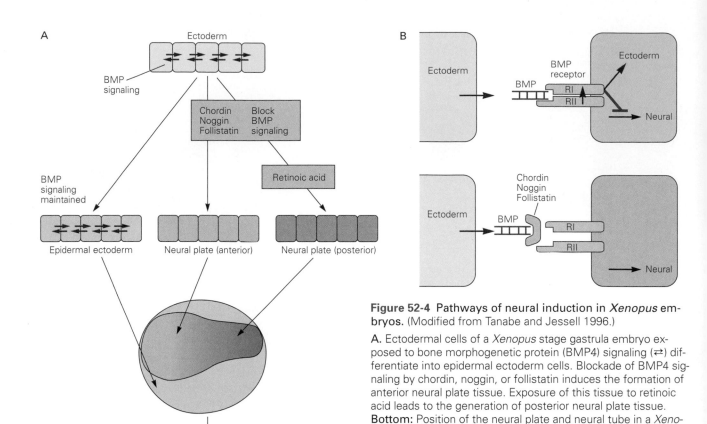

Figure 52-4 Pathways of neural induction in *Xenopus* embryos. (Modified from Tanabe and Jessell 1996.)

A. Ectodermal cells of a *Xenopus* stage gastrula embryo exposed to bone morphogenetic protein (BMP4) signaling (⇄) differentiate into epidermal ectoderm cells. Blockade of BMP4 signaling by chordin, noggin, or follistatin induces the formation of anterior neural plate tissue. Exposure of this tissue to retinoic acid leads to the generation of posterior neural plate tissue. **Bottom:** Position of the neural plate and neural tube in a *Xenopus* embryo and the anteroposterior gradient of neural positional character.

B. A potential mechanism of action of anterior neural inducers. Tonic BMP signaling between ectodermal cells directs the differentiation of epidermis and blocks neural differentiation. The secretion of chordin, noggin, and follistatin by organizer cells blocks BMP signaling and permits ectodermal cells to undergo a "default" program of neural differentiation. **RI** and **RII** indicate the two subunits of BMP receptors.

from other regions of the early gastrula did not induce a second body axis. This demonstration provided the first evidence that the nervous system is induced by signals from nonneural cells.

Neural Induction Involves Inhibition of Bone Morphogenetic Protein Signals

For decades, the identity of endogenous inducing factors remained obscure. However, recent studies in embryos of the frog *Xenopus laevis* have dramatically advanced our understanding of neural induction. The first breakthrough was the surprising finding that the potential for neural differentiation is actually the default state of the ectoderm. This possibility was first raised by a simple experiment. When early ectoderm is dissociated into single cells (so as to prevent any intercellular signaling) and

cultured in the absence of any added factors, these single cells form neural tissue. This observation suggested that in the embryo the capacity of ectodermal cells to undergo neural differentiation is suppressed by signals transmitted between neighboring cells.

The mediators of this suppressive signal appear to be members of the bone morphogenetic protein (BMP) subclass of transforming growth factor β (TGFβ)-related proteins. Evidence for this role of BMPs emerged from experiments in which a truncated so-called dominant-negative version of a BMP receptor, which blocks BMP signaling, was expressed in the ectodermal cells of *Xenopus*. Cells expressing this truncated receptor differentiated into neural tissue, suggesting that blocking BMP signaling is sufficient to trigger neural differentiation. Conversely, BMP signaling was found to promote the differentiation of ectoderm into epidermis.

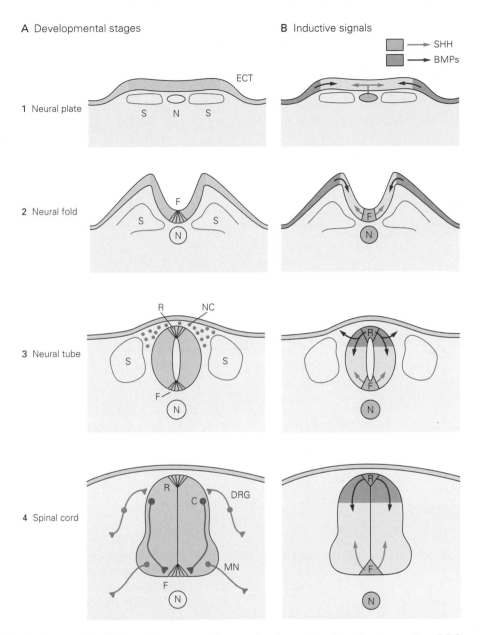

Figure 52-5 Sonic hedgehog and BMP signaling pattern the neural tube along its dorsoventral axis. (Modified from Tanabe and Jessell 1996.)

A. Four stages in the embryonic development of the spinal cord: (**1**) The neural plate is generated as a columnar epithelium under which lies the notochord (N) and paraxial mesoderm fated to give rise to the somites (S). The neural tube is flanked by the epidermal ectoderm (ECT). (**2**) During neurulation, the neural plate buckles at its midline to form the neural fold, and floor plate cells (F) form at the ventral midline. (**3**) The neural tube forms by fusion of the dorsal tips of the neural folds, and roof plate cells (R) form at its dorsal midline. Neural crest cells (NC) begin to migrate from the dorsal region of the neural tube. Neuroepithelial cells proliferate and then differentiate into neurons located at different dorsoventral positions. (**4**) As the spinal cord matures, subclasses of contralaterally projecting commissural (C) neurons differentiate dorsally, close to the roof plate, whereas motor neurons (MN) differentiate ventrally, near

the floor plate. Dorsal root ganglion (DRG) neurons are generated from neural crest cells.

B. Two classes of proteins provide inductive signals that control the pattern of cell differentiation along the dorsoventral axis of the spinal cord. Sonic hedgehog (SHH) patterns the ventral neural tube, and bone morphogenetic proteins (BMPs) pattern the dorsal neural tube. Sources of these inducing factors are shown at sequential stages of spinal cord development. Initially, SHH is expressed in the axial mesoderm, and BMPs originate in the epidermal ectoderm flanking the lateral edges of the neural plate. At the neural fold stage, SHH is expressed by floor plate cells at the midline and BMPs by cells in the dorsal tips of the neural folds. After neural tube closure BMPs are no longer expressed in the epidermal ectoderm but are expressed in the roof plate and in the adjacent dorsal neural tube. At the onset of neuronal differentiation, BMP expression persists in the dorsal neural tube, and SHH expression is maintained in the floor plate.

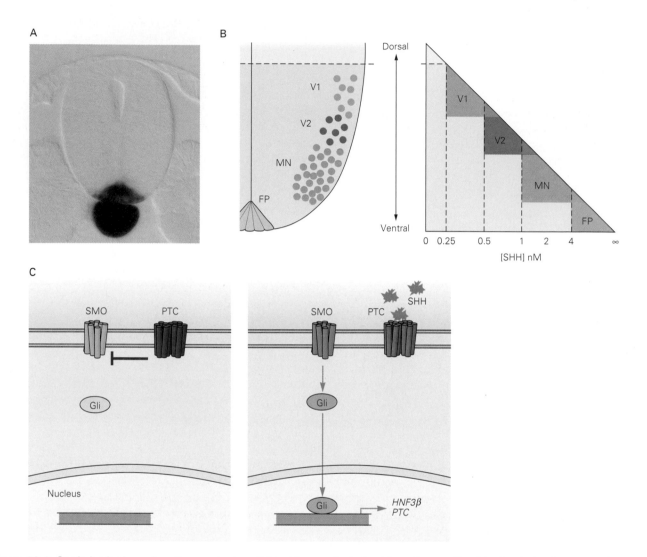

Figure 52-6 Sonic hedgehog signaling controls cell identity and pattern in the ventral neural tube.

A. Expression of sonic hedgehog mRNA in the notochord and floor plate of a chick embryo.

B. The dorsoventral position of motor neurons (**MN**) and two classes of ventral interneurons (**V1** and **V2** neurons) within the ventral spinal cord. The "French flag" model of Lewis Wolpert depicts the observed relationship between sonic hedgehog (**SHH**) concentration, neuronal and floor plate (**FP**) cell identity, and dorsoventral position in the ventral neural tube. This model

is derived from the results of in vitro induction assays in neural plate explants. (Adapted from Ericson et al. 1997.)

C. The sonic hedgehog signal transduction pathway. Sonic hedgehog binds to the protein patched (**PTC**), which has 12 transmembrane regions. The binding of sonic hedgehog relieves the patched-dependent inhibition of the protein smoothened (**SMO**), which has seven transmembrane regions. Once relieved from inhibition by PTC, smoothened activates members of the Gli class of zinc finger transcription factors, which enter the nucleus and induce expression of *HNF3β, PTC*, and other target genes.

These observations raised the possibility that the inductive signal from the organizer region could induce neural tissue by blocking BMP signaling. Direct support for this idea came with the finding that cells in the organizer region express three secreted proteins—follistatin, noggin, and chordin—each of which is able to induce *Xenopus* ectoderm to differentiate into neural tissue (Figure 52-4). All three proteins appear to act by binding

to BMPs and inhibiting their activity; these binding proteins therefore are strong candidates for endogenous neural inducers. The differentiation of neural plate cells triggered by inhibition of BMP signaling appears to involve the expression of transcription factors of the *Sox* gene family.

Once cells of the neural plate are induced they rapidly acquire specialized properties that depend on the position they initially occupy within the neural plate. The fate of induced neural cells is controlled by two independent signaling systems. One system patterns the neural plate along its medial-to-lateral axis; after neurulation this axis becomes the dorsoventral axis of the neural tube. The second system controls the pattern of the neural plate along the anteroposterior axis. Signals along this axis divide the neural tube into its four major rostrocaudal subdivisions: the spinal cord, hindbrain, midbrain, and forebrain. In the next section we discuss the signals that impose the dorsoventral pattern of the neural tube, focusing initially on caudal levels of the neural tube that give rise to the spinal cord.

The Neural Plate Is Patterned Along Its Dorsoventral Axis by Signals From Adjacent Nonneural Cells

The neurons of the mature spinal cord serve two major functions. They process sensory input, and coordinate motor output. The neuronal circuits that subserve these functions are segregated anatomically. Neurons involved in the processing of sensory input are located in the dorsal half of the spinal cord, whereas those involved in motor output are located in the ventral half.

These distinct cell types are generated at different positions along the dorsoventral axis of the neural tube at early stages in the development of the spinal cord. In the ventral half of the neural tube, a population of specialized glial cells, the *floor plate*, forms at the midline (Figure 52-5A). Motor neurons are generated lateral to the floor plate, and several classes of interneurons are formed dorsal to the position of motor neurons. In the dorsal half of the neural tube, two types of cells form initially: *neural crest cells*, which populate the peripheral nervous system; and specialized glial cells, which form the midline *roof plate*. At later stages, cells lateral to the roof plate differentiate into distinct classes of dorsal sensory interneurons.

How are the identity and dorsoventral positions of these cell types determined? The crucial signals for their initial differentiation come from nonneural cells that lie close to the neural plate. As with initial induction of the nervous system, the early differentiation of cell types in the ventral neural tube is controlled by signals from mesodermal cells that give rise to the notochord underlying the midline of the neural plate. In contrast, cell differentiation in the dorsal half is controlled by signals from nonneural cells of the epidermal ectoderm that flank the lateral margins of the neural plate (see Figure 52-5B).

The Ventral Neural Tube Is Patterned by Sonic Hedgehog Secreted From the Notochord and Floor Plate

Mesodermal cells in the organizer region and later in the notochord provide two types of inductive signals: a locally acting signal that induces the formation of the floor plate in the overlying midline neural plate, and a longer-range signal that induces the differentiation of both motor neurons and ventral interneurons. Once induced, the floor plate cells have the same short- and long-range signaling ability originally present in the notochord.

The short- and long-range signaling activities of the notochord are mediated by the same protein: sonic hedgehog (Figure 52-6A). Sonic hedgehog (SHH) is a member of a family of secreted proteins related to *Hedgehog*, a gene that controls many aspects of embryonic development in *Drosophila*. The inductive capabilities of the sonic hedgehog protein are impressive. By itself it can induce the differentiation of floor plate cells, motor neurons, and ventral interneurons. Elimination of sonic hedgehog function blocks the ability of the notochord to induce virtually all of the cell types normally generated in the ventral neural tube. Thus one protein is both necessary and sufficient for the induction of most cell types generated in the ventral half of the neural tube.

How does sonic hedgehog exert such a powerful influence on the development of the central nervous system? Some insight into its actions has emerged from studies of the mechanism by which the sonic hedgehog signal is perceived in target cells. This signaling pathway is triggered by the interaction of the sonic hedgehog protein with a heterodimeric receptor complex. Sonic hedgehog binds to one subunit of the receptor, a transmembrane protein called patched, and this binding relieves the repression by patched of the second subunit, a transmembrane protein named smoothened (see Figure 52-6C). Smoothened activity generates an intracellular signal that regulates several protein kinases and activates a class of transcription factors, the gli proteins, that mimic some of the signaling activities of sonic hedgehog.

How does a single protein, sonic hedgehog, determine the fate of many different cell types in the ventral half of the central nervous system? The answer appears to lie in the ability of sonic hedgehog to act not only as an inducer but also as a *morphogen*, a type of inductive signal that can direct different cell fates at different concentration thresholds. The exposure of ventral neural tube cells to low concentrations of sonic hedgehog induces ventral interneurons; exposure to a higher concentration induces motor neurons; and a further in-

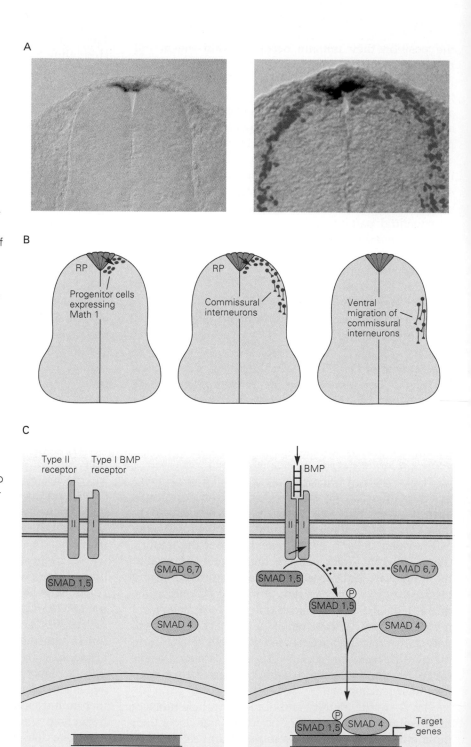

Figure 52-7 BMP signaling from the roof plate induces the formation of dorsal commissural interneurons.

A. The left image shows the expression of bone morphogenetic protein 4 (BMP4) in the roof plate of the spinal cord of a chick embryo. The right image shows the expression of growth and differentiation factor 7 (Gdf7) in the roof plate of a mouse embryonic spinal cord. The progenitors of dorsal commissural interneurons express the basic helix-loop-helix factor Math1 (**pink**), and postmitotic commissural neurons express the LH2A/B homeodomain proteins (**blue**). (Images provided by K. Lee)

B. Generation of dorsal commissural interneurons in response to BMP mediated signals from the roof plate (**RP**).

C. A simplified version of the BMP signal transduction pathway. BMP ligands bind to type II receptors and trigger the phosphorylation and activation of type I receptors. The type I receptors phosphorylate the SMAD 1,5 proteins. Activated SMAD 1,5 proteins associate with SMAD 4 the complex translocates to the nucleus and regulates the transcription of target genes. SMAD 6,7 act as inhibitors that can block this signaling pathway. (Modified from Whitman 1998.)

crease in concentration induces floor plate cells (see Figure 52-6B).

The ability of sonic hedgehog to act at different concentration thresholds depends on the formation of a gradient of sonic hedgehog activity in the ventral neural tube, apparently controlled by the rate of diffusion of sonic hedgehog from the notochord and floor plate. How then is the diffusion of sonic hedgehog controlled? Sonic hedgehog is synthesized as an inactive precursor, which is cleaved autocatalytically by a serine protease-like activity contained within the carboxy-terminal domain of the sonic hedgehog protein itself. This cleavage generates an amino terminal protein fragment that possesses the signaling activity of sonic hedgehog. Remarkably, during cleavage the amino terminal fragment of sonic hedgehog is modified by the covalent addition of a cholesterol molecule. The addition of a lipophilic cholesterol molecule is thought to tether most of the sonic hedgehog protein to the surface of notochord and floor plate cells but permits the diffusion of small amounts of sonic hedgehog from notochord and floor plate cells.

Disruption of different components of the sonic hedgehog signaling pathway results in a wide variety of diseases in humans. Mutations in the human sonic hedgehog gene result in a syndrome known as holoprosencephaly, in which ventral forebrain structures fail to develop. Mutations in the human patched, smoothened, and gli proteins also result in neurological defects such as spina bifida, in limb deformities, and even in cancer.

The Dorsal Neural Tube Is Patterned by Bone Morphogenetic Proteins Secreted From the Epidermal Ectoderm and Roof Plate

How are cell fates in the dorsal neural tube controlled? At first glance it would seem that because of the potency of sonic hedgehog signaling, dorsal cell types might also be induced by sonic hedgehog but at lower concentrations. Alternatively, cells might acquire dorsal fates by virtue of their lack of exposure to sonic hedgehog. Instead, a distinct class of secreted factors, the BMPs, involved earlier in the control of neural induction actively induce dorsal cell differentiation at a later stage. Like hedgehog proteins, the BMPs have homologs in *Drosophila*, and one of these proteins, decapentaplegic, patterns the dorsal region of the early fly embryo.

The differentiation of cell types—neural crest cells, roof plate cells, and dorsal interneurons—in the dorsal neural tube is initiated by BMP signals from ectodermal cells that flank the neural tube, the same cells that later give rise to the epidermis (see Figure 52-5). After the neural tube has closed, roof plate cells express several BMPs that are responsible for generating several classes of sensory interneurons in the dorsal spinal cord (Figure 52-7A,B).

BMPs in turn activate a relatively novel class of receptors, the transmembrane serine-threonine kinases (see Figure 52-7C). One subunit of the BMP receptor is involved in the specificity of ligand binding and the other in transducing intracellular signals. BMP signals are transduced from the surface membrane to the nu-

cleus by a class of transcription factors termed SMADs. In the absence of BMP signaling, SMAD proteins are found in the cytoplasm in an unphosphorylated state. Upon activation of BMP receptors, SMADs are phosphorylated and enter the nucleus, where they control the expression of transcription factors that specify the fate of individual dorsal cells (see Figure 52-7C).

Inductive Signaling in the Two Halves of the Neural Tube Depends on a Common Principle

Cell differentiation in both the dorsal and ventral halves of the neural tube is controlled by inductive signals. Ventral patterning is regulated by the activities of a single protein, sonic hedgehog, which generates different cell types at different concentrations. In contrast, dorsal patterning appears to involve several members of the BMP family, each of which may induce a particular set of cells. There is, however, one common feature to the patterning of the dorsal and ventral neural tube. In both halves inductive signals are initially expressed by nonneural cells (in the epidermal ectoderm dorsally and in the notochord ventrally). Then, through a process of *homeogenetic induction,* a process by which like begets like, these signals are transferred to specialized glial cells at the midline of the neural tube (the roof plate dorsally and the floor plate ventrally). This process presumably ensures that future cellular sources of inductive signals are positioned appropriately to control neural cell fate and pattern at later stages of development.

Dorsoventral Patterning Is Maintained Throughout the Rostrocaudal Length of the Neural Tube

The strategies used to establish the dorsoventral pattern in the spinal cord appear also to control cell identity and pattern along the dorsoventral axis of the hindbrain, midbrain, and much of the forebrain (Figure 52-8). For example, sonic hedgehog signals from the floor plate act on progenitor cells in mesencephalic regions of the neural tube to generate the dopaminergic neurons of the substantia nigra and ventral tegmental area. As we discuss in Chapter 43, these dopaminergic neurons degenerate in Parkinson disease. Thus an understanding of sonic hedgehog signaling may eventually help to design a treatment for Parkinson disease based on the de novo generation or regeneration of dopaminergic neurons.

In the forebrain, however, sonic hedgehog and BMPs appear to act in combination to induce certain ventral cell types. In particular, in the ventral region of the rostral diencephalon and telencephalon, both sonic hedgehog and BMPs are expressed in the axial mesoderm and appear to cooperate in establishing the fate of

A

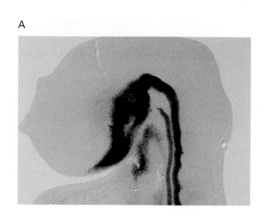

B

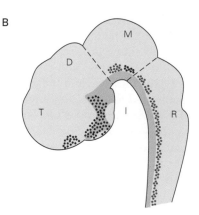

Figure 52-8 The sonic hedgehog protein induces formation of distinct classes of ventral neurons at different rostrocaudal levels.

A. Lateral view of the rostral part of a chick neural tube showing the expression of *Sonic hedgehog* RNA in the notochord and floor plate of the hindbrain and midbrain, and in the ventral diencephalon. Micrograph provided by T. Lints and J. Dodd.

B. Some of the distinct neuronal classes induced by SHH at dif-

ferent rostrocaudal positions of the neural tube. At different levels of the hindbrain and midbrain (**M**), motor neurons (**green**), serotonergic neurons (**blue**), and dopaminergic neurons (**purple**) differentiate close to cells that express sonic hedgehog. In the telencephalon (**T**), the ventral, or diencephalon (**D**), domain of sonic hedgehog expression is close to the position of ventral forebrain interneurons (**red**). I = region of the infundibulum; R = rhombencephalon. (Adapted from Lumsden and Graham 1995.)

midline cells (Figure 52-8). Thus at the most rostral region of the neural tube the source of BMP signals appears to be translocated from dorsal to ventral cells—from the epidermal ectoderm to the prechordal mesoderm—a shift that may contribute to the generation of the distinctive cell types found in the forebrain.

The Rostrocaudal Axis of the Neural Tube Is Patterned in Several Stages

We now turn to the mechanisms by which the identity of neural cells along the rostrocaudal axis is established. Rostrocaudal patterning begins at the neural plate stage and appears intimately linked with the process of neural induction itself. The neural tissue induced by follistatin, noggin, and chordin appears to express genes that are characteristic of forebrain but not of more posterior tissues. Thus additional signaling pathways may be required for the induction of posterior neural tissue, which later gives rise to the midbrain, hindbrain, and spinal cord.

One class of signals involved in the induction of more posterior neural tissue is the fibroblast growth factor (FGF) family of secreted proteins. In addition, an unrelated molecule with the ability to induce posterior neural tissue characteristic of the spinal cord and hindbrain is retinoic acid, which belongs to a class of steroid-like molecules expressed by cells surrounding the organizer region. Exposure of *Xenopus* embryos to retinoic acid does not itself induce neural tissue but instead

leads to the generation of posterior neural tissue at the expense of anterior neural cells (see Figure 52-4). Thus establishing the early anteroposterior identity of cells in the neural plate may require the combined actions of different neural inducers and patterning signals. Collectively, these patterning signals progressively subdivide the neural tube along its rostrocaudal axis; as a result, neurons at the same dorsoventral positions but at different rostrocaudal levels of the neural tube develop distinctive identities and functions.

How then is the finer-grained rostrocaudal pattern of the neural tube achieved? As examples, we shall first examine how neural cells are organized into distinct segmental units within the hindbrain and then consider how cell pattern is controlled at the more anterior levels of the neural tube that give rise to the midbrain and forebrain.

The Hindbrain Is Organized in Segmental Units by Hox Genes

As we have seen in Chapter 44, the hindbrain gives rise to cranial sensory ganglia and motor nuclei. An appreciation of the development of the hindbrain is important for understanding the basis of neurological disorders that affect these neurons, including amyotrophic lateral sclerosis (Lou Gehrig disease) and sensory neuropathies.

Moreover, cell patterning in the developing hindbrain provides a model for studying the more basic question of how the neural tube is subdivided into

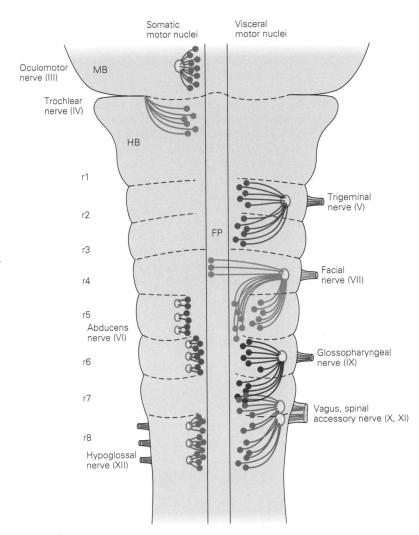

Figure 52-9 Organization of motor neurons in the developing hindbrain. A chick embryo hindbrain and caudal midbrain, viewed from the pial side, shows rhombomeres (r1 to r8) and the cranial motor nuclei. The motor neuron classes in each nucleus are somatic or visceral. Abbreviations: **MB** = midbrain; **HB** = hindbrain; **FP** = floor plate. The **dashed line** across the midline represents the boundary between the midbrain and hindbrain. The nerve exit points are shown as light ellipses. (Adapted from Keynes and Lumsden 1990.)

repetitive units, or segments. For over a century the neural tube had been known to exhibit periodic swellings, but the significance of these swellings was unclear. The swellings in the hindbrain, termed *rhombomeres,* are now known to be fundamental to many aspects of neuronal organization. The developmental importance of rhombomeres emerged from a detailed examination of the relationship between the organization of neurons in the hindbrain and the innervation of adjacent peripheral structures by cranial nerves. Adjacent pairs of rhombomeres were found to contain sensory and motor neurons that innervate individual branchial arches, the embryonic tissues representing the evolutionary derivatives of the gill structures of aquatic vertebrates (Figure 52-9). Many such observations—the precise register that exists between rhombomeres, the pattern of innervation of the branchial arches, and the organization of sensory and motor neurons in the hind-

brain—raised the question of how the identity of individual rhombomeres is established.

We first address how the distinct properties of cells in individual rhombomeres are established during the development of the hindbrain. One class of genes, the *Hox* genes, has been implicated in the control of rhombomere identity. These genes encode proteins that have a highly conserved 60-amino-acid DNA-binding domain termed the *homeodomain* (Box 52-1). Homeodomain proteins represent one of the major classes of transcription factors that regulate developmental process in organisms as diverse as yeast, plants, and mammals.

In mammals the *Hox* genes comprise a structurally divergent subset of homeobox genes that are organized into four separate chromosomal complexes or clusters, each of which is located on a different chromosome. The four *Hox* clusters are thought to derive from a common

Box 52-1   Conserved Homeobox Genes Regulate the Body Plan in Vertebrates and *Drosophila*

Studies of early development in *Drosophila* have provided fundamental insight into the mechanisms underlying the development of body form. In the early 1980s Christiane Nüsslein-Volhard and Eric Weischaus performed the first systematic screen for genes that affect the early pattern of the *Drosophila* embryo. This screen identified numerous genes that control different aspects of the embryonic body plan (Figure 52–10). These genes were then ordered into a hierarchy, by which specific genes organize individual regions of the embryo in progressively finer detail.

Earlier analyses by Ed Lewis had defined much of the genetic logic by which the later body plan of *Drosophila* is controlled. In particular, the genes of the *HOM-C* complex are responsible for body plan. These genes are clustered together in the genome, and the linear arrangement of these genes on the chromosome corresponds to the domains of expression and function of the genes in the embryo. Molecular cloning of the genes of the *HOM-C* cluster showed that they encode transcription factors—proteins that bind to DNA—and activate the transcription of downstream targets, many of which

are themselves transcriptional regulatory factors. Thus, the *HOM-C* genes act at a later stage in the genetic cascade defined by Nüsslein-Volhard and Weischaus.

A further key discovery was that many of these *Drosophila* regulatory genes contain a shared 180 bp nucleotide sequence, the *homeobox*, which encodes a 60-amino-acid sequence termed a homeodomain. The homeodomain forms three α-helical regions, one of which is involved in binding to specific DNA target sequences. The name "homeobox" derives from findings that mutations in some of these genes lead to homeotic transformations—perturbations in which one body structure develops in place of another.

In the mouse and human genomes there are four homeobox gene clusters (*Hoxa, Hoxb, Hoxc,* and *Hoxd*) located on different chromosomes (Figure 52–10). The *HOM-C* complex in *Drosophila* and the corresponding *Hox* clusters in mice are thought to have arisen from a common ancestor of vertebrates and insects. Moreover, in both *Drosophila* and vertebrates these homeodomain proteins are involved in specifying regional identity along the anteroposterior axis of the embryo.

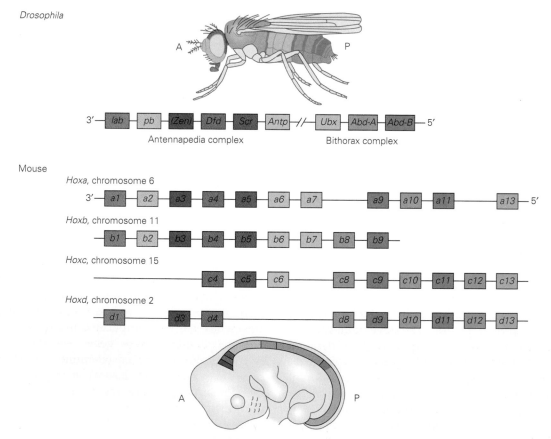

Figure 52-10 The clustered organization of *Hox* genes is conserved in flies and mammals. The diagram shows the chromosomal arrangement of structurally related *Hox* genes in the mouse and *HOM-C* genes in *Drosophila*. The mouse has four *Hox* gene clusters, as do humans. (Adapted from Wolpert et al. 1998.)

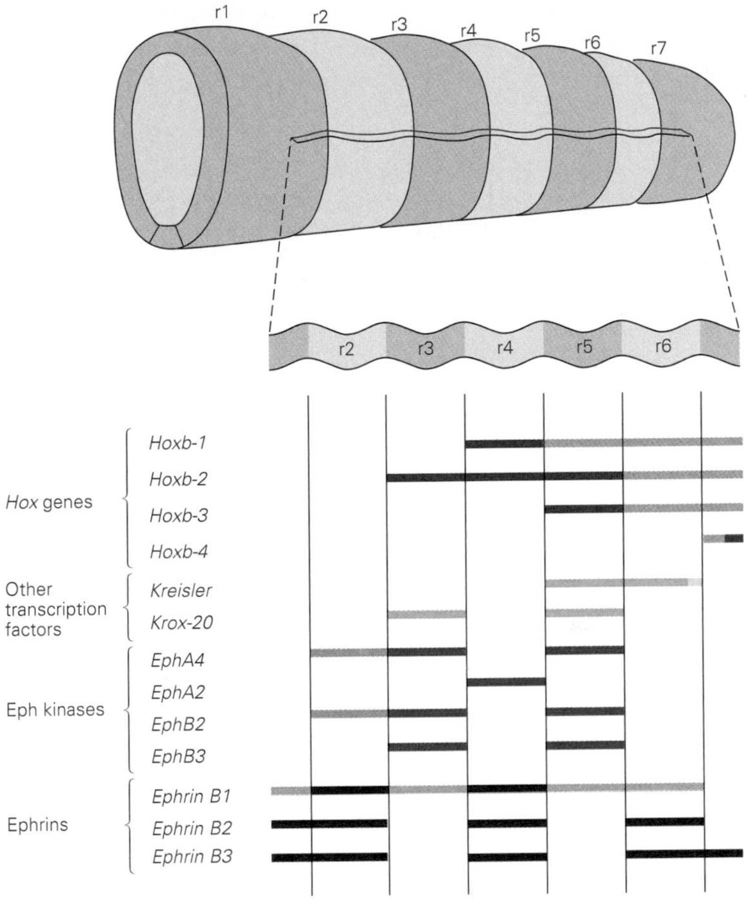

Figure 52-11 Genes involved in patterning the hindbrain are expressed segmentally. Gene expression is restricted to specific rhombomeres. **Vertical lines** indicate the boundaries between rhombomeres. Related genes are indicated by the same color: *Hoxb* homeobox genes (**red**), other transcription factors (**yellow**), Eph family tyrosine kinase receptors (**blue**), Ephrin ligands (**purple**). The darkest colors indicated the highest levels of gene expression. (Adapted from Lumsden and Krumlauf 1996.)

ancestral *Hox* complex that also gave rise to the *HOM-C* gene complex in *Drosophila*. The vertebrate *Hox* genes are expressed in overlapping domains along the antero-posterior axis of the developing hindbrain and spinal cord. As in *Drosophila* a striking relationship exists between the position of an individual *Hox* gene within its cluster and its anterior limit of expression. Those *Hox* genes located at the most 5' position of a cluster are expressed in the most posterior regions of the neural tube, whereas genes located at more 3' positions are expressed at progressively more anterior positions. Moreover, within the hindbrain the anterior limit of expression of many *Hox* genes appears to coincide with the boundaries of rhombomeres (Figure 52-11). *Hox* gene expression in the hindbrain is regulated in part by mechanisms that are intrinsic to the neural tube but is also influenced by signals from surrounding mesodermal cells.

Genetic studies of the mouse have shown that *Hox* genes control the identity of cells in individual rhombomeres. As one example, we describe here the role of the *Hoxb-1* gene in establishing cell identity in the hind-

brain. *Hoxb-1* is normally expressed at high levels in rhombomere 4, a region giving rise to facial motor neurons. Elimination of this *Hox* gene causes a change in the fate of cells in rhombomere 4, resulting in a switch in the identity of cranial motor neurons and their axonal projections: In such mutants cells in rhombomere 4 generate trigeminal rather than facial motor neurons (Figure 52-12). Similar genetic studies of many additional *Hox* genes have shown that the identity of other classes of neurons in the hindbrain is controlled by the expression of specific combinations of *Hox* genes.

The selective expression of *Hox* genes within different rhombomeres in the hindbrain is itself regulated by other transcription factors. For example, the zinc finger protein Krox20 is expressed in two strips of cells that give rise to rhombomeres 3 and 5 (see Figure 52-11) and controls the expression of *Hox* genes in these two rhombomeres. *Hox* gene expression in the hindbrain is also regulated by retinoic acid, which is expressed in mesodermal cells adjacent to the organizer region. Embryos treated with retinoic acid express *Hox* genes at more anterior levels of the hindbrain than normal. As a conse-

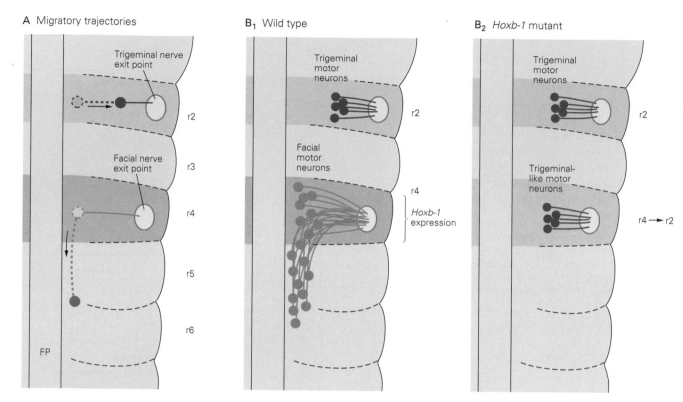

A Migratory trajectories

B₁ Wild type

B₂ *Hoxb-1* mutant

Figure 52-12 Mutations in *Hox* genes change motor neuron identity in the hindbrain. (Adapted from Studer et al. 1996.)

A. Migratory trajectories of the trigeminal and facial motor neurons in the hindbrain. Trigeminal motor neurons are generated in r2 and migrate laterally, whereas facial motor neurons are generated in r4 and migrate caudally.

B1, B2. In *Hoxb-1* mutant embryos, motor neurons generated in the domain of r4 fail to migrate caudally and instead migrate laterally in a manner reminiscent of trigeminal motor neurons in r2.

quence, neurons in these regions acquire a more posterior identity. Therefore, the patterned expression of *Hox* genes in the hindbrain may be controlled by the exposure of hindbrain cells to different levels of retinoic acid signaling from mesodermal cells. The teratogenic and craniofacial abnormalities found after exposure of mammalian embryos to retinoic acid may result in part from alteration in the pattern of *Hox* gene expression in the hindbrain.

The Midbrain Is Patterned by Signals From a Neural Organizing Center

Neurons in the midbrain serve many essential functions. In the ventral midbrain, for example, the dopaminergic neurons of the substantia nigra control aspects of motor function; dorsally, neurons in the superior colliculus (or tectum) have important roles in the processing of visual information from the retina.

How is the position of the midbrain established and how are cell groups patterned within it? The midbrain lies beyond the rostral limit of *Hox* gene expression and, in contrast to the hindbrain, is not subdivided into obvious segments. Instead, the pattern of cells in the midbrain is controlled by the long-range action of signals from the isthmus region, a secondary organizing center located at the junction of the mesencephalon and metencephalon. Two signaling molecules, Wnt-1 and FGF8, are secreted by isthmus cells and control the differentiation of the mesencephalon (Figure 52-13). FGF8 mimics the ability of signals from the isthmus to control the polarity of the mesencephalon. Thus grafting isthmus cells or cells expressing FGF8 in the posterior diencephalon causes surrounding cells to acquire a midbrain character.

The isthmus also controls the rostrocaudal patterning of cells within the midbrain. For example, the rostrocaudal polarity of midbrain tissue is inverted with respect to that of the host midbrain upon exposure to a transplanted isthmus or FGF8. FGF8, in turn acts through homeodomain proteins to set up a rostrocaudal axis. The involvement of homeodomain proteins in rostrocaudal patterning is thus a general feature of neural development. In the midbrain the expression of two homeodomain proteins, engrailed 1 and 2, is normally graded in a caudal-to-rostral direction (Figure 52-13). If the mesencephalon is reversed at a late stage, the gradient of engrailed protein expression, the cytoarchitecture of the tectum, and the pattern of retinal axon innervation are inverted. Moreover, these effects on cytoarchitecture and axonal patterning can be reproduced by experimentally altering the gradient of expression of engrailed proteins in the tectum. Thus, as in the hindbrain, the rostrocaudal pattern of the midbrain is also controlled by local inductive signals that regulate expression of homeodomain proteins.

The Developing Forebrain Is Subdivided Along Its Rostrocaudal Axis

The neurons in the mammalian forebrain mediate the most sophisticated cognitive behaviors. The forebrain comprises the cerebral cortices, basal ganglia, and the hypothalamus and thalamus. In contrast to other regions of the central nervous system, not much is known of the molecular events that underlie forebrain development. Nevertheless, the little that we do know indicates that early patterning of the forebrain is controlled in a manner similar to that at more caudal levels of the neural tube.

Analysis of the patterns of gene expression in the forebrain suggests that the embryonic forebrain is initially divided along its rostrocaudal axis into transversely organized domains or *prosomeres* (Figure 52-14). Prosomeres 1 to 3 develop into the caudal part of the diencephalon and prosomeres 4 to 6 into the rostral diencephalon and telencephalon. The ventral region of the rostral diencephalon gives rise to the hypothalamus and basal ganglia. As in the hindbrain, the boundaries of the prosomeres coincide with the boundaries of expression of inductive signals and transcription factors. For example, sonic hedgehog is expressed by a strip of cells located at the boundary between prosomeres 2 and 3, a region termed the *zona limitans intrathalamica*. Signals from this region may control cell pattern in the forebrain in much the same way that signals from the isthmus region control midbrain cell pattern.

The subdivision of the forebrain into prosomeres raises the question of whether each prosomere forms a separate developmental compartment. Early in the development of the telencephalon, a pronounced border exists between the regions that give rise to the neocortex and striatum. Because this border coincides with the domains of expression of several transcription factors, cells in the early subdivisions of the telencephalon might be

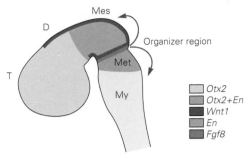

A Gene expression at the developing midbrain/hindbrain boundary

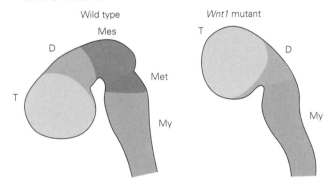

B Deletion of the mesencephalon and metencephalon in *Wnt1* mutants

Figure 52-13 Signals from cells of the isthmus pattern the midbrain. (Adapted from Joyner 1996.)

A. Patterns of expression of genes encoding transcription factors and secreted signaling factors in the mesencephalon of an embryonic day 10 mouse brain. Abbreviations: **T** = telencephalon; **D** = diencephalon; **Mes** = mesencephalon; **Met** = metencephalon; **My** = myelencephalon.

B. Deletion of the mesencephalon and metencephalon in *Wnt1* mutant embryos. The mesencephalon and metencephalon are also deleted in the absence of the *En1/En2* genes.

expected to develop independently. We now know, however, that some neurons in the neocortex develop from cells that migrate from the striatal subdivision of the telencephalon. These striatal progenitors express two ho-meodomain proteins, DLX-1 and DLX-2. In mice lacking these proteins, striatal progenitors fail to migrate into the neocortex (Figure 52-14), resulting in a marked depletion of γ-aminobutyric acid (GABA) expressing neurons in the neocortex. It is evident therefore that not all subdivisions of the telencephalon develop independently. Nevertheless, the basic principle that inductive signals control homeobox gene expression is conserved in the developing forebrain.

What principles have these molecular studies of rostrocaudal and dorsoventral patterning revealed?

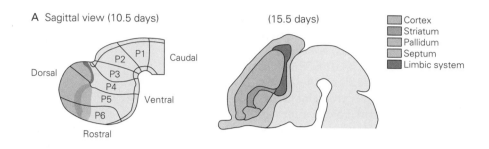

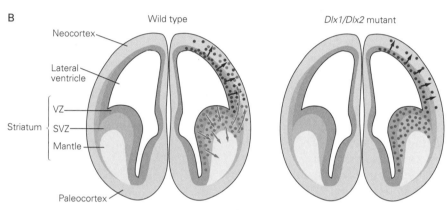

Figure 52-14 The developing forebrain is subdivided into distinct domains.

A. Sagittal views of the embryonic mouse brain at 10.5 days and 15.5 days. The sagittal view shows the six prosomeric divisions (P1–P6) that are thought to divide the forebrain. Individual prosomeres, however, do not give rise selectively to specific regions. Abbreviations: **VZ** = ventricular zone; **SVZ** = subventricular zone. (Adapted from Fishell 1997.)

B. Homeobox genes control cell fate and migration in the developing telencephalon. The diagram shows the location of cells expressing *Dlx1* and *Dlx2* that derive from the ventricular and subventricular zones (**orange**) of the striatal mantle. Neurons from these regions migrate into the neocortex where they mix with the descendants of cortical precursors (**purple**). In *Dlx-1/Dlx-2* mutant mice striatal mantle neurons are generated (**pale blue**), but they do not migrate into the cortex. (Adapted from Anderson et al. 1997 and Lumsden and Gulisano 1997.)

Studies of the *Hox* genes, of sonic hedgehog signaling, and of many other genes involved in embryonic development have led to one of the fundamental insights in modern biology. We have appreciated for some time that molecules are conserved across phylogeny, as are cellular functions. What emerged in the 1990s was the more surprising finding that developmental signals and even entire programs of nerve cell differentiation are conserved despite the enormous variety of body forms. The examples of *Hox* genes and sonic hedgehog provide dramatic evidence that the same transcription factors and secreted signals control body form in animals as different as vertebrates and insects. We now know of dozens of other conserved genes that have crucial roles in the development of invertebrate and vertebrate or-

ganisms. Moreover, this conservation of structure and function does not simply extend from flies to amphibians and mice: It is also evident in humans.

Regional Differentiation of the Cerebral Cortex Depends on Afferent Input As Well As Intrinsic Programs of Cell Differentiation

Finally, we turn to the issue of how regional specialization develops within the mammalian cerebral cortex. As we have seen in Chapters 17 and 19, functionally distinct areas in the adult cortex can be distinguished by differences in the layering pattern of neurons—the cytoarchitecture of the areas—and in their neuronal con-

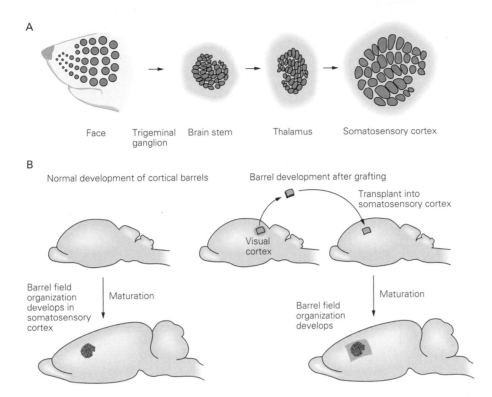

Face   Trigeminal   Brain stem   Thalamus   Somatosensory cortex
        ganglion

B

Normal development of cortical barrels   Barrel development after grafting

                                                Transplant into
                                                somatosensory cortex

                                Visual
                                cortex

Barrel field
organization   Barrel field
develops in   Maturation   organization   Maturation
somatosensory   develops
cortex

Figure 52-15 Thalamic input influences the organization of barrels in the somatosensory cortex of rodents. (Adapted from Schlagger and O'Leary 1991.)

A. The barrels in the somatosensory cortex of rodents are a somatotopic representation of the whiskers on the animal's face. Similar barrel representations of the whisker field are present in the brain stem and thalamic nuclei that relay somatosensory inputs from the face to the cortex.

B. A barrel field organization is induced when a region of the developing visual cortex is grafted into the site normally occupied by somatosensory cortex. The grafted region of visual cortex now acquires a barrel-like organization.

nections. At early stages of development, however, these anatomical features are lacking.

The development of regional differentiation within the cortex has been examined in the primary somatosensory cortex. The primary somatosensory cortex in rodents contains discrete structures termed *barrels*. The arrangement of the barrels reflects the organization of the whisker field on the body surface because the afferent inputs from the thalamus are organized somatotopically (Figure 52-15).

The barrels are normally evident soon after birth. During a critical period of development, barrel formation depends on input from the periphery; their formation is disrupted if the whisker field in the skin is eliminated during this critical period. Moreover, if prospective visual cortex tissue is transplanted in place of the somatosensory cortex around the time of birth, barrels form in the transplanted tissue in a pattern that closely resembles that of the normal somatosensory bar-

rel field (see Figure 52-15). Thus, many regions of the cortex are competent to develop features characteristic of specific areas, and new patterns are determined by local cues such as the inputs they receive.

Some aspects of regional differentiation of the neocortex, however, appear to be programmed intrinsically and independent of afferent innervation. One striking example has emerged from the study of a transgenic mouse line in which the β-galactosidase reporter gene is expressed only in the somatosensory cortex (Figure 52-16). When the prospective somatosensory cortex in this strain of mice is grafted into other regions of the cortex, the transplanted cells continue to express β-galactosidase, despite their new location. Thus although certain local features of the cortex are not specified until late in development, intrinsic differences between cortical areas also exist at early stages, and these differences may underlie important features of the regional specialization of the cortex.

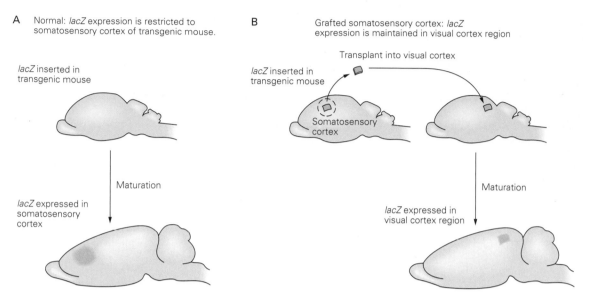

A Normal: *lacZ* expression is restricted to somatosensory cortex of transgenic mouse.

lacZ inserted in transgenic mouse

Maturation

lacZ expressed in somatosensory cortex

B Grafted somatosensory cortex: *lacZ* expression is maintained in visual cortex region

Transplant into visual cortex

lacZ inserted in transgenic mouse

Somatosensory cortex

Maturation

lacZ expressed in visual cortex region

Figure 52-16 Regional properties of the developing cerebral cortex are determined intrinsically. (Adapted from Cohen-Tannoudji et al. 1994.)

A. A transgenic mouse selectively expresses the *lacZ* gene in the somatosensory cortex region at postnatal day 7.

B. Tissue derived from the somatosensory cortex region of transgenic mouse begins to express the *lacZ* marker after grafting into the cerebellum or other regions of the cerebral cortex of wild-type mice.

An Overall View

The diverse functions of the mature vertebrate nervous system depend critically on the establishment of regionally distinct subdivisions of the neural tube. Establishment of these subdivisions is a complex process but one that can be analyzed in three major developmental steps: (1) the generation of progenitor cells in the neural plate, (2) the formation of the neural tube, and (3) the generation of regional differences within the neural tube.

The early pattern of cell differentiation in the neural tube can be viewed as a series of inductive interactions in which signals provided by one group of cells direct the fate of neighboring cells. The diversification of cell types is orchestrated by a relatively small number of inducing factors that control programs of gene expression in target cells. The developmental history of the cell determines its responsiveness to these inducing factors.

Despite differences in the organization of the nervous systems of invertebrates and vertebrates, the signaling molecules responsible for the differentiation and patterning of developing neurons have been conserved throughout animal evolution to a surprisingly high degree, reflecting an economical use of genetic information. Not only are the same signaling molecules used in many different organisms, but the receptors for these signals and the developmental programs they activate are also conserved. In addition, the same processes are used at many different developmental stages within one organism. Thus the analysis of the development of the vertebrate nervous system has benefited greatly from genetic studies of flies and worms.

It is also becoming apparent that studies of the inductive signaling pathways and transcriptional responses that control development of the vertebrate nervous system can provide important insights into the molecular basis of human neurological disorders.

Thomas M. Jessell
Joshua R. Sanes

Selected Readings

Chitnis AB. 1999. Control of neurogenesis—lessons from frogs, fish and flies. Curr Opin Neurobiol 9:18–25.

Fishell G. 1997. Regionalization in the mammalian telencephalon. Curr Opin Neurobiol 7:62–69.

Hamburger V. 1988. *The Heritage of Experimental Embryology. Hans Spemann and the Organizer.* New York: Oxford Univ. Press.

Hynes M, Rosenthal A. 1999. Specification of dopaminergic and serotonergic neurons in the vertebrate CNS. Curr Opin Neurobiol 9:6–36.

Joyner AL. 1996. *Engrailed, Wnt and Pax* genes regulate midbrain-hindbrain development. Trends Genet 12:15–20.

Lee KJ, Jessell TM. 1999. The specification of dorsal cell fates in the vertebrate central nervous system. Annu Rev Neurosci 22:261–294.

Maconochie M, Nonchev S, Morrison A, Krumlauf R. 1996. Paralogous Hox genes: function and regulation. Annu Rev Genet 30:529–556.

Rubenstein JL, Shimamura K, Martinez S, Puelles L. 1998. Regionalization of the prosencephalic neural plate. Annu Rev Neurosci 21:445–477.

Tanabe Y, Jessell TM. 1996. Diversity and pattern in the developing spinal cord. Science 274:1115–1123.

Wolpert L, Beddington R, Brockes J, Jessell TM, Lawrence PA, Meyerowitz E. 1998. *Principles of Development.* New York: Oxford Univ. Press.

References

Anderson SA, Eisenstat DD, Shi L, Rubenstein JL. 1997. Interneuron migration from basal forebrain to neocortex: dependence on D1x genes. Science 278:474–476.

Baker JC, Harland RM. 1997. From receptor to nucleus: the SMAD pathway. Curr Opin Genet Dev 7:467–473.

Belloni E, Muenke M, Roessler E, Traverso G, Siegel-Bartelt J, Frumkin A, Mitchell HF, Donis-Keller H, Helms C, Hing AV, Heng HH, Koop B, Martindale D, Rommens JM, Tsui LC, Scherer SW. 1996. Identification of *Sonic hedgehog* as a candidate gene responsible for holoprosencephaly. Nat Genet 14:353–356.

Chiang C, Litingtung Y, Lee E, Young KE, Corden JL, Westphal H, Beachy PA. 1996. Cyclopia and defective axial patterning in mice lacking *Sonic hedgehog* gene function. Nature 383:407–413.

Cohen-Tannoudji M, Babinet C, Wassef M. 1994. Early determination of a mouse somatosensory cortex marker. Nature 368:460–463.

Crossley PH, Martinez S, Martin GR. 1996. Midbrain development induced by FGF8 in the chick embryo. Nature 380:66–68.

Dale JK, Vesque C, Lints TJ, Sampath TK, Furley A, Dodd J, Placzek M. 1997. Cooperation of BMP7 and SHH in the induction of forebrain ventral midline. Cell 90:257–269.

Ericson J, Briscoe J, Rashbass P, van Heyningen V, Jessell TM. 1997. Graded sonic hedgehog signaling and the specification of cell fate in the ventral neural tube. Cold Spring Harb Symp Quant Biol 62:451–466.

Goddard JM, Rossel M, Manley NR, Capecchi MR. 1996. Mice with targeted disruption of *Hoxb-1* fail to form the motor nucleus of the VIIth nerve. Development 122:3217–3228.

Goodrich LV, Milenkovic L, Higgins KM, Scott MP. 1997. Altered neural cell fates and medulloblastoma in mouse patched mutants. Science 277:1109–1113.

Graham A, Papalopulu N, Krumlauf R. 1989. The murine and *Drosophila* homeobox gene complexes have common features of organization and expression. Cell 57: 367–378.

Guthrie S, Prince V, Lumsden A. 1993. Selective dispersal of avian rhombomere cells in orthotopic and heterotopic grafts. Development 118:527–538.

Hemmati-Brivanlou A, Melton DA. 1994. Inhibition of activin receptor signaling promotes neuralization in *Xenopus.* Cell 77:273–281.

Hynes M, Porter JA, Chiang C, Chang D, Tessier-Lavigne M, Beachy PA, Rosenthal A. 1995. Induction of midbrain dopaminergic neurons by *Sonic hedgehog.* Neuron 15:35–44.

Keeler RF. 1975. Teratogenic effects of cyclopamine and jervine in rats, mice and hamsters. Proc Soc Exp Biol Med 149:302–306.

Keynes R, Lumsden A. 1990. Segmentation and the origin of regional diversity in the vertebrate central nervous system. Neuron 4:1–9.

Lamb TM, Harland RM. 1995. Fibroblast growth factor is a direct neural inducer, which combined with noggin generates anterior-posterior neural pattern. Development 121:3627–3636.

Lamb TM, Knecht AK, Smith WC, Stachel SE, Economides AN, Stahl N, Yancopolous GD, Harland RM. 1993. Neural induction by the secreted polypeptide noggin. Science 262:713–718.

Liem KF Jr, Tremml G, Roelink H, Jessell TM. 1995. Dorsal differentiation of neural plate cells induced by BMP-mediated signals from epidermal ectoderm. Cell 82: 969–979.

Lumsden A, Graham A. 1995. Neural patterning: a forward role for hedgehog. Curr Biol 5:1347–1350.

Lumsden A, Gulisano M. 1997. Neocortical neurons: where do they come from? Science 278:402–403.

Lumsden A, Krumlauf R. 1996. Patterning the vertebrate neuraxis. Science 274:1109–1115.

Marigo V, Davey RA, Zuo Y, Cunningham JM, Tabin CJ. 1996. Biochemical evidence that patched is the Hedgehog receptor. Nature 384:176–179.

Marshall H, Nonchev S, Sham MH, Muchamore I, Lumsden A, Krumlauf R. 1992. Retinoic acid alters hindbrain *Hox* code and induces transformation of rhombomeres. Nature 360:737–741.

McMahon AP, Bradley A. 1990. The *Wnt-1 (int-1)* proto-oncogene is required for development of a large region of the mouse brain. Cell 62:1073–1085.

McMahon AP, Joyner AL, Bradley A, McMahon JA. 1992. The midbrain-hindbrain phenotype of *Wnt-1-/Wnt-1-* mice results from stepwise deletion of engrailed-expressing cells by 9.5 days postcoitum. Cell 69:581–595.

Nüsslein-Volhard C, Wieschaus E. 1980. Mutations affecting segment number and polarity in *Drosophila.* Nature 287:795–801.

O'Leary DD, Borngasser DJ, Fox K, Schlaggar BL. 1995. Plasticity in the development of neocortical areas. Ciba Found Symp 193:214–230.

Piccolo S, Sasai Y, Lu B, De Robertis EM. 1996. Dorsoventral patterning in *Xenopus*: inhibition of ventral signals by direct binding of chordin to BMP-4. Cell 86:589–598.

Porter JA, von Kessler DP, Ekker SC, Young KE, Lee JJ, Moses K, Beachy PA. 1995. The product of hedgehog autoproteolytic cleavage active in local and long-range signaling. Nature 374:363–366.

Porter JA, Young KE, Beachy PA. 1996. Cholesterol modification of hedgehog signaling proteins in animal development. Science 274:255–259.

Roelink H, Porter JA, Chiang C, Tanabe Y, Chang DT, Beachy PA, Jessell TM. 1995. Floor plate and motor neuron induction by different concentrations of the amino-terminal cleavage product of sonic hedgehog autoproteolysis. Cell 81:445–455.

Roessler E, Belloni E, Gaudenz K, Jay P, Berta P, Scherer SW, Tsui LC, Muenke M. 1996. Mutations in the human *Sonic hedgehog* gene cause holoprosencephaly. Nat Genet 14:357–360.

Sasai Y. 1998. Identifying the missing links: genes that connect neural induction and primary neurogenesis in vertebrate embryos. Neurons 21:455–458.

Schlaggar BL, O'Leary DD. 1991. Potential of visual cortex to develop an array of functional units unique to somatosensory cortex. Science 252:1556–1560.

Spemann H, Mangold H. 1924. Über Induktion von Embryonalangen durch Implantation artfremder Organisatoren. Wilhelm Roux Arch Entwicklungsmech Org 100:599–638.

Stone DM, Hynes M, Armanini M, Swanson TA, Gu Q, Johnson RL, Scott MP, Pennica D, Goddard A, Phillips H, Noll M, Hooper JE, de Sauvage F, Rosenthal A. 1996. The tumour-suppressor gene *patched* encodes a candidate receptor for sonic hedgehog. Nature 384:129–134.

Studer M, Lumsden A, Ariza-McNaughton L, Bradley A, Krumlauf R. 1996. Altered segmental identity and abnormal migration of motor neurons in mice lacking *Hoxb-1*. Nature 384:630–634.

Studer M, Popperl H, Marshall H, Kuroiwa A, Krumlauf R. 1994. Role of a conserved retinoic acid response element in rhombomere restriction of *Hoxb-1*. Science 265:1728–1732.

Whitman M. 1998. Smads and early developmental signaling by the TGFbeta superfamily. Genes Dev 12:2445–2462.

Xu Q, Alldus G, Holder N, Wilkinson DG. 1995. Expression of truncated Sek-1 receptor tyrosine kinase disrupts the segmental restriction of gene expression in the *Xenopus* and zebrafish hindbrain. Development 121:4005–4016.

Zimmerman LB, De Jesus-Escobar JM, Harland RM. 1996. The Spemann organizer signal noggin binds and inactivates bone morphogenetic protein 4. Cell 86:599–606.

53

The Generation and Survival of Nerve Cells

I N CHAPTER 52 WE SAW that local sources of inductive signals pattern the neural tube and establish the early regional subdivisions of the nervous system—the spinal cord, hindbrain, midbrain, and forebrain. We now turn to the question of how, within each of these regions, progenitor cells are directed to differentiate into neurons and glial cells, the two major cell types that populate the nervous system.

We first discuss the basic mechanisms of neurogenesis that endow cells with common neuronal properties (features that are independent of the region of the nervous system in which they are generated and the specific functions they perform). We next discuss some of the molecules that specify neuronal and glial cell fates and how they are regulated.

Cell differentiation, however, does not stop when a cell leaves the cell cycle and becomes a neuron. For a mature neuron to function it must express many highly specialized properties, particularly the transmitters that signal to other neurons and target organs and the receptors that permit the cell to respond to incoming synaptic inputs. In the second part of this chapter, we shall discuss the mechanisms by which neurons acquire some of these specialized properties.

Even after the identity and functional properties of the neuron have been fully established, developmental processes determine whether the neuron will live or die. Remarkably, almost half the neurons generated in the mammalian nervous system are lost through a process known as *programmed cell death*. We will therefore conclude the chapter by examining the factors that determine whether neurons survive or die and describing a conserved biochemical pathway that is responsible for the death of neural cells.

The Molecular Basis of Neuronal Generation Is Similar Throughout Phylogeny

Clues to the mechanisms controlling the differentiation of a dividing progenitor cell into a postmitotic neuron have emerged from molecular genetic studies of neurogenesis in *Drosophila melanogaster*. To understand the control of neuronal identity in vertebrates it is therefore

A Notch signalling between cells in proneural region is balanced

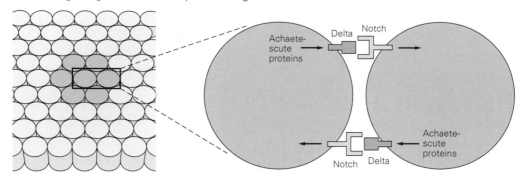

B A slight imbalance in notch signaling develops

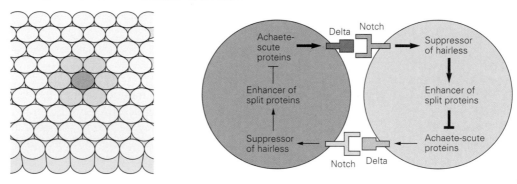

C The imbalance is quickly amplified, leading to development of a neuronal precursor

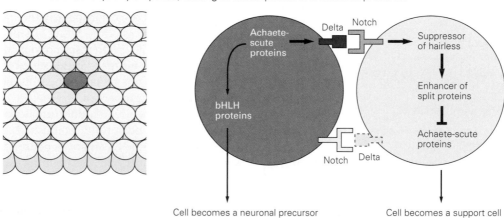

Cell becomes a neuronal precursor   Cell becomes a support cell

Figure 53-1 Notch signaling controls the specification of neural cell identity in *Drosophila*.

A. Notch signaling between cells is initially similar in the proneural region of the ectoderm that express *achaete-scute* class basic helix-loop-helix genes (**brown**).

B. A slight imbalance in notch signaling develops between cells in the proneural region. One cell begins to express higher levels of delta and thus activates notch to a higher level in the neighboring cell.

C. The initial imbalance in the level of notch signaling is rapidly amplified by a feedback pathway involving two transcription factors: suppressor of hairless and enhancer of split. Cells in which notch signaling is relatively low activate other basic helix-loop-helix (bHLH) proteins and progress to become neuroblast precursors, and cells in which notch signaling is high become support cells.

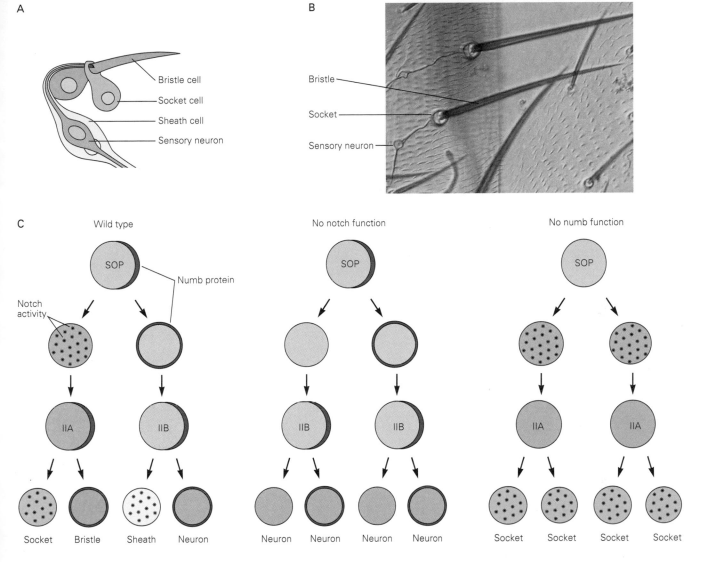

Figure 53-2 Numb inhibits notch signaling and controls neural fate in *Drosophila*.

A, B. A typical *Drosophila* sensory bristle comprises four cells—the hair cell, socket cell, sheath cell, and a sensory neuron. The development of these distinct cells depends on the asymmetric cell divisions of a sensory organ precursor (SOP) cell. (Image in B provided by Y. N. Jan.)

C. Within the SOP cell, the numb protein is localized to one side only. When the SOP divides, numb is inherited by only one of the daughter cells, cell IIB which gives rise to the sensory neuron and sheath cell. The cell that does not receive numb, cell IIA, expresses a high level of notch activity and gives rise to the bristle and socket cells. In the absence of notch function both daughters of the SOP cell acquire cell IIB-like properties, and the further division of these cells give rise to neurons. In mutants lacking *numb* gene function, notch activity is high and both daughters of the SOP cell acquire cell IIA properties, and the later division of these cells forms only socket cells. (From Lu et al. 1998.)

necessary to review briefly the key mechanisms and molecules used in *Drosophila*.

The selection of a single neuron from a large and initially uniform population of ectodermal cells in *Drosophila* involves a program of cell interactions that gradually restrict the fate of a cell. The initial step in this program is the recruitment of a small cluster of ectodermal cells that acquire the potential to give rise to neuronal precursors (Figure 53-1A). This region of the ectoderm is known as the *proneural region*. Within each

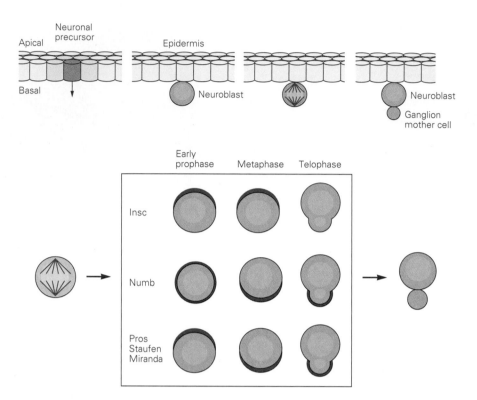

Figure 53-3 Subcellular localization of numb during mitosis of *Drosophila* neuroblasts. Neuroblasts in *Drosophila* arise by segregating basally from the overlying epithelial cell layer (**top**). The neuroblast then divides asymmetrically along its apical-basal axis to generate a larger apical cell that retains neuroblast characteristics and a smaller basal ganglion mother cell. During this division numb and several other proteins become segregated to the ganglion mother cell. The **bottom figure** illustrates the asymmetric localization of inscuteable (Insc), numb, prospero (Pros), staufen, and miranda. (From Knoblich 1997.)

Inscuteable is a cytoskeletal protein transiently localized to the apical side of the neuroblast. Inscuteable functions upstream of miranda, which appears to act as an adaptor protein that localizes prospero, numb, and staufen to the basal cortical membrane. Prior to mitosis a complex of inscuteable and

staufen appears to bind *prospero* RNA in the apical region of the neuroblast, where *prospero* RNA is translated. At the beginning of mitosis the *inscuteable-staufen-prospero* complex is translocated to the basal cortex perhaps by a microfilament-dependent mechanism that also depends on miranda activity. Numb, miranda, staufen, and prospero are then segregated to the ganglion mother cell.

This linkage between the cellular machinery for protein localization and the cell cycle in *Drosophila* ensures asymmetric inheritance of proteins that specify neuronal fates. It seems likely that similar mechanisms control protein segregation and neuronal fates in the vertebrate nervous system. Blue, brown and orange areas denote localization of the proteins. (Modified from Knoblich 1997.)

proneural region only a few cells will become neurons; the others will remain as nonneuronal support cells of the epidermis.

Neuronal fate is decided by a process of signaling between adjacent cells in the proneural region. This process depends on the interactions between two cell-surface proteins encoded by the neurogenic genes *delta* and *notch*. Both proteins span the cell membrane: delta functions as a ligand, and notch is its receptor. Initially all cells in the proneural region express both proteins at similar levels. The activation of notch by delta initiates a local feedback signal between adjacent cells whose purpose is to ensure that even a minor difference in the ini-

tial level of notch activity is amplified rapidly to generate a large discrepancy in the state of notch activation and consequently in cell fate. Cells in which notch is activated to high levels are inhibited from acquiring a neuronal fate, whereas cells with a relatively low level of notch signaling become neurons.

This feedback circuit functions in the following manner. Activation of notch in one cell (cell A) initiates an intracellular signaling cascade that involves proteolytic cleavage of the cytoplasmic domain of notch, the translocation of this domain into the nucleus, and the activation of a transcription factor, called suppressor of hairless (see Figure 53-1B). Suppressor of hairless is one

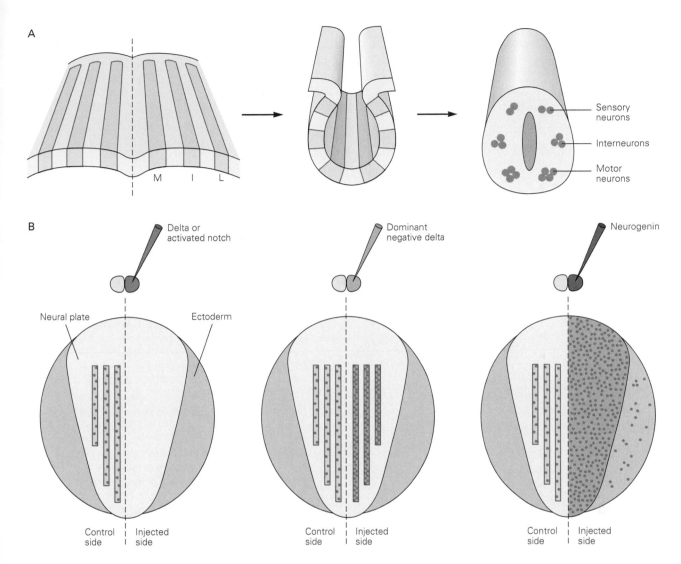

Figure 53-4 Notch signaling regulates neuronal fate in the vertebrate central nervous system. Primary neurogenesis in *Xenopus* and the effect of manipulation of notch signaling on expression of basic helix-loop-helix genes and neuronal differentiation.

A. Three domains of primary neuron differentiation in the neural plate develop as parallel stripes (L, lateral; I, intermediate; and M, medial). Cells in these three stripes become sensory neurons, interneurons, and motor neurons within the neural tube.

B. Activation of notch signaling by injection of delta or a constitutively active form of notch inhibits neuronal differentiation in these stripes. Inhibition of notch signaling by injection of a dominant negative form of delta increases the number of neurons generated within these stripes. Expression of neurogenin (or another basic helix-loop-helix protein neuroD) induces additional neuronal differentiation. Additional neurons are also found outside the three stripes and in the nonneural ectoderm. (Adapted from Chitnis et al. 1995 and Anderson and Jan 1997.)

of a large group of transcription factors of the basic helix-loop-helix class that are encoded by *proneural* genes and play critical roles in neurogenesis. Suppressor of hairless activates the expression of inhibitory basic helix-loop-helix proteins of the enhancer of split class, which represses expression of still other helix-loop-helix genes, *achaete-scute* genes. Finally the activation of achaete-scute proteins leads to a decrease in expression of delta on the cell surface. Although first recognized in the context of neurogenesis, notch signaling via helix-loop-helix proteins is now known to be a mechanism used throughout the *Drosophila* embryo to impose different fates upon initially equivalent cell populations.

Notch signaling is also regulated by other proteins, notably a cytoplasmic protein called numb that binds to

A Neural crest cells migrate from the dorsal
neural tube along different paths

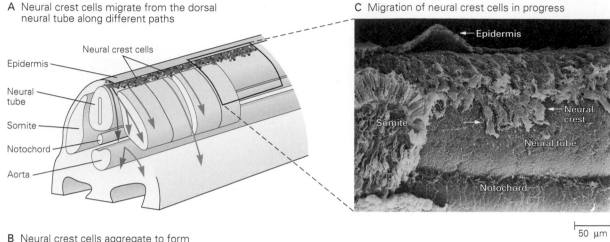

C Migration of neural crest cells in progress

B Neural crest cells aggregate to form
sensory and autonomic ganglia

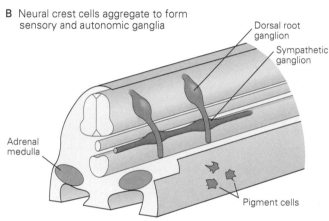

Figure 53-5 The main pathways of neural crest cell migration in a chick embryo. The diagram shows a section through the middle part of the trunk.

A. Neural crest cells that take a superficial migratory pathway, just beneath the ectoderm, form pigment cells of the skin. Those that take an intermediate pathway via the somites form sensory ganglia, and those that take a more medial pathway form sympathetic ganglia and the cells of the adrenal medulla.

B. Positions at which melanocytes, the sympathetic and sensory ganglia, and the adrenal gland are located after neural crest migration is complete.

C. Scanning electron micrograph showing neural crest cells migrating away from the dorsal surface of the neural tube of a chick embryo. (Courtesy of K. Tosney.)

the intracellular domain of notch and in doing so inhibits notch signaling (Figure 53-2). During the division of certain neural progenitor cells, only one of the two daughter cells receives the numb protein (Figure 53-3), and the cells that inherit the numb protein become neurons. What is the purpose of having notch regulated by numb? In the proneural cluster described above, the choice of which cell becomes a neuron may be made at random, by a so-called stochastic process. In other cases, however, a particular product of mitosis regularly acquires a specific fate—for example, the anterior daughter might become a neuron and the posterior one a glial cell. In these cases proteins such as numb could activate notch in one of the two daughters, thereby determining cell fate. Thus, the basic program of neurogenesis may underlie both indeterminate and determinate lineage decisions, depending on whether the outcome of the notch-delta competition is decided stochastically or biased by regulatory factors such as numb.

The basic mechanisms controlling vertebrate neurogenesis are similar to those operating in *Drosophila*. Vertebrate neural cells express both delta and notch pro-

teins. The roles of these proteins in the determination of neuronal fate have been analyzed most extensively in the frog *Xenopus laevis*. Early in the development of the *Xenopus* nervous system, primary (early-born) neurons are generated within three longitudinally arrayed stripes. Cells in the medial stripe become motor neurons, those in the intermediate stripe become interneurons, and those in the lateral stripe become primary sensory neurons. Before the onset of neuronal differentiation the *delta* gene is expressed only in these three stripes, whereas the *notch* gene is expressed in both the stripe and interstripe regions (Figure 53-4).

To reveal the roles of the delta and notch proteins in the generation of neurons the *delta* and *notch* genes were overexpressed in *Xenopus* embryos. Expression of *delta* or an activated version of *notch* markedly inhibits the generation of primary neurons. Conversely, expression of a truncated form of *delta,* one thought to inhibit notch signaling, generates additional primary neurons. Thus, notch-delta interactions regulate neurogenesis in vertebrates as they do in flies.

In all cases of notch-delta misexpression, primary

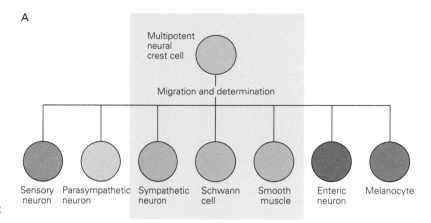

Figure 53-6 The progeny of the neural crest.

A. Many different classes of neurons, glial cells, and other cell types develop from the neural crest cells. (Adapted from Anderson 1989.)

B. Specific growth factors control the fate of certain neural crest cells. Bone morphogenetic proteins 2 and 4 (BMP2,4) promote the differentiation of sympathetic neurons, GGF represses neurogenesis and promotes Schwann cell differentiation, and TGFβ promotes smooth muscle cell differentiation. (Adapted from Shah et al. 1996.)

neurons are generated only within the three stripes (see Figure 53-4). These three stripes can therefore be viewed as equivalent to the proneural regions of the *Drosophila* ectoderm. Why is neurogenesis in the neural plate restricted to these stripes? Neural plate cells contain several basic helix-loop-helix proteins that are closely related in structure to the *Drosophila* proneural proteins and promote neurogenesis in a similar manner. To provide one example, we consider the role of *neurogenin,* a basic helix-loop-helix gene that is expressed prior to *delta* in the three proneural stripes. If *neurogenin* is overexpressed in the *Xenopus* neural plate, additional neurons are formed. Moreover, in contrast to the results obtained simply by inhibiting notch signaling, the additional neurons induced by *neurogenin* are not restricted to the three neural plate stripes (see Figure 53-4). Thus notch-and-delta control neurogenesis only in the domain that expresses neurogenic basic helix-loop-helix genes. Studies of defects

in neurogenesis that occur in mice lacking basic helix-loop-helix genes have confirmed that these genes have important roles in promoting the differentiation of neurons.

Neuronal and Glial Fates Are Controlled by Local Signaling

In most regions of the nervous system neural precursors develop into glial cells as well as neurons. Indeed, the number of glial cells vastly exceeds that of neurons. How are glial cells generated? One of the best understood systems for studying the distinction between neuronal and glial fates has been the *neural crest,* a migratory cell population that emerges from the dorsal neural tube and rapidly disperses along different pathways in the periphery (Figure 53-5). The extensive migration of neural crest cells and the ability of researchers to culture

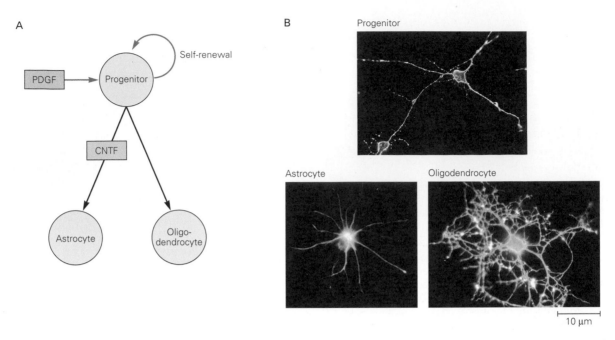

Figure 53-7 Growth factors control glial cell diversification in the rat optic nerve.

A. PDGF secreted by astrocytes maintains the proliferation of oligodendrocyte progenitor cells. Postnatally, these progenitor cells begin to lose sensitivity to PDGF, even though the factor is still present in the local environment and cells begin to differentiate into oligodendrocytes. Later, astrocytes begin to se-

crete CNTF, which helps to promote the differentiation of progenitor cells into astrocytes. (Adapted from Lillien and Raff 1990.)

B. Micrographs showing cultured progenitor cells, astrocytes labeled with an antibody against glial-fibrillary acidic protein, and oligodendrocytes labeled with an antibody against galacto-cerebroside. (From Raff et al. 1990.)

these cells at clonal density has made it possible to analyze in detail the role of local environmental signals in the control of neuronal and glial cell fate.

An early advance in analyzing the control of neural crest cell differentiation came from the studies of Nicole Le Douarin and her colleagues in the late 1960s. Le Douarin appreciated that the difference in condensation of chromatin within the nuclei of chick and quail cells could be exploited as a permanent cell lineage marker for tracing the fate of quail neural crest cells grafted into chick hosts. Le Douarin found that neural crest cells from the same position along the neural tube give rise to many distinct cell types, including neurons, Schwann cells, and melanocytes (Figure 53-6A). In addition, neural crest cells transplanted to a different rostrocaudal level of the neural axis often generated cell types characteristic of the level to which the graft was made rather than of the level from which the graft was taken. These findings led to the idea that the different environments encountered by neural crest cells as they migrate in the periphery—and the distinct signals produced by these environments—appear to have a critical role in controlling their fate.

Secreted Factors Direct the Differentiation of Neural Crest Cells into Neurons and Glia

What are the environmental signals that control the fate of neural crest cells? This question has been addressed in most detail for the subset of neural crest cells that migrate ventrally to form autonomic ganglia. One class of signals that impose neuronal identity on these cells are *bone morphogenetic proteins* (BMPs), the factors responsible at an earlier stage of development for inducing the differentiation of premigratory neural crest cells in the dorsal neural tube (see Figure 53-6B). The induction of autonomic neurons by BMP signals also requires the expression of a basic helix-loop-helix protein called mash-1; thus basic helix-loop-helix transcription factors are required for the generation of both peripheral and central neurons.

Why don't all neural crest cells become neurons? Here the execution of the neurogenic program described above may be regulated by additional local factors in the environment of the developing neuron. For example, the formation of neurons from neural crest cells appears to be under negative regulation by glial growth factor (GGF), a member of a family of neural cell surface proteins encoded by the *neuregulin* gene. GGF is expressed on the surface of autonomic neurons at the time they first differentiate and appears to act on nearby neural crest cells to prevent neurogenesis, directing them instead along a pathway of glial differentiation. The expression of GGF by newly differentiated neurons therefore may provide a feedback signal that ensures an appropriate balance of Schwann cells and neurons within each ganglion.

Glial Cell Differentiation in the Central Nervous System Is Also Controlled by Diffusible Factors

The generation of glial cells in the central nervous system is also controlled by secreted signaling factors. There are two major classes of glial cells in the central nervous system: astrocytes and oligodendrocytes. The program of oligodendrocyte differentiation is controlled by platelet-derived growth factor (PDGF). In the absence of PDGF, oligodendrocyte progenitors stop dividing and almost immediately differentiate. In the presence of PDGF, progenitor cells continue to proliferate for a prolonged period, resulting in an eventual increase in the number of oligodendrocytes (Figure 53-7). The differentiation of progenitor cells into astrocytes is, in contrast, promoted by ciliary neurotrophic factor (CNTF). Thus in the central nervous system the differentiation of progenitor cells into astrocytes and oligodendrocytes is also controlled by secreted growth factors. The PDGF that controls oligodendrocyte fate may be produced and secreted by astrocytes. Such interactions between glial subtypes would help to ensure that proper numbers of each cell type are generated.

Neuronal Fate in the Mammalian Cortex Is Influenced by the Timing of Cell Differentiation

Do the principles of neuronal differentiation that have emerged from studies of early neurogenesis in vertebrates also apply in higher centers of the human brain such as the cerebral cortex? The neurons of the cerebral cortex are generated in the ventricular zone, an epithelial layer of progenitor cells that lines the lateral ventricles. Once they have left the cell cycle, the immature neurons migrate out of the ventricular zone to form the cortical plate, which eventually becomes the gray matter of the cerebral cortex. To reach the cortical plate, the neurons migrate on radial glial cells, a specialized class of glial cells that retain contact with both the ventrical and pial surfaces (Figure 53-8).

Within the cortical plate, neurons become organized into well-defined layers. Remarkably, the final position of a cortical neuron, and therefore its final laminar position is correlated precisely with the birthday of the neuron. (The term *birthday* refers to the time at which a dividing precursor undergoes its final round of cell division and gives rise to a postmitotic neuron.) Cells that migrate from the ventricular zone and leave the cell cycle at early stages give rise to neurons that settle in the deepest layers of the cortex. In contrast, cells that leave the ventricular zone and exit the cell cycle at progressively later stages migrate over longer distances, past early-born neurons, and settle in more superficial layers of the cortex (Figure 53-8A). Thus, the layering of neurons in the cerebral cortex is established in an inside-first, outside-last manner.

When is the subtype identity of newly generated cortical neurons acquired? This question has been addressed in experiments in which progenitor cells from the ventricular zone of young animals were transplanted into older hosts. Normally, these cells migrate to deep layers, but in the older host the transplanted cells intermingled with cells on their way to superficial layers. Remarkably, the fate of the transplanted cells turns out to depend on the phase of the cell cycle they are in at the time of transplantation (see Figure 53-8B). Progenitor cells in S phase at the time of transplantation acquire the fate of neurons generated at later stages of cortical neurogenesis. That is, they give rise to neurons that settle in the superficial layers of the cortex. In contrast, cells that have passed through their final S phase prior to transplantation adopt the normal fate of neurons generated at early stages of cortical neurogenesis. That is, they migrate to layers 5 and 6. Thus young cortical progenitor cells remain sensitive to time-dependent environmental signals that direct their fate, but as they become postmitotic they become committed to a specific fate.

In contrast, progenitor cells present at later stages are not able to acquire the fate of younger neurons when transplanted in the ventricular zone of a younger host. Hence, not only do the signals that direct neurons to specific laminae change, but also the competence of the neurons to respond to those signals changes as development proceeds.

What controls the decision of a cortical progenitor cell to remain proliferative or to differentiate into a neuron? Early in neural development the progenitor cells that give rise to neurons of the mature cerebral cortex proliferate rapidly and give rise to additional progenitors, expanding the population of neuronal precursor cells. At later stages, however, progenitor cells alter their program of cell division and give rise both to neu-

A Cortical cells obey an inside-first outside-last program of neurogenesis

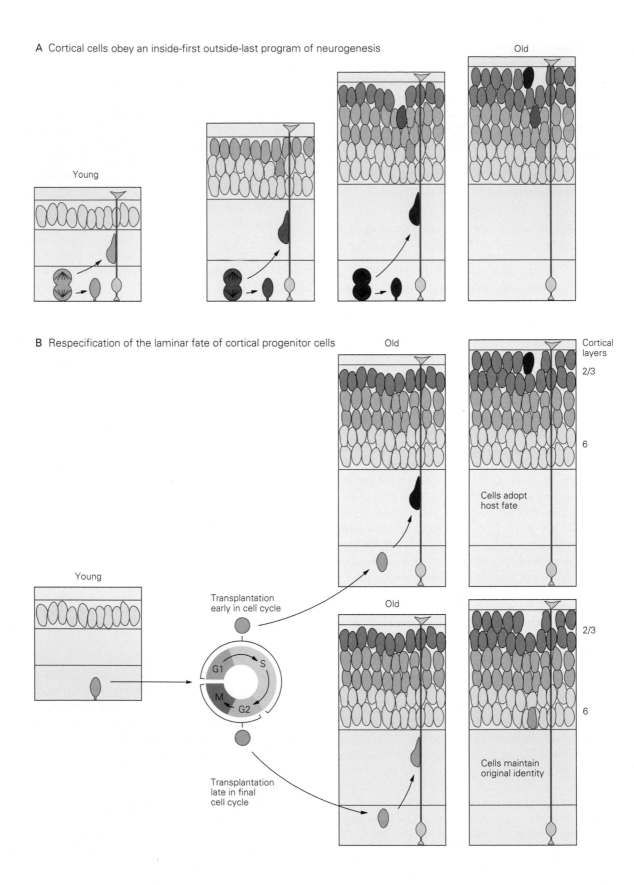

B Respecification of the laminar fate of cortical progenitor cells

rons and to additional progenitor cells. At a still later stage they generate only neurons.

By time-lapse monitoring of the ventricular zone in real time, progenitor cells in the cerebral cortex have been shown to divide in an asymmetric manner. The orientation of the plane of cleavage of cortical progenitor cells—and consequently whether the division of the cell is symmetric or asymmetric—correlates with the fate of the cell. Cells that undergo vertical cleavage—in a plane perpendicular to the ventricular surface—divide symmetrically and generate two similar daughter cells that remain in the ventricular zone. As a consequence, these cells undergo additional rounds of proliferation, expanding the population of progenitor cells in the ventricular zone. Cells that undergo horizontal cleavage—in a plane parallel to the ventricular zone—appear to divide asymmetrically, generating two daughter cells that have distinctive morphologies and migratory behaviors. The basal daughter cell loses its attachment to the ventricular surface of the cortex and migrates out of the ventricular zone to give rise to a young neuron. The apical cell, however, remains in the ventricular zone and undergoes further rounds of cell division (Figure 53-9). Regulation of the plane of division of progenitor cells may therefore help to determine the timing of neurogenesis in the cerebral cortex.

What molecules determine the distinct fates of the cells that have undergone asymmetric divisions? In

Drosophila one way of determining cell fate after an asymmetric division is through the unequal distribution of the numb protein to daughter cells during mitosis and the consequent modulation of Notch activity. Thus it is intriguing to find that in the ventricular zone of the forebrain a vertebrate numb-like protein becomes asymmetrically localized as progenitor cells enter mitosis. In contrast, notch expression is more uniform. The role of numb and notch in cortical progenitor cells is not well understood, but these observations suggest that the principles of neurogenesis defined in *Drosophila* may be at work in the cerebral cortex.

The Neurotransmitter Phenotype of a Neuron Is Controlled by Signals From the Neuronal Target

Neuronal differentiation does not stop when a cell leaves the cell cycle and migrates to its final position. For a mature neuron to participate in neuronal circuits it must express many specialized properties, the most important being a chemical transmitter that permits the cell to signal to other neurons.

The mechanisms that control the neurotransmitter phenotype have been studied in most detail in sympathetic neurons. Most sympathetic neurons use norepinephrine as their primary transmitter, but some—for example, those that innervate the exocrine sweat glands in the foot pads—use acetylcholine instead. These neurons express norepinephrine when they first innervate the sweat glands of the skin, but they stop synthesizing norepinephrine and switch to making acetylcholine once their axons have contacted the sweat glands.

The cells of the sweat gland target are critical in inducing cholinergic properties in sympathetic neurons. This influence was shown by transplanting the sweat glands from the foot pad of a newborn rat into a site in the skin that normally is innervated by noradrenergic sympathetic neurons. Those neurons that innervate the ectopic sweat glands acquired cholinergic transmitter properties. Other studies have shown that sympathetic neurons switch gradually from noradrenergic to cholinergic properties, passing through a stage in which the neuron releases both norepinephrine and acetylcholine.

The switch from noradrenergic to cholinergic neurotransmitter phenotype can be induced in cultured neurons by several factors, notably two members of the interleukin 6 class of cytokines: leukemia inhibitory factor (LIF) and CNTF. Sympathetic neurons that have been exposed to these factors undergo a coordinated change in their cellular properties. For example, factors that pro-

Figure 53-8 (Opposite) Generation and migration of neurons in the mammalian cerebral cortex. (Adapted from Chen et al. 1997.)

A. Cortical neurons are generated in an inside-first, outside-last order. Neurons born within the ventricular zone at early stages migrate to the deepest layers of the cortical plate. Neurons generated at later stages migrate past the earlier-generated neurons to form the more superficial layers of the cortex.

B. Respecification of the laminar fate of cortical progenitor cells. Transplantation of progenitor cells from young animals to older hosts changes the fate of cortical neurons. Ventricular zone progenitor cells destined to give rise to neurons in the deep layers adopt different fates when transplanted into the ventricular zone of older host brain at a time when upper-layer neurons are being generated. Those progenitors transplanted late during early S phase of the cell cycle generate daughters that migrate to upper layers 2 and 3, as do neurons being generated in the host environment. In contrast, cells transplanted during late S phase or in G2 or M phases of their final cell cycle retain their original laminar identity and migrate to the deeper layers (5 and 6).

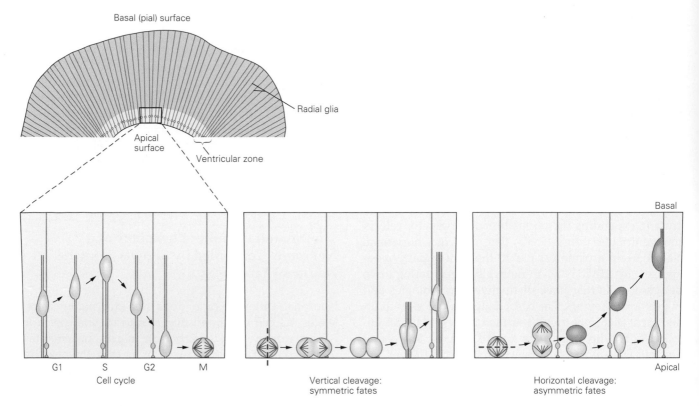

Figure 53-9 The plane of division of progenitor cells in the ventricular zone of the cerebral cortex influences their fate. The nuclei of ventricular zone precursors migrate during the cell cycle. During the G1 phase of the cell cycle, nuclei rise from the inner (apical) surface of the ventricular zone. During the S phase the nuclei reside in the outer (basal) third of the ventricular zone. During G2 the nuclei migrate apically, and mitosis occurs when the nuclei reach the ventricular surface.

The vertical cleavage (perpendicular to the ventricular surface) of progenitor cells generates two similar daughters that retain their apical connections. Following mitosis, the nuclei of both cells reenter the cell cycle.

The horizontal cleavage (parallel to the ventricular surface) produces an asymmetric division in which the apical daughter retains contact with the apical surface and the basal daughter loses its apical contact. The basal daughter migrates away from the ventricular zone and later becomes a postmitotic neuron. (Adapted from Chen and McConnell 1995.)

mote acetylcholine synthesis also cause a change in the molecular properties of their synaptic vesicles, from the large dense-core granules found in noradrenergic neurons to the small electron-translucent vesicles typical of cholinergic neurons (Figure 53-10). In vivo the sweat gland appears to secrete interleukin 6-like molecules that induce cholinergic properties in neurons that would otherwise become or remain adrenergic. Thus many, and perhaps all, of the neurotransmitter properties of these neurons are likely to be controlled by factors from the environment of the cell's synaptic target. This form of control may not be used universally, however, for many neurons in the brain the choice of neurotransmitter appears to be part of the cells' intrinsic neurogenic program.

The Survival of a Neuron Is Also Regulated by Signals From the Neuronal Target

We have seen that many biochemical properties of a neuron are imposed by signals from surrounding cells, even after the neuron has left the cell cycle and acquired the ability to synthesize its characteristic neurotransmitter. Apart from its identity, the very survival of the neuron itself depends on factors released from surrounding cells. As with the control of neurotransmitter phenotype, factors essential for neuronal survival are provided by the target of the neuron.

The discovery of the critical role of target cells in neuronal survival has its origins in studies in the 1920s

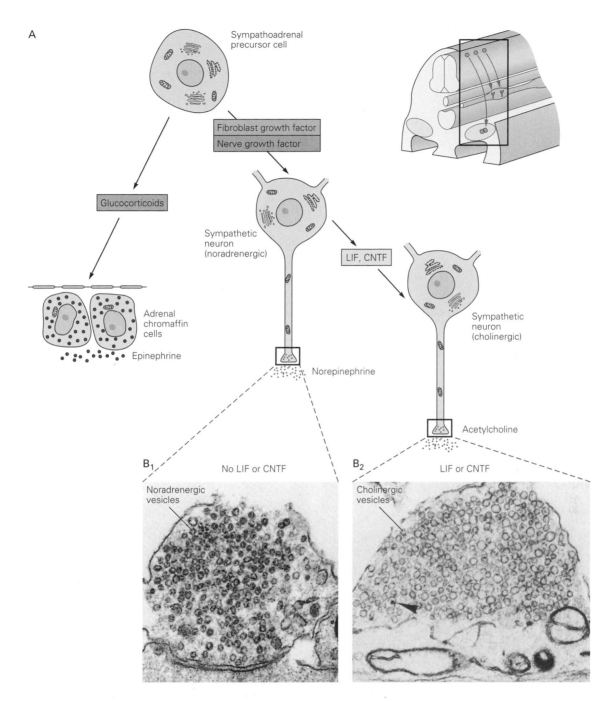

Figure 53-10 Target-dependent differentiation of neurons in the sympathoadrenal lineage of the neural crest.

A. The developmental potential of an undifferentiated precursor cell in the sympathoadrenal lineage. The differentiation of chromaffin cells from neural crest precursors is triggered by the migration of these cells into the adrenal gland, where they are exposed to high levels of glucocorticoids synthesized by the adrenal cortex. NGF induces precursor cells to differentiate into sympathetic neurons, which possess 50-nm electron-dense synaptic vesicles and synthesize norepinephrine as transmitter. If these neurons are cultured in medium containing LIF or other related cytokines, they acquire cholinergic properties, synthe-

size acetylcholine, and contain small (30–50 nm) electron-translucent synaptic vesicles. (Adapted from Doupe et al. 1985.)

B. The morphology of synaptic vesicles in cultured sympathetic neurons grown in the absence (**1**) or presence (**2**) of a cholinergic-inducing factor such as LIF or CNTF. In sympathetic neurons grown without these factors adrenergic differentiation is maintained and nerve terminals contain dense-core synaptic vesicles. Sympathetic neurons grown with medium containing cytokines have terminal varicosities that contain almost exclusively clear synaptic vesicles. (Adapted from Landis 1980.)

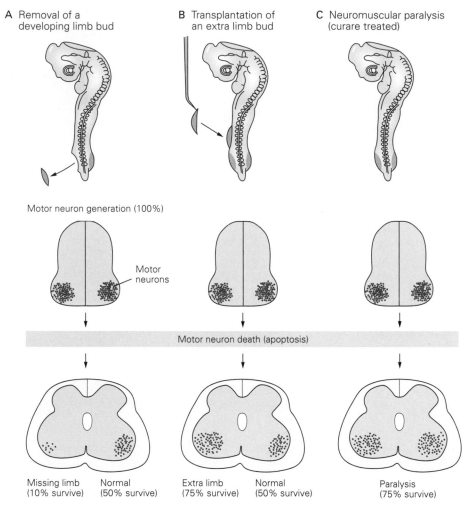

A Removal of a developing limb bud

B Transplantation of an extra limb bud

C Neuromuscular paralysis (curare treated)

Motor neuron generation (100%)

Motor neurons

Motor neuron death (apoptosis)

Missing limb (10% survive)   Normal (50% survive)

Extra limb (75% survive)   Normal (50% survive)

Paralysis (75% survive)

Figure 53-11 Changing the size or activity of the muscle target controls the survival of motor neurons. (Adapted from Purves 1988.)

A. Removing a developing limb results in a marked decrease in the number of motor neurons. Limb bud amputation is performed in a chick embryo at about 2.5 days. Although motor neurons are generated in normal numbers, later in development few motor neurons remain on the side of the spinal cord on the side of the missing limb. The number of motor neurons on the contralateral side is about 50% of the number generated originally.

B. Increasing the size of the limb target reduces the extent of naturally occurring neuronal death during development. Transplantation of an extra limb bud prior to the normal period of cell death in a chick embryo results in an increased number of limb motor neurons on the side with additional target tissue.

C. Blocking muscle activity prevents the developmental death of motor neurons. Neuromuscular transmission is blocked early in development by application of curare, a drug that blocks activation of acetylcholine receptors. Blockade of neuromuscular transmission with curare reduces the extent of motor neuron death in the lumbar spinal cord.

and 1930s by Samuel Detwiler and Viktor Hamburger, who showed that the number of sensory neurons in the dorsal root ganglion of amphibian embryos was increased by transplantation of an additional limb bud into the target field. Conversely, the number of neurons was markedly decreased by removing the normal target. At this time the target-evoked change in neuronal number was thought to reflect the influence of the target on the proliferation and differentiation of sensory neuroblasts.

In the 1940s, however, this interpretation was questioned by Rita Levi-Montalcini, prompted by her startling observation that the death of neurons is a normal occurrence during embryonic development. In key experiments, she and Victor Hamburger showed that removing the limb from a chick embryo led to excessive death of sensory neurons that would have innervated the limb.

Neuronal cell death also occurs during the development of the central nervous system. Hamburger showed

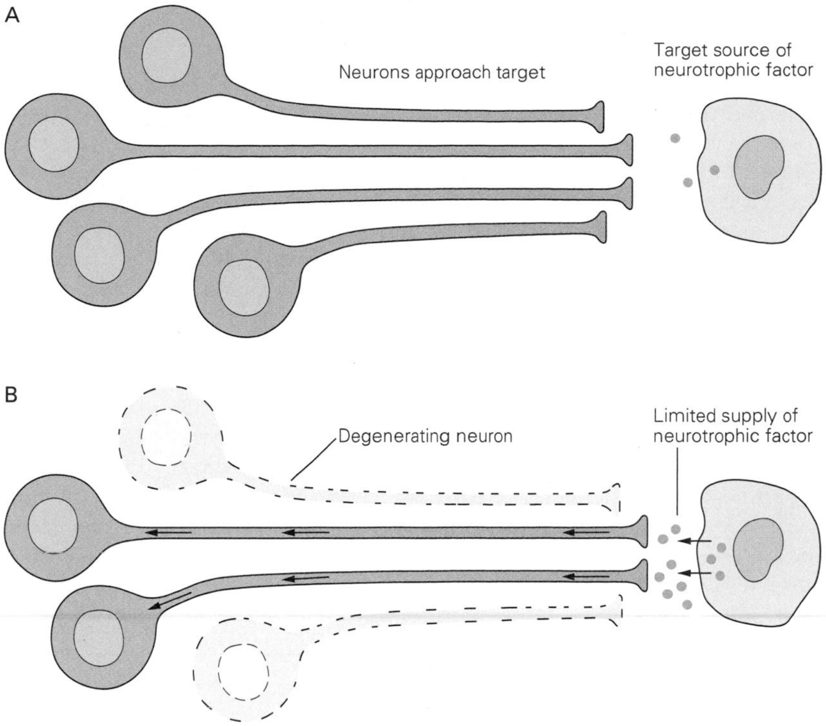

Figure 53-12 The neurotrophic factor hypothesis. (Adapted from Reichardt and Fariñas 1997.)

A. Neurons extend axons to the vicinity of target cells.

B. The target cells secrete limited amounts of neurotrophic factors. The neurotrophic factors bind to specific cell surface receptors. Neurons that do not receive adequate amounts of neurotrophic factor die by apoptosis with fragmented nuclei.

that about half of the motor neurons generated in the lateral motor column of the chick spinal cord are destined to die during embryonic development. Moreover, in experiments similar to those conducted on sensory ganglia, Hamburger found that the number of motor neurons that died was increased by removing the target and reduced by adding an additional limb (Figure 53-11). Thus the size of the muscle target is critical for the survival of spinal motor neurons. The process of neuronal overproduction followed by death is now known to occur in almost all regions of the central and peripheral nervous systems.

The findings of Hamburger and Levi-Montalcini led to the *neurotrophic factor hypothesis*, the idea that the target cells of developing neurons produce a limited amount of an essential nutrient or trophic factor that is taken up by the nerve terminals (Figure 53-12). On the strength of this hypothesis, Levi-Montalcini and Stanley Cohen isolated nerve growth factor (NGF), the first neurotrophic factor to be identified by assaying sensory neurons in cell culture (Box 53-1). The identification of NGF provided the first direct support for the neurotrophic hypothesis.

Studies of the development of spinal motor neurons showed that the survival of motor neurons depends on the state of muscle activity. Blockade of neuromuscular transmission by drugs such as curare produces a dramatic enhancement in the number of motor neurons that survive (Figure 52-11). Conversely, direct stimula-

tion of the muscle enhances the death of motor neurons.

The level of activity of a target cell or the neuron could, in turn, influence survival of the neuron in several ways. Activity in the target cell could inhibit production of the neurotrophic factor. Because the supply of the neurotrophic factor is thought normally to be limited, any reduction in the supply would lead to a greater degree of neuronal death. However, electrical activity in the neurons themselves also appears to be required for appropriate responses to neurotrophic factors. Thus, activity might regulate both production of and responsiveness to neurotrophic factors, thereby permitting the extent to which a neuronal population is used to shape its eventual number.

Target Cells Secrete a Variety of Neurotrophic Factors

The discovery of NGF was a milestone in the study of growth factors and prompted the search for other neurotrophic factors. We now know that NGF is merely one of a large array of secreted factors that have the ability to promote the survival of neurons (Table 53-1). The best studied class of trophic factors are the *neurotrophins*. Four major neurotrophins have been isolated from mammals: NGF, brain-derived neurotrophic factor (BDNF), neurotrophin 3 (NT3), and neurotrophin 4/5 (NT4,5) (Figure 53-13A). The neurotrophins are struc-

Box 53-1 Discovery of Nerve Growth Factor

Shortly after Viktor Hamburger and Rita Levi-Montalcini determined that target tissues have a critical role in regulating the number of surviving neurons, Elmer Bueker, Hamburger's former student, performed experiments to determine whether the implantation of various tumor tissues into mice might serve as a substitute peripheral target supporting the survival of sensory neurons. Bueker found that mouse sarcoma tissue evoked extensive growth of sensory fibers into the tumor. He also observed that dorsal root ganglia near the site of implanted tumors were significantly larger than the corresponding ganglia on the opposite side of the spinal cord.

These studies were extended by Levi-Montalcini and Hamburger, who noted a dramatic increase in the size of sympathetic ganglia in the vicinity of the sarcoma implant. Further experiments showed that the effect of sarcoma cells was caused by a diffusible factor. Levi-Montalcini developed quantitative assays to measure the effects of the tumor tissue on the survival and outgrowth of axons from sensory and sympathetic ganglia in vitro. Together with Stanley Cohen he began

to purify the diffusible molecule, which by this time had been named nerve growth factor (NGF).

In a key biochemical experiment, Cohen and Levi-Montalcini attempted to exclude DNA or RNA as a source of the neurotrophic activity. By chance they used a crude preparation of snake venom as a source of a phosphodiesterase activity intended to degrade any nucleic acids present in partially purified preparations of the factor. Instead they found that the snake venom itself produced a greater degree of axon outgrowth than did NGF itself.

Cohen then investigated a mammalian counterpart of the snake venom gland, the male mouse submaxillary gland, and found that it was a rich source of NGF. This insightful observation provided an abundant source of NGF for purification and protein sequencing. Subsequent work has shown that the protein exists as a complex of three subunits, with a molecular weight of 130,000. The active component is the β subunit, a 118-amino-acid sequence that exists in solution as a homodimer.

---

turally related to NGF, and the entire family exhibits a distant relationship to members of the transforming growth factor β (TGFβ) family.

The neurotrophins interact with two major classes of receptors. The major signal-transducing receptors are a family of three membrane-spanning tyrosine kinases

Table 53-1 A Partial List of Neurotrophic Factors

Neurotrophin class
  Nerve growth factor
  Brain-derived neurotrophic factor
  Neurotrophin 3
  Neurotrophin 4/5

Interleukin 6 class
  Ciliary neurotrophic factor
  Leukemia inhibitory factor
  Cardiotrophin

Transforming growth factor β class
  Transforming growth factor β 3
  Bone morphogenetic proteins
  Glial-derived neurotrophic factor
  Neurturin
  Persephin
  Artemin

Fibroblast growth factor class

Hepatocyte growth factor

named trkA, trkB, and trkC, each of which exists as a dimer (see Figure 53-13A). NGF interacts selectively with trkA, whereas brain-derived neurotrophic factor and neurotrophin 4/5 interact primarily with trkB. Neurotrophin 3 activates trkC and, to a lesser extent, trkB. As with other tyrosine kinase receptors, activation of the trk receptors depends on the dimerization of the receptor, a process initiated by the binding of the neurotrophin ligand. Phosphorylation of the cytoplasmic domain of trk receptors recruits specific signaling molecules within the neuron (Figure 53-14), many of which are also used by other tyrosine kinase receptors.

The neurotrophins also bind to a receptor called p75^{NTR} (see Figure 53-13). In contrast to the trk receptors, each neurotrophin binds to p75^{NTR} with similar affinity. The p75^{NTR} receptor is thought to have several functions. First, it can present NGF to trkA. Second, it transmits intracellular signals directly through activation of transduction pathways that depend on signals triggered by membrane lipids. Paradoxically, the activation of the p75^{NTR} receptor in cells that lack trk receptors has been shown to promote rather than prevent neuronal cell death.

In addition to the neurotrophins, other classes of proteins that promote neuronal survival include members of the TGFβ family, the interleukin 6-related cytokines, fibroblast growth factors, and sonic hedgehog. Thus the secreted proteins that have patterning roles at early stages of neural development are also active later in controlling the survival of neurons.

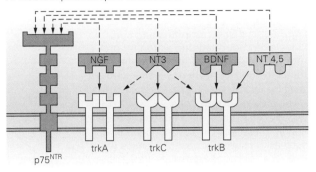

A Neurotrophin receptor interactions

Figure 53-13 Neurotrophic factors and their receptors.

A. Neurotrophins interact with tyrosine kinase receptors of the trk class. The figure illustrates the interactions of each member of the neurotrophin family with the trk proteins. Strong interactions are depicted with **solid arrows;** weaker interactions with **broken arrows.** In addition, all neurotrophins can bind to the low-affinity receptor p75^{NTR}. Abbreviations: **NGF** = nerve growth factor; **NT** = neurotrophin; **BDNF** = brain-derived neurotrophic factor. (Adapted from Reichardt and Fariñas 1997.)

B. Two related cytokines, CNTF and LIF, transduce signals via two common receptor subunits, gp130 and LIF receptor-β. In addition, CNTF activity depends on binding to a lipid-anchored subunit of the CNTF receptor-α.

C. The TGFβ proteins—glial-derived neurotrophic factor (GDNF), neurturin, artemin, and persephin—transduce signals via a common receptor subunit, c-ret. Each ligand appears to bind to a distinct lipid-anchored subunit of the receptor. (Adapted from Rosenthal 1999.)

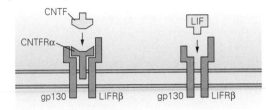

B Cytokine receptor interactions

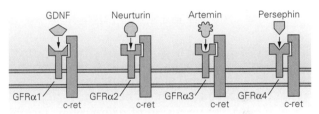

C GDNF receptor interactions

Elimination of Neurotrophic Factors and Their Receptors Leads to Neuronal Death

What evidence is there that trophic factors have essential functions in neuronal survival? The pioneering studies of Levi-Montalcini in the 1960s, using antibodies to NGF, first demonstrated that sympathetic and sensory neurons require neurotrophic factors for their survival. More recently, the analysis of mouse strains carrying mutations in the genes encoding neurotrophic factors and their receptors has provided extensive genetic evidence that sensory and sympathetic neurons require trophic support from neurotrophins secreted by their targets.

For example, sympathetic ganglia are virtually absent in mice carrying mutations in the *NGF* or *trkA* genes, confirming Levi-Montalcini's early studies. Importantly, a partial depletion of these neurons occurs in mice that lack one copy of the *NGF* gene, supporting the idea that neurotrophins are normally provided in limited amounts. In addition, mice that lack the *NT3* gene have a greatly reduced number of sympathetic neurons. Thus both NGF

and NT3 are required for the survival of sympathetic neurons. Gene targeting studies have shown that survival of sensory neurons is also dependent on the neurotrophins.

Do neurotrophins have an equivalent role in promoting the survival of neurons in the central nervous system? Here the picture is more complex. The survival of central neurons appears to depend on the actions of multiple neurotrophic factors. The survival of motor neurons in vitro can be promoted by the neurotrophins NT3 and BDNF. Despite this, the number of motor neurons in mutant mice lacking these neurotrophins or their receptors is normal, suggesting that other neurotrophic factors normally contribute to the survival of motor neurons. Candidates include the TGFβ proteins, such as glial-derived neurotrophic factor, interleukin 6-like proteins, such as cardiotrophin-1, and hepatocyte growth factors, all of which are expressed by muscles or by peripheral glial cells. Indeed, in mice lacking glial-derived neurotrophic factor 20–30% of motor neurons are lost. Figure 53-15 shows some of the many neu-

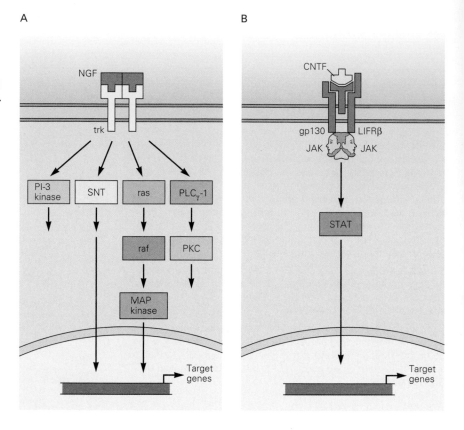

Figure 53-14 Neurotrophins and cytokines exert neurotrophic action by promoting the dimerization of receptors and the activation of protein tyrosine kinases.

A. Upon NGF binding, dimerization and phosphorylation of the (trk) receptor lead to tyrosine kinase activation and the association of the receptor cytoplasmic proteins, such as phosphatidylinositol 3-kinase (PI-3 kinase) and phospholipase $C\gamma$ (PLC_γ-1). These proteins then activate multiple downstream proteins, including ras. Activation of trk receptors also induces the phosphorylation of SNT, a protein whose phosphorylation is associated with neuronal differentiation and leads to activation of the ras/raf/MAP kinase pathway.

B. Upon activation by cytokines, the CNTF or LIF receptor-β (LIFRB) complex activates cytoplasmic JAK protein tyrosine kinases, which phosphorylate many substrates, including the STAT transcription factors. (Adapted from Reichardt and Fariñas 1997.)

rotrophic factors now known to promote the survival of motor neurons and peripheral neurons.

Although the provision of neurotrophic factors by target cells is a major influence on neuronal survival, it is also likely that some instances of neuronal death may obey different rules. Some proteins implicated in neuronal cell death such as p75 and Fas, may therefore be activated by target independent signals.

Deprivation of Neurotrophic Factors Activates a Cell Death Program in Neurons

Neurotrophic factors were originally believed to promote the survival of neural cells by stimulating their metabolism in beneficial ways—hence their name. Instead, it now appears that such factors act predominantly by suppressing a latent biochemical pathway present in all cells of the body. This biochemical pathway is in effect, a suicide program. Once activated it kills cells by *apoptosis,* a process characterized by four features: cell shrinkage, the condensation of chromatin, cellular fragmentation, and the phagocytosis of cellular remnants. Apoptotic cell deaths are distinguishable from *necrotic* cell deaths, which often result from acute

traumatic injury and characteristically involve rapid lysis of cellular membranes without activation of the endogenous cell death program.

The first evidence that the lack of neurotrophic factors kills neurons by releasing an active biochemical program emerged from studies that assessed the effects of inhibiting protein or RNA synthesis on the survival of sympathetic neurons in vitro. Such neurons are maintained in the continuous presence of NGF and die if NGF is removed from the culture media. Surprisingly, inhibiting protein or RNA synthesis at the time of NGF removal prevents removal death. The blockade of protein synthesis also rescues neurons in vivo. These results suggested that neurotrophins suppress an endogenous death program.

Many of the key insights into the biochemical components of the endogenous cell death program have emerged from genetic studies of the nematode worm *Caenorhabditis elegans.* During the normal development of *C. elegans* a precise and fixed number of cells is generated. About 15% of these identified cells, most of them neurons, undergo programmed cell death. This observation permitted the design of screens to identify genes that either block cell death or increase the number of dying cells. About a dozen cell death genes (*ced*) are

Distinct neuronal subtypes depend on different neurotrophic factors

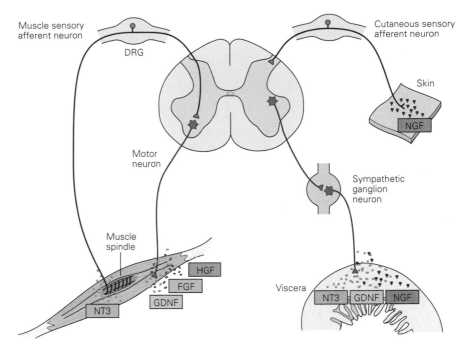

Figure 53-15 Differential dependence of neuronal populations of the peripheral and motor systems on neurotrophic factors. Diagram is based on the phenotypes of mouse mutations in which neurotrophic factors or their receptors have been inactivated by gene targeting. Abbreviation: **DRG** = dorsal root ganglion. (Adapted from Reichardt and Farinas 1997.)

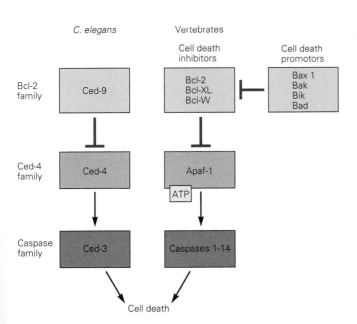

Figure 53-16 A genetic pathway for cell death in worms and vertebrates. In the nematode worm *C. elegans* the ced9 protein acts upstream of and inhibits the activity of ced4, which is responsible for activation of ced3. The activation of ced-3 results in the cleavage of protein substrates and results in cell death.

Many vertebrate homologs of ced9 have been identified and are members of the Bcl-2 family. Some of these proteins, such as Bcl-2 itself, inhibit cell death; but some promote cell death by antagonizing the actions of the Bcl2 subclass of death-preventing proteins. Bcl2 proteins act upstream of Apaf1 (a vertebrate homolog of ced4) and the caspases (vertebrate homologs of ced3).

known to control apoptosis in *C. elegans* (Figure 53-16). Two of these genes, *ced3* and *ced4,* are essential for cell death; in the absence of either gene all cells destined to die instead survive. The third key gene, *ced9,* functions in cells that normally survive; it antagonizes the activities of *ced3* and *ced4* and protects cells from apoptosis (see Figure 53-16). Thus in the absence of *ced9* activity, many additional cells die, although these additional deaths are still dependent on *ced3* and *ced4* activity.

Does the existence of a cell death pathway in a worm have any relevance to the developmental death of cells in the vertebrate nervous system? We now know that the nematode cell death pathway is conserved almost completely in vertebrates and underlies the apoptotic death of neurons, indeed of all cells, programmed to die during development. The discovery of this striking conservation came initially with the cloning of the *ced9* gene. This gene encodes a protein that is structurally and functionally related to members of the Bcl2 family of vertebrate proteins (see Figure 53-16), which had already been shown to protect lymphocytes and other cells from apoptotic death. The Bcl-2-like proteins function as dimers. Certain other members of this family bind to Bcl-2 and inhibit its function, thus promoting cell death. The molecular identification of other cell death genes soon followed. The *C. elegans ced3* gene encodes a protein closely related to a member of the vertebrate family of cysteine proteases, known as the cas-

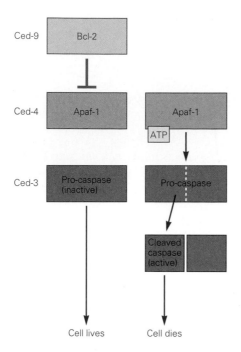

Figure 53-17 Caspases are generated in an inactive precursor form. Cleavage of the caspase precursor results in the removal of a prodomain and the subsequent assembly of a proteolytically active protein. Apaf1 is thought to interact with the caspase precursor via a caspase recruitment domain or death effector domain. Bcl-2-related proteins appear to inhibit caspase activation by binding directly to Apaf-1, preventing its ability to trigger pro-caspase cleavage.

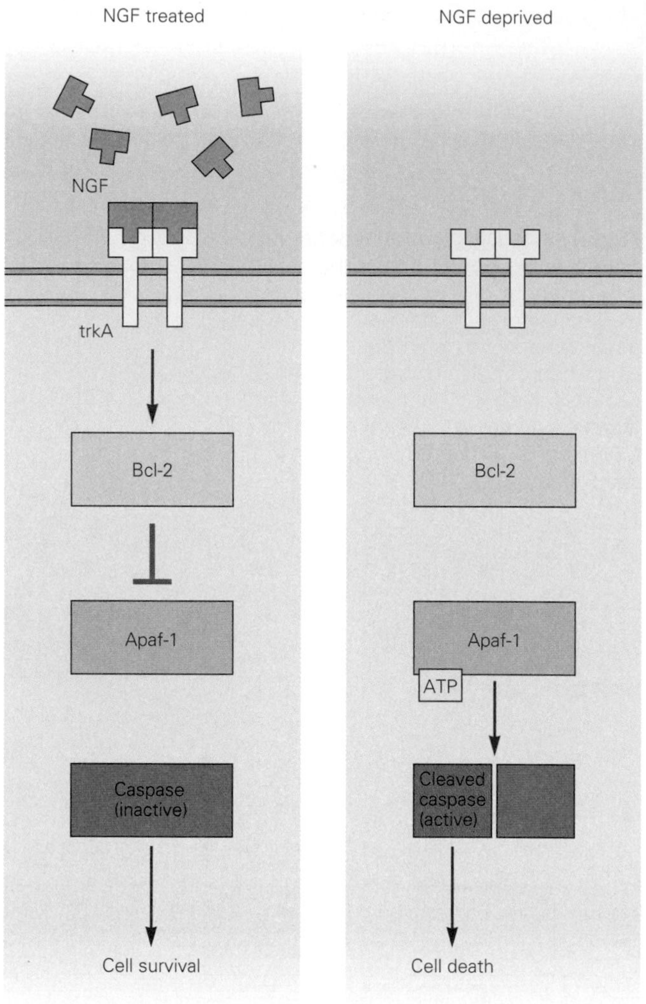

Figure 53-18 Neurotrophic factor deprivation triggers caspase activation and apoptotic cell death. In the presence of NGF, trk receptor signaling is thought to activate Bcl-2, which inhibits Apaf-1 activity and blocks caspase cleavage. Removal of NGF permits cleavage of pro-caspases and results in cell death. Many other stimuli can trigger apoptosis by activating caspases. Such stimuli include signaling via the p75[NTR]/tumor necrosis factor class of receptors, or damage to DNA. Each stimulus is thought to activate a distinct biochemical pathway that triggers one of a large family of caspases. In many cases the activation of a specific caspase leads to the proteolytic cleavage of other target caspases, thus initiating a cascade of caspase activation that leads eventually to the proteolysis of non-caspase proteins that are essential for cell viability.

pases, that have been implicated in apoptotic cell deaths (Figure 53-16). Finally, the *C. elegans ced4* gene encodes a protein that is structurally related to another vertebrate protein, apoptosis activating factor-1 (Apaf-1).

Caspases are enzymes that cleave substrate proteins at the amino acid carboxy-terminal to aspartate residues. The vertebrate caspase family contains more than a dozen members that can be divided into three subgroups on the basis of sequence analysis. Individual neuronal subtypes appear to express different caspase members. Nevertheless, there is evidence that caspase activity is central to the cell death program of all neurons. For example, viral proteins that function as caspase inhibitors, notably CrmA and p35, are effective at rescuing sensory and sympathetic neurons from neuronal death triggered by trophic factor degeneration.

How do these proteins interact to regulate cell death? The caspases (ced-3 in *C. elegans*) serve as the "executors" of cell death. The Apaf-1 and ced-4 proteins possess an ATP-dependent hydrolytic activity thought to promote the processing and activation of caspases/ced-3 (Figure 53-17). Thus if Apaf-1 and ced-4 proteins are absent, the processing of caspases and ced-3 does not occur and cells survive. The Bcl-2-like proteins (ced-9 in *C. elegans*) appear to prevent the activity of caspases and ced-3 by interacting directly with Apaf-1 and ced-4 to inhibit the processing of their precursors (Figure 53-17). This survival-promoting activity is mediated in part by inhibiting the ATPase activity of Apaf-1 and ced-4. Caspases cleave a wide variety of protein substrates, many of which are essential for cell viability.

What is the biochemical link between neurotrophic factor signaling and the activation of caspases? The binding of neurotrophic factors to their tyrosine kinase receptors is thought to lead to the phosphorylation of protein substrates that promote Bcl-2-like activities or inhibit caspase activity (Figure 53-18). The caspase pathway, and thus the cell death program, is also activated by many other cellular insults, including DNA damage and anoxia. Moreover, some instances of apoptotic deaths may not involve Bcl-2 and Apaf-1 related proteins but even in these cases, caspases may still serve as the final executors of apoptotic cell deaths. Because many neurodegenerative disorders result in apoptotic death, pharmacological strategies to inhibit caspases are being investigated.

An Overall View

The embryonic development of the nervous system involves the generation of an overabundance of neurons and glial cells and the programmed death of superfluous cells. From beginning to end, intercellular signals provide crucial direction to the developing nervous system. After many years of descriptive embryology, the past decade has seen the emergence of the first molecular insights into two fundamental issues in neurogenesis: (1) the mechanisms by which cells acquire neuronal and glial identities, and (2) the mechanisms by which certain young neurons and glial cells survive at the expense of others.

Major insights into these aspects of neurogenesis have emerged from genetic studies of two invertebrate organisms: the fruit fly *Drosophila* and the nematode worm *C. elegans*. This research has shown, once again, the striking phylogenetic conservation of the molecular machinery responsible for animal development. Yet, insight into the trophic factors that promote the development and survival of nerve cells came first from studies of vertebrates. Moreover, research on neurotrophic factor signaling and the biochemistry of cell death mechanisms is beginning to be applied to the search for treatment of neurodegenerative disorders such as Alzheimer disease and amyotrophic lateral sclerosis (Lou Gehrig disease).

Thomas M. Jessell
Joshua R. Sanes

Selected Readings

Anderson DJ. 1997. Cellular and molecular biology of neural crest cell lineage determination. Trends Genet 13:276–280.

Doe CQ. 1996. Asymmetric cell division and neurogenesis. Curr Opin Genet Dev 6:562–566.

Francis NJ, Landis SC. 1999. Cellular and molecular determinants of sympathetic neuron development. Ann Rev Neurosci 22:541–566.

Guo M, Jan LY, Jan YN. 1996. Control of daughter cell fates during asymmetric division: interaction of numb and notch. Neuron 17:27–41.

Hatten ME. 1999. Central nervous system neuronal migration. Ann Rev Neurosci 22:261–294.

Henderson CE. 1996. Programmed cell death in the developing nervous system. Neuron 17:579–585.

Le Douarin NM. 1998. Cell line segregation during peripheral nervous system ontogeny. Science 231:1515–1522.

Oppenheim RW. 1981. Neuronal cell death and some related regressive phenomena during neurogenesis: a selective historical review and progress report. In: WM Cowan (ed). *Studies in Developmental Neurobiology: Essays in Honor of Viktor Hamburger*, pp. 74–133. New York: Oxford Univ. Press.

Raff M. 1998. Cell suicide for beginners. Nature 396:119–122.

Simpson P. 1997. Notch signalling in development on equivalence groups and asymmetric developmental potential. Curr Opin Genet Dev 7:537–542.

References

Agapite J, Steller H. 1997. Neuronal cell death. In WM Cowan, TM Jessell, SL Zipursky (eds). *Molecular and Cellular Approaches to Neuronal Development*, pp. 264–289. New York: Oxford Univ. Press.

Anderson DJ. 1989. The neural crest cell lineage problem: neuropoiesis? Neuron 3:1–12.

Anderson DJ, Jan YN. 1997. The determination of the neuronal phenotype. In: WM Cowan, TM Jessell, SL Zipursky. *Molecular and Cellular Approaches to Neural Development*, pp. 26–63. New York: Oxford Univ. Press.

Chenn A, Braisted JE, McConnell SK, O'Leary DDM. 1997. Development of the cerebral cortex: Mechanisms controlling cell fate, laminar and areal patterning, and axonal connectivity. In: WM Cowan, TM Jessell, SL Zipursky. *Molecular and Cellular Approaches to Neural Development*, pp. 440–473. New York: Oxford Univ. Press.

Chenn A, McConnell SK. 1995. Cleavage orientation and the asymmetric inheritance of notch1 immunoreactivity in mammalian neurogenesis. Cell 82:631–641.

Chitnis A, Henrique D, Lewis J, Ish-Horowicz D, Kintner C. 1995. Primary neurogenesis in *Xenopus* embryos regulated by a homologue of the *Drosophila* neurogenic gene delta. Nature 375:761–766.

Detwiler SR. 1936. *Neuroembryology: An Experimental Study*. New York: Macmillan.

Doupe AJ, Landis SC, Patterson PH. 1985. Environmental influences in the development of neural crest derivatives: glucocorticoids, growth factors, and chromaffin cell plasticity. J Neurosci 5:2119–2142.

Fariñas I, Jones KR, Backus C, Wang XY, Reichardt LF. 1994. Severe sensory and sympathetic deficits in mice lacking neurotrophin-3. Nature 369:658–661.

Fariñas I, Yoshida CK, Backus C, Reichardt LF. 1996. Lack of neurotrophin-3 results in death of spinal sensory neurons and premature differentiation of their precursors. Neuron 17:1065–1078

Frise E, Knoblich JA, Younger-Shepherd S, Jan LY, Jan YN. 1996. The *Drosophila* numb protein inhibits signaling of the notch receptor during cell-cell interaction in sensory organ lineage. Proc Natl Acad Sci U S A 93:1925–1932.

Furshpan EJ, Potter DD, Landis SC. 1982. On the transmitter repertoire of sympathetic neurons in culture. Harvey Lect 76:149–191.

Hamburger V. 1975. Cell death in the development of the lateral motor column of the chick embryo. J Comp Neurol 160:535–546.

Hamburger V, Levi-Montalcini R. 1949. Proliferation differentiation and degeneration in the spinal ganglia of the chick embryo under normal and experimental conditions. J Exp Zool 111:457–501.

Hengartner MO, Horvitz HR. 1994. *C. elegans* cell survival gene *ced-9* encodes a functional homolog of the mammalian proto-oncogene *bcl-2*. Cell 76:665–676.

Hengartner MO, Horvitz HR. 1994. Programmed cell death in *Caenorhabditis elegans*. Curr Opin Genet Dev 4:581–586.

Jones KR, Fariñas I, Backus C, Reichardt LF. 1994. Targeted disruption of the BDNF gene perturbs brain and sensory neuron development but not motor neuron development. Cell 76:989–999.

Knoblich JA. 1997. Mechanisms of asymmetric cell division during animal development. Curr Opin Cell Biol 9:833–841.

Kraut R, Chia W, Jan LY, Jan Y, Knoblich JA. 1996. Role of inscuteable in orienting asymmetric cell divisions in *Drosophila*. Nature 383:50–55.

Landis SC. 1980. Developmental changes in the neurotransmitter properties of dissociated sympathetic neurons: a cytochemical study of the effects of medium. Dev Biol 77:349–361.

Lillien LE, Raff MC. 1990. Differentiation signals in the CNS: Type-2 astrocyte development in vitro as a model system. Neuron 5:111–119.

Lu B, Jan LY, Jan YN. 1998. Asymmetric cell division: lessons from flies and worms. Curr Opin Genet Dev 8:392–399.

Ma Q, Kintner C, Anderson DJ. 1996. Identification of neurogenin, a vertebrate neuronal determination gene. Cell 87:43–52.

Patterson PH, Chun LLY. 1974. The influence of nonneuronal cells on catecholamine and acetylcholine synthesis and accumulation in cultures of dissociated sympathetic neurons. Proc Natl Acad Sci U S A 71:3607–3610.

Purves D. 1988. *Body and Brain: A Trophic Theory of Neural Connections.* Cambridge: Harvard Univ. Press.

Raff MD, Hart IK, Richardson WD, Lillien LE. 1990. An analysis of the cell-cell interactions that control the proliferation and differentiation of a bipotential glial progenitor cell in culture. Cold Spring Hrb Symp Quant Biol 55:235–238.

Reichardt LF, Fariñas I. 1997. Neurotrophic factors and their receptors: roles in neuronal development and function. In WM Cowan, TM Jessell, SL Zipursky (eds). *Molecular and Cellular Approaches to Neuronal Development,* pp. 220–263. New York: Oxford Univ. Press.

Rhyu MS, Jan LY, Jan YN. 1994. Asymmetric distribution of numb protein during division of the sensory organ precursor cell confers distinct fates to daughter cells. Cell 76:477–491.

Rosenthal A. 1999. The GDNF protein family: Gene ablation studies reveal what they really do and how. Neuron 22:201–207.

Schotzinger RJ, Landis SC. 1988. Cholinergic phenotype developed by noradrenergic sympathetic neurons after innervation of a novel cholinergic target in vivo. Nature 335:637–639.

Shah NM, Groves AK, Anderson DJ. 1996. Alternative neural crest cell fates are instructively promoted by TGF beta superfamily members. Cell 85:331–343.

Shah NM, Marchionni MA, Isaacs I, Stroobant P, Anderson DJ. 1994. Glial growth factor restricts mammalian neural crest stem cells to a glial fate. Cell 77:349–360.

Spana EP, Doe CQ. 1996. Numb antagonizes notch signaling to specify sibling neuron cell fates. Neuron 17:21–26.

Vaux DL. 1997. Ced-4, the third horseman of apoptosis. Cell 90:389–390.

Zhong W, Jiang MM, Weinmaster G, Jan LY, Jan YN. 1997. Differential expression of mammalian numb, numb-like and notch1 suggests distinct roles during mouse cortical neurogenesis. Development 124:1887–1897.

Zou H, Henzel WJ, Lui X, Lutschg A, Wang X. 1997. Apaf-1, a human protein homologous to *C. elegans* ced-4 participates in cytochrome c-dependent activation of caspase-3. Cell 90:405–413.

54

The Guidance of Axons to Their Targets

IN THE PREVIOUS TWO CHAPTERS we have examined the molecular mechanisms that ensure the differentiation of appropriate numbers and types of nerve cells at correct times and places in the developing nervous system. These mechanisms, however, fail to explain the specificity of functional synaptic connections evident in the mature nervous system. Many neurons extend axons over great distances—up to several meters in a giraffe—bypassing billions of potential but inappropriate synaptic targets before terminating in the correct area and recognizing the appropriate targets. The topological relationships of neurons within a functional neural circuit are so complex that they require a special set of mechanisms to develop properly.

In essence, these mechanisms involve recognition of environmental cues by the growing axons. The pathways along which axons grow provide a large number of diverse molecular cues to guide axons to their targets, and the axons possess exquisitely specific receptors to recognize and interpret these cues. To illustrate this process, we first describe the molecular cues along one well-studied pathway, that connecting the retina to the brain. Second, we discuss how axons in this pathway respond to guidance cues. Third, we describe some of the main classes of molecules thought to mediate the interactions between the growing axon and its environment. Finally, we consider how families of axon guidance molecules work together to direct axons to their targets.

Specific Molecular Cues Guide Axons to Their Targets

For much of the twentieth century a debate raged between advocates of two very different views of how axons reach their targets. The molecular view of axonal pathfinding was first clearly articulated at the turn of the twentieth century by the physiologist J. N. Langley (who also was the first to map the autonomic nervous system). In contrast, some eminent developmental biol-

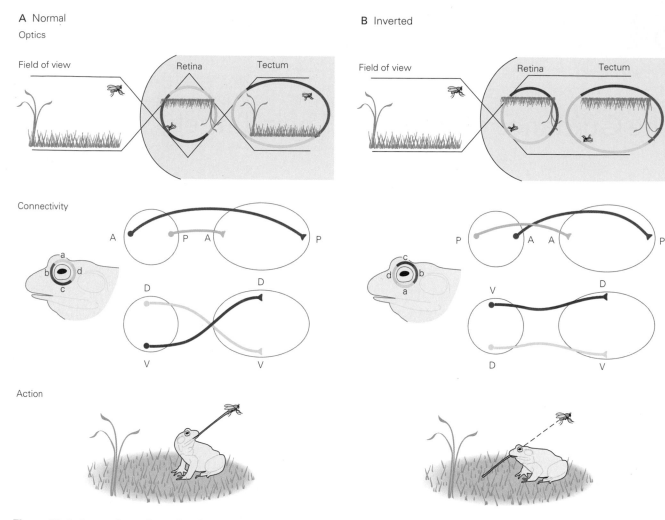

Figure 54-1 Axons from the retina form a topographic representation of the retina at their termination in the optic tectum.

A. The lens projects an inverted image onto the retina, and the optic nerve then transfers the image, with another inversion, to the optic tectum. An orderly arrangement of axons is responsible for transferring the image from retina to tectum. Neurons in the anterior retina extend axons that terminate in the posterior tectum, neurons in the posterior retina project to the anterior tectum, neurons in the dorsal retina project to the ventral tec-

tum, and neurons in the ventral retina project to the dorsal tectum. As a result, the animal (here, a frog) is capable of accurate visually guided behavior (here, catching a fly for its supper).

B. When the optic nerve regenerates following surgical rotation of the eye in its socket, visually guided behavior is maladaptive. When a fly is presented overhead, the frog seems to think it is below, and vice versa. The reversal of reflexes reflects the reconnection of retinal axons to their original targets, even though these connections now transfer an inverted map of the world onto the tectum. **P,** posterior; **A,** anterior; **D,** dorsal; **V,** ventral.

ogists, notably Paul Weiss, believed that axons received only general instructions on where to grow, and that much axonal outgrowth was random. Weiss proposed that appropriate connections survive because they are the ones in which the axon and target match patterns of electrical activity.

In our molecular age Weiss's ideas may seem farfetched. In fact, they were not unreasonable at the time. It had been shown that in tissue culture, axons grow preferentially along mechanical discontinuities (eg,

along scratches on a cover slip) and that nerve trunks often form along solid supports in embryos (eg, along blood vessels or cartilage). It seemed logical, therefore, that mechanical guidance, called *stereotropism,* might account for axonal patterning. Moreover, we are quite comfortable today with the idea that electrical signals can be used to change the way current flows in a computer without any need to resolder connections. Likewise, experience can strengthen or weaken neural connections without formation of new axonal pathways, as

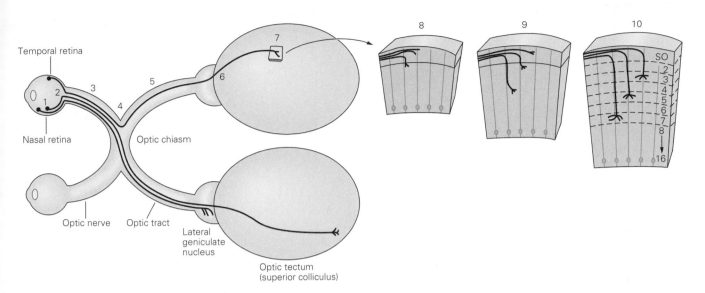

Figure 54-2 Axons of retinal ganglion cells follow a complex path to the optic tectum. Three axons are shown. One axon arises from a neuron carrying information from the nasal half of the retina; the axon crosses the optic chiasm to reach the contralateral optic tectum. A second axon also arises in the nasal hemiretina and crosses at the chiasm but terminates in the geniculate body. A third axon arises from a neuron carrying information from the temporal hemiretina; it remains ipsilateral at the chiasm and terminates in the ipsilateral tectum. The numbers indicate important steps in the axon's journey: (**1**) Directed growth toward the optic nerve head with the retina; (**2**) Entry into the optic nerve; (**3**) Extension through the optic nerve; (**4**) Swerving to remain ipsilateral or crossing to the contralateral side at the optic chiasm; (**5**) Extension through the optic tract; (**6**) Entry into the optic tectum or lateral geniculate nucleus; (**7**) Navigation to an appropriate rostrocaudal and dorsoventral position on the tectum; (**8**) Descent from the tectal surface; (**9**) Stopping at an appropriate layer and formation of a rudimentary terminal arbor; and (**10**) Refinement of the arbor.

occurs in learning. Why not, then, imagine that congruent activity, called *resonance* by Weiss, establishes the appropriate connections? Today, however, few scientists believe that stereotaxis or resonance are important forces in embryonic development. Key to the triumph of the molecular view was an experiment performed in the early 1940s by Roger Sperry, who, ironically was a student of Weiss.

Visual information is transmitted from the eye to the brain by axons of retinal ganglion cells (Chapter 26). These axons form an orderly map of the world onto their target areas, the lateral geniculate body in the thalamus and the superior colliculus (or optic tectum) in the midbrain (Figure 54-1A). In lower vertebrates, with which Sperry worked, the tectum is the main visual center in the brain. Retinal axons from the most nasal (anterior) part of the retina project to the most temporal (posterior) part of the tectum, axons from the temporal (posterior) edge of the retina project to the tectum's rostral (anterior) margin, and axons from each nasotemporal position in between project to a corresponding point along the tectum's rostrocaudal axis. Likewise, the dorsoventral retinal axis is mapped onto the tectum's mediolateral axis (Figure 54-1B). If the optic nerve is cut

the animal is blinded. In lower vertebrates, cut retinal axons can regenerate to the tectum, whereupon vision is restored. This is not the case in mammals (see Chapter 55).

Sperry performed a simple and stunning experiment that illuminated the mechanism by which retinotectal projections form. He severed the optic nerve in a frog but rotated the eye in its socket by 180° before allowing regeneration to occur. Remarkably, the frog exhibited orderly but maladaptive behavior: when presented with a fly on the ground it jumped up, and when offered a fly above its head it struck downward (Figure 54-1B). Moreover, it never learned to correct its mistakes. Sperry suggested—and later proved, using anatomical and physiological methods—that the retinal axons had returned to their original tectal targets, even though these connections now provided the brain with spatial misinformation and thereby led to maladaptive behavior. The inescapable conclusion was that axon-target recognition relied on chemical matching rather than functional validation of randomly formed connections. Sperry's idea, often called the *chemospecificity hypothesis*, motivated the next generation of developmental neurobiologists to initiate an intensive search for

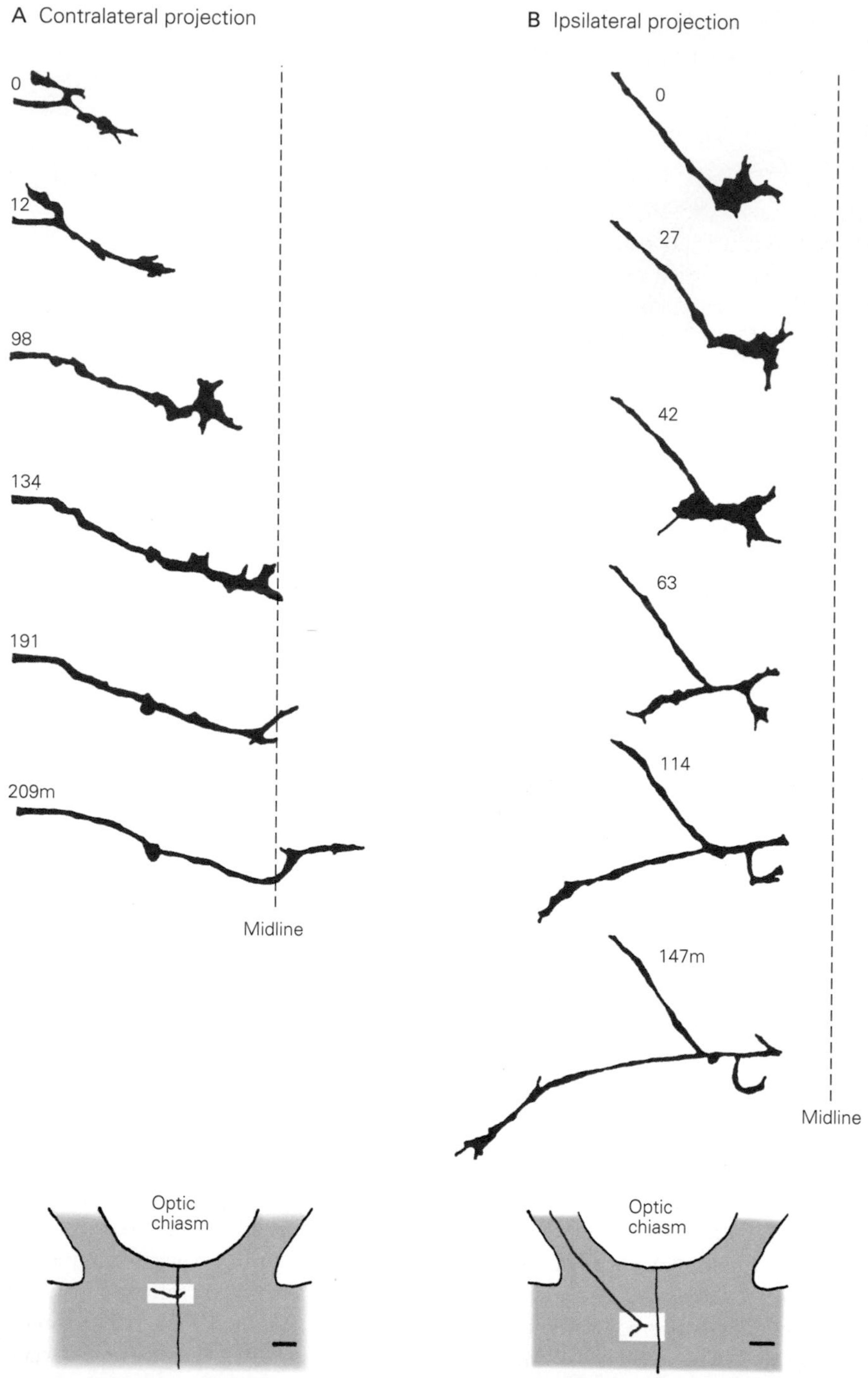

A Contralateral projection

B Ipsilateral projection

Figure 54-3 Ganglion cells from the nasal and temporal hemiretinas make divergent choices at the optic chiasm. Axons were labeled by application of a dye to the retina, then visualized by time-lapse video microscopy. **Numbers** indicate time in minutes, and **dotted lines** show the position of the optic chiasm. The axon in **A** arose from the nasal hemiretina and crossed the optic chiasm. The axon in **B** arose from the temporal hemiretina, reached the chiasm, but then turned back to remain ipsilateral. (From Godemont et al. 1994.)

these "recognition molecules." As we will see later in this chapter, this search has begun to be successful.

Before continuing, though, it is important to note that Weiss's ideas are by no means obsolete. Indeed, we now recognize that electrical activity in neural circuits can play a crucial role in shaping connectivity. The current view is that molecular matching predomi-

nates during embryonic development, and that activity (experience) modifies the circuits once they have been established. In this chapter we focus on the molecular cues that guide the initial establishment of neural connections. In Chapter 56 we examine the role of neuron-target activity in fine-tuning synaptic connections.

Axons Reach Their Destinations in a Series of Discrete Steps

Retinal Axons React to Intermediate Cues en Route to Their Targets

Sperry's experiment implied that axon guidance cues existed, but it did not indicate where they were or how they worked. For a time, a predominant view was that recognition occurred mostly at the target and that simple mechanical forces or long-range chemotactic factors sufficed to get axons to the right vicinity. We now know, however, that axons reach distant targets in a series of discrete steps, making decisions at relatively frequent intervals along the way. To illustrate this critical point, let us trace in greater detail the path a retinal axon follows to the optic tectum. Perhaps surprisingly, we can distinguish at least 10 steps on the journey and at least as many decision points (Figure 54-2).

The first task of a retinal ganglion cell axon is to leave the retina. To this end it enters the optic fiber layer and grows along the retinal basal lamina and the end-feet of glial cells. Growth is highly oriented from the outset, indicating that axons read directional cues in their terrain. Once they reach the central retina, axons come under the influence of attractants emanating from the optic nerve head and thereby enter the optic stalk. Having left the retina the axons follow the optic nerve toward the brain. The first axons to travel this route follow the cells of the optic stalk, the rudiment of the neural tube that connects the retina to the diencephalon from which it arose. These "pioneer" axons then serve as guides for subsequent axons, which can find their way simply by following their predecessors.

Although all retinal axons follow the same path during the first three steps of their journey, they make divergent choices at later stages. The divergence of axons is first apparent at the optic chiasm. The axons that arise from neurons in the nasal half of each retina cross the chiasm and proceed to the opposite (contralateral) side of the brain. In contrast, a sizable fraction of the axons from the temporal half of each retina turn before reaching the chiasm and remain ipsilateral (see Figure 54-2). This difference in behavior appears to reflect different responses of nasal and temporal retinal axons to special populations of cells that are localized in the midline at the chiasm. Nasal retinal axons contact and pass by these cells, whereas those temporal retinal axons destined to remain in the ipsilateral side are inhibited by the cells and are thereby deflected in their journey.

Having passed the optic chiasm, all retinal axons rejoin to form the optic tract, which runs along the ventral surface of the diencephalon. Subsets of axons leave the tract at different points, however. In most vertebrates the tectum of the midbrain—called the *superior colliculus* in mammals—is the major target, whereas a small number of axons project to the lateral geniculate nucleus of the thalamus. In humans, in contrast, most axons project to the lateral geniculate, but a sizable number still reach the colliculus and a smaller number project to the pulvinar and pretectal nuclei. In each case retinal axons need to leave the optic tract at an appropriate point and enter their target field. Then, within the target, different retinal axons project to different subregions. In the tectum, as Sperry showed, the retinal axons form a precise topographic map of the retina—and thereby the visual world—on the tectal surface.

Having reached a topographically appropriate site within the tectum, the retinal axons find themselves in a layer of axons and glial processes but not yet in direct apposition to a synaptic partner. Thus additional guidance steps are necessary. For the last leg of their journey the axons turn and dive into the tectal neuropil (see Figure 54-2). They descend along the surface of radial glial cells, which, as their name implies, provide a scaffold for radial growth. Although the radial glia span the entire neuroepithelium from its pial to its ventricular surface, each retinal axon confines its synaptic terminals to a single layer. Moreover, even though the dendrites of many postsynaptic cells extend through multiple layers and receive synapses along their whole length, the retinal synapses are restricted to a small fraction of the dendritic tree. These behaviors imply the existence of layer-specific cues that arrest elongation or trigger arborization.

The formation of a terminal arbor does not end the growth of the retinal axon. The size and shape of the arbor—and therefore the number and distribution of synapses that it forms—are regulated by interactions with synaptic targets and by patterns of neural activity in the circuits that form.

Numerous experimental approaches have been successful in localizing and characterizing the structures that present positional cues to growing axons. Perhaps the most powerful is direct observation of development in progress. By following live axons for example, the growth cones of nasal and temporal retinal axons have been shown to respond differently as they approach the optic chiasm (Figure 54-3). Careful analysis of these behaviors suggests that cells in the chiasm act as intermediate targets, bearing or releasing cues to retinal axons to continue (grow contralaterally) or swerve (remain ipsilateral). In fact, specialized populations of neurons and glia have been identified in the optic chiasm, and their interactions with axons are under active investigation.

B

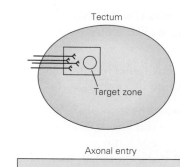

Tectum

Target zone

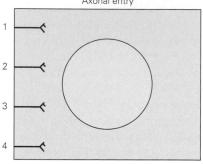

Axonal entry

1

2

3

4

Figure 54-4 Advancing axons correct their course to reach the appropriate domain of the optic tectum.

A. The surface of the optic tectum following application of a fluorescent dye to a small patch of the retina. Axons from the labeled region of the retina terminate and arborize in a restricted area of the tectum. Many axons can be seen growing along the tectum to their termination site. Some axons, however, appear to be initially misdirected and then change course. (Adapted from Nakamura and O'Leary 1989.)

B. Summary of paths taken by retinal axons. Although some axons project directly to and stop at their termination zone (**3**), many more grow past their target and then loop back (**2**) or extend a collateral branch (**4**). Still others are misdirected initially, then turn, swerve, or branch to correct course (**1**). Once in the correct region all form elaborate, definitive arbors. These patterns indicate that the surface of the optic tectum has graded positional cues to which the retinal axons respond with graded sensitivities.

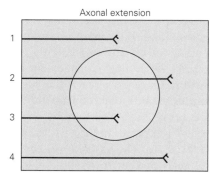

Axonal extension

1

2

3

4

A

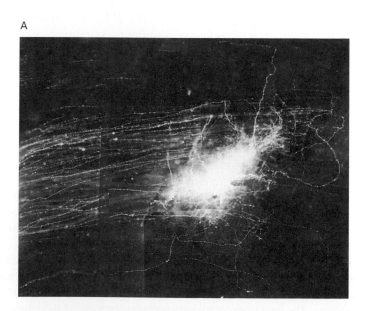

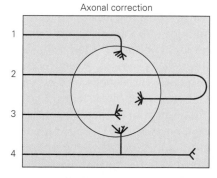

Axonal correction

1

2

3

4

Analysis of the trajectories of retinal axons also provides evidence for cues within the tectum. Nearly all axons that arise from a single region of the retina form terminal arbors in a single region of the tectum (Figure 54-4A), as was expected from Sperry's work. However, the axons take a variety of paths to reach their destination. Some grow directly to their termination site; but others make a variety of apparent "mistakes" and then change course or extend new branches (Figure 54-4B).

Thus although most axons enter the tectum at appropriate points, those that do not still have a chance to change course and reach proper targets. Such corrections imply the existence of positional cues in the tectum. As we discuss later in this chapter, molecules with such properties, the ephrins, have been discovered.

Microsurgical experiments on embryos have also been useful in identifying positional cues for growing axons. For example, when the patch of neural tube between the chiasm and tectum is rotated 90° before axons reach it, the axons nonetheless grow in proper relationship to the epithelial cells, even though this course causes them to bypass the tectum (Figure 54-5). This result suggests that the diencephalic neuroepithelium bears markers of position or polarity that guide developing axons.

Motor Axons Grow Through Peripheral Nerves to Muscles

We have seen that retinal axons reach distant targets in discrete steps. Other axons use similar strategies, but the cues they follow—axon bundles, epithelia, intermediate targets, and so on—are arranged in different ways. To illustrate this point we briefly consider the pathway that motor axons traverse on their way to skeletal muscles.

The motor neurons that innervate one muscle are clustered in a *motor pool* in the spinal cord. Motor pools are arranged in rostrocaudal columns according to the type of muscle innervated (eg, extensor, flexor, axial). The pathways between motor neurons and muscles are accurate from the outset. Because the distance from the spinal cord to muscles is great, even in early embryos, such accuracy early in the growth of axons cannot be the result of trial and error. Instead, the motor axons, like retinal axons, receive guidance along the way to their targets.

Some of the steps that motor axons take to reach limb muscles are summarized in Figure 54-6. First, motor axons leave the spinal cord all along its length but are gathered into segmental ventral roots by barriers present within the somites. Second, axons rearrange in a plexus region—roughly akin to the interchange at the convergence of freeways. Thus axons destined for dorsal or ventral muscles are gathered into discrete nerves by the time they enter the base of the limb. Third, the axons run through large nerves within the limb, avoiding cartilage and skin. Fourth, axons destined for one muscle gather together and leave the large nerves at discrete points to enter their target muscle. Finally, axons leave the intramuscular nerve to synapse on individual muscle fibers. Thus, motor axons like retinal axons are guided to their targets in a series of steps.

The Cellular Environment Provides a Complex Set of Commands to the Growing Axon

The options for a developing axon are limited: It can grow, turn, or stop. Nevertheless, the cellular environment of the growing axon can choreograph these behaviors with exquisite subtlety. Some of the strategies that have evolved to guide axons are illustrated in Figure 54-7.

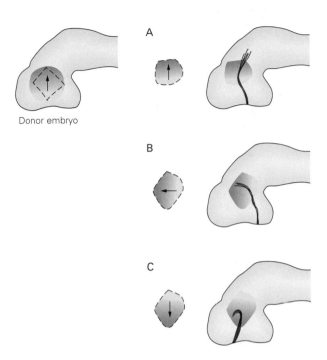

Figure 54-5 Local cues in the neuroepithelium guide formation of the optic tract. Patches of neuroepithelium from the embryonic optic tract were excised from a donor tadpole (**left**) and transplanted into the corresponding position of a host tadpole at the same stage (**right**). Grafts were placed in different orientations in the host. Retinal axons were labeled before they reached the optic chiasm, then viewed after they had crossed the chiasm and formed optic tracts. Grafts were placed into the host in the original orientation (**A**), rotated 90° counterclockwise (**B**), rotated 180° (**C**). In each case the axons grew toward the part of the graft that was originally caudal (shown as **shaded**). (From Harris 1989.)

A major problem to be solved is one of distance. In some cases the first axons reach their targets when the embryo is very small and the distance to be traversed is short. These axons, sometimes called "pioneers," respond to molecular cues embedded in cells or the extracellular matrix along their way. The first axons to exit the retina may fall within this class. Axons that arise later, when distances are longer and obstacles are more numerous, can reach their targets by following the pioneers.

Axons can also divide growth over a long distance into discrete short segments, recognizing and responding to intermediate targets along the way to their final targets. Some intermediate targets are especially useful at "decision" points where axons diverge, such as the optic chiasm or the limb plexus.

Figure 54-6 Motor axons make several decisions on their way to muscles. The two **greens** indicate motor neurons from two different motor pools, one in the medial and the other in the lateral portion of the lateral motor column. Axons from both pools mingle as they assemble to form ventral roots and enter the plexus. The axons then sort out in the plexus: The axons from the medial motor pool enter a ventral trunk, and those from the lateral pool enter the dorsal trunk at the base of the limb. Later, axons from each motor pool exit the trunk together to form the nerve that innervates a single muscle.

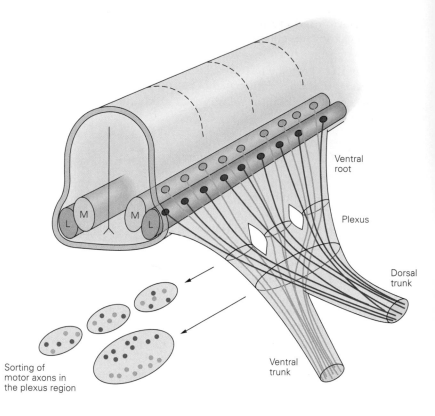

Sorting of motor axons in the plexus region

Another solution to the problem of long distance is to have the axon navigate along gradients. Along some pathways these are gradients of cell surface molecules, such as those in the tectum; on others soluble molecules released from a discrete source form gradients that evoke responses akin to chemotaxis.

Although the first axon guidance cues to be recognized were the positive or growth-promoting cues, it is now clear that numerous negative (inhibitory) cues also exist. Negative cues can repulse advancing axons, cause them to turn, or prevent them from entering the wrong territory. Together, combinations of positive and negative cues exercise finer control over the direction of the growing axon than either category could alone.

Another way of exerting fine directional control is through a combination of short- and long-range cues. Short-range cues include molecules embedded in cell membranes or the extracellular matrix; these molecules provide contact guidance that is precise to the submicron level. Long-range cues include soluble molecules that diffuse from producer cells and can attract or repel axons from afar, albeit with somewhat less precision. Together, the short- and long-range cues permit axons to circumvent obstacles and reach their targets (Figure 54-7).

The Growth Cone Is a Sensory-Motor Structure That Recognizes and Responds to Guidance Cues

Elongating axons terminate in a protuberance called the *growth cone.* In the 1890s Santiago Ramon y Cajal, the greatest of all developmental neurobiologists, proposed that the growth cone was responsible for axonal pathfinding. Building only on static images, he envisioned that it was ". . . endowed with exquisite chemical sensitivity, rapid ameboid movements and a certain motive force, thanks to which it is able to proceed forward and overcome obstacles met in its way . . . until it reaches its destination." Numerous studies over the intervening decades have demonstrated that Ramon y Cajal was correct. The growth cone is both a sensory structure that receives directional cues from the environment and a motor structure whose activity leads to axon elongation.

Cajal also considered "what mysterious forces precede the appearance of these processes . . . promote their growth and ramification . . . and finally establish those protoplasmic kisses . . . which seem to constitute the final ecstasy of an epic love story." In more modern and prosaic terms, we now assert that the growth cone guides the axon by transducing positive and negative cues into signals that regulate the cytoskeleton and thereby determine the course and rate of axon outgrowth.

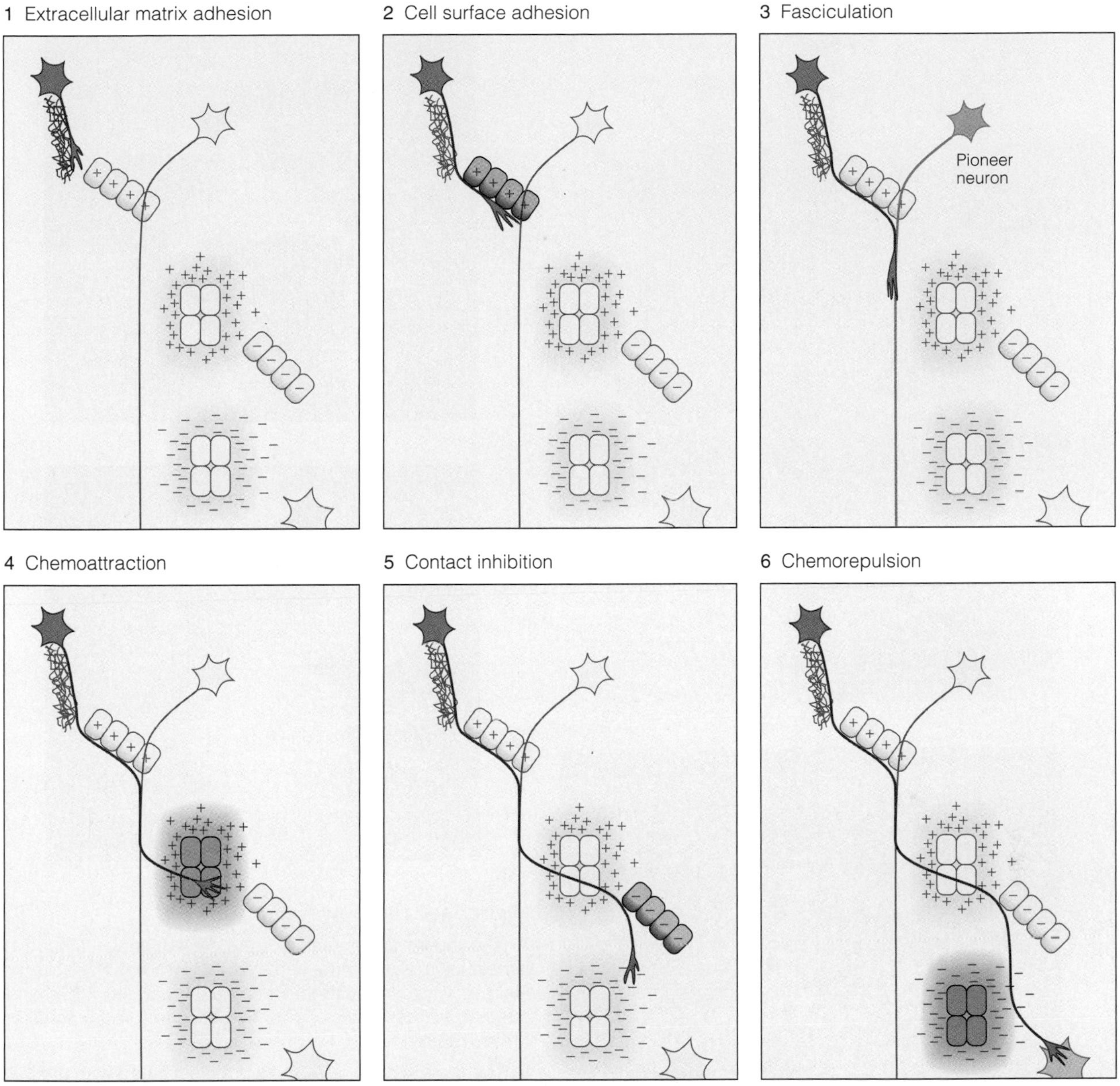

1 Extracellular matrix adhesion   2 Cell surface adhesion   3 Fasciculation

Pioneer
neuron

4 Chemoattraction   5 Contact inhibition   6 Chemorepulsion

Figure 54-7 Growth cones advancing to their synaptic targets encounter a variety of guidance cues. The diagrams illustrate some of them arrayed in a single hypothetical pathway. (1) The axon interacts with growth-promoting molecules in the extracellular matrix en route to its synaptic target. (2) Adhesive cell surface molecules on neuroepithelial cells promote the axon's growth. (3) The axon encounters another axon and fasciculates with it. (4) A soluble chemoattractant molecule directs the axon. (5) An intermediate target bears a repellent cue on its surface, which makes the axon turn. (6) A soluble inhibitory molecule biases the axon's trajectory to the right. Finally, after contact with the synaptic target the growth cone stops elongating and begins to form a terminal arbor.

Growth cones have three main regions. A central core is rich in microtubules, mitochondria, and a variety of other organelles. Projecting from the body are long slender extensions called *filopodia*. Between the filopodia are *lamellipodia*, which are also motile and give the growth cone its characteristic ruffled appearance (Figure 54-8A).

The sensory capability of the growth cone depends in large part on its filopodia. These rod-like, actin-rich, membrane-limited structures are highly motile. Their

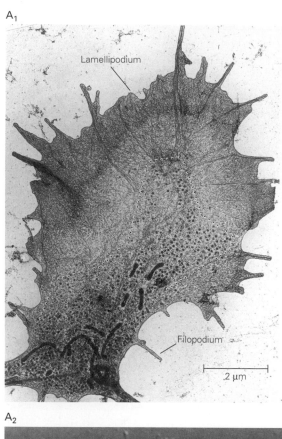

A₁

Lamellipodium

Filopodium

2 μm

A₂
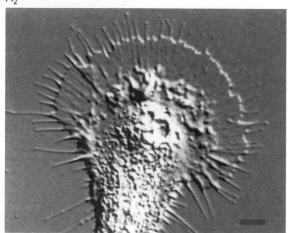

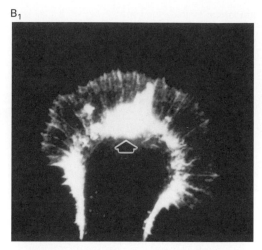

B₁

B₂

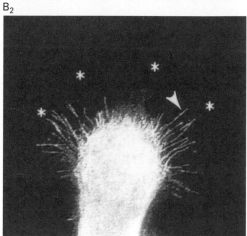

Figure 54-8 The growth cone.

A. The three main domains of the growth cone—filopodia, lamellipodia, and central core—are shown by (**1**) whole-mount electron microscopy (from Bridgman and Dailey 1989) and (**2**) differential interference light microscopy (from Forscher and Smith 1988).

B. The growth cone in **A2** was double-labeled with antibodies to actin and microtubules. Actin is concentrated in lamellipodia and filopodia (**1**), whereas microtubules are concentrated in the central core (**2**). (From Forscher and Smith 1988.)

membranes bear receptors for the molecules that serve as directional cues for the axon. The length of the filopodia (tens of microns in some cases) allows them to sample the environment far ahead of the central core, their rapid movements allow them to make a detailed inventory of the environment, and their flexibility allows them to navigate cells and other obstacles.

When receptors on the filopodia encounter signals in the environment, the growth cone is stimulated to ad-

vance, retract, or turn. Several motors involving actin, myosin, and membrane components power these reactions (Figure 54-9A), and the contribution of each molecular motor to the advance of the growth cone likely varies from one situation to another. With all of the motors, however, the final step involves the flow of microtubules from the central core into the newly extended protrusion, thus moving the growth cone ahead and leaving behind a new stretch of axon. Lamellipodia and

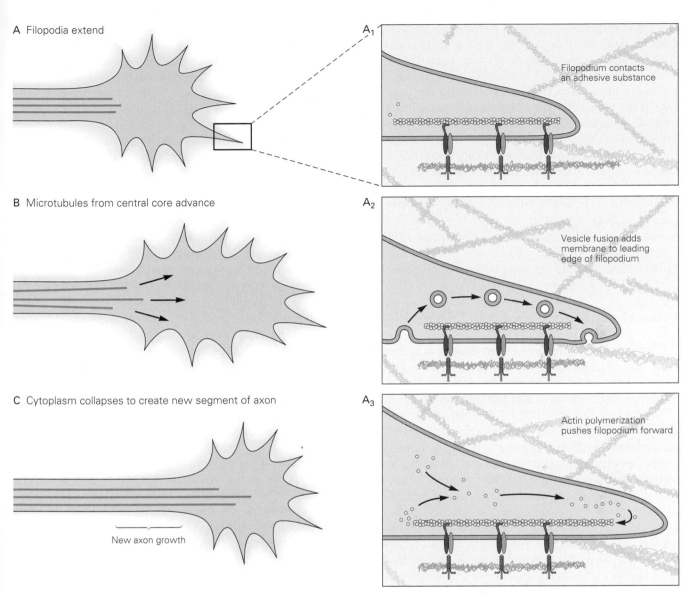

A Filopodia extend

B Microtubules from central core advance

C Cytoplasm collapses to create new segment of axon

New axon growth

A₁ Filopodium contacts an adhesive substance

A₂ Vesicle fusion adds membrane to leading edge of filopodium

A₃ Actin polymerization pushes filopodium forward

Figure 54-9 Many motors move the growth cone.

A. A filopodium contacts an adhesive cue and contracts, thus pulling the growth cone forward. Actin filaments assemble at the leading edge of a filopodium, disassemble at the trailing edge, and interact with myosin along the way. Force generated by the retrograde flow of actin pushes the filopodium forward. Exocytosis adds membrane to the leading edge of the filopodium and supplies new adhesion receptors to maintain traction. Membrane is recovered at the back of the filopodium.

Action polymerization pushes the filopodium forward. The actin polymer is linked to adhesion molecules on the plasma membrane.

B. The combined action of all the motors creates an actin-poor space into which the microtubules from the central core advance.

C. The microtubules form a bundle, and the cytoplasm collapses around them to create a new length of axonal shaft. (Modified from Heidemann 1996.)

filopodia form in the "new" growth cone, and the process begins anew (Figure 54-9B).

Particularly critical for axonal guidance is the coupling between the sensory and motor capabilities of the growth cone: Accurate pathfinding can occur only if the motor action is dependent on the sensory apparatus. In this regard it is crucial that the receptors on the filopodia are not merely binding moieties that mediate adhesion but rather are signal-transducing receptors coupled to numerous second-messenger pathways. Second messengers in turn affect the organization of the cytoskeleton, thereby regulating the direction and rate at which the growth cone moves.

One important second messenger is calcium. Growth cone motility is optimal at a specific calcium concentration called the *set point*. Activation of receptors on the filopodia can lead to changes in calcium concentration in either direction, thus affecting the organization of the cytoskeleton and modulating motility. Moreover, local activation of filopodia on one side of the growth cone can lead to a gradient of calcium concentration across the growth cone, a likely basis for changes in the direction of growth. Calcium is certainly not the only link between receptor and motor molecules; others include the cyclic nucleotides. All of these messengers then modulate the activity of a plethora of protein kinases, protein phosphatases, and rho-family GTPases. Finally, these molecular signals are integrated in the growth cone to guide the axon in a specific direction.

Pathway Guidance Cues Act in Diverse Ways

It will come as no surprise to learn that the numerous effects of the embryonic environment on the growing axon are mediated by hundreds of molecular species. Although these molecules are diverse in structure and each produces a constellation of effects, it is useful to categorize them by their primary effect and subcellular localization. First, in the most general of terms, guidance cues act by either promoting or inhibiting neurite outgrowth. Second, growth cones encounter some molecules on cell surfaces, others in the extracellular matrix, and still others in soluble form. In practice, these categories blur. For example, some molecules promote outgrowth of some axons but inhibit others. Likewise, some molecules exist in both membrane-bound and soluble isoforms. Nonetheless, we use this simple categorization to enumerate some of the most important environmental cues and growth cone receptors that interact to guide axons to their targets.

Integrins on Growth Cones Interact With Laminins in the Extracellular Matrix

In vertebrates and invertebrates many peripheral axons grow through connective tissue or along basal laminae. These patterns were initially thought to result from preferential extension through channels or along hard surfaces. Simple studies of axon outgrowth in vitro were instrumental in revising this view. For example, when neurons were grown on patterned substrates (ie, stripes of one substance alternating with patches of a second), the axons extended preferentially along pathways of the more adhesive substance, even when the less adhesive substance was quite capable of support-

ing neurite outgrowth on its own (Figure 54-10A). We now know that axonal preferences correlate only imperfectly with adhesiveness, but the main point stands: Growing axons recognize molecular differences among the substrates along which they grow, and these distinctions can regulate the direction and rate of their growth.

Those studies used substrates coated with molecules derived from the extracellular matrix and led to the idea that axon outgrowth is promoted by such molecules in vivo. Numerous substances capable of promoting outgrowth in vitro have now been identified, including collagens, fibronectin, and some proteoglycans. Of particular importance, however, are the heterotrimeric laminins, major components of all basal laminae in vertebrates and invertebrates alike. So far 14 trimers have been isolated, each with a unique distribution. This diversity permits all basal laminae to share a common structure yet present distinct position- or stage-dependent signals to advancing axons or other cells with which they interact.

How do axons recognize growth-promoting molecules in the extracellular matrix? A variety of matrix-binding proteins have been isolated from neural cells, but the main signaling receptors appear to be the integrins. These are heterodimers, drawn from a set of at least 16 α and 8 β chains. Essentially all cells in the body bear at least one integrin, and some express several. Each dimer recognizes a distinct set of ligands—$\alpha1\beta1$, for example, binds to collagens and laminins, $\alpha4\beta1$ binds to fibronectin, and so on. At least seven different integrin heterodimers bind to laminins, but they differ in the laminin isoforms they prefer and the domains on laminin that they recognize (see Figure 54-10B). Together, the multiplicity of integrins and matrix components provides the potential for considerable subtlety and specificity in the interactions of growth cones with the extracellular matrix.

Molecules That Mediate Cell-Cell Adhesion Also Promote Neurite Outgrowth

Early studies on dissociated cells showed that cells aggregate selectively, leading to the idea that groupings of cells in vivo result from selective adhesive interactions between adjoining membranes (Figure 54-11A). Later analysis showed that cell adhesive interactions are mediated by two sets of binding components, one requiring calcium ions and the other not. This distinction is a fundamental one, and it is now thought that the two types of adhesion are mediated predominantly by two families of transmembrane molecules, the cadherin and immunoglobulin-like adhesion molecules, which are re-

A Growth cone extension on an extracellular matrix component

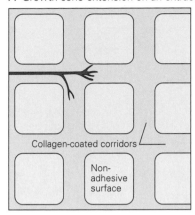
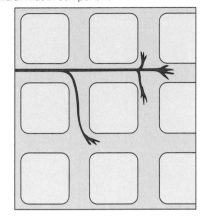

Collagen-coated corridors

Non-adhesive surface

B Laminins in basal laminae interact with integrins on growth cones

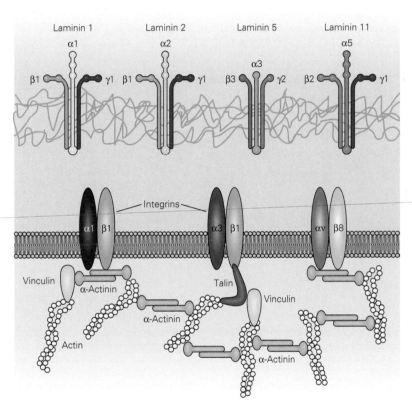

Figure 54-10 Extracellular matrix molecules promote neurite outgrowth.

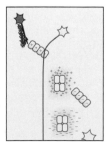

A. Diagram of two frames from a time-lapse film of neurons cultured on a patterned substrate in which corridors coated with collagens are separated by patches coated with an inert metal. Growth cones extend only on the collagen-coated surface. (From Letourneau 1975.)

B. Laminins are major components of basal laminae and account for much of the axon outgrowth-promoting ability of the extracellular matrix. Laminins are cruciform heterotrimers of related α, β, and γ subunits, drawn from

a family of at least 5 α, 4 β, and 3 γ genes. The diagram shows just 4 of the 11 trimers that have been isolated: laminin 1 is a component of many tumor matrices, laminin 2 is present on Schwann cells and muscle fibers, laminin 5 is abundant in skin basement membrane, and laminin 11 is present at the neuromuscular junction. Integrins are matrix-binding proteins in nerve cells. They are heterodimers of α and β subunits. The diagram shows just three of at least seven different dimers that recognize laminins. Integrins differ in the laminins (and other matrix molecules) with which they interact. The intracellular domain of integrins bind to cytoskeletal components such as α-actinin and talin. These interactions couple membrane-matrix adhesion to the cytoskeletal arrangements required for growth cone advance.

A   Cell adhesion assay

Dispersed cell suspension   Cell aggregation   Blockade of cell aggregation by NCAM antibodies

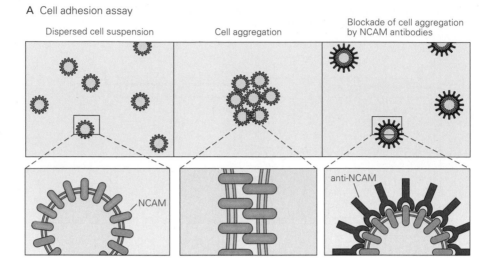

anti-NCAM

NCAM

B₁ Cadherin superfamily   B₂ Immunoglobulin superfamily

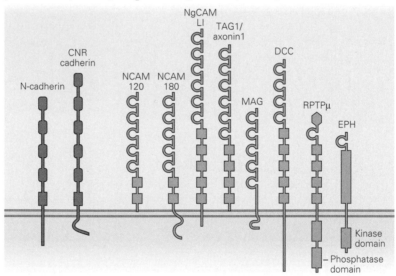

N-cadherin   CNR cadherin   NCAM 120   NCAM 180   NgCAM L1   TAG1/ axonin1   MAG   DCC   RPTPμ   EPH

Kinase domain

Phosphatase domain

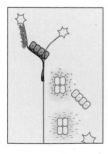

Figure 54-11 Cell adhesion molecules of the cadherin and immunoglobulin superfamilies promote outgrowth of the neurite.

A. A cell adhesion assay used to identify NCAM. Neurons (or other cells) aggregate when swirled gently. Antibodies to the cell surface block the aggregation if they are directed at the adhesive molecules responsible for aggregation. Antibodies with this property can then be used as reagents to isolate adhesion molecules.

B. Structure of some cell adhesion molecules. Classical cadherins (N-cadherin is shown) have extracellular segments that bind calcium and an intracellular domain that binds to catenins and thereby links to the cytoskeleton. Other cadherin-related molecules (protocadherins and cadherin-related neuronal re-

ceptors [CNR]) differ in the number of extracellular segments and structure of their cytoplasmic domains. The members of the immunoglobulin superfamily have disulfide-bonded immunoglobulin- like segments in the extracellular domain, but the number and arrangement of these segments varies among members. For example, some immunoglobulin superfamily molecules link to the cytoskeleton, like the cadherins, whereas others have phosphatase or kinase catalytic activities. Some genes, such as NCAM, even encode diverse proteins with different membrane attachment sites, generated by alternative splicing. Finally, the effects of different immunoglobulin superfamily molecules on neurons are also diverse. For example, NCAM and L1 promote neurite outgrowth, MAG sometimes inhibits neurite outgrowth, and DCC and EPH serve as receptors for netrins and ephrins. Approximately 100 immunoglobulin superfamily molecules have been identified in the nervous system; this diagram shows only a small sample.

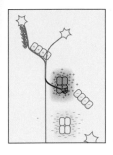

Figure 54-12 Netrins and their receptors mediate chemotropic responses of neurons to intermediate targets.

A. The floor plate, an intermediate target of spinal commissural axons, exerts a tropic effect on commissural axons in a spinal cord explant. (From Tessier-Lavigne et al. 1988.)

B. The netrins account for the tropic activity of the floor plate. Two netrin genes, *netrin 1* and *netrin 2*, have been identified in vertebrates. Their N-termini resembles the N-termini of the laminin γ subunits, but the C-termini are unique. The netrins act on two sets of receptors in the growth cone membrane—the DDC/neogenin family and the unc-5H family. Both are immunoglobulin superfamily members (see Figure 54-11) and interact via their cytoplasmic domains.

A

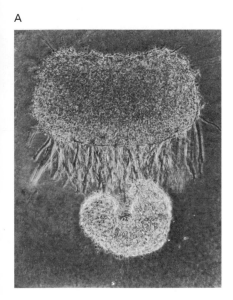

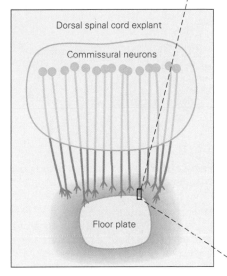

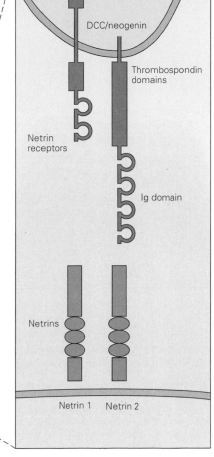

sponsible for calcium-dependent and independent adhesion, respectively. Members of both families serve not only to bind cells together, but also as short-range promotors of neurite outgrowth.

The cadherins are a group of at least 100 related membrane-spanning glycoproteins. The extracellular domains of prototypic cadherins include five related segments, each with about 100 amino acids, that bind calcium (see Figure 54-11B). Cells throughout the body express cadherins. One of the first family members to be isolated, N-cadherin, is abundant in the nervous system, but many other cadherins are expressed by neurons. Cadherins on adjoining membranes interact to form adhesive bonds. Each cadherin prefers to bind to its own kind, forming homophilic interactions. Because of this preference, which is quite strong though not absolute, the cadherins are able to selectively promote adhesion of subsets of embryonic cells. There are also groups of more distantly related proteins called proto-

cadherins and cadherin-related neuronal receptors that number in the dozens. These proteins expand the range of specific interactions mediated by cadherin-like molecules.

The immunoglobulin superfamily may be even larger and more diverse than the cadherins. Its extracellular domain includes one or more characteristic segments, each with about 100 amino acids. The structure of these segments is dominated by disulfide bridges that form a regular pattern. This pattern was first identified in the immunoglobulins made by lymphocytes, which accounts for the family name. Members of the family differ in the number of immunoglobulin segments they bear, and in the number and type of other domains with which the immunoglobulin segments are interspersed (see Figure 54-11B). Like cadherins, many members of the immunoglobulin superfamily bind to others of their own kind; however, many family members also interact with other family members or even with unrelated li-

A Evolutionary conservation in netrin receptor expression and function

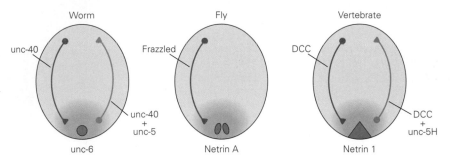

B PKA activation modifies growth cone responses to netrins

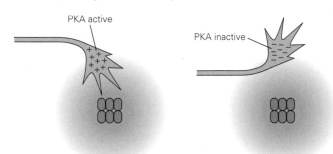

Figure 54-13 Molecules that direct the crossing of central axons at the midline are conserved in worms, flies, and vertebrates.

A. In all three phyla a specific factor secreted by cells at the midline interacts with receptors on axons that grow dorsally and ventrally. The factor (unc-6) and its receptors (unc-5 and unc-40) were discovered in worms. The unc-5 receptor plays a predominant role in axons that grow away from the midline, and the unc-40 receptor is responsible for growth toward the midline. Homologous midline factors (netrins) and receptors (frazzled or DCC on dorsal axons, unc-5h on ventral axons) have

been found in flies and vertebrates. Thus key components of the machinery responsible for circumferential axon guidance is phylogenetically conserved, even though the architecture of the nervous system varies drastically among phyla.

B. The state of protein kinase A (PKA) activation in growth cones can alter the response to a gradient of netrins. Under conditions of PKA activity, such as in the presence of a high cAMP concentration, growth cones are attracted; under conditions of PKA inactivation, growth cones are repelled. (Adapted from Ming et al. 1997.)

gands. The first identified and best characterized member of this family is the neural cell adhesion molecule (NCAM).

Cadherins and immunoglobulin superfamily molecules do not mediate adhesion merely by "sticking" cells together. Adhesion is weak if the intracellular portions of the proteins are removed, indicating that initial adhesion triggers a cytoplasmic reaction that strengthens the adhesion. The cytoplasmic domain is similar in all cadherins and seems to bind a set of proteins called the catenins, which interact with and affect the organization of cytoskeletal elements. In the immunoglobulin superfamily the intracellular domain is more diverse. Some molecules have intracellular domains with catalytic activities, notably protein tyrosine phosphatase or protein tyrosine kinase. In any case, the ability of any of the molecules in either family to promote neurite outgrowth depends critically on so-called

outside-in signaling, whereby the binding or aggregation of adhesion molecules leads to distinct effects within the cell. Although many of these molecules were discovered by use of adhesion assays, and are therefore called adhesion molecules, it may be more accurate to think of them as signaling molecules activated by membrane receptors.

Netrins Are Chemoattractant Factors

Soluble growth factors operate in at least two distinct ways to promote axon growth. One mechanism promotes the survival of the neuron and involves enhancing its ability to extend axons in directions determined by other factors. Crucial trophic factors include the neurotrophins (see Chapter 53).

The other mechanism is chemotaxis, in which the axon grows up or down a concentration gradient of a

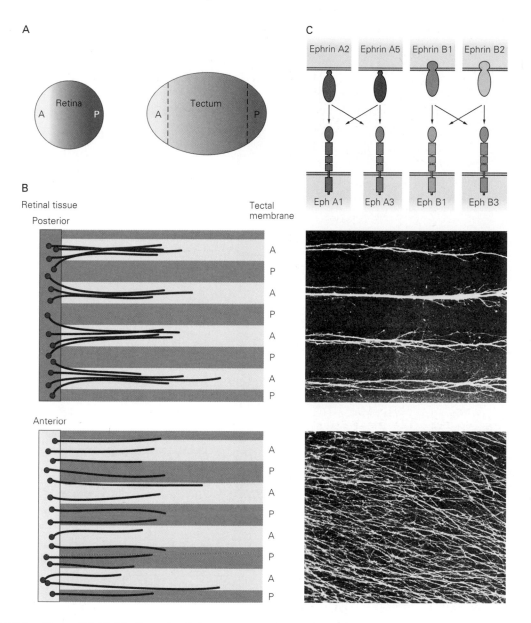

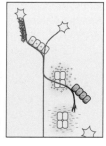

Figure 54-14 Binding of ephrins to eph kinases mediates an inhibitory signal that guides developing axons.

A. Membranes were prepared separately from anterior and posterior optic tectum and laid down in alternating stripes.

B. Axons from explants of posterior (temporal) retina grow selectively on the anterior membranes, thus exhibiting the same preference they show in vivo. In contrast, axons from anterior (nasal) retina grew on both anterior and posterior membranes. The preferential growth of axons on anterior membranes results from the presence of an inhibitory cue in the posterior membranes. (From Walter et al. 1987.)

C. Eph kinases and their ligands, called ephrins, account for at least some of the inhibitory interactions demonstrated in the experiment described in A. Kinases are present on growth cones, where their activation generates an inhibitory signal that reorients growth in a new direction. Ephrins are ligands present on tectal cells and also distributed broadly throughout the nervous system and in nonneural tissues. Kinases and ligands each form two subfamilies. Ephrin A molecules are glycosyl phosphatidyl inositol (GPI)-linked proteins that bind preferentially to the ephA kinases, whereas the ephrin B molecules are membrane-spanning proteins that bind preferentially to the eph B kinases.

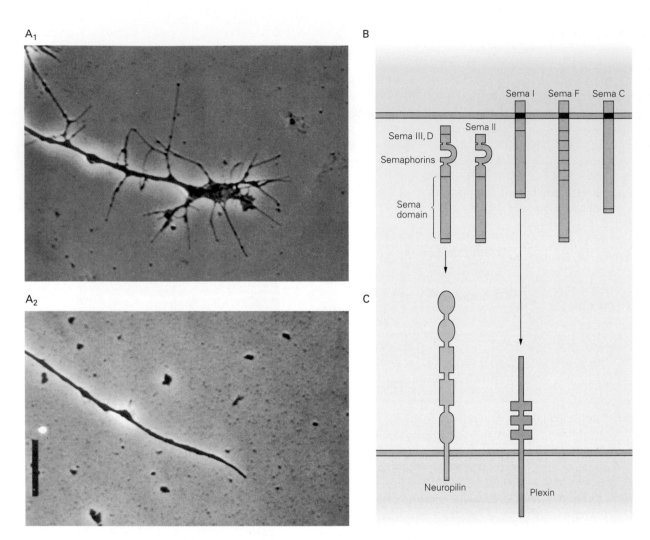

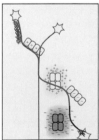

Figure 54-15 Binding of semaphorins to neuropilins causes growth cones to collapse.

A. The growth cone collapse assay used to isolate the semaphorin collapsin-1. A growth cone was imaged live (**1**), then a brain extract was applied locally. The filopodia and lamellipodia of the growth cone collapsed over the next 10 minutes (**2**) but then recovered over the next hour. If the collapsin is applied to only one side of the growth cone, filopodia collapse locally, and the growth cone turns. (Adapted from Raper and Kapfhammer 1992.)

B. At least 15 semaphorins have now been identified, of which five are shown here. All share a characteristic extracellular "sema" domain but differ elsewhere. The family includes membrane-bound and soluble molecules and plays roles both inside and outside the nervous system.

C. Cell adhesion molecules called neuropilins bind the semaphorin III class of proteins and comprise part of the semaphorin receptor complex. A separate class of receptors, the plexins, bind the semaphorin I class of proteins.

chemotropic factor and is thereby guided in a particular direction. This mechanism is called tropism. Some molecules can act as both tropic and trophic factors. In experimental situations axons can sense and grow toward localized sources of the neurotrophin nerve growth fac-

tor. However, clear examples of trophic factors that also act as tropic factors in vivo have not been found. Instead, directed searches for neuronal chemoattractants led to the isolation of two glycoproteins, the netrins, which are related to each other but not to known trophic factors. These secreted proteins are unique but include sequences that resemble the N-terminal portion of the laminin γ subunits (Figure 54-12).

Cloning of netrin genes revealed considerable similarity to the product of *unc-6*, a gene already known to regulate axon guidance in the nematode *Caenorhabditis elegans*. Two other *C. elegans* genes, *unc-5* and *unc-40*, were already thought to encode receptors for *unc-6*, implying that vertebrate netrin receptors would be related to *unc-5* and *unc-40*. As soon as the worm *unc-5* and *unc-40* genes were cloned, their mammalian orthologs were quickly isolated. The unc-5H proteins are homologs of *unc-5* and *DCC* and *neurogenin* are homologs of *unc-40* (see Figure 54-12C). These receptors are members of two subclasses of the immunoglobulin superfamily. The function as well as the structure of the netrins and their receptors has been remarkably conserved during evolution (Figure 54-13).

Ephrins and Semaphorins Guide Growth Cones by Providing Inhibitory Signals

Early evidence that growth cones are guided by inhibitory as well as growth-promoting signals came from studies of retinotectal topography. Friedrich Bonhoeffer and colleagues devised an elegant bioassay in which explants from defined portions of the retina were laid upon a substrate of tectal membrane fragments. The membrane fragments were taken from defined anteroposterior portions of the tectum and were arrayed in alternating stripes. Axons from temporal (posterior) retina grow preferentially on membranes from anterior tectum, displaying a preference reminiscent of that shown in vivo (Figure 54-14A). Remarkably, heat treatment of the anterior membranes, which might be expected to inactivate growth-promoting substances, had little effect on axon outgrowth in the stripe assay, whereas heat treatment of the posterior membranes led to random outgrowth. The preference of axons for anterior membranes thus reflects the presence of inhibitory material in posterior membranes rather than a concentration of attractive or adhesive substances in anterior membranes.

Using this stripe assay, Bonhoeffer and colleagues isolated an inhibitory cue present in membranes from posterior but not anterior tectum. They called it *repulsive axon guidance signal*, or RAGS. Independently, several groups of molecular biologists identified a large class of receptor tyrosine kinases, now called *eph kinases*, and a similar large family of membrane-associated ligands, now called *ephrins* (see Figure 54-14B). These two lines of research converged when molecular cloning revealed that RAGS is ephrin A5. The eph kinases and ephrins

appear to serve a multitude of purposes in neural and nonneural tissues alike. In the developing nervous system these proteins comprise a major group of inhibitory ligands and receptors.

A separate bioassay was used to isolate additional inhibitory molecules, capable of causing growth cones to stop growing, collapse, and then grow in a new direction. This strategy led to the isolation of collapsin-1, the first mammalian member of a family of inhibitory molecules now called the *semaphorins* (Figure 54-15A). At least 15 semaphorins are now known to exist (Figure 54-15B). Each is uniquely distributed and affects distinct types of neurons and many are present and active in nonneural tissues. Key receptors for the semaphorins are immunoglobulin superfamily molecules called *neuropilins* and a family of proteins called *plexins* that shows some structural features of the semaphorins themselves (Figure 54-15C).

Soluble Factors Attract Some Growth Cones and Repel Others

Axons are guided by long-range inhibitory as well as attractive cues, essentially negative chemotactic factors that axons grow away from. Two groups of molecules that provide such inhibitory cues are the semaphorins and netrins which we have already encountered as cell-associated inhibitory cues and soluble attractive cues respectively. Some semaphorins are membrane bound, and act at short range but others are secreted in soluble form and could serve as chemorepellents. Perhaps more surprisingly, the same netrins that attract some axons can inhibit others in vitro (Figure 54-16A). The particular response a growth cone makes to netrins may reflect the complement of netrin receptors it bears: DCC or neogenin appear to mediate attraction responses whereas unc-40 homologs can convert attraction responses into repellent ones. In addition, alterations in levels of intracellular messengers such as cyclic AMP can interconvert attraction and repulsion responses (Figure 54-13B). Finally, some neurotransmitters can arrest growth cone progress, raising the possibility that synaptic transmission in one pathway could exert an inhibitory effect on the formation of another pathway.

Molecules of Different Families Interact to Guide Axons to Their Destinations

So far we have seen that numerous guidance cues line the pathway that any one axon follows, that the growth cone can resolve multiple cues, and that several large

A₁ Netrin attracts commissural axons

A₂ Netrin repels trochlear motor axons

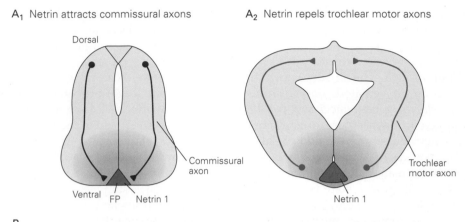

B

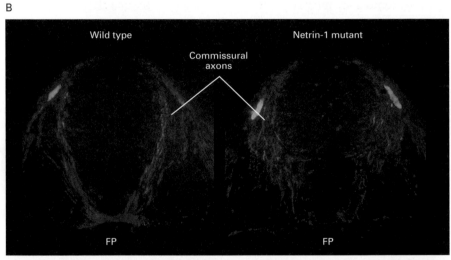

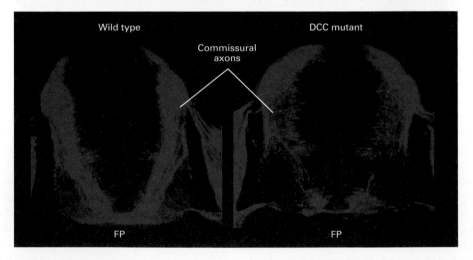

Figure 54-16 Netrin 1 acts as an attractant for some classes of advancing axons but as a repellent for others.

A1. Commissural axons in the spinal cord are attracted by netrins secreted from the floor plate (FP). **2.** Axons of trochlear motor neurons in the brain stem are repelled by the same cue. This repulsion may contribute to the dorsal injection of trochlear motor neurons, a course that is unusual for motor neurons.

B. The trajectories of the commissural axons are perturbed in mutant mice lacking either netrin 1 (**top;** from Serafini et al. 1996) or its receptor, DCC (**bottom;** Fazeli et al. 1997). In contrast, trochlear motor neurons have normal trajectories in mice lacking netrin 1 or DCC, indicating that other factors are involved in their repulsion.

families of molecules are involved in the transmission and reception of guidance cues. The task of assigning specific molecules to specific steps is a daunting one, and the task of understanding how multiple guides work together to get an axon to its target is even more challenging. Nonetheless, the recent convergence of studies in vitro and in vivo has begun to provide real insights into this crucial issue. To illustrate this point, we return to the phenomenon of retinotopic mapping.

Sperry's original surgical and behavioral experiment provided indirect but strong evidence that retinal axons and components of their pathway bear specific cues that promote position-dependent targeting of axons to appropriate tectal regions (see Figure 54-1). Subsequent physiological and anatomical studies provided direct evidence for matching of axons to specific target cells. It became clear that retinal axons reach the optic tectum in a series of steps, each of which is controlled in a distinct way (see Figure 54-2), and all of which are crucial for establishment of the topographic map. Both integrins and cadherins have been implicated in these processes.

In addition, analysis of growing retinal axons within the tectum suggested strongly that gradients of guidance molecules are present within the tectum itself (see Figure 54-4). Using the stripe assay, Bonhoeffer and his colleagues showed that the membranes of tectal cells bear molecules that inhibit axon outgrowth (see Figure 54-14). The concentration of the inhibitory influence varied with tectal position, and axonal sensitivity to it varied with retinal position. The stripe assay then became a critical tool both for purifying active factors and for testing putative factors initially isolated from other sources. Both approaches have converged on two membrane-bound ligands of receptor tyrosine kinases, ephrin A2 and ephrin A5. Both ligands are expressed in low-to-high gradients in the rostral direction in the tectum; both selectively inhibit outgrowth of temporal retinal axons in the stripe assay; and a kinase receptor that binds both of them, eph A3, is expressed in a low-to-high gradient in the temporal direction by retinal ganglion cells (Figure 54-17A). Thus ephrins A2 and A5 are strong candidates for the type of chemospecificity factors Sperry originally proposed.

Based on these discoveries, the role these ephrins play in the formation of the topographic map has been assayed in vivo (see Figure 54-16B, C). In one set of experiments, ephrin A2 was overexpressed in the developing optic tectum of chick embryos. This procedure generated small patches of cells in the rostral tectum that were abnormally rich in ephrin A2. Temporal retinal axons, which normally avoid the ephrin A2-rich caudal tectum also avoided these patches in the rostral tectum and thus terminated in abnormal positions. In contrast, nasal ax-

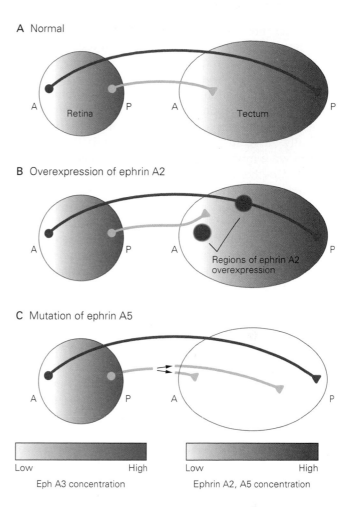

Figure 54-17 Ephrins and eph kinases are required for formation of the retinotopic map in the optic tectum.

A. Eph kinases are distributed in gradients in the retina, and ephrins are distributed in gradients in the optic tectum. These two molecular gradients may regulate retinotectal topography because ephrins bind to eph kinases and activation of eph kinases inhibits axon outgrowth. In particular, the levels of ephrin A2 and A5 are higher in the posterior tectum than in the anterior tectum, and this could inhibit extension of posterior retinal axons, which are rich in eph A3. However, eph kinases are expressed in the tectum as well as the retina, and ephrins are expressed in the retina as well as the tectum; thus the mapping functions are sure to be complex.

B. When ephrin A2 is expressed in portions of the chick optic tectum that normally have low levels of this ligand, posterior retinal axons avoid sites of overexpression and terminate in abnormal positions. In contrast, anterior retinal axons, which normally grow into the ephrin-rich posterior tectum, behave normally when they encounter excess ephrin A2. (Adapted from Nakamoto et al. 1996.)

C. In mutant mice lacking ephrin A5 some posterior retinal axons terminate in inappropriate regions of the tectum. (Adapted from Frisen et al. 1998.)

ons, which normally grow toward the caudal tectum, were not perturbed by encounters with excess ephrin. Conversely, in mice with targeted mutations in *ephrin A2* or *ephrin A5* genes some temporal retinal axons terminated in inappropriate tectal regions, and some transiently extended beyond the caudal boundary of the tectum, into the inferior colliculus, but nasal axons behaved normally. In double mutants lacking both ephrins, deficits were more severe than in either single mutant. Both studies therefore indicate that ephrins influence the targeting of temporal retinal axons.

A full account, however, is not going to be as simple because eph kinases are expressed in the tectum as well as in the retina, ephrins are expressed in the retina as well as in the tectum, and some ephrins as well as eph kinases are expressed in dorsoventral as well as in rostrocaudal gradients. Moreover, some activities observed in the stripe assay are not accounted for by known properties of the ephrins, suggesting that other molecules may contribute to the visuotrophic arrangement of retinal axons. Perhaps most important, the many discrete decisions that axons make on their way to the tectum and after they find the right spot on the tectum remain to be explained. Nonetheless, for the first time, we can see at least the outlines of a molecular explanation for a process that underlies the formation of specific connections in the brain.

This example emphasizes the impact of the use of genetically engineered mice to analyze axonal guidance. Two other genetic approaches also deserve mention. First, in several contexts we have indicated the value of using simple and genetically accessible invertebrates to unravel developmental complexities. In no area has this approach been more fruitful than in the analysis of axon guidance. Dozens of genes that affect this process have been identified and cloned in *Drosophila* and *C. elegans*. This approach has become even more compelling with the recent discovery that several guidance systems are conserved from vertebrates to invertebrates (Figure 54–13). Second, the zebrafish recently became the first vertebrate to which techniques of mutagenesis, so successful in flies and worms, have been applied. Already this approach has generated numerous mutations that affect axonal pathfinding in the retinotectal system.

An Overall View

The specificity of its neuronal connections is the most striking physical feature of the nervous system. Many developmental processes contribute to establishing these precise patterns of connections, but none is more important than the guidance of axons from their points of origin to their appropriate targets. The specificity re-

quired to achieve the correct wiring is quite extraordinary, in that many axons need to grow long distances, bypassing numerous targets along the way, before reaching and forming connections with functionally appropriate synaptic partners.

The nervous system has devised elaborate mechanisms to solve the wiring problem. At the cellular level one basic strategy is to break the long journey into manageable legs. Thus axons do not set off like explorers of old, crossing completely uncharted territory in search of distant goals. Instead, they receive guidance at intervals along the way. Some axons that grew early in the embryo, when distances were short, serve as scaffolds for later-growing axons. Other axons grow along epithelial surfaces or extracellular matrices. Sometimes so-called guidepost cells mark sites at which axons need to make divergent choices.

The axon receives and responds to these guidance clues with a specialized terminal apparatus, the growth cone. The growth cone is both a sensory and a motor structure. It bears numerous receptors to which environmental cues bind as well as cytoskeletal proteins and actin-based motors that propel it forward. And it contains signal transduction systems that convert ligand binding by the receptors into instructions that steer the growth cone. In this way the growing axon can integrate multiple cues to traverse complex terrain.

The past few years have witnessed extraordinary progress in the identification of molecules that guide axons. Guidance cues include soluble, membrane-bound, and extracellular matrix molecules. Many of the soluble molecules are members of large gene families, such as the netrins, semaphorins, laminins, and cadherins. Families of membrane-bound receptors on the growth cones include immunoglobulin superfamily adhesion molecules, cadherins, neuropilins, plexins, and integrins. Perhaps not surprisingly, some developmental neurological disorders are now known to result from mutations in genes that encode these ligands and receptors.

Joshua R. Sanes
Thomas M. Jessell

Selected Readings

Flanagan JG, Vanderhaegen P. 1998. The ephrins and eph receptors in neural development. Annu Rev Neurosci 21:309–345.

Kamiguchi H, Hlavin ML, Yamasaki M, Lemmon V. 1998. Adhesion molecules and inherited diseases of the human nervous system. Annu Rev Neurosci 21:97–125.

Mason CA, Sretavan DW. 1997. Glia, neurons, and axon pathfinding during optic chiasm development. Curr Opin Neurobiol 7:647–653.

Mueller BK. 1999. Growth cone guidance: first steps towards a deeper understanding. Annu Rev Neurosci 22:351–388.

O'Leary DD, Wilkinson DG. 1999. Eph receptors and ephrins in neural development. Curr Opin Neurobiol 9:65–73.

Redies C, Takeichi M. 1996. Cadherins in the developing central nervous system. Dev Biol 180:413–423.

Sanes JR, Yamagata M. 1999. Formation of lamina-specific synaptic connections. Curr Opin Neurobiol 9:79–87.

Shapiro L, Colman DR. 1998. Structural biology of cadherins in the nervous system. Curr Opin Neurobiol 8:593–599.

Song HJ, Poo MM. 1999 Signal transduction underlying growth cone guidance by diffusible factors. Curr Opin Neurobiol 9:355–363.

Tessier-Lavigne M, Goodman CS. 1996. The molecular biology of axon guidance. Science 274:1123–1133.

Varela-Echavarría A, Guthrie S. 1997. Molecules making waves in axon guidance. Genes Dev 11:545–557.

References

Baier H, Klostermann S, Trowe T, Karlstrom RO, Nusslein-Volhard C, Bonhoeffer F. 1996. Genetic dissection of the retinotectal projection. Development 123:415–425.

Bretscher MS. 1996. Getting membrane flow and the cytoskeleton to cooperate in moving cells. Cell 87:601–606.

Bridgman PC, Dailey ME. 1989. The organization of myosin and actin in rapid frozen nerve growth cones. J Cell Biol 108:95–109.

Burrill JD, Easter SS Jr. 1995. The first retinal axons and their microenvironment in zebrafish: cryptic pioneers and the pretract. J Neurosci 15:2935–2947.

Chien CB, Harris WA. 1994. Axonal guidance from retina to tectum in embryonic Xenopus. Curr Top Dev Biol 29:135–169.

Colamarino SA, Tessier-Lavigne M. 1995. The axonal chemoattractant netrin-1 is also a chemorepellent for trochlear motor axons. Cell 81:621–629.

Deiner MS, Kennedy TE, Fazeli A, Serafini T, Tessier-Lavigne M, Sretavan DW. 1997. Netrin-1 and DCC mediate axon guidance locally at the optic disc: loss of function leads to optic nerve hypoplasia. Neuron 19:575–589.

Fazeli A, Dickinson SL, Hermiston ML, Tighe RV, Steen RG, Small CG, Stoeckli ET, Keino-Masu K, Masu M, Rayburn H, Simons J, Bronson RT, Gordon JI, Tessier-Lavigne M, Weinberg RA. 1997. Phenotype of mice lacking functional deleted in colorectal cancer (DCC) gene. Nature 386:796–842.

Forscher P, Smith SJ. 1988. Actions of cytochalasins on the organization of actin filaments and microtubules in a neuronal growth cone. J Cell Biol 107:1505–1516.

Frisen J, Yates PA, McLaughlin T, Firedman GC, O'Leary DMD, Barbacid M. 1998. Ephrin-A5 (AL-1/RAGS) is essential for proper retinal axon guidance and topographic mapping in the mammalian visual system. Neuron 20:233–243.

Godement P, Wang LC, Mason CA. 1994. Retinal axon divergence in the optic chiasm: dynamics of growth cone behavior at the midline. J Neurosci 14:7024–7039.

Gundersen RW, Barrett JN. 1979. Neuronal chemotaxis: chick dorsal-root axons turn toward high concentrations of nerve growth factor. Science 206:1079–1080.

Harris WA. 1989. Local positional cues in the neuroepithelium guide retinal axons in embryonic Xenopus brain. Nature 339:218-221.

Harrison RG. 1910. The outgrowth of the nerve fiber as a mode of protoplasmic movement. J Exp Zool 9:787–846.

He ZG, Tessier-Lavigne M. 1997. Neuropilin is a receptor for the axonal chemorepellent semaphorin III. Cell 90:739–751.

Heidemann SR. 1996. Cytoplasmic mechanisms of axonal and dendritic growth in neurons. Int Rev Cytol 165:235–296.

Hynes RO. 1996. Targeted mutations in cell adhesion genes: What have we learned from them? Dev Biol 180:402–412.

Kapfhammer JP, Grunewald BE, Raper JA. 1986. The selective inhibition of growth cone extension by specific neurites in culture. J Neurosci 6:2527–2534.

Keino-Masu K, Masu M, Hinck L, Leonardo ED, Chan SS-Y, Culotti JG, Tessier-Lavigne M. 1996. Deleted in colorectal cancer (DCC) encodes a netrin receptor. Cell 87:175–185.

Kidd T, Brose K, Mitchell KJ, Fetter RD, Tessier-Lavigne M, Goodman CG, Tear G. 1998. Roundabout controls axon crossing of the CNS midline and defines a novel subfamily of evolutionarily conserved guidance receptors. Cell 92:205–215.

Klostermann S, Bonhoeffer F. 1996. Investigations of signaling pathways in axon growth and guidance. Perspect Dev Neurobiol 4:237–252.

Kolodkin AL, Levengood DV, Rowe EG, Tai Y-T, Giger RJ, Ginty DD. 1997. Neuropilin is a semaphorin III receptor. Cell 90:753–762.

Koppel AM, Feiner L, Kobayashi H, Raper JA. 1997. A 70 amino acid region within the semaphorin domain activates specific cellular response of semaphorin family members. Neuron 19:531–537.

Lance-Jones C, Landmesser L. 1981. Pathway selection by chick lumbosacral motoneurons during normal development. Proc R Soc Lond B 214:1–18.

Lance-Jones C, Landmesser L. 1981. Pathway selection by embryonic chick motoneurons in an experimentally altered environment. Proc R Soc Lond B 214:19–52.

Letourneau PC. 1975. Cell-to-substratum adhesion and guidance of axonal elongation. Dev Biol 44:92–101.

Lumsden AGS, Davies AM. 1983. Earliest sensory nerve fibres are guided to peripheral targets by attractants other than nerve growth factor. Nature 306:786–788.

Luo L, Jan LY, Jan YN. 1997. Rho family small GTP-binding proteins in growth cone signalling. Curr Opin Neurobiol 7:81–86.

Luo Y, Raible D, Raper JA. 1993. Collapsin: a protein in brain that induces the collapse and paralysis of neuronal growth cones. Cell 75:217-227.

Ming GL, Song HJ, Berninger B, Holt CE, Tessier-Lavigne M, Poo MM. 1997. cAMP-dependent growth cone guidance by netrin-1. Neuron 6:1225-1235.

Mitchison T, Kirschner M. 1988. Cytoskeletal dynamics and nerve growth. Neuron 1:761-772.

Nakamoto M, Cheng H-J, Friedman GC, McLaughlin T, Hansen MJ, Yoon CH, O'Leary DMD, Flanagan JG. 1996. Topographically specific effects of ELF-1 on retinal axon guidance *in vitro* and retinal axon mapping *in vivo*. Cell 86:755-766.

Nakamura H, O'Leary DDM. 1989. Inaccuracies in initial growth and arborization of chick retinotectal axons followed by course corrections and axon remodeling to develop topographic order. J Neurosci 9:3776-3795.

Püschel AW. 1996. The semaphorins: a family of axonal guidance molecules? Eur J Neurosci 8:1317-1321.

Raper JA, Kapfhammer JP. 1990. The enrichment of a neuronal growth cone collapsing activity from embryonic chick brain. Neuron 4:21-29.

Rehder V, Kater SB. 1996. Filopodia on neuronal growth cones: multi-functional structures with sensory and motor capabilities. The Neurosciences 8:81-88.

Serafini T, Colamarino SA, Leonardo ED, Wang H, Beddington R, Skarnes WC, Tessier-Lavigne M. 1996. Netrin-1 is required for commissural axon guidance in the developing vertebrate nervous system. Cell 87:1001-1014.

Serafini T, Kennedy TE, Galko MJ, Mirzayan C, Jessell TM, Tessier-Lavigne M. 1994. The netrins define a family of axon outgrowth-promoting proteins homologous to *C. elegans* UNC-6. Cell 78:409-424.

Taniguchi M, Yuasa S, Fujisawa H, Naruse I, Saga S, Mishina M, Yagi T. 1997. Disruption of semaphorin III/D gene causes severe abnormality in peripheral nerve projection. Neuron 19:519-530.

Tessier-Lavigne M, Placzek M, Lumsden AGS, Dodd J, Jessell TM. 1988. Chemotropic guidance of developing axons in the mammalian central nervous system. Nature 336:775-778.

Varela Echavarria A, Tucker A, Puschel AW, Guthrie S. 1997. Motor axon subpopulations respond differentially to the chemorepellents netrin-1 and semaphorin D. Neuron 18:193-207.

Walter J, Henke-Fahle S, Bonhoeffer F. 1987. Avoidance of posterior tectal membranes by temporal retinal axons. Development 101:909-913.

Weiss P. 1941. Nerve patterns: the mechanics of nerve growth. Growth 5(Suppl):163-203.

Winberg ML, Noordermeer JN, Tamagnone L, Comoglio PM, Spriggs MK, Tessier-Lavigne M, Goodman CS. 1998. Plexin A is a neuronal semaphorin receptor that controls axon guidance. Cell 95:903-916.

Zheng JQ, Poo M, Connor JA. 1996. Calcium and chemotropic turning of nerve growth cones. Perspect Dev Neurobiol 4:205-213.

Zinn K, Sun Q. 1999. Slit branches out: A secieted protein mediates both attractive and repulsive axon guidance. Cell 97:1-4.

55

The Formation and Regeneration of Synapses

I N THE THREE PREVIOUS chapters (52–54) we described the early events in the development of the mammalian nervous system: the formation of the neural tube, its subdivision along the anterior-posterior and dorsoventral axes, the birth and differentiation of neurons and glial cells, and the extension of axons. After axons reach appropriate targets they begin to form synapses, the structures that permit signaling between nerve cells. Synapse formation completes the hard wiring of the nervous system. Once synapses have formed, an information-processing circuit begins to function. Thereafter, the information-processing capacity of each circuit is refined through use. In this sense, the nervous system continues to develop throughout life.

Synapse formation involves three key events: the formation of selective connections between the developing axon and its target, the differentiation of the axon's growth cone into a nerve terminal, and the elaboration of a postsynaptic apparatus in the target cell. These steps depend critically on intercellular interactions. Indeed, the current consensus is that a series of signals between cells is responsible for the axon's recognition of an appropriate postsynaptic cell (and sometimes even a specific domain on the postsynaptic cell's surface) and the coordinated differentiation of pre- and postsynaptic elements of the synapse. In this chapter we therefore focus on the intercellular signaling that underlies formation of the synapse.

Most of what we know about these developmental interactions comes from studies of the neuromuscular junction, the synapse that motor neurons make on skeletal muscle fibers. The simplicity and accessibility of this synapse have made it a useful model for ultrastructural and electrophysiological studies of chemical synapses

A

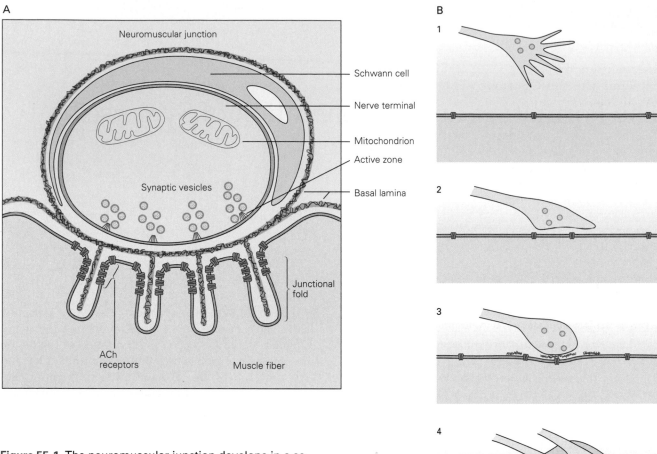

Neuromuscular junction

Schwann cell

Nerve terminal

Mitochondrion

Active zone

Basal lamina

Synaptic vesicles

Junctional fold

ACh receptors

Muscle fiber

B

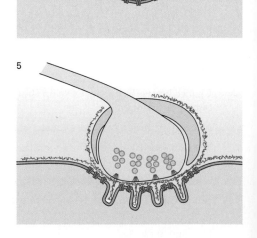

Figure 55-1 The neuromuscular junction develops in a series of steps.

A. At the mature neuromuscular junction, pre- and postsynaptic membranes are separated by a synaptic cleft containing extracellular material. Vesicles are clustered at a presynaptic release site, transmitter receptors are clustered in the postsynaptic membrane, and nerve terminals are coated by glial processes.

B. Stages in the development of the neuromuscular junction: (**1**) A growth cone approaches a newly formed myotube and (**2**) forms a morphologically unspecialized but functional contact. (**3**) The terminal accumulates synaptic vesicles and a basal lamina forms in the synaptic cleft. (**4**) As the muscle matures, multiple axons converge on a single site. (**5**) Finally, all axons but one are eliminated and the survivor matures. (Based on Hall and Sanes 1993.)

(see Chapter 11). These same features, as well as the wealth of information on the adult neuromuscular junction, have made it a powerful system for the analysis of synaptic development. We therefore use the neuromuscular synapse here to exemplify key features of synaptic

development. We then apply what has been learned from this model synapse to other, less tractable synapses that form between neurons in the peripheral and central nervous systems. Finally, we discuss the limited ability of the central nervous system to form new synapses after injury and consider new strategies to circumvent this limitation.

Interactions Between Motor Neurons and Skeletal Muscles Organize the Development of the Neuromuscular Junction

The mature neuromuscular junction comprises parts of three types of cells—a motor nerve terminal, a muscle fiber, and a few Schwann cells. All three cells are highly differentiated in their region of apposition (Figure 55-1A).

The terminals of the motor neuron are rich in synaptic vesicles that contain the neurotransmitter acetylcholine (ACh). Many of these vesicles are clustered at dense patches on the presynaptic membrane, called *active zones,* where they fuse with the plasma membrane of the nerve terminal and release their contents into the synaptic cleft (see Chapter 4). The nerve terminal is also rich in mitochondria, which provide the energy required to synthesize, package, and release neurotransmitter and to recover and recycle membrane after vesicle fusion. In contrast, the segments of the motor axon that lead to the terminals are rich in neurofilaments but contain few vesicles or mitochondria and no active zones.

Schwann cells are glial cells that insulate the entire motor axon, from the point at which it exits the spinal cord to its nerve terminals. Preterminal Schwann cells form the myelin sheath, whereas terminal Schwann cells extend thin processes that form a continuous nonmyelin layer over the nerve terminals.

The surface of the muscle fiber is indented directly opposite the active zones in the nerve terminal, forming a series of postsynaptic sites on the membrane called the *junctional folds.* The postsynaptic sites are rich in ACh receptors and include an elaborate cytoskeleton that holds the receptors in place, as well as a number of specialized adhesion and signaling molecules. In contrast, nonsynaptic portions of the muscle membrane are not folded, contain very few ACh receptors, and have a markedly different cytoskeleton.

A layer of extracellular material called *basal lamina* ensheaths the entire muscle fiber. The synaptic portion of the basal lamina is continuous with, and ultrastructurally similar to, the nonsynaptic portion, but the two regions have distinctive molecular structures. For example, synaptic basal lamina is rich in the enzyme acetylcholinesterase, which hydrolyzes released ACh and thus terminates transmitter action.

The process of synapse formation is initiated when a motor axon, guided by the multiple factors described in Chapter 54, reaches a developing skeletal muscle and

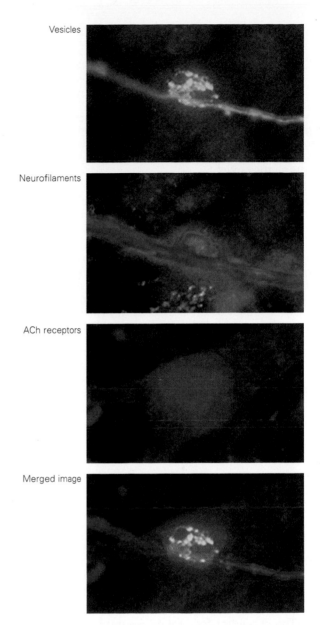

Vesicles

Neurofilaments

ACh receptors

Merged image

Figure 55-2 Nerve and muscle cells organize each other's differentiation at points of apposition. Images show embryonic neurons and muscle cells cultured together, then stained with antibodies to axonal neurofilaments (**blue**), synaptic vesicle proteins (**green**), and ACh receptors (**red**). In regions of nerve-muscle apposition, the neurons form vesicle-rich, filament-poor terminal arborizations and the muscle organizes clusters of ACh receptors. (Courtesy of Young-Jin Son.)

approaches an immature muscle fiber or *myotube.* Contact is then made and the process of differentiation begins. The growth cone begins its transformation into a nerve terminal while the portion of the muscle surface opposite the nerve terminal becomes distinct from the nonsynaptic regions. As development proceeds, synaptic components are added and ultrastructural signs of

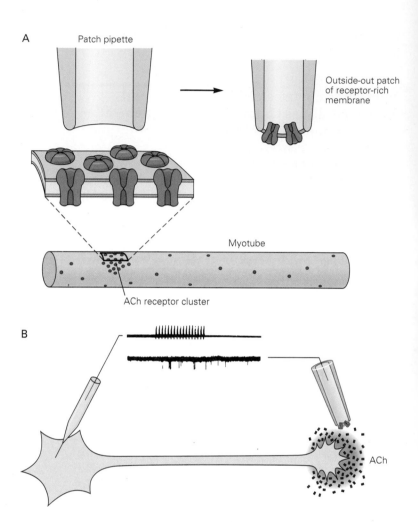

Figure 55-3 Although synaptic differentiation requires intercellular interactions, nerve and muscle cells can assemble synaptic components on their own.

A. Demonstration of the release of ACh from growth cones. An electrode tip is coated with an outside-out patch of muscle membrane containing a high density of ACh receptors.

B. A microelectrode is used to stimulate an isolated cultured motor neuron; the evoked action potentials are shown in the top trace. The membrane patch containing ACh receptors is activated by the ACh released from the neuron upon stimulation. Bottom trace shows ACh receptor activity within the membrane patch. The receptor-bearing micropipette serves as a sensitive biodetector of released ACh. Use of this method showed that motor axons synthesize and release ACh even in the absence of myotubes. (Based on Hume et al. 1983.)

synaptic differentiation become apparent in the pre- and postsynaptic cells and in the synaptic cleft. Eventually, the neuromuscular junction acquires its mature and complex form (see Figure 55-1B).

Three general features of neuromuscular development give us clues about the mechanisms that underlie synapse formation. First, nerve and muscle organize each other's differentiation. In principle, the precise apposition of pre- and postsynaptic specializations might be explained by independent programming of nerve and muscle properties. However, studies of cultured cells show that this is not how it happens. When motor neurons and myoblasts from embryonic chicks or rodents are cultured in isolation, the myoblasts fuse to form myotubes and the motor neurons extend axons to the myotubes. At sites where the two cells meet, both acquire specializations that are found at synapses in vivo (Figure 55-2). The initial contact of the cells is essentially random; thus the site of synaptic specialization is not predetermined. Such specializations are instead initi-

ated and organized by molecular signals that pass between the nerve and muscle.

The second key feature of neuromuscular development is that new synaptic components are added in a series of defined developmental steps. Thus the newly formed neuromuscular junction is not simply an immature version of the fully developed synapse. For example, although the nerve and muscle membrane form contacts at an early stage in synaptogenesis, only at a later stage does the synaptic cleft widen and the basal lamina appear. Similarly, ACh receptors accumulate in the postsynaptic membrane before acetylcholinesterase accumulates in the synaptic cleft. Active zones form in the nerve terminal only after vesicles have accumulated, and junctional folds form in the postsynaptic membrane only after the nerve terminal has matured. Around the time of birth several different axons innervate each myotube, but during early postnatal life all but one withdraw (see Figure 55-1B). This elaborate sequence is unlikely to be organized by simple contact between

A Nerve evoked redistribution of preexisting ACh receptors

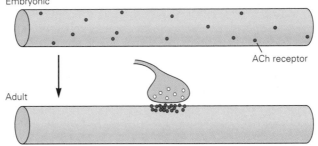

B Nerve evoked transcription of ACh receptor genes in subsynaptic nuclei leads to local receptor insertion

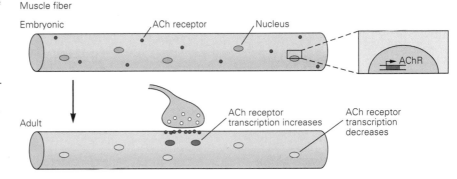

Figure 55-4 The clustering of ACh receptors at the neuromuscular junction is due to both translocation and transcriptional regulation of receptors.

A. ACh receptors are distributed diffusely on the surface of newly formed myotubes. As development proceeds, the number of receptors decreases in extrasynaptic regions but increases at the synapse. In part this redistribution reflects aggregation of existing receptors beneath the nerve terminal.

B. In addition, expression of ACh receptor genes is modulated as the myotube matures. Initially, the genes are expressed throughout the myotube. Subsequently, gene expression is upregulated in nuclei that lie directly beneath the nerve terminal. Later still, transcription of ACh receptor genes is downregulated in nuclei in extrasynaptic regions. This transcriptional pattern leads to localized synthesis of ACh receptors at synaptic sites of the muscle fiber.

nerve and muscle. More probably, signals pass between the cells: The nerve sends a signal to the muscle that triggers the first steps in postsynaptic differentiation, which generates a retrograde signal that triggers the initial steps of nerve terminal differentiation. The nerve then sends further signals to the muscle and this reverberative interaction continues.

The third critical feature of neuromuscular development is that most synaptic components of the motor neuron and myotube develop on their own. Motor axons, for example, can form synaptic vesicles and synthesize neurotransmitter in the absence of muscle. In fact, clever electrophysiological detection methods have revealed that vesicles in growth cones can release ACh in response to electrical stimulation, even before the growth cones have reached their target cells (Figure 55-3A). Similarly, uninnervated myotubes can synthesize functional ACh receptors. Moreover, some of these receptors cluster into high-density aggregates, much like those found in the postsynaptic membrane, and these aggregates become associated with components of the cytoskeleton and basal lamina that are localized at synapses in vivo (Figure 55-3B). When synapses form, however, these specializations disperse and new ones

are assembled at sites of nerve muscle contact. These observations tell us that the developmental signals that pass between nerve and muscle are unlikely to be signals that induce wholesale changes in cell properties, such as those that regulate neurogenesis at earlier stages (Chapter 52). Instead, the role of the developing nerve and muscle is to assure that components of the pre- and postsynaptic apparatus are formed at appropriate levels, at the correct time, and in correct places. For this reason, it is helpful to think of the intercellular signals that control synaptogenesis as organizers rather than inducers.

The Motor Nerve Organizes Differentiation of the Postsynaptic Muscle Membrane

To illustrate the ways in which axons organize postsynaptic differentiation, we will consider the development of the ACh receptors of the neuromuscular junction. As we have seen in Chapter 11, ACh receptors are pentamers, composed of α, β, δ, γ, or ε subunits encoded by related genes. The subunits form a barrel-like structure that spans the membrane; the channel formed by

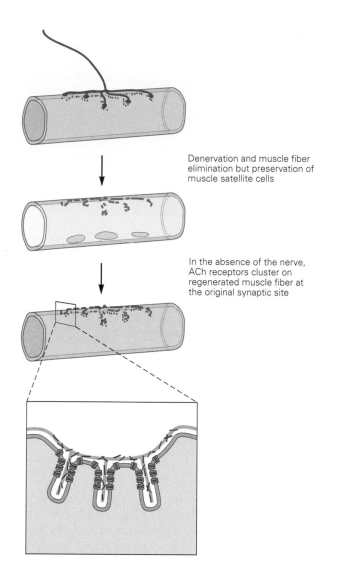

Denervation and muscle fiber elimination but preservation of muscle satellite cells

In the absence of the nerve, ACh receptors cluster on regenerated muscle fiber at the original synaptic site

Figure 55-5 Components in the synaptic basal lamina direct the clustering of ACh receptors on the muscle surface. Denervation of a skeletal muscle fiber and elimination of mature muscle fibers leaves the basal lamina sheath intact. Muscle satellite cells proliferate and differentiate to form new myofibers. The expression of ACh receptors on the regenerated myofiber surface is concentrated in the region of the synaptic basal lamina, even when reinnervation is prevented. These findings showed components of the basal lamina are sufficient to direct the localization of ACh receptors on the muscle membrane. (Based on McMahan 1990.)

the plasma membrane. Although some receptors spontaneously cluster into aggregates, the majority are distributed throughout the membrane at a density of about 1000 per μm^2. Once synapse formation is complete, the distribution of the receptors changes drastically: The receptors become highly concentrated in the synaptic sites of the membrane (to a density up to 10,000 per μm^2) and depleted in the nonsynaptic membrane (being present at 10 per μm^2 or less). This thousand-fold difference in ACh receptor density occurs within a few tens of microns at the edge of the nerve terminal (see Figure 55-4B).

The redistribution of ACh receptors is the result of the combined effects of three distinct processes: translocation of ACh receptors within the membrane from nonsynaptic to synaptic regions; a transcriptional activation of the expression of genes for the ACh receptor subunits in the few nuclei that lie directly beneath the postsynaptic membrane; and repression of the expression of receptor subunit genes in the nuclei of nonsynaptic regions. The motor nerve controls the entire redistribution program but uses distinct signals to regulate each process. We will consider each process in turn.

Agrin Triggers the Clustering of Acetylcholine Receptors

To analyze the distribution of ACh receptors on the muscle surface it is first necessary to label them. The most common means of visualizing ACh receptors on muscle cells is by use of a toxin, α-bungarotoxin, isolated from the venom of the poisonous snake *Bungarus bungaris*. This small protein binds specifically and almost irreversibly to ACh receptors, inactivating them. In the wild the snake uses α-bungarotoxin to paralyze its prey. In the laboratory neurobiologists conjugate a fluorophore to the toxin, creating a stain for ACh receptors.

Monroe Cohen, Gerald Fischbach, and their collaborators analyzed the distribution of labeled ACh receptors on muscle cells in vitro before and after innervation by motor neurons. Prior to innervation ACh receptors were distributed uniformly on the muscle surface, or in occasional patches, but after innervation prelabeled receptors were concentrated at synaptic sites. The simple observation that receptors present on the muscle surface before the nerve arrives later appeared at synapses indicates that axons can cause the redistribution of ACh receptors within the plane of the membrane. Based on these studies and denervation experiments indicating that the activity responsible for clustering ACh receptors resides in the basal lamina (Figure 55-5), Uel McMahan and colleagues searched for factors that might

this structure opens to let cations through when ACh binds.

Soon after myoblasts fuse to form myotubes the genes that encode ACh receptor subunits are activated. The subunits are synthesized, assembled into pentamers in the endoplasmic reticulum, and inserted into

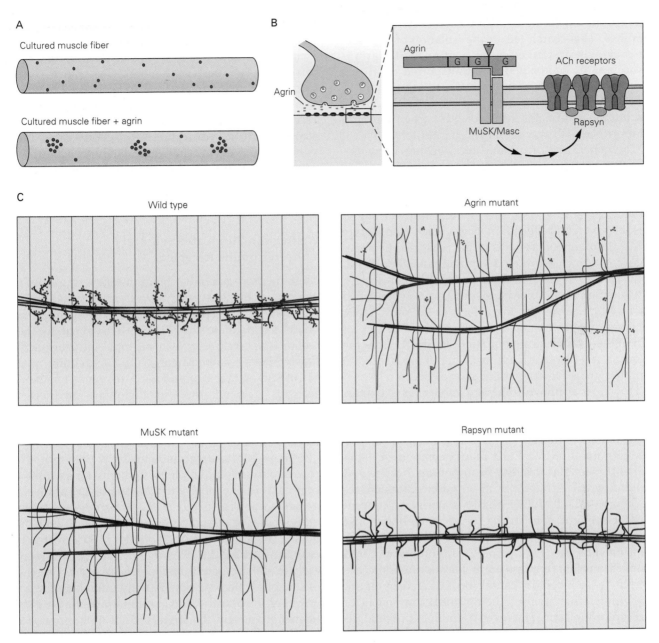

Figure 55-6 Agrin released by nerve terminals acts through MuSK and rapsyn to aggregate ACh receptors at synaptic sites in the muscle fiber.

A. ACh receptors on cultured myotubes were labeled with rhodamine-conjugated α-bungarotoxin. Few receptor clusters form under control conditions, but addition of basal lamina extract induces clustering. Researchers used this assay to purify agrin from the basal lamina extract.

B. Agrin is a large extracellular matrix proteoglycan. Alternative splicing at a site called "z" regulates ability of agrin to cluster ACh receptors. Only neurons synthesize the active isoform containing the z site. Agrin activates the membrane-associated receptor tyrosine kinase MuSK, triggering a cascade of intracellular reactions that results in clustering. Rapsyn, a cytoplasmic

ACh receptor-associated protein is essential for clustering.

C. Muscles from a wild-type neonatal mouse and from mutants lacking agrin, MuSK, or rapsyn. Muscles were double labeled for ACh receptors (**green**) and nerves (**brown**). By birth, ACh receptor clusters have formed beneath each nerve terminal. Few clusters are present in the agrin mutant, and none are present in the MuSK or rapsyn mutants. In the rapsyn mutant, however, ACh receptor levels are higher in the synaptic area than at the ends of myotubes, reflecting the preservation of synapse-specific transcription. All three mutants also have nerve abnormalities, reflecting the inability of the muscle to supply proper retrograde factors. (Based on Gautam et al. 1995, 1996; DeChiara et al. 1996.)

influence the clustering of ACh receptors in embryonic myotubes. This search led to the isolation of an ~400-kDa proteoglycan termed agrin (Figure 55-6). Agrin is synthesized by motor neurons, transported down the axon, released from nerve terminals, and incorporated into the synaptic cleft. Agrin is also made by muscle cells, but the neuronal isoforms of agrin are a thousand-fold more active in aggregating ACh receptors.

The generation of mutant mice lacking agrin provides strong evidence that agrin has a role in the organization of ACh receptors. Agrin mutants have grossly perturbed neuromuscular junctions and die at birth. The number, size, and density of ACh receptor aggregates is severely reduced in these mice (see Figure 55-6C). All other components of the postsynaptic apparatus—including cytoskeletal, membrane, and basal lamina proteins—are similarly reduced. Interestingly, differentiation of presynaptic elements is also perturbed in the mutant. However, the defects in the presynaptic element probably do not result directly from lack of agrin in the motor neuron but result indirectly from the failure of the disorganized postsynaptic apparatus to generate signals for presynaptic specialization.

How does agrin work? Several molecules that interact with agrin are present in myotube membranes, including dystroglycan, which is critical to maintaining muscle stability, and integrins, which mediate interactions with many extracellular matrix components. Any or all of these molecules may be important, but the best candidate as an agrin receptor is a muscle-specific tyrosine kinase called MuSK. MuSK is normally concentrated at synaptic sites in the muscle membrane, and muscles of mutant mice lacking MuSK have no ACh receptor clusters (see Figure 55-6C). Myotubes cultured from these mutants express normal levels of ACh receptors, but these receptors cannot be clustered by agrin. MuSK therefore appears to be a critical component of the receptor for agrin. However, agrin does not bind directly to MuSK, so the agrin receptor may contain an additional subunit.

One key component in the cascade of reactions initiated by MuSK is a cytoplasmic protein called rapsyn. Rapsyn is colocalized with ACh receptors in vivo and is present at ACh receptor clusters soon after they form. It can induce the aggregation of ACh receptors in vitro. In mice lacking rapsyn, muscles form normally and ACh receptors accumulate in normal numbers but fail to aggregate at the synaptic sites on the membrane (see Figure 55-6C). Thus rapsyn is an essential component of the cytoskeletal apparatus responsible for ACh receptor clustering.

Although many components of the synaptic membrane and cytoskeleton in muscle remain diffusely distributed in rapsyn-deficient mice, MuSK nevertheless becomes concentrated at synaptic sites. It is likely therefore, that MuSK is a critical component of a primary synaptic scaffold to which rapsyn recruits ACh receptors and other postsynaptic proteins. Agrin released from the nerve localizes MuSK to synaptic sites in addition to activating MuSK. MuSK in turn stimulates ACh receptor clustering via its kinase activity and plays a structural role in nucleating synapse assembly. In this way the nerve not only stimulates specialization at synaptic sites in the muscle, but also ensures that ACh receptor aggregates are precisely apposed to sites of ACh (and agrin) release from the nerve.

Neuregulin Stimulates Synthesis of Acetylcholine Receptors

Motor neurons not only trigger the clustering of ACh receptors in the postsynaptic cell membrane, but also stimulate ACh receptor synthesis. A search for the molecules that mediate this distinct activity of the nerve led to isolation of an ACh receptor–inducing activity (ARIA) later renamed neuregulin. Neuregulin is capable of stimulating expression of the genes for the ACh receptor subunit. Molecular cloning revealed that neuregulin is the product of the gene that encodes a protein previously purified as the ligand of a set of receptor tyrosine kinases called erbB2, erbB3, and erbB4.

Like agrin, neuregulin is made by both motor neurons and muscles; like MuSK, the erbB kinases are concentrated in the postsynaptic muscle membrane. Together, these results suggest that neuregulin activates erbB kinases to stimulate ACh receptor synthesis in the muscle (Figure 55-7A). Mutant mice lacking neuregulin, erbB2, or erbB4 die of cardiovascular malformations early in embryogenesis and so are not useful for studies of synaptic differentiation. In neuregulin heterozygotes, however, the density of ACh receptors in the postsynaptic membrane and the abundance of ACh receptor subunit RNA in muscle are both decreased by 50% (Figure 55-7B). These observations support the idea that neuregulin is an activator of postsynaptic specialization. They do not tell us, however, whether nerve- or muscle-derived neuregulin is more important.

Why would the nerve need to stimulate expression of ACh receptor genes when myotubes can express these genes on their own? The answer may lie in the peculiar geometry of the muscle fiber. Individual muscle fibers can be several centimeters long and contain hundreds of nuclei along their length. ACh receptors synthesized near the ends of fibers would never reach the synapse, despite the actions of agrin. However, several nuclei are clustered just beneath the synaptic membrane, and their products do not have far to go to reach

A Neuregulin controls ACh receptor gene transcription

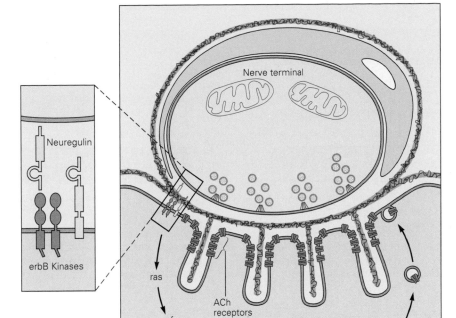

B A decrease in ACh receptors in neuregulin heterozygote mice

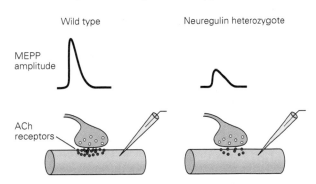

Figure 55-7 Neuregulin stimulates expression of the genes encoding the ACh receptors.

A. Neuregulins are synthesized and secreted by motor axons. Binding of neuregulin to erbB kinases in the postsynaptic membrane activates transcription of ACh receptor genes via a cascade of protein kinases. Neuregulins are also synthesized by muscle, and the neuregulin gene is subject to alternative splicing to generate more than 20 membrane- and matrix-bound forms. Thus neuregulins may influence ACh receptor synthesis both as a nerve-derived messenger and as a muscle-derived second messenger. In addition, three different erbB kinases

(erbB2, erbB3, and erbB4) are expressed by muscle, and erbB2 and erbB3 are also expressed by Schwann cells. Neuregulin may stimulate ACh receptor expression through transduction pathways that involve ras, and the raf, and the ETS class transcription factors.

B. A decrease in ACh receptors in heterozygos neuregulin mice. Both the density of the ACh receptors and the amplitude of the miniature end-plate potential (MEPP) is decreased around 50% in the heterozygote compared to wild type mice, suggesting that neuregulin is a rate-limiting factor for ACh receptor expression. (From Sandrock et al. 1997.)

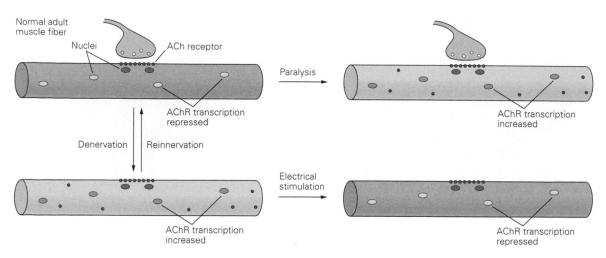

Figure 55-8 Nerve activity regulates expression of the ACh receptor in nonsynaptic areas of the muscle fiber. During development, electrical activity evoked by synaptic transmission represses ACh gene expression by nuclei in nonsynaptic regions of the embryonic muscle, leading to a lower density of ACh receptors in these regions. The nuclei near synaptic sites are immune to this repressive effect of activity. Following de- nervation, ACh receptor gene expression is upregulated in extrasynaptic nuclei, though not to the high level maintained by synaptic nuclei. Paralysis mimics the effect of denervation, whereas electrical stimulation of denervated muscle mimics the nerve and maintains low levels of ACh receptors in the extrasynaptic membrane.

the synapse. These subsynaptic nuclei express the genes encoding ACh receptor subunits (and those encoding some other components of the postsynaptic membrane as well) at far higher levels than nonsynaptic nuclei within the same cytoplasm (see Figure 55-4). The concentration of ACh receptor subunit mRNAs in synaptic areas leads to preferential synthesis and insertion of ACh receptors near synaptic sites. Thus, by acting locally, neuregulin and the erbB kinases activate transcription in synaptic nuclei and thereby stimulate synthesis of ACh receptors specifically in synaptic areas.

Neural Activity Represses Synthesis of Acetylcholine Receptors in Nonsynaptic Areas

Around the time of birth, the density of ACh receptors in nonsynaptic portions of the muscle membrane declines. Yet many more receptors in nonsynaptic areas of the membrane are lost than can be accounted for by clustering at the synapse. The loss of nonsynaptic receptors results primarily from a decrease in the expression of the ACh receptor subunit genes by nonsynaptic nuclei, which decreases the level of ACh receptor mRNA and thus receptor synthesis.

The decreased ACh receptor expression reflects a repressive effect of the nerve, as originally shown by studies of denervated muscle. When muscle fibers are dener- vated, as happens when the motor nerve is damaged, the density of ACh receptors in the postsynaptic membrane increases markedly, a phenomenon termed *denervation supersensitivity*. This suppressive effect of the nerve is mediated by electrical activation of the muscle rather than by a protein factor such as agrin or neuregulin. Under normal conditions the nerve keeps the muscle electrically active, and active muscle synthesizes fewer ACh receptors than inactive muscle. Indeed, direct stimulation of denervated muscle through implanted electrodes decreases ACh receptor expression, preventing or reversing the effect of denervation (Figure 55-8). Conversely, when nerve activity is blocked by application of a local anesthetic, the number of ACh receptors throughout the muscle fiber increases, even though the synapse is intact. Blockade of synaptic transmission by application of α-bungarotoxin to the muscle has a similar effect. Thus the number of ACh receptors in extrasynaptic regions of the muscle is controlled by the level of activity of the muscle cell.

In essence then, the nerve uses ACh to repress expression of the ACh receptor genes. Current that passes through the receptor leads to an action potential that propagates along the entire muscle fiber. This depolarization opens voltage-dependent Ca^{2+} channels, leading to an influx of Ca^{2+}. The Ca^{2+} influx activates a cascade of protein kinase reactions that transduces signals that reach the nonsynaptic nuclei and regulate the

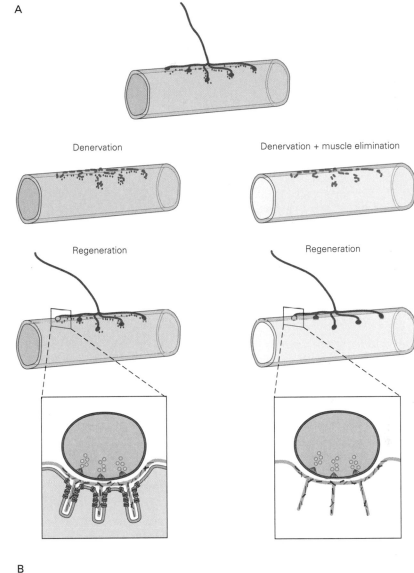

Figure 55-9 Components of the basal lamina at the synaptic site help organize the nerve terminal.

A. Following nerve damage motor axons regenerate and form new neuromuscular junctions. Nearly all of the new synapses form at the original synaptic sites (**left**). A strong preference for original sites persists even after the muscle fibers have been removed, leaving behind basal lamina "ghosts" (**right**). Moreover, the regenerating axons differentiate into nerve terminals when they contact original synaptic basal lamina. Thus components of synaptic basal lamina account for the selective reinnervation of synaptic sites and trigger the differentiation of growth cones into nerve terminals.

B. Micrograph showing a normal neuromuscular junction (**left**). Micrograph showing nerve terminals that differentiated following reinnervation of a basal lamina ghost (**right**). (From Glicksman and Sanes 1983.)

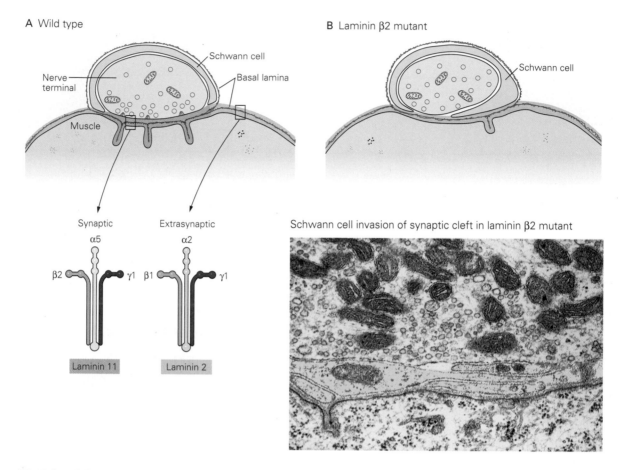

Figure 55-10 Laminins are major components of the basal lamina.

A. Different laminin isoforms are found in synaptic and extrasynaptic basal lamina. Laminin 11, composed of α5, β2, and γ1 subunits, is confined to the synaptic basal lamina, whereas laminin-2 (α2/β1/γ1) is confined to the extrasynaptic basal lamina.

B. Maturation of neuromuscular junctions is impaired in mice lacking the laminin-11 protein as a consequence of targeted inactivation of the laminin β2 gene. Few active zones form and Schwann cell processes invade the synaptic cleft. (From Noakes et al. 1995.)

transcription of ACh receptor genes. Thus the same voltage changes that produce muscle contraction over a period of milliseconds also regulate transcription of ACh receptor genes over a period of days.

Several Aspects of Postsynaptic Differentiation Are Controlled by the Motor Axon

Many components of the postsynaptic apparatus are subject to the organizing influences of the three neural signals (agrin, neuregulin, and ACh) that lead to clustering of ACh receptors. Mice lacking agrin, MuSK, or rapsyn are defective in nearly all aspects of postsynaptic specialization. Nevertheless, not all components are regulated in the same way, because postsynaptic specialization occurs in sequential steps. For example, agrin stimulates aggregation of acetylcholinesterase as well as

ACh receptors, but synthesis of acetylcholinesterase also requires muscle activity. The requirement of nerve-evoked muscle activity for the synthesis of acetylcholinesterase but not ACh receptors may explain the sequential expression of these two proteins at synapses.

The Muscle Fiber Organizes the Differentiation of Motor Nerve Terminals

Soon after the growth cone of a motor axon contacts a developing myotube a rudimentary form of neurotransmission begins. The axon releases ACh in vesicular packets, the transmitter binds to receptors, and the muscle responds with depolarization and weak contractions. The onset of transmission at the new synapse reflects the intrinsic capabilities of each synaptic partner.

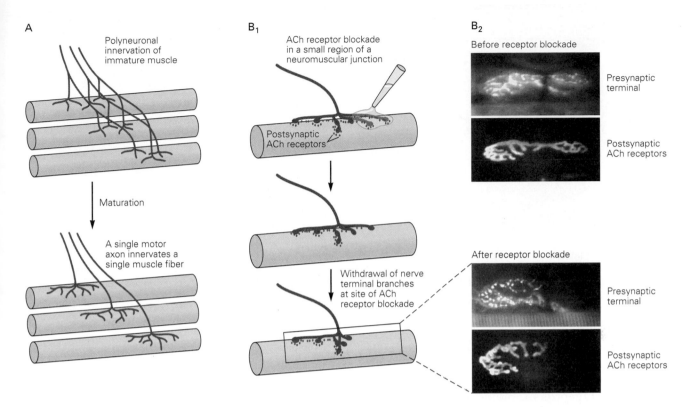

Figure 55-11 Some synapses are eliminated after birth.

A. As the neuromuscular junction develops, each myotube becomes innervated by several motor axons at a common synaptic site. After birth all terminals but one withdraw from each site, and the survivor grows. This elimination occurs without any overall loss of axons: The axons that "lose" at some muscle fibers "win" at others.

B. Diagrams (**B1**) and fluorescent images (**B2**) show that local postsynaptic inactivity can cause elimination of overlying nerve terminals. Some ACh receptors at an adult neuromuscular junction are blocked by focal application of α-bungarotoxin whereas

others are left unperturbed. Those nerve terminals opposite the blocked ACh receptors retracted, and those opposite the unblocked receptors maintained synaptic contact. In contrast, blockade of all ACh receptors had little effect (not shown). This result suggests that differential activity by competing inputs (but not activity per se) influences the survival of those inputs. This mechanism may be responsible for synapse elimination during development. In **B2**, a nerve terminal dye was used to image presynaptic terminals and rhodamine-α bungarotoxin labeling to map the distribution of ACh receptors. (Adapted from Balice-Gordon and Lichtman 1994.)

Nevertheless, cell-intrinsic behaviors cannot readily explain the marked increase in the rate of transmitter release that occurs after nerve-muscle contact is made, nor can they explain the accumulation of synaptic vesicles and assembly of active zones in the small portions of the motor axon that directly abut the muscle surface. These developmental steps require retrograde signals from muscle to nerve.

Evidence for the existence of such retrograde signals has come from studies on the reinnervation of adult muscle. Although axotomy leaves muscle fibers denervated, and leads to a proliferation of ACh receptors in nonsynaptic regions, the postsynaptic apparatus remains largely intact. It is still recognizable by its subsynaptic nuclei, junctional folds, and the ACh receptors, which remain far more densely packed in synaptic areas

than in extrasynaptic areas of the cell. Damaged peripheral axons regenerate readily (unlike those in the central nervous system) and form new neuromuscular junctions that look and perform much like the original ones. A century ago Fernando Tello, a student of Santiago Ramón y Cajal, noted that most such junctions form at preexisting synaptic sites on the denervated muscle fibers (Figure 55-8A) even though the postsynaptic membrane occupies only 0.1% of the muscle fiber surface (Figure 55-9). Thus motor axons must recognize signals associated with the postsynaptic apparatus. Moreover, presynaptic specialization in the axon occurs only at sites where it contacts the muscle. In fact, active zones form directly opposite the mouths of junctional folds, thus reconstituting normal synaptic geometry at a submicron level of precision.

Central synapse

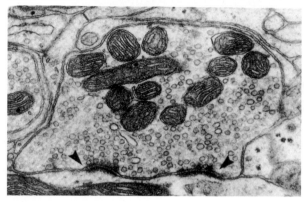

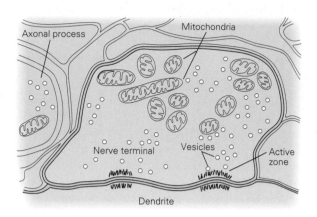

Figure 55-12 Ultrastructure of a synapse in the mammalian central nervous system. Interneuronal synapse from the cerebellum, showing synaptic vesicles in the nerve terminal clustered at an active zone that is directly opposite a thickened, receptor-rich patch of postsynaptic membrane. These features are similar to those seen in neuromuscular junctions.

What factors organize presynaptic differentiation? We know much less about them than we do about the nerve-derived organizers. Candidates include cell adhesion molecules of the type that promote neurite outgrowth. For example, two homophilic cell adhesion molecules, N CAM and N-cadherin (see Chapter 54), are present on both the motor axon growth cone and the surface of developing myotubes. Both molecules promote outgrowth of motor axons on myotubes, and the adhesive interactions they mediate might stabilize initial nerve-muscle contacts. Other candidates are soluble trophic factors of the type that promote neuronal survival and differentiation (see Chapter 53). Brain-derived neurotrophic factor and ciliary neurotrophic factor lead to a rapid increase in the rate of transmitter release, much like that seen at the early stages of synaptogenesis.

Additional candidates have been suggested by experiments exploring the ability of adult axons to reinnervate muscle fibers and form synapses at original postsynaptic sites. Muscles were damaged in vivo in ways that killed the muscle fibers but left their basal lamina intact. The necrotic fibers were phagocytized, leaving behind basal lamina sheaths on which synaptic sites were readily recognizable. The nerve was cut at the same time that the muscle was damaged, and time was allowed for regeneration. Under these conditions motor axons reinnervated the empty basal lamina sheaths and contacted synaptic sites as precisely as they had done when muscle fibers were present. Moreover, nerve terminals developed at regions of contact with synaptic basal lamina, and active zones even formed opposite struts of basal lamina that once lined junctional folds (see Figure 55-9).

Components of the basal lamina therefore appear to be organizers of presynaptic specialization.

One such organizer is an isoform of laminin. Laminins are major components of all basal laminae and are potent promoters of axon outgrowth from many neuronal types (see Chapter 54). They are heterotrimers of α, β, and γ chains, comprising a family of at least five α, four β, and three γ chains. Laminin 11 (α5/β2/γ1) is a major laminin of synaptic basal lamina; Laminin 2 (α2/β1/γ1) is the major laminin of nonsynaptic basal lamina (Figure 55-10).

Motor axons that encounter a deposit of synaptic laminin in vitro stop growing, accumulate synaptic vesicles, and acquire the ability to release neurotransmitter. Furthermore, the development of nerve terminals and Schwann cells is markedly aberrant in mutant mice that lack the laminin β2 chain (Figure 55-10B). Thus laminin-11 is a retrograde synaptic organizer. However, because presynaptic specialization does proceed to a considerable extent in the absence of laminin-11, additional retrograde organizers of axonal specialization must exist.

Many Neuromuscular Junctions That Form in the Embryo Are Eliminated After Birth

In adult mammals a one-to-one relationship exists between motor nerve terminals and muscle fibers. Each motor axon branches to contact tens of hundreds of muscle fibers, but each muscle fiber bears only a single synapse. However, this is not the condition in the embryo. At intermediate stages of development several axons converge on each myotube and form synapses at a common site. Soon after birth all inputs but one are eliminated.

This process of synapse elimination is not a consequence of neuronal death. In fact, synapse elimination takes place long after the period of naturally occurring cell death (see Chapter 53). Instead, each motor axon withdraws branches from some myotubes and strengthens its connections with others, thus focusing its increasing capacity for transmitter release on a decreasing number of targets. Moreover, the elimination process is not targeted at defective synapses; all the inputs to a neonatal myotube are morphologically and electrically differentiated and each can activate the postsynaptic cell (Figure 55-11).

The purpose of this transient polyneuronal innervation remains a mystery. One possibility is that it provides a way to ensure that each muscle fiber is innervated. A second is that it allows all axons to capture appropriate numbers of target cells. A third and more intriguing idea is that synapse elimination provides a means by which activity can change the strength of specific synaptic connections. We will revisit this idea in Chapter 56.

Like synapse formation, synapse elimination results from intercellular interactions. Two observations support this point. First, every muscle fiber ends up with exactly one input: none have zero and very few have more than one. It is difficult to imagine how this could occur without some feedback from the muscle cell. Second, if some axons are removed by partial denervation at birth, each remaining axon maintains a larger number of synapses. Thus synapse elimination must be in part a competitive process.

What does competition in synapse elimination mean: Who is competing for what? Jeff Lichtman has drawn a provocative analogy to athletic competitions, which can be of two types. In one, for example, a wrestling match, the participants compete by interacting with each other. In others, such as diving contests, participants compete by performing on their own.

Most students of synapse elimination have proposed models akin to the first type of competition. In these models the mechanisms that determine the maintenance and elimination of synapses are similar to those that determine whether neurons live or die. For example, the muscle might provide limited amounts of a trophic substance for which the axons compete. As the winner grows it either deprives the loser of its sustenance or gains enough strength to mount an attack on its competitor. Alternatively, the muscle might release a toxic or punitive factor. In these scenarios the muscle only contributes a factor in the competition; the outcome is entirely dependent on differences between axons. These differences could be related to activity. The more active axon might, for example, be better able to take up trophic factor or resist a toxin. Such positive and negative competitive interactions have been demonstrated in *Xenopus* nerve-muscle cocultures but not in vivo.

In vivo synapse elimination appears to be more akin to the second type of competition. In this model the axons need not interact directly with each other—that is, they are divers, not wrestlers—and muscle plays a selective role in synapse elimination rather than just providing a broadly distributed signal. This model is based on studies of living mice in which individual neuromuscular junctions were observed at close intervals during the process of synapse elimination. ACh receptors and components of the postsynaptic cytoskeleton begin to disappear from parts of the maturing neuromuscular junction before the nerve terminals actually withdraw. This observation suggests that differences in activity among competing axons may elicit different responses in the postsynaptic ACh receptors. For example, the more active axon might trigger the generation of a local retrograde signal that strengthens its adhesive interactions with the synaptic cleft, whereas the less active axon might elicit a retrograde signal that weakens its adhesive interactions. In support of this model, blockade of one synaptic region of ACh receptors by focal application of α-bungarotoxin leads to elimination of the portion of the nerve terminal arbor overlying the blocked receptors without obvious effects on other portions of the arbor (see Figure 55-11). One implication of this model is that components of synaptic basal lamina may regulate not only the assembly of the presynaptic nerve terminal but also its demise.

Central Synapses and Neuromuscular Junctions Develop in Similar Ways

Synapses in the central nervous system are structurally similar to neuromuscular junctions in many respects (Figure 55-12). Moreover, like neuromuscular junctions, central synapses develop in a series of steps that imply the exchange of signals between the synaptic partners. To what extent can insights into the development of the neuromuscular junction guide our understanding of synaptic development in the brain?

Central Nerve Terminals Develop Gradually and Are Subject to Elimination

Nerve terminals of neuromuscular junctions and central synapses are quite similar, perhaps reflecting the fact

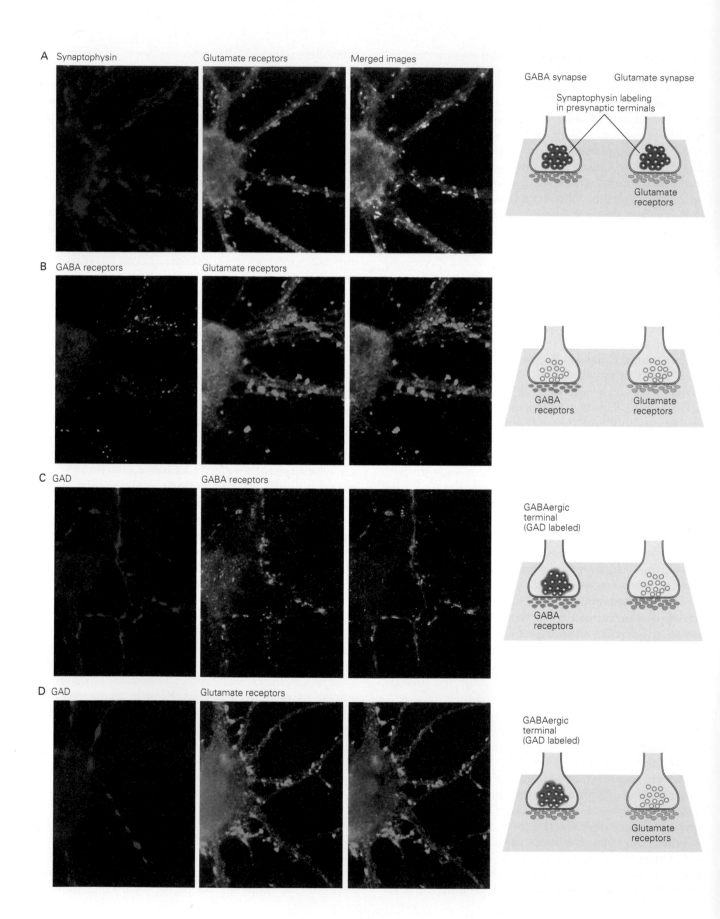

that the motor axon is part of a central neuron. Most of the major protein components of synaptic vesicles have now been isolated and appear to be identical at both types of synapses. Likewise, the mechanisms of transmitter release differ only quantitatively, not qualitatively. Because only a few active zone components and retrograde synaptogenetic signals have been identified, it is not yet clear whether the mechanisms that underlie presynaptic organization have been conserved.

The complexity of the brain makes direct demonstration of synapse elimination problematic, but electrophysiological evidence for elimination has been obtained in the cerebellum, and counts of synapse density as a function of developmental age suggest that a similar process occurs in the cerebral cortex. Synapse elimination in autonomic ganglia has been documented directly and is similar to that seen at neuromuscular junctions. Individual axons withdraw from some postsynaptic cells while simultaneously increasing the size of the synapses they form with other neurons.

Neurotransmitter Receptors Cluster at Central Synapses

The concentration of neurotransmitter receptors in the postsynaptic membrane is a feature shared by many synapses. In the brain, receptors for glutamate, glycine, γ-aminobutyric acid (GABA), and other neurotransmitters are concentrated in patches of membrane directly underlying nerve terminals that contain the corresponding transmitter. The processes by which these receptors become localized may be similar to those at the neuromuscular junction. In cultures of dissociated hippocampal neurons, for example, both glutamatergic and GABA-ergic nerve terminals appear to stimulate clustering of appropriate receptors in the postsynaptic

membrane (Figure 55-13). The mediators of these effects are unknown, but it is noteworthy that agrin, which triggers the clustering of ACh receptors at the neuromuscular junction, is abundant in the brain. Moreover, nerves can induce expression of genes encoding central glutamate receptors, much as occurs for ACh receptors in muscle, and neuregulin has been implicated as a mediator of this effect in cerebellum. Finally, electrical activity regulates neurotransmitter receptor expression in neurons as it does in muscle.

In forming receptor clusters central neurons face an obvious challenge that myotubes do not: They are contacted by a variety of inputs mediated by different neurotransmitter types. Thus it would seem essential that the nerve terminal have an instructive role in managing the clustering of appropriate receptors. Indeed, in cultures of the hippocampal neurons, where glutamatergic and GABA-ergic axons innervate adjacent regions of the same dendrite, initially dispersed glutamate and GABA receptors each cluster selectively beneath terminals that release the appropriate neurotransmitter. This implies the existence of multiple clustering signals with parallel pathways of signal transduction.

Consistent with this idea, several distinct proteins in central neurons have been found to play a role similar to that of rapsyn at the neuromuscular junction. One, gephyrin, is highly concentrated in the synaptic densities at glycinergic and some GABA-ergic synapses (Figure 55-14). Gephyrin is not structurally homologous to rapsyn but appears to be a functional analog: It links the receptors to the underlying cytoskeleton, its overexpression in nonneural cells leads to clustering of glycine receptors, and gephyrin-deficient mutant mice fail to form glycine receptor clusters at inhibitory synapses (Figure 55-14). Similarly, a class of proteins that share conserved segments called PDZ domains, the prototype being PSD-95 or SAP-90, facilitates clustering of NMDA-type glutamate receptors (Figure 55-14). Still other PD2 proteins interact with AMPA-class and metabotropic glutamate receptors. An attractive hypothesis is that distinct presynaptic signals activate the pathways that lead to the expression and localization of gephyrin, PSD-95, and other such proteins.

The Synaptic Cleft Differs at Central and Neuromuscular Synapses

Although the pre- and postsynaptic membranes of neuromuscular and central synapses are generally similar, the synaptic cleft differs dramatically. Whereas muscle fibers are ensheathed by a basal lamina that has a distinctive molecular structure at the neuromuscular junction, central neurons do not have a basal lamina. Central

Figure 55-13 (Opposite) Neurotransmitter receptors cluster at synaptic sites on central neurons. (Images provided by A. M. Craig 1994.)

A. Localization of glutamate receptors and synaptophysin at synapses formed between hippocampal neurons in culture. Glutamate receptors are clustered underneath synaptophysin-labeled nerve terminals, but not all nerve terminals are associated with clusters of glutamate receptors.

B. Localization of glutamate and GABA receptor cluster. These two classes of receptors cluster at different sites on the neuronal membrane.

C. GABA$_A$ receptors are clustered beneath GABA-releasing nerve terminals that express the (transmitter synthetic enzyme) glutamatergic acid decarboxylase (GAD).

D. Glutamate receptors are located at postsynaptic sites spatially distinct from GABA-releasing nerve terminals.

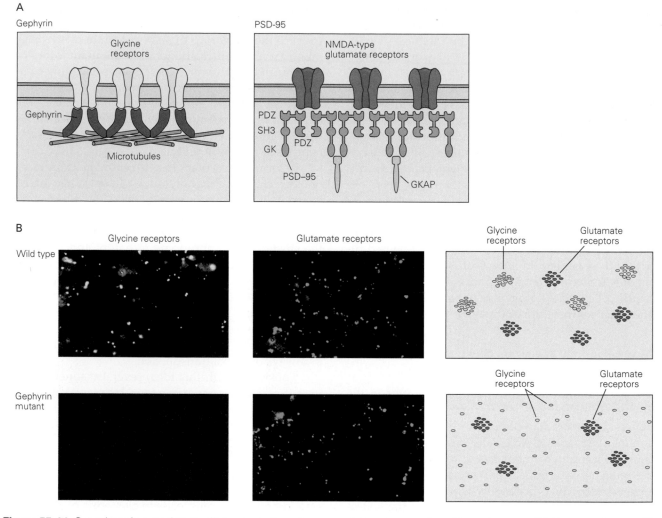

Figure 55-14 Cytoplasmic proteins mediate clustering of receptors at central synapses.

A. Gephyrin links glycine receptors to microtubules whereas PSD-95–related molecules link NMDA-type glutamate receptors to each other and to the cytoskeleton. The PSD family of molecules contains PDZ domains that interact with other synaptic proteins to assemble signaling complexes. Other PDZ-containing proteins interact with AMPA-type and metabotropic glutamate receptors. The existence of linking proteins specific for different receptor subclasses provides a means of separately regulating the localization of each receptor type.

B. In gephyrin mutant mice, glycine receptors (**yellow**) no longer cluster at synaptic sites on spinal motor neurons, and the animals show spasticity and hyperreflexia. The defect is specific in that glutamate receptor clusters on the same neurons are intact in the mutant. (Adapted from Feng et al. 1998.)

synaptic clefts contain no detectable laminin, or collagen. Instead, intercellular adhesion at central synapses may involve the interaction of matched adhesion molecules on pre- and postsynaptic membranes, with no intermediate matrix (Figure 55-15A). For example, the cell adhesion molecule N-cadherin is present in some central synaptic clefts, and the related E- and R-cadherins are present at others; both are homophilic adhesion molecules that adhere far better to their own kind than to each other. Proteins called neurexins and neuroligins that bind to each other are also present at synapses. The cytoplasmic segments of these proteins bind to PDZ-class proteins, such as PSD-95, which bind to neurotransmitter receptors (Figure 55-15B). Neurexin-neuroligin interaction could therefore provide a means of coupling the intercellular interactions required for synaptic recognition to the intracellular interactions required to cluster synaptic components within the cell membrane.

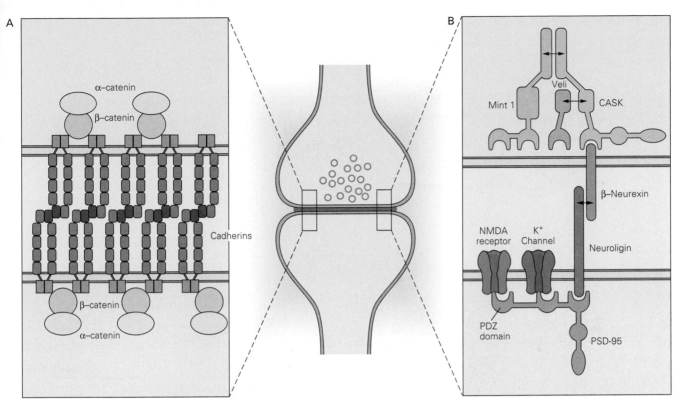

Figure 55-15 Macromolecular complexes link pre- and postsynaptic membranes at central synapses.

A. Cadherins are concentrated at synaptic sites in both pre- and postsynaptic membranes and link to the cytoskeleton via catenins. The model depicts cadherin-mediated bonds that could link pre- and postsynaptic membranes. Because cadherins bind homophilically (each preferentially to its own kind), the presence of distinct cadherins at different synapses could

play a role in the selectivity of synapse formation. (Adapted from D.R. Colman 1997.)

B. Neurexins and neuroligins are present in synaptic membranes and bind to each other. Moreover, both bind to PDZ domain-containing proteins, such as PSD-95, which also interact with neurotransmitter receptors and other synaptic components. Thus this macromolecular complex could link intercellular adhesive interactions to the machinery of synaptic transmission. (Adapted from Butz et al. 1998.)

The Recognition of Synaptic Targets Is Highly Specific

Perhaps the most amazing physical feature of the nervous system is the specificity of its connections. This specificity arises from several developmental processes, including the generation of appropriate numbers and types of neurons, their migration to appropriate nuclei or laminae, and the guidance of their axons to appropriate target areas. In addition, synapse formation is itself a selective process. Unfortunately, although we know an impressive amount about the molecular cues that guide axons (see Chapter 54) and the intercellular signals that regulate synapse formation, we know distressingly little about the molecules that drive target recognition. Nevertheless, we can at least enumerate some of the synaptic choices for which molecular explanations will need to be found.

The specificity with which connections form is particularly evident when intertwined axons select subsets of interspersed postsynaptic cells. For example, autonomic preganglionic axons that arise from distinct rostrocaudal levels of the spinal cord enter sympathetic ganglia together but then synapse on distinct ganglion cells. The axons of rostral cells synapse on ganglion cells that project their axons to relatively rostral targets, whereas those of caudal cells synapse on caudally projecting neurons. This preference is apparent from the initial stages of innervation, even though the postsynaptic cells are more or less randomly distributed within the ganglion. Moreover, this preference is reestablished during reinnervation in adults following nerve damage. Likewise, sensory axons contact specific motor neurons in the spinal cord, even though the dendrites of motor neurons that innervate neighboring muscles have over-

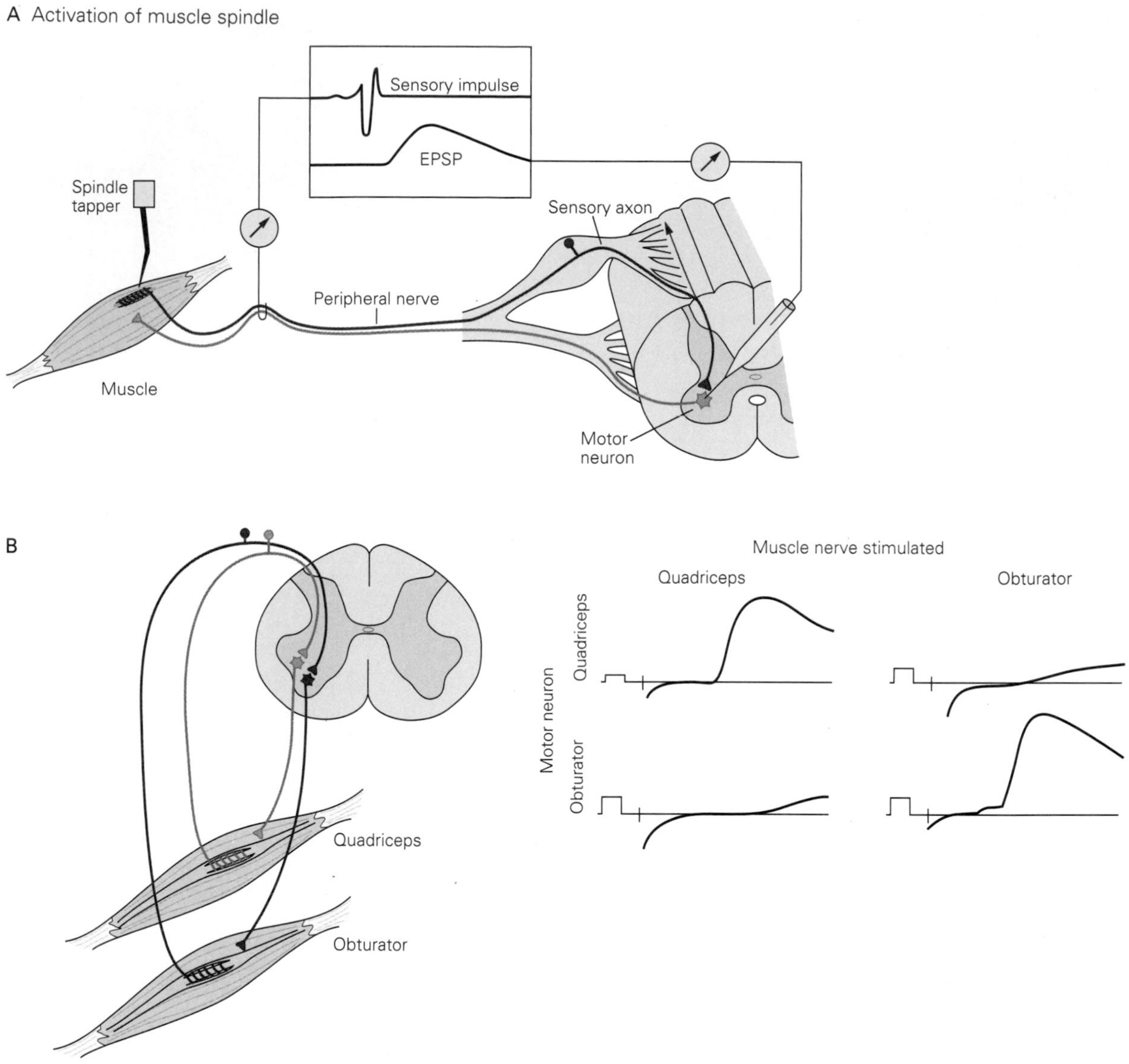

A Activation of muscle spindle

B

Figure 55-16 Sensory neurons that innervate muscle spindles selectively synapse on appropriate motor neurons. (Adapted from Mears and Frank 1997.)

A. Spindle afferents are activated by tapping the muscle. The resulting synaptic potential in the peripheral nerve is detected by intracellular recording from motor neurons in the spinal cord.

B. Although sensory neurons arborize in areas where dendrites from many types of motor neurons overlap, they preferentially synapse on motor neurons that project to their own muscles. In the example here, the quadriceps and obturator afferents make their most powerful synapses on quadriceps and obturator motor neurons, respectively. This selectivity is seen early in development and occurs even in the absence of activity.

lapping territories (Figure 55-16). The selectivity of these connections has also been demonstrated by reinnervation and transplantation experiments.

Another common type of synaptic selectivity is the preference of some nerve terminals for specific portions of the target cell's surface. The best-studied example of this type of selectivity is reinnervation of the original synaptic site in adult muscle, described earlier in this chapter. Similar cases abound in the brain. For example, several distinct types of axons terminate on distinct domains of the Purkinje cells in the cerebellum: granule cell axons on dendritic spines, climbing fiber axons on dendritic shafts, basket cell axons on cell bodies, and so on (see Chapter 42). This specificity is likely to be based

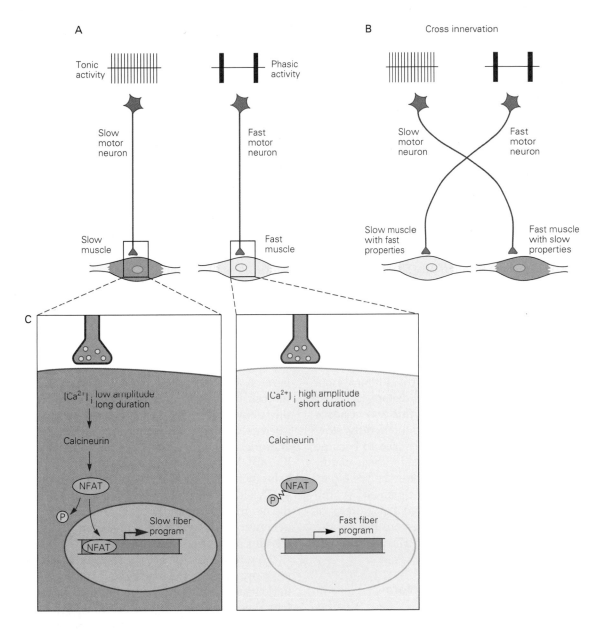

Figure 55-17 Synaptic input can profoundly influence the properties of the postsynaptic cell.

A. Motor neurons and muscles both have characteristic electrical properties that identify them as tonic (often called "slow") or phasic ("fast"). Fast and slow motor neurons connect exclusively with fast and slow muscle fibers, respectively. Thus muscles with a predominance of fast fibers are innervated mostly by fast motor neurons.

B. Cross-innervation can be produced by surgically connecting the fast axons to the predominantly slow muscle and vice versa. The properties of the motor neurons are essentially unchanged, but the properties of the muscle change profoundly: The fast nerve induces fast properties in the originally slow muscle and vice versa. (Adapted from Salmons and Sreter 1976.)

C. The effects of innervation by fast and slow nerves on muscle are mediated largely by their distinct patterns of activity. When a fast nerve is tonically stimulated in a slow pattern, the muscle acquires slow electrical and molecular properties. The selection of muscle fiber type is thought to involve the regulation of a Ca^{2+}-regulated protein phosphatase, calcineurin, and a transcription factor, NFAT. In this view, under conditions of tonic activity, when steady-state Ca^{2+} levels are high, calcineurin is active and the dephosphorylated form of NFAT enters the nucleus and activates the slow muscle fiber transcriptional program. Under conditions of phasic activity, when steady-state Ca^{2+} levels are low, NFAT fails to enter the nucleus permitting expression of the fast fiber program. (Adapted from Chin et al. 1998.)

on molecular cues, either on the postsynaptic cell surface or in its immediate environment, that the approaching axon discerns. Likewise, axons terminating in layered structures often confine their synapses to dendrites in one layer, even though the dendritic tree of the postsynaptic cell traverses numerous layers.

Finally, synaptic selectivity can arise when one synaptic partner induces new properties in the other. This mechanism has been most clearly demonstrated in muscle. In general, mammalian muscle fibers can be divided into several categories such as fast-twitch and slow-twitch, according to their contractile characteristics. Fibers of each type express genes for distinctive isoforms of the main contractile proteins—myosins, troponins, and so on. A few muscles are composed exclusively of a single type of fiber, but most muscles have fibers of both (or all) types. The branches of an individual motor neuron innervate exclusively muscle fibers of a single type, even in "mixed" muscles.

This matching does not come about solely because each motor axon recognizes fibers of the appropriate type. Instead, the motor axon converts muscle fibers to the appropriate type. This was demonstrated in an experiment by John Eccles and colleagues, in which muscles were cross-reinnervated at birth, before the fiber properties were fully established. In this way a nerve that would normally innervate a predominantly slow muscle came to innervate a muscle destined to become predominantly fast and vice versa. Under these conditions the contractile properties of the muscle were partially transformed in a direction determined by the nerve. Other studies have shown that the pattern of neural activity is at least partially responsible for the switch in muscle properties (Figure 55-17).

New Neural Connections Can Reform Following Nerve Injury

One reason that clinicians are interested in the development of synaptic connections is their hope that developmental principles may shed light on the mechanisms underlying the regeneration of connections following injury. Understanding developmental mechanisms may eventually help us restore synaptic function by improving regenerative capacity. Here we outline how neural cells respond to injury, discuss why their regeneration is limited, and consider some strategies for improving regenerative capacity.

Both Neurons and Cells Around Them Are Affected by Damage to the Axon

Because neurons have long axons and small cell bodies, most injuries to the central or peripheral nervous system involve damage to axons. Transection of the axon, either acutely by cutting or more slowly by crushing, is called *axotomy*, and its consequences are numerous (Figure 55-18).

First, axotomy divides the axon into a proximal segment that remains attached to the cell body and a distal segment that has lost that attachment. Because the capacity for protein synthesis is largely restricted to the cell body, axotomy dooms the distal segment. Generally, transmission fails rapidly at the terminals of the distal segment; physical degeneration of the axon, in contrast, may be a slow and gradual process but inevitably proceeds to completion. As this happens glial cells that ensheath the distal segment are also affected. The myelin sheath, which requires axonal contact for its maintenance as well as genesis becomes fragmented and is eventually enveloped, along with axonal debris, by phagocytic cells. This pattern of changes is called *Wallerian degeneration*.

The proximal portion of the neuron also suffers. In some cases the neuron dies by apoptosis, probably because axotomy cuts it off from its supply of target-derived trophic factors. Even when this does not occur the cell body may undergo a series of changes called the *chromatolytic reaction*: The cell body swells, the nucleus moves to an eccentric position, and the rough endoplasmic reticulum becomes fragmented (Figure 55-18B). Metabolic changes also accompany chromatolysis, including overall increases in protein and RNA synthesis as well as changes in the pattern of genes that the neuron expresses. These changes are reversible if regeneration is successful; if not, many neurons eventually die.

Axotomy also affects postsynaptic neurons. When axotomy disrupts the major inputs to a cell—as happens in denervated muscle, for example, or to neurons in the lateral geniculate when the optic nerve is cut—the consequences are severe. Usually the target atrophies and sometimes dies. When targets are only partially denervated their responses are more subtle.

Axotomy affects not only the targets of but also inputs to the injured neuron. Frequently, synaptic terminals withdraw from the neuronal cell bodies or dendrites of chromatolytic neurons and are replaced by the processes of glial cells—Schwann cells in the periphery and microglia or astrocytes in the central nervous system (see Figure 55-18B). This process, called *synaptic stripping*, depresses synaptic function and can impair recovery of function. The mechanism of synaptic stripping remains unclear, but two possibilities have been suggested. One is that axon terminals lose their adhesiveness to synaptic sites as a consequence of postsynaptic injury and are subsequently enwrapped by

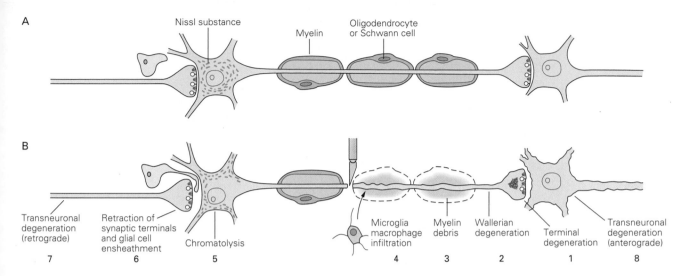

Figures 55-18 Axotomy affects not only the injured neuron but also its synaptic partners and neighboring cells.

A. A normal neuron with an intact functional axon.

B. (1) After axotomy the nerve terminals of the injured neuron fail rapidly. (2) The distal stump, separated from the cell body, undergoes Wallerian degeneration. (3) Myelin degenerates and (4) phagocytic cells invade. (5) The cell body undergoes chromatolysis, in which the nucleus moves to an eccentric position. (6) Presynaptic terminals on the chromatolytic neuron withdraw and are enwrapped by glial processes. (7, 8) The inputs to and targets of the injured neuron can atrophy and even degenerate.

glia. The other is that glia respond to factors released from the injured neuron or to changes in its cell surface and then initiate the process of synaptic stripping.

As a result of these trans-synaptic effects, neuronal degeneration can propagate through a circuit in both anterograde and retrograde directions. For example, a denervated neuron that becomes severely atrophic can fail to activate its target, which then becomes atrophic as well. Likewise, when synaptic stripping prevents an afferent neuron from obtaining sufficient trophic sustenance from its target neuron, the afferent neuron's inputs are placed at risk. Such chain reactions explain in part how an injury to one site in the central nervous system can affect sites distant from the injury.

Finally, axotomy indirectly affects a variety of non-neural cells. As noted earlier in this section, Wallerian degeneration destroys some myelin-forming glial cells. In many cases, however, axotomy also triggers generation of new oligodendrocytes or Schwann cells, presumably to supply new myelin if regeneration succeeds. In addition, axotomy of central neurons leads to the activation of microglia and astrocytes. Both cell types participate in synaptic stripping, and the so-called *reactive astrocytes* also contribute to formation of a scar (called a *glial scar*) near sites of injury. If the injury is of sufficient magnitude, cells of the immune system, including monocytes and macrophages, are also recruited.

Regenerative Capacity Is Greater in the Peripheral Than in the Central Nervous System

Damage to peripheral nerves can often be repaired. Although distal segments of axons degenerate, connective tissue elements of the so-called *distal stump* generally survive. Axonal sprouts grow from the *proximal stump*, enter the distal stump, and grow toward the nerve's end-organs. The mechanisms involved are related to those that guide embryonic axons: Chemotropic factors secreted by Schwann cells attract axons to the distal stump, adhesive molecules within the distal stump promote axon growth along cell membranes and extracellular matrices, and inhibitory molecules in the perineurium prevent the regenerating axons from going astray (see Chapter 54).

Once they return to their targets the regenerated axons can form new functional nerve endings. Motor axons, for example, form new neuromuscular junctions (see Figure 55-9). Likewise, autonomic axons can successfully reinnervate glands, blood vessels, and viscera, and sensory axons can reinnervate muscle spindles. Finally, those axons that were demyelinated become remyelinated, and chromatolytic somata regain their original appearance. Thus in all three divisions of the peripheral nervous system (motor, sensory, and autonomic) the effects of axotomy are reversible.

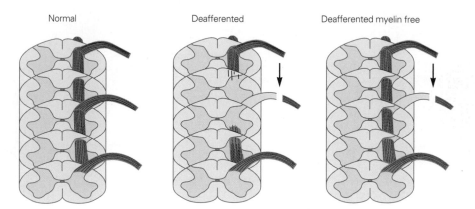

Figure 55-19 Myelin inhibits regeneration of central axons. (Adapted from Schwegler et al. 1995.)

Right dorsal roots were sectioned in 2-week-old normal rats and in littermates that had received local x-irradiation to block myelination. Regeneration of afferents was assessed histochemically 20 days later. In both groups of animals, the central branches of the sectioned sensory axons degenerated, leaving a portion of the spinal cord denervated (**center**). Denervation

elicited sprouting from afferents that entered the cord through neighboring uninjured roots.

In myelin-rich animals this regeneration was very limited in extent, so the central region remained deafferented (**center panel**). In the myelin-free animals, sprouts extended long distances into the denervated region of the dorsal spinal cord (**right panel**).

This is not to say that regeneration is perfect. In the motor system recovery of strength may be substantial but recovery of fine movements is impaired because some motor axons are guided to and form synapses on inappropriate muscle fibers. Some axons may never find a target at all, and some neurons die. Nonetheless, regenerative capacities in the peripheral nervous system are impressive.

In contrast, little regeneration occurs in the central nervous system following injury. The proximal stumps of damaged axons often form short sprouts, but long-distance regeneration is rare and the damaged axons make few new synapses. This failure of regeneration has led to the dismal view that injuries to the brain and spinal cord are largely irreversible, and that therapy must be restricted to rehabilitative measures. For some time, however, neurobiologists have been systematically seeking the reasons why regenerative capacity differs so dramatically between the central and peripheral nervous systems. The aim of this work is to identify the crucial barriers to regeneration so that they can be overcome. In addition, neurobiologists have asked why regeneration of central nerves is much greater in lower vertebrates such as fish and frogs than in mammals. These studies have begun to bear fruit, and there is now cautious optimism that the injured human brain and spinal cord have a latent regenerative capacity that can be exploited.

Therapeutic Interventions May Promote Axonal Regeneration in the Injured Central Nervous System

At least four factors may contribute to the superior regenerative capacities of the peripheral nervous system. First, peripheral nerves appear to provide a more favorable environment for regeneration than do central axons. In a seminal experiment performed a century ago, Tello transplanted a segment of peripheral nerve into the brain. The central axons were capable of growing into the peripheral nerve even though they were incapable of regeneration in their normal central environment. This result implied that Schwann cells provide growth-promoting factors, normally absent from the brain, to the injured areas.

Indeed, numerous studies over the succeeding century have revealed that several constituents of peripheral nerves and Schwann cells are potent promoters of neurite outgrowth. These include components of Schwann cell basal laminae, such as laminin, and cell adhesion molecules of the immunoglobulin superfamily, such as NgCAM/L1. In addition, denervated distal stumps upregulate production of neurotrophins and other trophic molecules. Central neurons are poor sources of these molecules. For example, they contain little laminin and typically produce only low amounts of trophic molecules. In the embryo both the central and peripheral nervous systems provide environments that promote axon outgrowth; it may be that only the peripheral environment retains that capacity in adulthood or is able to regain it following injury.

In the 1980s a radically different interpretation was offered to explain the finding that central axons can regenerate in peripheral but not central nerves. According to this view, both environments contain a sufficiency of growth-promoting elements, but central nerves also contain inhibitory components. In fact, central myelin is a potent inhibitor of axon outgrowth. This may be why myelination occurs late in development, after the major nerve tracts have already formed (Figure 55-19). Using myelin as a starting material, two potent inhibitors of axonal elongation have been purified. One is *myelin-associated glycoprotein,* a structural component of myelin that it is capable of promoting the outgrowth of some neurons and inhibiting the outgrowth of others. The second is a novel protein called *neurite inhibitor of 35kDa,* or NI-35. Central neurons in culture fail to grow on carpets of myelin or oligodendrocytes, but they can do so in the presence of antibodies to NI-35.

The two models described above emphasize differences in the native environments of peripheral and central axons. A third model emphasizes differences between peripheral and central neurons themselves. In fact, even though central axons can regenerate in peripheral nerves, a central axon is markedly inferior to a peripheral axon navigating the same path. It may be, therefore, that central axons are intrinsically incapable of regeneration. In support of this idea several experiments in culture have shown that the growth potential of central neurons decreases with age, whereas even mature peripheral neurons can extend axons in a favorable environment. An explanation for this difference may be found in the pattern of expression of some proteins thought to be critical for optimal axon elongation, such as the *growth-associated protein of 43kDa,* or GAP-43. This protein is expressed at high levels in both central and peripheral neurons in the embryo. In peripheral neurons the level of GAP-43 remains high in maturity and increases even more following axotomy, whereas in central neurons it decreases as development proceeds and does not increase greatly following axotomy.

Finally, a fourth model focuses not on intrinsic differences between central and peripheral neurons, or between their environments, but rather on secondary changes that occur following axotomy. As noted earlier in this chapter, a number of events are prominent following brain injury: astrocyte proliferation, activation of microglia, scar formation, inflammation, and invasion by immune cells. These changes may render an otherwise permissive environment inhospitable. In fact, when care is taken to sever central axons without trau-

matizing surrounding tissues, scar formation and inflammation are minimized, and far more regeneration occurs than is seen following injuries that result in scarring and inflammation.

All four of these models have served as starting points for designing therapeutic interventions. The idea that the central environment lacks growth-promoting factors that are present in the periphery leads naturally to the idea of supplementing the central environment. To this end, investigators have infused trophic factors, such as the neurotrophins, into areas of injury and inserted conduits rich in matrix molecules such as laminin. In some cases Schwann cells themselves have been grafted into sites of injury, and central axons have been shown to grow through these grafts. Based on the idea that the central environment is inhibitory, Martin Schwab and his colleagues have infused antibodies to NI-35 into sites of injury, and enhanced regeneration. Others have tried to uncover the second messengers that the inhibitory components use, with the aim of enhancing regeneration by interfering with the transduction apparatus downstream of the inhibitory signal. In view of the possibility that adult central neurons are intrinsically unable to regenerate well, transplantation of fetal neurons has been attempted. Finally, immunosuppressants, anti-inflammatory agents, and enzymes that degrade glial scars have all been administered following injury. Indeed, an anti-inflammatory steroid, methylprednisolone, is now routinely given as soon as possible to patients with spinal cord trauma, and the positive effects of this intervention have been documented convincingly.

In summary, analysis of axon outgrowth has led to a variety of possible ways to enhance regeneration of diseased or injured central axons. Current studies in many laboratories are now aimed at perfecting and combining these methods. The prospect of clinically useful intervention is, for the first time, a very real one.

Restoration of Function Requires Synaptic Regeneration

Efforts to enhance regeneration of central axons would be of little use if the regenerated axons were unable to form functional synapses on their targets. Therefore, the same fundamental questions asked about axon growth in adults apply to synaptogenesis: Can it happen, and if not, why not?

It has been difficult to address these questions, largely because in most cases axonal regeneration following experimental injury is so poor that the axons never reach appropriate target fields. However, several studies suggest that central axons may retain into

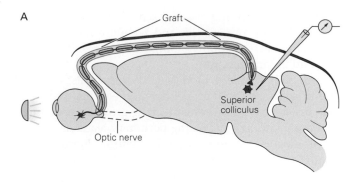

A

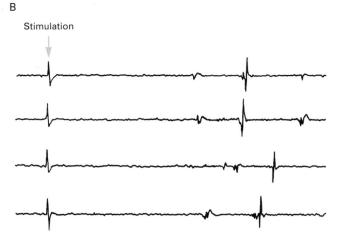

B

Figure 55-20 Peripheral nerves grafted to the brain provide a permissive environment for central axons to regenerate to their targets and form synapses. (From Keirstead et al. 1989.)

A. A segment of optic nerve in an adult rat was removed and a segment of sciatic nerve was grafted in its place. The other end of the sciatic nerve was attached to the superior colliculus. Some retinal ganglion cells axons regenerated through the sciatic nerve and entered the superior colliculus. In contrast, no substantial regeneration occurred through the optic nerve.

B. Once the axons of the retinal ganglion cells had regenerated, recordings were made from the superior colliculus. Flashes of light delivered to the eye elicited action potentials in the target neuron.

maturity their capacity to form synapses. For example, Albert Aguayo and his colleagues have carried out extensive studies on the regeneration of retinal axons that project to the superior colliculus. They first showed that a modest number of axons were capable of regenerating in a grafted peripheral nerve, thereby providing strong support for the theory that the central environment is inhospitable to regeneration (Figure 55-20A). They then recorded the electrical activity of neurons in the superior colliculus while flashing spots of light on the retina. Remarkably, at least some collicular neurons fired action

potentials when the eye was illuminated, proving that functional synaptic connections had been reestablished (Figure 55-20B). Moreover, electron microscopic studies showed that the new synapses had formed on appropriate target cells in appropriate laminae. The number of new synapses was small and retinotopic arrangement of inputs to the superior colliculus was not restored, but these and other results show that mature neurons retain their synaptogenetic abilities.

An Overall View

The formation of synapses completes the hard wiring of the nervous system and enables it to function. The requirements for an adequate synapse are stringent: The nerve terminal must recognize the proper target cell and often even a specific portion of the target cell's surface. The postsynaptic membrane must be highly responsive to the particular neurotransmitter that the nerve terminal releases. The apposition of pre- and postsynaptic elements must be spatially matched at a submicron level of precision, so that responses can occur on a time scale of milliseconds. And the whole structure must be sufficiently stable to last a lifetime yet sufficiently plastic to change with experience.

To meet these specifications, synaptogenesis is a highly interactive process. Although the pre- and postsynaptic cells can each synthesize synaptic components on their own, they exchange numerous signals to coordinate their activities in space and time. In this chapter we have used the neuromuscular junction to illustrate these interactions. Motor nerve terminals use a combination of electrical and chemical signals to sculpt the postsynaptic apparatus of the muscle fiber, and the muscle fiber in turn provides retrograde signals to organize synaptic specialization in the nerve terminal.

A key anterograde signal is agrin, which activates a tyrosine kinase called MuSK; MuSK in turn uses the cytoplasmic protein rapsyn to aggregate ACh receptors in the postsynaptic membrane. Simultaneously, neuregulins and electric activity regulate the synthesis of ACh receptors. Retrograde signals include both soluble trophic factors and matrix-associated proteins such as the laminins. Some of these molecules, such as neuregulin, also function at central synapses. In addition to the molecules that direct synaptic specialization, target recognition molecules must account for the selectivity of synapse formation, but few of these have been identified.

Finally, axons can regenerate and form new synapses following injury. This regeneration is far more effective in the peripheral than in the central nervous system. However, recent studies have identified several key factors that limit regeneration of central axons. By manipulating these factors it should be possible to enhance regeneration following injury and thus provide restoration of function to many patients for whom there is currently little hope.

Joshua R. Sanes
Thomas M. Jessell

Selected Readings

Buonanno A, Fields RD. 1999. Gene regulation by patterned electrical activity during neural and skeletal muscle development. Curr Opin Neurobiol 9:110–120.

Duclert A, Changeux JP. 1995. Acetylcholine receptor gene expression at the developing neuromuscular junction. Physiol Rev 75:339–368.

Fischbach GD, Rosen KM. 1997. ARIA: a neuromuscular junction neuregulin. Annu Rev Neurosci 20:429–458.

Ide C. 1996. Peripheral nerve regeneration. Neurosci Res 25:101–121.

Kirsch J. 1999. Assembly of signaling machinery at the postsynaptic membrane. Curr Opin Neurobiol 9:329–335.

Sanes JR, Lichtman JW. 1999. Development of the vertebrate neuromuscular junction. Annu Rev Neurosci. 22:389–442.

Vaughn JE. 1989. Fine structure of synaptogenesis in the vertebrate central nervous system. Synapse 3:255–285.

References

Anderson MJ, Cohen MW. 1977. Nerve-induced and spontaneous redistribution of acetylcholine receptors on cultured muscle cells. J Physiol 268:757–773.

Apel ED, Glass DJ, Moscoso LM, Yancopoulos GD, Sanes JR. 1997. Rapsyn is required for MuSK signaling and recruits synaptic components to a MuSK-containing scaffold. Neuron 18:623–635.

Balice-Gordon RJ, Lichtman JW. 1994. Long-term synapse loss induced by focal blockade of postsynaptic receptors. Nature 372:519-524.

Buller AJ, Eccles JC, Eccles RM. 1960. Interactions between motoneurons and muscles in respect of the characterisitc speeds of their responses. J Physiol (Lond) 150:419.

Butz S, Okamoto M, Sudhof TC. 1998. A tripartite protein complex with the potential to couple synaptic vesicle exocytosis to cell adhesion in brain. Cell 94:773–782.

Campagna J, Ruegg M, Bixby J. 1995. Agrin is a differentiation-inducing "stop signal" for motoneurons in vitro. Neuron 15:1365–1374.

Caroni P, Schwab ME. 1988. Antibody against myelin-associated inhibitor of neurite growth neutralizes nonper-missive substrate properties of CNS white matter. Neuron 1:85–96.

Chin ER, Olson EN, Richardson JA, Yang Q, Humphries C, Shelton JM, Wu H, Zhu W, Bassel-Duby R, Williams RS. 1998. A calcineurin-dependent transcriptional pathway controls skeletal muscle fiber type. Genes Dev 12:2499–2509.

Cohen I, Rimer M, Lomo T, McMahan UJ. 1997. Agrin-induced postsynaptic-like apparatus in skeletal muscle fibers in vivo. Mol Cell Neurosci 9:237–253.

Colman DR. 1997. Neurites, synapses, and cadherins reconciled. Mol Cell Neurosci 10:1–6.

Craig AM, Blackstone CD, Huganir RL, Banker G. 1994. Selective clustering of glutamate and gamma-aminobutyric acid receptors opposite terminals releasing the corresponding neurotransmitters. Proc Natl Acad Sci U S A 91:12373–12377.

Davies SJA, Fitch MT, Memberg SP, Hall AK, Raisman G, Silver J. 1997. Regeneration of adult axons in white matter tracts of the central nervous system. Nature 390:680–684.

DeChiara TM, Bowen DC, Valenzuela DM, Simmons MV, Poueymirou WT, Thomas S, Kinetz E, Compton DL, Rojas E, Park JS, Smith C, DiStefano PS, Glass DJ, Burden SJ, Yancopoulos GD. 1996. The receptor tyrosine kinase MuSK is required for neuromuscular junction formation in vivo. Cell 85:501–512.

Ehlers MD, Mammen AL, Lau L-F, Huganir RL. 1996. Synaptic targeting of glutamate receptors. Curr Opin Cell Biol 8:484–489.

Fannon AM, Colman DR. 1996. A model for central synaptic junctional complex formation based on the differential adhesive specificities of the cadherins. Neuron 17:423–434.

Feng G, Tintrup H, Kirsch J, Nichol MC, Kuhse J, Betz H, Sanes JR. 1998. Dual requirement for gephyrin in glycine receptor clustering and molybdoenzyme activity. Science 282:1321–1324.

Frank E, Mendelson B. 1990. Specification of synaptic connections between sensory and motor neurons in the developing spinal cord. J Neurobiol 21:33–50.

Gautam M, Noakes PG, Moscoso L, Rupp F, Scheller RH, Merlie JP, Sanes JR. 1996. Defective neuromuscular synaptogenesis in agrin-deficient mutant mice. Cell 85:525–535.

Gautam M, Noakes PG, Mudd J, Nichol M, Chu GC, Sanes JR, Merlie JP. 1995. Failure of postsynaptic specialization to develop at neuromuscular junctions of rapsyn-deficient mice. Nature 377:232–236.

Glass DJ, Bowen DC, Stitt TN, Radziejewski C, Bruno J, Ryan TE, Gies DR, Shah S, Mattsson K, Burden SJ, Distefano PS, Valenzuela DM, Dechiara TM, Yancopoulos GD. 1996. Agrin acts via a MuSK receptor complex. Cell 85:513–523.

Glicksman MA, Sanes JR. 1983. Differentiation of motor nerve terminals formed in the absence of muscle fibres. J Neurocytol 12:661–671.

Hall ZW, Sanes JR. 1993. Synaptic structure and development: the neuromuscular junction. Cell 72:99–121.

Hume RI, Role LW, Fischbach GD. 1983. Acetylcholine release from growth cones detected with patches of acetylcholine receptor-rich membranes. Nature 305:632–634.

Irie M, Hata Y, Takeuchi M, Ichtchenko K, Toyoda A, Hirao K, Takai Y, Rosahl TW, Südhof TC. 1997. Binding of neuroligins to PSD-95. Science 277:1511–1515.

Jones G, Meier T, Lichtsteiner M, Witzemann V, Sakmann B, Brenner HR. 1997. Induction by agrin of ectopic and functional postsynaptic-like membrane in innervated muscle. Proc Natl Acad Sci U S A 94:2654–2659.

Keirstead SA, Rasminsky M, Fukuda Y, Carter DA, Aguayo AJ, Vidal-Sanz M. 1989. Electrophysiologic responses in hamster superior colliculus evoked by regenerating retinal axons. Science 246:255–257.

Lomo T, Westgaard RH. 1976. Control of ACh sensitivity in rat muscle fibers. Cold Spring Harbor Symp Quant Biol 40:263–274.

Mears SC, Frank E. 1997. Formation of specific monosynaptic connections between muscle spindle afferents and motoneurons in the mouse. J Neurosci 17:3128–3135.

McMahan UJ. 1990. The agrin hypothesis. Cold Spring Harb Symp Quant Biol 55:407–418.

Noakes PG, Gautam M, Mudd J, Sanes JR, Merlie JP. 1995. Aberrant differentiation of neuromuscular junctions in mice lacking s-laminin/laminin-2. Nature 374:258–262.

Ozaki M, Sasner M, Yano R, Lu HS, Buonanno A. 1997. Neuregulin-β induces expression of an NMDA-receptor subunit. Nature 390:691–694.

Patton BL, Miner JH, Chiu AY, Sanes JR. 1997. Localization, regulation and function of laminins in the neuromuscular system of developing, adult and mutant mice. J Cell Biol 139:1507–1521.

Salmons S, Sreter FA. 1976. Significance of impulse activity in the transformation of skeletal muscle type. Nature 263:30–34.

Sandrock AW, Dryer SE, Rosen KM, Gozani SN, Kramer R, Theill LE, Fischbach GD. 1997. Maintenance of acetylcholine receptor number by neuregulins. Science 276:599–603.

Schwegler G, Schwab ME, Kapfhammer JP. 1995. Increased collateral sprouting of primary afferents in the myelin-free spinal cord. J Neurosci 15:2756–2767.

Svensson M, Aldskogius H. 1993. Synaptic density of axotomized hypoglossal motor neurons following pharmacological blockade of the microglial cell proliferation. Exp Neurol 120:123–131.

Uchida N, Honjo Y, Johnson KR, Wheelock MJ, Takeichi M. 1996. The catenin cadherin adhesion system is localized in synaptic. J Cell Biol 135:767–779.

Yamagata M, Herman JP, Sanes JR. 1995. Lamina-specific expression of adhesion molecules in developing chick optic tectum. J Neurosci 15:4556–4571.

56

Sensory Experience and the Fine-Tuning of Synaptic Connections

P ERCEPTION—THE BRAIN'S synthesis of a coherent mental image from discrete sensory signals—is mediated by the interconnections of tens of thousands of nerve cells. How is this precision of neural connections achieved? As we have seen in Chapters 54 and 55, the pathfinding of axons to their appropriate target cells within the nervous system and the formation of specific connections with those targets are controlled in large part by molecular programs that are genetically determined, independent of activity or experience. Such molecular cues are not, however, always sufficient to establish the final pattern of synaptic connections. The

precise matching of presynaptic neurons to specific postsynaptic targets depends at least in part on patterned neural activity evoked by sensory input. Activity-dependent fine-tuning of neural circuitry is not limited to early development. As we shall see in Chapter 63, neural circuits are adaptable even in the mature individual. Indeed, modification of synaptic connections is thought to be the physiological basis of learning.

We begin this chapter by examining the role of neural activity in the formation of visual circuitry during pre- and postnatal development, and consider the significance of this early neural activity for later visual perception. We focus on the visual system because studies of the effects of experience on visual perception have been particularly informative in furthering our understanding of how experience shapes neural circuitry throughout the brain.

Development of Visual Perception Requires Sensory Experience

Molecular cues guide the initial formation of the afferent pathways of the visual system: the axons of mammalian retinal ganglion neurons are directed in the optic nerve to their target cells in the lateral geniculate nucleus, and the axons of these cells are guided to specific layers of the visual cortex. Once formed, however, these visual circuits are refined by interactions between the organism and its environment. The influence of the environment is usually more profound at early stages of postnatal development than in adulthood.

The effect of sensory experience on the brain, and the ability of that experience to shape perception, first

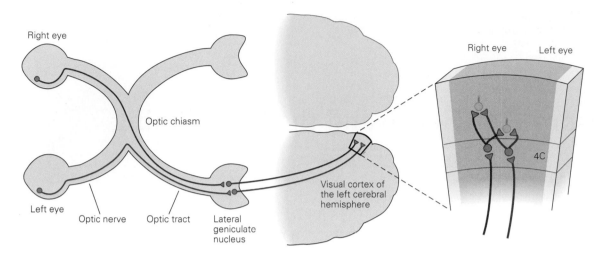

Figure 56-1 Afferent pathways from the two eyes remain segregated as they project to the visual cortex. Retinal ganglion neurons from each eye send axons to separate layers of the lateral geniculate nucleus. The axons of neurons in the lateral geniculate nucleus project to and form synaptic connections with neurons in layer 4C of the primary visual cortex, also known as area 17. Neurons in layer 4C are organized in alternating sets of ocular dominance columns; each column receives input from only one eye. The axons of the neurons in layer 4C project to neurons in adjacent columns (not shown) as well as to neurons in the upper and lower layers of the same column. As a result, most neurons in the upper and lower layers of the cortex receive information from both eyes.

became evident in people born with cataracts. Cataracts are opacities of the lens that interfere with the optics of the eye but do not interfere directly with the nervous system. Cataracts are easily removed surgically. In the 1930s it became apparent that the common practice of removing congenital binocular cataracts between the ages of 10 and 20 resulted in permanent impairment of the ability to perceive shape and form. Even long after the cataracts were removed, patients had difficulty recognizing shapes and patterns. Similar results were obtained in more controlled studies of newborn monkeys that had been raised in the dark for the first 3–6 months of their lives. When these monkeys were later introduced to a normal visual world they could not discriminate even simple shapes. It took weeks or months of training to teach them to distinguish a circle from a square, whereas normal monkeys learn this distinction in days. Today, partly as a result of such studies, congenital cataracts are usually removed in infancy.

In a series of studies performed in the 1960s, David Hubel and Torsten Wiesel examined the cellular mechanism by which patterned visual stimulation affects the development of visual perception. They recorded response characteristics of neurons in the visual cortex when visual stimuli were presented to one or both eyes of newborn kittens and monkeys. As we saw in Chapter 26, cells in layer 4C of the visual cortex of monkeys respond exclusively to inputs from a single eye. Cells acti-

vated by each eye then send inputs to common target cells above and below layer 4C of the visual cortex (Figure 56-1). Thus most cells above and below layer 4C respond to an appropriate stimulus presented to either eye. Only a small proportion of these cells respond exclusively to the left or right eye. This convergence is the anatomical substrate of binocular interaction.

In a key experiment Hubel and Wiesel raised a monkey from birth to six months of age with one eyelid sutured shut, thus depriving the animal of vision in that eye. When the sutures were removed and the eye was exposed to light, it became clear that the animal was blind in the deprived eye. The blindness was largely cortical. The retinal ganglion cells in the deprived eye and the cells in the lateral geniculate nucleus that received input from that eye responded well to visual stimuli and had relatively normal receptive fields, but most cells in the visual cortex no longer responded to visual input to the deprived eye (Figure 56-2). The few cortical cells that were responsive were not sufficient for visual perception. Not only had the deprived eye lost its ability to drive most cortical neurons, but this loss was irreversible. Thus proper vision was necessary for the maturation or maintenance of the connections from the lateral geniculate nucleus to the visual cortex.

Further analysis revealed two surprising results. First, whereas most cortical cells are driven only by the eye that remains open following monocular depriva-

Figure 56-2 Responses of neurons in area 17 of the monkey visual cortex to visual stimuli. (Adapted from Hubel and Wiesel 1977.)

A. A diagonal bar of light is moved leftward across the two eyes in the path of the receptive fields (**colored rectangles**) of two cells, each conveying input from one eye. The receptive fields of the two cells are similar in orientation, position, shape, and size, and they respond to the same form of stimulus. The center of the visual field falls on the fovea (**F**), the region of the retina with greatest acuity. Retinal images for the right and left eyes are drawn separately for clarity. The inputs from these cells converge on a single neuron in area 17 of the cortex. Recordings from the cortical neuron (**below**) show that the neuron responds more effectively to input from the ipsilateral eye than from the contralateral eye.

B. The responses of single cortical neurons in area 17 can be classified into seven groups. Neurons receiving input only from the contralateral eye (**C**) fall into group 1, whereas neurons that receive input only from the ipsilateral eye (**I**) fall into group 7. Other neurons receive inputs from both eyes, but the input from one eye may influence the neuron much more than the other (groups 2 and 6), or the differences may be slight (groups 3 and 5). Some neurons respond equally to input from both eyes (group 4). According to these criteria, the neuron shown in part A falls into group 6.

C. Responsiveness of neurons in area 17 to stimulation of one or the other eye. **1.** Responses of over 1,000 neurons in area 17 in the left cerebral cortex of normal adult and juvenile monkeys. The neurons in layer 4C that normally receive only monocular input have been excluded. Most neurons respond to input from both eyes. **2.** Responses of neurons in the left cerebral cortex of a monkey in which the contralateral (**right**) eye was closed from the age of 2 weeks to 18 months and then reopened. Most neurons respond only to stimulation of the ipsilateral eye.

tion, many cells remain responsive to both eyes following *binocular* deprivation. This result suggested that appropriate connections depend not only on activity in the afferent pathways but also on a proper balance between those inputs. Second, whereas deprivation of sight in one eye for as little as one week during the first six months of life results in a nearly complete loss of vision in that eye, a much longer period of visual deprivation in an adult has little effect on cortical responsiveness or visual perception. These results led to the concept of a *critical period* in the maturation of the cortical connections that control visual perception.

Development of Binocular Circuits in the Cortex Depends on Postnatal Neural Activity

Why do cells in the visual cortex fail to respond to sensory information from an eye in which vision has been transiently deprived early in postnatal life? Are these functional defects due to structural changes? As de-

A   Movement across the retina

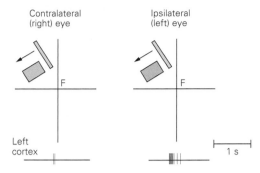

B   Categories of responses given by single cells

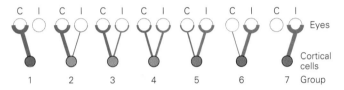

C₁   Normal area 17

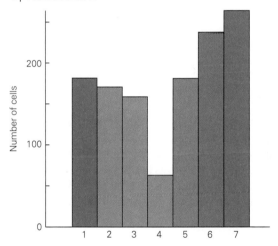

C₂   Area 17 after monocular closure of contralateral eye

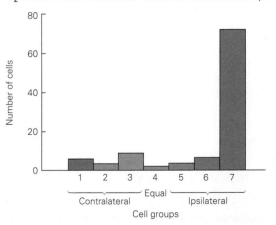

Figure 56-3 Visual deprivation of one eye during a critical period of development reduces the width of the ocular dominance columns for that eye. (A–C adapted from Hubel et al. 1977; D from LeVay 1980.)

A. A tangential section through area 17 of the right cerebral cortex 10 days after the right eye of a normal adult monkey was injected with a radiolabeled amino acid. The autoradiograph shows the radioactivity as localized stripes (**white areas**) in layer 4C of the visual cortex, indicative of areas innervated by afferents from the lateral geniculate nucleus that carry input from the injected eye. The alternating unlabeled **dark stripes** correspond to regions innervated by afferents from the uninjected eye. Labeled and unlabeled regions form stripes of equal width. (Scale bars in micrographs A, B, and C = 1 mm.)

B. A comparable section through the visual cortex of an 18-month-old monkey whose right eye had been surgically closed at 2 weeks of age. The label was injected into the left eye. The wider **white stripes** of label correspond to the terminals of afferent axons carrying signals from the open (left) eye; the narrower **dark stripes** correspond to inputs for the closed (right) eye.

C. A section comparable to that in part B from an 18-month-old monkey whose right eye had been shut at 2 weeks. In this case the label was injected into the closed right eye, giving rise to narrow white stripes and expanded dark stripes of label in the visual cortex.

D. Reconstruction of the ocular dominance columns in area 17 of the right brain hemisphere of a normal monkey, showing the intricate organization of the columnar map.

A Normal

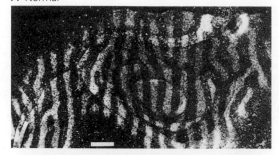

B Deprived: open eye labeled (white)

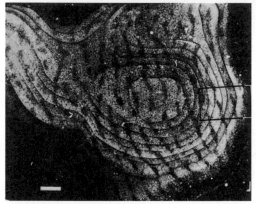

C Deprived: closed eye labeled

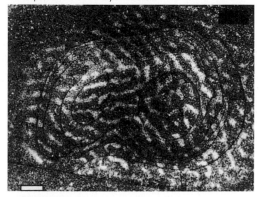

D Reconstruction: normal ocular dominance columns

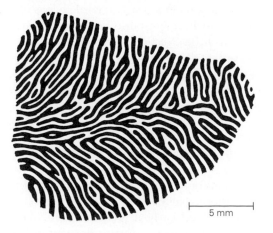

5 mm

scribed in Chapter 27, inputs from the two eyes to the cortex terminate in alternating *ocular dominance columns* in the primary visual cortex. To examine whether the architecture of these columns is affected by visual deprivation early in postnatal life, Hubel and Wiesel deprived newborn monkeys of input from one eye and then injected a labeled amino acid into the normal eye.

The injected label was incorporated into proteins in retinal ganglion cell bodies and transported along the retinal axons to the lateral geniculate nucleus, where it was transferred to the neurons of the nucleus and then transported to their synaptic terminals in layer 4C of the primary visual cortex. After closure of one eye the ocular dominance columns receiving input from the deprived eye were reduced in area, whereas the columns receiving input from the normal eye were expanded (Figure 56-3). Here, then, is direct evidence that sensory deprivation early in life can alter the structure of the cerebral cortex.

Ocular Dominance Columns Are Organized After Birth

How are these anatomical changes brought about? Does sensory deprivation interfere with the formation of the

Figure 56-4 Autoradiographs of four stages in the development of the visual cortex in a cat show the postnatal development of ocular dominance columns. The images show horizontal sections through columns ipsilateral to an eye that was injected with a radiolabeled amino acid. The afferent fibers from the lateral geniculate nucleus receiving input from the injected eye become labeled by transneuronal transport. At about 2 weeks (15 days) after birth the labeled afferent fibers have spread in a relatively uniform manner along layer 4 and are intermingled with unlabeled afferents receiving input from the contralateral eye. At 3 and 5.5 weeks some segregation of the fibers is visible but only as modest fluctuations in labeling density. At 13 weeks the borders of the labeled bands become more sharply defined as the afferent fibers from the two eyes segregate. (Adapted from LeVay et al. 1978.)

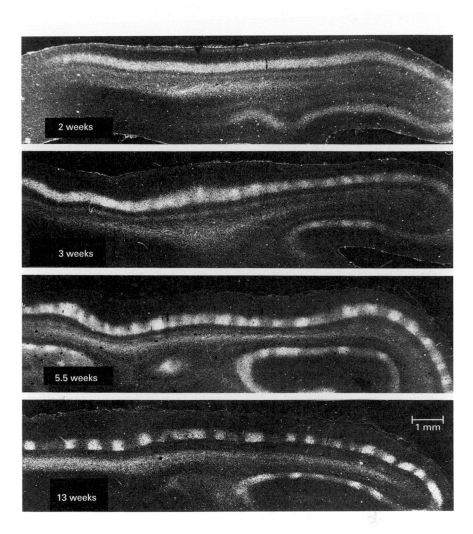

ocular dominance columns or does it alter already established columns? It is now clear that the mature pattern of ocular dominance columns in monkeys is not achieved until six weeks after birth. Only at this time do the afferent fibers from the lateral geniculate nucleus become completely segregated (Figure 56-4). Thus well-segregated columns do not exist at the time that visual deprivation exerts its effects. Instead, visual deprivation perturbs the segregation of afferent inputs into columns.

Understanding the effects of visual deprivation therefore requires us to learn how ocular dominance columns are formed. When developing axons from the lateral geniculate nucleus first reach layer 4C, their terminal endings overlap extensively. With further development the inputs from each eye become segregated to columnar arrays of cortical cells.

The development of afferent fibers from the lateral geniculate nucleus can be observed by labeling axons at different developmental stages. At first each fiber extends a few branches over an area of the visual cortex that spans several future ocular dominance columns. As each thalamic neuron matures, its axon in the visual cortex retracts some branches, expands others and even forms new axon branches. With time, the neuron becomes connected almost exclusively to a subset of cortical neurons (Figures 56-5 and 56-6). These two processes, axon retraction and local outgrowth, occur widely throughout the nervous system during development.

Synchronized Activity in the Pathways From Each Eye Organizes the Ocular Dominance Columns

Why, during the formation of ocular dominance columns, do some afferent fibers retract while others form more extensive synaptic contacts? Despite extensive study, the mechanisms are not known with certainty. One plausible hypothesis is based on the idea that minor differences exist in the proportion of axon terminals from each eye that contact a common target cell at birth. If afferents from one eye are initially, and by chance, more numerous in one local region of cortex,

Figure 56-5 The effects of eye closure on the formation of ocular dominance columns in layer 4C. The **red shapes** represent the terminals of geniculate afferents in layer 4C from one eye; the **blue shapes** represent the terminals from the other eye. The lengths of the shapes represent the density of the terminals at each point along layer 4C. For clarity, the columns are shown here as one above the other, whereas in reality they are side by side in the cortex. During normal development (**left**) layer 4C is gradually divided into an alternating group of fibers from each eye. The consequences of depriving one eye (**right**) depend on the timing of eye closure. Eye closure at birth leads to complete dominance by the open eye (**red**) because at this point little segregation has occurred. Closure at 2, 3, and 6 weeks has a progressively weaker effect on the formation of ocular dominance columns because the columns already have become more segregated with time. Bottom diagrams show that after deprivation of input from the right eye there is a more extensive arborization of the geniculate axons from the left eye. (Adapted from Hubel et al. 1977.)

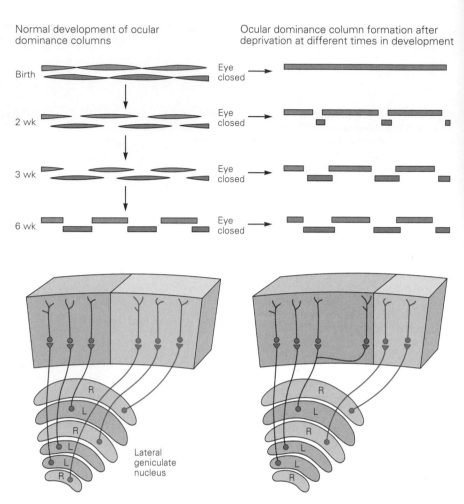

these axons could have an advantage in capturing that territory.

The advantage of the winning eye over the loser, in turn, appears to reflect an imbalance in their electrical activities. In kittens, ocular dominance columns fail to form if retinal activity is blocked before the critical period of development by injecting into each eye tetrodotoxin, a toxin that selectively blocks voltage-sensitive Na$^+$ channels. This situation also permits controlled stimulation of the afferent fibers from the two eyes. When the two optic nerves are stimulated synchronously, ocular dominance columns fail to form. Only when the optic nerves are stimulated *asynchronously* do ocular dominance columns form. Thus the formation and maintenance of segregated ocular dominance columns, and normal binocular vision, require more that just activity in general in the afferent pathways—they require asynchronous or patterned activity in the pathways from the two eyes.

How do multiple axons from one eye maintain connections with a cortical target while seemingly similar inputs from the other eye are eliminated? One possibility is that neighboring axons from the same eye cooperate in the excitation of a target cell through synchronization of their firing. In that view, cooperative action might strengthen the synaptic contacts formed by each cooperating axon at the expense of those formed by noncooperating axons. Cooperative activity promotes further branching of the participating axons and thus creates the opportunity for the formation of additional synaptic connections with cells in the target region. At the same time, the strengthening of synaptic terminals made by the axons of one eye impedes the growth of synaptic inputs from the opposite eye. In this sense, fibers from the two eyes compete for a target cell. Together, cooperation and competition between axons could ensure that two populations of afferent fibers eventually innervate distinct regions of the primary visual cortex with little local overlap.

Can cooperation and competition between axons explain the reorganization of ocular dominance columns after visual deprivation? Monocular deprivation

A   Young   Mature   B   Open eye   Deprived eye

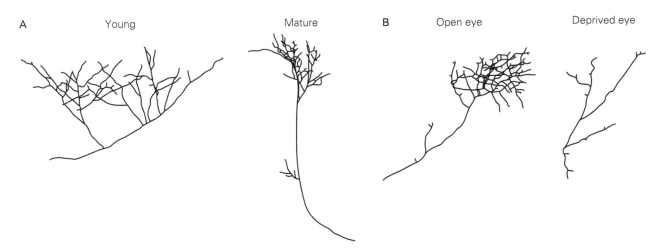

Figure 56-6 The branching pattern of geniculocortical fibers in normal development and after visual deprivation.

A. During postnatal development the axons of geniculocortical fibers branch extensively at several points. Later in development the axon terminals are concentrated in a single region.

B. After one eye had been closed in a kitten the terminal arbors of neurons from the deprived eye show a dramatic reduction in complexity as compared to that of the nondeprived eye. (Modified from Antonini and Stryker 1993.)

interferes with the normal development of ocular dominance columns by decreasing activity in the afferent fibers from the deprived eye. As a consequence of the imbalance in activity, an abnormally high proportion of fibers from the deprived eye will retract while fibers from the normal eye will form additional synaptic contacts in the areas that would have been occupied by afferent inputs from the other eye (Figure 56-6).

The specific consequences of this imbalance depend on the timing of visual deprivation. If an animal is deprived of the use of one eye early during the critical period of axonal segregation, the terminals of lateral geniculate neurons that receive input from the closed eye become less active and many of them retract. At the same time, afferent inputs from the normal eye that would normally have been relinquished are now maintained. If, however, an animal is deprived of the use of one eye later in this critical period, when the ocular dominance columns are almost fully segregated, then a second mechanism comes into play. The afferent axons in the pathway from the open eye begin to sprout and extend collateral branches into regions of the cortex that they had vacated earlier during the segregation of the inputs in columns (Figure 56-6).

If the development of ocular dominance columns depends on competition between afferent fibers, it might be possible to induce the formation of segregated columns where columns normally are not present by establishing competition between two sets of axons. This possibility has been tested in frogs. In frogs the retinal ganglion neurons from each eye project only to the contralateral side of the brain, so that the afferent fibers from

the two eyes do not compete for the same target cells in the brain. To generate a condition in which competition could occur, Martha Constantine-Paton and Thomas Reh transplanted a third eye into a region of the frog's head near one of the normal eyes early in larval development. The retinal ganglion cells of the extra eye extended axons to the contralateral optic tectum. Remarkably, axon terminals from the transplanted and normal eyes segregated, generating a pattern of regular alternating columns (Figure 56-7). This result suggests that competition between two sets of afferent neurons for the same population of target neurons is sufficient to segregate the terminals of the presynaptic cells into distinct territories.

Studies of the three-eyed frog have also provided us with one clue as to how cooperating presynaptic cells may gain an advantage over noncooperating inputs on the same target. As in the mammalian visual system, the segregation of afferent fibers into ocular dominance columns in the three-eyed frog appears to require synchronous activity among neighboring fibers. Retinal ganglion neurons release the neurotransmitter glutamate at synapses with tectal neurons, activating both the N-methyl-D-aspartate (NMDA) and non-NMDA classes of glutamate receptors on the postsynaptic neuron (see Chapter 26). Under resting conditions the ion channel of the NMDA-type receptor is blocked by Mg^{2+}. The Mg^{2+} is removed from the ion channel by intense depolarization, and synchronous activity in retinal afferents leads to a level of depolarization that is sufficient to open NMDA receptor channels. Once the channels are open, Ca^{2+} flows into the cell and activates calcium-dependent second-messenger systems.

A Normal

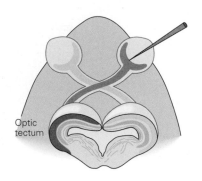

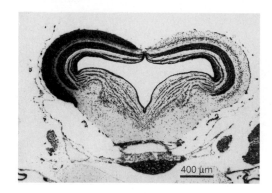

400 μm

B Transplanted eye induces ocular dominance columns

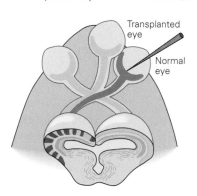

Transplanted
eye

Normal
eye

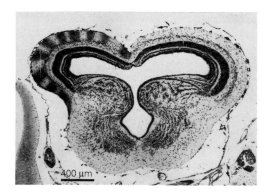

400 μm

Figure 56-7 Ocular dominance columns can be induced experimentally in a frog by the transplantation of a third eye. The radiographs show a coronal section through the midbrain of the frog. (Adapted from Constantine-Paton and Law 1978.)

A. The diagram shows injection of radiolabel into one eye and the corresponding transport of label into the contralateral optic tectum. The autoradiogaph was obtained after the right eye of a normal frog was injected with a radiolabeled amino acid 3 days before the transplant. The region filled with silver grains, the entire superficial neuropil of the left optic lobe (**left**), is the region that contains the synaptic terminals from the labeled

(contralateral) eye.

B. The diagram shows injection of radiolabel into one eye in a three-eyed frog and the appearance of stripes of label in the contralateral optic tectum. The autoradiograph (**right**) was obtained after transplantation of a third eye near the normal right eye, which was injected with a radiolabeled amino acid. The left optic lobe receives inputs from both the labeled eye and the supernumerary eye. The normally continuous synaptic zone of the contralateral eye has become divided into alternating zones occupied by the terminals of each eye.

The intracellular changes elicited by activation of NMDA-type receptors are thought to stabilize the synapse. Supporting this idea, the columnar segregation of retinal afferents in the frog brain can be blocked by exposing tectal neurons to antagonists of the NMDA-type glutamate receptors. Conversely, exposure of tectal neurons to NMDA, an agonist at this glutamate receptor, sharpens the columnar organization (Figure 56-8). The critical factor underlying competition and cooperation between retinal afferents in the frog brain appears to be patterned neural activity. Thus in both mammals and lower vertebrates neural activity seems to have a similar role in fine-tuning visual circuitry.

These findings can be interpreted as an example of an idea first proposed by Donald Hebb in the 1940s: Synapses are strengthened when the pre- and postsynaptic elements are synchronously active. Hebb's idea has been incorporated into many models of neuronal competition and cooperation. Indeed, we shall encounter it again in Chapter 63 in connection with the cellular mechanisms of learning and memory. It is also the basis of several mathematical models of activity-dependent competition between the afferent fibers from the two eyes. These models simulate with remarkable accuracy the segregation of ocular dominance columns during development.

A Normal development

Low power view

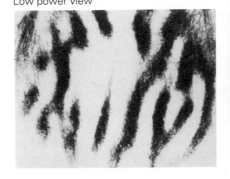

High power view

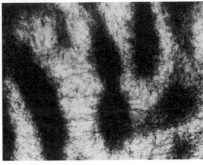

Figure 56-8 The activity of NMDA-type glutamate receptors controls the segregation of afferent input in the frog optic tectum. (From Constantine-Paton et al. 1990)

A. Segregated pattern of retinal projections in the optic tectum of an experimentally generated three-eyed frog.

B. Blockade of NMDA receptor activity by coadministration of the NMDA channel blocker MK801 and NMDA prevents the segregation of retinal ganglion axons.

C. Enhancing NMDA receptor activity by application of NMDA alone sharpens the segregation of the inputs from the graft and host eye (compare with the normal pattern shown in part A). In these experiments the segregation is revealed by labeling the axons of one eye with horseradish peroxidase tracer.

B NMDA receptor blockade

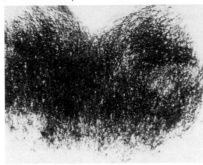

C NMDA receptor activation

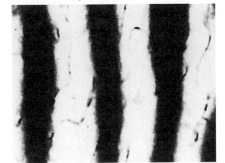

Segregation of Retinal Inputs in the Thalamus Is Driven by Spontaneous, Synchronized Neural Activity in Utero

As in the cortex, the organization of retinal inputs to the lateral geniculate nucleus in the thalamus also depends on neural activity. In the lateral geniculate nucleus the inputs from the two eyes are segregated into alternating layers, much as the axons from the lateral geniculate nucleus terminate in alternating ocular dominance columns in the cerebral cortex (Figure 56-9). Here, however, the segregation of inputs to geniculate layers is complete before birth. How does this come about?

As in the cortex, the segregation of the inputs from each eye can be disrupted by applying tetrodotoxin to the optic chiasm, indicating that activity is essential for the segregation. However, because segregation occurs before birth, the source of the neural activity essential for this segregation cannot be visual stimuli on the retina. Rather, as first demonstrated by Lucia Galli and Lamberto Maffei, the axons of retinal neurons are spontaneously active in utero, well before the eyes open.

In the embryo neighboring ganglion cells tend to be active together, firing in synchronous bursts that last a few seconds, followed by silent periods that last minutes (Figure 56-10). The spontaneous but synchronous firing of a select group of afferent fibers excites a local group of target neurons in the lateral geniculate nucleus, and such synchronized activity appears to strengthen those synapses. Nearby synapses with inactive or asynchronous inputs are placed at a disadvantage. The discovery that local clusters of retinal ganglion neurons are spontaneously active in utero may have important implications for the development of the visual system and of other functional pathways in the brain.

Synchronous Presynaptic Activity May Enhance the Release of Neurotrophic Factors From Target Neurons

How does synchronous activity in presynaptic fibers strengthen the synapses formed by those fibers? As noted above, activation of NMDA receptors on postsynaptic cells can generate chemical as well as electrical signals in those cells. How then, do these signals affect the fate of the inputs? An intriguing possibility is that

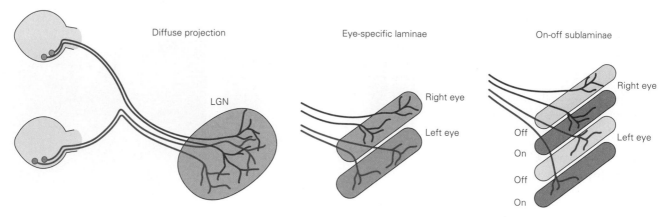

Figure 56-9 Segregation of retinal axon terminals in the lateral geniculate nucleus. At early stages the axons from each eye intermingle. At later stages the axons from the left and right eyes segregate. Later still, in some mammals such as ferrets, axons from the on and off cells of each eye segregate into distinct sublaminae. (Adapted from Sanes and Yamagata 1999.)

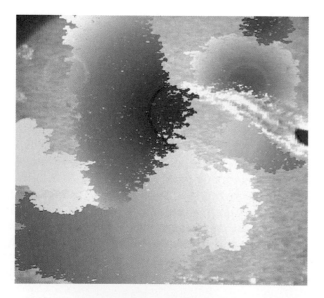

Figure 56-10 Spontaneous neural activity spreads over the retina in waves. Spontaneous waves of activity are detected with fluorescence imaging of local Ca^{2+} levels in a ferret retina labeled with a Ca^{2+}-sensitive indicator. The spatial and temporal properties of many consecutive waves, observed over several minutes, are shown. Different colors correspond to individual domains on the retina. (From Meister et al. 1991.)

the same neurotrophins that control neuronal survival early in development (see Chapter 53) affect the survival of synaptic connections at a later stage.

Neurons in the central nervous system can release neurotrophic factors upon depolarization, as occurs when multiple presynaptic inputs from one eye synchronously activate a cortical neuron. Synchronous inputs to the same target cell might therefore result in a level of depolarization sufficient to increase the amount of trophic factor released from the postsynaptic cell. Because competing axons from different eyes, or even axons from nonneighboring neurons in the same eye, fire asynchronously, they would not depolarize the postsynaptic cell sufficiently to increase the secretion of the neurotrophic factor. In support of this idea, widespread administration of brain-derived neurotrophic factor (BDNF) and NT-4, which bind to the trkB receptor, blocks the formation of ocular dominance columns (Figure 56-11). Likewise, interfering with the action of trkB receptors also blocks the formation of ocular dominance columns.

One problem with this view is that noncooperating nerve terminals near the terminals that fire synchronously might also be able to take up the neurotrophins released by the postsynaptic cell. This possibility could be minimized by transient enhancement of endocytosis and membrane retrieval in active terminals immediately after transmitter release. These processes would facilitate the uptake of factors released by the target neuron (see Chapter 14), putting the active (cooperating) neurons at an advantage over inactive (noncooperating) neurons. Thus, nerve terminals that do not fire in phase with the predominant inputs would more likely be eliminated (Figure 56-12). This hypothesis remains unproven at this point but does provide an example of how well-examined elements of early embryonic programs could, in combination, account for the plasticity detected at later developmental stages.

Early Intracortical Connections May Direct the Development of Orientation Columns

In addition to ocular dominance columns, the primary visual cortex has a distinct set of columns concerned with the orientation of visual stimuli (see Chapter 27). Orientation-specific columns are evident before the eyes open, suggesting that patterned visual activity is not necessary for the initial establishment of the preferred axis of orientation of cortical cells. Two studies support this idea. In one study the orientation-specific columns developed identically in normal cats and those deprived of vision in both eyes over the first three weeks of postnatal life. After this initial period, however, the orientation columns degenerated in the visually deprived cats.

In another study the eyelids of kittens were sutured shut on alternate weeks so that the two eyes never received simultaneous input during the critical period. Despite this, the orientation maps for the two eyes were virtually identical. These studies suggest that patterned visual activity is not required for the formation of the orientation maps but is required for their maintenance.

How is the early map of orientation columns formed? Neurons with similar orientation selectivity in different regions of the cortex are interconnected by both excitatory and inhibitory synapses, with relatively little input from cells with different orientation selectivity. Such intracortical connections exist prior to the formation of functional maps and may therefore lay down the basic organization of orientation-specific columns. These intracortical connections may provide the early information required to align the orientation maps from the two eyes. The development of these selective intracortical connections may itself depend on the spontaneous activity of axons that project to the cortex from the lateral geniculate nucleus.

Activity-Dependent Refinement of Connections Is a General Feature of Circuits in the Central Nervous System

We have seen that neural activity is critical for segregating projections from the two retinae into distinct lami-

A Normal

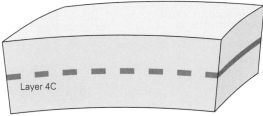

B NGF or NT3 administration

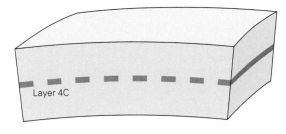

C NT4, 5 or BDNF administration

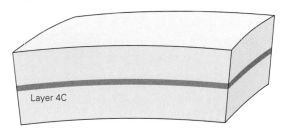

Figure 56-11 Neurotrophins modulate the formation of ocular dominance columns. Neurotrophins were administered in cats by intracortical infusion. Geniculocortical fibers become labeled after injection of proline into the eye ipsilateral to the neurotrophin-infused hemisphere. Infusion of NGF or NT3 does not affect ocular dominance column formation. By contrast, infusion of NT-4, 5 or BDNF leads to a loss of ocular dominance columns. (Modified from Cabelli et al. 1995.)

nae in the lateral geniculate nucleus and then into distinct columns in the visual cortex. Activity also sharpens the topographic mapping of retinal axons onto their central targets, a topic we introduced in Chapter 54.

Histological and physiological studies of lower vertebrates have shown that the map formed initially in the optic tectum is coarse, and that individual retinal axons have large, overlapping arbors in the tectum. Later these axonal arbors become smaller and the map becomes more precise. In Chapter 54 we described how molecular cues such as the eph kinases and the ephrins guide axons to appropriate tectal target sites. These cues are not, however, sufficient for formation of the refined

Axon from left eye fires alone, leading to a small depolarization of the target cell which is inadequate to activate the NMDA receptors. Small amounts of neurotrophic factor normally available do not sustain the axon.

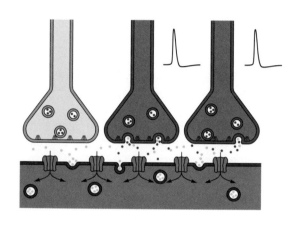

Axons from right eye fire synchronously, leading to a larger depolarization of the target cell and activation of the NMDA receptors. This causes the target cell to release increased amounts of neurotrophic factor which is taken up by the active presynaptic terminals from the left eye during endocytic retrieval of the plasma membrane.

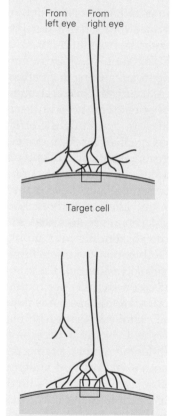

The inactive axon from the left eye, which has not taken up neurotrophic factor, retracts.

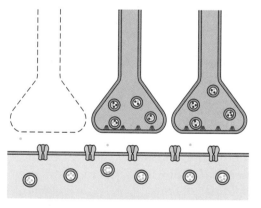

Axon branches from the right eye, stimulated by the neurotrophic factor, sprout and occupy the vacated target site.

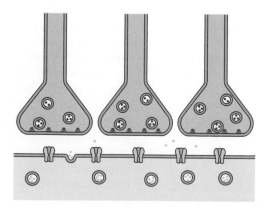

map. If retinal activity is inhibited by intraocular injection of tetrodotoxin, only the initial, coarse map forms. Thus in the absence of activity molecular cues can generate a coarse topographic matching of retinal axons with tectal targets, but refinement of such maps requires activity.

Do axons simply need to be active to express or respond optimally to molecular cues, or is the actual pattern of activity important? Many experiments have shown that the specific pattern of activity is critical. For example, the retinotectal map develops differently in fish raised in a normal laboratory environment or in a tank illuminated only by brief flashes from a strobe light. Although the total light intensity the fish are exposed to is similar under both conditions the resulting pattern is very different. In control fish the images fall on various parts of the retina as the fish swim around their tanks. This input produces local synchronous activity of the sort generated by the waves of spontaneous activity we encountered in our consideration of the mammalian retina. Neighboring ganglion cells tend to fire together, and there is little correlation in the firing of distant ganglion cells. In these control fish the map becomes precise. In contrast in fish exposed to stroboscopic illumination nearly all of the ganglion cells are synchronously activated, and, as a result, the retinotectal map remains coarse.

Presumably, the topographic map is refined by synchronous activity in neighboring afferent fibers. When all of the axons fire in synchrony, neurons in the tectum cannot judge which axons are neighbors, refinement fails, and the map remains coarse. Thus along with molecular cues synchronous activity is required to generate a proper topographic map.

The visual system is particularly dependent on activity for its patterning but it is by no means unique. Auditory connections can also be refined or modified by experience. Auditory inputs form orderly tonotopic maps on neurons in the cochlear nucleus, inferior colliculus, and auditory cortex, such that neurons that respond best to low frequencies lie at one edge of each structure and neurons tuned to high frequencies lie at the other edge. These maps underlie our sense of pitch. In addition, neurons vary in their sensitivity to sounds sensed by the contralateral and ipsilateral ears, with the balance helping us to determine the point in horizontal space from which a sound arises (see Chapter 30). These auditory patterns are analogous to the retinotopic maps and ocular disparity representations, respectively, in the visual system.

Although tonotopic maps can form in silence, exposure of an animal to "white noise" impairs refinement of the tuning curves of neurons in the inferior colliculus, and exposure to specific frequencies enhances representation of those frequencies in the map. Similarly, neurons in the inferior colliculus of birds acquire frequency-matched inputs from both ears in an experience-independent way, but attenuating sensitivity in one ear (with an ear plug) alters their binaural balance. Whether experience acts by way of synchronous activation in these cases, as it does in the visual system, has not yet been tested, but it is likely that it does.

There Is a Critical Period in the Development of Social Behavior

It has been difficult to demonstrate direct links between the development of the nervous system and the development of complex behavior. However, research on the formation of the ocular dominance columns has provided an important link between these two realms. The binocular vision necessary to perceive form and depth develops after birth. Psychophysical studies show that stereoscopic vision (*stereopsis*) develops during the same period as the maturation of the ocular dominance columns and that stereopsis is absent following manipulations that block the formation of appropriate binocular inputs on cortical neurons. This postnatal period is probably a critical period in the development of stereopsis because sensory experience is critical in the development of the neural structures underlying the behavior.

Just as the development of the brain's sensory apparatus depends on sensory experience at certain critical

Figure 56-12 (Opposite) A speculative model showing how competition between neurons might mediate the fine-tuning of synaptic connections in the developing visual cortex. In this model a geniculocortical synapse is stabilized when factors released from the postsynaptic cortical cell stimulate or stabilize the growth of active presynaptic terminals. In the absence of presynaptic activity there is only a low level of spontaneous release of the neurotrophic factor from cortical neurons. Release of the growth factors is enhanced when the postsynaptic cortical neuron is depolarized sufficiently to activate NMDA receptors. A high level of depolarization occurs only when there is synchronous activity among presynaptic terminals. The growth factor can be taken up in the presynaptic terminal only when the terminal itself is active, and endocytic retrieval of the vesicle membrane is under way. Thus inactive presynaptic terminals competing with active ones will fail to obtain adequate amounts of growth factor and consequently will shrink and eventually withdraw. Active presynaptic terminals that take up neurotrophic factors grow, increasing the strength of the contact with the cortical target neuron.

stages, so too does development of social behavior depend on social experience at specific periods of neural development. A particularly striking illustration of the close relationship between neural development and learning is evident in *imprinting,* a form of learning in birds that was examined in detail in the classical work of Konrad Lorenz. Just after birth, birds become indelibly attached, or imprinted, to almost any prominent moving object in their environment, typically their mother. The process of imprinting is important for the protection of the hatchling. Although the attachment is acquired rapidly and persists, such imprinting can occur only during a critical period soon after hatching. In some species this critical period lasts just a few hours.

The clearest way to show that certain social or perceptual experiences are important for human development is to study children who have been deprived of these stimuli early in life. Reliable histories of infants who were abandoned in the wild and who later returned to human society describe children without language who are socially maladjusted, usually in an irreversible way.

The first compelling evidence that early social interactions with other humans is essential for normal social development came in the 1940s from the work of the psychoanalyst René Spitz. Spitz compared the development of infants raised in a foundling home with the development of infants raised in a nursing home attached to a women's prison. Both institutions were clean and both provided adequate food and medical care. The babies in the prison nursing home were all cared for by their mothers, who, although in prison and away from their families, tended to shower affection on their infants in the limited time allotted to them each day. In contrast, infants in the foundling home were cared for by nurses, each of whom was responsible for several babies. As a result, children in the foundling home had much less contact with other humans than those in the prison's nursing home.

The two institutions also differed in another respect. In the prison nursing home the cribs were open, so that the infants could readily watch other activities in the ward; they could see other babies play and observe their mothers and the staff go about their business. In the foundling home the bars of the cribs were covered by sheets that prevented the infants from seeing outside. This dramatically reduced the infants' environment. In effect, the babies in the foundling home lived under conditions of sensory and social deprivation.

Groups of newborn infants at the two institutions were followed throughout their early years. At the end of the first four months the infants in the foundling home fared better on several developmental tests than those in the prison nursing home. However, by the end of the first year the motor and intellectual performance of the children in the foundling home had fallen far below that of children in the prison nursing home. Many of the children in the foundling home had developed a syndrome that Spitz called *hospitalism* (now often called *anaclitic depression*). These children were withdrawn and showed little curiosity or gaiety. Remarkably, they were also prone to infection.

By their second and third years children in the prison nursing home were similar to children raised in normal families at home: They walked well and talked actively. In contrast, the development of the children in the foundling home was still delayed. Very few children in the foundling home were able to walk and speak; those who could speak said only a few words. Normal children at this age are agile, have a vocabulary of hundreds of words, and speak in sentences.

This work was carried one important step further in the 1960s when two psychologists, Harry and Margaret Harlow, studied monkeys reared in isolation. They found that newborn monkeys isolated for 6–12 months were physically healthy but behaviorally devastated. These monkeys crouched in a corner of their cage and rocked back and forth like autistic children. They did not interact with other monkeys, nor did they fight, play, or show any sexual interest. Thus a 6-month period of social isolation during the first 18 months of life produced persistent and serious disturbances in behavior. By comparison, isolation of an older animal for a comparable period lacked such drastic consequences.

It is plausible that the devastating consequences of early social deprivation are caused by structural defects in brain development, much as early visual deprivation results in changes in the organization of the visual cortex.

An Overall View

Connections between neurons in the sensory areas of the brain are achieved by two fundamentally different development programs: molecular guidance cues and patterned neural activity. Molecular cues control neuronal identity, guide axons from specific regions of the periphery to broadly defined target regions, and initiate the formation of synaptic connections. Once synaptic contact is established, however, continued development depends on the coordination of neural activity between pre- and postsynaptic neurons.

In the visual system this patterned activity leads to cooperation between afferent fibers from the same eye and competition between afferent fibers from the opposite eye. Afferent fibers from the same local region of the retina of one eye that terminate on a common cortical neuron have an advantage if they fire in synchrony. Synchronous firing strengthens the synapses of all cooperating fibers, whereas the synapses of the noncooperating fibers decline until the axon terminals withdraw entirely. As a consequence, the overlap in inputs from the two eyes is eliminated, and the inputs from the two eyes become segregated into alternating columns in the cortex.

Cooperation and competition between axons influence the development of ocular dominance columns primarily during a critical period of development. During this period the segregation of afferent fibers and the establishment of ocular dominance columns is affected dramatically by changing the balance of activity in the fibers from the two eyes. After the critical period, existing connections become stable and are much less susceptible to such modification.

In addition to providing insights into the mechanisms governing development, the studies of cortical development reviewed in this chapter have clinical relevance. For example, the clinical treatment of strabismus, a misalignment of the visual axes of the two eyes, changed once the effects of strabismus on the development of visual perception was understood. Moreover, studies of the development of ocular dominance columns suggest how other, more complex sensory experiences early in development might change the circuitry and structure of the growing brain. Studies of sensory development in general provide a striking example of how genetic factors and experience acting at successive stages in the maturation of the brain can alter neural development.

Eric R. Kandel
Thomas M. Jessell
Joshua R. Sanes

Selected Readings

Constantine-Paton M, Cline HT, Debski E. 1990. Patterned activity, synaptic convergence, and the NMDA receptor in developing visual pathways. Annu Rev Neurosci 13:129–154.

Crair MC. 1999. Neuronal activity during development: permissive or instructive? Curr Opin Neurobiol 9:88–93.

Goodman CS, Shatz CJ. 1993. Developmental mechanisms that generate precise patterns of neuronal connectivity. Cell 72:77–98.

Katz LC, Schatz CJ. 1996. Synaptic activity and the construction of cortical circuits. Science 274:1133–1138.

Knudsen EI. 1984. The role of auditory experience in the development and maintenance of sound localization. Trends Neurosci 7:326–330.

Rakic P. 1981. Development of visual centers in the primate brain depends on binocular competition before birth. Science 214:928–931.

Shatz CJ. 1997. Neurotrophins and visual system plasticity. In: WM Cowan, TM Jessell, SL Zipursky (eds). *Molecular and Cellular Approaches to Neural Development*, pp. 509–524. New York: Oxford Univ. Press.

Wong ROL. 1999. Retinal waves and visual system development. Annu Rev Neurosci 22:29–47.

References

Antonini A, Stryker MP. 1993. Rapid remodeling of axonal arbors in the visual cortex. Science 260:1819–1821.

Bonhoeffer T. 1996. Neurotrophins and activity-dependent development of the neocortex. Curr Opin Neurobiol 6:119–126.

Cabelli RJ, Hohn A, Shatz CJ. 1995. Inhibition of ocular dominance column formation by infusion of NT 4/5 or BDNF. Science 267:1662–1666.

Cohen-Corey S, Fraser S. 1995. Effects of brain-derived neurotrophic factor on optic axon branching and remodeling in vivo. Nature 378:192–196.

Constantine-Paton M, Law MI. 1978. Eye-specific termination bands in tecta of three-eyed frogs. Science 202:639–641.

Crair MC, Gillespie DC, Stryker MP. 1998. The role of visual experience in the development of columns in cat visual cortex. Science 279:566–570.

Feller MB, Wellis DP, Stellwagen D, Werblin S, Shatz CJ. 1996. Requirement for cholinergic synaptic transmission in the propagation of spontaneous retinal waves. Science 272:1182–1187.

Frith V. 1989. *Autism: Explaining the Enigma*. Oxford: Basil Blackwell.

Galli L, Maffei L. 1988. Spontaneous impulse activity of rat retinal ganglion cells in prenatal life. Science 242:90–91.

Gödecke I, Bonhoeffer T. 1996. Development of identical orientation maps for two eyes without common visual experience. Nature 379:251–254.

Harlow HF. 1958. The nature of love. Am Psychol 13:673–685.

Hata Y, Stryker MP. 1994. Control of thalamocortical afferent rearrangement by postsynaptic activity in the developing visual cortex. Science 265:1732–1735.

Hebb DO. 1949. *Organization of Behavior: A Neuropsychological Theory*. New York: Wiley.

Held R. 1989. Perception and its neuronal mechanisms. Cognition 33:139–154.

Hubel DH, Wiesel TN. 1977. Ferrier lecture: functional architecture of macaque monkey visual cortex. Proc R Soc Lond B 198:1–59.

Hubel DH, Wiesel TN, LeVay S. 1977. Plasticity of ocular dominance columns in monkey striate cortex. Philos Trans R Soc Lond B Biol Sci 278:377–409.

Kang H, Schuman EM. 1995. Long-lasting neurotrophin-induced enhancement of synaptic transmission in the adult hippocampus. Science 267:1658–1662.

Leiderman PH. 1981. Human mother-infant social bonding: Is there a sensitive phase? In: K Immelmann, GW Barlow, L Petrinovich, M Main (eds). *Behavioral Development: The Bielefeld Interdisciplinary Project*, pp. 454–468. Cambridge, England: Cambridge Univ. Press.

LeVay S, Stryker MP, Shatz CJ. 1978. Ocular dominance columns and their development in layer IV of the cat's visual cortex: a quantitative study. J Comp Neurol 179:223–244.

LeVay S, Wiesel TN, Hubel DH. 1980. The development of ocular dominance columns in normal and visually deprived monkeys. J Comp Neurol 191:1–51.

Lindholm D, Castren E, Berzaghi MP, Blochl A, Thoenen H. 1994. Activity-dependent and hormonal regulation of neurotrophin mRNA levels in the brain—implications for neuronal plasticity. J Neurobiol 25:1362–1372.

Meister M, Wong ROL, Baylor DA, Shatz CJ. 1991. Synchronous bursts of action potentials in ganglion cells of the developing mammalian retina. Science 252:939–943.

Miller KD, Chapman B, Stryker MP. 1989. Visual responses in adult cat visual cortex depend on N-methyl-D-aspartate receptors. Proc Natl Acad Sci U S A 856:5183–5187.

Miller KD, Keller JB, Stryker MP. 1989. Ocular dominance column development: analysis and simulation. Science 245:605–615.

Moreau E. 1913. Histoire de la guerison d'un aveugle-ne. Ann Ocul 149:81–118.

Riddle DR, Lo DC, Katz LC. 1995. NT-4 mediated rescue of lateral geniculate neurons from effects of monocular deprivation. Nature 378:189–191.

Riesen AH. 1958. Plasticity of behavior: psychological aspects. In: HF Harlow, CN Woolsey (eds). *Biological and Biochemical Bases of Behavior*, pp. 425–450. Madison: Univ. Wisconsin Press.

Sanes JR, Yamagata M. 1999. Formation of lamina-specific synaptic connections. Current Opinion Neurobiology 9:79–87.

Shatz CJ. 1990. Impulse activity and the patterning of connections during CNS development. Neuron 5:745–756.

Shatz CJ, Stryker MP. 1988. Prenatal tetrodotoxin infusion blocks segregation of retino-geniculate afferents. Science 242:87–89.

Spitz RA. 1945. Hospitalism: an inquiry into the genesis of psychiatric conditions in early childhood. Psychoanal Study Child 1:53–74.

Spitz RA. 1946. Hospitalism: a follow-up report on investigation described in Volume 1, 1945. Psychoanal Study Child 2:113–117.

Udin SB, Fawcett JW. 1989. Formation of topographic maps. Annu Rev Neurosci 11:289–327.

Weliky M, Katz LC. 1997. Disruption of orientation tuning in visual cortex by artificially correlated neuronal activity. Nature 386:680–685.

57

Sexual Differentiation of the Nervous System

S EXUAL DIFFERENTIATION OF the brain has been conclusively demonstrated in many mammalian species. Are there also structural sex differences in the human brain? If so, are they determined prenatally or postnatally? What is the functional significance of these differences? Is sexual differentiation of the brain a factor in the development of behavior? If so, can variations in this differentiation explain homosexuality?

In many mammalian species the brain is inherently feminine (or perhaps neuter). Masculine characteristics of structure and function are imposed on the developing central nervous system by the action of testicular hormones during a critical period, or quite possibly several critical periods, of development. Although many hormonally dependent sex differences in the structure of the central nervous system have been identified, the functional significance of many of these differences is unknown. Certain differences, such as the control of gonadal function and of sexual behavior, are clearly related to reproduction. Other differences, such as those related to cognitive function in humans, are less easily explained.

Sexual Differentiation of the Reproductive System Is a Fundamental Characteristic of Development

We begin by discussing the sexual differentiation of the reproductive organs, which has been clearly documented in many mammalian species, including humans.

Figure 57-1 Schematic representation of sex determination.

A. The Y chromosome possesses a gene (or genes) called the *testis determining factor* (**TDF**). The chromosomally normal XY individual becomes phenotypically male.

B. The chromosomally normal XX individual develops ovaries. The black arrow here and in part C indicates "default programming," or development that takes place in the absence of TDF.

C. Crossing over occurs in a homologous region of the X and Y chromosome so that the TDF becomes located on the X chromosome. If these altered chromosomes are in a sperm cell that fertilizes an ovum, the resulting individual would be either an XX male or an XY female. **MIH** = mullerian duct inhibiting hormone.

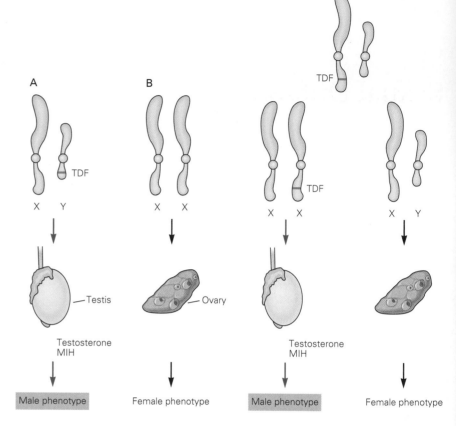

Development of the Testes Depends on a Testis Determining Factor

The mammalian gonad develops from the mesodermal lining of the coelomic cavity and the underlying mesenchyme. The mesodermal lining produces cords of cells that invade the mesenchyme. At an early stage in embryonic development the gonad is structurally identical in both males and females. It consists of an outer layer of mesodermal cells, the cortex of the indifferent gonad, and an inner layer of mesenchyme that constitutes the medulla of the indifferent gonad. This is the tissue that is invaded by cords of mesoderm (the sex cords). The sex cords, in turn, are invaded by the primordial germ cells, the source of the germ cell line (*spermatogonia* in males or *oogonia* in females), and differentiate into the seminiferous tubules (males) and follicles (females).

What determines the type of germ cell? The short arm of the Y chromosome contains a gene or genes, referred to as the testis determining factor (TDF), responsible for the differentiation of the indifferent gonad into a testis. The mechanisms by which TDF leads to the formation of the testes are unknown.

The region of the Y chromosome containing the TDF is homologous with a region of the X chromosome; crossing over of chromosomal material can occur. Thus, an XX chromosomal female will develop testes and become male if one of the X chromosomes carries the TDF, the prerequisite for masculine differentiation. Similarly, an XY individual, who otherwise should be male, will develop ovaries and become female if TDF has been deleted from the Y chromosome (Figure 57-1). Thus, chromosomal sex does not always accurately predict gonadal sex or, as will be seen, phenotypic sex. What is important is the presence on either chromosome of an active TDF.

In XX (or XY) individuals without the TDF, several weeks after the testes begin to differentiate, the sex cords are invaded by the primordial germ cells, which now form oogonia. Thus, without instructions provided by the TDF, ovaries develop.

Sexual Differentiation of the Internal and External Genitalia Depends on Hormones Produced by the Testes

Just as one cannot predict the sex of a mammalian embryo from the structure of the indifferent gonads, one cannot determine the sex of an animal from the precursors of the internal reproductive organs. For a time both

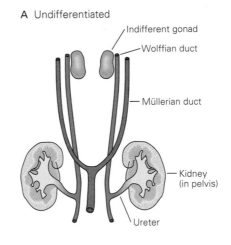

A Undifferentiated

Indifferent gonad

Wolffian duct

Müllerian duct

Kidney
(in pelvis)

Ureter

Figure 57-2 Sexual differentiation of the genital ducts.

A. Schematic representation of the wolffian and müllerian ducts in both sexes before the onset of testicular activity in males. Note that the ureters and eventually the collecting system of the kidneys are derived from the wolffian duct.

B. In the adult male the wolffian duct has formed the epididymis, seminal vesicle, and the ductus deferens. The müllerian duct has disappeared except for a small remnant in the prostatic urethra (not shown). The testes have descended into the scrotum and the kidneys have ascended into the upper abdominal region. (The ultimately separate openings of the ureter and ductus deferens are due to the manner in which the bladder develops.)

C. In the adult female the müllerian ducts have formed the oviducts, uterus, and the deepest part of the vagina. Without hormonal stimulation the wolffian duct has disappeared except for several small remnants (not shown). The kidneys ascend, as in the male, and the ovaries descend into the pelvis.

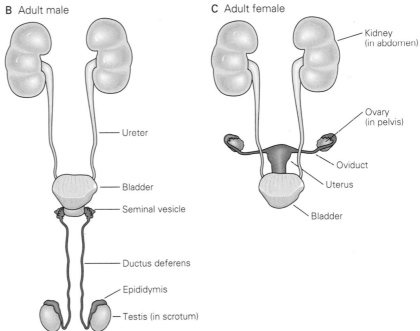

B Adult male

Ureter

Bladder

Seminal vesicle

Ductus deferens

Epididymis

Testis (in scrotum)

C Adult female

Kidney
(in abdomen)

Ovary
(in pelvis)

Oviduct

Uterus

Bladder

the mesonephric (or wolffian) duct, which gives rise to male structures (the ductus deferens, seminal vesicles, and epididymis), and the paramesonephric (or müllerian) duct, which gives rise to female structures, are present (Figure 57-2). What factors are initially responsible for these developmental decisions? The testes produce *müllerian duct inhibiting hormone* (MIH), which prevents the development and differentiation of the female internal reproductive organs, and *testosterone,* which stimulates the development and differentiation of the wolffian duct.

Development of the wolffian duct is not this simple, however. In both sexes the wolffian duct serves for a time as a functional urinary duct. The ureter and collecting system of the mature kidney develop as an outgrowth of the wolffian duct. This renal collecting system

remains functional throughout life in both sexes. Why this specific urinary derivative of the wolffian duct does not depend on testosterone for survival, while its reproductive derivatives do, is unknown. No hormone stimulus, like testosterone or estrogen, is necessary for the development and differentiation of the reproductive derivatives of the müllerian duct or the urinary derivatives of the wolffian duct.

The development of the external genitalia presents a similar picture but with an important difference. The potential internal reproductive ducts in the embryo are represented by two *anlagen,* one "female" and the other "male," whereas the potential external genitalia are represented by only a single midline phallic tubercle, bilateral urethral folds, and genital swellings. In response to testicular hormones these anlagen differentiate into the

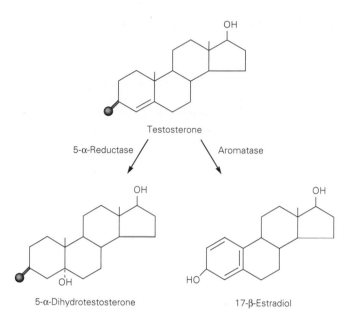

Figure 57-3 Testosterone is a prohormone for dihydrotestosterone and estradiol. The alternations in the steroid molecules seem unimpressive when represented in two dimensions but actually impart highly significant and functionally important changes in the three-dimensional structure, eg, in receptor binding.

penis, penile urethra, and scrotum; in the absence of this hormonal stimulus the same tissues develop into the clitoris and labia. Thus, the same tissues can develop into the external genitalia of either the female or the male. Interestingly, the masculine differentiation of the external genitalia is triggered by the hormone *dihydrotestosterone* (DHT), not testosterone, which serves only as the prohormone for DHT (Figure 57-3). As will be discussed below, testosterone is also a prohormone for estradiol, a hormone essential for the masculinization of the rat brain.

Three clinical syndromes are significant for understanding the sexual differentiation of the reproductive organs and perhaps also the brain (Table 57-1). In the *androgen insensitivity syndrome* XY individuals have TDF, and therefore develop testes that produce testosterone, but they lack functional androgen receptors because of autosomal gene mutations. As a result, tissues cannot respond to testosterone or dihydrotestosterone, and affected individuals develop feminine external genitalia. Because müllerian duct inhibiting hormone is a polypeptide, its action is not affected by the absence of androgen receptors, and the derivatives of this duct fail to develop. Thus, these XY women do not have oviducts, a uterus, or a cervix and the vagina is underdeveloped.

The second syndrome, *5-α-reductase deficiency*, also occurs in XY individuals. The enzyme 5-α-reductase converts testosterone to dihydrotestosterone. Individuals deficient in this enzyme have testes that are hormonally active but their external genitalia are not masculinized. These individuals are commonly initially classified as females.

The third syndrome, *congenital adrenal hyperplasia*, can occur in both males and females. In males this syndrome causes precocious puberty whereas in females it disrupts the normal development of the genitalia. In this condition the adrenal cortex lacks one or more specific enzymes required for the synthesis of cortisol, the levels of which are regulated by the hypothalamo–hypophyseal axis. Without cortisol the adrenals respond to increased levels of adrenocorticotropic hormone (ACTH) and release sufficient androgenic adrenal hormones to masculinize the genitalia. Genital masculinization can cause physicians to err in assigning sex, identifying a genetic female as a male with undescended testes!

These three syndromes are consistent with the concept that the reproductive system is feminine by default and that steroid hormone action is necessary for masculine differentiation.

The Brain Also Undergoes Hormonally Dependent Sexual Differentiation

If nature's default program for the reproductive system is female, does the same hold true for the brain? During the past several decades it has become clear that the reproductive system depends on the brain. Thus, those regions of the brain directly involved with reproduction might also be expected to undergo hormone-dependent sexual differentiation.

Specific regions of the brain play important roles in controlling reproductive behavior, gonadal function, and ovulation. In fact, the concept of the sexual differentiation of the brain began with studies of reproductive functions. In 1936 Carroll Pfeiffer demonstrated that testicular implants in neonatal female rats permanently blocked ovulation. Pfeiffer concluded, incorrectly, that there is a hormone-dependent sex difference in the anterior pituitary. It was later shown that the male pituitary transplanted beneath the hypothalamus of a hypophysectomized female does support ovulation. Thus, the sex difference resides in the brain, not in the pituitary.

Subsequently, Geoffrey Harris, Roger Gorski, and Jackson Wagnor demonstrated that the ability to ovulate is related to the absence of the testes at neonatal stages. In male rats castrated as adults, an ovarian graft in the

Table 57-1 Three Clinical Syndromes That Provide Insight Into Sexual Differentiation of the Reproductive System and Brain

	Androgen insensitivity (feminizing testis)	5-α-reductase deficiency	Congenital adrenal hyperplasia (adrenogenital syndrome)
Chromosomal sex	XY	XY	XX
Main feature	Lack functional androgen receptors	Lack the enzyme	Lack enzyme(s) needed for adrenal synthesis of cortisol and sometimes aldosterone
Gonad/function	Testes/normal	Testes/normal	Ovaries/normal
Appearance of genitalia			
At birth	Female	Female	Variable virilization
After puberty	Female	Minimal to marked virilization	Variable virilization (female, if corrected surgically and on cortisol therapy)
Internal sex organs	Wolffian derivatives only	Wolffian derivatives only	Müllerian derivatives only
Psychosexual identity	Female	Female or male	Female with some signs of masculinization

anterior chamber of the eye failed to ovulate. However, in males castrated within the first few days after birth, ovulation did occur in the ovarian graft when the animals became adults. Testosterone injected into female rats within the first week of postnatal life permanently alters the functional activity of the medial preoptic area of the hypothalamus. Treatment with testosterone induces anovulatory sterility that cannot be overcome by electrical stimulation of the medial preoptic area, even though such stimulation is successful in normal females in which spontaneous ovulation has been blocked pharmacologically.

These studies of so-called *androgenized* females suggested that the secretion of luteinizing hormone (LH) is regulated by both a cyclic and a tonic neural system (see Table 57-2, next page). Both genetic male and androgenized female rats appear to lack the neural control mechanisms that bring about the ovulatory discharge of luteinizing hormone release hormone (LHRH). As will be described later, this sex difference in the control of LHRH release may have a neuroanatomical basis.

Gonadal hormone exposure during development is also responsible for dimorphisms in the neural mechanisms that regulate sexual behavior. Although there is a marked sexual dimorphism in LHRH regulation, normal male rats occasionally exhibit components of female sexual behavior, such as the lordosis reflex, and females exhibit the mounting behavior typical of the male. However, castration of the male rat during early postnatal development suppresses masculine sexual behavior in the adult and markedly enhances feminine sexual behavior. Conversely, exposing neonatal female rats to testosterone permanently suppresses feminine sexual behavior and enhances masculine behavior. Sexual differentiation of the cyclic regulation of LHRH secretion, and to a lesser degree the different mechanisms that control sexual behavior, is comparable to that of other components of the reproductive system. Thus, the default pathway for these aspects of brain function also appears to be feminine.

The observation that occasionally males exhibit lordosis and females mounting led to the suggestion that

Table 57–2 Consequences of Hormonal Manipulation

Treatment	Age when treated	LH secretion pattern	Sexual behavioral responsiveness		Number of spine synapses in MPOA
			Female	Male	
Females					
Controls	—	Cyclic	High	Low	High
Testosterone	Postnatal day 4[a]	*Acyclic*	*Low*	*High*	*Low*
Testosterone	Postnatal day 16[b]	Cyclic	High	Low	High
Males					
Controls	—	Acyclic	Low	High	Low
Castration	Postnatal day 1[a]	*Cyclic*	*High*	*Low*	*High*
Castration	Postnatal day 7[b]	Acyclic	Low	High	Low

Abbreviations: LH = Luteinizing hormone; MPOA = medial preoptic area.
[a]During the critical period of sexual differentiation.
[b]After the critical period of sexual differentiation.

the observed functional sex differences were determined by the "threshold" of hormonal activation or disinhibition of neural circuits presumed to exist in both sexes. At that time there was no evidence for hormone-dependent structural sex differences in the central nervous system. However, as described below, there are many hormone-dependent sex differences in the structure of the brain, and these structural differences presumably underlie the many differences in sexual behavior that have been observed.

Gonadal Hormones Exert Permanent Effects on the Developing Central Nervous System and Transient Effects on the Adult Brain

The distinction between the transient (or *activational*) effects of gonadal steroids on the mature brain and the permanent (or *organizational*) effects of hormones during early development is conceptually important. This distinction was proposed in 1959 by Charles Phoenix and his colleagues based on studies of the effect on adult sexual behavior of exposure to testosterone during early development.

Testosterone is often thought of as the male sex hormone and estrogen and progesterone as female sex hormones. In reality, however, each sex has a particular balance of several hormones, although testosterone does predominate in males and estrogen or progesterone in females. Any sex differences in brain func-

tion or structure established during sexual differentiation should remain after gonadectomy in adulthood or after exposing adults of either sex to similar hormonal regimes. Conversely, sex differences due to the activational effects of different hormone environments, if not related to sexual differentiation of the brain per se, should disappear after gonadectomy or in the presence of similar hormonal environments in both sexes.

How do gonadal steroids exert permanent or transient actions on the brain? Steroids can act on neurons in at least two ways. One is the classical pathway involving steroid receptors that activate or inhibit specific genes upon binding steroid. This is the mechanism presumed to mediate the organizational effects of hormones. The second way in which steroids act on neurons involves direct action on the cell membrane but is less well understood.

Exposure to Testicular Hormones During Development Produces Sex Differences in the Central Nervous System

The variety of hormone-dependent sex differences in brain function is more extensive than the examples we have so far considered. Sex differences in maternal or parenting behavior as well as in aggressive and territorial behavior are found in many species. These behaviors are, of course, closely related to reproduction. There are, however, also sex differences in the regulation of food

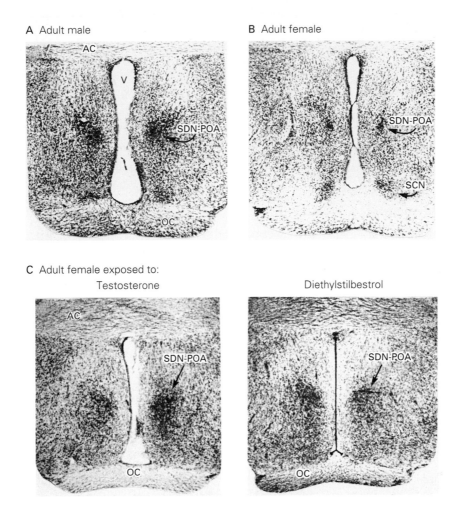

A Adult male

B Adult female

C Adult female exposed to:
Testosterone

Diethylstilbestrol

Figure 57-4 Hormones change neuronal morphology. (From Gorski 1987.)

A-B. The sexually dimorphic nucleus of the preoptic area in rats is larger in adult males than in adult females, as seen in these coronal sections. Abbreviations: **AC** = anterior commissure; **OC** = optic chiasm; **SCN** = suprachiasmatic nucleus; **SDN-**

POA = sexually dimorphic nucleus of the preoptic area ; **V** = ventricle.

C. Adult female rats were exposed perinatally to testosterone or the synthetic estrogen diethylstilbestrol. In both cases the volume and number of neurons of the sexually demorphic nucleus of the preoptic area increased after hormone exposure.

intake and body weight; open-field, play, and social behaviors; and learning behavior and performance.

Sex differences in brain function may, at least in part, result from sex differences in the structure of the central nervous system. In a region of the medial preoptic area of the hypothalamus there is a sex difference in the proportion of synapses found on dendritic spines versus shafts following transection of the afferent stria terminalis. In rats that have been hormonally manipulated after birth this structural sex difference goes in exactly the same direction (masculinization or feminization) as the neural control of LHRH release or sexual behavior (Table 57-2). Although this structural difference between the sexes is subtle, the effect of testicular hormones is profound.

In rats there is a striking sex difference in a group of neurons called the *sexually dimorphic nucleus of the preoptic area*. The volume of the nucleus is about five times larger in the male than in the female (Figure 57-4). As discussed below, the volume of the nucleus is determined by the perinatal action of gonadal hormones. There are also sex differences in the thickness of various regions of the cerebral cortex: The thickness of the left side of the male rat cortex is greater than that of the right, so that there is greater asymmetry in the male. Moreover, the number of neurons in the splenium of the corpus callosum is greater in female rats. There are also sex differences in neurotransmitters, neuropeptides, and neuromodulators in various brain regions. The sex differences in brain structures identified to date are listed in Table 57-3.

Table 57-3 Structural Sex Differences in the Rat Central Nervous System

Volume or size	
Male greater than female	**Female greater than male**
Accessory olfactory bulb	Anteroventral periventricular nucleus
Bed nucleus of olfactory tract	Locus coerulus
Bed nucleus of stria terminalis	Parastrial nucleus
Medial nucleus of amygdala	
Medial preoptic nucleus	
Sexually dimorphic nucleus of the preoptic area	
Spinal nucleus of the bulbocavernosus	
Supraoptic nucleus*	
Ventromedial nucleus	
Visual cortex*	
Vomeronasal organ	

Synaptic morphology
Arcuate nucleus
Corpus callosum*
Hippocampus*
Lateral septum
Medial nucleus of amygdala
Medial preoptic area
Sexually dimorphic nucleus of the preoptic area
Suprachiasmatic nucleus*
Ventromedial nucleus
Visual cortex*

*The perinatal influence of the hormonal environment on these sex differences has not been studied. Therefore it is possible that they reflect the activational effects of the hormonal milieu and not organizational effects.

Estradiol Is the Masculinizing Hormone for Many Sexually Dimorphic Brain Characteristics

Estrogen masculinizes brain function at doses lower than those of testosterone. In fact, aromatization of testosterone to estrogen is a prerequisite for masculinization. But what is the role of estrogen in the development of the female brain?

In newborn rats of either sex the plasma levels of estrogen are high. If estrogen is the masculinizing hormone and its plasma levels are high during the critical period of sexual differentiation in both males and females, why is the female's brain not masculinized?

In rats a liver protein that binds estrogen but not testosterone is present in the blood in high titers during the first several weeks of postnatal life. This protein, α-fetoprotein, binds physiological levels of plasma estrogen and sequesters this hormone, protecting the female's brain from exposure to this masculinizing hormone (although injection of exogenous estrogen is thought to overwhelm these protective mechanisms). In males testicular testosterone is not bound by α-fetoprotein and therefore can enter neurons, where it is aromatized to estrogen and exerts its masculinizing action. The *protection hypothesis* is consistent with the finding that ovariectomy of newborn female rats has no apparent effect on the regulation of LHRH release or on female sexual behavior. It is also consistent with the view that the default developmental pathway of the brain is feminine.

However, several experimental observations temper this interpretation. First, estrogen stimulates neurite outgrowth in explant cultures of the hypothalamus and in fact is required for the outgrowth of axons of estrogen-responsive neurons (Figure 57-5). Moreover, antiestrogen treatment of neonatal female rats inhibits normal ovulation and lordosis behavior without enhancing masculine sexual behavior (ie, the female is

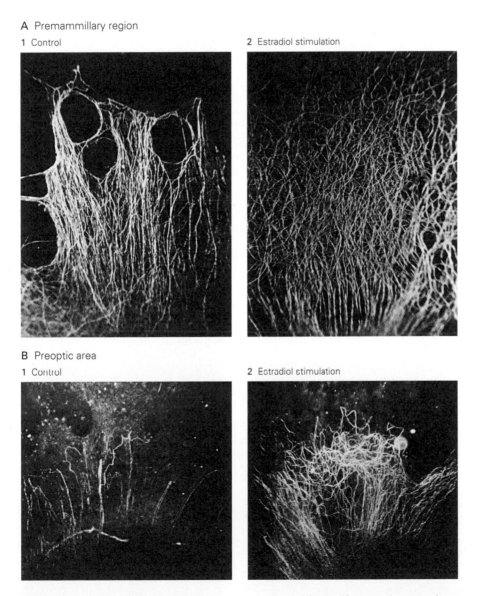

A Premammillary region

1 Control

2 Estradiol stimulation

B Preoptic area

1 Control

2 Estradiol stimulation

Figure 57-5 Neurite growth is stimulated by estradiol. These darkfield photomicrographs of silver-impregnated cultures of the hypothalamus of a newborn mouse were made after approximately three weeks in vitro. In all four panels the explants are located just below the area of neurite outgrowth. (From Toran-Allerand 1976.)

A. Culture of the premammillary region. **1.** Incubation in a control

medium of fetal calf serum that contains some estradiol. **2.** Incubation of the same region from the other side of the brain with additional estradiol. The field covered by neurite outgrowth is almost three times larger than that in the control culture.

B. Culture of the preoptic area. **1.** Incubation plus antibodies to estradiol. **2.** Culture incubated with antibodies to bovine serum albumin.

"defeminized" but not masculinized). As expected, antiestrogen treatment in neonates decreases the adult sex difference in the volume of the sexually dimorphic nucleus of the preoptic area in males, but it does so in females as well. Finally, α-fetoprotein may actually enter some neurons and deliver estrogen.

One interpretation of these findings is that the rat brain is not inherently feminine but instead is neuter. In species in which sexual differentiation of the brain occurs postnatally, α-fetoprotein may serve as a source of estrogen after parturition so that the brain of the female can develop normally. According to this *delivery hypothesis,* some level of exposure to estrogen is necessary for the normal development of the female brain. The estrogen required for masculine differentiation of the brain, derived from the aromatization of testosterone, is therefore additional to the plasma estrogen available.

Hormones Exert Diverse Actions on the Development of the Central Nervous System

Estradiol May Prevent Apoptotic Cell Death in the Sexually Dimorphic Nucleus of the Preoptic Area

The sexually dimorphic nucleus of the preoptic area of the rat is about five times larger in volume in the male than in the female. Most of the differences in this nucleus are due to a greater number of neurons in the male's nucleus. It is unlikely that this sex difference is programmed in the male genome since perinatal exposure to testosterone or the synthetic estrogen diethylstilbestrol completely reverses the difference (see Figure 57-4). Thus, hormones alone can fully masculinize the sexually dimorphic nucleus of the preoptic area.

How might this increase in the number of neurons occur? Steroids are known to prevent programmed cell death by apoptosis. In females the number of cells within the posterior component of the nucleus decrease significantly between postnatal days 4 and 10. This decrease does not occur in intact males or in females given the sex-reversing regime of testosterone. Moreover, the incidence of apoptotic cell death within a subregion of the nucleus is greater and more prolonged in the female. Furthermore, administration of exogenous testosterone in males castrated postnatally markedly suppresses apoptotic cell death (Figure 57-6).

Gonadal Hormones May Induce Apoptotic Cell Death in the Anteroventral Periventricular Nucleus

The anteroventral periventricular nucleus is one of the few nuclei that is larger in volume in the female rat than in the male. Castration of the newborn male eliminates

Figure 57-6 Exogenous testosterone in male rats castrated postnatally suppresses apoptosis. The plots compare the incidence of apoptosis in two regions of the hypothalamus in two groups of male rats at different ages (day of sacrifice). All rats were castrated on the day of birth. On postnatal day 5 one group was treated with oil and the other group with 500 µg testosterone propionate. Apoptosis was determined by the terminal deoxy-uridine triphosphate nick end-labeling method, which identifies fragmentation of DNA before the cells actually die. (Modified from Davis et al. 1996.)

A. The level of apoptosis in a subcomponent of the sexually dimorphic nucleus of the preoptic area (the central part of the medial preoptic nucleus). **Asterisks** indicate statistically significant differences from same-age males treated with oil.

B. The level of apoptosis in the lateral preoptic area, which is not known to be sexually dimorphic.

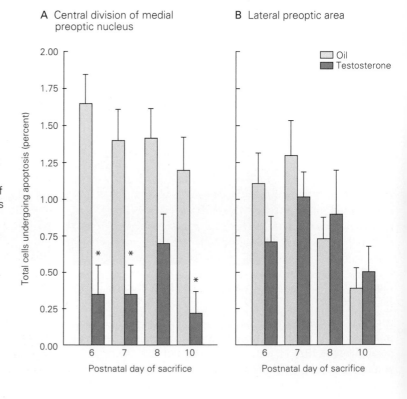

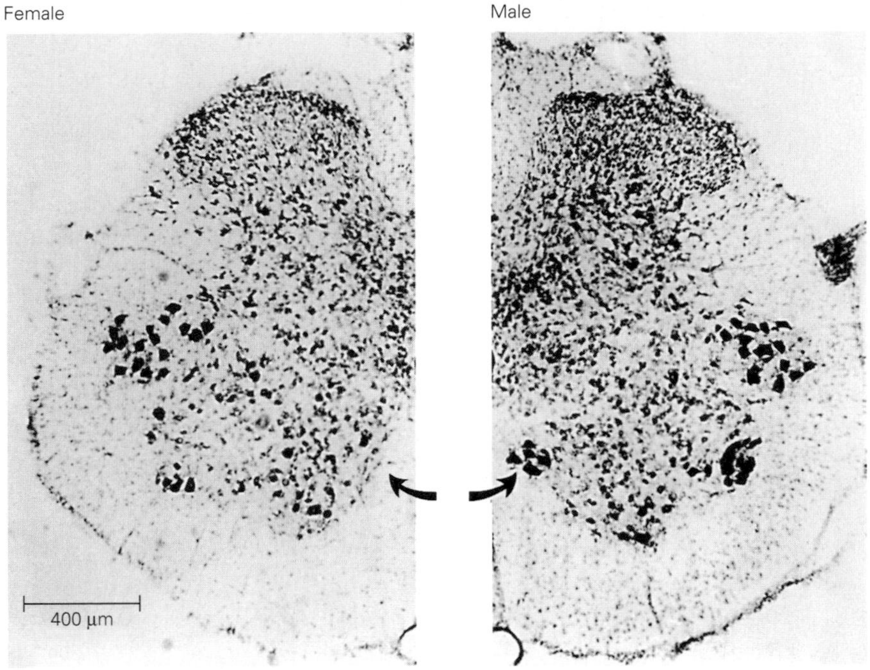

Figure 57-7 An important anatomical difference between female and male rats. These photomicrographs of the fifth lumbar segment of the spinal cord show that the spinal nucleus of the bulbocavernosus (**arrow**) is virtually absent in the female. (From Breedlove and Arnold 1981.)

this sex difference, as does the administration of testosterone to the female. Although a greater incidence of dying cells is evident in the male during late embryonic development, the sex difference in the volume of this nucleus is not detected until near the time of puberty. Thus, the development of the sex difference in this nucleus may be due to hormone-induced apoptosis during perinatal development coupled with further changes at the time of puberty.

The Action of Testosterone on Peripheral Muscles May Prevent Neuronal Death in the Spinal Nucleus of the Bulbocavernosus

A small number of motor neurons which form the spinal nucleus of the bulbocavernosus innervate penile muscles. This nucleus is almost completely absent in the female's spinal cord (Figure 57-7). In both sexes phallic musculature and neurons of the spinal nucleus of the bulbocavernosus are present at birth, but they disappear in female rats over the course of the first postnatal week of life. The results of several studies clearly indicate that testosterone, not estrogen, maintains the penile musculature. This enhanced degree of muscle differentiation appears to promote the survival of the motor neurons of this spinal nucleus.

Hormone-Induced Modifications in Brain Structure Are Not Limited to Development

Gonadal hormones produce structural changes in the brain not only during development but also in adults. Perhaps the most dramatic example of this is the marked seasonal change in singing behavior in young male birds. With the onset of testicular activity in a new breeding season, dendrites lengthen and new synapses form. In female rats there are significant changes in the number of hippocampal synapses over the four-day estrous cycle (Figure 57-8). In humans, given the marked changes in the body's structure, in personality, and sexual awareness during puberty, it is likely that structural changes in the central nervous system also occur during this period.

Specific Sex Differences in the Brain Control Behavior

What is the functional significance of sex differences in the brain? Sex differences in the anatomical structure of the song-control system in birds have a clear function. Females do not sing unless treated during development with gonadal hormones, which trigger the masculiniza-

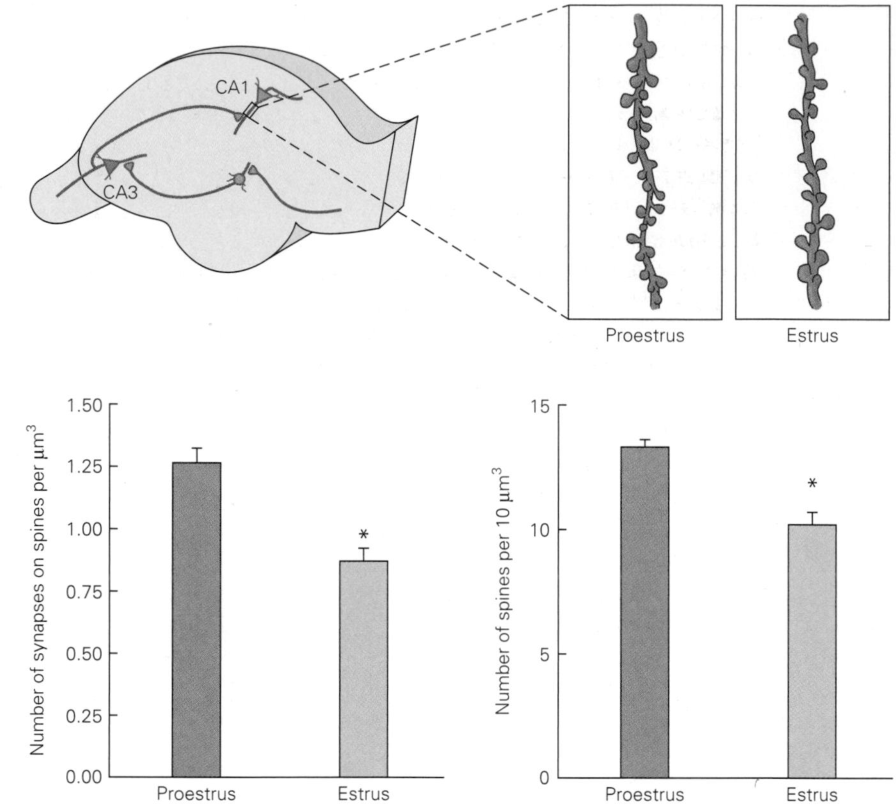

Figure 57-8 The estimated density of synapses on dendritic spines in the striatum radiatum (hippocampal CA1 region) changes with the stage of the estrous cycle. The **asterisk** indicates a statistically significant difference. (Modified from Woolley and McEwen 1992.)

tion of specific brain nuclei. Sex differences in brain structure in the frog *Xenopus laevis* also appear to be related to vocalization. In the gerbil the sexually dimorphic area of the preoptic area of the hypothalamus may have a role in territorial marking. In the rat the anteroventral periventricular nucleus may participate in the regulation of the cyclic secretion of LHRH, since lesions in this area disrupt ovulation.

A number of structural sex differences in the human brain have been reported (Table 57-4), but these differences and their functional significance are less well established than those in rodents. The sexually dimorphic nucleus of the preoptic area in humans has been reported to be significantly larger and to include more neurons in males than in females. The difference, however, develops only after about five years of age. One other hypothalamic nucleus, the interstitial nucleus of the anterior hypothalmus-3 (INAH-3), is also larger in men than women (Figure 57-9).

Certain sex differences in cognitive performance have been well demonstrated. Men perform better than women on visuospatial tasks, and women perform better than men on verbal tasks. Although these differences are statistically significant, they are often based on a large number of subjects, and there is significant overlap in performance between the sexes. One fairly robust sex difference is that boys outnumber girls 13:1 in advanced mathematical reasoning ability. In addition, brain function in men appears to be more lateralized than in women. This was first observed in a clinical setting; women are more likely than men to recover speech after a stroke that damages cortical speech areas.

Studies of individuals with clinical conditions that disturb the normal relationship between genetic sex and psychosexual identity have also proved informative. Genetic males with the androgen insensitivity syndrome (Table 57-1) are psychosexually female. These "women" develop feminine phenotypes at puberty because of their testicular activity and the aromatization of testosterone. Their feminine psychosexuality is seemingly in accord with the idea that the developmental default state of sexual differentiation is female. However, this interpretation is at odds with the general view that estrogen is actually the masculinizing hormone in sexual differentiation of the brain. Perhaps humans have some protective mechanism, akin to α-fetoprotein, that protects the developing brain from exposure to estrogen, or perhaps estrogen is not the masculinizing hor-

Table 57–4 Putative Structural Sex Differences in the Human Central Nervous System

Larger in the male than in the female
  Central component of the bed nucleus of the stria
    terminalis
  Darkly staining component of the bed nucleus of the stria
    terminalis
  Second interstitial nucleus of the anterior hypothalamus
  Third interstitial nucleus of the anterior hypothalamus
  Sexually dimorphic nucleus of the preoptic area
  Onuf's nucleus in spinal cord

Larger in the female than in the male
  Anterior commissure (midsagittal area)
  Corpus callosum (midsagittal area)
  Isthmus of the corpus callosum (compared only with that
    of consistently right-handed men)
  Massa intermedia (incidence and midsaggital surface
    area)

Greater asymmetry in the male
  Planum temporale

Shape differences
  Splenium of the corpus callosum (more bulbous in
    females)
  Suprachiasmatic nucleus (elongated in females, more
    spherical in males)

mone in humans. Studies of the cognitive abilities of such individuals or of their brain structure are lacking.

Chromosomal males (XY) with 5-α-reductase deficiency (Table 57-1) are an interesting group. Without this enzyme testosterone is not converted to dihydrotestosterone and the external genitalia do not become masculinized: Instead the urethra opens into a vagina-like urogenital sinus. Cursory examination of the appearance of the external genitalia leads to sex assignment as female, but careful examination of the genitalia reveals that the individual is not a normal female. A common treatment of this condition is castration and continued sex assignment as (an infertile) female.

When individuals with this enzyme defect reach puberty, the testes descend, the clitoris enlarges, and a masculine habitus develops. In a group of 18 individuals reportedly raised unambiguously as girls in the Dominican Republic, 17 "changed" their psychosexual identity from female to male, suggesting that even in humans hormone action during early development, and perhaps at puberty, can overcome the psychological effects of being raised as a female. This interpretation is in accord with the concept that sexual differentiation of the brain is dependent on hormones.

The clinical history of such individuals has generated controversy. The individuals were subjected over many years to ridicule, and some investigators seriously doubt that these individuals were raised unambiguously as girls, a conclusion that was actually drawn from retrospective analysis of studies that spanned decades. Moreover, in the Dominican Republic it is socially advantageous to be male, and adopting a male psychosexual identity is one way to adapt to the masculinization of one's body. In other parts of the world patients more readily accept castration and continue as women psychosexually. Perhaps what this syndrome teaches us is that humans react as individuals and that hormones, personal experiences, body appearance, and perhaps the attitude of physicians all play a role in that reaction. Again, there appear to be no studies of the cognitive abilities or brain structure of individuals with 5-α-reductase deficiency who have or have not adopted a male psychosexual identity.

In congenital adrenal hyperplasia one or several enzymatic defects interfere with the production of adrenal cortical hormones (eg, cortisol), and thus individuals are exposed to excess androgen. Compensatory elevation of adrenal secretion leads to the release of adrenal steroids with androgenic activity adequate to cause masculinization of the genitalia. When recognized, even at the hospital after birth, the condition can be alleviated by administering the missing adrenal hormones. These individuals exposed to excess androgen before birth must be treated with cortisol throughout life, a situation that might psychologically affect their behavior. These girls are often "tomboys" and play more frequently with toys ordinarily preferred by boys. In adulthood there is a greater incidence of lesbian behavior among these women.

To date, the study of these clinical conditions has not provided clear support for a role of hormones in the sexual differentiation of behavior in the human brain.

There May Be a Genetic and Anatomical Basis for Homosexuality

One of the most sexually dimorphic characteristics of human behavior is sexuality itself. Is the sexual differentiation of the brain responsible for this fundamental difference in human behavior? Once again, study of this question is difficult, but progress can perhaps be made by studying individuals who display atypical behavior.

One such behavior is transsexualism. A transexual is an individual of one genetic and phenotypic sex who believes that he or she is psychologically of the other sex and chooses to undergo a surgical sex change. Dick

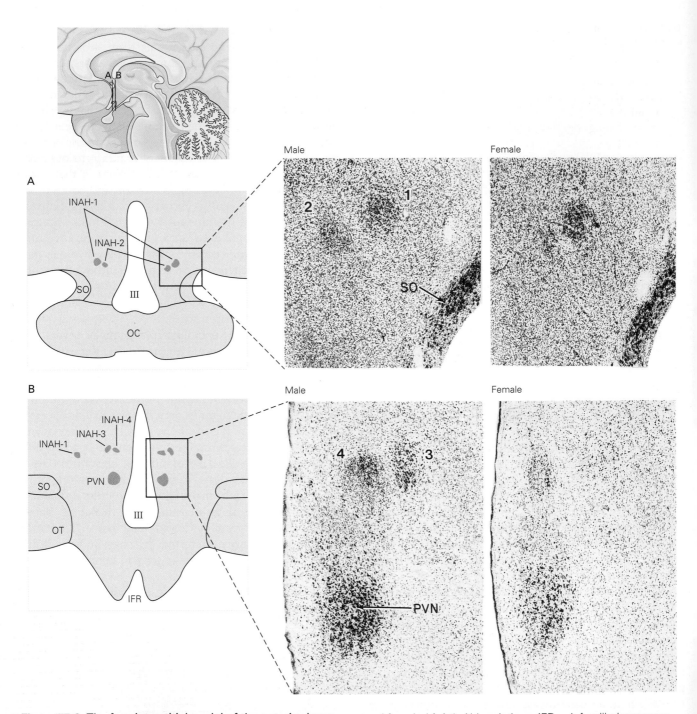

Figure 57-9 The four interstitial nuclei of the anterior hypothalamus (INAH-1 to INAH-4) in the human brain. The section shown in part A is about 800 μm anterior to the one in part B. Photomicrographs in parts A and B compare the male (**left**) and female (**right**). Abbreviations: **IFR** = infundibular recess; **OT** = optic tract; **OC** = optic chiasm; **PVN** = paraventricular nucleus; **SO** = supraoptic nucleus; **III** = third ventricle. (From Gorski 1988.)

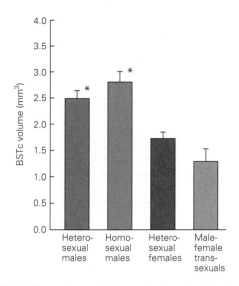

Figure 57-10 The volume of the central part of the bed nucleus of the stria terminalis (BSTc) in four sexually diverse groups: presumed heterosexual and homosexual men, presumed heterosexual women, and six postoperative male-to-female transsexuals. The volume of the nucleus was estimated by the density of vasoactive intestinal polypeptide innervation, which in turn was measured immunohistochemically.

*Indicates significantly greater than females or transexuals. (Based on Zhou et al. 1995.)

Swaab and his colleagues have studied the central nucleus of the bed nucleus of the stria terminalis, which in postmortem studies is larger in volume in men than in women. The volume of the nucleus does not vary with sexual orientation in men, but in postoperative male-to-female transsexuals the volume is reduced to that of the female (Figure 57-10). Although these findings are subject to the same difficulties as those based on postmortem examination of the human brain, they raise the possibility that disturbances in differentiation of the brain could lead to transsexualism.

Much recent research has focused on neural correlates of homosexuality. Homosexual men and women generally consider themselves male or female, respectively. Thus, unlike transsexualism, there is no discordance between "brain sex" and phenotypic sex. However, the process of the sexual differentiation of the brain need not be all or nothing. In fact, it appears to involve several independent processes, such as masculinization as opposed to defeminization, each with different temporal characteristics, hormonal dependencies, and neuroanatomical loci. It is conceivable that a change in hormonal production or response could alter sexual differentiation of one part of the brain but not another and thus contribute to a homosexual orientation.

Three structural differences between the brains of homosexual and apparently heterosexual men have been identified. The suprachiasmatic nucleus was found to be larger in volume and to contain more neurons in homosexual men than in a reference group of heterosexuals. The hypothalamic nucleus INAH-3, which is larger in volume in men than in women, is reportedly larger in heterosexual than in homosexual men. Finally, the midsagittal cross-sectional area of the anterior commissure, which is larger in women than in men, was found to be even larger in one group of homosexual men. In all three differences, however, there is considerable overlap between the groups being compared, and these data require confirmation.

Although it remains plausible that alterations in the hormone-dependent sexual differentiation of the brain contribute to homosexuality, there is also evidence that genetic factors may also be involved. The concordance rate for homosexuality is relatively high for both men and women. The concordance rate among twins—the occurrence of homosexuality in both twins of a pair—is much higher among identical twins than among nonidentical twins and is even smaller for adopted siblings of homosexual individuals (Table 57-5).

Using pedigree analysis, Dean Hamer and his colleagues found an unusually high incidence of homosexuality only among maternal uncles and male cousins of homosexual men. This led Hamer to perform a gene-linkage analysis of the X chromosome in 40 pairs of homosexual brothers. Of these 40 pairs, 33 pairs had inherited the same chromosomal markers of a region at one tip of the X chromosome labeled Xq28. Thus there

Table 57–5 Concordance for Homosexuality in Twins

	Males[a]	Females[b]
Monozygotic twins	(29/56) 52%	(34/71) 48%
Dizygotic twins	(12/54) 22%	(6/37) 16%
Adopted same-sex siblings	(6/57) 11%	(2/35) 6%
	Males[c]	Females[c]
Monozygotic twins	(22/34) 65%	(3/4) 75%
Dizygotic twins		
Male/male	(4/14) 29%	
Male/female	(3/9) 33%	

[a]Bailey and Pillard 1991.
[b]Bailey et al. 1993.
[c]Whitman, Diamond, and Martin, 1993.

may be one or more genes within Xq28 that predispose an individual to male homosexuality.

For many years the debate over the causes of homosexuality has been framed in terms of nature versus nurture: Is homosexuality determined by choice, that is by experiential factors, or by biological factors such as hormones or genes? It is likely that *both* are involved. A complex behavioral trait such as sexual orientation is unlikely to be caused by a single gene, a single hormone-induced alteration in brain structure, or a single experience in life. The etiology of homosexuality—and heterosexuality—must be multifactorial. Whether the sexual differentiation of the brain is an important factor remains to be determined.

An Overall View

In many laboratory animals the central nervous system appears to be inherently feminine, although a minimal exposure to estrogen may be necessary for completely normal development of the female brain. It is very clear, however, that for the mammalian brain to have the functional and structural characteristics typical of the male of the species, the developing brain *must* be exposed to testicular hormones and, in many species, specifically to estrogen derived from the aromatization of testosterone.

However, the morphological effects of gonadal steroids are not limited to developmental processes (the period of the classical organizational effects of gonadal steroids). Gonadal activity can produce seasonal and even more rapid changes in neuroanatomy, as with the four-day estrous cycle of the female rat. Marked changes in central nervous system structure, either permanent or transient, are also likely to occur at puberty. The influence of hormones on the central nervous system is therefore *dynamic*.

Studies in experimental animals strongly suggest that the human brain also undergoes hormonally induced sexual differentiation during development. Although at present the observed sex differences in human cognitive function appear unrelated to reproductive function, evolutionary biologists may some day be able to explain the rather widespread effect of testicular hormones on brain development by a coherent theory that accounts for the role of hormones in the development of cognitive as well as reproductive function.

Roger A. Gorski

Selected Readings

Byne W, Parsons B. 1993. Human sexual orientation. The biologic theories reappraised. Arch Gen Psychiatry 50:228–239.

De Vries GJ. 1990. Sex differences in neurotransmitter systems. J Neuroendocrinol 2:1–13.

De Vries GJ, De Bruin JPC, Uylings HBM, Corner MA (eds). 1984. Sex differences in the brain. Prog Brain Res 61:1–516.

Dörner G, Poppe I, Stahl F, Kolzsch J, Uebelhack R. 1991. Gene and environment-dependent neuroendocrine etiogenesis of homosexuality and transsexualism. Exp Clin Endocrinol 98:141–150.

Gorski RA. 1996. Gonadal hormones and the organization of brain structure and function. In: D Magnusson (ed). *Lifespan Development of Individuals: Behavioral, Neurobiological, and Psychosocial Perspectives*, pp. 315–340. New York: Cambridge Univ. Press.

Goy RW, McEwen BS. 1980. *Sexual Differentiation of the Brain*. Cambridge, MA: MIT Press.

Guillamón A, Segovia S. 1996. Sexual dimorphisms in the CNS and the role of steroids. In: TW Stone (ed). *CNS Neurotransmitters and Neuromodulators: Neuroactive Steroids*, pp. 127–152. Boca Raton, FL: CRC Press.

Hines M. 1993. Hormonal and neural correlates of sex-typed behavioral development in human beings. In: M. Havg (ed). *The Development of Sex Differences and Similarities in Behavior*, pp. 131–149. Netherlands: Kluwer.

Kelly DB. 1988. Sexually dimorphic behaviors. Annu Rev Neurosci 11:225–251.

Kawata M. 1995. Roles of steroid hormones and their receptors in structural organization in the nervous system. Neuroscience Res 24:1–46.

Kimura D. 1996. Sex, sexual orientation and sex hormones influence human cognitive function. Curr Opin Neurobiol 6:259–263.

Matsumoto A, Arai Y, Urano A, Hyodo S. 1995. Molecular basis of neuronal plasticity to gonadal steroids. Funct Neurol 10:59–76.

McCormick CM, Witelson SF, Kingstone E. 1990. Left-handedness in homosexual men and women: neuroendocrine implications. Psychoneuroendocrinology 15:69–76.

Nass R, Baker S. 1991. Androgen effects on cognition: congenital adrenal hyperplasia. Psychoneuroendocrinology 16:189–201.

Reinisch JM, Sanders SA. 1992. Prenatal hormonal contributions to sex differences in human cognitive and personality development. In: AA Gerall, H Moltz, IL Ward (eds). *Handbook of Behavioral Neurobiology*. Vol. 11, *Sexual Differentiation*, pp. 221–243. New York: Plenum.

References

Allen LS, Gorski RA. 1992. Sexual orientation and the size of the anterior commissure in the human brain. Proc Natl Acad Sci U S A 89:7199–7202.

Allen LS, Hines M, Shryne JE, Gorski RA. 1989. Two sexually dimorphic cell groups in the human brain. J Neurosci 9:497–506.

Allen LS, Richey MF, Chai YM, Gorski RA. 1991. Sex differences in the corpus callosum of the living human being. J Neurosci 11:933–942.

Arendash GW, Gorski RA. 1982. Enhancement of sexual behavior in female rats by neonatal transplantation of brain tissue from males. Science 217:1276–1278.

Bailey JM, Pillard RC. 1991. A genetic study of male sexual orientation. Arch Gen Psych 48:1089–1096.

Bailey JM, Pillard RC, Neale MC, Agyei Y. 1993. Heritable factors influence sexual orientation in women. Arch Gen Psych 50:217–223.

Barraclough CA, Gorski RA. 1961. Evidence that the hypothalamus is responsible for androgen-induced sterility in the female rat. Endocrinology 68:68–79.

Benbow CP, Benbow RM. 1984. Biological correlates of high mathematical reasoning ability. Prog Brain Res 61:468–490.

Berenbaum SA, Hines M. 1992. Early androgens are related to childhood sex-typed toy preferences. Psychol Sci 3:203–206.

Breedlove SM, Arnold AP. 1981. Sexually dimorphic motor nucleus in the rat lumbar spinal cord: response to adult hormone manipulation, absence in androgen-insensitive rats. Brain Res 225:297–307.

Davis EC, Popper P, Gorski RA. 1996. The role of apoptosis in sexual differentiation of the rat sexually dimorphic nucleus of the preoptic area. Brain Res 734:10–18.

Davis EC, Shryne JE, Gorski RA. 1996. Structural sexual dimorphisms in the anteroventral periventricular nucleus of the rat hypothalamus are sensitive to gonadal steroids, but develop peripubertally. Neuroendocrinology 63:142–148.

de Lacoste-Utamsing C, Holloway RL. 1982. Sexual dimorphism in human corpus callosum. Science 216:1431–1432.

DeVoogd TJ. 1991. Endocrine modulation of the development and adult function of the avian song system. Psychoneuroendocrinology 16:41–66.

Diamond MC. 1991. Hormonal effects on the development of cerebral lateralization. Psychoneuroendocrinology 16:121–129.

Dodson RE, Gorski RA. 1993. Testosterone propionate administration prevents the loss of neurons within the central part of the medial preoptic nucleus. J Neurobiol 24:80–88.

Döhler KD, Coquelin A, Davis F, Hines M, Shryne JE, Gorski RA. 1984. Pre- and postnatal influence of testosterone propionate and diethylstilbestrol on differentiation of the sexually dimorphic nucleus of the preoptic area in male and female rats. Brain Res 302:291–295.

Goldstein LA, Sengelaub DR. 1994. Differential effects of dihydrotestosterone and estrogen on the development of motoneuron morphology in a sexually dimorphic rat spinal nucleus. J Neurobiol 25:878–892.

Gorski RA. 1987. Sex differences in the rodent brain: their nature and origin. In: JM Reinisch, LA Rosenblum, SA Sanders (eds). Masculinity/Feminity: Basic Perspectives, pp. 37–67. New York: Oxford Univ. Press.

Gorski RA. 1988. Hormone-induced sex differences in hypothalamic structure. Bulletin of the Tokyo Metropolitan Institute of Neuroscience 16(Suppl 3):67–90.

Gorski RA, Harlan RE, Jacobsen CD, Shryne JE, Southam AM. 1980. Evidence for the existence of a sexually dimorphic nucleus in the preoptic area of the rat. J Comp Neurol 193(2):529–539.

Gorski RA, Wagner JW. 1965. Gonadal activity and sexual differentiation of the hypothalamus. Endocrinology 77:226–239.

Gubbay J, Collignon J, Koopman P, Capel B, Economou A, Munsterberg A, Vivian N, Goodfellow P, Lovell-Badge R. 1990. A gene mapping to the sex-determining region of the mouse Y chromosome is a member of a novel family of embryonically expressed genes. Nature 346:245–250.

Hamer DH, Hu S, Magnuson VL, Hu N, Pattatucci AML. 1993. A linkage between DNA markers on the X chromosome and male sexual orientation. Science 261:321–327.

Harris GW. 1964. Sex hormones, brain development and brain function. Endocrinology 75:627–648.

Hines M, Chiu L, McAdams LA, Bentler PM, Lipcamon J. 1992. Cognition and the corpus callosum: verbal fluency, visuospatial ability, and language lateralization related to midsagittal surface areas of callosal subregions. Behav Neurosci 106(1):3–14.

Imperato-McGinley J, Peterson RE, Gautier T, Sturla E. 1979. Androgens and the evolution of male-gender identity among male pseudohermaphrodites with 5-alpha-reductase deficiency. N Engl J Med 300:1233–1237.

Juraska JM. 1993. Sex differences in the rat cerebral cortex. In: M Haug (ed). Development of Sex Differences and Similarities in Behavior, pp. 377–388. Netherlands: Kluwer Academic.

LeVay S. 1991. A difference in hypothalamic structure between heterosexual and homosexual men. Science 253:1034–1037.

McPhaul MJ, Marcelli M, Tilley WD, Griffin JE, Wilson JD. 1991. Androgen resistance by mutations in the androgen receptor gene. FASEB J 5:2910–2915.

Money J, Schwartz M, Lewis VG. 1984. Adult erotosexual status and fetal hormonal masculinization and demasculinization: 46, XX congenital virilizing adrenal hyperplasia and 46, XY androgen-insensitivity syndrome compared. Psychoneuroendocrinology 9:405–414.

Nass R, Baker S. 1991. Androgen effects on cognition: congenital adrenal hyperplasia. Psychoneuroendocrinology 16:189–201.

Nottebohm F. 1981. A brain for all seasons: cyclical anatomical changes in song control nuclei of the canary brain. Science 214:1368–1370.

Nottebohm F, Arnold AP. 1976. Sexual dimorphism in vocal control areas of the songbird brain. Science 194:211–213.

Pfeiffer CA. 1936. Sexual differences of the hypophyses and their determination by the gonads. Am J Anat 58:195–226.

Phoenix CH, Goy RW, Gerall AA, Young WC. 1959. Organizing action of prenatally administered testosterone propionate on the tissues mediating mating behavior in the female guinea pig. Endocrinology 65:369–382.

Raisman G, Field PM. 1973. Sexual dimorphism in the neuropil of the preoptic area of the rat and its dependence on neonatal androgen. Brain Res 54:1–29.

Reinisch JM, Ziemba-Davis M, Sanders SA. 1991. Hormonal contributions to sexually dimorphic behavioral development in humans. Psychoneuroendocrinology 16:213–278.

Shaywitz BA, Shaywitz SE, Pugh KR, Constable RT, Skuklarski P, Fulbright RK, Bronen RA, Fletcher JM, Shankweller DP, Katz L, Gore JC. 1995. Sex differences in the functional organization of the brain for language. Nature 373:607–609.

Swaab DF, Fliers E. 1985. A sexually dimorphic nucleus in the human brain. Science 228:1112–1115.

Swaab DF, Gooren LJG, Hofman MA. 1992. The human hypothalamus in relation to gender and sexual orientation. Prog Brain Res 93:205–219.

Swaab DF, Hofman MA. 1990. An enlarged suprachiasmatic nucleus in homosexual men. Brain Res 537:141–148.

Terasawa E, Davis GA. 1983. The LHRH neuronal system in female rats: relation to the medial preoptic nucleus. Endocrinol Jpn 30:405–417.

Toran-Allerand CD. 1976. Sex steroids and the development of the newborn mouse hypothalamus and preoptic area in vitro: implications for sexual differentiation. Brain Res 106:407–412.

Toran-Allerand CD. 1984. On the genesis of sexual differentiation of the central nervous system: morphogenetic consequences of steroidal exposure and possible role of α-fetoprotein. Prog Brain Res 61:63–98.

Whitman FL, Diamond M, Martin J. 1993. Homosexual orientation in twins: a report on 61 pairs and three triplet sets. Arch Sex Behav 22:187–206.

Williams CL, Meck WH. 1991. The organizational effects of gonadal steroids on sexually dimorphic spatial ability. Psychoneuroendocrinology 16:155–176.

Witelson SF. 1991. Neural sexual mosaicism: sexual differentiation of the human-temporo-parietal region for functional asymmetry. Psychoneuroendocrinology 16:131–153.

Woolley CS, McEwen BS. 1992. Estradiol mediates fluctuation in hippocampal synapse density during the estrous cycle in the adult rat. J Neurosci 12:2549–2554.

Zhou J, Hofman MA, Gooren LJG, Swaab DR. 1995. A sex difference in the human brain and its relation to transsexuality. Nature 378:68–70.

58

Aging of the Brain and Dementia of the Alzheimer Type

A LTHOUGH THE MAXIMUM human life span has not increased in recent history, the average life expectancy has risen dramatically, especially since the turn of this century. In the United States in 1900 it was about 50 years; at present it is approximately 73 years for men and 78 for women (Figure 58-1). This increase is largely due to a reduction in infant mortality, the development of vaccines and antibiotics, better nutrition, improved public health measures, and advances in the treatment and prevention of heart disease and stroke. But the increase has revealed a new epidemic: the elderly are at significant risk for *dementia*, a syndrome characterized by impaired memory and cognitive capacities.

Lengthening the life span has little merit if the quality of life is not preserved. One of the principal goals of research on aging is not only to lengthen life but, equally importantly, to maintain and enhance its quality. In this chapter we review age-associated alterations in cognition, brain structure, and chemistry, and then discuss Alzheimer disease, the most common cause of severe memory loss and intellectual deterioration in the elderly.

Several Hypotheses Have Been Proposed for the Molecular Mechanisms of Aging

Several lines of evidence suggest that some features of senescence may result from changes in informational macromolecules (DNA, RNA, and proteins). According to one view, mutations and chromosome anomalies accumulate with age. Another hypothesis maintains that errors in the duplication of DNA increase with age because of random damage that occurs over time (wear and tear, radiation effects, etc); when a significant number of genetic errors accumulate, aberrant mRNA and proteins are formed, leading eventually to senescence. Other hypotheses suggest that there is a specific genetic program for senescence or that aging is part of a larger developmental process.

A particularly intriguing variant of these ideas, based on the work of Leonard Hayflick, is that a cell can divide only a limited number of times. Hayflick discov-

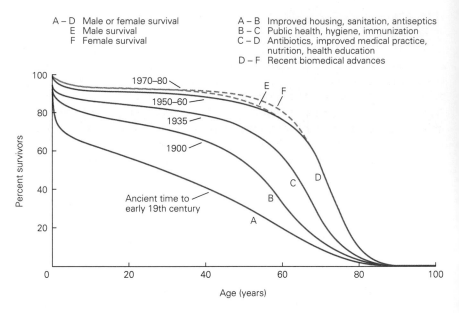

Figure 58-1 Trends in human longevity from ancient times to the present illustrate the rapid changes that have occurred during the past 150 years. The major factors responsible for these transitions are listed above the graph. In men 50 years or older the life expectancy has changed only slightly since 1950. However, female longevity has improved significantly during this period, in part because of better treatment of reproductive system malignancies. (Adapted from Strehler 1975.)

ered that normal human fibroblasts grown in culture divide regularly until they cover the entire surface of the culture flask. If the cells are subcultured into fresh medium, they divide until they again cover the surface of the flask. But the total number of divisions is limited: during a period of 7–9 months normal cultured human fibroblasts double only about 50 times. At approximately the thirty-fifth passage their ability to divide decreases; they eventually stop dividing and die. The number of cell doublings is roughly related to the age of the donor: fibroblasts from older people double significantly fewer times than those obtained from embryos.

The number of possible passages is also related to the longevity of the species from which fibroblasts are obtained. Fibroblasts from mouse embryos (whose expected life span is three years) divide about 15 times before they die; cells from Galapagos tortoises (with a life span of 175 years) divide about 90 times. Moreover, if a nucleus from a young fibroblast is interchanged with that of an old fibroblast, the newly formed hybrid cell's capacity to divide is governed by the age of the nucleus, not that of the cytoplasm. Thus, the biological clock of cells seems to be located in the nucleus.

A strong causal connection between genomic instability and aging has been established by Leonard Guarente and his colleagues in a model system in the yeast *Saccharomyces cerevisiae*. Cell division in these cells is asymmetric, yielding a small daughter cell and a large mother cell. Aging is evident in the phenotype of the mother cell prior to senescence as well as in the limited number of cell divisions. At some point in the life of the mother a circular copy of ribosomal DNA (rDNA) pops

out of the 100 to 200 tandem copies of rDNA present in chromosome XII by homologous recombination. During subsequent cell cycles this extrachromosomal rDNA replicates and segregates to the mother cell. Thus the mothers accumulate rDNA circles whereas the daughters are free of them. As the circles accumulate in the mother cell, reaching 100 in number, they shorten the life span of the cell by leading to fragmentation of the nucleolus, the site of rDNA transcription and ribosome assembly. How this fragmentation occurs is not known, but it may result from a titrating away of critical components required for transcription and DNA replication.

In Werner syndrome, a human disease characterized by premature aging, there is a loss-of-function mutation in a gene that encodes a DNA helicase. This helicase suppresses recombination of small rDNA in yeast and leads to a progressive build up of extrachromosomal small rDNA circles, thus shortening the life span of the cell.

Changes in the Function and Structure of the Brain Are Associated With Aging

Many old people remain intellectually intact, and some even make outstanding contributions late in life—Sophocles, Titian, Verdi, Eleanor Roosevelt, Picasso, Rebecca West, and Richard Strauss are well-known examples. Titian continued to paint masterpieces in his late 80s, and Sophocles is said to have written "Oedipus at Colonnus" in his 92nd year.

Nevertheless, many elderly people show a mild decline in memory and cognitive abilities, and some develop dementia. Thus, it is difficult after only one clinical examination to determine whether an individual with mild age-associated memory impairment will remain relatively stable or will progress to severe dementia. The most accurate approach to analyzing age-related abnormalities is to measure cognitive abilities and memory performance repeatedly in the same patient over a prolonged period.

In the Baltimore Longitudinal Study of Aging (National Institute on Aging) more than 2000 people have been tracked with repeated medical, neurological, and neuropsychological examinations for nearly 40 years. The results suggest that age-associated alterations in cognitive processes, such as the speed of learning and problem solving, are often mild and occur relatively late in life. In some people the ability to retain large amounts of new information declines. Visuo-spatial ability, such as arranging blocks into a design or drawing a three-dimensional figure, may also be impaired in older people. Verbal fluency (as measured by rapid naming of objects or naming as many words as possible that start with a specific letter of the alphabet) decreases with age. General intelligence scores may decline somewhat in the mid 60s and continue to fall with old age, but achievement on subtests of the verbal section of the Wechsler Adult Intelligence Scale (for example vocabulary, information, and comprehension) is often maintained well into the 80s.

Long-term studies such as the Baltimore study demonstrate wide variability between individuals in the rate and severity of cognitive decline with age. Moreover, mild changes in cognition and memory do not significantly impair the quality of life for many people.

Because longitudinal information is not available for most of the elderly, and because achievement on tests for cognitive ability and memory is not sufficiently sensitive or specific to diagnose the initial stages of dementia, the early diagnosis of a dementing illness often depends on interviews of family members who are familiar with the patient's day-to-day activities and can report even a subtle decline in the patient's abilities. Confirmation of an evolving dementia is best diagnosed by several examinations over time complemented by selected laboratory studies.

A variety of behavioral changes occur with age, but in general such changes do not seriously compromise the quality of life. For example, motor skills and sleep patterns change in the elderly. The posture of an old person is less erect than that of a young adult—gait is slower and stride length is shorter. Postural reflexes are often sluggish, making the individual more susceptible to loss of balance. These motor abnormalities may result from subtle processes that involve the peripheral or central nervous systems. As described in Chapter 47, sleep patterns change with age: older people sleep less and wake more frequently after falling asleep. Specifically, the amounts of time spent in stages 3 and 4 and in rapid eye movement sleep are reduced, while stage 1 of slow-wave sleep increases. These changes are troublesome and can produce chronic sleep deprivation.

Many age-related alterations of the brain occur in old age. Brain weight may decrease, and some populations of neurons may be reduced in number through cell death. In addition, several enzymes that synthesize various transmitters—dopamine, norepinephrine, and, to a lesser extent, acetylcholine—decrease with age, indicating abnormalities in the neurons that synthesize these transmitters. Microscopic examinations of the brains of elderly individuals reveal senile plaques and neurofibrillary tangles, two lesions that are abundant in Alzheimer disease (see below). Age-related abnormalities in specific neuronal circuits are believed to result in some of the clinical signs associated with aging—alterations in memory, motor activity, mood, sleep patterns, appetite, and neuroendocrine functions.

A Variety of Senile Dementias Afflict the Elderly

The term *senile dementia* refers to a clinical syndrome in elderly people that involves loss of memory and cognitive impairments of sufficient severity to interfere with social or occupational functioning. As described in the *Diagnostic and Statistical Manual* of the American Psychiatric Association *(DSM-IV)*, senile dementia must show at least two abnormalities: memory loss in an otherwise alert patient and impairments in at least one other area of cognition—language, problem solving, judgment, calculation, attention, perception, praxis, and so on.

In 1907 Alois Alzheimer described the first case of dementia that now bears his name. A middle-aged woman had developed memory deficits and progressive loss of cognitive abilities. One of the first noticeable symptoms of this woman's illness was unprovoked suspicion of her husband's behavior. Her memory became increasingly impaired. She could no longer orient herself, even in her own home, and she hid objects in her apartment. At times she believed that people intended to murder her. She was institutionalized in a psychiatric hospital and died less than five years after the onset of illness. An autopsy disclosed the now-recognized classical pathology of Alzheimer disease—neurofibrillary

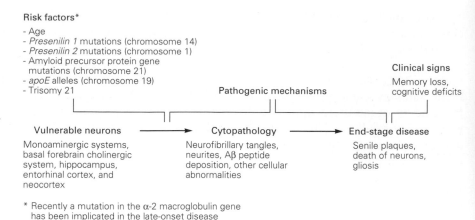

Figure 58-2 The relationships of risk factors, pathogenic processes, and clinical signs to cellular abnormalities in the brain during Alzheimer disease. The same brain abnormalities that occur in Alzheimer disease are also seen in Down syndrome.

tangles and senile plaques in the neocortex and hippocampus. After this case was reported, the term *Alzheimer disease* was given to this type of presenile dementia.

Alzheimer disease is the most common cause of dementia in the elderly. It affects approximately 7% of people older than 65 and perhaps 40% of people over the age of 80. Five million people in the United States now suffer from dementia. Because of increased life expectancy and the post-World War II baby boom, the elderly—the population at risk for Alzheimer disease—is the fastest growing segment of our society. During the next 25 years the number of people with Alzheimer disease in the United States will triple, as will the cost. Thus, Alzheimer disease is one of society's major public health problems.

The second most common cause of dementia in the elderly is cerebrovascular disease, alone or in combination with Alzheimer disease. Other causes of dementia include Lewy body dementia, Parkinson disease, frontotemporal dementia with parkinsonism, alcoholism, drug intoxications, infections such as AIDS and syphilis, brain tumor, vitamin deficiencies (eg, B_{12}), thyroid disease, and a variety of other metabolic disorders. Some of these problems are readily detected by laboratory studies; others must be diagnosed from the clinical examination.

It is extremely important for the physician to exclude other causes of dementia from Alzheimer disease in a given case because certain dementias respond to specific treatments, whereas at present, only the symptoms of Alzheimer disease are treatable. The accuracy of clinical diagnoses of specific causes of dementia, particularly Alzheimer disease, has greatly improved during the past two decades. In the 1970s diagnostic error rates were more than 30%. Experienced clinical centers now report autopsy confirmation of the clinical diagnosis of Alzheimer disease in more than 90% of cases.

Most patients with Alzheimer disease exhibit the first clinical signs during their seventh decade, but, as with the case described by Alzheimer, sometimes the condition develops in mid life. In these cases there may be a family history of the disease. In both the sporadic and familial forms of Alzheimer disease, patients show abnormalities of memory, problem solving, language, calculation, visuospatial perception, judgment, and behavior. Some patients develop psychotic symptoms, such as hallucinations and delusions. In all these patients mental functions and activities of daily living progressively become impaired; in the late stages these individuals are mute, incontinent, and bedridden and usually die of other medical illnesses.

Except for brain biopsy, there are no tests that definitively establish the diagnosis of Alzheimer disease in living subjects. To make the diagnosis of Alzheimer disease and to exclude other causes of dementia, clinicians rely on histories from patients and informants; physical, neurological, and psychiatric examinations; neuropsychological testing; laboratory assessments; and a variety of other diagnostic tests including neuroimaging. Alterations of levels of specific proteins in the serum or cerebrospinal fluid, such as the amyloid peptides and Tau, may prove useful in diagnosis. The inheritance of the *apoE4* allele is a risk factor in late-onset disease (see below) and is a useful research tool, but at present is not of great value for diagnostic purposes in the elderly.

Computerized tomography (CT) or magnetic resonance imaging (MRI) are performed on most patients with Alzheimer disease, so that other potentially treatable diseases and patterns consistent with Alzheimer disease can be identified. In these patients imaging may show abnormalities, particularly in the medial temporal lobe, that may have predictive value for establishing a diagnosis. Positron emission tomography (PET) and single photon emission computerized tomography usu-

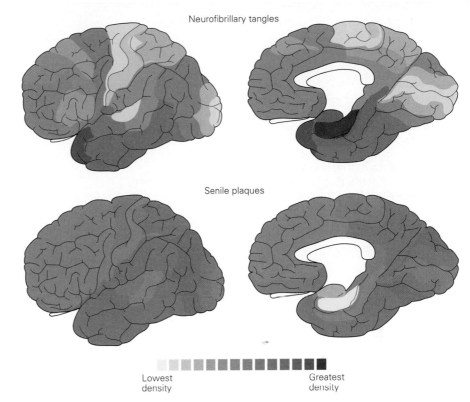

Neurofibrillary tangles

Senile plaques

Figure 58-3 The topography of neurofibrillary tangles and senile plaques (mean values). Lateral and medial views of the cerebral hemisphere show 37 of the 39 Brodmann areas examined. The amygdala and the nucleus basalis of Meynert are not shown. (Adapted from Arnold et al. 1991.)

Lowest density

Greatest density

ally show decreased regional blood flow in the parietal and temporal lobes and also in other cortical areas at later stages.

Alzheimer Disease Is Characterized by Several Structural Abnormalities in the Brain

Alzheimer disease is a prototypical neurodegenerative disease. It is characterized by a series of abnormalities in the brain that selectively affect neurons in specific regions, particularly in the neocortex, the entorhinal area, hippocampus, amygdala, nucleus basalis, anterior thalamus, and several brain stem monoaminergic nuclei (ie, the locus ceruleus and raphe complex) (Figures 58-2, 58-3, and 58-4).

In damaged regions of the brain, the dysfunction and death of neurons is associated with cytoskeletal abnormalities and results in a reduction in the level of synaptic proteins in the regions of the brain within which these neurons terminate. The distribution and the spread of these abnormalities follow characteristic patterns that are area-specific and even cell-specific. In the neocortex and entorhinal area the cells most severely affected are the large glutaminergic pyramidal neurons; in the neocortex interneurons also degenerate. Similarly, in the hippocampus, particularly in the CA1 and CA2 regions, pyramidal cells are selectively damaged. The

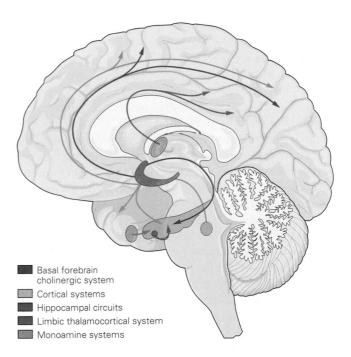

■ Basal forebrain cholinergic system
□ Cortical systems
■ Hippocampal circuits
■ Limbic thalamocortical system
■ Monoamine systems

Figure 58-4 Specific neuronal systems have been identified in morphological and neurochemical analyses as vulnerable in Alzheimer disease. Note that only one cortical system (i.e. entorhinal neurons) is shown; in fact many neocortical neurons, particularly those in association cortices, are affected by disease. The involvement of these brain regions and neural systems in Alzheimer disease is reflected in the clinical signs of the disease.

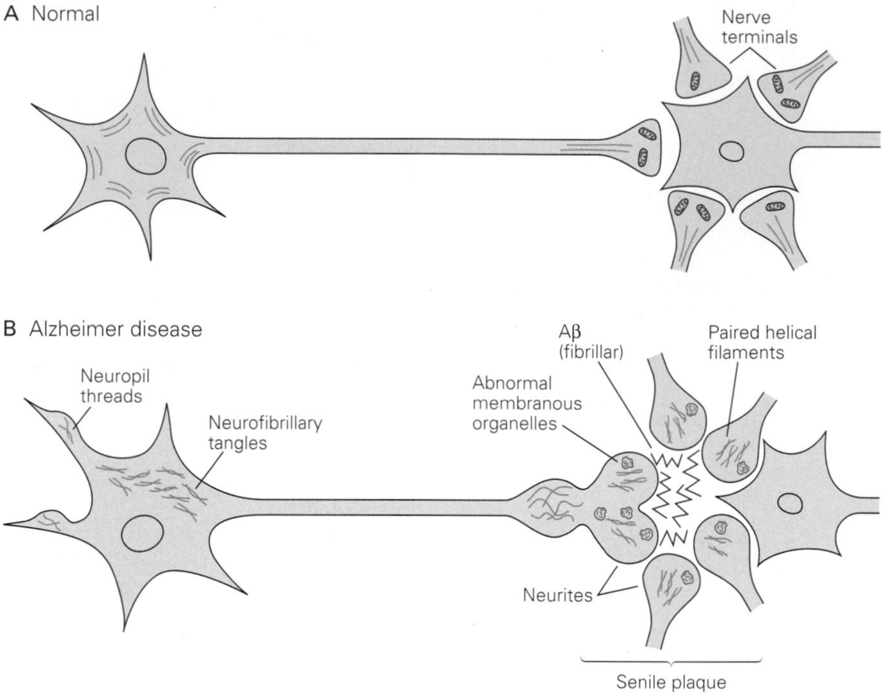

A Normal

Figure 58-5 Comparison of a normal nerve cell and a neuron exhibiting abnormalities that occur in Alzheimer disease. The principal components of senile plaques are neurofibrillary tangles in the cell bodies, neuropil threads, and neurites as well as extracellular Aβ amyloid. These lesions are surrounded by microglial cells and astrocytes.

cholinergic neurons in the nucleus basalis, medial septal nucleus, and diagonal band of Broca that provide the principal cholinergic pathways to the neocortex and hippocampus are destroyed, resulting in a reduction in the levels of acetylcholine and cholinergic markers (ie, activity of choline acetyltransferase) in the target areas of these cells. Other affected nerve cells include specific nuclei within the amygdala, the anterior nucleus of the thalamus, locus ceruleus, and raphe nuclei.

These lesions have profound clinical consequences. Abnormalities of the entorhinal cortex, hippocampus, and other circuits in the medial temporal cortex are presumed to be critical factors in memory impairment in Alzheimer disease. Abnormalities in the association areas of the neocortex (Chapter 20), believed to be related to alterations in the basal forebrain cholinergic systems, may also contribute to the memory difficulties and attention deficits of this disease. The behavioral and emotional disturbances that occur in some patients may reflect involvement of the limbic cortex, amygdala, thalamus, and several brain stem monoaminergic systems that project to the hippocampal cortex.

Alzheimer Disease Is Associated With Cytoskeletal Abnormalities in Neurons

In affected nerve cells the cytoskeleton is often altered. The most common cytoskeletal alteration is *neurofibril-*

lary tangles, filamentous inclusions in the cell bodies and proximal dendrites that contain paired helical filaments and 15 nm straight filaments. These abnormal inclusions are made up of poorly soluble hyperphosphorylated isoforms of tau, a microtubule-binding protein that normally is soluble (Figure 58-5). Neurofibrillary tangles often first become evident in neurons of the entorhinal cortex, which receives inputs from isocortex and projects to the hippocampus. Later the neurofibrillary pathology extends to the neocortex. Other fibrillar cytoskeletal abnormalities involve axons and terminals (dystrophic neurites) and dendrites (neuropil threads); both of these types of lesions include intracellular, paired helical filaments. It is likely that all of these fibrillar inclusions result from common mechanisms.

As described in Chapter 4, the cytoskeleton is essential for maintaining cell structure and intracellular trafficking of proteins and organelles, including transport along axons. Thus, disturbances of the cytoskeleton are likely to impair axonal transport and thereby compromise the functions of synaptic inputs and, eventually, the viability of neurons. The affected nerve cells eventually die and the extracellular neurofibrillary tangles are left behind as tombstones of the cells destroyed by disease. As these neurons die, the synaptic inputs in regions of the brain critical for normal cognitive and memory function are lost.

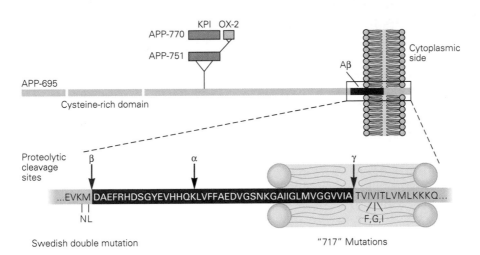

Figure 58-6 Synthesis and processing of the precursors of the Aβ amyloid peptide. The amyloid precursor proteins APP-751 and APP-770 contain a domain that is homologous with the Kunitz class of serine protease inhibitors (KPI). APP-695 lacks this domain. **Top:** The extracellular, transmembrane, and cytoplasmic domains of Aβ amyloid. **Bottom:** The detail of the peptide shows the sites of α-, β-, and γ-secretase cleavages and the nature and position of several APP mutations linked to familial Alzheimer disease. The endopeptidase α-secretase cleaves within the Aβ region, resulting in the secretion of the extracellular domain of APP; hence, the cleavage does not produce the Aβ peptide. In contrast, the β-secretase and γ-secretase cleavages do result in production of the peptide. (Courtesy of G. Thinakaran.)

Amyloid Deposits Are One of the Hallmarks of Alzheimer Disease

The brain regions affected by Alzheimer disease also contain neuritic or *senile plaques* in which extracellular deposits of amyloid are surrounded by dystrophic axons as well as the processes of astrocytes and microglia (inflammatory cells). Senile plaques occur throughout the neuropil as well as in the walls of cerebral blood vessels (Figure 58-5). *Amyloid* is the histological name for fibrillar peptides arranged as β-pleated sheets in aggregates that are doubly refractive when stained with Congo red (or thioflavin) and viewed in polarized light (or fluorescence). The principal constituent of amyloid is a 4 kDa peptide called Aβ amyloid. Aβ amyloid is cleaved from a larger precursor protein, *amyloid precursor protein* (Figure 58-6).

Amyloid precursor protein (APP) is a member of a family that includes the amyloid precursor-like proteins APLP1 and APLP2. It is encoded by a gene in the mid portion of the long arm of human chromosome 21. APP exists in three principal isoforms of 695, 751, and 770 amino acids, each of which contains Aβ amyloid. APP is present in the dendrites, cell bodies, and axons of neurons, and neuronal APP is likely the source of most of the Aβ amyloid deposited in the central nervous system in patients with Alzheimer disease. The functions of neuronal APP are not yet known.

APP is synthesized in the rough endoplasmic reticulum, glycosylated in the Golgi apparatus, and delivered to the cell surface as an integral membrane protein. Some of these molecules are cleaved within the Aβ sequence, thus preventing the formation of the Aβ peptide (Figure 58-6).

A fraction of the APP within the plasmalemma is internalized in the cell to generate various forms of amyloid Aβ (Aβ1–40, Aβ1–42, and Aβ1–43) as well as truncated forms of the Aβ peptide (β17–40), all of which are normally present in cerebrospinal fluid. According to one model, a β-secretase cleaves APP at the N terminus of the Aβ peptide sequence in endosomal compartments and a γ-secretase enzyme cleaves at the C terminus of the Aβ peptide at or near the cell surface (Figure 58-6).

The Aβ peptide is predominantly 40 amino acids in length, that is, Aβ1–40. However, Aβ1–42 and Aβ1–43 nucleate more rapidly into amyloid fibrils than Aβ1–40 does. In the cerebral cortices of individuals with Alzheimer disease or Down syndrome, Aβ amyloid deposition begins with Aβ1–42 and Aβ1–43, not Aβ1–40. The Aβ1–42 fragment of the Aβ peptide appears to be neurotoxic by mechanisms not yet fully understood.

Several Genetic Risk Factors for Alzheimer Disease Have Been Identified

Five principal genetic risk factors for Alzheimer disease are known: (1) mutations in the APP gene on chromosome 21; (2) mutations in the *presenilin 1* gene on chromosome 14; (3) mutations in the *presenilin 2* gene on chromosome 1; (4) alleles for the *ApoE* positioned on the proximal long arm of chromosome 19; and (5) possibly, a mutation or polymorphism in a gene on chromosome 12 that encodes alpha-2 macroglobulin. Any of the first three mutations is associated with early onset of the disorder in the third through sixth decades. In contrast, specific *apoE* alleles or alterations in alpha-2 macroglobulin predispose individuals to the early-onset sporadic Alzheimer disease and even more to the late-onset familial disease.

Certain Mutations Increase the Risk of Early-Onset Alzheimer Disease

Missense mutations have been identified in the APP gene on chromosome 21 (Figure 58-6) in a small fraction of the families in which Alzheimer disease has an early onset. These mutations encode amino acid substitutions flanking or within the Aβ region. In several families the normal valine residue at position 717 is replaced with either isoleucine, glycine, or phenylalanine (Figure 58-6). Cells that express an APP mutated at position 717 secrete increased levels of Aβ1–42 and Aβ1–43, which have a propensity to nucleate rapidly into amyloid fibrils and appear to be particularly toxic.

In two large, related Swedish families with early-onset Alzheimer disease a double mutation at residues 670 and 671 results in the substitution of Asn-Leu for the normal Lys-Met (Figure 58-6). Cells that express this mutant sequence secrete approximately six to eight times more Aβ peptide. Interestingly, in one patient with cerebral hemorrhage that resulted from amyloid deposition in blood vessels, a mutation leading to a Glu-to-Gln substitution at residue 693 (corresponding to amino acid 22 of Aβ peptide) is associated with deposition around blood vessels. In vitro studies of the effects of this mutation demonstrate that these Aβ peptides are prone to aggregate into fibrils.

Approximately 10% of patients with Alzheimer disease exhibit clinical syndromes before the age of 50, and these illnesses are inherited in an autosomal dominant manner. Nearly 30% of these cases are linked to the *presenilin 1* gene (on chromosome 14q). This gene encodes a 467-amino acid polypeptide of unknown function that contains eight transmembrane domains. In cultured cells and brains from humans, monkeys, and mice, frag-

ments of *presenilin 1* accumulate as an N-terminal (~28 kDa fragment) and a C-terminal (~18 kDa fragment), indicating that *presenilin 1* is subject to endoproteolytic processing in vivo.

In early-onset familial Alzheimer disease approximately 40 missense mutations and one exon deletion of *presenilin 1* cosegregate, and the majority of these mutations occur within or immediately adjacent to predicted transmembrane domains. Two mutations in the *presenilin 2* gene on chromosome 1 have been reported to cause autosomal dominant Alzheimer disease in two pedigrees. *Presenilin 2* has substantial homology to *presenilin 1*, and mutations in *presenilin 2* also reside within predicted transmembrane helices. The mechanisms by which the expression of mutant presenilin leads to Alzheimer disease are not fully understood. However, examination of serum from patients with *presenilin 1* and *presenilin 2* mutations shows that the levels of Aβ1–42 and Aβ1–43 are higher than in unaffected controls.

Although the biological functions of the presenilin genes are not well understood, there is a significant homology between presenilin and sel-12, a protein that plays a role in the determination of cell fates during development of the nematode *Caenorhabditis elegans*. Gene targeting studies have shown that *presenilin 1* is important in cell fate decisions in mammalian development, and that an absence of PS1 reduces levels of Aβ dramatically.

Missense mutations in either *APP* or presenilin genes promote the formation of more toxic forms of Aβ peptide. It is likely that these forms of Aβ peptide are central to the pathogenesis of Alzheimer disease. These mutations link Alzheimer disease to changes in the processing of APP, including increasing the formation of Aβ peptides, increasing the amounts of the longer Aβ forms, and promoting fibril formation. Additional evidence that some of these mutations are associated with amyloidogenesis comes from studies on transgenic mice (discussed below).

Alleles of Genes Increase the Risk of Late-Onset Alzheimer Disease

ApoE, a 34,000 molecular weight glycoprotein that carries cholesterol and other lipids in the blood, has been implicated as a risk factor for late-onset Alzheimer disease. At the single *apoE* locus three alleles are expressed: *apoE2, apoE3,* and *apoE4*. The allele *apoE3* has a cysteine at position 112 and an arginine at position 158; *apoE4* has arginine at both positions; and *apoE2* has cysteine at both positions. The *E3* allele is most common in the general population (frequency of 0.78), whereas the allelic frequency of *E4* is 0.14. The frequency of the *E4* allele is

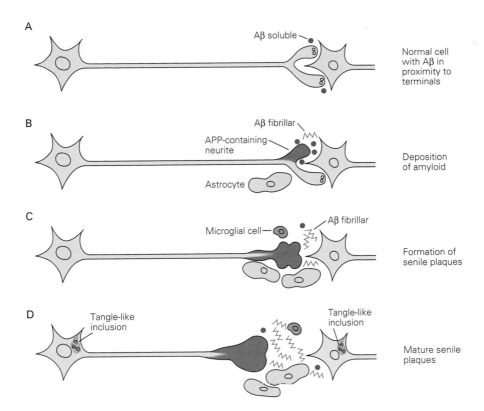

Figure 58-7 The evolution of cellular abnormalities in the brains of aged nonhuman primates. Similar abnormalities occur in transgenic mice with mutant *APP* and in individuals with Alzheimer disease (Figure 58-5).

A. A normal neuron and its target cell.

B. The enlarged axon terminal retracts from its target, and soluble Aβ1–40 and fibrillar Aβ1–42 and Aβ1–43 are present. Note the astrocyte. Other proteins in this lesion include α-antichymotrypsin and components of the complement cascade.

C. Mature senile plaques are formed when the fibrillar amyloid appears. Swollen axon terminals accumulate altered organelles, and astrocytes and microglia are activated.

D. In mature senile plaques, fibrillar Aβ amyloid deposits are surrounded by axon terminals, astrocytes, and microglia. Finally, filamentous inclusions, resembling neurofibrillary tangles, are present in the cell bodies of some neurons. Similar lesions occur in transgenic mice with *APP* mutations.

0.50 in patients with late-onset disease. Thus, the risk for late-onset Alzheimer disease is increased by the presence of *apoE4*.

The mechanism by which the *apoE* allele elevates the risk for late-onset disease is not known, but it has been hypothesized that specific *apoE* isoforms influence the biology of Aβ peptides. The *apoE4* allele appears to accelerate the disease in some families with mutations in the APP gene but not in families with mutations in the presenilin gene.

Another, less well studied risk factor for late-onset disease is the gene for alpha-2 macroglobulin, studied by Rudy Tanzi and his colleagues. Some patients with late-onset Alzheimer disease have a mutation (or polymorphism) in this gene which is thought to predispose the patient to the dementia by interfering with the normal scavenger functions that remove Aβ deposits from these synaptic regions.

Animal Models Provide Insight Into the Molecular Mechanisms of the Disease

Both spontaneously occurring and experimentally produced diseases in animals are used to model Alzheimer disease. Although several rodent species develop age-associated behavioral deficits, they do not exhibit the structural or biochemical lesions of Alzheimer disease. At present the rhesus monkey, *Macaca mulatta*, which has an estimated life span of more than 35 years, is the best available model of spontaneously occurring age-related behavioral and brain abnormalities.

In monkeys cognitive and memory deficits appear at the end of the second and the beginning of the third decade of life. Older monkeys of the same age may show significant variations in performance on behavioral tasks. Visuospatial performance declines in some animals that are 16–19 years of age, but performance on a visual recognition memory task is altered only in monkeys older than 25 years of age. In contrast, some tasks—the learning of object discriminations and simple motor skills—are performed satisfactorily at all ages. The variations in performance between tasks and between individuals are similar to variations in the abilities of a cohort of aged humans performing similar tasks.

Aged nonhuman primates develop many of the brain abnormalities observed in older humans. The cortex of rhesus monkeys older than 20 years often shows enlarged distal axons or nerve terminals as well as deposits of Aβ amyloid. Older monkeys show mature senile plaques with neurites in regions where amyloid is aggregated (Figure 58-7). As in aged humans, reactive astrocytes and microglia are associated with plaques. Moreover, as in humans, there are modest age-related alterations in cholinergic, peptidergic, and monoaminergic systems. The distribution and severities of various lesions differ among animals of the same age. The performance of specific behavioral tasks is postulated to be related to different patterns of these lesions in different animals.

The ability to introduce wild-type or mutant transgenes into mice provides an opportunity to determine whether overexpression of wild-type or mutant APP or presenilin genes causes any of the abnormalities associated with Alzheimer disease: behavioral abnormalities, Aβ amyloid deposits, the neurofibrillary abnormalities, cell death, and reductions in synaptic or transmitter markers.

During the past few years many models of Alzheimer disease in mice have been attempted by introducing a variety of transgenes into different strains. Lines of mice expressing a human APP gene harboring the familial Alzheimer disease-linked valine-to-phenylalanine mutation at residue 717 or the Swedish double mutation (Figure 58-6) have shown brain abnormalities, particularly amyloid deposits that share features with Alzheimer disease. In these mice the levels of the human APP proteins are significantly increased as are the levels of Aβ amyloid. Amyloid deposits ranging from diffuse irregular types to compacted plaques with cores are seen in the hippocampus and cerebral cortex, and these deposits increase in number over time and are associated with distorted neurites, astrocytes, and microglial cells. Some of the transgenic mice also develop behavioral abnormalities. Transgenic mice coexpressing *presenilin 1* mutations and mutant APP transgenes show elevated ratios of Aβ42:Aβ40 as compared with mice coexpressing wild-type *presenilin 1* and APP transgenes. Moreover, these double transgenic mice show accelerated Aβ deposition in the brain. The mouse models show that memory impairment may antedate overt Aβ amyloid deposition but not increases in levels of Aβ. Tau pathology is not a conspicuous part of the cellular pathology in these several lines of mice.

Such animal models are crucial for understanding the molecular mechanisms of the disease and for testing novel therapies.

Treatment of Alzheimer Disease

At present there is no cure for Alzheimer disease. Present-day therapies focus on treating associated symptoms, such as depression, agitation, sleep disorders, hallucinations, and delusions. One of the principal targets is the basal forebrain cholinergic system, a region of the brain that is severely damaged in Alzheimer disease. Several strategies have been developed to influence this cholinergic system. Unfortunately, the addition of precursors (choline, lecithin, etc) and muscarinic agonist have not proven effective. Similarly, the acetylcholinesterase inhibitor Tacrine (1,2,3,4-tetrahydro-9-acridinamine monohydrochloride monohydrate) has, at best, a very modest effect on cognitive functions and activities of daily living. Many research groups are working on strategies to prevent or ameliorate Aβ deposition and/or to influence the roles of inflamatory/immune mediated processes in the disease.

An Overall View

Alzheimer disease is one of the most complex and perplexing diseases encountered in clinical medicine and is the most common cause of morbidity and mortality in the elderly. In recent years, however, major advances in understanding this disease have been made. New approaches and instruments have improved diagnostic accuracy. In addition, there have been significant advances in understanding the pathophysiology of Alzheimer disease.

Mutations in several genes (*APP, presenilin 1, presenilin 2*) have been identified as central to the pathogenesis of some cases of familial Alzheimer disease, and an allele type of another gene (*apoE4*) can influence the onset of late-onset sporadic and familial disease. Significant progress has been made in understanding the biology of genes/proteins involved in the pathogenesis of amyloid deposits and cytoskeletal abnormalities in neurons.

Why particular regions of the brain and specific populations of neurons are selectively vulnerable in the disease remains unclear. Moreover, the pathways that lead to cell death need to be resolved. However, animal models, particularly those created by transgenic strategies, hold promise for investigations of the mechanisms of this disease.

In this chapter, we have focused primarily on Alzheimer disease, the most common cause of dementia in the elderly, but there are a number of other diseases that are manifest by dementia in mid and late life. The most interesting of these disorders are the *prion diseases*. This group of neurodegenerative diseases was first identified when Kuru, an illness occurring among the Fore tribe in New Guinea, was found to be transmissible by injection of brain tissue from affected humans into nonhuman primates. The prion disorders include three human diseases: Creutzfeldt-Jacob disease, Gerstmann-Sträussler-Scheinker syndrome, and fatal familial insomnia in humans. In addition, there is a prion disease in sheep called *scrapie* and a prion disease in cows called *bovine songiform*. All of these illnesses can take one of the three forms—sporadic, familial, or transmissible—and all involve modification of a protein discovered by Stanley Prunsiner called prion (for proteinaceous infectious organisms). The prion protein (PrP) is found in two isoforms: a normal cellular isoform (Prp^c) and an infectious (scrapie) isoform PrP^{sc}. The infectious form is found in human prion disease and differs from the normal cellular protein only in its physical conformation. The cellular prion has a high content of α-helix and essentially no β-sheet, whereas the infectious prion has a high content of β-sheet and a low content of α-helix. The conversion from α-helices into β-sheets underlies the capability of the protein to both replicate and produce infection.

These diseases are not only infectious, but can also be inherited. The heritable forms are associated with specific mutations in the gene that encodes the cellular prion protein (PrP^{sc}). Indeed, mice expressing the prion gene with specific point mutations characteristic of the syndrome develop a degenerative neurologic disease analogous to the human diseases. Both disorders involve a similar pathogenic mechanism. An abnormal version of the cellular prion protein carries information encouraging the PrP^c to adopt a PrP^{sc} conformation.

Thus, prion proteins represent a novel pathogenetic mechanism. Moreover, studies of these diseases clearly show that degenerative diseases of the human brain can be transmitted. In fact, recent evidence suggests that new variants in Creutzfeldt-Jacob disease in the United Kingdom are linked to consumption of meat from cows with spongiform encephalopathy. The fact that conformational changes encode sufficient information to produce brain degeneration in humans has given new direction to research on the molecular mechanisms responsible for many fatal degenerative neurological diseases. The possibility that prions or prionlike proteins could also play a role in a variety of other diseases must now be given serious consideration.

Donald L. Price

Selected Readings

Borchelt DR, Thinakaran G, Eckman CB, Lee MK, Davenport F, Ratovitsky T, Prada C-M, Kim G, Seekins S, Yager D, Slunt HH, Wang R, Seeger M, Levey AI, Gandy SE, Copeland NG, Jenkins NA, Price DL, Younkin SG, Sisodia SS. 1996. Familial Alzheimer disease-linked presenilin 1 variants elevate AA1–42/1–40 ratio *in vitro* and *in vivo*. Neuron 17:1005–1013.

Cai X-D, Golde TE, Younkin SG. 1993. Release of excess amyloid β protein from a mutant amyloid protein precursor. Science 259:514–516.

Corder EH, Saunders AM, Strittmatter WJ, Schmechel DE, Gaskell PC, Small GW, Roses AD, Haines JL, Pericak-Vance MA. 1993. Gene dose of apolipoprotein-E type 4 allele and the risk of Alzheimer disease in late onset families. Science 261:921–923.

Doan A, Thinakaran G, Borchelt DR, Slunt HH, Ratovitsky T, Podlisny M, Selkoe DJ, Seeger M, Gandy SE, Price DL, Sisodia SS. 1996. Protein topology of presenilin 1. Neuron 17:1023–1030.

Epstein CJ, Martin GM, Schultz AL, Motulsky AR. 1986. Werner syndrome: a review of its symptomatology, natural history, pathogenic features, genetics and relationship to the natural aging process. Medicine 45:177–221.

Haass C, Schlossmacher MG, Hung AY, Vigo-Pelfrey C, Mellon A, Ostaszewski BL, Lieberburg I, Koo EH, Schenk D, Teplow DB, Selkoe DJ. 1992. Amyloid β-peptide is produced by cultured cells during normal metabolism. Nature 359:322–325.

Hsiao K, Chapman P, Nilsen S, Eckman C, Harigaya Y, Younkin S, Yang F, Cole G. 1996. Correlative memory deficits. Aβ elevation and amyloid plaques in transgenic mice. Science 274:99–102.

Iwatsubo T, Odaka A, Suzuki N, Mizusawa H, Nukina N, Ihara Y. 1994. Visualization of Aβ42(43)-positive and Aβ40-positive senile plaques with end-specific Aβ-monoclonal antibodies: evidence that an initially deposited amyloid basic species is Aβ1–42(43). Neuron 13:45–53.

Johnson FB, Sinclair DA, Guarente L. 1999. The molecular biology of aging. Cell 96:291–302.

Kang J, Lemaire H-G, Unterbeck A, Salbaum JM, Masters CL, Grzeschik K-H, Multhaup G, Beyreuther K, Miller-Hill B. 1987. The precursor of Alzheimer disease amyloid

A4 protein resembles a cell-surface receptor. Nature 325:733–736.

Price DL, Sisodia SS. 1994. Cellular and molecular biology of Alzheimer disease and animal models. Annu Rev Med 45:435–446.

Price DL, Sisodia SS, Borchelt DR. 1998. Alzheimer's disease—when and why? Nature Genetics 19:314–316.

Rapp PR, Amaral DG. 1992. Individual differences in the cognitive and neurobiological consequences of normal aging. Trends Neurosci 15:340–345.

Rogaev EI, Sherrington R, Rogaeva EA, Levesque G, Ikeda M, Liang Y, Chi H, Lin C, Holman K, Tsuda T, Mar L, Sorbi S, Nacmias B, Piacentini S, Amaducci L, Chumakov I, Cohen D, Lannfelt L, Fraser PE, Rommens JM, St. George-Hyslop PH. 1995. Familial Alzheimer disease in kindreds with missense mutations in a gene on chromosome 1 related to the Alzheimer disease type 3 gene. Nature 376:775–778.

Selkoe DJ. 1996. Amyloid β-protein and the genetics of Alzheimer disease. J Biol Chem 271:18295–18298.

Sisodia SS, Koo EH, Beyreuther K, Unterbeck A, Price DL. 1990. Evidence that β-amyloid protein in Alzheimer disease is not derived by normal processing. Science 248:492–495.

Thinakaran G, Borchelt DR, Lee MK, Slunt HH, Spitzer L, Kim G, Ratovitsky T, Davenport F, Nordstedt C, Seeger M, Hardy J, Levey AI, Gandy SE, Jenkins N, Copeland N, Price DL, Sisodia SS. 1996. Endoproteolysis of presenilin 1 and accumulation of processed derivatives *in vivo*. Neuron 17:181–180.

Yankner BA. 1996. Mechanisms of neuronal degeneration in Alzheimer disease. Neuron 16:921–932.

References

American Psychiatric Association. 1987. *Diagnostic and Statistical Manual of Mental Disorders,* 3rd rev. ed. Washington, DC: American Psychiatric Association.

Arnold SE, Hyman BT, Flory J, Damasio AR, Van Hoesen GW. 1991. The topographical and neuroanatomical distribution of neurofibrillary tangles and neuritic plaques in the cerebral cortex of patients with Alzheimer disease. Cereb Cortex 1:103–116.

Bachevalier J, Landis LS, Walker LC, Brickson M, Mishkin M, Price DL, Cork LC. 1991. Aged monkeys exhibit behavioral deficits indicative of widespread cerebral dysfunction. Neurobiol Aging 12:99–111.

Borchelt DR, Ratovitski T, Van Lare J, Lee MK, Gonzales VB, Jenkins NA, Copeland NG, Price DL, Sisodia SS. 1997. Accelerated amyloid deposition in the brains of transgenic mice co-expressing mutant presenilin 1 and amyloid precursor proteins. Neuron 19:939–945.

Braak H, Braak E. 1994. Pathology of Alzheimer disease. In: DB Calne (ed). *Neurodegenerative Diseases,* pp. 585–613. Philadelphia: Saunders.

Davis KL, Thal LJ, Gamzu ER, Davis CS, Woolson RF, Gracon SI, Drachman DA, Schneider LS, Whitehouse PJ, Hoover TM, Morris JC, Kawas CH, Knopman DS, Earl NL, Kumar V, Doody RS, Tacrine Collaborative Study Group. 1992. A double-blind, placebo-controlled multicenter study of tacrine for Alzheimer disease. N Engl J Med 327:1253–1259.

Evans DA, Funkenstein HH, Albert MS, Scherr PA, Cook NR, Chown MJ, Hebert LE, Hennekens CH, Taylor JO. 1989. Prevalence of Alzheimer disease in a community population of older persons. Higher than previously reported. JAMA 262:2551–2556.

Farlow M, Gracon SI, Hershey LA, Lewis KW, Sadowsky CH, Dolan-Ureno J. 1992. A controlled trial of tacrine in Alzheimer disease. JAMA 268:2523–2529.

Glenner GG, Wong CW. 1984. Alzheimer disease: initial report of the purification and characterization of a novel cerebrovascular amyloid protein. Biochem Biophys Res Commun 120:885–890.

Games D, Adams D, Alessandrini R, Barbour R, Berthelette P, Blackwell C, Carr T, Clemens J, Donaldson T, Gillespie F, Guido T, Hagopian S, Johnson-Wood K, Khan K, Lee M, Leibowitz P, Lieberburg I, Little S, Masliah E, Mc-Conlogue L, Montoya-Zavala M, Mucke L, Paganini L, Penniman E, Power M, Schenk D, Seubert P, Snyder B, Soriano F, Tan H, Vitale J, Wadsworth S, Wolozin B, Zhao J. 1995. Alzheimer-type neuropathology in transgenic mice overexpressing V717F β-amyloid precursor protein. Nature 373:523–527.

Goate A, Chartier-Harlin M-C, Mullan M, Brown J, Crawford F, Fidani L, Giuffra L, Haynes A, Irving N, James L, Mant R, Newton P, Rooke K, Roques P, Talbot C, Pericak-Vance M, Roses A, Williamson R, Rossor M, Owen M, Hardy J. 1991. Segregation of a missense mutation in the amyloid precursor protein gene with familial Alzheimer disease. Nature 349:704–706.

Iwatsubo T, Mann DMA, Odaka A, Suzuki N, Ihara Y. 1995. Amyloid β protein (Aβ) deposition: Aβ42(43) precedes Aβ40 in Down syndrome. Ann Neurol 37:294–299.

Kitt CA, Price DL, Struble RG, Cork LC, Wainer BH, Becher MW, Mobley WC. 1984. Evidence for cholinergic neurites in senile plaques. Science 226:1443–1445.

Koo EH, Sisodia SS, Archer DR, Martin LJ, Weidemann A, Beyreuther K, Fischer P, Masters CL, Price DL. 1990. Precursor of amyloid protein in Alzheimer disease undergoes fast anterograde axonal transport. Proc Natl Acad Sci U S A 87:1561–1565.

Levy-Lahad E, Wasco W, Poorkaj P, Romano DM, Oshima J, Pettingell WH, Yu C-E, Jondro PD, Schmidt SD, Wang K, Crowley AC, Fu Y-H, Guenette SY, Galas D, Nemens E, Wijsman EM, Bird TD, Schellenberg GD, Tanzi RE. 1995. Candidate gene for the chromosome 1 familial Alzheimer disease locus. Science 269:973–977.

Levy-Lahad E, Wijsman EM, Nemens E, Anderson L, Goddard KAB, Weber JL, Bird TD, Schellenberg GD. 1995. A familial Alzheimer disease locus on chromosome 1. Science 269:970–973.

Lezak MD. 1995. *Neuropsychological Assessment,* 3rd ed. NY: Oxford Univ. Press.

Martin LJ, Sisodia SS, Koom EH, Cork LC, Dellovade TL, Weidemann A, Beyreuther K, Masters C, Price DL. 1991.

Amyloid precursor protein in aged nonhuman primates. Proc Natl Acad Sci U S A 88:1461–1465.

McKhann G, Drachman D, Folstein M, Katzman R, Price D, Stadlan EM. 1984. Clinical diagnosis of Alzheimer disease: report of the NINCDS-ADRDA Work Group under the auspices of the Department of Health and Human Services Task Force on Alzheimer Disease. Neurology 34:939–944.

Morris JC, McKeel DW Jr, Storandt M, Rubin EH, Price JL, Grant EA, Ball MJ, Berg L. 1991. Very mild Alzheimer disease: informant-based clinical, psychometric, and pathologic distinction from normal aging. Neurology 41:469–478.

Mullan M, Crawford F, Axelman K, Houlden H, Lillius L, Winblad B, Lannfelt L. 1992. A pathogenic mutation for probable Alzheimer disease in the APP gene at the N-terminus of β-amyloid. Nat Genet 1:345–347.

Price DL, Davis PB, Morris JC, White DL. 1991. The distribution of tangles, plaques and related immunohistochemical markers in healthy aging and Alzheimer disease. Neurobiol Aging 12:295–312.

Price DL, Sisodia SS, Borchelt DR. 1998. Genetic neurodegenerative diseases: the human illness and transgenic models. Science 282:1079–1083.

Roses AD. 1995. Apolipoprotein E genotyping in the differential diagnosis, not prediction, of Alzheimer disease. Ann Neurol 38:6–14.

Schellenberg GD, Bird TD, Wijsman EM, Orr HT, Anderson L, Nemens E, White JA, Bonnycastle L, Weber JL, Alonso ME, Potter H, Heston LL, Martin GM. 1992. Genetic linkage evidence for a familial Alzheimer disease locus on chromosome 14. Science 258:668–671.

Selkoe DJ, Bell DS, Podlisny MB, Price DL, Cork LC. 1987. Conservation of brain amyloid proteins in aged mammals and humans with Alzheimer disease. Science 235:873–877.

Shock NW, Greulich RC, Costa PT Jr, Andres R, Lakatta EG, Arenberg D, Tobin JD. 1984. *Normal Human Aging: The Baltimore Longitudinal Study of Aging.* Baltimore: U.S. Department of Health & Human Services.

Suzuki N, Cheung TT, Cai X-D, Odaka A, Otvos L Jr, Eckman C, Golde TE, Younkin SG. 1994. An increased percentage of long amyloid β protein secreted by familial amyloid protein precursor (APP717) mutants. Science 264:1336–1340.

Terry RD, Masliah E, Salmon DP, Butters N, DeTeresa R, Hill R, Hansen LA, Katzman R. 1991. Physical basis of cognitive alterations in Alzheimer disease: synapse loss is the major correlate of cognitive impairment. Ann Neurol 30:572–580.

Van Broeckhoven C, Haan J, Bakker E, Hardy JA, Van Hul W, Wehnert A, Vegter–Van der Vlis M, Roos RAC. 1990. Amyloid protein precursor gene and hereditary cerebral hemorrhage with amyloidosis (Dutch). Science 248:1120–1122.

Whitehouse PJ, Price DL, Struble RG, Clark AW, Coyle JT, DeLong MR. 1982. Alzheimer disease and senile dementia: loss of neurons in the basal forebrain. Science 215:1237–1239.

Wisniewski HM, Terry RD. 1973. Reexamination of the pathogenesis of the senile plaque. In: HM Zimmerman (ed). *Progress in Neuropathology,* 2:1–26. New York: Grune & Stratton.

Wong PC, Zheng H, Chen H, Becher MW, Sirinathsinghji DJS, Trumbauer ME, Chen HY, Price DL, Van der Ploeg LHT, Sisodia SS. 1997. Presenilin 1 is required for *Notch1* and *Dll1* expression in the paraxial mesoderm. Nature 387:288–292.

Part IX

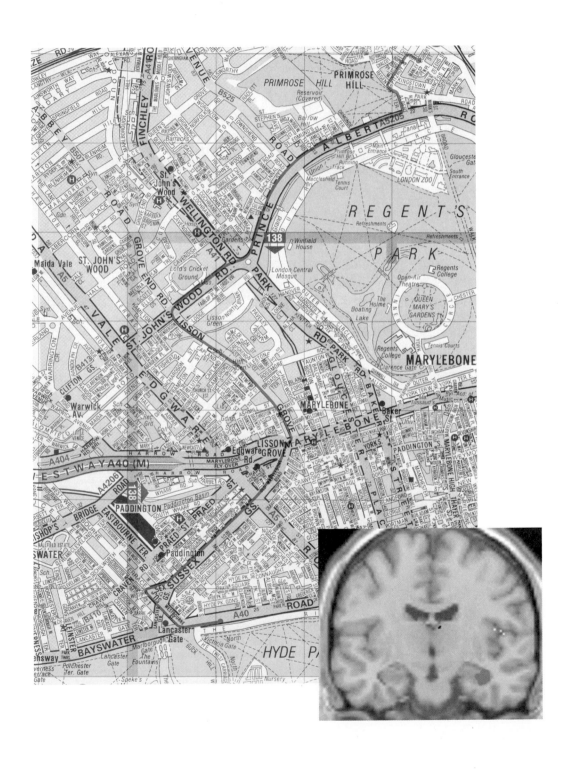

Preceding page

The Hippocampus Is Involved in Processing Spatial Memory in Humans. Much human behavior takes place in familiar environments in which knowledge of spatial layouts has become part of so-called semantic memory. In this study, positron emission tomography (PET) is used to examine the neural substrates of topographical memory retrieval by licensed London taxi drivers with many years' experience while they recalled complex routes around the city. Route recall, shown here from Hyde Park to Primrose Hill, results in activation of a network of specific brain regions, including the right hippocampus. Recall of famous landmarks for which the drivers had no knowledge of the topographical location activated similar parts of the brain, except for the right hippocampus. This suggests that the right hippocampus is used specifically for navigation in large-scale spatial environments. In contrast, nontopographical semantic memory retrieval involves the left inferior frontal gyrus. (Based on images from Maguire, EA, Frakowiak RS, Frith CD 1996. Learning to find your way: a role for the human hippocampal formation. Proc R Soc London B 263:1745–1750.)

IX Language, Thought, Mood, Learning, and Memory

OTOR AND SENSORY CENTERS take up less than one-half of the cerebral cortex in humans. The rest of the cortex is occupied by the association areas, which coordinate events arising in the motor and sensory centers. Three association areas—the prefrontal, parietal temporal occipital, and limbic—are involved in cognitive behavior planning, thinking, feeling, perception, speech, learning, memory, emotion, and skilled movements.

Most of the early evidence relating cognitive functions to the association areas came from clinical studies of brain-damaged patients. For example, the study of language in patients with aphasia has yielded important information about how human mental processes are distributed in the two hemispheres of the brain. More recently, studies using experimental animals, including genetically modified mice, have provided important insight into the neural mechanisms that underlie mental functions other than language.

Genetic manipulation in experimental animals also helps evaluate the relative contribution of genes and learning to specific types of behavior. Even the highest cognitive abilities have a genetic component. Composing music is an excellent example. Music conforms to complex, unusually abstract rules that must be learned, yet clearly it has genetic components intertwined with its learned aspects. The great composer Johann Sebastian Bach had many children, five of whom were distinguished musicians and composers. His only grandson also was a composer and harpsichordist to the Court of Prussia. In 1730 Bach proudly wrote that he was able to "put on a vocal and instrumental concert with my own family."

Today's neural science is *cognitive* neural science, a merger of neurophysiology, anatomy, developmental biology, cell and molecular biology, and cognitive psychology. This discipline is grounded in the idea, first stated by Hippocrates more than two thousand years ago, that the proper study of the mind begins with the brain. Until two decades ago the study of higher mental function was approached in two complementary ways: through psychological observation and through invasive experimental physiology. In the first part of the twentieth century, to avoid untestable concepts and hypotheses, psychology became rigidly concerned with behaviors defined strictly in terms of observable stimuli and responses. Orthodox behaviorists thought it unproductive to deal with consciousness, feeling, attention, or even motivation.

By concentrating only on observable motor actions behaviorists asked, What can an organism do and how does it do it? Indeed, careful quantitative analysis of stimuli and responses has contributed greatly to our understanding of the acquisition and use of "implicit" knowledge. However, humans and other higher animals also have "explicit" knowledge. Thus we also need to ask, What does the animal know about the world and how does it come to know it? How is that knowledge represented in the brain? And how does explicit knowledge differ from implicit knowledge?

The modern effort to understand the neural mechanisms of higher mental functions began at the end of the eighteenth century when Franz Joseph Gall, a German neuroanatomist, proposed that particular mental functions are discretely localized in the brain. By the mid nineteenth century clinical neurologists, who regarded their patients as "natural experiments" in brain function, studied brain lesions at autopsy to discover where particular brain functions are located. In 1861 Pierre Paul Broca, using evidence from the damaged brains of aphasic patients, convinced the scientific establishment that speech is controlled by a specific area of the left frontal lobe. Soon afterward the control of voluntary movement was localized and the various primary sensory cortices for vision, audition, somatic sensation, and taste were delineated.

Neural science is only beginning to analyze the nature of the internal representations that cognitive psychologists have insisted intervenes between stimulus and response, and the very real dynamic mental processes studied by psychoanalysts. Neural science has not yet been able to address directly the subjective sense of individuality, will, and purpose that is common to us all. In the past, ascribing a particular behavioral feature to mental process that could not be directly observed meant that the process must be excluded from study because no reliable techniques were available to examine brain function in the context of behavior. In this part of the book we show that, because the nervous system has become more accessible to behavioral experiments, internal representations of experience can be explored in a controlled manner.

A key concern of cognitive psychology and psychoanalysis is the relative importance of genetic and learned factors in forming a mental representation of the world. These disciplines can be strengthened by the insights into behavior that neurobiology now offers. The task for the years ahead is to produce a psychology that—though still concerned with problems of mental representation, cognitive dynamics, and subjective states of mind—is grounded firmly in empirical neural science.

Part IX

59

Language and the Aphasias

L ANGUAGE IS THE REMARKABLE system that allows people to communicate an unlimited combination of ideas using a highly structured stream of sounds (or, in signed languages, of manual and facial gestures). Language is the most accessible part of the mind, and for millennia it has been a central concern of scholars in many disciplines. Intensive scientific investigation by linguists and psycholinguists in the past 40 years has revealed that all languages are based on remarkably similar design principles and that language emerges spontaneously in all normal children in all societies. Language thus appears to be a species-wide adaptation and, as we shall see, is supported by neural circuitry of considerable complexity.

Language Is the Ability to Encode Ideas Into Signals and Must Be Distinguished From Thought, Literacy, and Correct Usage

The word *language* is used in many ways, and in undertaking a scientific investigation of language it is useful to distinguish the core faculty of language itself from other abilities that are often lumped with it.

First, language is often said to be inextricable from thinking, but in fact the two should be distinguished. *Thinking* is the ability to have ideas and to infer new ideas from old ones; *language* is the ability to encode ideas into signals for communication to someone else. Language, the code by which we transmit ideas, is different from ideas themselves. People do not think only in the words and sentences of their language; thinking can occur in the absence of language. Infants, nonhuman primates, aphasic individuals, and normal adult humans think when they use visual images, abstract concepts and propositions, and other nonlinguistic forms of thought. Moreover, language is too ambiguous and sketchy to express the totality of a person's knowledge.

Second, language should be distinguished from reading and writing. Written language is a recent invention in human history and must be explicitly taught, with uneven results. Finally, mastery of language is not the same as mastery of the *prescriptive* rules of "correct" usage spelled out by teachers and style manuals. These rules specify differences between standard and nonstandard dialects of a language (eg, *isn't* vs *ain't*) and the conventions of written prose. The scientific study of language is *descriptive*. It is concerned with how people do talk, not how they ought to talk. Thus, for linguists, "grammar" refers to the rules that allow people to connect thoughts in sentences, both when speaking and understanding.

Language Has a Universal Design

All human cultures have language, and everywhere people use it creatively to convey new ideas. How do they do it?

The design of language is based on two components: words and grammar. A *word* is an arbitrary association between a sound and a meaning. For example, English speakers use the word *cat* (as opposed to *chat, dog,* or *blicket*) to refer to a certain animal, not because the word has any natural connection with this animal but simply because it is a shared convention used by a community of speakers who have all, at some time in their lives, memorized the connection between that sound and that meaning. By age 6, children comprehend about 13,000 words, and high school graduates have mastered at least 60,000. This means that children connect a new sound and meaning about every 90 waking minutes. The connection is bidirectional: Children merely have to hear a word to use it themselves; they do not need molding or feedback.

Words in the huge open-class (or content) vocabulary refer to a vast number of concepts, such as objects, states, events, motions, qualities, people, paths, and places, and include nouns, verbs, adjectives, adverbs, and some prepositions. Words in the much smaller closed-class (or grammatical) vocabulary have a more restricted set of meanings related to time, logic, and the relationships among the content words. They are used primarily to define a sentence's structure and include articles, auxiliaries, prefixes and suffixes, particles, and prepositions not included in the open class.

Grammar is the system that specifies how vocabulary units can be combined into words, phrases, and sentences, and how the meaning of a combination can be determined by the meanings of the units and the way they are arranged. It allows us to distinguish, for example, between *Man bites dog* and *Dog bites man*, using the positions of the words *man* and *dog* with respect to *bites*. Because grammar is based on a set of rules for assembling words into new combinations, rather than on the storage and recall of fixed word sequences, the number of sentences a language speaker can produce and understand is vast. The number of possibilities grows exponentially with the length of the sentence; there are on the order of 10^{20} grammatically meaningful sentences of 20 words or fewer. Indeed, the number of possible sentences is in principle infinite, because one can embed one sentence inside another without limit: *I think that he thinks that she thinks that . . . .*

Grammar has three main components: morphology, syntax, and phonology. *Morphology* refers to the rules for combining words and affixes into larger words, as in *fax + able + ity* or *bite + s*. In many languages morphology plays a crucial role in conveying who did what to whom. Nouns are marked with suffixes that help indicate whether the noun is the agent, the affected party, or some other kind of participant in the event or state, and verbs are marked with suffixes that pin down various properties of those participants (such as person, number, and gender). Old English relied heavily on these devices, and modern English has vestiges of them in pronoun case (*I* versus *me, he* versus *him*) and subject-verb agreement (*He dawdles* versus *They dawdle*).

Syntax consists of rules for combining words into phrases and sentences and determining relations among words. These rules do not simply order words in a linear string. At heart, syntax involves three principles. First, sequences of words are grouped into phrases, which are grouped into larger phrases, and so on, defining a tree-like phrase structure. For example, in *Animal Crackers* Groucho Marx said, "I once shot an elephant in my pajamas. How he got into my pajamas I'll never know." The joke stems from the fact that two phrase structures are possible for the same sequence of words: "[I shot] [an elephant] [in my pajamas]," and "[I shot] [an elephant in my pajamas]."

Second, the verb determines how the meanings of the words in a phrase structure are to be integrated into a cohesive proposition. A person's "mental dictionary entry" for a word includes not just its sound, meaning, and grammatical category (noun, verb, adjective, preposition) but also a grammatical subcategory. Familiar examples of subcategories for verbs are those for transitive and intransitive verbs. A *transitive verb* requires an object (eg, we say *Maria devoured the pizza*, never just *Maria devoured*), while an *intransitive verb* does not have an object (eg, we say *Maria dined*, not *Maria dined the pizza*). The subcategory of a verb specifies the semantic roles of its *arguments*, the different participants in the action or state expressed by the verb. For example, in the sentences *Man fears dog* and *Man frightens dog*, *man* has a different role despite the fact that the word occupies the same position in both phrases. The word *fear* specifies "the subject is the experiencer, the object is the cause," whereas *frighten* specifies "the subject is the cause, the object is the experiencer." To understand either of these sentences, one must distinguish between the subject and the object; they can be identified by their positions in phrase structure, their case endings, or both.

The third syntactic principle is that two phrases in a sentence are sometimes linked so that they refer to the same entity in the world, a phenomenon called *anaphora*. For example, in *Sheila washed herself* the words *Sheila* and *herself* are understood to refer to the same person. Sometimes the process of anaphora links a word to a structural gap later in the sentence that provides a clue to the role of the word in the sentence. In the sentence *Which man did the dog bite _____* , the semantic role of *which man* (the man who was bitten) is determined not by the position of that phrase at the beginning of the sentence but by the empty object position after the word *bite*. That is, the position for the object is left empty and is not expressed overtly in the speaker's utterance. This phenomenon motivated Noam Chomsky to distinguish between the deep structure and the surface structure of a sentence. In the *deep structure* every phrase is in its proper position (for example, *which man* would follow *bite*). However, a movement rule or transformation can move a phrase to another position (such as the beginning of the sentence), leaving behind a gap (or *trace*). The resulting structure of the sentence is called the *surface structure*.

The third subsystem of grammar, *phonology*, consists of rules combining sounds into a consistent pattern in the language. For example, we recognize that *blicket* may be an English word, whereas *ngagat* probably is not. But unlike syntax and morphology, phonology does not assign a meaning to the elements it combines. Sound elements of phonemes, such as *t* and *i*, and their articulatory components, such as voicing and use of the tongue tip, do not themselves have meanings, nor does their arrangement correspond to some meaningful relation among entities. (There is nothing in the ordering of *d*, *o*, and *g* that predicts how the meaning of *dog* differs from the meaning of *god*.) The rules of phonology, then, are merely a way of taking a small set of basic articulatory gestures and using them to form a vast set of possi-

ble words, each with an arbitrary meaning that must be memorized. Phonology also embraces *prosody*: patterns of intonation, stress, and timing that span entire phrases and sentences. Prosody can have a grammatical role—for example, in distinguishing words (*blackboard* versus *black board*)—as well as a broader communicative function, differentiating questions from statements, supplying emphasis, indicating sarcasm, and expressing emotion.

Using grammar and lexicon alone does not allow one to produce or comprehend a sentence. Grammar and lexicon are merely codes, or protocols, that establish a relationship between meanings and signals for a given language. To produce a sentence one must choose words and use grammatical rules to encode ideas and intentions (that is, the message) and generate a set of articulatory commands to the motor system. To comprehend a sentence one must coordinate the sensory information that comes in through the auditory system (or the visual system in signing and reading) with the grammar and lexicon and send information about the resulting interpretation (the message) to the systems underlying memory and reasoning. Using language, then, requires complex patterns of information flow involving many parts of the brain.

Complex Language Develops Spontaneously in Children

According to Darwin, "Man has an instinctive tendency to speak, as we see in the babble of our young children; while no child has an instinctive tendency to brew, bake, or write." In the first year of life children work on sounds. They begin to make language-like sounds at 5–7 months, babble in well-formed syllables at 7–8 months, and gibber in sentence-like streams by the first year. In their first few months, they can discriminate speech sounds, including ones that are not used in their parents' language and that their parents do not normally discriminate (for example, Japanese babies can discriminate *r* and *l*). By 10 months they discriminate phonemes much as their parents do. This tuning of speech perception to the specific ambient language precedes the first words, so it must be based on the infant performing sophisticated acoustic analyses, rather than on the infant correlating the sounds of words with their meanings.

A child's first words are spoken around the time of his or her first birthday, and the rate of word learning increases suddenly around age 18 months, which is also the age at which children first string words into combinations such as *More outside* and *Allgone doggie*. Children at age 2 begin to speak in rich phrase structures and master the grammatical vocabulary of their language (articles, prepositions, etc). By age 3, children use grammatical words correctly most of the time, use most of the constructions of the spoken language appropriately, and in general become fluent and expressive conversational partners. Although children make many errors, their errors occur in a minority of the words they use and are highly systematic. Indeed, this fact confirms what we might have guessed from the fact that children are so fluent and creative: children must be engaging in sophisticated grammatical analysis of their parents' speech rather than merely imitating them.

Take, for example, this error of a 3-year-old: *Mommy, why did he dis it appear?* First, it shows that children do not merely record stretches of sound but are hyperalert for word boundaries. This child misanalyzed *disappear* as *dis appear*. Second, this error shows that children work to classify words in grammatical categories. The child's newly extracted *appear* is being used not as the verb an adult uses but as a unit of speech that the child has hypothesized from the context, namely, a particle (examples of particles are the second words in *blow away* and *take apart*). Third, it shows how children look for grammatical subcategories that determine the interaction between words and grammar. The child creatively converted an intransitive verb meaning "vanish" to a transitive verb meaning "cause to vanish," in conformity with a widespread pattern in English grammar: *The ice melted/She melted the ice; The ball bounced/She bounced the ball,* and so on.

Languages Are Learned and the Capacity to Learn Language Is Innate

Language, like other cognitive abilities, cannot be attributed entirely to either innate structure or learning. Clearly, learning plays a crucial role: any child will acquire any language he or she is exposed to. Likewise, "wild children" who are abandoned by parents to survive in forests, or who are raised in silent environments by deranged parents, are always mute. But learning cannot happen without some innate mechanism that does the learning, and other species exposed to the same input as a child fail to learn at all. In 1959 Chomsky proposed a then-revolutionary hypothesis that children possess innate neural circuitry specifically dedicated to the acquisition of language. The hypothesis is still controversial; some psychologists and linguists believe that the innate capacity for language is merely a general capacity to learn patterns, not a specific system for language, and that the brain areas subserving these skills have no properties that are tailored specifically to the design of language.

Several kinds of evidence have been adduced to support Chomsky's hypothesis. First, there are the gross facts of the distribution of language across the species. People in technologically primitive cultures, helpless 3-year-olds, and poorly educated adults in our culture all master complex grammar when they first acquire language, and they do so without special training sequences or feedback. Indeed, when children in a social environment are deprived of a bona fide language, they create one of their own; this is how the sign languages of the deaf arise. Similarly, in the eighteenth and nineteenth centuries, slave children living on plantations and children in other mixed-culture societies who were exposed to crude *pidgin* languages (choppy strings of words) used by their parents developed full-fledged languages, called *creoles,* from the pidgin languages. In all these cases the languages children master or create follow the universal design of language described earlier in this chapter.

In addition, language and more general intelligence are dissociated from one another in several kinds of pathological conditions. Children with a heritable syndrome called *specific language impairment* can have high intelligence, intact hearing, and normal social skills but have long-lasting difficulty in speaking and understanding according to the grammatical rules of their language. Conversely, children with certain kinds of mental retardation can express their confabulated or childlike thoughts in fluent, perfectly grammatical language and score at normal levels on tests of comprehension of complex sentences. These dissociations, in which complex language abilities are preserved despite compromised intelligence, can appear in people who have hydrocephalus caused by spina bifida and in people with Williams syndrome, a form of retardation associated with a defective stretch of chromosome 7.

Finally, grammar has a partly quirky design that cuts across the categories underlying concepts and reasoning. Consider the statements *It is raining* and *Pat is running.* Both "it" and "Pat" have the same grammatical function; both words serve as subjects of the sentence and both can be inverted with the verb to form a question (*Is it raining? Is Pat running?*) despite the fact that "it" is a grammatical placeholder without cognitive content. Though the sentence *The child seems to be sleepy* can be shortened to *The child seems sleepy,* the nearly identical sentence *The child seems to be sleeping* cannot be shortened to *The child seems sleeping.* Subtleties such as these, which emerge in all speakers without specially tailored training sequences or systematic feedback, are consequences of the design of grammar; they cannot be predicted from principles governing what makes sense or what is easy or difficult to understand.

In sum, children seem to acquire language using abilities that are more specific than general intelligence but not so specific as the capacity to speak a given language—English, Japanese, and so on. What, then, is innate? Presumably, it is some kind of neural system that analyzes communicative signals from other people, not as arbitrary sequences of sound or behavior but according to the design of language. By following this design a child learns a lexicon of bidirectional arbitrary pairings of sound and meaning and several kinds of grammatical rules. One kind assembles phonological elements into words; other kinds assemble words into bigger words, phrases, and sentences according to the principles of phrase structure, grammatical categories and subcategories, case and agreement, anaphora, long-distance dependencies, and movement transformations. Presumably all these abilities come from adaptations of the human brain that arose in the course of human evolution.

Other Animals Appear to Lack Homologs of Human Language, but Language May Nonetheless Have Evolved by Darwinian Natural Selection

One might think that if language evolved by gradual Darwinian natural selection it must have a precursor in other animals. But the natural communication systems of nonhuman animals are strikingly unlike human language. They are based on one of three designs: a finite repertoire of calls (eg, one to warn of predators, one to announce a claim to territory), a continuous analog signal that registers the magnitude of some condition (eg, the distance a bee dances signals the distance of a food source), or sequences of randomly ordered responses that serve as variations on a theme (as in birdsong). There is no hint of the discrete, infinite combinatorial system of meaningful elements seen in human language.

Some animals can be trained to mimic certain aspects of human language in artificial settings. In several famous and controversial demonstrations, chimpanzees and gorillas have been taught to use some hand signs based on American Sign Language (though never its grammar), manipulate colored switches or tokens, and carry out some simple spoken commands. Parrots and dolphins have also learned to recognize or produce ordered sequences of sounds or other signals. Such studies have taught us much about the cognitive categories of nonhuman species, but the relevance of these animal behaviors to human language is questionable.

It is not a matter of whether one wants to call the trained artificial systems "language." This is not a scientific question, but a matter of definition—how far are we willing to stretch the meaning of the word *language?* The scientific question, and the only one relevant to whether these trained behaviors can serve as an animal model for language, is whether the abilities are *homologous* to human language—whether the two cognitive systems show the same basic organization owing to descent from a single system in a common ancestor. For example, biologists do not debate whether the wing-like structures of gliding rodents (flying squirrels) may be called "genuine wings" or something else (an uninformative question of definition). These structures are not homologous to the wings of bats because they have a different anatomical plan reflecting a different evolutionary history. Bat wings are modifications of the hands of a common mammalian ancestor; the wings of a flying squirrel are modifications of its rib cage. The two structures are merely similar in function, or *analogous,* but not homologous.

Though artificial signaling systems taught to animals have some analogies to human language (eg, they are used in communication and sometimes involve combining basic signals), it seems unlikely that they are homologous. Chimpanzees require extensive teaching contrived by another species (humans) to acquire rudimentary abilities, mostly limited to a small number of signs, strung together in repetitive, quasirandom sequences, used with the intent of requesting food or tickling. The core design of human language—particularly the formation of words, phrases, and sentences according to a single plan that supports both production and comprehension—fails to emerge as the chimps interact with each other and, as far as we know, it cannot be taught to them.

All this contrasts sharply with human children, who learn thousands of words spontaneously; combine them in novel structured sequences in which every word has a role; respect the word order, case marking, and agreement of the adult language; use sentences for a variety of nonutilitarian purposes, such as commenting on interesting objects; and creatively interpret the grammatical complexity of the input they receive (reflected in their systematic errors or in their creation of novel sign languages and creoles).

Nevertheless, this lack of homology does not cast doubt on a Darwinian, gradualist account of language evolution. Humans did not evolve directly from chimpanzees. Both evolved from a common ancestor, probably around 6–8 million years ago. This time span leaves about 300,000 generations in which language could have evolved gradually in the lineage leading to humans after it split off from the lineage leading to chimpanzees. Presumably language evolved in the human lineage because of two related adaptations in our ances-

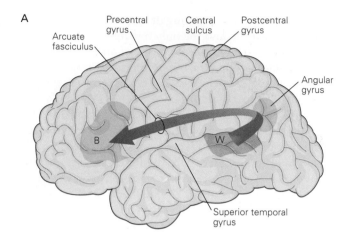

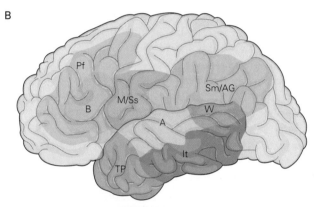

Figure 59-1 Language-related areas in the human brain.

A. A highly simplified view of the primary language areas of the brain are indicated in this lateral view of the exterior surface of the left hemisphere. Broca's area (**B**) is adjacent to the region of the motor cortex (precentral gyrus) that controls the movements of facial expression, articulation, and phonation. Wernicke's area (**W**) lies in the posterior superior temporal lobe near the primary auditory cortex (superior temporal gyrus). Wernicke's and Broca's areas are joined by a bidirectional pathway, the arcuate fasciculus (**brown arrow**). These regions are part of a complex network of areas that all contribute to normal language processing.

B. Modern and more elaborate view of the language areas in a lateral view of the left hemisphere. These language areas contain three functional language systems: the implementation system, the mediational system, and the conceptual system. Two of these are illustrated here. The *implementation system* is made up of several regions located around the left sylvian fissure. It includes the classical language areas (**B** = Broca's area; **W** = Wernicke's area) and the adjoining supramarginal gyrus (**Sm**), angular gyrus (**AG**), auditory cortex (**A**), motor cortex (**M**), and somatosensory cortex (**Ss**). The posterior and anterior components of the implementation system, respectively Wernicke's area and Broca's area, are interconnected by the arcuate fasciculus. The *mediational system* surrounds the implementation system like a belt (**blue areas**). The regions identified so far are located in the left temporal pole (**TP**), left inferotemporal cortex (**It**), and left prefrontal cortex (**Pf**). The left basal ganglia complex (not pictured) is an integral part of the language implementation system. (Courtesy of H. Damasio.)

tors: They developed technology to exploit the local environment in their lifetimes and were involved in extensive cooperation. These preexisting features of the hominid lifestyle may have set the stage for language, because language would have allowed evolving hominids to benefit by sharing hard-won knowledge with their kin and exchanging it with their neighbors.

The specific origins of language are obscure. *Homo habilis,* which lived about 2.5 to 2 million years ago, left behind caches of stone tools that may have served as home bases or butchering stations. The sharing of skills required to make the tools, and the social coordination required to share the caches, may have made it necessary for *H. habilis* to put simple language to use, though this is speculation. The skulls of *H. habilis* bear faint imprints of the gyral patterns of their brains, and some of the areas involved in language in modern humans (Broca's area and the supramarginal and angular gyri) are visible and are larger in the left hemisphere. We cannot be sure, of course, that these areas were used for language, since they have homologs even in monkeys, but the homologs play no role in the monkeys' vocal communication. *Homo erectus,* which spread from Africa across much of the Old World from 1.5 million to 500,000 years ago, controlled fire and used a stereotyped kind of stone hand ax. It is easy to imagine some form of language contributing to such successes, though again we cannot be sure.

The first *Homo sapiens,* thought to have appeared about 200,000 years ago and to have moved out of Africa 100,000 years ago, had skulls similar to ours and much more elegant and complex tools showing considerable regional variation. They almost certainly had language, given that their anatomy suggests they were biologically very similar to modern humans and that all modern humans have language. The major human races probably diverged about 50,000 years ago, which puts a late boundary on the emergence of language, because all modern races have indistinguishable language abilities.

The Study of Aphasia Led to the Discovery of Critical Brain Areas Related to Language

The lack of a homolog to language in other species precludes the attempt to model language in animals, and our understanding of the neural basis of language must be pieced together from other sources. By far the most important source has been the study of language disorders, known as *aphasias,* which are caused by focal brain lesions that result, most frequently, from stroke or head injury.

The early study of the aphasias paved the way for a number of important discoveries on the neural basis of language processing. First, it suggested that in a majority of individuals language depends principally on left hemisphere rather than on right hemisphere structures. All but a few right-handed individuals have left cerebral dominance for language, and so do most left-handed individuals. All told, about 96% of people depend on the left hemisphere for language processing related to grammar, the lexicon, phonemic assembly, and phonetic production. Even languages such as American Sign Language, which rely on visuomotor signs rather than auditory speech signs, depend primarily on the left hemisphere. Second, the early study of aphasia revealed that damage to each of two cortical areas, one in the lateral frontal region, the other in the posterior superior temporal lobe, was associated with a major and linguistically different profile of language impairment. The two cortical areas are Broca's area and Wernicke's area (Figure 59–1).

These findings allowed neurologists to develop a model of language that has become known as the Wernicke-Geschwind model. The earliest version of this model had the following components. First, two areas of the brain, Wernicke's and Broca's, were assumed to have the burden of processing the acoustic images of words and the articulation of speech, respectively. Second, the arcuate fasciculus was thought to be a unidirectional pathway that brought information from Wernicke's area to Broca's area. Third, both Wernicke's and Broca's areas were presumed to interact with the polymodal association areas. After a spoken word was processed in the auditory pathways and the auditory signals reached Wernicke's area, the word's meaning was evoked when brain structures beyond Wernicke's area were activated.

Similarly, nonverbal meanings were converted into acoustic images in Wernicke's area and turned into vocalizations after such images were transferred by the arcuate fasciculus into Broca's area. Finally, reading and writing ability both depended on Wernicke's and Broca's areas, which, in the case of reading, received visual input from left visual cortices and, in the case of writing, could produce motor output from Exner's area (in the premotor region above Broca's area).

This general model formed the basis for a useful classification of the aphasias (Table 59-1) and provided a framework for the investigation of the neural basis of language processes. However, several decades of new lesion studies and research in psycholinguistics and experimental neuropsychology have shown that the general model has important limitations. In particular, much progress has come from the advent of new methodologies, including positron emission tomography (PET), functional magnetic resonance imaging (fMRI), event-related electrical potentials (ERP), and the direct recording of electrical potentials from the ex-

posed cerebral cortex of patients undergoing surgery for the management of intractable epilepsy. Each of these techniques has contributed to a better definition of the areas important for the performance of language tasks.

As a result of these advances, it now is apparent that the roles of Wernicke's and Broca's areas are not as clear as they first appeared. Similarly, the arcuate fasciculus is now appreciated to be a bidirectional system that joins a broad expanse of sensory cortices with prefrontal and premotor cortices. Finally, a variety of other regions in the left hemisphere, both cortical and subcortical, have been found to be critically involved in language processing. These include higher-order association cortices in the left frontal, temporal, and parietal regions, which seem to be involved in mediating between concepts and language; selected cortex in the left insular region thought to be related to speech articulation; and prefrontal and cingulate areas that implement executive control and mediation of necessary memory and attentional processes. The processing of language requires a large network of interacting brain areas.

The modern framework that has emerged from this work suggests that three large systems interact closely in language perception and production. One system is formed by the language areas of Broca and Wernicke, selected areas of insular cortex, and the basal ganglia. Together, these structures constitute a *language implementation system.* The implementation system analyzes incoming auditory signals so as to activate conceptual knowledge and also ensures phonemic and grammatical construction as well as articulatory control. This implementation system is surrounded by a second system, the *mediational system,* made up of numerous separate regions in the temporal, parietal, and frontal association cortices (Figure 59-1). The mediational regions act as third-party brokers between the implementation system and a third system, the *conceptual system,* a collection of regions distributed throughout the remainder of higher-order association cortices, which support conceptual knowledge.

Broca Aphasia Results From a Large Frontal Lobe Lesion

Broca aphasia is not a single entity. True persisting Broca aphasia is a syndrome resulting from damage to Broca's area (the inferior left frontal gyrus, which contains Brodmann's areas 44 and 45); surrounding frontal fields (the external aspect of Brodmann's area 6, and areas 8, 9, 10, and 46); the underlying white matter, insula, and basal ganglia (Figure 59-2); and a small portion of the anterior superior temporal gyrus. The patient's speech is labored and slow, articulation is impaired, and the melodic intonation of normal speech is lacking (Table 59-2). Yet patients have considerable success at verbal

Table 59-1 Differential Diagnosis of the Main Types of Aphasia

Type of aphasia	Speech	Comprehension	Capacity for Repetition	Other Signs	Region Affected
Broca's	Nonfluent, effortful	Largely preserved for single words and grammatically simple sentences	Impaired	Right hemiparesis (arm > leg); patient aware of defect and may be depressed	Left posterior frontal cortex, and underlying structures
Wernicke's	Fluent, abundant, well articulated, melodic	Impaired	Impaired	No motor signs; patient may be anxious, agitated, euphoric, or paranoid	Left posterior, superior, and middle temporal cortex
Conduction	Fluent with some articulatory defects	Intact or largely preserved	Impaired	Often none; patient may have cortical sensory loss or weakness in right arm	Left superior temporal and supramarginal gyri
Global	Scant, nonfluent	Impaired	Impaired	Right hemiplegia	Massive left perisylvian lesion
Transcortical Motor	Nonfluent, explosive	Intact or largely preserved	Intact or largely preserved	Sometimes right-sided weakness	Anterior or superior to Broca's area
Transcortical Sensory	Fluent; scant	Impaired	Intact or largely preserved	No motor signs	Posterior or inferior to Wernicke's area,

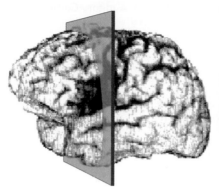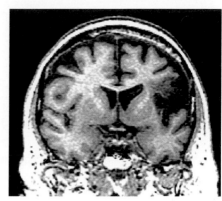

Figure 59-2 Broca aphasia. **Left:** A three-dimensional magnetic resonance imaging (MRI) reconstruction of a lesion (an infarction in the left frontal operculum, **dark gray area**) in a patient with Broca aphasia. **Right:** Coronal section of the same brain taken along the plane defined by the **blue slab.** The brain is viewed from the front, with the left hemisphere on the right half of the image. The infarct is visible in black.

communication even when their words are difficult to understand because the selection of words, especially nouns, is often correct. Verbs, as well as grammatical words such as conjunctions, are less well selected and may be missing altogether. Another major sign of Broca aphasia is a defect in the ability to repeat complex sentences spoken by the examiner. In general, patients with Broca aphasia appear to comprehend the words and sentences they hear, but the comprehension is only partial, as we shall see below.

When damage is restricted to Broca's area alone, or to its subjacent white matter, a condition now known as *Broca area aphasia*, the patient develops a milder and transient aphasia rather than true Broca aphasia.

People With Broca Aphasia Have Trouble Understanding Grammatically Complex Sentences

Broca aphasia was initially thought to be a deficit of production only, because most patients give the impression of understanding casual speech. Modern psycholinguistic studies have shown that people who have Broca aphasia comprehend sentences whose meaning can be pieced together from the individual meanings of content words and prior knowledge of how the world works. For example, these patients can understand *The apple that the boy is eating is red.* Boys eat apples, but apples do not eat boys; apples are red, but boys are not. But they cannot comprehend sentences in which meaning depends on complex grammar. They cannot understand *The boy that the girl is chasing is tall.*

Aphasic patients can understand the first sentence, as well as much casual conversation in general, based on vocabulary and general knowledge, without exercising grammatical abilities. But they have difficulty with the second sentence because either boys or girls can be tall and either one can chase the other. The only way to understand the second sentence is to recover its phrase structure, look up the lexical entry of *chase* to find the

positions of the chaser and the person being chased, and link the gap after *chasing* to *the boy.* People with Broca aphasia are tripped up by this demand, showing that their aphasia is not just a disorder of speech output but embraces deficits in syntactic processing.

Is Broca aphasia, then, a deficit of grammar, implying that Broca's area is the center for grammar? Not really. First, the speech of patients with Broca aphasia is not altogether devoid of grammatical structure. Their speech retains the phrase order of their particular language (eg, subject-verb-object in English, subject-object-verb in Turkish). Moreover, although grammatical suffixes such as *-ed*, *-ing*, and *-s* are often omitted in the speech of English-speaking aphasic patients, suffixes may be preserved in the speech of aphasic patients speaking other languages in which suffixes are obligatory to conform with the phonological structure of words. Second, people with Broca aphasia often can make surprisingly fine grammatical judgments, discriminating the grammatical and ungrammatical versions of sentences such as the following:

John was finally kissed by Louise.
John was finally kissed Louise.

I want you to go to the store now.
I want you will go to the store now.

For a sentence to be grammatically well formed, it needs certain functional *morphemes*—the smallest meaningful unit of a word. The ability of patients to recognize that a sentence needs these morphemes—combined with an inability to analyze those morphemes when understanding complex sentences—has been called the *"syntax-there-but-not-there"* paradox.

A possible resolution is that the major syntactic difficulty in Broca aphasia is linking up elements in different parts of the sentence that must refer to the same entity (anaphora and gap-filling). In *John was finally kissed by*

Table 59-2 Examples of Spontaneous Speech Production, Auditory Comprehension, and Repetition for the Primary Types of Aphasia

Type of aphasia	Spontaneous speech	Auditory comprehension	Repetition
	Stimulus (Western Aphasia Battery picnic picture): What do you see in this picture?	Stimulus: What seems to be the trouble?	Stimulus: The pastry cook was elated.
Broca	"O, yea. Det's a boy an' a girl . . . an' . . . a . . . car . . . house . . . light po' (pole). Dog an' a . . . boat. 'N det's a . . . mm . . . a . . . cofee, an' reading. Det's a . . . mm . . . a . . . det's a boy . . . fishin'." (Elapsed time: 1 min 30 s)	"Yea, but, ah, notes an', ah . . . an', ah . . . I don' know."	"Elated."
Wernicke	"Ah, yes, it's, ah . . . several things. It's a girl . . . uncurl . . . on a boat. A dog . . .'S is another dog . . . uh-oh . . . long's . . . on a boat. The lady, it's a young lady. An' a man a They were eatin'. 'S be place there. This . . . a tree! A boat. No, this is a . . . It's a house. Over in here . . . a cake. An' it's, it's a lot of water. Ah, all right. I think I mentioned about that boat. I noticed a boat being there. I did mention that before. . . . Several things down, different things down . . . a bat . . . a cake . . . you have a . . ." (Elapsed time: 1 min 20 s)	"Well, I jus' lost a lot a time"	"/I/ . . . no . . . In a fog."
Conduction	"Kay. I see a guy readin' a book. See a women / ka . . . he . . . /pourin' drink or somethin'. An' they're sittin' under a tree. An' there's a . . . car behind that an' then there's a house behind th' car. An' on the other side, the guy's flyn' a / fait . . . fait /(kite). See a dog there an' a guy down on the bank. See a flag blowin' in the wind. Bunch of /hi . . . a . . . /trees in behind. An a sailboat on th' river, river . . . lake. 'N guess that's about all . . . 'Basket there." (Elapsed time: 1 min 5 s)	"T: see if I can't talk straight, where I can have . . . not havin' trouble to say words an' sentences."	"The baker was . . . What was that last word?" ("Let me repeat it: The pastry cook was elated.") "The baker-er was /vaskerin/ . . . uh . . ."
Global	(Grunt)	(Gesturing)	(No response)

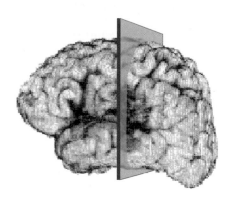 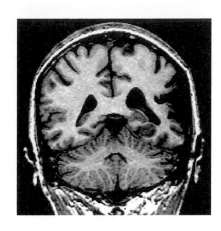

Figure 59-3 Wernicke aphasia. **Left:** A three-dimensional magnetic resonance imaging (MRI) reconstruction of a lesion in a patient with Wernicke aphasia. The infarction affected a large area of temporal lobe cortex as well as underlying white matter. Large, deep lesions are typically seen in severe cases. **Right:** Coronal section of the same brain taken along the plane defined by the **blue slab.** The brain is viewed from the front, with the left hemisphere on the right half of the image. The infarct is visible in black.

Louise, the failure to link *John* to the empty object position after *was kissed* would make the sentence incomprehensible. The aphasic person is able to detect the ungrammaticality of *John was finally kissed Louise* by simply noting that a passive verb *(was kissed)* appears illicitly with a direct object. This recognition does not depend on linking a gap with its filler. Indeed, people who have Broca aphasia *cannot* recognize that a sentence is ungrammatical if the ungrammaticality comes from an incorrect linkage between two separated elements in a sentence. That is, they are poor at discriminating between sentences such as the following pairs:

> *The woman is outside, isn't she?*
> *The woman is outside, isn't it?*
>
> *The girl fixed herself a sandwich.*
> *The girl fixed themselves a sandwich.*

Linking two elements (filler to gap, or antecedent to pronoun) requires keeping the first element in one's working memory (Chapters 19 and 62) until the second is encountered and the two can be joined. This suggests that Broca's area and associated regions may participate in the verbal short-term memory required for sentence comprehension. Recent functional brain imaging studies using PET show that the level of activation in a subregion of Broca's area increases when a subject has to understand a sentence in which there is a long gap in the middle compared with the level when the subject must understand similar sentences with shorter gaps in the middle.

The idea that Broca's area is related to short-term working memory fits with other findings. Working memory is thought to have a phonological loop consisting of a transient memory store for phonological information and a rehearsal process—a covert articulatory process in which commands are sent to the vocal tract muscles but not carried out—which repeatedly refreshes

the memory. Broca's area may participate in the rehearsal component of the loop, something that accords with the well-documented role of Broca's area in articulation.

The structures usually damaged in true Broca aphasia and in Broca area aphasia may be part of a neural network involved in both the assembly of phonemes into words and the assembly of words into sentences. This network is thought to be concerned with relational aspects of language, which include the grammatical structure of sentences and the proper use of grammatical vocabulary and verbs. The other cortical components of the network are located in external areas of the left frontal cortex (Brodmann's areas 47, 46, and 9), the left parietal cortex (areas 40, and 39), and sensorimotor areas above the sylvian fissure between Broca's and Wernicke's areas (the lower sector of areas 3, 1, 2, and 4) and the insula.

Wernicke Aphasia Results From Damage to Left Temporal Lobe Structures

Wernicke aphasia is usually caused by damage to the posterior sector of the left auditory association cortex (Brodmann's area 22), although in severe and persisting cases there is involvement of the middle temporal gyrus and deep white matter (Figure 59-3). The speech of patients with Wernicke aphasia is effortless, melodic, and produced at a normal rate and is thus quite unlike that of patients with true Broca aphasia. The content, however, is often unintelligible because of frequent errors in the choice of words and *phonemes,* the individual sound units that make up morphemes (Table 59-2).

Patients with Wernicke aphasia often shift the order of individual sounds and sound clusters and add or subtract them to a word in a manner that distorts the intended phonemic plan. These errors are called *phonemic paraphasias* (*paraphasia* refers to any substitution of an erroneous phoneme or entire word for the intended, correct one). When phoneme shifts occur frequently and close together, words become unintelligible and constitute neologisms. Even when words are put together with the proper individual sounds, patients with Wernicke aphasia have great difficulty selecting words that accurately represent their intended meaning (known as a *verbal* or *semantic paraphasia*). For example, a patient may say *headman* for *president*.

These patients also have difficulty comprehending sentences uttered by others. Although this deficit is suggested by the Wernicke-Geschwind model, Wernicke's area is no longer seen as the center of auditory comprehension. The modern view is that Wernicke's area is part of a processor of speech sounds that associates the sounds with concepts. This processing involves, in addition to Wernicke's area, the many parts of the brain that subserve grammar, attention, social knowledge, and knowledge of the concepts corresponding to the meanings of the words in the sentences.

Conduction Aphasia Results From Damage to Structures That Interact With Major Language Areas of the Brain

Patients with *conduction aphasia* comprehend simple sentences and produce intelligible speech but, like those with Broca and Wernicke aphasias, they cannot repeat sentences verbatim, cannot assemble phonemes effectively (and thus produce many phonemic paraphasias), and cannot easily name pictures and objects (the task called *confrontation naming*). Speech production and auditory comprehension are less compromised in conduction aphasia than in the two other major aphasias (Table 59-2).

Persistent conduction aphasia is caused by damage to the left superior temporal gyrus and the inferior parietal lobe (Brodmann's areas 39 and 40). The damage may extend to the left primary auditory cortex (Brodmann's areas 41 and 42), the insula, and the underlying white matter. There is no evidence that conduction aphasia is caused by a simple interruption or disconnection of the arcuate fasciculus alone, although the damage does destroy feed-forward and feedback projections that interconnect temporal, parietal, insular, and frontal cortices. This connectional system seems to be part of the network required to assemble phonemes into words and coordinate speech articulation.

Even though the exact anatomical correlates of conduction aphasia are being revised and the mechanism of the defect now appears not to be as proposed in the Wernicke-Geschwind model, Wernicke correctly predicted the main signs of the syndrome. This is a testimony to the considerable power of the early clinical observations in aphasia.

Transcortical Motor and Sensory Aphasias Result From Damage to Areas Near Broca's and Wernicke's Areas

The Wernicke-Geschwind model predicts that aphasias can be caused by damage not only to components of the language system but also to areas and pathways that connect those components to the rest of the brain. Patients with transcortical motor aphasia speak nonfluently but they can *repeat* even very long sentences. According to the Wernicke-Geschwind model, the aphasia is caused by a disconnection of the language areas from those that initiate and control spontaneous speech; repetition is preserved because the connection to Wernicke's area is intact.

The aphasia has been linked to damage to the left dorsolateral frontal area, a patch of association cortex anterior and superior to Broca's area, although there may be substantial damage to Broca's area itself. Dorsolateral frontal cortex is involved in the allocation of attention and the maintenance of higher executive abilities, including the selection of words. For example, part of the area is activated in PET studies when subjects have to produce the names of actions associated with particular objects (eg, saying *kick* in response to *ball*). Damage to this area leaves patients unable to perform such a task, although they can produce words in ordinary conversation.

The aphasia can also be caused by damage to the left supplementary motor area, located high in the frontal lobe, directly in front of the primary motor cortex and buried mesially between the hemispheres. Electrical stimulation of the area in nonaphasic surgery patients causes the patients to make involuntary vocalizations or be unable to speak, and neuroimaging studies have shown this area to be activated in tasks of speech production. Thus the supplementary motor area appears to contribute to the initiation of speech, whereas the dorsolateral frontal regions contribute to its ongoing control, particularly when the task is difficult.

People with transcortical sensory aphasia have fluent speech with impaired comprehension, and they also have great trouble naming things. This aphasia differs from Wernicke aphasia in the same way that transcortical motor aphasia differs from Broca aphasia: repetition is spared. In fact, patients with transcortical sensory aphasia may repeat and even make grammatical corrections in phrases and sentences they do not understand, and they can repeat words in foreign languages. The aphasia thus appears to be a deficit in semantic retrieval, with syntactic and phonological abilities still relatively intact.

Transcortical motor and sensory aphasias are believed to be caused by damage outside of the perisylvian area, in particular, outside the superior temporal and

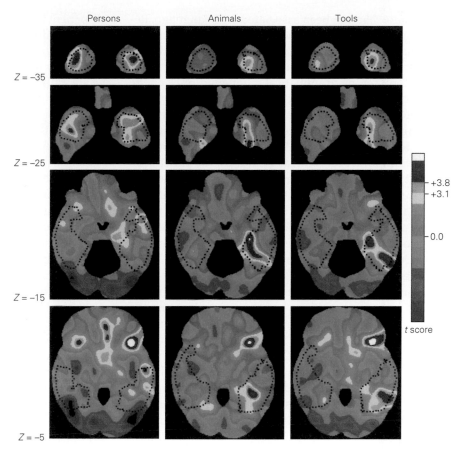

Figure 59-4 Positron emission tomography images compare the adjusted mean activity in the brain during separate tasks: naming of unique persons, animals, and tools. All sections are axial (horizontal) with left hemisphere structures on the right half of each image. The search volume (the section of the brain sampled in the analysis) includes inferotemporal and temporal pole regions (enclosed by the **dotted lines**). **Red areas** are statistically significant activity after correction for multiple comparisons. There are distinct patterns of activation in the left inferotemporal and temporal pole regions for each task. (Courtesy of H. Damasio.)

inferior parietal lobes, which explains the sparing of repetition skills. Transcortical aphasias are thus the complement of conduction aphasia, behaviorally and anatomically. Transcortical sensory aphasia itself appears to be caused by damage to parts of the junction of the temporal, parietal, and occipital lobes, which connect the perisylvian language areas with the parts of the brain underlying word meaning.

Global Aphasia Is a Combination of Broca, Wernicke, and Conduction Aphasias

Global aphasics have completely lost the ability to comprehend language, formulate speech, and repeat sentences, thus combining the features of Broca, Wernicke, and conduction aphasias. Speech is reduced to a few words at best. The same word may be used repeatedly, appropriately or not, in a vain attempt to communicate an idea. However, other abilities may be preserved: nondeliberate ("automatic") speech such as stock expletives (used appropriately and with normal phonemic, phonetic, and inflectional structures), routines such as counting or reciting the days of the week, and the ability to sing previously learned melodies and their lyrics. Au-

ditory comprehension is limited to a few words and idiomatic expressions.

Classic global aphasia is accompanied by weakness in the right side of the face and paralysis of the right limbs and is caused by damage in the anterior language region and the basal ganglia and insula (as in Broca's area), the superior temporal gyrus (as in conduction aphasia), and the posterior language regions (as in Wernicke aphasia). So much damage can only be caused by a large infarct in the region supplied by the middle cerebral artery.

Beyond the Classic Language Areas: Other Brain Areas Are Important for Language

The anatomical correlates of the classical aphasias comprise only a restricted map of language-related areas in the brain. The past decade of research on aphasia has uncovered numerous other language-related centers in the cerebral cortex and in subcortical structures. Some are located in the left temporal region.

For example, until recently the anterior temporal and inferotemporal cortices, in either the left or the right hemisphere, had not been associated with language. Recent studies reveal that damage to left temporal cortices (Brodmann's areas 21, 20, and 38) causes severe and pure naming defects—impairments of word retrieval without any accompanying grammatical, phonemic, or phonetic difficulty. When the damage is confined to the left temporal pole (Brodmann's area 38) the patient has difficulty recalling the names of unique places and persons but not names for common things. When the lesions involve the left midtemporal sector (areas 21 and 20) the patient has difficulty recalling *both* unique and common names. Finally, damage to the left posterior inferotemporal sector causes a deficit in recalling words for particular types of items—tools and utensils—but not words for natural things or unique entities. Recall of words for actions or spatial relationships is not compromised.

These findings suggest that the left temporal cortices contain neural systems that access words denoting various categories of things but not words denoting the actions of the things or their relationships to other entities. Localization of a brain region that mediates word-finding for classes of things has been inferred from two types of studies: examination of patients with lesions in their brain from stroke, head injuries, herpes encephalitis, and degenerative processes such as Alzheimer disease and Pick disease, and functional imaging studies of normal individuals and electrical stimulation of these same temporal cortices during surgical interventions (Figure 59-4).

Another area not included in the classical model is a small section of the insula, the island of cortex buried deep inside the cerebral hemispheres (Figure 59-5). Recent evidence suggests that this area is important for planning or coordinating the articulatory movements necessary for speech. Patients who have lesions in this area have difficulty pronouncing phonemes in their proper order; they usually produce combinations of sounds that are very close to the target word. These patients have no difficulty in perceiving speech sounds or recognizing their own errors and do not have trouble in finding the word, only in producing it. This area is also damaged in patients with true Broca aphasia and accounts for much of their articulatory deficits.

The frontal cortices in the mesial surface of the left hemisphere, which includes the supplementary motor area and the anterior cingulate region (also known as Brodmann's area 24), play an important role in the initiation and maintenance of speech. They are also important to attention and emotion and thus can influence many higher functions. Damage to these areas does not cause an aphasia in the proper sense but impairs the initiation of movement (akinesia) and causes *mutism*, the complete absence of speech. Mutism is a rarity in apha-

sic patients and is seen only during the very early stages of the condition. Patients with akinesia and mutism fail to communicate by words, gestures, or facial expression. They have an impairment of the drive to communicate, rather than aphasia.

The Right Cerebral Hemisphere Is Important for Prosody and Pragmatics

In almost all right-handers, and in a smaller majority of left-handers, linguistic abilities—phonology, the lexicon, and grammar—are concentrated in the left hemisphere. This conclusion is supported by numerous studies of patients with brain lesions and studies of electrical and metabolic activity in the cerebral hemispheres of normal people. In "split-brain" patients, whose corpus callosum has been sectioned to control epilepsy, the right hemisphere occasionally has rudimentary abilities to comprehend or read words, but syntactic abilities are poor, and in many cases the right hemisphere has no lexical or grammatical abilities at all.

Nonetheless, the right cerebral hemisphere does play a role in language. In particular, it is important for communicative and emotional prosody (stress, timing, and intonation). Patients with right anterior lesions may produce inappropriate intonation in their speech; those with right posterior lesions have difficulty interpreting the emotional tone of others' speech. In addition, the right hemisphere plays a role in the *pragmatics* of language. Patients with damage in the right hemisphere have difficulty incorporating sentences into a coherent narrative or conversation and using appropriate language in particular social settings. They often do not understand jokes. These impairments make it difficult for patients with right hemisphere damage to function effectively in social situations, and these patients are sometimes shunned because of their odd behavior.

When adults with severe neurological disease have the entire left hemisphere removed, they suffer a permanent and catastrophic loss of language. In contrast, when the left hemisphere of an infant is removed the child learns to speak fluently. Adults do not have this plasticity of function, and this age difference is consistent with other findings that suggest there is a critical period for language development in childhood. Children can acquire several languages perfectly, whereas most adults who take up a new language are saddled with a foreign accent and permanent grammatical errors. When children are deprived of language input because their parents are deaf or depraved, they can catch up fully if exposed to language before puberty, but they are strikingly inept if the first exposure comes later.

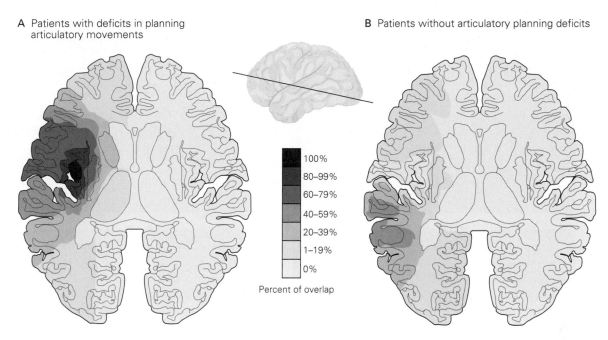

A Patients with deficits in planning articulatory movements

B Patients without articulatory planning deficits

100%
80–99%
60–79%
40–59%
20–39%
1–19%
0%

Percent of overlap

Figure 59-5

A. Lesions of 25 patients with deficits in planning articulatory movements were computer-reconstructed and overlapped. All patients had lesions that included a small section of the insula, an area of cortex underneath the frontal, temporal, and parietal lobes. The area of infarction shared by all patients is depicted here in **dark purple**.

B. The lesions of 19 patients without a deficit in planning articulatory movements were also reconstructed and overlapped. Their lesions completely spare the precise area that was infarcted in the patients with the articulatory deficit. (For this figure, left hemisphere lesions were reconstructed on the left side of the image.)

Despite the remarkable ability of the right hemisphere to take on responsibility for language in young children, it appears to be less suited for the task than the left hemisphere. One study of a small number of children in whom one hemisphere had been removed revealed that the children with only a right hemisphere were impaired in language (and other aspects of intellectual functioning), compared with children who had only a left hemisphere (these children were less impaired overall). Like people with Broca aphasia, children with only a right hemisphere comprehend most sentences in conversation but have trouble interpreting more complex constructions, such as sentences in the passive voice. A child with only a left hemisphere, in contrast, has no difficulty even with complex sentences.

Alexia and Agraphia Are Acquired Disorders of Reading and Writing

Certain brain lesions in adults can cause *alexia* (also known as word blindness), a disruption of the ability to

read, or *agraphia*, a disruption of the ability to write. The two disorders may appear combined or separately, and they may or may not be associated with aphasia, depending on the site of the causative lesion. Reading emerged only recently in history (less than 5000 years ago), and universal literacy is even more recent (less than a century ago). Therefore, pure alexia without aphasia cannot be attributed to impairment of a special "reading system" in the brain but must be caused by a disconnection between the visual and language systems.

Because vision is bilateral and language is lateralized, pure alexia results from disruptions in the transfer of visual information to the language areas of the left hemisphere. In 1892 the French neurologist Jules Dejerine studied an intelligent and highly articulate man who had recently lost the ability to read, even though he could spell, understand words spelled to him, copy written words, and recognize words after writing the individual letters. The patient could not see color in his right visual field, but his vision was otherwise intact in both visual fields. Postmortem examination revealed damage in a critical area of the left occipital region that

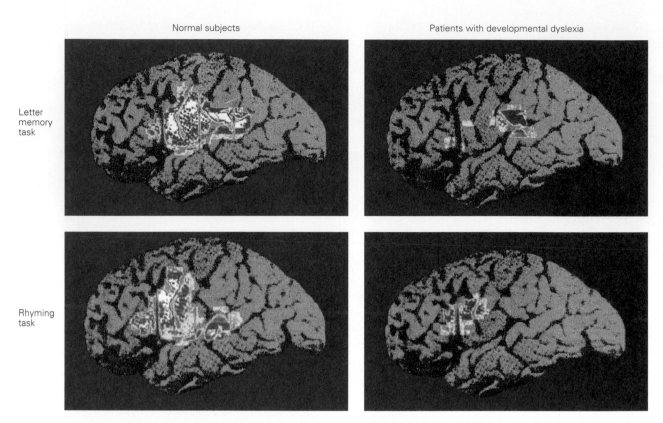

Figure 59-6 Areas of significant change in activity, indexed by perfusion, when subjects performed two language tests. The activated areas are superimposed on a lateral projection of the dominant left hemisphere with the frontal lobe to the left. The two pictures on the **left** are the results from normal subjects and the pictures on the **right** demonstrate results from patients with developmental dyslexia.

Memory task: The upper two images demonstrate activity associated with remembering short lists of letters. In the normal subject an extensive area involving the inferior left frontal cortex, the superior temporal cortex, and the inferior parietal cortex is activated. In dyslexic patients only the inferior parietal and superior temporal cortex are activated.

Rhyming task: During a rhyming task (lower images) that engages inner speech almost exclusively without taxing phonological memory, the inferior frontal and superior temporal cortex are activated in normal subjects, but only the inferior frontal cortex is activated in dyslexic subjects. Thus, dyslexic patients are able to activate each component of the verbal working memory system separately, but, unlike normal subjects, integrated activity between the precentral and postcentral structures appears defective. (Courtesy of R. Frackowiack.)

disrupted the transfer of visually related signals from *both* the left and right visual cortices to language areas in the left hemisphere. The postmortem examination also revealed some damage to the *splenium,* the posterior portion of the corpus callosum that interconnects left and right visual association cortices. This lesion is no longer believed to be involved in pure alexia, however. When the splenium is cut for surgical reasons without damaging visual cortices, the patient can read words normally in the right visual field but not those in the left.

PET studies have shown that reading words and word-like shapes selectively activates extrastriate left cortical areas anterior to the visual cortex. This suggests that the processing of word shapes, like other complex visual qualities, requires that general region.

Developmental Dyslexia Is a Difficulty in Learning to Read

A more prevalent form of reading disorder is seen in children who have difficulty in learning to read and spell despite normal eyesight and hearing, adequate education, and normal IQ. This syndrome, called *developmental dyslexia,* has been estimated to affect between 10 and 30% of the population. As mentioned earlier, reading is a complex and historically recent skill, and it is unlikely that there is a well-defined system in the brain dedicated to it. Many disorders of visual and language processing could disrupt reading, and dyslexia is probably a condition with several possible causes rather than a single syndrome.

Most children with dyslexia have not developed phonological awareness: the ability to attend to individual sounds, particularly phonemes, in the continuous speech wave and to associate them with letters. However, they understand other communicative symbols—such as traffic signs or words—that have a unique visual appearance, such as the Coca Cola trademark. Indeed, studies in the United States have shown that some dyslexic children can learn to read English when entire words are represented by single characters rather than a sequence of characters.

Defects in visual processing can also lead to developmental dyslexia. Similarities between dyslexia and alexia caused by stroke suggest that developmental dyslexia might sometimes result from abnormalities in connections between visual and language areas.

Some dyslexic children also exhibit a tendency to read words backward (eg, confusing *saw* and *was*) and have difficulty distinguishing letters that are mirror images of each other—such as *b* and *d*—both in reading and writing. These errors, together with the disproportionate number of left-handers among dyslexics, suggest that dyslexia might involve a deficit in the development of hemispheric specialization. In fact, in dyslexic males, unlike in normal males, the left planum temporale is not much larger than the right one, and it shows cytoarchitectonic abnormalities, including an incomplete segregation of cell layers and clusters of inappropriately connected neurons. Thus the migration of neurons to the left temporal cortex during development may have been slowed in some dyslexic patients.

Another possible problem in dyslexia is an inability to process transient sensory input quickly. The normally rapid conduction in the magnocellular pathway of the visual system (Chapter 27) is below average in people with dyslexia, whereas conduction in the parvocellular pathway is normal. In particular, dyslexic patients have difficulty processing fast, high-contrast, visual stimuli. A plausible anatomical correlate of this disorder is seen in some dyslexic patients examined at autopsy: the cells in the magnocellular layers of the lateral geniculate nucleus are abnormally small compared to parvocellular layers and compared to magnocellular layers in control subjects. A similar defect is sometimes evident in the fast-conducting component of the auditory pathways (Chapter 30).

In addition to these processing impairments, patients who have developmental difficulties with reading can have other neuropsychological deficits (Figure 59–6). Such linkages must be considered tentative, however, until there is finer delineation of the disorders currently lumped together as dyslexia.

An Overall View

The study of language processing in the brain has come a long way in a century, but the challenges to understanding it are formidable. Great progress has been made since Broca's and Wernicke's seminal discoveries, and that progress has brought a more complete understanding of linguistic processes and an appreciation of the complex ways in which they interconnect with systems for perception, motor control, conceptual knowledge, and attention.

Several developments offer the hope of even greater progress in the near future. Improvements in anatomical imaging will allow more precise and consistent delineation of lesions that affect specific features of language ability, and greater involvement by linguists and experimental psychologists will allow more precise and consistent delineation of the deficits in functioning.

Measurement of brain activity in normal subjects, using PET, functional MRI, and magnetoencephalography (MEG), will become more important in the next few years as the spatial and temporal resolution of these techniques improves and the most sophisticated experimental paradigms and linguistic analyses are systematically applied. Neurosurgical candidates, whose brain functions must be mapped by stimulation during surgery or recording from implanted electrode grids that remain in the skull during everyday activities, will be an important source of fine-grained information, especially if the language tasks administered to them are carefully constructed to isolate functions.

Progress in the understanding of language is important for the advancement of fundamental neuroscience and indispensable for the treatment of patients with aphasia, which is by far the most frequent impairment of higher function caused by stroke and head injury. The astonishing feat of language is too complex to be understood with the tools of any single academic or medical specialty, but as several disciplines come together to study the underlying neural processes, we can expect significant breakthroughs.

Nina F. Dronkers
Steven Pinker
Antonio Damasio

Selected Readings

Damasio AR, Damasio H. 1992. Brain and language. Sci Am 267:88–95.

Dronkers NF. 1999. The neural basis of language. In: R Wilson, F Keil (eds). *The MIT Encyclopedia of the Cognitive Sciences*, pp. 448–451. Cambridge: MIT Press.

Fromkin V, Rodman R. 1997. *An Introduction to Language*, 6th ed. New York: Harcourt Brace Jovanovich.

Goodglass H. 1993. *Understanding Aphasia*. San Diego: Academic.

Pinker S. 1994. *The Language Instinct*. New York: William Morrow.

References

Baddeley AD, Hitch GJ. 1994. Developments in the concept of working memory. Neuropsychology 8:485–493.

Basso A, Lecours AR, Moraschini S, Vanier M. 1985. Anatomoclinical correlations of the aphasias as defined through computerized tomography: exceptions. Brain Lang 26:201–229.

Bates E, Wulfeck B, MacWhinney B. 1991. Cross-linguistic research in aphasia: an overview. Brain Lang 41:123–148.

Baynes K. 1990. Language and reading in the right hemisphere: highways or byways of the brain? J Cogn Neurosci 2:159–179.

Bishop DV. 1983. Linguistic impairment after left hemidecortication for infantile hemiplegia? A reappraisal. Q J Exp Psychol [A]35:199–207.

Broca P. 1861. Remarques sur le siegè de la faculté du langage articulé, suivies d'une observation d'aphemie (perte de la parole). Bulletin Société Anatomique de Paris 6:330–357.

Caplan D. 1987. *Neurolinguistics and Linguistic Aphasiology: An Introduction*. Cambridge: Cambridge Univ. Press.

Caramazza A, Zurif EB. 1976. Dissociation of algorithmic and heuristic processes in language comprehension: evidence from aphasia. Brain Lang 3:572–582.

Chomsky N. 1991. Linguistics and cognitive science: problems and mysteries. In: A Kasher (ed). *The Chomskyan Turn*. Cambridge, MA: Blackwell.

Cornell TL, Fromkin VA, Mauner G. 1993. A linguistic approach to language processing in Broca's aphasia: a paradox resolved. Curr Direct Psychol Sci 2:47–52.

Damasio AR. 1992. Aphasia. N Engl J Med 326:531–539.

Damasio AR. 1990. Category-related recognition defects as a clue to the neural substrates of knowledge. Trends Neurosci 13:95–98.

Damasio AR, Geschwind N. 1984. The neural basis of language. Annu Rev Neurosci 7:127–147.

Damasio AR, Tranel D. 1993. Nouns and verbs are retrieved with differently distributed neural systems. Proc Natl Acad Sci U S A 90:4957–4960.

Damasio H, Damasio AR. 1989. *Lesion Analysis in Neuropsychology*. New York: Oxford Univ. Press.

Damasio H, Grabowski TJ, Tranel D, Hichwa RD, Damasio AR. 1996. A neural basis for lexical retrieval. Nature 380:499–505.

Darwin CR. 1874. *The Descent of Man and Selection in Relation to Sex*, 2nd ed, pp. 101–102. New York: Hurst.

Deacon TW. 1997. *The Symbolic Species: The Co-Evolution of Language and the Brain*. New York: Norton.

Dejerine J. 1892. Contribution a l'étude anatomopathologique et clinique des differentes varietés de cecité verbale. Memoires Societé Biologique 4:61–90.

Demonet JF, Chollet F, Ramsay S, Cardebat D, Nespoulous JL, Wise R, Rascol A, Frackowiak R. 1992. The anatomy of phonological and semantic processing in normal subjects. Brain 115:1753–1768.

Dennis M, Whitaker HA. 1976. Language acquisition following hemidecortication: linguistic superiority of the left over the right hemisphere. Brain Lang 3:404–433.

Dronkers NF. 1996. A new brain region for coordinating speech articulation. Nature 384:159–161.

Etcoff NL. 1989. Asymmetries in recognition of emotion. In: F Boller, J Grafman (eds). *Handbook of Neuropsychology*, 3:363–382. New York: Elsevier.

Etcoff NL. 1986. The neuropsychology of emotional expression. In: G Goldstein, RE Tarter (eds). *Advances in Clinical Neuropsychology*, 3:127–179. New York: Plenum.

Galaburda AM. 1994. Developmental dyslexia and animal studies: at the interface between cognition and neurology. Cognition 50:133–149.

Gardner H, Brownell H, Wapner W, Michelow D. 1983. Missing the point: the role of the right hemisphere in the processing of complex linguistic materials. In: E Perecman (ed). *Cognitive Processes in the Right Hemisphere*. New York: Academic.

Gardner RA, Gardner BT. 1969. Teaching sign language to a chimpanzee. Science 165:664–672.

Gazzaniga MS. 1983. Right hemisphere language following brain bisection: a 20-year perspective. Am Psychologist 38:525–549.

Geschwind N. 1965. Disconnexion syndromes in animals and man II. Brain 88:585–644.

Geschwind N. 1970. The organization of language and the brain. Science 170:940–944.

Grodzinsky Y. 1990. *Theoretical Perspectives on Language Deficits*. Cambridge, MA: MIT Press.

Hauser M. 1996. *The Evolution of Communication*. Cambridge, MA: MIT Press.

Jackendoff R. 1994. *Patterns in the Mind*. New York: Basic Books.

Lesser RP, Arroyo S, Hart J, Gordon B. 1994. Use of subdural electrodes for the study of language functions. In: A Kertesz (ed). *Localization and Neuroimaging in Neuropsychology*, pp. 57–72. San Diego: Academic.

Linebarger MC, Schwartz MF, Saffran EM. 1983. Sensitivity to grammatical structure in so-called agrammatic aphasics. Cognition 13:361–392.

Mazoyer BM, Tzourio N, Frak V, Syrota A, Murayama N, Levrier O, Salamon G, Dehaene S, Cohen L, Mehler J. 1993. The cortical representation of speech. J Cogn Neurosci 5:467–479.

Mazzocchi F, Vignolo LA. 1979. Localization of lesions in

aphasia: clinical CT scan correlations in stroke patients. Cortex 15:627–653.

Naeser MA, Hayward RW. 1978. Lesion localization in aphasia with cranial computed tomography and the Boston Diagnostic Aphasia Exam. Neurology 28:545–551.

Ojemann G. 1994. Cortical stimulation and recording in language. In: A Kertesz (ed). *Localization and Neuroimaging in Neuropsychology,* pp. 35–55. San Diego: Academic.

Paulesu E, Frith CD, Frackowiak RJ. 1993. The neural correlates of the verbal component of working memory. Nature 362:342–345.

Penfield W, Roberts L. 1959. *Speech and Brain Mechanisms.* Princeton, NJ: Princeton Univ. Press.

Petersen SE, Fox PT, Posner MI, Mintun M, Raichle ME. 1988. Positron emission tomographic studies of the cortical anatomy of single-word processing. Nature 331:585–589.

Pinker S, Bloom P. 1990. Natural language and natural selection. Behav Brain Sci 13:707–784.

Rapp BC, Caramazza A. 1995. Disorders of lexical processing and the lexicon. In: M Gazzaniga (ed). *The Cognitive Neurosciences.* Cambridge, MA: MIT Press.

Seidenberg MS. 1986. Evidence from the great apes concerning the biological basis of language. In: W Demopoulos, A Marras (eds). *Language Learning and Concept Acquisition: Foundational Issues.* Norwood, NJ: Ablex.

Seidenberg MS, Petitto LA. 1979. Signing behavior in apes: a critical review. Cognition 7:177–215.

Shaywitz SE. 1998. Dyslexia. New Engl J Med 338:307–312.

Stromswold K, Caplan D, Alpert N, Rauch S. 1996. Localization syntactic comprehension by using positron emission tomography. Brain Lang 52:452–473.

Terrace HS, Petitto LA, Sanders RJ, Bever TG. 1979. Can an ape create a sentence? Science 206:891–902.

Ullman M, Corkin S, Coppola M, Hickok G, Growdon JH, Koroshetz WJ, Pinker S. 1997. A neural dissociation within language: evidence that the mental dictionary is part of declarative memory, and that grammatical rules are processed by the procedural system. J Cogn Neurosci 9:289–299.

Wallman J. 1992. *Aping Language.* New York: Cambridge Univ. Press.

Wernicke C. 1874. *Der Aphasische Symptomencomplex.* Breslau: Kohn and Weigert.

Wertz RT, LaPointe LL, Rosenbek JC. 1984. *Apraxia of Speech in Adults: The Disorder and Its Management.* Orlando, FL: Grune & Stratton.

Zaidel E. 1990. Language functions in the two hemispheres following complete commissurotomy and hemispherectomy. In: F Boller, J Grafman (eds). *Handbook of Neuropsychology.* New York: Elsevier.

Zurif EB, Caramazza A, Myerson R. 1972. Grammatical judgments of agrammatic aphasics. Neuropsychologia 10:405–417.

60

Disorders of Thought and Volition: Schizophrenia

THE SUCCESS OF NEUROBIOLOGY in providing insights into perception and language has inspired biological investigation into thought and mood and their disorders. In this chapter and the next we examine the four most serious disorders of thinking and mood: schizophrenia, depression, mania, and the anxiety states. These disorders involve disturbances in thought, self-awareness, perception, affect, volition, and social interaction.

In addition to being scientifically challenging, mental illness is of great social importance. Fully 10% of people with schizophrenia commit suicide. Many more are homeless. Before the advent of psychopharmacologic agents, schizophrenia and the affective disorders accounted for more than half of all hospital admissions in the United States. Even now schizophrenia accounts for about 30% of *all* hospitalizations.

Mental Illnesses Can Be Diagnosed Using Classical Medical Criteria

In medicine the term *disease* refers to a cluster of symptoms and signs that results from a specific cause and leads through a defined course to a specific outcome. As with other diseases of the brain, the analysis of a mental disease requires good delineation of the symptoms and signs. Ideally, a diagnosis is based on two additional factors: (1) a clear and evident *causative agent* (whether the illness results from a genetic abnormality, a viral or bacterial infection, toxins, tumors, or stress) and (2) a plausible *pathogenesis* (a clear idea of the mechanism by which the causative agent produces the disease).

Unfortunately, unlike most other medical illnesses, the causes and pathogenesis of most mental illnesses have not, as yet, been determined with certainty. As a result, psychiatric disorders are to a large extent still grouped today as they were in other areas of medicine at the beginning of the twentieth century. In other areas of medicine diseases were once grouped according to organ systems: lung, heart, gastrointestinal system, etc.

Likewise, in psychiatry diseases were grouped according to which of the four major mental systems was affected: cognition, affect, intelligence, or social behavior. Thus the diseases are categorized as follows: (1) disorders of cognition (schizophrenia and delirium); (2) disorders of mood (affective disorders and anxiety states); (3) disorders of learning, memory, and intelligence (mental retardation and dementia); and (4) disorders of social behavior (personality disorders).

This classification derives importantly from the work at the turn of the century by Emil Kraepelin, the director of the Psychiatry Clinic at the University of Heidelberg in Germany. Before Kraepelin's initiative psychiatrists did not think of mental illnesses as diseases with a specific onset, progression, and outcome. They classified symptoms along arbitrary lines that had no medical significance. Influenced by Rudolf Virchow, the German pioneer of cellular pathology, and Thomas Sydenham, the English clinician who focused attention on the course of disease, Kraepelin began to study the disorders of mental faculties as specific disease processes. Kraepelin argued that even in the absence of empirical knowledge about etiology and pathogenesis, diseases of the mind could be distinguished descriptively on the basis of two classical approaches that had been followed in other areas of medicine.

First, mental disorders can be classified on the basis of signs (what the examiner sees) and symptoms (what the patient reports). Of course, the presentation of a single sign or symptom is not in itself evidence for disease, since it may occur in healthy people. But when certain signs and symptoms occur together in several patients, they are said to form a *syndrome,* a condition that can be distinguished from normal behavior or from other clusters of signs and symptoms.

Second, a mental disorder can be characterized on the basis of its *natural history,* by tracing the emergence of signs and symptoms at specific times in the patient's life and the evolution of these symptoms over time. Thus, a syndrome may be present at a characteristic age or be associated with a specific event, or it may follow a characteristic clinical course. For example, at least 33% of patients with schizophrenia deteriorate progressively, whereas most patients with the major affective disorders show cycles of relapse and recovery.

Since Kraepelin's pioneering work both approaches have been used to delineate a mental disease. The delineation of a mental disease can, in principle, be refined further by one of three measures:

1. *Response to specific treatment.* A disease may respond specifically to a class of drugs that are not effective against other diseases. For example, manic-depressive illness responds to lithium, but other mental illnesses do not.

2. *Pathologic condition.* The clinical diagnosis of diseases of the heart, lung, kidney, and intestines, and even many neurological diseases, can be confirmed by examining the structural and functional changes in the diseased tissue, and this examination in turn provides information about the pathogenesis of disease. The absence of anatomically demonstrable pathologic conditions distinguishes diseases of the mind from those of other areas of medicine, including neurology. Huntington disease, for example, is associated with a lesion in the head of the caudate nucleus.

3. *Causality.* To conclude that a syndrome is the manifestation of a specific disease, specific causative agents must be identified. A syndrome need not have a single cause and therefore need not be a unitary disease. For example, the syndrome of pneumonia can be caused by different bacteria or different viruses giving rise to different specific diseases. The discovery of a specific molecular abnormality can provide particularly powerful insight into the cause of a disease. For example, in Duchenne muscular dystrophy the membrane-associated protein dystrophin is always absent or abnormal because of abnormalities in the gene encoding the protein.

Unfortunately, the pathogenesis of most psychiatric disorders has yet to be demonstrated. The defects underlying most psychiatric disorders are thought to involve subtle genetic, molecular, and anatomical changes, and these changes have remained elusive.

Psychiatric diagnosis therefore must rely heavily on the individual patient's history and the patient's response to treatment. Yet these clinical features can be hard to determine and even harder to quantify. In the past these limitations made it difficult to achieve consensus in the evaluation of psychiatric symptoms and to investigate psychiatric illness systematically. Today, however, substantial progress has been made in diagnosing mental illness and, as we shall see later, there is reason to hope that a genuine neuropathology of mental illness may emerge soon.

Schizophrenia Is Likely to Be Several Related Disorders

Schizophrenia is perhaps the most devastating disorder of humankind. Fairly common, it strikes about 1% of the population worldwide, and it seems to affect men

Box 60-1 The Functional Neuroanatomy of Hallucinations in Schizophrenia

Imaging studies are beginning to shed light on the functional anatomy of hallucinations in schizophrenia. Frank Middleton and Peter Strick found that the basal ganglia, which are known to receive input from widespread areas of the cerebral cortex, including the frontal, parietal, and temporal lobes, project to both the frontal and the inferotemporal cortex.

The inferotemporal cortex is critically involved in the recognition and discrimination of visual objects and is the area disturbed in prosopagnosia, a disorder concerned with the recognition of faces (Chapters 25 and 28). The output nuclei of the basal ganglia—the substantia nigra pars reticulata—project via the thalamus to the inferotemporal cortex. Thus, the inferotemporal cortex is not only a source of input to the basal ganglia but also a target of basal ganglia output (Figure 60-1).

This result implies that the basal ganglia can influence higher-order visual processing, and that the basal ganglia loop may lead to alterations in visual perception, including visual hallucinations characteristic of schizophrenia. In fact, visual hallucinations are a major side effect of L-DOPA and other dopaminergic agents used in the treatment of Parkinson disease. Approximately 30% of patients with Parkinson disease treated in this manner experience this peculiar side effect.

The hallucinations in these patients may be due to excessive stimulation of the dopamine receptors in the visual striatum, which leads to a net increase in activity in the nucleus pars reticulata and thus abnormal increases in thalamic input to the inferotemporal cortex. Brain images of schizophrenic patients experiencing hallucinations support this hypothesis; the subjects display significant changes in blood flow at several brain sites that are part of the inferotemporal system (Figure 60-2).

Figure 60-1 Proposed loop between the basal ganglia and the inferotemporal cortex. In a series of PET studies five patients with classical auditory-verbal hallucinations received medication yet still hallucinated. PET scans taken during hallucinations demonstrated activation of thalamic and striatal nuclei as well as of the hippocampus, the paralimbic region, the cingulate cortex, and the orbitofrontal cortex. One patient who had never received drugs had visual as well as auditory hallucinations. That patient showed activation in visual and auditory language association cortices near Wernicke's area, part of a distributed cortical network involved in the hallucinations. The interaction of these distributed neural systems may provide a neuroanatomical basis for the bizarre behavior of patients with schizophrenia. The prominent feature in this group of patients is involvement of the thalamus and the lack of activation of Broca's area. **Shading** indicates the portion of each structure that contributes to the circuit. (Based on Silbersweig et al. 1995.)

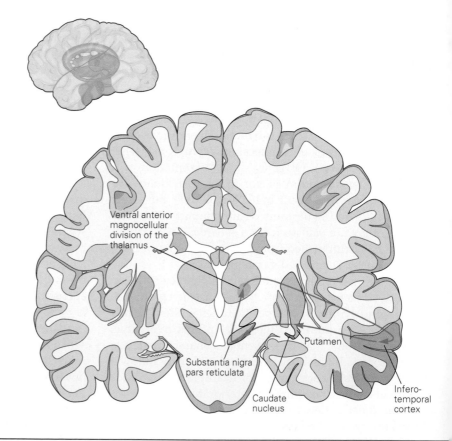

slightly more frequently and severely than it does women. In addition to the 1% with schizophrenia, another 2–3% of the general population have *schizotypal personality disorder,* which is often considered to be a milder form of the disease because patients do not manifest overtly psychotic behavior.

In 1990 the annual cost of caring for patients with schizophrenia in the United States was estimated to be $33 billion. This cost accounts for about 2.5% of the total annual expenditures for health care in the United States. Even more disturbing is the estimate that about 30% of all the homeless people in the United States have schizo-

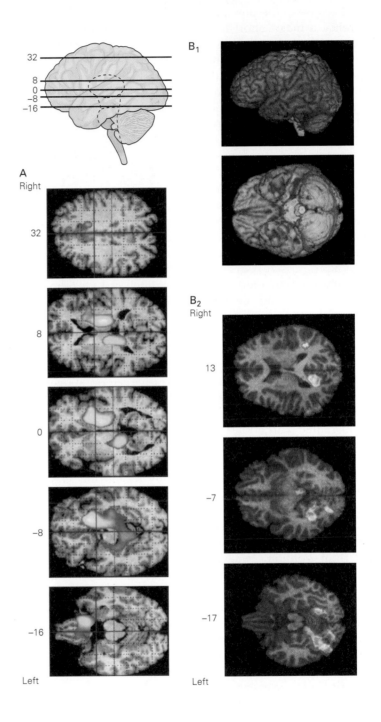

Figure 60-2

A. Increased activity in the brain during auditory-verbal hallucinations. Functional PET results (**yellow** and **orange**) are superimposed on a magnetic resonance image for anatomical reference. Section numbers refer to the distance from the anterior commissure–posterior commissure line, with positive numbers being superior to the line. Activation (**yellow**) extends into the amygdala bilaterally and the right orbitofrontal cortex. These regions are consistent with activation of limbic, paralimbic, and inferotemporal system during hallucinations.

B.1. Two surface projections (left lateral and ventral) show brain areas with significantly increased activity during visual and auditory-verbal hallucinations. **2.** Functional PET results (**yellow** and **orange**) are superimposed on the structural T_1 weighted MRI scan, illustrating several areas of activation.

phrenia, and the homeless are not likely to be beneficiaries of the health care system. Thus the substantial funds being spent on the treatment of schizophrenia reach only a fraction of those afflicted with the disease. The increase in the incidence of schizophrenia among the homeless in the United States dates to 1960, with the movement away from institutional treatment for schizophrenia. (Before 1960 patients with schizophrenia were almost routinely committed for long-term in-hospital care.) At the same time, adequate community outpatient facilities have not been developed to handle the social problems of patients with chronic schizophrenia.

Because of the prevalence and social cost of schizophrenia, a major effort has been expended to develop better criteria for diagnosing the illness. More precise criteria have emerged only recently. In the early 1900s two majors types of mental disorders had been well delineated: *senile dementia,* the loss of cognitive capacities in certain elderly people (a disease we now recognize as Alzheimer disease), and *personality disorders,* disorders of social behavior. Based on a review of the signs and symptoms as well as long-term progress of hundreds of patients with a variety of mental disorders, Kraepelin defined two new syndromes.

One new syndrome he called *dementia praecox* (early deterioration of the intellect) because of its early age of onset (typically in adolescence as compared to senile dementia). Kraepelin observed that this syndrome often follows a progressive course without remission, leading ultimately to a dramatic deterioration of intellect. Kraepelin called the second newly defined syndrome *manic-depressive psychosis.* This condition usually has different symptoms—disturbances of mood rather than intellect—but most important it also has a very different course. Characteristically, the onset is later and is marked by remissions and relapses without progressive deterioration.

Eugen Bleuler objected to the term *dementia praecox* because he saw some patients who became sick in adulthood rather than adolescence and other patients who occasionally experienced remission. He concluded that the symptoms described by Kraepelin did not reflect a single disease, but a group of closely related illnesses characterized by a specific disorder of cognition rather than a general deterioration of intellect (*dementia*). He proposed that the disorder was a fragmentation of the mind, with the result that cognitive processes were split off from volition, behavior, and emotion. Therefore Bleuler called this group of illnesses *schizophrenia,* a splitting of the mind. (This condition is not to be confused with multiple or split personalities, an uncommon disease in which a person alternately assumes two or more identities.) People with schizophrenia may show evidence of this splitting of the mind by having inappropriate *affect* (emotion). They may laugh while recounting a tragic event or may show no emotion (a flat affect) while describing a joyous occasion.

Schizophrenia is characterized by *psychotic episodes*—discrete, often reversible, mental states in which some of the patient's thought processes are not able to test reality correctly. During a psychotic episode patients are unable to examine their beliefs and perceptions realistically and to compare them to what is actually happening in the world. This *loss of reality testing* is accompanied by other disturbances of higher mental functioning, especially delusions (aberrant beliefs that fly in the face of facts and are not changed by evidence that the beliefs are unreasonable), hallucinations (Box 60-1), incoherent thinking, disordered memory, and sometimes confusion. For example, people with schizophrenia often hear internal voices (auditory hallucinations) that tell them things that are not true, for example that their parents are trying to poison them.

Psychotic episodes are not unique to schizophrenia and often also occur in affective disorders, brief reactive states, and states of toxic delirium (for example, psychosis resulting from the use of phencyclidine, also known as PCP or angel dust, which we shall learn about later). Using modern descriptive approaches, as given in the revised fourth edition of the *Diagnostic and Statistical Manual of the American Psychiatric Association* (DSM-IV), psychiatrists are now able to differentiate schizophrenia more clearly from other psychotic disorders with similar features that were formerly lumped with schizophrenia into a common diagnostic category. Modern diagnostic criteria include not only those features required to *make* the diagnosis (*inclusive criteria*) but also those that would cause one to *reject* it (*exclusive criteria*). Moreover, in actual clinical contexts independent observers agree on the usefulness of DSM-IV criteria in achieving accurate diagnoses.

Psychotic Episodes Are Preceded by Prodromal Signs and Followed by Residual Symptoms

The first psychotic episode of schizophrenia is often preceded by *prodromal signs.* These include social isolation and withdrawal, impairment in the normal fulfillment of expected roles, odd behavior and ideas, neglect of personal hygiene, and blunted affect. The prodromal period is then followed by one or more psychotic episodes that may include loss of reality testing, memory disturbances, delusions, and hallucinations. These episodes are sometimes separated by long periods in which the patient is not overtly psychotic but nonetheless behaves eccentrically, is socially isolated, and has a low level of emotional arousal (a flat affect), an impoverished social drive, poverty of speech, a poor attention span, and lack of motivation.

These symptoms of the nonpsychotic period are called *negative symptoms* because they reflect the absence of certain normal social and interpersonal behaviors. In contrast, the striking abnormalities of psychotic episodes are called *positive symptoms* because they reflect the presence of distinctively abnormal behaviors. The negative symptoms are chronic features of the illness and are the most difficult to manage.

Modern criteria for the diagnosis of schizophrenia require that a patient be continuously ill for at least six months and that there be at least one psychotic phase followed by a residual phase. During the psychotic episode one or more of the following three groups of positive symptoms must be present:

1. Delusions (for example, the belief that one is being persecuted or that one's feelings, thoughts, and actions are controlled by an outside force).
2. Prominent hallucinations, usually auditory (for example, hearing voices commenting on one's actions).
3. Disordered thoughts, incoherence, loss of the normal association between ideas, or marked poverty of speech accompanied by a loss of emotional expression (flattening of affect).

During psychotic episodes patients with schizophrenia may also exhibit unusual postures, mannerisms, or rigidity. On the basis of these criteria and other differences, schizophrenia is often divided into subtypes, of which three are most readily distinguished: *paranoid schizophrenia,* a form more often found in men, in which systematic delusions of persecution predominate; *disorganized schizophrenia* (hebephrenia), a form characterized by early age of onset, a wide range of symptoms, and a profound deterioration of personality; and *catatonic schizophrenia,* a rare form in which mutism and abnormal postures dominate.

In diagnosing schizophrenia it is important to exclude a disorder of mood, especially manic-depressive illness or a drug-induced psychosis resulting from the use of amphetamine, PCP, or other psychostimulants. The prognosis for schizophrenia is generally (but not always) poor. There are frequent relapses into psychotic behavior, and each relapse in turn results in greater deterioration.

Some students of schizophrenia view the psychotic episodes (positive symptoms) and nonpsychotic episodes (negative symptoms) as different phases of the same disease, with the negative symptoms representing the long-term outcome of positive symptoms. However, other students of schizophrenia view the two types of symptoms as independent, arguing that negative and positive symptoms reflect two distinctive courses and underlying psychopathologies. According to this second view, patients in whom the negative symptoms predominate have a more severe illness, one in which the prognosis is poorer and in which, as we shall see later, there is more of a disturbance in the anatomy of the brain, especially more prominently enlarged ventricles, and more loss of cortical tissue. Negative symptoms are often associated with a history of poor social development before the onset of the disease, and this history of

social withdrawal is perhaps the strongest predictor of a poor prognosis.

Genetic Predisposition Is an Important Factor

Identifying the causes of schizophrenia is one of the most challenging goals of psychiatric research. The only reliable clue as to cause comes from the finding that schizophrenia is due in part to a genetic abnormality.

The first direct evidence that genes are important in the development of schizophrenia was provided in the 1930s by Franz Kallmann. Kallmann was impressed when he discovered that the incidence of schizophrenia throughout the world is uniformly about 1%, even though social and environmental factors vary dramatically. He found, however, that the incidence of schizophrenia among parents, children, and siblings of patients with the disease is about 15%, strong evidence that the disease runs in families. A genetic basis for schizophrenia cannot simply be inferred from the increased incidence in families, however. Not all conditions that run in families are necessarily genetic—wealth and poverty and habits and values also run in families. In earlier times even the nutritional deficiency pellagra ran in families.

To distinguish genetic from environmental factors, Kallmann and other investigators developed several research strategies. One strategy was to compare the rates of illness in monozygotic (identical) and dizygotic (fraternal) twins. Monozygotic twins have essentially identical genomes; they share almost 100% of each other's genes. In contrast, dizygotic twins share only 50% of their genes and are genetically equivalent to siblings. If schizophrenia were caused entirely by genetic factors, monozygotic twins would have an identical tendency to have the disease develop. Even if genetic factors were necessary but not sufficient for the development of schizophrenia, because environmental factors were also involved, the monozygotic twin of a patient with schizophrenia would still be at significantly higher risk than a dizygotic twin. The tendency for twins to have the same illness is called *concordance.* Studies of twins have established that the concordance for schizophrenia in monozygotic twins is about 45%, but in dizygotic twins only about 15%, about the same as for other siblings.

However, the high concordance in identical twins is still insufficient evidence for a genetic basis for schizophrenia, which can be explained as being acquired by learning from the disturbed behavior of the parents. To address this issue, and to disentangle further the effects of nature and nurture, Leonard Heston studied the rate of schizophrenia among adoptees in the United States, and Seymour Kety, David Rosenthal, and Paul Wender

Table 60-1 Evidence for the Importance of Genetic Factors in Schizophrenia[a]

	Biological relatives		Adoptive relatives	
	With schizophrenia	Control	With schizophrenia	Control
Chronic schizophrenia	2.9%[b]	0%	1.4%	1.1%
Latent schizophrenia	3.5	1.7	0	1.1
Schizophrenia, uncertain subtype	7.5[a]	1.7	1.4	3.3
Total	14.0[a]	3.4	2.7	5.5

[a]Adapted from Kety et al. 1975.
[b]Statistically significant.

studied adoptees in Denmark. In both sets of studies the rate of schizophrenia was higher among the biological relatives of schizophrenic adoptees than among relatives of normal adoptees. The difference in rate, about 10–15%, was the same observed earlier by Kallmann (Table 60-1). In addition to documenting the importance of genetic factors in schizophrenia, these studies of adoptees in whom schizophrenia developed showed that rearing does not play a major role in the disease.

Studies of adoptees further revealed that some of the blood relatives of adoptees with schizophrenia show odd behavior even if they do not manifest signs of schizophrenia—they are socially isolated, have poor rapport with people, ramble in their speech, tend to be suspicious, have eccentric beliefs, and engage in magical thinking. This group of symptoms, called *schizotypal personality disorder,* is thought to be a mild form of the disease, a nonpsychotic condition related to schizophrenia.

The familial pattern of schizophrenia is most dramatically illustrated in an analysis by Irving Gottesman, who ranked the relatives of Danish schizophrenics by the percentage of genes shared with the patient. He found a higher incidence of schizophrenia among first-order relatives (those who share 50% of the patient's genes, including siblings, parents, and children) than among second-order relatives (those who share 25% of the patient's genes, including aunts, uncles, nieces, nephews, and grandchildren). Even the third-degree relatives, who share only 12.5% of the patient's genes, had a higher incidence of schizophrenia than the 1% found in the population at large (Figure 60-3). These data strongly support a genetic contribution to schizophrenia.

If schizophrenia were caused entirely by genetic abnormalities, then the concordance rate for monozygotic twins, who share almost 100% of each other's genes, would be nearly 100%. The finding that the concordance rate in monozygotic twins is only about 45% indicates that the genetic transmission is unusual and that genetic factors are not the only cause.

Relatively routine studies of pedigrees often are sufficient to decide whether the mode of transmission of a disease is the classical dominant or recessive Mendelian inheritance of a single gene controlling the critical trait that is disordered. For example, Huntington disease is expressed in nearly 100% of those who carry the gene mutations associated with the disease at a single allele of the gene, and there are only minor nongenetic influences in the expression of this disease. Thus it could be said from pedigree inspection of Huntington disease, even before the mutant gene was discovered, that the disease is rare and fully penetrant and that all the symptoms are due to the transmission of a single dominant gene.

Schizophrenia clearly does not have this mode of transmission. Nor does it have the simple recessive node of such diseases as phenylketonuria, in which both alleles of a single gene have to be defective for the clinical phenotype to be evident. In simple recessive disease neither parent may have the disease but one in four children will.

The most likely explanation for the unusual genetic transmission of schizophrenia—its high frequency of 1% and its partial penetrance—is that the illness is polygenic, involving in any given case perhaps as many as 3 to 10 genes. As with other polygenic diseases, such as diabetes and hypertension, it is possible that one or all of the critical genes are simply allelic variations— polymorphisms—of genes, each one of which by itself would not cause disease. Rather it is the *combination* of allelic polymorphisms in the context of a specific genetic background that is critical for the disease.

As this argument makes clear, in the case of polygenic diseases the distinction between mutations and allelic variations is not black and white. This is perhaps

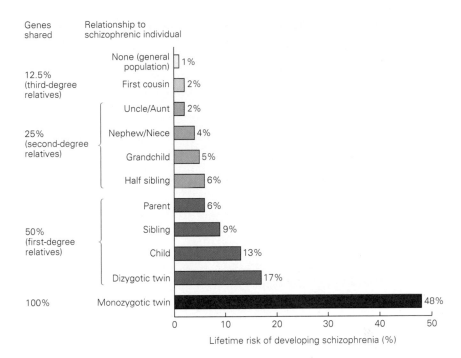

Figure 60-3 The lifetime risk for schizophrenia is correlated with genetic relatedness to a person with schizophrenia. (From Gottesman 1991.)

not surprising. With the exception of the genes that determine gender identity, people in the population at large do not differ from one another because they have different genes. We all have mainly the same genes. What distinguishes each of us from one another are a number of different alleles of the same genes.

The idea that schizophrenia is a polygenic disease is consistent with the evidence from other areas of behavioral genetics, which suggests that the normal range of variation for a given behavior or character type usually reflects the combined actions of many genes, each with only a small effect. Acting alone, most alleles alter behavior only subtly if at all. In fact, as we have learned, an allele that contributes to schizophrenia is not necessarily a mutation.

A search for particular allelic variations is now under way, applying genetic linkage analysis that makes use of both restriction fragment length polymorphisms and short tandem repeat polymorphisms that might contribute to schizophrenia. Recent studies of schizophrenia have uncovered two possible loci that correlate with schizophrenia. One locus is on the long arm of chromosome 22 (22q). The other is on chromosome 6 (6p). In each case the locus has been narrowed to a region containing about 50–100 genes.

Prominent Anatomical Abnormalities in the Brain Occur in Some Cases of Schizophrenia

Computerized tomography, magnetic resonance imaging, and cerebral blood flow studies have revealed that *some* patients with schizophrenia have one or more of four major anatomical abnormalities. First, early in the disease there is a reduction in the blood flow to the left globus pallidus (Figure 60-4), suggestive of a disturbance in the system that connects the basal ganglia to the frontal lobes. Second, there appears to be a disturbance in the frontal lobes themselves since blood flow does not increase during tests of frontal lobe function involving working memory, as it does in normal subjects. Third, the cortex of the medial temporal lobe is thinner and the anterior portion of the hippocampus is smaller than in normal people, especially on the left side, consistent with a defect in memory. Finally, the lateral and third ventricles are enlarged and there is widening of the sulci, especially in the thinner temporal lobe and in the frontal lobe, reflecting a reduction in the volume of this lobe as well.

The reduction in blood flow in the caudate nucleus and the frontal lobe, the reduced size of the hippocampus, the slightly enlarged ventricles, and the other structural changes of the brain are most commonly seen in patients who have prominent negative symptoms. These patients have a history of a prolonged prodromal period with poor social functioning before the onset of psychotic symptoms, suggesting that the disease starts early in life.

What is the relationship of these anatomical abnormalities to the genetic predisposition for schizophrenia? This question has been examined in a study of monozygotic twin pairs of which only one twin had schizophrenia. In 12 of 15 cases examined, the twin with

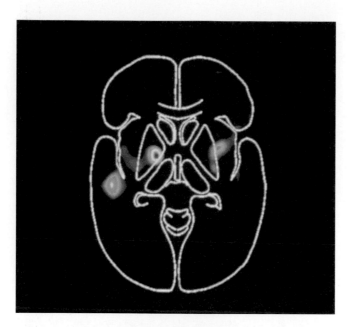

Figure 60-4 Reduced blood flow in the left globus pallidus is one of the first anatomical abnormalities to appear in brain scans of patients with schizophrenia. This defect is thought to reflect a disturbance in an attentional system that involves both the basal ganglia and the frontal lobes.

schizophrenia had larger ventricles compared to the normal twin (Figure 60-5). The twin with schizophrenia almost invariably also had a smaller anterior hippocampus on the left side, and this reduction in hippocampal mass correlated highly with the reduction in blood flow in the left prefrontal cortex. Moreover, the smaller the hippocampal volume of the affected twin, the less the left prefrontal cortex was activated during a cognitive task. These several anatomical findings therefore suggest that the hippocampus, the prefrontal cortex, and the globus pallidus are part of a cognitive system that is impaired in schizophrenia.

Indeed, the negative symptoms of schizophrenia, which include a loss of executive functions such as planning and working memory, involve activities that normally require the prefrontal association areas (Chapter 19). In monkeys, for example, activation of these executive functions is correlated with increased metabolism in a distributed network that includes the anterior hippocampus, parietal cortex, and dorsolateral prefrontal cortex. A disturbance in this network could contribute to the negative symptoms of schizophrenia.

A Two-Step Model Seems Most Consistent With the Pathogenesis of Schizophrenia

The fact that twins who share identical genes have anatomical differences in their brains suggests that

genes alone do not account for these structural changes. Rather, the structural changes presumably result from the combined actions of genes and some factors other than a genetic defect, perhaps a viral infection, a developmental abnormality, or a perinatal injury. Thus the development of schizophrenia may be a two-step process in which genetic predisposition is necessary but insufficient to produce the disease.

The possibility that developmental injury may be a causative agent in a two-step process that leads to schizophrenia is currently receiving much attention. Indeed, among the several anatomical defects that have been associated with schizophrenia, one developmental abnormality observed in a small group of patients by Edward Jones and his colleagues seems particularly interesting. This abnormality occurs in a population of neurons characterized histochemically by staining for the enzyme nicotinamide adenine dinucleotide phosphate diaphorase.[1] In normal people these neurons are found in white matter immediately below layer VI of the cortex. These neurons are part of the *cortical subplate,* a transitional structure that plays a key role in the formation of connections in the cerebral cortex (Chapter 53).

In patients with schizophrenia the number of these neurons in the superficial white matter of both the prefrontal and temporal lobe cortices is significantly reduced, whereas their number in the white matter deeper than 3 mm from the cortex is significantly greater compared to normal subjects. These differences suggest that, rather than remaining in the subplate region as they normally do, these neurons underwent abnormal migration during development. Since the subplate neurons are required for cortical development (Chapter 55), such a defect could lead to the establishment of abnormal patterns of cortical connections in the frontal and temporal lobes, the association areas thought to underlie the negative symptoms commonly observed in schizophrenia, and could contribute to their potential dysfunction.

What accounts for this disturbance in development? Some studies suggest that infants exposed to influenza during the second and third trimesters of gestation may have an increased risk for developing schizophrenia when they become adults, so that a viral infection during the mother's pregnancy might be responsible for the anatomical abnormalities. Alternatively, the migratory defect might reflect a premature switching off of genes involved in cell migration, genes that may respond to growth factors or their receptors. Thus, the genetic de-

---

[1] This enzyme colocalizes with and is thought to be identical to the enzyme nitric oxide synthase, which generates the gaseous transcellular messenger nitric oxide (Chapter 13).

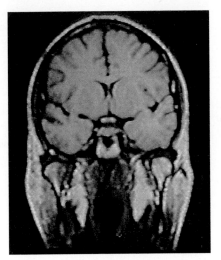
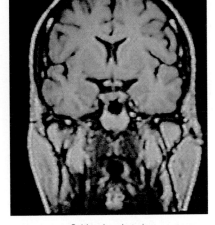

Unaffected twin   Schizophrenic twin

Figure 60-5 Magnetic resonance images of monozygotic twins show marked enlargement of the lateral ventricle in the twin with schizophrenia. Enlargement of the ventricles has been found to correlate strongly with the presence of schizophrenia. (Adapted from Suddath et al. 1990.)

fects in schizophrenia may reflect an underlying failure to maintain the expression of one or another gene required to complete the process of cortical neuronal migration.

It is likely, however, that these particular anatomical abnormalities in cortical development represent only one of a variety of basic anatomical defects that characterize the disease.

Antipsychotic Drugs Effective in the Treatment of Schizophrenia Act on Dopaminergic Systems

Until 1950 there was no effective treatment for schizophrenia. The first useful treatment was chlorpromazine, a drug that has a fascinating history. The French neurosurgeon Henri Laborit thought that anxiety experienced by patients before surgery led to the release of massive amounts of histamine from mast cells and that the histamines might contribute to the undesirable side effects of anesthesia, including sudden death. To block the release of histamine, Laborit examined various antihistaminics in an attempt to find one that would calm patients. Through trial and error he found chlorpromazine particularly effective.

Laborit was so impressed with the calming action of chlorpromazine that he began to think the drug might have a wider range of uses and soon appreciated that it might calm agitated patients with psychiatric conditions. In 1951 this idea was tested by John Delay and Pierre Deniker, who found that a high dosage of chlorpromazine calmed highly agitated and aggressive patients who had either schizophrenic or manic depressive symptoms.

Chlorpromazine was originally thought to act as a tranquilizer, calming patients without sedating them unduly. However, by 1964 it became clear that chlorpromazine and other related drugs of the phenothiazine class had specific effects on the psychotic symptoms of schizophrenia. The drugs mitigate or abolish delusions, hallucinations, and some types of disordered thinking (Table 60-2). Also, when patients who experience remission keep taking the antipsychotic medication throughout the period of remission, the rate of relapse is reduced.

These findings led to the delineation of a group of drugs, now called the *typical antipsychotics*, which include the phenothiazines (beginning with chlorpromazine), the

Table 60-2 Response of Schizophrenic Symptoms to Phenothiazines[1]

Response to Symptoms	Phenothiazines[2]
Schizophrenic symptoms	
Thought disorder	+++
Blunted affect	+++
Withdrawal	+++
Autistic behavior	+++
Hallucinations	++
Paranoid ideation	+
Grandiosity	+
Hostility, belligerence	0
Nonschizophrenic symptoms	
Anxiety, tension, agitation	0
Guilt, depression	0

[1]Adapted from Klein and Davis 1969.
[2]0, no response; +++, best response.

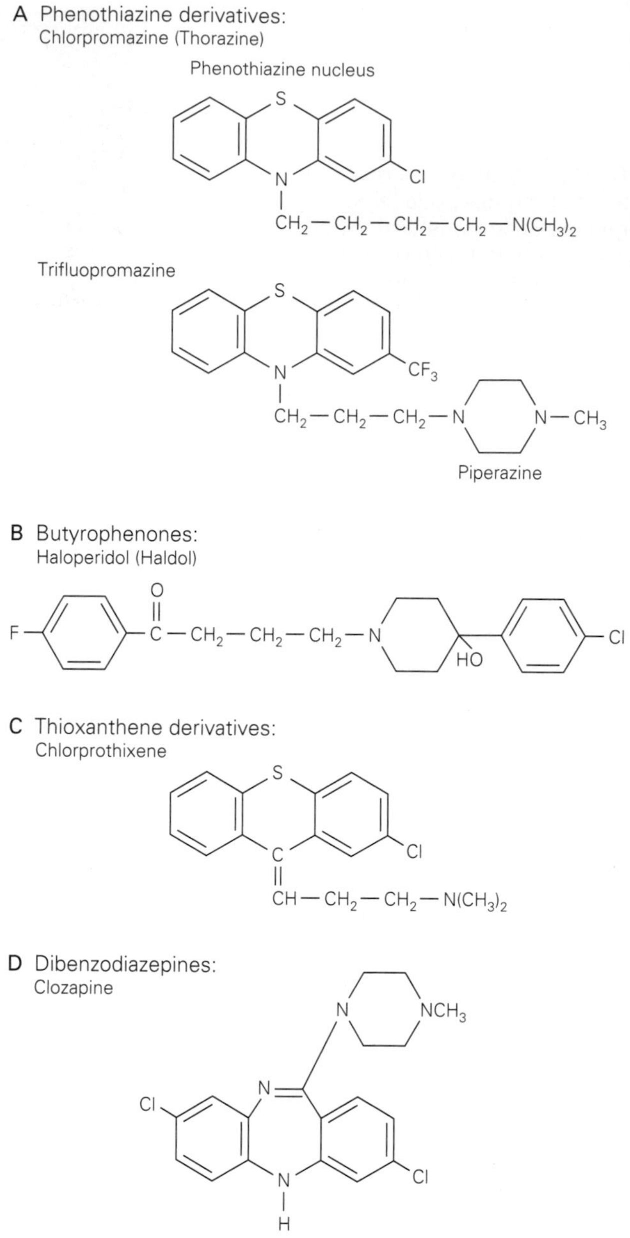

A Phenothiazine derivatives:
Chlorpromazine (Thorazine)

Phenothiazine nucleus

Trifluopromazine

Piperazine

Figure 60-6 The four major groups of antipsychotic drugs used to treat schizophrenia. The *typical antipsychotic* drugs—the phenothiazines (**A**), butyrophenones (**B**), and thioxanthenes (**C**)—bind to the dopaminergic D_2 receptors and have side effects in the extrapyramidal system, such as dry mouth and disorders of movement and gait. The *atypical antipsychotic* drugs, such as the dibenzodiazepine clozapine (**D**), bind primarily to dopaminergic D_3 and D_4 receptors and do not have extrapyramidal side effects.

B Butyrophenones:
Haloperidol (Haldol)

C Thioxanthene derivatives:
Chlorprothixene

D Dibenzodiazepines:
Clozapine

butyrophenones (haloperidol), and the thioxanthenes (Figure 60-6). More recently a second group of drugs, the *atypical antipsychotics* (clozapine, risperidone, olanzapine), have also proved useful in the treatment of schizophrenia. Atypical antipsychotics are better than typical antipsychotics in treating negative symptoms (and cognitive defects) in schizophrenia, and they produce fewer side effects on the extrapyramidal systems.

How do the typical and atypical antipsychotic agents produce their actions? Paradoxically, the first clue to the cellular action of the typical antipsychotic drugs came from analysis of their side effects. The drugs often produce a syndrome resembling parkinsonism, a group of disorders that result from a deficiency in

dopamine (Chapter 43). Following a suggestion by Arvid Carlsson, a number of studies soon found that many antipsychotic agents block dopamine receptors (Figure 60-7). This finding in turn suggested that perhaps excess dopamine transmission could be an important part of the pathogenesis of schizophrenia.

To determine whether dopaminergic transmission was excessive, it was important to identify the receptor sites at which the drugs exert their effect. At least six major types of dopamine receptors have now been cloned in humans: D_1, D_2, D_3, D_4, and D_5 (Figure 60-8). The amino acid sequences of each receptor subtype encode the seven membrane-spanning regions characteristic of G protein-coupled receptors (Table 60-3).

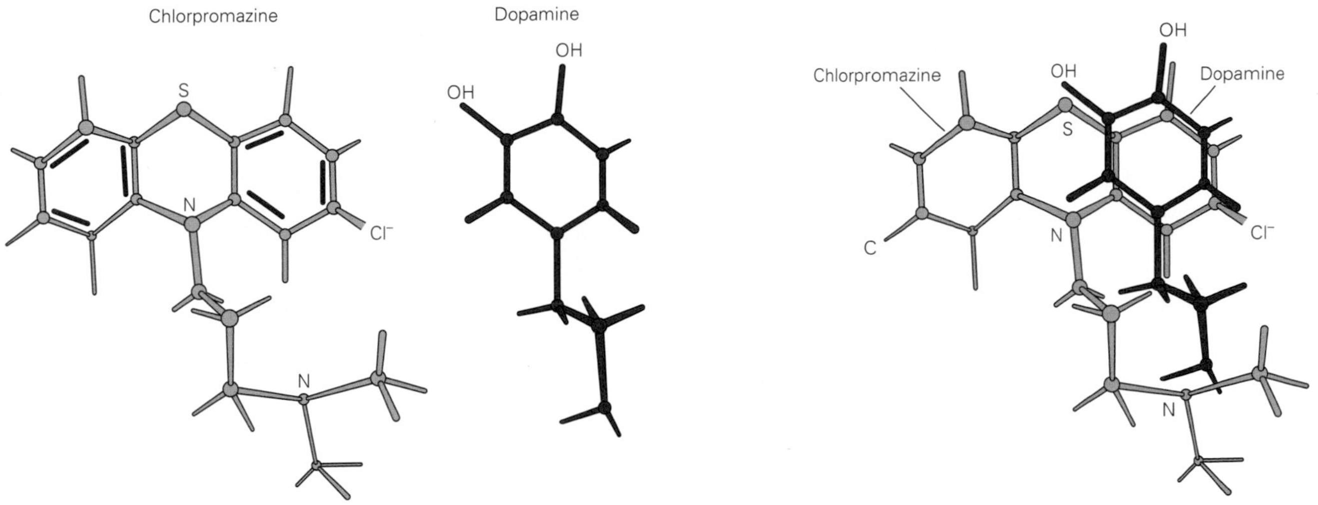

Figure 60-7 Chlorpromazine acts on dopamine receptors because it has a similar shape and therefore fits the receptor. However, because of differences in structure, chlorprom- azine simply sits on the receptor, blocking it without triggering a response. (Adapted from Snyder 1986.)

The D_1 and D_5 (also called D_{1b}) receptors are coupled to a G protein (G_s) that activates adenylyl cyclase, the enzyme that converts adenosine triphosphate (ATP) to cyclic adenosine monophosphate (cAMP) (Chapter 13). These receptors are expressed primarily in neurons of the cerebral cortex and hippocampus (although D_1 is also expressed in the caudate nucleus) and have a low affinity for most types of antipsychotic drugs.

The typical antipsychotic drugs have a high affinity for D_2 receptors, which are therefore thought to be one of the major sites of the therapeutic action of these drugs. Indeed, the clinical potency of the typical antipsychotic agents in patients with schizophrenia is closely correlated with the affinity of these drugs for the D_2 receptors (Figure 60-9).

The D_2 receptor is part of a family of related receptors (the D_2 group), which include D_3, and D_4. All three of these receptors are able to inhibit adenylyl cyclase (Figure 60-8). These receptors are expressed at particularly higher levels in neurons of the caudate nucleus, the

Table 60-3 Five Major Types of Known Postsynaptic Dopamine Receptors

	D_1	D_2	D_3	D_4	D_5
Molecular structure	Seven membrane-spanning regions	Seven membrane-spanning regions	Seven membrane-spanning regions	Seven membrane-spanning regions	Seven membrane-spanning regions
Effect on cyclic AMP	Increases	Decreases	Decreases	Decreases	Increases
Agonists	SKF 38393	Bromocriptitine	7-OH-DPAT	?	SKF 38393
Antagonists	SCH 23390 Phenothiazines Thioxanthenes Butyrophenones	Sulpiride Phenothiazines Thioxanthenes Butyrophenones Clozapine	UH232

Clozapine | Clozapine | SCH 23390 |

AMP = adenosine monophosphate.
SKF 38393 = Smith Kline French compound no. 38393.
7-OH-DPAT = 7-hydroxy-dipropylaminotetralin.
SCH 23390 = Scherring A. G. compound no. 23390.
UH232 = U. Hacksell compound no. 232.

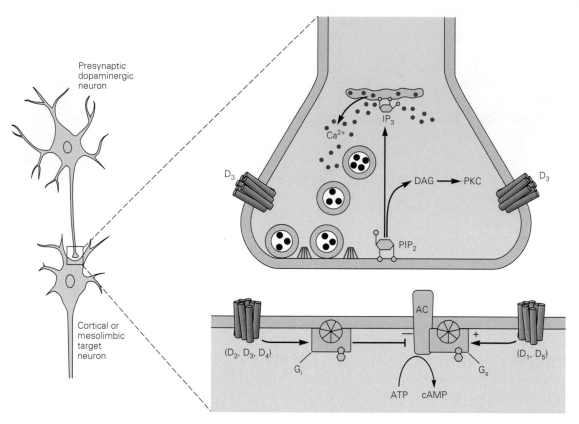

Figure 60-8 There are at least six types of dopamine receptors, four of which are illustrated here. The postsynaptic receptor D$_2$ inhibits adenylyl cyclase (**AC**) by an inhibitory G protein (**G$_i$**). The presynaptic inhibitory autoreceptor, thought to be D$_3$, regulates the amount of dopamine released in response to an action potential via a phosphoinositide second-messenger system (**DAG** = diacylglycerol; **IP$_3$** = inositol triphosphate; **PIP$_2$** = phosphoinositide diphosphate; **PKC** = protein kinase C). Both the presynaptic D$_3$ receptor and the postsynaptic receptor D$_2$ have a high affinity for the typical antipsychotic drugs (the phenothiazine, butyrophenone, and thioxanthene classes) and are thought to be key targets for the therapeutic actions of these drugs. The receptors D$_1$ and D$_5$ stimulate AC by a stimulatory G protein (**G$_s$**). These have a low affinity for the typical antipsychotic drugs and are therefore not thought to be involved in mediating the effects of these drugs on schizophrenic symptoms. The receptors D$_3$ and D$_4$ bind the atypical antipsychotic drugs.

putamen, and the nucleus accumbens, but D$_2$ receptors are also present in the amygdala, hippocampus, and parts of the cerebral cortex. Since the D$_2$ group is expressed in the caudate and putamen, these receptors presumably contribute to the side effects of the antipsychotic drugs on the extrapyramidal systems (Chapter 43). The amygdala, hippocampus, and neocortex, however, are possible sites of therapeutic action.

The atypical antipsychotic agents, such as clozapine, bind to D$_3$ and even more effectively to D$_4$ receptors. These two subtypes of the D$_2$ group are expressed primarily in the limbic system (Chapter 50) and cortex; they are only weakly expressed in the basal ganglia. This selective distribution may explain why the atypical antipsychotic agents do not give rise to side effects in the extrapyramidal systems. Both the D$_2$ and D$_3$ receptors are of further interest because they are present on

dopaminergic neurons themselves, on both the cell body and the terminals. Here they act as *inhibitory autoreceptors* (Chapter 14) to control both the rate of firing of the neuron and the release of dopamine by the action potential at the terminals (see Figure 60-8).

Abnormalities in Dopaminergic Synaptic Transmission Are Thought to Be Associated With Schizophrenic Symptoms

Excess Synaptic Transmission of Dopamine May Contribute to the Expression of Schizophrenia

The idea that excessive release of dopamine during synaptic transmission underlies at least some aspects of the pathogenesis of schizophrenia has received its primary support from pharmacologic studies. Drugs that increase the level of dopamine, such as L-dihydroxyphenylalanine (L-DOPA), cocaine, and amphetamine (Figure 60-10), can induce psychotic episodes resembling paranoid schizophrenia. Some of these drugs, such as amphetamine, also cause bizarre, repetitive, stereotyped behavioral acts in monkeys. Antipsychotic drugs reverse not only amphetamine psychosis in humans but also the bizarre behavioral syndrome in monkeys.

There is still no direct evidence, however, that excessive activity in dopaminergic neurons actually contributes to schizophrenia. The challenge in the study of schizophrenia, as with the depressive disorders that we shall consider in Chapter 61, is to advance from initial pharmacologic clues to precise physiological explanations of the pathogenesis of the disease. To explore further the role of dopaminergic transmission in schizophrenia we need to know which components of the dopamine system are altered in the disease and which of these alterations are related to specific neuroanatomic defects and clinical symptoms.

Distinct Anatomical Components of the Dopaminergic System Are Implicated in Schizophrenia

How are the dopaminergic neurons organized? Which particular grouping might contribute to schizophrenia? As we saw in Chapter 45, the dopaminergic neurons are not randomly distributed in the brain but are organized into four major systems: the tuberoinfundibular, nigrostriatal, mesolimbic, and mesocortical systems (Figure 60-11).

The dopaminergic *nigrostriatal system* contributes to the symptoms of Parkinson disease (Chapter 43). This system may also be involved in the short-term side effects of antipsychotic medication on the pyramidal system, such as hand tremor and rigidity of muscles, as well as the long-term side effect called *tardive dyskinesia*, a disorder involving involuntary movements that prominently affects the tongue.

The dopaminergic *mesolimbic system* has its origin in cell bodies in the ventral tegmental area, which is medial and superior to the substantia nigra. These cells project to the mesial components of the limbic system: the nucleus accumbens, the ventral striatum, the nuclei of the stria terminalis, parts of the amygdala and hippocampus, the lateral septal nuclei, the entorhinal cortex, the mesial frontal cortex, and the anterior cingulate cortex. In view of the role of the mesolimbic system in emotions and memory (see Chapters 50 and 62), and the similarity in disturbances of thought and perception

characteristic of schizophrenia and certain types of psychomotor (limbic system) epilepsy, Arvid Carlsson proposed that the positive symptoms of schizophrenia result from overactivity of the mesolimbic system. The idea that the mesolimbic dopaminergic system is affected in schizophrenia is supported by the finding that the earliest sign of brain disturbances in schizophrenia, detectable with positron emission tomography (PET) imaging, is a decrease in blood flow in a region of the basal ganglia (Figure 60-4). This disturbance is evident even before the prominent frontal lobe deficit becomes evident.

Among the projections of the mesolimbic system, those to the nucleus accumbens are thought to be particularly important because of the extensive connections of this nucleus to the limbic system. The nucleus accumbens receives and integrates inputs from the amygdala, hippocampus, entorhinal area, anterior cingulate area, and parts of the temporal lobe. The mesolimbic

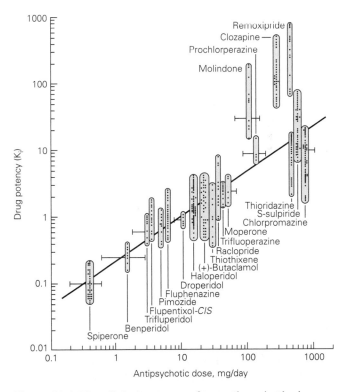

Figure 60-9 The clinical potency of an antipsychotic drug and the ability of the drug to block dopamine D₂ receptors are strongly correlated. On the horizontal axis is the average daily dose required to achieve the same clinical effect. On the vertical axis is the concentration of drug required to bind half the receptors. The higher the concentration required, the lower the affinity for the receptor. (Adapted from Seeman et al. 1976.)

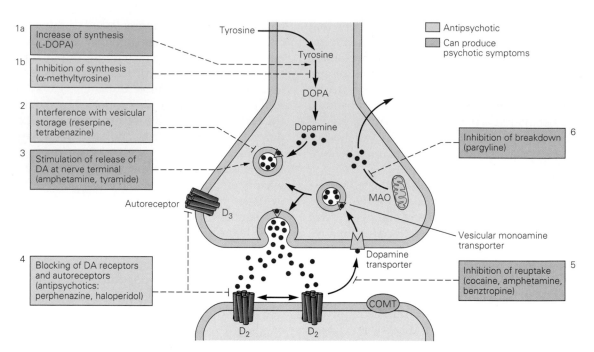

Figure 60-10 The key steps in the synthesis and degradation of dopamine and the sites of action of various psychoactive substances at the dopaminergic synapse. (Adapted from Cooper et al. 1996.)

1. Enzymatic synthesis. The dopamine precursor, dihydroxyphenylalanine (**DOPA**), is synthesized from tyrosine by tyrosine hydroxylase. This action is stimulated by L-DOPA and blocked by the competitive inhibitor α-methyltyrosine.

2. Storage. Reserpine and tetrabenazine interfere with the uptake and storage of dopamine by the storage granules. Reserpine is an effective antpsychotic drug; the depletion of dopamine by reserpine is long-lasting and the storage granules appear to be irreversibly damaged. Tetrabenazine also interferes with the uptake and storage mechanism of the granules, but only transiently.

3. Release. Amphetamine and tyramide enhance dopamine release from dopaminergic neurons.

4. Receptor interaction. Typical antipsychotics, such as perphenazine and haloperidol, are particularly effective in blocking the D$_2$ receptors and the presynaptic autoreceptors.

5. Reuptake. Dopamine activity is terminated when dopamine is taken up into the presynaptic terminal. Cocaine, amphetamine, and the anticholinergic drug benzotropine are potent inhibitors of this reuptake mechanism. Amphetamine induces a psychosis that is reversed by antipsychotic drugs.

6. Degradation. Dopamine in a free state within the presynaptic terminal can be degraded by the enzyme monoamine oxidase (**MAO**). Pargyline is an effective inhibitor of MAO. Dopamine can also be inactivated by the enzyme catechol-O-methyltransferase (**COMT**), which is believed to be localized in the postsynaptic cell.

dopaminergic projection to the nucleus accumbens is thought to modulate these inputs and thereby influence the output of the nucleus accumbens to its target regions: the ventral pallidum, septum, hypothalamus, anterior cingulate area, and frontal lobes. As we have seen, some of the input sources, in particular the hippocampus, and some of the output targets, such as the cingulate cortex and the frontal lobes are thought to be disturbed in schizophrenia. Overactive modulation of the integration of the inputs to the nucleus accumbens and of the output from it could contribute to positive symptoms of schizophrenia (Figure 60-12).

The dopaminergic *mesocortical system* originates in the ventral tegmental area and projects to the neocortex, in particular the prefrontal cortex. The prefrontal cortex is involved in the temporal organization of behavior, in

motivation, planning, attention, and social behavior (Chapter 20). The mesocortical system may be important in the negative symptoms of schizophrenia, symptoms that bear some resemblance to the defects seen after surgical disconnection of the frontal lobes, especially the dorsal prefrontal cortex. After loss of the dorsal prefrontal cortex, patients are poorly motivated, plan poorly, and have flattened affect.

The dopaminergic mesocortical system is essential for the normal cognitive functions of the dorsolateral prefrontal cortex. As is the case with ablating the prefrontal cortex, experimental depletion of dopamine in the prefrontal cortex (using the toxin 6-hydroxydopamine) impairs the performance of monkeys in cognitive tasks. This cognitive deficit can be reversed by giving the dopamine precursor L-DOPA or the agonist

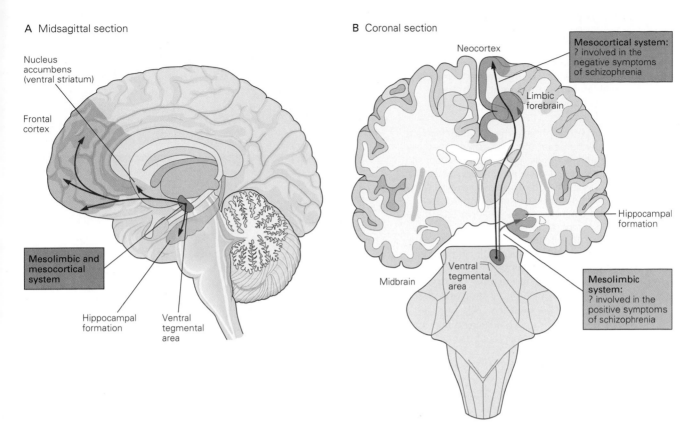

A Midsagittal section

Nucleus
accumbens
(ventral striatum)

Frontal
cortex

Mesolimbic and
mesocortical
system

Hippocampal
formation

Ventral
tegmental
area

B Coronal section

Neocortex

Mesocortical system:
? involved in the
negative symptoms
of schizophrenia

Limbic
forebrain

Hippocampal
formation

Midbrain

Ventral
tegmental
area

Mesolimbic
system:
? involved in the
positive symptoms
of schizophrenia

Figure 60-11 The four major dopaminergic tracts of the brain. The nigrostriatal system courses from the substantia nigra to the putamen and caudate. The tuberoinfundibular system originates in the arcuate nucleus of the hypothalamus and projects to the pituitary stalk. The mesolimbic system runs from the ventral tegmental area to many components of the limbic system. The mesocortical system projects from the ventral tegmental area to the neocortex, especially the prefrontal areas. We here only illustrate two of the four tracts. The mesolimbic system which may be involved in the positive symptoms of schizophrenia and the mesocortical system which may be involved in the negative symptoms.

apomorphine. In fact, patients with Parkinson disease, who have lost dopaminergic neurons, not only have a motor disorder (reflecting the deficit in the dopaminergic nigrostriatal system) but also lack motivation and have flat affect and reduced spontaneity, defects that may reflect a decrease in transmission in the dopaminergic mesocortical pathways. Similarly, lesions that destroy the ventral tegmental area, which gives rise to the dopaminergic mesolimbic system, cause dementia and psychotic symptoms.

These several findings led Daniel Weinberger to postulate that two dopaminergic systems are disturbed in different ways in schizophrenia. First, an increase in activity in the *mesolimbic* pathway (perhaps through the D_2 and D_3 receptors and particularly through the D_4 receptors) would account for the positive symptoms. Second, decreased activity of the *mesocortical* connections in the prefrontal cortex would account for the negative symptoms. According to this model, the imbalance between cortical and subcortical dopaminergic transmission un-

derlies the development of schizophrenia. Weinberger proposes that activity in the mesocortical pathway to the prefrontal cortex normally inhibits the mesolimbic pathway by feedback inhibition and that the primary defect in schizophrenia is a reduction in this activity, which leads to disinhibition and overactivity in the mesolimbic pathway (Figure 60-13).

Although Weinberger's scheme is still untested, there is experimental evidence for interaction between the mesolimbic and mesocortical pathways. Christopher Pycock and his colleagues found that chemical lesioning of the mesocortical pathway in experimental animals enhances synaptic responsiveness in the mesolimbic pathway, specifically in its terminations in the nucleus accumbens. It is not known how loss of dopaminergic terminals in the prefrontal cortex leads to increased activity of the mesolimbic pathway in the nucleus accumbens. However, Pycock and his collaborators suggest that reduced activity in one pathway may result in compensatory neuronal growth in the other.

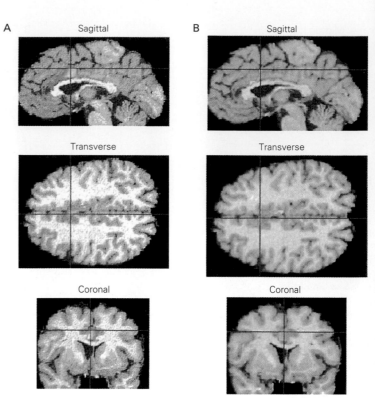

Figure 60-12 PET scans showing cerebral blood flow in schizophrenic patients during the performance of a cognitive task and after treatment with the dopamine agonist apomorphine. (From Dolan et al. 1995.)

A. In patients with schizophrenia the anterior cingulate cortex fails to activate when they perform an internally generated task such as thinking of a word (as opposed to a task where the response is specified by an environmental cue, eg, saying a word displayed visually). When normal subjects are engaged in internally generated tasks, the anterior cingulate cortex is activated and the modality-specific temporal cortex around the auditory area is deactivated (PET scans not shown). In patients with schizophrenia this integrated activity in the frontotemporal system is impaired and indeed reversed: there is inadequate activation of the anterior cingulate cortex and excessive activation of the temporal lobes.

B. After these same schizophrenic patients received apomorphine, a dopamine agonist, activity in their anterior cingulate is greater than in normal subjects for the same task.

Abnormalities in Dopaminergic Transmission Do Not Account for All Aspects of Schizophrenia

As these interesting but largely speculative arguments illustrate, we are far from understanding the role of dopaminergic transmission in normal mental function or in schizophrenia. The major argument for the involvement of dopaminergic pathways in schizophrenia comes from the analysis of the mechanisms of action of the antipsychotic drugs. It is difficult, in principle, to extrapolate from the mechanisms of action of a therapeutic agent to the causal mechanisms of a disease. Pharmacologic manipulation may produce changes that compensate for the disease without directly affecting the disordered mechanism itself. For example, the primary defect in Parkinson disease is a decrease in dopamine levels; but, as we have seen in Chapter 43, some symptoms can be alleviated by drugs that block *cholinergic* transmission.

This issue can be further illustrated by the hypothetical situation of three presynaptic neurons converging on a postsynaptic neuron, with each presynaptic neuron releasing a different transmitter. Transmitter A and dopamine reduce the excitability of the postsynaptic cell, whereas transmitter B directly excites it (Figure 60–14). If schizophrenia resulted from a defect in neuron

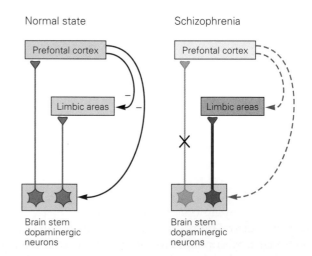

Figure 60-13 In this neuroanatomical model of schizophrenia the prefrontal cortex normally inhibits (through feedback inhibition) activity in the limbic areas and the dopaminergic mesolimbic pathway arising from the brain stem. A primary defect in schizophrenia may be depressed activity in the dopaminergic mesocortical projection from the brain stem to the frontal lobe, resulting in a loss of inhibitory feedback and consequent hyperactivity of the mesolimbic pathway. (Adapted from Weinberger 1987.)

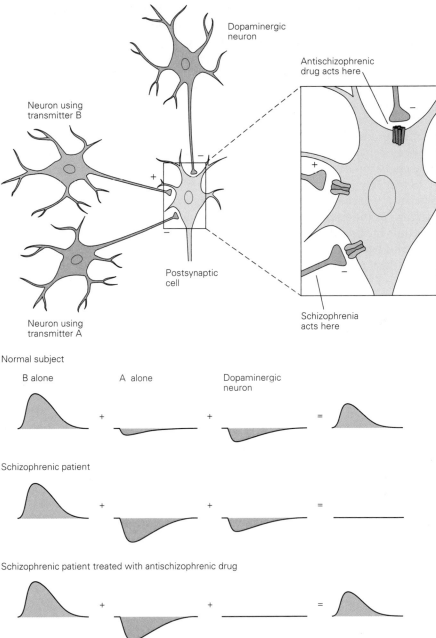

Figure 60-14 An antischizophrenic drug that acts by blocking a dopamine receptor could ameliorate symptoms without directly acting on the neurons responsible for the disease. Here a cell receives inputs from excitatory cells (using transmitter substance B) and two types of inhibitory cells (using transmitter A or dopamine). If schizophrenia is due to an imbalance of synaptic input, specifically overactivity in the inhibitory neurons that use transmitter A, blocking the effectiveness of the dopaminergic inhibitory neurons could ameliorate the disease by reducing the net inhibition in the postsynaptic cell. However, it would be incorrect to assume that, because the block partially restored the balance and thereby improved the patient's behavior, the dopaminergic neurons were the site of pathology. (Adapted from R. Zigmond, personal communication.)

A or its transmitter, causing an excess of this modulatory transmitter to act on the postsynaptic cell, one could improve the symptoms by simply blocking the action of dopamine, the other modulatory transmitter, because this intervention would reduce net inhibitory inputs to the postsynaptic cell.

However, this model could easily prove inadequate for determining the best treatment. For instance, the dopaminergic neuron and neuron A might have very different inputs converging on them. If so, inhibiting dopaminergic transmission might cause an imbalance in the inputs and therefore inappropriate signals in the postsynaptic neuron. Even this simple example illustrates that a correlation between excess dopaminergic activity and schizophrenia, however strong, is not sufficient to allow a conclusion about the underlying cause of the disease.

In addition, there are some reasons to question whether the affinity of antipsychotic agents for D_2 (as well as D_3 and D_4) receptors is the only basis of the clinical efficacy of these drugs. Although antipsychotic drugs occupy dopamine receptors very quickly after administration, the maximal therapeutic (antipsychotic) effects are often delayed several weeks. Thus the acute blockade of dopaminergic transmission is not likely to be sufficient for the therapeutic effect. The antipsychotic action may be secondary to other consequences in the brain that evolve over a period of several weeks. For example, activity in certain neural circuits may need to adjust to a new level of modulation. In addition, the drugs or the resulting alterations in neuronal activity might produce changes in gene expression, the consequences of which may not become manifest for one or more weeks.

One late consequence of long-term dopamine blockade, which may well involve gene regulation, is an increase in the number of dopamine receptors per cell, and thus increased sensitivity to dopamine in each cell. A second late consequence, supported by electrophysiological data, is a decrease in the activity of dopaminergic neurons. Third, the delayed actions might also reflect adjustments of other neuronal systems that interact with the dopaminergic systems (see Figure 60-10). For example, most typical antipsychotic agents also act on a class of serotonin receptors, the 5-HT$_2$ receptors at which lysergic acid diethylamide (LSD) and other psychedelic hallucinogens also act (see Chapter 61). Long-term administration of antipsychotic agents leads to a downregulation of 5-HT$_2$ receptors that parallels in time course the therapeutic action of the antipsychotic drugs. Finally, many antipsychotic agents also bind the D$_1$ receptor, although with low affinity, and this may enhance the action of dopamine at the receptors of the D$_2$ group.

At least 20% of patients with schizophrenia do not improve after treatment with dopaminergic blockers that act on the group of D$_2$ receptors. But these patients often respond to atypical antipsychotic agents such as clozapine (a dibenzodiazepine), which is only a weak blocker of D$_2$ receptors. Clozapine has the additional interesting property that it produces few, if any, parkinsonian (extrapyramidal) side effects, which characteristically occur with blockade of D$_2$ receptors. Clozapine and risperidone bind to D$_3$ receptors and even more effectively to D$_4$ receptors. As we have seen, D$_3$ and D$_4$ dopamine receptors are limited in their distribution to the limbic system.

Moreover, clozapine is not limited in its action to the dopamine system. It also blocks the serotonin receptor 5-HT$_{2a}$ as well as the α_1 epinephrine and H$_1$ histamine receptors. Just as schizophrenia is a multifactorial disease and perhaps affects more than one set of dopaminergic pathways in the brain (mesolimbic and mesocortical), so it is likely that antipsychotic drugs act on more than one molecular target.

Further evidence that disorders in pathways other than the dopaminergic system might contribute to schizophrenia comes from the finding that the addictive drug phencyclidine (PCP) produces a psychosis that resembles the psychosis in schizophrenia and exacerbates psychosis in patients with schizophrenia. Normal subjects given intravenous PCP experience depersonalization and feel disconnected from their environment. They also have delusions of being controlled by external agents and have auditory and visual hallucinations.

PCP binds to two identified molecular targets in the brain: (1) the dopaminergic terminals in the nucleus accumbens, and (2) the N-methyl-D-aspartate (NMDA) class of glutamate receptors. NMDA receptors are present on the dopaminergic axon terminals in the prefrontal cortex and enhance dopamine release from the terminals. PCP, when it binds to the NMDA receptors, inhibits release of dopamine. In contrast, at the dopaminergic terminals in the nucleus accumbens PCP increases dopamine release and inhibits reuptake, much like amphetamine.

Thus, the behavioral effects of PCP may be due in part to its ability to enhance release in the mesolimbic pathway while blocking dopamine release in the mesocortical pathway. Indeed, specific drugs developed to block NMDA receptors selectively (and used for the treatment of NMDA-induced neurotoxicity after stroke or prolonged seizure activity) have the undesirable side effect of producing psychosis, perhaps by reducing the release of dopamine in the mesocortical pathway to the frontal lobe.

The existence of drugs that produce psychotic behavior by binding to the NMDA receptor indicates that psychotic behavior can probably be produced by interfering with several transmitter systems that act either in parallel or in combination with dopamine.

An Overall View

In considering the biological defect in schizophrenia we have focused on current insights into the molecular mechanisms of the disease and not on the social and psychological factors that act on an individual before, during, and even after they have the disease. In this context it is useful to take note of two common misconceptions.

First, it is sometimes thought that in classifying mental disorders we are classifying *people*; in reality, we are classifying *disorders* that people have. A person is not a schizophrenic—one *has* schizophrenia. Second, even though all the people with a particular mental illness are similar in ways that are important and all of these people will, by definition, share the *defining* features of the disease, the individuals who have the disease will likely differ in quite fundamental ways that may influence both the course and the outcome of the disease.

In addition to social factors, further research on schizophrenia needs to explore other contributing factors. A particularly important question is the genetic component, although genetic factors seem only to predispose people to schizophrenia. Another factor to consider is developmental abnormalities in the brain. In fact, schizophrenia is sometimes associated with what appears to be aberrant cell migration in both frontal and temporal lobes as well as with enlarged lateral ventricles, widening of cortical sulci, and reduced blood flow to the frontal lobes.

Dopaminergic agonists are capable of producing psychosis, and the affinity of antischizophrenic drugs for the dopaminergic D_2 and particularly the D_4 receptors is directly correlated with their clinical potency in alleviating psychotic symptoms. Postmortem studies have indeed found increases in the number of dopamine receptors in these limbic areas.

Indeed, almost all patients with schizophrenia show attentional and motivational deficits similar to those in patients with deficits in prefrontal cortex function. How this prefrontal defect relates to the defect in the mesolimbic dopaminergic projection is unclear. Initial clues to the answers for these questions may come from cloning one or more of the allelic variations of genes involved in schizophrenia.

Eric R. Kandel

Selected Readings

Andreasen NC, Olsen SA, Dennert JW, Smith MR. 1982. Ventricular enlargement in schizophrenia: relationship to positive and negative symptoms. Am J Psychiatry 139:297–302.

Barondes SH. 1993. *Molecules and Mental Illness*. New York: Scientific American Library.

Bloom FE. 1993. Advancing a developmental origin of schizophrenia. Arch Gen Psychiatry 50:224–227.

Carpenter WT, Buchanan R. 1994. Schizophrenia. N Engl J Med 330:681–690.

Dawson E, Robin M. 1996. Schizophrenia: a gene at 6p. Curr Biol 6:268–271.

Early TS, Posner MI, Reiman EM, Raichle ME. 1989. Hyperactivity of the left striato-pallidal projection. II. Phenomenology and thought disorder. Psychiatric Dev 2:109–121.

Goodwin DW, Guze SB. 1989. *Psychiatric Diagnosis*, 4th ed. New York: Oxford Univ. Press.

Havens LL. 1973. *Approaches to the Mind: Movement of the Psychiatric Schools From Sects Toward Science*. Boston: Little, Brown.

Hyman SE, Nestler EJ. 1993. *The Molecular Foundations of Psychiatry*. Washington, DC: American Psychiatric Press.

LaFosse MJ, Mednick SA. 1991. A neurodevelopmental approach to schizophrenia research. In: SA Mednick (ed). *Developmental Neuropathology of Schizophrenia*, pp. 211–225. New York: Plenum.

Middleton FA, Strick PL. 1996. The temporal lobe is a target of output from the basal ganglia. Proc Natl Acad Sci U S A 93:8683–8687.

Plomin R, Owen MJ, McGuffin P. 1994. The genetic basis of complex human behaviors. Science 264:1733–1739.

Seeman P, Guan H-C, Van Tol HHM. 1993. Dopamine D_4 receptors elevated in schizophrenia. Nature 365:441–445.

Snyder SH. 1986. *Drugs and the Brain*. New York: Scientific American.

Suddath RL, Christison GW, Torrey EF, Casanova MF, Weinberger DR. 1990. Anatomical abnormalities in the brains of monozygotic twins discordant for schizophrenia. N Engl J Med 322:789–794.

Weinberger DR, Berman FB, Suddath R, Fuller-Torrey E. 1992. Evidence of dysfunction of a prefrontal-limbic network in schizophrenia: a magnetic imaging and regional cerebral blood flow study of discordant monozygotic twins. Am J Psychiatry 149:890–897.

References

Bassett AS. 1989. Chromosome 5 and schizophrenia: implications for genetic linkage studies. Schizophr Bull 15:393–402.

Benes FM, Davidson J, Bird ED. 1986. Quantitative cytoarchitectural studies of the cerebral cortex of schizophrenics. Arch Gen Psychiatry 43:31–35.

Bleuler E. [1911] 1950. *Dementia Praecox or the Group of Schizophrenias*. J Zinkin (transl). New York: International Universities Press.

Brozoski TJ, Brown RM, Rosvold HE, Goldman PS. 1979. Cognitive deficit caused by regional depletion of dopamine in prefrontal cortex of rhesus monkey. Science 205:929–932.

Carlsson A. 1974. Antipsychotic drugs and catecholamine synapses. J Psychiatr Res 11:57–64.

Cooper JR, Bloom FE, Roth RH. 1996. *The Biochemical Basis of Neuropharmacology*, 7th ed. New York: Oxford Univ. Press.

Dolan RJ, Fletcher P, Frith CD, Friston KJ, Frackowiak RSJ, Grasby PM. 1995. Dopaminergic modulation of impaired cognitive activation in the anterior cingulate cortex in schizophrenia. Nature 378:180.

Gottesman II. 1991. *Schizophrenia Genesis: The Origins of Madness*. New York: Freeman.

Havens LL. 1965. Emil Kraepelin. J Nerv Ment Dis 141:16–28.

Heston LL. 1970. The genetics of schizophrenic and schizoid disease. Science 167:249–256.

Ingvar DH. 1987. Evidence for frontal/prefrontal cortical dysfunction in chronic schizophrenia: The phenomenon of "hypofrontality" reconsidered. In: H Helmchen, FA Henn (eds). *Biological Perspectives of Schizophrenia*, pp. 201–211. Chichester, England: Wiley.

Jones EG. 1995. Cortical development and neuropathology in schizophrenia. In: Development of the Cerebral Cortex. Ciba Found Symp 193:277–295.

Kallmann FJ. 1938. *The Genetics of Schizophrenia*. New York: Augustin.

Kane J. 1987. Treatment of schizophrenia. Schizophr Bull 13:133–156.

Karayiorgou M, Morris MA, Morrow B, Shprintzen RJ, Goldberg R, Borrow J, Gos A, Nestadt G, Wolyneic PS, Lasseter VK, Eisen H, Childs B, Kazazian HH, Kucherlapati R, Antonarakis SE, Pulver AE, Housman DE. 1995. Schizophrenia susceptibility associated with interstitial deletions of chromosome 22q11. Proc Natl Acad Sci U S A 92:7612–7616.

Kety SS, Rosenthal D, Wender PH, Schulsinger F, Jacobsen B. 1975. Mental illness in the biological and adoptive families of adopted individuals who have become schizophrenic: A preliminary report based on psychiatric interviews. In: RR Fieve, D Rosenthal, H Brill (eds). *Genetic Research in Psychiatry*, pp. 147–165. Baltimore: Johns Hopkins Univ. Press.

Kirch DG, Weinberger DR. 1986. Anatomical neuropathology in schizophrenia: Post-mortem findings. In: HA Nasrallah, DR Weinberger (eds). *The Neurology of Schizophrenia*, pp. 325–348. Amsterdam: Elsevier.

Klein DF, Davis JM. 1969. *Diagnosis and Drug Treatment of Psychiatric Disorders*. Baltimore: Williams and Wilkins.

Klein DF, Gittelman R, Quitkin F, Rifkin A. 1980. *Diagnosis and Drug Treatment of Psychiatric Disorders: Adults and Children*, 2nd ed. Baltimore: Williams and Wilkins.

Kraepelin E. [1909] 1919. Dementia praecox and paraphrenia. RM Barclay (transl). In: *Kraepelin's Text-Book of Psychiatry*, 8th ed. Edinburgh: Churchill Livingstone.

Lipska BK, Jaskiw GE, Weinberger DR. 1993. Postpubertal emergence of hyperresponsiveness to stress and to amphetamine after neonatal excitotoxic hippocampal damage: a potential animal model of schizophrenia. Neuropsychopharmacology 9:67–75.

Nauta WJH, Smith GP, Faull RLM, Domesick VB. 1978. Efferent connections and nigral afferents of the nucleus accumbens septi in the rat. Neuroscience 3:385–401.

O'Dowd BF, Seeman P, George SR. 1994. Dopamine receptors. In: SJ Peroutka (ed). *Handbook of Receptors and Channels*, pp. 95–123. Boca Raton, FL: CRC.

Olney JW, Labruyere J, Price MT. 1989. Pathological changes induced in cerebrocortical neurons by phencyclidine and related drugs. Science 244:1360–1362.

Posner MI, Early TS, Reiman E, Pardo JP, Dhawan M. 1988. Asymmetries in hemispheric control of attention in schizophrenia. Arch Gen Psychiatry 45:814–821.

Pycock CJ, Kerwin RW, Carter CJ. 1980. Effect of lesion of cortical dopamine terminals on subcortical dopamine receptors in rats. Nature 286:74–77.

Reveley AM, Reveley MA, Clifford CA, Murray RM. 1982. Cerebral ventricular size in twins discordant for schizophrenia. Lancet 1:540–541.

Roberts PJ, Woodruff GN, Iversen LL (eds). 1978. *Advances in Biochemical Psychopharmacology*. Vol. 19, *Dopamine*. New York: Raven.

Seeman P, Lee T, Chau-Wong M, Wong K. 1976. Antipsychotic drug doses and neuroleptic/dopamine receptors. Nature 261:717–719.

Seeman P. 1995. Dopamine receptors: Clinical correlates. In: FE Bloom, PJ Kupter (eds). *Psychopharmacology: The Fourth Generation of Progress*, pp. 295–302. New York: Raven.

Shelton RC, Weinberger DR. 1986. X-ray computerized tomography studies in schizophrenia: A review and synthesis. In: HA Nasrallah, DR Weinberger (eds). *The Neurology of Schizophrenia*, pp. 207–250. Amsterdam: Elsevier.

Silbersweig DA, Stern E, Frith C, Cahill C, Holmes A, Grootoonk S, Seaward J, McKenna P, Chua SE, Schnorr L, Jones T, Frackowiak RSJ. 1995. A functional neuroanatomy of hallucinations in schizophrenia. Nature 378:176–179.

Snyder SH, Largent BL. 1989. Receptor mechanisms in antipsychotic drug action: focus on sigma receptors. J Neuropsychiatry Clin Neurosci 1:7–15.

Torack RM, Morris JC. 1988. The association of ventral tegmental area histopathology with adult dementia. Arch Neurol 45:497–501.

Van Tol HHM, Bunzow JR, Guan H-C, Sunahara RK, Seeman P, Niznik HB, Civelli O. 1991. Cloning of the gene for a human dopamine D_4 receptor with high affinity for the antipsychotic clozapine. Nature 350:610–614.

Weinberger DR. 1987. Implications of normal brain development for the pathogenesis of schizophrenia. Arch Gen Psychiatry 44:660–669.

61

Disorders of Mood: Depression, Mania, and Anxiety Disorders

MAKING THE DISTINCTION between a disturbance of cognitive faculties (a thought disorder) and a disturbance of emotion (a mood disorder) was an important step in the early development of the modern classification of mental illness. In clinical descriptions of emotional states the term *mood* refers to a sustained emotional state lasting weeks or more, while the term *affect* (or affective response) refers to immediate or momentary emotional state of a person. Affect is more directly responsive to external stimuli, although with significant mood disorders the range of affective responses is limited. Thus, affect is to mood as the weather (rainy or sunny) is to climate (tropical, moderate, or cold).

Normal affective responses serve important biological functions and range from euphoria to elation, pleasure, surprise, anger, anxiety, disappointment, sadness, grief, despair, and even depression. Three of these responses—euphoria, depression, and anxiety—can become so disordered, sustained, and dominant as to constitute a disease. We shall consider all three and discuss biological insights into these three disorders of mood. Although depression and euphoria (*mania*) have traditionally been referred to as disorders of affect, we use the more precise term mood. We shall then examine the anxiety states. Throughout we shall emphasize important interrelationships between the three mood disorders.

The Major Mood Disorders Can Be Either Unipolar or Bipolar

The most common mood disorder, unipolar depression, was described in the fifth century BC by Hippocrates. In the Hippocratic view moods were thought to depend on the balance of four humors—blood, phlegm, yellow bile, and black bile. An excess of black bile was believed to cause depression. In fact, the ancient Greek term for depression, *melancholia,* means black bile. Though this explanation of depression seems fanciful today, the underlying view that psychological disorders reflect physical processes is correct.

Modern efforts to update the Hippocratic formulation were, until very recently, hindered by a lack of precision in the classification of affective disorders. In his 1917 paper *Mourning and Melancholia,* Sigmund Freud wrote: "Even in descriptive psychiatry the definition of melancholia is uncertain; it takes on various clinical forms (some of them suggesting somatic rather than psychogenic affections) that do not seem definitely to warrant reduction to a unity." Only in the past two decades have relatively precise criteria for mood disorders been developed in parallel with those for cognitive disorders (see Chapter 60).

Unipolar Depression Is Most Likely Several Mood Disorders

The clinical features of unipolar depression are easily summarized. In Hamlet's words, "How weary, stale, flat, and unprofitable seem to me all the uses of this world!" Untreated, an episode of depression typically lasts 4–12 months. It is characterized by an unpleasant (*dysphoric*) mood that is present most of the day, day in and day out, as well as intense mental anguish, the inability to experience pleasure (*anhedonia*), and a generalized loss of interest in the world. The diagnosis also requires at least three of the following symptoms to be present: disturbed sleep (usually insomnia with early morning awakening, but sometimes oversleeping or hypersomnia), diminished appetite and loss of weight (but sometimes overeating), loss of energy, decreased sex drive, restlessness (psychomotoragitation), slowing down of thoughts and actions (psychomotor retardation), difficulty in concentrating, indecisiveness, feelings of worthlessness, guilt, pessimistic thoughts, and thoughts about dying and suicide. Other common symptoms, not required for diagnosis, are constipation, decreased salivation, and diurnal variation in the severity of symptoms, which are usually worse in the morning.

In addition to the inclusion criteria there are exclusion criteria; schizophrenia or other neurological diseases, for example, need to be excluded. There also should be no evidence of a recent death in the family or other traumatic events, since some of the symptoms of unipolar depression are also normal expressions of grief following trauma, personal loss, and mourning.

When the syndrome is defined in this manner, about 5% of the world's population have major unipolar depression. In the United States 8 million people at any given time are affected. Severe depression can be profoundly debilitating. In extreme cases patients stop eating or maintaining basic personal cleanliness. Although some people have only a single episode, usually the illness is recurrent. About 70% of patients who have one major depressive episode will have at least one more episode. The average age of onset is about 28 years, but the first episode can occur at almost any age. Indeed, depression also affects young children but is often unrecognized in them. Depression also occurs in the elderly; in fact, older people who become depressed often have not had an earlier episode. Women are affected about two to three times more often than men.

Unipolar depression is most likely not a single illness but a group of disorders. However, the attempt to distinguish three subtypes has been only partially successful so far. The subtypes that are commonly distinguished are melancholic depression, atypical depression, and dysthymia.

Melancholic depression represents the clearest subtype among the major depressions and accounts for 40–60% of people treated for unipolar depression. Because it often has no obvious external precipitating cause—no personal loss or rejection or obvious change in life events—it was formerly referred to as *endogenous depression.* The disorder is characterized by six symptoms: (1) depression with diurnal variations in mood (worse in the morning), (2) insomnia with early-morning wakening, (3) anorexia with significant weight loss, (4) psychomotor agitation and mental pain, (5) loss of interest in almost all activity and lack of response to pleasurable stimuli, and (6) when severe, a complete loss of the capacity for joy (anhedonia).

Patients with melancholic depression often have a history of one or more previous episodes of major depression with recovery. Many patients show characteristic abnormalities in sleep pattern, as measured by electroencephalography. These abnormalities occur primarily during the first half of the night, when the latency for the rapid eye movement (REM) phase of sleep is shortened. More than half of patients with melancholic depression have frequent awakenings. Melancholic depression sometimes leads to psychomotor retardation, to emotional or intellectual underactivity (*retardation*). At other times there is a rather painful state of agitation and an active and persistent preoccupation with perceived deficiencies and inadequacies of one's character. Patients with melancholic depression tend to respond preferentially to electroconvulsive therapy (ECT), tricyclic antidepressants, and selective serotonin reuptake inhibitors.

Atypical depression is slightly less common than melancholic depression; accounting for about 15% of patients hospitalized for major mood disorders. The disease is called atypical because symptoms are the opposite of melancholic depression: it first appears earlier in life and tends to be chronic rather than phasic. In addition, unlike patients with melancholic depression, patients with atypical depression cheer up temporarily when good things happen. Finally, patients with atypical depression do not have loss of appetite and weight loss but instead overeat and gain weight; they do not report insomnia but rather tend to sleep more; and their depression is worse, not better, in the evening. The patients also have prominent symptoms of anxiety. Patients with atypical depression tend to respond preferentially to monoamine oxidase inhibitors.

Finally, *dysthymia* is a persistent but milder depression lasting for at least two years with symptoms that fall short of the criteria of a major depression.

It is important to appreciate that we *normally* experience grief or despondency after loss of a family member, and this normal mourning can involve any of the individual symptoms of atypical or melancholic depression. Perhaps the most important distinction between bereavement and depression is that bereavement is rarely associated with persistent functional impairment. In addition, despondent or grief-stricken people have fewer suicidal thoughts and, more important, they have lower rates of suicide than patients with atypical or melancholic depression.

Most helpful in making a diagnosis of depression, however, is the finding of *reactive affect.* Unlike major depression, the depression normally experienced after a personal loss is not unrelenting and pervasive—*it does not persist every day, all day.* Two or three months after a personal loss, most people are able to experience and react to moments of pleasure and contentment that relieve the sadness, something a person with a major depression cannot do. Finally, normal mourning tends to remit after several months. It does not persist. When mourning does persist it usually reflects a transition to an episode of major depression, a transition that occurs in individuals with a genetic predisposition.

Bipolar Depressive (Manic-Depressive) Disorders Give Rise to Alternating Euphoria and Depression

About 25% of patients with major depression (or two million people in the United States) will also experience a manic episode, if only a mild one. Patients who experience both depressive and manic episodes have a distinct disorder called *bipolar mood disorder.* The illness affects men and women equally, and the average age of onset of the first episode is a decade younger than that of unipolar depression (the onset usually occurs at age 20 rather than 30).

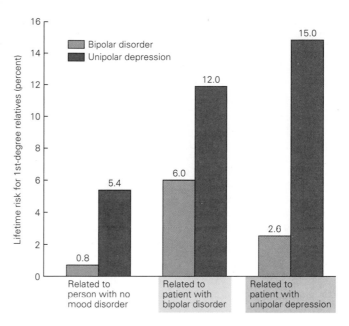

Figure 61-1 The incidence of bipolar and unipolar depression is higher among first-degree relatives of patients who have either disease than in the general population. (From Barondes 1993.)

Episodes of depression in bipolar disorders are clinically similar to those of the unipolar type. The manic episodes are characterized by an elevated, expansive, or irritable mood lasting at least one week, together with several of the following symptoms: over-activity, over-talkativeness (pressure of speech), social intrusiveness, increased energy and libido, flight of ideas, grandiosity, distractibility, decreased need for sleep, and reckless spending. In severe cases patients are delusional and hallucinate. Most episodes have no detectable psychosocial precipitant.

Bipolar disorder is typically recurrent. After an initial episode of euphoria, subsequent episodes of either depression or euphoria are likely to occur about twice as often in bipolar disorder as in unipolar disease. One of the most striking features of bipolar illness is that a subset of patients (*rapid cyclers*) may switch from depression to euphoria or vice versa quite rapidly, sometimes in a matter of minutes. Depression tends to become more pronounced with age and recur with greater frequency.

Mood Disorders Have a Strong Genetic Predisposition

As in schizophrenia, genetic factors are important in both unipolar and bipolar mood disorders. The morbidity rate of depression is modestly higher in first-degree relatives (parents, siblings, and children) of patients

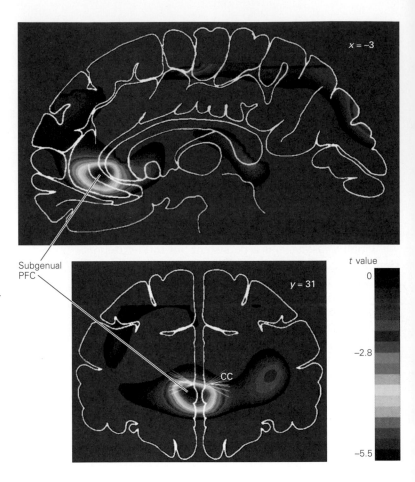

Figure 61-2 Some patients with unipolar and bipolar disease show a functional abnormality in the prefrontal cortex ventral to the genu of the corpus collosum. During the depressive phase of the bipolar disease activity is decreased, while during the manic phase it is increased. The two images show a decrease in metabolism in patients with depression relative to controls. Both phases of the illness localize to the agranular region of the anterior cingulate gyrus ventral to the corpus collosum. Anterior, or left, is to the left. (From Drevets et al. 1997.)

with depressive illness than in the general population (Figure 61-1). The overall concordance rate for monozygotic twin pairs with bipolar depression may reach 80%; the rate for dizygotic twins is approximately 10% (the same as for siblings).

Seymour Kety, Paul Wender, and David Rosenthal extended their studies of patterns of schizophrenia in the families of adoptees (Chapter 60) to include manic-depressive disorders. They found that the rate of mood disorders among the biological parents of adoptees with depressive or manic-depressive illness was higher than among the adoptive parents (and higher than the rate among biological and adoptive parents of mentally healthy adoptees). Particularly impressive was the finding that the incidence of suicide among biological relatives of adoptees with depressive illness was six times higher than among the biological relatives of normal adoptees. Furthermore, the concordance rate of affective illness in monozygotic twins reared apart is 40–60%, similar to the concordance in those reared together.

These concordance rates for unipolar and bipolar depression in monozygotic twin pairs indicate that, like schizophrenia, major depression is polygenic. Several genes are likely to be involved, each making a small contri-

bution. Nongenetic factors are also likely to be important in determining whether an affective disorder is expressed. Their importance is reflected in two important secular trends in depression over the past 50 years. Since 1940 the age of onset has become younger (28 years rather than 35), and the incidence of depression in the families of patients has increased. Perhaps people vulnerable to depression are now more likely to become depressed than they were half a century ago because of the increased stress of everyday life. In addition there may also be a genetic anticipation.

Genetic linkage analysis (see Chapter 3) has led to the identification of several loci that might contribute to affective illness. Although no specific gene has yet been identified, one locus on chromosome 18 (18q22-23) has the strongest supporting evidence.

Familial Unipolar and Bipolar Depressions May Reflect an Abnormality in the Functioning of the Subgenual Region of the Frontal Cortex

Positron emission tomography (PET) scanning and functional magnetic resonance imaging (fMRI) studies have recently defined a potential anatomical abnormality in

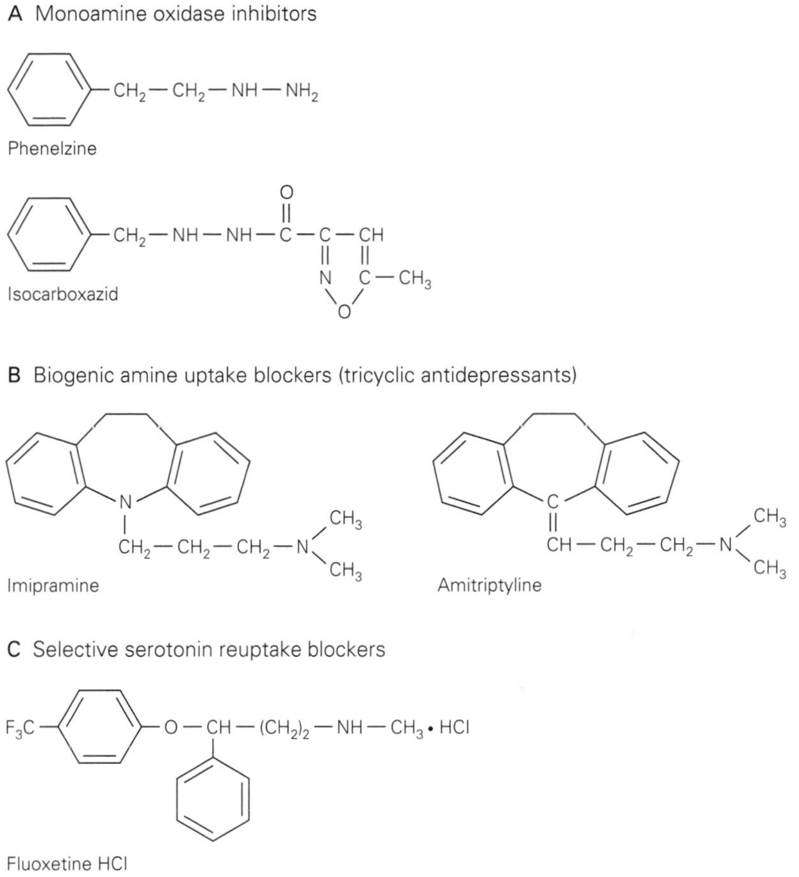

A Monoamine oxidase inhibitors

Phenelzine

Isocarboxazid

B Biogenic amine uptake blockers (tricyclic antidepressants)

Imipramine

Amitriptyline

C Selective serotonin reuptake blockers

Fluoxetine HCl

Figure 61-3 The three types of antidepressants.

A. Clinically useful monoamine oxidase inhibitors are chemically diverse. These drugs are thought to act by decreasing the breakdown of biogenic amines in the brain, thereby making more neurotransmitter available for release at aminergic synapses and prolonging the action of the aminergic transmitters. The anti-depressant effects of the drugs take several weeks to fully develop.

B. Tricyclic antidepressant drugs (see Figure 61-6) have immediate and long-term effects. Blockage of the reuptake of biogenic amine neurotransmitters from the synapse is evident soon after administration. The therapeutic action of antidepressants usually begins 4 days to 3 weeks after starting the medication.

C. Selective serotonin reuptake inhibitors are the most easily tolerated antidepressants.

the prefrontal cortex ventral to the genu in the corpus callosum that is affected in familial cases of unipolar and bipolar depression. During the depressive phase of the illness, activity in this region is decreased in patients who have either unipolar or bipolar depression. This decrease seems to be accounted for in large part by a reduction in the volume (by about 45%) of the gray matter of this part of the prefrontal cortex. In contrast, in patients with bipolar disease this region shows an increase in activity during the manic phase of the illness.

This finding is of interest because other clinical studies as well as studies in experimental animals have shown that the subgenual region of the prefrontal cortex is important for mood states (Figure 61-2). This region of the prefrontal cortex has extensive connections with other regions involved in emotional behavior, such as the amygdala, the lateral hypothalamus, the nucleus accumbens, and the noradrenergic, serotonergic, and dopaminergic systems of the brain stem (Chapter 50). People who have lesions in this area have difficulty experiencing emotion and have abnormal autonomic responses to emotionally arousing stimuli. Moreover, lesions in this area severely compromise the ability to reason and make intelligent, rational decisions. Conversely, Antonio Damasio and his colleagues have observed that small irritative lesions in this region cause episodes of anger and aggressive behavior.

Unipolar Depressive and Manic-Depressive Disorders Can Be Treated Effectively

There are four effective treatments for unipolar and bipolar illnesses: electroconvulsive therapy (ECT), antidepressant drugs, lithium, and anticonvulsants. Of the four, ECT has been used for the longest period of time, over 50 years. Although antidepressants are generally the first choice in the treatment of major depression, ECT is very effective. It produces full remission or marked improvement in about 85% of patients with well-defined major depression.

The critical therapeutic factor in ECT is the induction of a generalized brain seizure. Since the motor component of the seizure is not necessary for therapeutic results, modern ECT is always given under anesthesia with complete muscle relaxation. On average, six to eight treatments given at two-day intervals over a period of 2–4 weeks usually suffice to produce a complete remission of symptoms. As might be predicted from our knowledge of seizure activity (Chapter 46), ECT creates

A Pathways

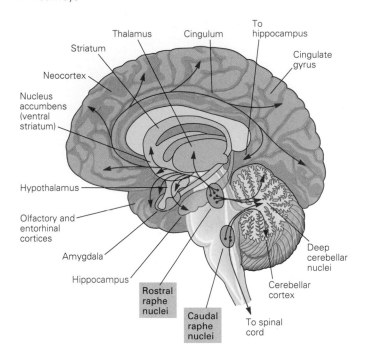

B Targets

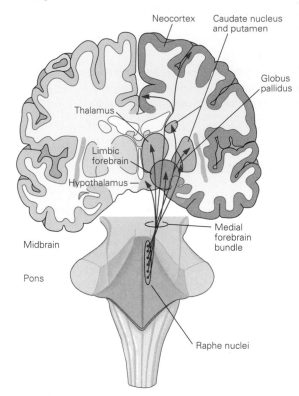

Figure 61-4 The major serotonergic pathways arise in the raphe nuclei. (Adapted from Heimer 1995.)

A. Lateral view of the brain illustrates that the raphe nuclei form a fairly continuous collection of cell groups close to the midline throughout the brain stem. For clarity, they are illustrated here in distinct rostral and caudal groups. The rostral

raphe nuclei project to a large number of forebrain structures (fibers that project laterally through the internal and external capsules to the neocortex are not shown here).

B. This coronal view of the brain illustrates some of the major targets of the serotonergic raphe nuclei neurons.

many temporary changes in brain functions. Although the therapeutic mechanism of ECT is not understood, it may be related to changes in aminergic receptor sensitivity, as we shall see later.

The most widely used antidepressant drugs fall into three major classes:

1. *Monoamine oxidase inhibitors*, such as phenelzine (Figure 61-3A). These were the first effective antidepressants to be used clinically but are now used only infrequently.
2. *Tricyclic compounds*, or general reuptake inhibitors of biogenic amines, such as imipramine, are so named for their three-ring molecular structure (Figure 61-3B). These compounds inhibit the uptake of both serotonin and norepinephrine and are probably the most effective drugs for patients who are *severely* depressed.
3. *Selective serotonin reuptake inhibitors*, such as fluoxetine (Prozac) (Figure 61-3C), paroxetine (Paxil), and

sertraline (Zoloft). These are the most commonly used antidepressants, and they work by selectively inhibiting the uptake of serotonin. They are most commonly used for patients who are only moderately depressed. These are, after the tricyclic compounds, the most commonly used drugs in severely ill patients.

The monoamine oxidase inhibitors and the tricyclic antidepressants produce remission or marked improvement in about 70% of patients with major depressions. When optimal doses are given, the success rate with tricyclic drugs and the specific serotonin reuptake inhibitors may reach 85%, almost as effective as ECT. Patients with bipolar depression occasionally become manic during treatment with either class of antidepressant drugs. Although a few patients with bipolar disease begin to improve immediately, there usually is a lag of 1–3 weeks before the symptoms of depression begin to improve, and 4–6 weeks are generally required for a full response.

Table 61-1 Serotonin Receptors

Receptors	Gene family
Receptors linked to second-message systems	Superfamily of receptors with seven transmembrane regions coupled to G proteins
5-HT$_{1A}$ linked to inhibition of adenylyl cyclase	
5-HT$_{1B}$ linked to inhibition of adenylyl cyclase	
5-HT$_{1D}$ linked to inhibition of adenylyl cyclase	
5-HT$_{1E}$ linked to inhibition of adenylyl cyclase	
5-HT$_{1F}$ linked to inhibition of adenylyl cyclase	
5-HT$_{2A}$ linked to phospholipase and PI turnover	
5-HT$_{2B}$ linked to phospholipase and PI turnover	
5-HT$_{2C}$ linked to phospholipase and PI turnover	
5-HT$_4$ linked to stimulation of adenylyl cyclase	
5-HT$_5$ unknown linkage	
5-HT$_6$ linked to stimulation of adenylyl cyclase	
5-HT$_7$ linked to stimulation of adenylyl cyclase	
Receptors linked to an ion channel	Superfamily of ligand-gated ion channels
5-HT$_3$	

5-HT = 5-hydroxytryptamine (serotonin); PI = Phosphatidylinositide.

A Pathways

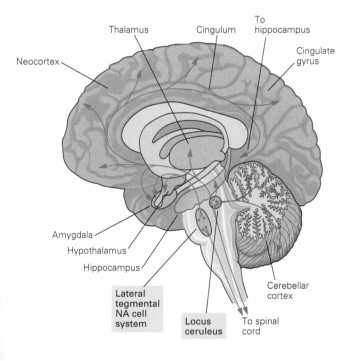

B Targets

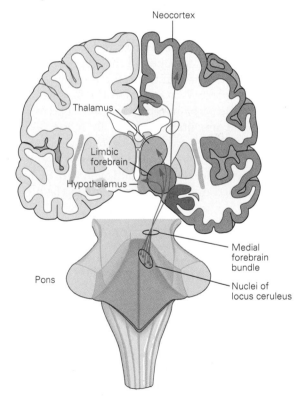

Figure 61-5 The noradrenergic pathways arise in the locus ceruleus. (Adapted from Heimer 1995.)

A. A lateral midsagittal view demonstrates the course of the major noradrenergic pathways from the locus ceruleus and lateral brain stem tegmentum. The pigmented locus ceruleus, located immediately beneath the floor of the fourth ventricle in the rostrolateral pons, is the best understood noradrenergic nu-cleus in the brain. Its projections reach many areas in the fore-brain, cerebellum, and spinal cord. Noradrenergic neurons in the lateral brain stem tegmentum innervate several structures in the basal forebrain, including the hypothalamus and the amygdaloid body.

B. A coronal section shows the major targets of neurons from the locus ceruleus. (Adapted from Heimer 1995.)

1215

Table 61-2 Noradrenergic Receptors Linked to Second-Messenger Systems

Type	Second-mesenger system	Location
β_1	Linked to stimulation of adenylyl cyclase	Cerebral cortex, cerebellum
β_2	Linked to stimulation of adenylyl cyclase	Cerebral cortex, cerebellum
α_1	Linked to phospholipase C, PI, PKC, DAG, Ca^{2+} in peripheral tissues	Brain, blood vessels, spleen
α_2	Linked to inhibition of adenylyl cyclase	Presynaptic nerve terminals throughout the brain

PI = Phosphatidylinositide; PKC = Protein kinase C; DAG = Diacylglycerol.

Lithium salts, first reported in the psychiatric treatment of manic-depressive illness in 1949 by John Cade, are effective in terminating manic episodes and are used as mood stabilizers. Moreover, maintenance therapy with lithium is of significant prophylactic value in preventing or attenuating recurrent manic and, to a lesser extent, depressive episodes. Lithium is rarely used by itself for treatment of unipolar depression. However, it is frequently used in conjunction with monoamine oxidase inhibitors, tricyclic compounds, or selective serotonin reuptake inhibitors to augment the response of these conventional antidepressants (see Figure 61-9).

Drugs effective as anticonvulsants (such as sodium valproate and carbamazepine) are also used as mood stabilizers and are quite effective in reducing psychotic symptoms in acute mania or severe depression. Antipsychotic drugs (Chapter 60) are also used frequently in combination with tricyclic drugs, and even with ECT when depression is accompanied by delusions and hallucinations.

Drugs Effective in Depression Act on Serotonergic and Noradrenergic Pathways

Drugs effective in treating depression act primarily on the serotonergic and noradrenergic systems of the brain (Chapter 45). The evidence is particularly impressive for serotonin—all selective serotonin reuptake inhibitors tested have been found to be effective against depression. The action of these drugs, therefore, provides the first clues to a neurochemical basis of depressive disorders. The major serotonergic pathways have their origin in the raphe nuclei in the brain stem (Figure 61-4). Cells from the rostral parts of these nuclei project to the forebrain; single serotonergic neurons project to hundreds of target cells in a large, diffuse distribution. (The cells of the caudal part of the raphe nuclei project to the spinal cord.)

The serotonergic receptors are traditionally classified into at least seven major types. Some types decrease

adenylyl cyclase, some increase adenylyl cyclase, others are coupled to phosphatidylinositide turnover, and still others are ligand-gated ion channels (Table 61-1).

The noradrenergic pathways originate in the locus ceruleus (Figure 61-5). The axons of some locus ceruleus neurons ascend to innervate the hypothalamus and all regions of the cerebral cortex, including the hippocampus. Other neurons have descending axons that reach the dorsal and ventral horns of the spinal cord. Like serotonergic cells, noradrenergic neurons innervate broad areas and act on a number of receptor types (Table 61-2). Certain components of the noradrenergic system appear to be involved with arousal and fear (Chapter 50), while others are thought to be involved, together with the mesolimbic components of the dopaminergic system, in positive motivation and pleasure (Chapter 51). The pervasive anxiety and loss of pleasure characteristic of melancholia and atypical depression might therefore be related to dysregulation of these two components of the noradrenergic system.

An Abnormality in Biogenic Amine Transmission May Contribute to the Disorders of Mood

Norepinephrine is synthesized from tyrosine, and serotonin from tryptophan (Chapter 15). The transmitters are packaged in synaptic vesicles and released into the synaptic cleft by means of exocytosis when the neuron fires an action potential. Both norepinephrine and serotonin interact with postsynaptic receptors, and this activity is limited by active reuptake of the released transmitter into the presynaptic terminals as well as into glial cells. Inside the presynaptic terminals the transmitters are packaged again into vesicles or catabolized primarily by the mitochondrial enzyme monoamine oxidase.

Until recently the consensus view—expressed first in the *catecholamine hypothesis* and then in the more general *biogenic amine hypothesis*—was that depression rep-

Table 61-3 Effects of Long-Term Administration of Antidepressant Drugs on the Serotonergic System

Antidepressant treatment	Responsiveness of somatodendritic 5-HT$_{1A}$ autoreceptors	Function of terminal 5-HT autoreceptors	Function of terminal α_2 adrenergic receptors	Responsiveness of postsynaptic receptors	Net serotonin transmission 5-HT receptors
Selective serotonin reuptake inhibitors	Decreased	Decreased	NC	NC	Increased
Monoamine oxidase inhibitors	Decreased	NC	?	NC or decreased	Increased
5-HT$_{1A}$ receptor agonists	Decreased	NC	ND	NC	Increased
Tricyclic antidepressants	NC	NC	ND	Increased	Increased
Electroconvulsive shocks	NC	NC	NC	Increased	Increased

From Blier and deMontigny 1994; NC = no change; ND = no data; 5-HT = 5-hydroxytryptamine (serotonin).

resented a decreased availability of either norepinephrine or serotonin or both. Mania was believed to result from the over-activity of noradrenergic systems. This hypothesis was derived from studies of the effects of various drugs on the serotonergic and noradrenergic systems of the brain. The idea originally came from the observation in 1950 that reserpine, a Rauwolfia alkaloid then used extensively in the treatment of hypertension, precipitated depressive syndromes in about 15% of treated patients. Reserpine also produced a depression-like syndrome, with motor retardation and sedation, in animals. Bernard Brodie and his colleagues found that reserpine depletes the brain of serotonin and norepinephrine (as well as dopamine) by inhibiting the uptake of the transmitter into synaptic vesicles in the presynaptic cell, thereby keeping the transmitter in the cytoplasm, where it undergoes degradation by monoamine oxidase (Figure 61-6).

Monoamine oxidase inhibitors, such as isoniazid, were later found to be effective antidepressants. Isoniazid was initially developed in the 1950s to treat tuberculosis. In the course of clinical trials it was noted that some patients who had depression as well as tuberculosis experienced elevations in mood when treated with the drug. Isoniazid was next tried in patients with depression who did not have tuberculosis and was found to be effective. Monoamine oxidase inhibitors increase the concentration of serotonin and norepinephrine in the brain by reducing the degradation of these transmitters by monoamine oxidase. In experimental animals monoamine oxidase inhibitors prevent reserpine's seda-

tive effects on behavior as well as its degradation of cytoplasmic monoamines.

Further support for the view that monoamine oxidase inhibitors act therapeutically by increasing the availability of serotonin and biogenic amines came with the discovery of a second class of effective antidepressants: the tricyclics. These agents *block* the active reuptake of serotonin and norepinephrine by presynaptic neurons, thereby prolonging the action of these transmitters in the synaptic cleft (see Figure 61-6). Finally, the third group of compounds that proved to be effective in depression, the selective serotonin reuptake inhibitors, affect *only* serotonin and not norepinephrine. Thus, all three major classes of antidepressants maximize synaptic transmission of serotonin by inhibiting the reuptake of the transmitter or its degradation (Table 61-3). Even electroconvulsive shock increases serotonergic transmission (Table 61-3). It does so by increasing the sensitivity of the 5-HT$_{1A}$ receptors in the hippocampus and increasing the number of 5-HT$_{2A}$ receptors.

The remarkable effectiveness of selective serotonin reuptake inhibitors on depression provides the most compelling evidence that enhancement of serotonergic transmission underlies the therapeutic response to some antidepressant treatments. However, the biogenic amine hypothesis fails to account for a number of important clinical phenomena. In particular, it fails to explain why the clinical response to all antidepressant drugs is so slow after administration of the drugs, whereas the tricyclic agents and the selective serotonin reuptake inhibitors rapidly block the high-affinity reuptake

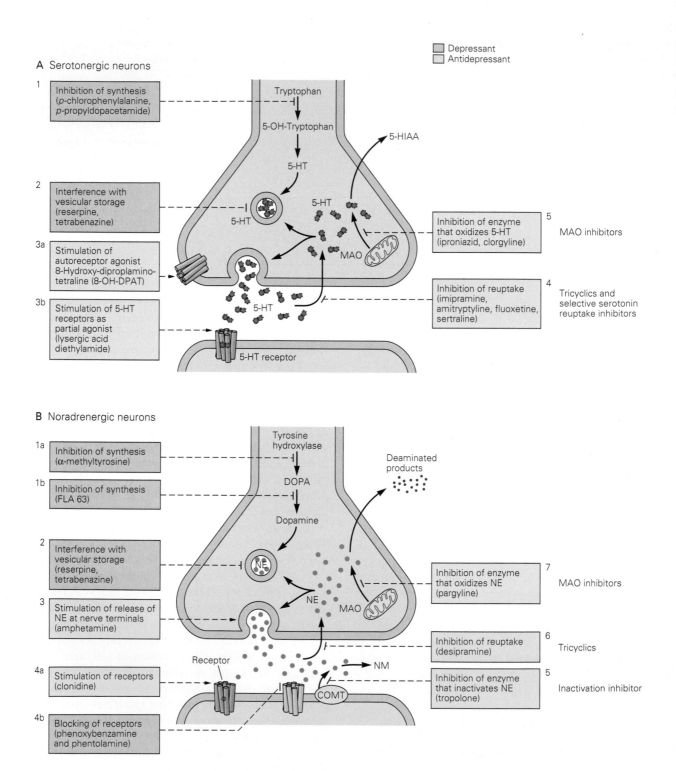

□ Depressant
□ Antidepressant

A Serotonergic neurons

1 Inhibition of synthesis (p-chlorophenylalanine, p-propyldopacetamide)

Tryptophan

5-OH-Tryptophan

5-HT

5-HIAA

2 Interference with vesicular storage (reserpine, tetrabenazine)

5-HT

5-HT

5 Inhibition of enzyme that oxidizes 5-HT (iproniazid, clorgyline)   MAO inhibitors

MAO

3a Stimulation of autoreceptor agonist 8-Hydroxy-diproplamino-tetraline (8-OH-DPAT)

3b Stimulation of 5-HT receptors as partial agonist (lysergic acid diethylamide)

4 Inhibition of reuptake (imipramine, amitryptyline, fluoxetine, sertraline)   Tricyclics and selective serotonin reuptake inhibitors

5-HT

5-HT receptor

B Noradrenergic neurons

1a Inhibition of synthesis (α-methyltyrosine)

Tyrosine hydroxylase

Deaminated products

DOPA

1b Inhibition of synthesis (FLA 63)

Dopamine

2 Interference with vesicular storage (reserpine, tetrabenazine)

NE

7 Inhibition of enzyme that oxidizes NE (pargyline)   MAO inhibitors

3 Stimulation of release of NE at nerve terminals (amphetamine)

NE

MAO

6 Inhibition of reuptake (desipramine)   Tricyclics

Receptor

NM

4a Stimulation of receptors (clonidine)

5 Inhibition of enzyme that inactivates NE (tropolone)   Inactivation inhibitor

COMT

4b Blocking of receptors (phenoxybenzamine and phentolamine)

Figure 61-6 (Opposite) Action of antidepressant and other drugs at serotonergic and noradrenergic synapses.

A. Antidepressant and other drugs have five possible sites of action at serotonergic synapses.

1. Enzymatic synthesis. Both p-chlorophenylalanine and p-propyldopacetamide can effectively inhibit the enzyme tryptophan nyroxylase, which converts tryptophan to 5-OH-tryptophan, the precursor of 5-hydroxytryptophan (5-HT, serotonin).

2. Storage. Reserpine and tetrabenazine interfere with the reuptake-storage mechanism of the amine granules, causing a marked depletion of serotonin.

3. Receptor interactions. These fall into two categories. a. Autoreceptor 8-hydroxy-diprolamino-tetraline (8-OH-DPAT) is an agonist of the 5-HT autoreceptor. b. Lysergic acid diethylamide (LSD) acts as a partial agonist at postsynaptic serotonergic receptors in the central nervous system. A number of specific compounds are now candidates to act as receptor-blocking agents at various serotonergic synapses.

4. Reuptake. Tricyclic drugs with a tertiary nitrogen, such as imipramine and amitryptyline, inhibit the reuptake of serotonin into the presynaptic terminal and thus increase the efficacy of transmission. Fluoxetine and sertraline are even more selective inhibitors of serotonin uptake.

5. Degradation by monoamine oxidase (**MAO**). Iproniazid and clorgyline are effective inhibitors of MAO, which is localized in the outer membrane of mitochondria and can degrade serotonin present in a free state within the presynaptic terminal. **5-HIAA** = 5-hydroxyindoleacetic acid.

B. Antidepressants and other drugs have seven possible sites of action at noradrenergic synapses.

1. Enzymatic synthesis. a. The competitive inhibitor α-methyltyrosine blocks the reaction catalyzed by tyrosine hydroxylase. b. A dithiocarbamate derivative, FLA 63, blocks the reaction catalyzed by dopamine β-hydroxylase, which converts DOPA to dopamine.

2. Storage. Reserpine and tetrabenazine interfere with the reuptake-storage mechanism of the amine granules. The depletion of norepinephrine (**NE**) by reserpine is long-lasting and the storage granules are irreversibly damaged, causing permanent depletion of NE available for release transmission. Tetrabenazine also interferes with the reuptake of free cytoplasmic NE into the granules.

3. Release. Amphetamine appears to cause an increase in the net release of NE, most likely because of its ability to block the reuptake.

4. Receptor interaction. a. Clonidine is a very potent α-receptor agonist. b. Phenoxybenzamine and phentolamine are effective α-receptor blocking agents. Recent experiments have indicated that these drugs also have a presynaptic site of action.

5. Degradation by COMT. Tropolone inhibits COMT, which inactivates NE. COMT is believed to be localized outside the postsynaptic neuron.

6. Reuptake. The tricyclic drug desipramine is a potent inhibitor of the reuptake of NE into the presynaptic terminal. As a result, NE remains in the synapse longer and has a greater postsynaptic effect.

7. Degradation by monoamine oxidase (**MAO**). Pargyline is an effective inhibitor of MAO, which appears to be localized in the outer membrane of mitochondria and can degrade the NE present in a free state within the presynaptic terminal. Normetanephrine (**NM**) is formed by the action of the enzyme catechol O-methyltransferase (**COMT**) on NE.

systems. This blockade is much more rapid than the clinical response. If the clinical response is a result of an increase in serotonergic synaptic transmission, what accounts for the delay in the response? In addition, the tricyclic drugs vary widely in their relative abilities to block serotonin or norepinephrine reuptake, yet their clinical efficacy in patients with depression is about the same. Finally, in some patients with depression the onset of the illness is associated not with a decrease but with an *increase* in the level of norepinephrine in spinal fluid and plasma, and treatment leads to reduction to a normal level.

Some clues are emerging that may help to resolve these issues. For example, it is now clear that antidepressant agents affect processes other than the reuptake and accumulation of serotonin. In addition to their rapid biochemical effects on reuptake, both monoamine oxidase inhibitors and tricyclic antidepressants produce a delayed but long-term increase in the sensitivity of serotonin receptors. Conversely, the selective serotonin reuptake inhibitors produce a delayed decrease in the sensitivity of $5HT_{1A}$ and $5HT_{1B}$ inhibitory autoreceptors present on many serotonergic cells, leading to increased release of serotonin. Both of these actions lead to a slow increase in the effectiveness of serotonergic synaptic transmission.

Given these findings, where does the biogenic amine hypothesis stand? The initial, simple form of the biogenic amine hypothesis, which states that reduction of biogenic amines leads to depression and elevation to mania, is no longer valid. There probably is no simple relationship between biogenic amines and depression. If a relationship exists at all, which seems likely, it is complicated by three factors.

First, the subtypes of major depression are most likely not single disorders, but a group of disorders with several underlying pathologies. Second, disturbances in one of several transmitter systems can lead to depression. Finally, the various modulatory systems of the brain—the serotonergic, dopaminergic, and adrenergic systems—do not function independently of each other but rather interact at several levels. Specifically, the distribution of the serotonergic system overlaps with and interacts with the noradrenergic system. Moreover, receptors for the two amines coexist on the same neurons, and there is cross-talk between second messengers activated by these transmitters. Long-term administration of antidepressants fails to downregulate the β-adrenergic receptors when serotonergic systems have been eliminated experimentally.

In addition, antidepressants act on the cholinergic and GABA-ergic systems. Cholinergic neurons excite the noradrenergic cells of the locus ceruleus through

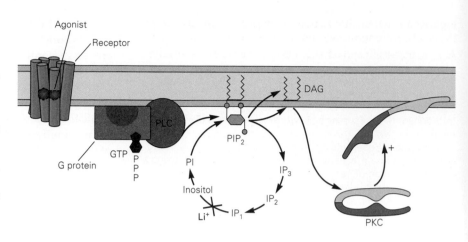

Figure 61-7 The exact therapeutic action of lithium, used to treat bipolar depression, is unknown. However, lithium has been shown to affect the phosphoinositide second-messenger system. Many synaptic receptors act through a G protein to mediate the conversion of phosphoinositol diphosphate (PIP_2), a membrane lipid, into diacylglycerol (**DAG**) and inositol triphosphate (IP_3). IP_3 is further broken down to inositol phosphate (**IP**), which is then converted to free inositol by the enzyme inositol-1-phosphatase. Lithium blocks this enzyme and therefore reduces the responsiveness of these neurons by causing IP_3 to accumulate in the cytoplasm. The roles of IP_3 and protein kinase C are discussed in Chapter 13.

muscarinic receptors, and cholinergic agonists can induce depression. Indeed, patients with a history of depression tend to be hyperresponsive to cholinergic agonists, even when their mood is normal.

Since most serotonergic and adrenergic receptors act on second-messenger pathways—activating or inhibiting adenylyl cyclase or stimulating phosphoinositide turnover—it is perhaps not surprising that drugs acting directly on these pathways are now being developed. For example, lithium salts, which are highly effective in bipolar disorder, block the enzyme inositol-1-phosphatase, which recycles inositol triphosphate back to inositol. This results in a buildup of inositol 1,4,5-triphosphate (IP_3), which is known to be active in regulating intracellular Ca^{2+} levels. Inhibition of this enzyme is thought to reduce the responsiveness of those neurons with transmitter receptors coupled to the IP_3 pathway (Figure 61-7). This could be the way lithium acts therapeutically, perhaps by dampening excessive neural activity in mania.

Unipolar Depression May Involve Disturbances of Neuroendocrine Function

As first pointed out by Edward Sachar, depression is associated with clinical signs of hypothalamic disturbance. The best-understood hypothalalmic disturbance in severe depression is neuroendocrine and is reflected in excessive secretion of adrenocorticotropic hormone (ACTH) by the pituitary, leading to excessive secretion of cortisol from the adrenal cortex. The hypersecretion of ACTH is so great that enlargement of the adrenal gland can be detected on computerized axial tomography (CAT) scans of some patients with depression.

In normal people the secretion of cortisol follows a circadian rhythm; secretion peaks at 8:00 AM and is rela-

tively lower in the evening and early morning hours. This circadian cycle is disturbed in about one-half of patients with depression, who secrete excessive amounts of cortisol throughout the day (Figure 61-8). The disturbance is not dependent on stress and is not found in other psychiatric disorders. Cortisol secretion returns to normal with recovery.

Philip Gold and his colleagues found that the increased secretion of cortisol results from hypersecretion of corticotropin-releasing hormone (CTRH) from the hypothalamus, and that the level of CTRH correlates positively with depression. Release of CTRH is stimulated by norepinephrine and acetylcholine, and release of CTRH induces anxiety in experimental animals. Thus, Gold and his colleagues have suggested that CTRH and the noradrenergic system may reinforce one another.

Hypersecretion of cortisol is sometimes resistant to feedback suppression by the potent synthetic corticosteroid dexamethasone, which depresses secretion of adrenocorticotropin. The *dexamethasone suppression test* has been used to diagnose depression because in at least 40% of rigorously diagnosed patients with depression hypersecretion of cortisol is resistant to feedback suppression by dexamethasone. However, the test is not specific; dexamethasone suppression is also abnormal in patients who have dementia, anorexia nervosa, bulimia, alcohol withdrawal, or weight loss.

There Are at Least Four Major Types of Anxiety Disorders

Just as grief is a normal response to personal loss, anxiety is a normal response to threatening situations. Perceived threats that generate anxiety may be active and direct or indirect, such as the absence of people or objects that represent security. Anxiety is adaptive; it signals potential danger and can contribute to the mastery of a difficult situation and thus to personal growth. Excessive anxiety, on the other hand, is maladaptive, either because it is too intense or because it is inappropriately provoked by events that present no real danger. Thus, anxiety is pathological when excessive and persistent, or when it no longer serves to signal danger.

The key feature of anxiety disorders is increased fearfulness accompanied by subjective as well as objective manifestations. The subjective manifestations range from a heightened sense of awareness to a deep fear of impending disaster and death. The objective manifestations are a racing heart, avoidance behavior and signs of restlessness, heightened responsiveness, palpitations, tremor, sweating, increased blood pressure, dry mouth, and a desire to run or escape. Depression and anxiety often occur together.

Anxiety disorders are the most common psychiatric disorders, found in 10–30% of the general population. Anxiety disorders can be subdivided into several types based on clinical characteristics and response to psychopharmacologic agents. These major categories include panic disorder, post-traumatic stress disorder, (PTSD), generalized anxiety disorder, social phobia, and obsessive-compulsive disorder (OCD).

Panic Attacks Are Brief Episodes of Terror

Panic attacks are brief, recurrent, unexpected episodes of terror without a clearly identifiable cause. The attacks are usually brief, most commonly lasting 15–30 minutes; occasionally, but only rarely, they last up to an hour. An essential feature of these attacks is that they are *unexpected*. They do not occur in situations that normally evoke fear or in which the patient is the focus of other people's attention. The attacks are characterized by a sense of impending doom accompanied by an intense over-activity of the sympathetic nervous system (referred to as a *sympathetic crisis*): The heart races, there is shortness of breath; dizziness; trembling or shaking of the hands and legs; flushes or chills; chest pain; and fear of dying, or of going crazy, or of doing something uncontrolled. Shortness of breath is characteristic of panic attacks but not of the acute terror evident in battle, suggesting that panic attacks may represent a false alarm for suffocation.

When panic attacks recur the resulting syndrome is called *panic disorder*. Attacks recur over a period ranging from months to several years and are often experienced several times a week. Panic disorders usually begin in adolescence.

An interesting aspect of panic attacks is that they can be induced in some patients who have this disorder, but not in most normal subjects, by the infusion of sodium lactate into the blood or the inhalation of carbon dioxide. Thus, sodium lactate infusion provides an approach for studying the mechanism underlying this disorder because the onset of an attack can be timed precisely. Moreover, regular use of antidepressants that are effective against spontaneous panic attacks also prevent the panic induced by the infusion. Similarly, yohimbine, a drug that activates central noradrenergic neurons (by blocking the α_2 adrenergic receptors that serve as inhibiting autoreceptors), precipitates panic attacks in patients but not in normal subjects, indicating that panic attacks involve an abnormality in the biogenic amine system of the brain.

A significant proportion of patients with panic disorders have a genetic predisposition. Half of patients

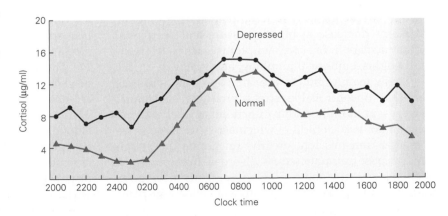

Figure 61-8 Many patients with depression secrete excess ACTH and cortisol during the day. In normal subjects there is a circadian rhythm to the secretion, which peaks at 8:00 AM and then decreases progressively from the early morning hours into the evening until 3:00 AM at night (0300). By contrast, in depressed patients the plasma cortisol concentration is elevated throughout much of the 24-hour period of the day, with only a slight decline in the evening (2000 to 0200). The plot shows the mean hourly plasma cortisol concentration over a 24-hour period for seven patients with unipolar depression compared with the mean for 54 normal subjects. Each point represents the mean cortisol concentration every 60 minutes.

with panic attacks also have depression, a finding that has led to the suggestion that panic attacks may be a variant of depressive illness or a precursor to it. This is consistent with the initially surprising finding that panic disorder is successfully treated with both tricyclic antidepressants and monoamine oxidase inhibitors. Now that more is known about the function of the locus ceruleus, this finding is perhaps less surprising. The noradrenergic cells in this nucleus respond most effectively to stimuli that produce intense fear. In fact, cognitive therapy for panic attacks trains patients not to act on their autonomic signals.

Post-Traumatic Stress Disorder Reflects Persistent Traces of Anxiety That Follow Traumatic Episodes

An interesting variant of panic attacks is *post-traumatic stress disorder*. Although now appreciated as fairly common, this disorder was not clearly recognized in its present form until the 1980s. Post-traumatic stress disorder occurs in people after an extremely stressful event, such as life-threatening combat or physical abuse. It is manifested in recurrent episodes of fear, often triggered by reminders of the initial trauma. One of the most striking features of this disorder is that the memory for the traumatic experience remains powerful for decades and is readily reactivated by a variety of stimuli and stressors. This is thought to be due to the recruitment of the noradrenergic system by these reactivating stimuli. As we shall learn in Chapter 63, biogenic amines are important in modulating various memory processes.

Vietnam War veterans with post-traumatic stress disorder show heightened noradrenergic functioning. They excrete high levels of norepinephrine in their urine, presumably reflecting high circulating catecholamine levels. When exposed to gunfire or other stimuli associated with combat, these veterans respond with dramatic increases in blood pressure and heart rate. When patients with post-traumatic stress disorder are given yohimbine, they experience a type of panic attack: An intense memory is accompanied by autonomic symptoms (increase in blood pressure and heart rate) and an increase in the core symptoms, such as frightening thoughts, emotional numbing, and grief.

These manifestations are all consistent with the idea that uncontrollable stress produces substantial increases in noradrenergic functioning in the brain. Propranolol and clonidine, which act to decrease noradrenergic transmission, greatly ameliorate the symptoms of post-traumatic stress disorder. Interestingly, a large percentage (about 50%) of patients with post-traumatic stress disorder also show a concurrent panic disorder.

Generalized Anxiety Disorder Is Characterized by Long-Lasting Worries

The key feature of generalized anxiety disorder is unrealistic or excessive worry, lasting not minutes but continuously for six months or longer. The symptoms are motor tension (trembling, twitching, muscle aches, restlessness), autonomic hyperactivity (palpitations, increased heart rate, sweating, cold hands), and vigilance and scanning (feeling on edge, exaggerated startle response, difficulty in concentrating). The disorder sometimes follows an episode of depression.

One group of drugs that is particularly effective in treating generalized anxiety disorder is the benzodiazepines, such as chlordiazepoxide (Librium) and its derivative, diazepam (Valium). Benzodiazepines produce their therapeutic effect by enhancing the activity of the $GABA_A$ receptor. GABA is the major inhibitory transmitter in the brain (Chapter 12). The $GABA_A$ receptor opens Cl^- channels and the resulting influx of Cl^- hyperpolarizes and thus inhibits target cells. Benzodiazepine increases the affinity of the receptor for GABA, resulting in an increase in Cl^- influx through the Cl^- channels and thereby prolonging the synaptic inhibition produced by GABA (Figure 61-9).

The $GABA_A$ receptor has separate binding sites for GABA, barbiturates, and benzodiazepines (Chapter 11). The protein is allosteric; binding of any one of the three ligands (GABA, benzodiazepine, or barbiturate) influences the binding of the other two and facilitates GABA's action. In particular, GABA will bind more tightly when a benzodiazepine also is bound to its site on the receptor. Nevertheless, all three sites are distinct. Analysis of the primary structure of the GABA receptor indicates that there are at least three subunits (α, β, γ); benzodiazepine binds to the γ subunit.

The calming effects of benzodiazepines are therefore best explained by an enhancement of certain of the inhibitory effects of GABA. Inverse agonists of benzodiazepine reduce rather than enhance GABA-ergic transmission and produce anxiety as well as predisposition to convulsions. Yet these inverse agonists bind to the benzodiazepine site on the GABA receptor and are blocked by benzodiazepine antagonists.

This has raised the possibility that endogenous inverse agonists might mediate naturally occurring anxiety states. High concentrations of GABA receptors have been found in the limbic system, specifically in the amygdala, an area thought to be of central importance for emotional behavior. However, as with other mental illnesses, it is unlikely that a single transmitter system is responsible for the illness. In fact, many patients with anxiety states respond extremely well to selective serotonin reuptake inhibitors and tricyclic antidepressants.

Figure 61-9 Benzodiazepines act on the GABA channel.

A. Structural model of the GABA$_A$ chloride channel. The channel protein contains at least five different subunit types, of which only three are illustrated here (α, β, γ). Benzodiazepines bind to the γ subunits, GABA to the α subunit, and barbiturates to the β subunit. All the subunits contribute to forming the Cl$^-$ channel. When GABA binds to GABA$_A$ receptors the Cl$^-$ channels open and the influx of Cl$^-$ hyperpolarizes the cell.

B. Diazepam, a benzodiazepine, is an effective drug in treating generalized anxiety disorders. The traces compare the responses of a mouse spinal cord neuron to GABA, the major inhibitory neurotransmitter in the brain, and to GABA in the presence of diazepam. Diazepam increases the affinity of the receptor for GABA and thus increases the Cl$^-$ conductance and the hyperpolarizing current.

C. Benzodiazepine (Benzo) modulates Cl$^-$ flux through the channel by enhancing the effect of GABA, which itself enhances the influx of Cl$^-$ into the nerve cell. As a result, basal levels of GABA become more effective in gating the channel. Benzodiazepine antagonists prevent enhancement of GABA effects but do not reduce the basal conductance of Cl$^-$. GABA antagonists prevent gating of Cl$^-$ channels in spite of the presence of benzodiazepines.

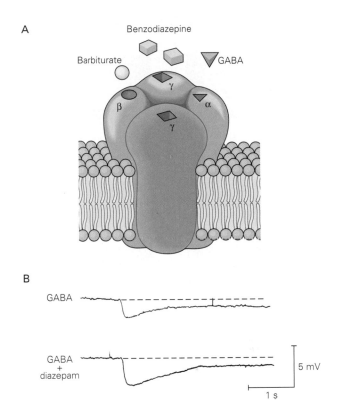

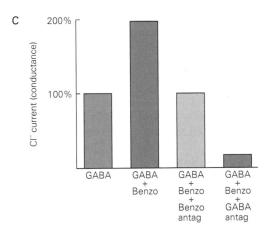

In Obsessive-Compulsive Disorder Obtrusive Thoughts Are a Source of Anxiety and Compulsion

Obsessive-compulsive disorders are usually chronic disorders with recurrent obsessions and compulsions as the predominant features. *Obsessions* are persistent and intrusive ideas, thoughts, images, or impulses that commonly fall into one of two categories: doubts or fears. Obsessive doubting can penetrate daily life, leaving patients repeatedly unsure whether the apartment door was locked, whether the stove was turned off, or whether their hands are clean enough. This preoccupation can result in excessive hand washing, sometimes to the extent of soreness or removal of skin. Obsessive fears focus on unrealistic and improbable dangers, such as the prospect of killing someone driving a car or lighting the stove. Interestingly, the person experiencing these fears typically views them as alien—senseless and unwanted invasions of consciousness. When the fears first become prominent, the patient attempts to ignore or suppress them, usually unsuccessfully. Later in the course of the illness the patient may no longer actively resist these fears.

To alleviate the anxiety and diminish the discomfort of the obsessive thoughts or urges, the patient often begins to carry out compulsive acts. In contrast to obsessions, which are repetitive ideas, *compulsions* are repetitive acts. To be defined as a compulsion a behavior must be repeated excessively and the repetition must not be realistically related to any environmental condition. The most common compulsions are handwashing, counting, checking, touching, and pulling out of hair.

The severe symptoms of obsessive-compulsive disorder are thought to represent the extreme end of a behavioral continuum that includes a compulsive lifestyle that typically begins between 18 and 25 years of age. Although the symptoms may disappear or become less severe for periods of time, the disorder rarely disappears.

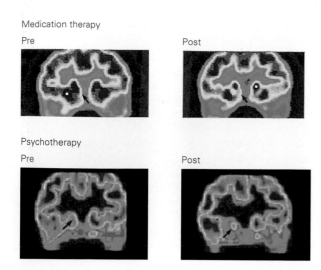

Medication therapy

Pre · Post

Psychotherapy

Pre · Post

Figure 61-10 Patients with obsessive-compulsive disorder tend to show hyperactivity in the head of the caudate. This hyperactivity can be reduced in one of two ways: by selective serotonin reuptake inhibitors (**top**), medication therapy, or cognitive therapy (**bottom**), psychotherapy.

Indeed, people with obsessive-compulsive disorder may also have other mental illness, such as depression, other anxiety disorders (panic attacks, eating disorders), or social phobias.

Obsessive-compulsive disorder is thought to reflect a disturbance of the basal ganglia. In fact, some forms of obsessive-compulsive disorder seem to be related to Tourette syndrome, a hereditary chronic motor tic disorder that has its locus in the basal ganglia. Patients with Tourette syndrome erupt in repetitive grunts, noises, and even obscenities that are not under the patient's control. Several other neurological syndromes that involve the basal ganglia, such as postencephalitic Parkinson disease, Sydenham chorea, bilateral necrosis of the globus pallidus, and Huntington disease, often are associated with a component of obsessive-compulsive disorder.

The head of the caudate nucleus and the pathway that connects the caudate with the prefrontal (orbitofrontal) cortex and cingulate gyrus seems to be hyperactive in obsessive-compulsive disorder. The caudate nucleus sends GABA-ergic inhibitory projections to the globus pallidus (one of the two major output elements of the striatum), which sends inhibitory projections to the thalamus, which then projects to the orbitofrontal cortex. The presence of serial inhibitory pathways—from the caudate nucleus to the globus pallidus, and from there to the thalamus—suggests the possibility

that a disease state produces a disinhibition, which could lead to reverberating activity in this circuit. Perhaps an increase in the first inhibitory pathway causes the second pathway to become less of an inhibitor of its targets, leading to the reverberatory state.

Obsessive-compulsive disorder is responsive to two types of treatments: (1) specific behavioral therapies based on conditioning (Chapter 62) and (2) specific serotonin reuptake inhibitors. The effectiveness of the serotonin reuptake inhibitors raises two questions: Is central serotonergic transmission abnormal in obsessive-compulsive disorder and, if so, can psychotherapy reverse this effect? In fact, serotonergic innervation of the striatum is extensive. This innervation is localized to the medial-ventral aspects of the head of the caudate nucleus and to the nucleus accumbens, regions that receive input from the orbitofrontal and cingulate cortex regions thought to be involved in emotional behavior. Surgical lesions of these tracts from the frontal cortex to subcortical sites has improved the symptoms of some otherwise intractable cases. After effective treatment of the disease with either serotonin reuptake inhibitors or behavioral therapy, hyperactivity of the caudate nucleus and orbitofrontal cortex decreases significantly (Figure 61-10). This suggests that psychotherapy and pharmacologic therapy lead to a similar biological change.

An Overall View

Certain major depressive illnesses may be the result of genetically determined defects in chemical synaptic transmission involving at least two major transmitter pathways of the brain: the serotonergic and noradrenergic systems. Although the mechanisms that cause the defects in transmission remain obscure, progress in studying allelic variations in the human genome provide hope that aspects of the molecular basis of affective disorders might soon be elucidated.

Because there are good animal models of anxiety and we now know a great deal about the amygdala and the neural circuitry in learned fear, it is likely that anxiety may soon be better understood. Like major depression and schizophrenia, two types of anxiety—panic disorder and generalized anxiety disorder—seem to reflect alterations in synaptic functioning. Since panic disorder responds well to certain antidepressants, it too may reflect an abnormality in the biogenic amine pathways of the brain. In contrast, generalized anxiety disorder may involve the $GABA_A$ receptor system, or more likely an abnormality in the interaction of the $GABA_A$ receptor and the serotonergic system.

Perhaps the most powerful insight into obsessive-compulsive disorders is the finding that psychotherapy and selective serotonin reuptake inhibitors are equally effective in reversing the symptoms and in so doing they also reverse the anatomical abnormalities.

Eric R. Kandel

Selected Readings

Barondes SH. 1993. *Molecules and Mental Illness.* New York: Scientific American Library.

Barondes SH. 1998. *Mood Genes: Hunting for the Origins of Mania and Depression.* New York: W.H. Freeman and Co.

Delgado PL, Charney DS, Price MD, Aghajanian GK, Landis H, Heninger GB. 1990. Serotonin function and the mechanism of antidepressant action. Arch Gen Psychiatry 47:411–419.

Gold PW, Goodwin FK, Chrousos GP. 1988. Clinical and biochemical manifestations of depression: relation to the neurobiology of stress. N Engl J Med 319:348–353 and 413–420.

Goodwin DW, Guze SB. 1989. *Psychiatric Diagnosis,* 4th ed. New York: Oxford Univ. Press.

Goodwin FK, Jamison KR. 1990. *Manic-Depressive Illness.* New York: Oxford Univ. Press.

Janowsky A, Sulser F. 1987. Alpha and beta adrenoreceptor in brain. In: HY Meltzer (ed). *Psychopharmacology: The Third Generation of Progress,* pp. 249–256. New York: Raven.

Klerman GL. 1983. The scope of depression. In: J Angst (ed). *The Origins of Depression: Current Concepts and Approaches,* pp. 5–25. Dahlem Konferenzen. Heidelberg: Springer.

Schwartz JM, Stoessel PW, Baxter LR, Martin KM, Phelps ME. 1996. Systematic changes in cerebral glucose metabolic rate after successful behavior modification treatment of obsessive-compulsive disorders. Arch Gen Psychiatry 53:109–113.

Triveldi MH. 1996. Functional neuroanatomy of obsessive-compulsive disorder. J Clin Psychiatry 57(Suppl 8):26–35.

References

Andén N-E, Dahlström A, Fuxe K, Larsson K, Olson L, Ungerstedt U. 1966. Ascending monoamine neurons to the telencephalon and diencephalon. Acta Physiol Scand 67:313–326.

Arango V, Ernsbverger P, Marzuk PM, Chen JS, Fierney H, Stanley M, Reiss DJ, Mann J. 1990. Autoradiographic demonstration of increased serotonin $5HT_2$ and β-adrenergic receptor binding in the brain of suicide victims. Arch Gen Psychiatry 47:1038–1047.

Åsberg M, Träskman L, Thorén P. 1976. 5-HIAA in the cerebrospinal fluid: a biochemical suicide predictor? Arch Gen Psychiatry 33:1193–1197.

Bench CJ, Friston KJ, Brown RG, Scott LC, Frackowiak RS, Dolan RJ. 1992. The anatomy of melancholia: focal abnormalities of cerebral blood flow in major depression. Psychol Med 22(3):607–615.

Blier D, deMontigny C. 1994. Current advances in the treatment of depression. Trends Pharmacol Sci 15:220–226.

Carroll BJ, Feinberg M, Greden JF, Tarika J, Albala AA, Haskett RF, James NMcI, Kronfol Z, Lohr N, Steiner M, de Vigne JP, Young E. 1981. A specific laboratory test for the diagnosis of melancholia. Arch Gen Psychiatry 38:15–22.

Charney DS, Woods SW, Goodman WK, Heninger GR. 1987. Neurobiological mechanisms of panic anxiety: biochemical and behavioral correlates of yohimbine induced attacks. Am J Psychiatry 144:1030–1037.

Cooper JR, Bloom FE, Roth RH. 1996. *The Biochemical Basis of Neuropharmacology,* 7th ed. New York: Oxford Univ. Press.

Davis JM, Maas JW (eds). 1983. *The Affective Disorders.* Washington, DC: American Psychiatric Press.

Drevets WC, Price JL, Simpson JR Jr, Todd RD, Reich T, Vannier M, Raichle ME. 1997. Subgenual prefrontal cortex abnormalities in mood disorders. Nature 386:824–827.

Everett GM, Toman JEP. 1959. Mode of action of Rauwolfia alkaloids and motor activity. In: JH Masserman (ed). *Biological Psychiatry,* pp. 75–81. New York: Grune & Stratton.

Freud S. [1917] 1959. Mourning and melancholia. In: *The Collected Papers,* Vol. 4, pp. 152–170. New York: Basic Books.

Heimer L. 1995. *The Human Brain and Spinal Cord,* 2nd ed. New York, Berlin: Springer-Verlag.

Hoyer D, Clarke DE, Fozard JR, Hartig PR, Martin GR, Mylecharane EJ, Saxena PR, Humphrey PPA. 1994. International union of pharmacology classification of receptors for 5-hydroxytryptamine (serotonin). Pharmacol Rev 46:157–203.

Kety SS. 1979. Disorders of the human brain. Sci Am 241(3):202–214.

Kety SS, Rosenthal D, Wender PH, Schulsinger F, Jacobsen B. 1975. Mental illness in the biological and adoptive families of adopted individuals who have become schizophrenic: a preliminary report based on psychiatric interviews. In: RR Fieve, D Rosenthal, H Brill (eds). *Genetic Research in Psychiatry,* pp. 147–165. Baltimore: Johns Hopkins Univ. Press.

Klein DF. 1974. Endogenomorphic depression: a conceptual and terminological revision. Arch Gen Psychiatry 31:447–454.

Klein DF. 1993. False suffocation alarm. Spontaneous panics, and related conditions: an integrative hypothesis. Arch Gen Psychiatry 50:306–317.

Kraepelin E. 1919. *Dementia praecox and paraphrenia.* Tr by RM Barclay from the 8th German ed. Edinburgh: Livingstone.

Nemeroff CB, Krishnan RR, Reed D, Leder R, Beam C, Dunnick R. 1992. Adrenal gland enlargement in major depression. Arch Gen Psychiatry 49:384–387.

Pletscher A, Shore PA, Brodie BB. 1956. Serotonin as a mediator of reserpine action in brain. J Pharmacol Exp Ther 116:84–89.

Sachar EJ, Asnis G, Halbreich U, Nathan RS, Halpern F. 1980. Recent studies in the neuroendocrinology of major depressive disorders. Psychiatr Clin North Am 3:313–326.

Schou M, Juel-Nielsen N, Strömgren E, Voldby H. 1954. The treatment of manic psychoses by the administration of lithium salts. J Neurol Neurosurg Psychiatry 17:250–260.

Styron W. 1990. *Darkness Visible: A Memoir of Madness.* New York: Random House.

Tallman JF, Gallagher DW. 1985. The GABA-ergic system: a locus of benzodiazepine action. Annu Rev Neurosci 8:21–44.

Van Praag HM. 1982. Neurotransmitters and CNS disease. Lancet 2:1259–1264.

62

Learning and Memory

BEHAVIOR IS THE RESULT OF the interaction between genes and the environment. In earlier chapters we saw how genes influence behavior. We now examine how the environment influences behavior. In humans the most important mechanisms by which the environment alters behavior are learning and memory. Learning is the process by which we acquire knowledge about the world, while memory is the process by which that knowledge is encoded, stored, and later retrieved.

Many important behaviors are learned. Indeed, we are who we are largely because of what we learn and what we remember. We learn the motor skills that allow us to master our environment, and we learn languages that enable us to communicate what we have learned, thereby transmitting cultures that can be maintained over generations. But not all learning is beneficial. Learning also produces dysfunctional behaviors, and these behaviors can, in the extreme, constitute psychological disorders. The study of learning therefore is central to understanding behavioral disorders as well as normal behavior, since what is learned can often be unlearned. When psychotherapy is successful in treating behavioral disorders, it often does so by creating an environment in which people can learn to change their patterns of behavior.

As we have emphasized throughout this book, neural science and cognitive psychology have now found a common ground, and we are beginning to benefit from the increased explanatory power that results from the convergence of two initially disparate disciplines. The rewards of the merger between neural science and cognitive psychology are particularly evident in the study of learning and memory.

In the study of learning and memory we are interested in several questions. What are the major forms of learning? What types of information about the environment are learned most easily? Do different types of learning give rise to different memory processes? How is memory stored and retrieved?

In this chapter we review the major biological principles of learning and memory that have emerged from clinical and cognitive/psychological approaches. In the next chapter we shall examine learning and memory processes at the cellular and molecular level.

Memory Can Be Classified as Implicit or Explicit on the Basis of How Information Is Stored and Recalled

As early as 1861 Pierre Paul Broca had discovered that damage to the posterior portion of the left frontal lobe (Broca's area) produces a specific deficit in language (Chapter 1). Soon thereafter it became clear that other mental functions, such as perception and voluntary movement, can be related to the operation of discrete neural circuits in the brain. The successes of efforts to localize brain functions led to the question: Are there also discrete systems in the brain concerned with memory? If so, are all memory processes located in one region, or are they distributed throughout the brain?

In contrast to the prevalent view about the localized operation of other cognitive functions, many students of learning doubted that memory functions could be localized. In fact, until the middle of the twentieth century many psychologists doubted that memory was a discrete function, independent of perception, language, or movement. One reason for the persistent doubt is that memory storage does indeed involve many different regions of the brain. We now appreciate, however, that these regions are not equally important. There are several fundamentally different types of memory storage, and certain regions of the brain are much more important for some types of storage than for others.

The first person to obtain evidence that memory processes might be localized to specific regions of the human brain was the neurosurgeon Wilder Penfield. Penfield was a student of Charles Sherrington, the pioneering English neurophysiologist who, at the turn of the century, mapped the motor representation of anesthetized monkeys by systematically probing the cerebral cortex with electrodes and recording the activity of motor nerves. By the 1940s Penfield had begun to apply similar methods of electrical stimulation to map the motor, sensory, and language functions in the cerebral cortex of patients undergoing brain surgery for the relief of focal epilepsy. Since the brain itself does not have pain receptors, brain surgery is painless and can be carried

out under local anesthesia in patients that are fully awake. Thus, patients undergoing brain surgery are able to describe what they experience in response to electrical stimuli applied to different cortical areas. On hearing about these experiments, Sherrington, who had always worked with monkeys and cats, told Penfield, "It must be great fun to put a question to the [experimental] preparation and have it answered!"

Penfield explored the cortical surface in more than a thousand patients. On rare occasions he found that electrical stimulation of the temporal lobes produced what he called an *experiential response*—a coherent recollection of an earlier experience. These studies were provocative, but they did not convince the scientific community that the temporal lobe is critical for memory because all of the patients Penfield studied had epileptic seizure foci in the temporal lobe, and the sites most effective in eliciting experiential responses were near those foci. Thus the responses might have been the result of localized seizure activity. Furthermore, the responses occurred in only 8% of all attempts at stimulating the temporal lobes. More convincing evidence that the temporal lobes are important in memory emerged in the mid 1950s from the study of patients who had undergone bilateral removal of the hippocampus and neighboring regions in the temporal lobe as treatment for epilepsy.

The first and best-studied case of the effects on memory of bilateral removal of portions of the temporal lobes was the patient called H.M., studied by Brenda Milner, a colleague of Penfield and the surgeon William Scoville. H.M., a 27-year-old man, had suffered for over 10 years from untreatable bilateral temporal lobe seizures as a consequence of brain damage sustained at age 9 when he was hit and knocked over by someone riding a bicycle. As an adult he was unable to work or lead a normal life. At surgery the hippocampal formation, the amygdala, and parts of the multimodal association area of the temporal cortex were removed bilaterally (Figure 62-1).

H.M.'s seizures were much better controlled after surgery, but the removal of the medial temporal lobes left him with a devastating memory deficit. This memory deficit (or *amnesia*) was quite specific. H.M. still had normal short-term memory, over seconds or minutes. Moreover, he had a perfectly good long-term memory for events that had occurred before the operation. He remembered his name and the job he held, and he vividly remembered childhood events, although he showed some evidence of a retrograde amnesia for information acquired in the years just before surgery. He retained a perfectly good command of language, including his normally varied vocabulary, and his IQ remained unchanged in the range of bright-normal.

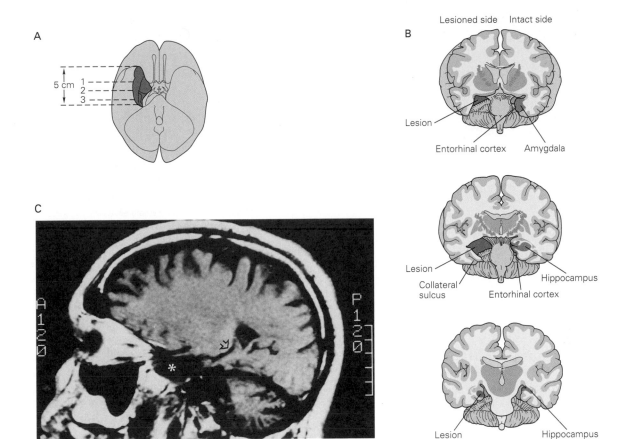

Figure 62-1 The medial temporal lobe and memory storage.

A. The longitudinal extent of the temporal lobe lesion in the patient known as H.M. in a ventral view of the brain.

B. Cross sections showing the estimated extent of surgical removal of areas of the brain in the patient H.M. Surgery was a bilateral, single-stage procedure. The right side is shown here intact to illustrate the structures that were removed. (Modified from Milner 1966.)

C. Magnetic resonance image (MRI) scan of a parasagittal section from the left side of H.M.'s brain. The calibration bar on the right side of the panel has 1 cm increments. The resected portion of the anterior temporal lobes is indicated with an **asterisk.** The remaining portion of the intraventricular portion of the hippocampal formation is indicated with an **open arrow.** Approximately 2 cm of preserved hippocampal formation is visible bilaterally. Note also the substantial cerebellar degeneration obvious as enlarged folial spaces. (From Corkin et al. 1997.)

What H.M. now lacked, and lacked dramatically, was the ability to transfer new short-term memory into long-term memory. He was unable to retain for more than a minute information about people, places, or objects. Asked to remember a number such as 8414317, H.M. could repeat it immediately for many minutes, because of his good short-term memory. But when distracted, even briefly, he forgot the number. Thus, H.M. could not recognize people he met after surgery, even when he met them again and again. For example, for several years he saw Milner on an almost monthly basis, yet each time she entered the room H.M. reacted as though he had never seen her before. H.M. had a similarly profound difficulty with spatial orientation. It took him about a year to learn his way around a new house. H.M. is not unique. All patients

with extensive bilateral lesions of the limbic association areas of the medial temporal lobe, from either surgery or disease, show similar memory deficits.

The Distinction Between Explicit and Implicit Memory Was First Revealed With Lesions of the Limbic Association Areas of the Temporal Lobe

Milner originally thought that the memory deficit after bilateral medial temporal lobe lesions affects all forms of memory equally. But this proved not to be so. Even though patients with lesions of the medial temporal lobe have profound memory deficits, they are able to learn certain types of tasks and retain this learning for as long as normal subjects. The spared component of

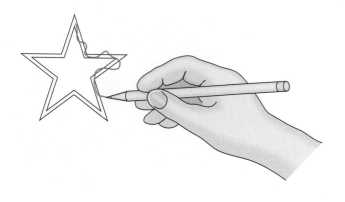

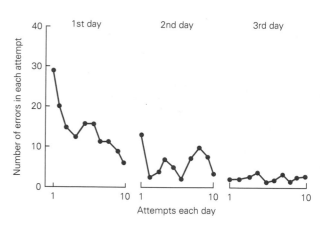

Figure 62-2 The patient H.M. showed definite improvement in any task involving learning skilled movements. He was taught to trace between two outlines of a star while viewing his hand in a mirror. He improved considerably with each fresh test, although he had no recollection that he had ever done the task before. The graph plots the number of times, in each trial, that he strayed outside the outlines as he drew the star. (From Blakemore 1977.)

memory was first revealed when Milner discovered that H.M. could learn new motor skills at a normal rate. For example, he learned to draw the outlines of a star while looking at his hand and the star in a mirror (Figure 62-2). Like normal subjects learning this task, H.M. initially made many mistakes, but after several days of training his performance was error-free and indistinguishable from that of normal subjects.

Later work by Larry Squire and others has made it clear that the memory capacities of H.M. and other patients with bilateral medial temporal lobe lesions are not limited to motor skills. Rather, these patients are capable of various forms of simple reflexive learning, including habituation, sensitization, classical conditioning, and operant conditioning, which we discuss later in this chapter. Furthermore, they are able to improve their performance on certain perceptual tasks. For example, they do well with a form of memory called *priming,* in which the recall of words or objects is improved by prior exposure to the words or object. Thus, when shown the first few letters of previously studied words, a subject with amnesia correctly selects as many previously presented words as do normal subjects, even though the subject has *no* conscious memory of having seen the word before (Figure 62-3).

The memory capability that is spared in patients with bilateral lesions of the temporal lobe typically involves learned tasks that have two things in common. First, the tasks tend to be reflexive rather than reflective in nature and involve habits and motor or perceptual skills. Second, they do not require conscious awareness or complex cognitive processes, such as comparison and evaluation. The patient need only respond to a stimulus

or cue, and need not try to remember anything. Thus, when given a highly complex mechanical puzzle to solve the patient may learn it as quickly and as well as a normal person, but will not consciously remember having worked on it previously. When asked why the performance of a task is much better after several days of practice than on the first day, the patient may respond, "What are you talking about? I've never done this task before."

Although these two fundamentally different forms of memory—for skills and for knowledge—have been demonstrated in detail in amnesia patients with lesions of the temporal lobe, they are not unique amnesiacs. Cognitive psychologists had previously distinguished these two types of memory in normal subjects. They refer to information about how to perform something as *implicit memory* (also referred to as *nondeclarative memory*), a memory that is recalled unconsciously. Implicit memory is typically involved in training reflexive motor or perceptual skills. Factual knowledge of people, places, and things, and what these facts mean, is referred to as *explicit memory* (or *declarative memory*). This is recalled by a deliberate, conscious effort (Figure 62-4). Explicit memory is highly flexible and involves the association of multiple bits and pieces of information. In contrast, implicit memory is more rigid and tightly connected to the original stimulus conditions under which the learning occurred.

The psychologist Endel Tulving first developed the idea that explicit memory can be further classified as *episodic* (a memory for events and personal experience) or *semantic* (a memory for facts). We use episodic memory when we recall that we saw the first flowers of spring yesterday or that we heard Beethoven's *Moonlight Sonata*

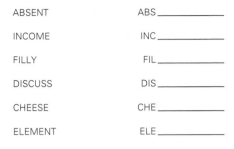

ABSENT	ABS_____
INCOME	INC_____
FILLY	FIL_____
DISCUSS	DIS_____
CHEESE	CHE_____
ELEMENT	ELE_____

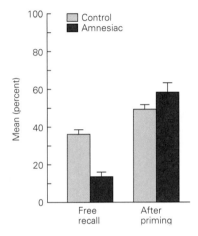

Figure 62-3 In a study of recall of words, amnesiacs and normal control subjects were tested under two conditions. First they were presented with common words and then asked to recall the words (free recall). Amnesiac patients were impaired in this condition. However, when subjects were given the first three letters of a word and instructed simply to form the first word that came to mind (completion), the amnesiacs performed as well as normal subjects. The baseline guessing rate in the word completion condition was 9%. (From Squire 1987.)

several months ago. We use semantic memory to store and recall objective knowledge, the kind of knowledge we learn in school and from books. Nevertheless, all explicit memories can be concisely expressed in declarative statements, such as "Last summer I visited my grandmother at her country house" (episodic knowledge) or "Lead is heavier than water" (semantic knowledge).

Animal Studies Help to Understand Memory

The surgical lesion of H.M.'s temporal lobe encompassed a number of regions, including the temporal pole, the ventral and medial temporal cortex, the amygdala, and the hippocampal formation (which includes the hippocampus proper, the subiculum, and the dentate gyrus) as well as the surrounding entorhinal, perirhinal, and parahippocampal cortices. Since lesions restricted to any one of these several sectors of the medial temporal lobe are rare in humans, experimental lesion studies in monkeys have helped define the contribution of the different parts of the temporal lobe to memory formation.

Mortimer Mishkin and Squire produced lesions in monkeys identical to those reported for H.M. and found defects in explicit memory for places and objects similar to those observed in H.M. Damage to the amygdala alone had no effect on explicit memory. Although the amygdala stores components of memory concerned with emotion (Chapter 50), it does not store factual information. In contrast, selective damage to the hippocampus or the polymodal association areas in the temporal cortex with which the hippocampus connects—the perirhinal and parahippocampal cortices—produces clear impairment of explicit memory.

Thus, studies with human patients and with experimental animals suggest that knowledge stored as explicit memory is first acquired through processing in one or more of the three polymodal association cortices (the prefrontal, limbic, and parieto-occipital-temporal cortices) that synthesize visual, auditory, and somatic information. From there the information is conveyed in series to the parahippocampal and perirhinal cortices,

Figure 62-4 Various forms of memory can be classified as either explicit (declarative) or implicit (nondeclarative).

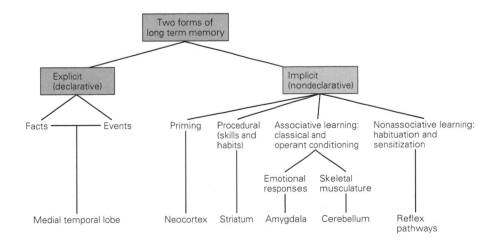

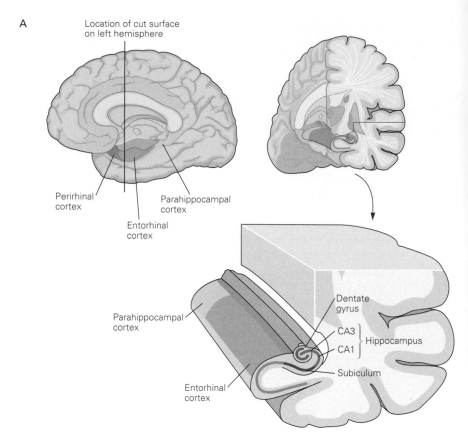

A

Location of cut surface
on left hemisphere

Perirhinal
cortex

Parahippocampal
cortex

Entorhinal
cortex

Parahippocampal
cortex

Dentate
gyrus

CA3
CA1   } Hippocampus

Subiculum

Entorhinal
cortex

Figure 62-5 The anatomical organization of the hippocampal formation.

A. The key components of the medial temporal lobe important for memory storage can be seen in the medial (**left**) and ventral (**right**) surface of the cerebral hemisphere.

B. The input and output pathways of the hippocampal formation.

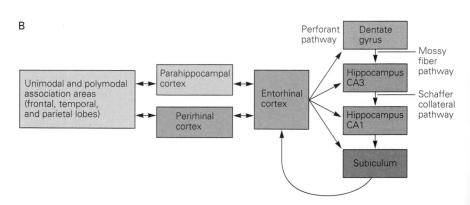

B

Unimodal and polymodal
association areas
(frontal, temporal,
and parietal lobes)

Parahippocampal
cortex

Perirhinal
cortex

Entorhinal
cortex

Perforant
pathway

Dentate
gyrus

Hippocampus
CA3

Hippocampus
CA1

Subiculum

Mossy
fiber
pathway

Schaffer
collateral
pathway

then the entorhinal cortex, the dentate gyrus, the hippocampus, the subiculum, and finally back to the entorhinal cortex. From the entorhinal cortex the information is sent back to the parahippocampal and perirhinal cortices and finally back to the polymodal association areas of the neocortex (Figure 62-5).

Thus, in processing information for explicit memory storage the entorhinal cortex has dual functions. First, it is the main input to the hippocampus. The entorhinal cortex projects to the dentate gyrus via the perforant pathway and by this means provides the critical input pathway through which the polymodal information from the association cortices reaches the hippocampus (Figure 62-5B). Second, the entorhinal cortex is also the major output of the hippocampus. The information coming to the hippocampus from the polymodal association cortices and that coming from the hippocampus to the association cortices converge in the entorhinal cortex. It is therefore understandable why the memory impairments associated with damage to the entorhinal cortex are particularly severe and why this damage affects not simply one but all sensory modalities. In fact, the earliest pathological changes in Alzheimer disease, the major degenerative disease that affects explicit memory storage, occurs in the entorhinal cortex.

Damage Restricted to Specific Subregions of the Hippocampus Is Sufficient to Impair Explicit Memory Storage

Given the large size of the hippocampus proper, how extensive does a bilateral lesion have to be to interfere with explicit memory storage? Clinical evidence from several patients, as well as studies in experimental animals, suggests that a lesion restricted to *any* of the major components of the system can have a significant effect on memory storage. For example Squire, David Amaral, and their collegues found that the patient R.B. had only one detectable lesion after a cardiac arrest—a destruction of the pyramidal cells in the CA1 region of the hippocampus. Nevertheless, R.B. had a defect in explicit memory that was qualitatively similar to that of H.M., although quantitatively it was much milder.

The different regions of the medial temporal lobe may, however, not have equivalent roles. Although the hippocampus is important for object recognition, for example, other areas in the medial temporal lobe may be even more important. Damage to the perirhinal, parahippocampal, and entorhinal cortices that spares the underlying hippocampus produces a greater deficit in memory storage, such as object recognition than do selective lesions of the hippocampus that spare the overlying cortex.

On the other hand, the hippocampus may be relatively more important for spatial representation. In mice and rats lesions of the hippocampus interfere with memory for space and context, and single cells in the hippocampus encode specific spatial information (Chapter 63). Moreover, functional imaging of the brain of normal human subjects shows that spatial memories involve more intense hippocampal activity in the right hemisphere than do memories for words, objects, or people, while the latter involve greater activity in the hippocampus in the dominant left hemisphere. These physiological findings are consistent with the finding that lesions of the right hippocampus give rise to problems with spatial orientation, whereas lesions of the left hippocampus give rise to defects in verbal memory (Figure 62-6).

Explicit Memory Is Stored in Association Cortices

Lesions of the medial temporal lobe in patients such as H.M. and R.B. interfere only with the long-term storage of *new* memories. These patients retain a reasonably good memory of earlier events, although with severe lesions such as those of H.M. there appears to be some retrograde amnesia for the years just before the operation. How does this come about?

The fact that patients with amnesia are able to remember their childhood, the lives they have led, and the factual knowledge they acquired before damage to the hippocampus suggests that the hippocampus is only a temporary way station for long-term memory. If so, long-term storage of episodic and semantic knowledge would occur in the unimodal or multimodal association areas of the cerebral cortex that initially process the sensory information.

For example, when you look at someone's face, the sensory information is processed in a series of areas of the cerebral cortex devoted to visual information, including the unimodal visual association area in the inferotemporal cortex specifically concerned with face recognition (see Box 28-1 and Chapter 28). At the same time, this visual information is also conveyed through the mesotemporal association cortex to the parahippocampal, perirhinal, and entorhinal cortices, and from there through the perforant pathway to the hippocampus. The hippocampus and the rest of the medial temporal lobe may then act, over a period of days or weeks, to facilitate storage of the information about the face initially processed by the visual association area of the inferotemporal lobe. The cells in the visual association cortex concerned with faces are interconnected with other regions that are thought to store additional knowledge about the person whose face is seen, and these connections could also be modulated by the hippocampus. Thus the hippocampus might also serve to bind together the various components of a richly processed memory of a person.

Viewed in this way the hippocampal system would mediate the initial steps of long-term storage. It would then slowly transfer information into the neocortical storage system. The relatively slow addition of information to the neocortex would permit new data to be stored in a way that does not disrupt existing information. If the association areas are the ultimate repositories for explicit memory, then damage to association cortex should destroy or impair recall of explicit knowledge that is acquired before the damage. This is in fact what happens. Patients with lesions in association areas have difficulty in recognizing faces, objects, and places in their familiar world. Indeed, lesions in different association areas give rise to specific defects in either semantic or episodic memory.

Semantic (Factual) Knowledge Is Stored in a Distributed Fashion in the Neocortex

As we have seen, semantic memory is that type of long-term memory that embraces knowledge of objects, facts, and concepts as well as words and their meaning. It includes the naming of objects, the definitions of spoken words, and verbal fluency.

Figure 62-6 The role of the hippocampus in memory. We spend much of our time actively moving around our environment. This requires that we have a representation in our brain of the external environment, a representation that can be used to find our way around. The right hippocampus seems to be importantly involved in this representation, whereas the left hippocampus is concerned with verbal memory.

A. The right hippocampus is activated during learning about the environment. These scans were made while subjects watched a film that depicted navigation through the streets of an Irish town. The activity during this task was compared with that in the control task where the camera was static and people and cars came by it. In the latter case there was no learning of spatial relationships and the hippocampus was not activated. Areas with significant changes in activity, indexed by local perfusion change, are indicated in **yellow** and **orange**. The scan on the left is a coronal section and the scan on the right is a transaxial section; in each panel the front of the brain is on the right and the occipital lobe on the left. (From Maguire et al. 1996.)

B. The right hippocampus also is activated during the recall by licensed taxi drivers of routes around the city of London. These people spend a long time learning the intricacies of the road network in the city and are able to describe the shortest routes between landmarks as well as the names of the various streets. The right parahippocampal and hippocampal regions are significantly activated when they do this task. The scan on the left is a coronal section and the scan on the right is a transaxial section; in each panel the front of the brain is on the right and the occipital lobe on the left. Areas with significant changes in activity, indexed by local perfusion change, are depicted in **yellow** and **orange**. (From Maguire et al. 1996.)

C. Three anatomical slices in the coronal (**left upper**), transverse (**right upper**), and sagittal (**right lower**) planes show activation (**red**) in the left hippocampus associated with the successful retrieval of words from long lists that have to be memorized. **A** = anterior, **P** = posterior, **I** = inferior.

A Learning about surroundings (right hippocampus)

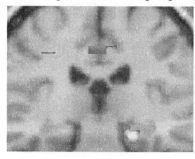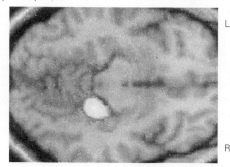

B Recall of taxi routes (right hippocampus)

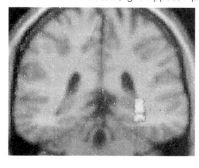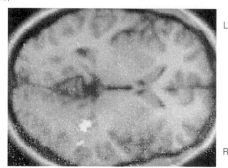

C Word recall (left hippocampus)

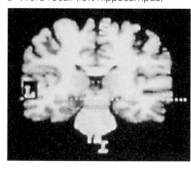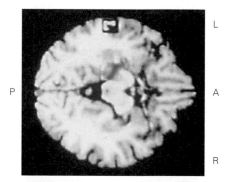

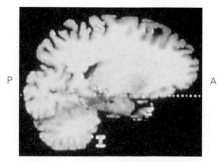

How is semantic knowledge built up? How is it stored in the cortex? The organization and flexibility of semantic knowledge is both remarkable and surprising. Consider a complex visual image such as a photograph of an elephant. Through experience this visual image becomes associated with other forms of knowledge about elephants, so that eventually when we close our eyes and conjure up the image of an elephant, the image is based on a rich representation of the concept of an elephant. The more associations we have made to the

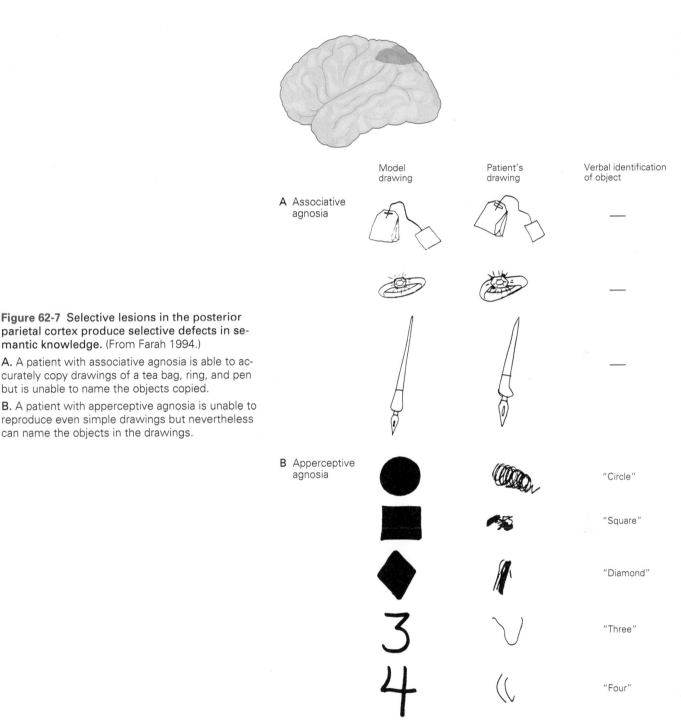

Model drawing | Patient's drawing | Verbal identification of object

A Associative agnosia

B Apperceptive agnosia

"Circle"

"Square"

"Diamond"

"Three"

"Four"

Figure 62-7 Selective lesions in the posterior parietal cortex produce selective defects in semantic knowledge. (From Farah 1994.)

A. A patient with associative agnosia is able to accurately copy drawings of a tea bag, ring, and pen but is unable to name the objects copied.

B. A patient with apperceptive agnosia is unable to reproduce even simple drawings but nevertheless can name the objects in the drawings.

image of the elephant, the better we *encode* that image, and the better we can recall the features of an elephant at a future time. Furthermore, these associations fall into different categories. For example, we commonly know that an elephant is a living rather than a nonliving thing, that it is an animal rather than a plant, that it lives in a particular environment, and that it has unique physical features and behavior patterns and emits a distinctive set of sounds. Moreover, we know that elephants are used by humans to perform certain tasks and that they have a specific name. The word *elephant* is associated with all of these pieces of information, and any one bit of information can open access to all of our knowledge about elephants.

As this example illustrates, we build up semantic knowledge through associations over time. The ability

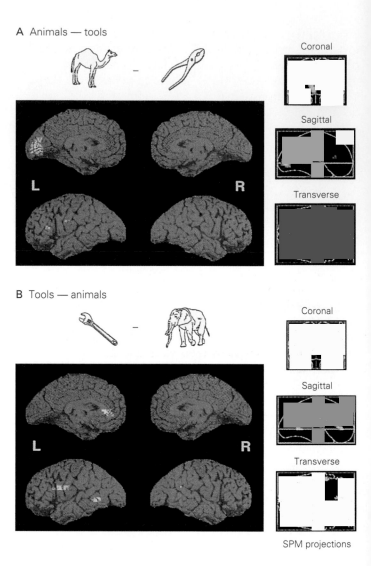

A Animals — tools

Coronal

Sagittal

Transverse

B Tools — animals

Coronal

Sagittal

Transverse

SPM projections

Figure 62-8 Neural correlates of category-specific knowledge are dependent on the intrinsic properties of the objects. (From Martin et al. 1996.)

Regions active when subjects silently named drawings of animals and tools include the calcarine sulcus, the left and right fusiform gyri of the temporal lobe, left thalamus, left insula and inferior frontal region (Broca's area), and right lateral and medial cerebellum. Active regions are identified by increased blood flow. In the statistical procedure regions that are active during the naming of both animals and tools cancel each other and do not show a signal. In both panels the top pair of brain images are medial views, the lower pair are lateral views. **SPM** = statistical parametric maps.

A. Regions selectively activated when subjects silently named animals are predominantly in the early visual area, the medial occipital cortex.

B. Regions selectively activated when subjects silently named tools are predominantly in areas of the left hemisphere associated with hand movements and the generation of action words.

to recall and use knowledge—our *cognitive efficiency*—is thought to depend on how well these associations have organized the information we retain. As we first saw in Chapter 1, when we recall a concept it comes to mind in one smooth and continuous operation. However, studies of patients with damage to the association cortices have shown that different representations of an object—say, different aspects of elephants—are stored separately. These studies have made clear that our experience of knowledge as a seamless, orderly, and cross-referenced database is the product of integration of multiple representations in the brain at many distinct anatomical sites, each concerned with only one aspect of the concept that came to mind. Thus, there is no general semantic memory store; semantic knowledge is not stored in a single region. Rather, each time knowledge about anything is recalled, the recall is built up from distinct bits of information, each of which is stored in spe-

cialized (*dedicated*) memory stores. As a result, damage to a specific cortical area can lead to loss of specific information and therefore a fragmentation of knowledge.

For example, damage to the posterior parietal cortex can result in *associative visual agnosia*; patients cannot *name* objects but they can *identify* objects by selecting the correct drawing and can faithfully reproduce detailed drawings of the object (Figure 62-7). In contrast, damage to the occipital lobes and surrounding region can result in an *apperceptive visual agnosia*; patients are unable to draw objects but they can name them if appropriate perceptual cues are available (Figure 62-7).

While verbal and visual knowledge about objects involve different circuitry, visual knowledge involves even further specialization. For example, visual knowledge about faces and about inanimate objects is represented in different cortical areas. As we have seen in Chapter 25, lesions in the inferotemporal cortex can result in *prosopagnosia*, the inability to recognize familiar faces or learn new faces, but these lesions can leave intact all other aspects of visual recognition. Conversely, positron emission tomography (PET) imaging studies show that object recognition activates the left occipitotemporal cortex and not the areas in the right hemisphere associated with face recognition. Thus, not all of our visual knowledge is represented in the same locus in the occipitotemporal cortex.

Category-specific defects in object recognition were first described by Rosaleen McCarthy and Elizabeth Warrington. They found that certain lesions interfere with the memory (knowledge) of living objects but not with memory of inanimate, manufactured objects. For example, one patient's verbal knowledge of living things was greatly impaired. When asked to define "rhinoceros" the patient responded by merely saying "animal." But when shown a picture of a rhinoceros he responded, "enormous, weighs over a ton, lives in Africa." The same patient's semantic knowledge of inanimate things was readily accessible through both verbal and visual cues. For example, when asked to define "wheelbarrow" he replied, "The thing we have here in the garden for carrying bits and pieces; wheelbarrows are used by people doing maintenance here on your buildings. They can put their cement and all sorts of things in it to carry it around."

To investigate further the neural correlates of category-specific knowledge for animate and inanimate objects, Alex Martin, Leslie Ungerleider, and their colleagues used PET scanning to map regions of the normal brain that are associated with the naming of animals and tools. They found that naming of animals and tools both involved bilateral activation of the ventral temporal lobes and Broca's area. In addition the naming of animals selectively activated the left medial occipital lobe, a region involved in the earlier stages of visual processing. In contrast, the naming tools selectively activated a left premotor area, an area also activated with hand movements, as well as an area in the left middle temporal gyrus that is activated when action words are spoken. Thus, the brain regions active during object identification are dependent in part on the intrinsic properties of the objects presented (Figure 62-8).

Episodic (Autobiographical) Knowledge About Time and Place Seems to Involve the Prefrontal Cortex

Whereas some lesions to multimodal association areas interfere with semantic knowledge, others interfere with the capacity to recall any episodic event experienced more than a few minutes previously, including dramatic personal events such as accidents and deaths in the family that occurred before the trauma. Remarkably, patients with loss of episodic memory still have the ability to recall vast stores of factual (semantic) knowledge. One patient could remember all personal facts about his friends and famous people, such as their names and their characteristics, but could not remember any specific events involving these individuals.

The areas of the neocortex that seem to be specialized for long-term storage of episodic knowledge are the association areas of the frontal lobes. These prefrontal areas work with other areas of the neocortex to allow recollection of when and where a past event occurred (Chapter 19). A particularly striking symptom in patients with frontal lobe damage is their tendency to forget how information was acquired, a deficit called *source amnesia*. Since the ability to associate a piece of information with the time and place it was acquired is at the core of how accurately we remember the individual episodes of our lives, a deficit in source information interferes dramatically with the accuracy of recall of episodic knowledge.

Explicit Knowledge Involves at Least Four Distinct Processes

We have learned three important things about episodic and semantic knowledge. First, there is not a single, all-purpose memory store. Second, any item of knowledge has multiple representations in the brain, each of which corresponds to a different meaning and can be accessed independently (by visual, verbal, or other sensory clues). Third, both semantic and episodic knowledge are the result of at least four related but distinct types of processing: encoding, consolidation, storage, and retrieval (Figure 62-9).

Encoding refers to the processes by which newly learned information is attended to and processed when first encountered. The extent and nature of this encoding are critically important for determining how well the learned material will be remembered at later times. For a memory to persist and be well remembered, the incoming information must be encoded thoroughly and deeply. This is accomplished by attending to the information and associating it meaningfully and systematically with knowledge that is already well established in memory so as to allow one to integrate the new information with what one already knows. Memory storage is stronger when one is well motivated.

Consolidation refers to those processes that alter the newly stored and still labile information so as to make it more stable for long-term storage. As we shall learn in the next chapter, consolidation involves the expression of genes and the synthesis of new proteins, giving rise to

A Encoding memory

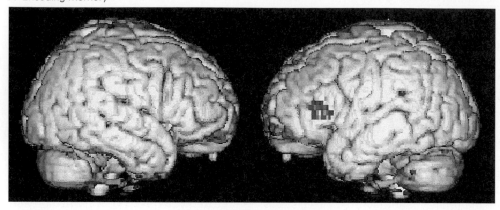

B Retrieving memory

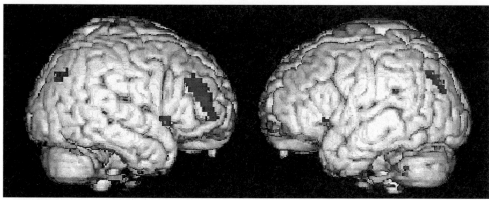

Figure 62-9 Encoding and retrieving episodic memories. Areas where brain activity is significantly increased during the performance of specific memory tasks are shown in **orange** and **red** on surface projections of the human brain (left hemisphere on the right, right hemisphere on the left).

A. Activity in the left prefrontal cortex is particularly associated with the encoding process. Subjects were scanned while attempting to memorize words paired with category labels:

country—Denmark, metal—platinum, etc.

B. Activity in the right frontal cortex is associated with retrieval. Four subjects were presented with a list of category labels and examples that were not paired with the category. The subjects were then scanned when attempting to recall the examples. In addition to right frontal activation a second posterior region in the medial parietal lobe (the precuneus) is also activated.

structural changes that store memory stably over time.

Storage refers to the mechanism and sites by which memory is retained over time. One of the remarkable features about long-term storage is that it seems to have an almost unlimited capacity. In contrast, short-term working memory is very limited.

Finally, *retrieval* refers to those processes that permit the recall and use of the stored information. Retrieval involves bringing different kinds of information together that are stored separately in different storage sites. Retrieval of memory is much like perception; it is a constructive process and therefore subject to distortion, much as perception is subject to illusions (Box 62-1).

Retrieval of information is most effective when it occurs in the same context in which the information was acquired and in the presence of the same cues (retrieval cues) that were available to the subject during learning. Retrieval, particularly of explicit memories, is critically dependent on short-term working memory, a form of memory to which we now turn.

Working Memory Is a Short-Term Memory Required for Both the Encoding and Recall of Explicit Knowledge

How is explicit memory recalled and brought to consciousness? How do we put it to work? Both the initial encoding and the ultimate recall of explicit knowledge (and perhaps some forms of implicit knowledge as well) are thought to require recruitment of stored information

Box 62-1 The Transformation of Explicit Memories

How accurate is explicit memory? This question was explored by the psychologist Frederic Bartlett in one series of studies in which the subjects were asked to read stories and then retell them. The recalled stories were shorter and more coherent than the original stories, reflecting reconstruction and condensation of the original. The subjects were unaware that they were editing the original stories and often felt more certain about the edited parts than about the unedited parts of the retold story. The subjects were not confabulating; they were merely interpreting the original material so that it made sense on recall.

Observations such as these lead us to believe that explicit memory, at least episodic (autobiographical) memory, is a constructive process like sensory perception. The information stored as explicit memory is the product of processing by our perceptual apparatus. As we saw in earlier chapters, sensory perception itself is not a faithful record of the external world but a constructive process in which incoming information is put together according to rules inherent in the brain's afferent pathways. It is also constructive in the sense that individuals interpret the external environment from the standpoint of a specific point in space as well as from the standpoint of a specific point in their own history. As discussed in Chapter 25, optical illusions nicely illustrate the difference between perception and the world as it is.

Moreover, once information is stored, later recall is not an exact copy of the information originally stored. Past experiences are used in the present as clues that help the brain reconstruct a past event. During recall we use a variety of cognitive strategies, including comparison, inferences, shrewd guesses, and suppositions, to generate a consistent and coherent memory.

---

into a special short-term memory store called *working memory*. As we learned in Chapter 19, working memory is thought to have three component systems.

An attentional control system (or *central executive),* thought to be located in the prefrontal cortex (Chapter 19), actively focuses perception on specific events in the environment. The attentional control system has a very limited capacity (less than a dozen items).

The attentional control system regulates the information flow to two rehearsal systems that are thought to maintain memory for temporary use: the articulatory loop for language and the visuospatial sketch pad for vision and action. The *articulatory loop* is a storage system with a rapidly decaying memory trace where memory for words and numbers can be maintained by subvocal speech. It is this system that allows one to hold in mind, through repetition, a new telephone number as one prepares to dial it. The *visuospatial sketch pad* represents both the visual properties and the spatial location of objects to be remembered. This system allows one to store the image of the face of a person one meets at a cocktail party.

The information processed in either one of these rehearsal, working memory systems has the possibility of entering long-term memory. The two rehearsal systems are thought to be located in different parts of the posterior association cortices. Thus, lesions of the extrastriate cortex impair rehearsal of visual imagery whereas lesions in the parietal cortex impair rehearsal of spatial imagery.

Implicit Memory Is Stored in Perceptual, Motor, and Emotional Circuits

Unlike explicit memory, implicit memory does not depend directly on conscious processes nor does recall require a conscious search of memory. This type of memory builds up slowly, through repetition over many trials, and is expressed primarily in performance, not in words. Examples of implicit memory include perceptual and motor skills and the learning of certain types of procedures and rules.

Different forms of implicit memory are acquired through different forms of learning and involve different brain regions. For example, memory acquired through fear conditioning, which has an emotional component, is thought to involve the amygdala. Memory acquired through operant conditioning requires the striatum and cerebellum. Memory acquired through classical conditioning, sensitization, and habituation—three simple forms of learning we shall consider later—involves charges in the sensory and motor systems involved in the learning.

Implicit memory can be studied in a variety of perceptual or reflex systems in either vertebrates or invertebrates. Indeed, simple invertebrates provide useful models for studying the neural mechanisms of implicit learning.

Implicit Memory Can Be Nonassociative or Associative

Psychologists often study implicit forms of memory by exposing animals to controlled sensory experiences. Two major procedures (or paradigms) have emerged from such studies, and these have identified two major subclasses of implicit memory: nonassociative and associative. In nonassociative learning the subject learns about the properties of a single stimulus. In associative learning the subject learns about the relationship between two stimuli or between a stimulus and a behavior.

Nonassociative learning results when an animal or a person is exposed once or repeatedly to a single type of stimulus. Two forms of nonassociative learning are common in everyday life: habituation and sensitization. *Habituation* is a decrease in response to a benign stimulus when that stimulus is presented repeatedly. For example, most people are startled when they first hear the sound of a firecracker on the Fourth of July, Independence Day in the United States, but as the celebration progresses they gradually become accustomed to the noise. *Sensitization* (or *pseudoconditioning*) is an enhanced response to a wide variety of stimuli after the presentation of an intense or noxious stimulus. For example, an animal responds more vigorously to a mild tactile stimulus after it has received a painful pinch. Moreover, a sensitizing stimulus can override the effects of habituation, a process called *dishabituation*. For example, after the startle response to a noise has been reduced by habituation, one can restore the intensity of response to the noise by delivering a strong pinch.

Sensitization and dishabituation are not dependent on the relative timing of the intense and the weak stimulus; no association between the two stimuli is needed. Not all forms of nonassociative learning are as simple as habituation or sensitization. For example, imitation learning, a key factor in the acquisition of language, has no obvious associational element.

Two forms of associative learning have also been distinguished based on the experimental procedures used to establish the learning. Classical conditioning involves learning a relationship between two stimuli, whereas operant conditioning involves learning a relationship between the organism's behavior and the consequences of that behavior.

Classical Conditioning Involves Associating Two Stimuli

Since Aristotle, Western philosophers have traditionally thought that learning is achieved through the association of ideas. This concept was systematically developed by John Locke and the British empiricist school of philosophy, important forerunners of modern psychology. Classical conditioning was introduced into the study of learning at the turn of the century by the Russian physiologist Ivan Pavlov. Pavlov recognized that learning frequently consists of becoming responsive to a stimulus that originally was ineffective. By changing the appearance, timing, or number of stimuli in a tightly controlled stimulus environment and observing the changes in selected simple reflexes, Pavlov established a procedure from which reasonable inferences could be made about the relationship between changes in behavior (learning) and the environment (stimuli). According to Pavlov, what animals and humans learn when they associate *ideas* can be examined in its most elementary form by studying the association of *stimuli*.

The essence of classical conditioning is the pairing of two stimuli. The *conditioned stimulus* (CS), such as a light, tone, or tactile stimulus, is chosen because it produces either no overt response or a weak response usually unrelated to the response that eventually will be learned. The reinforcement, or *unconditioned stimulus* (US), such as food or a shock to the leg, is chosen because it normally produces a strong, consistent, overt response (the *unconditioned response*), such as salivation or withdrawal of the leg. Unconditioned responses are innate; they are produced without learning. When a CS is followed by a US, the CS will begin to elicit a new or different response called the *conditioned response*. If the US is rewarding (food or water), the conditioning is termed *appetitive*; if the US is noxious (an electrical shock), the conditioning is termed *defensive*.

One way of interpreting conditioning is that repeated pairing of the CS and US causes the CS to become an anticipatory signal for the US. With sufficient experience an animal will respond to the CS as if it were anticipating the US. For example, if a light is followed repeatedly by the presentation of meat, eventually the sight of the light itself will make the animal salivate. Thus, classical conditioning is a means by which an animal learns to predict events in the environment.

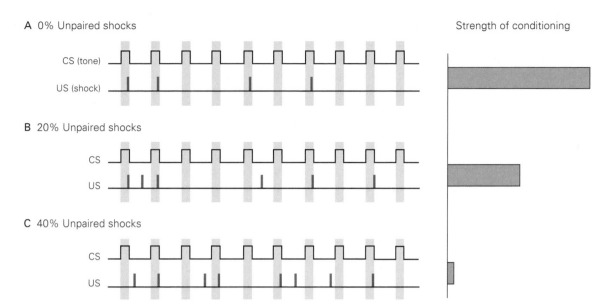

Figure 62-10 The capacity for a conditioned stimulus (CS) to produce a classically conditioned response is not a function of the number of times the CS is paired with an unconditioned stimulus (US) but rather the degree to which the CS and US are correlated. In this experiment on rats all animals were presented with a repeated tone (the CS) paired with an electric shock (the US) in 40% of the trials (**blue** vertical lines). Sometimes the shock was also presented when the tone was not present (**red** vertical lines). The percentage of these uncorrelated trials varied for different groups.

A. An experiment in which the US occurred only with the CS.

B-C. Examples in which the US was sometimes presented without the CS, either as often as the times the CS and US were paired (40%) or half as often (20%). After conditioning under the various circumstances, the degree of conditioning was evaluated by determining how effective the tone was in suppressing lever pressing to obtain food. Suppression of lever pressing is a sign of a conditioned emotional freezing response. The graph shows that in all three conditions the CS-US pairing was always 40%, but the percentage of US presentation with the absence of the CS pairing varied from 0% to 20% or 40%. When the shock occurred without the tone as often as with the tone (40%), little or no conditioning was evident. Some conditioning occurred when the shock occurred 20% of the time without the tone, and maximal conditioning occurred when the shock never occurred without the tone. (Adapted from Rescorla 1968.)

The intensity or probability of occurrence of a conditioned response decreases if the CS is repeatedly presented without the US (Figure 62-10). This process is known as *extinction*. If a light that has been paired with food is then repeatedly presented in the absence of food, it will gradually cease to evoke salivation. Extinction is an important adaptive mechanism; it would be maladaptive for an animal to continue to respond to cues in the environment that are no longer significant. The available evidence indicates that extinction is not the same as forgetting, but that instead something new is learned. Moreover, what is learned is not simply that the CS no longer precedes the US, but that the CS now signals that the US will *not* occur.

For many years psychologists thought that classical conditioning required only contiguity, that the CS precede the US by a critical minimum time interval. According to this view, each time a CS is followed by a reinforcing stimulus or US an internal connection is strengthened between the internal representation of the stimulus and the response or between one stimulus and another. The strength of the connection was thought to depend on the number of pairings of CS and US. This theory proved inadequate, however. A substantial body of empirical evidence now indicates that classical conditioning cannot be adequately explained simply by the temporal contiguity of events (Figure 62-10). Indeed, it would be maladaptive to depend solely on temporal contiguity. If animals learned to predict one type of event simply because it repeatedly occurred with another, they might often associate events in the environment that had no utility or advantage.

All animals capable of associative conditioning, from snails to humans, seem to associate events in their environment by detecting actual *contingencies* rather than simply responding to the *contiguity* of events. Why is this faculty in humans similar to that in much simpler animals? One good reason is that all animals face common problems of adaptation and survival. Learning provides a successful solution to this problem, and once a successful biological solution has evolved it continues to be selected. Classical conditioning, and perhaps all forms of associative learning, may have evolved to enable animals to distinguish events that reliably and predictably occur together from those that are only randomly associated. In other words, the brain seems to have evolved mechanisms that can detect causal relationships in the environment, as indicated by positively correlated or associated events.

What environmental conditions might have shaped or maintained such a common learning mechanism in a wide variety of species? All animals must be able to recognize prey and avoid predators; they must search out food that is edible and nutritious and avoid food that is poisonous. Either the appropriate information can be genetically programmed into the animal's nervous system (as described in Chapter 3), or it can be acquired through learning. Genetic and developmental programming may provide the basis for the behaviors of simple organisms such as bacteria, but more complex organisms such as vertebrates must be capable of flexible learning to cope efficiently with varied or novel situations. Because of the complexity of the sensory information they process, higher-order animals must establish some degree of regularity in their interaction with the world. An effective means of doing this is to be able to detect causal or predictive relationships between stimuli, or between behavior and stimuli.

Operant Conditioning Involves Associating a Specific Behavior With a Reinforcing Event

A second major paradigm of associational learning, discovered by Edgar Thorndike and systematically studied by B. F. Skinner and others, is operant conditioning (also called *trial-and-error learning*). In a typical laboratory example of operant conditioning an investigator places a hungry rat or pigeon in a test chamber in which the animal is rewarded for a specific action. For example, the chamber may have a lever protruding from one wall. Because of previous learning as well as innate response tendencies and random activity, the animal will occasionally press the lever. If the animal promptly receives a positive reinforcer (eg, food) when it presses the level, it will subsequently press the lever more often than the spontaneous rate.

The animal can be described as having learned that among its many behaviors (for example, grooming, rearing, and walking) one behavior (lever-pressing) is followed by food. With this information the animal is likely to take the appropriate action whenever it is hungry.

If we think of classical conditioning as the formation of a predictive relationship between two stimuli (the CS and the US), operant conditioning can be considered as the formation of a predictive relationship between a stimulus (eg, food) and a behavior (eg, lever pressing). Unlike classical conditioning, which tests the responsiveness of specific reflex responses to selected stimuli, operant conditioning involves behaviors that occur either spontaneously or without an identifiable stimulus. Operant behaviors are said to be *emitted* rather than elicited; when a behavior produces favorable changes in the environment (when it is rewarded or leads to the removal of noxious stimuli) the animal tends to repeat the behavior. In general, behaviors that are rewarded tend to be repeated, whereas behaviors followed by aversive, though not necessarily painful, consequences (punishment or negative reinforcement) are usually not repeated. Many experimental psychologists feel that this simple idea, called the *law of effect*, governs much voluntary behavior.

Because operant and classical conditioning involve different kinds of association—classical conditioning involves learning an association between two stimuli whereas operant conditioning involves learning the association between a behavior and a reward—one might suppose the two forms of learning are mediated by different neural mechanisms. However, the laws of operant and classical conditioning are quite similar, suggesting that the two forms of learning may use the same neural mechanisms.

For example, timing is critical in both forms of conditioning. In operant conditioning the reinforcer usually must closely follow the operant behavior. If the reinforcer is delayed too long, only weak conditioning occurs. The optimal interval between behavior and reinforcement depends on the specific task and the species. Similarly, classical conditioning is generally poor if the interval between the conditioned and unconditioned stimuli is too long or if the unconditioned stimulus precedes the conditioned stimulus. In addition, predictive relationships are equally important in both types of learning. In classical conditioning the subject learns that a certain stimulus predicts a subsequent event; in operant conditioning the animal learns to predict the consequences of a behavior.

Associative Learning Is Not Random But Is Constrained by the Biology of the Organism

For many years it was thought that associative learning could be induced simply by pairing any two arbitrarily chosen stimuli or any response and reinforcer. More recent studies have shown that associative learning is constrained by important biological factors.

As we have seen, animals generally learn to associate stimuli that are relevant to their survival. This feature of associative learning illustrates nicely a principle we encountered in the earlier chapters on perception. The brain is not a tabula rasa; it is capable of perceiving some stimuli and not others. As a result, it can discriminate some relations between things in the environment and not others. Thus, not all reinforcers are equally effective with all stimuli or all responses. For example, animals learn to avoid certain foods (called *bait shyness,* because animals in their natural environment learn to avoid bait foods that contain poisons). If a distinctive taste stimulus (eg, vanilla) is followed by a negative reinforcement (eg, nausea produced by a poison), an animal will quickly develop a strong aversion to the taste. Unlike most other forms of conditioning, food aversion develops even when the unconditioned response (poison-induced nausea) occurs after a long delay (up to hours) after the CS (specific taste). This makes biological sense, since the ill effects of naturally occurring toxins usually follow ingestion only after some delay.

For most species, including humans, food-aversion conditioning occurs only when taste stimuli are associated with subsequent illness, such as nausea and malaise. Food aversion develops poorly, or not at all, if the taste is followed by a nociceptive, or painful, stimulus that does not produce nausea. Conversely, an animal will not develop an aversion to a distinctive visual or auditory stimulus that has been paired with nausea. Evolutionary pressures have predisposed the brains of different species to associate certain stimuli, or a certain stimulus and a behavior, much more readily than others. Genetic and experiential factors can also modify the effectiveness of a reinforcer in one species. The results obtained with a particular class of reinforcer vary enormously among species and among individuals within a species, particularly in humans.

Food aversion may be a means by which humans ordinarily learn to regulate their diets to avoid the unpleasant consequences of inappropriate food. It may also be induced in special circumstances, as in the malaise associated with certain forms of cancer chemotherapy. Aversive conditioning to foods in the ordinary diet of patients might account in part for the depressed appetite of many patients who have cancer. The nausea that follows chemotherapy for cancer can produce aversion to foods that were tasted shortly before the treatment.

Certain Forms of Implicit Memory Involve the Cerebellum and Amygdala

Lesions in several regions of the brain that are important for implicit types of learning affect simple classi-

cally conditioned responses. The best-studied case is classical conditioning of the protective eyeblink reflex in rabbits, a specific form of motor learning. A conditioned eyeblink can be established by pairing an auditory stimulus with a puff of air to the eye, which causes an eyeblink. Richard Thompson and his colleagues found that the conditioned response (eyeblink in response to a tone) can be abolished by a lesion at either of two sites. Damage to the vermis of the cerebellum, even a region as small as 2 mm^2 abolishes the conditioned response, but does not affect the unconditioned response (eyeblink in response to a puff of air). Interestingly, neurons in the same area of the cerebellum show learning-dependent increases in activity that closely parallel the development of the conditioned behavior. Second, a lesion in the interpositus nucleus, a deep cerebellar nucleus, also abolishes the conditioned eyeblink. Thus, both the vermis and the deep nuclei of the cerebellum play an important role in conditioning the eyeblink, and perhaps other simple forms of classical conditioning involving skeletal muscle movement.

Maseo Ito and his colleagues have shown that the cerebellum is involved in another form of implicit memory. The vestibulo-ocular reflex keeps the visual image fixed by moving the eyes when the head moves (Chapter 41). The speed of movement of the eyes in relation to that of the head (the gain of the reflex) is not fixed but can be modified by experience. For example, when one first wears magnifying spectacles, eye movements evoked by the vestibulo-ocular reflex are not large enough to prevent the image from moving across the retina. With experience, however, the gain of the reflex gradually increases and the eye can again track the image accurately. As with eyeblink conditioning, the learned changes in the vestibulo-ocular reflex require not only the cerebellum (the flocculus) but also one of the deep cerebellar nuclei (the vestibular) in the brain stem (see Chapters 41 and 42). Finally, as we have seen in Chapter 50, lesions of the amygdala impair conditioned fear.

Some Learned Behaviors Involve Both Implicit and Explicit Forms of Memory

Classical conditioning, we have seen, is effective in associating an unconscious reflexive response with a particular stimulus and thus typically involves implicit forms of memory. However, even this simple form of learning may also involve explicit memory, so that the learned response is mediated at least in part by cognitive processes. Consider the following experiment. A subject lays her hand, palm down, on an electrified grill;

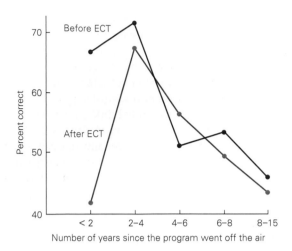

Figure 62-11 Recent memories are more susceptible than older memories to disruption by electroconvulsive treatment (ECT). The plot shows the responses of a group of patients who were tested on their ability to recall the names of television programs that were on the air during a single year between 1957 and 1972. Testing was done before and after the patients received ECT for treatment of depression. After ECT the patients showed a significant (but transitory) loss of memory for recent programs (1–2 years old) but not for older programs. (Adapted from Squire et al. 1975.)

a light (the CS) is turned on and at the same time she receives an electrical shock on one finger—she lifts her hand immediately (unconditioned response). After several light-shock conditioning trials she lifts her hand when the light alone is presented. The subject has been conditioned; but what exactly has been conditioned?

It appears that the light is triggering a specific pattern of muscle activity (a *reflex*) that lifts the hand. However, what if the subject now places her hand on the grill, palm up, and the light is presented? If a specific reflex has been conditioned the light should produce a response that moves the hand *into* the grill. But if the subject has acquired information that the light means "grill shock," her response should be consistent with that information. In fact, the subject often will make an *adaptive response* and move her hand away from the grill. Therefore, the subject did not simply learn to apply a fixed response to a stimulus, but rather acquired information that the brain could use in shaping an appropriate response in a novel situation.

As this example makes clear, learning usually has elements of both implicit and explicit learning. For instance, learning to drive an automobile involves conscious execution of specific sequences of motor acts necessary to control the car; with experience, however,

driving becomes an automatic and nonconscious motor activity. Similarly, with repeated exposure to a fact *(semantic learning)*, recall of the fact with appropriate clues can eventually become virtually instantaneous—we no longer consciously and deliberately search our memory for it.

Both Explicit and Implicit Memory Are Stored in Stages

It has long been known that a person who has been knocked unconscious selectively loses memory for events that occurred before the blow (retrograde amnesia). This phenomenon has been documented thoroughly in animal studies using such traumatic agents as electroconvulsive shock, physical trauma to the brain, and drugs that depress neuronal activity or inhibit protein synthesis in the brain. Brain trauma in humans can produce particularly profound amnesia for events that occur within a few hours or, at most, days before the trauma. In such cases older memories remain relatively undisturbed. The extent of retrograde amnesia, however, varies among patients, from several seconds to several years, depending on the nature and strength of the learning and the nature and severity of the disrupting event.

Studies of memory retention and disruption of memory have supported a commonly used model of memory storage by stages. Input to the brain is processed into short-term working memory before it is transformed through one or more stages into a more permanent long-term store. A search-and-retrieval system surveys the memory store and makes information available for specific tasks.

According to this model, memory can be impaired at several points. For example, there can be a loss of the contents of a memory store; as we have seen (Chapter 58), in Alzheimer's disease there actually is a loss of nerve cells in the entorhinal cortex. Alternatively, the search-and-retrieval mechanism may be disrupted by head trauma. This latter conclusion is supported by the observation that trauma sometimes only temporarily disrupts memory, since considerable memory for past events gradually returns. If stored memory were completely lost, it obviously could not be recovered.

Studies of memory loss in patients undergoing electroconvulsive therapy (ECT) for depression have confirmed and extended the findings from animal experiments. Patients were examined using a memory test that could reliably quantify the degree of memory for relatively recent events (1–2 years old), old events (3–9 years old), and very old events (9–16 years old). The patients were asked to identify, by voluntary recall, the names of television programs broadcast during a single year between 1957 and 1972. The patients were tested before ECT and then again afterward (with a different set of television programs). Both before and after ECT recall of the programs was more correct for more recent years. After ECT, however, the patients showed a significant but transitory loss of memory for more recent programs, while their recall of older programs remained essentially the same as it was before ECT (Figure 62-11).

One interpretation of these findings is that until memories have been converted to a long-term form, retrieval (recall) of recent memories is easily disrupted. Once converted to a long-term form, however, the memories are relatively stable. With time, however, both the long-term memory and the capacity to retrieve it gradually diminish, even in the absence of external trauma. Because of this susceptibility to disruption, the total set of retrievable memories changes continually with time.

Several experiments studying the effects of drugs on learning support the idea that memory is time-dependent and subject to modification when it is first formed. For example, subconvulsant doses of excitant drugs, such as strychnine, can improve the retention of learning of animals even when the drug is administered after the training trials. If the drug is given to the animal soon after training, retention of learning on the following day is greater. The drug has no effect, however, when given after a long delay (several hours) after training. In contrast, inhibitors of protein synthesis selectively block the formation of long-term memory but not short-term memory when given during the training procedure.

An Overall View

The neurobiological study of memory has yielded three generalizations: memory has stages, long-term memory is represented in multiple regions throughout the nervous system, and explicit and implicit memories involve different neuronal circuits.

Different types of memory processes involve different regions and combinations of regions in the brain. Explicit memory underlies the learning of facts and experiences—knowledge that is flexible can be recalled by conscious effort and can be reported verbally. Implicit memory processes include forms of perceptual and motor memory—knowledge that is stimulus-bound, is expressed in the performance of tasks without conscious effort, and is not easily expressed verbally. Implicit memory flows automatically in the doing of things, while explicit memory must be retrieved deliberately.

Long-term storage of explicit memory requires the temporal lobe system. Implicit memory involves the cerebellum and amygdala and the specific sensory and motor systems recruited for the task being learned. Moreover, the memory processes for many types of learning involve several brain structures. For example, learned changes of the vestibulo-ocular reflex appear to involve at least two different sites in the brain, and explicit learning involves neocortical structures as well as the hippocampal formation. Furthermore, there are reasons to believe that information is represented at multiple sites even within one brain structure.

This parallel processing may explain in part why a limited lesion often does not eliminate a specific memory, even a simple implicit memory. Another important factor that may account for the failure of small lesions to adversely affect a specific memory may reside in the very nature of learning. As we shall see in the next chapter, memory involves both functional and structural changes at synapses in the circuits participating in a learning task. Although such changes are likely to occur only in particular types of neurons, the complex nature of many tasks makes it likely that these neurons are widely distributed within the pathways that mediate the response. Therefore some components of the stored information (ie, some of the synaptic changes) could remain undisturbed by a small lesion. Furthermore, the brain can take even the limited store of remaining information and construct a good representation of the original, just as the brain normally constructs conscious memory.

Eric R. Kandel
Irving Kupfermann
Susan Iversen

Selected Readings

Corkin S, Amaral DG, González RG, Johnson KA, Hyman BT. 1997. H.M.'s medial temporal lobe lesion: findings from magnetic resonance imaging. J Neurosci 17:3964–3979.

Kamin LJ. 1969. Predictability, surprise, attention, and conditioning. In: BA Campbell and RM Church (eds). *Punishment and Aversive Behavior*, pp. 279–296. New York: Appleton-Century-Crofts.

Maguire EA, Frackowiak RS, Frith CD. 1996. Learning to

find your way: a role for the human hippocampal formation. Proc R Soc London B 263:1745–1750.

McClelland JL, McNaughton BL, O'Reilly RC. 1995. Why there are complementary learning systems in the hippocampus and neocortex: insights from the successes and failures of connectionist models of learning and memory. Psych Rev 3:419–457.

Milner B. 1966. Amnesia following operation on the temporal lobes. In: CWM Whitty and OL Zangwill (eds). *Amnesia*, pp. 109–133. London: Butterworths.

Milner B, Squire LR, Kandel ER. 1998. Cognitive neuroscience and the study of memory. Neuron 20:445–468.

Muller R. 1996. A quarter of a century of place cells. Neuron 17:813–822.

Schwartz B, Robbins SJ. 1994. *Psychology of Learning and Behavior.* 4th ed. New York: Norton.

Schacter D. 1996. *Searching For Memory. The Brain, the Mind and the Past.* New York: Harper Collins/Basic Books.

Squire LR, Kandel ER. 1999. *Memory: From Mind to Molecules.* New York: Freeman.

Squire LR, Zola-Morgan S. 1991. The medial temporal lobe memory system. Science 253:1380–1386.

Steinmetz JE, Lavond DG, Ivkovich D, Logan CG, Thompson RF. 1992. Disruption of classical eyelid conditioning after cerebellar lesions: damage to a memory trace system or a simple performance deficit? J Neurosci 12:4403–4426.

References

Bartlett FC. 1932. *Remembering: a Study in Experimental and Social Psychology.* Cambridge, England: The University Press.

Blakemore C. 1977. *Mechanics of the Mind.* Cambridge, MA: Cambridge Univ. Press.

Domjan M, Burkhard B. 1986. *The Principles of Learning and Behavior,* 2nd ed. Monterey, CA: Brooks/Cole.

Drachman DA, Arbit J. 1966. Memory and the hippocampal complex II. Is memory a multiple process? Arch Neurol 15:52–61.

du Lac S, Raymond JL, Sejnowski TJ, Lisberger SG. 1995. Learning and memory in the vestibulo-ocular reflex. Annu Rev Neurosci 18:409–441.

Farah M. 1990. *Visual Agnosia.* Cambridge, MA: MIT Press.

Frackowiak RS. 1994. Functional mapping of verbal memory and language. Trends Neurosci 17:109–115.

Hebb DO. 1966. *A Textbook of Psychology.* Philadelphia: Saunders.

Martin A, Wiggs CL, Ungerleider LG, Haxby JV. 1996. Neural correlates of category-specific knowledge. Nature 379:649–652.

McCarthy, RA, Warrington EK. 1990. *Cognitive Neuropsychology: A clinical Introduction.* San Diego: Academic Press.

McClelland JL, McNaughton BL, O'Reilly RC. 1995. Why there are complementary learning systems in the hippocampus and neocortex: insights from the successes and failures of connectionist models of learning and memory. Psychol Rev 102:419–457.

McGaugh JL. 1990. Significance and remembrance: the role of neuromodulatory systems. Psychol Sci 1:15–25.

Pavlov IP. 1927. *Conditioned Reflexes: Investigation of the Physiological Activity of the Cerebral Cortex.* Anrep GV, trans. London: Oxford University Press.

Penfield W. 1958. Functional localization in temporal and deep sylvian areas. Res Publ Assoc Res Ment Dis 36:210–226.

Rescorla RA. 1968. Probability of shock in the presence and absence of CS in fear conditioning. J Comp Physiol Psychol 66:1–5.

Rescorla RA. 1988. Behavioral studies of Pavlovian conditioning. Annu Rev Neurosci 11:329–352.

Skinner BF. 1938. *The Behavior of Organisms: An Experimental Analysis.* New York: Appleton-Century-Crofts.

Squire LR. 1987. *Memory and Brain.* New York: Oxford University Press.

Squire LR, Slater PC, Chace PM. 1975. Retrograde amnesia: temporal gradient in very long term memory following electroconvulsive therapy. Science 187:77–79.

Thorndike EL. 1911. *Animal Intelligence: Experimental Studies.* New York: Macmillan.

Tulving E, Schacter DL. 1990. Priming and human memory systems. Science 247:301–306.

Warrington EK, Weiskrantz L. 1982. Amnesia: a disconnection syndrome? Neuropsychologia 20:233–248.

63

Cellular Mechanisms of Learning and the Biological Basis of Individuality

THROUGHOUT THIS BOOK we have emphasized that all behavior is a function of the brain and that malfunctions of the brain give rise to characteristic disturbances of behavior. Behavior, in turn, is shaped by learning. How does learning act on the brain to change behavior? How is new information acquired and, once acquired, how is it retained? In the preceding chapter we saw that memory—the outcome of learning—is not a single process but has at least two forms. *Implicit* (nondeclarative) *memory* is unconscious memory for perceptual and motor skills, whereas *explicit* (declarative) *memory* is a memory for people, places, and objects that requires conscious recall.

In this chapter we examine the cellular and molecular mechanisms that contribute to these two forms of memory by exploring the mechanisms that underlie simple implicit forms of memory storage in invertebrates and the more complex explicit forms in vertebrates. We shall see that the molecular mechanisms of memory storage are highly conserved throughout evolution, and that the more complex forms of learning and memory depend on many of the same molecular mechanisms used in the simplest forms. Finally, we shall consider the idea that these mechanisms contribute to individuality by changing the connectivity of neurons in our brains.

A   Experimental setup

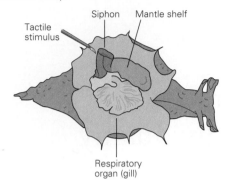

B   Gill-withdrawal reflex circuit

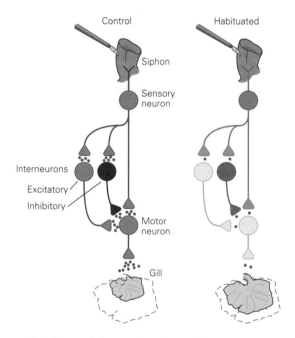

Figure 63-1 The cellular mechanisms of habituation have been investigated in the gill-withdrawal reflex of the marine snail *Aplysia.*

A. A dorsal view of *Aplysia* illustrates the respiratory organ (gill), which is normally covered by the mantle shelf. The mantle shelf ends in the siphon, a fleshy spout used to expel seawater and waste. A tactile stimulus to the siphon elicits the gill-withdrawal reflex. Repeated stimuli lead to habituation.

B. This simplified circuit shows key elements involved in the gill-withdrawal reflex as well as sites involved in habituation. In this circuit about 24 mechanoreceptors in the abdominal ganglion innervate the siphon skin. These glutaminergic sensory cells form synapses with a cluster of six motor neurons that innervate the gill and with several groups of excitatory and inhibitory interneurons that synapse on the motor neurons. (For simplicity, only one of each type of neuron is illustrated here.) Repeated stimulation of the siphon leads to a depression of synaptic transmission between the sensory and motor neurons as well as between certain interneurons and the motor cells.

Short-Term Storage of Implicit Memory for Simple Forms of Learning Results From Changes in the Effectiveness of Synaptic Transmission

Much progress in the cellular study of memory storage has come from examining elementary forms of learning: habituation, sensitization, and classical conditioning. These cellular modifications have been analyzed in the behavior of simple invertebrates and in a variety of vertebrate reflexes, such as flexion reflexes, fear responses, and the eyeblink. Most simple forms of implicit learning change the effectiveness of the synaptic connections that make up the pathway mediating the behavior.

Habituation Involves an Activity-Dependent Presynaptic Depression of Synaptic Transmission

In *habituation*, the simplest form of implicit learning, an animal learns about the properties of a novel stimulus that is harmless. An animal first responds to a new stimulus by attending to it with a series of orienting responses. If the stimulus is neither beneficial nor harmful, the animal learns, after repeated exposure, to ignore it.

Habituation was first investigated by Ivan Pavlov and Charles Sherrington. While studying posture and locomotion, Sherrington observed a decrease in the intensity of certain reflexes, such as the withdrawal of a limb, in response to repeated stimulation. The reflex response returned only after many seconds of rest. He suggested that this decrease, which he called habituation, results from diminished synaptic effectiveness within the pathways to the motor neurons that had been repeatedly activated.

This problem was later investigated at the cellular level by Alden Spencer and Richard Thompson. They found close cellular and behavioral parallels between habituation of the spinal flexion reflex in the cat and habituation of more complex behavioral responses in humans. They showed, through intracellular recordings from spinal motor neurons in cats, that habituation leads to a decrease in the strength of the synaptic connections between excitatory interneurons and motor neurons. The connections between the sensory neurons innervating the skin and the interneurons were unaffected.

Since the organization of interneurons in the spinal cord of vertebrates is quite complex, further analysis of the cellular mechanisms of habituation in the flexion reflex proved difficult. Progress in this effort required a simpler system. The marine sea slug *Aplysia californica*, which has a simple nervous system containing only about 20,000 central nerve cells, is an excellent simple system for studying implicit forms of memory. *Aplysia* has a repertory of defensive reflexes for withdrawing its gill and its siphon, a small fleshy spout above the gill used to expel seawater and waste (Figure 63-1A). These reflexes are similar to the leg withdrawal reflex studied by Spencer and Thompson. For example, a mild tactile stimulus delivered to the siphon elicits reflex withdrawal of both siphon and gill. With repeated stimulation these reflexes habituate. They can also be sensitized and classically conditioned, as we shall see later.

Gill withdrawal in *Aplysia* has been studied in detail. In response to a novel tactile stimulus to the siphon, firing in the sensory neurons innervating the siphon generates excitatory synaptic potentials in interneurons and motor cells (Figure 63-1B). The synaptic potentials from the sensory neurons and interneurons summate both temporally and spatially to cause the motor cells to discharge repeatedly, leading to strong reflexive withdrawal of the gill. If the stimulus is repeated, the direct monosynaptic excitatory synaptic potentials produced by sensory neurons in both the interneurons and the motor cells become progressively smaller. Thus, with repeated stimulation, several of the excitatory interneurons also produce weaker synaptic potentials in the motor neurons, with the net result that the motor neuron fires much less briskly and consequently the reflex response diminishes.

What reduces the effectiveness of synaptic transmission by the sensory neurons? Quantal analysis revealed that the decrease in synaptic strength results from a decrease in the number of transmitter vesicles released from presynaptic terminals of sensory neurons. These sensory neurons use glutamate as their transmitter. Glutamate interacts with two types of receptors in motor cells: one similar to the N-methyl-D-aspartate (NMDA) type of glutamate receptors of vertebrates and the other to a non-NMDA-type (Chapter 12). There is no change in the sensitivity of these receptors with habituation. How this decrease in transmitter release occurs is not yet understood; it is thought to be due in part to a reduced mobilization of transmitter vesicles to the active zone (see Chapter 14). This reduction lasts many minutes.

These enduring *plastic* changes in the functional strength of synaptic connections thus constitute the cellular mechanisms mediating the short-term memory for habituation. Since these changes occur at several sites in the reflex circuit, memory in this instance is distributed and stored throughout the circuit, not at one specialized site. Synaptic depression of the connections made by sensory neurons, interneurons, or both is a common mechanism for habituation and explains habituation of the several well-studied escape responses of crayfish and cockroaches as well as startle reflexes of vertebrates.

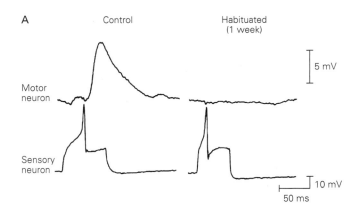

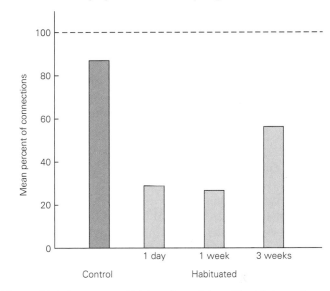

Figure 63-2 Long-term habituation of the gill-withdrawal reflex in *Aplysia* is represented on the cellular level by a dramatic depression of synaptic effectiveness between the sensory and motor neurons. (Adapted from Castellucci et al. 1978.)

A. Comparison of the synaptic potentials in a sensory and motor neuron in a control (untrained) animal and an animal that has been subjected to long-term habituation. In the habituated animal no synaptic potential is evident in the motor neuron one week after training.

B. The mean percentage of physiologically detectable connections in habituated animals at three points in time after long-term habituation training.

The synaptic mechanisms underlying habituation can vary in two ways. First, the locus of the depression can be situated at any of several synaptic sites. For example, in the flexion reflex of the spinal cord there is no depression of synaptic transmission at the direct connections made by the sensory neurons on interneurons.

Rather, depression is thought to occur at downstream sites: at the synapses made by certain classes of interneurons on the motor neurons of the reflex. Second, mechanisms other than homosynaptic depression, such as enhancement of synaptic inhibition, can contribute to habituation.

These studies illustrate that learning can lead to changes in synaptic strength and that the duration of the short-term memory storage is determined by the duration of the synaptic change. In turn, theses studies raise the question: How much can the effectiveness of a synapse change and how long can the change last? Whereas a single session of 10 tactile stimuli to the siphon leads to a short-term memory for habituation of the *Aplysia* gill-withdrawal reflex lasting minutes, four such sessions, separated by periods ranging from several hours to one day, produce a long-term memory that lasts for as long as three weeks! In naive *Aplysia* 90% of the sensory neurons make physiologically detectable connections onto identified gill motor neurons. In contrast, in animals trained for long-term habituation the number of such connections is reduced to 30%; this low incidence persists for a week and does not completely recover for three weeks after the training (Figure 63-2). As we shall see later, during this long-term inactivation of synaptic transmission the actual structure of the sensory neurons changes.

Not all synapses are equally adaptable. The strength of some synapses in *Aplysia* rarely changes, even with repeated activation. However, at synapses specifically involved in learning and memory storage, such as the connections between sensory and motor neurons and some interneurons in the withdrawal-reflex circuit, a relatively small amount of training, especially if it is appropriately spaced over many minutes or hours, can produce large and enduring changes in synaptic strength. Massed training, whereby the habituating stimuli are given one after the other without rest between training sessions, produces a robust short-term memory but long-term memory is seriously compromised. This illustrates a general principle of learning psychology: Spaced training is usually much more effective than massed training in producing long-term memory.

Sensitization Involves Presynaptic Facilitation of Synaptic Transmission

When an animal repeatedly encounters a harmless stimulus it learns to habituate to it. In contrast, with a *harmful* stimulus the animal typically learns to respond more vigorously not only to that stimulus but also to other stimuli, even harmless ones. Defensive reflexes for withdrawal and escape become heightened. This enhance-

ment of reflex responses, called *sensitization,* is more complex than habituation: A stimulus applied to one pathway produces a change in the reflex strength in another pathway. Like habituation, sensitization has both a short-term and a long-term form. Thus, whereas a single shock to an animal's tail produces short-term sensitization that lasts minutes, five or more shocks to the tail produce sensitization lasting days to weeks.

A noxious stimulus to the tail enhances synaptic transmission at several connections in the neural circuit of the gill-withdrawal reflex, including the connections made by sensory neurons with motor neurons and interneurons—the same synapses depressed by habituation. Thus a synapse can participate in more than one type of learning and store more than one type of memory. However, habituation and sensitization use different cellular mechanisms to produce synaptic change. Short-term habituation in *Aplysia* is a *homosynaptic process;* the decrease in synaptic strength is a direct result of activity in the sensory neurons and their central connections in the reflex pathway. In contrast, sensitization is a *heterosynaptic* process; the enhancement of

Figure 63-3 (Opposite) Short-term sensitization of the gill-withdrawal reflex in *Aplysia* involves presynaptic facilitation.

A. Sensitization of the gill is produced by applying a noxious stimulus to another part of the body, such as the tail. Stimuli to the tail activate sensory neurons in the tail that excite facilitating interneurons, which form synapses on the terminals of the sensory neurons innervating the siphon. At these axoaxonic synapses the facilitating interneurons enhance transmitter release from the sensory neurons (*presynaptic facilitation*).

B. Presynaptic facilitation in the sensory neuron is thought to occur by means of three biochemical pathways. The transmitter released by the presynaptic interneuron, here serotonin (5-HT, hydroxytryptamine), binds to two receptors. One engages a G protein (G_s), which increases the activity of adenylyl cyclase. The adenylyl cyclase converts adenosine triphosphate (ATP) to cyclic adenosine monophosphate (cAMP), thereby increasing the level of cAMP in the terminal of the sensory neuron. The cAMP activates the cAMP-dependent protein kinase A (PKA) by attaching to its inhibitory regulatory subunit, thus releasing its active catalytic subunit.

The catalytic subunit of PKA acts along three pathways. In **pathway 1** the catalytic subunit phosphorylates K^+ channels, thereby decreasing the K^+ current. This prolongs the action potential and increases the influx of Ca^{2+}, thus augmenting transmitter release. In **pathway 2** vesicles containing transmitter are mobilized to the releasable transmitter pool at the active zone, and the efficiency of the exocytotic release machinery is also enhanced. In **pathway 3** L-type Ca^{2+} channels are opened. Serotonin, acting through a second receptor, engages the G protein (G_o) that activates a phospholipase C (PLC), which in turn stimulates intramembranous diacylglycerol to activate protein kinase C (PKC). **Pathways 2-2a and 3-3a** involve the joint action of PKA and PKC.

A Gill sensitization

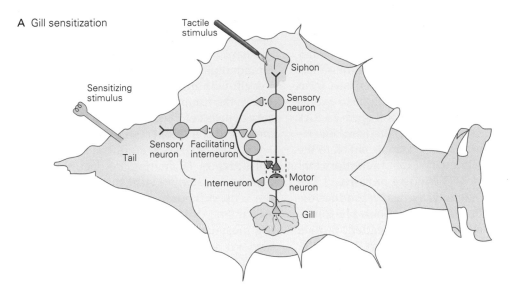

B Three molecular targets involved in presynaptic faciliation

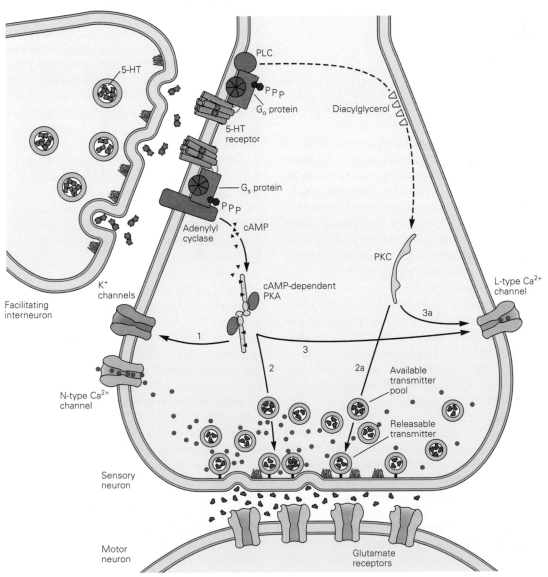

synaptic strength is induced by modulatory interneurons activated by stimulation of the tail.

There are at least three groups of modulatory interneurons, the best studied of which release serotonin. The serotonergic and other modulatory interneurons form synapses on the sensory neurons, including axo-axonic synapses on their presynaptic terminals (Figure 63-3A). The serotonin and other modulatory transmitters released from the interneurons after a single shock to the tail bind to specific membrane-spanning receptors that activate the heterotrimeric GTP binding protein $G_{\alpha s}$. The $G_{\alpha s}$ protein activates an adenylyl cyclase to produce the second messenger cyclic adenosine mono-phosphate (cAMP), which activates the cAMP-dependent protein kinase (PKA) (see the discussion of PKA in Chapter 13). PKA, together with protein kinase C, enhances release of transmitter from the sensory neurons' terminals for a period of minutes through the phosphorylation of several substrate proteins (Figure 63-3B). As we shall learn later, repeated sensitizing stimuli produce a strengthening of connections that lasts days.

Classical Conditioning Involves Presynaptic Facilitation of Synaptic Transmission That Is Dependent on Activity in Both the Presynaptic and the Postsynaptic Cell

Classical conditioning is a more complex form of learning than sensitization. Rather than learning only about one stimulus, the organism learns to associate one type of stimulus with another. As we have learned in Chapter 62, an initially weak conditioned stimulus can become highly effective in producing a response when paired with a strong unconditioned stimulus. In reflexes that can be enhanced by both classical conditioning and sensitization, classical conditioning results in a greater and longer-lasting enhancement.

The siphon- and gill-withdrawal reflexes of *Aplysia* are examples of reflexes that can be enhanced by both classical conditioning and sensitization. The gill-withdrawal reflex can be elicited in one of two ways: by stimulating either the siphon or a nearby structure called the *mantle shelf*. The siphon and the mantle shelf are separately innervated by distinct populations of sensory neurons. Thus, each reflex pathway can be conditioned independently by pairing a conditioned stimulus to the appropriate area (either the siphon or the mantle shelf) with an unconditioned stimulus (a strong shock to the tail). After such paired or associative training, the response of the conditioned (or paired) pathway to stimulation is significantly enhanced compared to that of the unpaired pathway (Figure 63-4).

In classical conditioning the timing of the conditioned and unconditioned stimuli is critical. The conditioned stimulus must *precede* the unconditioned stimulus, often within an interval of about 0.5 s. What cellular mechanisms are responsible for this requirement for temporal pairing of stimuli? In classical conditioning of the gill-withdrawal reflex of *Aplysia* one important feature is the timing of the convergence in individual sensory neurons of the conditioned stimulus (siphon touch) and the unconditioned stimulus (tail shock).

As we have seen, an unconditioned stimulus to the tail activates facilitating interneurons that make axo-axonic connections with the presynaptic terminals of the sensory neurons that carry information from the siphon and the mantle shelf (Figure 63-4A). The resulting presynaptic facilitation ordinarily gives rise to behavioral sensitization. However, if the unconditioned stimulus (to the tail) and the conditioned stimulus (to the siphon or mantle shelf) are timed so that the conditioned stimulus just precedes the unconditioned stimulus, then the modulatory interneurons engaged by the unconditional stimulus will activate the sensory neurons immediately *after* the conditioned stimulus has activated the sensory neurons. This sequential activation of the sensory neurons during a critical interval by the CS and the US leads to greater presynaptic facilitation than when the two stimuli are not appropriately paired (Figure 63-4B). This novel feature unique to classical conditioning is called activity dependence.

There are presynaptic and postsynaptic components to activity-dependent facilitation. Activity in the conditioned stimulus pathway leads to Ca^{2+} influx into the presynaptic sensory neuron with each action potential, and this influx activates the Ca^{2+}-binding protein calmodulin. The activated Ca^{2+}/calmodulin binds to adenylyl cyclase, potentiating its response to serotonin and enhancing its production of cAMP. Thus, the presynaptic cellular mechanism of classical conditioning in the monosynaptic pathway of the withdrawal reflex in *Aplysia* is in part an elaboration of the mechanism of sensitization in this same pathway. This is because adenylyl cyclase acts as a *coincidence detector*. That is, it recognizes the molecular representation of both the conditioned stimulus (spike activity in the sensory neuron and the consequent Ca^{2+} influx) and the unconditioned stimulus (serotonin released by tail stimuli), and it responds both to the conditioned stimulus (binding to the Ca^{2+}/calmodulin activated by the Ca^{2+} influx following action potentials) and the unconditioned stimulus (binding to the $G_{\alpha s}$ activated by the binding of serotonin to a receptor).

The postsynaptic component of classical conditioning is a retrograde signal to the sensory neuron. In the withdrawal reflex pathway in *Aplysia* the postsynaptic motor cell has two types of receptors to glutamate: non-NMDA and NMDA-type receptors. As we have learned in Chapter 11, the extracellular mouth of the NMDA-

Figure 63-4 Classical conditioning of the gill-withdrawal reflex in *Aplysia.* A conditioned stimulus (**CS**) applied to the mantle shelf is paired with an unconditioned stimulus (**US**) applied to the tail. As a control, a CS applied to the siphon is not paired with the US. (Adapted from Hawkins et al. 1983.)

A. A shock to the tail (US) excites facilitating interneurons that form synapses on the presynaptic terminals of sensory neurons innervating the mantle shelf and siphon. This is the mechanism of sensitization (A1).

B. When the mantle pathway is activated by a CS just before the US, the action potentials in the mantle sensory neurons prime them so that they are more responsive to subsequent stimulation from the (serotonergic) facilitating interneurons in the US pathway. This is the mechanism of classical conditioning; it both amplifies the response of the CS pathway and restricts the amplification to that pathway (B1).

Recordings of the excitatory postsynaptic potentials produced in an identified motor neuron by the mantle and siphon sensory neurons were made before training (**Pre**) and 1 hour after training (**Post**). After training the excitatory postsynaptic potential due to input from the mantle (paired) sensory neuron (B2) is considerably greater than the one due to the siphon (unpaired) neuron (A2).

C. The experimental protocol for classical conditioning compares the responses of paired and unpaired stimuli mediated by siphon and mantle sensory neurons. In the mantle sensory neurons the action potentials produced by the CS are paired with those produced by the US (tail stimulus). In a siphon sensory neuron the action potentials produced by the CS are not paired with the same US.

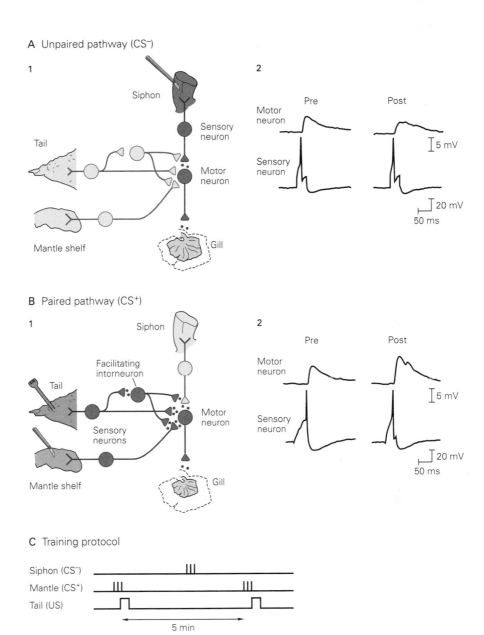

type receptor-channel is plugged by Mg^{2+} at the resting membrane potential. Thus, under normal circumstances and during habituation and sensitization only the non-NMDA receptor is activated because the NMDA receptor is blocked by Mg^{2+}. However, when the conditioned stimulus and unconditioned stimulus are paired appropriately during classical conditioning, the motor neuron fires a whole train of action potentials. The depolarization of the postsynaptic cell expels Mg^{2+} from the NMDA-type receptor-channel and Ca^{2+} flows into the

cell. The Ca^{2+} influx is thought to activate signaling pathways in the motor cell that give rise to a retrograde messenger that is taken up in the presynaptic terminals of the sensory cell, where it acts to enhance transmitter release even further.

Thus, three signals in a siphon sensory neuron must converge to produce the large increase in transmitter release that occurs with classical conditioning: (1) activation of adenylyl cyclase by Ca^{2+} influx, representing the conditioned stimulus; (2) activation of serotonergic receptors coupled to adenylyl cyclase, representing the unconditioned stimulus; and (3) a retrograde signal indicating that the postsynaptic cell has been adequately activated by the uncondtioned stimulus.

Long-Term Storage of Implicit Memory for Sensitization and Classical Conditioning Involves the cAMP-PKA-MAPK-CREB Pathway

Molecular Biological Analysis of Long-Term Sensitization Reveals a Role for cAMP Signaling in Long-Term Memory

As with habituation and most other forms of learning, practice makes perfect. Repeated experience consolidates memory by converting the short-term form into a long-term form. These physiological consequences of repeated training have been best studied for sensitization. In *Aplysia* a single training session (or a single application of serotonin to the sensory neurons) gives rise to short-term sensitization, lasting only minutes, that does not require new protein synthesis. However, five training sessions produce long-term sensitization, lasting several days, that requires new protein synthesis. Further spaced training produces sensitization that persists for weeks. These behavioral studies of *Aplysia* (and similar ones in vertebrates) suggest that short-term and long-term memory are two independent but overlapping processes that blend into one another. Several findings point to this interpretation.

First, both short- and long-term memory for sensitization of the gill-withdrawal reflexes involve changes in the strength of connections at several synaptic sites, including the synaptic connections between sensory and motor neurons (Figure 63-5A). Second, in both the long-term and short-term processes the increase in the synaptic strength of the connections between the sensory and motor neurons is due to the enhanced release of transmitter. Third, the same transmitter (serotonin) released by stimulation of the tail produces short-term facilitation after a single exposure and long-term facilitation after five or more repeated exposures. Finally, cAMP and PKA, intracellular second-messenger pathways that are critically involved in short-term memory, are also recruited for long-term memory (Figure 63-5B).

Despite these similarities, short- and long-term memory are distinct processes that can be distinguished by several criteria. In humans, epileptic seizure or head trauma affects long-term memory but not short-term memory. A similar dissociation between short- and long-term memory can be demonstrated in experimental animals using inhibitors of protein or mRNA synthesis to block long-term memory selectively.

As we saw in the preceding chapter, the process by which transient short-term memory is converted into a stable long-term memory is called *consolidation*. Consolidation of long-term implicit memory for simple forms

Figure 63-5 (Facing page) Persistent synaptic enhancement with long-term sensitization.

A. Long-term sensitization of the gill-withdrawal reflex of *Aplysia* involves facilitation of transmitter release at the connections between sensory and motor neurons. **1.** The recordings show representative synaptic potentials in a siphon sensory neuron and a gill motor neuron in a control animal and in an animal that received long-term sensitization training by repeated stimulation of its tail. The record was obtained one day after the end of training. **2.** The median amplitude of the postsynaptic potentials (**PSP**) in an identified gill motor neuron is greater in sensitized animals one day after training than in control animals. **3.** The effect of sensitization on the neural circuit of the gill- and siphon-withdrawal reflex is measured here by the median duration of withdrawal of the siphon (see Figure 63-1). (**Pre** = score before training; **post** = score after training.) The experimental group was tested one day after the end of training. (Adapted from Frost et al. 1985.)

B. Long-term sensitization of the gill-withdrawal reflex of *Aplysia* leads to two major changes in the sensory neurons of the reflex: persistent activity of protein kinase A and structural changes in the form of the growth of new synaptic connections.

Both the short-term and long-term facilitation are initiated by a serotonergic interneuron. Short-term facilitation (lasting minutes to hours), resulting from a single tail shock or a single pulse of serotonin, leads to covalent modification of preexisting proteins (short-term pathway). As shown in Figure 63-3, serotonin acts on a postsynaptic receptor to activate the enzyme adenylyl cyclase, which converts ATP to the second messenger cAMP. In turn, cAMP activates the cAMP-dependent protein kinase A, which phosphorylates and covalently modifies a number of target proteins, leading to enhanced transmitter availability and release. The duration of these modifications is a measure of the short-term memory.

Long-term facilitation (lasting one or more days) involves the synthesis of new proteins. The switch for this inductive mechanism is initiated by protein kinase A (**PKA**), which recruits the mitogen-activated kinase (**MAPK**) and together they translocate to the nucleus (long-term pathway), where PKA phosphorylates the cAMP-response element binding (**CREB**) protein. The transcriptional activators bind to cAMP response elements (**CRE**) located in the upstream region of two types of cAMP-inducible genes. To activate CREB-1, PKA needs also to remove the repressive action of CREB-2, which is capable of inhibiting the activation capability of CREB-1. PKA is thought to mediate the derepression of CREB-2 by means of another protein, MAPK. One gene activated by CREB encodes a ubiquitin hydrolase, a component of a specific ubiquitin protease that leads to the regulated proteolysis of the regulatory subunit of PKA. This cleavage of the (inhibitory) regulatory subunit results in persistent activity of PKA, leading to persistent phosphorylation of the substrate proteins of PKA, including both CREB-1 and the protein involved in the short-term process. The second gene activated by CREB encodes another transcription factor **C/EBP**. This binds to the DNA response element **CAAT**, which activates genes that encode proteins important for the growth of new synaptic connections.

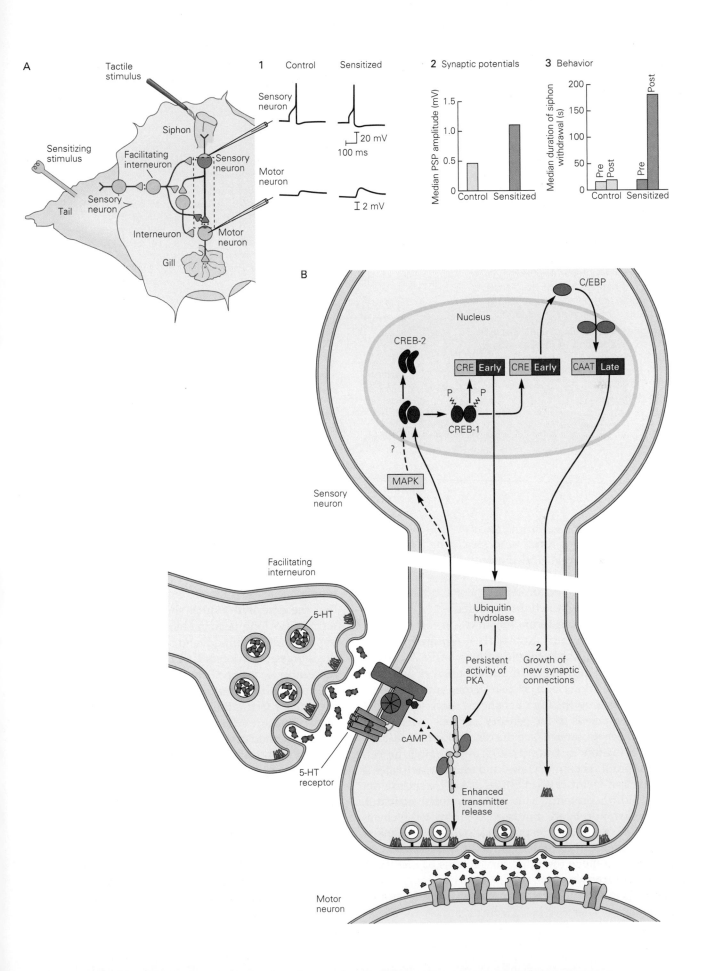

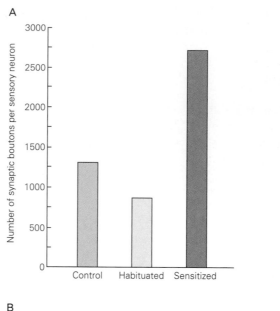

Figure 63-6 Long-term habituation and sensitization in *Aplysia* involve structural changes in the presynaptic terminals of sensory neurons. (Adapted from Bailey and Chen 1983.)

A. When measured 1 day or 1 week after training, the number of presynaptic terminals is highest in sensitized animals (about 2800) compared with control (1300) and habituated animals (800).

B. Long-term habituation leads to a loss of synapses and long-term sensitization leads to an increase in synapses.

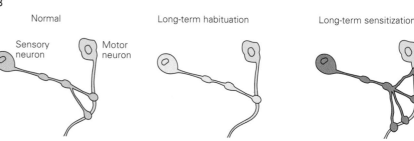

of learning involves three processes: gene expression, new protein synthesis, and the growth (or pruning) of synaptic connections.

How do genes and proteins operate in the consolidation of long-term functional changes?

Studies of long-term sensitization of the gill-withdrawal reflex indicate that with repeated application of serotonin the catalytic subunit of PKA recruits another second messenger kinase, the mitogen-activated protein (MAP) kinase, a kinase commonly associated with cellular growth. Together the two kinases translocate to the nucleus of the sensory neurons, where they activate a genetic switch (see the discussion of transcriptional regulation in Chapter 13). Specifically, the catalytic subunit phosphorylates and thereby activates a transcription factor called *CREB-1* (*cAMP response element binding* protein). This transcriptional activator, when phosphorylated, binds to a promoter element called *CRE* (the *cAMP response element*). By means of the MAP kinase the catalytic subunit of PKA also acts indirectly to relieve the inhibitory actions of *CREB-2*, a repressor of transcription.

The presence of both a repressor (CREB-2) and an activator (CREB-1) of transcription at the very first step in long-term facilitation suggests that the threshold for putting information into long-term memory is highly *regulated*. Indeed, we can see in everyday life that the ease with which short-term memory is transferred into long-term memory varies greatly depending on attention, mood, and social context. In fact, when the repressive action of CREB-2 is relieved (by injecting, for example, a specific antibody to CREB-2), a single pulse of serotonin, which normally produces only short-term facilitation lasting minutes, is able to produce long-term facilitation, the cellular homolog of long-term memory.

Under normal circumstances the physiological relief of the repressive action of CREB-2 and the activation of CREB-1 induce expression of downstream target genes, two of which are particularly important: (1) the enzyme ubiquitin carboxyterminal hydrolase, which activates proteasomes to make PKA persistently active, and (2) the transcription factor C/EBP, one of the components of a gene cascade necessary for the growth of new synaptic connections. The induction of the hydrolase is a key step in the recruitment of a regulated proteolytic complex: the ubiquitin-dependent proteosome. As in other cellular contexts, ubiquitin-mediated proteolysis also produces a cellular change of state, here by removing inhibitory constraints on memory. One of the substrates of this proteolytic process is the regulatory subunit of PKA.

PKA is made up of four subunits: two regulatory submits inhibit two catalytic subunits (Chapter 13). Long-term training and the induction of the hydrolase degrades about 25% of the regulatory (inhibitory) subunits in the sensory neurons. As a result, the catalytic subunits continue phosphorylating proteins important for enhancing transmitter release and strengthening the synaptic connections, including CREB-1, long after the second messenger, cAMP, has returned to its basal level (Figure 63-5B). This is the simplest mechanism for long-term memory: a second-messenger kinase critical for the short-term process is made persistently active for up to 24 hours by repeated training, without requiring a continuous signal of any sort. The kinase becomes autonomous and does not require either serotonin, cAMP, or PKA.

The second and more enduring consequence of the activation of CREB-1 is a cascade of gene activation that leads to the growth of new synaptic connections. It is this growth process that provides the stable, self-maintained state of long-term memory. In *Aplysia* the number of presynaptic terminals in the sensory neurons of the gill-withdrawal pathway increases and becomes twice as great in the long term in sensitized animals as in untrained animals (Figure 63-6). This structural change is not limited to the sensory neurons. In animals that have been sensitized for the long term, the dendrites of the motor neurons grow to accommodate the additional synaptic input. Such morphological changes do not occur with short-term sensitization. Long-term habituation, in contrast, leads to *pruning* of synaptic connections. The long-term inactivation of the functional connections between sensory and motor neurons reduces the number of terminals for each neuron by one-third (Figure 63-6), and the proportion of terminals with active zones from 40% to 10%.

Genetic Analyses of Implicit Memory Storage for Classical Conditioning Also Implicate the cAMP-PKA-CREB Pathway

How general is the role of the cAMP-PKA-CREB pathway in long-term memory storage? Does it apply to other species and other types of learning? The fruit fly *Drosophila* is particularly amenable to genetic manipulation. As first shown by Seymour Benzer and his students, *Drosophila* can be classically conditioned, and

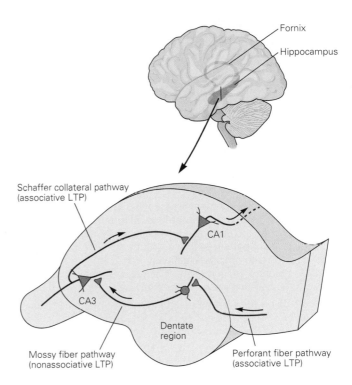

Figure 63-7 The three major afferent pathways in the hippocampus. (**Arrows** denote the direction of impulse flow.) The perforant fiber pathway from the entorhinal cortex forms excitatory connections with the granule cells of the dentate gyrus. The granule cells give rise to axons that form the mossy fiber pathway, which connects with the pyramidal cells in area CA3 of the hippocampus. The pyramidal cells of the CA3 region project to the pyramidal cells in CA1 by means of the Schaffer collateral pathway. Long-term potentiation (**LTP**) is nonassociative in the mossy fiber pathway and associative in the other two pathways.

four interesting mutations in single genes that lead to a learning deficit have been isolated: *dunce, rutabaga, amnesiac,* and *PKA-R1*. Studies of these mutants have given rise to two general conclusions. First, all of the mutants that fail to show classical conditioning also fail to show sensitization. Second, all four mutants have a defect in the cAMP cascade. *Dunce* lacks phosphodiesterase, an enzyme that degrades cAMP. As a result, this mutant has abnormally high levels of cAMP that are thought to be beyond the range of normal modulation. *Rutabaga* is defective in the Ca^{2+}/calmodulin–dependent adenylyl cyclase and therefore has a low basal level of cAMP. *Amnesiac* lacks a peptide transmitter that acts on adenylyl cyclase, and *PKA-R1* is defective in PKA.

More recently a reverse genetic approach has been used to explore memory storage in *Drosophila*. Various transgenes (see Chapter 3) are placed under the control

A Experimental setup

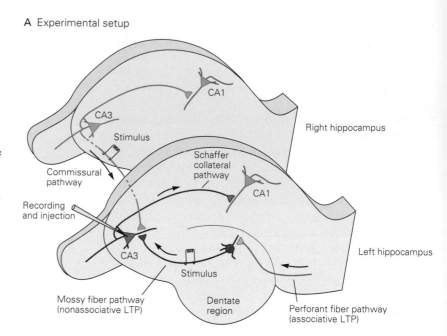

Figure 63-8 Long-term potentiation (LTP) of the mossy fiber pathway to the CA3 region of the hippocampus.

A. Experimental arrangement for studying LTP in the CA3 region of the hippocampus. Stimulating electrodes are placed so as to activate two independent pathways to the CA3 pyramidal cells: The commissural pathway from the CA3 region of the contralateral hippocampus and the ipsilateral mossy fiber pathway.

B. Whole-cell voltage-clamp recording allows injection of both fluoride and the Ca^{2+} chelator BAPTA into the cell body of the CA3 neuron. Together these two drugs are thought to block *all* second-messenger pathways in the postsynaptic cell. Despite this drastic biochemical blockade of the postsynaptic cell, LTP in the mossy fiber pathway is unaffected and is therefore thought to be presynaptically induced. In contrast, these injections do block LTP in the commissural pathway. This pathway requires activation of the *N*-methyl-D-aspartate (NMDA) receptor, and here induction of LTP is postsynaptic. (Adapted from Zalutsky and Nicoll 1990).

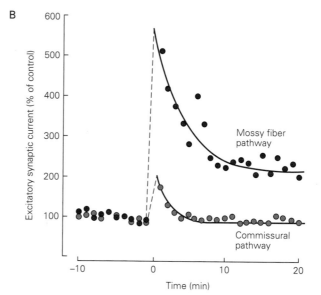

of an inducible promoter that is heat-sensitive, so that by heating and cooling the fly a particular gene can be turned on or off. This inducible control over gene expression, which we shall return to again later in the chapter, is useful for studying synaptic or behavioral plasticity in adult animals. It minimizes any potential effect that a transgene might produce on the development of the brain and therefore allows one to read out the selective effect of the gene on adult behavior.

The first such experiment involved inducing the expression of transgenes that blocked the catalytic subunit

of PKA. William Quinn and his colleagues found that blocking the action of PKA, even transiently, interferes with the fly's ability to learn and to form short-term memory. A similar disruption of learning and memory was observed in a mutant of a *Drosophila* homolog of the PKA catalytic subunit. These experiments indicate the importance of the cAMP signal transduction pathway is critical for associative learning and short-term memory in *Drosophila*.

Long-term memory after repeated training in *Drosophila* also requires new protein synthesis. *Drosophila* ex-

Figure 63-9 Long-term potentiation (LTP) in the Schaffer collateral pathway to the CA1 region of the hippocampus.

A. Experimental setup for studying LTP in the CA1 region of the hippocampus. The Schaffer collateral pathway is stimulated electrically and the response of the population of pyramidal neurons is recorded.

B. Comparison of early and late LTP in a cell in the CA1 region of the hippocampus. The graph is a plot of the slope (rate of rise) of the excitatory postsynaptic potentials (EPSP) in the cell as a function of time. The slope is a measure of synaptic efficacy. Excitatory postsynaptic potentials were recorded from outside the cell. A test stimulus was given every 60 s to the Schaffer collaterals. To elicit early LTP a single train of stimuli is given for 1 s at 100 Hz. To elicit the late phase of LTP four trains are given separated by 10 min. The resulting early LTP lasts 2–3 hours, whereas the late LTP lasts 24 or more hours.

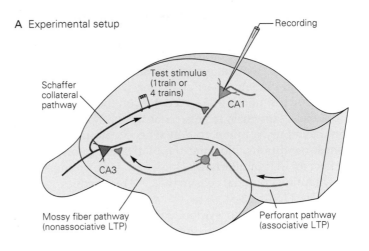

A Experimental setup

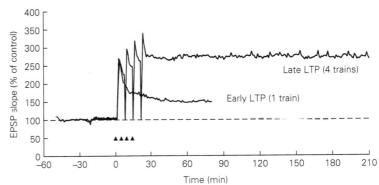

B LTP in the hippocampus CA1 area

presses both a CREB activator and a CREB-2 repressor. Jerry Yin, Tim Tully, and their colleagues found that overexpression of the repressor (CREB-2), which presumably prevents the expression of cAMP-activated genes, selectively blocks long-term memory without interfering with learning or short-term memory. Conversely, overexpression of the CREB activator results in immediate long-term memory, even with a training procedure that produces only short-term memory in wild-type flies.

Explicit Memory in Mammals Involves Long-Term Potentiation in the Hippocampus

What mechanisms are used to store explicit memory—information about people, places, and objects? One important component of the medial temporal system of higher vertebrates involved in the storage of explicit memory is the hippocampus (Chapter 62). As first shown by Per Andersen, the hippocampus has three major pathways: (1) the *perforant pathway*, which pro-

jects from the entorhinal cortex to the granule cells of the dentate gyrus; (2) the *mossy fiber pathway*, which contains the axons of the granule cells and runs to the pyramidal cells in the CA3 region of the hippocampus; and (3) the *Schaffer collateral pathway*, which consists of the excitatory collaterals of the pyramidal cells in the CA3 region and ends on the pyramidal cells in the CA1 region (Figure 63-7).

In 1973 Timothy Bliss and Terje Lomø discovered that each of these pathways is remarkably sensitive to the history of previous activity. A brief high-frequency train of stimuli (a tetanus) to any of the three major synaptic pathways increases the amplitude of the excitatory postsynaptic potentials in the target hippocampal neurons. This facilitation is called *long-term potentiation* (LTP). The mechanisms underlying LTP are not the same in all three pathways. LTP can be studied in the intact animal, where it can last for days and even weeks. It can also be examined in slices of hippocampus and in cell culture for several hours. We shall first consider the mossy fiber pathway.

Long-Term Potentiation in the Mossy Fiber Pathway Is Nonassociative

The mossy fiber pathway consists of the axons of the granule cells of the dentate gyrus. The mossy fiber terminals release glutamate as a transmitter, which binds to both NMDA and non-NMDA receptors on the target pyramidal cells. However, in this pathway the NMDA receptors have only a minor role in synaptic plasticity under most conditions; blocking the NMDA receptors has no effect on LTP. Similarly, blocking Ca^{2+} influx into the postsynaptic pyramidal cells in the CA3 region does not affect LTP (Figure 63-8).

Instead, LTP in the mossy fiber pathway region has been found to depend on Ca^{2+} influx into the *presynaptic* cell after the tetanus. The Ca^{2+} influx appears to activate Ca^{2+}/calmodulin-dependent adenylyl cyclase thereby increasing the level of cAMP and activating PKA in the presynaptic neuron, just as in the sensory neurons of *Aplysia* during associative learning. Moreover, mossy fiber LTP can be regulated by a modulatory input. This input is noradrenergic and engages β-adrenergic receptors, which activate adenylyl cyclase, as does the serotonergic input in *Aplysia*.

Long-Term Potentiation in the Schaffer Collateral and Perforant Pathways Is Associative

The Schaffer collateral pathway connects the pyramidal cells of the CA3 region of the hippocampus with those of the CA1 region (Chapter 5 and Figures 63-7 and 63-9A). Like the mossy fiber terminals, the terminals of the Schaffer collaterals also use glutamate as transmitter, but LTP in the Schaffer collateral pathway requires activation of the NMDA-type of glutamate receptor (Figures 63-9B and 63-10). Therefore, LTP in CA1 cells has two characteristic features that distinguish it from LTP in the mossy fiber pathway, both of which derive from the known properties of the NMDA receptor.

First, LTP in the Schaffer collateral pathway typically requires activation of several afferent axons together, a feature called *cooperativity*. This feature derives from the fact that the NMDA receptor-channel becomes functional and conducts Ca^{2+} only when two conditions are met: Glutamate must bind to the postsynaptic NMDA receptor *and* the membrane potential of the postsynaptic cell must be sufficiently depolarized by the cooperative firing of several afferent axons to expel Mg^{2+} from the mouth of the channel (Figure 63-10). Only when Mg^{2+} is expelled can Ca^{2+} influx into the postsynaptic cell occur. Calcium influx initiates the persistent enhancement of synaptic transmission by activating two calcium-dependent serine-threonine protein kinases—the Ca^{2+}/calmodulin-dependent protein ki-

nase and protein kinase C—as well as PKA and the tyrosine protein kinase fyn.

Second, LTP in the Schaffer collateral pathway requires concomitant activity in both the presynaptic and postsynaptic cells to adequately depolarize the postsynaptic cell, a feature called *associativity*. As we have seen, to initiate the Ca^{2+} influx into the postsynaptic cell, a strong presynaptic input sufficient to fire the postsynaptic cell is required.

The finding that LTP in the Schaffer collateral pathway requires simultaneous firing in both the postsynaptic and presynaptic neurons provides direct evidence for *Hebb's rule*, proposed in 1949 by the psychologist Donald Hebb: "When an axon of cell A . . . excites cell B and repeatedly or persistently takes part in firing it, some growth process or metabolic change takes place in one or both cells so that A's efficiency as one of the cells firing B is increased." As discussed in Chapter 56, a similar principle is involved in fine-tuning synaptic connections during the late stages of development.

The induction of LTP in the CA1 region of the hippocampus depends on four postsynaptic factors: postsynaptic depolarization, activation of NMDA receptors, influx of Ca^{2+}, and activation by Ca^{2+} of several second-messenger systems in the postsynaptic cell. The mechanisms for the expression of this LTP, on the other hand, is still uncertain. It is thought to involve not only

Figure 63-10 (Opposite) **A model for the induction of the early phase of long-term potentiation.** According to this model NMDA and non-NMDA receptor-channels are located near each other in dendritic spines.

A. During normal, low-frequency synaptic transmission glutamate (**Glu**) is released from the presynaptic terminal and acts on both the NMDA and non-NMDA receptors. The non-NMDA receptors here are the AMPA type. Na^+ and K^+ flow through the non-NMDA channels but not through the NMDA channels, owing to Mg^{2+} blockage of this channel at the resting level of membrane potential.

B. When the postsynaptic membrane is depolarized by the actions of the non-NMDA receptor-channels, as occurs during a high-frequency tetanus that induces LTP, the depolarization relieves the Mg^{2+} blockage of the NMDA channel. This allows Ca^{2+} to flow through the NMDA channel. The resulting rise in Ca^{2+} in the dendritic spine triggers calcium-dependent kinases (Ca^{2+}/calmodulin kinase and protein kinase C) and the tyrosine kinase Fyn that together induce LTP. The Ca^{2+}/calmodulin kinase phosphorylates non-NMDA receptor-channels and increases their sensitivity to glutamate thereby also activating some otherwise silent receptor channels. These changes give rise to a postsynaptic contribution for the maintenance of LTP. In addition, once LTP is induced, the postsynaptic cell is thought to release (in ways that are still not understood) a set of retrograde messengers, one of which is thought to be nitric oxide, that act on protein kinases in the presynaptic terminal to initiate an enhancement of transmitter release that contributes to LTP.

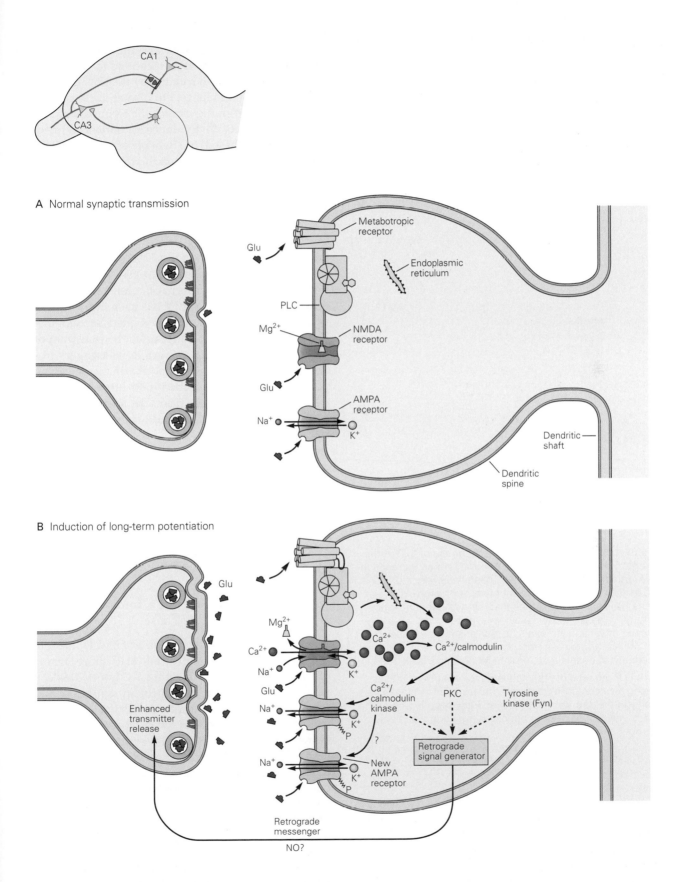

A Normal synaptic transmission

B Induction of long-term potentiation

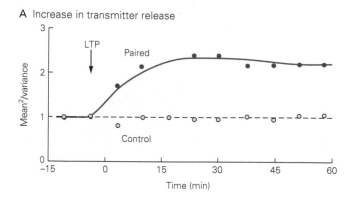

A Increase in transmitter release

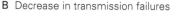

B Decrease in transmission failures

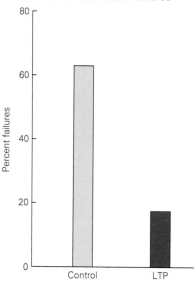

Figure 63-11 Maintenance of the early phase of LTP in the CA1 region of the hippocampus depends on an increase in presynaptic transmitter release. Quantal analysis of LTP in area CA1 is based on a coefficient of variation of evoked responses. This analysis assumes that the number of quanta of transmitter released follows a binomial distribution, where the coefficient of variation (mean squared/variance) provides an index of transmitter release from the presynaptic terminal that is independent of quantal size. (From Malinow and Tsien 1990.)

A. With LTP the ratio of mean squared to variance increases, indicating an increase in transmitter release. This increase occurs only in the pathway that is paired with depolarization of the postsynaptic cell. It does not occur in a control pathway that is not paired.

B. At normal rates of stimulation the number of failures in transmission is significant (60%). After LTP the percentage of failures decreases to 20%, another indication that LTP is presynaptic.

an increase in the sensitivity and number of the postsynaptic non-NMDA (AMPA) receptors to glutamate as a result of being phosphorylated by the Ca^{2+}/calmodulin-dependent protein kinase, but also an increase in transmitter release from the *presynaptic* terminals of the CA3 neuron (Figure 63-11). Evidence for enhanced presynaptic function is based on two observations. First, biochemical studies suggest that the release of glutamate is enhanced during LTP. Second, as we shall see later, quantal analysis indicates that the probability of transmitter release increases greatly during LTP.

Since induction of LTP requires events only in the postsynaptic cell (Ca^{2+} influx through NMDA channels), whereas expression of LTP is due in part to a subsequent event in the presynaptic cells (increase in transmitter release), the presynaptic cells must somehow receive information that LTP has been induced. There is now evidence that calcium-activated second messengers, or perhaps Ca^{2+} itself, causes the postsynaptic cell to release one or more retrograde messengers from its active dendritic spines. Recent pharmacological and genetic experiments have identified nitric oxide (NO), a gas that diffuses readily from cell to cell, as one of the possible candidate retrograde messengers involved in LTP.

These studies of the Schaffer collateral pathway indicate that LTP in CA1 uses two associative mechanisms in series: a Hebbian mechanism (simultaneous firing in both the pre- and postsynaptic cells) and activity-dependent presynaptic facilitation. A similar set of mechanisms is responsible for LTP in the perforant pathway. As we saw earlier, two associative mechanisms in series also contribute to classical conditioning in *Aplysia*.

Long-Term Potentiation Has a Transient Early and a Consolidated Late Phase

As with memory storage (Chapter 62), LTP has phases. One stimulus train produces an early, short-term phase of LTP (called *early LTP*) lasting 1–3 hours; this component does not require new protein synthesis. Four or more trains induce a more persistent phase of LTP (called *late LTP*) that lasts for at least 24 hours and requires new protein and RNA synthesis. As we have seen, the mechanisms for the early, short-term phase are quite different in the Schaffer collateral and mossy fiber pathways. However, the mechanisms for the late, long-term phase in the two pathways appear similar. In both pathways late-phase LTP requires the synthesis of new mRNA and protein and recruits the cAMP-PKA-MAPK-CREB signaling pathway.

What are the properties of this late phase of LTP? Does long-term explicit memory storage, like implicit

Figure 63-12 The early and late phases of LTP are evident in the synaptic transmission between a single CA3 cell and a single CA1 cell. (From Bolshakov et al. 1997.)

A. A single CA3 cell can be stimulated selectively to produce a single elementary synaptic potential in a CA1 cell. When the CA3 cell is stimulated repeatedly at low frequency, it gives rise to either an elementary response of the size of a miniature synaptic potential or a failure.

B. In control cells there are many failures; the synapse has a low probability of releasing vesicles. The distribution of the amplitudes of many responses can be approximated by two Gaussian curves, one centered on zero (the failures) and the other centered on 4 pA (the successful responses). These histograms are consistent with the type of synapse illustrated here, in which a single CA3 cell makes a single connection on a CA1 cell. This connection has a single active zone from which it releases a single vesicle in an all-or-none manner (failures or successes).

C. With the early phase of LTP the probability of release rises significantly, but the two Gaussian curves in the distribution of responses is consistent with the view that a single release site still releases only a vesicle but now with a high probability of release.

D. When the late phase of LTP is induced by a cAMP analog (**Sp-cAMPS**), the distribution of responses no longer fits two Gaussian curves but instead requires three or four Gaussian curves, suggesting the possibility that new presynaptic active zones and postsynaptic receptors have grown. These effects are blocked by anisomycin, an inhibitor of protein synthesis.

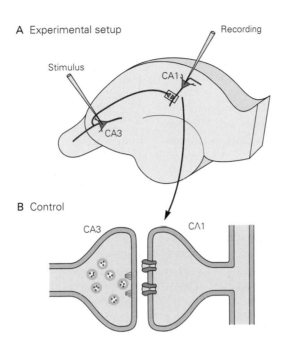

A Experimental setup

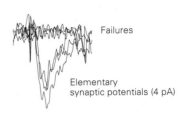

Failures

Elementary synaptic potentials (4 pA)

B Control

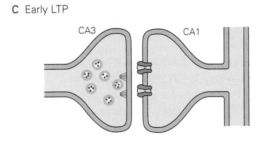

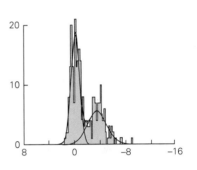

C Early LTP

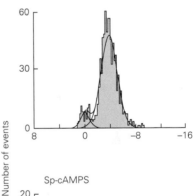

D Late LTP

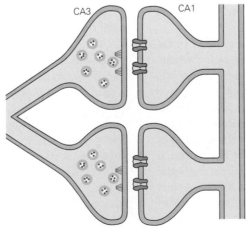

Sp-cAMPS

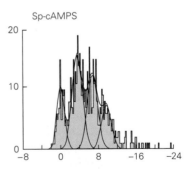

Sp-cAMPS + anisomycin

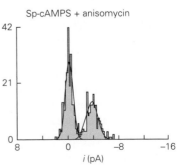

i (pA)

memory storage, also require the growth of new synaptic connections? In fact, cellular-physiological studies are beginning to suggest that the late phase of LTP involves the activation, perhaps the growth, of additional presynaptic machinery for transmitter release and the insertion of new clusters of postsynaptic receptors.

Charles Stevens and his colleagues and Steven Siegelbaum and Vadim Bolshakov have now examined LTP by stimulating a *single* presynaptic CA3 neuron and recording from a *single* CA1 postsynaptic cell. When the CA3 neuron is stimulated repeatedly at a low rate, most of the time the CA1 cell fails to respond with a synaptic potential. Only on occasion does activity in the presynaptic neuron lead to a small response, about 4 pA in amplitude, in the postsynaptic cell (Figure 63-12A). This response is approximately the size of a single spontaneous miniature synaptic potential (Chapter 14). When many failures and unitary responses are collected and measured, the failures of release and the unitary responses can be described by two random (Gaussian) distributions, one centered at zero, corresponding to the failures of release, and the other centered around 4 pA, corresponding both to successful responses and to the size of spontaneously released miniature synaptic potentials (Figure 63-12B). These distributions lend themselves to a surprisingly clear anatomical explanation. They suggest that a single CA3 neuron makes only a single functional synaptic contact on a CA1 neuron. This single synaptic contact appears to have only one active zone from which the transmitter content of only a single vesicle is released, in an all-or-none way, by a presynaptic action potential. In the basal state (where there are many more failures than responses) the probability of release of the vesicle is low. Thus, this situation is not very different from other central synaptic connections where a single release site typically releases only a single vesicle in an all-or-none fashion (Chapter 15).

What happens during the early phase of LTP? In the early phase the number of failures decreases and the number of successes increases, but the amplitude histograms of the responses and failures are still fit by two Gaussian distributions (corresponding to failures of release and successful responses). This indicates that the early phase of LTP produces no change in the number of synapses, the number of active zones, or the maximal number of vesicles released with each action potential (Figure 63-12C). Thus the early phase of LTP represents a functional change—an increase in the *probability* of transmitter release—without structural changes. An action potential still releases only one vesicle of transmitter from a single release site, but now it does so more reliably.

An equivalent of the late-phase LTP can be induced chemically, by exposing the neurons to permeant cAMP. After the late phase of LTP begins the distribution of successful responses changes dramatically and can no longer be approximated by two Gaussian functions. The responses now are not simply zero and 4 pA but are 8, 12, and even 20 pA in amplitude, so that several Gaussian curves are required to describe the distribution of responses (Figure 63-12D). This change suggests that during the late phase of LTP a single action potential in a single CA3 cell releases several vesicles of transmitter onto the CA1 neuron. Since each release site is thought to release only one vesicle in an all-or-none fashion, such an increase in the number of vesicles released would seem to entail growth of new presynaptic release sites as well as new clusters of postsynaptic receptors. Consistent with this idea, and with the properties of the late phase of LTP, the generation of these new distributions requires new protein synthesis (Figure 63-13).

Genetic Interference With Long-Term Potentiation Is Reflected in the Properties of Place Cells in the Hippocampus

LTP is an artificially induced change in synaptic strength produced by electrical stimulation of synaptic pathways. Does this form of synaptic plasticity exist naturally? If so, how does it affect the normal processing of information for memory storage in the hippocampus?

In 1971 John O'Keefe and John Dostrovsky made the remarkable discovery that the hippocampus contains a cognitive map of the spatial environment in which an animal moves. The location of an animal in a particular space is encoded in the firing pattern of individual pyramidal cells, the very cells that undergo LTP when their afferent pathways are stimulated electrically.

A mouse's hippocampus has about a million pyramidal cells. Each of these cells is potentially a *place cell*, encoding a position in space. When an animal moves around, different place cells in the hippocampus fire. For example, one cell will fire only when the animal's head enters a particular area in the north end of the space, while other cells will fire when the animal takes other positions at the south end of that space (Figure 63-14). Thus, the mouse's whereabouts are signaled by the discharge of a unique population of hippocampal place cells.

By this means the animal is thought to form a "place field," an internal representation of the space that it occupies. When the animal enters a new environment, new place fields are formed within minutes and are sta-

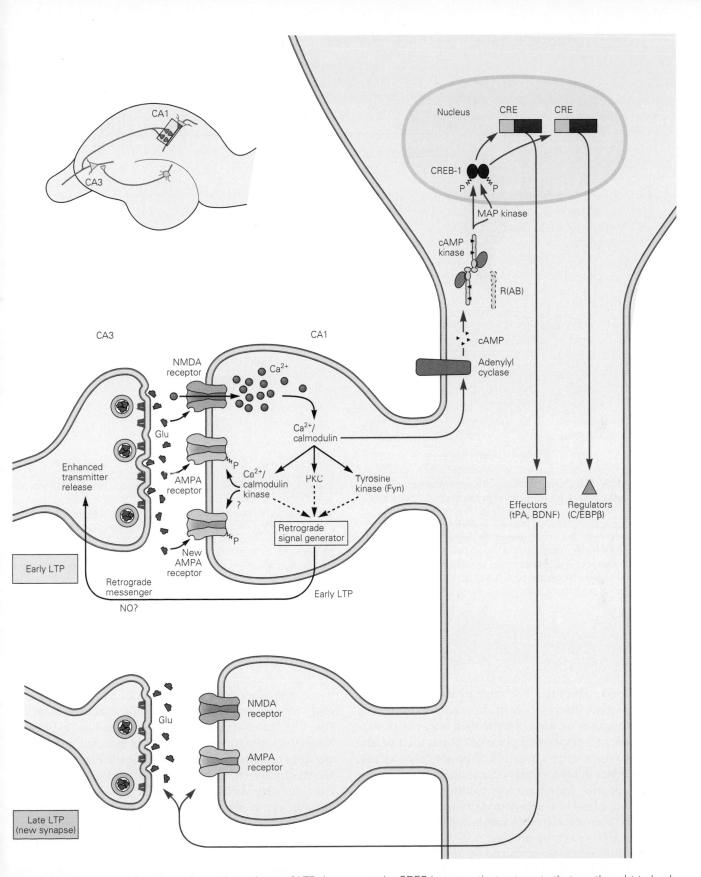

Figure 63-13 A model for the early and late phase of LTP. A single train of action potentials leads to early LTP by activating NMDA receptors, Ca²⁺ influx into the postsynaptic cell, and a set of second messengers. With repeated trains the Ca²⁺ influx also recruits an adenylyl cyclase, which activates the cAMP-dependent protein kinase (cAMP kinase) leading to its translocation to the nucleus, where it phosphorylates the CREB protein. CREB in turn activates targets that are thought to lead to structural changes. Mutations in mice that block PKA or CREB reduce or eliminate the late phase of LTP. The adenylyl cyclase can also be modulated by dopaminergic and perhaps other modulatory inputs. **BDNF** = brain-derived neurotrophic factor; **C/EBPβ** = transcription factor; **P** = phosphate; **R(AB)** = dominant negative PKA; **tPA** = tissue plasminogen activator.

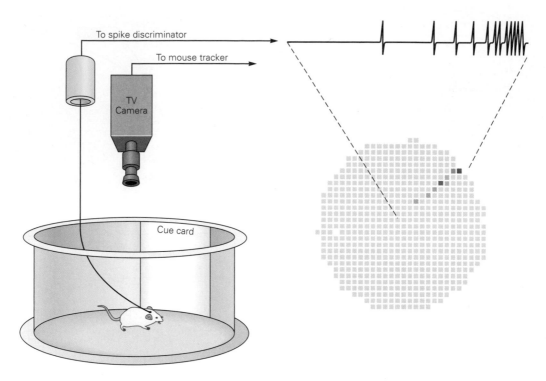

Figure 63-14A The firing patterns of pyramidal cells in the hippocampus create an internal representation of the animal's location within its surrounding. A mouse is attached to a recording cable and placed inside a cylinder (49 cm in diameter by 34 cm high). The other end of the cable goes to a 25-channel commutator attached to a computer-based spike-discrimination system. The cable is also used to supply power to a light-emitting diode mounted on the headstage the mouse carries. The entire apparatus is viewed with an overhead TV camera whose output goes to a tracking device that detects the position of the mouse. The output of the tracker is sent to the same computer used to detect spikes, so that parallel time series of positions and spikes are recorded. The occurrence of spikes as a function of position is extracted from the basic data and is used to form two-dimensional firing-rate patterns that can be numerically analyzed or visualized as color-coded firing-rate maps. (Based on Muller et al. 1987.)

ble for weeks to months. The same pyramidal cells may signal different information in different environments and can therefore be used in more than one spatial map.

The rapid formation of place fields and their persistence for weeks offer an excellent opportunity to ask, How are place fields formed and maintained? Is LTP important for the formation or maintenance of place fields? To address these questions two types of mutations have been examined in mice, each of which interferes with LTP in a different way.

One mutation was produced by Joe Tsien, Susumu Tonegawa, and their colleagues by selectively knocking out NMDA R1, one of the subunits of the NMDA receptor, in the pyramidal cells of the CA1 region. This restricted knockout, limited to just the CA1 region, disrupts LTP in the Schaffer collateral pathway completely (Box 63-1).

In the other mutation, produced by Mark Mayford and his colleagues, a persistently active form of the Ca^{2+}/calmodulin-dependent kinase is expressed throughout the hippocampus. This mutated gene product does not affect LTP produced at 100 Hz stimulation, the frequency commonly used in the laboratory, but it does interfere with LTP produced at low frequencies of stimulation, in the range of 1–10 Hz (Box 63-1). These lower frequencies are interesting because they are in the physiological range of a prominent spontaneous rhythm in the hippocampus, called the *theta rhythm*, that occurs in an animal as it moves in the environment.

In both types of mutants the interference with LTP does not prevent the formation of place fields. Although the place fields formed in the absence of LTP are larger and fuzzier in outline than normal, LTP is not required for the basic transformation of sensory information into

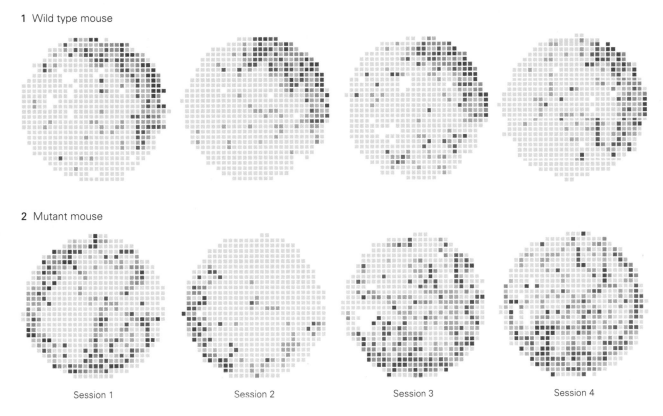

1 Wild type mouse

2 Mutant mouse

Session 1   Session 2   Session 3   Session 4

Figure 63-14B The firing-rate patterns from four successive recording sessions in a single cell from a wild-type mouse and a mouse carrying a gene for a persistently active Ca^{2+}/calmodulin-dependent kinase. Before each recording session the animal was taken out of the cylinder and reintroduced into it. In each of the four sessions the positional firing pattern for the wild-type cell is stable. By contrast, the pattern of the mutant cell is unstable in sessions 2 and 3.

place fields. LTP is required for fine-tuning the properties of place cells and ensuring their stability over time.

For example, pyramidal cells that encode for overlapping positions in space fire synchronously when the animal enters the space represented by those cells. Thomas McHugh and his colleagues found that this correlated firing is lost in mice lacking a functional NMDA receptor in the CA1 region. Alex Rotenberg found that the defect is more severe in mice that overexpress an activated form of the Ca^{2+}/calmodulin-dependent protein kinase. As noted earlier, in wild-type mice a place field forms within minutes after an animal enters a new environment and, once formed, remains stable in that environment for months. In contrast, when mutant mice are removed from a space and then put back into the same space, cells that were previously active in that space form *different* place fields. This instability of place cells is reminiscent of the memory defect in H.M. and other patients with lesions of the medial temporal lobe. Each time these patients enter the same space, they act as if they have never seen it before.

Associative Long-Term Potentiation Is Important for Spatial Memory

If LTP is a synaptic mechanism for maintaining a coherent spatial map over time, then defects in LTP should interfere with spatial memory. One spatial memory test is a water maze in which a mouse must find a platform hidden under opaque water in a pool. When released at random locations around the pool, the mouse must use contextual (spatial) cues—markings on the walls of the room in which the pool is located—to find the platform. This task requires the hippocampus. In a simple non-

Box 63-1 Restricting Gene Knockout and Regulating Transgene Expression

Biological analysis of learning requires the establishment of a causal relation between specific molecules and learning. This relationship, which has been difficult to demonstrate in mammals, can now be studied in mice either by the use of transgenes or the selective knockout of genes. With *transgenes* a new gene is introduced into the brain under the control of a promoter that expresses that gene in a specific region of the brain. With *gene knockout* specific gene deletions are induced in embryonic stem cells through homologous recombination (see Figure 3-8).

Experiments using transgenes and gene knockout have made it possible to examine the roles of NMDA receptors and different second-messenger kinases in a variety of learning mechanisms in the hippocampus, including long-term potentiation, spatial learning, and the development and maintenance of a cognitive map of space.

With conventional gene knockout techniques animals inherit the genetic deletions in all of their cell types. Global genetic deletion may cause developmental defects that interfere with the later functioning of neural circuits important for memory storage. As a result, interpretation of the results from conventional knockout mice runs into two types of difficulties. First, it is often difficult to exclude the possibility that the abnormal phenotype observed in mature animals results directly or indirectly from a developmental defect. Second, global gene knockout makes it difficult to attribute abnormal phenotypes to a particular type of cell within the brain.

To improve the utility of gene knockout and transgene technology, methods have been developed to restrict gene expression locally or temporally. One method for restricting gene knockout locally exploits the *Cre/loxP* system, a site-specific recombination system, derived from the P1 phage, in which the Cre recombinase catalyzes recombination between 34 bp *loxP* recognition sequences (Figure 63-15). The *loxP* sequences can be inserted into the genome of embryonic stem cells by homologous recombination such that they flank one or more exons of the gene one is interested in. Thus the gene encoding the R1 subunit of the NMDA receptor can be floxed and then ablated selectively in the CA1 region of the hippocampus. Loss of the R1 subunit leads to loss of LTP. Moreover, mice that lack this gene only in the CA1 region of the hippocampus show a deficiency in spatial memory (Figure 63-17). In contrast, these mice show no deficit in tasks that do not involve the hippocampus, such as learning simple visual discrimination.

In addition to regional restriction of gene expression, effective use of genetically modified mice requires control over the timing of gene expression. The ability to turn a transgene on and off gives the investigator an additional degree of flexibility and can exclude the possibility that any abnormality observed in the phenotype of the mature animal is the result of a developmental defect produced by the transgene. This can be done in mice by constructing a gene that can be turned on or off by giving a drug.

One starts by creating two lines of mice (Figure 63-16). One line carries a particular transgene, for example CaMKII-Asp 286, a mutated form of the gene CaMK-II coding for a constitutively active kinase (line 1). Instead of being attached to its normal promoter, the transgene is attached to the promoter *tet-O* that is ordinarily found only in bacteria. This promoter cannot, by itself, turn on the gene; it needs to be activated by a specific transcriptional regulator. Thus, a second transgene expressed in the second line of mice encodes a hybrid transcriptional regulator called *tetracycline transactivator* (tTA) that recognizes and binds to the *tet-O* promoter (line 2). Expression of tTA is placed under the control of a region-specific promoter, such as the promoter for CaMKII.

When the two lines of mice are mated some of the offspring will carry both transgenes. In these mice the tTA binds to the *tet-O* promoter and activates the mutated *CaMKII* gene. This mutant causes abnormalities in long-term potentiation. But when the animal is given doxycycline, the drug binds to the transcription factor tTA causing it to undergo a change in shape that makes it come off the promoter (Figure 63-16). The cell stops expressing *CaMKII* and long-term potentiation returns to normal, demonstrating that the transgene acts on the adult synapse and does not interfere with the development of the synapse.

One can also generate mice that express a mutant form of tTA called reverse tTA (rtTA). This transactivator will *not* bind to *tet-O* unless the animal is fed doxycycline. In this case the transgene is always turned off unless the drug is given.

Figure 63-15 (Opposite) Using the *Cre/loxP* system to restrict the region of gene knockout.

A. A mouse homozygous for the floxed R1 subunit of the NMDA receptor (**line 1**) is generated from embryonic stem cells by conventional techniques and is crossed to a second mouse that contains a *Cre* transgene under the control of a transcriptional promoter from the *CamKII* gene (**line 2**). In progeny that are homozygous for the floxed gene and that carry the *Cre* transgene, the floxed gene will be deleted by *Cre/loxP* recombination but only in those cell types in which the *Cre* gene-associated promoter is active. By this means efficient gene knockout is accomplished in postmitotic neurons in a highly restricted manner, limited to the CA1 pyramidal cells of the hippocampus.

B. LacZ staining reveals the region where recombination was successful and led to the removal of a floxed stopper sequence that allows LacZ to be expressed. When the Cre recombinase is combined with the promoter for the Ca^{2+}/calmodulin-dependent kinase, the transgene is restricted to the CA1 region. This is evident in the section of the brain illustrated here. (From Tsien et al. 1996a.)

A Regional restriction of gene expression

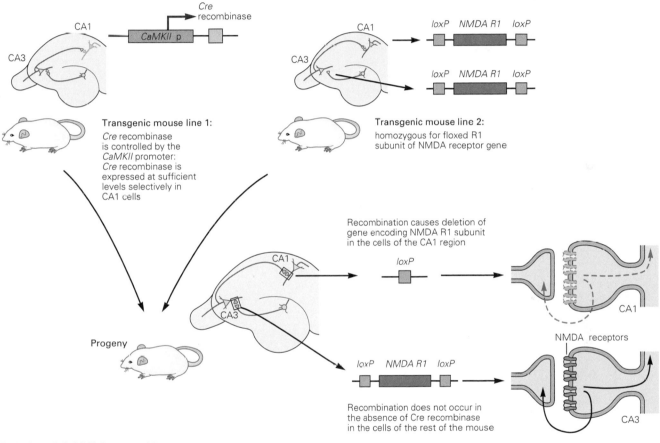

Transgenic mouse line 1:

Cre recombinase is controlled by the *CaMKII* promoter: *Cre* recombinase is expressed at sufficient levels selectively in CA1 cells

Transgenic mouse line 2: homozygous for floxed R1 subunit of NMDA receptor gene

Progeny

Recombination causes deletion of gene encoding NMDA R1 subunit in the cells of the CA1 region

NMDA receptors

Recombination does not occur in the absence of Cre recombinase in the cells of the rest of the mouse

B Action of *CaMKII-Cre* recombinase is restricted to CA1 region

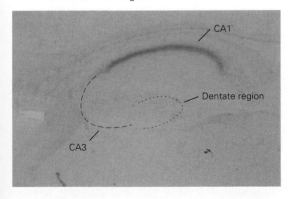

(continued)

Box 63-1 Restricting Gene Knockout and Regulating Transgene Expression (continued)

Temporal restriction of gene expression

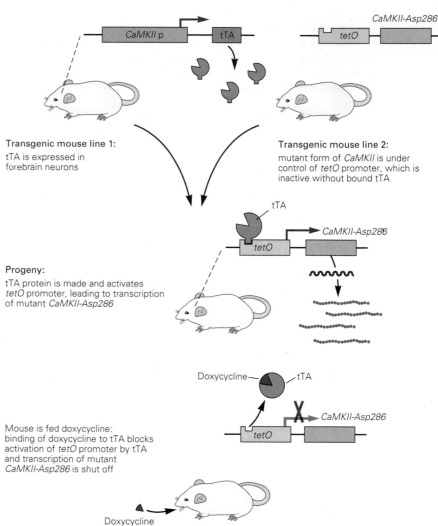

Transgenic mouse line 1:
tTA is expressed in
forebrain neurons

Transgenic mouse line 2:
mutant form of *CaMKII* is under
control of *tetO* promoter, which is
inactive without bound tTA

Progeny:
tTA protein is made and activates
tetO promoter, leading to transcription
of mutant *CaMKII-Asp286*

Mouse is fed doxycycline:
binding of doxycycline to tTA blocks
activation of *tetO* promoter by tTA
and transcription of mutant
CaMKII-Asp286 is shut off

Doxycycline

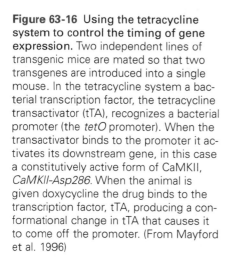

**Figure 63-16 Using the tetracycline
system to control the timing of gene
expression.** Two independent lines of
transgenic mice are mated so that two
transgenes are introduced into a single
mouse. In the tetracycline system a bacterial transcription factor, the tetracycline
transactivator (tTA), recognizes a bacterial
promoter (the *tetO* promoter). When the
transactivator binds to the promoter it activates its downstream gene, in this case
a constitutively active form of CaMKII,
CaMKII-Asp286. When the animal is
given doxycycline the drug binds to the
transcription factor, tTA, producing a conformational change in tTA that causes it
to come off the promoter. (From Mayford
et al. 1996)

Figure 63-17 (Opposite) Mice that lack the NMDA receptor
in the CA1 region of the hippocampus have a defect in LTP
and in spatial memory.

A. Field excitatory postsynaptic potentials (fEPSP) were
recorded in the stratum radiatum in the CA1 region of both mutant and wild-type mice. After a 30-min period of baseline
recording a tetanus (100 Hz for 1 s) was applied (**arrow**). Activity in the pathway remained unchanged in the mutant but became potentiated in the wild-type, indicating that knockout of
the NMDA receptor abolishes LTP.

B. Mice that lack the NMDA receptor in CA1 have impaired
spatial memory. **1.** In the Morris maze a platform is submerged
in one quadrant of an opaque fluid in a circular tank. To avoid remaining in the water the mice have to learn to find the platform
and climb onto it. **2.** Mutant mice are slower in learning to find

the submerged platform. The graph represents the escape latencies of mice trained to find the hidden platform using spatial
(contextual) cues. The mutant mice display a longer latency in
every block of trials (four trials per day) than do the wild-type
mice. Also, mutant mice do not reach the optimal performance
attained by the control mice, even though the mutants show
some improvement. **3.** After the mice have been trained in the
Morris maze, the platform is taken away and the mice are
given a transfer test for memory. A wild-type mouse focuses
its search in the quadrant that formerly contained the platform
because it remembers the platform as being there. The mutant
mouse, which does not remember where the platform was,
spends an equal amount of time (25%) in all quadrants. **a.** Illustrative examples. **b.** Actual data. (From Tsien et al 1996 b.)

A LTP defect in the Schaffer collateral pathway

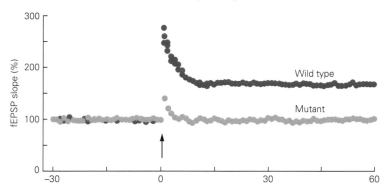

B Spatial memory defects

1 The Morris maze

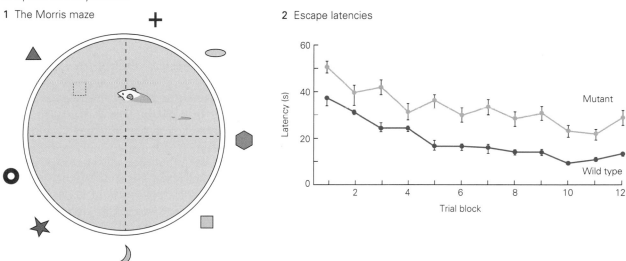

2 Escape latencies

3 Transfer test of Morris maze

a Movement patterns

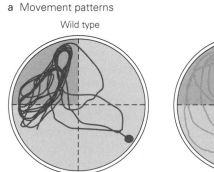

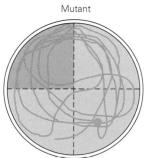

b Search time

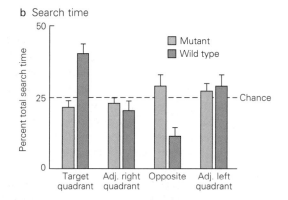

contextual (nonspatial) version of this test the platform is raised above the surface of the water or marked with a flag so that it is visible, permitting the mouse to navigate to the platform directly. This task does not require the hippocampus.

Richard Morris demonstrated that when NMDA receptors are blocked by the injection of a pharmacological antagonist into the hippocampus, the animal can navigate to the visible platform in the noncontextual version of the water maze test but cannot find its way to the submerged platform in the contextual version. These experiments suggested that some mechanism involving NMDA receptors in the hippocampus, perhaps LTP, is involved in spatial learning. More direct evidence for this correlation has come from genetic experiments with the two types of mutant mice described in Box 63-1.

In the first type of mutant the R1 subunit of the NMDA receptor of the pyramidal cells of the CA1 region is selectively knocked out. As a result, basal transmission is normal but LTP is completely disrupted (Figure 63-17A). Although this disruption is restricted to the Schaffer collateral pathway, these mice nevertheless have a serious deficit in spatial memory when tested in the water maze (Figure 63-17B and C). These findings provide the most compelling evidence so far that the NMDA channels and NMDA-mediated synaptic plasticity in the Schaffer collateral pathway are important for spatial memory.

In the second type of mutant, expression of the persistently active form of the Ca^{2+}/calmodulin-dependent protein kinase can be turned on and off at will. Expression of the kinase selectively interferes with LTP when the frequency of electrical stimulation is between 1 and 10 Hz, and this results in an instability in the hippocampal place cells (Figure 63-18). These mutant mice also do not remember spatial tasks. But when the transgene is turned off, the LTP becomes normal and the animal's capability for spatial memory is restored!

These two sets of experiments based on the restricted knockout of the NMDA receptor and the regulated expression of the Ca^{2+}/calmodulin-dependent kinase make it clear that LTP in the Schaffer collateral pathway is important for spatial memory.

How are defects in the various phases of LTP reflected in defects in the phase of memory storage? Indeed, the memory deficits are surprisingly selective. Selective expression in the hippocampus of the transgene that blocks cAMP-dependent protein kinase selectively disrupts the late phase of LTP in the Schaffer collateral pathway. Animals with this deficit have normal learning abilities and normal short-term memory when tested at

one hour, but they cannot convert short-term memory into stable long-term memory. They have defective long-term memory when tested at 24 hours after training. Essentially similar results are obtained in mice that have a knockout of several isoforms of CREB-1, as well as in normal wild-type mice that are exposed to pharmacological inhibitors of protein synthesis or cAMP-dependent protein kinase. These animals learn well and have normal short-term memory but poor long-term memory.

Thus, interference with the early and late component of LTP in the Schaffer collateral pathway interferes with both short- and long-term memory, whereas selective interference with the late component of LTP interferes only with the consolidation of long-term memory. Together, these experiments provide insight into the genetic chain of causation that connects molecules to LTP, LTP to place cells, and place cells to the outward behavior of the animal as reflected in both short- and long-term spatial memory.

Is There a Molecular Alphabet for Learning?

The changes in synaptic efficacy that we have encountered in studies of both implicit and explicit forms of storage raise three key issues in a neurobiological approach to learning.

First, the finding that the molecular mechanisms of some associative forms of synaptic plasticity are based on those of nonassociative forms in the same cell suggests that there may be a molecular alphabet for synaptic plasticity—simpler forms of plasticity might represent elements of more complex forms. Of course, all of these synaptic mechanisms are embedded in distributed neural circuits with considerable additional computational power, which can thus add substantial complexity to the actions of individual cells.

Second, the molecular mechanisms of elementary forms of associative memory storage used in both implicit and explicit learning are similar. In the two processes we have considered—activity-dependent presynaptic facilitation for storing implicit memory and associative LTP for storing explicit memory—the plasticity of neuronal function seems to derive from the associative properties of specific proteins: from the ability of proteins, such as adenylyl cyclase and the NMDA receptor, to respond conjointly to two independent signals.

Finally, despite clear differences in behavioral logic in the neural systems recruited for the task, implicit and explicit memory storage seem to use elements of a

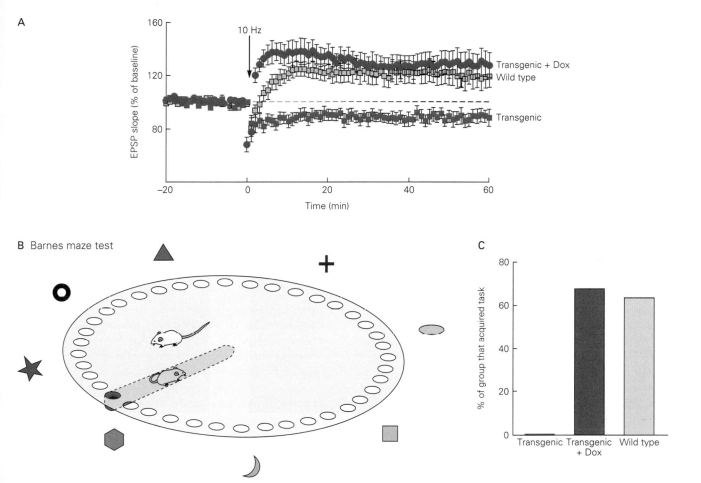

Figure 63-18 Reversal of the deficit in LTP and in spatial memory in the CA1 region of the hippocampus.

A. Field excitatory postsynaptic potentials (fEPSP) slopes before and after tetanic stimulation were recorded and expressed as the percentage of pretetanus baseline. Stimulation at 10 Hz (**arrow**) for 1.5 min induced a transient depression in activity followed by potentiation in wild-type mice but only a slight depression and no potentiation in transgenic mice. Doxycycline treatment (Dox) reversed the defect in the transgenic mice so that they show potentiation compared with wild type.

B. The Barnes maze measures the same spatial memory system explored in the Morris water maze. This maze consists of a platform with 40 holes, only one of which (marked in **black**)

leads to an escape tunnel that allows the mouse to exit the platform. The mouse is placed in the center of the platform. Because mice do not like open, well-lit spaces, they try to escape from the platform. The only way they can do that is to find the one hole that leads to the escape tunnel. The most efficient way of doing that (and the only way of meeting the criteria set for the task by the experimenter) is to use the distinctive markings on the four walls.

C. Percentage of transgenic and wild-type mice that met the learning criterion on the Barnes circular maze. Three groups of mice were tested: transgenics with and without doxycycline and wild-types. Transgenics that received doxycycline performed as well as wild-types, whereas those without the doxycycline did not learn the task.

A₁

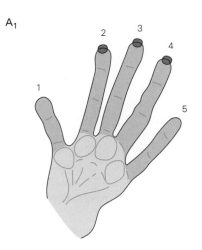

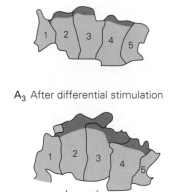

A₂ Before differential stimulation

A₃ After differential stimulation

1 mm

Figure 63-19 Training expands the existing representation of the fingers in the cortex.

A. A monkey was trained for 1 hour per day to perform a task that required repeated use of the tips of fingers 2, 3, and occasionally 4. After a period of repeated stimulation the portion of area 3b representing the tips of the stimulated fingers was substantially greater (**3**) than in untrained monkeys (**2**) measured 3 months before training). (Adapted from Jenkins et al. 1990.)

B. A human subject trained to do a rapid sequence of finger movements will improve in accuracy and speed after three weeks of daily (10–20 min) training. In these MRI scans of local blood oxygenation level-dependent signals in the primary motor cortex, the region activated in trained subjects (after three weeks of training) is larger than the region activated in control subjects who performed unlearned finger movements in the same hand. The change in cortical representation with the learned motor sequence persisted for several months.

B

Control

Trained

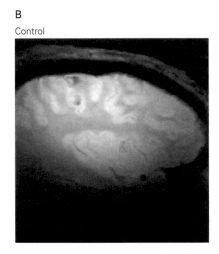

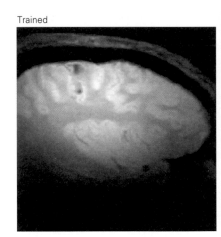

common genetic switch, involving cAMP-dependent protein kinase, MAP kinase, and CREB, to convert labile short-term memory into long-term memory.

Changes in the Somatotopic Map Produced by Learning May Contribute to the Biological Expression of Individuality

Learning, we have seen, can lead to structural alterations in the brain. How common are these changes in determining the functional architecture of the mature brain? This question has been examined in the somatosensory cortex.

The four maps of the body surface in the primary somatic sensory cortex vary among individuals in a manner that reflects different usage of sensory pathways. The connections of afferent pathways in the cortex can expand or retract depending on activity (see Chapter 20). Reorganization of afferent inputs is also evident at lower levels in the brain, specifically at the level of the dorsal column nuclei, which contain the first synapses of the somatic sensory system. Therefore, organizational changes probably occur throughout the somatic afferent pathway as well. As we grow up each of us is exposed to different combinations of stimuli and develops motor skills in different ways. Thus all brains—even the brains of identical twins who share the same genes—are uniquely modified by experience. This distinctive modification of brain architecture, along with a unique genetic makeup, constitutes a biological basis for individuality.

The process by which experience alters the somatosensory maps in the cortex is illustrated in an experiment in which adult monkeys were trained to use only their middle three fingers to obtain food. After several thousand trials of this behavior the area of cortex devoted to the middle finger expanded greatly (Figure 63-19). Practice alone therefore may strengthen the effectiveness of existing patterns of connections.

Experiments such as this one suggest that early development of the input connections to cortical neurons in the somatic sensory system may depend on correlated activity in different afferent axons. As we have seen, cooperative activity in different afferent fibers stabilizes the development of ocular dominance columns in the visual system (Chapter 56). In turn, the use of correlated firing to fine-tune cortical connections may depend on mechanisms that require correlated firing similar to those of LTP. For example, when the skin of two adjacent fingers of a monkey were surgically connected to ensure that the connected fingers were always used together, the correlation of inputs from the joined fingers abolished the normally sharp discontinuity between areas in the somatosensory cortex that receive inputs from these digits (see Figure 19-8).

Neuronal Changes Associated With Learning Provide Insights Into Psychiatric Disorders

The demonstration that learning produces changes in the effectiveness of neural connections has revised our view of the relationship between social and biological processes in the shaping of behavior. Until recently the majority view in medicine and psychiatry was that biological and social determinants of behavior act on separate levels of the mind. For example, psychiatric illnesses were traditionally classified as either organic or functional. Organic mental illnesses included the dementias, such as Alzheimer disease, and the toxic psychoses, such as those that follow the chronic use of alcohol or cocaine. Functional mental illnesses included the various depressive syndromes, the schizophrenias, and the neuroses.

This distinction dates to the nineteenth century, when neuropathologists examined the brains of patients coming to autopsy and found gross and readily demonstrable distortions in the architecture of the brain in some psychiatric diseases but not in others. Diseases that produce anatomical evidence of brain lesions were called *organic;* those lacking these features were called *functional.*

The experiments reviewed in this chapter show that this distinction is no longer tenable. Everyday events—sensory stimulation, deprivation, and learning—can effectively weaken synaptic connections in some circumstances and strengthen them in others. We no longer think that only certain diseases ("organic diseases") affect mentation through biological changes in the brain. The basis of contemporary neural science is that all mental processes are biological and therefore any alteration in those processes is necessarily organic.

In the attempt to understand the biological basis of a particular mental illness we must ask, to what degree is this biological process determined by genetic and developmental factors? To what degree is it determined by a toxic or infectious agent, or by a developmental abnormality? To what degree is it socially determined?

Even those mental disturbances that are considered most heavily determined by social factors must have a biological aspect, since it is the activity of the brain that is being modified. Insofar as social intervention works, whether through psychotherapy, counseling, or the support of family or friends, it must work by acting on the brain, quite likely on the strength of connections between nerve cells. Just because structural changes may not initially be detected following cognitive therapy does not rule out the possibility that important biological changes are nevertheless occurring. They may simply be below the level of detection with the limited techniques available to us.

Demonstrating the biological nature of mental functioning requires more sophisticated anatomical methodologies than the light-microscopic histology of nineteenth century pathologists. We must develop a neuropathology of mental illness based on functional as well as structural analysis. The new imaging techniques—positron emission tomography and functional magnetic resonance imaging, among others—have opened the door to the noninvasive exploration of the human brain on a cell-biological level, the level of resolution that is required to understand the physical mechanisms of mentation and therefore of mental disorders. This approach is now being pursued in the study of schizophrenia and depression.

It is intriguing to think that insofar as psychotherapy is successful in changing behavior, it may do so by producing alterations in gene expression. If so, successful psychotherapeutic treatment of neurosis or character disorders should also produce structural changes in the nervous system. Thus, we face the attractive possibility that as brain imaging techniques improve, these techniques might ultimately be useful not only for diagnosing various neurotic illnesses but also for monitoring the progress of psychotherapy.

A Alteration in gene structure in inherited psychiatric disease: Schizophrenia

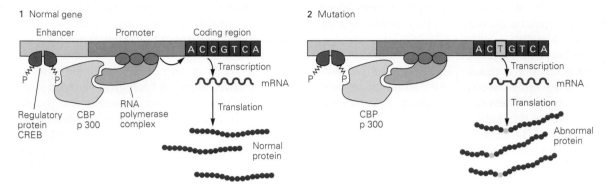

1 Normal gene

2 Mutation

B Alteration in gene regulation in acquired psychiatric disease: Post-traumatic stress syndrome

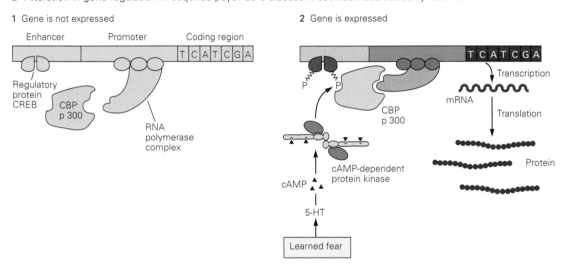

1 Gene is not expressed

2 Gene is expressed

Figure 63-20 Genetic and acquired illnesses both have a genetic component. Genetic illnesses result from the expression of altered genes or allelic variants, whereas acquired illnesses (*neuroses*) involve the modulation of gene expression by environmental stimuli as a result of learning, leading to the transcription of a previously inactive gene. The gene is illustrated as having two segments. A coding region is transcribed into a messenger RNA (mRNA) by an RNA polymerase. The mRNA in turn is translated into a specific protein. A regulatory segment consists of an enhancer region and a promoter region (see Chapter 13, Box 13-1). In this example the RNA polymerase can transcribe the gene when the regulatory protein binds to the enhancer region. For the regulatory protein must first be phosphorylated before it can act on the enhancer. Only when it is phosphorylated can CREB bind the adapter protein, the *CREB binding protein* (CBP), which allows the phosphorylated form of CREB to interact with the transcriptional machinery.

A. Inherited disease such as schizophrenia. **1.** Under normal conditions the phosphorylated regulatory protein binds to the enhancer segment, thereby activating the transcription of the structural gene, leading to the production of the normal protein. **2.** A mutant form of the coding region of the structural gene, in which a thymidine (T) has been substituted for a cytosine (C), leads to transcription of an altered messenger RNA. This in turn produces an abnormal protein, giving rise to the disease state. This alteration in gene structure becomes established in the germ line, is heritable, and contributes to the disease.

B. Acquired disease such as post-traumatic stress syndrome. **1.** If the regulatory protein for a normal structural gene is not phosphorylated, it cannot bind to the promoter site and thus gene translation cannot be initiated. **2.** In this case a specific experience leads to the activation of serotonin (5-HT) and cAMP, which activate the cAMP-dependent protein kinase. The catalytic unit translocates to the nucleus and phosphorylates the regulatory protein CREB, which then can bind to the enhancer segment and thus initiate gene transcription. By this means an abnormal learning experience could lead to the expression of a protein that gives rise to symptoms of a neurotic disorder.

In studying the specific molecular changes that underlie memory storage, we should look for altered gene expression in abnormal as well as normal mental states. There is now substantial evidence that the susceptibility to major psychotic illnesses—schizophrenia and manic-depressive disorders—is heritable and is due to allelic variations. The cell-biological data on learning and long-term memory reviewed here suggest that neurotic illnesses, acquired by learning, also are likely to involve alterations of gene expression but alterations due to disordered regulation (Figure 63-20).

Development, hormones, stress, drug addiction, alcoholism, and learning are all factors that alter gene expression by modifying the binding of transcriptional regulatory proteins to each other and to the regulatory regions of genes. It is likely that at least some neurotic illnesses (or components of them), as well as various forms of drug addiction, result from reversible defects in gene regulation.

An Overall View

Studies on synaptic plasticity suggest there are two overlapping stages in the development and maintenance of synaptic strength. The first stage, the initial steps of synapse formation, occurs primarily early in development and is under the control of genetic and developmental processes. The second stage, the fine-tuning of developed synapses by experience, begins during late stages of development and continues to some degree throughout life. An attractive possibility is that the activity-dependent cellular mechanisms involved in the associative learning of the mature organism may be similar to the activity-dependent mechanisms at work during critical periods of development.

The ongoing modification of synapses throughout life means that all behavior of an individual is produced by genetic and developmental mechanisms acting on the brain—that everything the brain produces, from the most private thoughts to the most public acts, should be understood as a biological process. Environmental factors and learning bring out specific capabilities by altering either the effectiveness or the anatomical connections of existing pathways.

The synthesis of neurobiology, cognitive psychology, neurology, and psychiatry that we have emphasized throughout this book is filled with promise. Modern cognitive psychology has shown that the brain stores an internal representation of the world, while neurobiology has shown that this representation can be understood in terms of individual nerve cells and their interconnections. This synthesis has given us a better perspective on perception, action, learning, and memory. It also provides us with a profound new biological insight into the nature of mental illnesses.

Although early behaviorist psychology led the way in exploring observable aspects of behavior, advances in modern cognitive psychology indicate that investigations that fail to consider brain mechanisms cannot adequately explain behavior. As recently as 10 years ago it would have been difficult to establish the existence of an internal representation directly, since internal mental processes were essentially inaccessible to experimental analysis. However, as we have seen throughout this book, cell biology, molecular biology, and brain imaging have now made biological experiments on elementary aspects of internal mental processes feasible.

Contrary to the expectations of some, biological analysis is unlikely to diminish our fascination with thinking or to make thinking trivial by reduction when we frame the issues in terms of molecular biology. Rather cell biology and molecular biology have expanded our vision, allowing us to perceive previously unanticipated interrelationships between biological and psychological phenomena.

The boundary between cognitive psychology and neural science is arbitrary and always changing. It has been imposed not by the natural contours of the disciplines, but by lack of knowledge. As our knowledge expands, the biological and behavioral disciplines will merge at certain points; it is at these points that our understanding of mentation will rest on more secure ground. As we have tried to illustrate in this book, the merger of biology and cognitive psychology is more than a sharing of methods and concepts. The joining of these two disciples represents the emerging conviction that scientific descriptions of mentation at several different levels will all eventually contribute to a unified biological understanding of behavior.

Eric R. Kandel

Selected Readings

Abel T, Nguyen PV, Barad M, Deuel TAS, Kandel ER, Bourtchouladze R. 1997. Genetic demonstration of a role for PKA in the late phase of LTP and in hippocampal-based long-term memory. Cell 88:615–626.

Dudai Y. 1989. *The Neurobiology of Memory: Concepts, Findings, Trends.* Oxford: Oxford Univ. Press.

Hawkins RD, Kandel ER, Siegelbaum SA. 1993. Learning to modulate transmitter release: themes and variations in synaptic plasticity. Annu Rev Neurosci 16:625–665.

Lisman J. 1994. The CaM kinase II hypothesis for the storage of synaptic memory. Trends Neurosci 17:406–412.

Merzenich MM, Recanzone EG, Jenkins WM, Allard TT, Nudo RJ. 1988. Cortical representational plasticity. In: PR Rakic, WR Singer (eds). *Neurobiology of Neocortex*, pp. 41–67. New York: Wiley.

Squire LR, Kandel ER. 1999. Memory: mind to molecules. New York: Sci Am Lib 1.

Tully T, Bolwig G, Christensen J, Connolly M, Del Vecchio J, DeZazzo J, Dubnau J, James C, Pinto S, Regulski M, Svedberg B, Velinzon K. 1997. A return of genetic dissection of memory in *Drosophila. Function and Dysfunction in the Nervous System.* Cold Spring Harb Symp Quant Biol 61:207–218.

References

Bailey CH, Chen MC. 1983. Morphological basis of long-term habituation and sensitization in *Aplysia*. Science 220:91–93.

Bliss TVP, Lomø T. 1973. Long-lasting potentiation of synaptic transmission in the dentate gyrus of the anesthetized rabbit following stimulation of the perforant path. J Physiol (Lond) 232:331–356.

Bonhoeffer T, Staiger V, Aertsen A. 1989. Synaptic plasticity in rat hippocampal slice cultures: local "Hebbian" conjunction of pre- and postsynaptic stimulation leads to distributed synaptic enhancement. Proc Natl Acad Sci U S A 86:8113–8117.

Bolshakov VY, Golan H, Kandel ER, Siegelbaum SA. 1997. Recruitment of new sites of synaptic transmission during the cAMP-dependent late phase of LTP at CA3-CA1 synapses in the hippocampus. Neuron 19:635–651.

Bourtchouladze R, Frenguelli B, Blendy J, Cioffi D, Schutz G, Silva A. 1994. Deficient long-term memory in mice with a targeted mutation of the cAMP responsive element-binding protein. Cell 79:59–68.

Castellucci VF, Carew TJ, Kandel ER. 1978. Cellular analysis of long-term habituation of the gill-withdrawal reflex in *Aplysia californica*. Science 202:1306–1308.

Chain DG, Casadio A, Schacher S, Hedge AN, Valbrun M, Yamamoto N, Goldberg AL, Bartsch D, Kandel ER, Schwartz JH. 1999. Mechanisms for generating the autonomous cAMP-dependent protein kinase for long-term facilitation in *Aplysia*. Neuron 22:147–156.

Frost WN, Castellucci VF, Hawkins RD, Kandel ER. 1985. Monosynaptic connections made by the sensory neurons of the gill and siphon withdrawal reflex in *Aplysia* participate in the storage of long-term memory for sensitization. Proc Natl Acad Sci U S A 82:8266–8269.

Grant SGN, O'Dell TJ, Karl KA, Stein PL, Soriano P, Kandel ER. 1992. Impaired long-term potentiation, spatial learning, and hippocampal development in *fyn* mutant mice. Science 258:1903–1910.

Gustafsson B, Wigström H, Abraham WC, Huang Y-Y. 1987. Long-term potentiation in the hippocampus using depolarizing current as the conditioning stimulus to single volley synaptic potential. J Neurosci 7:774–780.

Hawkins RD, Abrams TW, Carew TJ, Kandel ER. 1983. A cellular mechanism of classical conditioning in *Aplysia*: activity-dependent amplification of presynaptic facilitation. Science 219:400–405.

Hebb DO. 1949. *The Organization of Behavior: A Neuropsychological Theory.* New York: Wiley.

Hegde AN, Inokuchi K, Pei W, Casadio A, Ghirardi M, Chain DG, Martin KC, Kandel ER, Schwartz JH. 1997. Ubiquitin C-terminal hydrolase is an immediate-early gene essential for long-term facilitation in *Aplysia*. Cell 89:115–126.

Huang Y-Y, Kandel ER. 1994. Recruitment of long-lasting and protein kinase A-dependent long-term potentiation in the CA1 region of hippocampus requires repeated tetanization. Learning & Memory 1:74–82.

Huang Y-Y, Kandel ER, Varshavsky L, Brandon EP, Qi M, Idzerda RL, McKnight GS, Bourtchouladze R. 1995. A genetic test of the effects of mutations in PKA on mossy fiber LTP and its relation to spatial and contextual learning. Cell 83:1211–1222.

Huang Y-Y, Li X-C, Kandel ER. 1994. cAMP contributes to mossy fiber LTP by initiating both a covalently-mediated early phase and a macromolecular synthesis-dependent late phase. Cell 79:69–79.

Jenkins WM, Merzenich MM, Ochs MT, Allard T, Guic-Robles E. 1990. Functional reorganization of primary somatosensory cortex in adult owl monkeys after behaviorally controlled tactile stimulation. J Neurophsiol 63:82–104.

Kandel ER. 1989. Genes, nerve cells, and the remembrance of things past. J Neuropsychiatry 1:103–125.

Lin XY, Glanzman DL. 1994. Long-term potentiation of *Aplysia* sensorimotor synapses in cell culture: regulation by postsynaptic voltage. London: Proc R Soc 255:113–118.

Luscher C, Nicoll RA, Malenka RC, Muller D. 2000. Synaptic plasticity and dynamic modulation of the postsynaptic membrane. Nat. Neurosci 3:545–550.

Malenka RC, Nicoll RA. 1999. Long-term potentiation: a decade of progress? Science. 285:1870–1874.

Malinow R, Tsien RW. 1990. Presynaptic enhancement shown by whole cell recordings of LTP in hippocampal slices. Nature 357:134–139.

Mayford M, Bach ME, Huang Y-Y, Wang L, Hawkins RD, Kandel ER. 1996. Control of memory formation through regulated expression of a CaMKII transgene. Science 274:1678–1683.

McHugh TJ, Blum KI, Tsien JZ, Tonegawa S, Wilson MA. 1996. Impaired hippocampal representation of space in CA1-specific NMDAR1 knockout mice. Cell 87:1339–1349.

Muller RU, Kubie JL, Ranck JB Jr. 1987. Spatial firing patterns of hippocampal complex-spike cells in a fixed environment. J Neurosci 7:1935–1950.

O'Keefe J, Dostrovsky J. 1971. The hippocampus as a spatial map: preliminary evidence from unit activity in the freely-moving rat. Brain Res 34:171–175.

Pavlov IP. 1927. *Conditioned Reflexes: An Investigation of the Physiological Activity of the Cerebral Cortex.* GV Anrep (transl). London: Oxford Univ. Press.

Rotenberg A, Mayford M, Hawkins RD, Kandel ER, Muller RU. 1996. Mice expressing activated CaMKII lack low frequency LTP and do not form stable place cells in the CA1 region of the hippocampus. Cell 87:1351–1361.

Schuman EM, Madison DV. 1994. Locally distributed synaptic potentiation in hippocampus. Science 263:532–536.

Schuman EM, Madison DV. 1991. A requirement for the intercellular messenger nitric oxide in long-term potentiation. Science 254:1503–1506.

Sherrington CS. 1906. *The Integrative Action of the Nervous System.* New Haven, CT: Yale Univ. Press.

Silva AJ, Paylor R, Wehner JM, Tonegawa S. 1992. Impaired spatial learning in α-calcium-calmodulin kinase II mutant mice. Science 257:206–211.

Silva AJ, Stevens CF, Tonegawa S, Wang Y. 1992. Deficient hippocampal long-term potentiation in α-calcium-calmodulin kinase II mutant mice. Science 257:201–206.

Spencer AW, Thompson RF, Nielson DR Jr. 1966. Response decrement of the flexion reflex in the acute spinal cat and transient restoration by strong stimuli. J Neurophysiol 29:240–252.

Stevens C, Wang Y. 1994. Changes in reliability of synaptic function as a mechanism for plasticity. Nature 371:704–707.

Thompson RF, Spencer WA. 1966. Habituation: a model of phenomenon for the study of neural substrates of behavior. Psychol Rev 173:16–43.

Tsien JZ, Chen DF, Gerber D, Tom C, Mercer EH, Anderson DJ, Mayford M, Kandel ER, Tonegawa S. 1996a. Subregion- and cell type-restricted gene knockout in mouse brain. Cell 87:1317–1326.

Tsien JZ, Huerta PT, Tonegawa S. 1996b. The essential role of hippocampal CA1 NMDA receptor-dependent synaptic plasticity in spatial memory. Cell 87:1327–1338.

Tsien RW, Malinow R. 1990. Long-term potentiation: Presynaptic enhancement following postsynaptic activation of Ca^{2+}-dependent protein kinases. Cold Spring Harb Symp Quant Biol 55:147–159.

Weisskopf MG, Castillo PE, Zalutsky RA, Nicoll RA. 1994. Mediation of hippocampal long-term potentiation by cyclic AMP. Science 265:1878–1882.

Yin JCP, Wallach JS, Del Vecchio M, Wilder EL, Zhuo H, Quinn WG, Tully T. 1994. Induction of a dominant negative CREB transgene specifically blocks long-term memory in *Drosophila*. Cell 79:49–58.

Zalutsky RA, Nicoll RA. 1990. Comparison of two forms of long term potentiation in single hippocampal neurons. Science 248:1619–1624.

Appendix A

Current Flow in Neurons

THIS SECTION REVIEWS THE basic principles of electrical circuit theory. Familiarity with this material is important for understanding the equivalent circuit model of the neuron developed in Chapters 5 through 9. The section is divided into three parts:

1. The definition of basic electrical parameters.
2. A set of rules for elementary circuit analysis.
3. A description of current flow in circuits with capacitance.

Definition of Electrical Parameters

Potential Difference (V or E)

Electrical charges exert an electrostatic force on other charges: Like charges repel, opposite charges attract. As the distance between two charges increases, the force that is exerted decreases. *Work* is done when two charges that initially are separated are brought together: *Negative work* is done if their polarities are opposite, and *positive work* if they are the same. The greater the values of the charges and the greater their initial separation, the greater the work that is done (work $= \int_r^0 f(r)\ dr$, where f is electrostatic force and r is the initial distance between the two charges). Potential difference is a measure of this work. The potential difference between two points is the work that must be done to move a unit of positive charge (1 coulomb) from one point to the other, ie, it is the potential energy of the charge. One volt (V) is the energy required to move 1 coulomb a distance of 1 meter against a force of 1 newton.

Current (I)

A potential difference exists within a system whenever positive and negative charges are separated. Charge separation may be generated by a chemical reaction (as in a battery) or by diffusion between two electrolyte solutions with different ion concentrations across a permeability-selective barrier, such as a cell membrane. If a region of charge separation exists within a conducting medium, then charges move between the areas of potential difference: positive charges are attracted to the region with a more negative potential, and negative charges go to the regions of positive potential. The resulting movement of charges is *current flow*, which is defined as the net movement of positive charge per unit time. In metallic conductors current is carried by electrons, which move in the opposite direction of current flow. In nerve and muscle cells current is carried by positive and negative ions in solution. One ampere (A) of current represents the movement of 1 coulomb (of charge) per second.

Conductance (*g*)

Any object through which electrical charges can flow is called a conductor. The unit of electrical conductance is the siemen (S). According to Ohm's law, the current that flows through a conductor is directly proportional to the potential difference imposed across it.[1]

$$I = V \times g$$

Current (A) = Potential difference (V)
× Conductance (S).

As charge carriers move through a conductor, some of their potential energy is lost; it is converted into thermal energy due to the frictional interactions of the charge carriers with the conducting medium.

Each type of material has an intrinsic property called conductivity (σ), which is determined by its molecular structure. Metallic conductors have very high conductivities; they conduct electricity extremely well. Aqueous solutions with high ionized salt concentrations have somewhat lower values of σ, and lipids have very low conductivities—they are poor conductors of electricity and are therefore good insulators. The conductance of an object is proportional to σ times its cross-sectional area, divided by its length:

$$g = (\sigma) \times \frac{\text{Area}}{\text{Length}}$$

The length dimension is defined as the direction along which one measures conductance.

For example, the conductance measured along the cytoplasmic core of an axon is reduced if its length is increased or its diameter decreased (Figure A-1).

---

[1] Note the analogy of this formula for current flow to the other formulas for describing flow; eg, bulk flow of a liquid due to a hydrostatic pressure; flow of a solute in response to a concentration gradient; flow of heat in response to a temperature gradient, etc. In each case flow is proportional to the product of a driving force times a conductance factor.

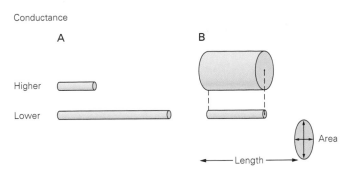

Conductance

Figure A-1 Geometric factors, together with intrinsic conductivity, determine the conductance of an object.

A. Conductance is inversely proportional to the length of a conductor.

B. Conductance is directly proportional to the cross-sectional area of a conductor.

Electrical resistance (*R*) is the reciprocal of conductance, and is a measure of the resistance provided by an object to current flow. Resistance is measured in ohms (Ω):

$$1 \text{ ohm} = (1 \text{ siemen})^{-1}.$$

Capacitance (*C*)

A capacitor consists of two conducting plates separated by an insulating layer. The fundamental property of a capacitor is its ability to store charges of opposite sign: positive charge on one plate, negative on the other.

A capacitor made up of two parallel plates with its two conducting surfaces separated by an insulator (an air gap) is shown in Figure A-2A. There is a net excess of positive charges on plate *x*, and an equal number of excess negative charges on plate *y*, resulting in a potential difference between the two plates. One can measure this potential difference by determining how much work is required to move a positive test charge from the surface of *y* to that of *x*. Initially, when the test charge is at *y*, it is attracted by the negative charges on *y*, and repelled less strongly by the more distant positive charges on *x*. The result of these electrostatic interactions is a force *f* that opposes the movement of the test charge from *y* to *x*. As the test charge is moved to the left across the gap, the attraction by the negative charges on *y* diminishes, but the repulsion by the positive charges on *x* increases, with the result that the net electrostatic force exerted on the test charge is constant everywhere between *x* and *y* (Figure A-2A). Work (*W*) is force (*f*) times the distance (*D*) over which the force is exerted:

$$W = f \times D.$$

Therefore, it is simple to calculate the work done in moving the test charge from one side of the capacitor to the

Capacitance

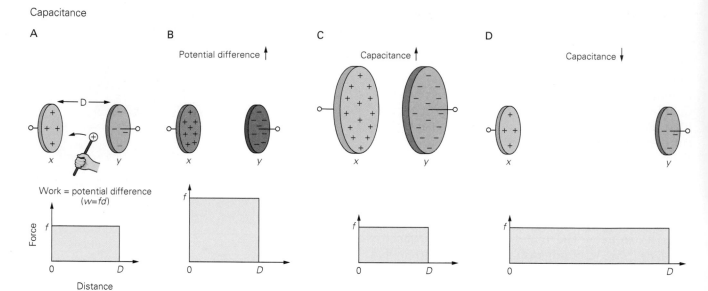

Figure A-2 The factors that affect the potential difference between two plates of a capacitor.

A. As a test charge is moved between two charged plates it must overcome a force. The work done against this force is the potential difference between the two plates.

B. Increasing the charge density increases the potential difference.

C. Increasing the area of the plates increases the number of charges required to produce a given potential difference.

D. Increasing the distance between the two plates increases the potential difference between them.

other. It is the shaded area under the curve in Figure A-2A. This work is equal to the difference in electrical potential energy, or potential difference, between x and y.

Capacitance is measured in farads (F). The greater the density of charges on the capacitor plates, the greater the force acting on the test charge, and the greater the resulting potential difference across the capacitor (Figure A-2B). Thus, for a given capacitor, there is a linear relationship between the amount of charge (Q) stored on its plates and the potential difference across it:

$$Q \text{ (coulombs)} = C \text{ (farads)} \times V \text{ (volts)} \quad \textbf{(A–1)}$$

where the capacitance, C, is a constant.

The capacitance of a parallel-plate capacitor is determined by two features of its geometry: the area (A) of the two plates, and the distance (D) between them. Increasing the area of the plates increases capacitance, because a greater amount of charge must be deposited on each side to produce the same charge density, which is what determines the force f acting on the test charge (Figure A-2A and C). Increasing the distance D between the plates does not change the force acting on the test charge, but it does increase the work that must be done to move it from one side of the capacitor to the other (Figure A-2A and D). Therefore, for a given charge separation between the two plates, the potential difference between them is proportional to the distance. Put another way, the greater the distance the smaller the amount of charge that must be deposited on the plates

to produce a given potential difference, and therefore the smaller the capacitance (Equation A–1). These geometrical determinants of capacitance can be summarized by the equation:

$$C \propto \frac{A}{D}.$$

As shown in Equation A–1, the separation of positive and negative charges on the two plates of a capacitor results in a potential difference between them. The converse of this statement is also true: The potential difference across a capacitor is determined by the excess of positive and negative charges on its plates. In order for the potential across a capacitor to change, the amount of electrical charges stored on the two conducting plates must change first.

Rules for Circuit Analysis

A few basic relationships that are used for circuit analysis are listed below. Familiarity with these rules will help in understanding the electric circuit examples that follow.

Conductance

The symbol for a conductor is:

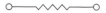

A variable conductor is represented this way:

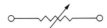

A pathway with infinite conductance (zero resistance) is called a short circuit, and is represented by a line:

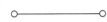

Conductances in parallel add:

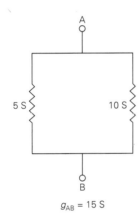

$$g_{AB} = 15\,S$$

$$g_{AB} = 15\,S$$

Conductances in series add reciprocally:

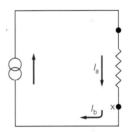

$$\frac{1}{g_{AB}} = \frac{1}{5} + \frac{1}{10} = \frac{3}{10}$$

$$g_{AB} = 3.3\,S.$$

Resistances in series add, while resistances in parallel add reciprocally.

Current

An *arrow* denotes the direction of current flow (net movement of positive charge). Ohm's law is

$$I = Vg = \frac{V}{R}.$$

When current flows through a conductor, the end that the current enters is positive with respect to the end that it leaves:

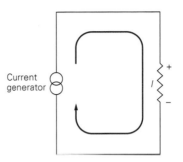

The algebraic sum of all currents entering or leaving a junction is zero (we arbitrarily define current approaching a junction as positive, and current leaving a junction as negative). In the following

the currents for junction x are:

$$I_A = +5\,A$$
$$I_B = -5\,A$$
$$I_A + I_B = 0.$$

In the following circuit

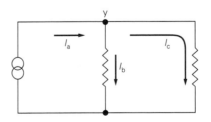

the currents for junction y are:

$$I_a = +3\,A$$
$$I_b = -2\,A$$
$$I_c = -1\,A$$
$$I_a + I_b + I_c = 0.$$

Current follows the path of greatest conductance (least resistance). For conductance pathways in parallel, the current through each path is proportional to its conductance value divided by the total conductance of the parallel combination:

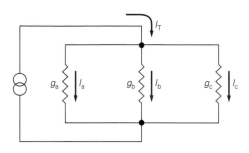

$$I_T = 10 \text{ A}$$
$$g_a = 3 \text{ S}$$
$$g_b = 2 \text{ S}$$
$$g_c = 5 \text{ S}$$

$$I_a = I_T \frac{g_a}{g_a + g_b + g_c} = 3 \text{ A}$$
$$I_b = I_T \frac{g_b}{g_a + g_b + g_c} = 2 \text{ A}$$
$$I_c = I_T \frac{g_c}{g_a + g_b + g_c} = 5 \text{ A}.$$

Capacitance

The symbol for a capacitor is:

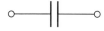

The potential difference across a capacitor is proportional to the charge stored on its plates:

$$V_C = \frac{Q}{C}.$$

Potential Difference

The symbol for a battery, or electromotive force is:

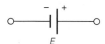

It is often abbreviated by the symbol E. The positive pole is always represented by the longer bar.

Batteries in series add algebraically, but attention must be paid to their polarities. If their polarities are the same, their absolute values add:

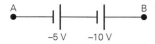

$$V_{AB} = -15 \text{ V}.$$

If their polarities are opposite, they subtract:

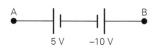

$$V_{AB} = -5 \text{ V}.$$

The convention used here for potential difference is that $V_{AB} = (V_A - V_B)$.

A battery drives a current around the circuit from its positive to its negative terminal:

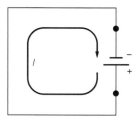

For purposes of calculating the total resistance of a circuit the internal resistance of a battery is set at zero.

The potential differences across parallel branches of a circuit are equal:

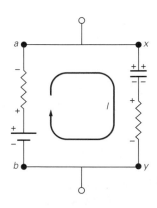

$$V_{ab} = V_{xy}.$$

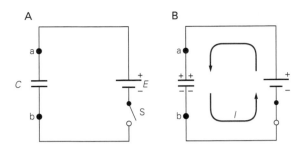

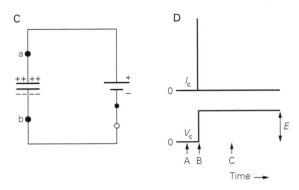

Figure A-3 Time course of charging a capacitor.

A. Circuit before the switch (**S**) is closed.

B. Immediately after the switch is closed.

C. After the capacitor has become fully charged.

D. Time course of changes in I_c and V_c in response to closing of the switch.

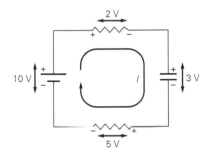

As one goes around a closed loop in a circuit, the algebraic sum of all the potential differences is zero:

$$2\,V + 3\,V + 5\,V - 10\,V = 0.$$

Current Flow in Circuits With Capacitance

Circuits that have capacitive elements are much more complex than those that have only batteries and conductors. This complexity arises because current flow varies with time in capacitive circuits. The time dependence of the changes in current and voltage in capacitive circuits is illustrated qualitatively in the following three examples.

Circuit With Capacitor

Current does not actually flow across the insulating gap in a capacitor; rather it results in a build-up of positive and negative charges on the capacitor plates. However, we can measure a current flowing into and out of the terminal of a capacitor. Consider the circuit shown in Figure A-3A. When switch S is closed (Figure A-3B), a net positive charge is moved by the battery E onto plate a, and an equal amount of net positive charge is withdrawn from plate b. The result is current flowing counterclockwise in the circuit. Since the charges that carry

this current flow into or out of the terminals of a capacitor, building up an excess of plus and minus charges on its plates, it is called a *capacitive current* (I_c). Because there is no resistance in this circuit, the battery E can generate a very large amplitude of current, which will charge the capacitance to a value $Q = E \times C$ in an infinitesimally short period of time (Figure A-3D).

Circuit With Resistor and Capacitor in Series

Now consider what happens if a resistor is added in series with the capacitor in the circuit shown in Figure A-4A. The maximum current that can be generated when switch S is closed (Figure A-4B) is now limited by Ohm's law ($I = V/R$). Therefore, the capacitor charges more slowly. When the potential across the capacitor has finally reached the value $V_c = Q/C = E$ (Figure A-4C), there is no longer a difference in potential around the loop, ie, the battery voltage (E) is equal and opposite to the voltage across the capacitor, V_c. The two thus cancel out, and there is no source of potential difference left to drive a current around the loop. Immediately after the switch is closed the potential difference is greatest, so current flow is at a maximum. As the capacitor begins to charge, however, the net potential difference ($V_c + E$) available to drive a current becomes smaller, so that current flow is reduced. The result is that an exponential change in voltage and in current flow occurs across the resistor and the capacitor. Note that in this circuit resistive current must equal capacitive current at all times (see Rules for Circuit Analysis, above).

Circuit With Resistor and Capacitor in Parallel

Consider now what happens if we place a parallel resistor and capacitor combination in series with a constant

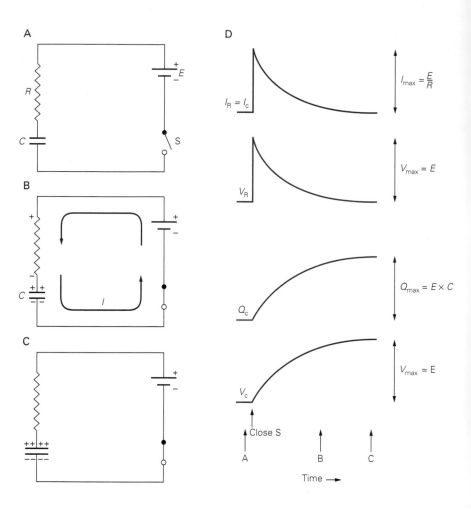

Figure A-4 Time course of charging a capacitor in series with a resistor from a constant voltage source (E).

A. Circuit before the switch (**S**) is closed.

B. Shortly after the switch is closed.

C. After the capacitor has settled at its new potential.

D. Time course of current flow, of the increase in charge deposited on the capacitor, and of the increased potential differences across the resistor and the capacitor.

current generator that generates a current I_T (Figure A-5A). When switch S is closed current starts to flow around the loop. Initially, in the first instant of time after the current flow begins, all of the current flows into the capacitor, ie, $I_T = I_c$. However, as charge builds up on the plates of the capacitor, a potential difference V_c is generated across it. Since the resistor and capacitor are in parallel, the potential across them must be equal; thus, part of the total current begins to flow through the resistors, such that $I_R R = V_R = V_c$ (Figure A-5B). As less and less current flows into the capacitor, its rate of charging will become slower; this accounts for the exponential shape of the curve of voltage versus time. Eventually, a plateau is reached at which the voltage no longer changes. When this occurs, all of the current flows through the resistor, and $V_c = V_R = I_T R$ (Figure A-5C).

John Koester

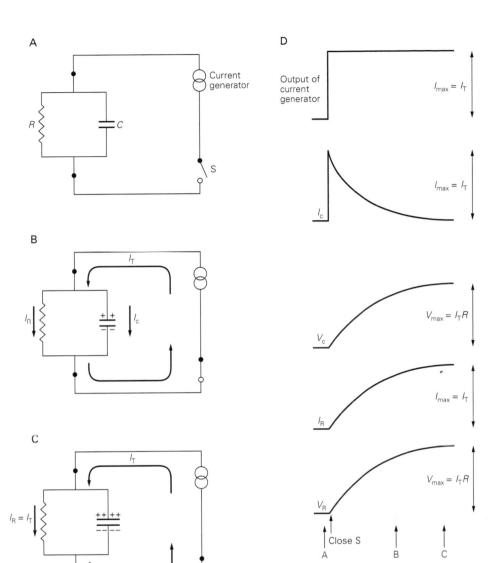

Figure A-5 Time course of charging a capacitor in parallel with a resistor from a constant current source.

A. Circuit before the switch (**S**) is closed.

B. Shortly after the switch is closed.

C. After the charge deposited on the capacitor has reached its final value.

D. Time course of changes in I_c, V_c, I_R, and V_R in response to closing of the switch.

Appendix B

Ventricular Organization of Cerebrospinal Fluid: Blood-Brain Barrier, Brain Edema, and Hydrocephalus

A BARRIER TO THE ENTRY of blood-borne substances to the brain has been recognized for at least a century. Evidence for the blood-brain barrier was first obtained in the nineteenth century, when it was observed that acidic vital dyes stain the brain if the dye is injected into the cerebrospinal fluid (CSF) but not if injected into the blood stream. This barrier maintains a stable environment for neurons to function effectively. It excludes many toxic substances and protects neurons from circulating neurotransmitters such as norepineph-

rine and glutamate, the blood levels of which can increase greatly in response to stress or even after a meal. Exclusion results primarily from specialized anatomic properties of brain endothelial cells that limit the passive diffusion of water-soluble substances across vessel walls. As a result, many metabolites required for brain growth and function must be transported selectively across the endothelial surface. Specific endothelial transporters deliver energy substrates, essential amino acids, and peptides from blood to brain and remove metabolites from the brain.

Differentiated Properties of Brain Capillary Endothelial Cells Account for the Blood-Brain Barrier

Anatomy of the Blood-Brain Barrier

Brain microvessels are composed of endothelial cells, pericytes with smooth muscle-like properties that reside adjacent to capillaries, and astroglial processes that ensheath more than 95% of the abluminal microvessel surface (Figure B-1). It was originally thought that the glial foot processes formed the blood-brain barrier, but electron-microscopic studies identified the endothelial cell as the principal anatomic site of the blood-brain barrier (Figure B-2).

The blood-brain barrier results from specialized properties of the endothelial cells, their intercellular junctions, and a relative lack of vesicular transport. In capillaries of peripheral organs and in the relatively few brain capillaries that do not form a barrier (eg, the circumventricular organs) blood-borne polar molecules

Figure B-1 The ultrastructural features of the capillary endothelial cells of the brain differ from those of general (systemic) capillaries. The endothelial cells of barrier capillaries are relatively lacking in pinocytotic vesicles, contain an increased number of mitochondria believed to support energy-dependent transport properties, and are interconnected by very complex interendothelial tight junctions. These anatomic features in conjunction with specific transport systems (see Figure B-5) result in highly selective transport of water-soluble compounds across the barrier endothelium. Astrocyte foot processes almost completely surround the blood-brain barrier capillaries and are thereby believed to influence barrier-specific endothelial differentiation. In contrast, systemic capillaries have interendothelial clefts, fenestrae, and prominent pinocytotic vesicles. These features of systemic capillaries allow relatively nonselective diffusion across the capillary wall. (From Goldstein and Betz 1986.)

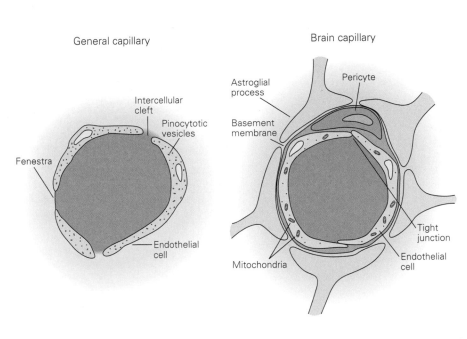

diffuse passively across vessels through spaces between endothelial cells, through specialized cytoplasmic fenestrations, or by fluid-phase or receptor-mediated endocytosis. *Fluid-phase endocytosis* is a relatively nonspecific process by which endothelial cells (and most other cells) engulf and then internalize molecules encountered in the extracellular space by vesicular endocytosis. *Receptor-mediated endocytosis* is a specific process in which a ligand first binds to a membrane receptor on the external surface of the cell, is internalized by means of clathrin-coated vesicles, and is transported across the cell membrane. Once within the cell, the vesicle may fuse with an endosome and release its ligand.

Endothelial cells of blood-brain barrier vessels are relatively deficient in vesicular transport. They also are not fenestrated. Instead they are interconnected by complex arrays of tight junctions (Figure B-2C). These junctions between the endothelial cells block diffusion across the vessel wall. All endothelial cells are interconnected by tight junctional complexes but normally have low resistance (5–10 Ω/cm^2). In the vessels of the blood-brain barrier, however, the resistance is very high (2000 Ω/cm^2), and molecules as small as K^+ ions are excluded (Figure B-3).

Selectivity of the Blood-Brain Barrier

Normal development and brain function require a large number of compounds that must be able to cross

brain microvessels. Entry into the CSF is achieved primarily in three ways: (1) by diffusion of lipid-soluble substances, (2) by facilitative and energy-dependent receptor-mediated transport of specific water-soluble substances, and (3) by ion channels.

Lipid-Soluble Substances

The brain is separated from blood only by a very large surface of endothelial cell membranes (approximately 180 cm^2/g in gray matter). This permits the efficient exchange of lipid-soluble gases such as O_2 and CO_2, an exchange limited only by the surface area of the blood vessel and by cerebral blood flow. Barrier vessels are impermeable to poorly lipid-soluble molecules such as mannitol, as compared to very lipid-soluble compounds such as butanol. The permeability coefficient of the blood-brain barrier for many substances is directly proportional to the lipid solubility of the substance as measured by the oil-water partition coefficient (Figure B-4).

An example of this effect is in the correlation between the relative abuse potential of psychoactive drugs such as nicotine and heroin and the high oil-water partition coefficients of these drugs. Increasing the lipid solubility of pharmacologic agents within strict limits will enhance their delivery to the brain. Drugs with very high oil-water partition coefficients are poorly soluble in blood and bind to serum protein albumin, properties that reduce delivery to the brain. However, the perme-

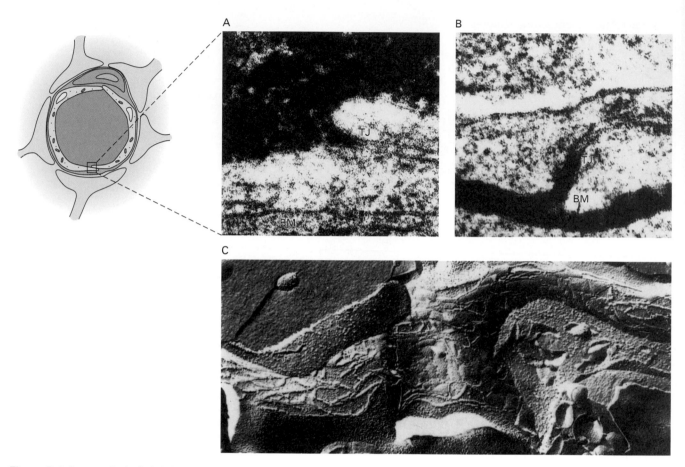

Figure B-2 Interendothelial tight junctions are the basis of the anatomic blood-brain barrier.

A. When injected into arteries that supply the brain, the electron-dense tracer horseradish peroxidase is easily visualized within the brain vessel lumens (**dark staining**) at top but is excluded from entering the brain by interendothelial tight junctions (**TJ**). (From Reese and Karnovsky 1967.)

B. When injected into the subarachnoid space, horseradish per-

oxidase readily diffuses between the perivascular astroglial foot processes and across the abluminal basement membrane (**BM**) but fails to penetrate interendothelial tight junctions (**TJ**). The luminal space appears at the top of the electron micrographs in both **A** and **B**. (From Brightman and Reese 1969.)

C. Freeze-fracture photomicrograph of isolated brain microvessels, showing complex arrays of interendothelial tight junctions. (From Shivers et al. 1984.)

ability of some substances, such as glucose and vinca alkaloids, is not predicted accurately by the lipid solubility of the substance. This observation is explained by the presence of selective endothelial transport or enzyme systems that increase or inhibit substrate permeability.

Blood-Brain Barrier Transport Properties

Most substances that must cross the blood-brain barrier are not lipid soluble and therefore cross by specific carrier-mediated transport systems (Figure B-5). Because the brain uses glucose exclusively as its source of energy, the hexose transporter (glucose transporter isotype-1, Glut1) of the blood-brain barrier endothelial cells has been particularly well characterized.

Glut1 consists of 492 amino acids and has 12 putative transmembrane domains, similar to other transporters. It is a facilitative, saturable, and stereospecific transporter that functions at both the luminal and the abluminal endothelial cell membranes. Because it is not energy dependent, it cannot move glucose against a concentration gradient. The net flux of glucose is driven by the relatively higher concentration of glucose in plasma. Transport is half-saturated at glucose concentrations of 5 to 10 mM. More than 99% of the glucose molecules that enter blood-brain barrier endothelial cells are shuttled across for use by neurons and glia. The gene that codes for Glut1 resides on human chromosome 1. Whereas the complete absence of Glut1 is likely to be incompatible with life, deficient Glut1 expression

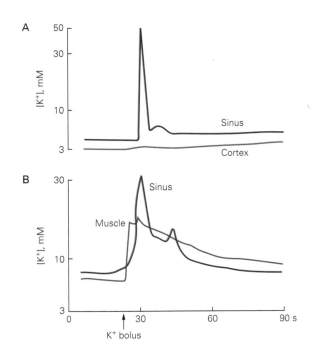

Figure B-3 Time course of K$^+$ concentration in the extracellular fluid of cerebral cortex (A), neck muscle (B), and sagittal sinus (A and B) following the bolus injection of KCl in the aortic arch. Note that the extracellular fluid K$^+$ concentration of cerebral cortex remains essentially unchanged because of the blood-brain barrier to ions. In contrast, K$^+$ diffuses rapidly across nonbarrier vessels into the extracellular space of muscle. (From Hansen et al. 1977.)

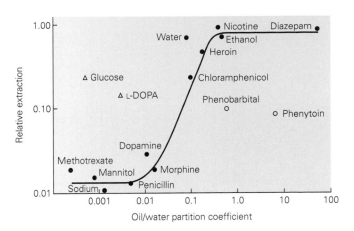

Figure B-4 The oil-water partition coefficient indicates the relationship between lipid solubility and brain uptake of selected compounds. The distribution into olive oil relative to water for each test substance serves as a measure of its lipid solubility. The brain uptake is determined by comparing the extraction of each test substance relative to a highly permeable tracer during a single passage through the cerebral circulation. In general, compounds with higher oil-water partition coefficients show increased entry into brain. Uptake of the anticonvulsants phenobarbital and phenytoin is lower than predicted from their lipid solubility partly because of their binding to plasma proteins. This explains the slower onset of anticonvulsant activity of these agents compared to diazepam. Uptake of glucose and L-DOPA is greater than predicted by their lipid solubility because specific carriers facilitate their transport into the brain capillary. (From Goldstein and Betz 1986.)

is thought to be responsible for a rare clinical syndrome consisting of mental retardation, epilepsy, and persistent low CSF glucose concentration (ie, hypoglycorrhachia).

Amino acids are transported across barrier endothelial cells primarily by three distinct carrier systems: the L system, the A system, and the ASC system. These carriers are characterized by their different patterns and mechanisms of transport, and by their preference for different amino acid analogs. Large neutral amino acids with branched or ringed side chains, such as leucine and valine, are transported primarily by the L system. The L system is a Na$^+$-independent, facilitative transporter and is located at luminal and abluminal endothelial membranes. It can be inhibited experimentally by 2-aminobicycloheptane-2-carboxylic acid (BCH). Like glucose, large neutral amino acids are transported from blood down a concentration gradient. This carrier system transports systemically administered L-DOPA, the dopamine precursor that is the mainstay for treating Parkinson disease. Competitive inhibition of the transport of large neutral amino acids by elevated levels of

phenylalanine may explain some of the neurotoxicity associated with untreated phenylketonuria, because phenylalanine is transported by the L system.

Glycine and neutral amino acids with short linear or polar side chains, such as alanine or serine, are preferentially transported by the A system. Unlike the L system, this carrier is energy dependent, Na$^+$ dependent, and experimentally inhibited by α-methylaminoisobutyric acid (MeAIB). The ASC system is also an energy-dependent and Na$^+$-dependent transporter that preferentially recognizes alanine, serine, and cysteine. ASC-mediated transport is insensitive to both BCH and MeAIB. In contrast to the L carrier, the A and ASC transport systems are located exclusively at the abluminal endothelial cell surface. The physiological consequence of this localization is that the small neutral amino acids are transported primarily out of the brain up a concentration gradient through these carriers. The A system may limit the accumulation of the inhibitory neurotransmitter glycine within the spinal cord and the excitatory neurotransmitter glutamate within the brain. The energy and Na$^+$ exchange required for these systems is supplied by Na$^+$-

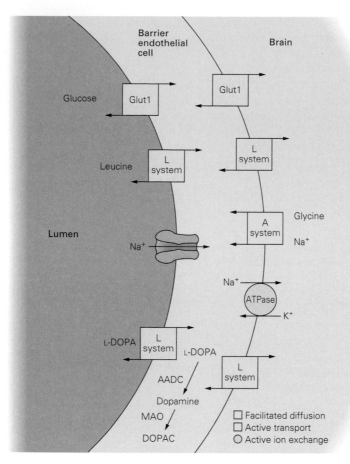

Figure B-5 A complex system of polarized transporter proteins and ionic channels determine the specific movement of water-soluble compounds and ions across barrier endothelial cells. Some transporters (eg, Glut1 and L system) facilitate the movement of substrates down concentration gradients, and others (eg, A system and Na$^+$-K$^+$-ATPase) actively transport substrates via energy-dependent mechanisms. Enzyme systems such as amino acid decarboxylase (AADC) and monoamine oxidase (MAO) function as a metabolic barrier by converting within the barrier endothelial cells substances such as L-DOPA to 3,4-dihydroxyphenylacetic acid.

K$^+$-ATPase, which also is localized to the abluminal endothelial membrane.

Another transport system found to be most abundant in the blood-brain barrier microvessels belongs to a family of transmembranous proteins initially described for their ability to impart multiple drug resistance (MDR) to tumor cells. These transmembranous transporters remove a broad range of natural and synthetic hydrophobic toxins from cells that express the transporters. The MDR transporter (ie, p-glycoprotein) in the blood-brain barrier influences the delivery to the brain of many compounds used for cancer chemotherapy (eg, vinca alkaloids, actinomycin-D) and for other therapeutic purposes (eg, cyclosporin). Because p-glycoproteins pump certain steroid hormones, they may also have a physiological role. MDR transporters are expressed by blood-brain barrier microvessels but not by vessels of most other tissues. Mice genetically engineered to lack MDR1a gene expression no longer express blood-brain barrier p-glycoprotein and are much more sensitive than wild-type controls to centrally acting toxic compounds, indicating that MDR gene expression at the blood-brain barrier protects the brain from circulating neurotoxins.

Ion Channels and Exchangers

Specific ion channels and ion transporters mediate electrolyte movement across the blood-brain barrier. Evidence from transport studies across brain microvessels in vivo and from patch-clamp studies of cultured brain microvessel endothelial cells support the existence of a nonselective luminal ion channel that is inhibited by both amiloride and atrial natriuretic peptide. The existence of luminal Na^+/H^+ and Cl^-/HCO_3^- exchangers has been suggested but is less well substantiated. The external membrane of brain endothelial cells has a relatively high concentration of Na^+-K^+-ATPase that exchanges extracellular K^+ with intracellular Na^+ in an energy-dependent manner. In conjunction with K^+ channels in astrocytes, this abluminal endothelial pump may play an important role in removing extracellular K^+ released during intense neuronal activity (see Chapter 2). In addition, the nonselective luminal ion channel, a distinct abluminal K^+ channel, and abluminal Na^+-K^+-ATPase may work together to regulate tightly the entry of Na^+ and the release or recycling of K^+.

The Metabolic Blood-Brain Barrier

Transport systems and carriers are not the only components that regulate the composition of the interstitial fluid. A similarly important role is also played by certain enzyme systems specific to the blood-brain barrier. The first recognized and still the best characterized example is the barrier to L-DOPA. Plasma L-DOPA enters brain endothelial cells by means of the L-system amino acid transporter. The relatively high amounts of DOPA decarboxylase and monoamine oxidase in endothelial cells of the barrier rapidly metabolize L-DOPA to 3,4-dihydroxyphenylacetic acid, thereby inhibiting the entry of L-DOPA to the brain (Figure B-5). This explains why effective Parkinson disease therapy requires that L-DOPA be given together with an inhibitor of DOPA decarboxylase. Other blood-borne amines, including catecholamines, are also inactivated by monoamine oxidases of the barrier endothelium. In addition to its proposed role in cystine transport, the abundant endothelial enzyme of the blood-brain barrier, γ-glutamyl transpeptidase, detoxifies glutathione-bound compounds and vasoactive leukotrienes.

Some Areas of the Brain Do Not Have a Blood-Brain Barrier

Not all cerebral blood vessels are entirely impermeable. Leaky areas include the posterior pituitary and circumventricular organs such as the area postrema, subfornical organ, the laminar terminalis, subcommissural organ,

median eminence, and neurohypophysis. In the posterior pituitary most of the capillaries are fenestrated. Capillaries that are not fenestrated contain many cytoplasmic vesicles that are thought to transport substances across the endothelial cell. These structural features account for the enhanced transport across these cells.

The absence of a blood-brain barrier in these regions is consistent with their physiological functions. In the pituitary, neurosecretory products have to pass across endothelial cells into the circulation. The subfornical organ is a chemoreceptive area that monitors blood angiotensin II levels to regulate water balance and other homeostatic functions.

These leaky regions are isolated from the rest of the brain by specialized ependymal cells called *tanycytes* located along the ventricular surface close to the midline. The tanycytes are coupled by tight junctions and prevent free exchange between the circumventricular organs and the CSF.

Brain-Derived Signals Induce Endothelial Cells to Express Blood-Brain Barrier Properties

The cellular and molecular signals that induce endothelial expression of the blood-brain barrier phenotype have been elusive. The neural anlagen of the brain is vascularized very early in development through the invasion of proliferating vessels derived from an extraneural vascular plexus. These perineural vessels are composed of fenestrated endothelial cells that have no blood-brain barrier. Soon after penetrating neural tissue (within 2–4 days in the rat), fenestrations are lost. The subsequent expression of different blood-brain barrier properties on the endothelium occurs gradually, suggesting a maturational cascade.

The blood-brain barrier properties expressed by brain endothelial cells are believed to be induced by cells within the surrounding brain. Thus, barrier properties will develop in peripheral endothelial cells that invade brain tissue transplants but not in brain endothelial cells that invade peripheral tissue transplants. The cellular origin and biochemical nature of the brain parenchymal signals that induce endothelial barrier formation are not known but may originate from perivascular astroglia. Consistent with an important role for such parenchymal signals is the observation that brain endothelial cells rapidly lose their blood-brain barrier properties when isolated in culture and reexpress barrier properties when reimplanted in the central nervous system. Of the principal cell types that comprise the brain—neurons, oligodendroglia, and astroglia—astroglia are thought to be particularly important for

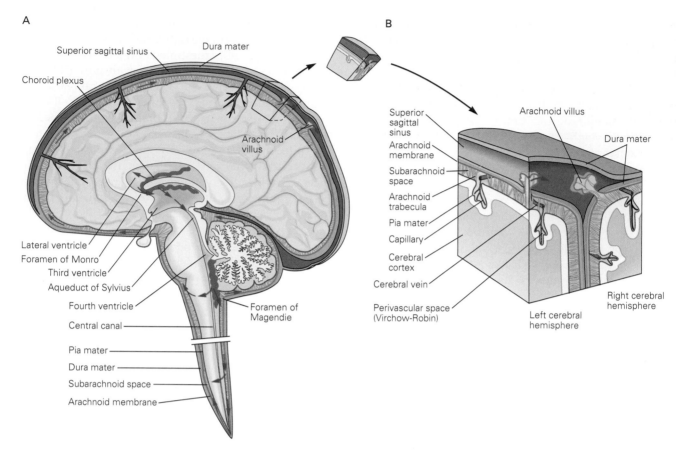

A

Superior sagittal sinus

Choroid plexus

Dura mater

Arachnoid villus

Lateral ventricle
Foramen of Monro
Third ventricle
Aqueduct of Sylvius
Fourth ventricle
Central canal
Pia mater
Dura mater
Subarachnoid space
Arachnoid membrane

Foramen of Magendie

B

Superior sagittal sinus
Arachnoid membrane
Subarachnoid space
Arachnoid trabecula
Pia mater
Capillary
Cerebral cortex
Cerebral vein
Perivascular space (Virchow-Robin)

Arachnoid villus

Dura mater

Right cerebral hemisphere

Left cerebral hemisphere

Figure B-6 Distribution of CSF. (Adapted from Carpenter 1978 and Fishman 1992.)

A. Sites of formation, circulation, and absorption of CSF. All spaces containing CSF communicate with each other. Choroidal and extrachoroidal sources of the fluid exist within the ventricular system. CSF circulates to the subarachnoid space and is absorbed into the venous system via the arach-

noid villi. The presence of arachnoid villi adjacent to the spinal roots supplements the absorption into the intracranial venous sinuses. (Adapted from Fishman 1992.)

B. The subarachnoid space is bounded externally by the arachnoid membrane and internally by the pia mater, which extends along blood vessels that penetrate the surface of the brain. (Adapted from Carpenter 1978.)

this function because of their close association with the abluminal endothelial surface in mature brain. Astroglial cells, particularly in conjunction with cyclic adenosine monophosphate agonists, specifically increase the complexity of interendothelial tight junctions.

Disorders of the Blood-Brain Barrier

A variety of pathological situations are associated with altered blood-brain barrier function. Many brain tumors contain vessels with a poorly developed blood-brain barrier. The least aggressive low-grade astrocytomas may contain vessels with close-to-normal barrier characteristics. In contrast, malignant primary tumors (ie, anaplastic astrocytoma, glioblastoma) and brain metastases of systemic cancers contain vessels that are excessively leaky and lack the differentiated transport prop-

erties of normal blood-brain barrier vessels. The abnormal vessel permeability accounts for the excessive accumulation of interstitial fluid (called *vasogenic edema*) commonly associated with brain tumors. The abnormal properties of tumor endothelial cells are presumably explained either by the absence of normal interactions between astrocytes and capillaries or by the secretion of factors by tumor cells. Vascular endothelial growth factor/vascular permeability factor is one such factor that may account for the excessive proliferation and permeability of the glioblastoma vessel.

Another condition in which the blood-brain barrier is altered is bacterial meningitis. The blood-brain barrier is normally impermeable to antibiotics such as penicillin. Bacterial meningitis, abscesses, and their associated inflammatory responses cause a partial breakdown of the barrier. This barrier response appears to be mediated in part by the accumulation of vasoactive eicosanoids and inflammatory cytokines such as tumor necrosis factor. Although this barrier dysfunction accounts for some of the adverse neurological effects of these infections, it also results in an enhanced ability to deliver antibiotics to the site of infection within the brain.

Because the development and function of the normal brain is linked closely to specific anatomical, biochemical, and transport properties of the blood-brain barrier, specific defects in genes that code for barrier endothelial proteins might account for inherited brain disorders. The first developmental disorder of blood-brain barrier transport has been described. Patients with this syndrome are normal at birth but soon develop poorly controlled seizures, diminished brain growth, and mental retardation in association with a substantially diminished concentration of glucose in the CSF. Glucose enters the CSF through Glut1. This transporter is also found in red blood cells. In these patients red blood cell Glut1 is reduced by approximately 50%, suggesting that this syndrome is due to reduced Glut1 gene expression and a subsequent decrease in blood-to-brain glucose transport. The genetic basis for this disorder has yet to be fully defined.

Cerebrospinal Fluid Has Several Functions

CSF communicates with brain interstitial fluid and is therefore important in maintaining a constant external environment for neurons and glia. The primarily one-way flow of CSF from the ventricular system, around the spinal cord, into the subarachnoid space around the brain, and into the venous sinuses is a major route for removing potentially harmful brain metabolites. CSF also provides a mechanical cushion to protect the brain from impact with the bony calvarium when the head moves. By its buoyant action, CSF allows the brain to float, thereby reducing its effective weight in situ to less than 50 g. CSF may also serve as a lymphatic system for the brain and as a conduit for polypeptide hormones that are secreted by hypothalamic neurons and that act at remote sites in the brain. The pH of CSF affects both pulmonary ventilation and cerebral blood flow—another example of the homeostatic role of CSF.

Cerebrospinal Fluid Is Secreted by the Choroid Plexus

CSF is secreted in the lateral ventricles mainly by the choroid plexus (Figure B-6A), which consists of capillary networks surrounded by cuboidal or columnar

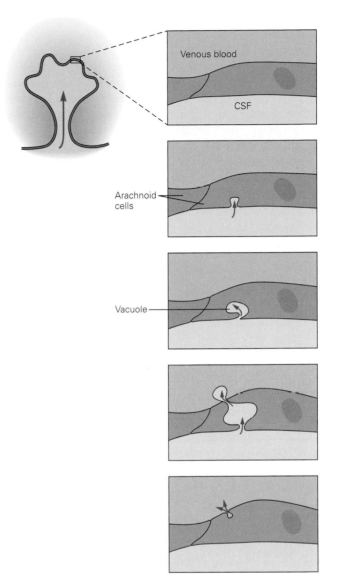

Figure B-7 Transport of CSF within the arachnoid villi is thought to be achieved by giant vacuoles. This mechanism could account for the one-way bulk flow of CSF from the subarachnoid space to the venous system. The arachnoid cells have tight intercellular junctions. Some vesicles are large enough to encompass red blood cells. (Adapted from Fishman 1992.)

epithelium. CSF flows from the lateral ventricles through the interventricular foramina of Monro into the third ventricle. From there it flows into the fourth ventricle through the cerebral aqueduct of Sylvius and then through the foramina of Magendie and Luschka into the subarachnoid space. The subarachnoid space lies between the arachnoid and the pia mater, which, together with the dura mater, form the three meningeal layers that cover the brain (Figure B-6B). Within the subarachnoid space, fluid flows down the spinal canal and also upward over the convexity of the brain (Figure B-6A).

CSF flowing over the brain extends into the sulci and the depths of the cerebral cortex in extensions of the subarachnoid space along blood vessels called *Virchow-Robin spaces*. Small solutes diffuse freely between the interstitial fluid and the CSF in these perivascular spaces and across the ependymal lining of the ventricular system, facilitating the movement of metabolites from deep within the hemispheres to cortical subarachnoid spaces and the ventricular system.

The total CSF volume has not been measured accurately but is estimated to be approximately 140 ml. The lateral and third ventricles contain approximately 12 ml, and the spinal subarachnoid space about 30 ml as measured by computerized tomography. The subarachnoid space and major cisterns (eg, cisterna magna and mesencephalic cistern) of the brain contain most of the CSF.

CSF is absorbed through the arachnoid granulations and villi. Arachnoid granulations consist of collections of villi. They are typically found in clusters that are visible herniations of the arachnoid membrane through

Table B-1 Comparison of Serum and Cerebrospinal Fluid

Component	CSF[1]	Serum[1]
Water content (%)	99	93
Protein (mg/dl)	35	7000
Glucose (mg/dl)	60	90
Osmolarity (mOsm/liter)	295	295
Na^+ (meq/liter)	138	138
K^+ (meq/liter)	2.8	4.5
Ca^{2+} (meq/liter)	2.1	4.8
Mg^{2+} (meq/liter)	0.3	1.7
Cl^- (meq/liter)	119	102
pH	7.33	7.41

[1]Average or representative values.
(From Fishman 1980.)

the dura and into the lumen of the superior sagittal sinus and other venous structures (see Figure B-6A). The villi themselves are visible microscopically and separate CSF from venous blood. Cells of the villus membrane may actively form vacuoles that transport fluid from one side of the cell to the other (Figure B-7).

The granulations appear to function as valves that allow one-way flow of CSF from the subarachnoid spaces into venous blood. This one-way flow of CSF is sometimes called *bulk flow* because all constituents of CSF leave with the fluid, including small molecules, proteins, microorganisms, and red blood cells. The rate of formation of CSF in adults is 0.35 ml/minute or about 500 ml/day, so that the entire volume of CSF is turned over three to four times per day (Figure B-8).

The choroid plexus is structurally similar to the distal and collecting tubules of the kidney, using capillary filtration and epithelial secretory mechanisms to maintain the chemical stability of the CSF. The capillaries that traverse the choroid plexus are freely permeable to plasma solutes. A barrier exists, however, at the level of the epithelial cells that make up the choroid plexus. This barrier is responsible for carrier-mediated active transport (Figure B-9). The secretory capacities of the choroid plexus are bidirectional, accounting for both continuous production of CSF and active transport of metabolites out of the central nervous system into the blood.

CSF and extracellular fluids of the brain are in a steady state under normal physiological circumstances. The concentrations of K^+, Ca^{2+}, bicarbonate, and glucose in CSF are lower than in blood plasma, and CSF is

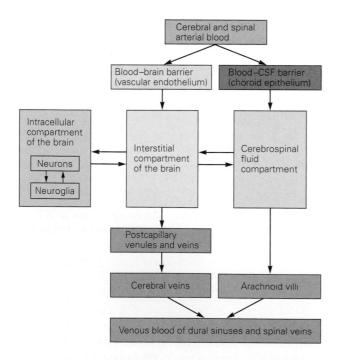

Figure B-8 Relationships between intracranial fluid compartments and the blood-brain and blood-CSF barriers. The tissue elements indicated in **parentheses** form the barriers. **Arrows** indicate the direction of fluid flow under normal conditions. (Adapted from Carpenter 1978.)

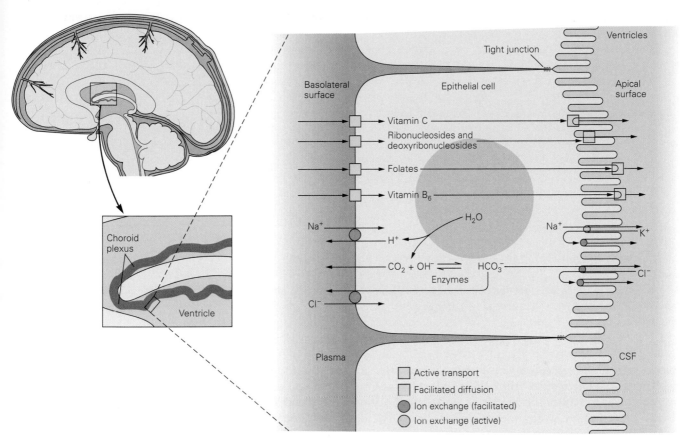

Figure B-9 Flow of molecules across the blood-CSF barrier is regulated by several mechanisms in choroid epithelial cells. Some micronutrients such as vitamin C are transported into epithelial cells by an energy-dependent active transporter located at the basolateral membrane and released into CSF at the apical surface by facilitated diffusion, which requires no energy. Essential ions are also exchanged between CSF and blood plasma. Transport of an ion in one direction is linked to the transport of a different ion in the opposite direction, as in the exchange of Na^+ ions for K^+ ions. (From Spector and Johanson 1989.)

also more acidic (Table B-1). These differences are due to regulation of the constituents of CSF by active transport. Under normal conditions, blood plasma and CSF are in osmotic equilibrium, because water follows the osmotic gradient created by active transport of solutes.

The Composition of Cerebrospinal Fluid May Be Altered in Disease

The gross appearance of the CSF has clinical significance. Normally it is clear and colorless. It may appear cloudy when it contains many leukocytes or has a high protein content. It may also appear grossly bloody or yellow (*xanthochromia*) when blood pigments are left behind after a hemorrhage or when its protein content is greater than 150 mg/dl, indicating that bilirubin (bound to albumin) has been brought from the plasma to the CSF.

Normal CSF does not contain red blood cells. White blood cell counts greater than $4/mm^3$ are pathological. In acute bacterial meningitis the count may be a thousandfold greater. Cells may be increased moderately in viral infections or in response to cerebral infarction, brain tumors, or other damage to cerebral tissue. Tumor cells in CSF can be collected and identified by their characteristic morphology and cell type–specific proteins.

Protein content may be increased by many pathological processes of the brain or spinal cord, because of changes in vascular permeability or changes in CSF dynamics due to altered function of choroid plexus or arachnoid granulations. In multiple sclerosis and a few other inflammatory diseases the γ-globulin content of CSF is disproportionately increased to more than 13% of total protein. When this increment in γ-globulin content of CSF is present without a corresponding increase in

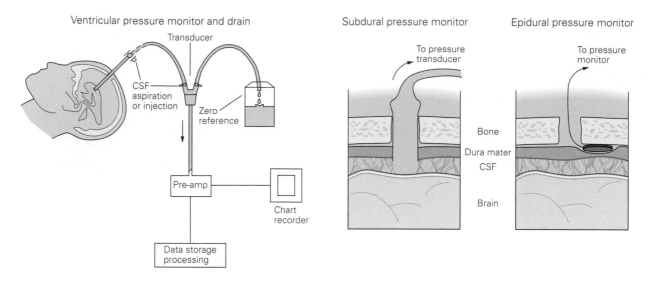

Figure B-10 Techniques for continuous measurement of intracranial pressure. (From Jennett and Teasdale 1981.)

blood γ-globulin, it cannot be attributed to vascular leak and instead results from the production of immunoglobulins within the central nervous system. Similarly, detection by immunoelectrophoresis of two or more oligoclonal immunological species in CSF that are not present in serum indicates immune-mediated brain disease. Oligoclonal immunoglobulins are present in CSF in about 90% of patients with multiple sclerosis. Protein content greater than 500 mg/dl is usually a manifestation of a block in the spinal subarachnoid space by a solid tumor, meningeal cancer, or other compressing lesion.

The concentration of glucose in the CSF is decreased in acute bacterial infections but only rarely in viral infections. In chronic diseases a CSF glucose content less than 40 mg/dl is a symptom of a tumor in the meninges; of fungal, yeast, or tuberculosis infection; or of sarcoidosis. The basis for the reduced CSF glucose content is not yet understood. It may be due to impaired transport into CSF; excessive glycolysis by organisms, blood cells, tumor cells, or the brain itself; or combinations of these mechanisms.

Increased Intracranial Pressure May Harm the Brain

In considering the factors that regulate intracranial pressure, the cranium and spinal canal can be regarded as a closed system. According to the Monro-Kellie doctrine, an increase in the volume of any one of the contents of the calvarium—brain tissue, blood, CSF, or other brain fluids—will produce increased intracranial pressure be-

cause the bony calvarium rigidly fixes the total cranial volume. Mass lesions and their frequently associated interstitial edema commonly increase intracranial pressure. Changes in arterial and intracranial venous pressures may also influence intracranial pressure by their actions on intracranial blood volume and CSF dynamics. Acute changes in arterial or venous pressures can change intracranial pressure dramatically. Chronic changes may be compensated for by several mechanisms, including venous collateralization and increased absorption or decreased formation of CSF.

CSF pressure is ordinarily measured by *lumbar puncture*, a procedure in which a needle is inserted through the skin, between the fourth and fifth lumbar vertebrae, and into the lumbar subarachnoid space, with the patient lying sideways (lateral decubitus position). Because the spinal cord extends only to the first lumbar vertebra, there is no risk of injuring the cord. When the CSF flows freely through the needle, the hub of the needle is attached to a manometer and the fluid is allowed to rise. The normal pressure is 65–195 mm CSF (or water) or 5–15 mm Hg.

In measuring the lumbar CSF pressure as a guide to intracranial pressure, it is assumed that pressures are equal throughout the neuraxis. Normally this is a reasonable assumption; however, in many disease states (eg, brain tumor or obstruction of CSF pathways) this may not be true. For this reason, and also because the lumbar needle cannot be left in place for prolonged periods, catheters are sometimes inserted into the lateral ventricles to measure the pressure there (Figure B-10).

Equally effective are pressure-sensitive transducers that can be inserted under the skull in the epidural or subarachnoid space for continuous monitoring of intracranial pressure. Continuous monitoring has the advantage of identifying transient elevations in intracranial pressure that can occur in certain disorders such as normal pressure hydrocephalus.

Brain Edema Is a State of Increased Brain Volume Due to Increased Water Content

Brain edema may be local (eg, from a surrounding contusion, infarct, or tumor) or generalized. The brain is divided into distinct compartments by relatively noncompliant membranes. Local brain edema may cause herniation of brain tissue across these membranes from one compartment into another. Specific examples include herniation of cingulate gyrus across the falx cerebri, temporal lobe uncus across the cerebellar tentorium, or the cerebral cortex through calvarial defects after surgery.

Vasogenic edema is the most common form of brain edema. It is attributed to increased permeability of brain capillary endothelial cells, which increases the volume of the extracellular fluid. White matter is generally affected more than gray because of the tendency of edema fluid to accumulate along tracts of white matter. Vasogenic edema is most easily visualized using T2-weighted magnetic resonance imaging. Pathological increases in blood-brain barrier permeability also can be visualized by computerized tomography and magnetic resonance imaging after intravenous administration of contrast agents that selectively enter the brain through the affected vessels. Pathologically increased blood-brain barrier permeability, particularly that associated with brain tumors, can be corrected by systemically administered glucocorticoids. The mechanism by which glucocorticoids enhance blood-brain barrier function is poorly understood.

Cytotoxic edema refers to the intracellular swelling of injured neurons, glia, and endothelial cells. It occurs in hypoxia from asphyxia or global cerebral ischemia after cardiac arrest because failure of the ATP-dependent Na^+-K^+ pump allows Na^+, and therefore water, to accumulate within cells. Another cause of cytotoxic edema is water intoxication, a consequence of the acute systemic hypoosmolarity caused by excessive ingestion of water or administration of hypotonic intravenous fluids. Acute hyponatremia, induced for example by inappropriate secretion of antidiuretic hormone or renal salt-wasting from secretion of atrial natriuretic hormone, can cause cellular swelling and brain edema. Under these circumstances water moves from extracellular to intracellular sites. Cytotoxic edema may also accompany vasogenic edema in encephalitis, trauma, and stroke.

Hydrocephalus Is an Increase in the Volume of the Cerebral Ventricles

Hydrocephalus has three possible causes: oversecretion of CSF, impaired absorption of CSF, or obstruction of CSF pathways.

Oversecretion of CSF is rare but is thought to occur in some functioning tumors of the choroid plexus (*papillomas*) because removal of the tumor may relieve the hydrocephalus. These tumors are associated with subarachnoid hemorrhage and high CSF protein content, which could also impair the absorption of CSF.

Impaired absorption of CSF may result from any condition that raises intracranial pressure, such as thrombosis of cerebral veins or sinuses. Impaired CSF absorption at the arachnoid villi is a common cause of *communicating hydrocephalus* (enlargement of the entire ventricular system without obstruction of CSF flow) following subarachnoid hemorrhage, trauma, or bacterial meningitis.

Impaired CSF absorption is also believed to be the cause of *normal-pressure hydrocephalus*, which is characterized by dementia, urinary incontinence, and a disorder of gait called *apraxia*. Brain imaging reveals communicating hydrocephalus, and routine lumbar puncture typically shows normal intracranial pressure. Continuous intracranial pressure monitoring reveals episodic elevations in intracranial pressure, however, suggesting that intermittent intracranial hypertension causes the condition.

Cisternography reveals alterations in the flow of CSF in these patients. In normal patients technetium-labeled albumin injected into the lumbar subarachnoid space can be traced by a gamma camera up to the cortical convexities where the arachnoid granulations are located; however, the label does not enter the ventricles. In patients with normal-pressure hydrocephalus the isotopic label reaches the cortical convexities after a prolonged delay and may reflux into the ventricles. If identified early, normal-pressure hydrocephalus can be treated surgically by shunting CSF using a ventriculoperitoneal catheter.

Obstruction of CSF pathways may result from tumors, congenital malformations, or scarring. A particularly vulnerable site for all three mechanisms is the narrow aqueduct of Sylvius. Aqueductal stenosis may result from congenital malformations or gliosis due to intrauterine infection or hemorrhage. Later in life the aqueduct may be occluded by tumor. The outlets of the fourth ventricle may be obstructed by congenital atresia of the foramina of Luschka and Magendie, which may lead to enlargement of all four ventricles (*Dandy-Walker syndrome*). In early life the cranial vault enlarges with the ventricles; after the sutures fuse, cranial volume is fixed and hydrocephalus develops at the expense of brain volume.

John Laterra
Gary W. Goldstein

Selected Readings

Bradbury MWB (ed). 1992. *Physiology and Pharmacology of the Blood-Brain Barrier.* New York: Springer.

Del-Bigio MR. 1993. Neuropathological changes caused by hydrocephalus. Acta Neuropathol (Berlin) 85:573–585.

Doczi T. 1993. Volume regulation of the brain tissue—a survey. Acta Neurochir (Wien) 121:1–9.

Doyle DJ, Mark PW. 1992. Analysis of intracranial pressure. J Clin Monit 8:81–90.

Fishman RA. 1975. Brain edema. N Engl J Med 293:706–711.

Fishman RA. 1992. *Cerebrospinal Fluid in Diseases of the Nervous System.* Philadelphia, PA: Saunders.

Goldstein GW, Betz AL. 1986. The blood-brain barrier. Sci Am 255(3):74–83.

Greer M. 1988. Carrier drugs: presidential address, American Academy of Neurology, 1987. Neurology 38:628–632.

Kalaria RN, Gravina SA, Schmidley JW, Perry G, Harik SI. 1988. The glucose transporter of the human brain and blood-brain barrier. Ann Neurol 24:757–764.

Katzman R, Pappius HM. 1973. *Brain Electrolytes and Fluid Metabolism.* Baltimore, MD: Williams & Wilkins.

Keep RF, Xiang J, Betz AL. 1993. Potassium transport at the blood-brain and blood-CSF barriers. Adv Exp Med Biol 331:43–54.

Laterra J, Stewart PA, Goldstein GW. 1991. Development of the blood-brain barrier. In: RA Polin, WW Fox (eds). *Neonatal and Fetal Medicine—Physiology and Pathophysiology*, pp. 1525–1531. Philadelphia, PA: Saunders.

Lyons MK, Meyer FB. 1990. Cerebrospinal fluid physiology and the management of increased intracranial pressure. Mayo Clin Proc 65:684–707.

Mooradian AD, Morin AM, Cipp LJ, Haspel HC. 1991. Glucose transport is reduced in the blood-brain barrier of aged rats. Brain Res 551:145–149.

Nilsson C, Lindvall-Axelsson M, Owman C. 1992. Neuroendocrine regulatory mechanisms in the choroid plexus—cerebrospinal fluid system. Brain Res Rev 17:109–138.

Pardridge W (ed). 1993. *The Blood-Brain Barrier: Cellular & Molecular Biology.* New York: Raven.

Rapoport SI. 1976. *Blood-Brain Barrier in Physiology and Medicine.* New York: Raven.

Ropper AH, Kennedy SF (eds). 1988. *Neurological and Neurosurgical Intensive Care.* Rockville, MD: Aspen.

Segal MB. 1993. Extracellular and cerebrospinal fluids. J Inherit Metab Dis 16:617–638.

References

Betz AL, Goldstein GW. 1986. Specialized properties and solute transport in brain capillaries. Annu Rev Physiol 48:241–250.

Borgesen SE, Gjetrris F. 1982. The predictive value of conductance to outflow of CSF in normal pressure hydrocephalus. Brain 105:65–86.

Borgesen SE, Gjetrris F. 1987. Relationships between intracranial pressure, ventricular size, and resistance to CSF outflow. J Neurosurg 67:535–539.

Brightman MW, Reese TS. 1969. Junctions between intimately apposed cell membranes in the vertebrate brain. J Cell Biol 40:648–677.

Carpenter MB. 1978. *Human Neuroanatomy*, 7th ed. Baltimore, MD: William & Wilkins.

DeVivo DC, Trifiletti R, Jacobson RI, Harik SI. 1990. Glucose transporter deficiency causing persistent hypoglycorrhachia: a unique cause of infantile seizures and acquired microcephaly. Ann Neurol 29:414–415.

Ehrlich P. 1885. *Das Sauerstoff-Bedörfnis des Organismus. Eine Farbenanalytische Studie.* Berlin: Hirschwold, cited by Friedemann 1942.

Friedemann U. 1942. Blood-brain barrier. Physiol Rev 22:125–145.

Goldman E. 1909. Die äussere und innere Sekretion des gesunden und kranken Organismus im Lichte der "vitalen Färbung." Beitr Klin Chirurg 64:192–265.

Guerin C, Laterra J, Hruban R, Brem H, Drewes LR, Goldstein GW. 1990. The glucose transporter and blood-brain barrier of human brain tumors. Ann Neurol 28:758–765.

Guerin C, Laterra J, Drewes L, Brem H, Goldstein GW. 1992. Vascular expression of glucose transporter in experimental brain neoplasms. Am J Pathol 140:114–125.

Hansen AJ, Lund-Andersen H, Crone C. 1977. K^+-permeability of the blood-brain barrier, investigated by aid of a K^+-sensitive microelectrode. Acta Physiol Scand 101:438–445.

Jennett B, Teasdale G. 1981. *Management of Head Injuries.* Philadelphia, PA: Davis.

Lal B, Indurti RR, Couraud P-O, Goldstein GW, Laterra J. 1994. Endothelial cell implantation and survival within experimental gliomas. Proc Natl Acad Sci U S A 21:9695–9699.

Reese TS, Karnovsky MJ. 1967. Fine structural localization of a blood-brain barrier to exogenous peroxidase. J Cell Biol 34:207–217.

Resnick L, Berger JR, Shapshak P, Tourtellotte WW. 1988.

Early penetration of the blood-brain barrier by HIV. Neurology 38:9–14.

Rubin LL, Hall DE, Porter S, Barbu K, Cannon C, Horner HC, Janatpour M, Liaw CW, Manning K, Morales J, Tanner LI, Toamselli KJ, Bard F. 1991. A cell culture model of the blood-brain barrier. J Cell Biol 115:1725–1735.

Schinkel AH, Smit JJM, Vantellingen O, Beijnen JH, Wagenaar E, Vandeemter L, Mol CAAM, Vandervalk MA, Robanusmaandag EC, Teriele HPJ, Berns AJM, Borst P. 1994. Disruption of the mouse *mdr1a* P-glycoprotein gene leads to a deficiency in the blood-brain barrier and to increased sensitivity to drugs. Cell 77:491–502.

Shivers RR, Betz AL, Goldstein GW. 1984. Isolated rat brain capillaries possess intact, structurally complex, interendothelial tight junctions; freeze-fracture verification of tight junction integrity. Brain Res 324:313–322.

Spector R, Johanson CE. 1989. The mammalian choroid plexus. Sci Am 261(5):68–74.

Stewart PA, Wiley MJ. 1981. Developing nervous tissue induces formation of blood-brain barrier characteristics in invading endothelial cells: a study using quail-chick transplantation chimeras. Dev Biol 84:183–192.

Svengaard N, Bjorklund A, Hardebo JE, Stenevi U. 1975. Axonal degeneration associated with a defective blood-brain barrier in cerebral implants. Nature 255:334–336.

Wahl M, Unterberg A, Baerthmann A, Schilling L. 1988. Mediators of blood-brain barrier dysfunction and formation of vasogenic brain edema. J Cereb Blood Flow Metab 8:621–634.

Wolburg H, Neuhaus J, Kniesel U, Kraub B, Schmid E-M, Ocalan M, Farrell C, Risau W. 1994. Modulation of tight junction structure in blood-brain barrier endothelial cells: Effects of tissue culture, second messengers, and cocultured astrocytes. J Cell Sci 107:1347–1357.

Appendix C

Circulation of the Brain

THE BRAIN IS HIGHLY vulnerable to disturbance of its blood supply. Anoxia and ischemia lasting only seconds cause neurological symptoms and when they last minutes they can cause irreversible neuronal damage.

Blood flow to the central nervous system must efficiently deliver oxygen, glucose, and other nutrients and remove carbon dioxide, lactic acid, and other metabolic products. The cerebral vasculature has unique anatomical and physiological features that protect the brain from circulatory compromise. When these protective mechanisms fail, the result is a stroke. Broadly defined, the term *stroke,* or *cerebrovascular accident,* refers to the neurological symptoms or signs, usually focal and acute, that result from diseases involving blood vessels.

The Blood Supply of the Brain Can Be Divided Into Arterial Territories

Each cerebral hemisphere is supplied by an *internal carotid artery,* which arises from a common carotid artery beneath the angle of the jaw, enters the cranium through the carotid foramen, traverses the cavernous sinus (giving off the *ophthalmic artery*), penetrates the dura, and divides into the anterior and middle cerebral arteries (Figure C-1).

The large surface branches of the *anterior cerebral artery* supply the cortex and white matter of the inferior frontal lobe, the medial surface of the frontal and parietal lobes, and the anterior corpus callosum. Smaller penetrating branches—including the so-called *recurrent artery of Heubner*—supply the deeper cerebrum and diencephalon, including limbic structures,

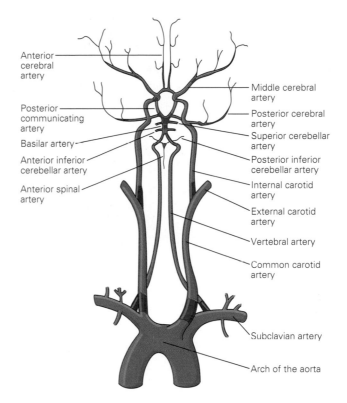

Figure C-1 The blood vessels of the brain. The circle of Willis is made up of the proximal posterior cerebral arteries, the posterior communicating arteries, the internal carotid arteries just before their bifurcations, the proximal anterior cerebral arteries, and the anterior communicating artery. **Dark areas** show common sites of atherosclerosis and occlusion.

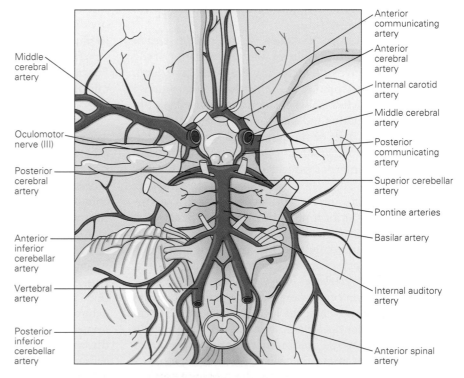

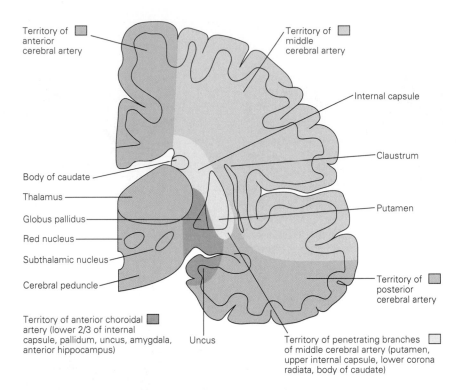

Territory of anterior cerebral artery

Territory of middle cerebral artery

Internal capsule

Claustrum

Body of caudate

Thalamus

Globus pallidus

Red nucleus

Subthalamic nucleus

Cerebral peduncle

Putamen

Territory of posterior cerebral artery

Territory of anterior choroidal artery (lower 2/3 of internal capsule, pallidum, uncus, amygdala, anterior hippocampus)

Uncus

Territory of penetrating branches of middle cerebral artery (putamen, upper internal capsule, lower corona radiata, body of caudate)

Figure C-2 Cerebral arterial areas.

the head of the caudate, and the anterior limb of the internal capsule.

The large surface branches of the *middle cerebral artery* supply most of the cortex and white matter of the hemisphere's convexity, including the frontal, parietal, temporal, and occipital lobes, and the insula. Smaller penetrating branches (the *lenticulostriate arteries*) supply the deep white matter and diencephalic structures, such as the posterior limb of the internal capsule, the putamen, the outer globus pallidus, and the body of the caudate. After the internal carotid emerges from the cavernous sinus, it also gives off the *anterior choroidal artery,* which supplies the anterior hippocampus and, at a caudal level, the posterior limb of the internal capsule.

Left and right vertebral arteries arise from the subclavian arteries and enter the cranium through the foramen magnum. Each gives off an *anterior spinal artery* and a *posterior inferior cerebellar artery.* The vertebral arteries join at the junction of the pons and the medulla to form the *basilar artery,* which at the level of the pons gives off the *anterior inferior cerebellar artery* and the *internal auditory artery* and at the midbrain the *superior cerebellar artery.* The basilar artery then divides into the two *posterior cerebral arteries,* which supply the inferior temporal and medial occipital lobes and the posterior corpus callosum. The smaller penetrating branches of these vessels

(the *thalamoperforate* and *thalamogeniculate arteries*) supply diencephalic structures, including the thalamus and the subthalamic nuclei, as well as parts of the midbrain.

These arterial territories are shown schematically in Figure C-2. Infarctions in the territories of the anterior, middle, and posterior cerebral arteries are shown in Figures C-3, C-4, and C-5.

Interconnections between blood vessels (*anastomoses*) protect the brain when part of its vascular supply is blocked (Figure C-6). At the *circle of Willis* the two anterior cerebral arteries are connected by the anterior communicating artery, and the posterior cerebral arteries are connected to the internal carotid arteries by the posterior communicating arteries. The circle of Willis provides an overlapping blood supply. A congenitally incomplete circle, which is common in the general population, is much more frequent among patients who have had strokes. Other important anastomoses include connections between the ophthalmic artery and branches of the external carotid artery through the orbit, and connections at the brain surface between branches of the middle, anterior, and posterior cerebral arteries (*sharing border zones* or *watersheds*). The small penetrating vessels arising from the circle of Willis and proximal major arteries tend to lack anastomoses. The deep brain regions they supply are therefore referred to as *end zones.*

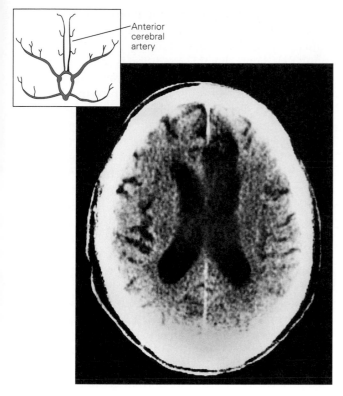

Figure C-3 CT scan showing infarction (dark area) in the territory of the anterior cerebral artery. (Courtesy of Dr. Allan J. Schwartz.)

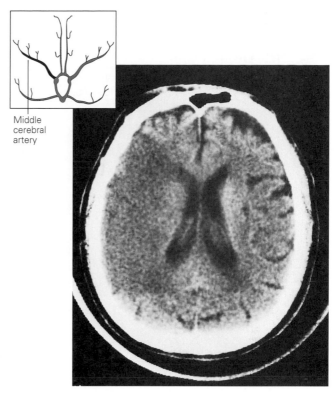

Figure C-4 CT scan showing infarction (dark area) in the territory of the middle cerebral artery. (Courtesy of Dr. Allan J. Schwartz.)

The Cerebral Vessels Have Unique Physiological Responses

Although the human brain constitutes only 2% of total body weight, it receives about 15% of the cardiac output and consumes approximately 20% of the oxygen used by the entire body. These values reflect the high metabolic rate and oxygen requirements of the brain. The total blood flow to the brain is about 750–1000 ml/min; about 350 ml of this amount flows through each carotid artery and about 100–200 ml flows through the vertebrobasilar system. Flow per unit mass of gray matter is approximately four times that of white matter.

Cerebral vessels are capable of altering their own diameter and can respond in a unique fashion to altered physiological conditions. Two main types of autoregulation exist. Brain arterioles constrict when the systemic blood pressure is raised and dilate when it is lowered. These adjustments help to maintain optimal cerebral blood flow. The result is that normal individuals have a constant cerebral blood flow between mean arterial pressures of approximately 60–150 mm Hg. Above or below these pressures cerebral blood flow rises or falls linearly.

The second type of autoregulation involves blood or tissue gases and pH. When arterial CO_2 is raised, brain arterioles dilate and cerebral blood flow increases; with hypocarbia, vasoconstriction results and cerebral blood flow decreases. The response is very sensitive: inhalation of 5% CO_2 increases cerebral blood flow by 50%; 7% CO_2 doubles it. Changing arterial O_2 causes an opposite and less pronounced response: Breathing 100% O_2 lowers cerebral blood flow by about 13%; 10% O_2 raises it by 35%. The mechanism of these responses is uncertain. The vasodilatory action of arterial CO_2 is probably mediated by alterations in extracellular pH. Local concentrations of K^+ and adenosine, both of which cause vasodilation in animals, may play a role.

Whatever the mechanism, these responses protect the brain by increasing the delivery of oxygen and the removal of acid metabolites in the presence of hypoxia, ischemia, or tissue damage. They also allow nearly instantaneous adjustments of regional cerebral blood flow to meet the demands of rapidly changing oxygen and glucose metabolism that accompany normal brain activities. For example, viewing a complex scene will increase oxygen and glucose consumption in the visual

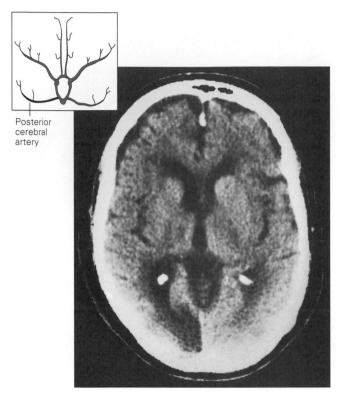

Posterior
cerebral
artery

Figure C-5 CT scan showing infarction (dark area) in the territory of the posterior cerebral artery. (Courtesy of Dr. Allan J. Schwartz.)

cortex of the occipital lobes. The resulting increased CO_2 concentration and lowered pH in the area cause an immediate local increase in blood flow.

A Stroke Is the Result of Disease Involving Blood Vessels

Diseases of the blood vessels are among the most frequent serious neurological disorders, ranking third as a cause of death in the adult population in the United States and probably first as a cause of chronic functional incapacity. Approximately two million people in the United States today are impaired by the neurological consequences of cerebrovascular disease. Many of them are between 25 and 64 years of age.

Strokes are either *occlusive* (due to closure of a blood vessel) or *hemorrhagic* (due to bleeding from a vessel). Insufficiency of blood supply is termed *ischemia;* if it is temporary, symptoms and signs may clear with little or no pathological evidence of tissue damage. Ischemia is not synonymous with *anoxia,* for a reduced blood supply deprives tissue not only of oxygen but also of glu-

cose. In addition, it prevents the removal of potentially toxic metabolites such as lactic acid. When ischemia is sufficiently severe and prolonged, neurons and other cellular elements die; this condition is called *infarction.*

Hemorrhage may occur at the brain surface (*extraparenchymal*), for example, from rupture of congenital aneurysms at the circle of Willis, causing subarachnoid hemorrhage. Alternatively, hemorrhage may be *intraparenchymal*—for example, from rupture of vessels damaged by long-standing hypertension—and may cause a blood clot or *hematoma* within the cerebral hemispheres, in the brain stem, or in the cerebellum. Hemorrhage may result in ischemia or infarction. The mass effect of an intracerebral hematoma may limit the blood supply of adjacent brain tissue. By mechanisms that are not understood, subarachnoid hemorrhage may cause reactive vasospasm of cerebral surface vessels, leading to further ischemic brain damage.

Although most occlusive strokes are due to atherosclerosis and thrombosis and most hemorrhagic strokes are associated with hypertension or aneurysms, strokes of either type may occur at any age from many causes, including cardiac disease, trauma, infection, neoplasm, blood dyscrasia, vascular malformation, immunological disorder, and exogenous toxins. Diagnostic strategies and treatment should vary accordingly; however, in this appendix we examine the anatomical and physiological principles relevant to *any* occlusive or hemorrhagic stroke.

Clinical Vascular Syndromes May Follow Vessel Occlusion, Hypoperfusion, or Hemorrhage

Infarction Can Occur in the Middle Cerebral Artery Territory

Infarction in the territory of the middle cerebral artery (cortex and white matter) causes the most frequently encountered stroke syndrome, with contralateral weakness, sensory loss, and visual field impairment (*homonymous hemianopsia*), and, depending on the hemisphere involved, either language disturbance or impaired spatial perception. Weakness and sensory loss affect the face and arm more than the leg because of the somatotopy of the motor and sensory cortex (pre- and postcentral gyri). The face- and arm-control areas are on the convexity, whereas the leg-control area is on the medial surface of the hemisphere. Motor and sensory loss are greatest in the hand, for the more proximal limbs and the trunk tend to have greater representation in both hemispheres. Paraspinal muscles, for example, are

Figure C-6 Angiograms demonstrating the importance of anastomoses in that they allow retrograde filling after occlusion of the middle cerebral artery.

A. Occlusion of the middle cerebral artery results in no filling in the middle cerebral distribution.

B. Retrograde filling of the middle cerebral artery has begun via distal anastomotic branches of the anterior cerebral artery.

C. Retrograde filling of the middle cerebral artery continues at a time when little contrast material is seen in the anterior cerebral artery. (Courtesy of Dr. Margaret Whelan and Dr. Sadek K. Hilal.)

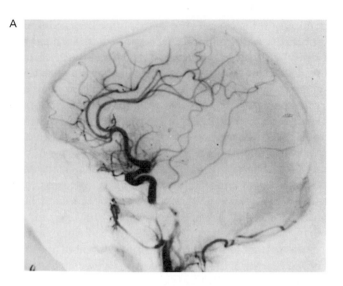

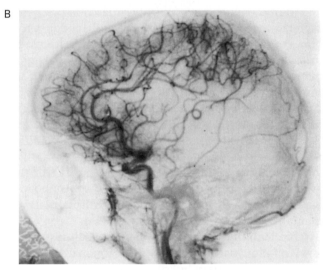

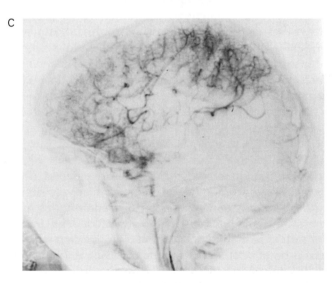

rarely weak in unilateral cerebral lesions. Similarly, the facial muscles of the forehead and the muscles of the pharynx and jaw are represented in both hemispheres and therefore are usually spared. Tongue weakness is variable. If weakness is severe (*plegia*), muscle tone is usually decreased at first but gradually increases over days or weeks to spasticity with hyperactive tendon reflexes. A Babinski sign, reflecting upper motor neuron disturbance (see Chapters 33 and 38), is usually present from the outset. When weakness is mild, or during recovery, there may be clumsiness or slowness of movement out of proportion to loss of strength; such motor disability may resemble parkinsonian bradykinesia or even cerebellar ataxia.

Acutely, paresis of contralateral conjugate gaze often occurs as a result of damage to the convexity of the cortex anterior to the motor cortex (the frontal eye field). The reason this gaze palsy persists for only 1 or 2 days, even when other signs remain severe, is not clear.

Sensory loss tends to involve discriminative and proprioceptive modalities more than affective modalities. Pain and temperature sensation may be impaired or altered but are usually not lost. Joint position sense, however, may be severely disturbed, causing limb ataxia, and there may be loss of two-point discrimination, *astereognosis* (inability to recognize a held object by tactile sensation), or *extinction* (failure to appreciate a touch stimulus if a comparable stimulus is delivered simultaneously to the unaffected side of the body).

Homonymous hemianopsia is the result of damage to the optic radiations, the deep fiber tracts connecting the thalamic lateral geniculate body to the visual (*calcarine*) cortex. If the parietal radiation is primarily affected, the visual field loss may be an inferior quadrantanopia, whereas in temporal lobe lesions quadrantanopia may be superior.

In more than 95% of right-handed persons and in the majority of those who are left handed, the left hemisphere is dominant for language. Destruction of left opercular (*perisylvian*) cortex in left-dominant individuals causes aphasia, which may take several forms depending on the degree and distribution of the damage. Frontal opercular lesions tend to produce particular difficulty with speech output and writing with relative preservation of language comprehension (*Broca aphasia*), whereas infarction of the posterior superior temporal gyrus tends to cause severe difficulty in speech comprehension and reading (*Wernicke aphasia*). When opercular damage is widespread, there is severe disturbance of mixed type (*global aphasia*).

Left-hemisphere convexity damage, especially parietal, may also cause motor apraxia, a disturbance of learned motor acts not explained by weakness or incoordination, with the ability to perform the act when the setting is altered (see Chapters 19 and 59). For example, a patient unable to imitate lighting a match might be able to perform the act normally if given a match to light.

Right-hemisphere convexity infarction, especially parietal, tends to cause disturbances of spatial perception. Patients may have difficulty in copying simple pictures or diagrams (*constructional apraxia*), in interpreting maps or finding their way about (*topographagnosia*), or in putting on their clothing properly (*dressing apraxia*). Awareness of space and the patient's own body contralateral to the lesion may be particularly affected (*hemi-inattention* or *hemineglect*). Patients may fail to recognize their hemiplegia (*anosognosia*), left arm (*asomatognosia*), or any external object to the left of their own midline. Such phenomena may occur independently of visual field defects and in patients otherwise mentally intact (see Chapter 20).

Particular types of language or spatial dysfunction tend to follow occlusion not of the proximal stem of the middle cerebral artery but of one of its several main pial branches. In such circumstances other signs (eg, weakness or visual field defect) may not be present. Similarly, occlusion of the rolandic branch of the middle cerebral artery may cause motor and sensory loss affecting the face and arm without disturbance of vision, language, or spatial perception.

Infarction Can Occur in the Anterior Cerebral Artery Territory

Infarction in the territory of the anterior cerebral artery causes weakness and sensory loss qualitatively similar to that of convexity lesions, but infarction in this territory affects mainly the distal contralateral leg. Urinary incontinence may be present, but it is uncertain whether this is because of a lesion of the paracentral lobule (medial hemispheric motor and sensory cortices) or of a more anterior region necessary for the inhibition of bladder emptying. Damage to the supplementary motor cortex may cause speech disturbance, considered aphasia by some and a type of motor inertia by others. Involvement of the anterior corpus callosum may cause apraxia of the left arm (*sympathetic apraxia*), which is attributed to disconnection of the left (language-dominant) hemisphere from the right motor cortex.

Bilateral anterior cerebral artery territory infarction (occurring, for example, when both arteries arise anomalously from a single trunk) may cause a severe behavioral disturbance, known as *abulia*, consisting of profound apathy, motor inertia, and muteness, and attributable to destruction, in variable combinations, of the inferior frontal lobes (orbitofrontal cortex), deeper limbic structures, supplementary motor cortices, and cingulate gyri.

Infarction Can Occur in the Posterior Cerebral Artery Territory

Infarction in the territory of the posterior cerebral artery causes contralateral homonymous hemianopsia by destroying the calcarine cortex. Macular (central) vision tends to be spared because the occipital pole, where macular vision is represented, receives blood supply from the middle cerebral artery. If the lesion is on the left and the posterior corpus callosum is affected, *alexia*—inability to read—may be present without aphasia or agraphia. A possible explanation for the alexia is the disconnection of the seeing right occipital cortex from the language-dominant left hemisphere. If infarction is bilateral (eg, following thrombosis at the point where both posterior cerebral arteries arise from the basilar artery), there may be cortical blindness with failure of the patient to recognize that he cannot see (*Anton syndrome*), or memory disturbance may occur as a result of bilateral damage to the inferomedial temporal lobes.

If posterior cerebral artery occlusion is proximal, the lesion may include, or especially affect, the following structures: the thalamus, causing contralateral hemisensory loss and sometimes spontaneous pain and dysesthesia (*thalamic pain syndrome*); the subthalamic nucleus, causing contralateral severe proximal chorea (*hemiballism*); or even the midbrain, with ipsilateral oculomotor palsy and contralateral hemiparesis or ataxia from involvement of the corticospinal tract or the crossed superior cerebellar peduncle (dentatothalamic tract).

The Anterior Choroidal and Penetrating Arteries Can Become Occluded

Anterior choroidal artery occlusion can cause contralateral hemiplegia and sensory loss from involvement of the posterior limb of the internal capsule and homonymous hemianopsia from involvement of the thalamic lateral geniculate nucleus.

As mentioned earlier in this chapter, the deeper cerebral white matter and diencephalon are supplied by small penetrating arteries, variously called the *lenticulostriates*, the *thalamogeniculates*, or the *thalamoperforates*, which arise from the circle of Willis or the proximal portions of the middle, anterior, and posterior cerebral arteries. These end-arteries lack anastomotic interconnections, and occlusion of individual vessels, usually in association with hypertensive damage to the vessel wall, causes small (less than 1.5 cm in diameter) infarcts (*lacunes*), which, if critically located, are followed by characteristic syndromes. For example, lacunes in the pyramidal tract area of the internal capsule cause *pure hemiparesis*, with arm and leg weakness of equal severity and with little or no sensory loss, visual field disturbance, aphasia, or spatial disruption. Lacunes in the ventral posterior nucleus of the thalamus produce pure hemisensory loss, with involvement of pain, temperature, proprioceptive, and discriminative modalities and with little motor, visual, language, or spatial disturbance. Most lacunes occur in redundant areas (eg, nonpyramidal corona radiata) and so are asymptomatic. If bilateral and numerous, however, they may cause a characteristic syndrome (*état lacunaire*) of progressive dementia, shuffling gait, and pseudobulbar palsy (spastic dysarthria and dysphagia, with lingual and pharyngeal paralysis and hyperactive palate and gag reflexes, plus lability of emotional response, with abrupt crying or laughing out of proportion to mood).

Infarction restricted to structures supplied by the recurrent artery of Heubner or other deep penetrating branches of the anterior cerebral artery (the anterior caudate nucleus and less predictably the anterior putamen and anterior limb of the internal capsule) results in varying combinations of psychomotor slowing, dysarthria, agitation, contralateral neglect, and, when left hemispheric, language disturbance.

The Carotid Artery Can Become Occluded

Atherothrombotic vessel occlusion often occurs in the internal carotid artery rather than the intracranial vessels. Particularly in a patient with an incomplete circle of Willis, infarction may include the territories of both the middle and anterior cerebral arteries, with arm and leg weakness and sensory loss equally severe. Alternatively, infarction may be limited to the distal shared territory (border zones of these vessels), producing, by destruction of the motor cortex at the upper cerebral convexity, weakness limited to the arm or the leg. Another cause of leg weakness and sensory loss in association with a convexity syndrome is occlusion of the middle cerebral artery at its proximal stem; the internal capsule and other diencephalic structures supplied by the middle cerebral artery's lenticulostriate branches are then affected in addition to the cortex of the cerebral convexity.

The Brain Stem and Cerebellum Are Supplied by Branches of the Vertebral and Basilar Arteries

Branches of the vertebral and basilar arteries consist of three sets: (1) Paramedian branches, including the anterior spinal artery, supply midline structures; (2) short circumferential branches supply more lateral structures, including the inferior, middle, and superior cerebral peduncles; and (3) long circumferential arteries—the posterior inferior, anterior inferior, and superior cerebellar arteries—also supply lateral brain stem structures and the cerebellar peduncles, as well as the cerebellum itself. Most of the midbrain is supplied by branches of the posterior cerebral artery. The interpeduncular branches, the most medial branches located between the basilar artery bifurcation and the posterior communicating arteries, supply paramedian midbrain structures. Lateral to this group are the thalamoperforate branches, which supply the inferior, medial, and anterior thalamus and the subthalamic nucleus. Further laterally are the thalamogeniculate branches, which supply lateral and dorsal structures in the midbrain and thalamus. In some people the midbrain also receives blood from the superior cerebellar, posterior communicating, and anterior choroidal arteries. After the posterior cerebral artery passes around the midbrain, it enters the middle fossa to supply the occipital and inferior temporal lobes. It does not supply the cerebellum.

Various syndromes resulting from damage to specific brain stem structures have been defined (Figure C-7). With the exception of the lateral medullary syndrome of Wallenberg, however, most of the original descriptions were based on patients with neoplasms. Brain stem infarction more often follows occlusion of the vertebral or basilar arteries themselves than of their medial or lateral branches; resulting syndromes and signs tend to be less stereotyped than classical descriptions imply.

Generally speaking, a lesion of the posterior fossa is suggested by (1) bilateral long tract (motor or sensory) signs, (2) crossed (eg, left face and right limb) motor or sensory signs, (3) cerebellar signs, (4) stupor or coma (from involvement of the ascending reticular activating system), (5) disconjugate eye movements or nystagmus, and (6) involvement of cranial nerves not usually affected by unilateral hemispheric infarcts (eg, unilateral

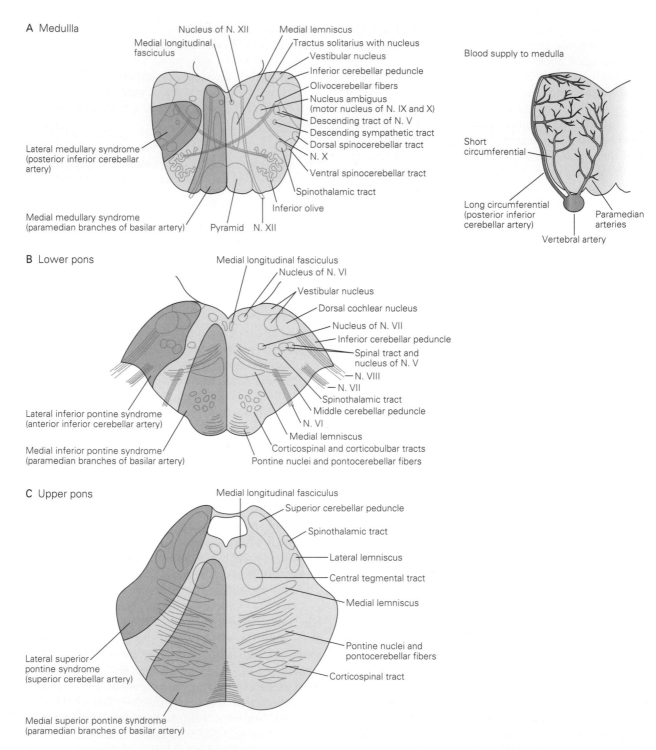

Figure C-7 Syndromes of brain stem vascular lesions (indicated on the left in each figure).

deafness or pharyngeal weakness). Sometimes a lesion involving only a single tiny structure can be localized accurately by symptomatology. For example, internuclear opthalmoplegia implicates a lesion of the median longitudinal fasciculus. Other lesions produce more ambiguous symptoms. For example, infarction limited to the upper pontine corticospinal tract can produce contralateral face, arm, and leg weakness indistinguishable from that caused by a small infarct in the internal capsule.

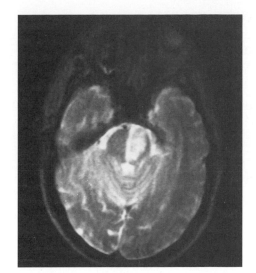

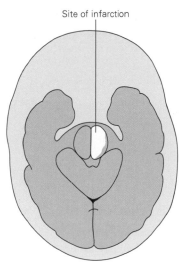

Site of infarction

Figure C-8 Magnetic resonance imaging shows a white highlight in the ventral portion of one half of the pons. The lesion stops abruptly at the midline, suggesting unilateral occlusion of one or more paramedian vessels.

Infarcts Affecting Predominantly Medial or Lateral Brain Stem Structures Produce Characteristic Syndromes

Infarction of the lateral medulla follows occlusion of the vertebral artery or less often the posterior inferior cerebellar artery. Symptoms and signs include (1) vertigo, nausea, vomiting, and nystagmus (from involvement of the vestibular nuclei); (2) ataxia of gait and ipsilateral limbs (inferior cerebellar peduncle or the cerebellum itself); (3) decreased pain and temperature (but not touch) sensation on the ipsilateral face (descending tract and nucleus of the trigeminal nerve) and the contralateral body (spinothalamic tract); (4) dysphagia, hoarseness, ipsilateral weakness of the palate and vocal cords, and ipsilaterally decreased gag reflex (nucleus ambiguus, or glossopharyngeal and vagus outflow tracts); and (5) ipsilateral Horner syndrome (descending sympathetic fibers). Involvement of the nucleus solitarius can cause ipsilateral loss of taste, and hiccups are often present (Table C-1).

Infarction of the medial medulla causes contralateral hemiparesis (from involvement of the corticospinal tract), ipsilateral tongue weakness with dysarthria and deviation toward the paretic side (hypoglossal nucleus or outflow tract), and contralateral impaired proprioception and discriminative sensation with preserved pain and temperature sensation (medial lemniscus).

Infarction of the lateral pons affects caudal structures when the anterior inferior cerebellar artery is occluded and rostral structures when the superior cerebellar artery is occluded (Figure C-8). Symptoms of caudal damage resemble those of lateral medullary infarction, with vertigo, nystagmus, gait and ipsilateral limb ataxia, crossed face-and-body pain and temperature loss, Horner syndrome, and ipsilateral loss of taste. There is also unilateral tinnitus and deafness (from involvement of the cochlear nuclei). Involvement of more medial structures can cause ipsilateral gaze paresis or facial weakness. Symptoms of rostral damage include gait and ipsilateral limb ataxia, Horner syndrome, and crossed sensory loss, which at this level includes touch, pain, and temperature sensation on the ipsilateral face (from involvement of the primary sensory nucleus or entering sensory fibers of the trigeminal nerve). There may also be ipsilateral jaw weakness with deviation to the paretic side (trigeminal motor nucleus and outflow tract). Vertigo, deafness, and face weakness are not present.

Infarction of the medial pons, whether caudal or rostral, causes contralateral hemiparesis (from involvement of the corticospinal tract). Caudal lesions affecting the facial nucleus or outflow tract cause ipsilateral facial weakness. Rostral lesions result in contralateral facial weakness. There may also be ipsilateral gaze paresis (paramedian pontine reticular formation or abducens nucleus, together comprising the *pontine gaze center*) or abducens paresis (sixth nerve outflow tract); internuclear ophthalmoplegia and limb and gait ataxia are often present. Contralateral impairment of proprioception and discriminative touch is most prominent with caudal lesions. Rapid involuntary movements of the palate—so-called *palatal myoclonus*—has been attributed to involvement of the central tegmental tract; the involuntary movements may spread to include the pharynx, larynx, face, eyes, or respiratory muscles.

Table C-1 Signs That Indicate the Level of Brain Stem Vascular Syndromes

Syndrome	Artery affected	Structure involved	Manifestations
Medial syndromes			
Medulla	Paramedian branches	Emerging fibers of twelfth nerve	Ipsilateral hemiparalysis of tongue
Inferior pons	Paramedian branches	Pontine gaze center	Paralysis of gaze to side of lesion
		Emerging fibers of sixth nerve	Ipsilateral abduction paralysis
Superior pons	Paramedian branches	Medial longitudinal fasciculus	Internuclear ophthalmoplegia
Lateral syndromes			
Medulla	Posterior inferior cerebellar	Emerging fibers of ninth or tenth nerves	Dysphagia; hoarseness; ipsilateral paralysis of vocal cord; ipsilateral loss of pharyngeal reflex
		Vestibular nuclei	Vertigo; nystagmus
		Descending tract and nucleus of fifth nerve	Ipsilateral facial analgesia
		Solitary nucleus and tract	Taste loss on ipsilateral half of tongue posteriorly
Inferior pons	Anterior inferior cerebellar	Emerging fibers of seventh nerve	Ipsilateral facial paralysis
		Solitary nucleus and tract	Taste loss on ipsilateral half of tongue anteriorly
		Cochlear nuclei	Deafness; tinnitus
Mid pons		Motor nucleus of fifth nerve	Ipsilateral jaw weakness
		Emerging sensory fibers of fifth nerve	Ipsilateral facial numbness

Syndromes of midbrain infarction are more conveniently characterized as peduncular (ventral), tegmental, or pretectal/tectal (dorsal) (Figure C-9). Unilateral peduncular lesions cause *Weber syndrome,* characterized by ipsilateral paresis of adduction and vertical gaze and pupillary dilation (involvement of oculomotor nerve outflow tract) and contralateral face, arm, and leg paresis (corticospinal and corticobulbar tracts). Unilateral tegmental lesions cause *Claude syndrome,* characterized by oculomotor paresis (oculomotor nucleus) and contralateral ataxia and tremor (often referred to as *rubral tremor* but probably the result of damage to the brachium conjunctivum). Lesions affecting both the peduncle and tegmentum produce combinations of oculomotor paresis, ataxia, and weakness (*Benedikt syndrome*). Dorsal midbrain lesions, which are infrequently vascu-

lar and rarely unilateral, cause *Parinaud syndrome,* characterized by impaired vertical gaze—especially upward (posterior commissure and the rostral interstitial nucleus of the median longitudinal fasciculus)—and loss of the pupillary light reflex (pretectal structures).

Bilateral Brain Stem Lesions Can Have Devastating Consequences

Bilateral paramedian infarction of the upper brain stem can involve the reticular activating system and cause obtundation or coma. Bilateral damage of the proximal posterior cerebral artery produces altered consciousness and various combinations of mesencephalic, diencephalic, and cortical signs (*top of the basilar artery syndrome*), affecting eye movements, pupils, vision (including, even without visual loss, vivid formed hallucinations), sensation, coordination, memory, and behavior (including agitated delirium).

Bilateral corticospinal tract infarction causes quadriparesis or quadriplegia; additional cranial weakness depends on how rostral or caudal the lesion is. Bilateral infarction of the rostral basis pontis (with sparing of the tegmentum) produces paralysis of all muscles except eye movements, the so-called *locked-in state*. Such a patient may appear comatose yet is awake and able to communicate through eye movements. Less severe damage to the corticospinal tracts in the rostral brain stem can cause pseudobulbar palsy, with spastic quadriparesis, dysarthria, dysphagia, a hyperactive gag reflex, and for reasons unclear, labile emotional responses with explosive crying or laughing.

Infarction Can Be Restricted to the Cerebellum

Infarcts of the inferior cerebellum, which has extensive vestibular connections, can cause vertigo, nausea, and nystagmus without other symptoms, suggesting disease of the inner ear or vestibular nerve. (Similar symptoms, with or without tinnitus or deafness, can occur following occlusions of the internal auditory artery, arising from the basilar artery and supplying the peripheral labyrinth.) More superior cerebellar infarcts produce gait and ipsilateral limb ataxia.

Infarction Can Affect the Spinal Cord

The ventral spinal cord is supplied by a single anterior spinal artery; the dorsal spinal cord is supplied by two or more posterior spinal arteries (Figure C-10). Except most rostrally, where the anterior spinal artery arises from the joining of two vertebral artery branches, the anterior and posterior spinal arteries are fed along their course by several radicular arteries, which arise from segmental branches of the aorta and iliac arteries. Moreover, whereas the posterior spinal arteries are longitudinally continuous and anastomotic, the anterior spinal artery's continuity is tenuous, making the anterior spinal cord more dependent on its segmental supply. The upper thoracic spinal cord is especially vulnerable in this regard.

Vascular anatomy explains the characteristic pattern of spinal cord infarction. Vessel occlusion is usually in a proximal segmental artery; because of the anastomotic continuity of the posterior spinal arteries, infarction tends to be limited to the anterior spinal artery territory. There is paraparesis or quadriparesis (corticospinal tracts), loss of bladder and bowel control, and loss of pain and temperature sensation below the lesion (spinothalamic tracts), but proprioception and discrimi-

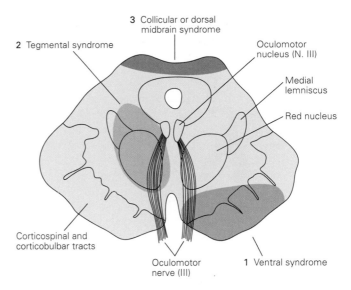

Figure C-9 The three midbrain syndromes.

native touch (dorsal columns) are spared. If the cervical or lumbar spinal cord is involved, atrophic weakness of upper or lower extremity muscles (anterior horns) can occur. Because the anterior spinal artery gives off sulcal arteries that alternately enter the left and right halves of the spinal cord, infarction can sometimes produce a *Brown-Séquard syndrome*, with ipsilateral weakness and contralateral loss of pain and temperature sensation.

Diffuse Hypoperfusion Can Cause Ischemia or Infarction

Brain ischemia or infarction may accompany diffuse hypoperfusion (shock). In such circumstances the most vulnerable regions are often the border zones between large arterial territories and the end zones of deep penetrating vessels. Whatever the cause of reduced cerebral perfusion, signs tend to be bilateral. Paralysis and sensory loss may be present in both arms (from bilateral infarction of the cortex at the junction of the middle and anterior arterial supply, affecting the arm-control area of the motor and sensory cortex).

Disturbed vision or memory may result (from infarction of the occipital or temporal lobes at the junction of the middle and posterior cerebral arterial supply). There may also be ataxia (from cerebellar border-zone infarction) or abnormal movements such as chorea or myoclonus (presumably from involvement of the basal ganglia). Such signs may exist alone or in combination and may be accompanied by a variety of aphasic or other cognitive disturbances.

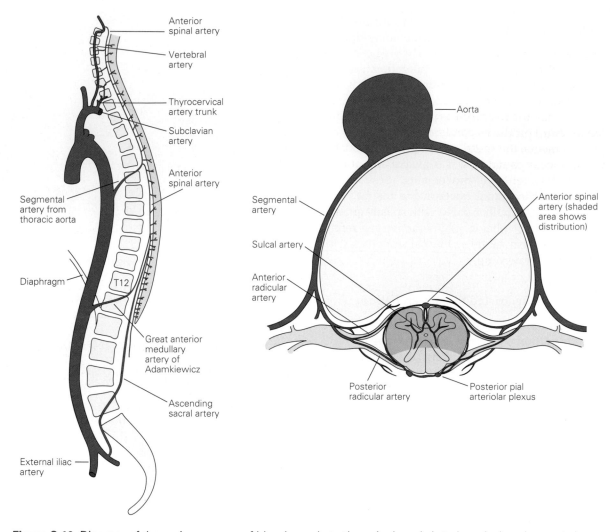

Figure C-10 Diagram of the major sources of blood supply to the spinal cord. Anterior spinal rami are not shown.

Hypotension can also cause spinal cord infarction, most often upper thoracic, affecting either the territory of the anterior spinal artery or the border zone between the anterior and posterior spinal arteries.

Cerebrovascular Disease Can Cause Dementia

Cerebral infarction causes dementia by a number of mechanisms, including:

1. Infarcts may be critically located. For example, thalamic or inferomedial temporal damage (posterior cerebral artery, usually bilateral) can cause amnesia; hemispheric convexity damage (middle cerebral artery) can cause cognitive or behavioral im-pairment not explained by disruption of language or spatial discrimination; and bilateral inferomedial frontal lobe damage (anterior cerebral artery) can cause abulia and impaired memory.

2. Multiple scattered infarcts, none sufficient to cause significant cognitive loss, can produce additive effects culminating in dementia. In such patients at least 100 cc of brain volume has usually been destroyed.

3. Small vessel disease, affecting especially the deep cerebral white matter, can cause either scattered lacunes or more diffuse ischemic lesions. When such lesions are severe enough to cause dementia—so-called *Binswanger disease*—altered behavior, pseudobulbar palsy, pyramidal signs, disturbed gait, and urinary incontinence usually occur.

The Rupture of Microaneurysms Causes Intraparenchymal Stroke

The two most common causes of hemorrhagic stroke, hypertensive intra-axial hemorrhage and rupture of a saccular aneurysm, tend to occur at particular sites and to cause recognizable syndromes. Hypertensive intercerebral hemorrhage is the result of damage to the same small penetrating vessels that, when occluded, cause lacunes; in the case of hemorrhage, however, the damaged vessels develop weakened walls (*Charcot-Bouchard microaneurysms*) that eventually rupture. The most common sites are the putamen, thalamus, pons, internal capsule and corona radiata, and cerebellum. Large diencephalic hemorrhages tend to cause stupor and hemiplegia and have a high mortality rate.

With lesions of the putamen the eyes are usually deviated ipsilaterally (because of disruption of capsular pathways descending from the frontal eye field), whereas with thalamic hemorrhage the eyes tend to be deviated downward and the pupils may not react to light (because of involvement of midbrain pretectal structures essential for upward gaze and pupillary light reactivity). Small hemorrhages may not impair alertness, and, with small thalamic hemorrhages, the motor sensory loss may exceed the weakness. Moreover, computerized tomography has shown that small thalamic hemorrhages may cause aphasia when on the left and hemi-inattention when on the right. Figures C-11 and C-12 show a large putamenal and a small thalamic hemorrhage, respectively.

Pontine hemorrhage, unless quite small, usually causes coma (by disrupting the reticular activating system) and quadriparesis (by transecting the corticospinal tracts). Eye movements, spontaneous or reflex (eg, to ice water in either external auditory canal) are absent, and pupils are pinpoint in size, perhaps in part from transection of descending sympathetic pathways and in part from destruction of reticular inhibitory mechanisms on the Edinger-Westphal nucleus of the midbrain. Pupillary light reactivity, however, is usually preserved, for the pathway subserving this reflex, from the retina to midbrain, is intact. Respirations may be irregular, presumably because of reticular formation involvement. These strokes are nearly always fatal.

Cerebellar hemorrhage, which tends to occur in the region of the dentate nucleus, typically causes a sudden inability to stand or walk (*astasia-abasia*), with ipsilateral limb ataxia. There may be ipsilateral abducens palsy, or horizontal gaze palsy, or facial weakness, presumably from pontine compression. Long-tract motor and sensory signs, however, are usually absent. As swelling increases, further brain stem damage may cause coma, ophthalmoplegia, miosis, and irregular respiration, with fatal outcome.

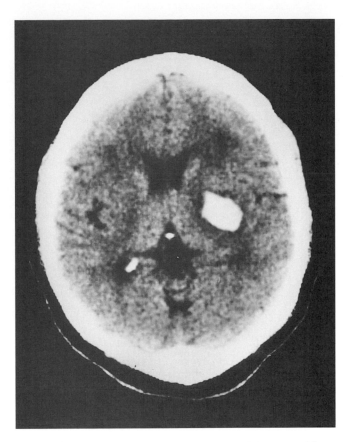

Figure C-11 CT scan showing hemorrhage (white area) in the putamen. (Courtesy of Dr. Allan J. Schwartz.)

The Rupture of Saccular Aneurysms Causes Subarachnoid Hemorrhage

Congenital saccular aneurysms (not to be confused with hypertensive Charcot-Bouchard microaneurysms) are most often found at the junction of the anterior communicating artery with an anterior cerebral artery, at the junction of a posterior communicating artery with an internal carotid artery, and at the first bifurcation of a middle cerebral artery in the sylvian fissure. Each aneurysm, upon rupture, tends to cause not only sudden severe headache but also a characteristic syndrome. By producing a hematoma directly over the oculomotor nerve as it traverses the base of the brain, a ruptured posterior communicating artery aneurysm often causes ipsilateral pupillary dilation with loss of light reactivity. A middle cerebral artery aneurysm may, by either hematoma or secondary infarction, cause a clinical picture resembling that of middle cerebral artery occlusion. After rupture of an anterior communicating artery aneurysm, there may be no focal signs but only decreased alertness or behavioral changes.

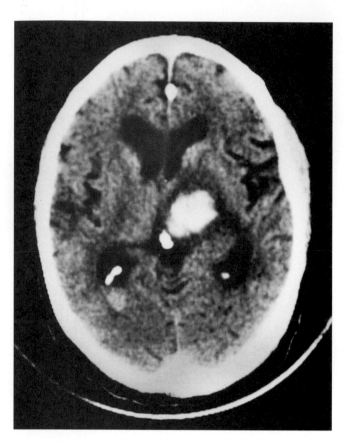

Figure C-12 CT scan showing thalamic hemorrhage. Hematoma is the **white area** surrounded by a darker zone of edema or infarction. (Courtesy of Dr. Allan J. Schwartz.)

brain infarction. Red venous blood may be seen draining infarcts (reflecting decreased oxygen extraction), and regional cerebral blood flow may or may not be absolutely increased. In addition, there may be vasomotor paralysis with loss of autoregulation to blood pressure changes and then blunted responses to alterations in arterial O_2 or CO_2. This kind of physiological abnormality occurs both within and around ischemic lesions.

In such patients CO_2 (or other cerebral vasodilators) may produce a paradoxical response, increasing cerebral blood flow in brain regions distant from the infarct without affecting the vessels around the lesion. Blood may therefore be shunted from ischemic to normal brain (*intracerebral steal*). In contrast, cerebral vasoconstrictors, by decreasing cerebral blood flow in normal brain without affecting the vessels of ischemic brain, may shunt blood into the area of ischemia or infarction (*inverse intracerebral steal*).

There is controversy about the frequency of these phenomena. Hyperperfusion is not invariable in infarcted brain, and it may coexist with adjacent hypoperfusion with increased oxygen extraction. Similarly, intracerebral steal, while probably most frequent with very large infarcts, is quite unpredictable (particularly in duration) in any single patient. It is also not clear whether increasing cerebral blood flow to infarcted or ischemic areas improves matters by increasing oxygen delivery and the removal of tissue-damaging metabolites or makes matters worse by increasing edema, mass effect, and anastomotic compromise.

Posterior fossa aneurysms most often occur at the rostral bifurcation of the basilar artery or at the origin of the posterior inferior cerebellar artery. They cause a variety of cranial nerve and brain stem signs. Rupture of an aneurysm at any site may cause abrupt coma; the reason is uncertain but may be related to sudden increased intracranial pressure and functional disruption of vital pontomedullary structures.

Stroke Alters the Vascular Physiology of the Brain

After a stroke, cerebral blood flow and cerebrovascular responses to changes in blood pressure or arterial gases are altered. The term *luxury perfusion* refers to the frequent appearance of hyperemia relative to demand after

John C. M. Brust

Selected Readings

Adams RD, Victor M, Ropper AH. 1996. *Principles of Neurology*, 6th ed., pp. 777–873. New York: McGraw-Hill.

Brust JCM. 1995. Cerebral infarction. In: LP Rowland (ed). *Merritt's Textbook of Neurology*, 9th ed., pp. 246–256. Philadelphia, PA: Lea & Febiger.

Feinberg TE, Farah MJ (eds). 1997. *Behavioral Neurology and Neuropsychology*. New York: McGraw-Hill.

Pulsinelli WA. 1996. Cerebrovascular diseases. In: JC Bennett, F Plum (eds). *Cecil Textbook of Medicine*, 20th ed., pp. 2057–2080. Philadelphia, PA: Saunders.

Appendix D

Consciousness and the Neurobiology of the Twenty-First Century

With the demise of behaviorism and the development of computers in the middle of the twentieth century, consciousness became increasingly interesting as a phenomenon for possible scientific analysis. As we enter the twenty-first century, discussion of consciousness amongst neuroscientists as well as philosophers has become popular, with a large number of papers, books, seminars, and even a journal (*Journal of Consciousness Studies*) devoted to the subject. The purpose of this appendix is to provide a guide to the most relevant literature about consciousness. As discussed in Chapter 20, we predict that cognitive neuroscientists will soon be designing and carrying out experiments to explain various aspects of the phenomenon. It would therefore be useful for the readers of this text to become familiar with the defining concepts.

Early Ideas About Consciousness Were Dualistic

Although the ancient Greek philosophers, notably Plato (circa 427–347 BC) and Aristotle (384–322 BC), developed important ideas about the nature of mind and soul (*psyche*), it is convenient to date modern discussions of consciousness to René Descartes (1596–1650). To arrive at certainty, Descartes discarded all ideas about which he could not be sure, and concluded that he could be absolutely certain only that he was a thinking being: *cogito, ergo sum*. Thus the only thing he could be certain of was the awareness of his own thoughts. Modern philosophers describe this introspective view of consciousness as a drama taking place in a personal Cartesian theater.

The British empiricists John Locke (1632–1704) and George Berkeley (1685–1753) and the Prussian philosopher Immanuel Kant (1724–1804), while contributing enormously to understanding the relationship between the external world and how we know it (epistemology), added very little to Descartes's basic concept of consciousness. They clearly assumed that the substance of mind is different from the substance of brain or of any other physical organ. This presumption, called dualism, was taken for granted in all accounts of consciousness until the nineteenth century. While these philosophers provided quite specific descriptions of consciousness, they were not concerned with explaining the way in which it worked. Thus no clear idea was offered about how the mental or spiritual component interacts with physical matter to result in mind and consciousness.

The Modern View of Consciousness Arose in the Nineteenth Century

The possibility of a physical explanation of consciousness became evident during the mid-nineteenth century with the rise of experimental psychology (Wilhelm Wundt [1832–1920]) and psychophysics (Gustav Fechner [1801–1887]; see Chapter 21), which presumed that mental activity correlates with distinct physical states (*psychophysical parallelism*). In 1890, William James (1842–1910) summarized the accomplishments of experimental psychology in his influential textbook *The Principles of Psychology*, and defined consciousness as a continuous stream that, although accessible only to the subject experiencing it, might be experimentally approached by analyzing its several functions. Thus the stream of consciousness is a continuous activity of the brain that involves attention, intentionality, and self-awareness. Self-awareness includes both perception *per se* and the awareness of experiencing perceptions, often referred to as "qualia."

Modern Thinking About Consciousness Is Materialistic

Most neuroscientists and philosophers now take for granted that all biological phenomena, including consciousness, are properties of matter. This physicalist stance breaks with the tradition of dualism stemming from ancient Greek philosophy. The break with the tradition that mind and consciousness arise from a mysterious interaction of spirit with body actually focused the problem of consciousness for the twentieth century neuroscientist. Philosophically disposed against dualism, we are obliged to find a solution to the problem in terms of nerve cells and neural circuits.

Is the problem of consciousness real, however? Some philosophers and many neuroscientists believe that consciousness is an illusion. This viewpoint is an example of radical functionalism, crudely illustrated by the assertion that mind and consciousness is to the brain as walking is to the legs. Patricia Churchland makes the argument that "electrical current in a wire is not caused by moving electrons; it *is* moving electrons. Genes are not caused by chunks of base pairs in DNA; they *are* chunks of base pairs." This point of view, called "eliminative materialism," is magisterially explicated in Daniel Dennett's *Consciousness Explained*.

Although the field of artificial intelligence has greatly influenced cognitive neuroscience, John Searle argues that consciousness cannot be reduced to a machine that can think, a physical computer with mind as a software program and consciousness as an emergent property. He maintains that the mind is not analogous to software being processed by the hardware of the brain. He argues that programs consist entirely of a set of rules (they are syntactic), whereas minds deal with values, sense, and meaning (semantics). Minds therefore differ from computer programs because a set of rules, no matter how complex, is not sufficient for semantics. Searle pleads for a scientific study of consciousness, rather than a denial of its evident existence.

Certain neurological disorders have cast some light on the problem of consciousness, as they have on other aspects of brain function as the aphasias added to our understanding of language. Especially influential is the phenomenon of blindsight as studied by Lawrence Weiskrantz and his colleagues at Oxford. Patients with lesions of the primary visual cortex (V1) are blind; but when forced to make a choice on the basis of what is shown before their eyes, they can make decisions almost as if they can see. Nevertheless, these patients insist that they cannot see. Thus, they perceive but are not conscious of perceiving. Martha Farah has reviewed these curious disorders—blindsight, prosopagnosia, and neglect—and their relevance to consciousness.

Two serious theoretical explanations derived from the known properties of neurons and neural circuits have been offered. Francis Crick and Christof Koch proposed that consciousness is an integration of neural activity similar in mechanism to the binding of different aspects of sensation that occurs to produce a unified perception. Like binding, consciousness would also depend on the synchronous firing of cortical neurons at frequencies around 40 Hz. Gerald Edelman has proposed that consciousness results from several crucial functions of brain activity: memory, learning, distinguishing self from nonself, and most important, re-entry—the recursive comparison of information by different brain regions. Giulio Tononi and Edelman suggest that this re-entry mechanism is localized in circuits of the thalamocortical system.

Can Consciousness Be Explained?

In a classic paper, Thomas Nagel argued that consciousness is first-person specific and unlike any other natural phenomenon. Because of its inherently subjective character, it poses a unique problem for scientific analysis. Colin McGinn took this argument a step further. Even though a materialist, McGinn believes that the human mind lacks the cognitive ability to understand the nature of consciousness, just as monkeys cannot understand particle physics. We agree that the problem of consciousness is difficult, perhaps the most difficult one that neuroscience has to face. As Crick and Koch and many others presume, consciousness must have a neural correlate. We are optimistic that future cognitive neural scientists will identify the neurons involved and characterize the mechanisms by which consciousness is produced.

James H. Schwartz

Selected Readings

Block N, Flanagan O, Güzeldere G (eds). 1997. *The Nature of Consciousness*. Cambridge, MA: MIT Press.

Churchland PM, Churchland PS. 1998. *On the Contrary: Critical Essays, 1987–1997*. Cambridge, MA: MIT Press.

Churchland PS. 1986. *Neurophilosophy: Toward a Unified Science of the Mind-Brain*. Cambridge, MA: MIT Press.

Churchland PS, Sejnowski T. 1992. *The Computational Brain: Models and Methods on the Frontier of Computational Neuroscience*. Cambridge, MA: MIT Press.

Crick F, Koch C. 1990. Towards a neurobiological theory of consciousness. Seminars in the Neurosciences 2:263–275.

Crick F, Koch C. 1998. Consciousness and neuroscience. Cerebral Cortex 8:97–107.

Dennett DC. 1991. *Consciousness Explained*. New York: Little Brown.

Descartes R. [1641] 1993. *Meditations on First Philosophy*. Cress DA (transl). Indianapolis, IN: Hackett Publishing Company.

Edelman GM. 1989. *The Remembered Present: A Biological Theory of Consciousness*. New York: BasicBooks.

Farah M. 1995. Visual perception and visual awareness after brain damage: A tutorial overview. In: C Umiltà, M Moscovitch (eds). *Attention and Performance XV: Conscious and Nonconscious Information Processing*, pp. 37–75. Cambridge, MA: MIT Press.

James W. 1890. *The Principles of Psychology*, Chap. IX. New York: Henry Holt and Company.

McGinn C. 1997. *The Character of Mind: An Introduction to the Philosophy of Mind*, 2nd ed. New York: Oxford Univ. Press.

Nagel T. 1974. What is it like to be a bat? Philosophical Review 83:435–450.

Searle JR. 1984. *Minds, Brains and Science*. Cambridge, MA: Harvard Univ. Press.

Searle JR. 1997. *The Mystery of Consciousness*. New York: A New York Review Book.

Shear J. 1997. *Explaining Consciousness: The Hard Problem*. Cambridge, MA: MIT Press.

Tononi G, Edelman GM. 1998. Consciousness and complexity. Science 282:1846–1851.

Weiskrantz L (ed). 1988. *Thought Without Language*. Oxford: Oxford Univ. Press.

Weiskrantz L. 1997. *Consciousness Lost and Found*. Oxford: Oxford Univ. Press.

Zeki S. 1993. *A Vision of the Brain*, pp. 321–336. Oxford: Blackwell Scientific Publishers.

Index

ISBN 0-07-112000-9